PROCEDURES

KINN'S
THE MEDICAL ASSISTANT

AN APPLIED LEARNING APPROACH

13TH EDITION

Deborah Proctor, EdD, RN
Adjunct Faculty Member
Butler County Community College
Butler, Pennsylvania

Brigitte Niedzwiecki, RN, MSN, RMA
Medical Assistant Program Director & Instructor
Chippewa Valley Technical College
Eau Claire, Wisconsin

Julie Pepper, BS, CMA (AAMA)
Medical Assistant Instructor
Chippewa Valley Technical College
Eau Claire, Wisconsin

Payel Bhattacharya Madero, MBA, RHIT
Adjunct Faculty
Cal State Fullerton University
Fullerton, California

Marti Garrels, MSA, MTA (ASCP), CMA (AAMA)
Medical Assisting Program Consultant
Retired Medical Assisting Program Director
Lake Washington Institute of Technology
Kirkland, Washington

Helen Mills, RN, MSN, RMA, LXMO, AHI
Clinical Educator
Martin Health System
Stuart, Florida

ELSEVIER

ELSEVIER

3251 Riverport Lane
St. Louis, Missouri 63043

KINN'S THE MEDICAL ASSISTANT: AN APPLIED LEARNING   ISBN: 978-0-323-35320-5
APPROACH, THIRTEENTH EDITION

Notices

Knowledge and best practice in this field are constantly changing. As new research and experience broaden our understanding, changes in research methods, professional practices, or medical treatment may become necessary.

Practitioners and researchers must always rely on their own experience and knowledge in evaluating and using any information, methods, compounds, or experiments described herein. In using such information or methods they should be mindful of their own safety and the safety of others, including parties for whom they have a professional responsibility.

With respect to any drug or pharmaceutical products identified, readers are advised to check the most current information provided (i) on procedures featured or (ii) by the manufacturer of each product to be administered, to verify the recommended dose or formula, the method and duration of administration, and contraindications. It is the responsibility of practitioners, relying on their own experience and knowledge of their patients, to make diagnoses, to determine dosages and the best treatment for each individual patient, and to take all appropriate safety precautions.

To the fullest extent of the law, neither the Publisher nor the authors, contributors, or editors, assume any liability for any injury and/or damage to persons or property as a matter of products liability, negligence or otherwise, or from any use or operation of any methods, products, instructions, or ideas contained in the material herein.

Previous editions copyrighted 2014, 2011, 2007, 2003, 1999, 1993, 1988, 1981, 1974, 1967, 1960, 1956

International Standard Book Number: 978-0-323-35320-5

Executive Content Strategist: Jennifer Janson
Content Development Manager: Ellen Wurm-Cutter
Senior Content Development Specialist: Becky Leenhouts
Publishing Services Manager: Julie Eddy
Senior Project Manager: Richard Barber
Design Direction: Paula Catalano

Printed in Canada

Last digit is the print number: 9   8   7   6   5   4   3   2

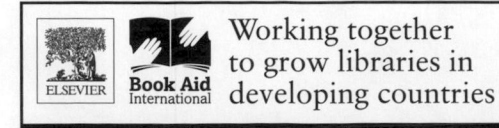

Working together to grow libraries in developing countries

www.elsevier.com • www.bookaid.org

PREFACE

Medical assisting as a profession has changed dramatically since *The Office Assistant in Medical and Dental Practice,* by Portia Frederick and Carol Towner, was first published in 1956. Each subsequent edition of this textbook has reflected the age in which it was published. Now, *Kinn's The Medical Assistant: An Applied Learning Approach,* thirteenth edition, in its 60th year of publication, continues to represent a long-standing commitment to high-quality medical assisting education with its engaging, straightforward writing style and demonstrated positive outcomes. Hundreds of instructors in classrooms across the country have used this text to teach thousands of students over the years. Many of these students have gone on to teach students of their own with this very same trusted resource. To continue the use and growth of this text and its features, the thirteenth edition continues to offer the most comprehensive, up-to-date, and innovative approach to teaching this subject today.

This textbook has endured throughout the years because it has been able to keep pace with an ever-changing profession while producing students who are well trained and qualified to enter medical practices across the country. This dependability is the reason the market continues to rely on this text, edition after edition. Underlying this dependability is a foundation of pedagogic features that has stood the test of time and that has been expanded and improved upon yet again in this latest edition. Such features include the following:

- An easy-to-read, highly interactive writing style that engages students through practical applications of medical assistant competencies.
- An emphasis on skill development, with procedural steps outlining each skill, supported by rationales that provide meaning to each step.
- A pedagogic framework based on the use of learning objectives, vocabulary terms, and supportive student supplements.
- A package of supportive materials to accommodate a wide variety of student learning types and instructor teaching styles.

NEW TO THIS EDITION

- **Updated Art Program.** The artwork throughout has been updated and modernized, providing a more attractive textbook for student use. Many new photographs and line drawings throughout support the revised content more effectively and are more relevant to the actual healthcare setting. New images show up-to-date equipment, provide more disease examples, and better illustrate key procedural steps.

- **New chapter on Competency-Based Education for Medical Assisting.** The emphasis of competency mastery is high to meet accreditation standards. This chapter helps set the stage for medical assisting students to understand their programming and how the road to mastery will affect their ability to attain a job.
- **New Chapter on The Health Record.** The manner in which the medical record is maintained in a medical office has changed dramatically with the move to the EHR. This chapter reviews how the medical assistant maintains and interacts with the medical record.
- **Learning Objectives are listed in the same order as the flow of content.** The learning objectives are tied to curriculum competencies. This feature makes it easy to see where the learning objectives are covered to aid in review of the material and measurement of competency coverage.
- **Procedures are integrated into the TOC.** Provides a quick reference to where the procedures will be covered and in what order.
- **Professional Behaviors boxes.** The medical assistant must develop the ability to interact professionally with patients, families, co-workers, and other members of the healthcare team. These boxes provide tips on professional behavior that are specific to each chapter's content.

EVOLVE

The Evolve site features a variety of student resources, including Chapter Review Quizzes, new Procedure Videos, Medical Terminology Audio Glossary, practice CMA and RMA exams, and much more! The instructors' Evolve Resources site consists of TEACH Instructor Resources, including Lesson Plans, PowerPoint Presentations, Answer Keys for Chapter Review Quizzes, and a retooled Test Bank with more than 5000 questions.

STUDY GUIDE AND PROCEDURE CHECKLIST MANUAL

The Study Guide provides students with the opportunity to review and build on information they have learned in the text through vocabulary reviews, case studies, workplace applications, and more. The updated Procedure Checklists include CAAHEP and ABHES competencies that can be traced to the online correlation grid.

FEATURES

A Scenario is presented at the beginning of each chapter so the student can envision a real-world situation when reading the chapter content.

Scenario questions provide a way for students to apply the concepts they are learning and think about decisions they would make in real situations.

Learning Objectives emphasize the cognitive and performance objectives presented in the chapter.

Each chapter contains a vocabulary list with definitions so students can first familiarize themselves with the important terms associated with each chapter.

11

THE HEALTH RECORD

SCENARIO

Susan Beezler has just begun her career in the medical assisting profession. She is attending medical assisting school in the morning and works part-time for a family practitioner in the afternoons as a clerical record assistant. Susan is eager to learn about medicine and looks forward to taking on more responsibility at the office.

The practice is growing swiftly and recently added a new provider, Dr. Alex Thomas. Dr. Thomas has enjoyed working with Susan and feels that her energy will be just what his patients need. He has taken a professional interest in Susan and often lets her assist him with patients when her other duties allow.

Susan knows that although she is a beginner in the office, she will gain trust from her supervisors and patients as long as she projects a teachable

attitude. The office has recently converted to an electronic records system but is still using paper records as well. Susan uses the information she learned in school about both types of health records. She cheerfully performs filing and even does some transcription for Dr. Thomas. The other staff members are pleased with her willingness to perform the most mundane tasks.

Susan enjoys sharing her experiences with her classmates. She is the only one currently working in the "real world" of medicine. She discusses situations at work, always mentioning patient confidentiality; she discusses situations, never mentioning any patients' names.

Susan feels a great sense of pride that she is a member of the healthcare team and able to contribute to the [...]

While studying this chapter, think about the following questions:
- Why would some patients have concerns about the healthcare facility using electronic health records (EHRs)?
- How can the medical assistant earn the patient's trust so that the person is comfortable revealing the very private information required by a health history?
- Why is it so important to have a sign[...] before sending patient information [...]
- Why is it important that the health[...]
- Why is it important to know both [...] provider's office?

LEARNING OBJECTIVES

1. Define, spell, and pronounce the terms listed in the vocabulary.
2. Name and discuss the two types of patient records.
3. State several reasons that accurate health records are important.
4. Differentiate between subjective and objective information in creating a patient's health record.
5. Explain who owns the health record.
6. Distinguish between an electronic health record (EHR) and an electronic medical record (EMR).
7. Do the following related to healthcare legislation and EHRs:
   - Explain how the American Recovery and Reinvestment Act (ARRA) applies to the healthcare industry.
   - Define meaningful use and relate it to the healthcare industry.
   - List the three main components of meaningful use legislation.
8. Explore the advantages, disadvantages, and capabilities of an EHR system, and explain how to organize a patient's health record.
9. Discuss the importance of nonverbal communication with patients when an EHR system is used.
10. Discuss backup systems for the EHR, as well as the transfer, destruction, and retention of health records as related to the EHR.

11. Describe how and when t[...] health information exch[...]
12. Identify and discuss the [...] medical record.
13. Discuss how to docu[...] record, and how to [...]
14. Discuss dictation a[...] and retention of [...]
15. Identify filing e[...] and maintain[...]
16. Describe ind[...] health rec[...]
17. Discuss t[...] file pati[...]
18. Discuss [...]
19. Discus[...] to [...]

VOCABULARY

age of majority The age at which a person is recognized by law to be an adult; can vary by state.

alleviate To partly remove or correct; to relieve or lessen.

alphabetic filing Any system that arranges names or topics according to the sequence of the letters in the alphabet.

alphanumeric Of or relating to systems made up of combinations of letters and numbers.

augment To increase in size or amount; to add to in order to improve or complete.

caption A heading, title, or subtitle under which records are filed.

computerized provider/physician order entry (CPOE) The process of entering medication orders or other provider instructions into the electronic health record (EHR).

continuity of care Continuation of care smoothly from one provider to another, so that the patient receives the most benefit and no interruption in care.

culpability Meriting condemnation, responsibility, or blame, especially as wrong or harmful.

dictation (dik-ta'-shun) The act or manner of uttering words to be transcribed.

direct filing system A filing system in which materials can be located without consulting an additional source of reference.

e-prescribing The use of electronic software to communicate with pharmacies and send prescribing information, taking the place of writing a prescription by hand and physically giving it to a patient; most new or refill prescriptions can be submitted electronically, cutting down on fraud and errors.

electronic health record (EHR) An electronic record of health-related information about a patient that conforms to nationally recognized interoperability standards and that can be created, managed, and consulted by authorized clinicians and staff from more than one healthcare organization.

electronic medical record (EMR) An electronic record of health-related information about an individual that can be created, gathered, managed, and consulted by authorized clinicians and staff within a single healthcare organization.

gleaned Gathered bit by bit (e.g., information or material); picked over in search of relevant material.

indirect filing system A filing system in which an intermediary source of reference (e.g., a card file) must be consulted to locate specific files.

interoperability The ability to work with other systems.

microfilm A film with a photographic record of printed or other graphic matter on a reduced scale.

numeric filing The filing of records, correspondence, or cards by number.

objective information Data obtained through physical examination, laboratory and diagnostic testing, and by measurable information.

obliteration (uh-blih-tuh-ra'-shun) The act of making undecipherable or imperceptible by obscuring or wearing away.

outguide A sturdy cardboard or plastic file-sized card used to replace a folder temporarily removed from the filing space.

parameters Any set of physical properties, the values of which determine characteristics or behavior.

patient portal A secure online Web site that gives patients 24-hour access to personal health information using a username and password.

personal health record (PHR) An electronic record of health-related information about an individual that conforms to nationally recognized interoperability standards and that can be drawn from multiple sources but that is managed, shared, and controlled by the individual.

pressboard A strong, highly glazed composition board resembling vulcanized fiber; heavy card stock.

provisional diagnosis A temporary diagnosis made before all test results have been received.

purging The process of moving active files to inactive files.

quality control An aggregate of activities designed to ensure adequate quality, especially in manufactured products or in the service industries.

reasonable cause Circumstances that would make it unreasonable for the covered entity, despite the exercise of ordinary business care and prudence, to comply with the administrative simplification provision (part of Health Information Technology for Economic and Clinical Health Act [HITECH]) that was violated.

reasonable diligence The business care and prudence expected from a person seeking to satisfy a legal requirement under similar circumstances.

requisites (reh'-kwuh-zihts) Entities considered essential or necessary.

retention schedule A method or plan for retaining or keeping health records and for their movement from active to inactive to closed filing.

reverse chronologic order Arranged in order so that the most recent item is on top and older items are filed further back.

subjective information Data or information elicited from the patient, including the patient's feelings, perceptions, and concerns; obtained through interview or questions.

subpoena duces tecum A court order to produce documents or records.

tickler file A chronologic file used as a reminder that something must be dealt with on a certain date.

transcription A written copy of something made either in longhand or by machine.

vested Granted or endowed with a particular authority, right, or property; to have a special interest in.

willful neglect Conscious, intentional failure or reckless indifference to the obligation to comply with the administrative simplification provision violated.

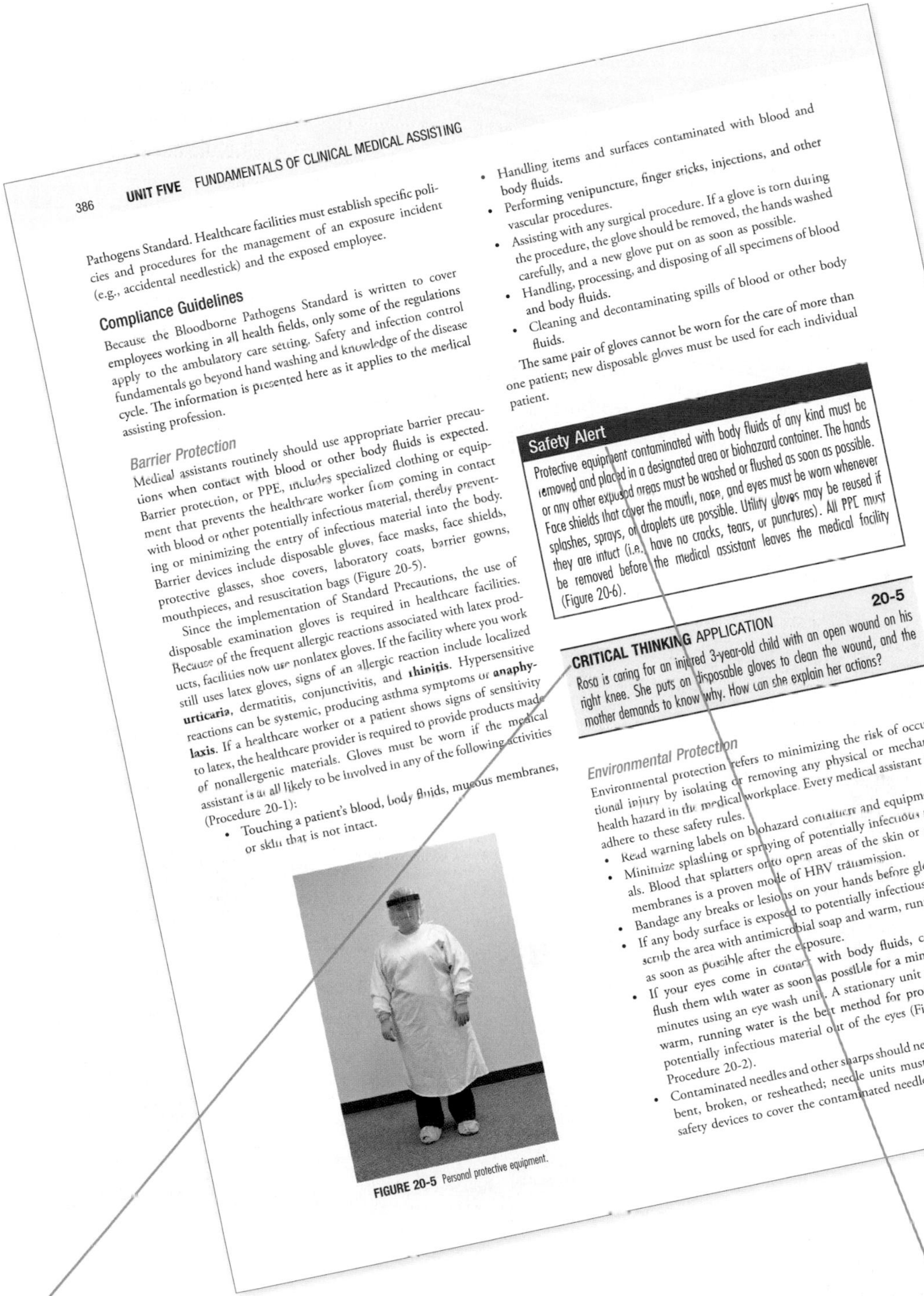

Pathogens Standard. Healthcare facilities must establish specific policies and procedures for the management of an exposure incident (e.g., accidental needlestick) and the exposed employee.

Compliance Guidelines

Because the Bloodborne Pathogens Standard is written to cover employees working in all health fields, only some of the regulations apply to the ambulatory care setting. Safety and infection control fundamentals go beyond hand washing and knowledge of the disease cycle. The information is presented here as it applies to the medical assisting profession.

Barrier Protection

Medical assistants routinely should use appropriate barrier precautions when contact with blood or other body fluids is expected. Barrier protection, or PPE, includes specialized clothing or equipment that prevents the healthcare worker from coming in contact with blood or other potentially infectious material, thereby preventing or minimizing the entry of infectious material into the body. Barrier devices include disposable gloves, face masks, face shields, protective glasses, shoe covers, laboratory coats, barrier gowns, mouthpieces, and resuscitation bags (Figure 20-5).

Since the implementation of Standard Precautions, the use of disposable examination gloves is required in healthcare facilities. Because of the frequent allergic reactions associated with latex products, facilities now use nonlatex gloves. If the facility where you work still uses latex gloves, signs of an allergic reaction include localized **urticaria**, dermatitis, conjunctivitis, and **rhinitis**. Hypersensitive reactions can be systemic, producing asthma symptoms or **anaphylaxis**. If a healthcare worker or a patient shows signs of sensitivity to latex, the healthcare provider is required to provide products made of nonallergenic materials. Gloves must be worn if the medical assistant is at all likely to be involved in any of the following activities (Procedure 20-1):

- Touching a patient's blood, body fluids, mucous membranes, or skin that is not intact.

FIGURE 20-5 Personal protective equipment.

- Handling items and surfaces contaminated with blood and body fluids.
- Performing venipuncture, finger sticks, injections, and other vascular procedures.
- Assisting with any surgical procedure. If a glove is torn during the procedure, the glove should be removed, the hands washed carefully, and a new glove put on as soon as possible.
- Handling, processing, and disposing of all specimens of blood and body fluids.
- Cleaning and decontaminating spills of blood or other body fluids.

The same pair of gloves cannot be worn for the care of more than one patient; new disposable gloves must be used for each individual patient.

Safety Alert

Protective equipment contaminated with body fluids of any kind must be removed and placed in a designated area or biohazard container. The hands or any other exposed areas must be washed or flushed as soon as possible. Face shields that cover the mouth, nose, and eyes must be worn whenever splashes, sprays, or droplets are possible. Utility gloves may be reused if they are intact (i.e., have no cracks, tears, or punctures). All PPE must be removed before the medical assistant leaves the medical facility (Figure 20-6).

CRITICAL THINKING APPLICATION 20-5

Rosa is caring for an injured 3-year-old child with an open wound on his right knee. She puts on disposable gloves to clean the wound, and the mother demands to know why. How can she explain her actions?

Environmental Protection

Environmental protection refers to minimizing the risk of occupational injury by isolating or removing any physical or mechanical health hazard in the medical workplace. Every medical assistant must adhere to these safety rules.

- Read warning labels on biohazard containers and equipment.
- Minimize splashing or spraying of potentially infectious materials. Blood that splatters onto open areas of the skin or mucous membranes is a proven mode of HBV transmission.
- Bandage any breaks or lesions on your hands before gloving.
- If any body surface is exposed to potentially infectious material, scrub the area with antimicrobial soap and warm, running water as soon as possible after the exposure.
- If your eyes come in contact with body fluids, continuously flush them with water as soon as possible for a minimum of 15 minutes using an eye wash unit. A stationary unit connected to warm, running water is the best method for properly flushing potentially infectious material out of the eyes (Figure 20-7 and Procedure 20-2).
- Contaminated needles and other sharps should never be recapped, bent, broken, or resheathed; needle units must have protective safety devices to cover the contaminated needle after injection.

Critical Thinking Application boxes prompt students to apply what they have learned as they read and study the chapter.

Safety Alert boxes alert students to important safety information and reinforce the importance of safety in the profession.

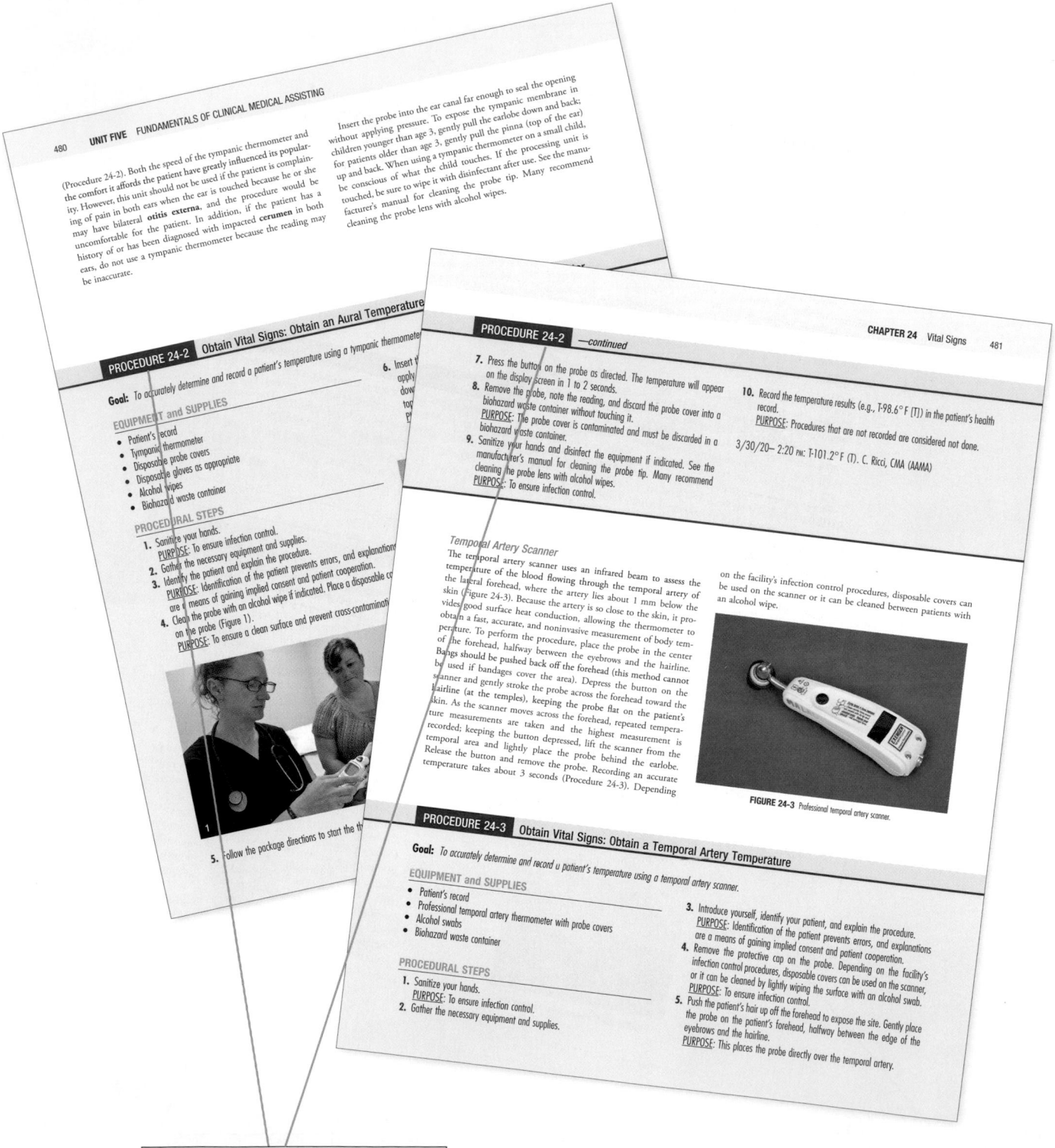

UNIT FIVE FUNDAMENTALS OF CLINICAL MEDICAL ASSISTING

480

(Procedure 24-2). Both the speed of the tympanic thermometer and the comfort it affords the patient have greatly influenced its popularity. However, this unit should not be used if the patient is complaining of pain in both ears when the ear is touched because he or she may have bilateral **otitis externa**, and the procedure would be uncomfortable for the patient. In addition, if the patient has a history of or has been diagnosed with impacted **cerumen** in both ears, do not use a tympanic thermometer because the reading may be inaccurate.

Insert the probe into the ear canal far enough to seal the opening without applying pressure. To expose the tympanic membrane in children younger than age 3, gently pull the earlobe down and back; for patients older than age 3, gently pull the pinna (top of the ear) up and back. When using a tympanic thermometer on a small child, be conscious of what the child touches. If the processing unit is touched, be sure to wipe it with disinfectant after use. See the manufacturer's manual for cleaning the probe tip. Many recommend cleaning the probe lens with alcohol wipes.

PROCEDURE 24-2 Obtain Vital Signs: Obtain an Aural Temperature

Goal: To accurately determine and record a patient's temperature using a tympanic thermometer

EQUIPMENT and SUPPLIES

- Patient's record
- Tympanic thermometer
- Disposable probe covers
- Disposable gloves as appropriate
- Alcohol wipes
- Biohazard waste container

PROCEDURAL STEPS

1. Sanitize your hands.
   PURPOSE: To ensure infection control.
2. Gather the necessary equipment and supplies.
3. Identify the patient and explain the procedure.
   PURPOSE: Identification of the patient prevents errors, and explanations are a means of gaining implied consent and patient cooperation.
4. Clean the probe with an alcohol wipe if indicated. Place a disposable cover on the probe (Figure 1).
   PURPOSE: To ensure a clean surface and prevent cross-contamination.

5. Follow the package directions to start the thermometer.

6. Insert the probe into the ear canal far enough to seal the opening without applying pressure. To expose the tympanic membrane, pull the earlobe down and back for children younger than age 3 and up and back for patients older than age 3 (top of the ear up and back). Insert the probe.

PROCEDURE 24-2 —continued

CHAPTER 24 Vital Signs 481

7. Press the button on the probe as directed. The temperature will appear on the display screen in 1 to 2 seconds.
8. Remove the probe, note the reading, and discard the probe cover into a biohazard waste container without touching it.
   PURPOSE: The probe cover is contaminated and must be discarded in a biohazard waste container.
9. Sanitize your hands and disinfect the equipment if indicated. See the manufacturer's manual for cleaning the probe tip. Many recommend cleaning the probe lens with alcohol wipes.
   PURPOSE: To ensure infection control.

10. Record the temperature results (e.g., T-98.6° F [T]) in the patient's health record.
    PURPOSE: Procedures that are not recorded are considered not done.

3/30/20– 2:20 PM: T-101.2° F (T). C. Ricci, CMA (AAMA)

Temporal Artery Scanner

The temporal artery scanner uses an infrared beam to assess the temperature of the blood flowing through the temporal artery of the lateral forehead, where the artery lies about 1 mm below the skin (Figure 24-3). Because the artery is so close to the skin, it provides good surface heat conduction, allowing the thermometer to obtain a fast, accurate, and noninvasive measurement of body temperature. To perform the procedure, place the probe in the center of the forehead, halfway between the eyebrows and the hairline. Bangs should be pushed back off the forehead (this method cannot be used if bandages cover the area). Depress the button on the scanner and gently stroke the probe across the forehead toward the hairline (at the temples), keeping the probe flat on the patient's skin. As the scanner moves across the forehead, repeated temperature measurements are taken and the highest measurement is recorded; keeping the button depressed, lift the scanner from the temporal area and lightly place the probe behind the earlobe. Release the button and remove the probe. Recording an accurate temperature takes about 3 seconds (Procedure 24-3). Depending on the facility's infection control procedures, disposable covers can be used on the scanner or it can be cleaned between patients with an alcohol wipe.

FIGURE 24-3 Professional temporal artery scanner.

PROCEDURE 24-3 Obtain Vital Signs: Obtain a Temporal Artery Temperature

Goal: To accurately determine and record a patient's temperature using a temporal artery scanner.

EQUIPMENT and SUPPLIES

- Patient's record
- Professional temporal artery thermometer with probe covers
- Alcohol swabs
- Biohazard waste container

PROCEDURAL STEPS

1. Sanitize your hands.
   PURPOSE: To ensure infection control.
2. Gather the necessary equipment and supplies.

3. Introduce yourself, identify your patient, and explain the procedure.
   PURPOSE: Identification of the patient prevents errors, and explanations are a means of gaining implied consent and patient cooperation.
4. Remove the protective cap on the probe. Depending on the facility's infection control procedures, disposable covers can be used on the scanner, or it can be cleaned by lightly wiping the surface with an alcohol swab.
   PURPOSE: To ensure infection control.
5. Push the patient's hair up off the forehead to expose the site. Gently place the probe on the patient's forehead, halfway between the edge of the eyebrows and the hairline.
   PURPOSE: This places the probe directly over the temporal artery.

Step-by-step Procedure boxes demonstrate how to perform and document procedures encountered in the healthcare setting.

- Write out the entire word and refrain from using abbreviations and emoticons.
- Use proper capitalization, grammar, sentence structure, and punctuation. Check the spelling of the e-mail before sending it. Most e-mail software has a spell-checker.
- Be concise, accurate, and clear in your message.
- Always end your e-mail with "Thank you" or "Sincerely" and your complete name. For business e-mails, include contact information after your name, including the agency's address, phone number, and fax number.
- Leave white space (i.e., one blank line) between the salutation, paragraphs, and your complete name.
- Zip large attachments before sending the files. **Zip** is a computer program that compresses a file or folder, making it smaller and easier to send. The receiver uses an unzip program to extract the contents.
- Many e-mail programs have features such as (!) urgent or a response box that sends an e-mail back to the sender when the e-mail is opened by the recipient. Use the urgent feature only for crucial e-mails.

CRITICAL THINKING APPLICATION   7-14

Christiana receives an e-mail from a patient that is in all capital letters. How might she perceive the situation with the patient? How could she verify her perceptions? How should she handle this situation?

Some healthcare facilities may also include language in e-mails related to confidentiality and whom to contact if the e-mail was sent to the wrong address. Medical assistants must adhere to the facility's confidentiality rules when communicating with or about patients. Copies of e-mail communications should be uploaded to the patient's EHR for a permanent record of the electronic communication.

EHR software frequently contains clinical messaging or clinical e-mail features. This feature is an e-mail within the EHR. The clinical messaging feature provides secure communication for healthcare employees to converse about the patient. For instance, the message may be sent from the receptionist to the medical assistant regarding a patient who called requesting a refill. The medical assistant can then follow up with the provider regarding the refill.

Faxed Communication

Fax (short for facsimile) machines send and receive documents using the phone lines. In the healthcare facility, the fax machine may be part of a copy machine, or the computers may have software that allows faxes to be sent and received. As communications technology has advanced, the use of fax machines has decreased, but they are still an important piece of equipment in the ambulatory care center.

When sending a fax, you must adhere to HIPAA and HITECH rules. Healthcare facilities usually have a required face sheet (the first sheet) that includes confidentiality language, which instructs the recipient, if he or she is not the intended party, to destroy the fax and contact the medical facility. Besides the confidentiality statement, the face sheet should include the contact information for sender and recipient, the date, and the total number of pages.

CLOSING COMMENTS

Patient Education

If the medical assistant is responsible for preparing patient education materials using the computer's word processing program, it is important that these materials contain correct grammar, spelling, punctuation, and sentence structure. The appearance of brochures and documents created by the ambulatory care center staff reflects on the medical practice. The medical assistant should proofread all documents carefully before printing them.

Legal and Ethical Issues

The medical assistant should keep a copy of all documents produced using word processing. A copy of any document sent to a patient must also be uploaded into the patient's EHR. All patient-related documents are confidential, and the medical assistant must ensure the security and privacy of the information.

Professional Behaviors

Written communication in any form requires the medical assistant to be respectful, polite, and professional. It is important to proofread all written communication before it is sent to the recipient. Spell-checker tools can help identify misspelled words and sometimes incorrect usage of grammar and punctuation. However, these tools cannot always identify a word used incorrectly; only proofreading can capture those errors. Proofreading also allows the reader to reassess the tone of the communication, making sure it is appropriate. Finally, the medical assistant should recheck the spelling of the person's name and address for accuracy. A well-composed message gives the reader a reassuring sense of the accuracy and professionalism of the healthcare facility's staff.

NEW! Professional Behaviors boxes provide tips on professional behavior that are specific to each chapter's content.

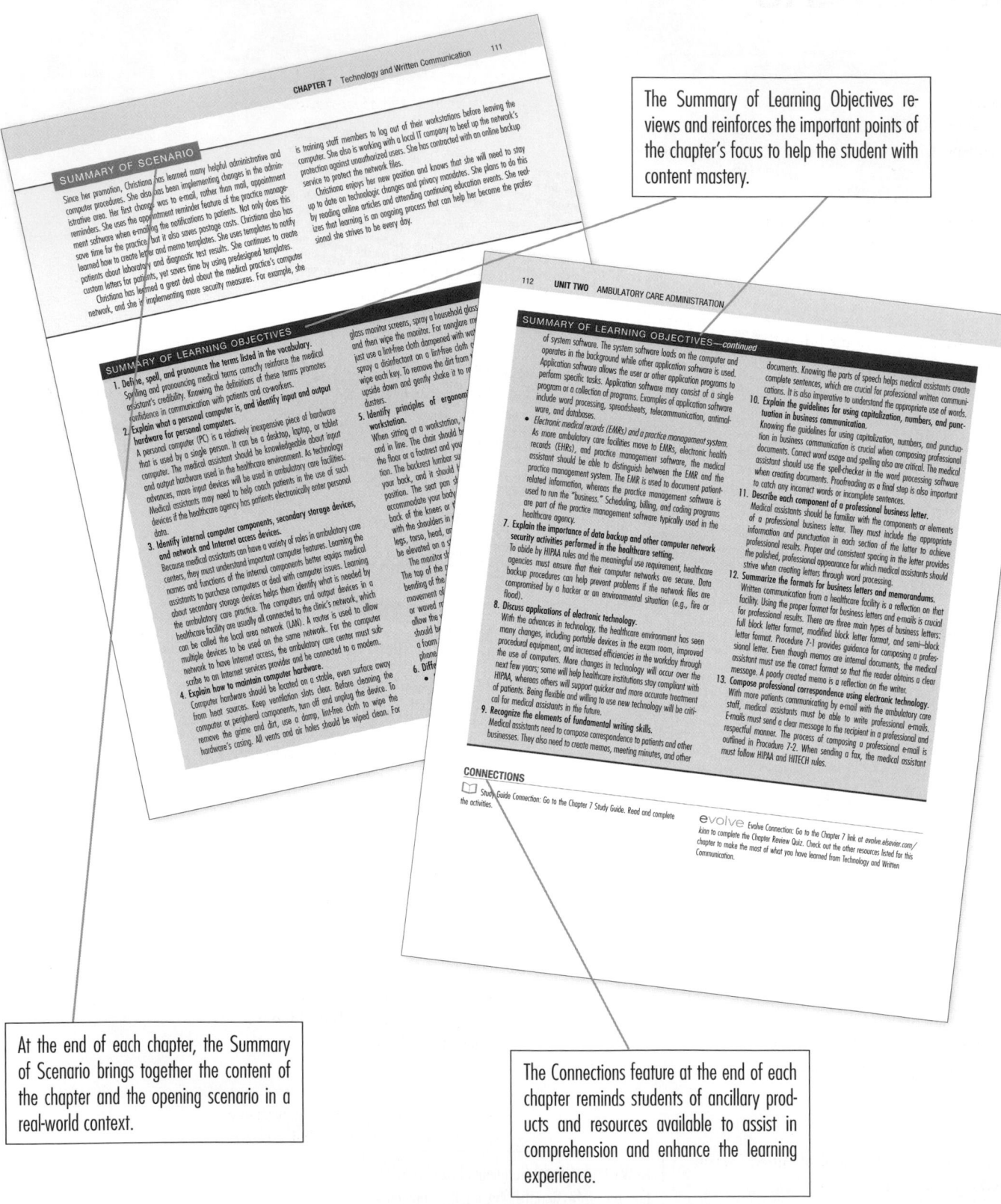

The Summary of Learning Objectives reviews and reinforces the important points of the chapter's focus to help the student with content mastery.

At the end of each chapter, the Summary of Scenario brings together the content of the chapter and the opening scenario in a real-world context.

The Connections feature at the end of each chapter reminds students of ancillary products and resources available to assist in comprehension and enhance the learning experience.

REVIEWERS

Brenda G. Abplanalp, RN, BSN, MSEd
Director
Pennsylvania College of Technology
Williamsport, Pennsylvania

Pam Alt, RN, MSN, RMA
Medical Assistant Program Director
Mid-State Technical College
Marshfield, Wisconsin

Deborah A. Balentine, MEd, RHIA, CCS, CCS-P, CHTS-TR
Adjunct Instructor—Adult Education
City Colleges of Chicago
Chicago, Illinois

Janet K. Baumann, BS, CMA (AAMA), EMT-B
Medical Assistant Program Director
Northcentral Technical College
Wausau, Wisconsin

Cynthia A. Bloss, AA, RMA, BMO
Instructor, Clinical Liaison
Southeastern College
Clearwater, Florida

Marquitta Breeding, CMA (AAMA)
Wallace State Community College
Hanceville, Alabama

Leon Deutsch, RMA, BS, MEd
Dean of Teaching & Learning
Grayson College
Denison, Texas

Jennifer Dietz, BS, CMA (AAMA), PBT (ASCP) [CM]
Assistant Professor
Cuyahoga Community College—Metropolitan Campus
Cleveland, Ohio

Tracie Fuqua, BS, CMA (AAMA)
Medical Assistant Program Director
Wallace State Community College
Hanceville, Alabama

Deborah S. Gilbert, RHIA, MBA, CMA
Assistant Professor of School of Allied Health
Dalton State College
Dalton, Georgia

Kimberly Annette Head, DC, BS, BA
Director of CE Healthcare Programs
Collin College
Plano, Texas

Judith K. Kline, RMA, NCMA, CCMA, CMAA, AHI, NCET, NCICS, NCPT
Professor
Miami Lakes Educational Center & Technical College
Miami Lakes, Florida

Jennifer K. Lester, BA, NHA, AMT
Medical Administrative Instructor
Charleston Job Corps Center & Bridge Valley Community & Technical College Workforce Program
Charleston, West Virginia

Michelle C. Maus, MBA, BS, PhD, ABD
Department Chair/Assistant Professor
Tiffin University
Tiffin, Ohio

Tammy McClish, MEd, CMA (AAMA), RTARRT
Allied Health Instructor
The University of Akron
Akron, Ohio

Brigitte Niedzwiecki, RN, MSN, RMA
Medical Assistant Program Director & Instructor
Chippewa Valley Technical College
Eau Claire, Wisconsin

Cynthia B. Orlando, CAHI, OBT, NRCMA
Instructor
Eastern College of Health Vocations
New Orleans, Louisiana

Julie Pepper, BS, CMA (AAMA)
Medical Assistant Instructor
Chippewa Valley Technical College
Eau Claire, Wisconsin

Melanie Shearer, MS, MT (ASCP) PBT [CM]**, CMA (AAMA)**
Medical Assisting Associate Professor
Cuyahoga Community College
Cleveland, Ohio

Paula Denise Silver, BS, PharmD
Medical Instructor
ECPI University: Medical Careers Institute
Newport News, Virginia

Rayona Mullen Staniec, CMA—AC
Medical Assisting Instructor
Santa Cruz County Regional Occupational Program
Santa Cruz, California

Roelabeth de Leon Villa, MD, RMA
Goodman Career Institute
Rockford, Illinois

Karon G. Walton, CMA (AAMA), AAS, BS
Program Director
Augusta Technical College
Augusta, Georgia

P. Ann Weaver, MSEd, MT (ASCP)
Instructor
Chippewa Valley Technical College
Eau Claire, Wisconsin

Barbara Westrick, AAS, CPC, CMA (AAMA)
Program Chair—Medical Assisting and Medical Insurance
    Billing/Office Administration
Ross Education, LLC
Brighton, Michigan

Nicole Ellen Zahuranec, CMA (AAMA), AOS
Elmira Business Institute
Elmira, New York

CONTENTS

UNIT SIX

Assisting with Medications

Deborah Proctor

UNIT NINE

Assisting with Surgeries
Deborah Proctor

UNIT TEN

Career Development
Brigitte Niedzwiecki and Julie Pepper

COMPETENCY-BASED EDUCATION AND THE MEDICAL ASSISTANT STUDENT

SCENARIO

Shawna Long is a newly admitted student in a medical assistant (MA) program at your school. Shawna is anxious about starting classes and very concerned that she may not be a successful student. She had trouble with some of her classes in high school and must continue to work part time while taking medical assistant classes. Based on what you discover about the learning process in this chapter, see whether you can help Shawna take steps toward success.

While studying this chapter, think about the following questions:

- What is competency-based education and how can it help Shawna learn and achieve skills?
- Why is it important for Shawna to understand how she learns best?
- Time management is a crucial part of being a successful student and a successful medical assistant. What are some methods Shawna can implement to help her manage her time as effectively as possible?

- Shawna will face many problems and challenges while working through the MA program. How can she develop workable strategies for dealing with these issues?
- What is the role of assertiveness in effective professional communications?
- Studying may be a challenge for Shawna. What skills can she use to help her learn new material and prepare for examinations?

LEARNING OBJECTIVES

1. Define, spell, and pronounce the terms listed in the vocabulary.
2. Discuss competency-based education and adult learners.
3. Summarize the importance of student portfolios in proving academic success and skill competency.
4. Examine your learning preferences and interpret how your learning style affects your success as a student.
5. Differentiate between adaptive and nonadaptive coping mechanisms.
6. Apply time management strategies to make the most of your learning opportunities.
7. Integrate effective study skills into your daily activities.
8. Design test-taking strategies that help you take charge of your success.
9. Incorporate critical thinking and reflection to help you make mental connections as you learn material.
10. Analyze healthcare results as reported in graphs and tables.
11. Apply problem-solving techniques to manage conflict and overcome barriers to your success.
12. Relate assertiveness, aggressiveness, and passive behaviors to professional communication and discuss the role of assertiveness in effective communication.

VOCABULARY

competencies Mastery of the knowledge, skills, and behaviors that are expected of the entry-level medical assistant.

critical thinking The constant practice of considering all aspects of a situation when deciding what to believe or what to do.

empathy (em'-puh-the) Sensitivity to the individual needs and reactions of patients.

learning style The way an individual perceives and processes information to learn new material.

mnemonic A learning device (e.g., an image, a rhyme, or a figure of speech) that a person uses to help him or her remember information.

perceiving (pur-sev'-ing) How an individual looks at information and sees it as real.

processing (pro'-ses-ing) How an individual internalizes new information and makes it his or her own.

reflection (re-flek'-shun) The process of thinking about new information so as to create new ways of learning.

stressor An event, activity, condition, or other stimulus that causes stress.

For many years the curriculum for medical assistant programs has been based on student achievement of specific **competencies**. According to the Medical Assisting Education Review Board (MAERB):

> Medical assistants graduating from programs accredited by the Commission on Accreditation of Allied Health Education Programs (CAAHEP) will demonstrate critical thinking based on knowledge of academic subject matter required for competence in the profession. They will incorporate the cognitive knowledge in performance of the psychomotor and affective domains in their practice as medical assistants in providing patient care.

The Accrediting Bureau of Health Education Schools (ABHES) also bases its recommended curriculum on student achievement of identified competencies:

> The depth and breadth of the program's curriculum enables graduates to acquire the knowledge and competencies necessary to become an entry-level professional in the medical assisting field. Competencies required for successful completion of the program are delineated, and the curriculum ensures achievement of these entry-level competencies through mastery of coursework and skill achievement. Focus is placed on credentialing requirements and opportunities to obtain employment and to increase employability.

National curriculum standards for the education of medical assistants are based on recognized competencies that employers expect entry-level medical assistants to have. The 2015 Core Curriculum for Medical Assistants established by the MAERB must be followed for programs accredited by CAAHEP. Those completing a CAAHEP-accredited program must demonstrate core entry-level competencies in knowledge of subject matter, be able to perform the psychomotor skills needed in an ambulatory care center, and have appropriate behavioral competencies to respond professionally and with **empathy** toward patients and their families. The 12 academic subjects in a CAAHEP-approved curriculum are as follows:

- I. Anatomy and Physiology
- II. Applied Mathematics
- III. Infection Control
- IV. Nutrition
- V. Concepts of Effective Communication
- VI. Administrative Functions
- VII. Basic Practice Finances
- VIII. Third Party Reimbursement
- IX. Procedural and Diagnostic Coding
- X. Legal Implications
- XI. Ethical Considerations
- XII. Protective Practices

ABHES also offers accreditation for medical assisting programs. The organization focuses its curriculum requirements on student competency achievement with 11 required areas of study:

1. General Orientation [to the field of medical assisting]
2. Anatomy and Physiology
3. Medical Terminology
4. Medical Law and Ethics
5. Psychology of Human Relations
6. Pharmacology
7. Records Management
8. Administrative Procedures
9. Clinical Procedures
10. Medical Laboratory Procedures
11. Career Development

What does this mean for you, the medical assistant student? To meet national standards, your MA program must comply with competency-based learning in multiple areas. The most important characteristic of competency-based education is that it measures learning and skill achievement over time. Students progress through the program by demonstrating their competence, which means they prove they have mastered the knowledge, skills, and professional behaviors required to achieve competency in a particular task. For example, one of the basic skills you must achieve as a medical assistant student is taking an accurate blood pressure. Some students will have more difficulty consistently achieving this goal than others, but each student must be able to take a blood pressure accurately before he or she can move on in the curriculum.

ADULT LEARNERS AND COMPETENCY-BASED EDUCATION

Competency-based learning is ideal for adult learners who are attempting to understand new information and achieve new skills. Educators recognize that adult learners come to the classroom with different work-related experiences and educational backgrounds. Therefore, adult students have a wide range of understanding about the knowledge and skills that must be achieved in the program. Adult students also learn material at different rates. Competency-based education recognizes these qualities of adult learners and takes advantage of them. Let's go back to the blood pressure example. Perhaps you took a healthcare lab in high school, in which you learned to take blood pressures; another student may have worked in a long-term care facility, where he was responsible for monitoring vital signs throughout the day. You both may need just a review of the anatomy and physiology aspects of a patient's blood pressure. However, other students in the class will not know anything about this skill. With competency-based education, your instructor can design laboratory activities that meet all students' needs, including your own.

CRITICAL THINKING APPLICATION   **1-1**

Can you think of any examples of how competency-based education might help you succeed as a medical assistant student? Come up with two possibilities and share them with your classmates.

PORTFOLIOS

Have you taken a class in the past that required you to develop a portfolio? Portfolios are frequently used in an Art or English class to demonstrate student skills and learning achievements. Generally, a portfolio is a collection of student materials that demonstrates learning. An advantage of developing a portfolio for a medical assistant program is that you can decide which pieces of your work best demonstrate your learning and skill achievement over time. Why would this be beneficial to you?

In a competency-based program, you must achieve a series of skills, not only to complete the program, but also to prove to future employers that you are competent in all the identified skills an entry-level medical assistant should have. Once you complete the program and are looking for your first medical assistant position, how can you prove to potential employers that you are competent in all required skills? What can you bring to an interview that summarizes your abilities? A comprehensive portfolio that you develop throughout the courses you take in your MA program contains materials that you can use to demonstrate the knowledge and skills you have accumulated throughout your course of study. A comprehensive portfolio includes examples of work completed in each course and proof of the skills achieved.

A comprehensive portfolio can be used to create an interview portfolio that is tailored to prove your competency in the skills outlined in a specific job description. (Interview portfolios are discussed in more detail in the chapter, Career Development and Life Skills.) For example, as a new graduate, you see an ad for a medical assistant position in a local pediatrician's office that is looking for an individual who is competent in electronic health records (EHRs), knowledgeable about immunizations, and who knows how to perform basic coding skills. If you have retained copies of all of your achievements in those designated areas in a comprehensive portfolio, you can pull out those specific copies to create a job interview portfolio that demonstrates your knowledge base and skill level. Items that you can feature in a comprehensive portfolio include:

- Samples of projects completed throughout your courses of study, to demonstrate your learning in a variety of subjects. For example, perhaps in one of your courses, you developed a list of community resources that could help patients with a variety of needs. Including this project demonstrates your knowledge of local agencies that might prove useful to the patient population of a healthcare facility where you are seeking employment. Another project may require you to investigate a specific disease process, including expected signs and symptoms, diagnostics, and treatment details. This project would demonstrate your knowledge of a disease process, management of patients, diagnostic studies, and medications. Other assignments may require you to demonstrate your administrative knowledge and skills, such as EHR skills, basic practice finances, and coding capabilities.
- Samples of key procedural checklists that show evidence of your achievement of skills in measuring and recording vital signs and performing hands-on skills, such as electrocardiography (ECG), phlebotomy, medical laboratory procedures, infection control, administration of medication, therapeutic communication, third-party reimbursement, medical law and ethics applications, and emergency preparedness and practices. Collecting copies of competency achievement documentation in all these areas will help you demonstrate entry-level job readiness during an interview.
- Copies of awards (e.g., scholarships, dean's list), to demonstrate your academic achievements.
- Copies of any certifications you have achieved (e.g., cardiopulmonary resuscitation [CPR] and First Aid and Safety), to demonstrate your readiness for employment in a healthcare facility.
- Letters of recommendation from current employers, faculty members, and others, to highlight your personal and work-related qualities.

Collecting material for a comprehensive portfolio should start with the very first course in the MA program in which you are enrolled. Choose examples of work that demonstrate your completion of core requirements, in addition to competency achievement across the curriculum. You then will have all the materials needed to create a specific interview portfolio for each job interview you earn.

WHO YOU ARE AS A LEARNER: HOW DO YOU LEARN BEST?

You have taken the first step toward becoming a successful student by choosing your profession and field of study. The medical assistant profession is both challenging and rewarding. Becoming a medical assistant opens the doors to a wide variety of opportunities in both administrative and clinical practice at ambulatory or institutional healthcare facilities. To become a successful medical assistant, you first must become a successful student. This chapter helps you discover the way you learn best and provides multiple strategies to assist you in your journey toward success.

CRITICAL THINKING APPLICATION   **1-2**

Consider your history as a student. What do you think helped you succeed? What do you think needs improvement? Create a plan for improvement that includes two or three ways you can become a more successful student. Be prepared to share this plan with your classmates.

Think about what you do when you are faced with something new to learn. How do you go about understanding and learning the new material? Over time you have developed a method for **perceiving** and **processing** information. This pattern of behavior is called your **learning style**. Learning styles can be examined in many different ways, but most professionals agree that a student's success depends more on whether the person can "make sense" of the information than on whether the individual is "smart." Determining your individual learning style and understanding how it applies to your ability to learn new material are the first steps toward becoming a successful student (Figure 1-1).

Learning Style Inventory

For you to learn new material, two things must happen. First, you must perceive the information. This is the method you have developed over time that helps you examine new information and recognize it as real. Once you have developed a method for learning about the new material, you must *process* the information. Processing the information is how you internalize it and make it your own. Researchers believe that each of us has a preferred method for learning new material. By investigating your learning style, you can figure out how to combine different approaches to perceiving and processing information that will lead to greater success as a student.

The first step in learning new material is determining how you perceive it, or as some experts explain, what methods you use to learn the new material. Some learners opt to watch, observe, and use **reflection** to think about and learn the new material. These students are *abstract perceivers,* who learn by analyzing new material, building

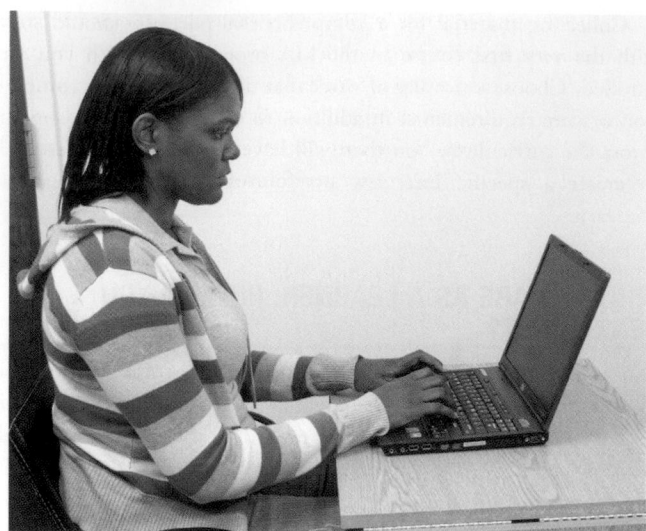

FIGURE 1-1 Student learning.

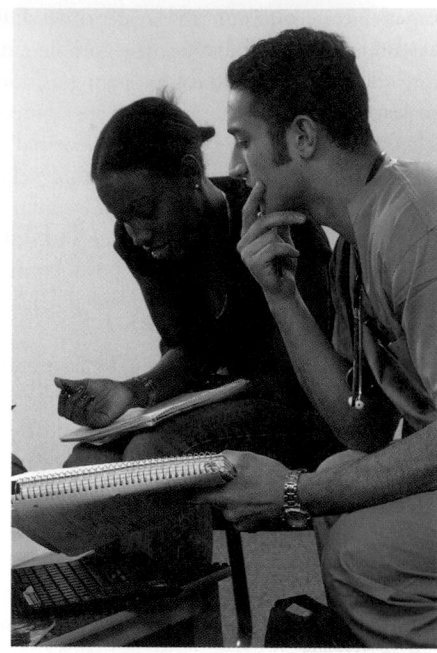

FIGURE 1-2 Learning in a small group.

theories about it, and using a step-by-step approach to learning. Other students need to perform some activity, such as rewriting notes from class, making flash cards, and outlining chapters, to learn new information. Students who learn by "doing" are called *concrete perceivers*. Concrete learners prefer to learn things that have a personal meaning or that they believe are relevant to their lives. So, which type of perceiver do you think you are? Before you actually learn new material, do you need time to think about it, or do you prefer to "do" something to help you learn the material?

The second step in learning new material is information processing, which is the way learners internalize the new information and make it their own. New material can be processed by two methods. *Active processors* prefer to jump in and start doing things immediately. They make sense of the new material by using it *now*. They look for practical ways to apply the new material and learn best with practice and hands-on activities. *Reflective processors* have to think about the information before they can internalize it. They prefer to observe and consider what is going on. The only way they can make sense of new material is to spend time thinking and learning a great deal about it before acting. Which type of information processor do you think you are? Do you prefer to jump in and start doing things to help you learn, or do you need to analyze and consider the material before you can actually learn it?

Using Your Learning Profile to Be a Successful Student: Where Do I Go From Here?

No one falls completely into one or the other of the categories just discussed. However, by being aware of how we generally prefer first to perceive information and then to process it, we can be more sensitive to our learning style and can approach new learning situations with a plan for learning the material in a way that best suits our learning preferences.

Your preferred perceiving and processing learning profile will fall into one of the following four stages of the Learning Style Inventory, which was created by David Kolb of Case Western Reserve University.

- *Stage 1* learners have a *concrete reflective* style. These students want to know the purpose of the information and have a personal connection to the content. They like to consider a situation from many points of view, observe others, and plan before taking action. They feel most comfortable watching rather than doing, and their strengths include sensitivity toward others, brainstorming, and recognizing and creatively solving problems. If you fall into this stage, you enjoy small-group activities and learn well in study groups.

- *Stage 2* learners have an *abstract reflective* style. These students are eager to learn just for the sheer pleasure of learning, rather than because the material relates to their personal lives. They like to learn lots of facts and arrange new material in a clear, logical manner. Stage 2 learners plan studying and like to create ways of thinking about the material, but they do not always make the connection with its practical application. If you are a stage 2 learner, you prefer organized, logical presentations of material and therefore enjoy lectures and readings and generally dislike group work. You also need time to process and think about new material before applying it.

- *Stage 3* learners have an *abstract active* style. Learners with this combination learning style want to experiment and test the information they are learning. If you are a stage 3 learner, you want to know how techniques or ideas work, and you also want to practice what you are learning. Your strengths are in problem solving and decision making, but you may lack focus and may be hasty in making decisions. You learn best with hands-on practice by doing experiments, projects, and laboratory activities. You enjoy working alone or in small groups (Figure 1-2).

- *Stage 4* learners are *concrete active* learners. These students are concerned about how they can use what they learn to make a difference in their lives. If you fall into this stage, you like to relate new material to other areas of your life. You have leadership capabilities, can create on your feet, and usually are vocal in a group, but you may have difficulty completing your work on time. Stage 4 learners enjoy teaching others and working in groups and learn best when they can apply new information to real-world problems.

To get the most out of knowing your learning profile, you need to apply this knowledge to how you approach learning. Each of the learning stages has pluses and minuses. When faced with a learning situation that does not match your learning preference, see how you can adapt your individual learning profile to make the best of the information. For example, if you are bored by lectures, look for an opportunity to apply the information being presented to a real problem you are facing in the classroom or at home. If you are an abstract perceiver, take time outside of class to think about new information so that you are ready to process it into your learning system. If you benefit from learning in a group, make the effort to organize review sessions and study groups. If you learn best by teaching others, offer to assist your peers with their learning. By taking the time now to investigate your preferred method of learning, you will perceive and process information more effectively throughout your school career.

COPING MECHANISMS

Have you ever thought about how you deal or cope with stressful situations? We each have our own ways of managing stress or conflict. We've developed these methods over time, and whether they are effective depends on the individual's personality and life experiences; the environment or situational specifics that surround the

issue; and the type of stress involved. For example, perhaps you have other demands on your time besides those related to school. Perhaps you are worried about money, house work, children, jobs, and so on. All these things can contribute to individual stress levels. Coping strategies are the methods we consciously use to solve problems and attempt to minimize the stress associated with them.

Strategies used to reduce stress are called *adaptive*, or *constructive*, *coping mechanisms*. For example, if finding time to study for an exam is stressful, an adaptive response to this stress is to use time management strategies, such as planning study hours in advance to avoid the stress of last-minute preparation. However, some coping strategies may actually increase stress levels. These are identified as *nonadaptive coping mechanisms*. Therefore, if you have a big project due and you procrastinate to the last minute to start working on it, your anxiety over the project may result in even more stress.

Adaptive coping mechanisms can help a person gain control over a stressful situation. Negative, or nonadaptive, strategies may be effective short term but often lead to long-term stress. The good news is that coping mechanisms are learned behaviors. It is possible to replace coping mechanisms that do not work with ones that are more successful.

One of the keys to managing stress in your life is to maintain your health. If you are eating properly, exercising regularly, and consistently getting enough sleep, you are much more capable of managing stress. Mentally managing your stress levels is also really important. Learning relaxation techniques, using positive self-talk, implementing time management strategies, expressing how you feel, and honestly communicating with others are all factors that can help you manage your stress levels more effectively.

Adaptive and Nonadaptive Coping Mechanisms

Adaptive Coping Mechanisms:
- Using humor to cope with a painful situation
- Gathering information about the cause of a problem
- Learning new skills to manage a problem
- Trying to derive meaning from a stressful situation
- Accepting the responsibility or blame
- Using distraction to manage negative feelings
- Practicing relaxation methods
- Using positive self-talk
- Seeking social support for the issue
- Anticipating a stressful situation and planning a coping strategy
- Getting adequate nutrition, exercise, and sleep

Nonadaptive Coping Mechanisms
- Compartmentalizing thoughts and emotions
- Anticipating or rehearsing stressful events
- Avoiding anxiety by relying on something (e.g., alcohol or drugs) or someone to cope with stress
- Doing everything you can to avoid stressful situations
- Running away, either physically or mentally, to escape a stressful situation

CRITICAL THINKING APPLICATION   1-6
Look back on the list of **stressors** in your life and how you typically responded to each. Is there anything you have learned from your reading that might help you better cope with stress? Next to each stressor, add an adaptive coping mechanism that could help.

TIME MANAGEMENT: PUTTING TIME ON YOUR SIDE

One of the most complicated tasks for a professional medical assistant is to manage time effectively. No other workplace can compete with the distractions and demands of a busy healthcare facility. Do you think you practice effective time management skills? Do you believe that you are in control of your time, or do you think that other people or situations control it? How frequently do you say that you just do not have enough time to do what you are supposed to do, let alone those things you would like to do? Time management gives you the opportunity to spend time in the way you choose. Effective time management is also crucial to your success as a student and as a future healthcare professional (Figure 1-3).

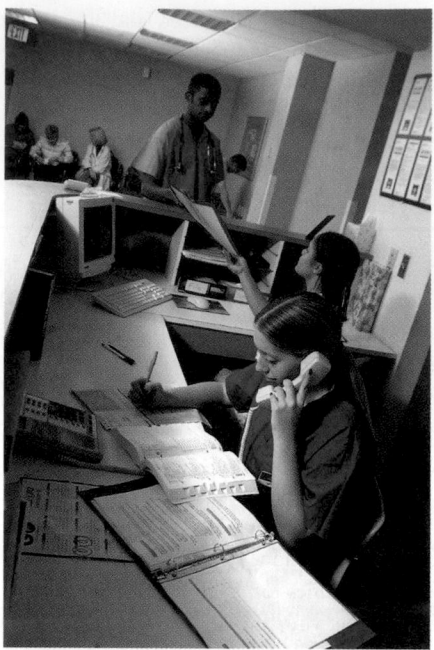

FIGURE 1-3 Time management in a busy medical practice.

How to Put Time on Your Side
The following time management skills are designed to help you deal effectively with the demands on your time. Highlight the ones you think will be most useful in helping you deal with your situation.
1. **Determine your purpose.** What do you want to accomplish this semester, in this course, or in this unit of study? What do you want to achieve as a student? What is one thing you can do to help achieve your goals?
2. **Identify your main concern.** Besides school, what other demands do you have on your time? Based on the learning goals you have established, what do you need to do to accomplish your goals?
   - *Plan time:* Schedule projects in advance, and make notes to yourself on deadlines.
   - *Guard time:* Avoid distractions (e.g., television, music, cell phones, social media) that interfere with your concentration. Notice how others abuse your time. Learn to say no to outside demands on your time.
   - *Discover time:* Think about what you do with your time all day long. Are there instances where you could "steal" time from something to "create" more time in your schedule? For example, maybe you spend time carpooling kids to activities or waiting for a class to start. Can you keep your books with you and use that downtime to highlight part of a chapter or create flash cards for an upcoming test?
   - *Assign time:* Ask for help when you need it from friends and family.
3. **Be organized.** What materials (e.g., books, research, supplies) do you need to have an effective study session? What preparation is needed to make the most of your time?
   - *Record time:* Use a day planner or calendar, either paper or electronic, to note the due dates for assignments and tests. If a paper or project is due on a specific date, put a reminder in your day planner to start the project on a specific date so that you are sure to have it done when it is due.

- *Optimal time:* Take advantage of the time of day when you study and learn the best. Schedule study time during your peak performance time. If you are an early riser, make time for homework first thing in the day; if you are a night owl, do your homework at night. Plan on dedicating at least some of your optimal time to your school work.

4. **Stop procrastinating.** If you avoid working on your goals, you may not achieve them. Examine the following suggestions as ways to break the procrastination cycle.

   - *Make the work meaningful:* What is important about the work you are putting off and what are the benefits of getting it done? Reflect on your long-range goals. Is it important to do a good job on the work so you can earn an acceptable grade, do well in the course, complete the medical assisting program, and ultimately find employment?
   - *Plan work deadlines:* Break assignments into achievable sections that can be completed in the time slots available. Schedule those work sections in your day planner so that you do not forget deadlines for assignments.
   - *Ask for help:* Let your support system know you have work to get done. Ask them for encouragement to stay on track. If you have school-age children, you can set an excellent example by planning "family" homework sessions. You can get some of your work done while acting as a role model for learning behaviors for your children. Let your partner know when due dates are looming or tests are scheduled. Ask for help in meeting day-to-day demands so that you can study or prepare for school.
   - *Prioritize:* If you keep avoiding a certain task, re-evaluate its priority. If it is really worth worrying about, get started now, not later. Don't waste time worrying about how you are going to get things done. Spend that time actually working on the projects that worry you the most.
   - *Reward yourself:* Create a reward that is meaningful and something for which you will work. If you want to spend time with your family or friends on the weekend, develop a plan and stick to it so that you can share that special time as a reward.

5. **Remember you.** It is very easy to become overwhelmed with responsibilities both in school and at home. Part of successful time management includes setting aside time to do things you enjoy. You have chosen a profession that can be very demanding. Now is the time to remember that you have to take care of yourself in addition to meeting your professional and personal responsibilities.

CRITICAL THINKING APPLICATION   **1-7**

How do you spend your time? For 3 days this week, write down the amount of time you spend on each activity. How much television do you watch? How much time do you spend talking or texting on the phone and checking social media? How about driving time, visiting time, work time, time for family and friends, and so on? At the end of the 3-day period, add up the amount of time you spent on your daily activities. Do you recognize any time you might be wasting? Can you implement any of the suggested time management strategies to make more time available?

STUDY SKILLS: TRICKS FOR BECOMING A SUCCESSFUL STUDENT

So far in this chapter, we have looked at the influence of individual learning styles and time management on learning success. Now we will investigate some ideas that are useful for learning new material. These study skills include memory techniques, active learning, brain tricks, reading methods, and note-taking strategies.

Several techniques can help you store and remember information. The first of these involves organizing information into recognizable groups so that the brain can find it easily. You can organize information by getting the big picture first before trying to learn the details. One way to implement this strategy is to skim a reading assignment before actually reading and taking notes on the material, thus getting a general impression of what you need to learn before tackling the details. Depending on your learning style, it may also help to find a way of making the new information meaningful. Think about your educational goals and how the new material will help you achieve those goals.

Another way of remembering material is to create an association with something you already know. If new material is grouped with already stored material, the brain remembers it much more easily. For example, maybe you took a biology class in high school and learned the basics about human anatomy and physiology. Try to create a link between what you previously learned and the detail of the new information you are expected to learn now. Or maybe you have a family member who suffers from a particular disease. Think about that individual's signs and symptoms while learning more details about the disease so that you can apply your learning to his or her situation.

A useful study skill for some learners is to be physically active while learning. Some students learn best if they walk or talk out loud while studying. Besides encouraging learning, moving and talking while studying relieves boredom and keeps you awake. Another way to be actively involved in learning is to use pictures or diagrams to represent the material you are studying. Some people are visual learners, and creating pictures of the material is the easiest method for them to retain the information. Other students find that rewriting notes, making lists of information, creating flash cards, color-coding notes, or highlighting important material in a textbook helps them retain the material. Writing also helps students who need to "do" something to learn.

Studying goes much more smoothly if you work with your brain rather than against it. If you tend to get anxious and worried while studying, you may be acting as your own worst enemy. One way of dealing with a topic you are anxious about is to overlearn it. If material is overlearned, you are much less likely to experience test anxiety. Another method for remembering material is to review it quickly after class. This mini-review helps the new information become part of your long-term memory system.

Many students find creating songs, dances, or word associations an effective way to learn and remember new material. Putting details into a familiar song and moving to it can help trick the brain into remembering the information. This is especially helpful when trying to learn anatomy and physiology. For example, think about one of your favorite songs and "dance" your way through the blood flow through the heart. Or, if you are finding the organization of the body especially tricky to remember, such as the movement of food through the gastrointestinal (GI) system, create a **mnemonic** that helps you remember the information. The most common one suggested for the parts of the intestines is: **D**ow **J**ones **I**ndustrial **C**limbing **A**verage **C**losing **S**tock **R**eport. The first letter of each word stands for an anatomic part of the intestines—*d*uodenum, *j*ejunum, *i*leum, *c*ecum, *a*ppendix, *c*olon, *s*igmoid, and *r*ectum. You can make up your own mnemonics or memory tricks to help you learn complicated material.

Another excellent way of learning information is to actually teach it to someone else. Teaching requires you to have a good understanding of the material and the ability to describe it for others. It can be an effective reinforcement of complicated material.

A great deal of the learning process is expected to take place from assigned readings. You can use several methods to make reading assignments more meaningful. If you find a reading assignment challenging or difficult to understand, the first step is to take the time to read it again. Sometimes the first time through the material is not enough to gain understanding. As you read, highlight important words or thoughts and stop periodically to summarize the material. Some students find outlining new material helpful. This is another way to use active learning to help you make the information "your own."

If you get bored while reading, use your body; walk or talk your way through the assignment. Take the time to look up words or terms you do not understand or ask your instructor or tutor for help. The best way to determine whether you have learned anything from your reading is to try to explain the material to someone else. For example, you can meet with other students and explain to them what you learned. If you can do that effectively, you know you have acquired the knowledge needed from the reading assignment.

Many students find effective note taking a challenge. The big question is, "How much of what the instructor says do I actually need to write down?" The first step in effective note taking is to come to class prepared. The more familiar you are with the material, the easier it will be to determine the important parts of the instructor's lecture. Pay attention to the instructor and look for clues to what he or she thinks is important. Ask questions about the material if you do not understand it, rather than writing down information that makes no sense to you. Think critically about what you hear before you write it down so you can start to build relationships among the things you want or need to know.

If your instructor uses PowerPoint presentations to teach a lesson, request copies of the slides before the lecture so you have an opportunity to review them as you are doing your reading. Many courses have an online website where PowerPoints or other lecture materials are available for review. Take advantage of these added materials to be prepared for each class so that you can ask questions about anything you don't understand. In addition, this textbook has an extensive online site (i.e., Evolve) that you can access for learning resources. Investigate the site and see whether something there can help you reach your learning goals.

When it comes to actual note taking, some strategies can make the process of recording notes an active learning tool. Organize the information as much as possible while you are writing or typing, either in an outline or a paragraph format. If you take notes on a laptop or tablet, make sure your typing skills are good enough for you to keep up with the flow of information and that you review

your notes shortly after class to fill in any missing details. If you take notes on paper, use only one side of the page (for easier reading) and leave blank spaces where needed to fill in details later. Use key words to help you remember the material, and create pictures or diagrams to help visualize it. If permitted, use tape recorders and make sure you have copies of any handouts or notes distributed by your instructor that cover material written on the board or provided in a PowerPoint presentation. If your instructor refers the class to a YouTube video or other website, transcribe the site address correctly to refer to it at a later time. Another helpful tool is to develop your own system of abbreviations to help simplify the note-taking process.

The most effective way to use your notes is to review them shortly after class. This is the time to add details, clarify information, or make notes about asking the instructor for explanations during the next class. You could even exchange notes with students you trust to compare information (Figure 1-4). Some students find it beneficial to create a computerized copy of their notes (if they wrote them out on paper) or to rewrite them. This gives you an opportunity to learn the material as you transcribe it. As you are reviewing your notes, you also can draw mind maps of the information or diagram outlines to help you better understand and remember the material.

Creating mind maps is a way of representing the main idea of a topic and supporting important details with a figure or picture. Healthcare textbooks present complicated concepts with multiple main ideas, each with its own important details. Mind maps are a way of combining complex details and organizing them into a format that is easier to remember. The spider map (Figure 1-5)

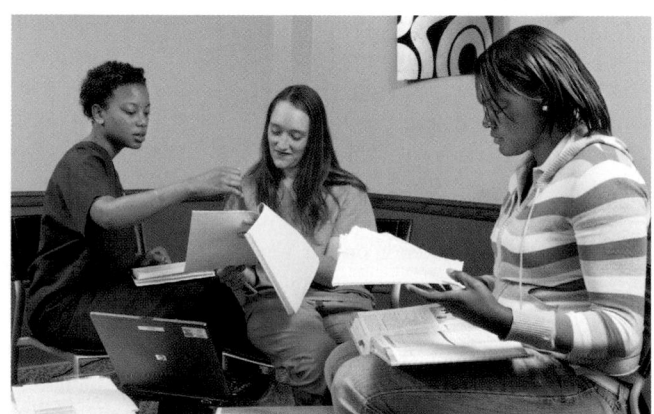

FIGURE 1-4 Sharing notes.

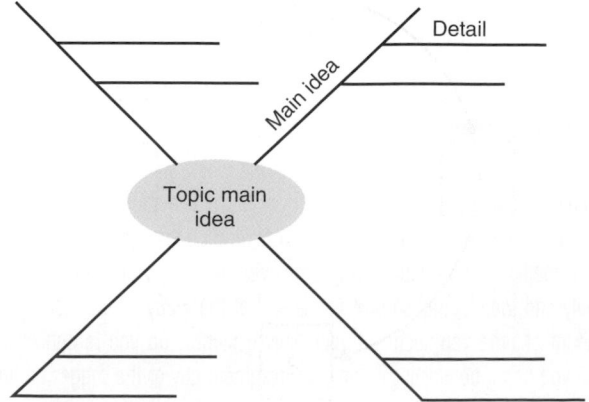

FIGURE 1-5 Spider map showing multiple main ideas with supporting details.

presents a method for including several main ideas with details in one study guide. The fishbone map (Figure 1-6) can be used to learn complicated causes of disease. The chain-of-events map (Figure 1-7) displays the cause and effect of events, such as infection control or the history of medicine. The cycle map (Figure 1-8) shows the connection between factors, such as in the chain of infection. Creating your own mind maps is a way of making the information more meaningful and easier for you to understand and remember.

Although many techniques can help you study, perhaps the most important one is your attitude toward learning. Some students fall into the "I can't possibly learn this material" trap. That type of attitude only leads to self-defeat. The way to overcome barriers is first to recognize that they exist. Once you know your weak spots, use the suggested study skills to improve in those areas. Do not be afraid to ask questions or to ask for help if you do not understand the material. Use as many different strategies as necessary to become a successful student.

CRITICAL THINKING APPLICATION   **1-8**

Write down at least two barriers to learning that you face. Review the study skills suggestions and choose four to try out. Use them over the next week to help you learn new material. Reflect on whether the chosen study skills helped you learn the material better.

TEST-TAKING STRATEGIES: TAKING CHARGE OF YOUR SUCCESS

What happens when you do not know the answer to the first question on a test? What if you do not know the next one? Are you able to go on without panicking? Many people find taking tests the most challenging part of being a successful student. Multiple approaches are available that you can use to take charge of your success and improve your ability to take tests. These include such strategies as adequate preparation, controlling negative thoughts during test time, and understanding ways to manage various types of questions.

The first step is to go into a test adequately prepared. Use the time management skills already outlined in this chapter to prepare for the big day. Recognize and use your preferred learning style to overlearn the material and increase your confidence. Use memory tools (e.g., flash cards, checklists, and mind maps) to help you visualize the material. Form a study group if you are the type of learner who benefits from studying in groups. Schedule and plan study time, and reward yourself for your hard work. It also is important to go into the test rested and relaxed; therefore, you should eat, exercise to relieve stress, and sleep before the test so that you are as alert as possible.

Before you start the test, make sure you read the directions carefully. If possible, begin with the easiest or shortest questions to build your confidence. Be aware of the amount of time allotted for the examination, and pace yourself accordingly. As you go through the test, look for clues to answers in other questions. During test time, remember to use positive self-talk at the first indication of panic. Repeatedly remind yourself that you are well prepared; relax and think about the material before you get worried. You need to stop negative thoughts as soon as they arise and instead visualize yourself being successful. Use slow, deep breathing to relax and, if helpful, close your eyes for a minute and visualize a relaxing place before you go on with the test.

Certain strategies are useful for answering different types of questions. With multiple choice questions, try to identify key words or clues in each question. Read the question carefully and answer it in your head before you review the provided answers. If you are not absolutely sure of the answer, make an educated guess or follow your instincts in choosing an answer. If there are answers that you know are not correct, that can eliminate the "all of the above" answer choice. By eliminating the answers that you know are incorrect, you can focus on the other answer choices.

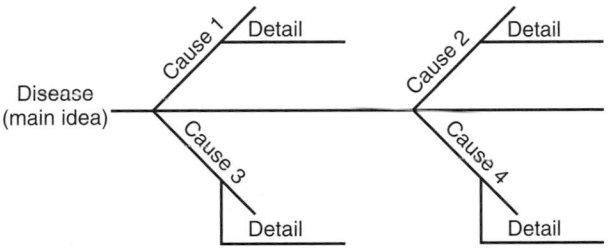

FIGURE 1-6 Fishbone map used to describe causes of disease.

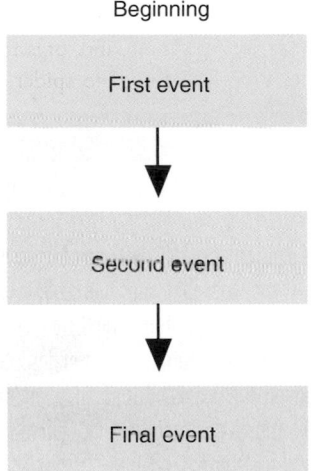

FIGURE 1-7 Chain-of-events map showing the cause and effect of events.

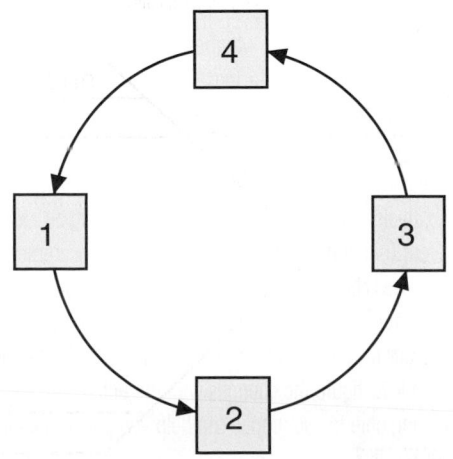

FIGURE 1-8 Cycle map illustrating the way one action leads to another.

"True or false" questions give you a 50/50 chance of being correct. Remember that if any part of the question is not true, then the statement is false. Again, check the statements for key words that help indicate the direction of the answer. Look for qualifying terms (e.g., *always, never, sometimes*) that are the key to understanding the meaning of the true or false statement.

CRITICAL THINKING APPLICATION   **1-9**

Think about a time you experienced test anxiety. Write down the details of the situation and how you felt. Choose four test-taking strategies you think would be beneficial in handling similar situations in the future.

BECOMING A CRITICAL THINKER: MAKING MENTAL CONNECTIONS

The ability to process information and arrive at reasonable conclusions is crucial to all healthcare workers. The process of **critical thinking** involves (1) sorting out conflicting information, (2) weighing your knowledge about that information, (3) ignoring or letting go of personal biases, and (4) deciding on a reasonable belief or action. Critical thinking is actually an active search for the truth.

Critical thinking could be described as thorough thinking, because it requires learners to keep an open mind to all possibilities. Successful students are thorough thinkers because they must determine the facts about a topic and come to logical conclusions about the material. Critical thinkers also are inquisitive learners; they constantly analyze and sort out conflicting information to reach conclusions.

A crucial step in critical thinking is evaluating the results of your learning. Reflection is the key to critical thinking. "How did I learn what I learned?" and "What does it mean in my life?" are questions that must be asked consistently to continue to learn. Becoming a successful student, and ultimately a successful member of the allied health team, requires critical thinking skills.

Tables and Graphs

Tables and graphs can be helpful tools in many aspects of healthcare, but you must take the time to analyze the information they include so that you process it accurately. For example, the body mass index (BMI) table you will learn about in the chapter, Nutrition and Health Promotion, and the growth chart graphs you will learn to use in the chapter, Assisting in Pediatrics, provide significant information about the health status of individual patients. In addition, tables throughout this textbook outline and summarize details about coding, health insurance, disease processes, medications, and treatments. To maximize your learning throughout the medical assistant program, you should use the information in tables and graphs to help prepare yourself to work as an entry-level medical assistant.

A graph is a diagram or picture that represents information and its relationships. Analyzing graphs is useful for determining a general

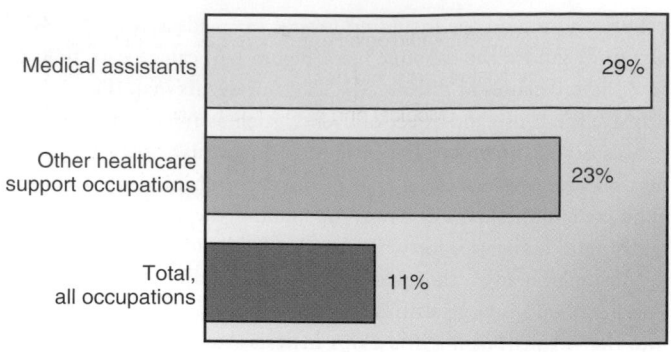

FIGURE 1-9 Projected percentage change in employment of medical assistants (2012 to 2022).

trend; for example, Figure 1-9 shows the projected increase in employment opportunities for medical assistants from 2012 to 2022. The bar graph clearly demonstrates the projected percentage of changes in employment opportunities for medical assistants. Figure 1-10 shows the projected change in total employment of select healthcare occupations. Can you see how graphs can help you understand a concept much easier than if the data were written out in paragraph form? More than one type of graph can be used to represent a single set of information.

How to Analyze a Graph

1. *Read the title and the axes of a graph to determine the information included.*

   The *x*-axis is the line on a graph that runs horizontally (left to right), and the *y*-axis is the line that runs vertically (up and down). For example, in Figure 1-10, different healthcare occupations are listed along the *y*-axis, and projected job opportunities (in hundreds of thousands) are listed on the *x*-axis. Based on your interpretation of this information, how many positions did the Bureau of Labor Statistics project for medical assistants?

2. *Determine the general trend of the graph.*

   For example, if you review the growth chart graph of a 2-year-old girl, you would be able to see whether her height and weight have consistently increased over time or whether she has had a sudden increase (maybe a growth spurt) or a decrease that might reflect a recent illness.

3. *Graphs can also be useful in visualizing information that doesn't seem to fit.*

   For example, if you are responsible for measuring the length and weight of a 4-month-old infant and the measurements that you took are markedly different (either larger or smaller) than the measurements recorded at the last well-child examination, perhaps your measurements are incorrect. If you check them again and come up with the same numbers, document your results but inform the provider of the differences so the provider can investigate the changes with the baby's caregiver. Can you see how being able to use graphs can help you gain insight into patient healthcare results?

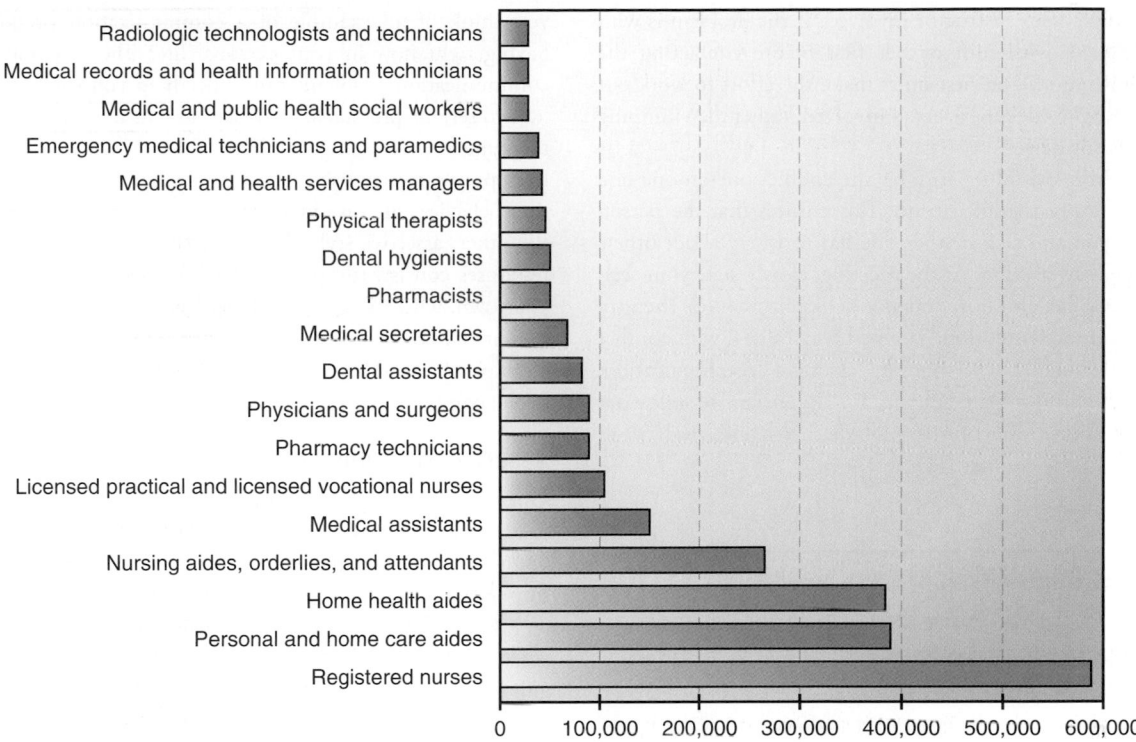

FIGURE 1-10 Projected change in total employment of select health care occupations, 2006-2016. Bureau of Labor Statistics, http://www.bls.gov/spotlight/2009/health_care/home.htm. Accessed August 31, 2015.

PROBLEM SOLVING AND CONFLICT MANAGEMENT

As a future member of the healthcare team, you frequently will face problems and conflict. Although we usually look at these situations as negative factors in our lives, problem solving and conflict management actually give us the opportunity to affect a potentially negative situation in a positive way. Learning how to manage problems can be very useful for your practice as a medical assistant and for your success as a student.

The first step in reaching an equitable solution to a problem or conflict is to identify the central issue. How many times have you known that you were upset about something but were not really sure why you felt that way? You cannot solve a problem or resolve a negative situation unless you are sure of what is at the root of your feelings. You need to understand the problem and gather as much information about the situation as possible before you decide to act. One way to do this is to ask yourself these questions:

- When does the situation occur and under what circumstances?
- How does it make me feel?
- Is someone else involved? Who? Is it the same person every time?
- What interferes with making a decision or resolving the conflict?

Once you understand the situation and how you feel about it, you need to decide whether it is worth the effort to resolve it. Prioritize your involvement. Sometimes situations and problems may arise that you are unable to resolve or that you may decide are not important enough to act on. For example, one of the students in your class occasionally checks her phone during lectures. You find her behavior distracting at times, but does it bother you enough to

do something about it? If it does, then you need to try to resolve the conflict. However, if it is a minor problem, then maybe it isn't worth the effort to talk to her about it. After you have gathered the details about the problem or conflict and you have decided it is important enough to act on, it is time to determine possible solutions. One way to do this is to ask for advice or brainstorm ideas with individuals you respect. Sometimes another person can give you special insight into the problem that you were unable to see on your own. After brainstorming for possible solutions, you should get feedback on the workability of the suggested solutions. An alternative to brainstorming possible solutions to the problem is to list the pros and cons of possible solutions on a piece of paper. Simply looking at a list of the positive and negative aspects of the solution may clarify how you could solve the problem. Before deciding on a particular solution, make sure you critically analyze the consequences of each proposed solution: Which one best meets your needs and has the potential for providing an outcome you can live with?

Finally, you are ready to implement the chosen solution. However, your work is not over yet. You need to evaluate the outcome of your decision and see whether it truly did meet your needs. If not, it may be time to review other possible solutions and try another approach.

Conflict management requires some additional consideration. If you are in conflict with a peer, an instructor, or a co-worker, it is important to follow certain guidelines. First of all, regardless of the situation, you should follow the chain of command to reach a reasonable resolution to the conflict. If you are in conflict with another student, then you should attempt to work it out with that person before trying to get your instructor involved. If the problem is with an instructor, meet with him or her first before contacting the school's administration. You first must make the effort to work out the issue directly with the other person involved, rather than jumping to another level for help.

In addition, you should try to solve the conflict one-on-one in a private place at a prescheduled time. This ensures that the person will meet with you and that neither one has to worry about others overhearing the conversation. At the meeting, clearly state your feelings about the conflict and how you would like it resolved. Then try to come to an agreeable solution. The best way to deal with conflict situations is through open, honest, assertive communication. However, just as with problem solving, it is important to follow up on the decided course of action to see whether it effectively dealt with the source of the conflict (Figure 1-11).

CRITICAL THINKING APPLICATION   1-10

Think about a serious problem you are currently facing. Use the brainstorming and/or pros and cons method for creating solutions to the problem. Implement your chosen solution, and follow up on its effectiveness. Did the problem-solving process help you manage the situation more effectively?

ASSERTIVE, AGGRESSIVE, AND PASSIVE COMMUNICATION

Effective communication is crucial in the healthcare environment. As a medical assistant, you are expected to communicate clearly and empathetically with patients, families, peers, and other healthcare professionals. Your ability to display professional communication behaviors will determine your success in this new profession. Can

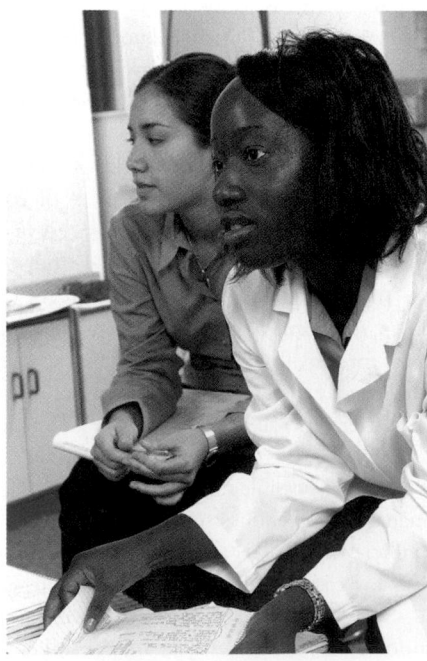

FIGURE 1-11 Dealing with conflict.

you think of an example of a communication problem you are having right now in your personal life? The way you respond to communication problems can either help you solve them fairly or lead to serious problems. We learn how to respond to conflict from the time we are young children. This learned behavior can range from passive to aggressive to assertive behaviors. Passive communication behaviors are on one extreme, and aggressive responses are on the other; assertive styles balance responses in the middle. Passive responses consistently protect the interests of another person over your own, whereas aggressive behaviors demand that your needs be met at the expense of another. Assertive communication strategies attempt to defend both your rights and those of the other individual in the conflict.

Assertive Communication

One of the challenges faced by workers in a healthcare environment is acting assertively when necessary. Assertive communication allows you to express your thoughts and feelings honestly and enables you to stand up for yourself in a reasonable, rational manner without an emotional scene. However, most of us are not born assertive; it is a behavior that must be learned, and many of us must practice it over and over again before it becomes a natural response.

Passive, or nonassertive, individuals often feel hurt when they are taken advantage of or are anxious about dealing with conflict. Just because they comply with what they are told to do or do not argue when they are treated unfairly does not mean that they are not upset about the situation. Often these individuals internalize their hurt and anxiety and eventually have an angry outburst because of built-up stress. Aggressive individuals, on the other hand, take advantage of others, appear self-righteous, and act in a superior way to get what they want. People who act aggressively may humiliate or hurt others to achieve their goals or to have their own needs satisfied.

Passive and Aggressive Behaviors and Language

An individual with passive or nonassertive body language displays the following behaviors when attempting to deal with conflict:
- Keeps the eyes downcast
- Shifts his or her weight when talking
- Has a slumped posture or wrings the hands
- Whines or uses a hesitant tone of voice
- May use the following phrases:
  - "Maybe" or "I guess"
  - "I wonder if you could…"
  - "Would you mind very much if…"
  - "It's not really important."

An aggressive person displays the following behaviors:
- Leans forward and points a finger when talking
- Raises the voice or sounds arrogant
- May use the following phrases:
  - "You'd better…"
  - "If you don't watch out…"
  - "Do it or else!"
  - "You should do it this way!"

Learning how to respond assertively in a potentially challenging situation enables us to be honest and direct with others while at the same time being emotionally honest with ourselves. The goal of assertive behavior is to treat others with respect while acknowledging our own feelings about the problem.

The first step in becoming assertive is to describe the situation and how it makes you feel. Perhaps you have a co-worker who is taking advantage of you; coming to work late, taking long breaks, not answering the phones, and so on. How does that make you feel? Are you angry, hurt, or disappointed? Decide which word best describes your feelings and, using an "I" sentence, clearly state how you feel about the situation. Be specific about the problem. If your statement is too general (e.g., "I am very hurt when you act like that"), the person you are confronting can either misunderstand or ignore you because he or she does not know specifically what is wrong. A statement such as, "I am very hurt that you take advantage of me by consistently being late for work, taking long breaks, and not helping with answering the phones," makes the problem very clear and expresses your feelings when the behavior occurs.

Acting assertively takes practice, practice, practice. In addition, just because you deliver a clear, concise, assertive message does not mean that the problem will be solved that quickly. Your assertive words must be combined with assertive body language to deliver a clear message about how serious you consider the situation. Remember, 80% to 90% of a message is nonverbal. Therefore, your "I" message must be accompanied by assertive behavior, including establishing eye contact and slightly raising your voice to get the individual's attention. And just because you deliver the perfect message does not mean you will always get what you want. The message may have to be repeated; do you really think someone who is habitually late for work is going to start showing up on time because of one assertive message? However, regardless of the outcome, you will feel better because you have honestly communicated how you feel about the situation, and you are actively working on a resolution of the problem.

CRITICAL THINKING APPLICATION 1-11

Do you consider yourself passive (nonassertive), assertive, or aggressive? Think about a recent conflict situation. How did you respond? Could assertive behaviors help you solve the problem while making you feel better about yourself?

Professional Behaviors Box

Perhaps the most difficult thing for you to learn is the art of assertiveness; that is, honestly informing others how you feel about a conflict situation, why you feel that way, and what changes you would like to see. The professional medical assistant faces many challenging situations. Communicating assertively helps you therapeutically resolve those conflicts. In addition, as a professional medical assistant, you are expected to act as the patient's advocate. To perform this crucial duty adequately, you must learn to communicate assertively with other individuals and organizations to meet the needs of your patients.

SUMMARY OF SCENARIO

One of the things Shawna can do to improve her learning is to determine her individual learning style. By understanding how she typically perceives and processes new information, she can plan the best methods for learning new material. In addition to understanding who she is as a learner, Shawna needs to practice successful coping mechanisms and time management skills to keep up with school and work responsibilities. Assertive communication, effective problem solving, and developing study skills that work for her are also keys to her success as a student.

SUMMARY OF LEARNING OBJECTIVES

1. **Define, spell, and pronounce the terms listed in the vocabulary.**
   Spelling and pronouncing medical terms correctly reinforce the medical assistant's credibility. Knowing the definitions of these terms promotes confidence in communication with patients and co-workers.

2. **Discuss competency-based education and adult learners.**
   The most important characteristic of competency-based education is that it measures learning and skill achievement over time. Students progress by demonstrating their competence, which means they prove that they have mastered the knowledge, skills, and professional behaviors required to achieve competency in a particular task.

3. **Summarize the importance of student portfolios in proving academic success and skill competency.**
   A portfolio is a collection of student materials that demonstrates learning. A comprehensive portfolio is developed throughout the courses in a medical assistant program and contains materials that demonstrate the knowledge and skills achieved by the student throughout the course of study. A comprehensive portfolio includes examples of work completed in each course and proof of the skills achieved. It can be used to create individual interview portfolios that demonstrate knowledge and skill achievement.

4. **Examine your learning preferences and interpret how your learning style affects your success as a student.**
   Learning preferences are the ways you like to learn and that have proven successful in the past. Your learning style is determined by your individual method of perceiving or examining new material and the way you process it or make it your own. People are either concrete or abstract perceivers and either active or reflective processors.

5. **Differentiate between adaptive and nonadaptive coping mechanisms.**
   Adaptive coping mechanisms help a person gain control over a stressful situation; negative or nonadaptive strategies may be effective short term but often lead to long-term stress.

Continued

SUMMARY OF LEARNING OBJECTIVES—*continued*

6. **Apply time management strategies to make the most of your learning opportunities.**

   Using effective time management strategies, such as setting goals, prioritizing, getting organized, and avoiding procrastination, results in a more successful student and an effective medical assistant.

7. **Integrate effective study skills into your daily activities.**

   Study skills, such as memory techniques, active learning, brain tricks, effective reading methods, note-taking strategies, and mind maps, all help students to be more successful.

8. **Design test-taking strategies that help you take charge of your success.**

   Test-taking strategies include preparing adequately for the examination, controlling negative thoughts during the examination, and understanding how to deal with different types of questions.

9. **Incorporate critical thinking and reflection to help you make mental connections as you learn material.**

   Critical thinking can be defined as *thorough thinking* because it considers all sides of the information without bias. Reflection is the process of thinking about or reviewing information before acting.

10. **Analyze healthcare results as reported in graphs and tables.**

    Tables and graphs can be helpful tools in many aspects of healthcare, but you must take the time to analyze the information they present so that you process it accurately. Tables are used to outline and summarize significant healthcare information, and graphs diagram or create a picture that represents information and its relationships. To maximize your learning throughout the medical assistant program, you should use the information in tables and graphs to help prepare you to perform as an entry-level medical assistant.

11. **Apply problem-solving techniques to manage conflict and overcome barriers to your success.**

    Problem-solving and conflict management techniques are crucial to your success. First, identify the central issue and how you feel about it; then, consider possible solutions and their potential results, implement the chosen solution, and analyze the results.

12. **Relate assertiveness, aggressiveness, and passive behaviors to professional communication and discuss the role of assertiveness in effective communication.**

    Passive responses consistently protect the interests of another person over your own, whereas aggressive behaviors demand that your needs be met at the expense of another. Assertive communication strategies attempt to defend both your rights and those of the other individual in the conflict.

    Assertive communication allows you to express your thoughts and feelings honestly and enables you to stand up for yourself in a reasonable, rational manner without an emotional scene. Learning how to respond assertively in a potentially challenging situation enables us to be honest and direct with others while at the same time being emotionally honest with ourselves. The goal of assertive behavior is to treat others with respect while acknowledging our own feelings about the problem.

CONNECTIONS

Study Guide Connection: Go to the Chapter 1 Study Guide. Read and complete the activities.

evolve Evolve Connection: Go to the Chapter 1 link at *evolve.elsevier.com/kinn* to complete the Chapter Review Quiz. Check out the other resources listed for this chapter to make the most of what you have learned from Competency-Based Education and the Medical Assistant Student.

THE MEDICAL ASSISTANT AND THE HEALTHCARE TEAM

2

SCENARIO

Carmen Angelos is a new student in a medical assisting program accredited by the Commission on Accreditation of Allied Health Education Programs (CAAHEP) at Butler County Community College. Carmen is returning to school after working at a local pharmacy for 5 years, where she became very interested in pursuing a career in medical assisting. She has been out of high school for a few years but is very excited about her new career choice.

While studying this chapter, think about the following questions:

- Why is it important to learn about professional medical assisting organizations?
- What is a typical job description for an entry-level medical assistant?
- What allied health professionals might you work with as a medical assistant?

- Why is it important for medical assisting students to learn about the various healthcare facilities and medical specialties?
- How will scope of practice and standards of care determine your role as a medical assistant?

LEARNING OBJECTIVES

1. Define, spell, and pronounce the terms listed in the vocabulary.
2. Summarize the history of medicine and its significance to the medical assisting profession.
3. Identify national departments and agencies that focus on health.
4. List professional medical assisting organizations.
5. Discuss the typical job description of a medical assistant and describe the role of the medical assistant as a patient navigator.
6. Identify a variety of allied health professionals who are part of the healthcare team.
7. Summarize the various types of medical specialties and healthcare facilities.
8. Define a patient-centered medical home (PCMH) and discuss its five core functions and attributes.
9. Differentiate between scope of practice and standards of care for medical assistants, and compare and contrast provider and medical assistant roles in terms of standard of care.

VOCABULARY

accreditation (uh-kre-duh-ta'-shun) The process by which an organization is recognized for adherence to a group of standards that meet or exceed the expectations of the accrediting agency.

allopathic (al-o-path'-ik) A system of medical practice that treats disease by the use of remedies, such as medications and surgery, to produce effects different from those caused by the disease under treatment; medical doctors (MDs) and osteopaths (DOs) practice allopathic medicine; also called *conventional medicine.*

complementary and alternative medicine (CAM) A group of diverse medical and healthcare systems, practices, and products that are not generally considered part of conventional medicine. Complementary medicine is used in combination with conventional medicine (allopathic or osteopathic); alternative medicine is used instead of conventional medicine.

contamination (kun-ta-mu-na'-shun) The process by which something becomes harmful or unusable through contact with something unclean.

holistic (ho-lis'-tik) A form of healing that considers the whole person (i.e., body, mind, spirit, and emotions) in individual treatment plans.

hospice (hos'-pus) A concept of care that involves health professionals and volunteers who provide medical, psychological, and spiritual support to terminally ill patients and their loved ones.

indicator An important point or group of statistical values that, when evaluated, indicates the quality of care provided in a healthcare facility.

negligence Conduct that falls below the standards of behavior established by law; a *negligent act* is one that does not meet the standards of what is expected of a reasonably prudent person acting under similar circumstances.

subluxations (sub-luk-sa'-shuns) Slight misalignments of the vertebrae or a partial dislocation.

triage The process of sorting patients to determine medical need and the priority of care.

Medical assistants are multiskilled healthcare workers who function under the direction of a licensed provider and are primarily employed in outpatient or ambulatory care facilities, such as medical offices and clinics. According to the U.S. Bureau of Labor Statistics, medical assisting is one of the nation's fastest growing careers, and employment opportunities are projected to grow 29% through 2022.

This growth in job opportunities for medical assistants is due to multiple factors, including a steady increase in the aging population as baby-boomers spur demand for preventive health services from physician offices and ambulatory care centers. Since medical assistants are trained in both administrative and clinical skills they are perfect employees to meet the needs of this increasing population. In addition, the Affordable Care Act has given millions of uninsured Americans the opportunity to have health insurance, which means physician practices and clinics will be caring for an ever-increasing number of patients. The switch to electronic health records (EHRs) in ambulatory care centers will also open up employment opportunities for medical assistants who are trained in EHR computer software.

THE HISTORY OF MEDICINE

Although religious and mythologic beliefs were the basis for care for the sick in ancient times, evidence suggests that drugs, surgery, and other treatments based on theories about the body were used as early as 5,000 BC. Moses presented rules of health to the Hebrews in approximately 1205 BC. He was the first advocate of preventive medicine and is considered the first public health officer. Moses knew that some animal diseases could be passed to humans and that **contamination** existed; therefore, a religious law was developed forbidding humans to eat or drink from dirty dishes. The people of that era believed that doing so would defile their bodies, and they would lose their souls.

Hippocrates, known as the Father of Medicine, is the most famous of the ancient Greek physicians. He was born in 450 BC on the island of Cos in Greece. He is best remembered for the Hippocratic Oath, which has been administered to physicians for more than 2,000 years. To this day, most graduating medical school students swear to some form of the oath (Figure 2-1). Hippocrates is credited with taking mysticism out of medicine and giving it a scientific basis. During this period of history, most believed that illness was caused by demonic possession; to cure the illness, the demon had to be removed from the body. Hippocrates' clinical descriptions of diseases and his volumes on epidemics, fevers, epilepsy, fractures, and instruments were studied for centuries. He believed that the body had the capacity to heal itself and that the physician's role was to help nature. He described four "humors": blood, phlegm, yellow bile, and black bile, which he believed must be in balance for the body to maintain a healthy state.

Medical knowledge developed slowly, and distribution of such knowledge was poor. In the seventeenth century, European academies or societies were established, consisting of small groups of men who met to discuss subjects of mutual interest. One of the earliest academies was the Royal Society of London, formed in 1662. In the United States, medical education was greatly influenced by the Johns Hopkins University School of Medicine in Baltimore, Maryland, established in the early 1890s. The school admitted only college graduates with at least one year's training in the natural sciences. The clinical education at Johns Hopkins was superior because the school partnered with Johns Hopkins Hospital, which had been created expressly for teaching and research by members of the medical faculty. Table 2-1 presents selected medical pioneers and their achievements.

I swear to fulfill, to the best of my ability and judgment, this covenant:

I will respect the hard-won scientific gains of those physicians in whose steps I walk, and gladly share such knowledge as is mine with those who are to follow.

I will apply, for the benefit of the sick, all measures [that] are required, avoiding those twin traps of overtreatment and therapeutic nihilism.

I will remember that there is art to medicine as well as science, and that warmth, sympathy, and understanding may outweigh the surgeon's knife or the chemist's drug.

I will not be ashamed to say "I know not," nor will I fail to call in my colleagues when the skills of another are needed for a patient's recovery.

I will respect the privacy of my patients, for their problems are not disclosed to me that the world may know. Most especially must I tread with care in matters of life and death. If it is given me to save a life, all thanks. But it may also be within my power to take a life; this awesome responsibility must be faced with great humbleness and awareness of my own frailty. Above all, I must not play at God.

I will remember that I do not treat a fever chart, a cancerous growth, but a sick human being, whose illness may affect the person's family and economic stability. My responsibility includes these related problems, if I am to care adequately for the sick.

I will prevent disease whenever I can, for prevention is preferable to cure.

I will remember that I remain a member of society, with special obligations to all my fellow human beings, those sound of mind and body as well as the infirm.

If I do not violate this oath, may I enjoy life and art, respected while I live and remembered with affection thereafter. May I always act so as to preserve the finest traditions of my calling and may I long experience the joy of healing those who seek my help.

Written in 1964 by Louis Lasagna, Academic Dean of the School of Medicine at Tufts University, and used in many medical schools today.

FIGURE 2-1 Modern version of the Hippocratic Oath.

TABLE 2-1   Medical Pioneers and Their Achievements

NAME	ACHIEVEMENT	NAME	ACHIEVEMENT
Andreas Vesalius (1514-1564)	Father of modern anatomy; wrote first anatomy book	Robert Koch (1843-1910)	Developed Koch's postulates, a theory of causative agents for disease; discovered the cause of cholera
William Harvey (1578-1657)	Discovered the circulatory system	William Roentgen (1845-1923)	Discovered the x-ray
Anton van Leeuwenhoek (1632-1723)	First to observe microbes through a lens; developed the first microscope	Walter Reed (1851-1902)	Proved that yellow fever was transmitted by mosquito bites while in the U.S. Army serving in Cuba
John Hunter (1728-1793)	Founder of scientific surgery	Paul Ehrlich (1854-1915)	Injected chemicals for the first time to treat disease (syphilis)
Edward Jenner (1749-1823)	Developed smallpox vaccine	Marie Curie (1867-1934)	Discovered radium and polonium
Ignaz Semmelweis (1818-1865)	First physician to recommend hand washing to prevent puerperal fever; believed there was a connection between performing autopsies and then delivering babies that caused puerperal fever in new mothers	Alexander Fleming (1881-1955)	Discovered penicillin
Florence Nightingale (1820-1910)	Founder of nursing	Albert Sabin (1906-1993)	Developed the oral live-virus vaccine for polio 10 years after Salk developed the first injected vaccine
Clara Barton (1821-1912)	Established the American Red Cross	Virginia Apgar (1909-1974)	Founded neonatology; developed the Apgar score, which assesses the status of newborns
Elizabeth Blackwell (1821-1910)	First woman in the United States to earn a Doctor of Medicine degree	Jonas Salk (1914-1955)	Developed the first safe and effective injectable vaccine for polio
Louis Pasteur (1822-1895)	Father of bacteriology and preventive medicine; developed pasteurization and established the connection between germs and disease	Christiaan Barnard (1922-2001)	Performed the first human heart transplant
Joseph Lister (1827-1912)	Father of sterile surgery; developed antiseptic methods for surgery	Edwin Carl Wood (1929-2011)	Pioneered the technique of in vitro fertilization (IVF)
		David Ho (1952-)	Research pioneer in acquired immunodeficiency syndrome (AIDS)

The History of Medical Assisting

As the practice of medicine became more organized and more complicated, some physicians hired nurses to help in their office practices. Gradually, the administrative part of running a practice became increasingly complicated and time-consuming, and physicians realized that they needed an assistant with both administrative and clinical training. Nurses were likely to have training only in clinical skills; therefore, many physicians began training individuals—medical assistants—to assist with all the office duties.

The first medical assistants started working in individual physicians' offices with on-the-job training to help out when an extra pair of hands was needed. Today medical assisting is one of the most respected allied health fields in the industry, and training is readily available through community colleges, junior colleges, and private educational institutions throughout the United States.

CRITICAL THINKING APPLICATION   2-1
- In Table 2-1, review the list of individuals who have made significant contributions to medicine. Which one do you believe had the greatest impact on modern healthcare?
- Consider how the medical assisting profession began. How do you think advances in medicine throughout history have affected the current practice of medical assisting?

NATIONAL DEPARTMENTS AND AGENCIES THAT FOCUS ON HEALTH

In the United States, the following agencies focus primarily on health and on safety in the workplace.

- *Department of Health and Human Services (HHS):* The principal U.S. department for providing essential human services and protecting the health of all Americans, especially those unable to help themselves. The HHS is made up of more than 300 programs covering research; child services, including immunizations; financial assistance for low-income families; programs for the elderly; and oversight of Medicare and Medicaid programs.
- *Centers for Disease Control and Prevention (CDC):* The principal U.S. federal agency concerned with health. It conducts research on health-related issues and serves as a clearinghouse for information and statistics associated with healthcare. The divisions of the CDC focus on specific health-related issues; some of these divisions are the National Center for HIV, STD, and TB Prevention; the Public Health Practice Program Office; the National Center on Birth Defects and Developmental Disabilities; and the National Center for Health Statistics. The CDC establishes regulations that affect all healthcare facilities.
- *National Institutes of Health (NIH):* The NIH is part of the HHS and seeks to improve the health of the American people. It supports and conducts biomedical research into the causes and prevention of diseases and uses a modern communications system to furnish biomedical information to the healthcare professions. It consists of 27 different institutes and centers, in addition to the National Library of Medicine. Thousands of research projects are under way in NIH laboratories and clinics at any given time. The NIH also provides funding for research projects conducted at universities, medical schools, and hospitals.
- *Occupational Safety and Health Administration (OSHA):* An agency of the Department of Labor responsible for establishing and enforcing regulations to protect individuals in the workplace. OSHA's influence in the healthcare setting is far-reaching, especially in the areas of infection control and the development of the Bloodborne Pathogens Standard to protect healthcare workers and patients from contracting infectious diseases in a healthcare setting.

PROFESSIONAL MEDICAL ASSISTING ORGANIZATIONS

In 1955 the Kansas Medical Assistants Society initiated a meeting to consider the creation of a national organization. This resulted in the formation of the American Association of Medical Assistants (AAMA) in 1956, which remains the only association devoted exclusively to the medical assisting profession. Maxine Williams, CMA-A, was elected the first AAMA president in 1957. In 1959 a Certification Committee was appointed to develop the AAMA Certification Program, and the first certification examinations were administered in 1963.

In 1974 the U.S. Office of Education recognized AMA/AAMA as an official accrediting agency for medical assisting programs in public and private institutions. In 1993 the **accreditation** process was restructured and became the responsibility of the Commission on Accreditation of Allied Health Education Programs (CAAHEP). Only graduates of CAAHEP-accredited programs or of programs accredited by the Accrediting Bureau of Health Education Schools (ABHES) can sit for the National Certification Examination to become Certified Medical Assistants (CMA [AAMA]). The AAMA has continued to grow; in 2014, it reported that the number of certified medical assistants (CMA [AAMA]) with current credentials exceeded 75,000. More information about the AAMA is available on the organization's website: *www.aama-ntl.org/.*

The American Medical Technologists (AMT) was founded in 1939 as a nationally recognized certification agency for multiple allied health professionals, including Medical Laboratory Technician (MLT), Phlebotomy Technician (RPT), Medical Assistant (RMA), Medical Administrative Specialist (CMAS), and Dental Assistant (RDA). The AMT certification examinations are developed, administered, and analyzed by a committee of subject matter experts. Once certification has been granted, applicants automatically become members of the AMT and earn the credential RMA. AMT is accredited by the National Commission for Certifying Agencies (NCCA). Additional information on the AMT is available on the organization's website: *www.americanmedtech.org/.*

The National Healthcareer Association (NHA) was established in 1990 to offer certification examinations in a number of allied health programs; for example, certification is granted for pharmacy, phlebotomy, and electrocardiography (ECG) technicians. The NHA also offers two different medical assisting certifications: Certified Clinical Medical Assistant (CCMA) and Certified Medical Administrative Assistant (CMAA). The NHA is not involved in program curriculum standards or program accreditation. It simply offers certification if the applicant can successfully pass the NHA examination developed for each particular medical discipline. You can find out more about the certifications offered through the NHA at the company's website: *www.nhanow.com/.*

MEDICAL ASSISTANT JOB DESCRIPTION

Medical assistants are the only allied health professionals specifically trained to work in ambulatory care settings, such as physicians' offices, clinics, and group practices. That training includes both clinical and administrative skills, covering a multitude of medical practice needs. The skills performed by an entry-level medical assistant depend on his or her place of employment, but all graduates of accredited programs are taught a similar skill set.

Clinical skills include:

- Assisting during physical examinations
- Performing patient screening procedures
- Assisting with minor surgical procedures, including sterilization procedures
- Performing electrocardiograms (ECGs)
- Obtaining and recording vital signs and medical histories
- Performing phlebotomy
- Performing tests permitted by the Clinical Laboratory Improvement Amendments (i.e., CLIA-waived tests)
- Collecting and managing laboratory specimens
- Following OSHA regulations on infection control
- Administering vaccinations and medications as ordered by the practitioner

- Performing patient education and coaching initiatives within the scope of practice
- Documenting accurately in a paper record or an EHR
- Performing first aid procedures as needed
- Performing infection control procedures
- Applying therapeutic communication techniques
- Adapting to the special needs of a patient based on his or her developmental life stage, cultural diversity, and individual communication barriers
- Acting as a patient advocate or navigator, including referring patients to community resources
- Acting within legal and ethical boundaries

Administrative skills include:

- Answering telephones
- Managing patient scheduling
- Creating and maintaining patient health records
- Documenting accurately in a paper record and an EHR
- Performing routine maintenance of facility equipment
- Performing basic practice finance procedures
- Coordinating third-party reimbursement
- Performing procedural and diagnostic coding
- Communicating professionally with patients, family members, practitioners, peers, and the public
- Managing facility correspondence
- Performing patient education and coaching initiatives within the scope of practice
- Following legal and ethical principles
- Complying with facility safety practices

These lengthy lists of capabilities that make up the basic skill set are not all that is expected of entry-level medical assistants; they also play a significant role as the patient's advocate (Figure 2-2). Current research describes this role as being a "patient navigator." If you have ever had a loved one who was very ill and required medical attention from a number of different practitioners and allied health specialty groups, you understand what a complex and overwhelming task it can be to make decisions and coordinate a loved one's care. Dr. Harold P. Freeman, a surgical oncologist at Harlem Hospital, pioneered the concept of patient navigation in 1990. His goal was to eliminate the barriers to timely cancer screening, diagnosis, treatment, and supportive care so often experienced by medically underserved or minority communities. These individuals consistently faced finan-

cial, cultural, healthcare system, and communication barriers. In 2005 policymakers in Congress passed the Patient Navigator Outreach and Chronic Disease Prevention Act, which authorized the Secretary of Health and Human Services to make grants through 2010 for the development of patient navigator programs. A total of $25 million was awarded over 5 years to develop community-based navigation programs, and the Center to Reduce Cancer Health Disparities was created at the NIH.

Data from navigator programs show that they can improve the diagnosis of cancer and treatment outcomes. Studies of the original navigation program at Harlem Hospital showed that patient 5-year survival rates for breast cancer improved from 39% before development of the program to 70%.

Since its origin at Harlem Hospital, the program designed to help cancer patients has expanded and spread to other medical disciplines. The Affordable Care Act (ACA) requires that "insurance navigators" be available to help consumers research and enroll in health insurance through the law's health insurance marketplace.

CRITICAL THINKING APPLICATION   **2-2**

Medical assistants have long been encouraged to act as patient advocates in the ambulatory care setting. Given their multilevel training, medical assistants can help patients navigate through a wide variety of confusing issues. Let's think about how you could help a patient and family navigate the following scenario:

Mrs. Kate Glasgow is an 82-year-old patient in the primary care practice where you work. Mrs. Glasgow recently suffered a mild cerebrovascular accident (CVA), and her son is trying to help coordinate her care. Mrs. Glasgow does not understand when or how to take her new medications; she is concerned about whether her health insurance will cover the cost of frequent clinic appointments and assistive devices; she doesn't understand how to prepare for an MRI the provider ordered; and she dislikes having to have blood drawn every week. Based on what you have learned about the job description of a medical assistant, how can you help navigate Mrs. Glasgow and her family through this complex and challenging medical regimen? What specific actions could help Mrs. Glasgow and her son mange her care?

ALLIED HEALTH PROFESSIONALS

The definition of an allied health professional can vary, but it loosely refers to those who can act only under the authority of a licensed medical practitioner (e.g., MD, DO, optometrist, dentist, pharmacist, podiatrist, or chiropractor). Allied health professionals include respiratory therapists, radiation therapists, occupational therapists, physical therapists, technologists of various types, dental hygienists, medical assistants, phlebotomists, pharmacy technicians, and other professionals who do not independently diagnose and prescribe treatment, but perform diagnostic procedures, therapeutic services, and provide care.

The allied health professions fall into two broad categories: technicians (assistants) and therapists. Technicians are trained to perform procedures, and their education lasts 2 years or less. They are required to work under the supervision of medical providers or licensed therapists. This part of the allied health field includes, among others,

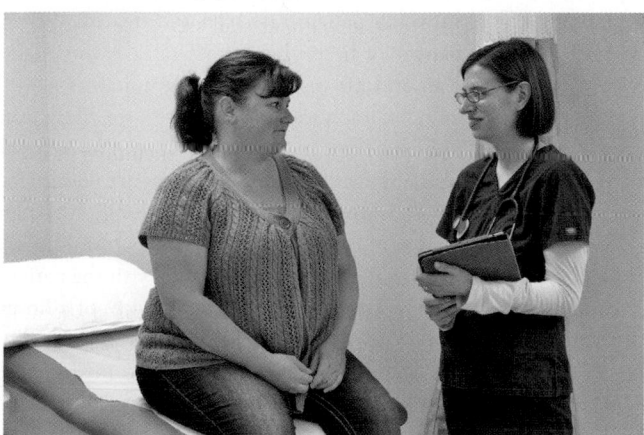

FIGURE 2-2 Medical assistant counseling a patient.

physical therapy assistants, medical laboratory technicians, radiology technicians, occupational therapy assistants, recreational therapy assistants, respiratory therapy technicians, and medical assistants (Table 2-2).

The educational process for nurses and therapists is more intensive. These professions require a state-issued license and an advanced degree, showing that the individual is trained to evaluate patients, diagnose conditions, develop treatment plans, and understand the rationale behind various treatments (Table 2-3).

Allied health professionals typically work as part of a healthcare team, which is what you will do as a professional medical assistant.

As a new medical assistant, you will enter the ranks of an ever-growing group of allied health professionals that provide services for patients in a variety of settings in today's healthcare system. Allied health professionals comprise nearly 60% of the healthcare workforce. The term "allied health" is used to identify a cluster of health professions, encompassing as many as 200 careers. In the United States, about 5 million allied health professionals work in more than 80 different professions; they represent approximately 60% of all healthcare providers.

MEDICAL PROFESSIONALS

Physicians and providers (e.g., nurse practitioners and physician assistants) are portals of entry or first contacts for patients seeking medical care. After the initial assessment or with the diagnosis of a more complex health issue, patients may be referred to a medical specialist for further examination and treatment. Primary care providers (PCPs) are often referred to as "gatekeepers," because most insurance policies require that patients first must be assessed and, if possible, treated by the PCP before they are referred to a specialist for more advanced assessment and care.

Doctors of Medicine

Medical doctors (Doctor of Medicine [MD]) are considered **allopathic** physicians. They are the most widely recognized type of physician. They diagnose illness and disease and prescribe treatment for their patients. MDs have a wide variety of rights, including writing prescriptions, performing surgery, offering wellness advice, and performing preventive medicine procedures. Becoming an MD requires 4 years of undergraduate university training (premed) and 4 years of medical school. Regardless of where premed students attend college, a national standard of course work is required to apply to medical school. They must take entry and advanced levels of biology, physics, organic and inorganic chemistry, mathematics, English, humanities, and social sciences. The United States has approximately 125 allopathic medical schools. After medical school, the student faces 3 to 8 years of residency programs, depending on the medical specialty he or she pursues. After completion of a residency program, a physician can obtain board certification in one or more of 37 different specialty areas recognized by the American Board of Medical Specialties (Table 2-4). An MD must have a state license to practice, and continuing education is required to maintain the license. Graduates of foreign medical schools usually can obtain a license in the United States after passing an examination and completing a residency program in this country.

Doctors of Osteopathy

Osteopathic physicians (Doctor of Osteopathy [DO]) complete requirements similar to those of MDs to graduate and practice medicine. Osteopaths use medicine and surgery, in addition to osteopathic manipulative therapy (OMT), in treating their patients. Andrew Taylor Still is considered the father of osteopathic medicine, which he established in 1874. He believed in a more **holistic** approach to medicine, and although he was an MD, he founded the American School of Osteopathy in Kirksville, Missouri. The school originally was chartered to offer an MD degree but later focused more on the osteopathic approach. DOs stress preventive medicine and holistic patient care, in addition to a special focus on the musculoskeletal system and OMT. Premed students moving toward osteopathic medicine complete the same undergraduate course work as allopathic candidates and 4 years of medical studies at a school for osteopathic medicine. Over the years there have become fewer differences between allopathic and osteopathic programs, with many DO physicians earning residency programs in the same institutions as MDs.

Doctors of Chiropractic

Chiropractors (Doctor of Chiropractic [DC]) typically are thought of as "bone doctors," but they actually focus on the nervous system to help patients live healthier lives. The nervous system is the master system of the body, controlling and coordinating all the other systems. Information from the environment, both internal and external, moves through the spinal cord to get to the brain, and in the same manner, information from the brain moves through the spinal cord to reach the body in a two-way flow of communication. The intention of the chiropractic adjustment is to remove any disruptions or distortions of this energy flow that may be caused by slight misalignments, which chiropractors call **subluxations**. Chiropractic colleges require undergraduate studies in biology, organic and inorganic chemistry, physics, English, and the humanities and then 3 to 4 years studying chiropractic services. Chiropractic care is one of the most common fields of **complementary and alternative medicine (CAM)**.

Hospitalists

Hospitalists are physicians whose primary professional focus is the general medical care of hospitalized patients. Most hospitalists are employed by the healthcare facility instead of having individual freestanding offices in which patients are seen and treated. Perhaps the most attractive benefit of becoming a hospitalist is the quality of life for the physician and his or her family. Hospitalists work a specific, set number of hours each week and receive a set salary from their employers. In addition, most institutions that employ hospitalists cover these physicians with blanket malpractice insurance, saving the practitioner the expense of costly premiums. Although the hospitalist is in charge of the patient while the person is in the hospital, if the patient has a PCP, he or she may still visit the patient. Of course, the patient is not required to use the services of a hospitalist and may be cared for by the attending physician of his or her choice. The hospitalist would still refer the patient to medical specialists as needed for more advanced care.

Text continued on p. 25

TABLE 2-2   Allied Health Occupations Recognized by the American Medical Association

TITLE	CREDENTIAL	JOB DESCRIPTION
Anesthesiology assistant	AA	Functions as a specialty physician assistant under the direction of a licensed and qualified anesthesiologist; assists in developing and implementing the anesthesia care plan.
Art therapist	ATR	Uses drawings and other art and media forms to assess, treat, and rehabilitate patients with mental, emotional, physical, and/or developmental disorders.
Athletic trainer	ATC	Provides a variety of services, including injury prevention, assessment, immediate care, treatment, and rehabilitation after physical injury or trauma.
Audiologist	CCC-A	Identifies individuals with symptoms of hearing loss and other auditory, balance, and related neural problems; assesses the nature of those problems and helps individuals manage them.
Blood bank technology specialist	SBB	Performs routine and specialized tests in blood center and transfusion services, using methods that conform to the accepted standards in the blood bank industry.
Diagnostic cardiovascular sonographer/ technologist	RDCS, RVT	Using invasive or noninvasive techniques (or both), performs diagnostic examinations and therapeutic interventions for the heart and blood vessels at the request of a physician.
Clinical laboratory science/medical technologist	MT, MLT	In conjunction with pathologists, performs tests to diagnose the causes and nature of disease; also develops data on blood, tissues, and fluids of the human body using a variety of methodologies.
Counseling-related professional	LPC, LMHC	Deals with human development through support, therapeutic approaches, consultation, evaluation, teaching, and research; practices the art of helping people to grow.
Cytotechnologist	CT	Works with pathologists to evaluate cellular material from all body sites, primarily through use of the microscope; examines specimens for normal and abnormal cytologic changes, including malignancies.
Dance therapist	DTR, ADTR	Uses the psychotherapeutic properties of movement as a process that furthers the emotional, cognitive, social, and physical integration of the patient as a tool for healing.
Dental assistant, dental hygienist, dental laboratory technician	CDA, RDH, CDT	Performs a wide range of tasks, from assisting the dentist to teaching patients how to prevent oral disease and maintain oral health.
Diagnostic medical sonographer	RDMS	Uses medical ultrasound to gather sonographic data, which can aid the diagnosis of a variety of conditions and diseases; also monitors fetal development.
Dietitian, dietetic technician	DTR	Integrates and applies the principles of food science, nutrition, biochemistry, physiology, food management, and behavior to achieve and maintain good health.
Electroneurodiagnostic technologist	REEG-T	Records and studies the electrical activity of the brain and nervous system; obtains interpretable recordings of patients' nervous system function.
Genetics counselor	IGC	Provides genetic services to individuals and families seeking information about the occurrence or risk of a genetic condition or birth defect.
Health information management professional	RHIA, RHIT	Provides expert assistance in the systems and processes for health information management, including planning, engineering, administration, application, and policy making.
Kinesiotherapist	RKT	Provides rehabilitation exercise and education designed to reverse or minimize debilitation and enhance the functional capacity of medically stable patients.

Continued

TABLE 2-2   Allied Health Occupations Recognized by the American Medical Association—*continued*

TITLE	CREDENTIAL	JOB DESCRIPTION
Massage therapist	MT	Applies manual techniques, and may apply adjunctive techniques, with the intention of positively affecting the health and well-being of a patient or client.
Medical assistant	CMA, RMA, CCMA, CMAA	Functions as a member of the healthcare delivery team and performs both administrative and clinical procedures and duties; a multiskilled health professional.
Medical illustrator	MI	Specializes in the visual display and communication of scientific information; creates visuals and designs communication tools for teaching both medical professionals and the public.
Music therapist	MT-BC	Uses music in a therapeutic relationship to address the physical, emotional, cognitive, and social needs of individuals of all ages; assesses the strengths and needs of clients and patients.
Nuclear medicine technologist	RT	Uses the nuclear properties of radioactive and stable nuclides to make diagnostic evaluations of anatomic or physiologic conditions of the body; also provides therapy with unsealed radioactive sources.
Ophthalmic laboratory technician, medical technician/technologist	COT, COMT	Collects data and performs clinical evaluations; performs tests and protocols required by ophthalmologists; assists in the treatment of patients.
Orthoptist	CO	Performs a series of diagnostic tests and measurements on patients with visual disorders; helps design a treatment plan to correct disorders of vision, eye movements, and alignment.
Orthotist/prosthetist	RTO, RTP, RTPO	Designs and fits devices (orthoses) to patients who have disabling conditions of the limbs and spine and/or partial or total absence of a limb.
Perfusionist	CCP	Operates extracorporeal circulation and autotransfusion equipment during any medical situation in which the patient's respiratory or circulatory function must be supported or temporarily replaced.
Pharmacy technician	CPhT	Assists pharmacists with duties that do not require the expertise or judgment of a licensed pharmacist.
Radiation therapist, radiographer	RRTD	Delivers prescribed dosages of radiation to patients for therapeutic purposes; provides appropriate patient care and maintains accurate records of the treatment provided.
Rehabilitation counselor	CRC	Determines and coordinates services to assist people with disabilities in moving from psychological and economic dependence to independence.
Respiratory therapist, respiratory therapy technician	RRT, CRT, RPFT, CPFT	Evaluates, treats, and manages patients of all ages with respiratory illnesses and other cardiopulmonary disorders. Advanced respiratory therapists exercise considerable independent judgment.
Surgical assistant	CSA	Assists in exposure, hemostasis, closure, and other intraoperative technical functions that help surgeons carry out a safe operation with optimal results for the patient.
Surgical technologist	ST, CST	Helps prepare patients for surgery and maintain the sterile field in the surgical suite, making sure all members of the surgical team follow sterile technique.
Therapeutic recreation specialist	CTRS	Uses treatment, education, and recreation services to help people with illnesses, disabilities, and other conditions develop and use their leisure in ways that enhance their health.

TABLE 2-3   Licensed Healthcare Professions

TITLE	CREDENTIAL	JOB DESCRIPTION
Certified nurse midwife	CNM	RN with additional training and certification; performs physical exams; prescribes medications, including contraceptive methods; orders laboratory tests as needed; provides prenatal care, gynecologic care, labor and birth care, and health education and counseling to women of all ages.
Diagnostic cardiac sonographer or vascular technologist	DCS or DVT	Assists in the diagnosis and treatment of cardiac and vascular diseases and disorders; performs noninvasive tests, including echocardiographs and electrocardiographs.
Emergency medical technician	EMT	Progresses through several levels of training, each providing more advanced skills. EMT's medical education encompasses managing respiratory, cardiac, and trauma cases and often emergency childbirth. Some states also recognize specialties in the EMT field, such as EMT-Cardiac, which includes training in cardiac arrhythmias, and EMT-Shock Trauma, which includes starting intravenous fluids and administering specific medications.
Licensed practical or vocational nurse	LPN or LVN	Provides bedside care, assisting with the day-to-day personal care of inpatients; assesses patients, documents their progress, and administers medications and intravenous fluids when allowed by law; often works in hospitals or skilled nursing facilities and in physicians' offices.
Medical technologist	MT	Performs diagnostic testing on blood, body fluids, and other types of specimens to assist the provider in arriving at a diagnosis.
Nurse anesthetist	NA	RN who administers anesthetics to patients during care provided by surgeons, physicians, dentists, or other qualified health professionals.
Nurse practitioner	NP	Provides basic patient care services, including diagnosing and prescribing medications for common illnesses; must have advanced academic training, beyond the registered nurse (RN) degree, and also must have extensive clinical experience.
Occupational therapist	OT	Assists in helping patients compensate for loss of function.
Paramedic	Paramedic	Specially trained in advanced emergency skills to aid patients in life-threatening situations.
Physical therapist	PT	Assists patients in regaining their mobility and improving their strength and range of motion. They devise treatment plans in conjunction with the patient's physician.
Physician assistant	PA	Provides direct patient care services under the supervision of a licensed physician; trained to diagnose and treat patients as directed by the physician, and in most states are allowed to write prescriptions; take patient histories, order and interpret tests, perform physical examinations, and make diagnostic decisions.
Radiology technician	RT	Uses various machines to help the provider diagnose and treat certain diseases; machines may include x-ray equipment, ultrasonographic machines, and magnetic resonance imaging (MRI) scanners.
Registered dietitian	RD	Thoroughly trained in nutrition and the different types of diets patients require to improve or maintain their condition. They design healthy diets for patients during hospital stays and can help plan menus for home use. They also teach patients about their recommended diet.
Registered nurse	RN	Provides direct patient care, assesses patients, and determines care plans; they have many career options.
Respiratory therapist	RT	Commonly uses oxygen therapy to assist with breathing; also performs diagnostic tests that measure lung capacity. Most RTs work in hospitals. All types of patients receive respiratory care, including newborns and geriatric patients.

TABLE 2-4   Examples of Medical Specialties

SPECIALTY	PRACTITIONER'S TITLE	DESCRIPTION
Allergy and immunology	Allergist/immunologist	Allergists/immunologists are trained to evaluate disorders and diseases of the immune system. This includes conditions such as adverse reactions to drugs and food, anaphylaxis, and problems related to autoimmune diseases, asthma, and insect stings.
Anesthesiology	Anesthesiologist	Anesthesiologists provide pain relief and pain management during surgical procedures and also for patients with long-standing conditions accompanied by pain.
Colon and rectal surgery	Colorectal surgeon	Colorectal surgeons diagnose and treat conditions affecting the intestines, rectum, and anal area, in addition to organs affected by intestinal disease.
Dermatology	Dermatologist	Dermatologists work with adult and pediatric patients in treating disorders and diseases of the skin, hair, nails, and related tissues. Dermatologists are specially trained to manage conditions such as skin cancers, cosmetic disorders of the skin, scars, allergies, and other disorders, both malignant and benign.
Emergency medicine	Emergency physician	Emergency physicians are experts in assessing and treating a patient to prevent death or serious disability. They provide immediate care to stabilize the patient's condition, and then refer the patient to the appropriate professional for further care.
Family medicine	Primary care provider (PCP)	PCPs offer care to the whole family, from newborns to elderly adults. They are familiar with a wide range of disorders and diseases, and preventive care is their primary concern.
General surgery	Surgeon	General surgeons correct deformities and defects and treat diseases or injured parts of the body by means of operative treatment.
Genetics	Medical geneticist	Geneticists are physicians trained to diagnose and treat patients with conditions related to genetically linked diseases. They provide genetic counseling when indicated.
Internal medicine	Internist	Internists are concerned with comprehensive care, often diagnosing and treating those with chronic, long-term conditions. They must have a broad understanding of the body and its ailments.
Neurologic surgery	Neurosurgeon	Neurosurgeons provide surgical care for patients with conditions of the central, autonomic, and peripheral nervous systems.
Neurology/psychiatry	Neurologist/psychiatrist	Neurologists diagnose and treat disorders of the nervous system. Psychiatrists are physicians who specialize in the diagnosis and treatment of people with mental, emotional, or behavioral disorders. A psychiatrist is qualified to conduct psychotherapy and to prescribe medications.
Nuclear medicine	Nuclear medicine specialist	These specialists use radioactive substances to diagnose, treat, and detect disease.
Obstetrics and gynecology	Obstetrician/gynecologist	Obstetricians provide care to women of childbearing age and monitor the progress of the developing child. Gynecologists are concerned with the diagnosis and treatment of the female reproductive system.
Ophthalmology	Ophthalmologist	Ophthalmologists diagnose, treat, and provide comprehensive care for the eye and its supporting structures. These physicians also offer vision services, including corrective lenses.

TABLE 2-4   Examples of Medical Specialties—*continued*

SPECIALTY	PRACTITIONER'S TITLE	DESCRIPTION
Otolaryngology	Otolaryngologist	Otolaryngologists treat diseases and conditions that affect the ear, nose, and throat and structures related to the head and neck. Problems that affect the voice and hearing are also referred to this specialist.
Pathology	Pathologist	Pathologists study the causes of diseases. They study tissues and cells, body fluids, and organs themselves to aid in the process of diagnosis.
Pediatrics	Pediatrician	Pediatricians promote preventive medicine and treat diseases that affect children and adolescents. They monitor the child's growth and development and provide a wide range of health services.
Physical medicine and rehabilitation	Physiatrist	Physiatrists assist patients who have physical disabilities. This may include rehabilitation, patients with musculoskeletal disorders, and patients suffering from pain as a result of injury or trauma.
Plastic surgery	Plastic surgeon	Plastic surgeons work with patients who have a physical defect as a result of some type of injury or condition. They perform reconstructive cosmetic enhancements and elective procedures.
Preventive medicine	Preventive medicine specialist	Preventive medicine specialists are concerned with preventing mental and physical illness and disability. They also analyze current health services and plan for future medical needs.
Radiology	Radiologist	Radiology is a specialty in which x-rays are used to diagnose and treat disease. A diagnostic radiologist specializes in using x-rays, ultrasound, nuclear medicine, computed tomography, and magnetic resonance imaging to detect abnormalities throughout the body.
Thoracic surgery	Thoracic surgeon	Thoracic surgeons are concerned with the operative treatment of the chest and chest wall, lungs, heart, heart valves, and respiratory passages.
Urology	Urologist	Urologists are concerned with the treatment of diseases and disorders of the urinary tract. They diagnose and manage problems with the genitourinary system and practice endoscopic procedures related to these structures.

CRITICAL THINKING APPLICATION   2-3

- Investigate the different philosophies of medicine among allopathic, osteopathic, and chiropractic physicians. Discuss with your class the similarities and differences among these three approaches to medicine.
- What experiences have you had with medical doctors (MDs), osteopaths (DOs), or chiropractors (DCs)? How does their training or expertise differ?

Dentists

There is no difference in training between dentists with a "DDS" or a "DMD." The two degrees mean the same thing: the dentist graduated from an accredited dental school. DDS stands for Doctor of Dental Surgery, and DMD stands for Doctor of Medicine in Dentistry or Doctor of Dental Medicine. The university where each dental school is based determines the degree in den-tistry that is awarded. The level of education and clinical training required to earn a dental degree are similar to those expected by medical schools. Upon completion of general dentistry training, additional postgraduate training is required to become a dental specialist, such as an orthodontist or periodontist.

Optometrists

The optometrist (OD) is trained and licensed to examine the eyes, to test visual acuity, and to treat vision defects by prescribing correctional lenses and other optical aids. Optometrists study at accredited schools of optometry for 4 years after completing undergraduate studies in the sciences, mathematics, and English. They must be licensed in the state in which they practice. Optometrists should not be confused with ophthalmologists, who are licensed MDs.

Podiatrists

Podiatrists (Doctors of Podiatric Medicine [DPMs]) are educated in the care of the feet, including surgical treatment. Podiatrists are trained to find pressure points and weight-distribution problems. These physicians must complete an undergraduate bachelor's degree in addition to 4 years of training in a podiatric medical school and 3 years of hospital residency training. This training is similar to that of other doctors.

Nurse Practitioners

Nurse practitioners (NPs) provide basic patient care services, including diagnosing and prescribing medications for common illnesses, or they may have additional training and expertise in a specialty area of medicine. These professionals must have advanced academic training beyond the registered nurse (RN) degree and also have vast clinical experience. An NP is licensed by individual states and can practice independently or as a part of a team of healthcare professionals.

Nurse Anesthetists

Nurse anesthetists are registered nurses (RNs) who administer anesthetics to patients during surgical or inpatient diagnostic procedures. They practice in many different healthcare settings, including hospital surgical areas, labor and delivery units, ophthalmology offices, plastic surgery offices, and many others. Certified Registered Nurse Anesthetist (CRNA) must have a Bachelor of Science in Nursing (BSN) or other appropriate baccalaureate degree; a current license as a registered nurse; and at least 1 year's experience in an acute care nursing setting. They also must have graduated from an accredited graduate school of nurse anesthesia program, which can range from 24 to 36 months, and must pass a national certification examination after graduation.

Physician Assistants

A physician assistant (PA) is a certified healthcare professional who provides diagnostic, therapeutic, and preventive healthcare services under the supervision of a medical doctor. Physician assistants must be licensed, which requires completion of a physician assistant program that is typically at the master's degree level. Physician assistants must pass the Physician Assistant National Certifying Examination to practice in any state. They may also complete advanced training to focus on a particular specialty practice.

TYPES OF HEALTHCARE FACILITIES

Hospitals

Hospitals are classified according to the type of care and services they provide to patients and by the type of ownership. There are three different levels of hospitalized care, which are interconnected.

Primary Level of Care
- Smaller city or community hospitals
- Usually serve as the first level of contact between the community members and the hospital setting

Secondary Level of Care
- Both PCPs and specialists provide care
- Larger municipal or district hospitals that provide a wider variety of specialty care and departments

Tertiary Level of Care
- Referral system for primary or secondary care facilities
- Provide care for complicated cases and trauma
- Medical centers, regional and specialty hospitals

Private hospitals are run by a corporation or other organization and usually are designed to produce a profit for the owners or stockholders. *Nonprofit* hospitals exist to serve the community in which they are located and are normally run by a board of directors. The term *nonprofit* sometimes is misleading, because "profit" is different from "making money." A nonprofit hospital or organization may make money in a campaign or fundraiser, but all of the money is returned to the organization. Nonprofit hospitals and organizations must follow strict guidelines in the area of finance and must account to the government for the money brought in and the purposes for which it is used.

A *hospital system* is a group of facilities that are affiliated and work toward a common goal. Hospital systems may include a hospital and a cancer center in a small community or may consist of a group of separate hospitals in a specific geographic region. Many hospital systems are designed as integrated health delivery systems. An integrated delivery system (IDS) is a network of healthcare providers and organizations that provides or arranges to provide a coordinated continuum of services to a defined population and is willing to be held clinically and fiscally accountable for the clinical outcomes and health status of the population served. An IDS may own or could be closely aligned with an insurance product, such as a type of insurance policy. Services provided by an IDS can include a fully equipped community and/or tertiary hospital, home healthcare and **hospice** services, primary and specialty outpatient care and surgery, social services, rehabilitation, preventive care, health education and financing, and community provider offices. An IDS can also be a training location for health professional students, including physicians, nurses, and allied health professionals.

Accreditation is considered the highest form of recognition for the quality of care a facility or organization provides. Not only does it indicate to the public that the facility is concerned with providing high-quality care, it also provides professional liability insurance benefits and plays a role in regulatory agency relicensure and certification efforts. Hospitals and other healthcare facilities are accredited by The Joint Commission, an organization that promotes and evaluates the quality of care in healthcare facilities. Standards or **indicators** have been developed that help determine when patients are receiving high-quality care. The term *quality* refers to much more than whether the patient liked the food served or had to wait to have a procedure or test performed. Categories of compliance include:
- Assessment and care of patients
- Use of medication
- Plant, technology, and safety management
- Orientation, education, and training of staff
- Medical staff qualifications
- Patients' rights

Accreditation by The Joint Commission is required to obtain reimbursement from Medicare, managed care organizations, and insurance companies. Besides accrediting healthcare facilities, The Joint Commission carefully evaluates patient safety. It has established the National Patient Safety Goals, which must be addressed by member facilities. The 2015 safety goals for ambulatory organizations took effect January 1, 2015. They included:

- Identifying patients correctly
- Using medicines safely
- Preventing infection
- Preventing mistakes in safety

All these safety factors are addressed in future chapters.

CRITICAL THINKING APPLICATION   2-4

- What types of hospitals are found in your local area, and what services do they provide?
- Are there any patient populations in your area that are underserved? Why might this be the case?

Ambulatory Care

Ambulatory care centers include a wide range of facilities that offer healthcare services to patients who seek outpatient health services. Physicians' offices, group practices, and multispecialty group practices are common types of ambulatory care facilities, and medical assistants can be employed in all of these practices. Group practices may involve a single specialty, such as pediatrics, or may be multispecialty. A multispecialty practice might consist of an internal medicine specialist, an oncologist, a primary care provider, and an endocrinologist.

Usually the providers in the practice refer patients to each other when indicated. This is not only more convenient for the patients, but also more profitable for the members in the practice. A patient seeing a provider for the first time is considered a *new* patient, whereas a patient who has seen the provider on previous occasions is called an *established* patient. Most providers charge new patients more than established patients because the levels of decision making, the extent of the physical examination, and the complexity of the medical history require that more time be directed toward the new patient.

Occupational health centers are concerned with helping patients return to work and productive activity. Often, physical therapy is used in conjunction with rehabilitation services to assist the patient in regaining as much of his or her previous level of ability as possible. Also, freestanding rehabilitation centers can assist patients with a wide range of services. Pain management centers help patients deal with discomfort associated with their condition. Sleep centers diagnose and treat people with sleep problems. Freestanding urgent or emergency care centers provide patients with an alternative to hospital emergency departments (EDs) and are typically open when traditional provider offices are closed.

Surgery has become more convenient because of the number of ambulatory surgical centers that exist today. Many insurance companies now prefer day surgery because it is more cost-effective. A wide variety of outpatient surgical facilities is available, offering procedures in ophthalmology, plastic surgery, and gastrointestinal concerns, including colonoscopies.

Dialysis centers offer services to patients with severe kidney disorders, and many of the larger cities across the country have cancer centers for patients who need treatment by oncologists. Among the many other types of ambulatory care facilities are centers that provide

magnetic resonance imaging (MRI), student health clinics, dental clinics, community health centers, and women's health centers.

Other Healthcare Facilities

Several other types of healthcare facilities deserve attention in the broad overview of the healthcare industry. Diagnostic laboratories offer testing services for patients referred by their providers. The enactment of CLIA in 1967 and its amendment in 1988 established that the only laboratory tests that can be performed in a physician's office lab are those designated as *CLIA-waived*. You will learn how to perform many CLIA-waived tests in your medical assistant program. Larger ambulatory care centers may contain an on-site advanced diagnostic laboratory where all studies can be completed. Smaller or independent practices typically have to send non-CLIA-waived tests to an outside diagnostic facility.

Home health agencies or hospital-affiliated home healthcare organizations provide crucial services to patients who require medical follow-up but are not in a hospital setting. Home healthcare includes therapy services, administration of and assistance with medications, wound care, and other services so that the patient can remain at home, yet still obtain consistent medical attention. Hospice care is a type of home health service that provides medical care and support for patients facing end-of-life issues and their families. The goal of hospice is to provide peace, comfort, and dignity while controlling pain and promoting the best possible quality of life for the patient. Some communities have inpatient hospice services available either in a special unit in a hospital or in an independent hospice center.

The Patient-Centered Medical Home

According to the Agency for Healthcare Research and Quality (AHRQ), which is part of the HSS, "The patient-centered medical home is a way of organizing primary care that emphasizes care coordination and communication to transform primary care into what patients want it to be."

The Patient-Centered Medical Home (PCMH) model, sometimes referred to as the *primary care medical home,* is one of the most exciting healthcare delivery reforms occurring today, and it is transforming the organization and delivery of primary care. Research indicates that PCMHs are saving money by reducing hospital and ED visits while at the same time improving patient outcomes. The AHRQ believes that improving our primary care system is the key to achieving high-quality, accessible, efficient healthcare for all Americans. The agency recognizes that health information technology (IT) plays a central role in the successful implementation of the key features of the primary care medical home. According to the AHRQ, the PCMH has five core functions and attributes:

1. *Comprehensive care:* The primary care practice has the potential to provide physical and mental healthcare, prevention and wellness, acute care, and chronic care to all patients in the practice. However, comprehensive care cannot be provided by only the practicing physician. It requires a team of care providers. The healthcare team for a PCMH includes physicians, nurse practitioners, physician assistants, nurses, pharmacists, nutritionists, social workers, educators, and medical assistants. If these specialty individuals are not readily available to smaller physician practices, virtual teams can be created online to link providers and patients to services in their communities.

2. *Patient-centered care:* The PCMH provides primary healthcare that is holistic and relationship-based, always considering the individual patient and all facets of his or her life. However, establishing a partnership with patients and their families requires understanding and respect of each patient's unique needs, culture, values, and preferences. Medical assistants are trained to provide respectful patient care regardless of individual patient factors. The goal of PCMH is to encourage and support patients in learning how to manage and organize their own care. Patients and families are recognized as core members of the care team.

3. *Coordinated care:* The PCMH coordinates care across all parts of the healthcare system, including specialty care, hospitals, home healthcare, and community services. Coordination is especially important when patients are transitioning from one site of care to another, such as from hospital to home. The PCMH works at creating and maintaining open communication among patients and families, the medical home, and members of the broader healthcare team.

4. *Accessible services:* The PCMH is designed to deliver accessible care. This is achieved through establishing policies that create shorter wait times for urgent needs, more office hours, around-the-clock telephone or electronic access to a member of the care team, and alternative methods of communication, such as e-mail and telephone care.

5. *Quality and safety:* The PCMH is committed to delivering quality healthcare by providing evidence-based medicine and shared decision making with patients and families; assessing practice performance and working on improvements; collecting safety data; and measuring and responding to patients' experiences and satisfaction. All of this information is made public to allow an open assessment of the practice and suggestions for possible methods of improvement.

For further information about the PCMH model, refer to the Patient Centered Medical Home Resource Center, Department of Health and Human Services: *http://pcmh.ahrq.gov*

SCOPE OF PRACTICE AND STANDARDS OF CARE FOR MEDICAL ASSISTANTS

Scope of practice is defined as the range of responsibilities and practice guidelines that determine the boundaries within which a healthcare worker practices. What is the scope of practice of a medical assistant? There is no single definition of the scope of practice for medical assistants throughout the United States, but some states have enacted scope of practice laws covering medical assistant practice. These states include Alaska, Arizona, California, Florida, Georgia, Illinois, Maine, Maryland, Montana, Nevada, New Hampshire, New Jersey, New York, Ohio, South Dakota, Virginia, Washington, and West Virginia. Medical assistants working in those states must refer to the identified roles specified in the law. However, for those employed in states without scope of practice laws, medical assistant practice is guided by the norms of that particular location, facility policies and procedures, and individual physician-employers. In some states, medical assistants are overseen by the board of nursing, whereas in others, the board of medicine oversees medical assistants. Make sure you are aware of your state's rules governing medical assistant scope

of practice. Procedure 2-1 outlines how to locate a state's legal scope of practice for medical assistants.

One factor is absolutely true about all practicing medical assistants—they are not independent practitioners. Whether certified or not, regardless of length of training or experience, every medical assistant must practice under the direct supervision of a physician or other licensed provider (e.g., nurse practitioner or physician assistant).

Earlier in this chapter we discussed the typical tasks performed by a medical assistant, so you already know generally what duties medical assistants perform in ambulatory care centers; however, some specific tasks are beyond the scope of practice of medical assistants, including the following:

• Performing telephone or in-person **triage**; medical assistants are not legally authorized to assess or diagnose symptoms
• Prescribing medications or making recommendations about over-the-counter drugs and remedies
• Giving out drug samples without provider permission
• Automatically submitting refill prescription requests without provider orders
• Administering intravenous (IV) medications and starting, flushing, or removing IV lines unless permitted by state law
• Analyzing or interpreting test results
• Operating laser equipment

What is the difference between scope of practice and standards of care? The *scope of practice* for a medical assistant is what has been established by law in some states or by practice norms, institutions, or physician-employers in states without scope of practice laws. *Standards of care,* however, is a legal term that refers to whether the level and quality of patient service provided is the same as what another healthcare worker with similar training and experience in a similar situation would provide. Standards of care set minimum guidelines for job performance. They define what the expected quality of care is and provide specific guidelines on whether the care standard has been met. Medical assistants not meeting the expected standard of care may be charged with professional **negligence** (discussed in greater detail in the chapter, Medicine and Law).

The following are examples of breaks in the standards of care in medical assisting.

• A patient calls reporting a persistent headache for 3 days. You tell the patient to get some rest and take ibuprofen, without referring the call to a provider. What standard of care has been broken?
• A patient asks you to explain his lab report. You do your best to explain what his blood count levels mean. What is the problem here?
• An elderly patient tells you she cannot afford to get her prescriptions filled. The provider is busy, but you know there are samples of the prescribed drug in the medication cupboard, so you give her several packets. Does this follow standard of care?
• A patient tells you her son fell on the playground yesterday, and he is complaining that his arm hurts. You tell the mother it is probably just a strain and suggest she wrap the arm with an elastic bandage. Why is this a problem?
• You overhear a patient calling one of your co-workers "nurse." Should your co-worker correct the patient? Why?

Hopefully you are beginning to see that the practice of medical assisting is limited not only by individual state laws or norms, but also by the standards and scope of practice established by the supervising providers where the medical assistant is employed. Remember, the scope of practice and expected standards of care for licensed medical professionals are quite different from those for medical

assisting practice. The medical assistant must refer to the provider for orders and guidance on what behaviors are expected for medical assistants in that facility. The medical assistant can *never* independently diagnose, prescribe, or treat patients. She or he must *always* have the written order of a provider or follow established policies and procedures when performing clinical skills.

PROCEDURE 2-1   Locate a State's Legal Scope of Practice for Medical Assistants

Goal: *To determine the legal scope of practice for medical assistants employed in your home state.*

No single definition of the scope of practice for medical assistants applies throughout the United States. However, some states have enacted scope of practice laws that cover medical assistant practice (i.e., Alaska, Arizona, California, Florida, Georgia, Illinois, Maine, Maryland, Montana, Nevada, New Hampshire, New Jersey, New York, Ohio, South Dakota, Virginia, Washington, and West Virginia). Medical assistants working in those states must refer to the identified roles specified in the law.

In states that do not have scope of practice laws, three main elements guide medical assistant practice: the norms of the particular location; the healthcare facility's policies and procedures; and the instructions of the individual physician employer. In some states medical assistants are overseen by the board of nursing, whereas in others, the board of medicine oversees medical assistants. Make sure you have closely studied and clearly understand your state's rules governing the medical assistant's scope of practice.

EQUIPMENT and SUPPLIES

- Computer with Internet access

PROCEDURAL STEPS

1. Google "medical assistant state scope of practice laws", or refer to the American Association of Medical Assistants website (*www.aama-ntl.org/employers/state-scope-of-practice-laws*).
   PURPOSE: To research scope of practice laws in your home state.
2. Summarize the scope of medical assistant practice in your state, and give details on where you found this information.
   PURPOSE: To learn the legal scope of practice in the state where you are employed.
3. Discuss the scope of practice for medical assistants in your home state with your peers.
   PURPOSE: To reinforce your learning about the legal scope of practice in your home state.

CLOSING COMMENTS

Medical assisting has developed over the years into a profession that makes considerable contributions to quality patient care in ambulatory care centers. Medical assistants are uniquely trained to manage both the administrative and clinical needs of patients in physicians' offices, clinics, and outpatient facilities. One of the crucial roles of medical assistants is to act as the patient's navigator; that is, to help patients understand and comply with complex care issues. The medical assistant joins a wide range of allied health professionals as part of a healthcare team in which all members work together to best meet the needs of patients. Medical assistants can work in a variety of healthcare facilities and alongside medical specialists to care for patients. They also can act as core members of the patient-centered medical home and, along with a variety of community resources, can help provide holistic care to patients in the healthcare system. However, medical assistant practice must align with state and regional scope of practice laws and must meet expected standards of

care. Medical assistants must always act under the direction of a physician or provider; they cannot diagnose, prescribe, or treat patients independently.

Patient Education

Some patients have very little knowledge about the healthcare industry and may need instruction and explanations about details important to their healthcare. They often call the healthcare facility with questions; therefore, medical assistants must understand the wide variety of healthcare facilities and medical resources available in the community. Become familiar with community resources to make provider-approved referrals for patients who need help from various sources. If a patient seems to have a need, speak with him or her privately and determine whether any agency or organization might help with the issues at hand. The patient-centered medical home model relies on all healthcare workers to participate in the care of patients.

Legal and Ethical Issues

Medical assistants are responsible for understanding and following the scope of practice in their communities and for always meeting the expected standards of care. Not meeting these responsibilities can result in serious liability for themselves and their employers. Remember, the medical assistant must act under the direct supervision of a physician or licensed provider. You must know the limitations placed on your practice by the state in which you live or by the facility or provider who employs you. There is nothing more important than patient safety, so always act within the guidelines of the law and according to the policies and procedures of the facility where you work. Medical assistants are multiskilled healthcare workers who can have a lasting positive effect on patient outcomes. However, never forget that you do not have the authority or education to diagnose, prescribe, or treat patient clinical problems.

Professional Behaviors

Much of this chapter has focused on an introduction to what it means to be a medical assistant and what you will need to learn so you can perform all the skills expected of an entry-level medical assistant. However, working with patients and providing quality care goes beyond being able to perform administrative and clinical skills. Each patient must be viewed holistically. This means considering the following patient factors:
- What is the patient's physical condition, and how is it affecting his or her life?
- What is the patient's psychological state; is it preventing the person from following treatment regimens?
- Are any communication barriers preventing the patient from understanding the diagnosis or suggested treatment?
- Is the patient's culture, age, or lifestyle preventing him or her from following the provider's orders?
- Are insurance issues or financial problems preventing the patient from following through with treatment plans?

These are just a few of the factors that can affect patient outcomes. Again, because you will be trained in both administrative and clinical duties, you will be in a unique position to understand all the factors that might affect patient care. It is your responsibility to treat all patients with respect and empathy and to do whatever you can to support them throughout the healthcare experience.

SUMMARY OF SCENARIO

Carmen is a bit overwhelmed but very excited about what she has learned about the role of medical assistants in ambulatory care. She finds it hard to believe that she will become competent in all aspects of the typical medical assistant's job description, but she anticipates learning both administrative and clinical skills. She is looking forward to joining the local AAMA chapter so that she can take advantage of professional development opportunities and networking with other medical assistant professionals and students in her community. Carmen now appreciates the significance of scope of practice and of meeting standards of care, and she is researching the laws affecting medical assistant practice in her state. She can't wait until she is actually able to work with the healthcare team to meet the holistic needs of patients in the practice where she will be employed.

SUMMARY OF LEARNING OBJECTIVES

1. **Define, spell, and pronounce the terms listed in the vocabulary.**
   Spelling and pronouncing medical terms correctly reinforce the medical assistant's credibility. Knowing the definitions of these terms promotes confidence in communication with patients and co-workers.

2. **Summarize the history of medicine and its significance to the medical assisting profession.**
   The history of medicine can be traced to ancient practices as far back as 5,000 BC. In 1205 BC Moses presented rules of health to the Hebrews, thus becoming the first advocate of preventive medicine. Hippocrates, known as the father of medicine, is the most famous of the ancient Greek physicians and is best remembered for the Hippocratic Oath, which has been administered to physicians for more than 2,000 years. The medical assistant profession relies on previous medical discoveries to provide patients with safe care in today's healthcare environment. Table 2-1 summarizes medical pioneers and their achievements.

3. **Identify national departments and agencies that focus on health.**
   The Department of Health and Human Services (HHS) is the principal U.S. department for providing essential human services and protecting the health of all Americans, especially those unable to help themselves. The Centers for Disease Control and Prevention (CDC) is the federal agency concerned with health; it conducts research on health-related issues and serves as a clearinghouse for information and statistics associated with healthcare. The CDC establishes regulations that affect all healthcare facilities. The National Institutes of Health (NIH) is part of the HHS and seeks to improve the health of the American people; it also supports and conducts biomedical research into the causes and prevention of diseases and uses

a modern communications system to furnish biomedical information to the healthcare professions. The Occupational Safety and Health Administration (OSHA), an agency of the Department of Labor, is responsible for establishing and enforcing regulations to protect individuals in the workplace, including those employed in healthcare.

4. List professional medical assisting organizations.

The American Association of Medical Assistants (AAMA) was formed in 1956 and is the only association devoted exclusively to the medical assisting profession. The AAMA is involved in accreditation of medical assisting programs through its association with the Commission on Accreditation of Allied Health Education Programs (CAAHEP), managing the CMA (AAMA) exam, providing professional development opportunities for medical assistants, and supporting and researching issues affecting practicing medical assistants. The American Medical Technologists (AMT) is a nationally recognized certification agency for multiple allied health professionals, including medical assistants (who earn the credential Registered Medical Assistant [RMA]). The National Healthcareer Association (NHA) is a company that offers certification examinations to a number of allied health programs, including two different medical assisting certifications: Certified Clinical Medical Assistant (CCMA) and Certified Medical Administrative Assistant (CMAA). The NHA is not involved in program curriculum standards or program accreditation.

5. Discuss the typical job description of a medical assistant and describe the role of the medical assistant as a patient navigator.

Medical assistants are the only allied health professionals specifically trained to work in ambulatory care settings, such as physicians' offices, clinics, and group practices. That training includes both clinical and administrative skills, covering a multitude of medical practice needs. The skills performed by an entry-level medical assistant depend on his or her place of employment, but all graduates of accredited programs are taught a similar skill set.

Medical assistants have long been encouraged to act as patient advocates in the ambulatory care setting. That role is now described as acting as a patient navigator to help patients manage the complexities of their care. Given their multilevel training, medical assistants can help patients navigate through a wide variety of confusing issues.

6. Identify a variety of allied health professionals who are part of the healthcare team.

The definition of an allied health professional can vary, but it loosely refers to those who can act only under the authority of a licensed medical practitioner. Allied health professions fall into two broad categories: technicians (assistants) and therapists. Allied health professionals, including professional medical assistants, typically work as part of a healthcare team. Table 2-2 presents a list of allied health occupations, and Table 2-3 shows a list of licensed healthcare professions.

7. Summarize the various types of medical specialties and healthcare facilities.

Physicians and other providers (e.g., nurse practitioners and physician assistants) are portals of entry or first contacts for patients seeking medical care. Medical professionals include physicians (MDs, DOs), dentists, chiropractors, optometrists, podiatrists, pharmacists, nurse practitioners, and physician assistants. Table 2-4 presents a list of medical specialties. Healthcare facilities include different levels of hospitals, ambulatory care facilities, and a variety of other institutions that provide specialty care for patients.

8. Define a patient-centered medical home (PCMH) and discuss its five core functions and attributes.

The PCMH is also referred to as the *primary care medical home,* a concept that is transforming the organization and delivery of primary care. Improving our primary care system is the key to achieving high-quality, accessible, efficient healthcare for all Americans. The PCMH has five core functions and attributes: (1) comprehensive care, (2) patient-centered care, (3) coordinated care, (4) accessible services, and (5) evidence-based, high-quality, safe care.

9. Differentiate between scope of practice and standards of care for medical assistants, and compare and contrast provider and medical assistant roles in terms of standards of care.

Scope of practice is defined as the range of responsibilities and practice guidelines that determine the boundaries within which a healthcare worker practices. The scope of practice for a medical assistant is what has been established by law in some states or by practice norms, institutions, or physician-employers in states without scope of practice laws (see Procedure 2-1). *Standards of care* is a legal term that refers to whether the level and quality of patient service provided is the same as what another healthcare worker with similar training and experience in a similar situation would provide. Standards of care set minimum guidelines for job performance.

The scope of practice and expected standard of care for licensed medical professionals are quite different from those acceptable for a medical assistant. The medical assistant must refer to the provider for orders and guidance on what behaviors are expected for medical assistants in that facility. The medical assistant can never independently diagnose, prescribe, or treat patients. He or she must always have the written order of a provider or follow established policies and procedures when performing clinical skills.

CONNECTIONS

Study Guide Connection: Go to the Chapter 2 Study Guide. Read and complete the activities.

evolve Evolve Connection: Go to the Chapter 2 link at *evolve.elsevier.com/kinn* to complete the Chapter Review Quiz. Check out the other resources listed for this chapter to make the most of what you have learned from The Medical Assistant and the Healthcare Team.

3

PROFESSIONAL BEHAVIOR IN THE WORKPLACE

SCENARIO

Karen Yon has wanted to work in the medical field for most of her adult life. She studied very hard in high school and graduated with honors. She volunteered in a local hospital and then, after working as a server in restaurants for 3 years, she enrolled in medical assisting classes. After her externship, she was offered an entry-level medical assistant position at a primary care practice.

Karen strives to perform all of her duties professionally and compassionately. She maintains a professional image for patients and co-workers. She had found it difficult to learn to be professional at all times and show compassion to patients through just the classroom experience. However, she knew that these were important aspects of her job, and she was able to gain valuable experience in these areas during her externship. Because this is her first job in the medical field, she wants to make a good impression on her employer and contribute to the healthcare team.

While studying this chapter, think about the following questions:

- Why is professionalism an important attribute in the field of medical assisting?
- How can Karen show professional behavior toward all patients in the healthcare setting?
- How can time management strategies help Karen prioritize her responsibilities as a member of the healthcare team?
- Would it benefit Karen to become a member of her local AAMA chapter?

LEARNING OBJECTIVES

1. Define, spell, and pronounce the terms listed in the vocabulary.
2. Explain the reasons professionalism is important in the medical field, and describe work ethics.
3. Discuss the attributes of professional medical assistants, and project a professional image in the ambulatory care setting.
4. Identify obstructions to professional behaviors.
5. Define the principles of self-boundaries.
6. Describe the dynamics of the healthcare team.
7. Apply time management strategies to prioritize the medical assistant's responsibilities as a member of the healthcare team.
8. Summarize the role of professional medical assistant organizations.

VOCABULARY

characteristics Distinguishing traits, qualities, or properties.
demeanor (dih-me′-nur) Behavior toward others; outward manner.
detrimental (deh-truh-men′-til) Obviously harmful or damaging.
disseminate (dih-seh′-muh-na-te) To disburse; to spread around.

reflection A therapeutic communication technique in which a person responds with a feeling term that indicates how the individual feels about a problem. For example, "You sound angry about being scheduled for this diagnostic test."

What is professional behavior? We tend to hold medical personnel to a higher standard of professionalism than those in most other career fields. The medical assistant who works to improve his or her professional approach in the workplace is an asset to the employer and will quickly be promoted to positions of more responsibility in the healthcare industry. Some employers are just as concerned about medical assistants' professional behavior as they are about their ability to perform administrative and clinical skills, because the way the medical assistant approaches and interacts with patients is critical to the success of the practice. Professionalism is useful not only in the workplace; it also is a valuable skill when dealing with other business professionals in everyday life.

THE MEANING OF PROFESSIONALISM

Professionalism is defined as having a courteous, conscientious, and respectful approach to all interactions and situations in the workplace. It is characterized by or conforms to the recognized standard

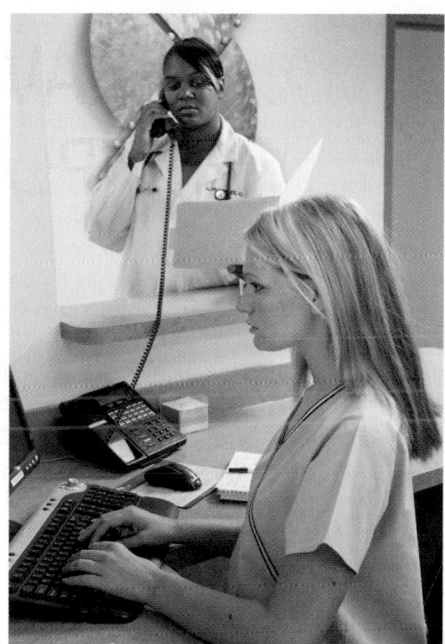

FIGURE 3-1 The professional medical assistant is an asset to the healthcare facility.

of care for the profession. Conducting themselves in a professional manner is essential for successful medical assistants. The attitude of those in the medical profession generally is more conservative than that seen in other career fields. Patients expect professional behavior and base much of their trust and confidence in those who show this type of **demeanor** in the healthcare facility (Figure 3-1).

WORK ETHICS

Work ethics are sets of values based on the moral virtues of hard work and diligence. They involve a whole range of activities, from individual acts to the philosophy of the entire facility. The medical assistant should always display initiative and be reliable. A person who has a good work ethic is one who arrives on time, is rarely absent, and always performs to the best of his or her ability. Co-workers become frustrated if another employee consistently arrives late or is absent. This forces the co-workers to take on additional duties and may prevent them from completing their own work. One missing employee can disrupt the entire day; phones may not be answered promptly, and patients may have to wait for appointments because the staff is shorthanded. Also, lunch and other breaks may be shortened because the staff cannot process cases as quickly when an employee does not show up. All employees should know, and follow, the attendance policies of the facility as outlined in the policies and procedures manual.

Most new hires have a probationary period that may last 30 to 90 days. Any absences or tardiness during the probationary period can be grounds to terminate the employee once the probationary period is up or even before that if multiple attendance issues arise. If the medical assistant has an emergency and must be absent or tardy, he or she should make sure to notify the supervisor according to office policy. All employees must be on time and in attendance every day in the healthcare facility. Providers and patients alike expect this reliability.

ATTRIBUTES OF PROFESSIONAL MEDICAL ASSISTANTS

Patients often see the medical assistant as an extension of the provider and healthcare facility. Therefore, the behavior and attitude of the medical assistant can either positively or negatively affect patients' perception of the quality of care they can expect to receive. As representatives of the healthcare facility, medical assistants must consistently display professionalism through their attitude, appearance, and behavior. Regardless of the situation, the medical assistant must always act professionally.

Many **characteristics** make up the professionalism required of medical assistants. Student medical assistants should begin developing these attributes while in school; these qualities do not appear magically when the student begins working with actual patients. Although we might think that we would always behave appropriately during an externship or in a job setting, the habits developed in school carry over into these experiences. If the behavior is unacceptable, it will be **detrimental** to the medical assistant's professional career. If the medical assistant wishes to advance and receive wage increases, promotions, and the trust of the employer, the attributes discussed in the following sections must be a part of his or her professional behavior.

CRITICAL THINKING APPLICATION   **3-1**
- How can students practice professional behavior while still in the classroom situation?
- When students are practicing administrative and clinical skills, how can they demonstrate proficiency in professional behavior?

Courteous and Respectful

Treating patients with courtesy and dignity are crucial to interacting with patients professionally. Courteous behavior is polite, open, and welcoming. Just the simple act of establishing eye contact, greeting patients with a smile, saying "Nice to see you"; "Can you please …"; and "Thank you …" can make a patient feel welcome and respected. Despite patient attitudes or the stressors in your personal and professional life, you must always treat patients with respect. Patients expect to be treated as individuals, not just another health problem. How can the medical assistant achieve the goals of treating others with courteous regard and thoughtful consideration?
- If you are working with an angry or unhappy patient, use therapeutic communication skills to find out about the real issues the patient is concerned about.
- Display positive nonverbal behaviors, including using an even, calm tone of voice; establishing eye contact; and taking the patient into a private area to discuss problems.
- Always use proper grammar, without slang words, to demonstrate your respect for the individual.
- If the patient is from another culture or speaks another language, communicate as best you can, but try either to have a family member present who understands English or to use an interpreter.

- Explain medical treatments and conditions with simple lay language rather than expecting the patient to understand medical terminology.
- Demonstrate interest in patients as individuals.
- Recognize the personal biases that you bring to the field of medical assisting and how they can affect respectful patient care.
- Respect the role of other members of the healthcare team in meeting the needs of patients and families.
- Demonstrate sensitivity to the patient's and the family's needs.
- Maintain patient confidentiality.

Diplomatic and Tactful

A diplomatic and tactful person always attempts to interact honestly without giving offense. The medical assistant must be sensitive to the needs of patients and co-workers, especially if the person you are communicating with is upset. How can you honestly and effectively communicate with someone who is asking you a difficult question or who may become angry about a particular situation? Could your personal belief system and biases affect how you interact with co-workers, patients, and families? What methods can the professional medical assistant use to communicate diplomatically and tactfully with co-workers and patients?

- Respond calmly to problematic situations with **reflection**, making sure the patient knows you recognize how he or she feels about the problem.
- Consistently communicate politely and honestly.
- Gather feedback about the possible causes of the problem.
- Recognize the needs and rights of others and attempt to reach a mutually beneficial resolution to the problem.
- Assess your personal response to the situation and do not allow your personal beliefs and biases prevent you from interacting diplomatically and tactfully with patients, families, and co-workers.
- Provide patient- and family-centered care.
- Show sensitivity to the needs of healthcare team members.

Responsible and Honest

A responsible medical assistant is one who is dependable. The healthcare team must be able to rely on the medical assistant to perform all his or her duties within the accepted standards of care. Practice managers should be confident that once given a task to do, the medical assistant will carry it out accurately and in a timely manner. At the same time, if an error is made or there is a problem performing a particular task, the medical assistant must honestly report these issues to the immediate supervisor. Patient safety is the number one priority, and anytime it is compromised, the medical assistant must report the problem so that the patient can be safeguarded against any further injury. This is true whether the issue is an administrative or a clinical one. Clearly, if you make a mistake when administering a medication, you must immediately report this error. However, an administrative error (e.g., inaccurate coding, making a mistake on an insurance document, or neglecting to make a follow-up appointment for a patient) also can result in significant negative effects on the practice and the patients involved. In addition, your co-workers depend on you to help out as needed and honestly share any problems noted in the workings of the facility. Dependability and honesty are critical components in earning the trust and respect of others.

How can an entry-level medical assistant perform his or her duties with responsibility, integrity, and honesty?

- Interact with patients in a straightforward, honest manner while supplying all the facts, using lay terms so the patient understands and can make educated decisions.
- Be thorough and pay close attention to detail so that the patient is confident you are a responsible professional.
- Never misrepresent yourself or the medical practice.
- Honestly recognize your own limitations and do not hesitate to seek guidance or assistance if you are not sure of a particular administrative or clinical procedure.
- Accept responsibility for your failures or errors and determine how to prevent them from occurring in the future.
- Take on responsibilities that are within your job description willingly and with the intent to perform them to the best of your ability.

Response to Criticism

A reliable way to improve professional behavior is by showing a willingness to respond to constructive criticism. It can be very difficult to receive negative feedback in the workplace. Being told we are doing something wrong can threaten our confidence and self-esteem. However, constructive criticism is a way for us to recognize that there are areas in which we need to improve our skills and develop more professional methods. To grow beyond entry-level skills, the medical assistant must be willing to recognize any weaknesses in practice and use this feedback to go beyond minimal expectations. Becoming defensive or blaming others only causes more problems. Learn to honestly evaluate your own behavior and be willing to use criticism as a means to excel in your profession.

Professional Image

How do you think a professional medical assistant should look? What visually marks an individual as a professional? How you appear affects the way you are treated and what others think of you. Think of the last time you had to go to a doctor's office. What did you like or dislike about the way employees were dressed or their general appearance? Important assumptions are made within seconds of meeting someone, based only on how they look. Let's consider some standard guidelines for the appearance of the professional medical assistant.

Most medical facilities require medical assistants to wear a uniform or scrubs; this gives patients a way to immediately identify employees of the clinic. Besides providing a consistent appearance for everyone who works at the facility, wearing scrubs can be an infection control measure to prevent the passage of "street germs" in the facility. However, scrubs must be clean and pressed and fit properly to establish a professional demeanor. If administrative staff members are permitted to wear street clothes, they must choose professional clothing that is not too tight and projects a professional, businesslike appearance. All staff members should wear the facility's name badge in a clearly visible location so that patients and visitors to the clinic can identify each employee and his or her title.

In addition, hair should be clean and not overly styled. Longer hair must be tied back to prevent it from interfering with patient procedures. Shoes should be clean (most facilities require white athletic shoes), and nails should be cut short and without nail polish (no artificial nails). Longer nails, artificial nails, and polish are an infection control problem because microbes can grow and multiply under the surface of the nails and in the cracks of the polish. Jewelry is another infection control factor, especially rings. Because microorganisms can invade the cracks and crevices of jewelry, facilities typically restrict employees from wearing anything but a plain wedding ring and watch. Tattoos and body piercings are not considered professional, so medical assistants must follow office policy about their appearance. Be careful with makeup; a moderate amount might enhance your appearance, but too much might be offensive to some patients. You also must be careful with the use of colognes or perfumes. Patients might be allergic to strong odors, and many facilities state that employees should not wear any strong scents, to avoid patient discomfort.

OBSTRUCTIONS TO PROFESSIONALISM

At times it is not easy to be a professional. Sometimes patients, co-workers, and supervisors try our patience, and it can be difficult to maintain a professional attitude in these cases. Some of the obstructions to professional behavior are discussed in this section.

Personal Problems and "Baggage"

Everyone has a life outside the workplace, and sometimes we face challenges and difficult times that are hard to put aside. During working hours, our thoughts should be on the job at hand, especially when we are dealing with patients. However, some situations in our lives may be so critical or distracting that we find ourselves thinking of them constantly. This personal baggage can interfere with our ability to perform job duties properly.

When a situation intrudes on our thoughts at work, it often is best to take the time to talk with a supervisor. It is not always necessary to share the intimate details, but a quick explanation that some difficulties are occurring outside of work helps the supervisor understand any changes in habit or attitude. Regardless of whether your supervisor understands your situation, it is always best to be honest about what is happening to you personally so your employer is at least aware of your personal stressors. The professional medical assistant never transfers personal problems or baggage to anyone at the medical facility, especially patients. The workday should be focused on delivering quality patient care; therefore, do not allow personal business to interfere with the time that should be spent assisting patients and the provider. The patient must be the prime concern of all the employees in a medical facility.

CRITICAL THINKING APPLICATION   3-2

It often is difficult to keep from thinking about a personal problem while you are working. How can Karen do this if she is concerned about an issue at home?

Rumors and the "Grapevine"

A rumor is talk or widely **disseminated** opinion with no discernible source, or a statement that is not known to be true. The definition alone suggests that spreading rumors should be avoided. Most people enjoy working in an environment in which employees cooperate and get along with each other, but rumors can cause problems with

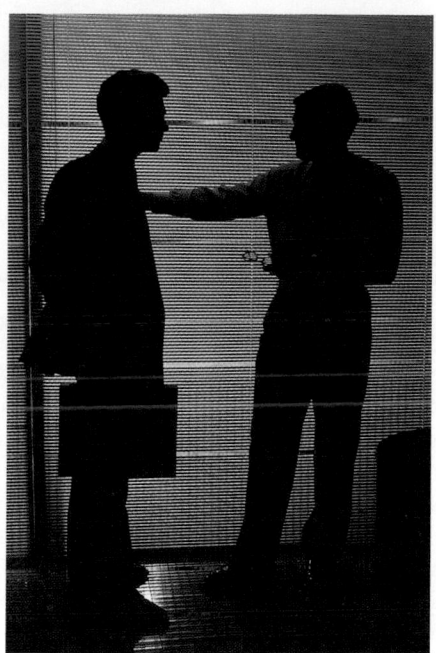

FIGURE 3-2 Gossip and rumors have no place in the medical profession. Avoid employees who participate in this type of activity.

employee morale and often are great exaggerations or manipulations of the truth. By promoting the grapevine, rumors are passed along and become more and more outrageous with each retelling. A medical assistant should refuse to participate in the office rumor mill and should attempt to be cordial and friendly to everyone at work (Figure 3-2). Supervisors regard those who spread or discuss rumors as unprofessional and untrustworthy. In addition, you should always avoid passing along work-related rumors to patients, family, and friends.

Personal Phone Calls and Business

The medical assistant should not take unnecessary phone calls from friends and family at the office. The office phone is a business line and must be used as such, except in emergencies. Using personal cell phones during working hours is not acceptable. Use breaks and lunch hours to take care of business on the phone. Never take a personal call or respond to text messages on a cell phone while working with a patient. If a phone must be carried, place it on the vibrate setting and always step into a hall or break area if a call absolutely must be taken. This should happen only in rare cases. Visitors should not frequent the office, especially the area where the medical assistant is working. If someone must come to the office, always offer the reception area as a waiting room. Visitors should never be allowed to enter patient areas.

Checking personal e-mail also should be avoided in the workplace. Any type of personal business, such as studying, looking up information on the Internet for personal use, Internet shopping, or using social media should be done at home and not in the office. All of these actions distract the medical assistant from the job at hand; the focus should be on serving the patients in the office at all times. Many employees are fired each year for surfing or shopping on the Internet for personal reasons or for checking personal e-mail. Make sure all personal business is handled outside of business hours.

ESTABLISHING HEALTHY SELF-BOUNDARIES

Personal or self-boundaries are extremely individual. We all determine our physical, emotional, and mental limits and use them to protect ourselves in both our personal and professional lives. Personal boundaries are developed to protect us from being manipulated or used by others. Each individual's personal boundaries help identify the person as a particular individual with certain thoughts and feelings that separate him or her from others. Self-boundaries help identify each of us as a unique individual. For example, you may not have a problem with a co-worker who refuses to take out the facility garbage at the end of the shift because she is willing to clean the examination rooms, but another co-worker may have a real issue with her refusal to share in all of the facility's jobs.

We must recognize our individual self-boundaries and appreciate their presence in others to develop healthy relationships in both our personal and professional lives. In other words, we expect those we live and work with to recognize and understand our personal limits, but at the same time we must respect the self-boundaries of others. Personal boundaries allow us to preserve our integrity and take responsibility for who we are and how we treat others. Even though we have the right to determine our own self-boundaries, we do not have the right to expect that everyone we interact with will feel the same way we do.

One way of protecting your personal boundaries is to clearly identify and explain them to others. For example, perhaps you enjoy the clinical side of the facility—interacting with patients about their health issues or helping to find community resources for patients in need—more than you enjoy the administrative responsibilities, such as coding and basic practice finances. Share this with your supervisor and co-workers and see whether you can work out a solution. Perhaps you can perform most of the clinical skills needed while another worker who likes to perform administrative skills can do so without interruption. Working out personal differences requires honest communication and compromise so that everyone understands your position and recognizes that you are willing to be a team member. This process starts with you recognizing that your needs and feelings are not more important than those of anyone else, but also that your preferences are just as important and deserve to be recognized. You have a right to personal boundaries, but you must also recognize this right in others.

Awareness of personal boundaries helps us determine the actions and behaviors that we find unacceptable. Healthy self-boundaries make it possible to respect our strengths, abilities, and individuality and those of others. Establishing healthy self-boundaries results in:

- Improved self-confidence
- Better ability to communicate honestly with others
- Relationships based on honesty and respect

THE HEALTHCARE TEAM

To deliver comprehensive quality care, everyone who interacts with patients, from the time they enter the facility to the time they leave, must work as a cooperative member of the healthcare team. If managers were asked to name the most important attributes for medical professionals, teamwork would be high on the list (Figure 3-3). Staff members must work together for the good of the patients. They must be willing to perform duties outside a formal job description if they are needed in other areas of the office. Many supervisors frown on employees who state, "That's not in my job description." A professional medical assistant should perform the duty and later discuss with the supervisor any valid reasons that the task should have been assigned to someone else. However, if the task is illegal, unethical, or places the patient or anyone else in danger, it should not be done. If you are ever concerned about patient safety, you should discuss the situation with your supervisor before performing the task.

Although we all would enjoy working in an office where everyone gets along and likes every other employee, this does not always happen. Personal feelings must be set aside at work, and all employees must cooperate with others to get the job done efficiently. If a medical assistant has an issue with another employee, the first move would be to discuss it privately with the other person. If the situation does not improve, perhaps a supervisor (office or practice manager) should be involved for further discussions. Do not bring the provider into the discussion unless there is no choice because the facility manager is expected to deal with personnel issues (Figure 3-4).

TIME MANAGEMENT

The time management strategies for students discussed in Chapter 1 can also be applied when you begin your work as a professional medical assistant. You often hear the expression to "work smart." This means that we are to use our time efficiently and concentrate on the most important duties first. To do this, we must first prioritize our duties and arrange our schedules to ensure that these duties can be performed. The first way to improve time management is to plan the tasks that need to be done that day. Taking 10 minutes to write down the tasks for the day helps ensure that they are done. Then, stay on schedule throughout the day, unless you are interrupted by

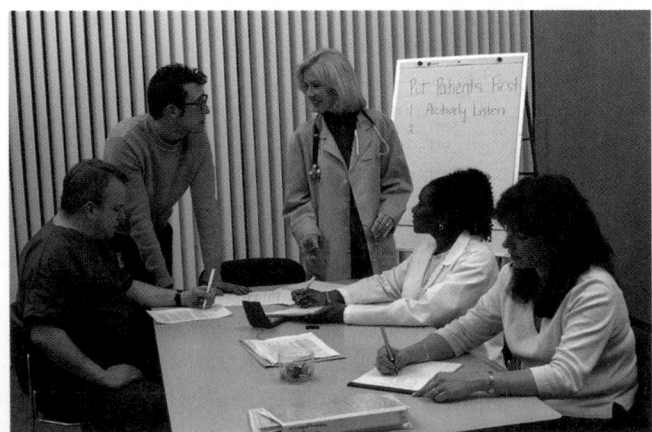

FIGURE 3-3 Teamwork is a vital part of the medical profession. All staff members must work together to care for the patient and perform required duties in the healthcare facility.

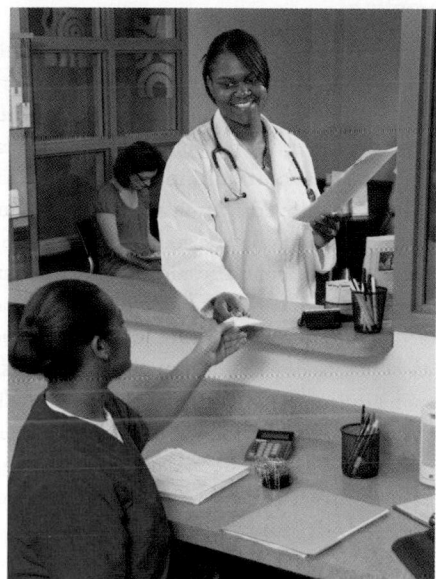

FIGURE 3-4 Knowing which employee to call when help is needed promotes goodwill among employees and often gets a task done more efficiently.

- Brainstorm with your peers about ways to achieve all the tasks facing everyone each day. Maybe someone can come up with a unique way to solve a problem; but if not, at least all of you will be on the same page.
- Make a master list of important tasks so nothing is forgotten.
- Try to accomplish like tasks in the same block of time. If you have phone calls to return or insurance referrals to complete, do each at the same time to be more efficient.
- Multitask as much as possible to accomplish a variety of responsibilities throughout the day.
- At the end of each day, create a new "to do" list for the next day so that nothing important is forgotten.

CRITICAL THINKING APPLICATION   **3-4**

How can Karen prioritize her tasks in the administrative medical office? Based on what you know about the typical job description for an administrative medical assistant, what tasks do you think should be a priority?

---

emergencies. Even then, when days are well planned, allowances can be made for emergencies and most tasks can still be completed. The key to managing time is prioritizing.

Prioritizing

Prioritizing is simply deciding which tasks are most important. Many people make a "to do" list for the day's activities, but the secret to success is prioritizing those activities into categories that give order to the tasks.

Most tasks can be prioritized into three general categories: those that must be done that day, those that *should* be done that day, and those that *could* be done if time permits. Once a general list of tasks has been established, review the list and further prioritize it, using a code such as *M* for must, *S* for should, and *C* for could (or this might be further simplified by using the letters *A, B,* and *C*). Once the tasks have been divided into these categories, they can be further classified in each section. For instance, if category *A* (must be done that day) has six tasks, they can be numbered in the order they should be performed. The same process is completed with the tasks in categories *B* and *C*. As the tasks are completed, they are checked off for that day. Other categories can be added to customize the list. For example, an *H* category can be used for duties to perform at home, *P* could represent phone calls that need to be made, *E* could represent errands to run, and *EM* might represent e-mails to be sent. Customizing the categories makes the list more user-friendly and helps the user to meet his or her individual needs.

Time Management Strategies

- Organize and review your daily "to do" list. If you honestly believe you can't possibly get everything that is a priority done, ask for help. It is better to admit you can't do it all than to ignore a task that is important.

MEDICAL ASSISTANT ORGANIZATIONS

Participation in a professional medical assistant organization has multiple benefits. According to the American Association of Medical Assistants (AAMA) website (*www.aama-ntl.org*), becoming a member includes the following benefits:

- AAMA legal counsel represents medical assistants across the United States to fight for the rights of medical assistant practice; in addition, the counsel stays abreast of federal and state laws regarding medical assisting.
- Membership shows a level of seriousness about your chosen profession.
- Members receive a complimentary subscription to *CMA Today,* an informative magazine devoted entirely to the medical assistant profession; each issue (six per year) offers continuing education unit (CEU) articles, medical assisting news, and healthcare information.
- The CMA (AAMA) Exam is one of the credentialing exams offered to medical assistants; members can take the exam at a reduced rate.
  - To be eligible for the CMA (AAMA) Certification/Recertification Examination, the candidate must be a graduate of a medical assisting program accredited by the Commission on Accreditation of Allied Health Education Programs (CAAHEP) or the Accrediting Bureau of Health Education Schools (ABHES).
  - The CMA (AAMA) certification must be renewed every 5 years

Another possible credential for medical assistants is the Registered Medical Assistant (RMA). This credential is awarded by the American Medical Technologists (AMT) organization and is accredited by the National Commission for Certifying Agencies.

Becoming credentialed as a medical assistant has definite benefits. Because credentialed medical assistants have had to pass a national standardized exam, they have the knowledge that allows them to perform well at their jobs and also a credential that is either preferred or required by employers in many facilities. For many new medical assistants, an earned credential improves their chances of getting and keeping a job in today's healthcare environment.

CLOSING COMMENTS

Patients expect and deserve professional behavior from those who work in medical facilities. Display courtesy and respect toward patients, families, and peers. A diplomatic and tactful person always attempts to interact honestly without giving offense. By displaying these attributes, the medical assistant earns the respect of co-workers and becomes indispensable to his or her employer. Behaving in a professional manner in the medical office helps gain the patient's trust. Trust is one of the most important factors in preventing cases of medical liability. Treating patients with care and not subjecting them to negative behaviors keeps the patient-provider relationship strong and conducive to the health and recovery of the patient. Performing as a cooperative team member goes a long way in promoting a positive healthcare environment for the patient. Incorporating time management strategies into each day not only helps you perform tasks more efficiently, but also ensures that no important tasks are left uncompleted. The entry-level medical assistant can promote professional behavior by joining one of the professional medical assistant organizations and seeking national credentialing.

Patient Education

Remember that most patients do not have any medical background and do not understand many of the phrases used by the medical community. Always be patient and courteously explain any aspect of the instructions or details the patient does not understand. Project a professional attitude of diplomacy and respect. If the patient seems concerned about revealing pertinent information, assure the person that medical assistants and the rest of the staff in the facility are bound by rules of patient confidentiality. Before the patient leaves the exam room, make sure to ask, "Do you have any questions?" This gives patients the opportunity to get all their questions answered before they leave the facility. A professional medical assistant does not share personal information with anyone at the medical facility. Refrain from passing along rumors of any type to patients or their families.

Legal and Ethical Issues

The workday should be centered around patient care, so never allow personal business to intrude on time that should be spent assisting patients and the provider. Otherwise, the patient may be left with the impression that the medical assistant, or the entire staff, is unprofessional, and this often leads to trust issues with the individuals employed at the facility. Professional credentialing is becoming more important each year. To safeguard future practice rights, medical assistants should become credentialed as either a CMA (AAMA) or an RMA.

SUMMARY OF SCENARIO

Karen is happy to be employed in a primary care practice in which providing quality patient care is paramount. She is learning to be careful about what she says and to remain focused on the patient instead of any personal difficulties she may be having. Karen knows it is her responsibility to be a team player and to assist the other staff members as much as possible. She maintains a good attitude and gets a strong sense of pride from being a member of the medical profession. She is meticulous about presenting a neat appearance and arrives on time for each workday. She always asks others whether they need help when she has any extra time throughout the day. Karen looks forward to a long relationship with her employer. The rewards she feels as a member of the health team are second to none.

SUMMARY OF LEARNING OBJECTIVES

1. **Define, spell, and pronounce the terms listed in the vocabulary.**
   Spelling and pronouncing medical terms correctly reinforce the medical assistant's credibility. Knowing the definitions of these terms promotes confidence in communication with patients and co-workers.

2. **Explain the reasons professionalism is important in the medical field, and describe work ethics.**
   Professionalism is the characteristic of conforming to the technical or ethical standards of a profession. Professionalism is vital in the medical profession because patients expect and deserve to be treated in a professional way. When the medical assistant acts in a professional way, he or she establishes trust with the patient. Patients notice professional behavior, even when it is not directed at them specifically. They notice how others are treated in the reception room and in other areas of the office. Always act in a professional manner while at work. Work ethics are sets of values

based on the moral virtues of hard work and diligence, involving a whole range of activities, from individual acts to the philosophy of the entire facility.

3. **Discuss the attributes of professional medical assistants, and project a professional image in the ambulatory care setting.**
   Professional medical assistants display courteous, respectful behaviors and communicate with tact and diplomacy. They demonstrate responsible and honest behaviors and always act with integrity. Professional medical assistants view constructive criticism as a way of improving their skill level. Important assumptions are made within seconds of meeting someone based only on how they look. Most medical facilities require that medical assistants wear a uniform or scrubs or professional clothing that is not too tight and projects a professional, businesslike appearance. In addition, name badges should be visible; hair should be clean, and longer hair should

SUMMARY OF LEARNING OBJECTIVES—*continued*

be tied back; shoes should be clean; nails should be short and without nail polish (no artificial nails); and no jewelry should be worn.

4. **Identify obstructions to professional behaviors.**

   Everyone has a life outside the workplace, and sometimes we face challenges and difficult times that are hard to put aside. The professional medical assistant never transfers personal problems or baggage to anyone at the medical facility. The medical assistant should refuse to participate in the office rumor mill and should be cordial and friendly to everyone at work. Avoid personal phone calls and visits unless it is an absolute emergency.

5. **Define the principles of self-boundaries.**

   Awareness of personal boundaries helps us determine the actions and behaviors that we find unacceptable. Healthy self-boundaries make it possible to respect our strengths, abilities, and individuality and those of others.

6. **Describe the dynamics of the healthcare team.**

   To deliver comprehensive quality patient care, everyone who interacts with patients, from the time they enter the facility to the time they leave, must work as a cooperative member of the healthcare team.

7. **Apply time management strategies to prioritize the medical assistant's responsibilities as a member of the healthcare team.**

   Medical assistants need to use time efficiently, prioritize duties, and arrange schedules to ensure that duties can be performed in a timely manner. This can be done by planning tasks that need to be done that day. Most tasks can be prioritized into three general categories: those that must be done that day, those that should be done that day, and those that could be done if time permits.

8. **Summarize the role of professional medical assistant organizations.**

   There are definite benefits to becoming credentialed as a medical assistant. Because credentialed medical assistants (i.e., those with a CMA [AAMA] or AMT certificate) have had to pass a national standardized exam, they have proven they have the knowledge to perform well at their jobs. These individuals also have a credential that may be required by healthcare employers.

CONNECTIONS

Study Guide Connection: Go to the Chapter 3 Study Guide. Read and complete the activities.

evolve Evolve Connection: Go to the Chapter 3 link at *evolve.elsevier.com/kinn* to complete the Chapter Review Quiz. Check out the other resources listed for this chapter to make the most of what you have learned from Professional Behaviors in the Workplace.

4 THERAPEUTIC COMMUNICATION

SCENARIO

Many types of patients seek medical attention and care in an ambulatory care setting. Each patient has different needs and different concerns, even if the diagnoses are similar. Communication and interpersonal skills are vital in meeting those needs and providing optimum care to the patient. However, the patient is not the only individual who must be considered; family members often are crucial to the patient's health and well-being.

Lucille Cloyd is an 83-year-old patient who has been diagnosed with heart disease and is seeing Dr. Neill for treatment. Her daughter, Sarah Smithson,

helps care for her and frequently accompanies her mother to Dr. Neil's office. Mrs. Cloyd is widowed and visits the physician once a month, in addition to receiving home care services. The medical assistant must consider not only the needs of Mrs. Cloyd, but also those of her extended family. Compassion and sensitivity are necessary to care for this patient, in addition to excellent therapeutic communication skills.

While studying this chapter, think about the following questions:

- What communication barriers might exist between patients and healthcare workers?
- How does the medical assistant effectively communicate with a patient's family members?
- How will developing good therapeutic communication skills make the medical assistant more effective?

LEARNING OBJECTIVES

1. Define, spell, and pronounce the terms listed in the vocabulary.
2. Discuss first impressions and patient-centered care.
3. Do the following related to communication paths:
   - Identify styles and types of verbal communication.
   - Identify types of nonverbal communication.
   - Recognize and respond to verbal and nonverbal communication.
4. Recognize communication barriers.
5. Summarize factors that should be considered when communicating with diverse patient populations.
6. Identify techniques for overcoming communication barriers.
7. Do the following related to communication during difficult times:
   - Recognize the elements of oral communication using the sender-receiver process.
   - Apply feedback techniques, including reflection, restatement, and clarification, to obtain information.
   - Discuss open and closed questions or statements
8. Discuss important factors about therapeutic communication across the life span.
9. List and explain the levels of Maslow's hierarchy of needs.

VOCABULARY

congruence Being in agreement, harmony, or correspondence; conforming to the circumstances or requirements of a situation.

stereotype Something conforming to a fixed or general pattern; a standardized mental picture that is held in common by many and represents an oversimplified opinion, prejudiced attitude, or uncritical judgment.

Therapeutic communication skills developed by the medical assistant help set the tone of care in a healthcare facility. Patients who visit the healthcare facility may not be at their best, and the way the medical assistant reacts to and interacts with them can make an incredible difference in whether they view the facility and those who care for them positively or negatively. These interactions may also affect the patient's treatment and recovery.

FIRST IMPRESSIONS

The opinions formed in the early moments of meeting someone remain in our thoughts long after the first words have been spoken. The first impression involves much more than just physical appearance or dress; it includes attitude, compassion, and therapeutic communication skills that clearly help the patient and family members realize that the medical assistant is interested in who they are and what they need (Figure 4-1).

Delivering quality patient care is the primary objective of the professional medical assistant. Patients are the reason the facility exists. Each patient should be welcomed warmly by name and with a polite greeting. Think for a moment about how it feels to be a new patient entering the unknown territory of a healthcare facility. Staff members of the facility are in familiar surroundings and already have some information about the new patient. However, the patient knows nothing about the staff members. One way to break that barrier is to have all staff members wear name badges, with letters large enough to be read at a distance of 3 feet. Include the staff position if several divisions of responsibility exist (e.g., "medical assistant," "administrative specialist," and "practice manager"). When the patient approaches, make introductions and smile. Smiles should show in the voice and the eyes. Genuinely welcome the patient to the facility. This small effort helps put the patient at ease in the healthcare environment.

To provide high-quality patient care, we must communicate effectively with the patient and provide a warm, caring environment. Positive reactions and interactions with the patient are vital. Because

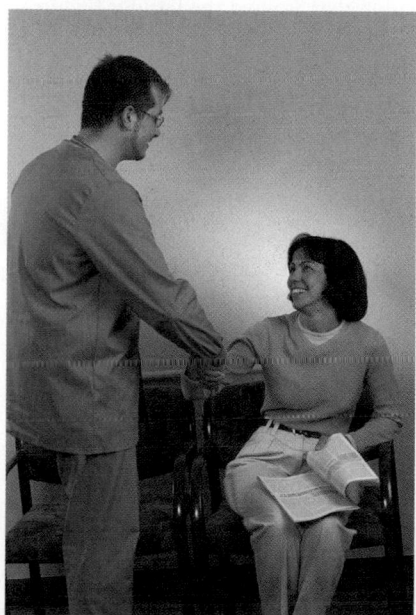

FIGURE 4-1 First impressions are critical in gaining the patient's trust.

medical care by nature is extremely personal, a medical assistant must always remember that each patient is an individual with certain anxieties. These anxieties often cause people to act and react in different ways; therefore, effective verbal and nonverbal communication with each patient is absolutely essential.

Healthcare professionals accept the responsibility of developing helping relationships with their patients. The interpersonal nature of the patient–medical assistant relationship carries with it a certain amount of responsibility to forget one's self-interest and focus on the patient's needs. A medical assistant can elicit either a positive or a negative response to patient care simply by the way he or she treats and interacts with patients. You usually are the first person with whom the patient communicates; therefore, you play a vital role in initiating therapeutic patient interactions.

PATIENT-CENTERED CARE

Healthcare professionals have embraced patient-centered care, an innovative approach to the planning, delivery, and evaluation of healthcare that is grounded in mutually beneficial partnerships among healthcare providers, patients, and families. Patient- and family-centered care applies to patients of all ages and may be practiced in any healthcare setting. Each patient who seeks care has a unique set of needs, including clinical symptoms that require medical attention and issues specific to the individual that can affect his or her care. As patients navigate the healthcare delivery system, providers and their employees must be prepared to identify and address not just the clinical aspects of care, but also the spectrum of each patient's demographic and personal characteristics. Good communication skills are vital to meeting the needs of the patient and his or her support system.

COMMUNICATION PATHS
Verbal Communication

When we communicate verbally with our patients, we use words to deliver the intended message. The two major forms of verbal communication are oral communication and written communication.

Most of us consider talking the only form of verbal communication. However, there are many different styles and methods of sending a patient a voice-related message, including face-to-face discussions, telephone conversations, voicemail, television or radio advertisements, and videos. Verbal communication occurs when we express our thoughts with words. Verbal communication is affected by many factors, including our tone of voice, enunciation of words, use of therapeutic pauses, emphasis on certain terms, and choice of words, including whether we use medical or lay language. Nonverbal behaviors (i.e., the tone of voice we use, facial expressions, and so on) can drastically affect how words are interpreted. All of these factors affect the patient's understanding of our verbal message.

The other form of verbal communication is the written word. When we put our thoughts to paper, such as writing down instructions for a patient, our verbal words are now in written form. A wide variety of written communication is used in the healthcare setting on a routine basis. Examples include patient education handouts, written provider orders (e.g., prescriptions), e-mails describing laboratory results or appointment reminders, letters, faxes, articles, hand-written notes, and text messages. A type of written communication used routinely for all patients is documentation in the health record. Just as with oral communication, we must be careful that written communication is both accurate and comprehensive to prevent patient confusion or medical errors. All written communication carries an added legal burden, so it is crucial that everything that is documented or written down for patient referral is accurate and comprehensive.

Electronic communication, such as e-mails or text messages, is an efficient way of delivering a written message to the patient, but several cautionary notes apply to the use of these methods. First, patient confidentiality must always be secured; for example, messages should be sent only to an e-mail address or cell phone number the patient has approved. Second, there is no way to confirm the patient actually received the message unless he or she is required to respond with a receipt of message or the message is flagged electronically to show that it was received. If the healthcare facility relies on e-mail or text messages to communicate with patients, these systems must be in place to make sure the patient is actually receiving the information. Text messages should be completely written out, without abbreviations or shortcuts; for example, do not use "u" for "you." In addition, it is important to use lay language rather than medical terminology so that the patient can understand the meaning of the message. You also must be careful of the writing style used in an e-mail. Using all capital letters in an e-mail can be interpreted as screaming at the person receiving the e-mail, which can lead to misunderstanding and communication problems.

Nonverbal Communication

Much of what we communicate to our patients is conveyed through the use of conscious or unconscious body language. Our nonverbal actions, such as gestures, facial expressions, and mannerisms, are learned behaviors that are greatly influenced by our family and cultural backgrounds. The body naturally expresses our true feelings; in fact, experts say that more than 90% of communication is nonverbal. This means that, even though the verbal message is an important method of delivering information, the *way* we deliver those words determines how the patient interprets them.

Most of the negative messages communicated through body language are unintentional; therefore, it is important to remember while conducting patient interviews that nonverbal communication can seriously affect the therapeutic process. You can do much to put a patient at ease by the tone of your voice. Your facial expression and the ease and confidence of your movements demonstrate a sincere interest in the patient. Therapeutic use of space and touch also are important ways of sending nonverbal messages to your patients. You should establish eye contact (in most cases), sit in a relaxed but attentive position, and avoid using furniture as a barrier between you and the patient. Give the patient your undivided attention and let your body language inform each patient that you are interested in his or her medical problems (Procedure 4-1).

The key to successful patient interaction is **congruence** between the words used and the body language observed. In other words, if you say to a patient who had an emergency that made him late for his appointment, "I understand you had an unexpected problem that prevented you from getting here on time," but you say it in a doubting or sarcastic tone of voice with your arms crossed and your face disapproving, what message did that patient receive? Effective therapeutic communication means we need to constantly be aware of our body language and work at making sure our nonverbal language matches our words. To be viewed as honest and sensitive to the needs of your patients, you must be aware of your nonverbal behavior patterns. The nonverbal message the patient receives from the medical assistant's listening behavior should be "You are a person of worth, and I am interested in you as a unique individual" (Figure 4-2).

Observing your patient fosters mutual understanding. The purpose of observing nonverbal communication is to become sensitive to or aware of the feelings of others as conveyed by small bits of behavior rather than words. This sensitivity enables you to adapt your behavior to these feelings; to deliberately select your response, either verbal or nonverbal; and thereby to have a favorable effect on others. The favorable effect may consist of providing emotional support, conveying that you care, defusing the patient's fear or anger, or providing an invitation to release pent-up feelings by talking about the situation that aroused the feelings (Figure 4-3). Table 4-1 lists some nonverbal behaviors by patients that may indicate anxiety, frustration, or fear.

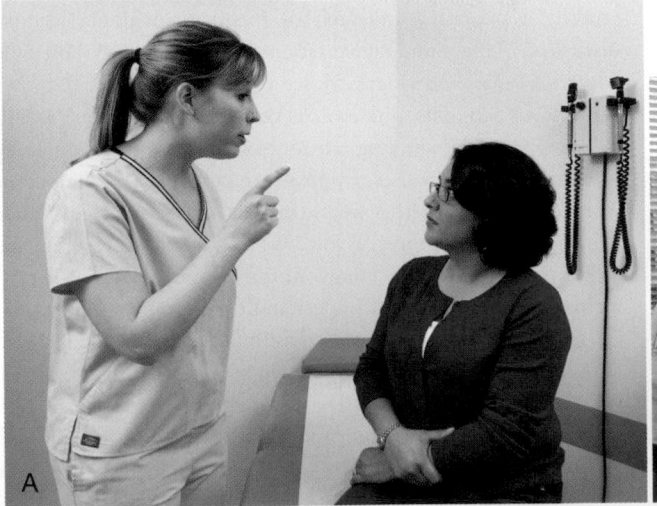
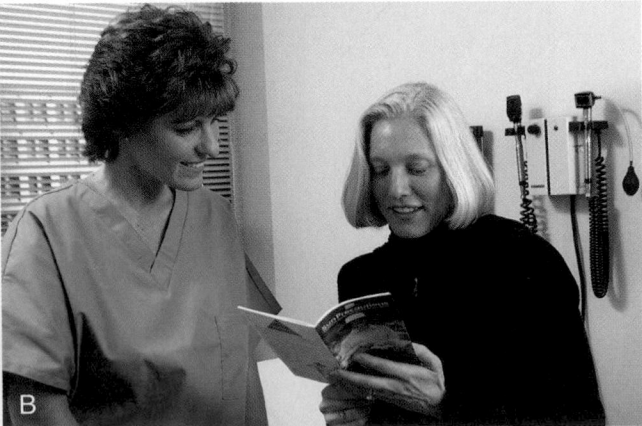

FIGURE 4-2 A, Pointing often is an accusatory gesture and causes discomfort. B, A bright smile helps to put the patient at ease and to relax.

Nonverbal Language Behaviors

Nonverbal behavior—that is, your body language—can have either a positive or negative effect on patient interactions. Positive nonverbal behaviors enhance the patient's experience in the healthcare setting. Communication experts recommend the following:

- When gathering information from a patient, lean toward the patient to show interest.
- Face the patient squarely and at eye level to help make the patient more comfortable and to demonstrate sensitivity and empathy.
- Eye contact is essential for therapeutic communication unless the patient is from a culture that discourages this; many Asian cultures consider eye contact during a conversation very rude.
- A closed posture (crossed arms or legs) may indicate disinterest.
- Be sensitive to the patient's personal space when possible. Maintain a comfortable distance, at least an arm's length away, when interacting with a patient.

- Be careful with body gestures such as hand and arm movements. Gestures, such as nodding your head when the patient talks, can display interest, but too much body movement can be distracting.
- Your tone of voice should reflect your interest in the patient. Speaking too quietly or too loudly can detract from therapeutic communication.
- Continually observe the patient's body language; watch for signs of confusion, boredom, worry, and other emotions so that you can respond appropriately.
- Documenting in an electronic health record can be distracting to both the medical assistant and the patient. Remind yourself to look at the patient frequently, and use encouraging body language to maintain a personal interaction with him or her.

PROCEDURE 4-1 | Respond to Nonverbal Communication

Complete this procedure with another student playing the role of the patient. To make the experience more realistic, choose a student about whom you know very little. To maintain the student's privacy, he or she does not have to share any confidential information.

Goal: *To observe the patient and respond appropriately to nonverbal communication.*

Scenario: *Tanya Williams, 36, is a new patient with the CC of intermittent abdominal pain with alternating diarrhea and constipation. Ms. Williams has experienced this discomfort for several months and appears very frustrated. You are working in the administrative side of the practice today and have to gather initial information from Ms. Williams about the history of her complaints, in addition to collecting her insurance information and having her sign several forms. She is sitting with her arms wrapped around her abdomen, tapping her right foot on the floor, and refusing to maintain eye contact. What is her nonverbal behavior telling you, and how can you establish therapeutic communication with this patient?*

EQUIPMENT and SUPPLIES

- Appropriate intake forms for a new patient
- Patient's health record

PROCEDURAL STEPS

1. Greet the patient pleasantly, introduce yourself, and verify her ID and date of birth (DOB). Explain your role.
   PURPOSE: To make the patient feel comfortable and at ease.
2. Ask the patient the purpose of her visit and the onset, duration, and frequency of her symptoms. Pay close attention to her body language to determine whether what she is telling you is congruent with her body language.
   PURPOSE: Nonverbal language naturally expresses the patient's true feelings. Closely observing body language helps you reach more detailed conclusions about patient information.
3. Use restatement, reflection, and clarification to gather as much information as possible about the patient's CC. Make sure all medical terminology is adequately explained.

PURPOSE: Therapeutic communication techniques help the medical assistant gather complete information; using feedback techniques and making sure the patient understands medical terms helps relieve anxiety.

4. Speak in a pleasant, distinct manner, remembering to maintain eye contact with your patient.
   PURPOSE: Positive nonverbal behaviors create a friendly, caring atmosphere. Remain sensitive to the diverse needs of your patient throughout the interview process.
5. Continue to observe the patient's nonverbal behaviors and select the appropriate verbal response to demonstrate your sensitivity to her discomfort, frustration, and anxiety.
   PURPOSE: Displaying sensitivity to and awareness of the patient's nonverbal body language demonstrates your concern for the patient and helps defuse the patient's concerns.

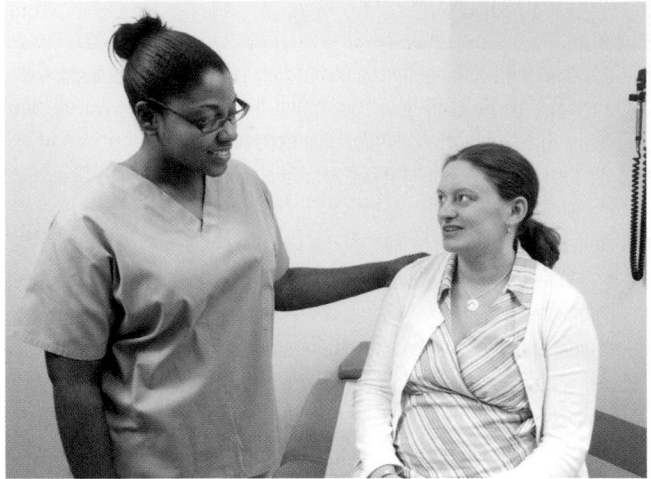

FIGURE 4-3 Touching the patient communicates care and compassion. Careful listening and asking questions helps the patient express thoughts and feelings.

TABLE 4-1 Observation of Nonverbal Communication in Patients		
AREA OBSERVED	OBSERVATION	INDICATION
Breathing patterns	Rapid respirations, sighing, shallow thoracic breathing	Anxiety, boredom, pain
Eye patterns	Side-to-side eye movements, looking down at the hands	Anxiety, distrust, embarrassment
Hands	Tapping fingers, cracking knuckles, continuous movement, sweaty palms	Anxiety, worry, fear
Arm placement	Folded across chest, wrapped around abdomen	Anxiety, worry, fear, pain
Leg placement	Tension, crossed and/or tucked under, tapping foot, continuous movement	Frustration, anger

Recognizing and Responding to Verbal and Nonverbal Communications

The medical assistant not only must implement therapeutic communication skills, he or she also must observe the patient to interpret the person's message and level of understanding. In the following critical thinking exercise, the medical assistant uses the therapeutic communication skills discussed in the chapter, including active listening techniques, open and closed questions and statements, positive nonverbal skills, and effective observation of the patient's body language. How would you answer each question?

Communication factors that should be considered in this exercise include the following:

• What nonverbal language is being used by the patient, Mr. Anderson, and how should it be interpreted?
• Mr. Anderson tells the medical assistant he is not following that crazy diet and never will. What therapeutic communication skills can be used to get more information out of Mr. Anderson and to reinforce the physician's recommendations?
• During the discussion Mr. Anderson says he stopped taking the blood pressure medicine because of the side effects. What communication techniques and therapeutic body language can be used to emphasize the need for Mr. Anderson to take his medicine as prescribed?

CRITICAL THINKING APPLICATION   **4-1**

Toby Anderson, a 52-year-old patient, was recently diagnosed with hypertension and prescribed Lotensin bid for treatment. He is being seen today for follow-up measurement of his blood pressure. Mr. Anderson also has issues with his bill, which he wants to discuss with the "woman in charge." He is 45 pounds overweight and was given information about a reduced-calorie, low-sodium diet 1 month ago, but he has not lost any weight. He tells the medical assistant who is trying to help him understand his bill that he is just going to quit coming to the doctor since he isn't getting any better and he can't afford it anyway. He is sitting with his arms across his chest, tapping his foot, and occasionally cracking his knuckles.

COMMUNICATION BARRIERS

Effective therapeutic communication requires the delivery of a clear message to the patient. However, along the way, many communication barriers can cause misunderstanding and misinterpretation of your message. Successful communication relies on knowing what barriers to communication exist and how to navigate around these roadblocks. By understanding what barriers may stand in the way of your attempts at effective communication, you can more successfully sidestep these challenges and engage in patient-centered communication. Communication barriers can arise from both medical assistants and patients. The following sections discuss just some of the communication barriers that the medical assistant might use when interacting with patients.

Providing Unwarranted Assurance

Mrs. Miller says to you, "I know this lump is going to turn out to be cancer." The typical reply is almost automatic: "Don't worry, I'm sure everything will be fine." This type of answer indicates that her anxiety is insignificant and denies her the opportunity to discuss her fears further. A reflective response, such as "You sound really worried about…" acknowledges her feelings and demonstrates empathy and a willingness to listen to her concerns.

Giving Advice

Mrs. Thompson has just finished talking to the physician. She looks at you and says, "Dr. Rowe says I need surgery to get rid of these gallstones. I just don't know. What would you do?" If you tell her how you would handle the situation, you may have shifted the accountability for decision making from her to you, and she has not worked out her own solution. Does this woman really want to know what you would do? Probably not. You could respond to her question with, "Based on what the doctor told you, what do you think you should do?" or "Do you need further information to make your decision?" If the patient continues to question recommendations, the medical assistant should encourage further discussion with the provider.

Using Medical Terminology

You must adjust your vocabulary to fit the patient. The more the patient understands about what is happening and the management of the problem, the better the outcome. Misinterpreted communication is the most common error in patient care. One of the biggest problems for the patient is understanding medical terminology. Closely observe the patient's body language while he or she receives instructions or patient education. If the patient shows signs of not understanding the procedure, ask the patient to repeat back to you the information or instructions. This demonstration–return demonstration form of providing feedback ensures that the patient completely understands what is happening. It also gives the medical assistant the opportunity to clarify any misconceptions.

Leading Questions

While gathering patient information, you ask the patient, "You don't smoke, do you?" By asking questions in this manner, you indicate the preferred answer. Telling you that he or she does smoke would surely meet with your disapproval. Keep your questions positive. A better way of asking would be "Have you ever smoked?" or "Do you use tobacco?"

Talking Too Much

Some medical assistants associate helpfulness with verbal overload. The patient may let you talk at the expense of his or her own need to explain what is wrong. Always remember that when interacting with a patient, you should listen more than you talk. Pay close attention to the patient's body language to make sure you are giving the patient ample opportunity to discuss the health problem or issue.

Stereotyping

Stereotyping is defined as the application of a standardized mental picture that is held in common by members of a group; it represents an oversimplified opinion or a prejudiced attitude. It is unfair to stereotype anyone or categorize the person based on preconceived and often incorrect assumptions. Although sometimes an assumption based on stereotypic categories may have a degree of truth, people should not be judged before you have gotten to know them as individuals. The medical assistant should push preconceived notions aside and look at the individual when forming and building a relationship. In the medical profession, stereotypic categories should not be considered when caring for patients.

Other communication barriers are caused by problems the patient might have. By being sensitive to such problems, the medical assistant can use therapeutic communication techniques to help these patients.

Physical Impairment

Patients may have physical conditions that impair their ability to communicate effectively. This could be a vision or hearing problem or one of many other conditions that make communicating a bit more difficult than usual. The medical assistant should use more descriptive language when speaking with the patient who has a visual disturbance. This helps the patient "see" what is being discussed. A person with diminished hearing may be very sensitive and in denial of the condition. Make sure you have his or her attention and that you are face-to-face with the person while speaking. People who are hearing impaired often are very dependent on lip reading for comprehension. In either case, involve family members or assistive devices to help communicate effectively with the patient.

> **CRITICAL THINKING** APPLICATION   4-2
> - What must be considered when communicating verbally with an elderly patient?
> - How can the medical assistant demonstrate patience with an elderly patient during her appointment when the office is extremely busy?

Language

With non-English-speaking patients, the medical assistant may need to use gestures and more body language to convey messages. In such cases, be alert to the possibility of misunderstanding. Confirm that the message sent is the message the listener received by asking for feedback. Ask the listener to repeat the message, and if family members are present, make sure they, also, have a good understanding of what was communicated. The clinic may employ a bilingual staff member to reduce the chance of miscommunication with those who speak a different language.

SENSITIVITY TO DIVERSITY

Practicing respectful patient care is extremely important when working with a diverse patient population. *Empathy* is the key to creating a caring, therapeutic environment. Empathy goes beyond sympathy. A medical assistant who is empathetic respects the individuality of the patient and attempts to see the person's health problem through his or her eyes, recognizing the effect of all holistic factors on the patient's well-being. Empathetic sensitivity to diversity first requires those interested in healthcare to examine their own values, beliefs, and actions; you cannot treat all patients with care and respect until you first recognize and evaluate your personal biases. We think and act a certain way for many reasons. The first step in understanding the process is to evaluate your individual value system. Why do you have certain attitudes or beliefs about the worth of individuals or things?

> **CRITICAL THINKING** APPLICATION   4-3
> What do you value most in life? What is important to you? What influences you to act in a certain way? Make a list of five things you value the most and share them with the class. Try to determine why you feel so strongly about those particular things.

Many different factors influence the development of a value system. Value systems begin as learned beliefs and behaviors. Families and cultural influences shape the way we respond to a diverse society. Other factors that influence reactions include socioeconomic and educational backgrounds. To develop therapeutic relationships, you must recognize your own value system to determine whether it could affect your method of interaction. Preconceived ideas about people because of their race, religion, income level, ethnic origin, sexual orientation, or gender can act as barriers to the development of a therapeutic relationship. You will be unable to treat your patients empathetically unless you can connect with them in some way. Personal biases or prejudices are monumental barriers to the development of therapeutic relationships.

CRITICAL THINKING APPLICATION　　4-4

Honestly evaluate your personal biases. What do you find unacceptable in people? Do you prejudge an individual based on his or her affiliation with a particular group or because of a certain lifestyle decision? Do these biases create barriers to the development of therapeutic relationships? If so, how can you get beyond these barriers?

Consider the following scenarios and discuss them with your classmates:

- While you are gathering a patient's insurance information, the patient tells you that he has tested positive for the human immunodeficiency virus (HIV). Do you think this will affect your therapeutic relationship?
- A homeless person with very poor hygiene stops in to make an appointment to see the provider. Will this cause a problem with your professional manner?
- You are told by your office manager that an inmate of the county prison is being brought in this afternoon for an examination. Do you think his status will affect your interaction with the patient?
- You are attempting to register a 20-year-old patient who brought her two young children with her to the clinic today. She is a single mother who is pregnant with her third child and receives public assistance. What do you think? Will you have difficulty being empathetic and communicating therapeutically with this young woman?

Sensitivity to Diversity

Regardless of the type of healthcare facility in which you work, you will care for a wide variety of patients. The following are some points to consider when communicating with diverse groups of patients.

- Patients of Asian backgrounds may have been raised in a culture that considers it extremely rude to establish eye contact. Americans view an unwillingness to establish eye contact as a sign of distrust or embarrassment; however, for individuals from Japan or China, lack of eye contact may be a way of demonstrating respect.
- Personal space may be an issue for patients from diverse backgrounds. If a patient appears very uncomfortable with touch or lack of personal space, attempt to accommodate him or her as much as possible.
- Research has shown that older people face unique communication problems in the healthcare environment. When you are caring for

an aging individual, it is important to focus patient teaching and information on the patient rather than the family member who may be present.
- Patients may use their religious beliefs and values to understand and cope with their health problems. However, using religion to guide healthcare decisions may result in a conflict with the provider's recommendations. Healthcare workers may need to find a balance between respect for a patient's beliefs and the delivery of high-quality healthcare.

OVERCOMING BARRIERS TO COMMUNICATION

We know that communication barriers exist, but how do we overcome them? Most people who enter the medical field have a natural sense of caring and empathy, but the medical assistant can nurture communication skills by using patience, observation, and sensitivity to patient needs, in addition to therapeutic listening skills. If a patient has a physical impairment, being observant helps with communication issues. Often these patients want to be self-sufficient, so they may not appreciate help with simple tasks. Be patient with them and with those who have a language barrier. Encourage these patients to bring an interpreter so that accurate, quality information can be placed into the health record. Prejudice can be overcome with facts about the source of social bias, and the same is true for stereotyping issues. Even highly abrasive patients can be tolerated when the medical assistant wants to be an effective communicator with all patients. If nothing seems to work, talk to the office manager or provider. In severe cases, the provider may have to speak to the patient, or even suggest that he or she seek a different facility for care.

Communication during Difficult Times

Communication is not an art that comes easily to everyone. It often is difficult to express feelings in an honest, open way. When a crisis occurs, it is much harder to communicate effectively, and we sometimes say things we do not mean. Medical assistants must develop communication skills that can be used in times of trouble. They must be able to understand the reason or reasons a patient or co-worker is unable to communicate.

Patience is important, too, because people are not always at their best when they are concerned about their condition or that of a loved one. Always remain calm when dealing with a person who is experiencing a traumatic event or has any depressive condition. Remember that he or she may be reacting to strong emotions, including fear, anger, doubt, inadequacy, or many others. The key is to listen, to determine the best way to help the patient out of any immediate danger, and to help him or her establish some type of support system (Figure 4-4).

Therapeutic Techniques

The linear communication model describes communication as an interactive process involving the sender of the message, the receiver, and the crucial component of feedback to confirm reception of the message. When two people interact, both usually act as senders and

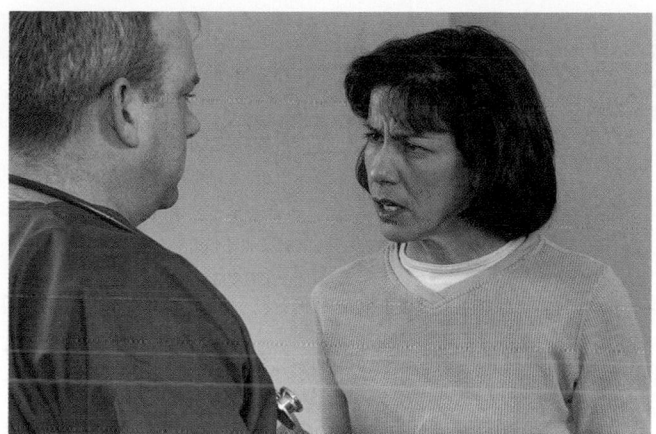

FIGURE 4-4 Remain calm even if a patient becomes verbally aggressive. Attempt to calm the person by listening and expressing empathy whenever possible.

as receivers (or communicators). The *sender* is the person who sends a message through a variety of different channels. *Channels* can be spoken words, written or e-mailed messages, and body language. The sender *encodes* the message, which simply means that he or she chooses a specific means of expression using words and other channels. The receiver *decodes* the message according to his or her understanding of what is being communicated. The message can be sent by a number of different methods or channels, such as face-to-face communication, telephone, e-mail, and letter; however, there is no way to confirm that the message was actually received unless the patient provides *feedback* about what he or she interpreted from the message. Feedback completes the communication cycle by providing a means for us to know exactly what message the patient received and therefore whether it requires clarification.

For example, as a medical assistant, one of your responsibilities will be to provide patient education on how to prepare for diagnostic studies. Let's say you have to explain to an elderly patient how to prepare for a colonoscopy. Even though you provide a detailed explanation of the preparation procedure, in addition to a handout explaining the step-by-step process, how do you really know whether the patient understands (has received the message you sent)? You ask the patient to provide feedback by explaining the process back to you. As a member of the healthcare team, you must become an effective communicator. You will play a vital role in collecting and documenting patient information. If your methods of collection or recording are faulty, the quality of patient care may be seriously impaired.

In summary, the verbal messages you send are only part of the communication process. You have a specific context in mind when you send your words, but the receiver puts his or her own interpretations on them. The receiver attaches meaning determined by his or her past experiences, culture, self-concept, and current physical and emotional states. Sometimes these messages and interpretations do not coincide. Feedback from the patient is crucial in determining whether the patient understood the message. Successful communication requires mutual understanding by both the interviewer and the person being interviewed.

Active Listening Techniques

Listening is just as important to good communication as the spoken word. *Hearing* is the process, function, or power of perceiving sound, whereas *listening* is defined as paying attention to sound or hearing something with thoughtful attention. Patients need to know that the medical assistant is listening. Sometimes it is hard to listen. We may not be able to listen effectively because we are distracted by our own thoughts. Perhaps the situations occurring in our own lives make the conversation we are hearing seem meaningless and unimportant. Or so many messages may be attacking at once that we are unable to focus on any specific one to listen to what is being communicated. At other times, we may simply be too tired to listen, or we may have prejudged the speaker and decided that we do not need to listen. However, while working with patients, the medical assistant must be diligent not only in hearing the words being spoken, but also in listening to them and to what the patient is attempting to communicate.

Active listeners go beyond hearing the patient's message to concentrating, understanding, and listening to the main points in the discussion. Active listening techniques encourage patients to expand on and clarify the content and meaning of their messages. They are very useful communication tools to implement when a patient is agitated or upset because these methods help the medical assistant clarify the important details of the patient's chief complaint.

Three processes are involved in active listening: restatement, reflection, and clarification.

- *Restatement* is simply paraphrasing or repeating the patient's statements with phrases such as "You are saying…" or "You are telling me the problem is…"
- *Reflection* involves repeating the main idea of the conversation while also identifying the sender's feelings. For example, if the mother of a young patient is expressing frustration about her child's behavior, a reflective statement identifies that feeling with the response "You sound frustrated about…" Or, if a patient expresses concern about being able to pay surgical bills, an appropriate reflective statement recognizes the patient's feelings: "You appear anxious about…" Reflective statements clearly demonstrate to patients that you are not only listening to their words; you also are concerned and are attending to their feelings.
- *Clarification* seeks to summarize or simplify the sender's thoughts and feelings and to resolve any confusion in the message. Questions or statements that begin with "Give me an example of…" or "Explain to me about…" or "So what you're saying is…" help patients focus on their chief concern and give you the opportunity to clear up any misconceptions before documenting patient information.

Listening is not a passive role in the communication process; it is active and demanding. You cannot be preoccupied with your own needs, or you will miss something important. For the duration of a patient interaction, no one is more important than this particular patient. Listen to the way things are said, the tone of the patient's voice, and even to what the patient may not be saying out loud but is saying very clearly with body language (Procedure 4-2).

Helpful Listening Guidelines

- Listen to the main points of the discussion.
- Attend to both verbal and nonverbal messages.
- Be patient and nonjudgmental.
- Do not interrupt.

- Never intimidate your patient.
- Use active listening techniques—restatement, reflection, and clarification.

PROCEDURE 4-2   Apply Feedback Techniques, Including Reflection, Restatement, and Clarification, to Obtain Patient Information

Complete this procedure with another student playing the role of the patient. To make the experience more realistic, choose a student about whom you know very little. To maintain the student's privacy, he or she does not have to share any confidential information.

Goal: *To use restatement, reflection, and clarification to obtain patient information and document patient care accurately.*

EQUIPMENT and SUPPLIES

- History form or computer with the patient history window open
- If using a paper form, two pens: a red pen for recording the patient's allergies and a black pen to meet legal documentation guidelines
- Quiet, private area

PROCEDURAL STEPS

1. Greet the patient pleasantly, introduce yourself, and verify the person's ID and date of birth (DOB). Explain your role.
   PURPOSE: To make the patient feel comfortable and at ease.
2. Take the patient to a quiet, private area for the interview and explain why the information is needed.
   PURPOSE: A quiet, private area is necessary to protect confidentiality and prevent interruptions. An informed patient is more cooperative and therefore more likely to provide useful information.
3. Complete the history form by using therapeutic communication techniques, including restatement, reflection, and clarification. Make sure all medical terminology is adequately explained.
   PURPOSE: Therapeutic communication techniques help the medical assistant gather complete information.
4. Speak in a pleasant, distinct manner, remembering to maintain eye contact with your patient.
   PURPOSE: Positive nonverbal behaviors create a friendly, caring atmosphere.
5. Remain sensitive to the diverse needs of your patient throughout the interview process.
   PURPOSE: Maintaining awareness of your personal biases, treat all patients with respect despite their diverse backgrounds.

6. State the message to your patient. Demonstrate sensitivity appropriate to the message being delivered.
   PURPOSE: To send a clearly communicated message.
7. Allow your patient to respond to the sent message. Apply active listening skills.
   PURPOSE: To make sure your patient understood your message and to allow him or her to communicate a response.
8. Restate your patient's response.
   PURPOSE: To make sure you understand the patient's message and to give the patient the opportunity to expand on the information.
9. Use reflection as appropriate to communicate your acknowledgement of the patient's feelings.
   PURPOSE: Use a "feeling" word in your response to demonstrate to the patient that you are attending to his or her emotions and words.
10. Clarify any issues that are unclear.
    PURPOSE: To make sure the meaning of each message sent is understood. You can use clarification to summarize the information you learned. This could serve as a final check on the accuracy of the information you gathered from the patient.
11. Continue to communicate back and forth, using active listening techniques to make sure that your message is understood correctly.
12. Analyze communications in providing appropriate responses and feedback.
    PURPOSE: To continually improve the communication process between healthcare professionals, other staff members, and patients.
13. Thank the patient for sharing the information and direct him or her back to the reception area.
    PURPOSE: To demonstrate respectful patient care.

Open and Closed Questions or Statements

When you gather information from a patient, it is helpful to use a combination of open and closed questions or statements.

An *open* question or statement asks for general information or states the topic to be discussed, but only in general terms. Use this communication tool to begin a conversation with a patient, to introduce a new section of questions, or whenever the person introduces a new topic. It is a very effective method of gathering more details from the patient about his or her problem. Example questions include:

"Why do you need to make an appointment to see Dr. Neill?"
"How have you been getting along?"
"You mentioned having problems with your insurance. Tell me more about it."

This type of question or statement encourages patients to respond in a manner they find comfortable. It allows patients to express themselves fully and provide comprehensive information about their chief complaint.

Direct, or *closed,* questions ask for specific information. In many cases, this form of questioning limits the patient's answer to one or two words: yes or no. Use this form of question when you need confirmation of specific facts, such as when asking about demographic information. For example:

"What is the name of your insurance carrier?"
"What is your birth date?"
"What pharmacy do you prefer for prescription refills?"

COMMUNICATION ACROSS THE LIFE SPAN

The key to communicating effectively with patients is using an age-specific approach. Given the age and developmental level of your patient, how can you best interact with the person and with significant family members?

For example, Tasha, a 2-year-old patient, is scheduled for a physical examination. How can you best interact with her and her father to ensure that the history phase of the visit is complete and accurate? Therapeutic use of nonverbal language is essential to interacting with children of all ages. Getting down on the child's level, establishing eye contact, and using a gentle but firm voice are ways of gaining the child's confidence and cooperation. Children fear the unknown, so explaining all procedures in language the child understands is important. At the same time, the medical assistant must communicate with the child's caregiver so that he or she can contribute to the intake process. The following are some important guidelines for communicating with children and their caregivers.

- Make sure the environment is safe and attractive.
- Do not keep children and their caregivers waiting any longer than necessary because children become anxious and distracted quickly.
- Do not offer a choice unless the child can truly make one. If part of the treatment requires an injection, asking the child whether she'd like her shot now is most likely to get an automatic "No!" However, giving her a choice of stickers after the injection is appropriate.

- Praising the child during the examination helps reduce anxiety and increase self-esteem. When possible, direct questions to the child so that he or she feels like part of the process.
- Involving the child in procedures by permitting him or her to manipulate the equipment may help relieve anxiety. If possible, use your imagination and make a game of what needs to be done.
- A typical defense mechanism seen in sick or anxious children is regression. The child may refuse to leave the mother's lap or may want to hold a favorite toy during the procedure as a comfort measure. Look for signs of anxiety, such as thumb-sucking or rocking during the assessment, and encourage caregivers to be involved in the process to help make the child feel as safe as possible.
- Listen to parents' concerns and respond truthfully to questions.

Older children may also have difficulty during the health visit. To help school-aged children gain a sense of control, give them the opportunity to make certain decisions about treatment. For example, Heather, a 13-year-old patient with diabetes, could be given the choice of having her father present during the visit. Or, if she requires an insulin injection, she could choose the site of the injection or perhaps administer the medication herself. This gives the medical assistant an opportunity to observe her technique and allows Heather to exert her independence.

Privacy is an important issue to consider with older children, especially adolescents. Respect their privacy by keeping body exposure to a minimum and adequately preparing the child for procedures and positions. In addition, older children want to know what is going on, what to expect, and what the findings mean; therefore, keeping them informed in a language they can understand is important. Teen patients should always be encouraged to ask questions, which should be answered as completely and clearly as possible. Take every opportunity to teach your patients, regardless of their age, about their disease and to share information about related wellness factors.

Therapeutic communication is extremely important when interacting with adult patients (Figure 4-5). Using language the adult patient understands and involving the patient in treatment decisions as much as possible are essential to developing a helping relationship with your older patients. Adults are bombarded by multiple responsibilities, which means that stress-related health problems are not unusual in these patients. Get to know your adult patients and

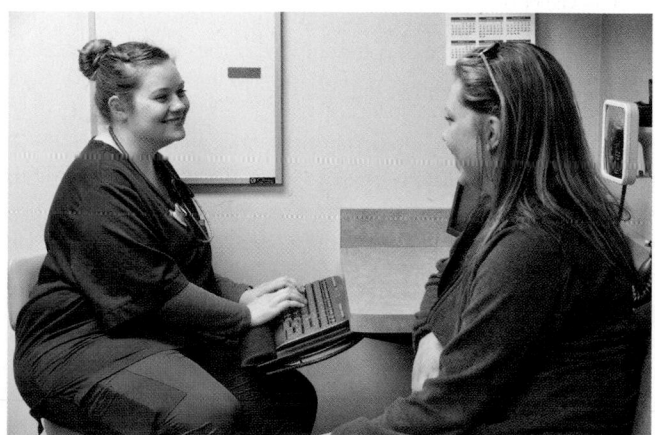

FIGURE 4-5 *Medical assistant communicating with an adult patient.*

emphasize preventive healthcare when possible. Coaching patients based on their cultural diversity, developmental age, and communication style is a key approach to effective communication and patient education (also see the chapter, Patient Education).

Suggestions for Effective Communication with Aging Patients

- Address the patient by Mr., Mrs., or Miss unless the patient has given you permission to use his or her first name.
- Introduce yourself and explain the purpose of a procedure before performing the procedure.
- Face the aging person and softly touch the individual to get his or her attention before beginning to speak.
- Use *expanded speech* by lowering the pitch or tone of your voice and speaking firmly, making sure to sound out each word clearly.
- Use gestures and demonstrations to clarify communication and print out instructions in block print using a larger font size to be sure aging individuals can read the information.
- If the message must be repeated, paraphrase or find other words to say the same thing.
- Observe the patient's nonverbal behavior for cues indicating whether he or she understands.
- Provide adequate lighting without glare.
- Allow patients time to process information and take care of themselves unless they ask for assistance.
- Conduct communication in a quiet room without distractions.
- Involve family members as needed for continuity of care.
- When leaving a telephone message, remember to speak slowly and clearly and repeat the message in the same manner. It is difficult to interpret a message, and even more difficult to write it down, if the message was delivered in a hurried manner.
- Use referrals and community resources for support.

MASLOW'S HIERARCHY OF NEEDS

Psychologist Abraham Maslow created what he called the "hierarchy of needs" (Figure 4-6). A *hierarchy* is defined as things arranged in order, rank, or a graded series. Maslow believed that our human needs can be categorized into five levels and that the needs on each level must be satisfied before we can move to the next level. These levels often are depicted as a triangle, with the most basic needs at the bottom and the highest potential for growth as a human being at the top.

The needs we have as humans, at the most basic level, are those that involve our physical well-being: food, rest, sleep, water, air, and sex. The second level includes issues related to our safety: we need to feel safe and secure in our homes, our environments, and the places where we work. The third level involves our social needs for love, a sense of belonging, and interaction with others. The fourth level relates to our self-esteem: we have an inner need to feel good about ourselves and to know that others view us in a positive manner. The highest level is the self-actualization stage, in which we maximize our potential. At this level, we attempt to be at our best and to live our lives to the fullest extent possible.

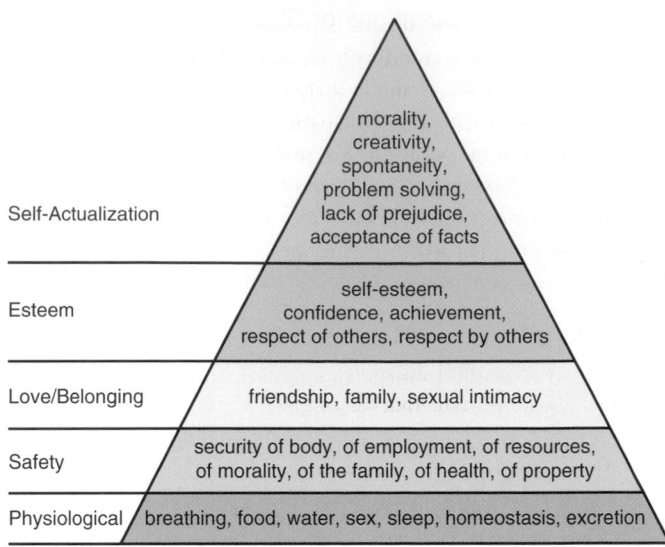

FIGURE 4-6 Maslow's hierarchy of needs.

People adapt to life based on their individual needs, and many factors influence that adaptation, including family history, culture, relationships, and socioeconomic status. The medical assistant should actively investigate the community resources available to help patients adapt to situations that affect their health status. Therapeutic communication techniques should be used to help gather information about current patient needs, especially those related to feeling safe in the healthcare environment. The medical assistant can play an important role in recognizing patient needs and helping to meet those needs in the ambulatory care center.

CLOSING COMMENTS

Developing therapeutic communication skills is critical to your success as a medical assistant. Communication is a part of all interactions throughout the day, and the better developed these skills are, the better the medical assistant can serve the patients in the facility and relate with co-workers. Every attempt should be made to enhance the interpersonal and human relations skills the medical assistant currently has and to strive continually to better these skills. This ensures that effective communication is part of the relationship with patients and with others with whom the medical assistant interacts.

Patient Education

The medical assistant has the opportunity to provide an educational service to every patient who enters the healthcare facility. Patients often have questions about their care or treatment, and the medical assistant with good communication skills can assist the patient in understanding a diagnosis and treatment protocol.

Patients must have a clear knowledge of the role they play in their own care. The medical assistant can communicate information to the patient in many ways other than verbally. Handouts and brochures can help patients understand their illness better and can educate them, but the medical assistant should always explain each piece of literature given to a patient. Never just hand out printed information and expect it to be read. Have the patient repeat instructions to clarify whether he or she understands.

Remember that physical care is not the only aspect of patient care; patients also have emotional needs. Often the very things we take for granted, such as food, shelter, or the ability to pay for healthcare, are a struggle for some patients. The resulting stress can worsen their physical condition. Ask questions and observe nonverbal behaviors to remain aware of what the patient is communicating to the staff and what is not being said. This helps the medical assistant to best serve the patient.

Legal and Ethical Issues

Patients see the medical assistant as an extension of the provider; therefore, it is important that all communication with the patient be professional and accurate. Never give a patient advice that is not approved by the provider, to prevent accusations of practicing medicine without a license. Always discuss with the provider any issues that might affect the patient's care. Never agree to withhold any information from the provider because even a small piece of information could completely change the plan of treatment. When you give instructions to patients, it is always best to have them in writing and to document the patient education intervention in the health record so that a record exists of what was communicated to the patient. Remember that all the patients in the facility deserve to be treated with respect and compassion. Help providers establish trust with the patient. An open, trusting relationship helps prevent legal issues in the future.

SUMMARY OF SCENARIO

Mrs. Cloyd and her daughter both face significant issues in dealing with Mrs. Cloyd's chronic heart condition. Both patients and their families need compassion and caring from the medical team. They want to feel as if they are being heard and that their opinions are important. Some of their needs are similar, but they also have differing needs. A gentle touch and laughter can brighten their day, and these nonverbal expressions are critical to a person experiencing a serious illness.

The medical assistant must ensure that Mrs. Cloyd understands her medications and treatments. She should assist Mrs. Cloyd and her daughter in finding community resources for which Mrs. Cloyd might be eligible. Be sure to directly interact with Mrs. Cloyd, but at the same time, make sure her daughter understands any directions her mother should follow. Even on the busiest of days, patients and their families deserve warmth from the staff and should be made as comfortable as possible when they seek medical care.

Although the ambulatory care center is always a busy place, medical assistants can take a moment to individualize the care they provide to patients. Establishing eye contact and genuinely asking how the person has been getting along demonstrate interest. Call patients by their name, and ask about their families. These techniques allow the medical assistant to develop rapport, which results in a more pleasant healthcare visit for the patient.

Listening is a skill that must be practiced and refined. Patients need to know that the medical assistant is focusing attention on them, listening to their concerns, and responding with restatement, reflection, and clarification to make sure the patient is understood correctly. Active listening is one of the most important skills the medical assistant can develop.

SUMMARY OF LEARNING OBJECTIVES

1. **Define, spell, and pronounce the terms listed in the vocabulary.**
   Spelling and pronouncing medical terms correctly reinforce the medical assistant's credibility. Knowing the definitions of these terms promotes confidence in communication with patients and co-workers.

2. **Discuss first impressions and patient-centered care.**
   First impressions are very important and are formed based on attitude, appearance, compassion, and therapeutic communication skills. Delivering patient-centered care is imperative for the professional medical assistant. To provide high-quality patient care, we must communicate effectively with the patient and provide a warm, caring environment. Good communication skills are vital to meeting the needs of the patient and his or her support system.

3. **Do the following related to communication paths:**
   - *Identify types of verbal communication.*
     When we are communicating verbally with our patients, we are using words to deliver the intended message. The two major forms of verbal communication are oral and written communication. Verbal communication is the expression of thoughts with words. When we put our thoughts to paper, such as writing down instructions for a patient, our oral words are now in written form.

   - *Identify types of nonverbal communication.*
     Much of what we communicate to our patients is conveyed through the use of conscious or unconscious body language. Our nonverbal actions, such as gestures, facial expressions, and mannerisms, are learned behaviors that are greatly influenced by our family and cultural backgrounds. The body naturally expresses our true feelings; in fact, experts say that more than 90% of communication is nonverbal. This means that, even though the verbal message is an important method of delivering information, the way we deliver those words is how the patient interprets them.

   - *Recognize and respond to verbal and nonverbal communication.*
     Procedure 4-1 presents an example of how to respond to nonverbal communication. The key to successful patient interaction is congruence between the words used and the body language observed. The medical assistant should use therapeutic communication skills to interpret the person's message and level of understanding.

Continued

SUMMARY OF LEARNING OBJECTIVES—*continued*

4. Recognize communication barriers.

Effective therapeutic communication requires the delivery of a clear message to the patient. However, along the way are many communication barriers that can create misunderstanding and misinterpretation of your message. Successful communication relies on knowing what barriers to communication exist and how to navigate around these roadblocks. By understanding what barriers may stand in the way of your attempts at effective communication, you can more successfully sidestep these challenges and engage in patient-centered communication. Communication barriers can occur with both medical assistants and patients.

5. Summarize factors that should be considered when communicating with diverse patient populations.

Practicing respectful patient care is extremely important when working with a diverse patient population. *Empathy* is the key to creating a caring, therapeutic environment. Empathy goes beyond sympathy. A medical assistant who is empathetic respects the individuality of the patient and attempts to see the person's health problem through his or her eyes, recognizing the effect of all holistic factors on the patient's well-being. Empathetic sensitivity to diversity first requires those interested in healthcare to examine their own values, beliefs, and actions; you cannot treat all patients with care and respect until you first recognize and evaluate your personal biases.

6. Identify techniques for overcoming communication barriers.

Most people who enter the medical field have a natural sense of caring and empathy, but the medical assistant can nurture communication skills by using patience, observation, and sensitivity to patient needs, in addition to therapeutic listening skills. If a patient has a physical impairment, being observant helps with communication issues. Often these patients want to be self-sufficient, so they may not appreciate help with simple tasks. Encourage these patients to bring an interpreter so that accurate, quality information can be placed in the health record. Prejudice can be overcome with facts about the source of the social bias, and the same is true for stereotyping. Even highly abrasive patients can be tolerated when the medical assistant wants to be an effective communicator with all patients.

7. Do the following related to communication during difficult times:

- *Recognize the elements of oral communication using the sender-receiver process.*

  The linear communication model describes communication as an interactive process involving the sender of the message, the receiver, and the crucial component of feedback to confirm reception of the message. The sender is the person who sends a message through a variety of different channels. Channels can be spoken words, written or e-mailed

messages, and body language. The sender encodes the message, which simply means that he or she chooses a specific means of expression using words and other channels. The receiver decodes the message according to his or her understanding of what is being communicated. There is no way to confirm that the message was actually received unless the patient provides feedback about what he or she interpreted from the message.

- *Apply feedback techniques, including reflection, restatement, and clarification, to obtain information.*

  Three processes are involved in active listening: restatement, reflection, and clarification. Restatement is simply paraphrasing or repeating the patient's statements; reflection involves repeating the main idea of the conversation while also identifying the sender's feelings; clarification seeks to summarize or simplify the sender's thoughts and feelings and to resolve any confusion in the message (see Procedure 4-2).

- *Discuss open and closed questions or statements.*

  When gathering information from a patient, it is helpful to use a combination of open and closed questions or statements. Open questions ask for general information, whereas closed questions typically limit the patient's answer to yes or no.

8. Discuss important factors about therapeutic communication across the life span.

The key to communicating effectively with patients is using an age-specific approach. Therapeutic use of nonverbal language is essential to interacting with children of all ages. Getting down on the child's level, establishing eye contact, and using a gentle but firm voice are ways of gaining the child's confidence and cooperation. To help school-aged children gain a sense of control, give them the opportunity to make certain decisions about treatment. Privacy is an important issue to consider with older children, especially adolescents. In addition, older children want to know what is going on, what to expect, and what the findings mean; therefore, keeping them informed in a language they can understand is important. Using language the adult patient understands and involving the patient in treatment decisions as much as possible are essential to developing a helping relationship with your older patients.

9. List and explain the levels of Maslow's hierarchy of needs.

Psychologist Abraham Maslow created what he called the "hierarchy of needs." A *hierarchy* is defined as things arranged in order, rank, or a graded series. Maslow believed that our human needs can be categorized into five levels and that the needs on each level must be satisfied before we can move to the next level. These levels often are depicted as a triangle, with the most basic needs at the bottom and the highest potential for growth as a human being at the top.

CONNECTIONS

Study Guide Connection: Go to the Chapter 4 Study Guide. Read and complete the activities.

evolve Evolve Connection: Go to the Chapter 4 link at *evolve.elsevier.com/kinn* to complete the Chapter Review Quiz. Check out the other resources listed for this chapter to make the most of what you have learned from Therapeutic Communication.

MEDICINE AND LAW

5

SCENARIO

Barbara Johnson is the new office manager for two neurologists in an urban area. Recently she was subpoenaed to appear in court with medical records to testify about a patient. This particular patient was referred to one of the providers in the clinic, Dr. Rebecca Patrick. Dr. Patrick saw the patient several years ago, and the patient has brought a medical professional liability case against a surgeon in another city. Barbara is considered the custodian of medical records and will take them to court and answer questions about the information in them.

One of Barbara's first priorities at her new job is to make sure the office is operating in compliance with the legal regulations that affect the facility. She is knowledgeable about the requirements of the Health Insurance Portability and Accountability Act (HIPAA) and the Health Information Technology for Economic and Clinical Health Act (HITECH), in addition to other legal issues. Two of the employees Barbara supervises, Samantha and Lynda, are newly graduated from medical assisting school and are anxious to learn more about the statutes and laws that affect the providers' office. Barbara is more than happy to share what she has learned with them.

While studying this chapter, think about the following questions:

- How can the medical assistant comply with legal regulations in the ambulatory care facility?
- How can new graduates learn about the laws that affect them in their state?
- What are some risk management strategies that will help prevent medical liability suits?

LEARNING OBJECTIVES

1. Define, spell, and pronounce the terms listed in the vocabulary.
2. Compare criminal and civil law as they apply to the practicing medical assistant; also discuss contract law.
3. Summarize the anatomy of a medical professional liability lawsuit and explain the four essential elements of a valid contract.
4. Discuss the various parts of a medical professional liability lawsuit.
5. Discuss the advantages of mediation and arbitration.
6. Do the following related to medical liability and negligence:
   - Differentiate malfeasance, misfeasance, and nonfeasance.
   - Explain the four Ds of negligence.
   - Define the types of damages.
7. Discuss risk management and describe liability, malpractice, and personal injury insurances, including the importance of informed consent.
8. Define statutes of limitation and confidentiality.
9. Discuss compliance reporting, the Patient Self-Determination Act, the Uniform Anatomical Gift Act, and the Patients' Bill of Rights.
10. Describe the important features of the ADAA and GINA Acts.
11. Explain the components of the Health Insurance Portability and Accountability Act (HIPAA).
12. Identify HITECH and its impact on electronic transmission of patient records.
13. Summarize the primary features of the Affordable Care Act.

VOCABULARY

abandonment The withdrawal of protection or support; in medicine, to discontinue medical care without proper notice after accepting a patient.

act The formal action of a legislative body; a decision or determination of a sovereign state, a legislative council, or a court of justice.

arbitration (ar-buh-tra'-shun) A type of alternative dispute resolution that provides parties to a controversy with a choice other than going to court for resolution of a problem. Arbitration is either court ordered to resolve a conflict, or the two sides select an impartial third party, known as an *arbitrator*, and agree in advance to comply with the arbitrator's award. The arbitrator's decision is usually final.

assault An intentional attempt to cause bodily harm to another; a threat to cause harm is an assault if it is combined with a physical action (e.g., a raised fist) so that the victim could reasonably assume there would be an assault.

VOCABULARY—*continued*

battery An intentional act of contact with another that causes harm or offends the individual being touched or injured.

contributory negligence A law that recognizes there may be some instances in which the individual contributes to the injury or condition; the injury or condition is partly due to the individual's own unreasonable action.

damages Money awarded by a court to an individual who has been injured through the wrongful conduct of another party. Damages attempt to measure in financial terms the extent of harm the victim has suffered. Harm may be an actual physical injury but can also be damage to property or the individual's reputation.

defendant A person required to answer in a legal action or suit; in criminal cases, the person accused of a crime.

due process A fundamental constitutional guarantee that all legal proceedings will be fair; that one will be given notice of the proceedings and an opportunity to be heard before the government acts to take away life, liberty, or property; a constitutional guarantee that a law will not be unreasonable or arbitrary.

emancipated minor A person under the age of majority (usually 18) who has been legally separated from his or her parents by the courts. The person is responsible for his or her own care.

expert witnesses People who provide testimony to a court as experts in certain fields or subjects to verify facts presented by one or both sides in a lawsuit. They typically are compensated and used to refute or disprove the claims of one party.

guardian ad litem An individual who is assigned by the court to be legally responsible for protecting the well-being and interests of a ward, typically a minor or a person who has been declared legally incompetent.

healthcare clearinghouses Businesses that receive healthcare transactions from healthcare providers, translate the data from a given format into one acceptable to the intended payer, and forward the processed transaction to designated payers. They include billing services, community health information systems, and private network providers or "value-added" networks that facilitate electronic data interchanges.

implied contract A contract that lacks a written record or verbal agreement but is assumed to exist. For example, if a patient is being seen in a physician's office for the first time, it is assumed that the patient will provide a comprehensive and accurate health history and that the provider will diagnose and treat the patient in good faith to the best of his or her ability.

incompetent Refers to a person who is not able to manage his or her affairs because of mental deficiency low IQ, deterioration, illness, or psychosis) or sometimes physical disability. The individual cannot comprehend the complexities of a situation and therefore cannot provide informed consent.

informed consent Voluntary agreement, usually written, for treatment after being informed of its purpose, methods, procedures, benefits, and risks. The patient must understand the details of the procedure and give his or her consent without duress or undue influence, and the patient must have the right to refuse treatment or voluntarily withdraw from treatment at any time.

law A binding custom or practice of a community; a rule of conduct or action prescribed or formally recognized as binding or enforceable by a controlling authority.

liable (li'-uh-buhl) Obligated according to law or equity; responsible for an act or a circumstance.

libel A written remark that injures another's reputation or character.

litigious (luh-tih'-juhs) Prone to engage in lawsuits.

malpractice A type of negligence in which a licensed professional fails to provide the standard of care, causing harm to a person.

negligence (neh'-glih-jents) Conduct expected of a reasonably prudent person acting under similar circumstances; it falls below the standards of behavior established by law for the protection of others against unreasonable risk of harm.

ordinance (or'-dih-nens) An authoritative decree or direction; a law set forth by a governmental authority, specifically, municipal regulation.

perjured testimony The voluntary violation of an oath or vow, either by swearing to what is untrue or by omission to do what has been promised under oath; false testimony.

plaintiff The person or group bringing a case or legal action to court.

precedent (preh'-suh-dent) A person or thing that serves as a model; something done or said that may serve as an example or rule to authorize or justify a subsequent act of the same kind.

prudent Marked by wisdom or judiciousness; shrewd in the management of practical affairs.

relevant Having significant and demonstrable bearing on the matter at hand.

slander An oral defamation or insult; a harmful, false statement made about another person.

subpoena duces tecum A subpoena for the production of records or documents that pertain to a case as evidence.

verdict The finding or decision of a jury on a matter submitted to it in trial.

The **law** is a fascinating subject. When law is applied to medicine, it can provoke interesting case studies and complex decisions. In today's **litigious** society, medical assistants, in addition to providers and other staff members, must take steps to protect themselves from lawsuits. Legal issues underlie many aspects of the provision of healthcare in a provider's office. Although the wording of statutes and regulations often is long and complicated, medical assistants must stay abreast of the rules governing medical facilities and do everything possible to remain in compliance with the standards and regulations for all organizations that oversee the medical industry.

Generally, the law holds that every person is **liable** for the consequences of his or her own **negligence** when another person is injured as a result. In some situations, this liability also extends to the employer. Providers may be held responsible for the mistakes of those who work in their healthcare facility, and sometimes they must pay **damages** for the negligent acts of their employees.

Under the doctrine of *respondeat superior* (Latin for "let the master answer"), providers are legally responsible for employees acting within the scope of their employment duties. In healthcare, this principal states that the physician-employer is legally responsible for the actions of his or her employees, including medical assistants, when they are performing duties as outlined in their job descriptions. Medical assistants guilty of negligence are liable for their own actions, but the injured party generally sues the provider because the chance of collecting damages is greater. However, medical assistants, regardless of their financial worth, can be held liable for negligent acts; this fact illustrates the continuing importance of exercising extreme care in performing all duties in the healthcare environment.

JURISPRUDENCE AND THE CLASSIFICATIONS OF LAW

Jurisprudence is the science and philosophy of law. The term *jurisprudence* comes from the Latin words *juris,* which means "law, right, equity, or justice," and *prudentia,* which means "skill or good judgment."

Law is a custom or practice of a community. It is a rule of conduct or action prescribed or formally recognized as binding or enforceable by a controlling authority. Law is the system by which society gives order to our lives. The U.S. Constitution is the supreme law of the United States (Figure 5-1); the rules established by the Constitution take priority over federal statutes, court opinions, and state constitutions. The state constitution is the supreme law within the boundaries of each state unless it conflicts with the U.S. Constitution. States cannot pass laws that conflict with the U.S. Constitution, nor can local governments pass laws that conflict with the state constitution.

A law enacted at the federal level, which must be passed by Congress, is called an **act**. *Statutes* are laws that have been enacted by state legislatures. Local governments create and enact **ordinances**. Much of our law is based on previous judge and jury decisions, which are called **precedents**. Often judges and juries follow precedents when making a decision on a case. The two basic categories of jurisprudence are criminal law and civil law.

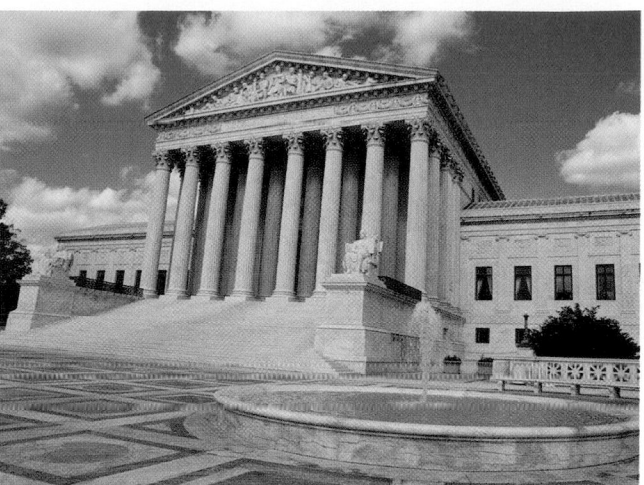

FIGURE 5-1 The U.S. Supreme Court. The Supreme Court decides cases that involve interpretation of the U.S. Constitution.

Criminal Law

Criminal law governs violations of the law punishable as offenses against the state or the federal government. Such offenses involve the welfare and safety of the public as a whole, rather than of one individual. A medical assistant can be prosecuted for criminal acts such as **assault** and **battery**, fraud, and abuse. Criminal offenses are classified into three basic categories: misdemeanors, felonies, and treason. To ensure fair treatment under the law, all individuals are entitled to **due process**, which guarantees that the accused will have an opportunity to defend himself or herself against any charges brought in opposition.

Misdemeanors

A minor crime is called a misdemeanor. Punishment for misdemeanors can include payment of a fine, probation, community service, and restitution. These cases are tried in the lowest local court, such as municipal, police, or justice courts. Typical misdemeanors include petty theft, disturbing the peace, simple assault and battery, and drunk driving without injury to others. If convicted of a misdemeanor, individuals may spend up to a year in jail. Some states have created a subcategory of misdemeanors for infractions, which often are called *violations*. Infractions are minor offenses, such as traffic tickets, which are punishable only by a fine.

Felonies

A *felony* is a major crime, such as murder, rape, or burglary. A felony charge can end with imprisonment for 1 or more years or even death for more serious crimes. An individual convicted of a felony may lose the right to vote, cannot be employed in certain professions (e.g., teachers and social workers), are not allowed certain types of licenses (e.g., medicine or nursing), and cannot buy or carry firearms. Felonies often are divided into subgroups, or degrees, such as first degree, second degree, and third degree. A first-degree offense is normally the most serious.

Civil Law

Civil law is concerned with acts that are not criminal in nature but involve relationships with other individuals, organizations, or government agencies. Many types of civil law exist to address numerous issues. The three that most directly affect the medical profession are tort law, contract law, and administrative law.

Tort Law

Tort law provides a remedy for a person or group that has been harmed by the wrongful acts of others. For example, a defamation case would be judged under tort law. *Defamation* is an intentional false statement, either written or spoken, that harms a person's reputation, diminishes the respect in which a person is held, or creates negative opinions toward another person. **Libel** (written) and **slander** (oral) are acts that fall into the category of defamation.

When a person is liable for an act, he or she is obligated or responsible according to the law. Professional and personal injuries are types of torts, meaning that a person or group has injured someone or something else. Medical professional liability, or medical **malpractice**, falls into this category. Providers carry professional liability insurance to help guard them from liability costs. Medical assistants can also invest in liability insurance. Remember, the terms *libel* and *liable* are defined differently, although they sound much the same.

CRITICAL THINKING APPLICATION   5-1
- What is the difference between libel and slander?
- Give an example of how a medical assistant might commit each of these actions against tort law?

Contract Law

A contract is an agreement that creates an obligation. Contract law touches our lives in many ways practically every day, but we usually do not give much thought to its influences. If a person parks a car in a parking garage for a monthly fee and signs a contract for a year, and then begins parking elsewhere and refuses to pay the fee, the person may be liable for the fees for the duration of the entire contract. If the person's vehicle is damaged while parked in the garage, the garage may be responsible for reimbursement if the contract does not specify otherwise.

A contract does not have to be formalized in writing to be binding on the parties involved. Oral contracts also are valid in many states in most situations. For example, an oral contract is created when the medical assistant makes an appointment for a new patient visit. Simply as a result of the scheduling of that first appointment, the patient and provider now are in an oral contract that requires the provider to care for the patient and the patient to comply with treatment protocols and payment of services. This is why most ambulatory care facilities require the medical assistant to gather payment information (e.g., the type of health insurance the patient has) before an appointment is scheduled.

ANATOMY OF A MEDICAL PROFESSIONAL LIABILITY LAWSUIT

A medical liability case often stems from a breach of trust or miscommunication between the provider and the patient. These cases fall into the category of tort law. Even when the provider has made an error, often the level of trust between the provider and patient determines whether a lawsuit is pursued. First, the provider-patient relationship must be formed. However, before this relationship can be discussed, you must understand the requirements for a valid, enforceable contract.

What Constitutes a Valid Contract?

A valid legal contract has four essential elements: agreement, legality, competence, and consideration.
1. The two parties must have a mutual understanding and *agreement* on the intent of the contract.
2. The contract must involve something that is *legal*.
3. Both parties must be legally *competent*.
4. *Consideration* must be involved; consideration is an exchange of something of value (e.g., money) for the provider's time.

CRITICAL THINKING APPLICATION   5-2
Barbara works for Dr. Rebecca Patrick, who saw the patient bringing the lawsuit against the surgeon as a referral patient. Does Dr. Patrick have a contract with the patient, based on a provider-patient relationship? Why or why not?

The provider-patient relationship is generally held by courts to be a contractual relationship that is the result of three steps:
1. The provider invites an offer by establishing availability (e.g., posting office hours).
2. The patient accepts the appointment and makes an offer by arriving for or requesting treatment.
3. The provider accepts the patient's offer by examining the patient and beginning treatment. Before accepting a patient, the provider is under no obligation, and no contract exists. However, once the provider has accepted the patient, an **implied contract** exists (Figure 5-2). An implied contract in this case assumes that the provider will treat the patient using reasonable care and that the provider has a degree of knowledge, skill, and judgment that might be expected of any other provider in the same locality and under similar circumstances.

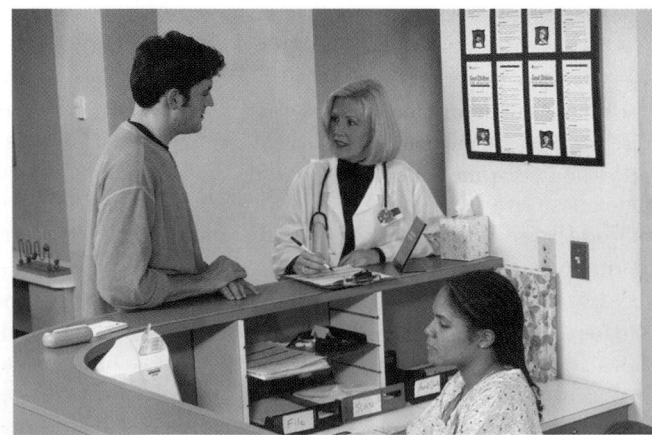

FIGURE 5-2 The provider-patient relationship is built on a strong foundation of trust, but it also is a contractual relationship.

It is extremely important that no express promise of a cure be made by anyone in the office, including the provider, because this would become a part of the contract.

The patient's responsibility in this agreement includes the liability of payment for services and a willingness to follow the advice of the provider. Most provider-patient contracts are implied contracts. Although the patient may complete many forms before he or she is accepted by the provider, these forms do not in most cases constitute a formal contract.

CRITICAL THINKING APPLICATION   **5-3**

- If the patient does not pay for the services rendered by the provider, does this negate the provider-patient contract?
- How might Barbara, Samantha, and Lynda ensure that patients understand that they are expected to follow the advice of the provider?

After the provider-patient relationship has been established, the provider is obligated to attend the patient as long as attention is required, unless the provider or patient terminates the contract. When a provider terminates the contract, the patient must be given notice of the provider's intentions so that the patient has sufficient time to arrange for another healthcare provider. The provider must write a letter of withdrawal from medical care of the patient, and it should be delivered by certified mail, return receipt requested. A copy of the letter and the return receipt should be included in the patient's health record. Reasonable time should be allowed for the patient to find other medical care.

To protect the provider against a lawsuit for **abandonment**, the details of the circumstances under which the provider is withdrawing from the case should be included in the patient's health record. To specify the withdrawal of care, a letter should be sent to the patient that includes a brief reason for the withdrawal of care, such as missing appointments or failing to comply with treatment orders. The letter should state the following:

- That professional care is being discontinued as of a particular date
- That the provider will supply copies of the patient's records to another provider on request
- That the patient should seek the attention of another provider as soon as possible

A patient who wants to terminate the provider-patient relationship simply no longer sees the provider for treatment. The patient does not have to inform the office; however, if she or he does so, the office manager or provider should follow up with a confirmation letter, stating that the patient has ended the relationship.

Breach of Contract

A breach of contract occurs if there is a failure to perform any term of a contract, written or oral, without a legitimate legal excuse. For example, if a plastic surgeon prepares an estimate for services and it states that the fee will be no more than $9,000, but then charges the patient $10,200, a breach of contract exists. Although most providers state that the document is just an estimate, this particular provider stated a clear amount that the surgery costs would not exceed.

CRITICAL THINKING APPLICATION   **5-4**

- For what reasons might a provider not want to accept a patient?
- Must the provider treat every patient who attempts to make an appointment?
- How might Barbara tactfully explain that the provider will not accept the patient into treatment?

MEDICAL PROFESSIONAL LIABILITY LAWSUIT

Medical professional liability suits are far from rare, and every provider faces the probability of being sued at least once during his or her career. A medical assistant may be involved in preparing materials for court and scheduling or participating in depositions. The best advice for a medical assistant in this position is to remember to tell the truth. Attorneys help prepare the defense of the provider and the staff, but everyone should be truthful in answering in court to prevent the loss of his or her credibility in the trial and charges of perjury. Be especially careful to present a true, complete statement to the representing attorney. Unless he or she knows the whole truth, an appropriate defense cannot be prepared.

Interrogatories

Before the trial, the provider may be asked to complete an *interrogatory*, which is a list of questions from each party to the other in the lawsuit. Answers to the interrogatory must be provided within a specified time, and the answers are considered to be given under oath. Only the parties named in the lawsuit may be questioned through interrogatories.

Depositions

A *deposition* is an oral testimony of a party or witness in a civil or criminal proceeding taken before trial. A witness who is not a party to the lawsuit may be summoned by subpoena for a deposition. If you are called to be deposed in a case, the attorney will prepare you for questions from opposing attorneys and will be present during the process. A deposition is taken in the presence of a court reporter and under oath. The transcribed deposition is sent to the witness for review, and the witness has the right to request changes or corrections in the document before it goes into the record. Depositions are a discovery tool. *Discovery* is the pretrial disclosure of pertinent facts or documents by one or both parties to a legal action or proceeding. Many states have extensive discovery statutes that require each side to reveal to the other the facts that they "discover" while investigating the case.

Subpoenas

A *subpoena* is a document issued by a court that requires a person to be present at a specific time and place to testify as a witness in a lawsuit, either in a court proceeding or in a deposition (Figure 5-3). A **subpoena duces tecum** is a court order to produce identified documents or records. This type of subpoena does not require the person named in it to give testimony at a deposition or trial.

In medical practice, a subpoena duces tecum typically is ordered for patient records needed in a malpractice suit. The facility may charge a fee for the time spent in compiling the records and for

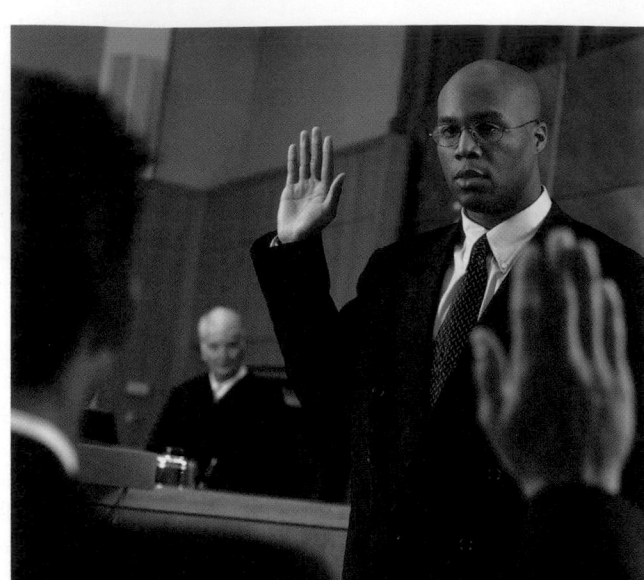

FIGURE 5-3 Witnesses must be credible and must tell the truth on the stand in court to avoid charges of perjury.

photocopying charges, but this fee must be requested at the time the subpoena duces tecum is served or it is considered to be waived. Original records should never be released under any circumstances. If an original record is demanded in the subpoena, it usually is taken to court or to mediation by the provider or an employee of the provider's office. Copies can be released in advance of the court date. Release only the information requested in the subpoena and provide only information that originated in the provider's office. Do not provide records sent from previous or consulting providers. Those records must be subpoenaed separately from the originating office.

Before responding to a subpoena, make sure it is valid. Although variances may occur from state to state, some general rules can be used to judge the validity of a subpoena:

- A subpoena issued in one state court generally is not valid in another state. Always verify the state in which the subpoena was issued.
- A subpoena issued by a federal court in one state generally is not valid in another state unless a federal statute authorizes nationwide service of process.
- Any duly authorized law officer may execute a valid subpoena anywhere in the same state. The officer notifies the issuing court once the subpoena has been served.
- Generally, the person or entity subpoenaed has 21 days to respond, but this period can differ from place to place.
- A subpoena duces tecum should be filed no less than 15 days before a trial. One served less than 15 days before a trial should not be honored.

Read the subpoena carefully to determine exactly what records are requested. The provider should always be notified of subpoenas served to the medical facility. Never copy records required in a subpoena without bringing the matter to the attention of the provider or office manager, or both. It also is advisable to keep a log of

subpoenas served to the office, what records were involved, and the disposition of the request, including when the records were presented to the court. Always inform the provider about the subpoena because he or she may want to present the document to an attorney for review before any information is released.

Inside the Courtroom

Knowing the role of each person in a court of law can be helpful. The person or body bringing the lawsuit to court is referred to by different terms, depending on the type of case. In a criminal court, the government brings the case and is represented by a prosecutor. In civil court, the person or group bringing the case to court is called the **plaintiff** (or *complainant* in some court systems), and the opposite party is called the **defendant**, or *respondent.* A judge presides over the case, giving instructions concerning the law to the jury, if a jury is present. If no jury is present, the judge decides the case; this is called a *bench trial.*

Burden of Proof

In a criminal case the burden of proof is on the prosecution, which must prove guilt beyond any reasonable doubt. *Reasonable doubt* is defined as the level of certainty a juror must have to find a defendant guilty of a crime. It is real doubt, based on reason and common sense after careful and impartial consideration of all the evidence, or lack of evidence, in a case.

Civil cases must be proven by a preponderance of the evidence. This means that the greater weight of evidence must point to the defendant or respondent as being responsible for the act involved in the case.

Outcome of the Case

Once both sides have presented their case to the judge or jury, they usually are given the opportunity to present a final summation of their case. The jury then retires to consider the **verdict**. This can take minutes, hours, days, or weeks. After the jury reaches a decision, the judge may enter it as a final verdict or may disregard it if the evidence does not support the jury's decision. The judge may also revise the verdict to comply with statutes, such as statutory limits on the amount of punitive damages. The final decision of the trial court is reflected in the judgment, signed by the judge.

MEDIATION AND ARBITRATION

Mediation and **arbitration** are two examples of alternative dispute resolutions that share the goal of avoiding litigation in court. In mediation, a neutral third party, the mediator, helps those involved in a dispute solve their own problems. The mediator facilities the parties' decisions by helping them communicate and move through the more difficult parts of their differences in search of a compromise that both parties can live with. Once the parties reach a resolution, a final settlement agreement is signed. Successful mediation enables the parties to design and retain control of the process at all times and, ideally, eventually strike their own bargain.

Arbitration is an alternative to trial in which a third party (an arbitrator) is chosen to hear evidence and make a decision about a case. The patient and the provider both have the opportunity to agree on who will arbitrate the case so that one side is not favored over the other. The arbitrator renders a legally binding decision based on very specific rules. Many providers and attorneys see mediation and arbitration as ways to solve the crisis of litigation in this country. Court battles can take years and can be extremely expensive, and much of the money reverts to the attorneys rather than the victors in the lawsuit.

MEDICAL LIABILITY AND NEGLIGENCE

When a patient is injured as a result of a provider's negligence, the patient may initiate a malpractice lawsuit to recover financial damages. However, experience has shown that the incidence of malpractice claims is directly related to the personal relationship and trust that exist between the provider and the patient. Deterioration of the provider-patient relationship is a common reason patients sue providers for malpractice, even when the patient has sustained no real injury.

Medical professional liability, commonly called *medical malpractice,* is governed by the law of torts. Medical malpractice occurs when a provider treats a patient in a way that does not meet the expected medical standard of care in the same medical community and because of this, the patient suffers harm. The medical standard of care is considered the type and level of care that a reasonably competent healthcare professional, in the same field and with similar training, would have provided in the same situation. Medical professional liability is much more easily prevented than defended.

To understand medical malpractice, the term *negligence* first must be understood. Negligence, in general, implies inattention to one's duty or business, or a lack of necessary diligence or care. In medicine, *negligence* is defined as the performance of an act that falls below the standards of behavior established by law, or the failure to perform an act that a reasonable and **prudent** provider would perform in a similar situation. The standard of prudent care and conduct is not defined by law; it is left to the determination of a judge or jury, usually with the help of **expert witnesses**. Expert witnesses are members of the profession involved (in this case, medicine). To be considered an expert witness, the individual has knowledge beyond that of the ordinary lay person, which enables him or her to give testimony that requires expertise to understand.

Professional negligence in medicine falls into one of three general classifications:

- *Malfeasance:* Intentionally doing something either dishonest or illegal. For example, a physician performs a surgical procedure for higher insurance payment when the patient could be treated with a nonsurgical method, such as medication. Another example would be if the wrong surgical procedure is performed on a patient.
- *Misfeasance:* Performing an act that is legal but not properly performed. For example, the surgeon performs abdominal surgery that is indicated and necessary to help the patient recover but does not do it properly, and the patient dies of complications that could have been avoided.
- *Nonfeasance:* Failure to perform an act that should have been performed. For example, diagnostic findings indicate that a patient has a tubal pregnancy, but the physician opts not to perform laparoscopic surgery to remove the tube.

A provider who performs an operation carelessly or fails to render care that should have been given may be found negligent. The doctrine of *res ipsa loquitur* (a Latin term meaning "the thing speaks for itself") presumes negligence if the individual or group being sued had exclusive control over whatever caused the injury, even though there is no specific evidence of negligence. For example, if a patient suffers an injury during surgery that is not connected to the actual surgical procedure (e.g., he has a reaction to the anesthetic or the provider amputated the left leg instead of the right leg). All those connected to the operation may be found negligent.

Although a medical assistant acts as an agent of the provider in carrying out most of his or her duties, the medical assistant may perform an act that can result in litigation. For instance, if the medical assistant gives a patient the wrong medication or the wrong dose of medication, both the provider and the medical assistant can be held liable for the error. Some states limit the scope of practice of medical assistants where medications are involved. However, if medical assistants are performing within the realm of duties for which they have received training, and the provider is accepting responsibility for the actions of those in the medical office, medical assistants usually are allowed to dispense and administer medications unless prohibited by state law. The medical assistant should always practice within the legal scope of practice of the state (see the chapter, The Medical Assistant and the Healthcare Team).

CRITICAL THINKING APPLICATION 5-5

Lynda asks Barbara whether a provider, as a medical professional, is liable if he or she makes a mistake in diagnosing a patient. When might this be considered malpractice and when might it not be considered malpractice?

What if the patient makes his or her own condition worse? Perhaps the patient does not take the medicine prescribed or refuses to schedule surgery as recommended by the physician. Is the provider responsible for the bad outcome? **Contributory negligence** exists when the patient contributes to his or her own condition, and it can lessen the damages that can be collected or even prevent them from being collected altogether. Some states have adopted a *comparative negligence* approach in which each party's negligence that resulted in an injury is considered when damages are determined.

The Four Ds of Negligence

Negligence is not presumed; it must be proven. The Committee on Medicolegal Problems of the American Medical Association (AMA) has determined that patients must present evidence of four elements before negligence has been proven. These elements have become known as the four Ds of negligence:

1. *Duty:* Duty exists when the provider-patient relationship has been established. Providers have a duty to provide the most accurate diagnosis and care and the duty to inform patients of potential problems they observe.
2. *Dereliction:* Dereliction refers to the failure of a provider to perform his or her duty; there must be proof that the provider somehow neglected the duty.

3. *Direct cause:* The patient must prove that the provider was aware of potential risks but did not inform the patient and as a result the patient was injured.
4. *Damages:* A physical, mental, emotional, or financial harm caused by the breach of duty.

If all four of these elements exist, the patient may obtain a judgment against the provider in a medical professional liability case.

Types of Damages

Five types of damages are common in tort cases: nominal, punitive, compensatory, general, and special damages.

- *Nominal damages* are small awards that are token compensations for the invasion of a legal right in which no actual injury was suffered. For instance, if an unauthorized medical facility employee accesses a patient's health record and is discovered but has not revealed any of the information in the record, the patient has not actually been harmed but may be awarded nominal damages in a lawsuit for the invasion of his or her privacy.
- *Punitive damages* are designed to punish the party who committed the wrong in such a way so as to deter repetition of the act; these are sometimes called *exemplary damages.* These damages historically were set so that the amounts would discourage intentional wrongdoing, misconduct, and outrageous behavior. The amount of damages awarded coincides in some percentage with the wealth of the defendant. Tort reform would cap the amount of money that could be collected during personal injury litigation, including medical malpractice cases. A specific monetary figure (e.g., $500,000) has been suggested as a limit on punitive damages; some believe that plaintiffs should be allowed to collect only up to three times the amount of compensatory damages. Some states have passed legislation that caps one or more of the categories of damages.

CRITICAL THINKING APPLICATION   5-6

Samantha and Lynda disagree on whether punitive damages should be awarded in medical professional liability cases. Samantha believes that nothing compensates for certain losses, but Lynda believes that monetary compensation is reasonable when a loss has been suffered. Discuss both sides of the issue.

- *Compensatory damages* are designed to compensate for any actual damages caused by the negligent person. They are intended to make the injured person "whole." Of course, nothing can substitute for the loss of an arm or a leg, for example, but compensatory damages help the patient or the family recover from the loss.
- *General damages* include compensation for pain and suffering, for loss of a bodily member or faculty, for disfigurement, or for other similar direct losses or injuries. The fact of the losses has to be proven, but the monetary value does not.
- *Special damages* are awarded for injuries or losses that are not a necessary consequence of the provider's negligent act or omission. These may include the loss of earnings or costs of travel. Both the fact of these losses and the monetary value must be proven.

RISK MANAGEMENT PRACTICES

Risk management practices are a combination of different approaches in the healthcare facility that reduces the likelihood that either an individual healthcare professional or the healthcare facility will be sued. The primary focus should be on delivering quality, safe patient care, but a secondary goal is to avoid the potential financial consequences of a malpractice suit. Each facility should have a plan for risk management that covers patient-specific risks. These plans might include the following features:

- Adequately trained providers and staff members.
- Open lines of communication among staff members regarding potential risky practices.
- Specific policies on how expired prescriptions are refilled to prevent prescription medication abuse.
- Policies on patient test results; making sure patients follow up with ordered diagnostic procedures; making sure the results are reviewed by the attending provider, and the patient is contacted with the results.
- Tracking missed appointments; implementing systems to follow-up with patients who miss appointments but fail to reschedule.
- Communication issues with patients; medical assistants can follow up with patients to make sure they understand information received from providers so that orders are not misinterpreted.
- Making sure that the facility is safe for patient use; this includes adequate lighting, grab bars, exit signs, assisting patients as needed, and a safe exterior area.
- Documentation procedures are strictly followed; all pertinent information is documented in the correct format in the patient's record.

LIABILITY, MALPRACTICE, AND PERSONAL INJURY INSURANCES

Individual providers and healthcare facilities typically purchase several different types of insurance. The administrative medical assistant may be involved in either researching or renewing these insurance policies for their employers. The following are types of insurance that are purchased by medical practices.

- *Liability insurance* protects the healthcare facility if there is an accident in the facility that causes bodily injury or property damage. For example, if a patient falls in the parking lot of the facility and suffers a broken arm, liability insurance covers this injury and protects the facility from financial loss.
- *Medical malpractice insurance* protects the provider and/or healthcare facility if there is a judgment against them for medical negligence, malfeasance, or malpractice. Most states require that providers have some form of medical malpractice insurance to protect them from a faulty or negligent action. The provider can either choose individual coverage or be part of a policy that incorporates the practice or institution where the provider is employed. The premiums for malpractice insurance are determined by the provider specialty. Each specialty area of practice has an insurance rate that is based on the probability of medical malpractice occurring. For example, orthopedic surgeons are more susceptible (because of the skill

required to perform surgery and the likelihood of patient complications) to negligent actions or mistakes, and as a result, are more likely to face a medical malpractice suit than a primary care provider (PCP). Therefore orthopedic surgeons have higher premiums for their medical malpractice insurance policies. Malpractice insurance rates also vary according to the location of the medical facility. For example, malpractice rates are higher in the Northeast than they are in the Midwest.

- *Personal injury insurance* covers both bodily harm and non-physical, noneconomic harm. Examples of nonphysical harm are libel or slander, discrimination, and invasion of privacy, which can cause psychological harm or damage the individual's reputation. Personal injury insurance is most commonly seen in auto insurance coverage for bodily injury if there is a car accident or in home owner's insurance if someone has an injury in or around personal property.

Consent

A provider must have consent to treat a patient, even though this consent usually is implied by the patient's appearance at the facility for treatment. This *implied consent* is sufficient for common or simple procedures generally understood to involve little risk. However, the medical assistant should always ask the patient's permission to perform procedures, even those as simple as taking vital signs. You can do this by using expressed consent. *Expressed consent,* sometimes known as general consent, is consent given after the patient is asked a question such as "Can I gather your health history?" If the patient replies, "Yes," you have been given expressed consent to perform that procedure.

When more complex procedures are involved, the provider must obtain the patient's **informed consent**. A provider who fails to secure consent could be charged with the crime of battery. A case for battery can be established if an individual is physically harmed or injured or if an illness occurs because of the contact. Battery may also occur if there is no physical harm but an act is considered offensive or insulting to the victim, such as touching a person without consent. If the patient refuses to consent to treatment and the treatment is performed anyway, the patient can sue for battery.

Informed consent involves a full explanation of the plan for treatment, including the potential for complications and the potential risks or side effects. Informed consent is not satisfied merely by having the patient sign a form. A discussion must occur during which the provider gives the patient or the patient's legal representative enough information to decide whether the patient will undergo the treatment or seek an alternative. The medical assistant cannot legally provide the information for the patient about informed consent. It is the provider's responsibility to make sure that each patient understands the treatment or procedure and has had all questions answered satisfactorily before the patient signs a consent form. However, the medical assistant can witness the document and ask the patient to sign the consent form. After consideration, the patient either consents to the proposed therapy and signs a consent form or refuses to consent. According to the AMA's standards for informed consent, the discussion about informed consent should include at least the following elements:

- Patient's diagnosis, if known
- Nature and purpose of the proposed treatment or procedure

- Risks and benefits of the proposed treatment or procedure
- Alternative treatments or procedures, regardless of the cost or the extent to which the treatment options are covered by health insurance
- Risks and benefits of the alternative treatment(s) or procedure(s)
- Risks and benefits of not receiving or undergoing a treatment or procedure

The discussion should be fully documented in the patient's health record, and a copy of the signed form should be placed in the record. Treatment may not exceed the scope of the consent that the patient has given. Often consent forms are lengthy and mention excessive possibilities and complications. Some language may attempt to be all inclusive (e.g., "included, but not limited to") when risks are listed. It is wise to have an attorney review the forms used for informed consent, because those that are too broad or too specific can be detrimental to the provider in a medical professional liability case.

Patients cannot be forced to undergo any type of medical treatment or care. The ultimate decision about care must be left to the patient or the legal guardian, and although medical professionals should disclose information to help the patient make a sound, informed decision, the patient should never be persuaded to act in any manner or accept any treatment with which he or she does not agree. Should the patient decide not to undergo treatment the provider feels is necessary, the patient should sign an informed refusal of treatment or care. This should be a statement similar to the informed consent, but it indicates that the patient has elected not to undergo treatment. Some providers discontinue all treatment if a patient does not participate in the care the provider recommends. This document, once signed, should be added to the patient's health record.

Each state has its own consent laws. Some states and insurance programs require a certain period to pass between the signing of the consent and the actual medical procedure; for instance, Medicaid sometimes requires a 30-day waiting period between the signing of consent for a tubal ligation and performance of the procedure. Medical assistants should be familiar with the laws in their own state that apply to their particular facility. Most of the laws can be found easily by searching on the Internet.

CRITICAL THINKING APPLICATION   **5-7**

Barbara stresses to Samantha and Lynda that at some time in their professional career, a patient will ask for their advice on whether the patient should undergo a certain procedure or treatment. Barbara explains that patients often consider advice from the medical assistants in the office to be an extension of the provider's opinions. How might they handle such questions from patients? Should a medical assistant offer any type of advice?

Giving Consent to Medical Procedures

Mentally competent adults (i.e., individuals capable of legally making their own decisions) can give consent to medical procedures. However, if an act is unlawful, the consent is invalid. For instance, a provider cannot prescribe medical marijuana for a patient who gives consent for the treatment unless it is legal to do so in that state.

Consent is also invalid if it is given by a person who is unauthorized to do so or if it is obtained by misrepresentation or fraud. For example, an adult child cannot give consent for a parent's treatment unless that individual has been declared **incompetent**. If a person is confused and unable to understand informed consent, a court of law can declare the individual mentally incompetent and appoint a guardian to give consent for treatment. If this is the case, the only care that can be given without the guardian's consent is emergency treatment. The patient's ability to give informed consent can also be compromised if the person is receiving pain medication or under the influence of alcohol or drugs. If the patient is not able to pay attention to the details of a procedure, or to understand those details or the need for care, or the risks of and alternatives to treatment, it is impossible for the patient to give informed consent.

Providers sometimes are reluctant to render aid in an emergency to someone who is not their patient for fear they will later be charged with negligence or abandonment. Under Good Samaritan laws, volunteers at the scene of an accident are given immunity to liability for any civil damages resulting from the rendering of emergency care. Most states now have either Good Samaritan or Volunteer Protection statutes. As long as the emergency care is given in good faith and without gross negligence, and the healthcare worker provides only emergency care that he or she has been trained to provide, the likelihood of a successful lawsuit against that individual is very slim.

Generally, when the patient is a minor, consent for surgery or treatment must be obtained from a parent, guardian, or **guardian ad litem**, except in an emergency requiring immediate treatment. If the parents are legally divorced or separated, consent should be obtained from the custodial parent, but if the child is visiting the second parent, consent may be obtained from that parent because in such a situation that parent has temporary custody.

Consent is not required for minors in the following circumstances:

- When consent may be assumed, such as in a life-threatening situation
- When a court order has been issued, as in a situation in which parents withhold consent for a necessary treatment because of religious reasons

In many states, treatment of sexually transmitted infections, drug abuse, alcohol dependency, pregnancy, or providing contraceptive methods does not require parental consent. Even if there are age of consent laws, providers can still treat minors with these issues.

An area of potential confusion regarding consent to treatment is the *mature minor doctrine,* which allows minors to give consent to medical procedures if they can show that they are mature enough to make a decision on their own. The mature minor doctrine is recognized in only a few states as law, but where it does exist it has been applied in cases where the minor is 16 years or older and demonstrates understanding of the consequences of the proposed surgical or medical treatment or procedure.

An exception to the need for parental consent is if the individual is an **emancipated minor**. Eligibility for emancipation varies, depending on state laws; however, it can be sought by those younger than the age of majority (usually 18 years of age) who meet one or more of the following conditions:

- Married
- In the armed forces
- Living separately and apart from parents or a legal guardian
- Self-supporting

Unless state law declares otherwise, an emancipated minor has the right to consent to treatment and the right to complete patient confidentiality, even from parents.

Statute of Limitations

A *statute of limitations* is a period after which a lawsuit cannot be filed. The statute of limitations for medical malpractice issues varies from state to state, ranging from 1 to 5 years. Most states have a separate deadline for minor children in medical malpractice cases. To research the limitations for minors in your state, see the National Conference of State Legislatures website: *www.ncsl.org/research/financial-services-and-commerce/medical-liability-malpractice-statutes-of-limitation.*

The statute of limitations may be extended because of a delay in the discovery of an injury. For example, a patient has surgery to replace a heart valve, and the surgery seems successful. One year later, the patient undergoes a routine echocardiogram, and the provider discovers that the valve was not implanted properly by the surgeon. Although it has been over a year since the surgery, the statute of limitations begins at the point of discovery of the injury; therefore the patient could now bring suit against the surgeon for the error.

Confidentiality

Confidentiality is one of the most sacred trusts the patient places in the hands of the provider and staff (Figure 5-4). Breach of patient confidentiality is grounds for immediate dismissal of a healthcare professional. The strictest care must be taken when handling patient records and discussing information about patients.

In special cases, patient confidentiality plays a vital role. A patient who tests positive for the human immunodeficiency virus (HIV) may face discrimination if the information surfaces. Providers who treat such patients may want to take extra care when leaving phone messages, texting, or sending e-mail or regular mail. Instead of leaving a message for a patient from "Dr. Watson's office," the medical assistant could say that the message is from "Terry Watson's office." This type of message does not identify the message as coming from a healthcare facility. Curious co-workers or relatives may not

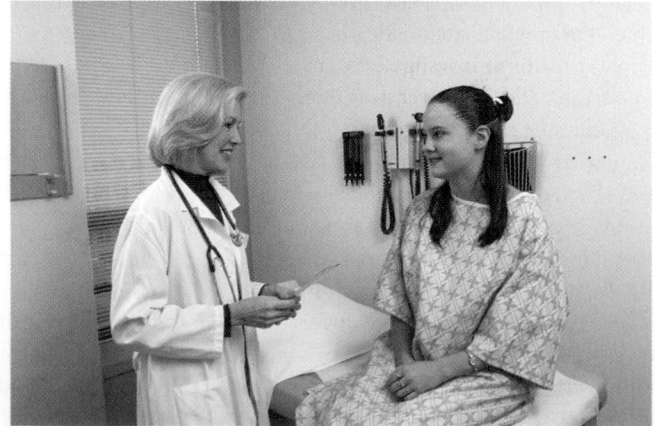

FIGURE 5-4 Patient confidentiality is the most important trust that exists between the provider and the patient.

grow as suspicious as they might if they were to encounter a message from a provider's office.

Patients receiving treatment for substance abuse are protected by federal statutes. Confidentiality also is of utmost importance to patients receiving treatment for mental health issues, sexually transmitted infections, sexual assault, and any type of abuse.

LAW AND MEDICAL PRACTICE

Law affects the provider's day-to-day practice. Some of the ways the medical assistant encounters legal issues in a healthcare setting are discussed in this section. Medical assistants must comply with both state and federal laws and regulations while performing the duties associated with their job.

Compliance Reporting

The provider is charged with safeguarding patient confidences within the constraints of the law, but according to state laws, which vary somewhat across the nation, certain disclosures must be made. Frequently the medical assistant is involved with the responsibility for compliance reporting.

Births and deaths must be reported. In some states, detailed information about stillbirths is required. Public health statutes also require compliance with wounds of violence reporting including gunshot wounds, knife injuries, or poisonings. Any death from accidental, suspicious, or unexplained causes must also be reported. In some states, occupational diseases and injuries must be reported within specific time limits.

Sexually transmitted infections are reportable in every state. All 50 states require that patients with confirmed cases of acquired immunodeficiency syndrome (AIDS) be reported by name to the local health department. Furthermore, most states require that patients who test positive for HIV be reported. Individuals are reported either by name or by unique identifiers. A continuing controversy exists as to whether the reporting prompts patients to receive care or deters individuals in high-risk groups from seeking care.

Child abuse is a leading cause of death among children younger than 5 years of age, and healthcare professionals are required by law to report any suspected cases of child abuse. The report should be made as soon as evidence is discovered that gives the provider "cause to believe" that abuse, neglect, or exploitation has occurred. Even if the evidence is uncertain, the provider should report it and allow the government to investigate and determine what action to take to protect the child. However, it is essential to make every attempt to ensure that the report is legitimate because it could lead to the child's being removed from the home and placed in foster care. Cases of spousal and elder abuse are difficult, because the person being abused often is reluctant to report the situation for fear of further mistreatment. The law requires that suspected cases of abuse of children, the elderly, or any others at risk be reported to the authorities.

Local health departments publish lists of reportable diseases and the method to use in reporting them. Reports are typically filed electronically to local public health officials or the state public health department. County and state health departments periodically issue bulletins that are sent to healthcare providers with information about disease outbreaks and various statistics. Local health departments should be consulted for specific procedures and reporting protocols.

Laws Having a Significant Impact on Healthcare
Patient Self-Determination Act

The Patient Self-Determination Act of 1990 brought the term *advance directive* to the forefront of medical care. This act requires healthcare facilities to develop and maintain written procedures that ensure that all adult patients receive information about advance directives and medical durable powers of attorney. Advance directives are legal documents that allow individuals to make decisions about end-of-life care ahead of time. They are a way for patients to communicate their wishes to family, friends, and healthcare professionals so that there is no confusion about what type of care they would like to receive or not receive when their condition is terminal. Advance directives specify which treatments you want if you are dying or permanently unconscious. Before completing an advance directive, patients should consider the following questions:

- What are your values about death and dying?
- Would you want treatment to extend your life by any means in any situation?
- If you are suffering from a terminal illness, would you want life-saving measures taken?

Patients can exert their right to accept or refuse treatment when they complete an advance directive form. Forms may be provided by healthcare facilities, hospitals, or long-term care facilities, but they can also be accessed online.

Advance directive forms ask patients to make decisions about a number of different treatment options, such as those in the following list. Patients may need assistance from medical personnel to understand the ramifications of each.

- The use of cardiopulmonary resuscitation (CPR) or a defibrillator; this means the heart has stopped and needs to be artificially stimulated with drugs and machines.
- Whether a mechanical ventilator or respirator should be used if breathing complications occur; this means the patient would have to have an airway put in place or be intubated.
- If, when, and for how long artificial feeding should be done; tube feeding supplies the body with nutrients and fluids intravenously or via a tube in the stomach.
- If, when, and for how long renal dialysis should be done to remove waste materials from the blood if the kidneys stop functioning.
- Antibiotics or antiviral medications can be used to treat infections. Many debilitated individuals develop pneumonia near the end of life. Should infections be treated aggressively, or should they be allowed to run their course?
- Decisions about palliative care measures to keep individuals comfortable and manage pain; these may include being allowed to die at home, pain medications, and avoiding invasive tests or treatments.
- Organ and tissue donations can be specified in a living will; if organs are removed for donation, the individual is kept on life-sustaining treatment temporarily until the procedure is complete.
- Donating the body for scientific study to a local medical school or university can be specified in the living will.

When completing an advance directive, the individual may also identify a *medical durable power of attorney* or a healthcare proxy; this is someone the person trusts to make health decisions for him or her if he or she is unable to do so. The patient may choose a spouse, family member, friend, or member of a faith community. This can be a different person from the one chosen to be the executor of a will. According to the American Bar Association, a person chosen as a medical durable power of attorney should:

- Meet your state's requirements for a healthcare agent
- Not be your doctor or a part of your medical care team
- Be willing and able to discuss medical care and end-of-life issues with you
- Be trusted to make decisions that follow your wishes and values
- Be trusted to be your advocate if disagreements arise about your care

Advance directives need to be in writing. Each state has different forms and requirements for creating legal documents. In some states the title of an advance directive can be different, such as a Living Will or an Advanced Health Care Directive. Depending on where you live, a form may need to be signed by a witness or notarized. A lawyer can assist with the process, but it is generally not necessary. Links to state-specific forms can be found on the National Hospice and Palliative Care Organization website: *www.caringinfo.org/i4a/pages/index.cfm?pageid=3289*. The American Bar Association also has a basic, easy to use advance directive form that can be used in most states. All adults should prepare an advance directive because unexpected end-of-life situations can develop at any age.

After completing the form, the patient should share it with his or her healthcare provider. A copy should be given to all providers involved in the patient's care, and this copy should be included in the patient's health record. An advance directive can be changed at any time. However, a new form must be created and witnessed as required by the state of residence, and revisions must be shared with family members and healthcare providers.

In most states, a Physicians Orders for Life Sustaining Treatment (POLST) form can also be completed to plan for the type of care desired if the patient has a medical emergency, such as respiratory or cardiac failure. POLST forms are created by the patient and physician to inform emergency care providers, such as emergency medical technicians (EMTs) and ambulance workers, what treatments you want and don't want in a medical emergency. The form must be signed by a physician and must instruct emergency medical personnel whether to perform CPR or an intubation, administer antibiotics, or start a feeding tube.

Uniform Anatomical Gift Act

The Uniform Anatomical Gift Act was developed to make sure that all states have the same laws about organ donation. The law states:

- A competent individual who is 18 years of age or older may donate all or any part of his or her body after death for research, transplantation, or placement in a tissue bank.
- A donor's valid statement of organ or tissue donation is enacted except when an autopsy is required by law or requested by the family.

- The donor's family can give permission for organ or tissue donation after the individual dies, even if the person did not do so.
- Providers who accept organs or tissues for transplant are protected from lawsuits.
- The time of death must be determined by a provider who is not part of a transplant team.
- The donor may change his or her mind about organ or tissue donation at any time.

The most important clause of the act permits the donation to be made by a written or witnessed document, such as an advance directive, organ donor identification on a driver's license, and/or possession of a donor card (Figure 5-5). This allows for immediate donation of the organs and/or tissues. The Uniform Donor Card is considered a legal document in all 50 states but must be signed by two witnesses.

The provisions of the Uniform Anatomical Gift Act are designed so that the donation occurs only after death. Therefore, donors should reveal their intentions to as many of their relatives and friends as possible and to their providers. Because the human body and its parts are not commodities in commerce, no money can be exchanged in making an anatomic donation itself. Fees are charged for performing the transplant and various procedures, but organs cannot be bought and sold. It also is important to note that family members should be prepared to receive the body of the person who has donated his or her entire body to research once the research facility has completed its study. This can often be a traumatic experience that rekindles the grief process, so the procedures and final disposition of the body should be decided at the time of the donation to avoid this difficult situation.

Patients' Bill of Rights

The Consumer Bill of Rights and Responsibilities, more commonly known as the Patients' Bill of Rights, outlines the relationship patients should have with their insurers, health plans, and care providers. The Patients' Bill of Rights was designed to strengthen confidence in the healthcare system, to encourage the development of quality provider-patient relationships, and to clarify that healthcare consumers also have a responsibility to participate in their care. Most healthcare facilities have adopted a Patients' Bill of Rights that is a condensed version of the entire bill. This information typically is

DONOR   DONOR CARD

I _____, have spoken to my family about organ and tissue donation. I wish to donate:
__ any needed organs and tissue
__ only the following organs and tissue: _____
The following people have witnessed my commitment to be a donor.
donor signature _____ date _____
witness_____
witness_____
next of kin _____ ph _____

FIGURE 5-5 Organ donation card.

shared with patients when they are admitted to healthcare facilities, or it may be posted in a prominent place in the facility. For medical assistants, every time you interact with a patient, you should keep the Patients' Bill of Rights in mind. For example, you should explain procedures to patients and make sure they understand treatments. Printed information about the facility should contain details about how and where a patient can make a complaint about the care received. Policies and procedures should honor the provisions of the Patients' Bill of Rights that apply in that particular medical facility (Procedure 5-1).

CRITICAL THINKING APPLICATION   **5-8**

Summarize how the medical assistant can apply the Patients' Bill of Rights to everyday practice in the healthcare setting.

Patients' Bill of Rights

I. Information Disclosure

You have the right to receive accurate and easily understood information about your health plan, healthcare professionals, and healthcare facilities. If you speak another language, have a physical or mental disability, or just don't understand something, assistance will be provided so you can make informed healthcare decisions.

II. Choice of Providers and Plans

You have the right to a choice of healthcare providers that is sufficient to provide you with access to appropriate high-quality healthcare.

III. Access to Emergency Services

If you have severe pain, an injury, or a sudden illness that convinces you your health is in serious jeopardy, you have the right to receive screening and stabilization emergency services whenever and wherever needed, without prior authorization or financial penalty.

IV. Participation in Treatment Decisions

You have the right to know all your treatment options and to participate in decisions about your care. Parents, guardians, family members, or other individuals whom you designate can represent you if you cannot make your own decisions.

V. Respect and Nondiscrimination

You have the right to considerate, respectful, and nondiscriminatory care from your doctors, health plan representatives, and other healthcare providers.

VI. Confidentiality of Health Information

You have the right to talk in confidence with healthcare providers and to have your healthcare information protected. You also have the right to review and copy your own medical record and request that your provider amend your record if it is not accurate, **relevant**, or complete.

VII. Complaints and Appeals

You have the right to a fair, fast, and objective review of any complaint you have against your health plan, doctors, hospitals, or other healthcare personnel. This includes complaints about waiting times, operating hours, the conduct of healthcare personnel, and the adequacy of healthcare facilities.

VIII. Consumer Responsibilities

In a healthcare system that protects consumer rights, it is reasonable to expect and encourage consumers to assume reasonable responsibilities. Greater individual involvement by consumers in their care increases the likelihood of achieving the best outcomes and helps support a quality-improvement, cost-conscious environment.

PROCEDURE 5-1 | **Apply the Patients' Bill of Rights in Choice of Treatment, Consent for Treatment, and Refusal of Treatment**

Goal: *To ensure that the patient's rights are honored in the daily procedures performed and policies enacted in the ambulatory healthcare setting.*

Case Study: *With a partner, role-play the following case study, which requires the application of the Patients' Bill of Rights to treatment choices, consent for treatment, and refusal of treatment.*

Dr. Patrick recommends that Mr. Tim Shields start taking Lipitor for his elevated blood cholesterol levels. She provides informed consent to Mr. Shields about the risks and benefits of Lipitor, including a decrease in total blood cholesterol levels, an increase in his "good" cholesterol and a decrease in his "bad" cholesterol. She also informs him of the possible side effects of the drug, including liver complications, leg cramps, and photosensitivity (increased risk of sunburn). Mr. Shields states he understands the information but is hesitating to give consent because he has a history of elevated liver enzymes and he works outside most of the year. Mr. Shields opts to refuse the Lipitor treatment. Dr. Patrick tells him that he might be able to lower his blood cholesterol by reducing saturated fat in his diet and exercising (aerobic exercise at least 4 or 5 days a week). Although Mr. Shields admits he may have trouble sticking to those recommendations, he chooses to try diet and exercise rather than medication at this time. Based on your knowledge of the Patients' Bill of Rights, has Dr. Patrick complied with the provider part of the agreement? Does Mr. Shields have the right to refuse the recommended medication? Because he has refused it, is it important to document his refusal of the recommended treatment in his health record? How can the medical assistant help both the provider and the patient in this situation?

PROCEDURE 5-1   *—continued*

EQUIPMENT and SUPPLIES

- Copy of the Patients' Bill of Rights
- Notice of Privacy Practices form

PROCEDURAL STEPS

1. Review the eight points of the Patients' Bill of Rights.
   PURPOSE: To become familiar with the points and content of the document.
2. The patient has the right to receive information about his health plan, professionals, facilities, and personal care. Role-play the information the physician gave Mr. Shields about his treatment choices.
   PURPOSE: To comply with the first article of the Patients' Bill of Rights.
3. Patients have the right to choose a healthcare provider, but their insurance plans may restrict those choices. Role-play the fact that Dr. Patrick's services are covered by Mr. Shields' insurance.
   PURPOSE: To comply with the second article of the Patients' Bill of Rights.
4. The patient has the right to receive emergency treatment and to be informed about the procedures for referral to emergency facilities and for emergency treatment in the office. Role-play a discussion with Mr. Shields about how he can contact the facility or Dr. Patrick if he has a medical emergency.
   PURPOSE: To comply with the third article of the Patients' Bill of Rights.
5. The patient has the right to know all treatment options and to participate in decisions about care. Role-play the information that Dr. Patrick gave Mr. Shields about his care and treatment choices.
   PURPOSE: To comply with the fourth article of the Patients' Bill of Rights.

6. The patient has the right to considerate, respectful, and nondiscriminatory care by all healthcare staff. Role-play respectful care for Mr. Shields.
   PURPOSE: To comply with the fifth article of the Patients' Bill of Rights.
7. Patients have the right to review their records and to expect confidential treatment of their healthcare information. Review methods of enforcing patient confidentiality in the facility. Role-play the patient completing a Notice of Privacy Practices form. Role-play a scenario in which Mr. Shields' girlfriend calls and asks you to tell her what Dr. Patrick suggested for treatment. She is not identified on the patient's Notice of Privacy Practices form. Can you give her that information?
   PURPOSE: To comply with the sixth article of the Patients' Bill of Rights.
8. The patient has the right to a fair and objective review of complaints. During your interaction with Mr. Shields, he complains about how long he had to wait for his appointment and that the receptionist was rude. Role-play how you should manage Mr. Shields' complaints.
   PURPOSE: To comply with the seventh article of the Patients' Bill of Rights.
9. The patient has the responsibility to be involved in care. Mr. Shields has opted to try exercise and dietary changes to manage his elevated cholesterol. Does he have a responsibility to follow through with this care plan? Role-play your interaction with Mr. Shields about his responsibilities.
   PURPOSE: To comply with the eighth article of the Patients' Bill of Rights.
10. Demonstrate sensitivity to patients' rights through empathy, use of therapeutic communications, and respect for individual diversity.
    PURPOSE: To reassure patients so that they know healthcare professionals are sensitive to their needs and desires.

Americans with Disabilities Act

In 1990 the Americans with Disabilities Act (ADA) was signed into law with the intent of eliminating discrimination against individuals with disabilities. The act addressed many areas in which a person might experience discrimination, including telecommunications, housing, public transportation, air carrier access, voting accessibility, education, and rehabilitation.

In 2008, Congress passed the ADA Amendments (ADAA) Act to broaden the definition of disability, which had been narrowed by U.S. Supreme Court decisions. The ADAA Act emphasizes that the definition of disability should be interpreted broadly to include any individual with a physical or mental impairment that substantially limits one or more of his/her major life activities; the individual has a record of such an impairment; or is thought to have an impairment. All individuals meeting this broad definition of disability should be provided the rights associated with the ADAA Act. To clarify the public accommodations requirement, the ADAA Act requires that all new construction and building modifications must be accessible to individuals with disabilities. For existing facilities, barriers that make services inaccessible must be removed if possible. Healthcare facilities fall under the category of public accommodations that must comply with specific requirements related to architectural standards for new and altered buildings; reasonable modifications to policies, practices, and procedures; effective communication with people with hearing, vision, or speech disabilities; and other access requirements.

Individuals with disabilities must be able to enter and exit the facility without difficulty. This means that individuals in wheelchairs need a ramp to enter and exit the building. They also must be able to navigate throughout the facility without major barriers. The law requires that public medical facilities must allow people with disabilities to easily and safely:

- Reach door handles for opening and closing
- Enter and exit buildings
- Move through doors and hallways
- Use drinking fountains, phones, and restrooms
- Move from floor to floor (elevators are required for multilevel buildings)
- Do everything the general public can do in a public place
- Have access to communication devices if they have a problem with vision, hearing, reading, or comprehension.

Genetic Information Nondiscrimination Act

The Genetic Information Nondiscrimination Act (GINA) of 2008 prohibits discrimination in health coverage and employment based on genetic information. Regardless of family history or personal genetic studies, individuals cannot be denied health insurance and employers cannot make job-related decisions based on an individual's genetic history. For example, if genetic testing reveals that an individual carries the gene for Huntington's disease (HD), an inherited neurologic illness that causes involuntary movements, severe emotional disturbance, and cognitive decline and ultimately leads to the need for complete care and an early death, statutes in GINA prevent insurance companies from cancelling coverage and employers from firing the affected individual. Many states already have laws that protect against genetic discrimination in health insurance and employment situations; however, the degree of protection varies widely. All entities subject to GINA must, at minimum, comply with all applicable GINA requirements, and they may also need to comply with more protective state laws.

CRITICAL THINKING APPLICATION   5-9

How do the ADAA and GINA acts affect the physical structure of a healthcare facility and the release of patient information to health insurance companies?

Health Insurance Portability and Accountability Act

The original Health Insurance Portability and Accountability Act (HIPAA) was signed into law in 1996. HIPAA sets national standards for how healthcare plans, **healthcare clearinghouses**, and most healthcare providers protect the privacy of a patient's health information. The law has two provisions: Title I (Insurance Reform) and Title II (Administration Simplification). HIPAA's primary purpose was to limit the administrative costs of healthcare, protect patient privacy, and prevent medical fraud and abuse in the Medicare and Medicaid systems.

Notice of Privacy Practices. The HIPAA Privacy Rule requires healthcare providers to distribute a notice that provides a clear, user-friendly explanation of individual personal health information rights. The law requires that patients sign a statement acknowledging they have received the Notice of Privacy Practices (NPP) (Figure 5-6). This document must be filed in the patient's health record. Signing the statement does not mean that patients have agreed to disclosure of health information. The signed statement simply means that the patient has been informed of the privacy practices of that particular facility. Even though patients have the right to refuse to sign the facility's NPP, the practice can use or disclose the patient's health information as long as the Privacy Rule is followed. However, if the patient does refuse to sign the form, that refusal must be documented in the patient's health record. The NPP describes the ways the practice will use and disclose protected health information. It must also explain that the practice will obtain the patient's permission before using individual health records for any other reason. The notice must include information about the patient's right to complain to the Department of Health and Human Services (HHS) and to the healthcare facility if privacy rights are violated. Most healthcare providers give the NPP to patients at their first service encounter (usually at the first appointment). The notice must also be posted in an easy to find location in the facility. If the practice has a website, the privacy notice must be included there.

Title I, which deals with insurance reform, includes several provisions that protect individuals and their insured dependents if they change jobs or lose a job. Individuals can no longer be prevented from getting insurance coverage because of their previous health history. However, most of the regulations in Title I consider the Privacy Rule, which protects all health information that can identify a specific individual and that is held by a covered entity or an entity's business associate. Covered entities must follow strict procedures to keep all patient information confidential. *Covered entities* include health insurance plans that provide or pay the cost of medical care, providers, healthcare facilities, pharmacies, home health agencies, healthcare clearinghouses, and so on.

A *business associate* is a person or an organization that uses or discloses individually identifiable health information in the process of filing insurance claims, billing, or performing business-related functions for the covered entity. Business associates include insurance claim processors, accounting or legal firms whose service includes access to protected health information, utilization review consultants for a hospital, medical transcriptionists, and a healthcare clearinghouse that performs insurance functions. A written agreement or contract must be in place addressing how the business associates will protect patient information before confidential information can be given to the business associate. This includes information about a patient's health history, the patient's diagnosis, the care provided, and payment information.

The Privacy Rule also defines how covered entities use individually identifiable health information, or personal health information (PHI). PHI is also referred to as protected health information, which includes the patient's demographic information (e.g., name, Social Security number, age, gender, and address), medical history, test and laboratory results, insurance information, and other items collected to identify a patient and determine appropriate care. A major purpose of the Privacy Rule is to define and limit the circumstances in which an individual's PHI may be used or disclosed by covered entities. A covered entity can disclose protected health information only if the Privacy Rule permits or requires it or if the patient authorizes its release in writing. PHI must be protected in all forms of communication, including telephone, fax, e-mail, text, and others.

However, according to the Centers for Disease Control and Prevention (CDC), the Privacy Rule allows covered entities to disclose PHI to public health authorities when required by federal, tribal, state, or local laws. This includes state laws for reporting certain diseases or infections, reportable injuries (e.g., gunshot wounds, child abuse), births, or deaths. PHI may also be used to perform public health studies or treatments. This process may include procedures to de-identify PHI through two different methods:

1. Removal of all information that could lead to the identification of the individual, including address, birth or death date, telephone numbers, e-mail addresses, medical record numbers, health plan account numbers, and so on, so that no reasonable method remains of identifying the person.

PATIENT HIPAA ACKNOWLEDGEMENT

I.   Acknowledgement of Practice's *Notice of Privacy Practices*:
By subscribing my name below, I acknowledge that I was provided a copy of the Notice of Privacy Practices and that I have read (or had the opportunity to read if I so chose) and understand the Notice of Privacy Practices and agree to its terms.

_____   _____   _____

Name of Patient   Date of Birth   Signature of Patient/Parent/Guardian   Date

II.   Designation of Certain Relatives, Close Friends and other Caregivers as my Personal Representative:
I agree that the practice may disclose certain pieces of my health information to a Personal Representative of my choosing, since such person is involved with my healthcare or payment relating to my healthcare. In that case, the Physician Practice will disclose only information that is directly relevant to the person's involvement with my healthcare or payment relating to my health care.

Print Name: _____   Last four digits of SSN or other identifier: _____
Print Name: _____   Last four digits of SSN or other identifier: _____
Print Name: _____   Last four digits of SSN or other identifier: _____

III.   Request to Receive Confidential Communications by Alternative Means:
As provided by Privacy Rule Section 164.522(b), I hereby request that the Practice make all communications to me by the alternative means that I have listed below.

Home or Cell Telephone Number: **Written Communication Address:**
_____   _____
____ OK to leave message with detailed information   ____ OK to mail to address listed above
____ Leave message with call back numbers only   ____ E-mail me at:
Work Telephone Number: **Email Communication:**
_____   _____
____ OK to leave message with detailed information   ____ OK to text at the number listed above
____ Leave message with call back numbers only   ____ E-mail me at:
Other:
_____

IV.   The following person(s) are not authorized to receive my Patient Health Information (PHI):
Print Name: _____   Print Name: _____
Print Name: _____   Print Name: _____

V.   The HIPAA Privacy rule requires healthcare providers to take reasonable steps to limit the use or disclosure of, and requests for PHI. I understand that this accounting will not reflect disclosures that are made in the course of the Practice's ordinary health care activities related to providing patient treatment, obtaining payment for its services or its internal operations. Also, the Practice does not have to account for disclosures for which I have executed an Authorization permitting disclosures of my PHI.

Date of disclosure request	Disclosed to whom: address/email	Description of disclosure	Purpose of disclosure	Dates of service of disclosure	Person completing request	Date completed

1. The above authorizations are voluntary and I may refuse to agree to their terms without affecting any of my rights to receive healthcare at the Practice.

2. These Authorizations may be revoked at any time by notifying the Practice in writing at the Practices mailing address marked to the attention of "HIPAA Compliance Officer."

3. The revocation of this authorization will not have any effect on disclosures occurring prior to the execution of any revocation.

4. I may see and copy the information described in this form, if I ask for it, and I will get a copy of this form after I sign it.

5. This form was completely filled in before I signed it and I acknowledge that all of my questions were answered to my satisfaction, that I fully understand this authorization form, and have received an executed copy.

6. This authorization is valid as of the date I have signed below and shall remain valid until changed or revoked.

Name of Patient (Printed) _____Signature of Patient _____Date _____

FIGURE 5-6 Example of a privacy practices acknowledgment form. (Department of Health and Human Services. *http://www.hhs.gov/ocr/ privacy/hipaa.* Accessed June 28, 2015.)

2. Determination by an expert with knowledge of statistical and scientific principles that the risk is very small that the information could be used to identify an individual.

Definitions of HIPAA Terms

Covered transactions: A transaction is covered under the regulations of the Health Insurance Portability and Accountability Act (HIPAA) if it involves the processing of healthcare claims, such as a request for payment by a healthcare provider to a health plan; an inquiry about the patient's benefit plan; a request for authorization for patient referrals; or any electronic communication about a patient's healthcare claim status. The enrollment or termination of health plan coverage is also a covered transaction.

Minimum necessary standard: The minimum necessary standard requires covered entities to take reasonable steps to limit unnecessary access to and disclosure of protected health information (PHI). The amount of personal information released should be the minimum amount necessary to accomplish the intended purpose.

State's preemption of HIPAA regulations: The HIPAA Privacy Rule provides federal privacy protections for PHI with covered entities or business associates. The federal Privacy Rule takes precedence over state laws unless the state law provides greater privacy protections; the information involves reporting of disease or injury, child abuse, birth, death, or data for public health purposes; or, if the reported information is to be used for financial audits.

TPO: HIPAA permits use and disclosure of PHI for treatment, payment, and healthcare operations (TPO). Treatment is the care provided to patients; payment includes billing and collection activities; and healthcare operations include administrative and business activities.

Medical assistants must be aware of the rights of individual patients regarding the use of and access to PHI. These include the following (for complete details you can refer to the CDC site at *www.cdc.gov/mmwr/preview/mmwrhtml/m2e411a1.htm*):

- Individuals have the right to access their own PHI. As long as the healthcare facility maintains the patient's records, individuals can request those records and receive copies of them. The only exceptions are psychotherapy notes and records that have been gathered for legal action. Psychotherapy notes are those recorded by a mental health professional that document conversations that occur during counseling sessions. The only time a provider can disclose psychotherapy notes without the express authorization of the patient is if the information can prevent serious harm to another person. Psychotherapy notes are kept in a separate record from the patient's health record. Covered entities must also release PHI if requested by patients, but only the part of the patient record that is requested, nothing more.
- Individuals can request changes or amendments to PHI and the covered entity must inform individuals if PHI changes have been made.
- Individuals have the right to be notified about the uses and disclosures of their PHI by a covered entity.

- Individuals have the right to know who the covered entity shared their PHI with and a brief description of the information disclosed.
- Individuals have the right to request restrictions on the use of PHI by covered entities.

Limited Data Sets

With the controls established by the Health Insurance Portability and Accountability Act (HIPAA) and the rules that apply to protected health information (PHI), medical researchers must follow specific protection guidelines to use patient data. A *limited data set* is a limited set of identifiable patient information that may be disclosed to an outside party without a patient's authorization. Before the patient data is released, all identifiers must be removed. These include the patient's name and address; any identifiable numbers (e.g., phone, fax, and medical record and account numbers, and also the Social Security number); e-mail addresses; and all biometric identifiers, including full face photos.

The reason for the disclosure may be only for research or public health purposes, and the person receiving the information must sign a data use agreement that must be kept on file. It is important to note that this information is still PHI under HIPAA rules; it is not just de-identified information, and it is still subject to the requirements of the Privacy Rule.

The HIPAA Security Rule (SR) covers the use and transmission of electronic protected health information (ePHI). The Security Rule requires three types of safeguards for protection of ePHI:

1. *Administrative safeguards:* Actions, policies, and procedures put into place to manage and maintain security measures to protect ePHI at both the healthcare facility and at the covered entity.
2. *Physical safeguards:* Actions, policies, and procedures taken to protect a covered entity's electronic information systems from natural and environmental hazards and unauthorized access.
3. *Technical safeguards:* The use of technology to secure PHI and limit its access. Covered entities are required to provide each individual who has access to PHI a Unique User Identification name and/or number that identifies and tracks that individual each time he or she accesses patient PHI.

Covered entities must also have in place procedures for obtaining ePHI during an emergency for healthcare employees with the authority to access the information. For example, if there is a natural disaster, healthcare workers who need individual PHI must know how to access it. The Security Rule recommends automatic log-off to prevent unauthorized access of ePHI. Another recommendation is to have encryption and decryption systems in place to protect ePHI.

Anyone can file a health information privacy complaint through the complaint portal of the Office for Civil Rights at the HHS: *https://ocrportal.hhs.gov/ocr/cp/wizard_cp.jsf*. The complaint also can be filed in writing by mail, fax, or e-mail. The complaint must include the name of the covered entity or business associate involved and describe the act or omission that violated HIPAA regulations. Under HIPAA an entity cannot retaliate against the individual filing a complaint.

Overview of the HIPAA Privacy Rule

- Gives patients control over the use of their health information
- Defines rules that covered entities must follow either to use or to disclose patients' health records
- Establishes national standards for safeguarding protected health information (PHI)
- Establishes limits to the use of PHI and minimizes the chance of its inappropriate disclosure
- Strictly investigates compliance-related issues and holds violators accountable with civil or criminal penalties for violating the privacy of an individual's PHI

Title II of HIPAA details the process of administrative simplification. Standardization of the exchange of healthcare data is one way HIPAA promotes computer-to-computer transactions. Standard 1 reduces the number of forms and methods used in insurance claim processing, including electronic transactions and standard code sets (e.g., diagnosis, procedure, and supply codes). Standard 4 provides for national identifiers for providers, employers, health plans, and patients. Medical professionals who access medical information must use log-in and password systems that prevent unauthorized individuals from accessing PHI. HIPAA standards have increased the use of electronic data interchange. All healthcare organizations that transmit any health information electronically must comply with HIPAA; fines and prison terms can be imposed on those who do not comply with the regulations (Procedure 5-2).

CRITICAL THINKING APPLICATION   5-10

What parts of the HIPAA Privacy Rule will the medical assistant have to practice? Give four examples of how the management of patient information must comply with HIPAA rules.

PROCEDURE 5-2   **Apply HIPAA Rules on Privacy and Release of Information and Report Illegal Activity in the Healthcare Setting**

Goal: To be aware of HIPAA privacy and release of information rules and apply them in the ambulatory care center.

Although not specifically required by HIPAA, a medical practice may want to use a routine Patient Consent form that specifies methods by which a patient agrees to let the practice notify the patient of routine treatment, payment, and healthcare operations (TPO) purposes. Figure 1 is an example of a routine consent form.

With a partner, role-play the following case study, which requires the application of the HIPAA privacy and release of information rules.

You recently graduated from a CAAHEP-accredited medical assisting program and just passed the certification exam to earn the CMA (AAMA) credential. You learned a great deal about HIPAA applications in your medical assisting program and are confident that you can apply these regulations in the family practice where you work. A patient comes to the office today very upset because a message about her laboratory test results was left on her home answering machine, even though she specifically requested in her disclosure consent form that messages be left only on her cell phone. Her mother then called the facility and requested information about her diagnosis. How should this situation be handled? The office manager does nothing to correct this error. Can the patient and/or the medical assistant report this infraction of the Privacy Rule to the Office for Civil Rights (OCR)? How can this be done? The patient decides to switch physicians because of her dissatisfaction with the management of her personal health information. Role-play the completion of a release of medical records form.

EQUIPMENT and SUPPLIES

- Computer with Internet access
- Copy of facility's protected health information (PHI) consent form
- Notice of Privacy Practices form
- Authorization for Release of Medical Records form

PROCEDURAL STEPS

1. Consistently review and apply HIPAA regulations that apply to the facility.
   <u>PURPOSE:</u> To ensure compliance with the law.
2. Identify the ramifications of noncompliance with HIPAA's Privacy Rule. Role-play the scenario presented. Did the facility comply with the Privacy Rule and the proper release of information?
   <u>PURPOSE:</u> To ensure full compliance in the medical facility.
3. Routinely apply Privacy Rule regulations to all operations in the medical office. Role-play how the patient's confidentiality and privacy should have been maintained.
   <u>PURPOSE:</u> To be in compliance with HIPAA regulations and to safeguard patients' health information.
4. Follow patient-directed methods of contact when TPO information must be left on an answering machine, mailed, or e-mailed. Role-play the correct way of contacting the patient about personal health information.
   <u>PURPOSE:</u> To be in compliance with HIPAA regulations and to safeguard patient health information.
5. Always follow office policy when performing any action that is covered under HIPAA rules.
   <u>PURPOSE:</u> To ensure full compliance in the medical facility.
6. Report HIPAA violations as you see fit to the appropriate supervisor in the medical facility. Role-play the methods for reporting HIPAA violations in the facility.

PROCEDURE 5-2 *—continued*

PURPOSE: To follow the chain of command in the medical facility and incorporate new regulations or changes into the office policy manual.

7. If appropriate, report HIPAA violations to the Office for Civil Rights at the Department of Health and Human Services (*https://ocrportal.hhs.gov/ocr/cp/wizard_cp.jsf*) or file a complaint in writing by mail, fax, or e-mail. Role-play how you could assist the patient in reporting a privacy violation.
PURPOSE: To ensure full compliance with laws and regulations that affect patient privacy issues.

8. The patient decides to switch providers because of her dissatisfaction with the care provided in the facility. Role-play the completion of an Authorization for Release of Medical Records form.
PURPOSE: To comply with the legal requirements for release of medical information.

9. Demonstrate sensitivity to patients' rights through empathy, use of therapeutic communication, and respect for individual diversity.
PURPOSE: To demonstrate your support of the patient's privacy issues and to act as a patient advocate/navigator in a complicated situation.

Kennedy Family Practice
414 Jacksonia St., Armandale, VA. 26004

Patient Consent for Use and Disclosure
of Protected Health Information

I hereby give my consent for Kennedy Family Practice to use and disclose protected health information (PHI) about me to carry out treatment, payment and health care operations (TPO).

I have the right to review the Notice of Privacy Practices prior to signing this consent. Kennedy Family Practice reserves the right to revise its Notice of Privacy Practices at any time. A revised Notice of Privacy Practices may be obtained by forwarding a written request to Sophia Viero, 414 Jacksonia St., Armandale, VA. 26004.

With this consent, a representative of Kennedy Family Practice may call my home or other alternative location and leave a message on voice mail or in person; may e-mail me on my approved email site; and/or may mail to my home or other alternative location any items that assists the practice in carrying out TPO such as appointment reminders, insurance items and any calls pertaining to my clinical care, including laboratory test results.

I have the right to request that Kennedy Family Practice restrict how it uses or discloses my PHI to carry out TPO. By signing this form, I am consenting to allow Kennedy Family Practice to use and disclose my PHI to carry out TPO.

I may revoke my consent in writing however previous disclosures are considered valid based on my prior consent.

_____
Signature of Patient or Legal Guardian

_____   _____
Print Patient's Name   Date

_____   _____
Patient Approved Telephone number   Patient Approved Email address

1

HITECH Act

The Health Information Technology for Economic and Clinical Health Act (HITECH) was signed into law in 2009 to promote the adoption and meaningful use of health information technology. The law encourages providers and healthcare entities to comply with HIPAA regulations by enacting stiff penalties for noncompliance. According to this law, providers who do not adopt electronic medical records in their practices will be penalized in Medicare payments.

The HITECH Act also requires that patients be notified if there is a breach that exposes their PHI. The HITECH Act allocated funds through the Medicare and Medicaid reimbursement systems as incentives for hospitals and providers who are "meaningful users" of EHR systems.

Under HITECH, mandatory penalties are imposed for "willful neglect" of the HIPAA Privacy Rule. Medical assistants who do not comply with HITECH guidelines can be fined. Civil penalties can be as high as $250,000, with repeated violations costing up to $1.5 million. In addition, HITECH requires the HHS to conduct periodic audits of covered entities and business associates.

Affordable Care Act of 2010

The Affordable Care Act (ACA), signed into law in March, 2010, was designed to provide better health security by enacting comprehensive health insurance reforms that hold insurance companies accountable, lower healthcare costs, guarantee more choice, and enhance the quality of care for all Americans. The law restricts the use of annual limits and bans lifetime limits on healthcare benefits. For example, if a patient has cancer, the insurance company cannot put a limit on the amount of coverage provided to that patient, even if it is a catastrophic amount.

Health insurers and employers are required to provide clear and consistent information about health plans, including an easy-to-understand Summary of Benefits and Coverage and a uniform Glossary of terms commonly used in health insurance coverage. Benefits from the act have taken effect over the last 5 years.

Healthcare Changes Resulting From the Affordable Care Act

2010: Stopped denial of healthcare insurance coverage based on pre-existing conditions; eliminated lifetime limits on insurance coverage; provided free preventive care, including mammograms and colonoscopies; allowed young adults to stay on their parents' plan until they turn 26 years old unless offered insurance at work; allowed states to cover more people on Medicaid.

2011: Made changes to Medicare, including free preventive services and a 50% discount on brand-name drugs; provided older adults with community care transition programs; increased access to services for disabled individuals through Medicaid.

2012: Established Accountable Care Organizations and other programs to help physicians and healthcare providers work together to deliver better care.

2013: Started open enrollment in the Health Insurance Marketplace.

2014: Implemented tax credits for middle- and low-income families that covered a significant portion of the cost of healthcare coverage; expanded the Medicaid program to cover more low-income Americans; prevented insurance companies from charging higher rates because of gender or health status.

2015: Modified provider payments so that practitioners who provide higher-value care receive higher payments.

CRITICAL THINKING APPLICATION   **5-11**

Summarize five details of the Affordable Care Act that have changed access to healthcare for all Americans.

CLOSING COMMENTS

Most patients never entertain the thought of taking legal action against their providers, and a medical assistant should not develop an attitude of skepticism. However, a medical assistant can play an important role in risk management in the healthcare setting.

- Give scrupulous attention to the needs of each patient and do not leave patients alone for long periods. This especially applies to young children and elderly patients. Do not criticize other providers or healthcare facilities. Never give out any information about the patient without the patient's written consent.
- Use discretion in phone and office conversations. One never knows who may be standing nearby. Be aware of tone of voice and attitude during spoken conversations. Communicate office policies and procedures to patients clearly before treatment whenever possible.
- Keep accurate records that show exactly what was done to the patient and when it was done. The medical assistant must never make any promises as to the outcome of treatment. Record cancelled and no-show appointments and record the facts if a patient discontinues treatment.
- Perform only the tasks for which you are trained and keep abreast of new findings and procedures in healthcare. Correctly follow all federal and state regulations.

Patient Education

Perhaps the most important detail to remember with regard to patient education and the law is patience. Many medical forms are complicated, and regulations change often. Patients usually are not as well educated as the medical assistant on matters concerning legal policies and procedures. Often patients become frustrated with the number of changes they have to deal with, and they unintentionally may project this frustration onto the medical assistant. Remain calm and answer questions, offering as much assistance to the patient as possible.

Legal and Ethical Issues

Generally, the law holds that every person is liable for the consequences of his or her own negligence when another person is injured as a result. In some situations, this liability extends to the employer. Providers may be held responsible for the mistakes of those who work in their healthcare facility, and sometimes they must pay damages for the negligent acts of their employees.

Under the doctrine of *respondeat superior,* providers are legally responsible for the acts of their employees when they are acting within the scope of their duties or employment. Providers also are responsible for the acts of assistants who are not their own employees if they commit acts of negligence in the presence of the provider while under the provider's immediate supervision. When providers practice as partners, they are liable not only for their own acts and those of their partners, but also for the negligent acts of any agent or employee of the partnership.

Medical assistants guilty of negligence are liable for their own actions, but the injured party generally sues the provider because the chances of collecting damages are better. However, even assistants with no money can be held liable for any negligent action, and liens can be placed on their property in anticipation of its sale and potential profit. This fact illustrates the continuing importance of exercising extreme care in performing all duties accurately and professionally in the healthcare facility.

Professional Behaviors

As professionals, medical assistants are responsible for their own actions and must adhere to the laws that guide healthcare practice. Medical assistants typically make the first appointment for new patients. In doing so, they initiate an unspoken contract between a new patient and the providers in the healthcare facility. Therefore, office policy must be strictly followed when establishing new patients. Most facilities want basic demographic information before accepting the patient into the practice, including insurance information and/or proof of the individual's ability to pay. As an agent of the provider, medical assistants are the first employee to interact with patients and must always present themselves as knowledgeable and caring individuals.

Medical assistants may work for a facility that occasionally uses temporary staff. The Latin term *locum tenens* means "to hold a place." *Locum tenens* physicians, nurse practitioners, and physician assistants are examples of professional staff that may be employed by a facility to temporarily fill open positions. The medical assistant is responsible for providing assistance to these individuals so that quality patient care is delivered seamlessly and professionally.

SUMMARY OF SCENARIO

Barbara is enthusiastic about her new job and duties. She is confident about appearing in court to represent Dr. Patrick and discuss the contents of the medical record of the patient suing his surgeon. Dr. Patrick is not a party to the lawsuit but has a provider-patient relationship with the patient just the same. An offer existed, as did the acceptance of that offer. The relationship was based on legal subject matter, and the provider and the patient had the legal capacity to enter into a contract. Consideration also existed, because the patient paid for services and the provider treated the patient. Both received something of value. Samantha and Lynda would like to accompany Barbara to the court proceedings to watch and learn.

Even if a patient does not pay for treatment, a contract still exists. The provider may elect to terminate the provider-patient relationship if the patient does not pay, but the trust that the patient places in the provider can be considered a thing of value.

Patients should understand their role in treatment and their responsibilities to the provider. Often this information is communicated in the patient policy brochure, or it may be discussed orally with the patient. Providers are not required to accept all patients; for instance, not all providers deliver babies. Some providers do not treat patients with workers' compensation claims. Providers have the right to see the types of patients they want to and are competent to treat, but they should never discriminate on the basis of race, gender, or any other protected status.

A provider may not always be correct in his or her diagnoses, but this does not mean that the provider has committed malpractice. However, if expert witnesses feel that the provider should have made a different diagnosis based on the case, the provider might be held liable for negligence. If an employee has information about a case that is damaging to the provider, he or she is ethically obligated to report the information, but rarely legally liable to speak up unless a law has been broken.

Medical assistants can help the provider comply with legal regulations in the office by making sure that they understand the policies and procedures required by the facility. Rules are made to ensure compliance so that both patients and employees are kept safe and risks in the office are kept to a minimum. Patient confidentiality is one of the most important rules to remember. New graduates can learn about the laws that affect medical facilities in their area by discussing them with their supervisors and by attending seminars and training. Much information is available on the Internet regarding legal issues.

Trust is a critical factor in avoiding medical professional liability lawsuits. When the patient trusts the provider, he or she is much more likely to work through issues that otherwise might lead to legal action. Keeping accurate patient records and documenting all information required helps prove that the provider adequately cared for the patient. Clearly, legible handwriting is vital in this process.

The medical assistant may find that the provider is not in compliance with certain rules and regulations. Never jump to conclusions and assume that the provider has no intention of complying. There are various reasons for noncompliance, and any issues should be brought to the attention of the office manager or the provider for clarification. It is the medical assistant's responsibility to question noncompliance and make every effort to bring the facility into compliance with the cooperation of supervisors, co-workers, and providers. As a team, medical professionals can remain in compliance and deliver excellent care to all patients.

SUMMARY OF LEARNING OBJECTIVES

1. **Define, spell, and pronounce the terms listed in the vocabulary.**
   Spelling and pronouncing medical terms correctly reinforce the medical assistant's credibility. Knowing the definitions of these terms promotes confidence in communication with patients and co-workers.

2. **Compare criminal and civil law as they apply to the practicing medical assistant; also discuss contract law.**
   Criminal law governs violations of the law punishable as offenses against the state or the federal government. A medical assistant can be prosecuted for criminal acts such as assault and battery, fraud, and abuse. Misdemeanors are minor crimes and include simple assault and battery or drunk driving without injury to others. If convicted of a misdemeanor, individuals may spend up to a year in jail. Felonies are major crimes that can result in imprisonment for one or more years or even death for more serious crimes. An individual convicted of a felony loses many rights including the ability to work in healthcare. Civil law is concerned with acts that are not criminal but involve relationships between individuals and other individuals, groups, or government agencies. Tort law is the division of civil law that deals with medical professional liability. Contract law involves contracts and a contract is an agreement that creates an obligation.

3. **Summarize the anatomy of a medical professional liability lawsuit and explain the four essential elements of a valid contract.**
   Four elements are essential to a valid legal contract: (1) Mutual understanding and agreement; (2) the contract must involve legal subject matter; (3) the parties to the contract must be legally competent; and (4) some type of consideration must be involved.
   A medical assistant may be involved in preparing materials for court including completing interrogatories and scheduling or participating in depositions. Discovery is the pretrial disclosure of pertinent facts or documents by one or both parties to a legal action or proceeding. Attorneys help prepare the defense of the provider and the staff.

4. **Discuss the various parts of a medical professional liability lawsuit.**
   Medical professional liability suits are far from rare, and they involve interrogatories, depositions, and subpoenas. Knowing the role of everyone inside the courtroom is imperative, and, in a criminal case, the burden of proof must prove guilt beyond any reasonable doubt. The final decision of the trial court is reflected in the judgment, signed by the judge.

5. **Discuss the advantages of mediation and arbitration.**
   Mediation and arbitration are two examples of Alternative Dispute Resolutions that share the goal of avoiding litigation in court. In mediation a neutral third party, the mediator, helps those involved in a dispute solve their own problems. Arbitration involves the use of a third party familiar with law or the issues at hand. The arbitrator renders a legally binding decision based on very specific rules. Many providers and attorneys see mediation and arbitration as a way to solve the crisis of litigation in this country.

6. **Do the following related to medical liability and negligence:**
   - **Differentiate malfeasance, misfeasance, and nonfeasance.**
     Malfeasance, misfeasance, and nonfeasance are types of negligence often involved in medical professional liability cases. *Malfeasance* is performing an act that is completely wrong or unlawful. *Misfeasance*, comparable to a mistake, is the improper performance of a lawful act. *Nonfeasance* is the failure to perform some act that should have been performed.
   - **Explain the four Ds of negligence.**
     The four Ds of negligence are (1) the duty to care for the patient; (2) dereliction, or failure to perform that duty; (3) proof that this failure was the direct cause of a patient's injury; and (4) proof that the patient suffered damages from the injury.
   - **Define the types of damages.**
     Nominal damages are token compensations for invasion of a legal right. Punitive damages are designed to punish an offender and discourage repetition of an act. Compensatory damages are designed to compensate for the actual damages suffered, whereas general damages include compensation for pain and suffering, loss of a body member, disfigurement, and other similar losses. Special damages can include such losses as earnings or travel costs.

7. **Discuss risk management and describe liability, malpractice, and personal injury insurances, including the importance of informed consent.**
   Risk management practices are a combination of different approaches in the healthcare facility that reduces the likelihood that either an individual healthcare professional or the healthcare facility will be sued.
   General liability insurance protects the healthcare facility if there is an accident in the facility that causes bodily injury or property damage. Medical malpractice insurance protects the provider and/or healthcare facility if there is a judgment against them for medical negligence, malfeasance, or general malpractice. Personal injury insurance covers both bodily harm and nonphysical, noneconomic harm.
   Informed consent gives the patient a full understanding of the condition that has been diagnosed, including what could happen if the patient undergoes treatment, refuses treatment, or delays treatment. It provides the patient with information on the advantages and risks of a medical procedure and alternative treatments the patient may want to consider. Informed consent places control in the hands of the patient, who is given the opportunity to make the decisions about his or her healthcare.

8. **Define statutes of limitation and confidentiality.**
   A statute of limitations is a period after which a lawsuit cannot be filed. Confidentiality is one of the most sacred trusts the patient places in the hands of the provider and staff. It is of the utmost importance to patients receiving treatment for mental health issues, sexually transmitted infections, sexual assault, and any type of abuse.

SUMMARY OF LEARNING OBJECTIVES—*continued*

9. Discuss compliance reporting, the Patient Self-Determination Act, the Uniform Anatomical Gift Act, and the Patients' Bill of Rights.

The provider is charged with safeguarding patient confidences with the constraints of the law, but according to state laws, which vary somewhat across the nation, certain disclosures must be made, like births and deaths, sexually transmitted diseases, and child abuse.

The Patient Self-Determination Act of 1990 brought the term "advance directives" to the forefront of medical care. This act requires healthcare facilities to develop and maintain written procedures that ensure that all adult patients receive information about advance directives and medical durable powers of attorney.

The Uniform Anatomical Gift Act was developed to make sure that all states have the same laws regarding organ donation.

The Patients' Bill of Rights was designed to (1) strengthen consumer confidence by ensuring that the healthcare system is fair and responsive to consumers' needs; (2) provide consumers with credible and effective mechanisms to address their concerns; (3) encourage consumers to take an active role in improving and ensuring their health; (4) affirm the importance of a strong relationship between patients and their healthcare professionals; and (5) affirm the critical role consumers play in safeguarding their health by establishing rights and responsibilities for all participants in improving patients' health.

10. Describe the important features of the ADAA and GINA Acts.

The ADAA Act broadens the definition of disability and emphasizes that the definition of disability should be interpreted broadly to include any individual with a physical or mental impairment that substantially limits one or more of his/her major life activities, the individual has a record of such an impairment, or is thought to have an impairment. GINA is a federal law that prohibits discrimination in health coverage and employment based on genetic information. Regardless of family history or personal genetic studies, individuals cannot be denied health insurance and employers cannot make job-related decisions based on individual genetic history.

11. Explain the components of the Health Insurance Portability and Accountability Act (HIPAA).

HIPAA is a federal law that sets national standards for how healthcare plans, healthcare clearinghouses, and most healthcare providers protect the privacy of a patient's health information. The law has two provisions: Title I (Insurance Reform) and Title II (Administration Simplification). HIPAA's primary purpose was to limit the administrative costs of healthcare, protect patient privacy, and prevent medical fraud and abuse in the Medicare and Medicaid systems.

12. Identify HITECH and its impact on electronic transmission of patient records.

The Health Information Technology for Economic and Clinical Health Act (HITECH) was signed into law in 2009 to promote the adoption and meaningful use of health information technology. Providers who do not adopt electronic medical records in their practices will be penalized in Medicare payments. The HITECH Act also requires that patients be notified if there is a breach that exposes their PHI. The HITECH Act allocated funds through the Medicare and Medicaid reimbursement systems as incentives for hospitals and providers who are "meaningful users" of EHR systems.

13. Summarize the primary features of the Affordable Care Act.

The Affordable Care Act, signed into law in March of 2010, was designed to provide better health security by enacting comprehensive health insurance reforms that hold insurance companies accountable, lower healthcare costs, guarantee more choice, and enhance the quality of care for all Americans. The law restricts the use of annual limits and bans lifetime limits on healthcare benefits. Health insurers and employers are required to provide clear and consistent information about health plans, including an easy-to-understand summary of benefits and coverage and a uniform glossary of terms commonly used in health insurance coverage. Benefits from the Act have taken effect over the last 5 years.

CONNECTIONS

Study Guide Connection: Go to the Chapter 5 Study Guide. Read and complete the activities.

evolve Evolve Connection: Go to the Chapter 5 link at *evolve.elsevier.com/kinn* to complete the Chapter Review Quiz. Check out the other resources listed for this chapter to make the most of what you have learned from Medicine and Law.

6

MEDICINE AND ETHICS

SCENARIO

Monica Johnson has been employed for 6 months as a medical assistant in a primary care practice. She works as the clinical medical assistant for Dr. Richard Wray. One of Dr. Wray's patients, Anna Walsh, recently adopted a baby after 8 years of trying to conceive a child. The baby, Delaney Gracelia, was born to a single mother, Susan, who participated in an open adoption in which she and the Walshes met and got to know each other during her pregnancy. Susan dated the baby's father for about 6 months before discovering that she was pregnant, and they are no longer dating. Susan wanted to make a good decision for the baby and decided to place her for adoption. Dr. Wray performed some genetic testing on Delaney, and the adoptive parents were involved throughout the pregnancy, even meeting Delaney's birth mother for physician appointments from time to time. Monica observed both Susan and the Walshes and saw many benefits from the arrangement, noticing that everyone was primarily concerned with Delaney and her happiness and well-being. However, some periods were difficult for both sides. This prompted Monica to give some thought to her own feelings and ideas about many different ethical situations and issues and how she would react in the face of having to make ethical decisions.

While studying this chapter, think about the following questions:

- How can personal values affect an ethical relationship with diverse patients?
- How can the medical assistant separate her personal beliefs from her professional behaviors?
- Should the medical assistant discuss personal beliefs about ethical situations with patients?

LEARNING OBJECTIVES

1. Define, spell, and pronounce the terms listed in the vocabulary.
2. Do the following related to medicine and ethics:
   - Define ethics and morals.
   - Identify the effect of personal morals and values on professional performance.
   - Differentiate between personal and professional ethics.
   - Recognize the effect personal ethics and morals have on the delivery of healthcare.
   - Develop a plan for separation of personal and professional ethics.
   - Demonstrate appropriate responses to ethical issues.
3. Discuss the history of ethics in medicine.
4. Do the following related to making ethical decisions:
   - List and define three general elements of ethics.
   - List and define the four types of ethical problems.
   - Discuss the five-step process used to make an ethical decision.
5. Summarize the ethical opinions reached by the Council on Ethical and Judicial Affairs (CEJA).
6. Describe the process of compliance reporting of conflicts of interest.

VOCABULARY

advocate (ad'-vuh-kat) A person who pleads the cause of another; one who defends or maintains a cause or proposal.

procurement (pro-kuhr'-ment) The act of getting possession of, obtaining, or acquiring; in medicine, this term relates to obtaining organs for transplant.

public domain A classification of information that indicates the information is open for public review; information or technology that is not protected by a patent or copyright and is available to the public for use without charge.

ramifications (ra-muh-fuh-ka'-shuns) Consequences produced by a cause or following from a set of conditions.

reparations (reh-puh-ra'-shuns) Acts of atonement for a wrong or injury.

sociologic Oriented or directed toward social needs and problems.

upcoding A fraudulent practice in which provider services are billed for higher procedural codes than were actually performed, resulting in a higher payment.

veracity (vuh-ra'-suh-te) A devotion to or conformity with the truth.

Ethics can be defined as the thoughts, judgments, and actions on issues that have implications of moral right and wrong. Ethics guides society's moral principles, which govern a person's or group's behavior. Various beliefs exist about what is and is not ethical in everyday life and in the medical profession. The decisions that people make based on ethical beliefs can quite possibly alter the course of human existence.

Ethics are different from legal issues mainly because something that is legal is not necessarily ethical. Ethics is considered a higher authority than legality. The American Medical Association's Council on Ethical and Judicial Affairs (CEJA) clarifies the relationship between law and ethics as follows: "Ethical values and legal principles are usually closely related, but ethical obligations typically exceed legal duties." In some cases, the law mandates unethical conduct. In general, when healthcare professionals believe a law is unjust, they should work to change the law. In exceptional circumstances of unjust laws, ethical responsibilities should supersede legal obligations. Ethics and morals are more closely related, although ethics often are attributed to professional interactions, whereas morals and values are usually personal in nature. An individual's morals are defined as his or her standards for behavior or beliefs about what is right and what is wrong. Individual morals are closely tied with value systems and help us judge others and conflict situations as being either acceptable or unacceptable. Medical assistants not only must have a strong knowledge base about ethical issues they might face throughout their careers, they also must come to terms with some of the deeply rooted morals and value systems that have been a part of their lives since youth.

To be able to treat all people ethically, you first must examine your own values, beliefs, and actions; you cannot treat all patients with care and respect until you first recognize and evaluate your personal biases. We think and act a certain way for many reasons. The first step in understanding the process is to evaluate your individual value system. Why do you have certain attitudes or beliefs about the worth of individuals or things?

Many different factors influence the development of a value system. Value systems begin as learned beliefs and behaviors. Families and cultural influences shape the way we respond to a diverse society. Other factors that influence reactions include socioeconomic and educational backgrounds. To develop ethical behaviors and therapeutic relationships, you first must recognize your own value system to determine whether it could affect how you interact or treat others. Preconceived ideas about people because of their race, religion, income level, ethnic origin, sexual orientation, or gender can act as barriers to the development of ethical behaviors. You will not be able to provide nonjudgmental, ethical treatment to your patients unless you can connect with them in some way. Personal biases or prejudices are monumental barriers to the development of ethical behaviors.

CRITICAL THINKING APPLICATION   **6-2**

Honestly evaluate your personal biases. What do you find unacceptable in people? Do you prejudge an individual based on his or her affiliation with a particular group or because of a certain lifestyle decision? Do these biases create barriers to ethical care? If so, how can you get beyond these barriers?

Personal, professional, and organizational ethics all contribute to the way the medical assistant approaches the patient. For instance, if a medical assistant personally believes that each child should receive immunizations, he or she must understand that, professionally, this decision must be left to the child's caregivers. The medical assistant must not force his or her personal ethical beliefs on the patient or family members. Personal and professional ethics must be kept separate so that patients can make their own decisions about their healthcare (Procedure 6-1). Professional organizations offer ethical guidelines; for example, each medical assistant is required to maintain patient confidentiality. This practice reflects the ethical belief that all patients have the right to confidentiality of their information and records (Procedure 6-2).

CRITICAL THINKING APPLICATION   **6-1**

What do you value most in life? What is important to you? What influences you to act in a certain way? Make a list of five things you value the most and share them with the class. Try to determine why you feel so strongly about those particular things.

PROCEDURE 6-1	**Develop a Plan for Separating Personal and Professional Ethics: Recognize the Impact Personal Ethics and Morals Have on the Delivery of Healthcare**

Goal: *To determine one's ethical and moral views before having to confront an ethical decision.*

Using the following case studies, role-play with your partner issues of personal and professional ethical behavior and how personal ethics and morals can affect the delivery of healthcare.

(1) While you are gathering information from a new patient, he informs you he is HIV positive. Do you think this will affect your therapeutic relationship?

(2) You are responsible for performing an in-depth diabetic education intervention with an individual with very poor hygiene. Will this cause a problem with your professional manner?

(3) You are told by your office manager that an inmate of the county prison is scheduled for an appointment this afternoon. Do you think his status will affect your reaction to this patient?

(4) You are attempting to gather insurance information from a 20-year-old patient who brought her two young children with her to the office today. She is a single mother who is pregnant with her third child and receives public assistance. What do you think? Will you have difficulty being empathetic?

PROCEDURE 6-1   —continued

EQUIPMENT and SUPPLIES

- Pen and paper
- Copy of the AAMA's Medical Assisting Code of Ethics

PROCEDURAL STEPS

1. Set aside time to study and consider the ethical issues outlined in this chapter.
   PURPOSE: To make any ethical decision, research the subject and give thought to each issue so that the decision is credible.
2. For each issue, make notes on your personal thoughts, paying particular attention to whether you agree with the AAMA's Medical Assisting Code of Ethics.
   PURPOSE: To examine the impact that personal ethics and morals may have on your practice.
3. Look at each issue as a separate ethical problem and apply the ethical decision-making process to each.
   PURPOSE: To consider each issue in an organized way.
4. Gather relevant information by researching each problem.
   PURPOSE: To make sure that you consider all facts in determining your personal views about each issue.
5. Identify the type of ethical problem each issue represents.
   PURPOSE: By accumulating information about the issue and matching it with an ethical problem, you will be able to apply knowledge and determine your personal views more easily.
6. Determine your personal view on each issue.
   PURPOSE: To recognize how personal ethics and morals can affect the delivery of quality patient care.
7. Determine the ethical approach to use.
   PURPOSE: Knowing the type of problem that each ethical issue represents helps you determine the best approach to each decision.

8. Explore practical alternatives.
   PURPOSE: Considering all practical alternatives helps you make the best ethical decisions.
9. Decide your personal stand on each issue.
   PURPOSE: By gathering information, identifying the problem and the best ethical approach to use, and then considering all practical alternatives, you can arrive at a sound ethical decision about your personal stand on each issue.
10. Determine the position of the Medical Assisting Code of Ethics on each issue.
    PURPOSE: By determining your personal stance and learning the professional position on each ethical issue, you will not be faced with having to make a decision on the spot.
11. Continue the process until each ethical issue has been addressed.
12. Refrain from inflicting personal ethical views on any patient.
    PURPOSE: To ensure that patients determine their own ethical views and make medical decisions based on their own views rather than those of the medical staff.
13. Interact with patients in a professional way, regardless of their or your ethical views.
    PURPOSE: All patients must be treated in a professional way, regardless of their ethical views or healthcare choices.
14. Re-evaluate personal ethical views periodically and apply new knowledge and experience to determine whether ethical views have changed.
    PURPOSE: To be open to change based on experience in the medical field and new discoveries or technology. Healthcare is an ever-changing profession; therefore, you must develop the attitude of being a lifelong learner. New trends or experiences may change your position on ethical issues.

PROCEDURE 6-2   Respond to Issues of Confidentiality

Goal: *To ensure that medical assistants treat all information on patient care as completely confidential.*

EQUIPMENT and SUPPLIES

- Patient's health record
- Copy of the Medical Assisting Code of Ethics
- Copy of the Medical Assisting Creed
- Copy of the Oath of Hippocrates (see the chapter, The Medical Assistant and the Healthcare Team)
- Copy of HIPAA guidelines (see the chapter, Medicine and Law)
- Notepad and pen
  Using the following case studies, role-play issues of patient confidentiality with your partner.

  (1) You work for a local OB/GYN. Your best friend tells you her brother's wife is having an affair, and your friend wants you to find out if she is pregnant. You saw the woman in the office today and know that her pregnancy test was positive. How would you manage this situation?

  (2) An attorney calls the office today and requests you send copies of a patient's health records to her office ASAP for a liability case. The patient has not signed a release form, but the attorney tells you she doesn't need one because this is a legal matter. What would you do?

  (3) The mother of an 18-year-old patient calls and asks you to release her son's laboratory test results. The son lives with her and is covered by her medical insurance. Does the mother have the right to this information?

PROCEDURE 6-2 —continued

PROCEDURAL STEPS

1. Read through each document, paying particular attention to the references to confidentiality.
PURPOSE: To gain insight into documents that stress confidentiality as a critical aspect of the healthcare process, to reinforce the importance of patient confidentiality, and to understand the roots of ethical behavior.
2. Select a student with whom to role-play as a patient. The patient should present with a situation or an illness he or she wants to keep confidential.
PURPOSE: Apply ethical behaviors, including honesty and integrity, in medical assisting practice.
3. Identify each patient by name and date of birth.
4. Take the patient to a private exam room or other area suitable for a private conversation and attend to his or her needs and questions.
PURPOSE: To restrict the conversation to medical personnel and the patient.
5. Listen carefully to what the patient says, taking notes if necessary, asking clarifying questions, and using restatement to clear up any misunderstandings.
PURPOSE: To demonstrate to patients an interest in what they say and to make sure all their concerns are addressed and answered.

6. Assure the patient that his or her concerns and health issues are confidential.
PURPOSE: To put the patient at ease, so that he or she feels comfortable in sharing each detail of the condition or of the concerns that need to be discussed.
7. Explain to the patient that information shared with you cannot be kept from the provider.
PURPOSE: To make sure you will not be asked to withhold information from the provider.
8. Discuss the information with the practitioner or ask the provider to speak personally with the patient, depending on which is appropriate to the circumstances.
PURPOSE: To act only with authorization from the provider.
9. Instruct the patient according to the provider's orders, if necessary.
10. Document the patient's concerns, information given by the patient, and the provider's orders in the health record.
PURPOSE: To provide a record of the conversation and the circumstances of the patient's concerns and the provider's plan for resolution.
11. Do not share information about the patient with anyone not directly related to the patient's care.
PURPOSE: To ensure complete patient confidentiality.

HISTORY OF ETHICS IN MEDICINE

From earliest recorded history, humans have pondered ethics, or the judgment of right and wrong. Ethics should not be confused with etiquette. Etiquette refers to courtesy, customs, and manners, whereas ethics explores the moral right or wrong of an issue. It is not surprising that for centuries, the field of medicine has set for itself a rigid standard of ethical conduct toward patients and professional colleagues.

The earliest written code of ethical conduct for medical practice was devised in approximately 2250 BC by the Babylonians. It was called the *Code of Hammurabi*. It elaborated on the conduct expected of a physician and even set the fees a physician could charge. The code was quite lengthy and detailed, which is probably the reason it did not survive the ages. In approximately 400 BC, Hippocrates developed a brief statement of principles that remains an inspiration to the physicians of today. The most significant contribution to medical ethics after Hippocrates was made by Thomas Percival, an English physician, philosopher, and writer. In 1803 he published his Code of Medical Ethics. Percival was very concerned about **sociologic** matters and took great interest in the study of ethical concepts as they related to the medical profession.

In 1846, as the American Medical Association (AMA) was being organized in New York City, medical education and medical ethics already were considered important aspects of the profession. At the first annual AMA meeting in 1847, a Code of Ethics was formulated and adopted. It specifically acknowledged Percival's code as its foundation, and this document became a part of the fundamental standards of the AMA and its components. Even

today, sections of the AMA Code of Ethics stem from Percival's writings.

The medical assisting profession has followed suit. The American Association of Medical Assistants (AAMA) has published the Medical Assisting Code of Ethics, which identifies ethical and moral principles as they relate to the practice of medical assisting (Figure 6-1).

Medical Assisting Code of Ethics

Members of AAMA dedicated to the conscientious pursuit of their profession, and thus desiring to merit the high regard of the entire medical profession and the respect of the general public which they serve, do pledge themselves to strive always to:

1. Render service with full respect for the dignity of humanity.

2. Respect confidential information obtained through employment unless legally authorized or required by responsible performance of duty to divulge such information.

3. Uphold the honor and high principles of the profession and accept its disciplines.

4. Seek to continually improve the knowledge and skills of medical assistants for the benefit of patients and professional colleagues.

5. Participate in additional service activities aimed toward improving the health and well-being of the community.

FIGURE 6-1 Medical Assisting Code of Ethics of the AAMA. (http://www.aama-ntl.org/about/overview#.VY2at_m6e7Q. Accessed 6/26/2015.)

Medical assistants are agents of the physicians who employ them and therefore should follow a code of ethics similar to that established by the AMA. Medical assistants facing ethical issues, such as managing confidential patient information, can use the AAMA code of ethics as a guide to help them make ethical decisions.

The AAMA has also written a Medical Assisting Creed, which can be used as a guideline for medical assistants facing complex ethical and moral issues in the course of their work. The Medical Assisting Creed supports the code of ethics by asking members to abide by ethical statements of belief. These include:

- I believe in the principles and purposes of the profession of medical assisting.
- I endeavor to be more effective.
- I aspire to render greater service.
- I protect the confidence entrusted to me.
- I am dedicated to the care and well-being of all people.
- I am loyal to my employer.
- I am true to the ethics of my profession.
- I am strengthened by compassion, courage, and faith.

To promote professionalism and ethical behaviors in those seeking the AAMA certification, individuals who are applying to or who have earned the CMA (AAMA) credential are expected to follow a Code of Conduct for CMAs (AAMA), which can be found on the AAMA website: *www.aama-ntl.org*. The following are provisions of the code:

- Act with integrity and adhere to the highest standards for personal and professional conduct.
- Accept responsibility for your actions.
- Continually seek to enhance your professional capabilities.
- Practice with fairness and honesty.
- Abide by all federal, state, and local laws and regulations.
- Encourage other medical assistants to act in a professional manner consistent with the certification standards and responsibilities of your profession.

CRITICAL THINKING APPLICATION   6-3

As you can see, a number of documents support ethical decision making and behaviors in those pursuing a career in medical assisting. How can you apply these statutes to your practice? Consider the following scenarios and discuss with the class how they can be ethically managed.

1. You discover a co-worker taking a controlled substance from the locked medicine cabinet. She begs you not to report her and promises never to do it again. She tells you she is having horrible back pain and has to continue to work to support her two young children.
2. You are working in the practice's billing department and realize that one of the providers is routinely **upcoding** office visits and patient procedures. There is no documentation in patient health records to support these coding charges.

MAKING ETHICAL DECISIONS

An understanding of a few of the elements of ethics, the different types of ethical problems, and how an ethical decision is made can help when entry-level medical assistants are faced with complicated issues in the workplace. This section enables the medical assistant to recognize the types of ethical problems that might arise in the ambulatory care center and provides a pattern to follow in making an ethical decision.

Elements of Ethics

Dr. Ruth Purtilo is an authority on ethics in medicine and has written a book on the subject, *Ethical Dimensions in the Health Professions*. She presents three general elements of ethics: duties, rights, and character traits. A *duty* is an obligation a person has or perceives himself or herself to have. For example, a daughter may feel the obligation to care for her elderly parents, or a husband who has hurt his spouse may feel an obligation to somehow make up for his act.

Purtilo mentions several types of duties related to the medical profession. *Nonmaleficence* is a principle of bioethics that states that healthcare professionals have an obligation not to inflict harm intentionally. *Beneficence* is a moral obligation to act for the benefit of others. In the case of healthcare professionals, the principle of beneficence asserts that those who pursue a profession in healthcare have an obligation to help others and that it furthers their interests to do so. *Fidelity* is the duty to follow through with obligations and keep promises, and **veracity** is the duty to tell the truth. In the practice of medical ethics, *justice* is the fair distribution of benefits to those who have legitimate claims on them. When a person has wronged another, he or she has a duty to make **reparations**, or right the wrong. Last, a person should feel grateful if he or she is a beneficiary of someone else's goodness; this also is a type of duty.

Rights are defined as claims made on society, a group, or an individual. The Bill of Rights appended to the U.S. Constitution guarantees certain liberties that we enjoy as American citizens. For instance, Americans have the "right" to vote, regardless of whether they choose to exercise that right. A *right* applies to all people within a group, without prejudice.

Purtilo defines *character traits* as a tendency to act a certain way. A person who values honesty as an important character trait usually can be trusted to speak the truth. One who feels comfortable with taking small items from work for use at home may not be able to resist an opportunity to take something more valuable. Character traits certainly do not always indicate how a person will react in all situations. No human being is perfect, and we sometimes are unpredictable. Stress also can interfere with our normal reactions, and other factors, such as depression or anger, influence how we act. The phrase that someone is acting "out of character" usually means that the person is deviating from his or her normal behavior patterns.

With an understanding of these basic elements of ethics, we have a good foundation to help us look more objectively at ethical problems and solve them to the best of our ability.

Types of Ethical Problems

Purtilo presents four basic types of ethical problems:

- Ethical distress
- Ethical dilemmas
- Dilemmas of justice
- Locus of authority issues

Ethical distress is a problem in which a certain course of action is indicated, but some type of problem or barrier prevents that action. A professional in ethical distress knows the right thing to do but for some reason cannot do it.

An *ethical dilemma* is a situation in which an individual must make a decision about two or more acceptable choices; however, choosing one course of action means that the person cannot follow the other course of action. A choice must be made, and something of value may be lost if a second choice is eliminated. This could be viewed as the saying, "being caught between a rock and a hard place," when the effect of a choice made may be greater than is immediately obvious.

The third type of ethical problem is the *dilemma of justice*. This problem focuses on the fair distribution of benefits to those who are entitled to them. Choices must be made about who receives these benefits and in what proportion. Examples include organ donation and distribution of scarce or costly medications.

In *locus of authority issues,* two or more authority figures have their own ideas about how a situation should be handled, but only one of those authorities can prevail. If one physician feels that a patient should have surgery and another does not, how does the patient decide?

Recognizing the type of ethical problem is not always easy. Sometimes an issue is a mixture of one or more types of ethical problems. When possible, it is wise to take time to weigh the courses of action before making an important decision. Unfortunately, with the fast pace of the medical profession, this is not always possible. Some decisions must be made in a split second; therefore, having a thorough grasp of ethical decision making before the need arises is important.

The Ethical Decision-Making Process

Purtilo proposes a five-step process for ethical decision making:
1. Gathering relevant information
2. Identifying the type of ethical problem
3. Determining the ethical approach to use
4. Exploring the practical alternatives
5. Completing the action

To gather information, a medical professional should ask questions, review records, talk to the patient and other professionals, and search for other data so that the entire situation is available for review. Once the information has been gathered, the medical professional must decide which ethical problem or problems are presented. In determining the ethical approach to use, we must consider the duties, rights, and character traits of all the individuals involved, paying close attention to the **ramifications** of all possible decisions. All of the alternatives must be considered and evaluated, after which an action should be taken.

Although taking time to give these areas some thought is best, it may not be possible. Therefore, those entering the medical profession should take stock of their core beliefs. Scan the newspapers and search professional journals for ethical situations, think about the facts, then decide how you would react to each one. This is excellent preparation for the day you are faced with making a quick ethical decision.

CRITICAL THINKING APPLICATION   **6-4**
- What are the ramifications of an open adoption, such as occurred with Delaney? What problems might occur during the first year of her life?
- How might these problems be prevented?
- What are the positive aspects of the adoption?

THE COUNCIL ON ETHICAL AND JUDICIAL AFFAIRS

The Council on Ethical and Judicial Affairs (CEJA) develops ethics policy for the AMA by analyzing and addressing ethical issues that confront physicians and the medical profession. The recommendations from the council ultimately are used to update the AMA's Code of Medical Ethics, which can be found at *http://www. ama-assn.org/ama/pub/physician-resources/medical-ethics/code-medical-ethics.page.* The part of the code that is perhaps most pertinent to medical assistants is the section that deals with allied health professions. An excerpt follows:

> When physicians practice medicine with allied health professionals, they should be guided by the following principles:
> 1. It is ethical for a physician to employ allied health professionals, as long as they are trained to perform the assigned activities.
> 2. Physicians have an ethical obligation to the patients for whom they are responsible to ensure that medical and surgical conditions are evaluated and treated appropriately.
> 3. The physician should not substitute the services of an allied health professional for those of a physician when the allied health professional is not adequately trained.

What do these principles mean to the medical assistant working in a healthcare facility? As the physician's agent, the medical assistant must be trained to perform assigned tasks. The entry-level medical assistant who has earned a nationally recognized credential, such as the CMA (AAMA) or the RMA, has proven that she or he has met national standards of medical assisting excellence, and healthcare facilities can be assured that these individuals have entry-level competency in all identified areas.

The AMA's Code of Ethics consists of nine separate categories of ethical concerns. The medical assistant can refer to these categories for guidance if he or she faces an ethical dilemma in the workplace. This chapter provides a short summary of AMA ethical policies with applications to the field of medical assisting.

Opinions on Social Policy Issues
Preventing, Identifying, and Treating Violence and Abuse
All patients may be at risk of interpersonal violence and abuse, regardless of socioeconomic issues. Therefore, providers should routinely inquire about physical, sexual, and psychological abuse as part of the medical history. These questions are often part of the initial intake form that is completed either by the patient or the medical assistant during the patient interview process. If the medical assistant suspects that a patient may be a victim of abuse, he or she should report this concern to the provider immediately. In addition, the clinic should keep a current list of community and health care resources available to abused or vulnerable individuals and share this information with suspected victims. The clinic also should follow up with whatever the state requirements are for reporting violence or abuse.

Healthcare professionals should do the following to address acts of violence and abuse:
- Providers must treat the immediate symptoms and results of violence and abuse and provide continued care to affected patients.

- Providers should be aware of cultural differences in response to abuse and public health measures that are effective in preventing violence and abuse.
- The practice should have policies and procedures in place for dealing with a suspected or confirmed abuse case.

HIV Testing

Providers must protect individual patient's rights while at the same time safeguarding the public's welfare. The AMA recommends the following ethical and legal guidelines on HIV testing. For a complete summary of AMA guidelines refer to *www.ama-assn.org/ama/pub/ physician-resources/medical-ethics/code-medical-ethics/opinion 223.page.*

1. Physicians should promote routine HIV screening for all adult patients.
2. Written consent for HIV testing is not required in most states. However, when considering the ethics of testing, providers should ask patients for consent before testing is done. This conversation should be documented in the patient's record, even if the patient refuses testing.
3. If a healthcare worker has an accidental exposure, such as a needlestick, HIV testing can be done on the patient without informed consent.
4. Providers must help HIV-positive patients access suitable follow-up care and counseling.
5. Providers must comply with state and federal reporting guidelines for infectious diseases while at the same time ensuring patient confidentiality.
6. Providers must attempt to prevent HIV-positive individuals from infecting third parties. If an HIV-positive individual is not compliant with infection control guidelines, the provider should:
   a. Notify local public health officials
   b. Counsel the HIV-positive patient about the risks of exposing others to the disease
   c. If permitted by state law, contact any third party who is in danger of infection while still maintaining patient confidentiality

---

CRITICAL THINKING APPLICATION   **6-5**

You have just had an accidental needlestick exposure. Does the source patient have to give legal consent to have a test done for the human immunodeficiency virus (HIV)? How should HIV information be managed in a busy healthcare practice?

Withholding or Withdrawing Life-Prolonging Treatment

A physician is committed to saving life and relieving suffering. Sometimes these two goals are incompatible, and a choice between them must be made. If possible, the patient should decide what treatment is given. Often the patient makes his or her wishes known to a responsible relative or other representative in case the patient becomes incapacitated. Some patients want a "do not resuscitate" (DNR) or "no code" order added to their health records. Usually such an order is established so that no heroic measures are taken in

a situation in which a patient would be unable or incompetent to make a decision. The decision to withdraw life support should be made before any mention of organ donation is made by the medical professionals tending the patient. In the best situation, the patient has formally completed an advance directive.

Organ Donation

Organ donation is not only considered ethical by the AMA, it is encouraged. However, it is considered unethical to participate in proceedings in which the donor receives payment, except reimbursement of expenses directly incurred in the removal of the donated organ. The rights of the patient and the donor must be protected equally. If the donor is deceased, the death must be certified by a physician other than the recipient's physician.

Because the need for donated organs is so extreme, protocols have been established by healthcare facilities to determine when it is proper to harvest organs. Organ **procurement** may be performed immediately after a person has died, or it may be done after a patient has been kept alive artificially for a time. Hospitals also have specific guidelines for the donation of organs from living donors, such as a kidney donation. When donations are made from one living person to another, both patients must have an **advocate** team that includes a physician so that the interests and well-being of each patient are addressed. Blood donations probably are the most common form of organ donation.

CRITICAL THINKING APPLICATION   **6-6**

- Monica has often thought about being an organ donor. Her parents are very opposed to the idea because of their religious beliefs. How can Monica deal with this conflict within her family?
- If Monica dies before her parents do, how can she ensure that her wishes are carried out?

Allocation of Health Resources

Sometimes society must decide who receives care when serving all who need care is not possible. Decisions must be made fairly and should be weighed carefully. The criteria to consider when allocating health resources include urgency of need, likelihood of benefit, duration of benefit, amount of resources required for successful treatment, and potential for change in the quality of life. Nonmedical criteria should not be considered; these include the ability to pay, the social worth of the individual, age, obstacles to treatment, and the patient's contribution to the illness. The provider must remain the patient's advocate and should not be involved in making allocation decisions for that patient. For example, individual providers do not decide who receives an organ donation. There are established national protocols for matching needy patients with available organs that help determine the potential success of the transplant rather than someone deciding which patient is more worthy.

Opinions on Confidentiality, Advertising, and Communications

Confidentiality is one of the cardinal rules of the medical profession. It is completely unethical to divulge any information about a patient to any other person not directly related to the patient's care. The places where confidentiality often is breached are elevators, hallways, waiting or reception areas, break rooms, and lunch rooms. A relative may be standing behind the medical assistant, listening to conversations that are inappropriate for those not personally involved in the patient's care to hear. Breach of patient confidentiality is grounds for immediate termination from a healthcare facility.

Confidentiality restrictions apply to information documented in a patient's record and also to anything the medical assistant is told by the patient or the patient's family. Never investigate a patient's record strictly for curiosity. All information in the record must be kept in confidence. Never share information about patients with anyone outside the medical facility or office, including your own immediate family (Figure 6-2).

Individuals accompanying the patient to the healthcare facility should be in the examination room only if the patient gives approval. In addition, students should not be permitted to observe in patient examination rooms unless the patient gives permission. Never discuss one patient's case with another patient. If curious patients ask questions about others, simply explain that medical assistants are obligated to keep all patient information confidential. Patients who ask questions of a medical nature about their own case should be referred to the provider for information and instructions unless the medical assistant is authorized to provide this information. When minors request confidential services and the law does not require otherwise, providers should allow competent minors to consent to medical care and should not notify the parents without the minor's consent.

Remember that the Health Insurance Portability and Accountability Act (HIPAA) has established strict regulations for patient confidentiality and disclosure of private health information. Make sure the healthcare facility is abiding by its own privacy policy and that all patients have been given a chance to review that policy. A document stating that the patient has read and understands the privacy policy or that he or she has refused to sign should be part of the patient's record.

Patients may not always understand the ethical standards to which providers and medical assistants adhere. They may ask questions about their own health or the health of a fellow patient.

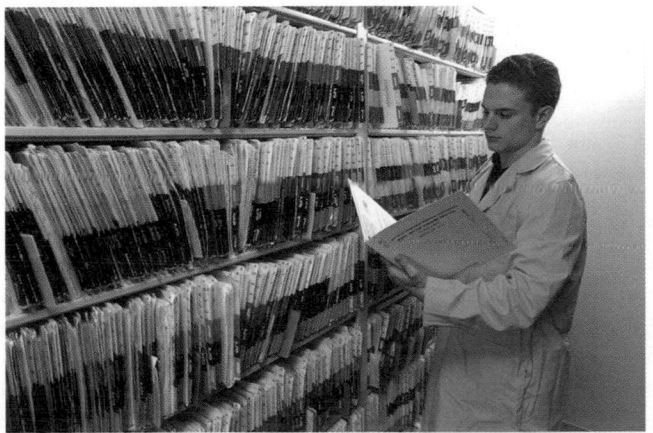

FIGURE 6-2 Confidentiality applies to all information about the patient, including what is documented and what is said between the patient and the medical assistant.

Medical assistants must educate patients about the issues of confidentiality in such a way that they are not offended; they should explain that all patients deserve to have their medical and personal information kept private. Now more than ever, the medical assistant's obligation to keep information private is not only an ethical but also a legal responsibility. All patients should understand that they are entitled to confidential treatment of their records and that the facility is dedicated to that principle.

CRITICAL THINKING APPLICATION   **6-7**

Patient confidentiality must be safeguarded at all times in the healthcare setting. You are working in an infectious disease facility, and your sister calls you very upset; she just heard a rumor that her daughter's boyfriend is HIV positive. She thought you might be able to find out for her. How should you manage this situation? Is there anything that the provider can do to safeguard others who may be infected by an HIV-positive person?

Advertising and Publicity

Advertising. There are no restrictions on advertising by physicians; the key issue is whether advertising or publicity is true and not misleading. The advertisement should be free of medical terminology so that the public can readily understand the message. Testimonials of patients should not be used in advertising because they are difficult to verify or measure by objective standards. Statements regarding the quality of medical services are highly subjective and difficult to verify. All advertised claims must be supported by actual data and facts.

Communication with the Media. Although information about some patients, such as celebrities and politicians, may be considered news, the provider cannot discuss any patient's condition with the press without authorization from the patient or the patient's legal representative. The provider may release only authorized information or that which is public knowledge. Certain kinds of news are part of public records; such news in the **public domain** includes births, deaths, accident reports, and police cases.

A medical assistant must be aware that only the provider is authorized to release information, and under no circumstances should the medical assistant violate the confidential nature of the provider-patient relationship. It is unethical to even verify that a patient is under the provider's care without the patient's permission. A policy must be in place for every medical office on how media inquiries should be handled and to whom they should be referred. Communication with the media falls under the HIPAA guidelines. Do not release a patient's health information without written permission.

Opinions on Practice Matters
Fees and Charges

Charging or collecting an illegal or excessive fee is unethical. The medical assistant is responsible for keeping informed about current billing regulations and for seeing that these regulations are followed conscientiously. However, requesting payment at the time of treatment is appropriate and very common in today's medical offices.

Often, managed care patients are asked to remit their co-payment before seeing the provider on the day of the visit. If the patient is notified in advance, adding interest or other reasonable charges to delinquent accounts also is considered ethical. In addition, a reasonable fee may be charged for duplicating patients' records. Most facilities use a patient information booklet which provides a written reference for all policies.

Providers should never base decisions about whether to order a diagnostic test or a procedure on the patient's insurance coverage. If an expensive diagnostic test is needed, such as a magnetic resonance imaging (MRI) scan, the provider cannot withhold it because of financial reasons. However, if the physician is aware of a way the patient could obtain financial assistance with the test, he or she should relay that information to the patient.

Fee Splitting and Contingent Fees

According to the AMA's Code of Ethics, "Payment by or to a physician solely for the referral of a patient is fee splitting and is unethical." This practice is unethical whether it involves another physician, a clinic, a laboratory, or a drug company.

Although attorneys often accept a case on a contingency fee basis, it is unethical for a provider to engage in this practice. The fee in this case is contingent on a successful outcome, but a provider should never set his or her fee on the successful outcome of medical treatment. A provider's fee must always be based on the value of service provided to the patient.

Waiver of Insurance Co-Payments

Providers may opt to write off or waive co-payments to help a patient who cannot afford care. If access to care is directly threatened because the patient cannot make the co-payment, the provider may forgive the payment. However, routine waiver of co-payments may violate the policies of some insurance companies. Providers need to make sure that their policies about co-payments follow applicable laws and are within the legal boundaries of their contracts with insurers. To avoid conflicts, providers may discount the entire service and all related fees to avoid potential legal conflicts with co-payment collection.

Professional Courtesy

Providers may opt not to charge or may offer a reduced rate for care given to other physicians, staff, or family members. This practice is called *professional courtesy.* This is a long-standing tradition but certainly not an ethical requirement. Providers make the decision as to who receives professional courtesy in their offices, and this should be written into the office policy manual. In some cases, extending professional courtesy is contrary to insurance and/or managed care contracts. In addition, some providers have stopped offering professional courtesy because of the rising costs of healthcare and shrinking reimbursements.

Conflicts of Interest

Questions about healthcare professionals and conflicts of interest can occur when providers or their employees accept gifts, including meals and drug samples, from pharmaceutical representatives; when the provider acts as a spokesperson on behalf of medical device companies; or when the professional has a financial interest in a

medical product company whose products they prescribe, use, or recommend. The AMA recommends that physicians not meet with pharmaceutical and medical device sales representatives except by documented appointment and at the physician's express invitation. It also recommends that physicians not accept drug samples except in specified situations for patients who lack financial access to medications.

If you work in a medical office, you soon learn that gifts from pharmaceutical and medical device representatives are commonplace. These gifts range from free drug samples to lunch for all employees, in addition to pens, notebooks, and other giveaways. A recent national survey revealed that more than 90% of physicians had received free drug samples and more than 60% had received meals, tickets to entertainment events, or free travel. What does that mean for the medical assistants working in the facility? It is always nice to get a free lunch, and it certainly helps patients to have access to free drug samples when approved by the physician. However, all employees must make sure that decisions on patient care are based on ethical matters, rather than as a result of gifts.

CRITICAL THINKING APPLICATION   6-8

A pharmaceutical representative who frequently requests appointments with the providers in your office to discuss new products brings lunch for the staff every Wednesday. Is this a conflict of interest? Is it more likely that the staff will treat this individual differently and make sure the provider blocks off time to meet with the sales rep?

Compliance With Conflicts of Interest Standards

The American College of Physicians recommends the following for all physicians:

Do not accept items of material value from pharmaceutical, medical device, and biotechnology companies unless it is part of a payment for a legitimate service.

Do not make educational presentations or publish scientific articles that are controlled by the industry.

Do not act as a consultant unless you are being paid for your expertise.

Do not meet with pharmaceutical and medical device sales representatives unless you have invited them and the appointment is documented.

Do not accept drug samples except in specified situations for patients who lack financial access to medications.

http://www.ncbi.nlm.nih.gov/books/NBK22944/. Accessed February 5, 2016.

Unethical Conduct by Members of the Health Professions

In rare instances, a medical assistant is faced with a situation in which the physician-employer's conduct appears to violate established ethical standards. Before making any judgments, the medical assistant must be absolutely sure of all the information and circumstances. If unethical conduct occurs, the medical assistant must then make his or her own decision about continued employment in the facility and whether the unethical behavior should be reported to a law enforcement agency or the local medical society. Would it be wise to remain in the practice under the circumstances? Would it be better to seek other employment? Would remaining adversely affect future opportunities for employment in another facility?

These decisions are difficult, especially if the relationship and employment conditions have been favorable and congenial. An ethical medical assistant does not want to participate in known substandard or unlawful practices, especially those that might be harmful to patients. In addition, the medical assistant must never make inaccurate reports about unethical behavior and should realize that some states can prosecute individuals who file a false report. Be absolutely certain of the facts before making such accusations against any health professional. When the provider's ethical standards conflict with those of the medical assistant, the medical assistant must decide whether staying with the provider is the best option. However, if the medical assistant believes that patient safety is at risk, he or she is ethically compelled to report provider actions to the local authorities and the state Medical Board.

CLOSING COMMENTS

Medical assistants have an ethical obligation to keep up with current developments that affect the practice of medicine and the care of patients. Membership in a professional organization provides access to continuing education to help you keep current in your knowledge and skills in medical assisting and to stay up-to-date on the latest ethical topics.

The study of ethics requires considerable thought and honest appraisal of what the medical assistant believes. Sometimes reflection at this level is difficult. Often our beliefs are a result of our environment, upbringing, and other factors that have influenced our thinking and actions from the time we were small children. It is important that our belief system is one that we developed personally, not just a set of beliefs and values that we learned from our families or were influenced by our friends. Medical assistants should take a serious look at the thoughts and concepts that make up their own ethical beliefs. With personal insight into how we feel about complex ethical issues, we are better prepared to recognize the difference between professional and personal ethics.

Patient Education

Patients may not always understand the ethical standards to which providers and medical assistants adhere. They may ask medical assistants questions about the health of a fellow patient or a friend or family member who are also patients at the facility. Medical assistants must educate patients about confidentiality in such a way that the patient does not take offense, explaining that all patients deserve to have their medical and personal information kept private. Now more than ever, ethical obligations for privacy, in addition to legal ones, are imperative. A medical assistant must make sure that all patients understand that they are entitled to confidential treatment of their records and that the facility is dedicated to that principle.

Legal and Ethical Issues

The prime objective of the healthcare profession is to render service and provide quality care to all individuals, regardless of race, gender, age, sexual orientation, or socioeconomic status. The importance of respecting the confidentiality of information learned from or about patients in the course of employment cannot be overemphasized. It is unethical to reveal the patient's identity or information to anyone, including family members, a spouse, best friends, and other medical assistants.

This chapter summarized a wide range of potential ethical conflicts. Regardless of the situation, the medical assistant is bound by ethical standards to treat all patients with respect and to make ethical decisions based on principles rather than personal beliefs and values. As members of the healthcare team, medical assistants are also responsible for reporting ethical infractions to their supervisors. In addition, legal requirements may exist for the reporting of ethical issues to local or state authorities. One of the roles of each medical assistant is to serve as the patient's advocate. In this role, it may be necessary to use legal means to protect the rights of patients in the practice.

Professional Behaviors

Ethics guides society's moral principles. The decisions that medical assistants make based on ethical beliefs can drastically alter how they treat individual patients. Ethics is considered a higher authority than legality since something that is legal may not necessarily be ethical. It is crucial that each person working in healthcare take the time to evaluate his or her own belief system and core values. Regardless of how we believe a particular situation should be handled, we must always provide our patients with respectful patient care. The AAMA Code of Ethics serves as a guide for the ethical responsibilities of the professional medical assistant.

SUMMARY OF SCENARIO

Pregnancy usually is a joyous time, but Monica has learned that even such an anticipated event can bring ethical issues to light. She has realized that every situation has two or more sides and that she must be open and willing to look at all sides when making an ethical decision.

Medical assisting is a rewarding career, but sometimes the decisions medical professionals face are quite difficult. Monica must learn to be nonjudgmental and not to inflict her opinions on her patients. They must make their own decisions about their health and emotional well-being, and the medical assistant should not influence their thinking unfairly.

Monica must continue to evaluate her own ideas and beliefs throughout her career as a medical assistant. Periodic self-evaluation is good for everyone, and she will grow both personally and professionally by always providing her patients ethical care.

SUMMARY OF LEARNING OBJECTIVES

1. **Define, spell, and pronounce the terms listed in the vocabulary.**
Spelling and pronouncing medical terms correctly reinforce the medical assistant's credibility. Knowing the definitions of these terms promotes confidence in communication with patients and co-workers.

2. **Do the following related to medicine and ethics:**
- *Define ethics and morals.*
  Ethical issues are not as strict as laws and vary from person to person, but most physicians follow the ethical guidelines set forth by the AMA. *Moral* issues are related to a person's concept of right and wrong. An individual's morals are defined as their standards for behavior or their beliefs about what is right and what is wrong.
- *Identify the effect of personal morals and values on professional performance.*
  Morals and values are usually personal in nature. Medical assistants not only must have a strong knowledge base about ethical issues they might face throughout their careers, they also must come to terms with some of the deeply rooted morals and value systems that have been a part of their lives since childhood. Interacting ethically requires you to examine your own values, beliefs, and actions; you cannot treat all patients with care and respect until you first recognize and evaluate personal biases.
- *Differentiate between personal and professional ethics.*
  Personal ethics are the beliefs or values held by an individual. *Professional* ethics are the beliefs or values generally held by most people in a profession; they typically are guided by established codes of ethics.
- *Recognize the effect personal ethics and morals have on the delivery of healthcare.*
  Medical assistants must avoid judging a situation or a patient based on the values they learned as a child or in their personal lives. If a patient makes a decision or performs in a way we do not approve, we still must treat him or her with respect and deliver the highest quality patient care.
- *Develop a plan for separation of personal and professional ethics.*
  Using the case studies in Procedure 6-1, role-play with your partner issues of personal and professional ethical behavior and how personal ethics and morals can affect the delivery of healthcare.
- *Demonstrate appropriate responses to ethical issues.*
  Using the case studies in Procedure 6-2, role-play with your partner issues of patient confidentiality.

3. **Discuss the history of ethics in medicine.**
The earliest written code of ethical conduct for medical practice was created in approximately 2250 BC by the Babylonians. It was called the Code of Hammurabi. In 1846, the American Medical Association (AMA) was organized, and a Code of Ethics was formulated at its first meeting in 1847. The American Association of Medical Assistants (AAMA) has published its own version of a Code of Ethics for Medical Assistants and has also created a Medical Assisting Creed that can be used as a guideline by medical assistants.

4. **Do the following related to making ethical decisions:**
- *List and define three general elements of ethics.*
  The three general elements of ethics, according to Dr. Ruth Purtilo, are duties, rights, and character traits. A duty is an obligation a person has or perceives himself or herself to have; rights are defined as claims made on society, a group, or an individual; character traits are a tendency to act a certain way.
- *List and define the four types of ethical problems.*
  Purtilo presents four basic types of ethical problems. *Ethical distress* is a situation in which an individual knows what should be done, but for some reason the action cannot be accomplished. An *ethical dilemma* exists when a situation can be handled in different ways, but only one way can be chosen, regardless of the benefit of the others. A *dilemma of justice* exists when a conflict arises over how limited resources can be distributed fairly. A *locus of authority* problem occurs when authority figures differ in their opinions on how a medical problem should be managed.
- *Discuss the five-step process used to make an ethical decision.*
  Making an ethical decision is a five-step process that begins with gathering information about the situation; determining which ethical problem or problems are presented; considering the duties, rights, and character traits of all the individuals involved; paying close attention to the ramifications of all possible decisions; and then making a decision to act in a particular way.

5. **Summarize the ethical opinions reached by the Council on Ethical and Judicial Affairs (CEJA).**
The CEJA develops ethics policy for the AMA by analyzing and addressing ethical issues that confront physicians and the medical profession. The recommendations from the council ultimately are used to update the AMA's Code of Medical Ethics, which can be found at *www.ama-assn.org/ama/pub/physician-resources/medical-ethics/code-medical-ethics.page.* AMA ethical opinions have been published to address social policy issues (e.g., preventing, identifying, and treating violence and abuse; HIV testing; withholding or withdrawing life-prolonging treatment; organ donation; and allocation of health resources), confidentiality, advertising, and communication (e.g., advertising and publicity), and public matters (e.g., fees and charges, fee splitting and contingent fees, waiver of insurance co-payments, professional courtesy, conflict of interest, and unethical conduct by members of the health professions).

6. **Describe the process of compliance reporting of conflicts of interest.**
The American College of Physicians has made specific recommendations for physicians regarding conflicts of interest. If the physician's ethical standards conflict with those of the medical assistant, the medical assistant must decide whether staying with the physician is the best option. However, if the medical assistant believes that patient safety is at risk, he or she is ethically compelled to report the physician's actions to the local authorities and the state medical board.

CONNECTIONS

📖 Study Guide Connection: Go to the Chapter 6 Study Guide. Read and complete the activities.

evolve Evolve Connection: Go to the Chapter 6 link at *evolve.elsevier.com/kinn* to complete the Chapter Review Quiz. Check out the other resources listed for this chapter to make the most of what you have learned from Medicine and Ethics.

7

TECHNOLOGY AND WRITTEN COMMUNICATION

SCENARIO

Christiana has been a medical assistant in Dr. Zachary Brown's family practice clinic for 5 years. She had been working as a clinical medical assistant, helping with diagnostic tests and treatment procedures. Christiana enjoyed providing patient care, but she wanted to use more of the administrative skills she learned in college 5 years ago. She is organized and enjoys challenges and technology. When a front office position opened up, Christiana transitioned into the administrative role. She is now the lead administrative medical assistant. Her role entails answering phones, scheduling appointments, greeting patients, and processing correspondence to patients. She also is responsible for reviewing the clinic's e-mails. Patients are encouraged to use e-mail to communicate with Dr. Brown. Christiana has seen the number of daily e-mails increase. She answers those that pertain to appointments, and the others are forwarded to Dr. Brown or to his clinical medical assistant. Besides performing her administrative duties, Christiana is now responsible for the clinic's computer system. She is excited to continue to learn the administrative role and the computer system.

While studying this chapter, think about the following questions:
- How does a computer system help with efficiency and accuracy in the ambulatory care center?
- What steps can a medical assistant take to ensure that written communication is professional?
- What are the benefits of providing professional communication to patients, whether by letter or e-mail?
- How can a medical assistant safeguard the privacy of medical records when using electronic health records?

LEARNING OBJECTIVES

1. Define, spell, and pronounce the terms listed in the vocabulary.
2. Explain what a personal computer is, and identify input and output hardware for personal computers.
3. Identify internal computer components, secondary storage devices, and network and Internet access devices.
4. Explain how to maintain computer hardware.
5. Identify principles of ergonomics that apply to a computer workstation.
6. Differentiate between:
   - System software and application software.
   - Electronic medical records (EMRs) and a practice management system.
7. Explain the importance of data backup and other computer network security activities performed in the healthcare setting.
8. Discuss applications of electronic technology.
9. Recognize the elements of fundamental writing skills.
10. Explain the guidelines for using capitalization, numbers, and punctuation in business communication.
11. Describe each component of a professional business letter.
12. Summarize the formats for business letters and memorandums.
13. Compose professional correspondence using electronic technology.

VOCABULARY

audit trail A record of computer activity used to monitor users' actions within software, including additions, deletions, and viewing of electronic records.

back up The process of copying and archiving computer data so that the duplicate files can be used to restore the original data if a compromise occurs.

computer network A system that links personal computers and peripheral devices to share information and resources.

computer on wheels (COW) Wireless mobile workstation; also called workstation on wheels (WOW).

data server Computer hardware and software that perform data analysis, storage, and archiving; also called a *database server*.

decryption The computer process of changing encrypted text to readable or plain text after a user enters a secret key or password.

dumb terminal A personal computer that doesn't contain a hard drive and allows the user only limited functions, including access to software, the network, and/or the Internet.

electronic health record (EHR) An electronic record of health-related information about a patient that conforms to nationally recognized interoperability standards and that can be created, managed, and consulted by authorized clinicians and staff members from more than one healthcare organization.

electronic medical record (EMR) An electronic record of health-related information about an individual that can be created, gathered, managed, and consulted by authorized clinicians and staff members within a single healthcare organization. An EMR is an electronic version of a paper record.

e-prescribing The use of electronic software to communicate with pharmacies and send prescribing information. It takes the place of writing a prescription by hand and giving it to a patient; most new or refill prescriptions can be submitted electronically, cutting down on fraud and errors.

ethernet A communication system for connecting several computers so information can be shared.

firewall A program or hardware that acts as a filter between the network and the Internet.

magnetism The attraction of materials to magnets; strong magnets can damage magnetic storage devices, such as hard drives.

Meaningful use requirements Requirements established by the Centers for Medicare and Medicaid Services (CMS) as part of the Electronic Health Records (EHR) Incentives Program. The program provides financial incentives for healthcare organizations that "meaningfully used" their certified EHR technology. The requirements include implementing security measures to ensure the privacy of patients' EHRs.

media A type of communication (e.g., social media sites); with computers, the term refers to data storage devices.

modem Peripheral computer hardware that connects to the router to provide Internet access to the network or computer.

operating system Software that acts as the computer's administrator by managing, integrating, and controlling application software and hardware.

output device Computer hardware that displays the processed data from the computer (e.g., monitors and printers).

point of care Something designed to be used at or near where the patient is seen; point-of-care tools and apps are resources for the provider to use when working directly with the patient.

portrait orientation The most common layout for a printed page; the height of the paper is greater than its width.

practice management software Computer programs used to run business operations, including scheduling, billing, and accounting tasks.

privacy filters Devices attached to the monitor that allow visualization of the screen contents only if the user is directly in front of the screen; also called *monitor filters* or *privacy screens.*

secondary storage devices Media (e.g., jump drive, hard drive) capable of permanently storing data until it is replaced or deleted by the user.

security risk analysis Identification of potential threats of computer network breaches, for which action plans are devised.

software A set of electronic instructions to operate and perform different computer tasks.

stylus A pen-shaped device with a variety of tips that is used on touch screens to write, draw, or input commands.

USB port The most common type of connector device that allows hardware to be plugged into the computer.

Zip Software that compresses a file or folder, making it smaller.

The uses for technology in healthcare facilities are growing. Technology was first introduced in the ambulatory care setting to help promote efficiency and accuracy in business functions. Many healthcare facilities used computer software to help with billing and accounting procedures. Registration and scheduling software were implemented to help limit the number of times patient information was collected and entered into computer programs. As technology advanced, the federal government provided incentives for healthcare organizations to use electronic health records instead of paper medical records to increase accuracy and efficiency, which in turn helped reduce the cost of healthcare. More recently, healthcare workers have been using "smart" devices for quicker access to information to help provide better patient care.

The format of communication also has changed over the years. Many people have moved from letter writing to sending e-mails and text messages. Social **media** sites have gained in popularity. Many of these changes have affected the ambulatory care center environment. Patients are communicating with their providers via e-mails and text messages instead of phone calls. To help ensure confidentiality, administrators have instituted tighter network security procedures and restrictions on employee social media postings.

Medical assistants in today's healthcare facilities must be more computer savvy than ever before to meet these technologic demands.

They must follow procedures to safeguard the privacy and security of patients' records. The need for correct grammar, punctuation, and word use is greater than ever as medical assistants communicate using letters and electronic technology.

CRITICAL THINKING APPLICATION   **7-1**

Christiana answers e-mails from patients. How might her response differ from her personal e-mails to her family and friends?

ELECTRONIC TECHNOLOGY IN THE AMBULATORY CARE CENTER

For many clinics, technology was first used in administrative departments for scheduling and billing procedures. This helped increase the efficiency and accuracy of those activities. Processes that previously had taken hours to perform now took minutes with technology. Information was entered once and then used for many purposes.

Today, many clinics use electronic technology in both administrative and patient care areas. Most clinics have replaced paper medical charts with electronic health records (EHRs). Technology has increased the efficiency of the office environment and has made patient information and resources quickly accessible to healthcare staff. Regardless of the medical assistant's duties, knowledge about computers is crucial in today's healthcare environment.

Personal Computer Hardware

A personal computer (PC) is a relatively inexpensive piece of hardware that is used by a single person. A personal computer is considered a *system unit,* and all other pieces of hardware used are considered *peripheral devices.* The personal computer is an electronic data processing device that accepts, stores, and processes data. After processing the information, it generates the data output in a specific form.

A personal computer can be a desktop, laptop, or tablet computer. A desktop computer is designed for use on a desk. In the ambulatory care center, desktop computers are typically used for employees who primarily perform word processing, data entry, and business tasks, such as scheduling, bookkeeping, and billing (Figure 7-1). Laptop computers have evolved over the years into thinner, lighter weight models with more functionality (Figure 7-2). Many laptop and tablet computers have a touch screen panel (Figure 7-3). Users can enter data on the touch screen panel or use the keyboard. Laptop and tablet computers are portable, allowing healthcare staff to be more mobile while accessing technology.

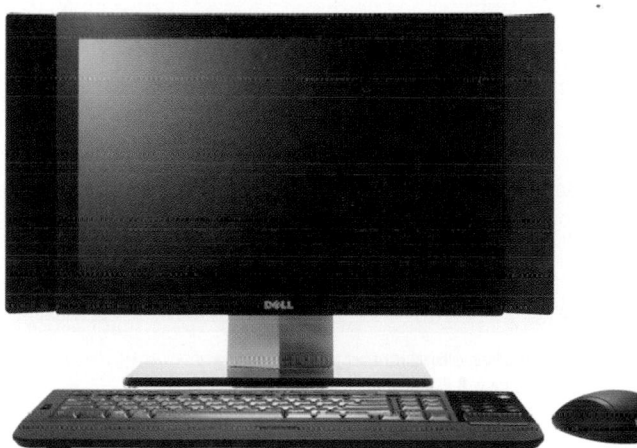

FIGURE 7-1 Many healthcare employees, including receptionists, clinical medical assistants, and providers, use desktop computers. (Courtesy Dell, Round Rock, Texas.)

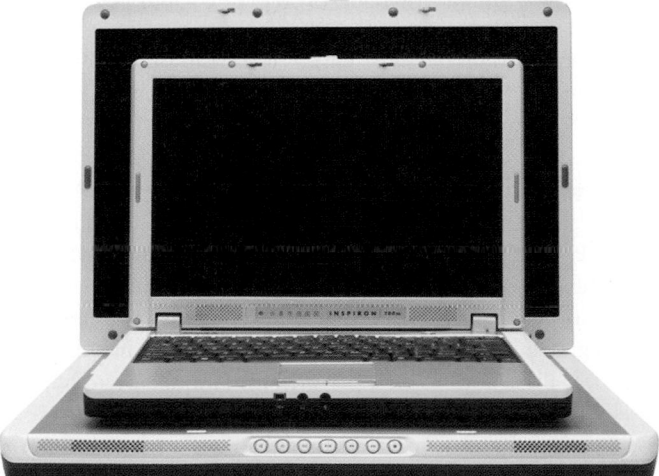

FIGURE 7-2 Laptop computers are available in thinner, lighter weight models with more functionality than older models. (Courtesy Dell, Round Rock, Texas.)

The hardware of a computer system includes the physical equipment required for communication and data processing functions. Computer hardware can be divided into the following categories: input devices, **output devices**, internal components, secondary storage devices, and network and Internet access devices.

CRITICAL THINKING APPLICATION   **7-2**

When Christiana transitioned into the administrative role, Dr. Brown hired Michaela as the new clinical medical assistant. Recently the medical practice switched from using desktop computers to tablet computers when working with patients in the exam rooms. How might Christiana's experience using the desktop computer in the exam rooms be different from Michaela's use of the tablet computer? Thinking of the patient's perception, which technology might a patient prefer the medical assistant to use? Why?

Input Devices

An *input device* is any peripheral hardware that allows the user to provide data to the computer. Many types of input devices are available on the market, but this discussion focuses on those typically used in the ambulatory care setting. Common input devices include keyboards, mice and other pointing devices, touch screens, webcams, microphones, scanners, and signature pads.

Keyboards are the most common input devices. The QWERTY keyboard is the standard keyboard for computers. (Q-W-E-R-T-Y are the first six letters, from left to right, just below the number keys on the keyboard.) A wide variety of keyboards is available, including standard, Internet, wireless, and ergonomic. Keyboards may have special keys that perform the same functionality as the buttons on Web pages. Numeric keypads are also a feature on many keyboards. Ergonomic keyboards help reduce repetitive strain injuries by minimizing muscle strain; these keyboards allow the user's hands to be in a natural position when typing. The two most common ergonomic keyboards are the split-key models and the "waved" or "curved" key layout (Figure 7-4).

CRITICAL THINKING APPLICATION   **7-3**

Christiana's keyboard looks different from Dr. Brown's keyboard in his office. Why might Christiana have a different keyboard?

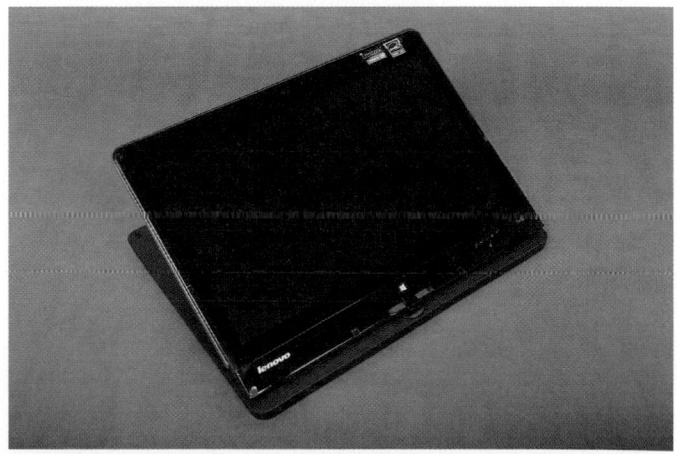

FIGURE 7-3 Tablet computers and other new computers have touch screen panels that allow users to easily enter data.

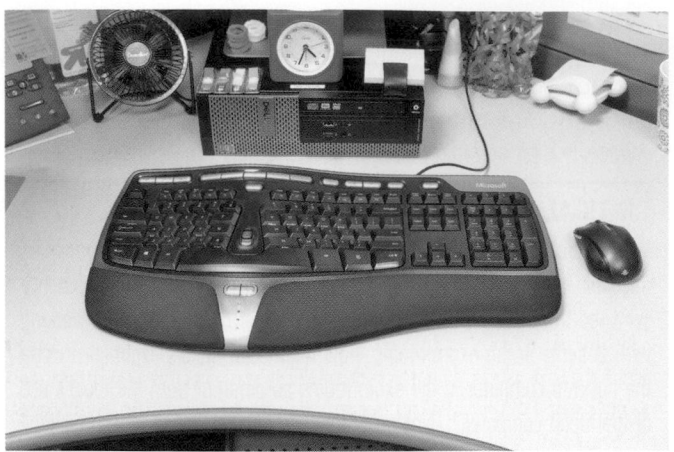

FIGURE 7-4 Ergonomic keyboards have different appearances, yet they all help reduce repetitive strain injuries.

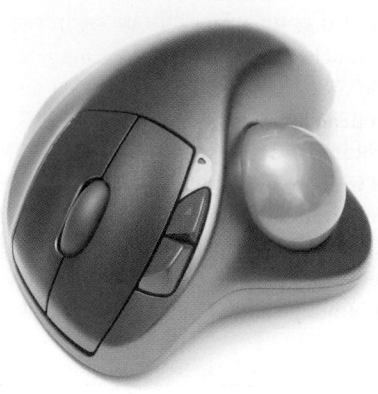

FIGURE 7-5 A trackball mouse uses a large ball to control the movement of the cursor/pointer.

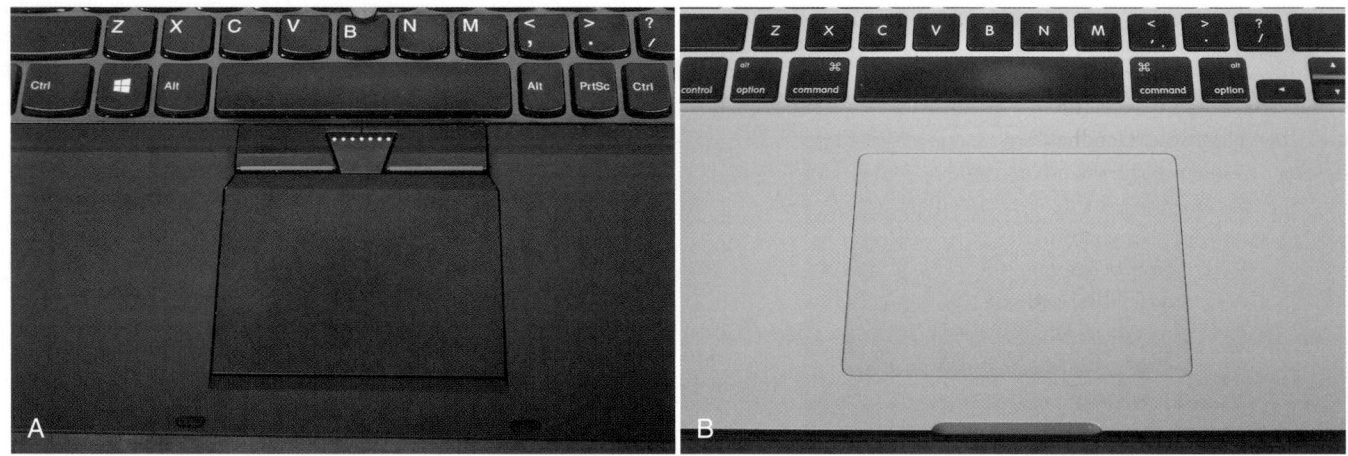

FIGURE 7-6 A touch pad is built into a computer, and its functions are similar to those of a mouse, although different touch pads may have different functions. For example, the device in **A** has a left and right click button, whereas the device in **B** does not.

Keyboards typically have the following categories of keys: typing, numeric, function, control, and special purpose keys. Typing keys include the numeric and alphabetic keys used for typing. Numeric keypads have the numeric keys in the same position as calculators. The twelve keys at the top of the keyboard are function keys, and each key has a specific purpose. Some software allows the function keys to be programmed by the user. When these programmed function keys are used, a specific task is performed by the computer. Control keys move the cursor and the screen. They include the following keys: Home, End, Insert, Delete, Page Up, Page Down, Control, Escape, Alternate, and four arrow keys. Special purpose keys include Enter, Shift, Caps Lock, Num Lock, Space Bar, Print Screen, and Tab.

The mouse is one of the most common input devices, making screen navigation much simpler than using the keyboard. A mouse is a palm-sized box with a laser sensor that tracks the user's movement of the mouse and sends those messages back to the computer. The mouse is used to move the pointer (cursor) on the screen. Many mice have a left and right button with a wheel between to help with cursor/pointer navigation and functionality. With a trackball mouse, the user moves the enlarged ball on the top of the mouse to control the pointer (Figure 7-5).

Touch pads are becoming more popular on laptops because they are portable and compact. Touch pads are touch sensitive; they move the pointer based on the user's finger movements on the touch pad. Touch pads' functionality can vary, but many include a left and right click button similar to a mouse (Figure 7-6).

A touch screen is different from a touch pad. A touch screen allows a person to interact with the computer by touching the display screen with a finger or **stylus**. The touch screens on computers and other electronic devices can vary, which means the compatible stylus can vary.

- Resistive Touch Screen: Responds to the touch of almost anything that can generate pressure (e.g., finger, plastic stylus, rubber-tip stylus). These screens are found in many handheld electronic devices.
- Capacitive Touch Screen: Responds to the electrical characteristics of a finger and is found in smart phones and other electronic devices. It requires a specialized stylus that has more surface area in the point.

- Surface Acoustic Wave Touch Screen: Responds to an inaudible wave of sound that is created on the screen from a finger. Like the resistive touch screen, it is very common and can be found in kiosks and ordering screens. A stylus with a rubber or soft tip the size of a pencil eraser is required.

Wireless webcams and microphones are becoming more popular. To see patients who are not able to come to the healthcare agency, providers can use webcams, microphones, and Internet video chat software. Webcams and microphones are also used for meetings and continuing education opportunities. Microphones can be used for dictating notes into a patient's health record.

CRITICAL THINKING APPLICATION   7-4

Dr. Brown works with a home health agency. Patients and nurses can communicate with him using the Internet, microphones, and webcams. How does this technology benefit the patients?

Scanners convert images to digital text through a process called *optical character recognition* (OCR). Handheld, sheet-fed, and flatbed scanners are available. Handheld scanners are used to scan bar codes. Sheet-fed scanners may be stand-alone units or include other features such as duplicating and faxing. Flatbed scanners have a glass panel on which the documents are placed for scanning. Scanners in the healthcare setting have become more popular since the use of electronic health records (EHRs) has increased. Old medical records are scanned, and the images are uploaded into the patient's new EHR. Receptionists use small, sheet-fed scanners to scan insurance cards when patients check in for appointments. The insurance card images are then uploaded into the patient's record and are referenced for billing activities.

In the ambulatory care setting, signature pads are used in the reception area. Patients need to sign a number of documents, including release forms, consent forms, and the Notice of Privacy Practices. Patients sign the signature pad, and the signatures are imported into the EHR as part of the patient's permanent health record (Figure 7-7).

Output Devices

The data entered into the computer with the input devices are processed by the computer. The processed data are displayed using output devices. Common output devices in the healthcare setting include monitors, printers, and speakers.

Monitors display the output as images, which are created by tiny dots called *pixels*. The higher the number of pixels used in the monitor, the sharper the image. The most common monitor in the healthcare setting is the liquid crystal display (LCD) monitor. These monitors are easier on the eyes and use less electricity, and they are smaller and lighter than older monitors. Some clinics use LCD monitors in the reception area so that patients can read documents before signing the signature pad.

Printers produce the output on paper. The two most common types of printers used in the ambulatory care center are inkjet and laser printers. Inkjet printers create images by spraying small drops of ink on the paper. Inkjet printers can create high-quality printing but are slower to print a document. Inkjet printers are inexpensive to purchase, but the maintenance costs are high because of the need for frequent ink cartridge changes. A laser printer uses a laser, electrical charges, and toner to produce images on paper. The advantages of laser printers include high-speed printing, high-quality output, quality graphics, and support of many fonts and font sizes. The initial cost of a laser printer is higher than that of an inkjet printer, but the maintenance costs may be less because the toner cartridges are changed less often compared to inkjet printers.

CRITICAL THINKING APPLICATION   7-5

Christiana frequently prints documents, including billing statements, appointment reminders, and receipts for payment. What type of printer might be the most economical to use in the reception area? Why?

Speakers for electronic devices come in all shapes and sizes. Typically in the ambulatory care center, speakers are built into the devices used (e.g., monitor, laptop, tablet).

Internal Components

For a desktop personal computer, the internal components are found in the tower or case. The central processing unit (CPU), or processor, is the "brains" of the computer. It is responsible for interpreting and executing commands from the software or the program. The CPU sits on the motherboard. The motherboard is a platform where all the internal computer parts attach, including the primary memory, hard drive, optical drive, sound and video cards, and ports.

The primary memory is accessed directly by the CPU and includes read-only memory (ROM), cache memory, and random access memory (RAM). ROM contains hardwired instructions that are used when the computer boots up or starts. The cache memory contains data and instructions for opened programs. When the computer needs to read memory or instructions, it first scans the cache memory to see if the data exist there before looking at the RAM or main memory. If the data exist in the cache memory, the computer doesn't look at the RAM. The cache memory is quicker than the main memory and allows programs to operate more quickly and efficiently. The limitations of cache memory include limited size and expense, and it provides only temporary use of information.

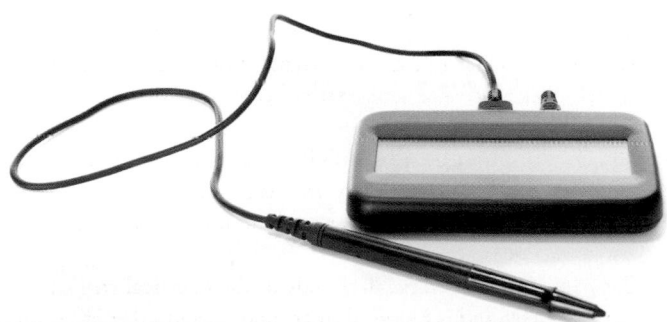

FIGURE 7-7 Signature pads allow patients' signatures to be imported into the electronic health record or practice management software.

RAM is the working memory of the computer, which is needed for the computer to operate. It holds the data that are currently being used. When a program is opened, the instructions are stored temporarily in RAM for easy access. The main memory has limited capacity and can be lost if the power is turned off. Before installing new software, make sure the computer has the required RAM. If there is not enough RAM for the program, the computer must go to the hard drive to read the data, which is a slower process.

The hard disk drive (HDD) is often referred to as the "hard drive." The HDD reads and writes on the hard disk, which provides the largest amount of permanent storage for the computer. Because the HDD and the hard disk are packaged together, "HDD" or "hard drive" is used to reference the entire unit. The hard drive is considered a secondary storage device and is not required to operate the computer. When you save a file on the computer, the file is saved on the C drive, which is the internal hard drive of the computer. Because of their low cost, hard drives are found in most desktop and laptop computers. A solid-state drive (SSD) can replace a hard drive in a computer, but an SSD is more expensive than an HDD. However, compared to an HDD, an SSD has faster access speed and better performance and reliability, and it is not affected by **magnetism**.

Optical drives can read or read and save data on optical discs, such as compact discs (CDs), digital versatile/video discs (DVDs), and Blu-Ray discs (BDs), which are removable storage devices. The sound card, also called the *audio card* or *audio adapter,* allows audio information to be sent to speakers or headphones. The video card is also called a *graphic card* or *video adapter.* It allows the computer to send graphic information to output devices, such as projectors or monitors. On many computers the sound and video card features are integrated into the motherboard; this limits the sound and graphic systems but lowers the overall computer cost. Most desktop computers and laptops have a number of **USB ports** that allow hardware (e.g., printers, mice, keyboards, and external hard drives) to connect to the computer.

Secondary Storage Devices

A **secondary storage device**, or **medium**, is capable of permanently storing data until it is replaced or deleted by the user. These devices can be considered removable, internal (such as the hard drive previously discussed), or external. The computer needs a secondary storage device to allow the user to save data. Without a storage device, the computer would be considered a **dumb terminal**. Dumb terminals provide the user access to software, the network, and/or the Internet but don't allow the user to save data to the C drive of the computer.

The types of computer storage devices are categorized as magnetic, optical, and flash (Table 7-1). One of the oldest types of storage is magnetic storage, which uses magnetic technology to read and write data to the device. Optical drives use lasers and lights to read and write data onto optical storage devices. Some optical devices are just recordable; for example, a CD-R disc allows only one opportunity to save data to the device. Other optical devices allow Read/Write (RW), which means discs allow data to be written and erased multiple times. Flash memory devices, which are becoming cheaper and have larger storage capacity, are replacing the older magnetic media. The jump drive is a portable device that connects to the USB port in the computer (Figure 7-8).

Besides storage hardware, the use of cloud storage is becoming more popular. Cloud storage, also known as *file sharing* or *online storage,* allows individuals to store computer files using the Internet and a third-party service. To get started, an individual signs up with a cloud storage service. Many companies allow free minimal storage, while others charge monthly fees or fees based on storage size. After signing up, individuals use the Internet to send computer files to the service company's **data servers**. The files are copied onto many servers in various locations. This is called redundancy and allows the information to be accessible even if one site goes down and needs repairs. With Internet access and a password, an individual has access to the files anytime and can share the files with others.

TABLE 7-1	Data Storage Devices
DEVICE	**EXAMPLES**
Magnetic storage device	Internal hard drive, portable hard drive
Optical storage device	Blu-Ray Disc (BD), Compact Disc (CD), Digital Versatile/Video Disc (DVD)
Flash memory device	Jump drive (also called USB flash, data stick, pen drive, keychain drive, travel drive, or thumb drive), memory card, memory stick, solid-state disk or drive (SSD)

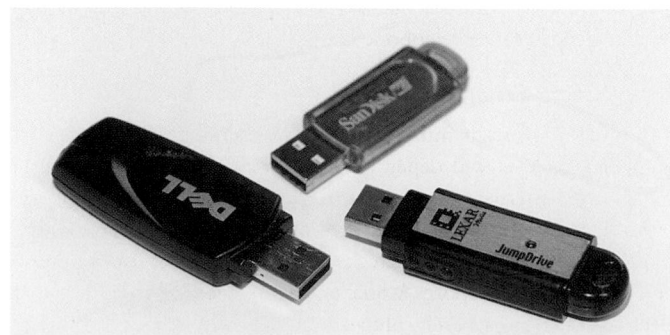

FIGURE 7-8 Jump drives, known by many different names, allow users to store documents and files for use on other computers.

TABLE 7-2 Terms for Data Storage Capacity on Electronic Devices	
1 kilobyte (KB)	1,024 bytes
1 megabyte (MB)	1,024 KB (about 1 million bytes)
1 gigabyte (GB)	1,024 MB (about 1 billion bytes)
1 terabyte (TB)	1,024 GB (about 1 trillion bytes)

The capacity of storage devices also must be considered. The storage capacity of such devices is measured in bytes. Most computers consider a byte to be a character, such as a number, letter, or symbol. To simplify communication, the storage size often is estimated. For instance, 1,024 bytes might be stated as 1,000 bytes. Over the years, the size of storage devices has increased, and the cost of additional storage has decreased (Table 7-2). Flash drives range in size, and some now can hold more than 250 gigabytes (GB), or 268,435,456,000 bytes.

Network and Internet Access Devices

The computers and output devices in a healthcare facility are usually all connected to the clinic's network, which can also be called the *local area network* (LAN). The local area network can span one building or multiple buildings. Some healthcare facilities that have clinics at a distance may have wide area network (WAN) technology, which consists of two or more LANs. LAN and WAN technology can use telephone lines or fiberoptic cables that increase the speed of transmission.

A router must be used to allow multiple devices to be on the same network. Most routers used today have wireless connectivity. This peripheral hardware is a small box that may have antennas, and it uses the **ethernet**, a standard communication protocol for hardware and software. The router allows multiple computers and other devices (e.g., smart devices) to use the same network to send and receive information.

For the **computer network** to have Internet access, the medical office must subscribe with an Internet services provider (ISP) and the facility's router must be connected to a **modem**. A modem provides access to the Internet. Most routers have a specific port that is designed to connect to the ethernet port of a cable or digital subscriber line (DSL) modem. DSL is a high-speed Internet service that uses a modem to translate the computer's digital signals into voltage that is then sent over telephone lines.

Maintaining Computer Hardware

The medical assistant must maintain the computer hardware. The maintenance level will depend on the size of the ambulatory care center and whether the ambulatory care center has information technology (IT) internal or external support. The medical assistant should always do a quick check of the malfunctioning hardware before calling IT support. A quick check to see that the cables and electric cords are securely plugged in can help reduce additional downtime. Primarily, the medical assistant's role is to prevent issues from arising and to do routine cleaning.

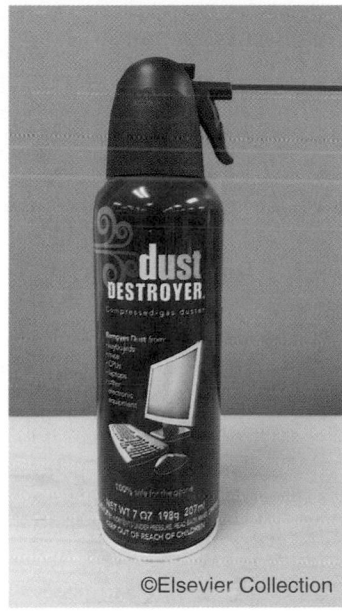

©Elsevier Collection

FIGURE 7-9 Compressed air dusters provide an efficient means of removing the dust and dirt from keyboards.

To prevent problems, the computer and all peripheral devices should be located on a stable, even surface away from heat sources. Ventilation slots should be clear, allowing air to flow into the computer to cool the components. Liquids and food should be kept away from the devices. If liquids spill on the keyboard, unplug the keyboard and tip the keyboard upside down to drain out the liquid. Let the keyboard dry overnight. Sticky liquids are more apt to damage the keyboard.

Before cleaning the computer or peripheral components, turn off and unplug the device. To remove the grime and dirt, use a damp lint-free cloth to wipe the hardware's casing. All vents and air holes should be wiped clean. For glass monitor screens, spray a household glass cleaner on a lint-free cloth and then wipe the monitor. Do not spray liquid directly on a component as the liquid may drip into the device. For nonglare monitors or antiglare screens, just use a lint-free cloth dampened with water. The keyboard usually contains a lot of bacteria. To disinfect the keyboard, spray a disinfectant on a lint-free cloth or use a disinfectant cloth and wipe each key. Avoid spraying or dripping liquids into the keyboard. To remove the dirt from the keyboard some people turn the keyboard upside down and gently shake it to remove dirt. Using compressed air dusters (i.e., pressurized air in a can) is a more efficient way to blow the dirt out of the keyboard (Figure 7-9). Air dusters can be purchased at many office supply stores. To clean the hardware, disconnect the cords and cables. Attach the extension tube to the duster and apply pressure on the trigger. Quick little bursts of air are enough to blow the dirt and dust from the hardware. Keeping the hardware clean and preventing complications help increase its useful life.

A disc should be handled with care; grasp its outer edges or center hole. Keep discs clean and dust free and store them in cases. Use a clean lint-free cloth to clean a disc, wiping in a straight line from the center of the disc toward the outer edge. Keep discs and flash drives out of sunlight and extreme heat or high-humidity environments. To prevent flash drive data loss, make sure you never unplug the flash drive while it is writing or reading data.

Computer Workstation Ergonomics

For people working on computers, it is important to arrange the workstation correctly to avoid the risk of repetitive stress injuries. Poor posture and straining can cause physical stress and injury to the body. Ergonomics is the field of study that involves reducing strain and injuries by improving the workstation design.

When you sit at a workstation, your torso and neck should be vertical and in line. The chair should be adjusted so that your feet are flat on the floor or a footrest (Figure 7-10, *A*) and your legs are comfortably below the workstation. The backrest lumbar support area should be fitted to the small of your back (Figure 7-10, *B*). The backrest should help support the upper body in the upright position. The seat pan should be the appropriate size and height to accommodate your body build so that there is no added pressure on the back of the knees or thighs. The armrest should support the forearms with the shoulders in a relaxed position (Figure 7-10, *C*). For standing workstations, your legs, torso, head, and neck should be vertical and in line. One foot can be elevated on a step.

The top of the monitor should be at or just below eye level, to prevent bending of the head or neck. The monitor should be directly in front of you and tilted to avoid glare. Use a document holder, so documents are placed at the same distance and height of the monitor, to prevent continual movement of the head as you look at the document and then at the monitor (see Figure 7-10, *D*). The keyboard should be an ergonomic split-key or waved model if possible and placed at a height and an angle that allow the wrists to be in a neutral position. The work surface and mouse should be at elbow level for

typing. Your wrist should be supported by a foam wrist rest (see Figure 7-10, *E*). Headsets should be used for those answering frequent phone calls to prevent muscle strain. Laptop computers and tablets are not ergonomically designed for prolonged use.

Whether you are standing or sitting at a workstation, it is important to change positions every 30 minutes. If you are sitting, adjustments can be made to chairs or backrests. Stretching your fingers, arms, and torso is important. Frequently look away from the computer to a distant object to prevent eye strain. Stand up and walk around for a few minutes. Preventing repetitive stress injuries is important for all computer users.

Software Used in the Ambulatory Care Center

For hardware to work, the computer must have **software**, or a set of electronic instructions to operate and perform different tasks. The terms "software" and "program" are mostly synonymous. Programs existed before software. A program is a sequence of instructions, written in a language understood by the computer that directs the computer to perform a specific task. Software contains several programs that together perform a function; Web browser, e-mail, games, spreadsheet, and word processor are all types of software.

The two main categories of software are system software and application software. System software is a collection of programs that operate and control the computer. **Operating systems** and utility software are two types of system software. Operating systems, such as Windows, act as the computer's software administrator by managing, integrating, and controlling application software and hardware. Utility software helps the computer function and can include file managers, screensavers, backup software, and clipboard managers. The system software loads on the computer and operates in the background while other application software is used.

Application software (also called an *application, app,* or *application program*) allows the user or other application programs to perform specific tasks. Application software may consist of a single program or a collection of programs, called a *software package* or

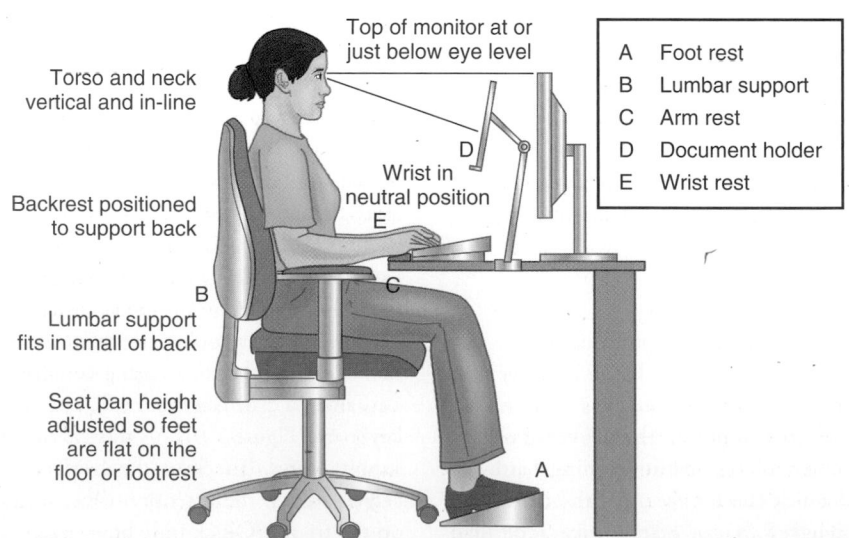

FIGURE 7-10 *Medical assistants should use an ergonomically correct workstation to prevent repetitive stress injuries. Equipment that helps create this type of workstation includes a foot rest* **(A),** *lumbar support* **(B),** *arm rest* **(C),** *document holder* **(D),** *and wrist rest* **(E).**

system. In the ambulatory care center, several types of application software are used. Word processing software (e.g., Microsoft Word) is used to compose letters and documents. Spreadsheet software (e.g., Microsoft Excel) is used to manage numbers, data, and expenses. Telecommunication software allows employees to e-mail patients and vendors. Antimalware software is used to protect computers against viruses (malware), which are programs that can damage the computer. (Additional security applications are discussed later in the chapter.) Database software allows the user to work with large amounts of data stored in the program. Microsoft Access, **practice management software** systems, and EHR software are examples of database software. Practice management software can include programs for scheduling, registering, billing, coding, and managing finances. Practice management software features can include appointment reminder e-mail or letter tools, bookkeeping programs, and financial analysis tools. Managers use practice management software for running their business, making processes more efficient.

The terms **electronic medical record (EMR)** and **electronic health record (EHR)** are used interchangeably by many people. However, there is a significant difference between these two types of software. When patients' records became electronic (or computerized), they were called *electronic medical records.* The EMR software contains limited information, usually related to medical treatment for one healthcare facility. The EMR was a digital version of the paper medical record. The *electronic health record* has advantages over the EMR. The EHR allows sharing of information with other providers outside the facility, including medical laboratories, nursing homes, hospitals, and specialists. The information from all types of healthcare providers can be managed in the EHR, making the EHR more of a health record than just a medical record.

It is important for the medical assistant to be aware of the differences between the practice management software and the EHR. You may use both during your day as a medical assistant, but the EHR contains a record of patient interactions and health history, whereas the practice management software allows the facility to operate the business side of the practice by maintaining schedules and financial information.

Computer Network Security

Electronic security is becoming more important in today's society as we store vast quantities of confidential and personal information in computer files. Several hospitals and clinics have had their network computer systems compromised by hackers and malware, potentially exposing patient and employee confidential information, which can lead to identity theft and other criminal actions. The Privacy Rule under the Health Insurance Portability and Accountability Act (HIPAA) and the Health Information Technology for Economic and Clinical Health Act (HITECH) require privacy and confidentiality of patient records. These acts mandate training and policies and procedures to be implemented in healthcare facilities to keep electronic records safe. Employers must provide medical record privacy and security training to new employees and periodic refreshers for current staff. Most clinics also need to comply with the **Meaningful use requirements**, which include developing a security risk analysis process to monitor for potential threats to privacy of the EHR and network files. (This process is explained in more detail later in the

chapter.) Administrators and employees must work together to keep the computer network safe.

Common network security procedures used by employees include authentication, frequent password changes, and logging out of the network when leaving a workstation. Authentication means that each employee with network access must log in using a unique password. Strong passwords have more than eight characters and use a random combination of upper and lower case letters, numbers, and symbols. It is important to use different passwords and to change them frequently. Employees need to log out of the computer programs when leaving their workstation to prevent unauthorized users from viewing confidential information. Leaving the EHR open and unsupervised can allow others to document in the patient's health record using someone else's electronic signature. To prevent others from seeing the information on the screen, computer users can apply **privacy filters** to the monitor. These filters diminish the viewing angle and require the user to be directly in front of the monitor to see the content on the screen.

Administrators have additional security responsibilities. To help manage these responsibilities, many medical clinics appoint an information technology (IT) employee to oversee the security and privacy of the network. This person, who is considered the "security officer," helps the facility meet federal regulations related to electronic technology security and monitors the network for suspected breaches. Many clinics have banned employees from downloading files, which can lead to malware being introduced into the network. Some of the software and procedures used to uphold the security include encryption, firewalls, virus protection, security risk analysis, audit trails, monitoring of log-in activity, automatic log-off, and access restrictions.

Encryption software is used to encode or change the information into nonreadable or encrypted data. Another name for encrypted data is *cipher text.* This prevents unauthorized users from reading the information. An authorized user must enter a password for **decryption** to occur and make the text readable again. A **firewall** is a program or hardware device that acts as a barrier or filter between the network and the Internet. Data coming from the Internet must pass through the firewall. Data that do not meet the firewall criteria are not allowed into the network. Virus protection software (also called *antivirus* or *antimalware software*) is used in the clinic to protect against malware. This software detects and removes malicious programs. Many types of virus protection software are available, including Norton and AVG Anti-Virus.

Healthcare agencies' IT departments manage **audit trails** to track the activity of users in the software (e.g., practice management and EHRs). They can identify who has been looking at a specific patient's record or what files a person looked at while on the computer. IT also performs **security risk analysis**, which means potential threats of network breaches are identified and action plans are instituted to prevent the breaches. Log-in activity is monitored, and multiple incorrect log-in attempts are flagged. With just a few incorrect log-in attempts, some systems lock out the user. This is to prevent hackers, unauthorized users that attempt to break into networks, from cracking passwords. The security officer is responsible for managing passwords, reminding staff to change passwords, and providing staff with the adequate access levels needed for each job. Automatic log-offs are also used in the healthcare facility to safeguard records. After a period of inactivity, the workstation logs off. *Access restrictions* limit what staff members can see on the computer. The information a receptionist can view would be different from that accessible to the medical assistant, who assists the provider. Not all staff members have the same access in software programs, such as EHRs and practice management software. Those with more responsibilities typically have more access.

CRITICAL THINKING APPLICATION   7-8

Like many small healthcare facilities without an IT department, Christiana must assume a leadership role with the EHRs. She has administrator rights, which means she can assign different levels of access for the various staff members. In such a small practice, what other security measures should she consider using to ensure the privacy of EHRs? What resources might she use to implement the security measures identified?

Another important role in securing the network is to perform data backup procedures. Depending on the size of the medical facility, the network may be backed up once to several times a day. **Back up** is a process in which the network files are copied and the copy is stored in a secure off-site location. Many healthcare facilities contract with cloud backup services, which back up all the data on the network to protect against data loss. Cloud backup services are similar to cloud storage services with regard to the access of the data anytime, anywhere, but file sharing is not a typical service provided by the backup companies. When computer data are compromised, either by errors, natural causes (e.g., floods, storm damage), or human causes (e.g., fires, hackers, and malware), the data can be restored using the backup copy.

CRITICAL THINKING APPLICATION   7-9

Some healthcare facilities store network backup copies in fireproof safes on site. Why is it important to store the backup copy off site? What would be the advantage of using a data backup Internet service that has several data storage locations around the country?

Technology Advances in Healthcare

Patients are seeing more technology in healthcare settings today compared to 10 years ago. Receptionists are wearing Bluetooth headsets, which allow them to be more mobile when answering phone calls (Figure 7-11). Bluetooth is a short-range wireless communication technology that uses short-wave radio frequencies to interconnect wireless electronic devices, such as phones and headsets.

Some of the technology changes in the reception area have been instituted for HIPAA compliance. Sign-in sheets are being replaced by sign-in kiosks. Some clinics have patients enter health information using the kiosk or a tablet computer. This information is then incorporated into the EHR. For copayment collection, receptionists have card readers for credit and debit cards. The card reader machines can be mounted on the computer monitor or stand-alone units. Many have a printer feature, allowing the receptionist to print a receipt for the patient.

Clinics are using the common hospital procedure of providing patients with wristbands with bar codes. Before diagnostic tests and

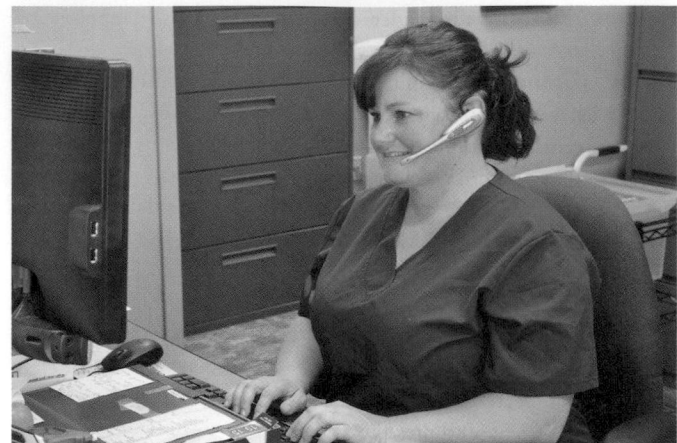

FIGURE 7-11 Bluetooth headsets are helpful for receptionists and other healthcare employees who frequently answer or make phone calls.

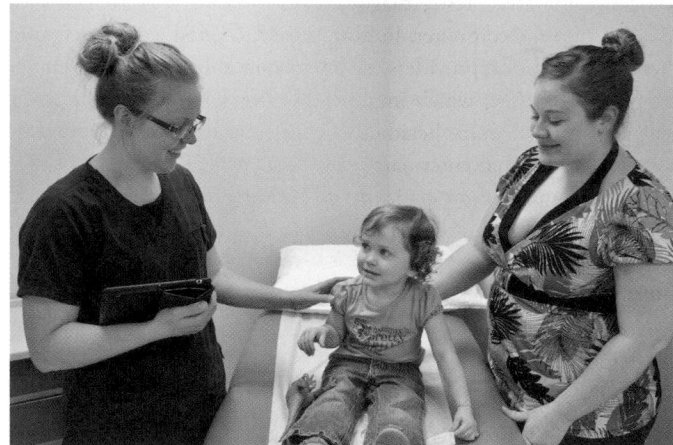

FIGURE 7-12 Medical assistants can use tablets to enter information into the electronic health record.

administration of medications, the patient's bar code is scanned, along with codes for the test or medications. This scanning process creates an automatic entry or note in the patient's EHR. This process is another step in ensuring patient safety and accuracy in billing.

Medical laboratories, ambulatory surgery centers, walk-in clinics and urgent-care centers are using patient tracking systems in both the reception area and the patient care area. Patients sign in or are signed into the system and their names go into the queue. For confidentiality purposes, patients may be given a unique number. As patients move from one area of the clinic to another, their progress shows on monitors in the reception area so family members can keep informed of their progress. Patients awaiting appointments or laboratory services can easily identify when their number moves up in the queue and/or current wait times. These tracking systems provide cost-effective ways to promote patient satisfaction while improving flow and efficiency.

In the exam room, healthcare workers are using more technology to help provide better patient care. Some clinics use wireless mobile workstations, such as **computers on wheels (COWs)** and workstations on wheels (WOWs). Providers and medical assistants use tablets, smart devices, and wearable computing devices to access EHRs and online resources (Figure 7-12). **Point-of-care** tools and apps are available for providers to use in the exam room with the patients. This technology gives providers the latest clinical information on diagnostic test results and treatments. Apps are available to help provide patients with visuals of surgical procedures, disease processes, and anatomic structures. Wearable computing devices allow healthcare employees to access medical records and information while moving around and providing patient care. Mobile devices and apps are helping providers make quicker decisions with a lower rate of error and improved patient care outcomes. With advances in Bluetooth smart technology, more medical equipment can work with apps on smart devices.

With advancements in EHR software and practice management software, new features and programs are being used. **E-prescribing** allows providers to send prescriptions to the pharmacy electronically (Figure 7-13). With voice recognition software, providers can dictate notes directly into the patient's EHR. Computerized provider/physician order entry (CPOE) is software that allows orders for medical laboratory tests, diagnostic tests, and medications to be entered into the computer. In many healthcare facilities, physicians, licensed healthcare providers, or credentialed medical assistants are able to use CPOE, which improves the efficiency of ordering tests and medications. Some healthcare agencies are hiring scribes, healthcare employees that enter data into the EHR for providers who are examining and treating patients. With all the advances in technology, medical assistants need to remain flexible and willing to adapt to changes in the workplace, while ensuring the privacy and confidentiality of patient records.

CRITICAL THINKING APPLICATION   **7-10**

Christiana had considered applying for a scribe position at a local healthcare facility before she was promoted to the lead administrative medical assistant. Why would a strong background in EHR be important for a scribe position?

FUNDAMENTALS OF WRITTEN COMMUNICATION

Whether electronic or paper, written communication from an ambulatory care center is a reflection of the provider and the clinic. Medical assistants commonly compose e-mails and letters to patients and vendors. A poorly worded message or incorrect punctuation in a letter or e-mail gives the reader a negative impression of the sender and thus the clinic. A medical assistant needs to know how to correctly write a letter or message to others. It is important that the sentence structure and tone of the message are professional.

Parts of Speech

A noun is a word or phrase for a person, place, thing, or idea (Table 7-3). A common noun is a general group of people, places, things, and ideas (e.g., desk, office) and a proper noun names a specific person, place or thing (e.g., Zachary, Boston). A proper noun should start with a capital letter. A pronoun is a word that takes the place of a noun (e.g., I, he, she, it, and they).

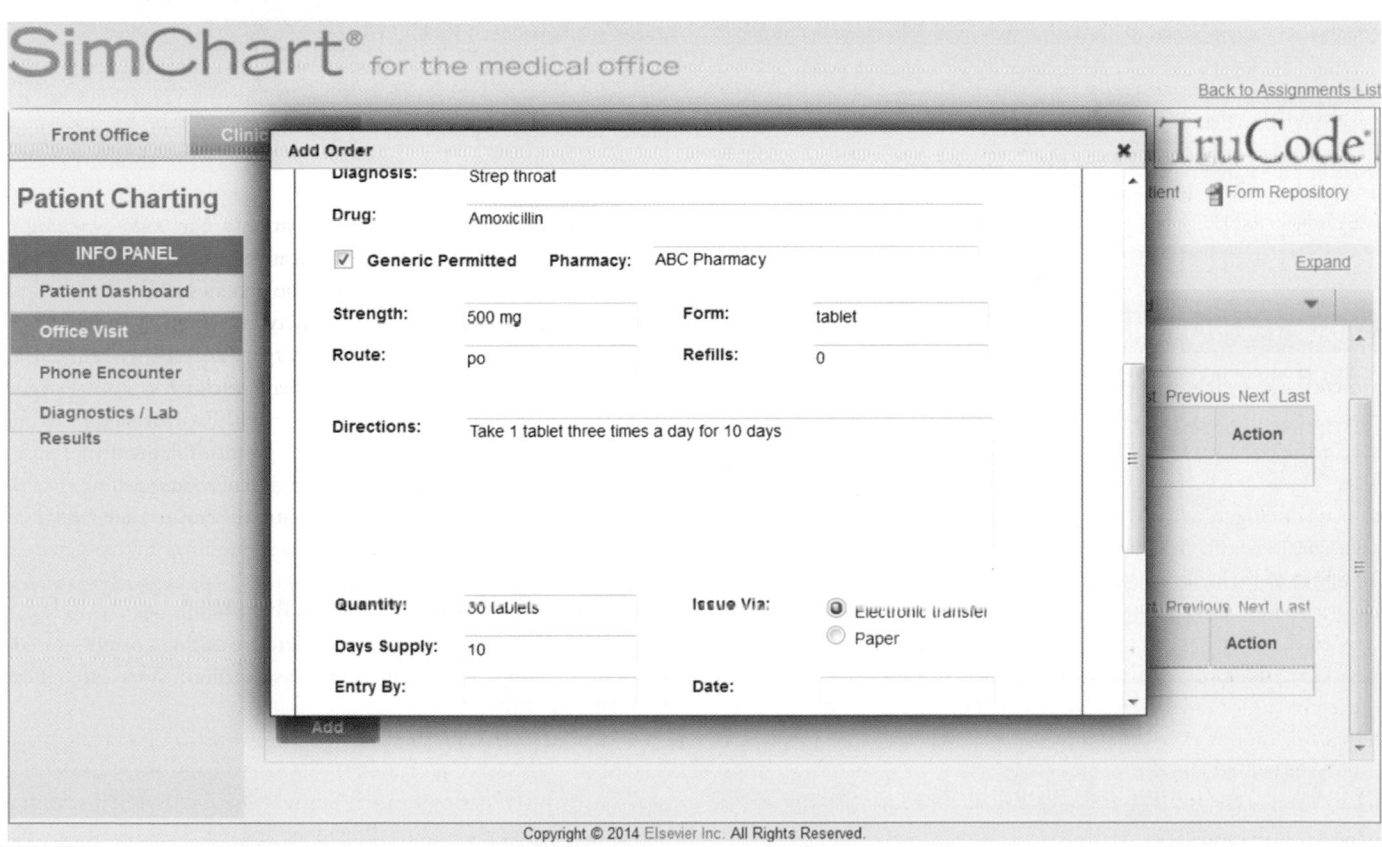

FIGURE 7-13 With e-prescribing, providers can enter the prescription information into the EHR and send it to the pharmacy. The pharmacist can easily read the information, which reduces the chance of errors.

A verb is a word or a phrase that shows action or a state of being (e.g., talks, walks, is, and are) (see Table 7-3). In a sentence the subject is a noun, pronoun, or set of words that performs the verb action (see Table 7-3). A sentence requires at least one main clause, which contains an independent subject and verb that expresses a complete thought. A fragment is a phrase without a main clause and is a major error in writing (Table 7-4). When the medical assistant composes written communication, it is important to make sure the subject and verb agree. A singular subject (e.g., provider, patient) must be matched with a singular verb (e.g., is, reads, goes). A plural subject (e.g., providers, patients) must be paired with a plural verb (e.g., are, read, go) (Table 7-4).

Many sentences also include dependent clauses, phrases, adjectives, adverbs, and prepositions. Dependent clauses often begin with words such as although, since, when, because, and if. Dependent clauses need an independent clause (e.g., subject and verb) to be a complete sentence (see Table 7-3). A phrase is a group of words without a subject or verb (see Table 7-3). An adjective is a word or group of words that describes a noun or pronoun. Adjectives come before or after the noun or pronoun they describe (see Table 7-3). An adverb is a word or group of words that answers how, where, when, or to what extent, thus further describing a verb, adjective, or other adverbs (see Table 7-3). A preposition is a word that indicates a relationship or a location between a noun or pronoun and the rest of the sentence. Examples of prepositions include near, beside, about, to, with, by, after, and in. A preposition must be accompanied by a related pronoun or noun (see Table 7-3).

CRITICAL THINKING APPLICATION   7-11

Christiana needs to compose a letter. How can she be sure she doesn't have any incomplete sentences in her letter? What parts of speech are required for a complete sentence?

Appropriate Use of Words

When you compose professional communications in the ambulatory care center, it is important to use language the reader will understand. Refrain from slang, generational terms, and abbreviations used with electronic communication. These can cause miscommunication with the reader. The medical assistant should know the proper use of commonly confused words and misspelled phrases (Table 7-5). Homonyms (i.e., words that sound alike) can lead to mistakes and may not always be identified by word processing software's spell-checker (Table 7-6).

A common mistake when communicating is a mismatch between the noun and pronoun number. When referring to plural nouns, use plural pronouns, such as *we, us, you, they,* and *them.* Singular pronouns, such as *I, me, you, she, her, he, him,* and *it,* should be used when referring to a singular noun. For example, "When the receptionist answers the phone, they need to be polite." The *receptionist* is a singular noun, but *they* is a plural pronoun. The noun and pronouns should agree in number, as in this example: "When receptionists answer the phones, they need to be polite."

To ensure that the message is clear to the reader, refrain from using two negatives in the same sentence. Refrain from using vague expressions or overusing the same words within a paragraph. Avoid using run-on sentences, which contain several independent clauses together without the required punctuation. Proper spelling, use of words, and sentence structure are important because they reflect on the writer and the healthcare practice.

Capitalization, Numbers, and Punctuation

Part of composing written communication is using correct capitalization and punctuation. As mentioned earlier, errors can reflect

---

TABLE 7-3	Parts of Speech	
PART	EXAMPLE	USE
Noun	computer	The medical assistant used the *computer.*
Verb	greeted	The receptionist *greeted* the patient.
Subject	receptionist	The *receptionist* of the Orthopedic and Pediatric departments answers the phone.
Dependent clause	because the patient felt sick	The receptionist immediately notified the clinical medical assistant *because the patient felt sick.*
Phrase	warm exam room	A *warm exam room* helps keep the patient comfortable during a physical exam.
Adjective	warm	The *warm* room was full of patients.
Adverb	softly	The patient spoke *softly.*
Preposition	beside	The student sat *beside* the receptionist.

TABLE 7-4	Common Grammatical Errors	
ERROR	INCORRECT	CORRECT
Fragment or incomplete sentence	*Greeted patients before she updating their information.*	*The receptionist always* greeted patients before she updated their information.
Nonagreement of subject and verb	The medical assistant talk to the patient.	The medical assistant *talks* to the patient.
	The patients is waiting for the doctor.	The patients *are* waiting for the doctor.

Commonly Misspelled Words and Phrases	
Anyway (not *anyways*)	Toward (not *towards*)
Supposed to (not *suppose to*)	Used to (not *use to*)

TABLE 7-5 Commonly Confused Words

WORDS	EXAMPLES
As: used in comparisons Has: to possess, own, or experience	She is *as* fast as he is on the keyboard. The medical assistant *has* increased his keyboarding speed by using the computer every day.
Lie: to recline or rest on a surface Lay: to put or place	I *lie* down to sleep. I *lay* down the book.
Set: to put or place Sit: to be seated	She *set* the gown on the table for the patient. *Sit* on the table when you have changed into a gown.
Who: refers to people; he or she did an action Whom: refers to him or her	*Who* placed the order for supplies? Mike saw *whom* yesterday?
That: refers to people, things, and groups of people Which: refers to things or groups	The letters *that* are on the printer need to be signed. The letters, *which* are on the printer, need to be signed.
Like: means "similar to" As: means "in the same manner" and requires a verb	The child is *like* her mother. He works *as* a phlebotomist.
Farther: refers to a measurable distance Further: refers to an abstract length	The clinic is *farther* away than I thought. *Further* research is needed before we purchase a new computer.

TABLE 7-6 Meanings of Common Homonyms

HOMONYMS	EXAMPLES
Affect (verb): to influence or transform Effect (noun): a result, outcome, consequence, or appearance	The outbreak of influenza will *affect* our patients. The *effect* of influenza was devastating to the city.
Accept (verb): to receive Except (preposition): excluding	Will you *accept* this certified letter? She mailed all the envelopes, *except* the certified letter.
Than (conjunction): used to compare Then (adverb): tells when	The receptionist was busier *than* the clinical medical assistant. The receptionist finished registering the patient and *then* she scheduled the appointment.
There (adverb): indicates place Their (pronoun): indicates possession They're (contraction): they are	*There* were 25 chairs in the reception area. *Their* children remained in the reception area. *They're* the only patients in the reception area.
Your (pronoun): indicates possession You're (contraction): you are	*Your* new job is in Pediatrics. *You're* working in Pediatrics today.
To (preposition): indicates direction, action, or condition Too (adverb): means "also" Two (noun): number	She went *to* answer the phone. The medical assistant's phone was ringing, *too*. Her phone has *two* lines.
Where: to, at, or in what place Were (verb): past tense plural of "be" Wear (verb): to have something on your body	*Where* did the patient go? *Were* you finished? *Wear* the gown, please.

poorly on the writer and the ambulatory care center. Professional documents should contain correct capitalization, appropriate punctuation, and the right number format.

The first letter of the first word in a sentence or question should be capitalized. The pronoun "I" should be capitalized. The first letter of proper nouns, including names of people, months, institutions, organizations, countries, and national nouns and adjectives (e.g., French, British) should be capitalized. Common nouns (e.g., girls, women, boys, men) should not be capitalized unless the word is the first word of a sentence.

A few rules apply to writing numbers. Spell out all numbers at the beginning of a sentence. Hyphenate all compound numbers from 21 to 99 (e.g., twenty-three) and all written-out fractions (e.g., two-thirds). Use commas for figures with four or more digits (e.g., 1,234). It is not advised to include a decimal point or a dollar sign when writing out sums less than a dollar (e.g., 23¢). Use noon and midnight, instead of 12:00 PM and 12:00 AM. The format for AM and PM can vary: a.m. and p.m., am and pm, AM and PM, and with or without a space between the time and AM or PM.

A sentence can end with one of three types of punctuation, a period (.), a question mark (?), or an exclamation point (!). For a sentence that makes a statement, use a period. A period goes inside a closing quotation mark (e.g., "Thank you for coming in today."). Use a question mark after a direct question. For sentences that express strong emotion, use an exclamation point. An exclamation point is rarely used in professional written communication.

Commas are frequently used in written communication (Table 7-7). A semicolon (;) is a common punctuation mark used in professional letters and documentation. The semicolon is used before certain words (however, therefore, for example) and when separating phrases in a series (e.g., "The provider is running late; however, our first two patients cancelled this morning."). A colon (:) is used to introduce a series of items either in the sentence or bulleted. A colon is also used after the greeting or salutation in a professional letter. Quotation marks (" ") are used to set off direct quotes. These are used frequently when documenting a patient's chief complaint, the main reason for the patient's visit. When using quotation marks, the periods and commas go inside the quotation marks. An apostrophe (') is used to show ownership. To show plural possession, the apostrophe is placed after the "s" (e.g., patients'). These are the most common punctuation marks used in professional correspondence and in charting in a patient's health record.

Using the correct words and punctuation marks is important when composing written correspondence. To reduce the risk of errors, the medical assistant should also perform a spelling and grammar check and proofread the document before sending it out to the recipient. Many times the reader develops an impression of the writer, the employer, and the agency based solely on written correspondence.

WRITTEN CORRESPONDENCE

Medical assistants are responsible for communicating with vendors or supply companies. They are also required to send written communication to patients and other providers as directed by their provider-employers. Knowing how to compose a professional letter is an important skill for medical assistants. To compose a letter, you must know the correct content and location for the parts of the letter. Creating an e-mail requires the writer to follow business etiquette while composing the e-mail.

TABLE 7-7   Use of Commas

RULE	EXAMPLE
Use before a coordinator (*and, but, yet, nor, for, or, so*) that links two main clauses. Do not use a comma before a coordinator that links two names, words, or phrases.	The last patient left, and the receptionist locked the door.
Use to separate items in a list.	The medical assistant escorted the mother, the father, and the child to the exam room.
Use to separate two interchangeable adjectives.	The patient was a strong, healthy child.
Use after certain words at the start of a sentence (i.e., yes, no, hello).	Yes, the bill was correct.
Use to set off the name or title or an expression that interrupts the flow of the sentence.	Will you, Michaela, want an appointment in two weeks? I am, by the way, very excited about the job opportunity.
Use after a dependent clause that starts a sentence.	If you have any questions, let me know.
Use to separate the day from the year.	May 24, 20–
Use to separate the city from its state. (*This rule does not apply when addressing envelopes.*)	Madison, Wisconsin
Can be used to separate Sr. or Jr. from the person's name, but this is not mandatory.	Bob Smith, Sr. or Bob Smith Sr. Bob Smith, Sr., has arrived for his appointment.
Use after a degree or title and to enclose the degree or title if it appears in a sentence.	John Williams, M.D. John Williams, M.D., will be the speaker for the event.
Use to set off nonessential words or phrases.	Catherine, the newest secretary, has arrived. My brother, Keith, has an appointment to see Dr. Smith.
Use with direct quotations.	She stated, "I have waited too long." "Why," I asked, "do you want tomorrow off?"

Parts of a Professional Letter

A professional letter is produced on 8.5 × 11-inch paper or letterhead paper. The letter typically has 1 inch margins on all four sides. The entire letter should be written using single line spacing. Consistency in line spacing is important for a professional appearance. The font should be a simple, easy to read one, such as Times New Roman or Arial, in a 10- or 12-point size. Limit the use of boldface and italics in the letter.

Sender's Address

The sender's address is usually located in the letterhead (Figure 7-14). Most facilities use letterhead, either preprinted or created at the top of the document using the word processing software's header tool. Depending on the ambulatory care center, the letterhead may or may not include the provider's name. It should have the clinic's name, street address or post office box, city, state, and ZIP code. Some letterheads have additional clinic contact information, such as phone numbers, website address, and an e-mail address. If letterhead is not used for a professional letter, the sender's address is placed at the left margin, 1 inch from the top of the document. Use single spacing and include the facility's address, but not the sender's name because that is located in the closing section of the letter.

Date

All professional letters must include a date. The date location is either at the left or right margin or starts at the center point of the document (see Figure 7-14). The location depends on the type of letter format used (this is discussed later in the chapter). When using letterhead, the date line starts on the second line after the letterhead. If letterhead is not used, the date line starts on the second line below the sender's address. In either situation, there should be one blank line between the date and the last line of the letterhead or sender's address.

When typing the date, write out the name of the month, then the number of the day, followed by a comma and the four-digit year. Make sure to have a blank space between the month and the day and after the comma (e.g., May 14, 20–). Do not use "th" or "st" after the day (e.g., May 14th, 20–).

Inside Address

The inside address starts between the second to the tenth line below the date line, depending on the length of the letter (see Figure 7-14). If the body of the letter is long, leave one blank line between the date and the inside address. If the body is short, add up to nine blank lines between the date line and the first line of the inside address. The goal is to have the body of the letter centered vertically on the page.

The inside address is always left-justified, regardless of your letter style. It includes the recipient's name and title on the first line, department and agency follow, and the last lines include the street address, followed by the city, state, and ZIP code. Always address the letter to a specific person. If the letter relates to a minor patient, address the letter to the guardian of the patient. When writing out the person's name, include the person's personal title (e.g., Miss, Ms., Mrs., Mr., or Dr.). If you are unsure of a woman's title preference, use Ms. Use the U.S. Postal Service format and abbreviations for the address (Table 7-8). No comma is needed between the city and state.

TABLE 7-8	U.S. Postal Service Standard Street Suffix Abbreviations		
Alley	ALY	Drive	DR
Avenue	AVE	Estate	EST
Boulevard	BLVD	Highway	HWY
Bridge	BRG	Parkway	PKWY
Bypass	BYP	Road	RD
Center	CTR	Route	RTE
Circle	CIR	Street	ST
Court	CT	Terrace	TER
Crossing	XING	Way	WAY

Use the two-letter abbreviations for the states. For all other abbreviations in the address, use only approved abbreviations. For international addresses, type the name of the country in capital letters on the last line.

Reference Line

The reference line may be used occasionally. It starts on the second line below the inside address at the left margin. The salutation then is placed on the second line below the reference line. The purpose of the reference line is to refer to a specific item, such as a file, case number, or product number, and provides easy reference for the reader and sender (e.g., Reference: Invoice #44549).

Salutation

The salutation is the greeting. It starts on the second line below the inside address and is always left-justified (see Figure 7-14). For business letters, the salutation should be formal. "Dear" is followed by the person's title and name and then ends with a colon (e.g., Dear Mr. Smith:). Some clinics, when addressing patient letters, also include the person's first name (e.g., Dear Mr. Ted Smith:). If the person's gender is not known, use the first and last name without the title (e.g., Dear Chris Smith:). The phrase "To Whom It May Concern" can also be used if a person's name is not known.

Subject Line

This notation, which is not used very often, would be left-justified and placed on the second line below the salutation. The body of the letter starts on the second line below the subject line. The purpose of the subject line is to state the main subject of the letter. The subject line should be composed using bold face, underlining, or all capital letters because this would draw the reader's attention (SUBJECT: ORDER NO. 45677-93).

Body of the Letter

The body of the letter starts on the second line below the salutation (see Figure 7-14). Depending on the type of letter, the body may be either left-justified or left-justified with each paragraph indented. There should be one blank line between paragraphs. The body of the

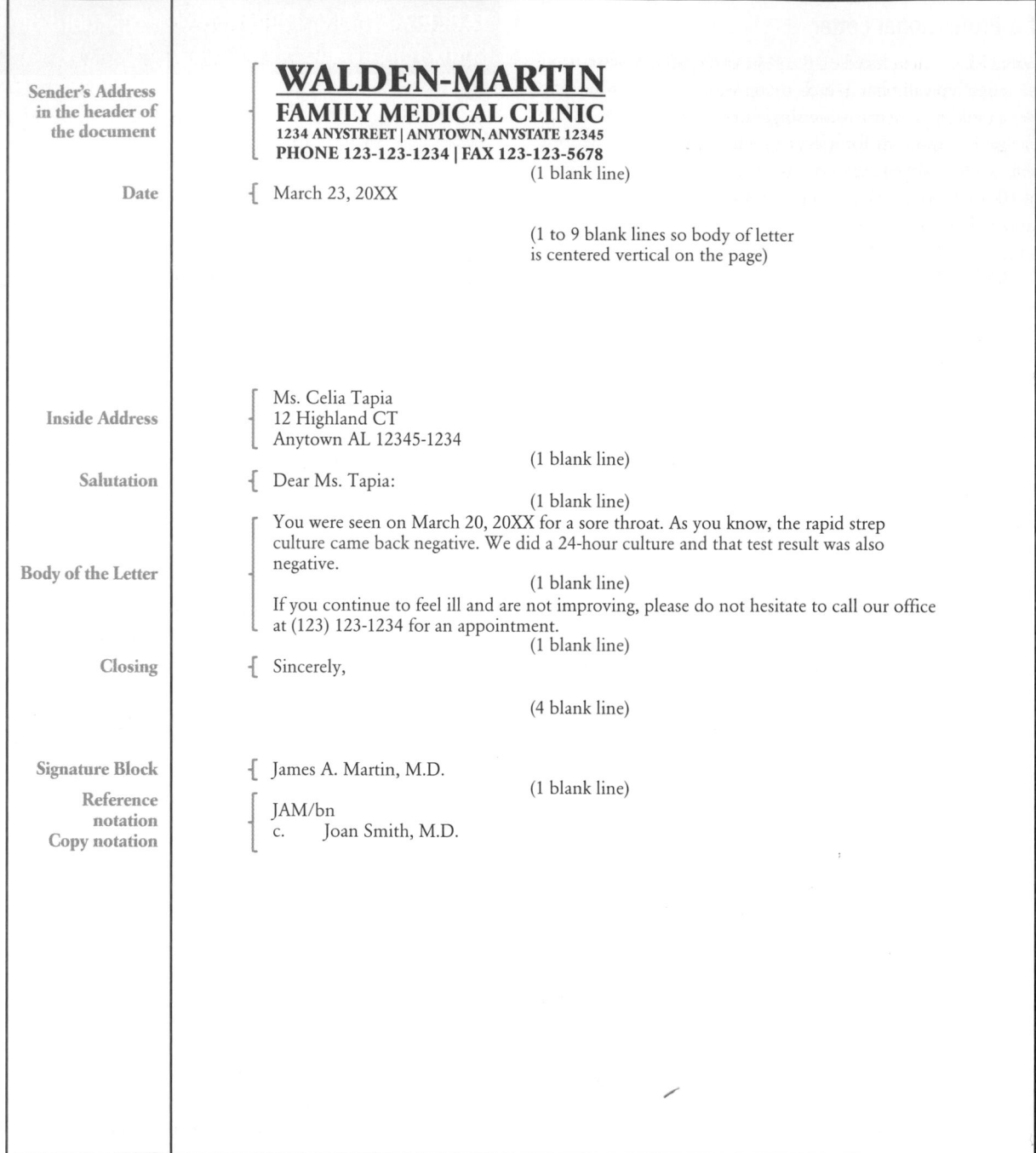

Sender's Address in the header of the document	**WALDEN-MARTIN** **FAMILY MEDICAL CLINIC** **1234 ANYSTREET | ANYTOWN, ANYSTATE 12345** **PHONE 123-123-1234 | FAX 123-123-5678**
	(1 blank line)
Date	March 23, 20XX
	(1 to 9 blank lines so body of letter is centered vertical on the page)
Inside Address	Ms. Celia Tapia 12 Highland CT Anytown AL 12345-1234
	(1 blank line)
Salutation	Dear Ms. Tapia:
	(1 blank line)
Body of the Letter	You were seen on March 20, 20XX for a sore throat. As you know, the rapid strep culture came back negative. We did a 24-hour culture and that test result was also negative.
	(1 blank line)
	If you continue to feel ill and are not improving, please do not hesitate to call our office at (123) 123-1234 for an appointment.
	(1 blank line)
Closing	Sincerely,
	(4 blank line)
Signature Block	James A. Martin, M.D.
	(1 blank line)
Reference notation **Copy notation**	JAM/bn c. Joan Smith, M.D.

FIGURE 7-14 Business letter format. When a medical assistant types a letter for a provider, the letter must be signed by that provider after it has been printed.

letter should be vertically in the middle of the page. Depending on the size of the letter, additional blank lines may be added after the date and before the inside address to move the body to the center of the page.

The body of the letter contains the content of the letter. The first paragraph is a friendly opening and states the purpose of the letter. The remaining paragraphs support the purpose of the letter and should be concise. The final paragraph may give a request for a specific action.

Closing

The closing is positioned vertically in the same position as the date (see Figure 7-14). There should be one blank line between the last line of the body of the letter and the closing. The first word should include a capital letter, although remaining words in the closing should be in lower case. Typically, "Sincerely" is used; more formal closings include "Yours truly" or "Very truly yours." The word or phrase is followed by a comma.

Signature Block

The signature block includes the signature, typed name, and title of the sender. There should be four blank lines between the closing and the typed name and credentials of the sender. This space allows the person to sign the letter. The person's title is capitalized and on the line directly below the typed name (e.g., Director of Walden-Martin Family Medicine Clinic). If the medical assistant typed the letter for a provider, the letter must be signed by that individual after it has been printed (see Figure 7-14).

CRITICAL THINKING APPLICATION   **7-12**

Christiana is composing several letters. Who would sign each letter?
- A letter to a patient indicating her test results.
- A letter to a vendor asking for specific pricing for a new computer.
- A letter to a referring physician, thanking him for the patient referral.

End Notations

Several items may be noted on the letter after the signature block. This may vary from agency to agency.
- The reference notation notes the initials of the person who composed the letter (e.g., MR) followed by the initials of the person who typed the letter (e.g., bn) (see Figure 7-14). A colon (:) or a forward slash (/) divides the two sets of initials (e.g., MR:bn, MR/bn). This notation should be left-justified on the second line below the last line of the signature block.
- The enclosure/attachment notation indicates the number of documents or attachments that accompany the letter. The enclosure notation is left-justified and starts on the second line below the reference notation. If the reference notation is not present, the enclosure notation is placed on the second line below the last line of the signature block. The enclosure notation can be typed in several ways. It can be indicated with either "Enclosure" or "Enc." If more than one enclosure is sent, the number of enclosures or the names of the enclosures should be indicated.
- The copy notation (c.) is used to notify the letter's recipient who also received a copy of the letter. The "c" is left-justified and goes on the line immediately following the last notation. It is then followed by a period. Use the tab tool to move ½ inch before typing the person's name (e.g., c. John Smith). Additional names should be aligned vertically on the document. You may still see letters that have "cc:," which means carbon copy or courtesy copy. Before computers and copy machines, duplicate letters were created by using carbon sheets placed between papers, thus creating carbon copies. With computers, "c." means "copy."
- Blind copy (bc.) is used if the sender does not want the recipient to know a copy was sent to another person. The format is the same as "c.," but the "bc." is added only to the office copy of the letter, not to the letter going to the recipient.

CRITICAL THINKING APPLICATION   **7-13**

For the letters that Christiana will sign, should she include a reference notation at the bottom of the letter? Why or why not? For the letters prepared by Christiana and signed by Dr. Brown, should she add the reference notation? Why or why not?

Suggested Styles for an Enclosure Notation

Any of the following three formats can be used to indicate that an enclosure is included with the letter:

Enclosures: 2

Enclosures (2)

Enclosures:
1. Draft of the policy statement
2. Invoice #45433

Continuation Pages

If the letter requires more than one page, the subsequent pages should be on paper that matches the letter but does not have the letterhead printing. Usually, letterhead paper is 20 to 24 lb bond paper (e.g., the thicker the paper, the larger the lb bond number). Each sheet after the letterhead must have a heading that includes these elements on separate lines: the recipient's name, the page number, and the date. The name should be on the first line below the top margin, and all three elements should be left-justified.

> Ms. Celia Tapia
> Page 2
> March 23, 20–

Business Letter Formats

Three main formats are used to compose a business letter. The formats vary slightly in the position of certain elements of the letter. Although the location of the elements may change, the spacing between the elements remains the same (Table 7-9). It is important for a medical assistant to be able to compose a professional letter (Procedure 7-1).

Full Block Letter Format

The full block format is the most common type of business letter (Figure 7-15). All elements are left-justified, meaning the elements start at the left margin of the document. Typically for business letters, "closed" punctuation is used. Closed punctuation means the document is typed using the punctuation marks described earlier in this chapter. Closed punctuation gives the letter a professional appearance.

Informal full block–formatted letters can use open punctuation, which means minimal punctuation is used in the letter. The body is the only part of the letter that contains the normal grammatical punctuation. No punctuation appears in the sender's or inside addresses, date, salutation, and the closing. This is a current

TABLE 7-9   Business Letter Formats

LETTER TYPE	FORMAT WITH VARIATIONS
Full block format	• Left-justified: All elements • Professional business letters use "closed" punctuation • Informal letters can use "open" punctuation
Modified block format	• Left-justified: Sender's address (if not using letterhead) and inside address • Center point or right-justified: Date, closing, and signature block start
Semi-block format (or modified block with indented paragraphs)	• Left-justified: Sender's address (if not using letterhead) and inside address • Center point or right-justified: Date, closing, and signature block start • Indented paragraphs 5 spaces

trend with electronic technology and letters produced by word processing, although it should not be used with professional letters.

Modified Block Letter Format

With the modified block format, the body and the inside address are left-justified. If letterhead is not used, the sender's address is also left-justified. The date, closing, and the signature block start either at the center point of the document or are right justified. If the center point is used, all three elements must start at that point (Figure 7-16). The text flows toward the right margin, and the three elements vertically line up in the document. When you use the right justified technique, the text for these three elements finish in a vertical line at the right margin (Figure 7-17).

Semi–Block Letter Format

The semi–block letter format can also be called the modified block with indented paragraphs (see Figure 7-17). The semi–block format resembles the modified block format with the three elements (i.e.,

---

PROCEDURE 7-1	Compose Professional Correspondence Using Electronic Technology: Compose a Professional Business Letter

Goal: *To compose a professional letter using technology.*

Scenario: *Create a letter for the following scenario: Jean Burke, NP, has requested that you compose a letter to Janine Butler (DOB 04/25/1968) and let her know that her mammogram from last Wednesday was negative. She should make a follow-up appointment in 6 months. If she has any questions, she should call the office. Janine's address is: 37 Park West Avenue, Anytown, AL 12345-1234. You are working at Walden-Martin Family Medical Clinic. The practice's address is: 1234 Anystreet, Anytown, AL 12345. The phone number is 123-123-1234 and the fax number is 123-123-5678.*

EQUIPMENT and SUPPLIES

- Patient's health record
- Computer with word processing software and printer
- Paper or letterhead paper
- #10 envelope

PROCEDURAL STEPS

1. Obtain the intended recipient's contact information and determine the message to convey to the recipient.
   PURPOSE: This gives you a focus when composing the letter. You will need the recipient's information to create the letter.
2. Using the computer and word processing software, compose the letter using one of the three business letter formats. If using blank paper, create a letterhead in the header of the document and include the clinic's name, street address or Post Office box, city, state, and ZIP code.
   PURPOSE: The information in the letterhead provides the reader contact information for the clinic.
3. Type the date in the correct location using the correct format. Have one blank line between the date line and the last line of the letterhead.
   PURPOSE: All letters require a date for legal purposes.

4. Type the inside address using the correct spelling, punctuation, and location for the information. Leave 1 to 9 blank lines between the date and the inside address, depending on the location of the body of the letter.
   PURPOSE: The body of the letter must be centered vertically from the top to the bottom of the document. More blank lines can be added to move the body to the correct location (see Figure 7-14).
5. Starting on the second line below the inside address, type the salutation, using the correct format.
   PURPOSE: A proper greeting helps set the tone of the letter.
6. Use your critical thinking skills to compose a concise, accurate message. Type the message in the body of the letter using the proper location and format. There should be a blank line after the salutation and between each paragraph. The message should be clear, concise, and professional. Use proper grammar, punctuation, capitalization, and sentence structure.
   PURPOSE: Proper grammar helps convey the message accurately and professionally.
7. Type a proper closing, leaving one blank line between the last line of the body and the closing. Use the correct format and location.
   PURPOSE: The closing helps end the message with a professional tone.

PROCEDURE 7-1 *—continued*

8. Type the signature block using the correct format and location. If a typist is preparing the letter for a provider, he or she must include a reference notation. There should be four blank lines between the closing and the signature block.
   <u>PURPOSE</u>: The signature block provides the reader with the name of the sender of the letter. The reference notation identifies who typed the letter.

9. Spell-check and proofread the document. Check for proper tone, grammar, punctuation, capitalization and sentence structure. Check for proper spacing between the parts of the letter.
   <u>PURPOSE</u>: The spell-checker identifies only certain errors; proofreading helps you find incorrect word use, improper tone, and errors in formatting.

10. Make any final corrections. Print the document on letterhead or on regular paper on which you have inserted the letterhead.

11. Address the envelope, using either the computer and word processing software or a pen and following the correct format. After addressing the envelope, give the letter with the envelope
    <u>PURPOSE</u>: Following the Post Office guidelines on format helps prevent a delay in delivery of the letter. The provider is the sender of the letter and should have the opportunity to review it before it is mailed to the patient.

12. File a copy of the letter in the paper medical record or upload an electronic copy of the letter to the electronic health record (EHR).
    <u>PURPOSE</u>: A copy of all correspondence should be kept in the patient's health record.

13. Fold the letter using the correct technique and place it in the envelope.

WALDEN-MARTIN
FAMILY MEDICAL CLINIC
1234 ANYSTREET | ANYTOWN, ANYSTATE 12345
PHONE 123-123-1234 | FAX 123-123-5678

March 23, 20XX

Ms. Celia Tapia
12 Highland CT
Anytown AL 12345-1234

Dear Ms. Tapia:

You were seen on March 20, 20XX for a sore throat. As you know, the rapid strep culture came back negative. We did a 24-hour culture and that test result was also negative.

If you continue to feel ill and are not improving, please do not hesitate to call our office at (123) 123-1234 for an appointment.

Sincerely,

James A. Martin, M.D.

JAM/bn
c.   Joan Smith, M.D.

FIGURE 7-15 Full block letter format.

WALDEN-MARTIN
FAMILY MEDICAL CLINIC
1234 ANYSTREET | ANYTOWN, ANYSTATE 12345
PHONE 123-123-1234 | FAX 123-123-5678
(1 blank line)
March 23, 20XX

(1 to 9 blank lines so body of letter
is centered vertical on the page)

Ms. Celia Tapia
12 Highland CT
Anytown AL 12345-1234
(1 blank line)
Dear Ms. Tapia:
(1 blank line)
You were seen on March 20, 20XX for a sore throat. As you know, the rapid strep
culture came back negative. We did a 24-hour culture and that test result was also
negative.
(1 blank line)
If you continue to feel ill and are not improving, please do not hesitate to call our office
at (123) 123-1234 for an appointment.
(1 blank line)
Sincerely,

(4 blank line)

James A. Martin, M.D.
(1 blank line)
JAM/bn
c.   Joan Smith, M.D.

FIGURE 7-16 Modified block letter format, showing the date, closing, and signature block starting at the center point of the document.

date, closing, and signature block) right-justified or starting at the center point of the document. The difference with the semi–block format is the indented paragraph or paragraphs in the body of the letter. The paragraphs should be indented five spaces.

Letter Templates

Using one of the business letter formats, a medical assistant can design a letter template, which is a sample letter that can be personalized for the patient. For routine communication with patients (e.g., normal laboratory results or appointment reminders), a letter template can be created. You can use the practice management software, EHR, or word processing software to merge the patient data into the letter template, creating an individualized letter for the patient. This is an efficient method of providing a customer-friendly document for a patient.

Preparing the Letter for Delivery

Business letters should be enclosed in business-sized envelopes, the standard #10 envelope, which is 4.125 × 9.5 inches. Business envelopes are available with a few variations, including the type of flap, preprinted return address, and a window envelope. The window envelope and the #6¾ envelope may be used for statements to patients. The envelopes can be white, manila, or made of recycled paper.

When the automated mail processing machine at the post office reads the envelope, it reads the bottom line of the recipient's address (i.e., city, state and ZIP code) before moving up and reading the next line. To ensure timely delivery, use the following tips when addressing mail:

- Type the envelope using a simple black font of at least 10-point size. Use all capital letters and no punctuation marks (Figure 7-18).
- Put one space between the city and state and two spaces between the state and ZIP code.
- If you can't fit the suite or apartment number on the same line as the delivery address, put it on the line above the delivery address, not below it.
- Use ZIP code + 4 code (e.g., 55555-1111) as often as possible. This allows the piece of mail to be directed to a more precise location than when just using the ZIP code.
- Do not put anything (e.g., logo, slogan, attention line) below the last line of the delivery address. The machine will read that and your letter may get misrouted or delayed.
- Use only approved U.S. Postal Service abbreviations.

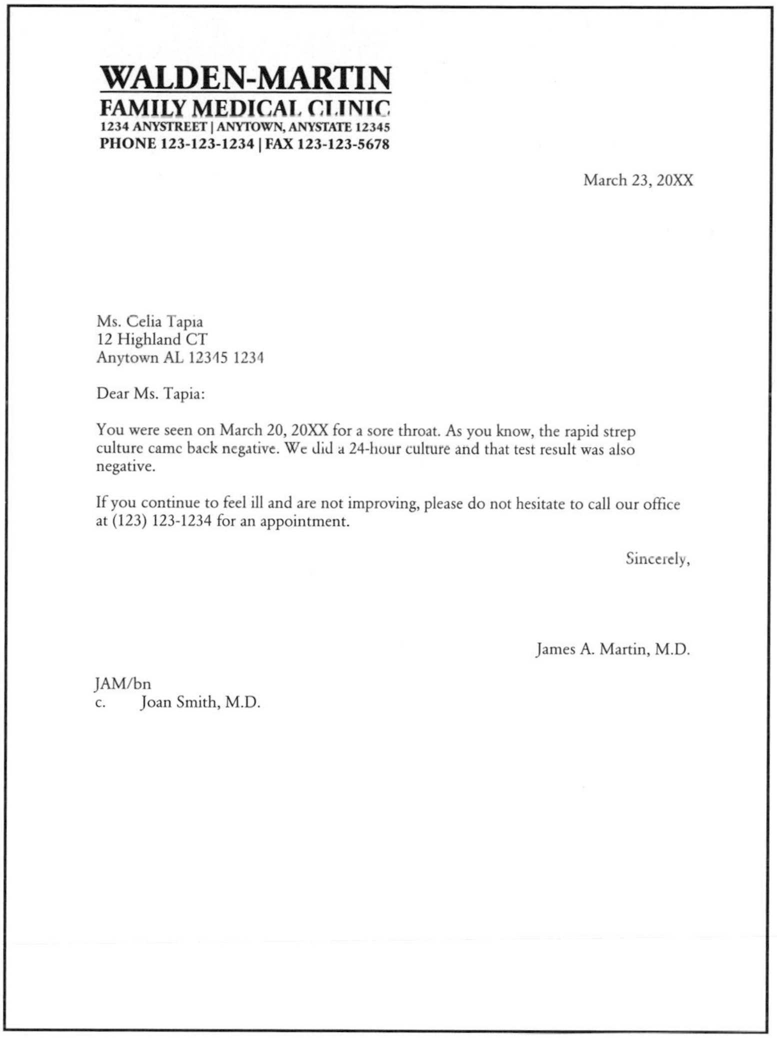

WALDEN-MARTIN
FAMILY MEDICAL CLINIC
1234 ANYSTREET | ANYTOWN, ANYSTATE 12345
PHONE 123-123-1234 | FAX 123-123-5678

March 23, 20XX

Ms. Celia Tapia
12 Highland CT
Anytown AL 12345 1234

Dear Ms. Tapia:

You were seen on March 20, 20XX for a sore throat. As you know, the rapid strep culture came back negative. We did a 24-hour culture and that test result was also negative.

If you continue to feel ill and are not improving, please do not hesitate to call our office at (123) 123-1234 for an appointment.

Sincerely,

James A. Martin, M.D.

JAM/bn
c.   Joan Smith, M.D.

FIGURE 7-17 Semi–block letter format (also called modified block with indented paragraph letter format). This letter uses right justification for the date, closing, and signature block.

The medical assistant should fold the letter by pulling up the bottom end of the letter until it reaches just below the inside address or two-thirds of the way up the letter. Crease the paper. Then fold the top of the letter down so it is flush with the bottom fold and crease the paper. For windowed business envelopes, fold the letter in a **Z** pattern. With the letter's print side facing up, place the envelope over the top third of the letter. Fold the bottom edge of the paper up to the bottom edge of the envelope and crease the paper. Then remove the envelope and flip the letter over so the backside of the document is facing up. Fold the top of the letter down to the prior crease line and crease the paper. The letterhead and recipient's addresses should then be visible. Place the letter in the envelope so that the recipient's address shows through the window.

Memorandums

Memorandums, or memos, are communication documents within an agency. They address one topic and provide a message to the reader. Use the **portrait orientation** for the document and 1-inch margins. Memorandums typically have four headings:

- **To**: Include the name of the recipient or recipients and omit the titles (e.g., Mr., Mrs.). For a number of recipients, each name can be followed by a comma, or each name can be on its own line.
- **From**: Include the name of the sender of the memo. It is optional if the sender initials the memo before it is sent.
- **Date**: Spell out the month and follow it with the day and year (e.g., May 23, 20–).
- **Subject**: Include the topic of the memo.

The headings are left-justified (Figure 7-19). Boldface and capital letters are used for the headings, and a colon (:) follows the heading. The information should be in regular font, with a mix of capital and small letters. The information should be aligned vertically down the page, using the tab tool in the word processing software. The date should be written out as indicated for professional letters.

The headings may be separated from the body of the memo by a centered black line that extends from 2 inches to the entire width of the page. Regardless if the line is used or not, there should be two to three blank lines separating the headers from the body of the memo. The body of the memo should be single-spaced and

Return Address
Use same format as the
delivery address

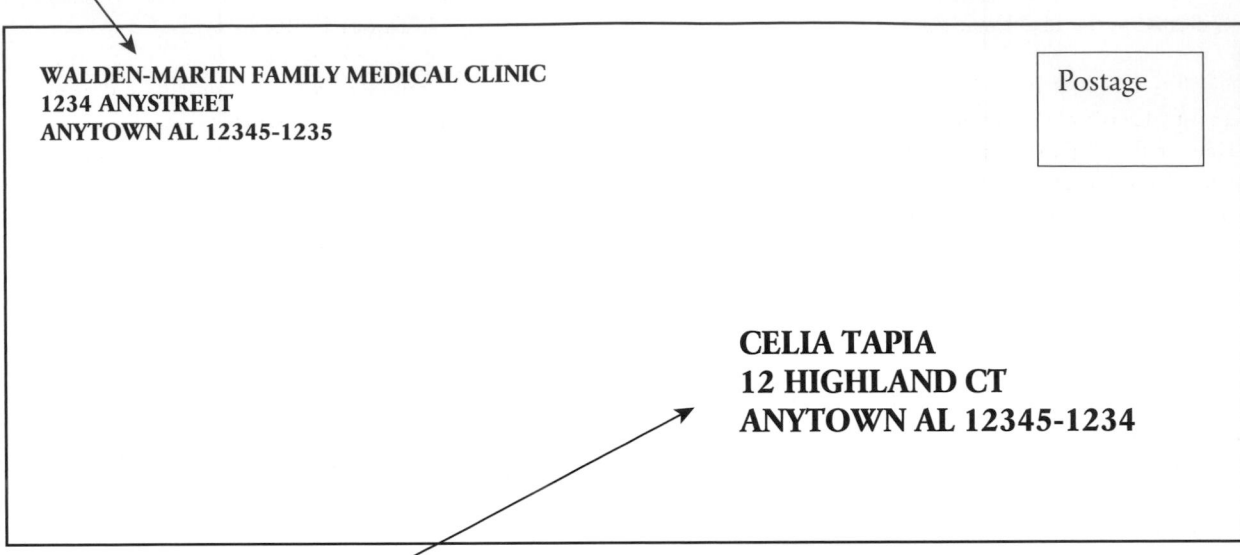

WALDEN-MARTIN FAMILY MEDICAL CLINIC
1234 ANYSTREET
ANYTOWN AL 12345-1235

Postage

CELIA TAPIA
12 HIGHLAND CT
ANYTOWN AL 12345-1234

Delivery Address
1st line: Recipient's Name
2nd line: Company name
3rd line: Post Office box or street address, including Apartment or Suite number
4th line: City, State (2 letter abbreviation), zip code

FIGURE 7-18 Address format for an envelope.

TO:	Staff
FROM:	James Martin, M.D.
DATE:	December 15, 20XX
SUBJECT:	Holiday Office Hours

The office will be closed at noon on December 24, 20XX through December 26th. We will reopen at our normal time on December 27, 20XX. We will then close at 3 p.m. on December 31st for the holiday and will reopen at our normal time on January 2, 20XX.

FIGURE 7-19 Format for a memorandum.

left-justified. If it consists of multiple paragraphs, skip a single line between paragraphs. The content in the body of the letter should be clear, concise, and informative. The writer does not need to add a closing or signature. Special notations, including reference, copy, and enclosures, can be added to the bottom of the memo and are formatted as indicated in the End Notations section.

Professional E-Mails

The use of electronic communication between the ambulatory care center staff and patients is increasing, and medical assistants need to know how to compose a professional e-mail (Procedure 7-2). Following e-mail etiquette is important for maintaining a customer-friendly environment. Tips on writing customer-friendly e-mails include:

- If you are sending the e-mail to several people, separate each e-mail address by a semicolon (;).
- Add an e-mail address to the cc line if another person needs to receive a courtesy copy of the e-mail.
- Make sure to include a subject on the subject line. Delete any messy FWD: or RE: RE: strings.
- Start with a greeting (salutation), which includes a formal greeting followed by the person's title and name (e.g., "Good morning, Mr. Jones," "Dear Mr. Jones,").
- Be courteous, polite, and respectful in your words and tone. Maintain the appropriate level of formality in the e-mail. Be gracious, using expressions such as "please" and "thank you."
- Refrain from using all capital letters because many people consider that to be "shouting" in e-mails.

PROCEDURE 7-2 | **Compose Professional Correspondence Utilizing Electronic Technology: Compose a Professional E-Mail**

Goal: *To compose a professional e-mail that conveys the message to the reader clearly, concisely, and accurately.*

Scenario: *Create an e-mail for the following scenario: Johnny Parker (DOB 06/15/2010) has an appointment at 10:00 AM. next Tuesday. Send his guardian an appointment reminder via e-mail. Johnny will be seeing Jean Burke, NP. The guardian should bring in any medications Johnny is currently taking. You are working at Walden-Martin Family Medical Clinic. The practice's address is: 1234 Anystreet, Anytown, AL 12345. The phone number is 123-123-1234 and the fax number is 123-123-5678. Your instructor will supply you with the guardian's name and e-mail address.*

EQUIPMENT and SUPPLIES

- Patient's health record
- Computer with e-mail software

PROCEDURAL STEPS

1. Obtain the intended recipient's contact information and determine the message to convey to the recipient.
   PURPOSE: This gives you a focus when composing the e-mail. You will need the recipient's information to create the e-mail.
2. Using the computer and e-mail software, type in the recipient's e-mail address. If the e-mail has two recipients, use a semicolon (;) after the name of the first recipient. Double-check the e-mail addresses for accuracy.
   PURPOSE: If the e-mail address is incorrect, the e-mail will not get to the recipient.
3. Type in a subject, keeping it simple but focused on the contents of the e-mail.
   PURPOSE: In many e-mail software packages, the user can search for e-mails using the subject field. Keeping the subject simple and focused makes it easier for the user to find the message.
4. Type a formal greeting, using correct punctuation.
   PURPOSE: A proper greeting helps set the tone of the letter.
5. Type the message in the body of the e-mail using proper grammar, punctuation, capitalization, and sentence structure. Avoid abbreviations. The message should be clear, concise, and professional.
   PURPOSE: Using proper grammar and avoiding abbreviations help convey the message accurately and professionally.

6. Finish the e-mail with closing remarks.
   PURPOSE: In the closing, you can thank the recipient or encourage him or her to follow up with concerns or questions. This gives the e-mail a professional tone.
7. Type a closing, followed by your name and title on the next line. Include the clinic's name and contact information below your name.
   PURPOSE: The e-mail clearly states who is sending it.
8. Spell-check and proofread the e-mail. Check for proper tone, grammar, punctuation, capitalization, and sentence structure. Check for proper spacing between the parts of the e-mail.
   PURPOSE: White space or spacing between the elements of an e-mail helps separate the parts of the e-mail, making it easier to read.
9. Make any final revisions, select any features to apply to the e-mail, and then send it.
   PURPOSE: If the e-mail is urgent (!), that feature should be selected before you send the e-mail. If you require a confirmation e-mail when the e-mail is opened, this can also be selected.
10. Print a copy of the e-mail to be filed in the paper medical record or upload an electronic copy of the e-mail to the patient's electronic health record (EHR).
    PURPOSE: A copy of all correspondence should be kept in the patient's health record.

- Write out the entire word and refrain from using abbreviations and emoticons.
- Use proper capitalization, grammar, sentence structure, and punctuation. Check the spelling of the e-mail before sending it. Most e-mail software has a spell-checker.
- Be concise, accurate, and clear in your message.
- Always end your e-mail with "Thank you" or "Sincerely" and your complete name. For business e-mails, include contact information after your name, including the agency's address, phone number, and fax number.
- Leave white space (i.e., one blank line) between the salutation, paragraphs, and your complete name.
- Zip large attachments before sending the files. **Zip** is a computer program that compresses a file or folder, making it smaller and easier to send. The receiver uses an unzip program to extract the contents.
- Many e-mail programs have features such as (!) urgent or a response box that sends an e-mail back to the sender when the e-mail is opened by the recipient. Use the urgent feature only for crucial e-mails.

CRITICAL THINKING APPLICATION   **7-14**

Christiana receives an e-mail from a patient that is in all capital letters. How might she perceive the situation with the patient? How could she verify her perceptions? How should she handle this situation?

Some healthcare facilities may also include language in e-mails related to confidentiality and whom to contact if the e-mail was sent to the wrong address. Medical assistants must adhere to the facility's confidentiality rules when communicating with or about patients. Copies of e-mail communications should be uploaded to the patient's EHR for a permanent record of the electronic communication.

EHR software frequently contains clinical messaging or clinical e-mail features. This feature is an e-mail within the EHR. The clinical messaging feature provides secure communication for healthcare employees to converse about the patient. For instance, the message may be sent from the receptionist to the medical assistant regarding a patient who called requesting a refill. The medical assistant can then follow up with the provider regarding the refill.

Faxed Communication

Fax (short for facsimile) machines send and receive documents using the phone lines. In the healthcare facility, the fax machine may be part of a copy machine, or the computers may have software that allows faxes to be sent and received. As communications technology has advanced, the use of fax machines has decreased, but they are still an important piece of equipment in the ambulatory care center.

When sending a fax, you must adhere to HIPAA and HITECH rules. Healthcare facilities usually have a required face sheet (the first sheet) that includes confidentiality language, which instructs the recipient, if he or she is not the intended party, to destroy the fax and contact the medical facility. Besides the confidentiality statement, the face sheet should include the contact information for sender and recipient, the date, and the total number of pages.

CLOSING COMMENTS

Patient Education

If the medical assistant is responsible for preparing patient education materials using the computer's word processing program, it is important that these materials contain correct grammar, spelling, punctuation, and sentence structure. The appearance of brochures and documents created by the ambulatory care center staff reflects on the medical practice. The medical assistant should proofread all documents carefully before printing them.

Legal and Ethical Issues

The medical assistant should keep a copy of all documents produced using word processing. A copy of any document sent to a patient must also be uploaded into the patient's EHR. All patient-related documents are confidential, and the medical assistant must ensure the security and privacy of the information.

Professional Behaviors

Written communication in any form requires the medical assistant to be respectful, polite, and professional. It is important to proofread all written communication before it is sent to the recipient. Spell-checker tools can help identify misspelled words and sometimes incorrect usage of grammar and punctuation. However, these tools cannot always identify a word used incorrectly; only proofreading can capture those errors. Proofreading also allows the reader to reassess the tone of the communication, making sure it is appropriate. Finally, the medical assistant should recheck the spelling of the person's name and address for accuracy. A well-composed message gives the reader a reassuring sense of the accuracy and professionalism of the healthcare facility's staff.

SUMMARY OF SCENARIO

Since her promotion, Christiana has learned many helpful administrative and computer procedures. She also has been implementing changes in the administrative area. Her first change was to e-mail, rather than mail, appointment reminders. She uses the appointment reminder feature of the practice management software when e-mailing the notifications to patients. Not only does this save time for the practice, but it also saves postage costs. Christiana also has learned how to create letter and memo templates. She uses templates to notify patients about laboratory and diagnostic test results. She continues to create custom letters for patients, yet saves time by using predesigned templates.

Christiana has learned a great deal about the medical practice's computer network, and she is implementing more security measures. For example, she is training staff members to log out of their workstations before leaving the computer. She also is working with a local IT company to beef up the network's protection against unauthorized users. She has contracted with an online backup service to protect the network files.

Christiana enjoys her new position and knows that she will need to stay up to date on technologic changes and privacy mandates. She plans to do this by reading online articles and attending continuing education events. She realizes that learning is an ongoing process that can help her become the professional she strives to be every day.

SUMMARY OF LEARNING OBJECTIVES

1. **Define, spell, and pronounce the terms listed in the vocabulary.**
   Spelling and pronouncing medical terms correctly reinforce the medical assistant's credibility. Knowing the definitions of these terms promotes confidence in communication with patients and co-workers.

2. **Explain what a personal computer is, and identify input and output hardware for personal computers.**
   A personal computer (PC) is a relatively inexpensive piece of hardware that is used by a single person. It can be a desktop, laptop, or tablet computer. The medical assistant should be knowledgeable about input and output hardware used in the healthcare environment. As technology advances, more input devices will be used in ambulatory care facilities. Medical assistants may need to help coach patients in the use of such devices if the healthcare agency has patients electronically enter personal data.

3. **Identify internal computer components, secondary storage devices, and network and Internet access devices.**
   Because medical assistants can have a variety of roles in ambulatory care centers, they must understand important computer features. Learning the names and functions of the internal components better equips medical assistants to purchase computers or deal with computer issues. Learning about secondary storage devices helps them identify what is needed by the ambulatory care practice. The computers and output devices in a healthcare facility are usually all connected to the clinic's network, which can be called the local area network (LAN). A router is used to allow multiple devices to be used on the same network. For the computer network to have Internet access, the ambulatory care center must subscribe to an Internet services provider and be connected to a modem.

4. **Explain how to maintain computer hardware.**
   Computer hardware should be located on a stable, even surface away from heat sources. Keep ventilation slots clear. Before cleaning the computer or peripheral components, turn off and unplug the device. To remove the grime and dirt, use a damp, lint-free cloth to wipe the hardware's casing. All vents and air holes should be wiped clean. For glass monitor screens, spray a household glass cleaner on a lint-free cloth and then wipe the monitor. For nonglare monitors or antiglare screens, just use a lint-free cloth dampened with water. To disinfect the keyboard, spray a disinfectant on a lint-free cloth or use a disinfectant cloth and wipe each key. To remove the dirt from the keyboard, turn the keyboard upside down and gently shake it to remove dirt or use compressed air dusters.

5. **Identify principles of ergonomics that apply to a computer workstation.**
   When sitting at a workstation, your torso and neck should be vertical and in line. The chair should be adjusted so that your feet are flat on the floor or a footrest and your legs are comfortably below the workstation. The backrest lumbar support area should be fitted to the small of your back, and it should help support the upper body in the upright position. The seat pan should be the appropriate size and height to accommodate your body build so that there is no added pressure on the back of the knees or thighs. The armrest should support the forearms with the shoulders in a relaxed position. For standing workstations, your legs, torso, head, and neck should be vertical and in line. One foot can be elevated on a step.

   The monitor should be directly in front of you and tilted to avoid glare. The top of the monitor should be at or just below eye level, to prevent bending of the head or neck. Use a document holder to prevent continual movement of the head. The keyboard should be an ergonomic split-key or waved model if possible and placed at a height and an angle that allow the wrists to be in a neutral position. The work surface and mouse should be at elbow level for typing. The wrists should be supported by a foam wrist rest. Headsets should be used for those answering frequent phone calls to prevent muscle strain.

6. **Differentiate between:**
   - *System software and application software.*
     System software is a collection of programs that operate and control the computer. Operating systems and utility software are two types

Continued

SUMMARY OF LEARNING OBJECTIVES—*continued*

of system software. The system software loads on the computer and operates in the background while other application software is used. Application software allows the user or other application programs to perform specific tasks. Application software may consist of a single program or a collection of programs. Examples of application software include word processing, spreadsheets, telecommunication, antimalware, and databases.

- *Electronic medical records (EMRs) and a practice management system.* As more ambulatory care facilities move to EMRs, electronic health records (EHRs), and practice management software, the medical assistant should be able to distinguish between the EMR and the practice management system. The EMR is used to document patient-related information, whereas the practice management software is used to run the "business." Scheduling, billing, and coding programs are part of the practice management software typically used in the healthcare agency.

7. **Explain the importance of data backup and other computer network security activities performed in the healthcare setting.**
   To abide by HIPAA rules and the meaningful use requirement, healthcare agencies must ensure that their computer networks are secure. Data backup procedures can help prevent problems if the network files are compromised by a hacker or an environmental situation (e.g., fire or flood).

8. **Discuss applications of electronic technology.**
   With the advances in technology, the healthcare environment has seen many changes, including portable devices in the exam room, improved procedural equipment, and increased efficiencies in the workday through the use of computers. More changes in technology will occur over the next few years; some will help healthcare institutions stay compliant with HIPAA, whereas others will support quicker and more accurate treatment of patients. Being flexible and willing to use new technology will be critical for medical assistants in the future.

9. **Recognize the elements of fundamental writing skills.**
   Medical assistants need to compose correspondence to patients and other businesses. They also need to create memos, meeting minutes, and other

documents. Knowing the parts of speech helps medical assistants create complete sentences, which are crucial for professional written communications. It is also imperative to understand the appropriate use of words.

10. **Explain the guidelines for using capitalization, numbers, and punctuation in business communication.**
    Knowing the guidelines for using capitalization, numbers, and punctuation in business communication is crucial when composing professional documents. Correct word usage and spelling also are critical. The medical assistant should use the spell-checker in the word processing software when creating documents. Proofreading as a final step is also important to catch any incorrect words or incomplete sentences.

11. **Describe each component of a professional business letter.**
    Medical assistants should be familiar with the components or elements of a professional business letter. They must include the appropriate information and punctuation in each section of the letter to achieve professional results. Proper and consistent spacing in the letter provides the polished, professional appearance for which medical assistants should strive when creating letters through word processing.

12. **Summarize the formats for business letters and memorandums.**
    Written communication from a healthcare facility is a reflection on that facility. Using the proper format for business letters and e-mails is crucial for professional results. There are three main types of business letters: full block letter format, modified block letter format, and semi–block letter format. Procedure 7-1 provides guidance for composing a professional letter. Even though memos are internal documents, the medical assistant must use the correct format so that the reader obtains a clear message. A poorly created memo is a reflection on the writer.

13. **Compose professional correspondence using electronic technology.**
    With more patients communicating by e-mail with the ambulatory care staff, medical assistants must be able to write professional e-mails. E-mails must send a clear message to the recipient in a professional and respectful manner. The process of composing a professional e-mail is outlined in Procedure 7-2. When sending a fax, the medical assistant must follow HIPAA and HITECH rules.

CONNECTIONS

📖 Study Guide Connection: Go to the Chapter 7 Study Guide. Read and complete the activities.

evolve Evolve Connection: Go to the Chapter 7 link at *evolve.elsevier.com/kinn* to complete the Chapter Review Quiz. Check out the other resources listed for this chapter to make the most of what you have learned from Technology and Written Communication.

TELEPHONE TECHNIQUES

8

SCENARIO

Ashlynn McDowell, a recent graduate of a medical assisting program, has begun her first position as a receptionist in an obstetrician's office. Ashlynn's lifelong goal has been to work in obstetrics, and she is determined to perform to the best of her abilities. However, she has never held a job in a professional office. She knows that she needs to practice all the skills she learned in school to be an effective receptionist.

Ashlynn works for Dr. Stella Frank, who is customer service–oriented and wants her patients to feel cared for and special. She insists that all their concerns be taken seriously. Ashlynn is anxious to build trust with the patients and offer them help with the problems they encounter that fall within her realm of responsibility.

Dr. Frank recently purchased computer software that allows Ashlynn to record telephone messages on the computer, and these messages are automatically routed both to an inbox for the provider and as an entry in the patient's health record. Although the system is new to everyone in the office, Ashlynn is determined to become proficient in its use as quickly as possible.

She knows that she must speak clearly and distinctly and must be adept at follow-up skills. She plans to dress professionally each day so that she projects the right image to the patients with whom she comes in contact. Ashlynn will strive to be the type of employee who has a willingness to learn, an ability to adapt, and a heart full of compassion for the patient. She is a team player who sincerely wants to cooperate with other staff members who might need her help.

Dr. Frank is pleased that she has found such an eager person to add to her staff and will assist and guide Ashlynn as she learns how to make the patients feel like part of the clinic family. Ashlynn's self-esteem has increased because she feels she is making a great contribution to healthcare.

While studying this chapter, think about the following questions:
- Why does tone of voice play an important role in patient perception?
- What can a medical assistant do to promote a positive image of the healthcare facility when using the telephone with patients?
- How can the medical assistant reduce patients' frustration with telephone issues?

LEARNING OBJECTIVES

1. Define, spell, and pronounce the terms listed in the vocabulary.
2. Identify and explain the features of a multiple-line telephone system, and also explain how each can be used effectively in a healthcare facility.
3. Do the following related to effective use of the telephone:
   - Discuss the telephone equipment needed by a healthcare facility.
   - Summarize active listening skills.
   - Demonstrate effective and professional telephone techniques.
   - Consider the importance of tone of voice and enunciation.
4. Explain the importance of thinking ahead when managing telephone calls; also, describe the correct way to answer the telephone in the office.
5. Discuss the screening of incoming calls, and list several questions to ask when handling an emergency call.
6. Do the following related to taking a message:
   - Document telephone messages accurately.
   - List the seven elements of a correctly handled telephone message.
   - Report relevant information concisely and accurately.
7. Discuss various types of common incoming calls and how to deal with each.
8. Discuss various types of special incoming calls and how to deal with each.
9. Discuss how the medical assistant should handle various types of difficult calls.
10. Discuss typical outgoing calls, including why knowledge of time zones and long distance calling is necessary.
11. Discuss the use of a telephone directory, and describe how answering services and automatic call routing systems are used in a healthcare facility.
12. Discuss the legal and ethical issues related to telephone techniques.

VOCABULARY

answering service A commercial service that answers telephone calls for its clients.

automatic call routing A system that distributes incoming calls to a specific group or person based on customer need; for example, the customer presses 1 for appointments, 2 for billing questions, and so on.

call forwarding A telephone feature that allows calls made to one number to be forwarded to another specified number.

caller ID A feature that identifies and displays the telephone numbers of incoming calls made to a particular line.

conference call A telephone call in which a caller can speak with several people at the same time.

emergency An unexpected, life-threatening situation that requires immediate action.

enunciation The use of articulate, clear sounds when speaking.

headset A set of headphones with a microphone attached, used especially in telephone communication.

intercom A two-way communication system with a microphone and loudspeaker at each station; often a feature of business telephones.

jargon The technical terminology or characteristic idioms of a particular group or special activity, as opposed to common, everyday terms.

monotone A succession of syllables, words, or sentences spoken in an unvaried key or pitch.

multiple-line telephone system A business telephone system that allows for more than one telephone line.

participating provider A physician or other healthcare provider who enters into a contract with a specific insurance company or program and by doing so agrees to abide by certain rules and regulations set forth by that particular third-party payer.

pitch The depth of a tone or sound; a distinctive quality of sound.

provider An individual or company that provides medical care and services to a patient or the public.

screen Something that shields, protects, or hides; to select or eliminate through a screening process.

speakerphone A telephone with a loudspeaker and a microphone; it can be used without having to pick up and hold the handset.

speed dialing A telephone function in which a selected stored number can be dialed by pressing only one key.

STAT The medical abbreviation for the Latin term *statum,* meaning immediately; at this moment.

tactful The quality of having a keen sense of what to do or say to maintain good relations with others or to prevent offense.

triage The process of assigning degrees of urgency to patients' conditions.

urgent An acute situation that requires immediate attention but is not life-threatening.

voice mail An electronic system that allows messages from telephone callers to be recorded and stored.

The telephone is one of the most important pieces of equipment used in a healthcare facility (Figure 8-1). It is used to communicate with patients, other healthcare organizations, and suppliers. It would be difficult to run an office without a telephone. It is often the first point of contact with patients, and this is an opportunity to make an outstanding first impression. Developing good telephone techniques will make you a valuable asset to your employer.

TELEPHONE EQUIPMENT

Multiple-Line Telephone

Familiarity with a **multiple-line telephone system** (Figure 8-2) is a must for the medical assistant. Even the smallest healthcare facility has at least two telephone lines so that patients rarely get a busy signal when they try to contact the office. The multiple-line telephone has a button for each line, and the button flashes when a call comes in on that line. The button also flashes, although in a different rhythm, when a caller is on hold on that line; this can serve as a reminder for the medical assistant to check back with the caller to see whether he or she would like to remain on hold or leave a message.

The multiple-line telephone also allows you to transfer calls and possibly to set up conference calls, which involve two or more callers. You should familiarize yourself with the multiple-line telephone system used in your healthcare practice.

Headset

Most business telephones have a handset that can be used to answer the telephone. However, the medical assistant who most frequently is responsible for answering the telephone may want to consider using a **headset** instead (Figure 8-3). Use of a headset can improve your ergonomics and help prevent neck strain. Also, having a headset frees your hands to use the computer or take a message.

A headset is a combination earphone and microphone that is attached to the telephone by a cord or is wireless. You can adjust the volume in the earpiece, and you may be able to adjust the volume of your voice through the microphone for callers who may have difficulty hearing. Bluetooth, a type of short-range wireless technology, allows you to be more mobile while on the telephone. Because this type of headset is not as visible, people may not be aware that you are on the telephone and may start a conversation with you. You should politely indicate that you are on the telephone and you will respond to the person when you can. Some healthcare facilities have a light system that indicates to a patient that you are on the phone and you will be with them when the call is complete. Many headsets can be muted so that you can speak with someone without the caller hearing you.

Features

Most multiple-line business telephones have many features that allow you to perform a number of different tasks in the healthcare facility.

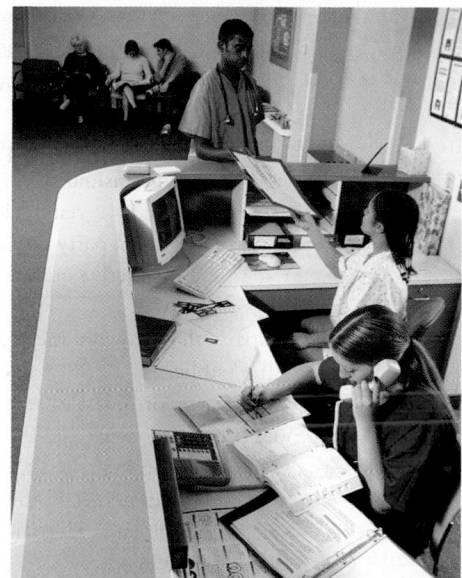

FIGURE 8-1 The telephone plays a vital role in the success of a medical practice.

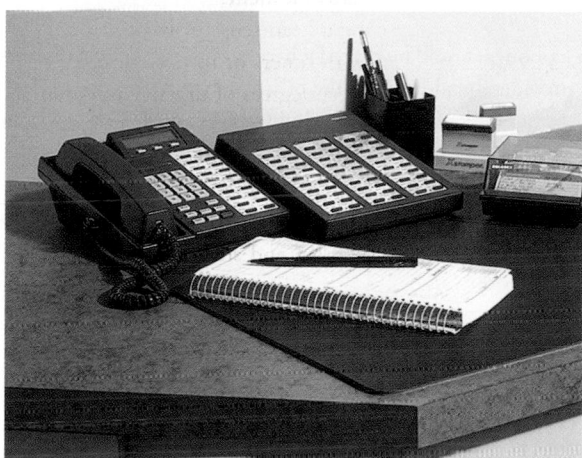

FIGURE 8-2 Multiple-line telephones allow numerous calls to come into the office at once. Each call deserves the same kind of attention and care from the medical assistant.

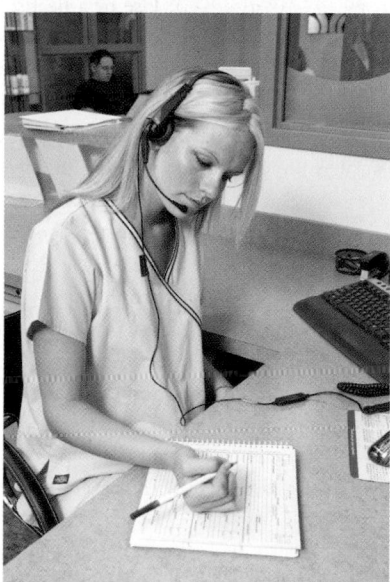

FIGURE 8-3 A headset allows the medical assistant to keep the hands free while using the telephone and is better ergonomically.

Speakerphone

The **speakerphone** function allows you to hear and speak to the caller without using the handset or a headset. Generally, a button on the telephone is labeled "speaker" (or is indicated with an icon), and once you push it, you can hang up the handset. This can be useful if you need to have more than two people on the call using the same phone.

You should always inform the caller that you will be putting him or her on speakerphone, and let the person know who else will be listening in. You must also be conscious of protecting patient information when using a speakerphone. The speakerphone function should not be used in areas such as the patient check-in area or anywhere a conversation can be overheard. The door or reception window should be closed so that no one just walking by can overhear the conversation.

Conference Calls

As mentioned, many multiple-line telephones allow you to set up **a conference call**, in which you can have multiple people on the call from different locations. The person initiating the call calls one person, puts that person on hold, and continues the sequence until all parties are on the call. Conference calls can be used when the healthcare facility has more than one location and people from all the locations must be involved in a conversation. For example, a committee may want to discuss policies and procedures for the practice. It is a much better use of time to set up a conference call than to have many people travel to one location.

Caller ID

Caller ID allows the user to see who is calling before he or she picks up the handset to answer the telephone. The caller's telephone number and name appear on a screen, and the user can decide whether to take the call. If the user subscribes to call-waiting services, another benefit, called *call-waiting caller ID,* is often available. This function allows the user to see who is calling even when the user is already on the telephone.

Voice Mail

Voice mail is widely used in today's business offices because it affords an around-the-clock method for receiving patient messages. Unfortunately, it can prove frustrating to those who find themselves speaking to an electronic device more often than a human being. Voice mail allows the caller to hear a recorded message that may also provide information about what to do in case of an emergency. Similar to an answering machine, voice mail records a caller's message, which can later be retrieved, and allows special temporary greetings when the user is away from the office. You can keep patients happy by answering voice mail messages promptly.

Call Forwarding

Call forwarding allows the user to forward calls to another designated number, such as an answering service. Usually a code is entered, then the telephone number to which the calls should be forwarded. If the medical assistant is going to be busy with a patient, the calls can be forwarded to another employee until the task is completed. This prevents the user from missing important calls when away from the main telephone.

Intercom

The business telephone in the healthcare facility may also have **intercom** capabilities. This feature allows for two-way communication, but it does not require you to pick up the handset or use a headset. This type of communication is not confidential, but it can be used to notify staff members of an emergency or to ask the provider to come out of the exam room.

CRITICAL THINKING APPLICATION   8-1

Ashlynn hears an employee using the speakerphone function to talk about a patient with another employee. How should she handle this situation? To whom, if anyone, should Ashlynn report this activity? What problems might be caused if this type of conversation is overheard?

Call Hold

The multiple-line business telephone has a hold button that allows you to interrupt a call temporarily. This often is used when you have answered an incoming call and then another line rings. You can put the first call on hold, answer the second call and put that person on hold, and then return to the first call. It is very important to be courteous and respectful of the caller. You should always ask if you can put the caller on hold and wait for a response before you push the hold button. You can also use this feature if you need to retrieve some information or speak to someone else to get some information.

Speed Dialing

Speed dialing allows you to program keys on the telephone keypad to automatically call a stored telephone number by just pressing one key. For example, if the healthcare facility uses a particular laboratory for specimen testing, the telephone number for that laboratory can be programmed for the numeral 1 on the telephone keypad; then, when you want to call that laboratory, you only need to press 1 and the call will be made. Speed dialing can be a time-saver; however, all staff members must know which telephone numbers have been programmed into particular keypad numbers.

Cell Phones

Considered a luxury item only 10 years ago, cell (or cellular) phones have become commonplace. Many people no longer have a landline because of the expenses of having two phones, and the cell phone usually is the better buy for the money. Several of the more popular cell phone companies offer free long distance calls in the United States and may provide users free night and weekend minutes. Most of today's smart phones even allow the user to access the Internet and check e-mail on their telephone. Cell phone companies usually offer a text messaging service, which allows the user to enter a message with cell phone keys, usually one that is a full QWERTY keyboard, which then is sent directly to a cell phone number.

Many people have a personal cell phone or smart phone. It is a great way to be accessible at all times, but it also can present some issues in a healthcare facility, particularly in regard to patient confidentiality. Most cell phones have a camera that could be used to take pictures of confidential information, and that information can be transmitted quickly to someone else or put on the Internet. Calls can be made or taken at inopportune times and may affect the care of patients. Most healthcare facilities have a policy that prohibits employees from having their personal cell phones with them during working hours.

TELEPHONE EQUIPMENT NEEDS OF A HEALTHCARE FACILITY

Number and Placement of Telephones

Few healthcare facilities can get along with just one telephone line. Two incoming lines, along with a private outgoing line with a separate number for the **provider's** exclusive use, is the minimum recommended number of lines.

One medical assistant can handle no more than two incoming lines; therefore, the addition of more lines may involve additional staffing. If a staff member is assigned solely to dealing with insurance and billing, a separate line and listing in the telephone directory for this service may considerably lessen the load on the main incoming lines.

Telephones should be placed where they are accessible but private. Each provider, in addition to the office manager, requires a telephone at his or her desk. A telephone should be available in the laboratory area and the clinical area, and multiple phones should be present in reception and business office areas. Many healthcare facilities also have a telephone available for patients to use. This telephone often has a separate line so that patient use does not interfere with the staff members' work.

EFFECTIVE USE OF THE TELEPHONE

Active Listening

It may seem odd to start out discussing listening instead of speaking in the Telephone Techniques chapter, but listening well while on the telephone is just as important as speaking well when it comes to communicating on the telephone. When you are on the telephone, you have fewer nonverbal cues to help you determine the message; therefore, it is very important that you use good listening skills. When you use active listening skills, your patients realize that you think they are important and that you respect the message they are communicating to you, whether you are on the telephone or face-to-face.

Active Listening

- Be present in the moment.
- Focus solely on the conversation.
- Don't interrupt.
- Don't start forming your response before the person has finished speaking.
- Confirm what the speaker has said, and ask if your interpretation is correct.
- Always be respectful and professional.

Active listening involves listening to what the speaker is saying, interpreting what the message is, and restating the message to make sure that you have received the intended message. For example, you receive a telephone call from a distraught mother. Using active listening skills, you pick up on the nonverbal cues, such as her tone of voice and rate of speech, and you can tell she is upset. The mother states that her child has been very sick for the past several days, and nothing she has done has helped with the fever her child has had for 2 days. Your response should be to restate what you have heard: the child has been ill with a fever for the past 2 days, and nothing she has tried has brought the fever down. This gives the caller the opportunity to correct any misinformation or to confirm that the information is correct. If it is correct, you should follow the healthcare practice's procedures for handling this situation; most likely, you will schedule an appointment for that same day.

Developing a Pleasing Telephone Personality

Each time a medical assistant answers the telephone, he or she is representing the healthcare practice (Procedure 8-1). The manner in which the telephone is answered can influence the caller's impression of the whole office and whether the person wants to be seen there. When patients call the healthcare facility, they should hear a friendly yet professional voice. Just as active listening is an important skill to receive the message being sent, a pleasing telephone personality facilitates the sending of the message.

Although it may seem silly, you should always smile when you answer the telephone. The physical act of smiling affects how your words sound. It is as if your caller can hear you smile, and you have created a positive impression.

It is also important to be aware of nonverbal communication that occurs during a telephone conversation. Be aware of your tone of voice. Is it helping to send the message that you want to send? Your callers can tell if you are preoccupied and not focused on the current conversation. You should vary the **pitch** of your voice and avoid speaking in a **monotone**.

Nonvisual/Nonverbal Communication

- Tone of voice
- Speed of speech
- Pitch
- Volume
- Enunciation
- Pausing or hesitation

Enunciation is crucial when speaking on the telephone. You should speak very clearly and distinctly so that the caller can understand what you are saying. Many letters of the alphabet sound very similar on the telephone, such as B, P, T, and F and S. You may need to clarify with the caller by saying, "That is B as in bravo."

Phonetic Alphabet

A	Alpha	N	November
B	Bravo	O	Oscar
C	Charlie	P	Papa
D	Delta	Q	Quebec
E	Echo	R	Romeo
F	Foxtrot	S	Sierra
G	Golf	T	Tango
H	Hotel	U	Uniform
I	India	V	Victor
J	Juliet	W	Whiskey
K	Kilo	X	X-ray
L	Lima	Y	Yankee
M	Mike	Z	Zulu

It is important to always be courteous and **tactful**. Think about the words you will be using before actually speaking them. For those of us working in a healthcare facility, it is easy to integrate medical terminology into our conversations. However, we must be careful not to use medical **jargon** when speaking with patients because this makes the message more difficult for them to understand. For example, if you are giving a male patient preprocedural instructions, advise him that he must not eat or drink anything for 12 hours before the procedure; do not tell him he should "stay NPO" (nothing by mouth).

To create a pleasant, friendly, and professional image of the healthcare facility, you must give the caller your full attention. Do not become distracted by other things going on around you. In addition, you should never eat, chew gum, or drink when on the telephone. Use a normal volume and tone of voice, and speak directly into the mouthpiece. Be sure to speak at a moderate rate of speed because speaking too quickly makes it difficult for the caller to understand you.

CRITICAL THINKING APPLICATION   8-2

Ashlynn has a tendency to speak a little fast in her normal conversations. How will she need to adjust as she is answering phones in the healthcare facility? She also is a friendly person and enjoys talking on the phone. What precautions should she take so that this does not become an issue on the job?

PROCEDURE 8-1 Demonstrate Professional Telephone Techniques

Goal: *To answer the telephone in a provider's office in a professional manner and respond to a request for action.*

Case Study: *Charles Johnson, DOB 3/3/1958, an established patient of Dr. Martin, has called to schedule an appointment to have his blood pressure checked. This will be a follow-up appointment that is 15 minutes long. He is requesting that the appointment be on a Friday during his lunchtime between 11:00 and 12:00.*

EQUIPMENT and SUPPLIES

- Telephone
- Pen or pencil
- Appointment book or EHR with appointment scheduling abilities
- Computer
- Notepad

PROCEDURAL STEPS

1. Demonstrate telephone techniques by answering the telephone by the third ring.
   PURPOSE: To convey interest in the caller by answering promptly. This makes a positive impression on the caller.
2. Speak distinctly with a pleasant tone and expression, at a moderate rate, and with sufficient volume for the person to understand every word.
3. Identify the office and/or provider and yourself.
   PURPOSE: To assure the caller that the correct number has been reached and to identify the staff member.
4. Verify the identity of the caller, and if using an electronic health record, bring the patient's health record to the active screen of the computer.
   PURPOSE: To confirm the origin of the call.
5. Screen the call if necessary.

PURPOSE: To determine whether the caller has an emergency and needs immediate attention or referral to a hospital emergency department.
6. Apply active listening skills to assess whether the caller is distressed or agitated and to determine the concern to be addressed.
   PURPOSE: To make sure the medical assistant hears and understands the message being sent by the patient and to show that the patient has the medical assistant's full attention.
7. Determine the needs of the caller and provide the requested information or service if possible. Provide the caller with excellent customer service. Be as helpful as possible. Check the appointment schedule and determine the first Friday that would have an open appointment between 11:00 and 12:00.
   PURPOSE: To allow the medical assistant to handle many calls and conserve the provider's and staff members' time and energy.
8. Obtain sufficient patient information to schedule the appointment, including the patient's full name, DOB, insurance information, and preferred contact method. Repeat the date and time of the appointment to ensure that the patient has the correct information.
9. Terminate the call in a pleasant manner and replace the receiver gently, always allowing the caller to hang up first.
   PURPOSE: To promote good public relations, provide excellent customer service, and ensure that the caller has no further questions.

MANAGING TELEPHONE CALLS

Thinking Ahead

Whether you are answering incoming calls or placing outgoing calls, it is important to be completely prepared. Before you start answering calls, make sure you have all the supplies needed to do your job. For example, for taking messages, you should have access to a computer (if your office documents telephone messages electronically) or a paper message form, in addition to working pens and a watch or clock to record the time. Many offices also keep a list of commonly used telephone numbers. Such a list includes poison control, other emergency numbers, community resources to which patients can be referred, and so on.

For outgoing calls, have all the information you need, such as the patient's health record, the telephone number of the person you will be calling, a list of questions, and a pad and a pen to make notes during the conversation.

Confidentiality

All communication in a healthcare facility must maintain patient confidentiality. When using the telephone, you must be aware of what is going on around you and who may be able to overhear your conversation. If patient-sensitive information will be discussed, place the call in an area where others cannot hear, especially other patients. Be careful when using a speakerphone because the sound can travel farther than you might think, and someone might overhear private medical information—this is a violation of the law, specifically the Health Insurance Portability and Accountability Act (HIPAA).

Answering Promptly

As mentioned earlier, telephone contact is often the first interaction with a patient. If the person's call is not answered promptly, this can create a negative impression before he or she even talks to someone. It is important that a call be answered within three rings. To accomplish this, you may need to do the following: (1) interrupt the call you are on by asking if you can place the person on hold for a moment; (2) answer the second call; if it is not an emergency, ask that person if you may place him or her on hold; and (3) return to the first caller.

An incoming call should never be answered with "Please hold." You should always find out the nature of the call before placing the person on hold. If it is an emergency, the second call is handled promptly, before you return to the first call. If it is not an emergency, you should always ask if you can place the person on hold and wait for an answer before pushing the hold button. If the person refuses to be placed on hold, determine the reason why and assure them that you will return to his or her call quickly.

The medical assistant who routinely answers the telephone should know how to activate emergency medical services (EMS) in his or her area. Generally, this means dialing 911. You may need to make this call for a patient who has called the healthcare facility and is now unable to contact EMS on her own. If your phone system allows it, you can set up a conference call that includes the patient, EMS, and yourself. It is important to get a telephone number where the caller can be reached if you get disconnected. It also is important to keep the patient and/or caregivers on the line while contacting EMS.

Identifying the Facility

When answering incoming telephone calls, the medical assistant should identify the facility first, state his or her name, and then follow with an offer of help. For example: "Good morning, Walden-Martin Family Medical Clinic. This is Ashlynn. How may I help you?" Medical assistants must always follow the policy of the healthcare facility when answering incoming calls. Speaking slowly and smoothly, with good enunciation, ensures that your callers understand whom they have reached.

CRITICAL THINKING APPLICATION   **8-3**

Most offices dictate how the phone is to be answered. What should Ashlynn do if she is very uncomfortable with the way she is asked to answer the phone? Who ultimately should decide how the phone is answered?

Identifying the Caller

If the caller does not offer a name, the medical assistant should ask, "May I ask who is calling?" It can be helpful to write down the caller's name and try to use it at least three times during the conversation, if it does not compromise patient confidentiality. This helps make a strong connection with the patient and assures the person that he or she has been identified correctly.

Occasionally callers refuse to identify themselves to the medical assistant and insist that they speak with the provider. You must be clear, in a professional manner, that you cannot connect the caller to the provider without knowing who the caller is. The caller may be a sales representative who knows that if she identifies herself, she will not get the opportunity to talk with the provider. When it becomes clear that the caller will not give a name but still insists on speaking with the provider, you can tell the person that the provider is busy with patients and has asked that messages be taken; if the caller cannot leave a name for the message, then he or she may want to write a letter and mark it Personal. Most people do not want to wait for a response to a letter and will then give you their names so that a message can be taken.

Screening Incoming Calls

Most healthcare facilities expect the medical assistant answering the telephone to **screen** the calls. You must determine which calls should be routed directly to the provider, which to the **triage** area, or which to the billing office. The provider, office manager, and staff members who will be answering the telephone should work together to develop policies for screening calls.

The first step in screening calls is to determine who the caller is and the nature of the call. If the call is from a patient with a question about a statement he or she just received in the mail, the call can be transferred to the appropriate area. If the call involves determining whether a patient should be seen that day, it can be transferred to the triage area. If the caller asks to speak directly to the provider, the situation can become more complicated, and healthcare facility policies should be created to address these cases.

Healthcare facility policies often state that calls from other providers are put through immediately. If that is not possible, assure the caller that the provider will return the call as soon as possible. Some providers may also ask that calls be put through immediately for certain family members. If the provider does not want to take the calls, the medical assistant must tactfully tell the caller that the provider cannot be disturbed at this time.

Screening policies also should address how calls should be handled when the provider is out of the office. If the provider is to be out of the office for an extended period (e.g., for a conference or vacation), another provider usually is designated to handle calls. It should be explained to the patient that the provider that he or she asked for is out of the office, but another provider is taking the calls. If the call is not an emergency, take a message, and the designated provider can return the call.

If a call is an **emergency**, the policies for handling emergency calls apply. Many emergency calls require judgment on the part of the person answering the telephone in the medical practice. Good judgment comes from experience and proper training by the provider with regard to what constitutes a real emergency in each type of practice and how such calls should be handled. The person answering the telephone first should determine whether the call is truly urgent. If so, never hang up the telephone until an ambulance reaches the patient or other help arrives. When necessary, ask another staff member to call 911 while remaining on the line with the patient. Emergency calls may include such conditions and/or symptoms as chest pain, profuse bleeding, severe allergic reactions, cessation of breathing, injuries resulting in loss of consciousness, and broken bones. An **urgent** call may be an adult patient with a fever over 102°F (38.9°C), an animal bite, or an increasingly painful ear infection. Emergency calls are life-threatening, whereas an urgent call requires prompt attention but is not life-threatening. In the case of emergencies, often the provider instructs the patient to go straight to the closest hospital emergency department instead of the office. Policies and procedures manuals should indicate the action to take in emergency situations. When in doubt, always ask the office manager and/or the provider.

If the provider is in, the call may need to be transferred to him or her immediately. All offices should have a written plan of action for the times the provider is not physically present in the office. These policies should include typical questions to ask the caller to determine the validity and disposition of an emergency. Some examples of questions to ask include:

- At what telephone number can you be reached?
- Where are you located?

- What are the chief symptoms?
- When did they start?
- Has this happened before?
- Are you alone?
- Do you have transportation?

Screening Guidelines

In a facility with multiple employees, the provider may designate one individual, such as a nurse or an experienced and trained medical assistant, as the telephone screener. Every healthcare facility would be wise to have a written telephone protocol for handling urgent situations and emergencies. The protocol should state that employees are bound by the written guidelines and that unauthorized personnel may give no advice. If advice is given, it may be grounds for dismissal.

A special sheet of instructions listing specific medical emergencies (e.g., chest pain, heavy bleeding, fainting, seizure, and poisoning) should be posted by each telephone. The telephone numbers for the nearest poison control center, hospital, and ambulance should be listed.

Emergency calls should be routed to a provider immediately. Additional instructions should include what action to take if no provider is available (e.g., sending the patient to an emergency department or calling for an ambulance). Most offices have some means of constant contact with the provider, whether by pager, cell phone, or another method.

Getting the Information the Provider Needs

As the medical assistant gains experience and knows the provider better, he or she begins to have a sense of the questions the provider will have for patients who call the facility. For example, the provider is interested in how long the patient has had symptoms, what makes the symptoms better or worse, what remedies have been tried, what has worked and not worked, and other specifics about the condition. If the patient complains of painful urination, the medical assistant learns to ask about pain in the back or blood in the urine. One way to learn about questions to ask is to listen to the provider carefully as he or she questions patients about their symptoms. This can help you learn more about signs and symptoms and enable you to be a better assistant to the provider.

Remember to always be "patient with your patients." Those who call the healthcare facility for help are almost never at their best. When feeling ill, people often are short tempered and even display poor manners. Some can be verbally abusive. Care for patients as if they were family members, and they will feel care and compassion in the medical facility.

If the provider is unavailable for only part of the day, take a message and inform the caller that the provider currently is out of the office but will return calls when he or she returns. It is important to give the caller the time frame in which the provider will be returning those calls so that the patient's time is not wasted in sitting by the phone, waiting for the call. It should be stressed that the time frame is approximate because emergencies cannot be predicted. If the caller is unavailable when the provider usually returns calls, ask what would be a convenient time and let the caller know you will try to work with that time frame.

Screening calls is an important task for medical assistants who answer the telephone. It can keep the healthcare facility running on schedule and ensure that calls that need to get to the provider do so immediately.

Placing Callers on Hold

The medical assistant should always ask before placing a caller on hold. If it has been determined through the screening process that this is a call that does not need to be put through to the provider right away, or if the call needs to be transferred to someone else in the healthcare facility and that person is not immediately available, you should ask if the caller would like to be put on hold, or if he or she would prefer to be called back. If you know that the person with whom the caller needs to speak may be busy for quite a while, inform the caller of that. The caller may still want to wait. You should check back periodically to make sure the caller still wants to remain on hold. No longer than 1 minute should pass before you check back with the caller. When you return to the call, you can use a statement such as, "Thank you for waiting. Would you like to continue to hold, or should I take a message?"

Minimizing the wait for the caller shows concern, and freeing up the telephone lines is important for other people trying to contact the healthcare facility.

Transferring a Call

During the screening process, the medical assistant may determine that the call should be transferred to the provider or to another person in the facility. Consider the following example: Ms. Fields calls your office because she has a billing question. You should ask Ms. Fields' permission before placing her on hold, and wait for a response. It is also helpful to give Ms. Fields the name and extension of the person to whom you will be transferring her call (if it is not the provider); this way, if Ms. Fields' call happens to get disconnected, she will have that information when she calls back. Once you have Ms. Fields' permission to put her on hold, you should contact the person to whom the call is being transferred; in this case, that is Mr. Lewis in the billing department. Tell Mr. Lewis who is calling and the reason for the call; this allows Mr. Lewis to be prepared to help Ms. Fields when the connection is made. Mr. Lewis may ask for a moment to pull up information before you put Ms. Fields' call through. You should stay on the line to introduce Ms. Fields to Mr. Lewis and to make sure the connection is made. If Mr. Lewis is unavailable, you should ask Ms. Fields if she would like to be connected to his voice mail. Some callers may prefer that you take a message in written form and bring it to the proper person.

Medical assistants who answer telephone calls must know who does what in the healthcare facility. An organizational chart with telephone extensions can be helpful, but it must be kept up to date so that calls can be transferred successfully.

Taking a Message

Telephone messages, whether taken in a handwritten or an electronic format, are an important part of patient care (Procedure 8-2). The patient relies on the medical assistant to get the message to the appropriate person. Taking messages allows information to be delivered to a provider or an appropriate person, who can make a decision (then or later), which can be communicated back to the patient without interrupting the flow of patients through the healthcare facility. You should be sure to let the caller know when to expect a call back; for example, explain that the provider usually returns calls between 3 and 4 PM.

Whether the message is taken in a handwritten or an electronic format, the information needed for a complete message is the same:

1. The name of the person calling
2. The name of the person to whom the call is directed
3. The caller's daytime, evening, and/or cell phone number
4. The reason for the call, including the telephone number of the caller's pharmacy if a medication is requested
5. The action to be taken
6. The date and time of the call
7. The initials of the person who took the call

PROCEDURE 8-2	**Document Telephone Messages and Report Relevant Information Concisely and Accurately**

Goal: *To take an accurate telephone message and follow up on the requests made by the caller.*

Case Study: *Norma Washington, DOB 8/1/1944, an established patient of Dr. Martin, has called to report her blood pressure readings that she has been taking at home. Dr. Martin had made a recent change in her medication and wanted her to monitor her BP at home for 3 days and call in with the results. She has taken her blood pressure in the morning and in the evening for the past three days, with the following results:*

Day 1 : 144/92 in the AM, 156/94 in the PM
Day 2: 136/84 in the AM, 142/86 in the PM
Day 3: 132/80 in the AM, 138/82 in the PM

EQUIPMENT and SUPPLIES

- Telephone
- Computer
- Message pad
- Pen or pencil
- Notepad Health record

PROCEDURAL STEPS

1. Demonstrate telephone techniques by answering the telephone using the guidelines in Procedure 8-1.
   PURPOSE: To answer promptly and courteously, which conveys interest in the caller and promotes good customer service.
2. Using a message pad or the computer, take the phone message (either on paper or by data entry into the computer) and obtain the following information:
   - Name of the person to whom the call is directed
   - Name of the person calling
   - Caller's telephone number
   - Reason for the call
   - Action to be taken
   - Date and time of the call
   - Initials of the person taking the call
   PURPOSE: To have accurate information, which allows the staff member or provider to address the caller's issues quickly and efficiently.
3. Apply active listening skills and repeat the information back to the caller after recording the message.
   PURPOSE: To verify that all the information was recorded accurately.
4. End the call and wait for the caller to hang up first.
5. Document the telephone call with all pertinent information in the patient's health record.
   PURPOSE: To ensure that the patient's health record is kept up to date.
6. Deliver the phone message to the appropriate person.
7. Follow up on important messages.
   PURPOSE: To make sure important issues are addressed in a timely manner.
8. If using paper messaging, keep old message books for future reference. Carbonless copies allow the facility to keep a permanent record of phone messages. If using an electronic system, the message will be saved to the patient's record automatically.
   PURPOSE: To have a permanent source of messages in case the information is needed after the paper message has been discarded. This can also serve as a telephone log.
9. File pertinent phone messages in the patient's health record. Make sure the computer record is closed after the documentation has been done.
   PURPOSE: To keep a permanent record of important information in the patient's chart.

Messages Taken on Paper

Many types of message pads or books are available (Figure 8-4). Many are pressure-sensitive, making a copy of the message and serving as a telephone call log. The original is given to the person the message is for and the medical assistant will have a copy to use

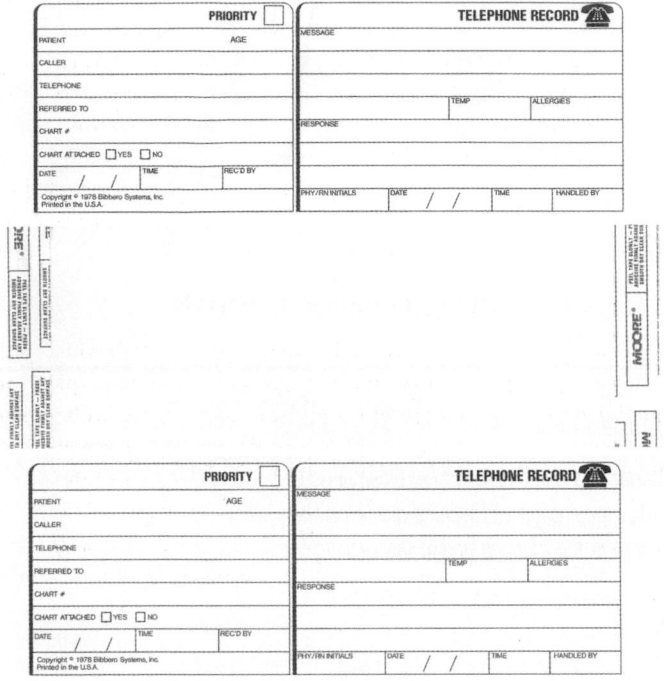

FIGURE 8-4 Phone message forms with self-adhesive backing make charting calls easier and more time efficient. (Courtesy Bibbero Systems, Petaluma, Calif.)

for follow-up. Having legible handwriting is a must when taking a manual, handwritten message.

Messages Recorded Electronically

Most electronic health record (EHR) systems can record telephone messages (Figure 8-5). The EHR automatically saves a copy of the message to the patient's health record and sends the message to the provider, who can either call the patient directly or give the medical assistant directions to respond to the patient. The electronic system may also be able to flag a message, to indicate its urgency, or that it requires a call back, or that a prescription refill is requested.

Taking Action on Telephone Messages

The message process is not complete until the necessary action has been taken. If a handwritten system is used, use an identifying mark to indicate a message that requires action. If an electronic system is used, check periodically during the day to be sure you do not have to complete the response to the message, such as calling the patient back or contacting the pharmacy. For risk management purposes, the healthcare facility should have a policy on the documentation of telephone messages and the specific information that must be included. Medical assistants should become familiar with that policy.

Retaining Records of Telephone Messages

If a handwritten system is used for recording telephone messages, the healthcare facility must establish a policy on the retention of telephone message records. If the message relates to patient care, a copy of the message should be added to the patient's health record. If the health record is electronic, this may mean scanning in a copy of the paper message and attaching it to the EHR. The copy in the

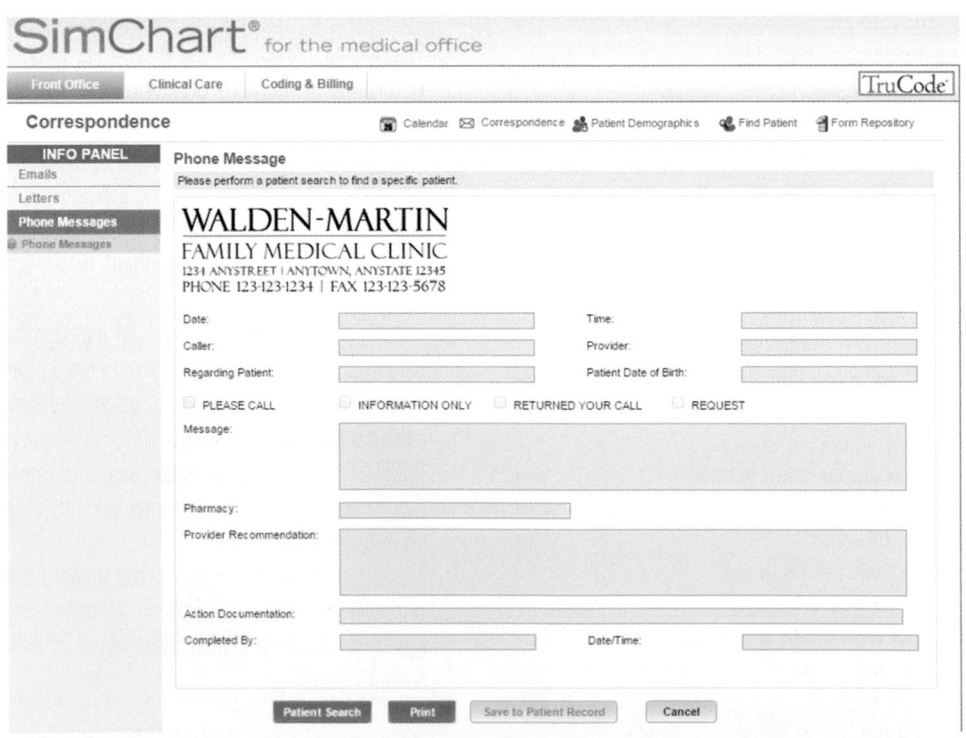

FIGURE 8-5 Phone message screen in an electronic health record system. (Elsevier: SimChart for the Medical Office, St Louis, 2015, Elsevier.)

message book usually is retained for the same period that the statute of limitations runs for medical professional liability cases.

If an electronic system is used, the message is automatically saved to the patient's record, along with the response to the message. The message record can show whether the patient contacted the office, if the office responded to that contact, and what the response was. All of these are key points if a medical professional liability case is brought against the provider. In addition, accurate telephone records can ensure quality patient care and customer service.

TYPICAL INCOMING CALLS

Handling incoming calls is often the responsibility of the medical assistant. You can handle many calls directly, but some will require the assistance of others. Knowing how to respond to the different types of calls will make you a valuable asset to the healthcare facility.

Requests for Directions

Each office should have a clear set of written directions that can be read to a caller who wants to know how to get to the office. Prepare the directions from various points in the area; for instance, one set for a patient coming from the north, and another for a patient coming from the south. Place these directions close to the telephone so that all employees can find them easily. Not all employees live close to the clinic or are familiar with the area; therefore, the written set of directions will be helpful both to staff members and to patients. Put a map on the office website and direct patients there for printable directions. Never simply suggest that callers refer to an Internet map when they ask for directions.

Inquiries About Bills

A patient may ask to speak with the provider about a recent bill. Ask the caller to hold for a moment while the ledger is obtained from the computer or files. If nothing irregular is found in the ledger, return to the telephone and say, "I have your account in front of me now. Perhaps I can answer your question." Most likely the caller will have some simple inquiry (e.g., whether the insurance company has paid its portion), or the person may want to delay making a payment until the next month. Not all patients realize that the medical assistant usually makes such decisions and is the best person with whom to discuss these matters. If the healthcare facility uses an external billing service, you may need to provide the caller with that agency's telephone number. When an external billing service is used, that telephone number is often shown on the patient's statement. When necessary, post a note in the EHR or to the physical ledger card about the patient's call, such as a promise to pay on a certain date.

A patient may have questions about a statement that came in the mail. If billing matters are handled by another employee, tell the patient that the call will be transferred to the billing office. If you are responsible for billing, politely ask the patient to hold the line while you obtain the patient ledger. On returning to the line, thank the patient for waiting and explain the charges carefully. If an error has occurred, apologize and say that a corrected statement will be sent out at once. Always remember to thank the patient for calling. If patients are properly advised about charges at the time services are rendered, the number of these calls can be reduced considerably.

Inquiries About Fees

Fees vary widely in each healthcare facility, and quoting an exact fee before the provider sees the patient can be difficult. However, a good estimate should be given to patients as to what they can expect to pay, especially on the first visit. Asking a patient to just appear at the office without having any idea of the cost is unreasonable. Discuss with the provider or office manager what range should be quoted to the patient, and then follow your quote with the statement that the fees vary, depending on the patient's condition and tests the provider orders. Most healthcare facilities require patients to pay the health insurance co-payment (or co-pay) on the day service is provided, and the caller should be informed of this. If fees are regularly discussed on the telephone, a suggested script should be included in the policies and procedures manual. Do not be evasive; have a list of fees available you can discuss with patients.

Questions About Participating Providers

Patients may call the office to inquire whether the provider is a **participating provider** with their particular insurance plan or managed care organization. A list of the insurance plans with which the provider has a contract should be readily available to the medical assistant who answers the telephone. This is important because insurance benefits vary widely for patients based on whether they see a participating provider or a nonparticipating provider. A claim may even be denied if the provider is not a provider for the patient's insurance company.

Requests for Assistance With Insurance

In the ever-changing world of health insurance, patients often are confused about their coverage, how payment is determined, and what they are actually financially responsible for when it comes to their bill from the healthcare facility. A solid understanding of the basics of health insurance, including managed care, allows you to answer patient questions about insurance. If the question is beyond your knowledge, you should know to whom to transfer the call so that the patient can get an answer.

Radiology and Laboratory Reports

Because of the increased use of EHRs, radiology and laboratory results often are available to providers as soon as the technician has completed the test. When the patient calls for those results, a message is taken, and the provider decides whether the medical assistant can relay the results or the provider needs to speak to the patient directly.

When tests are done at a facility that is not linked to the healthcare facility's EHR, the findings usually are delivered by mail to the provider's office. If the test has been marked **STAT**, which means the provider wants the results immediately, reports may be telephoned, faxed, or e-mailed to the provider's office and an original report delivered by mail.

It is helpful to have blank laboratory results forms available that list the various tests, with their normal values, so that you can easily and accurately document results telephoned to the healthcare facility. This can save time, and you can be assured that the test name is spelled correctly. You should repeat the results you have been given to make sure you have written them down correctly. This report must be documented in the patient's health record and sent to the provider for review.

Satisfactory Progress Reports from Patients

Providers sometimes ask patients to telephone the office to report on their condition a few days after the office visit. The medical assistant can take such calls and relay the information to the provider if the report is satisfactory. Assure the patient that you will inform the provider of the call. The report should be documented in the health record. The provider should always be informed immediately about unsatisfactory progress reports, and he or she should give instructions for the patient to follow in such situations. The provider may discuss this directly with the patient, or the medical assistant may be instructed to relay the information to the patient. All instructions given should also be documented in the health record.

Routine Reports from Hospitals and Other Sources

Routine calls may be received from hospitals and other sources reporting a patient's progress. Take the message carefully and make sure the provider sees it. The message should be placed in the patient's health record after the provider has reviewed and initialed it.

Requests for Referrals

Well-respected providers, especially primary care providers, are often asked for recommendations for referrals to other specialists. If the provider has furnished the medical assistant with a list of practitioners for this purpose, these inquiries may be handled without consulting the provider, unless the patient's insurance plan requires a written referral. However, the provider should always be informed of such requests. Referrals should also be documented in the patient's health record.

Some managed care organizations require a provider referral before a patient may see a specialist; this referral should come from the provider unless he or she has authorized automatic referrals. Most providers require the patient to come in for an office visit to discuss the referral. Afterward, a staff member calls the referral provider and notifies the office staff of the referral. This process may also be done electronically. A managed care organization may offer the option of using its website to enter the referral information and then electronically forwarding the information to the new provider. Handle these calls as quickly as possible so that the patient may make an appointment to see the referral provider.

Office Administration Matters

Not all calls concern patients. Calls may come from the accountant or the auditor or about banking procedures, office supplies, or office maintenance, most of which the medical assistant can handle or refer to the appropriate person. For some of these calls, the medical assistant may need to gather additional information and return the call.

SPECIAL INCOMING CALLS

Patients Refusing to Discuss Symptoms

Occasionally patients call and want to talk with the provider about symptoms they are reluctant to discuss with a medical assistant. Patients have the right to privacy, but the provider cannot be expected to take numerous calls from patients who do not want to speak to the medical assistant. If the patient refuses to discuss any symptoms, follow the healthcare facility's procedures, which may

include suggesting that the patient make an appointment with the provider to discuss the problem in person.

Unsatisfactory Progress Reports

If a patient under treatment reports that he or she is still not feeling well or that the prescription the provider provided is not helping, do not practice medicine illegally by giving the patient medical advice. Make detailed notes about the patient's comments and then give your notes to the provider. He or she may make a medication change or may decide that the patient should return to the office. Follow up with the patient and convey the provider's instructions.

CRITICAL THINKING APPLICATION   8-4

A patient calls the healthcare facility to report that she has been taking her prescribed antibiotic for 3 days and still isn't feeling any better. She says she might even be feeling worse than before she started taking the pills. She asks Ashlynn if she should stop taking the pills.

- How should Ashlynn respond to this patient?
- What actions should Ashlynn take in response to this telephone call?
- What should Ashlynn document in the patient's record?

Requests for Test Results

When the provider orders special tests, the patient may be told to call the office in a couple of days for the results. It is ultimately the responsibility of the provider to notify the patient of test results, especially if they are abnormal. When a patient calls for the results, make sure the provider has seen them and has given permission before sharing the results with the patient. If specified in the office policy, the medical assistant can give test results to the patient. Patients do not always understand that the medical assistant cannot give out information without the provider's permission. If the results are unfavorable, the provider should be the one to inform the patient and give further instructions. This call must be handled tactfully; otherwise, the patient may feel as if the staff is concealing information.

Most providers prefer that medical assistants give only normal test results to patients. However, the medical assistant may give abnormal test results if authorized by the provider. For example, when a patient has an abnormal Pap test result, the medical assistant usually is the person who calls the patient with the result and further instructions from the provider. If the patient has any questions about the test result, she must be referred to the provider. The medical assistant needs good communication skills to relay information such as this without crossing the line of practicing medicine without a license.

The best policy for dealing with more serious abnormal test results is to schedule an appointment for the patient to see the provider. These results are best relayed in person instead of on the telephone.

Patients who call the office for test results must be appropriately identified before the results are given. Some offices use a special code that is written in the patient's health record, and knowledge of this code or password gives the person access to the information. Other offices may use the patient's date of birth or other information that is known only to the patient and has been shared with the healthcare facility. You should always use at least two different methods of identifying patients.

Medical assistants must know and follow federal regulations and the laws in their state regarding the release of any information to someone other than the patient, this includes information about a minor. Make sure the right individual is on the line before offering results by verifying name and date of birth. It is considered a breach of confidentiality and of the Privacy Rules of the Health Insurance Portability and Accountability Act (HIPAA) if the patient is not identified correctly and information is released to the wrong individual.

Requests for Information from Third Parties

The patient must give permission before any member of the provider's staff can give information to third-party callers; this includes insurance companies, attorneys, relatives, neighbors, employers, and any other third party. HIPAA is very specific about the information that should be included in the release of information form. The patient must specify who can receive the information and exactly what information can be released. The release of information form also must include an expiration date. The medical assistant must carefully review the patient's form before releasing any information to third parties.

Complaints About Care or Fees

A medical assistant may be able to offer a satisfactory explanation to a patient who complains about the care he or she received or the fee charged. Often the patient simply does not understand a charge, and the medical assistant can provide assistance by reviewing the bill. If a patient seems angry, offer to pull the health record, research the problem and if needed, discuss it with the provider. Four magic words often calm the angry patient: "Let me help you." This reassures the patient that someone is willing to talk about the problem. However, if you are unable to appease the patient easily, the provider or office manager may prefer to talk directly to the patient.

When callers complain, do not attempt to blame someone else, and never argue with the patient. Find the source of the problem, and then present options to the caller as to how the situation can be resolved. Remember to treat callers in the same manner that you would wish to be treated. A complaint may seem small and insignificant to the office staff, but to the patient it may be a serious issue. Provide good customer service to patients, and complaints will be few and far between.

Calls from Staff Members' Families or Friends

The telephone lines should never be burdened with an excess of personal calls to the staff. A call is necessary in emergencies, but staff members should never monopolize the telephone for personal business and conversations. Emergency calls could be coming through, and the lines must be clear. Keep personal calls and texting to an absolute minimum.

HANDLING DIFFICULT CALLS

Angry Callers

No matter how efficient the medical assistant is on the telephone or how well liked the provider might be, sooner or later an angry caller will be on the line. The anger may have a legitimate cause, or the caller's irritation may have resulted from a misunderstanding. Handling such calls is a real challenge. First, take the required actions, even if it is to say that the matter will be discussed with the provider as soon as possible and the patient will be called back later. If answers are not readily available, a friendly assurance that the situation is important and that every attempt will be made to find the answer quickly usually calms the angry feelings.

The medical assistant may find that lowering his or her tone of voice and volume of speech may force the angry caller to do the same. This method does not always work, but it usually is true that when dealing with an angry person, calm promotes calm. Some patients may misread this method and become even angrier, thinking that their complaint is not being taken seriously. Interpersonal skills are critical when dealing with other individuals because the more skilled the medical assistant becomes, the better able he or she is to deal with multiple types of personalities.

Always avoid getting angry or defensive in response to an angry caller, and try to get to the root of the real problem. Express interest and understanding, take careful notes, and follow through with the problem to the most appropriate resolution. Never "pass the buck" by saying, "That's not my job," or "I am not the person who filed that insurance claim." No matter whose fault the problem is, it is best to deal with it and find a solution instead of placing blame. It is important to respond to the patient when you said you would, even if the call is to tell him or her that you need a bit more time to work on the problem. Keeping the patient in the loop shows that you want to come up with a solution.

CRITICAL THINKING APPLICATION   **8-5**

An angry caller raises his voice at Ashlynn over an issue that happened before she began to work at the facility. She suggests that he speak with the office manager, but he refuses and continues to berate Ashlynn.
- What choices does Ashlynn have in this situation?
- Should she simply hang up on the patient?
- How can the call be handled diplomatically?

Aggressive Callers

Aggressive callers insist that they receive whatever action they feel is necessary, and they usually insist on action immediately. Treat these callers with a calm, poised attitude, but do not allow the caller's aggression to initiate inappropriate action. Reassure the caller that his or her concern is valid and will receive the full attention of the right person. Explain when the caller can expect a response from the office, and be sure to follow up with the patient.

Unauthorized Inquiry Calls

Some individuals call the provider's office requesting information to which they are not entitled. These callers must be told politely but firmly that such information cannot be provided to them because of privacy laws. Insistent callers should be referred to the office manager or provider.

Sales Calls

Sales calls often are thought of as an interruption to the provider's busy day, but some salespersons may have important information on products, equipment, or services the office uses regularly. Do not completely disregard salespeople, but do not allow them to monopolize time or telephone lines, either. Keep these calls quick and to the point. Most professional salespeople realize that the provider's and staff's time is extremely valuable and respect this. It may be the healthcare facility policy to give the salesperson an appointment, possibly over the lunch hour, to discuss the new product or service with the provider and/or office manager. Developing a rapport with representatives of the companies whose products the practice uses frequently may result in a discounted price and first news of sales and promotions. In turn, these professionals rarely waste the time of office personnel.

CRITICAL THINKING APPLICATION   8-6

Ashlynn answers the phone; the caller is a pharmaceutical representative who has been visiting the clinic for several months. She cheerfully greets him and asks if he is calling to make an appointment. He states that he wants to make an appointment with Ashlynn—for a date. How should she handle this call? What problems could arise if this were a patient and Ashlynn were to accept the date?

Callers With Difficulty Communicating

Occasionally calls come into the office from patients or family members who have difficulty with the English language. In some cases English is not the caller's primary language, so the medical assistant must use listening skills to ensure understanding. If a certain language is predominant in the area, the healthcare facility should consider hiring a medical assistant who is bilingual. Some patients speak English but have a heavy accent, so you should listen carefully and ask questions to be sure you have understood the person correctly. Many resources are available to assist with translation. The healthcare facility may contract with a translator who would be available to help with telephone calls and patient visits in the office. Many online services also offer translation. If the healthcare facility has a number of patients who speak a specific language other than English, it would be helpful to have commonly used phrases available in that language, especially the phrase that would refer the patient to the specific translation service used by the healthcare facility.

Some providers may have a number of patients who are deaf or hard of hearing. These patients may use a relay system to communicate with healthcare facilities over the telephone. Some relay systems have the patient use a keyboard to enter the information to an operator, who calls the office and reads the information to you; your response is then typed back to the patient. Newer technology uses an online captioned telephone service, much like closed captioning for television. Many smart phones can use a translation app to assist the caller. You should be familiar with the way this system works so that you can engage in these conversations in a professional manner.

TYPICAL OUTGOING CALLS

Most outgoing calls in the healthcare facility are responses to incoming calls. The same rules for courtesy and diction apply to calls made from the office to patients, other individuals, and businesses.

It is helpful to plan outgoing calls in advance. For instance, if the medical assistant is placing an order for office supplies, a list should be made that includes the product, the price, the quantity needed, and a catalog page number, if applicable. Questions about the various products ordered should be noted so that they can be asked while the sales representative is on the telephone.

Some medical assistants find it helpful to make all outgoing calls at once, when possible. This way the calls can be made one after another, and if a call back is necessary, the medical assistant is likely to still be by the telephone. Organizing calls helps increase office efficiency.

Never be rude to an individual on the telephone. Remember to treat those on the other end of the telephone as you would wish to be treated. Do not forget that you are a representative of the provider and that you must behave in a professional manner at all times.

Time Zones

When making outgoing calls, it is important to keep time zones in mind, especially when calling patients. If you are trying to contact a patient who is spending the winter somewhere else, you should place that call at an appropriate time for the patient. If you are trying to get information from an insurance company, you should call when someone is available to answer your questions. The continental United States is divided into four standard time zones: Pacific, Mountain, Central, and Eastern (Figure 8-6). When it is noon Pacific time, it is 3 PM Eastern time. If you will be calling from San Francisco to a business or professional office in New York, plan to make the call no later than 1 PM. When it is 2 PM on the West Coast, it is 5 PM on the East Coast.

Long Distance Calling

Long distance calls are simple to place, usually inexpensive, and efficient. When information is needed in a hurry, telephoning is much more expedient than written communication. Before placing a long distance call, have the correct number ready. If you do not have the number, you may access directory assistance by dialing 1, then the area code of the party you want to call, followed by 555-1212. In some areas, numbers are available by calling 1-411. Directory assistance is now an automated service in many regions, and you will be asked for the name of the city and person you are calling. Often a fee is charged for using directory assistance, so look for the telephone number using free sources whenever possible.

Some Internet services, such as Skype, Jajah, or magicJack, allow the user to call long distance, and sometimes even internationally, through the computer with no long distance charges.

USING A TELEPHONE DIRECTORY

The primary purpose of a telephone directory is to provide lists of those who have telephones, their telephone numbers and, in most cases, their addresses. In addition, the directory is an aid in checking the spelling of names and in locating certain types of businesses through the Yellow Pages. Directories are found on the Internet and in print format.

The Internet makes searching for telephone numbers much easier. Try to find telephone numbers through websites such as *www.yellowpages.com* or *www.whitepages.com,* or use a printed telephone

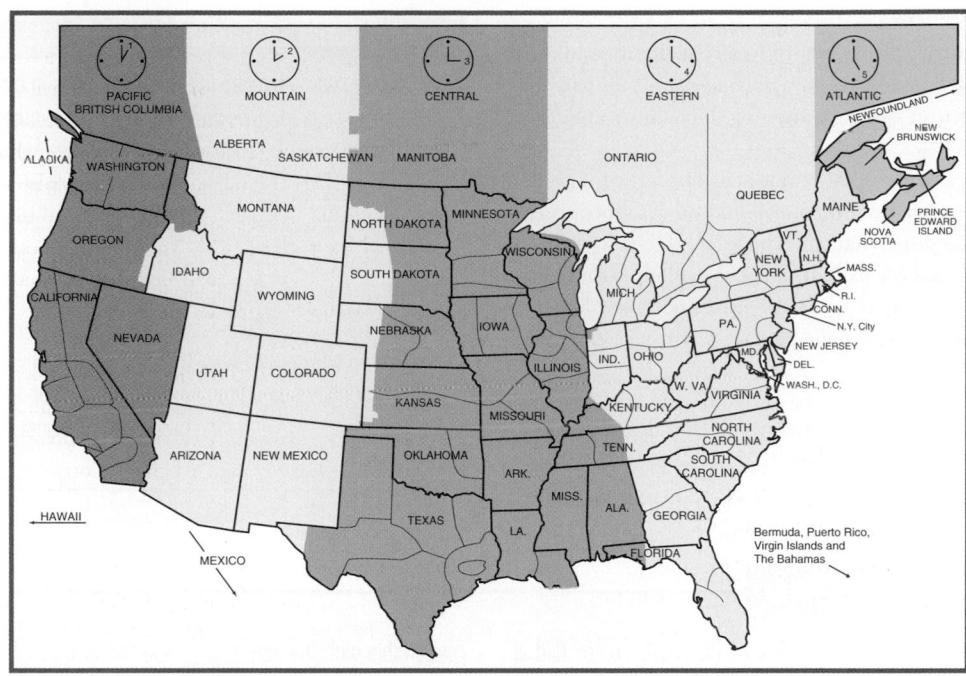

FIGURE 8-6 Time zones across the United States.

book to avoid directory assistance charges on the monthly phone bill. A Web search for the business or provider needed may yield the information. Companies with websites usually have a "Contact Us" page that directs the user to the individual departments.

In a print telephone directory, color coding is often used to differentiate between residence listings and business listings. Governmental offices usually have their own section (commonly blue). Some directories include ZIP code maps for the local area.

TELEPHONE SERVICES
Answering Services

Patients expect to be able to contact their provider if an emergency arises. This means that the telephone in the healthcare facility must be answered at all times, day and night, weekends and holidays. During normal office hours, the medical assistant is available to answer the telephone. After office hours, most healthcare facilities use an **answering service** or an answering machine that directs the caller to the answering service if there is an urgent issue.

With an answering service, an actual person answers the call, which can be comforting for patients. The staff at the answering service can act as a buffer for the provider after hours by screening the calls. By following the criteria given to them by the healthcare facility, they can determine whether the provider (or on-call person) should be contacted or the patient directed to the hospital emergency department, or whether a message can be taken and relayed to the healthcare facility in the morning.

It is common courtesy to call the answering service in the morning to let them know that you will be answering the calls and also to retrieve any messages taken overnight or over the weekend. You should also call the answering service when you are leaving for the day. Answering services also can be used to cover the telephone if all staff members need to be away from the telephones at the same time.

Automatic Call Routing

Many healthcare facilities have started using an **automatic call routing** system. The caller is given a menu of choices; he or she then presses a number on the telephone keypad to direct the call to the correct department. This can be an efficient way to handle a large volume of calls, but it can also be frustrating for some patients, especially elderly adults who may have trouble hearing and remembering the options. Some of the frustration can be minimized by providing a number option that connects the caller with a person (e.g., "Press 0"), who can then transfer the call to the appropriate department.

CRITICAL THINKING APPLICATION   8-7

Ashlynn has had many complaints from patients about the new call routing system because it takes so long to "get to a human being." How can she help make modern call routing systems easier for her patients?

CLOSING COMMENTS
Patient Education

Today's telephone systems allow providers to educate patients while they are on hold; recordings may be played that offer health information on subjects from A to Z. These messages can be professionally recorded and/or custom designed by the provider and staff. Special events may be announced, with the option to press a certain number for more information about the event.

Legal and Ethical Issues

The guidelines for medical confidentiality apply equally to telephone conversations; therefore, take care that no one overhears sensitive information. Use discretion when mentioning the name of the caller or patient.

Do not place or receive personal phone calls during work hours. Time limitations for personal phone use should be described in the office policies and procedures manual. The telephone is a business line and should be reserved for patients and others conducting business with the office. Personal cell phones also should not be used during working hours; this takes the medical assistant's time and attention away from patient care.

Telephone message records may be brought into court as evidence; make sure all messages are complete and legible. Most offices should keep these records for at least the same period as the statute of limitations in that state.

Professional Behaviors

We have talked on telephones and cell phones in our own lives, and most of us have used at least some of the special features on our phones. It is important to recognize that the way we present ourselves on the phone in our professional lives is different from the style of communication we use in our personal lives. The way we speak in our personal lives may not be appropriate in the healthcare facility. We must maintain a professional tone in communications with our patients and other contacts. For example, slang should not be used; "Hello" is not a proper way to answer a business telephone; and we must take care how we use medical terminology when on the telephone (jargon should not be used when speaking with patients). The goal is always to present a positive professional image of the healthcare facility we represent.

SUMMARY OF SCENARIO

Ashlynn is quickly becoming a part of the team at Dr. Frank's office and is developing into a well-liked asset to the staff. She has learned to slow down when speaking on the phone and to adjust her volume and pitch, depending on the patient with whom she is speaking. Although she tends to be quite talkative, she is balancing just the right amount of friendly chatter with the business at hand. She does this by offering a friendly greeting to callers, getting to the point of the call, then being affable before ending the call. By expressing her concern and asking how she can be of help to the patients, Ashlynn shows them that she sincerely cares about their problems. She is careful about her tone of voice, realizing that patients may take her comments the wrong way if she does not treat them in a cordial manner. Dr. Frank is very pleased with her performance.

Ashlynn takes care when she speaks to patients and others on the phone so that she does not breach confidentiality in any way. She has become comfortable with the way she is expected to answer the telephone. The pace of her speech and the wording are now a habit. Ashlynn is determined to maintain a professional relationship with all the people related to her work environment. She is adept now at handling calls from angry patients and can maintain control with even the most aggressive callers. She leaves callers on hold for a minimum time and reassures them frequently that she is attending to their situation. By treating callers as she would want to be treated, Ashlynn reduces frustration, and she feels that the office is more efficient at handling the large volume of calls that come in each day. She shows much promise for a long and rewarding career in the medical field and is satisfied with the current track of her career. As she continues to settle into her position, she looks forward to learning more about efficiency and time management. Her positive attitude and desire to learn will only enhance her performance at work, making her a valuable employee and one worth promoting.

SUMMARY OF LEARNING OBJECTIVES

1. **Define, spell, and pronounce the terms listed in the vocabulary.**
   Spelling and pronouncing medical terms correctly reinforce the medical assistant's credibility. Knowing the definitions of these terms promotes confidence in communication with patients and co-workers.

2. **Identify and explain the features of a multiple-line telephone system, and also explain how each can be used effectively in a healthcare facility.**
   A multiple-line telephone system has many features; most obviously, more than one telephone line comes into the office. This means that callers are less likely to get a busy signal when calling the healthcare facility. Additional features, such as speed dial, voice mail, and call forwarding, can increase efficiency.

   Medical assistants must understand how each feature of the telephone system works. For example, knowing when to use the speakerphone function and when not to helps protect patient confidentiality.

Knowing how to use the conference call feature helps facilitate telephone meetings with satellite offices. Understanding how the voice mail system works is crucial to the medical assistant's work life.

3. **Do the following related to effective use of the telephone:**
   * *Discuss the telephone equipment needed by a healthcare facility.*
     Two incoming lines is the minimum recommended number of lines for a healthcare facility. Telephones should be placed where they are accessible but private. One medical assistant can handle no more than two incoming lines; this means that the addition of more lines may involve the need for more employees.
   * *Summarize active listening skills.*
     A big part of communication is being able to listen. Honing your active listening skills also will increase your communication skills. Focus on the conversation by being present in the moment. Not only is interrupting rude, it also shows that you were not listening, truly listening,

because you were coming up with your response. Part of active listening is confirming what you heard to be sure that you have received the intended message.

- *Demonstrate effective and professional telephone techniques.*
  Medical assistants should answer the telephone promptly and professionally. A pleasing telephone personality conveys a favorable impression of the healthcare facility. Enunciate, pronouncing words clearly and distinctly. Vary the pitch of your voice, and avoid a monotonous or droning manner. Courtesy to patients and other callers is vital. First impressions are important, and a medical assistant's telephone manner sets the tone for the caller's perception of the healthcare facility. Be courteous and polite to all callers. (Refer to Procedure 8-1.)

- *Consider the importance of tone of voice and enunciation.*
  Tone of voice can completely change the message sent. Make sure you use the correct tone of voice so that the message is not misunderstood. Enunciation also ensures that your message is not misunderstood. Communicating over the telephone has its own issues, and enunciation is crucial. Speaking clearly helps your caller to hear your message.

4. **Explain the importance of thinking ahead when managing telephone calls; also, describe the correct way to answer the telephone in the office.**
   Before you start answering calls, make sure you have all of the supplies you need to do your job. Confidentiality in a healthcare facility must always be a priority.

   Medical assistants should answer the telephone promptly and professionally. The provider's image is affected by the way telephone calls are handled. Be courteous and polite to all callers. The medical assistant should identify the facility first when picking up the phone, followed by his or her name, followed by an offer of help. If the caller does not offer a name, the medical assistant should ask who is calling.

5. **Discuss the screening of incoming calls, and list several questions to ask when handling an emergency call.**
   Most healthcare facilities expect the medical assistant answering the telephone to screen the calls; this is an important task. The facility's screening policies should address how calls should be handled when the provider is out of the office, and the medical assistant should always ask before placing a caller on hold or transferring a call.

   If a phone call is an emergency, the policies for handling emergency calls apply. Ask for a phone number where the caller can be reached in case of a sudden disconnection. Ask about the chief symptoms and when they started. Find out whether the patient has had similar symptoms in the past and what happened in that situation. Determine whether the patient is alone, has transportation, or needs an ambulance. In severe cases, do not hang up the phone until the ambulance or police arrive. A special sheet of instructions listing specific medical emergencies (e.g., chest pain, heavy bleeding, seizure, fainting, poisoning) should be posted by each telephone.

6. **Do the following related to taking a message:**
   - *Document telephone messages accurately.*
     When taking a telephone message, either in a handwritten or electronic format, strive for accuracy. Be sure to get all the information the provider will need to act. Repeat any words or numbers that are not heard clearly. (Refer to Procedure 8-2.)

   - *List the seven elements of a correctly handled telephone message.*
     The seven elements of a correctly handled phone message are (1) the name of the person to whom the call should be directed; (2) the name of the person calling; (3) the caller's telephone number; (4) the reason for the call; (5) the medical assistant's description of the action to be taken; (6) the date and time of the call; and (7) the initials of the person taking the call, so that if any question arises that person can be consulted.

   - *Report relevant information concisely and accurately.*
     If a handwritten system is used for recording telephone messages, a policy must be developed on the retention of the telephone message records. Accurate records can ensure quality patient care and customer service. (Refer to Procedure 8-2.)

7. **Discuss various types of common incoming calls and how to deal with each.**
   Knowing how to respond to the different types of calls received will make you a valuable asset to the healthcare facility. Common types of incoming calls include the following: requests for directions; inquiries about bills; inquiries about fees; inquiries about participating providers; requests for assistance with insurance; inquiries about radiology and laboratory reports; progress reports; routine report calls from hospitals or other sources; requests for a referral; and questions about office administration matters.

8. **Discuss various types of special incoming calls and how to deal with each.**
   If a patient refuses to discuss symptoms with a medical assistant, follow the healthcare facility's policies and procedures, which may suggest that the patient make an appointment with the provider to discuss the problem in person. Other types of special calls a medical assistant must know how to handle include unsatisfactory progress reports, requests for test results, requests for information from third parties, complaints about care or fees, and calls from a staff member's family or friends.

9. **Discuss how the medical assistant should handle various types of difficult calls.**
   With angry callers, never return the anger. Remain calm and speak in tones that are perhaps slightly quieter than those of the caller. This often prompts the caller to lower his or her tone of voice. Offer to help the angry person and ask questions to gain control of the conversation, moving it toward resolution. Do not argue with angry callers.

   Callers who have a complaint should be handled in a manner similar to that for angry callers. Remain calm and offer to help. Take a serious interest in what the caller has to say. Let the caller know that his or her

Continued

SUMMARY OF LEARNING OBJECTIVES—*continued*

concerns are important to the staff and the provider. Find the source of the problem and determine exactly what the caller wants or expects as a resolution. Always follow up on complaints and make sure they were resolved as much to the caller's satisfaction as possible.

Other types of difficult callers that medical assistants must know how to handle include aggressive callers, unauthorized inquiry calls, sales calls, and callers with difficulty communicating.

10. **Discuss typical outgoing calls, including why knowledge of time zones and long distance calling is necessary.**

Most outgoing calls in the healthcare facility are made in response to incoming calls. It is helpful to plan outgoing calls in advance. Organizing calls helps increase office efficiency.

The continental United States is divided into four standard time zones. Long distance calls are simple to place, usually inexpensive, and efficient. Knowledge of both concepts are important for a medical assistant handling the telephone.

11. **Discuss the use of a telephone directory, and describe how answering services and automatic call routing systems are used in a healthcare facility.**

The primary purpose of a telephone directory is to provide lists of those who have telephones, their telephone numbers and, in most cases, their addresses. The Internet makes searching for telephone numbers much easier.

Answering services are used to answer the telephone in the healthcare facility when the staff is not available. This could be during the overnight hours or during regular office hours when the staff is at lunch or in a meeting. Automatic call routing systems allow the patient to select a number from a menu to reach specific departments in the healthcare facility. The system should have an option that allows patients to choose to speak to a person if they are not sure what number to press.

12. **Discuss the legal and ethical issues related to telephone techniques.**

The guidelines for medical confidentiality apply equally to telephone conversations; therefore, take care that no one overhears sensitive information. Telephone records may be brought to court as evidence.

CONNECTIONS

Study Guide Connection: Go to the Chapter 8 Study Guide. Read and complete the activities.

evolve Evolve Connection: Go to the Chapter 8 link at *evolve.elsevier.com/kinn* to complete the Chapter Review Quiz. Check out the other resources listed for this chapter to make the most of what you have learned from Telephone Techniques.

SCHEDULING APPOINTMENTS AND PATIENT PROCESSING

9

SCENARIO

Ramona West is the medical assistant in charge of scheduling appointments and patient processing for Dr. Charlotte Brown. Ramona is an extremely organized person who thinks quickly and creatively. Two of her professional goals are to ensure that the healthcare facility remains on schedule throughout the day with minimal wait time for the patients and that patient flow through the office is done in an efficient manner. She is fortunate that Dr. Brown is cooperative and time oriented, and they work well together to reach these common goals.

Ramona usually arrives at work at least 15 minutes early to begin her preparations for the day. She reviews the electronic health record for each patient to make sure test results from previous visits are available to the provider and that the medical record is complete. She pays special attention to the patients who arrive in the healthcare facility as she completes her daily tasks, remembering the importance of providing patients with good customer service. Ramona greets each patient by name and carries on a brief but cordial conversation. Patients appreciate that she goes the extra mile to remember something about them, and this promotes excellent patient relations.

Ramona leaves a little time in the morning and afternoon for emergency appointments. The healthcare facility uses an automatic call routing system to contact patients to confirm appointments in advance, which increases her show rate. She is always pleasant to the patients as they go through the check-in and checkout procedures. Her friendly, caring attitude makes her a favorite among the patients, and Dr. Brown is pleased with the relationship-building skills Ramona has developed.

While studying this chapter, think about the following questions:
- How can the medical assistant contribute to an efficient daily routine?
- How does the medical assistant contribute to keeping the daily schedule on track?
- How can the schedule be put back on track when emergencies disrupt the day?
- How does the flexibility of the medical assistant contribute to office efficiency?
- What are some ways to develop good rapport with patients?
- Why is the sign-in register a potential breach of patient confidentiality?
- What is the value of knowing some information about patients' personal lives?

LEARNING OBJECTIVES

1. Define, spell, and pronounce the terms listed in the vocabulary.
2. Describe guidelines to establishing an appointment schedule and creating an appointment matrix.
3. Discuss the advantages of computerized appointment scheduling.
4. Discuss appointment book scheduling and explain how self-scheduling can reduce the number of calls to the healthcare facility.
5. Discuss the legality of the appointment scheduling system.
6. Discuss pros and cons of various types of appointment management systems.
7. Discuss telephone scheduling and identify critical information required for scheduling appointments for new patients.
8. Discuss scheduling appointments for established patients.
9. Discuss how the medical assistant should handle scheduling other types of appointments.
10. Do the following related to special circumstances in scheduling:
    - Discuss several methods of dealing with patients who consistently arrive late.
    - Recognize office policies and protocols for rescheduling appointments.
    - Discuss how to deal with emergencies, provider referrals, and patients without appointments.
11. Discuss how to handle failed appointments and no-shows, as well as methods to increase appointment show rates.
12. Discuss how to handle cancellations and delays.
13. Discuss patient processing, including the importance of the reception area.
14. Describe how to prepare for patient arrival, including patient check-in procedures.
15. Explain why using the patient's name as often as possible is important, as well as how the medical assistant can make patients feel at ease.
16. Describe registration procedures, including obtaining a patient history.

LEARNING OBJECTIVES—*continued*

17. Do the following related to patient reception and processing:
    - Show consideration for patients' time.
    - Properly treat patients with special needs.
    - Escort and instruct the patient.
    - Describe where health records should be placed.

18. Describe how the medical assistant should deal with challenging situations, such as talkative patients, children, angry patients, and patients' relatives and friends.
19. Discuss the friendly farewell, patient checkout, and planning for the next day.
20. Discuss patient education, as well as legal and ethical issues, for scheduling appointments and patient processing.

VOCABULARY

amenity (uh-me'-nih-te) Something conducive to comfort, convenience, or enjoyment.

automatic call routing A software system that answers phones automatically and routes calls to staff after the caller responds to prompts; also used to call a large number of patients to remind them of appointments or make announcements.

demographics Statistical data of a population. In healthcare this includes patient name, address, date of birth, employment, and other details.

disruption An unexpected event that throws a plan into disorder; an interruption that prevents a system or process from continuing as usual or as expected.

established patients Patients who are returning to the office who have previously been seen by the provider.

expediency (ek-spe'-de-en-se) A means of achieving a particular end, as in a situation requiring haste or caution.

follow-up appointment An appointment type used when a patient needs to see the provider after a condition should have been resolved or to monitor an ongoing condition, such as hypertension. Also known as a recheck appointment.

harmonious Marked by accord in sentiment or action; having the parts agreeably related.

incidental disclosure A secondary use or disclosure that cannot reasonably be prevented, is limited in nature, and occurs because of another use or disclosure that is permitted.

intercom A two-way communication system with a microphone and loudspeaker at each station for localized use.

integral (in'-tih-grul) Essential; being an indispensable part of a whole.

interaction A two-way communication; mutual or reciprocal action or influence.

interval Space of time between events.

matrix Something in which a thing originates, develops, takes shape, or is contained; a base on which to build.

no-show When a patient fails to keep an appointment without giving advance notice.

Notice of Privacy Practices (NPP) A written document describing the healthcare facility's privacy practices. The patient must be provided with the NPP and sign an acknowledgment of receipt.

perception A quick, acute, and intuitive cognition; a capacity for comprehension.

phonetic (fuh-neh'-tik) Constituting an alteration of ordinary spelling that better represents the spoken language, uses only characters of the regular alphabet, and is used in a context of conventional spelling.

practice management software A type of software that allows the user to enter demographic information, schedule appointments, maintain lists of insurance payers, perform billing tasks, and generate reports.

preauthorization A process required by some insurance carriers in which the provider obtains permission to perform certain procedures or services or refers a patient to a specialist.

precertification A process required by some insurance carriers in which the provider must prove medical necessity before performing a procedure.

prerequisite (pre-reh'-kwih-zut) Something that is necessary to an end or to carry out a function.

proficiency (pruh-fih'-shun-se) Competency as a result of training or practice.

progress notes Notes used in the medical record to track the patient's progress and condition.

recheck appointment An appointment type used when a patient needs to see the provider after a condition should have been resolved or to monitor an ongoing condition, such as hypertension. Also known as a follow-up appointment.

screening A system for examining and separating into different groups; in the medical office, it means determining the severity of illness that patients experience and prioritizing appointments based on that severity.

sequentially (se-kwen'-shuh-le) Of, relating to, or arranged in a sequence.

The provider's time is the most valuable asset of a medical practice. The person responsible for scheduling this time must understand the practice, be familiar with the working habits and preferences of the provider (or providers), and have clear guidelines for time management in the practice.

Appointment scheduling is the process that determines which patients the provider sees, the dates and times of appointments, and how much time is allotted to each patient based on the complaint and the provider's availability. Time management involves the realization that unforeseen interruptions and delays always occur and must be handled appropriately. In addition, the medical assistant must assign the appropriate appointment time length for the complaint along with ensuring that the appointments are scheduled so that there are minimal gaps in the schedule. Most healthcare providers find that efficient appointment scheduling is one of the most important factors in the success of the practice. Scheduling can be done in a number of ways, and each facility must find the way that suits it best.

ESTABLISHING THE APPOINTMENT SCHEDULE

Developing a schedule that meets the needs of both the providers and the patients is key to keeping the office running smoothly and efficiently. The scheduling team, along with the provider, should come up with scheduling parameters to both meet the needs of the patient population and keep the providers' preferences and habits in mind.

Patient Needs

Consider the **demographics** of the patients that are being served when determining office hours and appointment times. The staff should answer the following questions:

- Is the office in a busy metropolitan area or a rural agricultural community?
- What type of patients are seen? Are they of a specific age or gender? Do they have common diagnoses? Is the provider a general practitioner?
- Are evening and weekend appointments essential for most of the patients served?

Knowing when the providers need to be available for patients is one of the factors in creating the patient schedule.

Provider Preferences and Habits

Consider the preferences and habits of the providers in the practice before establishing and implementing a scheduling plan. Ask the following questions:

- Does the provider become restless if the reception room is not packed with waiting patients?
- Does the provider worry if even one patient is kept waiting?
- Is the provider methodic and careful about being in the facility when patient appointments are scheduled to begin?
- Is the provider habitually late?
- Does the provider move easily from one patient to another?
- Does the provider require a "break time" after a few patients?

- Would the provider rather see fewer patients and spend more time with each one or schedule more patients each day?

All of these preferences and habits become an **integral** part of the scheduling process. Keep in mind that the provider cannot spend every moment of the day with patients. The provider also has telephone calls to make and receive, reports to examine and dictate, meetings to attend, mail to answer, and many other business responsibilities. An experienced staff can handle many but not all of these tasks.

Next the office hours and the length of appointment time **intervals** need to be determined. Keeping in mind patients' needs and the provider's preferences and habits, decide what would be the shortest time possible for an appointment. Most healthcare facilities use 10- or 15-minute time intervals for the appointment schedule. Paper-based appointment books can be purchased with various time intervals. A computerized appointment system can also be set to the specific time interval that has been decided on. A computerized system can be customized for different providers, so that one provider could have 10-minute time slots and another could have 15-minute time slots. If an appointment, such as a complete physical, needs longer than 15 minutes, multiple time slots are used to cover that appointment. Once the minimum time period has been set, then the appointment matrix can be established.

CREATING THE APPOINTMENT MATRIX

Setting up the appointment **matrix** (Procedure 9-1) involves blocking out the times when the provider is not available to see patients, such as lunch time, hospital rounds, conferences, and vacation (Figure 9-1). In a paper-based appointment book the matrix is usually established for 6 months at a time. In a computerized system the matrix can be set up indefinitely.

Establishing Guidelines for Appointment Scheduling

Before establishing the appointment matrix, decide the length of the shortest office visit type. This visit type would usually be for a **follow-up** or **recheck appointment** for an established patient. Other specific appointment types should now be determined. General categories for appointment types are: follow-up or recheck, wellness examination, complete physical examination, urgent visit, new patient visit, and comprehensive visit. Each category has a specific amount of time assigned to it; for example, a follow-up or recheck appointment could be 15 to 20 minutes and a comprehensive visit could be 30 to 40 minutes. The providers and scheduling team should work together to come up with these time periods to ensure that the office runs smoothly and efficiently.

If it is decided that a complete physical examination should be scheduled for 30 minutes, yet the provider routinely spends 45 minutes with the patient for a complete physical, then the scheduling guidelines need to be adjusted. Well-planned scheduling and adherence to that schedule allow the provider to do more than run in and out of examination rooms with little time for the patient to talk with the provider. There will be a bit of trial and error when developing the priorities for the appointment schedule.

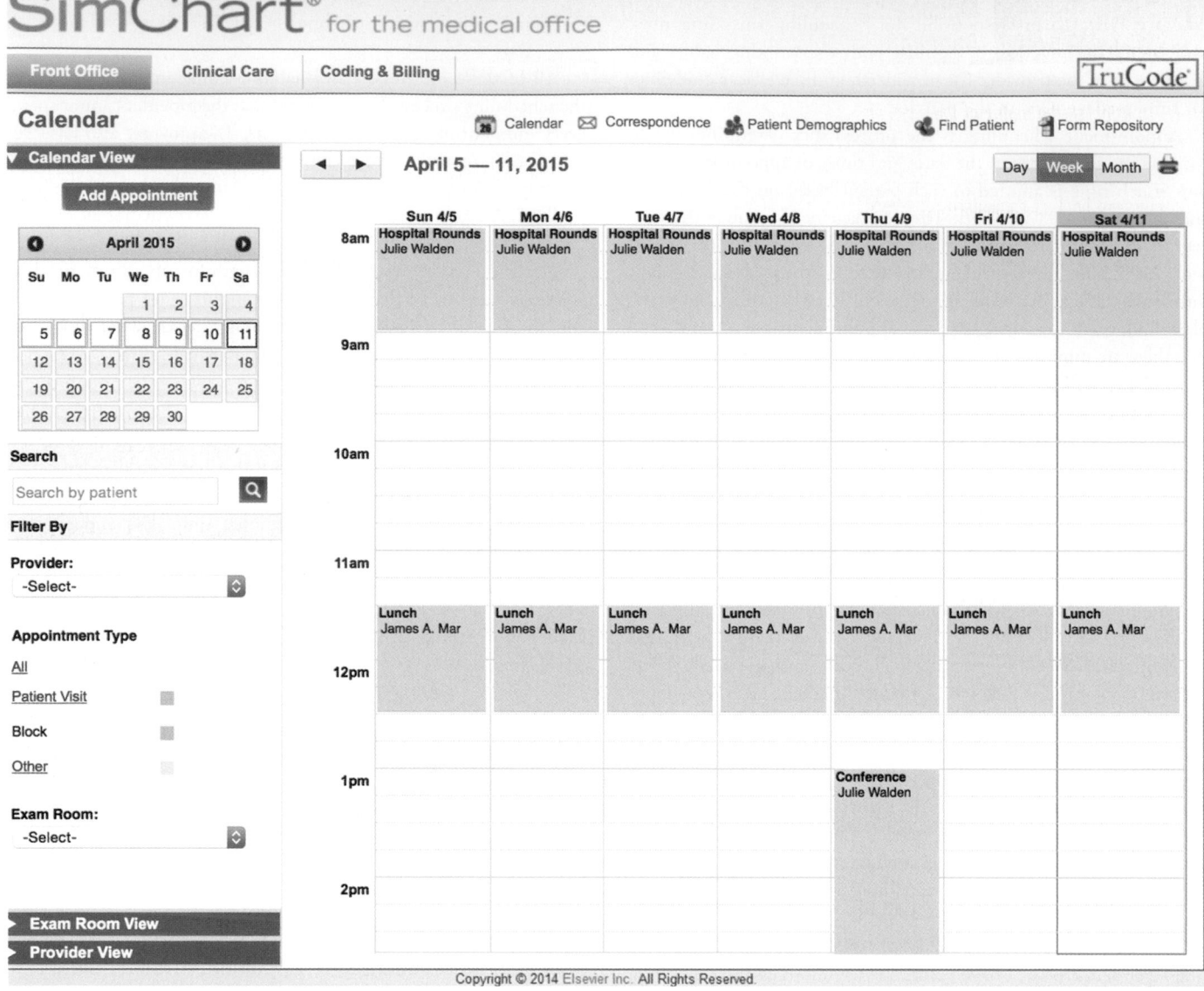

FIGURE 9-1 Schedule matrix showing provider availability.

Some providers need prompting to end the patient visit and move to the next patient. If there is a medical assistant in the examination room, he or she can help the provider remain on schedule by letting the provider know that the end of the appointment time is near. They may work out some type of signal, such as a hand gesture or phrase. A pager may be used when the medical assistant is not in room with the provider. When the provider's pager vibrates he or she will know that it is time to wind things up with that patient. The clinical medical assistant and the administrative medical assistant must work together to keep the healthcare facility running smoothly and efficiently.

CRITICAL THINKING APPLICATION   **9-1**

- Ramona has noticed that Dr. Brown is taking a little longer with patients than normal and that she is running consistently behind schedule by approximately 5 to 15 minutes. How can Ramona help rectify this situation?
- Discuss ways of approaching the provider when he or she is the cause of the delays in the schedule. What opening remarks can the medical assistant use to start the discussion in a positive way?

PROCEDURE 9-1	Manage Appointment Scheduling Using Established Priorities: Establish the Appointment Matrix

Goal: *To establish the matrix of the appointment schedule.*

EQUIPMENT and SUPPLIES

- Appointment book or computer with scheduling software
- Office procedure manual (optional)
- List of providers' availability and preferences
- Black pen, pencil, and highlighters
- Calendar

PROCEDURAL STEPS

1. Using the calendar, determine when the office is not open (e.g., holidays, weekends, evenings). If using the appointment book and a black pen, draw an *X* through the times the office is not open. If using the scheduling software, block the times the office is not open.
   PURPOSE: Blocking the closed times of the office helps prevent patients from being scheduled when the office is closed.

2. Identify the times each provider is not available. If using the appointment book, write in the providers' names on each column and then draw an *X* through their unavailable times. If using the scheduling software, select each provider and block the times the provider is unavailable.
   PURPOSE: Many providers do rounds in the hospital or long-term care facilities and cannot see patients in the clinic during those times. Providers also attend meetings and conferences during the workday. These events, along with vacations and lunch times, should be blocked on their schedules.

3. Using the office procedure manual or providers' preferences, determine when each provider performs certain types of examinations. In the appoint-

ment book, indicate these examinations either by writing the examination time or by highlighting the examination times. Follow the office's procedure on indicating these examination times in the appointment book. When using scheduling software, set up the times for the examinations or use the highlighting feature if available.
PURPOSE: Some providers perform a variety of examinations. It can be more time efficient to have the same types of examinations on the same day. For instance, a provider in a women's health department may perform both gynecologic and prenatal examinations. The provider may prefer to set aside certain days to do prenatal examinations and other days to do gynecologic examinations.

4. Using the office procedure manual or the list of providers' preferences and availability, identify other times to block on the scheduling matrix. Some providers require catch-up times and these time slots are blocked. Some medical facilities save appointment times for same-day appointments. When saving time blocks for same-day appointments, make sure to use pencil so it can be erased and the patient's information entered on the day of the appointment. For the scheduling software, block those times when patients cannot be booked and indicate the times for the same-day appointments.
PURPOSE: Allowing appointment times to be saved for same-day appointments provides the opportunity for the provider to see a patient who needs to get in immediately and prevents the patient from being turned away or double-booked.

Available Facilities

Another factor to keep in mind when scheduling appointments is the availability of facilities needed for the particular appointment type. Getting a patient into the office at a time when no facilities are available for the services needed is pointless. For example, suppose that a healthcare facility with two providers has only one room that can be used for minor surgery. Do not schedule two patients requiring minor surgery for the same time interval, even if both doctors could be available. If the healthcare facility has only one electrocardiograph, do not book two electrocardiograms (ECGs) at the same time. As the medical assistant gains **proficiency** in scheduling, it becomes easier to pair patient needs with the available facilities according to the provider's preference. Major equipment frequently used or a certain room with such equipment may need its own scheduling column in the appointment book or software system.

METHODS OF SCHEDULING APPOINTMENTS

The two most common methods of appointment scheduling are computerized scheduling and appointment book or paper-based

scheduling. Each has advantages and disadvantages, and the healthcare facility should weigh the benefits and choose the method that best suits the provider and the staff.

Computerized Scheduling

The computer has replaced the appointment book in many practices. Software for appointment scheduling, often referred to as **practice management software**, ranges from relatively simple programs that merely display available and scheduled times to more sophisticated systems that perform several other functions. Many programs can display such information as the length and type of appointment required and the patient's day or time preferences. The computer then can select the best appointment time based on the information entered into the computer.

Another advantage of a computerized scheduling system is the ability to search for future appointments. For example, when a patient calls and inquires about an appointment, the system can search by his or her name to find the time and date. With computerized scheduling, multiple users can access the appointment schedule at the same time, minimizing the wait time for patients. Another advantage of computerized schedules is the reports that can be generated. A hard copy of the provider's daily schedule can be created, showing the patients' names, telephone numbers, and the reason for the visit. Some healthcare facilities print these out, and others use them on screen. Healthcare facilities must have scheduling procedures to follow when the technology is down; some keep an appointment book as a backup to computer scheduling.

Appointment Book Scheduling

Office suppliers carry a variety of appointment book styles. Some appointment books show an entire week at a glance; many are color coded, with a special color used for each day of the week (Figure 9-2). This is very helpful when the provider asks the patient to return, for instance, in 2 weeks. If Wednesdays are colored yellow, the medical assistant can flip quickly to the correct day 2 weeks later and schedule the appointment. Multiple columns may be available to correspond with the number of doctors in a group practice, and the time can be divided according to their preferences.

Self-Scheduling

Allowing patients to schedule their own appointments using the Internet and the healthcare facility's Web site is becoming much more common. The patient is given limited access to the schedule, seeing only the available appointment times, not the other patients who are scheduled, thus protecting patient confidentiality. Other patients' names should never be visible on an online system.

Software is available that allows the patient to self-schedule through secure links to the provider's appointment book. The software or Internet site for the healthcare facility should give the patient guidelines as to the amount of time needed for certain appointments or should allow only a certain length of time to be self-scheduled, such as 15 minutes. These systems will reduce the number of calls and are available to the patient 24 hours a day. Some of these systems also send an automatic e-mail reminder to the patient the day before the appointment, requesting a reply to confirm. These systems are less frustrating to patients, who do not have to wait on hold to speak to the person who does scheduling for the healthcare facility. However, lengthy or complicated appointments should be scheduled through the staff.

Although this type of system for making appointments appeals to most technologically savvy people, some patients may not be comfortable using it. It does require minimal skills and Internet access. Others may object to online scheduling because they do not want their names anywhere on the Internet. This is a valid concern, and the facility should allow these patients to schedule over the telephone. If this system is used, some allowance must be made for patients who choose not to use it.

CRITICAL THINKING APPLICATION   **9-2**

The software used in Dr. Brown's office can allow patients to self-schedule. Ramona has heard about patient self-scheduling and would like to try this method in the office, but Dr. Brown is concerned that her patients will miss the personal contact and is not sold on the idea.

- What can Ramona say to convince Dr. Brown to try this new, time-saving method of scheduling?
- What challenges might the use of this system bring?

LEGALITY OF THE APPOINTMENT SCHEDULING SYSTEM

Because the paper-based appointment book can be used as a legal record, it must be accurate and maintained so that it provides correct information about the patients at the healthcare facility. Patients are expected to follow the provider's orders; this includes keeping appointments. If a patient does not show up for an appointment or cancels it and does not reschedule, a notation of this fact should be placed in the patient's health record. If a patient reschedules an appointment and subsequently keeps it, there is no need to document that it was rescheduled.

Pens are permanent, but the appointment book can become illegible if a number of patients change or cancel their appointments. Pencil is used in the appointment book so that making changes is easier. The information in the book includes the patient's name and a phone number where the patient can be reached. Some healthcare facilities list the reason for the appointment, but most note only the name and phone number. Listing the reason for the visit is not necessary if the medical assistant references the time needed for the appointment and blocks off that amount of time. Because the appointment book could be produced in litigation as a legal record, it should be kept for the number of years that constitute the statute of limitations in that individual state. If the appointment book is discarded, its contents should be shredded to protect patient privacy. Although the appointment book can be used as a legal record, actual medical records are more likely to be used in matters of litigation. Because **progress notes** are dated, a copy of the medical record shows all pertinent information about the patient's adherence to the provider's orders, including the appointments with the provider.

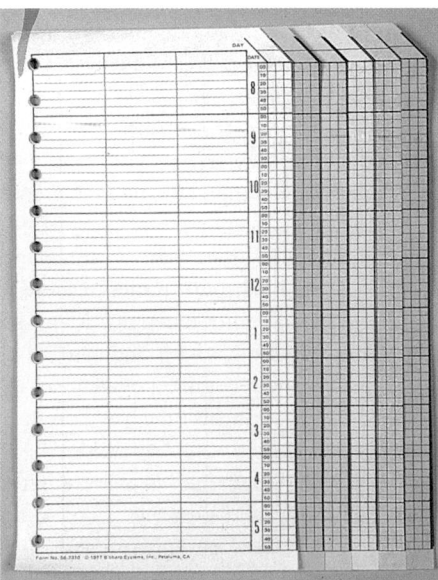

FIGURE 9-2 Color-coded appointment book pages help the medical assistant flip to the right day of the right week quickly. Appointments for multiple providers can be color-coded in the book.

Computerized scheduling systems can also be used to track patient appointments. Most computerized scheduling systems will allow the user to indicate if the patient has checked in, canceled, or missed the scheduled appointment. When a patient misses or cancels an appointment it should be documented in the electronic patient record for legal purposes.

TYPES OF APPOINTMENT SCHEDULING

Different types of appointment scheduling are used to meet the various needs of the medical facility, the providers, and the patients. Some offices use a combination of methods to create the right mix of activity during the day and to ensure that the day runs smoothly and efficiently. The medical assistant should become proficient at managing appointments. The following section presents several methods of appointment scheduling.

Time-Specified (Stream) Scheduling

When each patient is given a specific time for their appointment, this is referred to as time-specified or stream scheduling as it keeps a steady flow of patients moving through the office. This is the most common type of scheduling used in healthcare facilities. Studies have shown that providers can see more patients with less pressure when patient appointments are scheduled for a specific time slot. The medical assistant who is scheduling patients using this method should know the amount of time needed for each appointment type and keep time slots available for urgent visits.

Wave Scheduling

Wave scheduling is an attempt to create short-term flexibility within each hour. Wave scheduling assumes that the actual time needed for all the patients seen will average out over the course of the day. Instead of scheduling patients at each 15-minute interval, wave scheduling places three patients in the office at the same time, and they are seen in the order of their arrival. This way, one person's late arrival does not disrupt the entire schedule.

Modified Wave Scheduling

The wave schedule can be modified in several ways. For example, one method is to have two patients scheduled to come in at 10 AM and a third at 10:30 AM. This hourly cycle is repeated throughout the day. In another version, patients are scheduled to arrive at given intervals during the first half of the hour, and none are scheduled to arrive during the second half of the hour. This would allow time for urgent or walk-in patients to be seen.

Double-Booking

Booking two patients to come in at the same time is sometimes used to work in a patient with an acute illness or injury when there are no open appointments. This works out best if one of the patients needs laboratory work or another procedure done before seeing the provider. The provider can see one of the patients while the other one is being prepared.

Open Office Hours

With the open office hours method, the facility is open at given hours of the day or evening, and the patients are told that they can come in at any time. This type of system is often used in an urgent care setting. Patients are then seen in the order in which they arrive, although a patient with an urgent condition may be seen ahead of those who arrived before them.

The open office hours system can have many disadvantages. The office may already be crowded when the provider arrives, resulting in an extremely long wait for some patients. Patients may arrive in waves throughout the day, which causes parts of the day to be very busy and other parts to be slow. This makes accomplishing other office duties difficult. Without planning, the facilities and staff can be overburdened.

CRITICAL THINKING APPLICATION   **9-3**

Dr. Brown would like to implement evening appointments one night each week and open the office every other Saturday morning. She feels this will better serve her patients with children who have difficulty making daytime appointments. If this is her primary goal, should other types of patients be seen during these time slots? Why or why not?

Grouping Procedures

Grouping or categorizing of procedures is another method of scheduling that appeals to many practitioners. For instance, an internist might reserve all morning appointments for complete physical examinations, or a pediatrician might keep that time for well-baby visits. A surgeon might devote 1 day each week to seeing only referral patients. Obstetricians often schedule pregnant patients on different days from gynecology patients. The providers and staff can experiment with different groupings until the plan that works best for the practice eventually becomes evident. In applying a grouping system of appointments, the medical assistant may find it helpful to color-code the sections of the appointment book reserved for designated procedures.

Advance Booking

Often appointments are made months in advance. When any appointment is made, an appointment card should be completed and given to the patient. All appointment cards should mention that patients must give 24 hours' notice if they are unable to keep the time reserved. Most offices have some type of confirmation procedure by which patients are notified the day before to verify that they intend to keep the appointment. E-mail and text messages are becoming common methods of reminding patients of upcoming appointments. The medical assistant should be aware of the policies for his or her facility regarding patient reminders.

TIME PATTERNS

When booking appointments, the medical assistant should make it a policy to leave some open time during each day's schedule so that if a patient calls with a special problem that is not an immediate emergency, time will be available to book the patient for at least a brief visit. Mondays and Fridays generally are the most hectic days of the week. Keeping one time slot available in the morning and the afternoon specifically for emergencies also is a wise practice. A busy provider always fills these open slots, and having them in the schedule causes the least **disruption** during the day. If possible, set aside time in the morning and afternoon for a break. Even 15 minutes can give the provider time to return calls from patients, verify prescription calls, or answer questions.

TELEPHONE SCHEDULING

A pleasant manner and expressing a willingness to help are just as important on the telephone as when meeting patients face to face. This is especially true when making appointments, because the telephone contact may be the patient's first impression of the facility. Often the manner in which the booking is made makes more of an effect than the convenience of the appointment time.

Be especially considerate if the time requested for an appointment must be refused. Briefly explain why the time is not available and offer a substitute date and time. Comply with the patient's desires as much as possible, and do not show annoyance if the patient does not understand the scheduling process. Most people, however, understand the need for a well-managed office and are willing to cooperate.

Many offices offer the patient a choice when scheduling the appointment and let the patient decide which option is best for him or her. For example, the following dialog might take place during the scheduling call:

Medical assistant:	*"Mrs. Thomas, Dr. Stern is available to see you in the office next Tuesday or Wednesday, January 6 or 7. Which day is better for you?"*
Patient:	*"I will be working on Wednesday, so I would like to come in on Tuesday."*
Medical assistant:	*"Do you prefer a morning or afternoon appointment?"*
Patient:	*"The afternoon is best for me."*
Medical assistant:	*"Great. Would 1:30 or 3:30 be a better time?"*
Patient:	*"I can be there at 1:30."*
Medical assistant:	*"Then Dr. Stern will see you at 1:30 next Tuesday, January 6. Thank you for calling, Mrs. Thomas. We'll see you then!"*

These small courtesies give patients the feeling that they control their time. Always repeat the time to reinforce the appointment and do not hesitate to ask the patient if he or she has a pen ready to jot down the time and date. While repeating the information to the patient, check the appointment book or computer screen to ensure that it was posted correctly. When scheduling appointments over the telephone it is not possible to give the patient a reminder card for the appointment. Be sure to ask if they would like a telephone, e-mail, or text message reminder of the appointment.

Write legibly when using an appointment book. These records could be called into court, and the medical assistant must be able to read his or her own writing if asked to testify. Form the habit of entering the patient's daytime telephone number after every entry. The appointment may need to be canceled or the schedule

rearranged in a hurry, and many precious minutes can be saved if the telephone number is handy. Cell phone numbers also are quite useful for tracking down a patient quickly.

SCHEDULING APPOINTMENTS FOR NEW PATIENTS

Arranging the first appointment for a new patient requires time and attention to detail (Procedures 9-2 and 9-3). This encounter provides the first impression of the healthcare facility and may set the tone for all subsequent visits. Tact, courtesy, and professionalism are extremely important. During the conversation with the new patient, request preliminary information to help determine how much time to allow for the visit on the appointment schedule. The provider may also expect the medical assistant to give general instructions to patients seeking care for specific complaints. For example, the patient may be required to be fasting for certain laboratory tests. Patient demographic information should be collected during the conversation, including the type of insurance the patient has. Some insurance carriers restrict which providers can be used.

After the necessary information has been collected, offer the patient the first available appointment. Whenever possible, offer a choice between two dates and times. Ask the patient to arrive 15 minutes before their scheduled appointment time to complete any paperwork necessary. Also ask whether he or she knows the directions to the healthcare facility or offer the physical address for those who use a GPS or want to obtain exact directions from one of the many Internet direction sites, such as MapQuest. Tell the patient whether any special parking conveniences are available and whether the healthcare facility provides a token or parking validation. The patient's options for the first payment should also be discussed. If payment is expected immediately, inform the patient. The staff should expect patient concerns about the amount of the first bill and should address this issue before the appointment so that there are no surprises or misunderstandings. Before ending the conversation, repeat the appointment date and time and then thank the patient for calling.

Some healthcare facilities mail an information packet/brochure to new patients, especially if the appointment is several days away. With the patient's permission and e-mail address, such information can also be sent via the Internet. An ideal tool to use to deliver this information is a new patient brochure (Procedure 9-3). This brochure can be printed with graphics and images to promote a professional impression of the healthcare facility. This brochure should include the following:

- Description of the practice
- Location or a map
- Telephone numbers
- E-mail and Web site addresses
- Staff names and credentials
- Services offered
- Hours of operation
- How appointments can be scheduled

In addition to the brochure, the packet could include a health history form, the **Notice of Privacy Practices (NPP),** and release of information form (to obtain records from their previous provider).

If another provider has referred the patient, the medical assistant may need to call the referring provider's office to obtain additional information before the patient's appointment. This information should be printed out and given to the attending provider before the patient arrives. Remember to send a thank you note to anyone who refers a patient to the facility.

Often, the medical assistant will need to conduct **preauthorization** or **precertification** to determine whether a patient is eligible for treatment or for certain procedures. The office manager must make certain that these procedures are being done and assign these duties to a specific person(s). More about preauthorization and precertification is included in the Basics of Health Insurance chapter.

PROCEDURE 9-2	**Manage Appointment Scheduling Using Established Priorities: Schedule a New Patient**

Goal: *To schedule a new patient for a first office visit and identify the urgency of the visit using established priorities.*

Role Play Scenario: Patricia Black, a new patient, calls. She just moved to the area and her asthma has flared up over the last 24 hours, but her albuterol inhaler is empty and she needs a new prescription for it. She states that she is doing okay, but without the albuterol she knows it will get worse within the next few days. According to your screening guidelines, she needs to be seen today and scheduling guidelines indicate she needs a 45-minute appointment.

EQUIPMENT and SUPPLIES

- Appointment book or computer with scheduling software
- Scheduling and screening guidelines
- Pencil

PROCEDURAL STEPS

1. Obtain the patient's demographic information (e.g., full name, birth date, address, and telephone number). Write this information down or enter it into the scheduling software. Verify the information.
   PURPOSE: It is important to verify the information. If you have difficulty hearing the patient, use a system to verify the spelling (e.g., "A" as in apple).

2. Determine whether the patient was referred by another provider.
   PURPOSE: You may need to request additional information from the referring provider and your provider will want to send a consultation report.

3. Determine the patient's chief complaint and when the first symptoms occurred. Utilize the scheduling and screening guidelines as needed.
   PURPOSE: You must know the amount of time that will be required for the visit and how quickly the patient needs to be seen based on the chief complaint.

4. Search the appointment book or scheduling software for the first suitable appointment time and an alternate time. Offer the patient a choice of these dates and time. Be open to alternative times if the patient cannot make the initial options you gave. Provide additional appointment options as needed.
   PURPOSE: Providing the patient with a choice of dates and times and additional options as needed helps to demonstrate sensitivity when managing appointments. It is an important customer service technique (Figure 1).

5. Enter the mutually agreeable time into the schedule. Enter the patient's name, telephone number, and add *NP* for new patient.
   PURPOSE: The *NP* in the appointment book indicates the patient is a new patient. Having the phone number available helps increase your efficiency if you need to contact the patient.

6. Obtain the patient's insurance information. If new patients are expected to pay at the time of the visit, explain this financial arrangement when the appointment is made.
   PURPOSE: Obtaining the patient's insurance information now ensures that the patient is seeing a provider covered by his or her insurance carrier. By explaining the payment policy before the appointment, the patient can come to the appointment prepared to pay.

7. Provide the patient with directions to the healthcare facility and parking instructions if needed.
   NOTE: Many facilities will e-mail or mail new-patient paperwork to the patient, who is instructed to complete the forms before the appointment and bring them to the appointment.

8. Before ending the call, ask if the patient has any questions. Reinforce the date and time of the appointment. Politely and professionally end the call, making sure to thank the patient for calling.
   PURPOSE: It is important to restate the appointment time and date to ensure the patient knows the correct information before ending the call.
   NOTE: For legal and safety reasons, many healthcare practices encourage patients with urgent same-day appointments to seek emergency care immediately if the condition worsens before the appointment time.

PROCEDURE 9-2   *—continued*

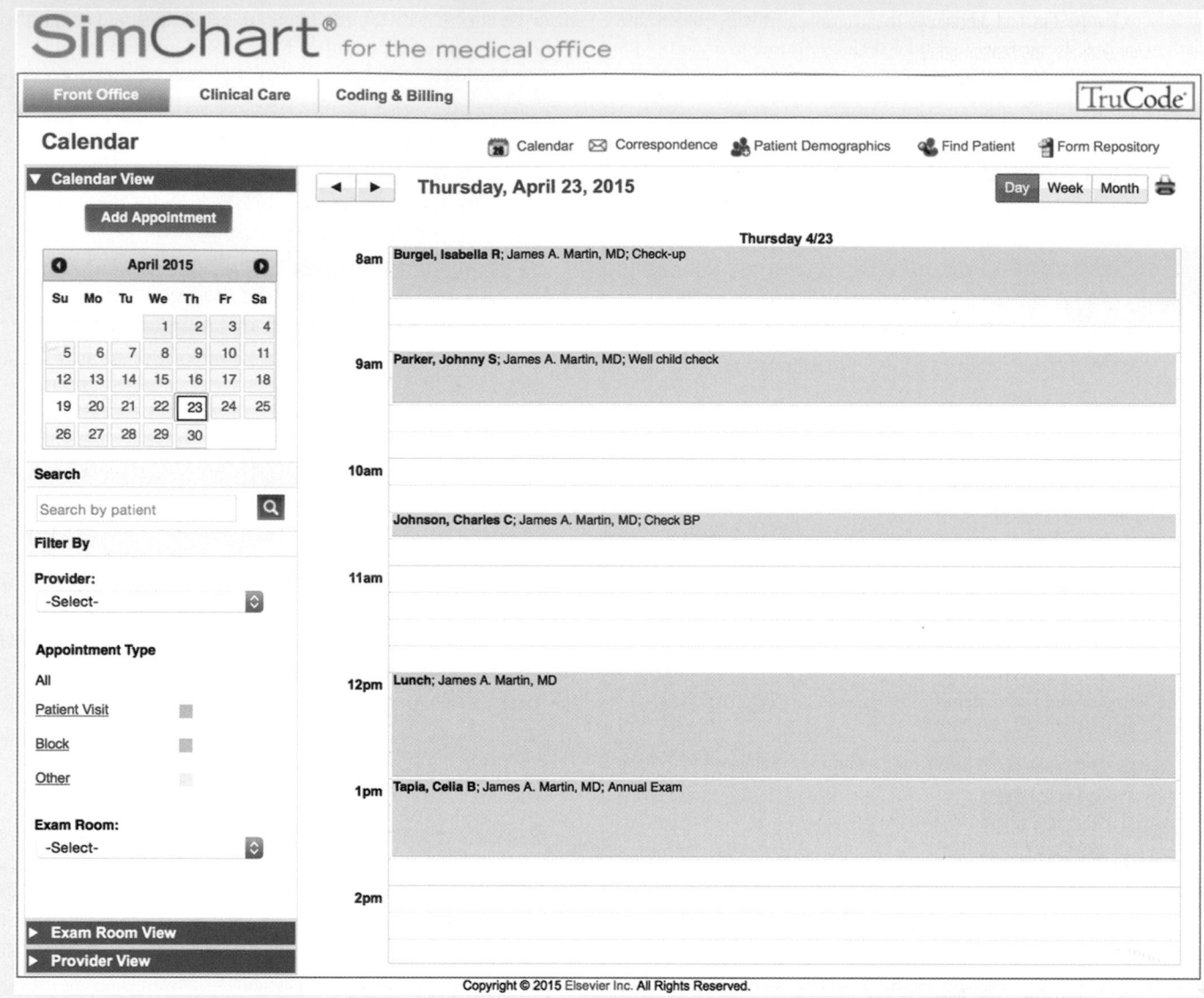

1

PROCEDURE 9-3   Coach Patients Regarding Office Policies: Create the New Patient Brochure

Goal: *Create a new patient brochure that provides an orientation to the practice and the office's policies and procedures.*

Role Play Scenario: Adam Burns stops by the office and he is interested in establishing a relationship with a provider. You need to coach him on the office's information, policies, and procedures.

EQUIPMENT and SUPPLIES

- Computer with word processing software
- Office procedure manual (optional)

PROCEDURAL STEPS

1. Using word processing software, design an informational brochure for patients that provides information about the practice and describes practice procedures. At a minimum, the information should include:

- Description of the practice (e.g., type of practice, mission statement)
- Location or a map of the practice
- Contact information (i.e., telephone numbers, e-mails, and Web site addresses)
- Staff names and credentials
- Services offered
- Hours of operation
- How appointments can be scheduled

- Practice policies and procedures (e.g., payment policies, appointment cancellations, medication refills, assistance after hours)
  PURPOSE: Providing patients with a written brochure listing the practice's information, policies, and procedures enables patients to use it as a reference.
2. Give a brief summary of the different parts of the brochure, including how appointments are scheduled and the practice's policies and procedures.
   PURPOSE: By discussing each part of the brochure with the potential patient, you can help explain what is stated. Summarize the information without reading the sections to the other person.

3. During the summary, use active listening skills by listening to what is said and how the message is said.
   PURPOSE: By actively listening to the other person's responses, you can understand more about what the person is unclear about or what the person wants. Actively listening helps to ensure you provide the necessary answers to the other person.
4. Ask if the person has any questions and listen to the person's questions and needs/wants. Address the questions and clarify any information that is required. Watch and listen for verification of the person's understanding.
   PURPOSE: Again, by using active listening skills, you can better understand what the person is unclear about and then address those areas.

SCHEDULING APPOINTMENTS FOR ESTABLISHED PATIENTS

In Person

Most return appointments for **established patients** are arranged when the patient is leaving the office. A good policy is to have all patients stop by the front desk to check out before leaving in case any information is needed from the patient or any outside scheduling must be done. The patient's health record can be reviewed to see whether the provider ordered any laboratory tests or procedures, and these can be scheduled and discussed with the patient. When making a return appointment, follow the same procedures as for scheduling any appointment by phone, offering the patient choices in the day and time slots (Procedure 9-4). If a certain time the patient specifically requests is not available, offer two alternatives. Always give the patient an appointment card and any necessary instructions at this time, along with a bright smile. Never forget to provide excellent customer service.

PROCEDURE 9-4 Manage Appointment Scheduling Using Established Priorities: Schedule an Established Patient

Goal: *To manage the provider's schedule by scheduling appointments for an established patient and handling rescheduling and a no-show appointment.*

Role Play Scenario: Celia Tapia has just completed seeing Dr. Martin and is checking out at your desk. You see that she needs to schedule a follow-up appointment in 2 weeks. The scheduling guidelines indicate a follow-up appointment is 15 minutes long.

EQUIPMENT and SUPPLIES

- Appointment book or computer with scheduling software
- Scheduling guidelines
- Pencil, red pen
- Reminder card
- Patient's health record

PROCEDURAL STEPS

1. Obtain the patient's name and information, purpose of the visit, the provider to be seen, and any scheduling preferences. If using the scheduling software, enter the patient's name and date of birth (DOB). Verify the correct patient is selected.
   PURPOSE: To schedule an appointment, the patient's information is required, along with the provider to be seen and the type of appointment

required. Knowing any scheduling preferences or limitations will help you efficiently find an acceptable appointment time for the patient.
2. Identify the length of the appointment by using the scheduling guidelines.
   PURPOSE: Depending on the appointment type, each provider may require a different length of time for that appointment. Ensuring you schedule the appropriate amount of time will help facilitate the flow of patients on that day.
3. Search the appointment book or scheduling software for the first suitable appointment time and an alternate time. Offer the patient a choice of these dates and time. Be open to alternative times if the patient cannot make the initial options you gave. Provide additional appointment options as needed.
   PURPOSE: Providing the patient with a choice of dates and times and additional options as needed helps to demonstrate sensitivity when managing appointments. It is an important customer service technique (Figure 1).

PROCEDURE 9-4   *—continued*

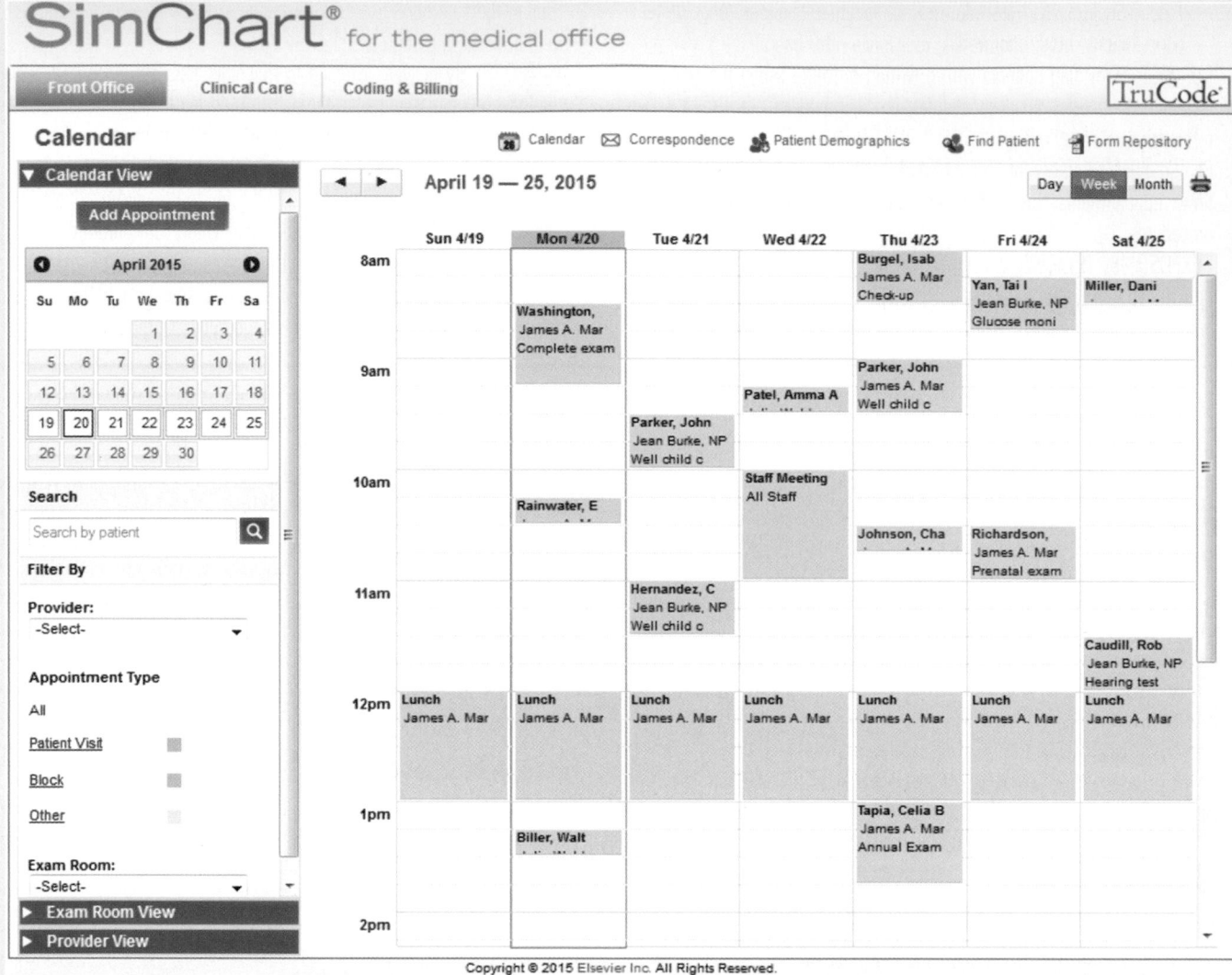

1

4. Using a pencil, write the patient's name and phone number in the appointment book and block out the correct amount of time. Add in any other relevant information per the facility's procedures. If using the scheduling software, create the appointment per the facility's guidelines.

   PURPOSE: By adding the patient's phone number to the appointment book, if the patient needs to be contacted, it saves time. Using pencil to write down the information in the book allows it to be erased if the patient cancels or reschedules for another time.

5. Complete the appointment reminder card and ensure the date and time on the card matches the appointment time. Give the card to the patient.

   PURPOSE: Using appointment reminder cards helps patients remember when their appointments are and helps decrease the number of no-show appointments.

Continuation of Scenario: Later that day, Mary Jones calls and needs to reschedule her appointment for the next day at the same time.

6. When a patient calls to reschedule an appointment, follow steps #1 through #4. When the new appointment is made, make sure to erase the old appointment from the appointment log. With the scheduling software, ensure the old appointment time is removed from the schedule. Repeat the appointment date and time to the patient.

   NOTE: It is important to erase the old appointment so the patient is not expected on two different days. By erasing or deleting the old appointment, it opens up that time for another patient.

Continuation of Scenario: Mary Jones no-shows for her follow-up appointment.

7. In the appointment book, using red pen, indicate the patient no-showed. Using the patient's health record, document that the patient failed to show for the follow-up examination with the provider. In an electronic system change the appointment status to no-show and ensure that it is documented in the health record.

   PURPOSE: For legal purposes, the healthcare facility must keep a record of patients who no-show for appointments. By indicating it in the appointment book and in the health record, the practice is covered if any issues should arise. Some medical practices have procedures that include contacting the patient regarding the no-show appointment and finding out the reason. This is then also charted in the health record.

By Telephone

Usually the medical assistant needs only to determine when the patient must return and to find a suitable time in the schedule. Established patients do not usually need directions and parking information unless the office has recently moved. The patient's address, telephone number, and insurance should always be verified and any changes documented in the health record. If an e-mail address and/or cell phone number is not on file, obtain one so as to have a quick, easy way to notify the patient of appointments and other events.

SCHEDULING OTHER TYPES OF APPOINTMENTS

The medical assistant may also schedule services other than appointments at the healthcare facility, and these will appear on the appointment schedule. This includes surgeries the provider will perform at a hospital or other facility, consultations, outside appointments and meetings, and even house calls if the provider makes them. The provider also must have time to get from one location to another, so driving time must be considered when arranging all appointments.

Some critical information is required when scheduling admission or treatments in other facilities. Always provide the facility with the patient's name, address, phone numbers (both home and cell), Social Security number, and insurance information and relay the procedures that are to be performed. Patient allergies should be mentioned if the patient is being admitted. Additionally, the facility may have forms that the patient needs to complete, so an e-mail address is helpful in such cases. Always provide the admitting diagnosis and orders to the healthcare facility before admission time. Some facilities require a history form before admission. The patient will be required to bring a form of picture identification, such as a state driver's license, and his or her insurance card.

Inpatient Surgeries

When scheduling a surgery, call the facility where the procedure will be performed as soon as the operation is planned. Provide all necessary information and state any special requests the provider may have, such as the amount of blood to have available for the patient. The facility may want the patient's insurance information and

certainly will want a phone number so that the patient can be contacted before the surgery if necessary. Make sure all this information is available before placing the call.

Outpatient and Inpatient Procedure Appointments

A medical assistant often is asked to arrange laboratory or radiography appointments for patients. Before calling the facility to schedule the appointment, be sure all necessary information is available. Inform the patient of the time and place of the appointment, relay any special instructions, and then note these arrangements in the patient's health record. Some offices make a reminder call to the patient or send a reminder e-mail or text message.

Outpatient testing is common because most providers do not have extensive x-ray or laboratory equipment in their offices. Magnetic resonance imaging (MRI), computed tomography (CT) scans, numerous x-ray evaluations, ultrasonography, and simple blood tests all may need to be scheduled (Procedure 9-5). Provide the patient with the name, address, and phone number of the facility where the tests will be done.

Some patients may require a series of appointments (e.g., at weekly intervals). Try to set up these appointments on the same day each week at the same time of day. This considerably reduces the risk of the patient forgetting an appointment.

In some cases the medical assistant may be responsible for scheduling inpatient admissions or inpatient surgical procedures. This is similar to scheduling outpatient testing, but the medical assistant coordinates with a hospital rather than an outside facility and should also be documented in the patient's health record.

It is often the medical assistant's responsibility to provide the patient with any special instructions for the procedure or test that is going to be performed. The patient should be provided with written instructions as well. A patient undergoing general anesthesia will need to fast for approximately 12 hours before the procedure. If medications are to be taken the morning of the procedure the patient may take them with a small sip of water. The provider will instruct the patient about which medications to take. The patient should also be instructed to leave valuables at home. If it is an outpatient procedure and the patient will be sedated in any way, he or she should be instructed to have someone drive them home.

PROCEDURE 9-5 | **Schedule a Patient Procedure**

Goal: *To schedule a patient for a procedure within the time frame needed by the provider, confirm with the patient, and issue all required instructions.*

Role Play Scenario: Monique Jones has just completed seeing Dr. Walden and is checking out at your desk. She gives you an order from the provider that states she needs to have a magnetic resonance image (MRI) of her left ankle within a week. The radiology department in your facility performs MRIs.

EQUIPMENT and SUPPLIES

- Provider's order detailing the procedure required
- Computer with order entry software (optional)
- Name, address, and telephone number of facility where procedure will take place

- Patient's demographic and insurance information
- Patient's health record
- Procedure preparation instructions
- Telephone
- Consent form (if required for procedure)

PROCEDURE 9-5 —*continued*

PROCEDURAL STEPS

1. Obtain an oral or written order from the provider for the exact procedure to be performed.
   PURPOSE: For you to schedule the procedure, you will need an order from the provider for the procedure to be performed.
2. Gather the patient's demographic and insurance information. If using an electronic health record, verify you have the correct patient.
   NOTE: For some procedures and diagnostic tests, precertifications or pre-authorizations need to be completed before scheduling the patient. This will be discussed in a later chapter.
3. Determine the patient's availability within the time frame provided by the provider for the procedure (Figure 1).
   PURPOSE: Make sure the patient will be able to comply with the arrangements for the test.

4. Contact the diagnostic facility and schedule the patient's procedure. If you are using a computerized provider order entry (CPOE) system and your facility performs the procedure, you also need to enter the order using the CPOE system.
   - Provide the patient's diagnosis and provider's exact order, including the name of procedure and time frame.
   - Establish the date and time for the procedure.
   - Give the patient's name, age, address, telephone number, and insurance information (i.e., insurance policy numbers, precertification information, and addresses for filing claims).
   - Determine any special instructions for the patient or special anesthesia requirements.
   - Notify the facility of any urgency for test results.
   PURPOSE: Schedule the procedure and provide needed information.

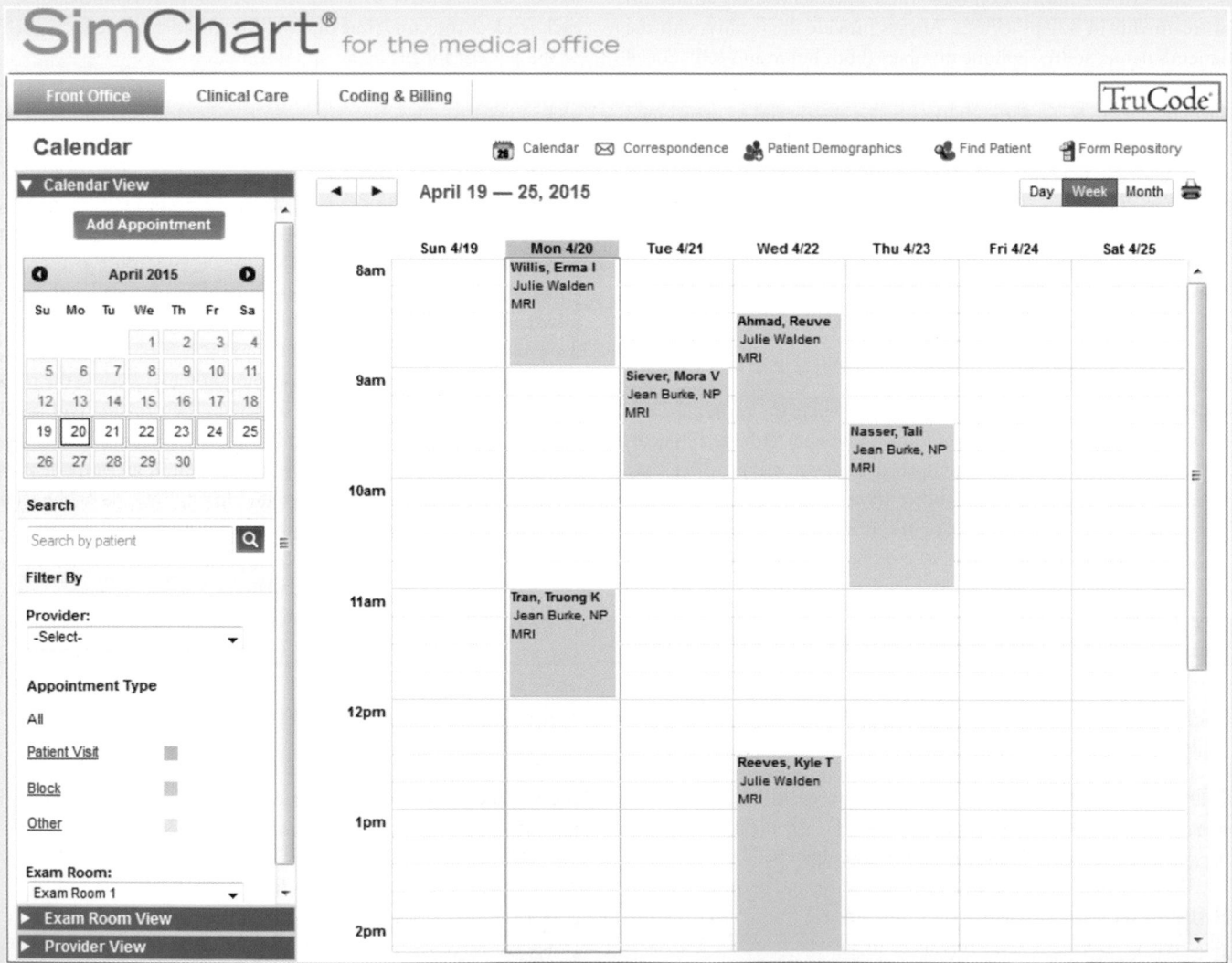

PROCEDURE 9-5 *—continued*

5. Notify the patient of the arrangements and provide the information in a written format.
- Give the name, address, and telephone number of the diagnostic facility.
- Specify the date and time to report for the procedure.
- Give instructions on preparation for the test (e.g., eating restrictions, fluids, medications, enemas).
- If using another facility, the patient will need to bring a form of picture identification and the insurance card.
- If not using a CPOE system, explain whether the patient needs to pick up orders or whether the order will be sent to the facility in advance.
- Ask if the patient has any questions and answer the questions.

PURPOSE: Make sure the patient understands the necessary preparations and the importance of keeping the appointment. Providing written instructions to the patient will help reinforce what was discussed and give the patient a reference for the information.

6. If a consent form is required for the procedure, ensure the provider has reviewed the form with the patient and the patient has signed the consent form. A copy of the consent form may be required by the diagnostic facility before the procedure. The consent form should be scanned and uploaded into the electronic health record or placed in the paper record.

PURPOSE: The consent form is used to make sure the patient understands the risks, benefits, and alternatives to the procedure.

7. Document the details of the scheduled procedure in the patient's health record. If applicable, create a reminder to check on the procedure results after the appointment date.

PURPOSE: Document that the procedure was scheduled. It is legally important to show that what was ordered was scheduled. Creating a reminder for you to check up on the results of the procedure is also important in assisting the provider. 2/27/20XX Patient scheduled for colonoscopy on 3/10/20XX 8:00 am at Anytown Hospital. Patient preparations instructions given and patient verbalized understanding.

Outside Visits

If the provider regularly makes house calls or visits patients in skilled nursing facilities, a special block of time must be reserved in the appointment schedule. There has been an increase in the number of providers who are making house calls again, especially if they have an elderly patient base that are still living independently. The provider needs demographic information, such as addresses, room numbers, and the best route to each home or facility. Remember to allow for travel time.

There are a number of other situations that may have to be added to the schedule, sometimes without much advance warning. Handle all of these situations with care and courtesy.

Providers

Another provider dropping into the facility should be ushered in to see the provider as soon as possible, regardless of the appointment schedule. If the provider is seeing a patient, explain the situation and, if possible, take the visiting provider into a private room, such as the provider's office, to wait. Then notify the provider as soon as possible. Visits from other providers are usually brief and do not appreciably affect the schedule.

Pharmaceutical Representatives

Representatives from pharmaceutical companies are frequent visitors to healthcare facilities and generally are welcomed when the schedule permits. They are well trained and bring the provider valuable information on new drugs. The medical assistant often is expected to screen such visitors and turn away those whose products would not be used in that practice. If the representative or the pharmaceutical company is unknown to the office, ask for a business card and then check with the provider, who will decide whether to see the caller.

Pharmaceutical representatives will often bring samples of the medications that they are going to talk to the provider about. It is important for the medical assistant to understand the policies and procedures for the handling and dispensing of the samples. Most healthcare facilities will require that these samples be stored in a locked cabinet or closet and are given to patients only with provider approval.

Specialists usually limit their conferences with pharmaceutical representatives to their line of practice. The medical assistant, together with the provider, can prepare a list of the representatives with whom the provider is willing to spend time; the list is the determining factor in future conferences. The medical assistant can say whether the provider will be available that day and give an estimate of the waiting time or suggest a later time at which the representative may return. The representative then can decide whether to wait or return later. The pharmaceutical representative usually is quite understanding and cooperative and willing to wait patiently for a long time for just a brief visit with the provider. In turn, the medical assistant should treat the representative with courtesy, showing as much cooperation as possible.

Salespeople

Salespeople from medical, surgical, and office supply houses call regularly at healthcare facilities. Sometimes they want to see the provider, but the office manager or the medical assistant in charge of ordering supplies usually can handle these calls.

Unsolicited salespeople sometimes can present a problem in the professional office. If the provider does not want to see such callers, the medical assistant must firmly but tactfully send them away. Suggest that they leave their literature and cards for the provider to study and say that the provider will contact them if further information is desired.

SPECIAL CIRCUMSTANCES

Late Patients

Every medical practice has a few patients who are habitually late for appointments. This seems to be a problem for which no cure has been found. Emergencies and small delays can happen to anyone, but a patient who constantly arrives late can put a strain on the practice. Such patients can be booked as the last appointment of the day. Then, if closing time arrives before the patient does, the staff has no obligation to wait and other patients have not been inconvenienced. Some medical assistants tell the patient to come in 30 minutes before the appointment time actually scheduled. Make an attempt to work with patients who have occasional difficulties arriving on time, but do not allow the schedule to be constantly disrupted by late patients.

CRITICAL THINKING APPLICATION   **9-4**

Seth Jones is always late for his appointments. How might Ramona approach him about this? What can Ramona do to assist Mr. Jones in arriving for appointments on time?

Rescheduling Appointments

Changes sometimes must be made in the appointment schedule. Unexpected conflicts might arise that force a patient to change the appointment time. When rescheduling an appointment, make sure the first appointment is removed from the appointment book, and then set the new appointment. Otherwise, the patient will be expected in the office on 2 days, and time will be wasted with calls and follow-up, only to discover that the appointment was rescheduled. Most computerized scheduling systems will allow the medical assistant to open the appointment and change the date and time or to cut and paste the appointment into the new date and time.

Emergency Situations

Periodically, emergency or urgent calls come into the office, and an appointment needs to be scheduled. To some extent, all calls that come in go through a **screening** process to evaluate the urgency of the need to see the provider, and emergencies are prioritized. Screening is an extremely important function that requires experience, knowledge of signs and symptoms, and tact.

Emergencies may involve emotional crises in addition to the more obvious physical problems. Patients with emergencies and those who are acutely ill should be seen the same day. The urgency of the call initially can be determined by having a list of questions prepared for reference. The provider should help with this list; he or she should determine what is considered an emergency (life-threatening) or urgent (serious but not life-threatening). The patient may need to be referred directly to a hospital emergency department, or the provider may want to see the patient that day in the office. If patients are unable to get themselves to the hospital the medical assistant may need to contact the emergency medical services in your area. Remember to keep the patient on the phone until emergency medical technicians (EMTs) or other help arrives at the patient's location. Never place an emergency call on hold. Always obtain the name, phone number, and location at the start of the call so that the patient can be found if he or she loses consciousness or is disconnected.

Provider Referrals

If another provider telephones and requests that a patient be seen on the same day, most offices honor that request if at all possible. It is important to keep a schedule that is not intolerant of this type of request.

Patients Without Appointments

The provider and scheduling team should come up with a policy for patients without appointments, also referred to as walk-in patients. A patient who requires immediate attention most likely will be accommodated in the schedule somehow. If the patient does not need immediate care, a scheduled appointment at a later time may be the answer. Be sure to follow established office policy.

FAILED APPOINTMENTS

Why do patients fail to keep appointments? Some are simply forgetful. Once this tendency is detected in a patient, form the habit of telephoning or e-mailing a reminder the day before the appointment. **Automated call routing** offers the patient the option of canceling an appointment and can be programmed to keep calling until the patient responds and confirms or cancels the appointment.

A patient who has been pressed for payment may stay away because of an inability to pay for medical services. Do not make the mistake of classifying all such patients as "deadbeats." Many have every desire to pay, but they cannot afford to and feel embarrassed about their situation, so they avoid their appointments.

Patients also may fail to keep appointments because they are in a state of denial about their condition. For instance, if a patient recently tested positive for the human immunodeficiency virus (HIV), he or she may avoid appointments because going to see the provider forces the patient to face the reality of the disease. Take special care with such patients, and if denial is suspected, discuss this with the provider, who may want to refer the patient for counseling.

It is important to determine the reason for failed appointments and to do whatever is possible to remedy the situation. Telephone the patient to make sure no misunderstanding has occurred. If the patient's health is such that medical care must continue, the provider may write a letter explaining this to the patient. Send the letter by certified mail with return receipt requested. A copy of the letter needs to be added to the patient's medical record for legal protection.

Failed appointments need to be documented in the patient's health record and the appointment schedule for legal purposes. A patient may try to claim abandonment, when he or she has actually been the one to miss the appointments.

NO-SHOW POLICY

Some patients may not realize the importance of keeping their appointments. The patient who does not arrive for a scheduled appointment or reschedule it is called a **no-show**. A busy practice must have a very specific policy on appointment no-shows and must enforce it effectively. The first time a patient fails to show, note the fact on the health record and/or ledger card. The second time, warn the patient, and if a third no-show occurs, consider dropping the patient by using the customary methods that provide legal protection for the provider. Another option, instead of dropping a patient, is to only allow the patient to schedule for same day appointments.

The provider may wish to charge patients for not showing up for the appointment. Be understanding whenever possible, but do not let a patient take advantage of the provider's time. The office policy manual must state that patients may be charged for missed appointments and this should be explained to new patients when their first appointment is made. Because the time slot was scheduled and the provider was ready and available to treat the patient, it is ethical to charge the patient for missing an appointment, especially if he or she did not call to cancel or reschedule. Many providers do not press this issue, but it is an available tool if needed.

INCREASING APPOINTMENT SHOW RATES

Everyone benefits from a full schedule of kept appointments. Appointment show rates can be increased in several ways.

Automated Call Routing

As mentioned earlier, automated call reminders can contact patients scheduled for appointments. The patient is asked to press a certain key on the phone to confirm the appointment and a different key to cancel the appointment. This same tool can be used to send messages to patients (e.g., a reminder that it is the time of year to get a flu vaccination), to introduce a new provider at the office, or announce the availability of a new procedure. The provider can even record the call so that it sounds more personal. These systems can also be set up to send text messages to remind patients of their upcoming appointments.

Appointment Cards

Most healthcare facilities use appointment cards to remind patients of scheduled appointments and to eliminate misunderstandings about dates and times (Figure 9-3). Make a habit of reaching for an appointment card while writing an entry in the appointment book or scheduling it on the computer. After the date and time have been written on the card, double-check with the book/computer to make sure the entries agree.

Confirmation Calls

Patients who have made appointments in advance may appreciate a confirmation call to remind them they have a time set aside to see the provider. Always note the phone number the patient prefers the office to use for such calls. Many individuals have a home phone, cell phone, and work phone numbers; however, they may want calls from the provider to go only to their home phone. Highlight the preferred phone number in the medical record or indicate it on the computer. The office must use caution in making calls to patients because of the significance of privacy guidelines and standards. Some offices may want to prepare a release form in which the patient grants the office staff permission to contact the patient. Many providers

insist that messages left on voice mail not mention the term "doctor" or "doctor's office" for confidentiality reasons. The medical assistant might say, "This is Pam at Robert Welch's office confirming your appointment tomorrow at 2 PM. Please call us if you cannot make the appointment. Our number is 555-212-0909. Thank you!"

If the patient has signed the privacy policy and the policy states that messages from the provider's office may be left at certain numbers, the office certainly can leave messages at that number and mention that the call is from the healthcare facility. Still, it is a good idea to have an established policy on leaving messages that does not breach the patient's confidentiality.

E-Mail Reminders

Many computer scheduling programs can send an e-mail to patients the day before an appointment to remind them of it. This is a great timesaver for the office staff, because no time is taken to perform this duty other than the original scheduling of the appointment.

Mailed Reminders

The office staff may mail reminder letters to patients. This method is a bit time-consuming with a paper-based appointment system but worth the effort if the patients show up for their appointments. Computer scheduling systems can be set up to generate the reminder letters for scheduled appointments and also to remind patients that they are due for their annual physical or influenza vaccination.

HANDLING CANCELLATIONS AND DELAYS

When the Patient Cancels

Inevitably, cancellations occur. If a list is kept of patients with advance appointments who would like to come in sooner, the medical assistant can begin calling to try to get one of them in to fill the available opening. By keeping a list of patients willing to take the first canceled appointment, the medical assistant can readily identify which patients to call to fill the vacancy. Each cancellation should be noted in the medical record, along with a reason for the cancellation if that information is available. If the patient simply reschedules an appointment, a notation need not be made in the health record unless a pattern develops that might be significant to the patient's medical treatment.

When the Provider Is Delayed

Some days the provider will be delayed in reaching the office. If advance notice of the delay is received, start calling patients with early appointments and suggest that they come later. If some patients arrive before the office learns of the delay, explain that an emergency has detained the provider.

Show concern for the patient, but do not be overly apologetic, which might imply some degree of guilt. Most patients realize that a provider has certain priorities. The patient in the office may be inconvenienced, but it is not a "life or death" matter. If this kind of situation occurs frequently, however, consider devising a different scheduling system.

When the Provider Is Called to an Emergency

Providers are conscious of their responsibilities for responding to medical emergencies, and most patients understand if the medical

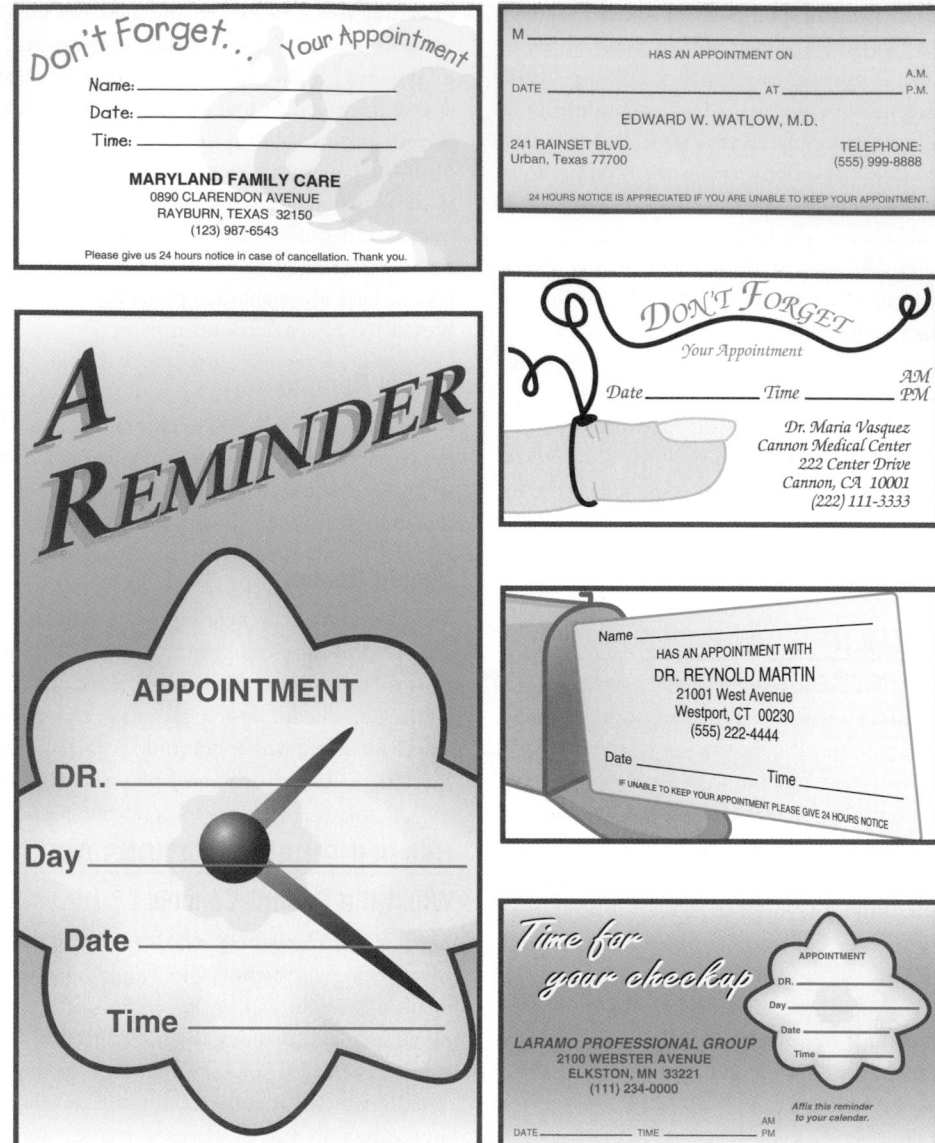

FIGURE 9-3 Examples of appointment cards.

assistant takes time to explain what has happened. The medical assistant may say, "Dr. Wright has been called away due to an emergency. She asked me to tell you she is very sorry to keep you waiting. There will be at least a 1-hour delay." The medical assistant should then ask the patient, "Would you like to wait? If that is inconvenient, I'll be glad to give you the first available appointment on another day. Or perhaps you'd like to have some coffee or do some shopping and return in an hour." It is also possible that another provider may be able to see the patient.

As quickly as possible, call the patients scheduled for a later hour. In many offices, especially those of obstetricians, surgeons, and general practitioners, a whole day's appointments must be canceled. For this reason, it is particularly important to have the daytime telephone number of each patient available so that the appointment can be rescheduled. If at all possible, cancel appointments before the patient arrives in the office to find that the provider is not available.

The **expediency** of the office staff in contacting patients who will be affected by an emergency is appreciated.

When the Provider Is Ill or Out of Town

Providers get ill, too, and patients scheduled to be seen during the course of the provider's recovery must be informed of this and their appointments rescheduled. They need not be told the nature of the illness.

When the provider is called out of town for personal or professional reasons, appointments must be canceled or rescheduled. Customarily, the patient is given the name of another provider, or possibly a choice of several, who will provide care during such absences. For security reasons, merely state that the doctor is unavailable. Stating over the telephone that the provider is out of town could lead to attempted burglary or other unauthorized intrusion on the premises.

PATIENT PROCESSING

The patient reception area should be an inviting place where patients feel comfortable. Visits to the provider can be times of great stress, and the staff must do everything possible to make the experience pleasant for patients. A patient usually has a choice of healthcare providers and should be given excellent customer service. Good patient relations result in referrals to the provider, and this helps the practice grow. When patients have a good experience with a provider, they are likely to tell others. When the staff is committed to making the patient feel welcome and the focus is on care of the patient, success of the practice is inevitable.

THE RECEPTION AREA

A first impression is a lasting one. Nowhere is this more important than in the healthcare facility, where the environment must appear orderly and faultlessly clean. The facility may be a provider's office, a hospital, a health maintenance organization, or one of the many other healthcare establishments. No matter the type of facility, the appearance of the reception room and the front desk, as well as a cordial greeting from the medical assistant, influence patients' **perception** of the entire facility and of the care they will receive.

The reception room is just that—a place to receive patients and visitors. The area should be planned for patients' comfort; it should be as attractive and cheerful as possible and kept clean and uncluttered. Some medical assistants have the opportunity to assist in the design and decoration of this very important area. Consider the traffic flow (i.e., the movement of patients from place to place) both in the reception room and through the rest of the facility so that it is unhindered and logical (Figure 9-4).

CRITICAL THINKING APPLICATION   9-5
Ramona believes that her patients enjoy a homey atmosphere, which is less intimidating than the sterile, clinical feel of some healthcare facilities. How might she give her facility this type of ambiance?

Fresh, **harmonious** colors and cleanliness are the foundation of an attractive room (Figure 9-5). Select comfortable furniture appropriate to the patients seen (e.g., higher chairs with arms for orthopedic patients, wider chairs for larger patients, small chairs for pediatric patients). Furniture should accommodate the peak load of patients seen each day; arrange it in conversational groups. Individual seating usually is the best choice for the provider's office. Provide good lighting, ventilation, and a regulated temperature. Reduce room clutter by providing a place to hang coats, rainwear, and umbrellas.

Most providers' offices are well supplied with recent magazines, and some have various books. Publications with short items of popular interest, such as *Reader's Digest,* are favorites. Any reading material placed in the reception room should be of interest to the general public; *Good Housekeeping, U.S. News and World Report, Real Simple, Oprah,* and *People* are examples of interesting magazines that most people enjoy reading. Some patients may donate magazines to the healthcare facility; if there is a name in the subscription area, be sure to mark through it so that the patient's name cannot be read.

The reception room is not the place for the provider's professional journals or pharmaceutical company's flyers.

A writing desk with writing paper in the reception area for the convenience of patients is a nice touch. A selection of tea and coffee is also appreciated by patients. Music from a concealed speaker is often used to make patients feel more comfortable while waiting and also provides white noise to help maintain patient confidentiality. A lighted aquarium or an educational display of some sort enhances the attractiveness and individuality of the reception area in the professional practice. Patients often are interested in health-related brochures. The provider also may have a DVD or healthcare book library that allows patients to check out items of interest to them. A telephone in the reception area is an asset and can be programmed by the telephone company not to allow long distance calls. A television or DVD player can help the time pass much faster, especially in pediatric practices. Children enjoy Disney movies and cartoon programs, and these hold their interest until it is time to see the provider. A children's corner equipped with small-scale furniture and some playthings works well. Youngsters who might otherwise get into mischief are kept pleasantly occupied. Toys should be easily cleanable; plastic washable items are especially good. Take extra care to ensure that no toy has sharp corners that could cause injury or small parts that could be swallowed. When selecting toys, make sure they will not stimulate the child toward noisy activity. Never place any type of ball in the reception area, because small children tend to throw them, and the balls can injure a patient or visitor.

CRITICAL THINKING APPLICATION   9-6
Ramona has a few patients who bring young children to their appointments. Sometimes the children are a bit disruptive and make other patients feel uncomfortable. How might Ramona handle this problem in the healthcare facility? Some children misbehave in public, and the parents do not respond or correct them. How might Ramona deal with this situation if it arises?

Many healthcare facilities offer a computer for patients to use while waiting to see the provider. This is a great **amenity**, because patients can make good use of their time in the reception area. Some patients may bring their personal laptop computers and use their wait time to complete projects. Providing Internet access for patients also is helpful; an amazing amount of work can be done just by checking e-mail. If patients are allowed to connect to the facilities network, the wise course is to provide one specific log-on name and password just for them so as to maintain control over access to private health information.

Periodically, take an objective look around the reception room. Could it use a little brightening or freshening up? Try to look at the room as if seeing it for the first time. The medical assistant is responsible for the appearance of the area by making sure the room remains neat and orderly throughout the day. Check the temperature and lighting for comfort. Scan the room at intervals during the day to ensure that it is in good order.

If the medical assistant's desk is in the reception area or in open view of patients, it should be free of clutter. In particular, patients' medical and financial records should not be in sight. To protect patient confidentiality, keep computer monitors turned so that those

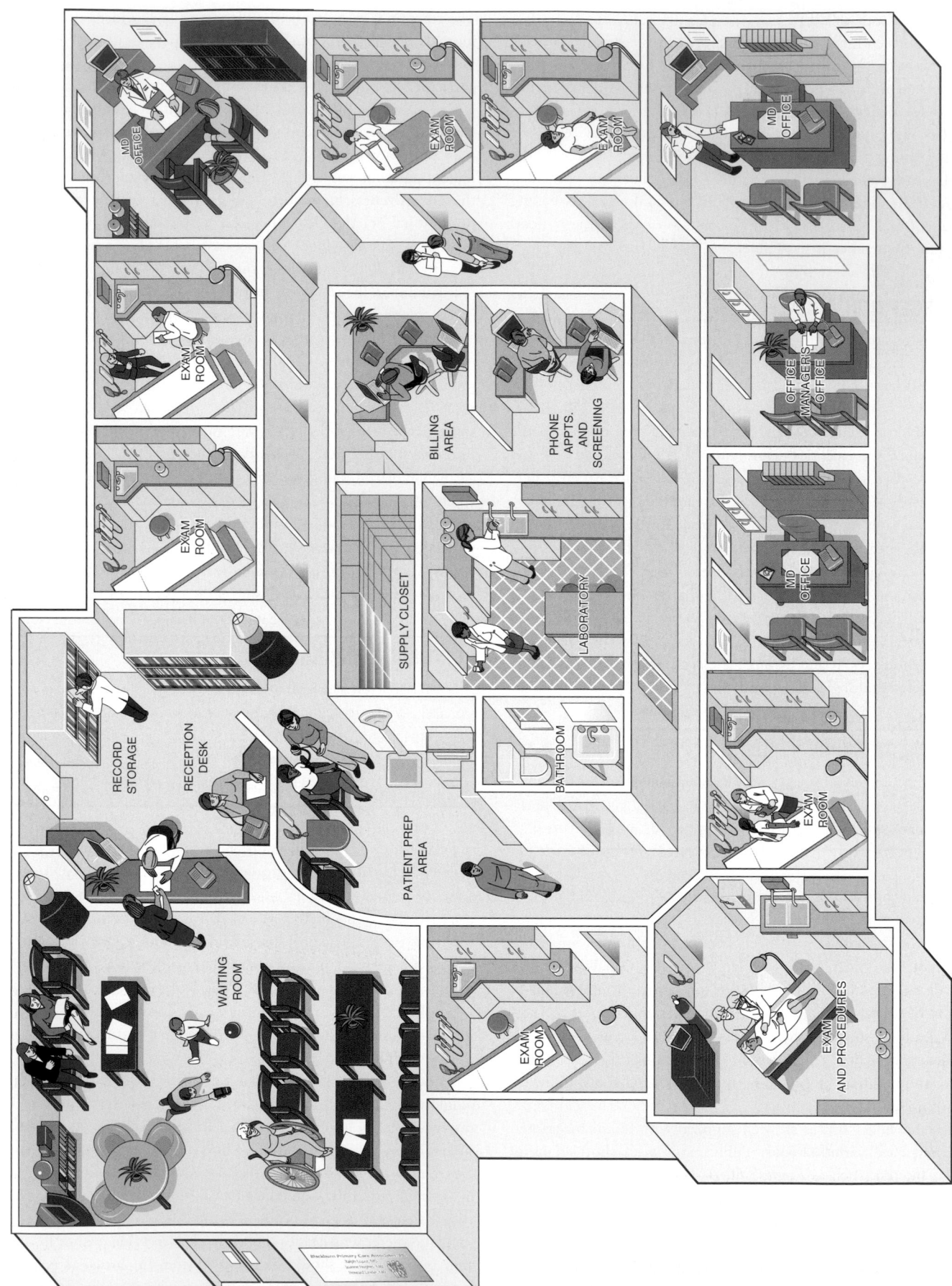

FIGURE 9-4 The medical office should be arranged so that the flow of traffic is conducive to the movement of patients throughout the office.

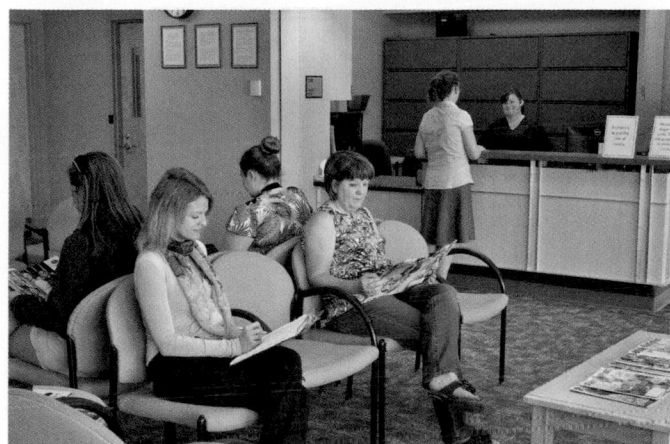

FIGURE 9-5 Patients appreciate cleanliness, restful colors, good ventilation, and light to read by when waiting in the reception area.

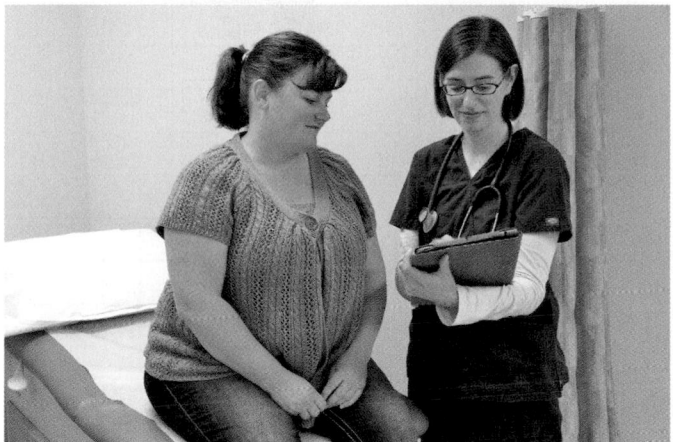

FIGURE 9-6 More providers and their staff members use electronic medical records to reduce paperwork and provide better, more efficient patient care.

waiting cannot view them. Some healthcare facilities use privacy screens that allow only the user to see the monitor, or they use a screen saver that activates after being idle for a few minutes. Medical assistants should not keep personal items on their desks.

PREPARING FOR PATIENT ARRIVAL

Advanced preparation helps make the day go smoothly and contributes to a more relaxed atmosphere for all. Some healthcare facilities prepare for the next day on the evening before, whereas others prepare each morning. The healthcare facility should be consistent, and the same routine should always be performed so that important preparations are not left undone.

Preparing Health Records

Review a list of patients who will visit the provider during the next appointment period. If an electronic health record system is used, this task could be as simple as pulling up and printing a report (Figure 9-6). If a paper-based appointment book system is used, pull the medical records for the day (or the next day if this is done in the evenings) and check off the patient's name on a copy of the appointment schedule; this helps ensure that all the records have been

located and are ready. Occasionally two or more patients may have the same or a similar name. Check the patient's Social Security number, date of birth, or other pertinent information to make sure the right medical record has been pulled. Review each record to verify that any recently received information (e.g., laboratory reports, radiograph readings) has been entered correctly and permanently attached to the record; if a document is missing, attempt to obtain it before the patient's arrival using a fax or other electronic means. Arrange the medical records **sequentially** in the order in which the patients are scheduled. The medical assistant may be expected to place the records of all the patients to be seen that day on the provider's desk, but the provider is more likely to prefer reviewing each record just before entering the examination room. Make sure enough space is available on the **progress notes** for the provider to write in the record. If not, place additional progress notes pages in the record.

Patient Check-in

The reception desk should be in clear view of all visitors who come into the office. If only one medical assistant is present, welcoming each new visitor personally sometimes is impossible. Develop an announcement system that alerts the staff when people enter the office. Patients who enter an empty reception room do not know whether to sit down, knock on the glass partition, or try to announce themselves in some other way. Glass partitions are used to maintain some privacy; however, some providers have eliminated them because they are so impersonal and they send the signal that the provider and staff are off limits to patients. If the partition is used, the policy and procedure manual should dictate when the glass should remain open and when it should be closed.

Make sure no patient medical records are on the reception desk and that the computer monitor is positioned so that it cannot be viewed by patients at the desk. This prevents violation of the regulations established by the Health Insurance Portability and Accountability Act (HIPAA).

The medical assistant should check the reception room each time he or she has been away from the desk to see whether more patients have arrived. Greet these patients by name; if you do not know the person who has entered the reception area, ask the individual's name. Use a sign-in register that promotes patients' privacy (Figure 9-7). Although patients can read the names of others who are in the healthcare facility to visit the provider, this is not considered a violation of HIPAA policy as long as the information disclosed is appropriately limited. This is one type of **incidental disclosure**. Pressure-sensitive labels printed with lines for the patient's name, the appointment time, and a "yes" or "no" question about changes in insurance coverage are a practical, inexpensive solution for confidential patient registers. Patients should not be expected to provide details of the reason for their visit in a public area.

During the patient check-in process it is vital that the medical assistant takes steps to protect the other patients in the reception area. One of the first questions that must be asked, according to the Centers for Disease Control and Prevention (CDC), is whether in the last 21 days, the patient has traveled to a country with widespread transmission or uncertain control for Ebola (e.g., Guinea, Liberia, or Sierra Leone) or had contact with someone with confirmed Ebola virus disease (EVD). If the patient answers yes, he or she should be isolated immediately. The medical assistant should

Patient Sign-In   Date: _____

Please sign-in and notify us if:

• New patient   • Phone/address change   • Insurance change

No.	Patient Name print	Appt. Time	Arrival Time	Appt. with	New patient (✓)	Phone/address change (✓)	Insurance change (✓)
1	P L E A S E						
2	2						
3	3						
4	4						
5	5						
6	6						
7	7						
8	8						
9	9						
10	10						
11	11						
12	12						
13	13						
14	14						
15	15						
16	16						
17	17						
18	18						
19	19						
20	20						
21	21						
22	22						
23	23						
24	24						
25	25						

FIGURE 9-7 Sign-in sheets contain very basic information about the patient and provide information for the medical assistant about changes that need to be edited on the patient's record.

follow the procedures of the facility for this process. During periods of increased respiratory infection activity (e.g., flu season) the health-care facility should make masks available for patients in the reception area. At check-in the medical assistant may need to ask patients to put on a mask while they are waiting if they are coughing. Tissues, along with waste containers and hand sanitizer, should be available for patients in the reception area.

GREETING THE PATIENT

Every patient has the right to expect courteous treatment in a pro-vider's office. Regardless of the patient's economic or social status, each person who enters the reception room should receive a cordial,

friendly greeting (Figure 9-8). A personal touch, such as greeting the patient by name, is an easy way to develop patient rapport. Use the patient's last name and title unless the patient insists on the use of his or her first name or prefers a nickname. For example, the medical assistant may say:

"How are you today, Mr. Roberts?"

"Ms. Nelson, the doctor will be in to see you shortly."

If the healthcare facility has a policy of obtaining a copy of all patients' photo identification cards, such as the driver's license, these can be used to identify patients and greet them by name, even if they do not visit the healthcare facility often. Some EHR systems allow for a patient's picture to be added so the medical assistant can be assured that they have the correct patient record opened during

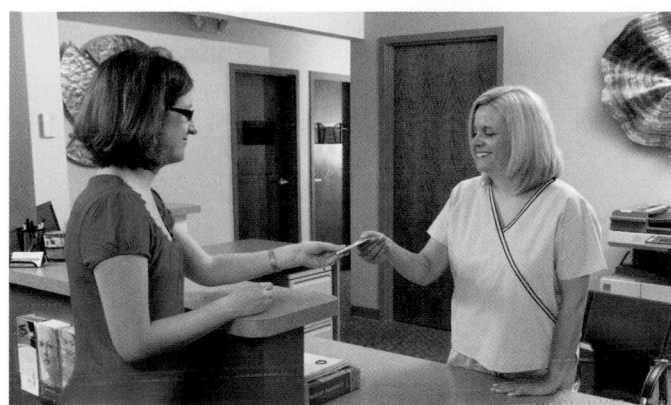

FIGURE 9-8 Greet all patients with a warm smile and assist them with forms they need to complete for the medical record.

check-in. Requesting a photo identification card or having the patient's picture on file also ensures that the person requesting benefits is actually the person covered by the insurance policy.

Patient Interaction

Although the healthcare facility can make patients feel uncomfortable, the medical assistant should try to make everyone feel at ease. Cultivate the habit of greeting each patient immediately in a friendly, self-assured manner. Establish eye contact and smile while introducing yourself to the patient. For example, "Good morning. I'm Elizabeth, Dr. Wade's medical assistant." Remember to ask about why the patient is here before asking about insurance coverage; no patient wants to feel that the provider's main interest is the collection of an insurance check.

Patients like to be acknowledged when they arrive. All staff members should review the day's schedule in the morning to be prepared to greet patients by name and to know whether the patient is new or established. Learn how to pronounce each patient's name correctly; incorrect pronunciations may offend or irritate some people. If the name is unusual, make a note of the **phonetic** spelling in the health record for reference. Note if the patient prefers a nickname. Documenting this information in the health record can help staff members remember names when talking to patients on the phone or in person. By using the patient's name often, the medical assistant also ensures that the correct patient is being treated.

Providers and staff members sometimes make brief notes in the health record about the current events in the patient's life. With this information, the medical assistant and the provider can read those notes before entering the examination room and share a short dialog with patients at the beginning of their visits. For example:

Medical assistant:	"Hello, Mrs. Williams, how are you today?"
Mrs. Williams:	"I am doing very well, Ramona, how are you?"
Medical assistant:	"I'm fine. How was the cruise you took with your husband last month?"
Mrs. Williams:	"It was wonderful! The water was the bluest I have seen!"
Medical assistant:	"You went to Cozumel, didn't you?"

Mrs. Williams:	"Yes, we did! I'm surprised you remember, as many patients as you see each day!"

This brief chat confirms that the staff members care about the individual patient, because they take an interest in their personal lives. Because the patient does not see the medical assistant or provider look at the notes before entering the patient room, the patient assumes that the information is recalled from memory. This is an impressive customer service technique. Most patients appreciate the provider and staff's interest in their families, hobbies, and work. Computer-based health records systems usually have a notes option where such information can be recorded.

Patients may feel somewhat anxious when visiting the provider's office, especially if they know they may be receiving bad news; perhaps a tumor has been discovered to be cancerous, or a family member may have been diagnosed with Alzheimer's disease. Watch the patient's body language. If a patient does not maintain good eye contact or seems otherwise uneasy, a gentle touch or a reassuring smile may be helpful as the office visit progresses. Remember to keep the patient's safety in mind and make certain that he or she has some type of support that will assure a safe arrival back home or at a family or friend's home after the office visit.

Some state regulations prohibit the placement of information other than health details in the health record; however, most health professionals agree that a patient's mental and emotional health are connected to the person's physical health. Details about what is happening in patients' lives provide clues to their physical problems. As a simple example, a patient going through a divorce may experience depression that needs to be treated with medication. Without knowledge of the divorce, the provider does not have all the information needed to make a sound medical decision. Providers can treat patients more effectively when such information is available in the health record.

REGISTRATION PROCEDURES

On a patient's first visit to the provider's office, the staff performs certain registration procedures. Most providers use a patient information or registration form to gather demographic information about the patient. The form may be attached to a clipboard and handed to the patient with instructions to complete sections. The medical assistant must be ready and willing to answer any questions

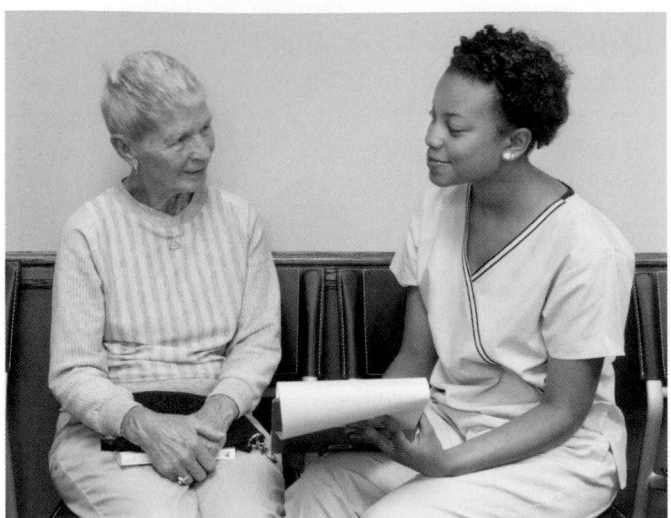

FIGURE 9-9 The medical assistant should take time to explain forms the patient does not understand and should always be willing to answer questions.

(Figure 9-9). The patient's name should appear prominently at the top of the form, followed by other pertinent facts in logical order. Most information sheets contain the following:
- Patient's full name and date of birth
- Responsible person's name and relationship to the patient
- Address and telephone number
- Name, address, and telephone number of contact person
- Occupation
- Place of employment
- Social Security number
- Driver's license number
- Nearest relative not living with the patient and his or her relationship
- Source of referral, if any

When the completed form is returned, check carefully to verify that all the necessary information has been provided. At this time the medical assistant should scan or obtain a copy of both sides of the patient's insurance card, verify the subscriber's date of birth, and collect any copayments. Ask the patient for payment, using phrases such as, "Your copay today is $15, Mrs. Williams. Will you be writing a check or would you like to charge this visit to your Visa?"

Some healthcare facilities insist that copays be collected before the office visit; this matter is handled according to the provider's discretion. Some patients do not believe they should have to pay before seeing the provider; they simply are not used to paying at the start of the visit. The medical assistant can say, "Mr. Thomas, would you like to go ahead and pay your copay now?" By giving the patient the option, it seems as if the medical assistant is helping the patient save time instead of insisting on collecting before seeing the provider. Follow the procedures outlined in the policy.

If this is a new patient, he or she will need to be given the healthcare facility's NPP document and sign an acknowledgment of receipt of the NPP that will need to be added to the patient's health record. In addition to scanning or copying the insurance card, many healthcare facilities also require the scanning or copying of patient's legal photo identification.

Some practices place their registration paperwork on their Web site, and the patient can download, complete, and print the paperwork before the first office visit. If a good length of time will pass between making the appointment and arriving for the office visit, the paperwork can be mailed to the patient with instructions to bring the completed documents to the office visit.

CRITICAL THINKING APPLICATION   **9-8**

Often some time is needed to complete forms when a new patient arrives in the healthcare facility. How might Ramona keep the healthcare facility on schedule when new patients arrive who require health record construction and form completion? What are some ways to trim time from these activities?

Obtaining a Patient's History

The patient's personal history, medical history, and family history may be obtained by asking him or her to complete a questionnaire. The questionnaire could be in a paper or electronic format. The paper form can be mailed to the patient to complete before they arrive for their appointment and the medical assistant may enter the information into the EHR. The electronic form can be completed at a private computer station once the patient has arrived at the healthcare facility, or the medical assistant may gather the information and enter it into the EHR. Another electronic option is for the patient to go to the healthcare facility's Web site and complete the form before the appointment. The provider can augment this information during the patient interview. Some experienced medical assistants conduct the interview to obtain the patient's personal and medical history, family history, and chief complaint.

SHOWING CONSIDERATION FOR PATIENTS' TIME

The patient expects to see the provider or practitioner at the appointed time. The medical assistant should bring the patient to the examination room for treatment or consultation as close to the appointment time as possible or explain delays. All patients want to be kept informed about how long they should expect to wait to see the provider. Any delay longer than 10 to 15 minutes should be explained (Figure 9-10). The medical assistant can also offer to reschedule the appointment for the patient. A crowded reception room is not always an indication of a provider's popularity. It may simply mean that the provider or assistant is inefficient at scheduling patients. Always consider the patient's time and make every effort to streamline the office visit.

A solo or small practice should seldom have more than three to five patients in the reception room. Patients complain that the wait time in medical facilities is one of the most frustrating aspects of the medical profession. The patient who complains about medical fees or the care received may first have become agitated during a long wait to see the provider. Many patients are fearful and tense; long wait times intensify these feelings. The medical assistant can often put patients in a better frame of mind with just a friendly smile and a show of concern.

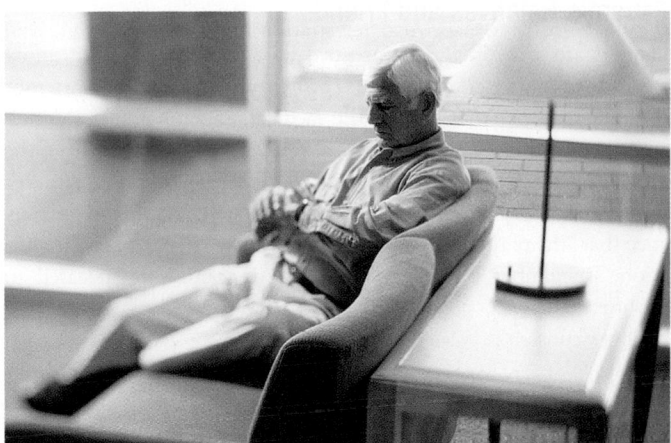

FIGURE 9-10 One of the most common patient complaints is the time spent in the reception area.

CRITICAL THINKING APPLICATION   9-9

Ramona offers to reschedule patient appointments if the schedule ever falls more than 15 minutes behind. If a patient becomes belligerent about the delays, how can Ramona handle the situation in a professional manner?

Patients With Special Needs

Some patients are physically challenged, some are very ill, and some are severely uncomfortable. Language or cultural barriers may exist. Observe the patient's appearance and behavior. Is the patient pale? Do the eyes or voice reflect pain or discomfort? Find out how the patient is feeling before suggesting that he or she be seated to wait for the provider. The patient may need to lie down in a cool room or perhaps be seen as an emergency case. Patients with disabilities, such as those who use a wheelchair, cane, walker, or crutches, may need extra attention. Some patients may need help disrobing even if a disability is not obvious. Always ask if the patient needs assistance and how you can actually help them. If there is a language barrier, having translation assistance available will help. This could be an actual person who does the translation or technology can be used do the translation. There are many online programs that can assist with translation in many different languages. In all special needs cases it is important to remain professional and treat everyone with respect.

ESCORTING AND INSTRUCTING THE PATIENT

While in the healthcare facility, most patients prefer to be escorted rather than simply told where to go. This usually is the clinical medical assistant's responsibility, but the task may be assigned to an administrative medical assistant. Pronounce the patient's name correctly when calling the person to the clinical area. If unsure of the pronunciation, ask the patient. Write the name phonetically on the health record for quick retrieval at the next appointment.

Some patients bring a family member or friend with them to the appointment. On occasion, several people want to accompany the patient when the person sees the provider. The healthcare facility policy and procedure manual should address the maximum number of patients allowed in. If the patient insists on more visitors, explain that the examination rooms are small and have only two chairs and suggest that the additional people may be uncomfortable standing in such a small room. If the patient still insists, make every attempt to satisfy the patient's needs.

Remember that, to an employee of the practice, the healthcare facility surroundings may become as familiar as home. A stranger to the practice's environment may be confused or disoriented by all the hallways, doors, and rooms. Uncertainty creates anxiety. Take the time to escort the patient personally to the appropriate examination or treatment room; do not point to the room and expect the patient to find the way. If a urine specimen is needed, direct the patient to the restroom and always explain how to collect the specimen and what to do with it. Having signs on the wall with room numbers and directions can be helpful to patients also.

HEALTH RECORD CARE

Health records should never be left in the examination room to be picked up and read by a patient. Doing so can cause misunderstandings, because patients rarely know medical terms and abbreviations. A number of methods are used to signal that a patient is ready to be seen. Often file holders are located on the doors of the examination rooms, and the health record can be placed in the holder horizontally when the patient is ready to be seen. The provider can signal the medical assistant that he or she is finished examining the patient by placing the health record in an upright position on leaving the examination room. Place the health record so that other patients in the hallway cannot see the patient's name. HIPAA considers names on health records to be incidental disclosures; however, protecting patient privacy by simply turning the record so that the name cannot be read is a good habit to cultivate.

With an EHR system, it is important to remember to log out of the computer when you are ready to leave the room. This will prevent any additions or deletions to the record and prevent the patient from viewing the record without a healthcare professional with them to explain any questions or concerns.

Some healthcare facilities have call light systems, by which a provider can press a button to call the medical assistant for help with the examination. Others have a flag system outside the door that signals what that particular patient needs next. Other healthcare facilities place patients in examination rooms in a certain order, and the provider knows, for instance, that when he or she has finished with the patient in room 1, the next patient will be waiting in room 2. The healthcare facility should develop a method that allows the most efficient use of time, provides high-quality care, and protects patient confidentiality.

CHALLENGING SITUATIONS
Talkative Patients

Any professional office has problem patients. Talkative patients, for example, take up far more of the provider's time than is justified. An alert medical assistant usually can spot this tendency during the initial interview. The patient's history can be flagged with a symbol to alert the provider. The medical assistant can buzz the provider's **intercom** and remind him or her that the next patient is ready. Once the medical assistant has learned which patients take extra time, they can be booked for the end of the day, or more time can be allowed for them.

CRITICAL THINKING APPLICATION   9-10
Ramona has one patient who insists on sitting close to her desk and attempting to chat the entire time she is waiting to see the provider. Even worse, she comes to her appointments at least an hour early. How might Ramona subtly deal with this patient?

Children

Children frequently present special management challenges, whether they are patients or they accompany a patient. Usually, the parent or guardian accompanies the child into the examination room, but some exceptions exist, such as cases of suspected child abuse. Older children certainly can see the doctor without a parent, especially for routine visits, such as a school sports physical. However, minors still need a parent to consent to treatment in most cases. The provider cannot force the parent to leave the examination room by any means. Although this practice of separating children from their parents to treat their needs is not always feasible, it sometimes can be applied with great success. By explaining to the parent that the child needs to develop a sense of independence and control of his or her own health care, they will often agree that they do not need to be in the exam room for the whole visit. Often there can be compromise by having the parent in the room before the examination to talk to the provider; the parent would then leave the room for the actual physical examination.

Parents are responsible for their children's behavior while at the healthcare facility. If children are doing something that could harm them or other patients, quietly speak to the parents and allow them to handle the situation. When children behave badly, the medical assistant can go to the child, kneel down to his or her level, and offer a book or toy, leading the child away from any objects that could be broken or from other patients. The medical assistant can say, "Let's come over here and play next to your mom!" The medical assistant should not discipline the child. If the child continues to behave badly, call the parent to the examination room early so that others in the reception area can relax and enjoy a pleasant office visit. Some patients may be anxious about receiving test results or have other issues, and an unruly child can make the situation even worse.

Angry Patients in the Reception Area

Every medical assistant eventually is confronted with an angry patient. The anger may simply reflect the patient's pain or fear of what the provider may discover during the examination. If possible, invite the patient into a room out of the reception area. Usually the best course is to let the patient talk out the anger. Present a calm attitude and speak in a low tone of voice. Under no circumstances should the medical assistant return the anger or become argumentative. Medical assistants must use good listening skills with angry people and must be empathetic.

There should be a policy in place for dealing with potentially dangerous individuals. Policies can include making sure that you can reach the exit if you take the patient to another room; having another employee close by; and knowing under what circumstances you should contact the police or building security for assistance.

Patient's Relatives and Friends

Patients are sometimes accompanied by a relative or well-meaning friend who may become restless waiting for the patient and attempt to discuss the patient's illness. The medical assistant should sidestep any discussion of a patient's medical care, except by direction of the provider. Avoid a "too casual" attitude, such as, "I'm sure there's nothing to worry about." A show of moderate concern and reassurance that "the patient is in good hands" usually takes care of the situation. Remember that health information cannot be released to anyone, including concerned friends and relatives, without the patient's consent.

THE FRIENDLY FAREWELL

The medical assistant can help convey a sense of caring by terminating the visit cordially. If the patient will return for another visit, the assistant can say something like, "We'll see you next week." If the patient will not be returning soon, a pleasant "I hope you'll be feeling better soon" is appropriate. Whatever words of goodbye are chosen, all patients should leave the facility feeling that they have received top-quality care and were treated with friendliness, respect, and courtesy.

PATIENT CHECKOUT

When the patient returns to the front office for checkout, greet him or her with a friendly smile and call the individual by name. Form the habit of asking patients whether they have any questions. Check the health record to determine when the provider wants the patient to return. Most providers note this information on the encounter form. Make the return appointment, remembering the technique of giving the patient choices for days, morning or afternoon, and specific times.

Be sure to thank the patient for coming and wish the person well as he or she leaves the facility.

PLANNING FOR THE NEXT DAY

As the day is winding down, look over the appointments scheduled for the next day. Review the health records for scheduled patients. If laboratory tests or other procedures were scheduled on the patient's last visit, determine whether the reports are available in the health record. If the patient is scheduled for specific procedures on this visit, make sure everything needed for the procedure is on hand and available. Planning can save many precious moments at the time of the patient visit.

CLOSING COMMENTS

The administrative medical assistant has a huge effect on the efficiency of the healthcare facility. A friendly, helpful attitude is a **prerequisite** for cordial **interaction** with patients, as is the ability to make compromises that benefit both the provider and patient. A personal touch is vital to projecting a sense of caring to the patients seen in the healthcare facility. Many healthcare facilities are not concerned enough about the customer service aspect of the business. Patients talk about their experiences with their friends and relatives and may be an excellent source of referrals if they are treated with dignity and courtesy. If they have a good experience, they tell several people. If they have a poor experience, they tend to tell everyone they know. Make sure to play a part in having each patient feel a sense of satisfaction as he or she leaves the office. All patients should feel that their time and money have been well spent. An office that runs smoothly and stays on schedule indicates professionalism and competence and is greatly appreciated by all who come in contact with it.

Patient Education

Providing patients with an information booklet about the healthcare facility can familiarize them with policies and procedures. Many providers compile an extensive booklet that even provides tips as to when the provider should be called immediately, listing symptoms and signs of emergencies.

Educating the patient about the healthcare facility's policies helps the facility run smoothly from day to day. All patients should be familiar with the policies about appointments. This leads to fewer misunderstandings and conflicts over bills that might include a charge for a missed appointment.

If the facility offers Internet-based appointment scheduling or forms completion, patients must be taught how to use the system. A printed pamphlet or information sheet is helpful for providing instructions to the patient. A wise option is to have a special phone number patients can call if they have problems with the system. For best results, choose a program that is simple to use, easy to understand, and does not breach patient confidentiality.

Legal and Ethical Issues

As mentioned earlier, the appointment schedule may be used as a legal record and could be brought by subpoena into a court of law. Make sure all handwriting in the book is completely legible and that information is routinely collected in a consistent manner for each entry. Do not fail to note a no-show both in the patient's health record and the appointment schedule. This often is helpful when a provider must prove that the patient did not follow medical advice or that the patient contributed to his or her poor condition by missing appointments. Old appointment schedules should be kept for a time equal to that of the statute of limitations in the state where the practice is located.

A medical assistant must never offer medical advice to a patient unless specifically instructed to do so by the provider. The patient sees the medical assistant as an extension of the provider and tends to weigh advice and comments by the medical assistant with the same validity as if they came from the provider. Provide only information the provider has approved or that is included in the healthcare facility's policy and procedure manual.

When a patient complains, listen carefully and try to resolve the problem or assure the patient that the issue will be discussed with the appropriate staff member to find a solution. If someone other than the patient asks for information about the patient, refrain from discussion unless the patient or provider has authorized the release of information.

Professional Behaviors

When working in scheduling and helping patients move through the healthcare facility, there are many opportunities to demonstrate professionalism. It is important to remember that we are often seeing patients when they are not at their best, so we must learn not to take all of the responses personally. When an angry patient approaches the reception desk you should smile politely, ask how you can help the person, and respond in a soothing tone of voice. When a patient calls for an appointment and demands a day and time when the provider is not available, you should remain calm and explain why that day and time is not an option. As a medical assistant in the front office you have the opportunity to make an amazing first impression on patients. Remember to always behave professionally.

SUMMARY OF SCENARIO

Ramona is an asset to the healthcare facility because her dedication and customer service skills help her interact with patients in a positive way. She genuinely cares about the patients and makes every effort to meet their needs while following Dr. Brown's preferences. She has found that her bright smile is a valuable aid when patients have been waiting and are growing restless.

Ramona cooperates with other staff members to get the patients seen as quickly as possible and to minimize wait time. She is flexible and can change the order of the patients soon, if needed, to maximize the use of time and facilities in the office. Because she is so cheerful and friendly, patients do not seem to mind when she asks for their cooperation. She keeps current phone numbers and cell phone information so that she can notify a patient quickly if Dr. Brown is running behind schedule. Ramona's proficiency on the computer also is an asset, and she makes frequent use of e-mail to take care of patient problems or rescheduling requests.

Because of the cooperation she receives from staff and patients alike, Ramona successfully runs an efficient office. She contributes to that efficiency by constantly refining her knowledge about her job. She pays attention to the times during the day that do not run as smoothly as others, evaluates the problems at those times, and then corrects them. Ramona also keeps the schedule moving by communicating with the clinical medical assistants, keeping them informed about arriving patients and those who have come early or are running late. She can quickly adjust and substitute a patient who already has arrived. Ramona has learned how to manipulate the schedule to accommodate an emergency. She knows that by making minor adjustments and keeping the waiting patients informed, the staff can handle any emergency.

All medical assistants need to develop skills in flexibility. Establishing a system that works and using it correctly makes patients and staff members more content with their experience in the healthcare facility.

SUMMARY OF LEARNING OBJECTIVES

1. **Define, spell, and pronounce the terms listed in the vocabulary.**
Spelling and pronouncing medical terms correctly bolster the medical assistant's credibility. Knowing the definition of these terms promotes confidence in communication with patients and co-workers.

2. **Describe guidelines to establishing an appointment schedule and creating an appointment matrix.**
When appointments are scheduled, a medical assistant must consider (1) the patients' needs, (2) the provider's preferences and habits, and (3) the available facilities. Make every attempt to schedule a patient at his or her most convenient time; this helps prevent no-shows. The provider will outline his or her preferences, which should be a high priority to the medical assistant. However, most providers are flexible and make adjustments according to the needs of the office. The availability of facilities in the office is perhaps the most inflexible factor. If a certain room or piece of equipment is being used for one patient, it usually cannot be used for another.
Refer to Procedure 9-1 to create an appointment matrix.

3. **Discuss the advantages of computerized appointment scheduling.**
Computerized scheduling programs are in demand because they are easy to operate and simplify both scheduling and changing of appointments. The computer can find the first available time much faster than a person scanning an appointment book. Most programs can prepare reports and even notify patients of the impending appointment automatically by e-mail, telephone, or text message. Web-based self-scheduling programs are becoming popular; these allow a patient to see the provider's available appointments and book his or her own date and time.

4. **Discuss appointment book scheduling and explain how self-scheduling can reduce the number of calls to the healthcare facility.**
Office suppliers carry a variety of appointment book styles; many are color-guided.
Self-scheduling can vastly reduce the number of calls to the office because a high number of everyday calls are requests to schedule appointments. With self-scheduling, patients can even make an appointment at midnight if they desire.

5. **Discuss the legality of the appointment scheduling system.**
Because the paper-based appointment book can be used as a legal record, it must be accurate and maintained. Computerized scheduling systems can also be used to track appointments; missed or canceled appointments should be documented in the electronic system for legal purposes.

6. **Discuss pros and cons of various types of appointment management systems.**
Scheduling of specific appointments is the most popular method of seeing patients. Wave and modified wave scheduling brings two or three patients to the office at the same time, and they are seen in the order of their arrival. This type of scheduling can be modified in many ways to suit the needs of the facility. Open office hours allow patients to come to the healthcare facility when it is convenient and wait their turn to see the provider. Other scheduling methods include double-booking and grouping of like procedures.

7. **Discuss telephone scheduling and identify critical information required for scheduling appointments for new patients.**
Extend small courtesies to patients when on the phone with them to schedule an appointment. Write legibly when using an appointment book.
Arranging the first appointment for a new patient requires time and attention to detail. Tact, courtesy, and professionalism are all extremely important. Collect patient demographic data and offer the patient the first available appointment. Some healthcare facilities mail an information packet/brochure to new patients; this can also be sent via e-mail. Often, the medical assistant will need to conduct preauthorization and precertification to determine whether a patient is eligible for treatment or for certain procedures.
Refer to Procedure 9-2 to see how to schedule a new patient and to Procedure 9-3 to see how to coach patients regarding office policies and how to create a new patient brochure.

8. **Discuss scheduling appointments for established patients.**
Most return appointments for established patients are arranged when the patient is leaving the healthcare facility. Refer to Procedure 9-4. Others are reserved by telephone, and the patient's address, telephone number, and insurance should always be verified and any changes documented in the health record.

9. **Discuss how the medical assistant should handle scheduling other types of appointments.**
The medical assistant could be responsible for setting up other appointments such as inpatient surgeries, outpatient and inpatient procedure appointments, outside visits, providers, pharmaceutical representatives, and salespeople. Refer to Procedure 9-5 for specific procedures on how to schedule outpatient and inpatient procedure appointments.

10. **Do the following related to special circumstances in scheduling:**
   - Discuss several methods of dealing with patients who consistently arrive late.
   Patients who are habitually late for appointments might be told to arrive 15 minutes before the time written in the book. Some offices book these patients as the last appointment of the day, so that if they do not arrive promptly, they do not see the provider. Usually talking with the patient and gaining an understanding of why the patient arrives late improves the situation. The office can work with the patient to choose the best times that will result in a kept appointment.
   - Recognize office policies and protocols for rescheduling appointments.
   Changes sometimes must be made in the appointment schedule. When rescheduling an appointment, make sure the first appointment is removed from the appointment book, and then set the new appointment.
   - Discuss how to deal with emergencies, provider referrals, and patients without appointments.
   Periodically, emergency or urgent calls come into the office, and an appointment needs to be scheduled. Follow office procedures. Provider

referrals and patients without appointments should also be scheduled according to office policy.

11. Discuss how to handle failed appointments and no-shows, as well as methods to increase appointment show rates.

It is important to determine the reason for failed appointments and to do whatever is possible to remedy the situation. Failed appointments need to be documented. A busy practice must have a very specific policy on appointment no-shows and must enforce it effectively. Methods to increase appointment show rates include automated call routing, appointment cards, confirmation calls, e-mail reminders, and mailed reminders.

12. Discuss how to handle cancellations and delays.

Cancellations will occur because of a variety of reasons (e.g., when the patient cancels, when the provider is delayed, when the provider is called to an emergency, or when the provider is ill or out of town). All situations should be handled in accordance with office policy.

13. Discuss patient processing, including the importance of the reception area.

The patient reception area should be an inviting place where patients feel comfortable. A first impression is a lasting one. Consider the traffic flow when designing the reception area, as well as fresh, harmonious colors and cleanliness. A writing desk with writing paper in the reception area for the convenience of patients is a nice touch. Some offices offer a computer for patients to use while waiting to see the provider.

14. Describe how to prepare for patient arrival, including patient check-in procedures.

Advanced preparation helps make the day go smoothly and contributes to a more relaxed atmosphere for all. Health records should be prepared for the provider, arranged sequentially. The reception desk should be in clear view of all visitors who come to the office. Use a sign-in register that promotes patients' privacy. During the patient check-in process, it is vital that the medical assistant takes steps to protect the other patients in the reception area.

15. Explain why using the patient's name as often as possible is important, as well as how the medical assistant can make patients feel at ease.

Using a patient's name as often as possible shows that the interaction is about the individual patient. By using the patient's name often, the medical assistant also ensures the correct patient is being treated. Providers and staff members make brief notes in the health record about the current events in the patient's life, which allows them to make friendly conversation.

16. Describe registration procedures, including obtaining a patient history.

On a patient's first visit to the provider's office, the staff performs certain registration procedures. Most providers use a patient information or registration form to gather demographic information. The patient may also need the NPP document and to sign an acknowledgment of receipt

of the NPP. The patient's personal history, medical history, and family history may be obtained by asking him or her to complete a questionnaire, which could be paper or electronic.

17. Do the following related to patient reception and processing:
- Show consideration for patients' time.
  The medical assistant should bring the patient to the examination room for treatment or consultation as close to the appointment time as possible or explain delays.
- Properly treat patients with special needs.
  In all special needs cases, it is important to remain professional and treat everyone with respect.
- Escort and instruct the patient.
  While in the provider's office, most patients prefer to be escorted rather than simply told where to go, and this is usually the medical assistant's responsibility.
- Describe where health records should be placed.
  Health records should never be left in the examination room to be picked up and read by a patient. When using EHRs, it is important to remember to log out of the computer when you are ready to leave the room.

18. Describe how the medical assistant should deal with challenging situations, such as talkative patients, children, angry patients, and patients' relatives and friends.

For talkative patients, the patient's history could be flagged with a symbol to alert the provider. Parents are responsible for their children's behavior while at the provider's office. The medical assistant should not discipline the child. Medical assistants should use empathy and good listening skills when dealing with angry patients, and there should be a policy in place for dealing with potentially dangerous individuals. Avoid a "too casual" attitude with patients' relatives and friends; show moderate concern and empathy.

19. Discuss the friendly farewell, patient checkout, and planning for the next day.

The medical assistant can help convey a sense of caring by terminating the visit cordially. Be sure to thank the patient for coming and wish the person well as he or she leaves the office. As the day winds down, look over the appointments scheduled for the next day and plan ahead where possible.

20. Discuss patient education, as well as legal and ethical issues, for scheduling appointments and patient processing.

The administrative medical assistant has a huge effect on the efficiency of the medical office. Educating the patient about office policies helps the facility run smoothly day to day. The appointment schedule may be used as a legal record and could be brought by subpoena into a court of law. When a patient complains, listen carefully and try to resolve the problem and assure the patient. If someone other than the patient asks for information about the patient, refrain from discussion unless the patient or provider has authorized the release of information.

CONNECTIONS

Study Guide Connection: Go to the Chapter 9 Study Guide. Read and complete the activities.

evolve Evolve Connection: Go to the Chapter 9 link at *evolve.elsevier.com/kinn* to complete the Chapter Review Quiz. Check out the other resources listed for this chapter to make the most of what you have learned about scheduling appointments and patient processing.

DAILY OPERATIONS IN THE AMBULATORY CARE SETTING

10

SCENARIO

Marie Van Bakel, CMA (AAMA), is a new medical assistant in a small orthopedic clinic. She was hired by Dr. Carol Schmidt and Dr. Michael Michalski to be their clinical medical assistant. Marie just graduated from a medical assistant school and this is her first job. She is excited to work in orthopedics, which was the same specialty she worked in during her medical assistant practicum. In a small practice, Marie has a variety of different responsibilities compared with a medical assistant in a larger practice. She and the receptionist, Catherine, will be the only staff members in the office four out of five mornings a week because the doctors will be making hospital rounds and will be in surgery. Marie and Catherine need to open the office and prepare for the patients. Marie is also responsible for the inventory of clinical supplies and equipment. During Marie's interview, Dr. Schmidt expressed her concern about the lack of procedures for ordering and maintaining inventory and would like Marie to develop those procedures. As part of her job, Marie is to manage ordering supplies and ensuring the proper quantities are in stock at all times. Not having much exposure to supplies and ordering during her practicum, Marie realizes she needs to learn about these procedures.

While studying this chapter, think about the following questions:

- What are the medical assistant's responsibilities when opening and closing the healthcare facility?
- What strategies are utilized to help keep the medical environment safe and secure?
- How do you perform a supply and equipment inventory?
- How does the healthcare facility utilize the United States Postal Service (USPS) and other delivery companies?
- How can a medical assistant practice proper body mechanics?

LEARNING OBJECTIVES

1. Define, spell, and pronounce the terms listed in the vocabulary.
2. Describe the administrative and clinical opening duties performed by the medical assistant.
3. Discuss the administrative and clinical closing responsibilities performed by the medical assistant, as well as daily and monthly duties.
4. Explain safety and security procedures important in the healthcare facility.
5. Do the following related to equipment in a medical practice:
   - Describe the elements of an equipment inventory list.
   - Explain the purpose of routine maintenance of administrative and clinical equipment.
   - Explain the steps of creating a maintenance log, performing maintenance, and documenting the maintenance.
   - Describe the medical assistant's role in ordering equipment.
6. Do the following related to supplies in the medical practice:
   - Discuss the elements on a supply inventory list.
   - List the steps involved in completing an inventory.
   - Perform an inventory with documentation.
   - Prepare a supply order.
7. Describe how the healthcare facility utilizes USPS and other delivery agencies.
8. Use proper body mechanics.

VOCABULARY

accounts payable Money owed by a company to other companies for services and goods; pertains to paying the bills of the facility.

answering service A business that receives and answers telephone calls for the healthcare facility when it is closed.

authorized agent A person who has written documentation that he or she can accept a shipment for another individual.

backordered An order placed for an item that is temporarily out of stock and will be sent at a later time.

billable service Assistance (i.e., service) that is provided by a healthcare provider that can be billed to the insurance company and/or patient.

bonded When an employer obtains a fidelity bond from an insurance company, which will cover losses from employee dishonest acts (e.g., embezzlement, theft).

buying cycle Refers to how often an item is purchased; depends on frequency of the use of the item and storage space available for the item.

VOCABULARY—*continued*

continuing medical education (CME) Activities (e.g., conferences, seminars) that promote further education for physicians and providers.

crash cart Emergency medications and equipment (e.g., oxygen, intravenous [IV], and airway supplies) stored in a cart, ready for an emergency.

depreciate To diminish in value (of an item) over a period of time; concept used for tax purposes.

discrepancies A lack of similarity between what is stated and what is found; for instance, when what is stated on the packing slip is different than what is found in the box.

disinfected The state of having destroyed or rendered pathogenic organisms inactive; does not include spores, tuberculosis bacilli, and certain viruses.

e-prescribing The ability of the provider to electronically send a prescription directly to the pharmacy.

girth The measurement around something; when referring to mail, it is the measurement around the middle of the package that is being shipped.

inventory The stored medical and administrative supplies that are used in the medical office. It is also the process of counting the supplies in stock.

invoices Billing statements that list the amount owed for goods or services purchased.

packing slip A document that accompanies purchased merchandise and shows what is in the box or package.

purchase order number Unique number assigned by the ordering facility that allows the facility to track or reference the order. Many vendors will add this number to the order documents (e.g., packing slip and statement).

quality control Manufactured samples with known values used to see if a test method is reliable by consistently producing accurate and precise results.

quantity to reorder The amount of supplies that need to be ordered.

restock Process of replacing the supplies that were used.

sanitized The state of having cleaned equipment and instruments with detergent and water, removing debris and reducing the number of microorganisms.

sterilized The state of having removed all microorganisms.

termination letters Documents sent to patients explaining that the provider is ending the physician-patient relationship and the patients need to see other providers.

vendor A company that sells supplies, equipment, or services to another company or individual.

white noise The sounds from a television or stereo that muffle or mute the conversation of others, thus helping to protect the confidentiality of patients.

zone A region or geographic area used for shipping.

MEDICAL OFFICE ENVIRONMENT

Opening the Healthcare Facility

In the healthcare facility, employees must arrive before patients to prepare for the patients. The preparation can differ based on the size of the facility and the practice's policies on preparation.

In smaller agencies, a few reliable employees are given keys to unlock the doors and the code to deactivate the alarm system. In larger facilities, employees must use the employee entrances, which are locked. Employees can unlock the doors by entering unique codes into a keypad or by using unique keycards (Figure 10-1, *A, B*). Both systems are developed to monitor who enters the building. Usually security, custodial, or supervisory personnel have the responsibility to deactivate the alarm system in larger facilities. The main patient doors are then opened by staff at a set time.

Regardless of the size of the agency, the medical assistant will be responsible for preparing the department or office for patients. For the administrative staff, voice mails need to be checked or messages from the **answering service** need to be obtained. The answering service may e-mail or fax the messages to the office, and these messages need to be addressed by staff and documented in the patients' health records. The phone voice mail message may need to be updated, and in some facilities the phones need to be "turned on" so patients can reach the healthcare facility and not get the answering service.

Computers, copy machines, and other equipment must be turned on. Some facilities require the medical assistant to print schedules of the day's appointments, keeping one for chart preparation and placing the other on the provider's desk. With the use of electronic health records (EHRs), providers and staff can utilize the software to see the appointments instead of having to rely on the paper schedule. Along with the list of appointments for the day, the medical assistant needs to pull the required paperwork for the patients. For practices without EHRs, the patients' medical records need to be pulled and prepared with any required documents. For practices with EHRs, required patient education literature (e.g., well-child visit documents) and preprinted paper screening forms may be prepared.

The administrative medical assistants need to prepare the reception area for patients. Magazines should be neatly displayed. Toys for children should be **disinfected** on a routine basis for infection control. Tissue boxes, hand sanitizer, and face masks should be well stocked and available for sick patients. Televisions and/or "**white noise**" music should be turned on. If the reception area includes beverages for patients, the medical assistant should prepare those and ensure they are adequately stocked.

CRITICAL THINKING APPLICATION   **10-1**

Catherine, the receptionist, utilizes low-volume music from a stereo as white noise in the reception area, which is near the reception desk. What are the benefits of the music?

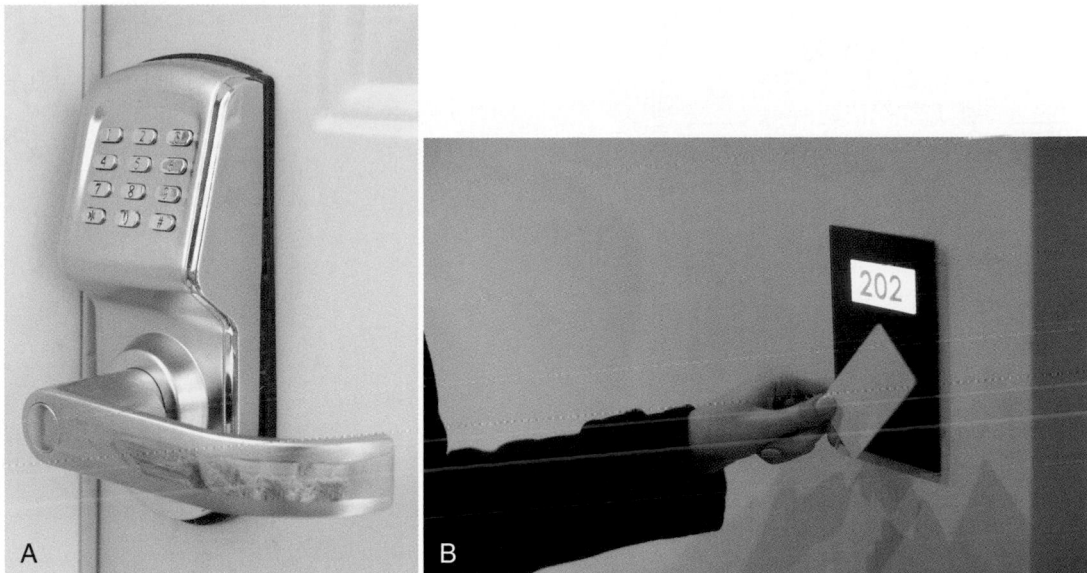

FIGURE 10-1 A, Keyless Access Locks allow employees to enter unique numbers that open the door and track who has keyed in. Once a person is no longer employed, the number is deleted. **B,** Employees can unlock doors using their unique key card. This system can track which keycard was used to open the door. (Photos copyright iStock.com.)

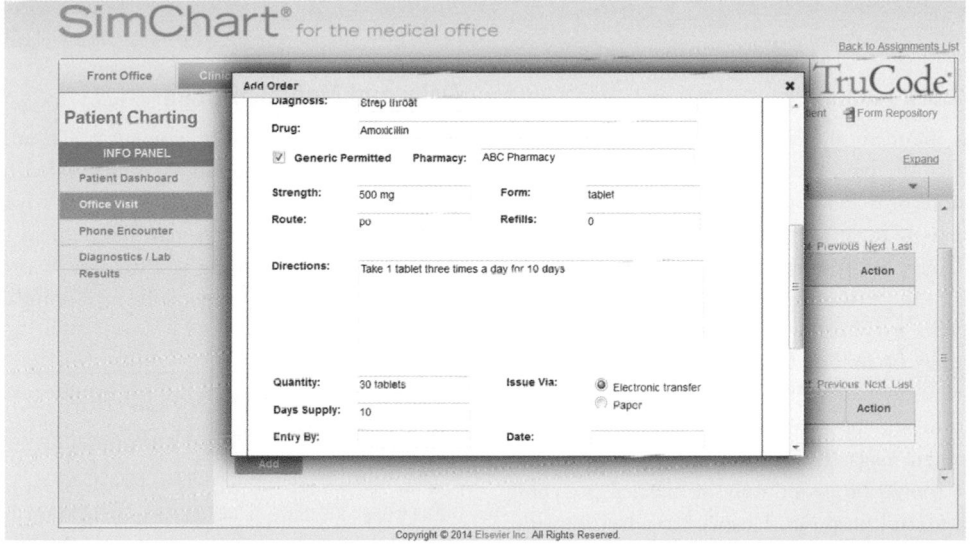

FIGURE 10-2 With e-prescribing, providers can enter the prescription information into the electronic health record (EHR) and send it to the pharmacy.

Medical assistants must also prepare the patient examination rooms by turning on the lights, checking that the supplies are stocked, and ensuring the rooms are cleaned appropriately. The medical assistant should scan the room, making sure it is neat, orderly, and safe for patients and children. For practices that do not use **e-prescribing**, prescription pads should not remain in examination rooms (Figure 10-2 and Figure 10-3). The provider should keep a pad in his or her pocket and the extra prescription pads should be stored in a locked cabinet. Prescription pads should never be accessible to patients because some might take the pads and try to forge a prescription, which is illegal.

Supply cabinets must be unlocked, except the narcotic cabinet. Narcotic medications should remain locked up at all times. The medical assistant must ensure restrooms have adequate supplies for patients (e.g., urine specimen containers, cleansing towelettes).

Quality control tests must be done on laboratory equipment. Outstanding patient issues from the prior day and any new reports on patients' diagnostic tests, including radiology tests and medical laboratory tests, need to be followed up. For facilities using paper records, the patient's record must be matched with the diagnostic report and then given to the provider to review. For facilities with EHRs, many times this process is completed electronically through the use of messaging systems in the software.

CRITICAL THINKING APPLICATION   **10-2**

When opening the orthopedic office, what jobs does Marie, the clinical medical assistant, need to do? What jobs does Catherine, the receptionist, need to do to prepare for the day?

FIGURE 10-3 One prescription pad should be kept by the provider and extra pads should be locked up.

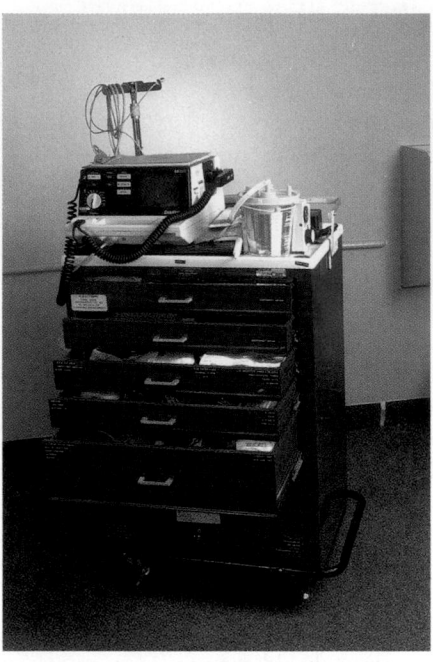

FIGURE 10-4 Crash carts must be inventoried monthly, ensuring medication and supplies have not expired and all the required supplies are available for an emergency.

Closing the Healthcare Facility

At the end of the day, the medical assistant needs to help with the closing duties. Some facilities have the administrative medical assistant prepare the patient records and documents for the next day. The administrative medical assistant must turn off the computers, copy machine, and other office equipment. The phones need to be switched to voice mail or the answering service. If the medical assistant handles co-payments from patients, the office procedures for handling the money must be followed. Any patient documents on the desk need to be put away for confidentiality purposes.

The medical assistant should clean up the reception area by gathering up the scattered magazines and returning them to their proper locations. Toys should be periodically disinfected per clinic protocol for infection control purposes. Unsolicited advertisements (e.g., pharmaceutical) and garbage need to be removed from the tables and chairs. The lights, television, stereo, and other devices should be turned off.

The clinical medical assistant must ensure that all the patients have left by checking the examination and treatment rooms. The medical assistant should **restock** the rooms and organize any reading materials in the room. The examination table, writing table, counters, computer keyboards, and chairs (i.e., those made of plastic, metal, or wood) should be disinfected. Patient-related documents should be put away. Computers and other devices should be shut down. Equipment and instruments should be **sanitized**, disinfected, or **sterilized**. Supply and medication cabinets need to be locked. If the department stocks narcotic medications, some facilities require the medications be counted by two staff members to verify the stock.

Depending on the facility, the medical assistant may be responsible for turning off the lights, activating the alarms, and locking the doors. In larger facilities, the custodial or security staff handles these responsibilities.

Daily and Monthly Duties

Medical facilities either employ custodial staff or hire cleaning services to clean. This cleaning takes place after hours each day. Larger facilities that employ custodial staff will have the staff clean high-traffic areas several times a day. These areas include the restrooms and the entrances. During wet weather, it is critical that the floors are kept dry to prevent people from slipping and falling.

CRITICAL THINKING APPLICATION   **10-3**

The orthopedic office utilizes a local cleaning service to clean the practice's rooms. The staff arrives after hours and are gone by the time Catherine and Marie open the office in the morning. Over the last month, Marie has noticed that the rooms do not look as clean as they should. Should she address this? If so, with whom should she discuss this?

The medical assistant also has responsibilities for cleaning and organizing the reception area and the examination rooms. During slow times, medical assistants are expected to do extra duties, including restocking medical and office supplies, forms, and patient literature. Just like at home, the cabinets and drawers in a medical office need to be straightened and reorganized. Medications and supplies that have expiration dates need to be checked monthly. **Crash carts** and other emergency supplies need to be inventoried monthly (Figure 10-4).

It is important that the medical practice be clean and organized. By taking the initiative to perform those tasks during quiet times, you will be considered a more valuable employee. Supervisors and providers value employees that look for additional activities to do during quiet times.

SECURITY IN THE HEALTHCARE FACILITY

Security and safety is important to the wellbeing of the medical practice staff, patients, and visitors. The healthcare facility can draw unwanted attention from those seeking drugs and money. Having plans in place that can be implemented when security is in question is critical for all.

Medical assistants need to stay alert for suspicious people. If a situation or a person makes you feel strange or on edge, listen to your instincts. Try to alert another staff person of the situation. Keep yourself at a distance from the person, including separating yourself from the person by a desk or piece of furniture if possible. If you are rooming a patient, position yourself so you are the closest to the door. If you feel uncomfortable rooming the patient, discuss the situation with the provider.

Medical facilities can be a target for those wanting to steal money, narcotic medications, and prescription pads. The staff should implement measures to limit the amount of money available in the building. Cash and checks from patients should be deposited daily to limit large quantities of money in the facility. Cash drawers should be stored out of sight of patients and visitors. Narcotic medications, if present in the agency, should always be in a double-locked cabinet with the keys hidden. Depending on the type of clinic, some will post signs stating there are no narcotic medications on site. As mentioned in a prior section, prescription pads are used in clinics that do not use e-prescribing. The prescription pads should remain out of view and reach of patients. They should not be stored in the patient examination rooms.

CRITICAL THINKING APPLICATION   **10-4**

Over the last 6 months, crime and break-ins have increased in the local area around the clinic. Many people believe the clinic has a supply of narcotic medication in stock, which is not true. What strategies can the staff implement to increase the security of the practice?

The healthcare facility should have procedures in place for dealing with suspicious people or potential robberies. Some clinics have code words that indicate specific situations. When these words are used by staff, they alert other staff members of the potential situation. Some clinics have installed alarm buttons under countertops and workstations. In a robbery situation or other security risk situation, the medical assistant can activate the alarm, which will trigger a notification to the clinic administration and the local police department. Remember it is always better to err on the side of caution and notify the police.

Many facilities have moved to locking employee entrance doors at all times during business hours and require either a key card or unique code to enter the building. In high crime areas, low-staffed clinics, or rural clinics, the doors to the patient care areas are also locked. This prevents unauthorized entry of people from the reception area to the patient care areas in the back, increasing the security.

After hours the facility should utilize alarms that are triggered when break-ins occur. When the alarm is triggered, an employee of the alarm company notifies the police department and the administrative personnel listed as emergency contacts. The police and the administrative personnel must determine what was the target and if anything was taken.

EQUIPMENT AND SUPPLIES

One of the most important responsibilities of the medical assistant is to manage the equipment and supplies in the medical office. In smaller facilities, the medical assistant may have more duties, including ordering and maintaining an inventory control system. In larger facilities, employees are hired for such roles in the purchasing department.

Equipment

In a medical practice, administrative and clinical equipment are used. The medical assistant needs to know how to operate, maintain, and handle issues with the equipment. For financial and tax purposes, the medical practice must know details about the equipment owned, including the purchase cost and age of each item. The process of gathering and creating a list of the equipment in the facility is called managing inventory.

Equipment Inventory

Each piece of equipment in the medical practice should be identified and records need to be maintained. The healthcare facility must be able to account for all of the equipment used and owned by the practice. In case of disaster or theft, the practice can provide these details to the insurance company to help facilitate the replacement of the equipment. In case of theft, equipment details can also be shared with the police to help identify equipment if it is found.

CRITICAL THINKING APPLICATION   **10-5**

Marie needs to learn more about managing inventory. She reviews her medical assistant textbook and reads articles online. She decides to start by creating an inventory list of the equipment in the medical office. What are some advantages of having an updated list of administrative and clinical equipment?

The practice's accountant utilizes the equipment inventory list while preparing the tax paperwork for the practice. Small equipment (e.g., thermometers, glucose monitors) is deducted as a practice expense for the year in which it is purchased. Computer hardware, calculators, and copiers are considered larger office equipment and **depreciate** over 5 years. Office furniture items (e.g., desks, files, safes, examination tables) depreciate over 7 years.

The equipment inventory list also helps the providers and supervisors identify equipment that needs to be replaced. Preplanning equipment purchases is a financial strategy for the practice. It allows the practice to be prepared and plan ahead for future investments.

To create an equipment inventory list, the medical assistant should create a spreadsheet and include all the administrative and clinical equipment (Figure 10-5). For each item, the medical assistant should document the following:

- Equipment name, manufacturer, and serial number
- Purchase date, cost, and supplier

Equipment Name	Manufacturer / Serial Number	Location / Facility Number	Purchase Date / Supplier	Cost	Warranty Information
Laser Printer	HP / HP3598XA	Medical Assistant Desk / LP59483	08/01/20XX / Best Office Supplies	$325	Parts and labor expires 07/31/20XX
AT2 Plus ECG / Spirometry	Schiller / WA4893X	Treatment Room / ES00012	05/02/20XX / Medical Equipment Supplies	$2987	Parts and Labor expires 05/01/20XX

FIGURE 10-5 An equipment inventory list can be created in a spreadsheet and provides useful information on the administrative and clinical equipment in the facility.

- Warranty information (e.g., start and end date, warranty coverage)

Larger facilities will also include the location of the equipment and the unique facility number of the equipment on the inventory list. For tracking purposes, larger facilities will place a sticker on the equipment and give each item a unique number. Procedure 10-1 explains how to create an equipment inventory.

The owner's or operation manual and warranty information for each item should be kept at a central location, available to users. Many manufacturers have the operation manuals available online as a convenience for users. The manuals are used to problem-solve performance issues, identify service schedules and routine maintenance, and identify parts or supplies needed for the operation of the machine.

PROCEDURE 10-1   Perform an Inventory with Documentation: Equipment Inventory

Goals: *Perform an equipment inventory and document the inventory on the equipment inventory form.*

EQUIPMENT and SUPPLIES

- Pen
- Administrative and/or clinical equipment
- Purchase information (e.g., date, cost, and supplier) and warranty information (e.g., start and end date, warranty coverage)
- Equipment inventory form

PROCEDURAL STEPS

1. For the equipment to be inventoried, gather the following information for each piece of equipment:
   - Name of equipment, manufacturer, and serial number
   - Location and facility number (if applicable)
   - Purchase date, cost, supplier, and warranty information

PURPOSE: To have the essential information required when creating the spreadsheet.

2. Complete an equipment inventory form by adding the gathered information for each item inventoried (see Figure 10-5).

PURPOSE: Creating an equipment inventory list on the computer will help you organize the information and also help you maintain the information easily.

3. Review the document created. Make any necessary revisions.

Equipment Safety and Maintenance

The medical assistant is responsible for monitoring equipment safety and proper functioning. Potential issues should not be overlooked and action should be taken to prevent injury to staff or patients and costly damage to the equipment. For administrative and clinical equipment, electrical cords should be checked for damage. Any suspected overheating issues should be immediately addressed. Any unusual noise or change in performance should be investigated. Equipment should be routinely cleaned and maintained in accordance with the operation manual, which will help promote the life of the machine.

CRITICAL THINKING APPLICATION   **10-6**

Marie realized that the practice did not have maintenance logs for the various pieces of equipment. She decided to start making logs, but realized there were a lot of logs she would have to make. How could she create logs in a very time-efficient manner? For a small office, describe options that she could use to organize all the logs so they are easy to locate and use.

Equipment operation manuals include information on cleaning, routine maintenance, service schedules, and how to troubleshoot common problems. The medical assistant should follow the cleaning procedures and the routine maintenance for the equipment utilized. Routine maintenance varies with the equipment. Copiers and printers may entail changing toner or cartridges. For clinical equipment, maintenance may include changing filters or batteries. Making a schedule as a reminder for routine maintenance can be helpful. Many facilities utilize logs to help track routine maintenance and service calls (Figure 10-6). The logs should include:

- Equipment name, serial number, location of machine, and facility's unique equipment number (if applicable)

- Manufacturer's name
- Date of purchase
- Warranty information (e.g., start and end date, warranty coverage)
- Service provider contact information
- Date and time maintenance activities performed
- Maintenance activities performed
- Signature of person performing maintenance

Procedure 10-2 explains the steps involved in creating a maintenance log, performing the maintenance, and then documenting the maintenance.

Maintenance Log

Equipment Name: **Laser Printer**   Serial #: **HP3598XA**   Location: **Medical Assistant Desk**

Facility #: **LP59483**   Manufacturer: **HP**   Purchased: **08/01/20XX**

Warranty Information: **Parts and labor expires 07/31/20XX**

Freqency of Inspections: **Every 6 months**

Service Provider: **Best Office Supplies**

Date	Time	Maintenance Activities	Signature
12/15/20XX	0956	**Replaced toner cartridge**	**Marie Van Bakel, CMA (AAMA)**
02/11/20XX	1235	**Service call: Office Repair Company – to fix stray ink marks on copies**	**Catherine Black, RMA**

Maintenance Log

Equipment Name: **AT2 Plus ECG/Spirometry**   Serial #: **WA4893X**   Location: **Treatment Room**

Facility #: **ES00012**   Manufacturer: **Schiller**   Purchased: **05/02/20XX**

Freqency of Inspections: **Every 12 months**

Warranty information: **Parts and Labor expires 05/01/20XX**

Service Provider: **Medical Equipment Suppliers**

Date	Time	Maintenance Activities	Signature
10/23/20XX	1123	**Replaced battery**	**Marie Van Bakel, CMA (AAMA)**
05/02/20XX	1445	**No tracing, cleaned stylus with alcohol**	**Marie Van Bakel, CMA (AAMA)**

FIGURE 10-6 Equipment maintenance logs are utilized to track maintenance activities by the staff and outside repair agencies.

PROCEDURE 10-2 | **Perform Routine Maintenance of Administrative or Clinical Equipment**

Goals: *To perform routine maintenance of administrative or clinical equipment and document the maintenance on the log.*

EQUIPMENT and SUPPLIES

- Maintenance log(s)
- Administrative or clinical equipment (e.g., oral thermometers)
- Supplies for routine maintenance (e.g., battery)
- Operation manual if needed

- Pen
- Information regarding the equipment (i.e., name, serial number, location, facility number, manufacturer, purchase date, warranty information, frequency of inspections, and service provider)

PROCEDURE 10-2   —continued

PROCEDURAL STEPS

1. Gather information on the piece of equipment identified for routine maintenance, including: name, serial number, location, facility number, manufacturer, purchase date, warranty information, frequency of inspections, and service provider.
   PURPOSE: To have the essential information required when completing the log.
2. Fill in the equipment details on the log (see Figure 10-6).
   PURPOSE: Adding the equipment details helps identify the machine and provides a quick reference to useful information that might be asked by the service provider. The form serves as a log for documenting the maintenance activities that are performed.
3. To perform the maintenance activities, gather the required supplies. If you are not familiar with the procedure or the required supplies, refer to the operation manual.

PURPOSE: You need to be familiar with the supplies and the procedure before you start the maintenance.
4. Perform the maintenance activities as directed in the operation manual. Take any required safety precautions necessary to protect yourself and others.
   PURPOSE: Following the outlined procedure in the operation manual will help you successfully complete the maintenance without injuring yourself and others or doing damage to the machine.
5. Clean up the work area.
6. Using a pen, document the date, time, the maintenance activity performed, and your signature on the log.
   PURPOSE: Completing the log indicating the activities performed will serve as a communication tool for future reference and services needed on that piece of equipment.

Service Calls and Warranties

When equipment is purchased, a warranty is given for a period of time. The warranty is the manufacturer's guarantee that if the piece of equipment needs to be repaired or has a defective part, the manufacturer will pay for the cost of the repair and in some cases replace the item. Typically the warranty language includes details on what is covered and what is not covered. Some warranties are not honored if someone other than a "recognized" service person attempts to fix the machine. Extended warranties can be purchased for some machines, which lengthens the protection time.

Typically for complex and/or expensive equipment, the medical practice will contract with a service provider for repairs and routine service checks, which are explained in the operation manual. This assistance with equipment maintenance is necessary for some equipment and also helps to extend the lifetime of those machines. For repairs on other equipment, it might be necessary to ship or bring the machine to the repair service. Usually the cost for on-site repairs is more than if the machine is brought or shipped to the service provider for repairs. One of the main concerns when a piece of equipment breaks down is the effect on the medical practice. Some service providers will also loan equipment to healthcare facilities while the repairs take place. This service greatly lessens the burden on the practice.

Purchasing Equipment

Depending on the size of the medical organization, the process of purchasing equipment can vary. Large agencies typically have staff in purchasing departments who research the needs of the organization, identifying the best equipment to purchase. For smaller practices, the medical assistant may be involved with the process.

If a provider or supervisor is considering replacing a piece of equipment, a number of factors are taken into consideration. The age of the machine and the availability of parts are considered. Sometimes repair parts are not available or are very expensive for older machines. The frequency and cost of repairs is a factor. Is the practice spending more on the repair costs compared with purchasing a new model? The utilization of the machine will be examined. If the machine is used often, it needs to be reliable. Does the new model have features that will enhance the practice or can the features provide extra **billable services** for the business? These factors are considered when a piece of equipment needs to be replaced.

CRITICAL THINKING APPLICATION   **10-7**
Currently, the providers are using an off-site radiology service. They are contemplating creating a small radiology room where they could take x-rays. How could Marie assist the providers with their plans for a potential purchase of x-ray equipment?

The provider and/or supervisor may also consider leasing a piece of equipment. With the frequency of technology changes in the medical field, leasing medical equipment is becoming a popular option for smaller facilities. Monitoring equipment, diagnostic testing equipment, examination tables, computer systems, and furniture are just some of the items that can be leased. The healthcare facility pays a fee to lease the machine or the furniture, which is less than what would be paid out if the item is purchased. The lease fees are tax deductible and allow the agency the ability to provide extra billable services.

The medical assistant may help the provider or supervisor identify potential new models. Using the Internet and contacting salespeople representing the models of interest are two ways to get additional information. Some salespeople will meet with the staff, demonstrating the product and answering any questions they may have. In addition to research, the medical assistant may need to explain the usage of the machine and the frequency of repair checks. Usually the

Item Name	Size	Quantity	Item Number	Supplier's Name	Reorder Point	Quantity to Reorder	Cost	Stock Available	Order (✓)
Nonsterile gauze sponges, 8 ply	2″x 2″	100/pkg	NG0022	Midwest Medical	5	25	$2.31/pkg		
Sterile gauze sponges, 12 ply, 2/pkg	2″x 2″	25 pkg/box	NG0042	Midwest Medical	4	20	$3.99/box		

FIGURE 10-7 A supply inventory list shows details for items in inventory. For efficiency, use two extra columns ("Stock Available" and "Order") as shown. This list can be duplicated and utilized when performing inventory.

supervisor or provider has the final say on the new model and if the purchase should occur.

Supplies

There are many supplies required to run the medical office and treat patients. Supplies can include administrative items such as pens, paper, envelopes, and paperclips. Supplies can also include bandages, vaccines, medications, slings, and splints. The medical assistant needs to ensure the practice has enough supplies to treat patients. Running out of supplies can greatly affect the services provided to patients and can be more expensive for the healthcare facility because of last-minute ordering at higher prices. On the other hand, overstocking supplies can be a financial waste to the practice. Many supplies have expiration dates and cannot be used beyond that date. Having adequate amounts of supplies in **inventory** is crucial.

Inventory Management

Inventory management involves ordering, tracking inventory, and identifying the quantity of product to purchase. The goal of inventory management is to have adequate supplies on hand to use in the healthcare facility, yet not have too much stock that will expire or take a long time to use.

The medical assistant in charge of ordering and managing supplies must keep a record on each item in inventory. The record can be a manual recording written in a notebook or on index cards, or it can be computerized in a spreadsheet or inventory control system software (Procedure 10-3 explains how to create the supply inventory list using a spreadsheet). For each inventory item, the medical assistant must record the following:

- Item details: Item name, size, quantity, item number, supplier's name, and cost (Figure 10-7).
- **Quantity to reorder**: Amount of product used during the **buying cycle**. For instance, the healthcare facility's buying cycle for 2x2 nonsterile gauze (100 per pack) is 1 month. The facility typically goes through 25 packs in 1 month. This would be the quantity used during the buying cycle and would be the quantity to reorder (see Figure 10-7).
- Reorder point: When the quantity of the item gets to a specific number, indicating that it needs to be reordered. For instance, when the inventory of 2x2 nonsterile gauze packs gets to 5 packs, the medical assistant must reorder (see Figure 10-7). Five is the reorder point or the quantity that triggers an order to be placed to replenish the inventory. The reorder point for

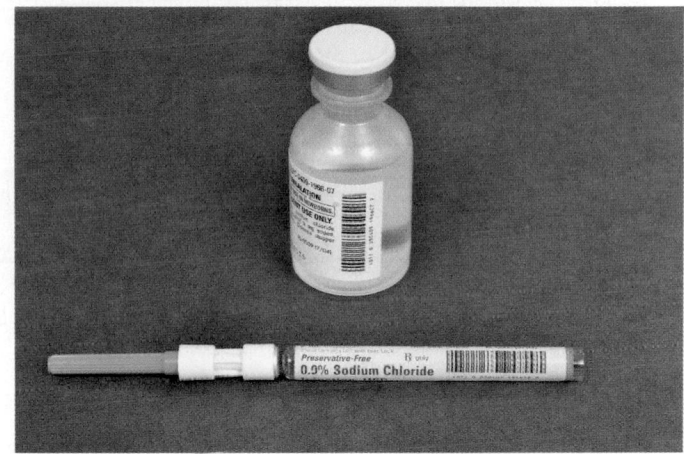

FIGURE 10-8 Using bar codes can make inventory control more efficient.

medical and administrative supplies can be different for each item because of the usage rate and the time it takes to receive the item after it is ordered. The reorder point for an item can be calculated based on the number used per day and the number of days it takes to order and receive the product. For instance, the practice uses half a pack of 2x2 nonsterile gauze per day. It takes 4 days to receive the order from the medical supply company. The medical practice may also want 6 extra days' worth of supplies on hand to prevent issues of running out of the item. Here is how you would figure out the reorder point:

Stock to cover order time: 0.5 pack per day × 4 days to receive order = 2 packs

Extra stock: 6 days × 0.5 pack per day = 3 packs

Reorder point: 2 packs (stock to cover order time) + 3 packs (6-day supply) = 5 packs

Inventory Control Systems

To make inventory management work well, an inventory control system should be in place. Large medical facilities may utilize computerized inventory control systems, which monitor usage and inventory in stock, and also identify items that need to be ordered. Smaller facilities may utilize simple computerized or manual systems.

To help create an efficient computerized system, many medical facilities utilize bar codes to track inventory and for billing for supplies (Figure 10-8). With this system, each item has a unique bar code. The bar code is scanned with a bar code reader when items are added or taken from inventory. Software can then help monitor the inventory quantity. For bar codes to work successfully, the staff must be diligent in scanning the bar codes when taking a product from stock. Bar code inventory control systems work successfully in large and small practices.

There are several manual systems utilized for identifying what supplies need to be ordered. The following are some of the more common methods utilized in medical facilities.

- When staff identify a product needs to be ordered, the item is written in a log. This process is similar to making a list of what you need at the grocery store. The person responsible for ordering supplies then prepares the order based on the information in the log.
- Another system includes using product identification slips, which contain the name of the product. The slips or cards are attached to the product or a box/package of items. When the

product is used, the slip is put in a special location like a box or plastic pocket. The slips in the box or pocket are then used by the medical assistant who prepares the supply order.

- The two-bin system consists of having a main bin for each item in inventory and then a backup bin for each. When the main bin is emptied, the backup bin is used and the product is reordered.
- The medical assistant responsible for ordering performs a hand count of the items in stock, identifying what needs to be ordered. This system is explained in the next section (see Procedure 10-3).

CRITICAL THINKING APPLICATION   10-8
Marie decided to implement a manual system for inventory. Of the manual systems discussed, which method might work best in the small orthopedic practice? Discuss your answer.

PROCEDURE 10-3   Perform an Inventory with Documentation: Perform an Inventory of Supplies While Using Proper Body Mechanics

Goals: *Perform a supply inventory using correct body mechanics. Document the inventory on the supply inventory form.*

EQUIPMENT and SUPPLIES

- Pen
- Administrative and/or clinical supplies to be inventoried
- Purchase information (e.g., item number, cost, and supplier) for supplies in inventory
- Reorder point and quantity to reorder for each item in inventory
- Supply inventory form

PROCEDURAL STEPS

1. For the supplies in inventory, gather the following information for each item:
   - Name, size, quantity (e.g., purchased individually, 100 per box)
   - Item number, supplier's name, cost
   - Reorder point and quantity to reorder
   PURPOSE: To have the essential information required when creating the spreadsheet.
2. Enter each supply's information on the inventory form, making sure the appropriate entry is in the right location (see Figure 10-7).
   Note: The "Stock Available" column will be empty for now.
   PURPOSE: Creating a supply inventory list on the computer will help you organize the information and also help you maintain the information easily.
3. Review the document. Make any necessary revisions.
   PURPOSE: Using a copy of the supply inventory list when counting the stock available will save time and help increase the accuracy of the information.

4. Using the supply inventory list, inventory the supplies in the department. Identify how the supply should be counted (e.g., individually, by the box) and count the number of items in stock.
   PURPOSE: By identifying the correct quantity that the item is inventoried by, you will increase the accuracy of the inventory. Counting an item by "each" when it comes as a package can cause confusion when identifying what needs to be ordered.
5. Add the number in the appropriate row under the "Stock Available" header.
6. Indicate which supplies need to be reordered by checking the appropriate columns.
7. After counting the item, place the stock neatly back, making sure the oldest stock is in the front.
   PURPOSE: It is important to clean up your workspace. The oldest stock must be moved to the front to ensure it is used first.
8. Continue steps 5 through 7 until all supplies are inventoried.
9. Use proper body mechanics when lifting and moving supplies by maintaining a wide, stable base with your feet. Your feet should be shoulder-width apart and you should have good footing. Bend at the knees, keeping your back straight. Lift smoothly with the major muscles in your arms and legs. Use the same technique when putting the item down.
   PURPOSE: Correct body mechanics will decrease your risk for injury when carrying or lifting heavy objects. See Figure 10-13 and 10-14 for proper body mechanics when lifting boxes.
10. Use proper body mechanics when reaching for an object. Clear away barriers and use a step stool if needed. Your feet should face the object. Avoid twisting or turning with a heavy load.
    PURPOSE: Straining when reaching or standing on tiptoes can increase your risk for injury.

Taking Inventory

No matter if a healthcare facility has an automated inventory control system or not, taking inventory at periodic times is critical. Many businesses that utilize automated inventory control systems hand count their inventory at least once a year, usually around the close of the business year. These companies compare their hand counts to the computer counts and identify discrepancies. The discrepancies are followed up on. The manual inventory procedure provides the company with information on the actual number of items in stock. With this information, the financial value of the inventory can be calculated and used for financial reports and taxes at the close of the business year.

For medical offices that do not implement inventory control systems, performing inventory or counting the items in stock is important before each buying cycle. See Procedure 10-3 for instructions on performing an inventory. One of the most frequent errors when performing inventory is to report a different quantity than what is on the supply inventory list, spreadsheet, or cards. For instance, if a medical assistant is counting nonsterile sponges, each package should be counted as 1 and not as 100 each. Looking at Figure 10-8, if there were 6 packages of sponges left in the supply cabinet, it should be noted as 6 packages, not 600 sponges or 600 each. Counting each item in a box or package when the product is inventoried by box or package creates conflict and confusion when looking at the reorder point.

To be most efficient when performing an inventory count, the medical assistant should utilize a supply inventory list (Figure 10-9). The supply inventory list shows all the items in stock. When using this document, the medical assistant can mark down the inventory counts for each item (see Procedure 10-3). If the supply inventory list is not available, then the medical assistant needs to write down the item number, size, quantity (e.g., 100/box), manufacturer, and any other identifying information. This process takes a lot more time.

When performing an inventory in the medical practice, the medical assistant should work in a systematic manner. The medical assistant starts with one supply cabinet, working from top to bottom, before moving onto another cabinet. All stock areas should be inventoried before preparing the supply order.

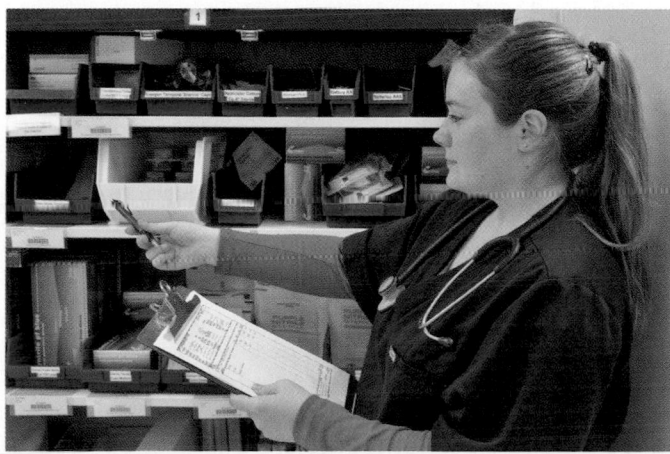

FIGURE 10-9 A medical assistant performing an inventory.

Price Consideration When Ordering Supplies

When ordering supplies, price comparison shopping is important, but it also takes time. The medical practice must balance the time it takes to the money saved. Some medical offices compare prices only on more expensive items or items that are used in vast quantities. They may compare prices every 6 to 12 months, instead of comparing prices with each order. When comparing prices, it is important to consider shipping and handling changes, as well as ensuring the products compared are the same quantity and quality.

Quantity discounts or price breaks are also a way to save money when ordering. The more of an item purchased, the cheaper the product becomes. For instance:

- Quantity 1 to 5, $1.50 per each item
- Quantity 6 to 15, $1.25 per each item

If the medical assistant purchased a quantity of 6, the price per each would be cheaper than if 4 were purchased. The medical assistant must consider storage space, how quickly the item will be used, and the shelf life (or expiration date) of the item. Buying too much just to get a price break may not be in the best interest of the medical practice if there is not adequate storage space or if the product will expire before it can all be used.

Some medical facilities join group purchasing organizations (GPOs), which combine orders from many different medical facilities and thus receive volume discounts from specific vendors. GPOs typically purchase both supplies and medications. Physician buying groups (PBGs) offer providers favorable pricing for vaccines, but the provider must only use the vaccines from the contracted manufacturers.

Ordering Supplies

If the medical practice does not join a GPO, then the medical assistant who orders typically identifies a couple of **vendors** from which to purchase administrative and medical supplies. The medical assistant can utilize the supplier's printed catalog, if available, or the company's online Web site store. Many medical and business supply companies only print the complete catalogs once or twice a year and they can become outdated between printings. The catalog provides a reference for supplies, but the Web site shows all the products available with the most updated prices and sale prices (Procedure 10-4).

Many suppliers require the medical assistant to create an account before ordering products. The account is set up using the practice's information. In some states, ordering sterile solutions (e.g., intravenous [IV] bags, normal saline vials), medications, and needles requires the provider's license number. The setup of the account will only be complete when a copy of the license is faxed to the company. If the medical assistant is ordering narcotics, the physician must authorize the order and provide a copy of his or her Drug Enforcement Administration (DEA) registration. Narcotics require special tracking documentation and thus a high level of authorization when purchasing them.

Some medical facilities utilize **purchase order numbers**, giving each order a unique reference number. This reference number should be included on the order sheets, added to the online information, or provided during the phone order. Vendors add the purchase order number to the order documentation and it can be used as a reference for both parties when discussing the order. The healthcare facility uses the purchase order number to track the order.

Payment terms may vary with suppliers, including credit cards, check, money order, or a line of credit. Typically, the line of credit is good for 30 to 60 days and **invoices** are sent to the ambulatory care clinic to be paid after the purchases have been received. Orders can typically be placed via fax, mail, or phone or online. If the medical assistant is faxing or mailing the order, the vendor usually requires the order to be placed on the vendor's order sheet. A copy of the phone, mailed, or fax order or a printout of the online order should be kept by the medical assistant to verify the order was correctly filled.

CRITICAL THINKING APPLICATION   **10-9**
Currently the practice has been ordering clinical supplies from two vendors. Marie would like to do some cost comparisons to get the best deals on supplies. She does not have a lot of time to spend on the research. How might she approach this situation? Where should she start first? What might be a long-term goal for her?

PROCEDURE 10-4   Prepare a Purchase Order

Goal: *Create an accurate purchase order for supplies.*

EQUIPMENT and SUPPLIES

* Pen
* Supply inventory list showing item name, size, quantity, item number, supplier's name, reorder point, quantity to reorder, cost, and current stock available
* Computer
* Internet
* Printer

PROCEDURAL STEPS

1. Review the supply inventory list with the current stock counts and determine what supplies need to be reordered.
   PURPOSE: By determining what needs to be reordered, you are preventing having too much or too little stock of a particular item.
2. Using the Internet, find the online store used for ordering the needed supplies.
3. Using the search box, type in the item number or description. Verify that the item from the search results is what you need to order.
   PURPOSE: It is important to verify you have the correct product before you add the product to your basket/cart.

4. Apply critical thinking skills as you identify the quantity to reorder for that item and order this amount.
   PURPOSE: The "Quantity to Reorder" column will indicate how much to reorder to prevent too many or too few of the product in inventory.
5. Repeat steps 3 and 4 until all items are ordered.
6. When you have finished, verify the contents in your basket/cart. Review the supply inventory list to ensure you have ordered everything that needs to be reordered and have ordered the correct quantity of each item.
   PURPOSE: Rechecking the order before finalizing the order will prevent costly mistakes.
7. Print a copy of the order.
   Note: For a real order, the payment information would be added and the order would be submitted at this time.
   PURPOSE: When ordering products, the copy of the order is then compared with the packing slips to ensure you have received the complete order. The copy and the packing slips are then stapled together and verified against the invoice when it is received. For prepaid orders, the packing slips and copy of the order are then filed once the entire order has been received.

Receiving the Order

Orders can arrive via the mail, a national delivery service (e.g., FedEx, United Parcel Service [UPS]), or a local delivery service. These services are discussed in a later section. The delivery person may require a signature from an employee. This signature is used to track who received the delivery.

The medical assistant must check the delivery as soon as possible to see if it needs immediate attention. Some medications are shipped on ice to maintain a constant cool temperature. These medications need to be immediately placed in the refrigerator or freezer upon arrival. If the temperature in the package warms up too much, the medication must be discarded. Storage information for medications can be found in the package insert or on the manufacturer's Web site.

For all orders, remove the **packing slip** from the box and compare the items in the package to the packing slip (Figure 10-10). Check off all items received. Some supply companies also indicate items that are **backordered** and will be arriving at a later time. Note any **discrepancies** or differences on the packing slip. Any items damaged should also be noted on the packing slip. The copy of the original order should be compared against the packing slip and any differences should be noted. Any discrepancies or damaged items should be addressed with the supply company as soon as possible.

Once the supplies have been reviewed, the packing slip should be attached to the copy of the order. When the complete order has been received, the copy of the order with the packing slips attached should be filed if the order was prepaid. If a line of credit was used, place the copy of the order with the attached packing slips in the

Vaccine Storage Guidelines

Frozen Vaccines
- Ideal temperature for frozen vaccines: −58° F to 5° F.
- Diluent storage directions are different from those for frozen vaccines.

Refrigerated Vaccines
- Each type of vaccine should be placed in its own container, which allows for air flow. Place newer vaccines behind older vaccines. Keep vaccine vials in their original boxes to prevent light exposure.
- Ideal temperature for refrigerated vaccines: 35° F to 46° F.
- Do not store vaccines next to the wall, top shelf, door, or floor of the refrigerator.
- Do not put food or beverages in the vaccine storage refrigerator.

Monitoring Guidelines
- To monitor temperatures, use a thermometer with a minimum and maximum reading. It will indicate the warmest and coldest temperatures since the thermometer was last reset.
- Read the thermometer when opening and closing the medical office.
- Document the readings and include the date, time, and your initials on the log.
- Leave a blank line if readings were not done.
- Report any out-of-range temperatures immediately.

Example of a Temperature Log

DATE	TIME	REFRIGERATOR TEMPERATURE			FREEZER TEMPERATURE			INITIALS
		MAX	MIN	CURRENT	MAX	MIN	CURRENT	
10/11/xx	0750	40° F	37° F	39° F	3° F	−13° F	−12° F	MVB
10/11/xx	1722	38° F	35° F	38° F	−8° F	−28° F	−19° F	BMN
10/12/xx	0752	42° F	36° F	39° F	−13° F	−23° F	−18° F	MVB
10/13/xx	0748	47° F	38° F	38° F	−8° F	−27° F	−22° F	MVB

Vaccine Storage and Handling, accessed 10/11/2015, http://www.cdc.gov/vaccines/recs/storage/default.htm.

CRITICAL THINKING APPLICATION   10-10
Using the Vaccine Storage Guidelines box, answer the following questions:
- Did all the refrigerator temperatures fall within the required range? Explain.
- Did all the freezer temperatures fall within the required range? Explain.
- If a temperature was outside the required range, what should be done?
- Why was a blank line left on the log?

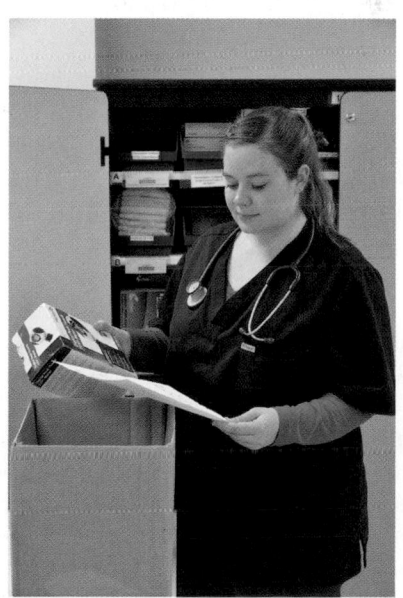

FIGURE 10-10 Comparing the packing slip to the contents in the box is an important step in receiving supplies.

accounts payable folder to wait for the invoice's arrival. The person responsible for paying the medical practice's bills will match the invoice with the copy of the order, ensuring everything is in order before paying the bill.

The items received should be put away as soon as possible and the boxes should be discarded. When putting supplies away, it is important to rotate stock. This means the new stock should go in the back and the older stock needs to be moved forward so it can be used first. Any items with expiration dates should be placed so the items expiring first are in front so they are used first. For stock without expiration dates, consider following the saying "First in, first out," which means when new stock comes in, it is placed behind the older stock. The older stock needs to be used first.

Common Inventory and Purchase Abbreviations

BTL: Bottle | PO: Purchase Order
BX: Box | PPD: Pre-Paid
CS: Case | PYMT: Payment
EA: Each | QTY: Quantity
PKG: Package

HANDLING MAIL

Depending on the size of the medical practice, medical assistants will have varying responsibilities with the mail. If the healthcare facility is large, there may be employees hired to prepare the mail for the United States Postal Service (USPS) and other shipping agencies. These employees also sort incoming mail and deliver the mail to the different departments in the facility. The medical assistant in the department is responsible for addressing the outgoing mail and sorting incoming mail. In smaller practices, the medical assistant is responsible for handling all the mail duties.

United States Postal Service

The USPS is an independent branch of the federal government that handles domestic and international mail services. Domestic mail includes items mailed and received within the United States, its territories and possessions, the military (i.e., Army Post Offices [APOs], Fleet Post Offices [FPOs], and Diplomatic Post Offices [DPOs]), and the United Nations in New York. International mail includes mail sent from a foreign country or to a foreign country. The majority of mail sent by a healthcare facility is domestic mail and the discussion will focus on these services.

To prepare mail to be sent, you will need to address the envelopes and packages following the USPS guidelines discussed in the Technology and Written Communication chapter. The postage is dependent on the:

- Weight and size of the item
- Urgency for arrival
- Delivery **zone**
- Services required

See Table 10-1 for domestic shipping sizes. Postage can be added to the item either by utilizing the USPS Web site or a local Post Office. The USPS Web site (www.usps.com) provides valuable resources for addressing and shipping mail. It allows you to buy stamps, schedule a pickup, calculate the shipping cost, look up ZIP codes, and track sent mail.

Domestic United States Postal Services

The medical assistant will utilize different types of mail services for the healthcare facility's business. It is crucial to understand the different services. For routine mail, the healthcare facility will use First-Class Mail, but for packages or urgent letters, other options are available (Table 10-2).

Priority Mail Express provides a 7-day-a-week delivery service. It guarantees overnight scheduled deliveries. This service is used for time-sensitive letters and packages up to 70 pounds (lb.) that need to get to the recipient quickly. The cost of this service is based on the item's weight and the delivery zone. Insurance is provided as part

of the service. Priority Mail Express envelopes and boxes are available at the Post Office and a flat rate fee is available.

Priority Mail provides delivery of letters and packages up to 70 lb. within 1 to 3 days. The cost of this service is based on the item's weight and the delivery zone. Priority Mail envelopes and boxes are available at the Post Office and a flat rate fee is available based on the size of the envelope or box for items up to 70 lbs. Priority Mail is cheaper than Priority Mail Express and insurance is part of the service.

First-Class Mail service provides delivery in 3 days or less. Envelopes and packages weighing up to 13 ounces (oz.) can be mailed using this service. This is the most common service used by the healthcare facility. The postage is based on the item's size, shape, and weight. Insurance and additional services can be added for an extra fee.

TABLE 10-1 United States Postal Service Domestic Shipping Sizes

DOMESTIC SHIPPING	SIZE
Postcard	Height: 3.5"–4.25" Length: 5"–6" Maximum thickness: 0.016"
Letter	Height: 3.5"–6.125" (6⅛") Length: 5"–11.5" Maximum thickness: 0.25"
Large Envelopes	Height: 6.125"–12" Length: 11.5"–15" Maximum thickness: 0.75"
Packages	Maximum length plus girth: 108" (130" for Standard Post)

TABLE 10-2 Summary of the United States Postal Service's Domestic Services

Priority Mail Express	Very expensive; 7-days-a-week delivery service with guaranteed overnight scheduled delivery. Insurance is included.
Priority Mail	Expensive; delivery within 3 days. Insurance is included.
First-Class Mail	Most commonly used service. Cost based on size, shape, and weight. Add-on services are available for an extra fee.
Standard Post	Used for oversized packages, with delivery in 2–8 days.
Media Mail	Use for sending books and educational material, with delivery in 2–8 days.

Standard Post service is an economical ground service for oversized, less urgent packages. This service can be used for larger packages weighing up to 70 lbs. and measuring up to 130 inches in combined **girth** and length. The cost is based on the item's weight and shape and the delivery zone. Insurance can be added with an extra fee.

Media Mail replaced the Book Rate and is used for sending books, electronic media, and educational materials. The cost is based on the weight of the item and insurance can be added for an additional fee.

Insurance and Additional Services

The USPS also has a host of optional services that can be added onto the standard services for an additional fee. In general, these services include insurance, shipping confirmation, delivery confirmation, and tracking. Some of these services, including Certified Mail and Return Receipt, are the options used more commonly by medical facilities.

The Standard Insurance option can be added to the postage to insure against loss or damage. The cost is based on the item's declared value. Priority Mail Express and Priority Mail insure the item to a point and additional coverage can be purchased.

Registered Mail can be added to First-Class and Priority Mail. This optional service can provide insurance for items valued up to $25,000. A mailing receipt is provided, and upon request, an electronic verification can be sent to the sender showing the item was delivered or an attempted delivery was made. If the healthcare facility was shipping an expensive machine to a repair service, Registered Mail may be used to help protect against loss or further damage.

Certified Mail is available for First-Class and Priority Mail. With Certified Mail, a mailing receipt showing the date when the item was mailed is included (Figure 10-11, *A*). It can be combined with Return Receipt to get additional information on when the delivery occurred and the recipient's signature (Figure 10-11, *B*). Many state laws mandate that **termination letters** be sent by Certified Mail with Return Receipt. The mailing receipt showing the letter was mailed and the Return Receipt along with a copy of the letter are uploaded into the EHR or filed in the paper medical record. These items provide proof the law was followed if there is ever a question.

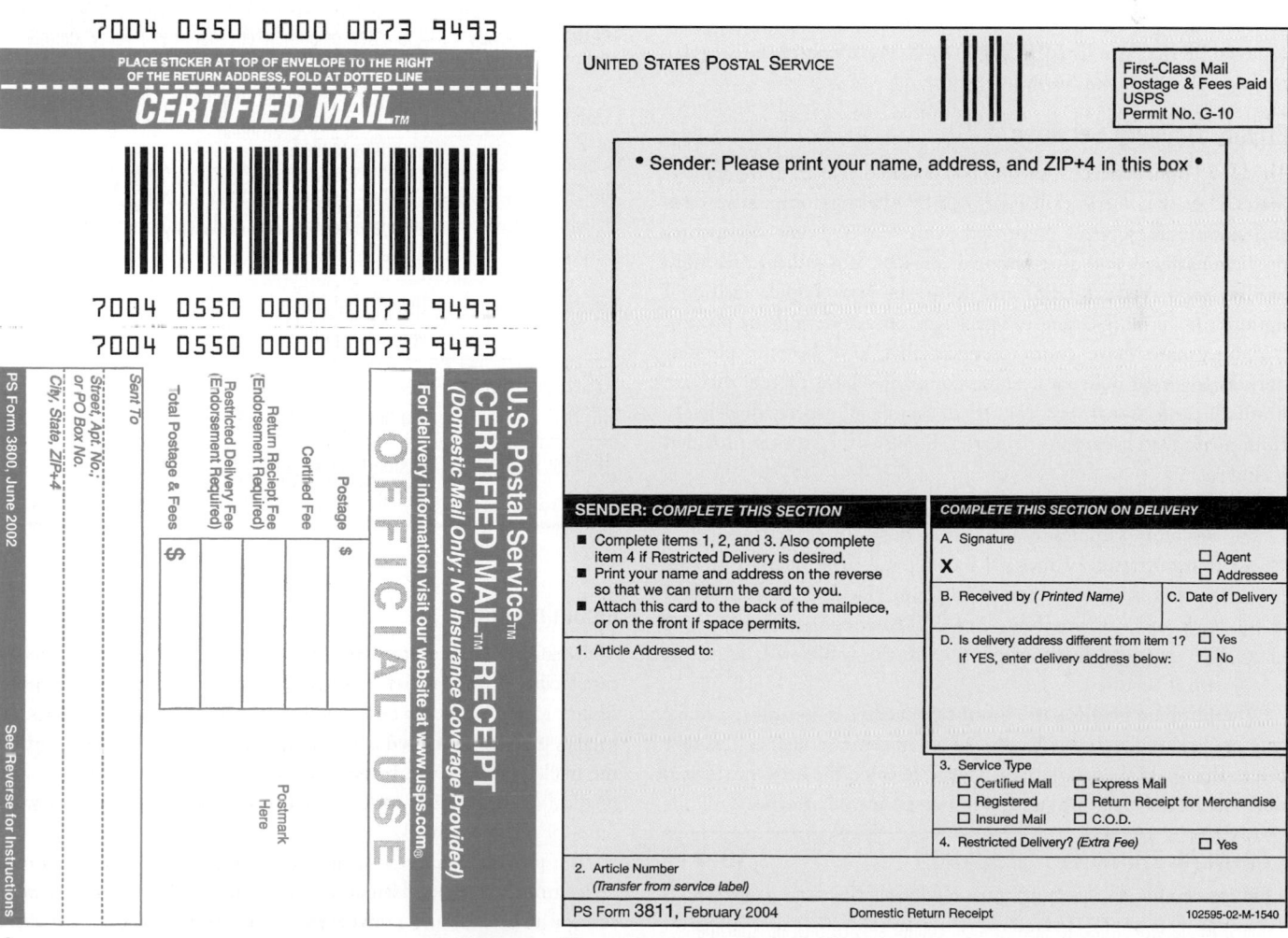

FIGURE 10-11 A, Receipt for Certified Mail. Attach the bottom portion of the receipt to the top of the package or envelope, just to the right of the return address. **B,** Return Receipt used to provide an automatic electronic or hardcopy record showing the recipient's signature.

Signature Confirmation is an optional service that can be added to First-Class, Priority Mail, and Media Mail. This service provides information about the date and time an item was delivered or a delivery attempt was made. The delivery record, which includes the recipient's signature, is kept by the USPS and is available electronically or by e-mail upon request.

The healthcare facility utilizes the Return Receipt more often than the Signature Confirmation (see Figure 10-11, *A*). The advantage of the Return Receipt service is that it provides an automatic e-mail or hardcopy mail delivery record showing the recipient's signature. The hardcopy is more expensive than the e-mail. Return Receipt can be added to the five domestic delivery services mentioned in the prior section.

With Restricted Delivery service and Adult Signature Restricted Delivery service, the mailed item can only be delivered to the addressee, an **authorized agent** of the addressee, or a parent/guardian. The receiver must verify his or her identity and must sign for the delivery. With the Adult Signature Restricted Delivery service, the person signing must also show proof that he or she is over 21.

The Certificate of Mailing provides evidence that the item was mailed. It shows the date and time the item was mailed. This service is limited because it doesn't show evidence of the delivery. It can be combined with other services for additional information. Additional optional services are listed in Table 10-3. For a complete list, refer to the USPS Web site (www.usps.com).

Private Delivery Services

The USPS only handles a portion of the mail delivered in the United States. Private companies have grown by offering competitive rates and additional services compared with USPS. Some companies provide national and international services, but others are more locally based. FedEx, UPS, and DHL are very popular national options for shipping letters and packages. Some offer on-site pickup.

Larger cities have courier services that have become popular options for local deliveries. Some companies have drivers that are **bonded**, professional, and trained to handle all aspects of delivery from medical to hazardous deliveries. Some of the services provided include:

- Pickup and delivery of medical specimens (e.g., take patient laboratory samples to a medical laboratory for testing).
- Transportation of medical records and documents from one location to another, complying with Health Insurance Portability and Accountability Act (HIPAA) requirements.
- Pickup and delivery of deposits to the bank, with return of cash if required.

The ultimate goal for the healthcare facility is to utilize a mail/courier service that provides the most efficient service at the best price. The medical assistant may have to research the delivery services available in the area to identify the best fit for the practice.

CRITICAL THINKING APPLICATION　　10-11
The providers would like to utilize an off-site laboratory to process specimens. Marie would like to have a local courier service pick up specimens and deliver them to the off-site laboratory. When researching potential delivery couriers for this activity, what factors should Marie consider?

TABLE 10-3　Optional Services Provided by United States Postal Service

Standard Insurance	Protects against loss or damage. Cost is based on the item's declared value.
Registered Mail	Used to protect expensive items. A mailing receipt is given; upon request an electronic verification of delivery can be sent.
Certified Mail	Mailing receipt provides evidence the letter was mailed and the Return Receipt shows delivery information and the recipient's signature.
Signature Confirmation	Provides date and time of delivery, along with the recipient's signature. Copy of delivery record is available upon request.
Return Receipt	Provides an automatic electronic or mailed delivery record showing the recipient's signature.
Adult Signature Restricted Delivery	Addressee or authorized agent must verify identity and age (i.e., must be over 21); must sign for delivery.
Restricted Delivery	Addressee or authorized agent must verify identity and must sign for delivery.
Certificate of Mailing	Provides evidence (i.e., date and time) when an item was mailed.
United States Postal Service Tracking	Provides updates as an item is being shipped. Will include date and time of delivery or attempted delivery.
Special Handling	Used to get preferential handing when shipping very unusual items or items that need extra care.
Collect on Delivery (COD)	Recipient pays for merchandise and shipping when the package is received.
Hold for Pickup	Option to pick up item from a specified Post Office within 15 days, depending on service selected.

Incoming Mail

Mail can be collected at the post office or be delivered to the healthcare facility. If the facility is large, some employees have the responsibility to sort and deliver the mail to the different departments. In smaller practices, the medical assistant may be responsible for sorting the mail. Mail received by the healthcare facility greatly varies. The medical assistant must sort the mail following the practice's procedure for incoming mail.

The provider receives all mail marked *Personal* and correspondence from lawyers and accountants. Professional journals, pharmaceutical materials, and convention/**continuing medical education (CME)** events flyers are also given to the provider. Bills are given to the provider if he or she is responsible for paying them. If not, then the bills are given to the person responsible for the accounts payable

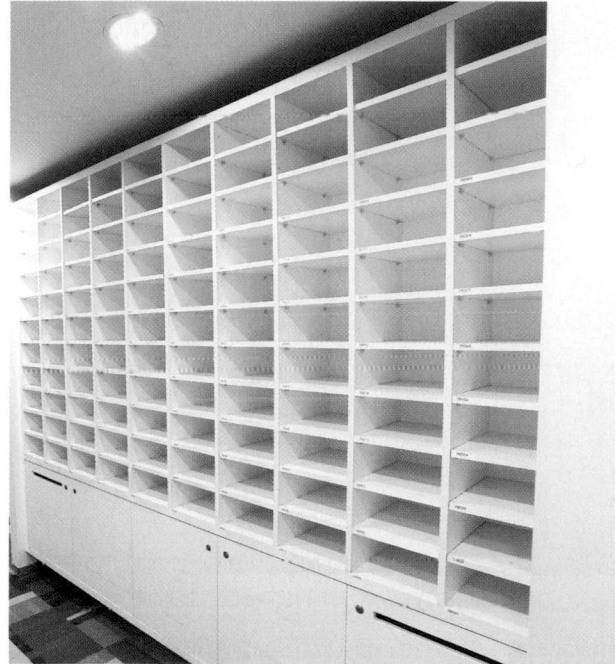

FIGURE 10-12 Mailboxes are efficient ways of sorting and storing mail for individuals in the department. (Photo copyright iStock.com.)

TABLE 10-4 Principles of Proper Body Mechanics

- To lift an object, maintain a wide, stable base with your feet. Your feet should be shoulder-width apart and you should have good footing. Bend at the knees, keeping your back straight. Lift smoothly, using the major muscles in your arms and legs. Use the same technique when putting the item down. Bending over to lift or to set down a heavy object will increase your risk of injury.
- When lifting and carrying heavy items, keep the item directly in front of you to avoid rotating your spine.
- Keep your movements smooth. Jerky or uncoordinated movements increase the risk for injury.
- When reaching for an object, your feet should face the object. Twisting or turning with a heavy load can cause injury.
- Prevent reaching and straining to get an object. Clear away barriers and utilize a firm and level surface (e.g., step stool) to get close to the object. Avoid standing on tiptoes.
- Get help if the item is too heavy to lift by yourself.
- Store heavy objects at waist-level or below.

activities. A provider may request the incoming mail be placed on his or her desk. In larger departments, mailboxes are utilized for each person in the department (Figure 10-12). The medical assistant can easily sort the mail and place it in the individual mailboxes.

CRITICAL THINKING APPLICATION 10-12

Catherine sorts the mail for the practice. Because the practice is small, they do not use the mailbox system. Mail has gotten lost when she has placed it on the providers' desks. What are some other options that Catherine can implement to prevent mail from getting lost or misplaced on providers' desks?

Mail related to patients, like diagnostic test and laboratory results and consultation letters, are opened and dated. If the practice uses paper medical records, the document should be clipped to the chart. If the ambulatory care facility uses an EHR, some practices have the medical assistant identify the patient in the system and write the patient's EHR number on the document. The provider can just type in this number, verify the patient's name, and proceed to reviewing the document and the EHR notes. This helps save time for the provider. Eventually the received document needs to be scanned and uploaded into the patient's EHR or filed in the paper record.

The medical assistant handles the magazines for the reception area, supply shipments, and correspondences from insurance companies. Payments from insurance companies and patients should be recorded immediately in the day's receipts.

The practice are procedures on handling mail that is not addressed to a specific person. Typically it is given to the department supervisor, office manager, or medical director. If a medical assistant has a question regarding who should get a specific piece of

mail, it is important to ask. If the medical assistant questions if a letter should be opened, it is better to not open it and ask the provider or office manager. When a provider is on vacation, the practice will have a procedure for handling the mail. If something is urgent or relates to a patient, procedures are in place to guide the medical assistant.

BODY MECHANICS

The Occupational Safety and Health Act (OSHA) of 1970 requires that employers provide a workplace that is free from serious recognized hazards and the employer must comply with OSHA standards. In the healthcare environment, the majority of injuries are sprains, strains, and tears. Back injuries are one of the most common injuries and can result from microtrauma related to repetitive activity over time or from one traumatic experience. Typically, improper lifting or lifting items too heavy for the back to support are the main reasons for acute back injuries. Other reasons for back injuries include:

- Reaching, twisting, or bending when lifting
- Bad body mechanics when lifting, pushing, pulling, or carrying items
- Poor footing or constrained posture

Medical assistants need to protect themselves from bodily harm while lifting, reaching, and carrying heavy boxes and equipment associated with supplies and equipment (Figure 10-13 and Figure 10-14). Using proper body mechanics is important to prevent injuries (Table 10-4). Proper body mechanics entails utilizing the appropriate muscles and body movements to maintain correct posture and body alignment. By utilizing proper body mechanics, coordination and endurance will be increased and the risk of strain and injury to the body will be decreased. See Procedure 10-3, which explains how to use correct body mechanics when performing a supply inventory.

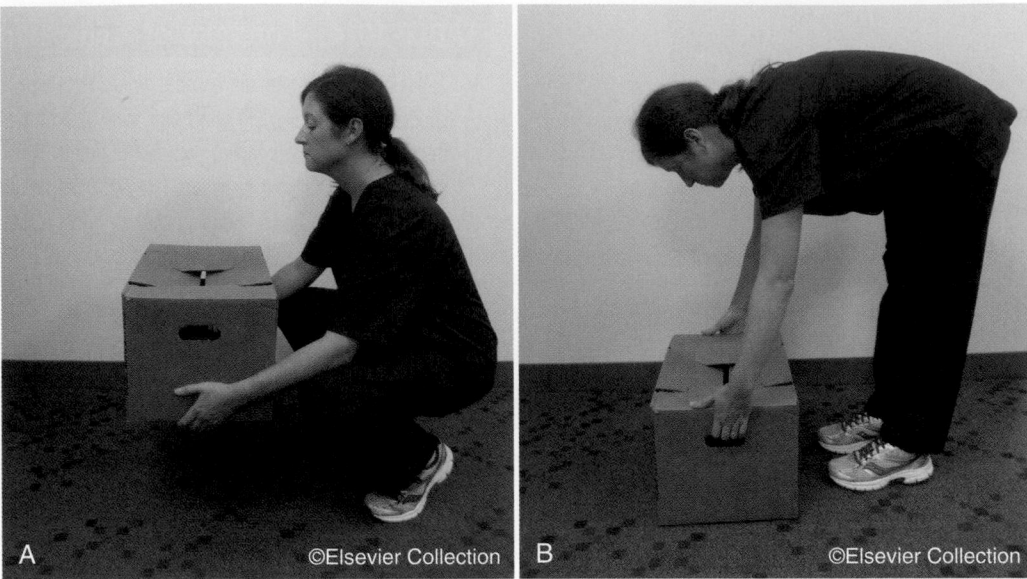

FIGURE 10-13 A, Bend knees for proper lifting technique. **B,** Improper lifting technique.

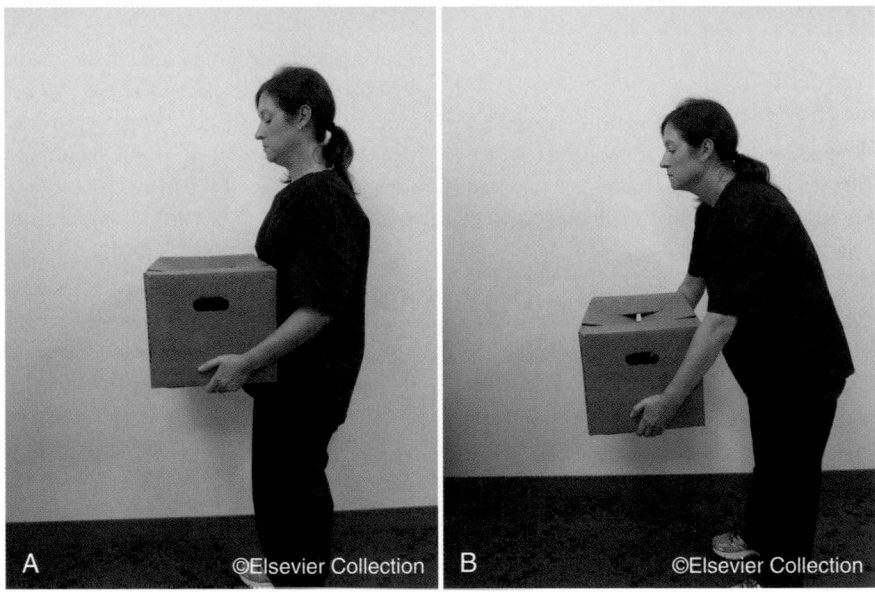

FIGURE 10-14 A, Carrying an item close to the body. **B,** Improper carrying technique.

CLOSING COMMENTS

Patient Education

The principles of body mechanics utilized by the medical assistant for tasks in the medical office can also be used in everyday life. The medical assistant may need to coach a patient on the correct techniques for lifting, reaching, and carrying heavy objects to prevent injury. With the frequency of back injuries, it is important to emphasize proper body alignment, proper posture, and good footing when moving heavy objects. Encourage patients to use a safe step stool when reaching high objects. The step stool should be sturdy and needs to accommodate the weight of the patient. Some step stools have a handle or grab bar, which can provide extra safety. Using proper body mechanics all the time is the key to preventing injuries that may last a lifetime.

Legal and Ethical Issues

The medical assistant must help to protect the medical practice from lawsuits. For any document sent to a patient, it is important for the medical assistant to file a copy in the medical record or to upload an electronic copy to the EHR. When using Certified Mail is required for what is being sent, the medical assistant needs to ensure that all the required paperwork is added to the health record, thus providing evidence that the laws were followed. Without evidence that a letter was sent and received, the medical practice could face a lawsuit.

Professional Behaviors

In the healthcare facility there is an abundance of administrative and clinical supplies. The medical assistant may be tempted to take some supplies for his or her personal use. This action could be looked upon as theft and is not professional.

Medical and administrative supplies cost the practice money. The medical assistant needs to appreciate the cost of supplies and help look for ways to decrease supply expenses. Being wasteful can cost the employer money. Making sure to rotate and use supplies before their expiration date will help prevent wasting money. Providers and supervisors appreciate staff that are cost conscientious.

SUMMARY OF SCENARIO

Marie has started to implement an inventory management process that is helping her identify when to reorder and how much to reorder. She initially started by hand counting the inventory, and then she identified how much was utilized each buying cycle. It took a few months for her to identify trends; even then, she found certain times of the year can affect the quantity of orthopedic products used. For instance, providers tend to use more casting products in the winter and summer months, which means Marie will need to increase her stock of those items during these times of the year. Marie knows that she can become more efficient with the inventory with the more she learns. She has already helped the practice save money by identifying cheaper vendors for commonly used expensive items. Marie loves her new job and the variety of responsibilities she has. She looks forward to continuing to learn in the future.

SUMMARY OF LEARNING OBJECTIVES

1. **Define, spell, and pronounce the terms listed in the vocabulary.**
   It is important to spell and pronounce terms commonly used in the healthcare setting. By using these terms correctly, the medical assistant will demonstrate professional traits and be credible when discussing the topics with others.

2. **Describe the administrative and clinical opening duties performed by the medical assistant.**
   The medical assistant has administrative and clinical duties that need to be performed to prepare the office for patients and the activities for the coming day. Some of the administrative responsibilities include preparing the reception area, turning on lights and equipment, and preparing the paperwork for patients' visits. In the clinical area, examination rooms need to be opened and stocked, supply cabinets need to be unlocked, quality control tests need to be completed, and outstanding patient issues need to be handled.

3. **Discuss the administrative and clinical closing responsibilities performed by the medical assistant, as well as daily and monthly duties.**
   At the end of the business day, the administrative duties include closing the office, cleaning and restocking the reception area as needed, turning off the equipment, switching the phones over to the answering service or voice mail, and following the facility's procedures for handling the money collected during the day. The medical assistant in the clinical area must clean and restock the examination rooms, turn off equipment, and lock cabinets. All patient information should be put away. During slow times, medical assistants need to do extra duties, including restocking medical and office supplies, forms, and patient literature. Crash carts need to be inventoried monthly.

4. **Explain safety and security procedures important in the healthcare facility.**
   The medical assistant must keep at a distance from a suspicious person. Being behind the desk or closest to the door in the examination room are a few ways to protect yourself. Healthcare facilities have implemented various strategies, including code words, alarms, and locked doors to help increase security.

5. **Do the following related to equipment in a medical practice:**
   - Describe the elements of an equipment inventory list.
     The equipment inventory list provides information about the administrative and clinical machines in the facility. This information is used by the provider, supervisor, and/or accountant for future planning and tax paperwork. Procedure 10-1 describes how to create an equipment inventory list and Figure 10-5 provides an example of an equipment inventory list.
   - Explain the purpose of routine maintenance of administrative and clinical equipment.
     Routine maintenance is crucial for the equipment to run correctly. The medical assistant should inspect equipment for unsafe issues. Equipment should be routinely cleaned as specified in the operation manual. The manual will also indicate routine maintenance and service schedules. Following these directions will help prevent problems with the equipment and will extend the machine's longevity.
   - Explain the steps of creating a maintenance log, performing maintenance, and documenting the maintenance.
     See Procedure 10-2 for the steps in creating a maintenance log. The procedure also provides directions for performing and documenting

Continued

maintenance. Figure 10-6 provides an example of an equipment maintenance log.

- Describe the medical assistant's role in ordering equipment.
  The medical assistant can help research potential equipment by utilizing the Internet and meeting with the salesperson. Leasing or buying the equipment are options to investigate, along with what additional billable services might be provided by using that machine. The provider or supervisor will make the final decision regarding the purchase or lease.

6. **Do the following related to supplies in the medical practice:**

- Discuss the elements on a supply inventory list.
  The supply inventory list can be created in a notebook, on index cards, or by using the computer and a spreadsheet or inventory control processing software. The elements on the list include the details about the item (i.e., name, size, quantity, item number, supplier's name, and cost), quantity to reorder, and reorder point. Procedure 10-3 describes how to create a supply inventory list and how to utilize it for inventory. See Figure 10-7 for an example of a supply inventory list.
- List the steps involved in completing an inventory.
  Procedure 10-3 describes how to perform an inventory by hand counting supplies.
- Perform an inventory with documentation.
  Procedure 10-3 discusses how to perform a supply inventory and document the inventory counts on the supply inventory list.
- Prepare a supply order.
  Procedure 10-4 describes how to identify which items need to be ordered. The steps on creating an online order using a supplier's Web site are described.

7. **Describe how the healthcare facility utilizes USPS and other delivery agencies.**
   The majority of the mail sent by the healthcare facility will be sent through the USPS. The USPS has a number of different types of mail services available to meet the needs of the healthcare facility. First-Class Mail is the most common service used in the healthcare facility to mail letters. Depending on the packages mailed or the urgency of the item, other services may be utilized. The USPS also offers insurance, shipping confirmation, delivery confirmation, and tracking services. These services can be added to other mail services for an additional fee. In some situations the medical office will need to use Certified Mail to send termination letters to patients.

   The facility may also use other national delivery agencies for urgent letters or large packages. Local delivery agencies' services can vary by location, but many assist healthcare facilities by transporting patients' medical records and laboratory samples to other agencies for processing or patient appointments. The medical assistant needs to be knowledgeable about the mail services available and the correct service to use to meet the needs of the healthcare facility.

8. **Use proper body mechanics.**
   The medical assistant must use proper body mechanics and posture to help decrease the risk of injury. See Table 10-4 for the principles of proper body mechanics when reaching, lifting, and carrying heavy items. Using proper body mechanics is important when performing inventory in the healthcare environment. Procedure 10-3 describes how to implement proper body mechanics when taking an inventory of supplies in the healthcare facility.

CONNECTIONS

Study Guide Connection: Go to the Chapter 10 Study Guide. Read and complete the activities.

evolve Evolve Connection: Go to the Chapter 10 link at *evolve.elsevier.com/kinn* to complete the Chapter Review Quiz. Check out the other resources listed for this chapter to make the most of what you have learned from Daily Operations in the Ambulatory Care Setting.

THE HEALTH RECORD

SCENARIO

Susan Beezler has just begun her career in the medical assisting profession. She is attending medical assisting school in the morning and works part-time for a family practitioner in the afternoons as a clerical record assistant. Susan is eager to learn about medicine and looks forward to taking on more responsibility at the office.

The practice is growing swiftly and recently added a new provider, Dr. Alex Thomas. Dr. Thomas has enjoyed working with Susan and feels that her energy will be just what his patients need. He has taken a professional interest in Susan and often lets her assist him with patients when her other duties allow.

Susan knows that although she is a beginner in the office, she will gain trust from her supervisors and patients as long as she projects a teachable attitude. The office has recently converted to an electronic records system but is still using paper records as well. Susan uses the information she learned in school about both types of health records. She cheerfully performs filing and even does some transcription for Dr. Thomas. The other staff members are pleased with her willingness to perform the most mundane tasks.

Susan enjoys sharing her experiences with her classmates. She is the only one currently working in the medical field, and the other students ask her lots of questions about the "real world" of medicine. She is very careful not to breach patient confidentiality; she discusses situations only in general terms, never mentioning any patients' names.

Susan feels a great sense of pride that she is already a member of the healthcare team and able to contribute to the lives of her patients.

While studying this chapter, think about the following questions:

- Why would some patients have concerns about the healthcare facility using electronic health records (EHRs)?
- How can the medical assistant earn the patient's trust so that the person is comfortable revealing the very private information required by a health history?
- Why is it so important to have a signed release of information form before sending patient information out?
- Why is it important that the health record be legible?
- Why is it important to know both administrative and clinical skills in the provider's office?

LEARNING OBJECTIVES

1. Define, spell, and pronounce the terms listed in the vocabulary.
2. Name and discuss the two types of patient records.
3. State several reasons that accurate health records are important.
4. Differentiate between subjective and objective information in creating a patient's health record.
5. Explain who owns the health record.
6. Distinguish between an electronic health record (EHR) and an electronic medical record (EMR).
7. Do the following related to healthcare legislation and EHRs:
   - Explain how the American Recovery and Reinvestment Act (ARRA) applies to the healthcare industry.
   - Define *meaningful use* and relate it to the healthcare industry.
   - List the three main components of meaningful use legislation.
8. Explore the advantages, disadvantages, and capabilities of an EHR system, and explain how to organize a patient's health record.
9. Discuss the importance of nonverbal communication with patients when an EHR system is used.
10. Discuss backup systems for the EHR, as well as the transfer, destruction, and retention of health records as related to the EHR.
11. Describe how and when to release health record information; discuss health information exchanges (HIEs).
12. Identify and discuss the two methods of organizing a patient's paper medical record.
13. Discuss how to document information in an EHR and a paper health record, and how to make corrections/alterations to health records.
14. Discuss dictation and transcription, and discuss transfer, destruction, and retention of medical records as related to paper records.
15. Identify filing equipment and filing supplies needed to create, store, and maintain medical records.
16. Describe indexing rules, and how to create and organize a patient's health record.
17. Discuss the pros and cons of various filing methods, as well as how to file patient health records.
18. Discuss organization of files, as well as health-related correspondence.
19. Discuss patient education, as well as legal and ethical issues, related to the health record.

VOCABULARY

age of majority The age at which a person is recognized by law to be an adult; can vary by state.

alleviate To partly remove or correct; to relieve or lessen.

alphabetic filing Any system that arranges names or topics according to the sequence of the letters in the alphabet.

alphanumeric Of or relating to systems made up of combinations of letters and numbers.

augment To increase in size or amount; to add to in order to improve or complete.

caption A heading, title, or subtitle under which records are filed.

computerized provider/physician order entry (CPOE) The process of entering medication orders or other provider instructions into the electronic health record (EHR).

continuity of care Continuation of care smoothly from one provider to another, so that the patient receives the most benefit and no interruption in care.

culpability Meriting condemnation, responsibility, or blame, especially as wrong or harmful.

dictation (dik-ta′-shun) The act or manner of uttering words to be transcribed.

direct filing system A filing system in which materials can be located without consulting an additional source of reference.

e-prescribing The use of electronic software to communicate with pharmacies and send prescribing information, taking the place of writing a prescription by hand and physically giving it to a patient; most new or refill prescriptions can be submitted electronically, cutting down on fraud and errors.

electronic health record (EHR) An electronic record of health-related information about a patient that conforms to nationally recognized interoperability standards and that can be created, managed, and consulted by authorized clinicians and staff from more than one healthcare organization.

electronic medical record (EMR) An electronic record of health-related information about an individual that can be created, gathered, managed, and consulted by authorized clinicians and staff within a single healthcare organization.

gleaned Gathered bit by bit (e.g., information or material); picked over in search of relevant material.

indirect filing system A filing system in which an intermediary source of reference (e.g., a card file) must be consulted to locate specific files.

interoperability The ability to work with other systems.

microfilm A film with a photographic record of printed or other graphic matter on a reduced scale.

numeric filing The filing of records, correspondence, or cards by number.

objective information Data obtained through physical examination, laboratory and diagnostic testing, and by measurable information.

obliteration (uh-blih-tuh-ra′-shun) The act of making undecipherable or imperceptible by obscuring or wearing away.

outguide A sturdy cardboard or plastic file-sized card used to replace a folder temporarily removed from the filing space.

parameters Any set of physical properties, the values of which determine characteristics or behavior.

patient portal A secure online Web site that gives patients 24-hour access to personal health information using a username and password.

personal health record (PHR) An electronic record of health-related information about an individual that conforms to nationally recognized interoperability standards and that can be drawn from multiple sources but that is managed, shared, and controlled by the individual.

pressboard A strong, highly glazed composition board resembling vulcanized fiber; heavy card stock.

provisional diagnosis A temporary diagnosis made before all test results have been received.

purging The process of moving active files to inactive status.

quality control An aggregate of activities designed to ensure adequate quality, especially in manufactured products or in the service industries.

reasonable cause Circumstances that would make it unreasonable for the covered entity, despite the exercise of ordinary business care and prudence, to comply with the administrative simplification provision (part of Health Information Technology for Economic and Clinical Health Act [HITECH]) that was violated.

reasonable diligence The business care and prudence expected from a person seeking to satisfy a legal requirement under similar circumstances.

requisites (reh′-kwuh-zihts) Entities considered essential or necessary.

retention schedule A method or plan for retaining or keeping health records and for their movement from active to inactive to closed filing.

reverse chronologic order Arranged in order so that the most recent item is on top and older items are filed further back.

subjective information Data or information elicited from the patient, including the patient's feelings, perceptions, and concerns; obtained through interview or questions.

subpoena duces tecum A court order to produce documents or records.

tickler file A chronologic file used as a reminder that something must be dealt with on a certain date.

transcription A written copy of something made either in longhand or by machine.

vested Granted or endowed with a particular authority, right, or property; to have a special interest in.

willful neglect Conscious, intentional failure or reckless indifference to the obligation to comply with the administrative simplification provision violated.

Health records can be found in basically two different formats, electronic and paper. Most healthcare facilities have switched to **electronic health records (EHRs)** for a number of reasons. The advantages of EHRs include easy storage of patient information, accessibility by multiple users at the same time, and making electronic claim submission a more efficient process, to name a few. The federal government has also offered financial incentives for providers to implement EHRs. Although most providers are using EHRs there are still some who are using paper records and others who are using a combination of both electronic and paper. When a provider is making a switch to an EHR he or she may decide to keep the patient's previous records in the paper format and just use the electronic format from now forward. Some providers may decide to scan in the last 3 to 5 years of the patient's record into the electronic record. Whatever the scenario the healthcare facility has chosen, it is important for the versatile medical assistant to be knowledgeable about both systems and able to perform well with either.

TYPES OF RECORDS

The two major types of patient records are the paper health record and the EHR. With the advances in computer technology, the paper health record has been shown to be much less efficient than the EHR. In most cases, only one person at a time can use the paper record. It is fairly common for information to be filed in the incorrect record, and the entire record also can be misfiled. Data cannot be accessed easily for research and **quality control,** and in facilities with multiple departments or locations, the information is difficult to share. The paper-based record is good evidence of patient care, but it is not nearly as useful in other capacities.

The EHR is much more efficient than the paper record. Multiple users can access the record at the same time. There are fewer errors because handwritten notes do not have to be interpreted. In addition, most EHRs also link the clinical information needed for billing purposes, and include practice management capabilities that allow for patient scheduling and generation of reports needed for research and quality control.

CRITICAL THINKING APPLICATION   **11-1**

Some of Dr. Thomas' patients are concerned that computer-based health records may not be completely private. They are worried that unauthorized individuals could access their information on the computer and do them harm. Should patients be allowed to decide whether their records are kept on computer or on paper?

THE IMPORTANCE OF ACCURATE HEALTH RECORDS

Health records are kept for five basic reasons. First, the health record helps the provider provide the best possible medical care for the patient. The provider examines the patient and enters the findings in the patient's health record. These findings are clues to the diagnosis. The provider may order many types of tests to confirm or **augment** the clinical findings. As the reports of these tests come in, the findings fall into place, much like the pieces of a jigsaw puzzle.

Then, with the confirmation data to support the diagnosis, the provider can prescribe treatment and form an opinion about the patient's chances of recovery, assured that every resource has been used to arrive at a correct judgment. The health record provides a complete history of all the care given to the patient.

Second, the health record also provides critical information for others. By reading through the record and discovering the methods used to treat the patient, healthcare professionals can provide **continuity of care.** Each person knows what the patient has experienced and can provide continuous care, even from one facility to another. For example, when a patient is transferred from a hospital to a skilled nursing facility, the information from the patient's hospital record helps the nursing facility staff to better care for the patient. When patients move from place to place or caregivers change, copies of the pertinent information should move with the patient to provide this continuity of care.

Third, health records are kept as legal protection for those who provided care to the patient. A documented health record is excellent proof that certain procedures were performed or that medical advice was given. An accurate record is the foundation for a legal defense in cases of medical professional liability. This is one reason that writing legibly in the paper record to document exactly what happened to the patient and the provider's response are critical. Remember: If it is not documented, it did not happen.

Fourth, health records provide statistical information that is helpful to researchers. The patient's record provides information about medications taken and the reactions to them. Health records may be used to evaluate the effectiveness of certain kinds of treatment or to determine the incidence of a given disease. Providers often take part in drug studies that track adverse reactions and side effects. The effects of various treatments and procedures also can be tracked and statistics **gleaned** from the information in patients' records. In tracking statistical information the information that would identify specific patients is removed. Correlation of such statistical information may result in a new outlook on some phases of medicine and can lead to revised techniques and treatments. The statistical data from health records also are valuable in the preparation of scientific papers, books, and lectures.

Fifth, health records are vital for financial reimbursement. The information in the health record supports claims for reimbursement and is required by most third-party payers.

CONTENTS OF THE HEALTH RECORD

The patient's health record is the most important record in a provider's practice. For completeness, each patient's record should contain **subjective information** provided by the patient and **objective information** obtained by the provider and staff of the healthcare facility. If all entries are completed, the health record will stand the test of time. No branch of medicine is exempt from the need to keep patient health records.

Subjective Information
Personal Demographics

The patient's health record begins with routine personal data, which the patient usually supplies on the first visit when the health record is established. Most patients are required to complete a patient information form (Figure 11-1 and Procedure 11-1). The basic facts needed are:

- Patient's full name, spelled correctly
- Names of parents/guardians if the patient is a child
- Patient's gender
- Date of birth
- Marital status
- Name of spouse if married
- Home address, telephone number, and e-mail address
- Occupation
- Name of employer
- Business address and telephone number
- Employment information for spouse

- Healthcare insurance information
- Source of referral
- Social Security number

Past Health, Family, and Social History

The past health, family, and social history is often obtained by having the patient complete a questionnaire. The medical assistant may review the form for completeness and clarify any questions or missing information with the patient before the patient is seen by the provider. The provider will also augment this history with information provided during the patient interview. The responses provide information about any past illnesses (including injuries and/or physical defects, whether congenital or acquired), hospitalizations, or

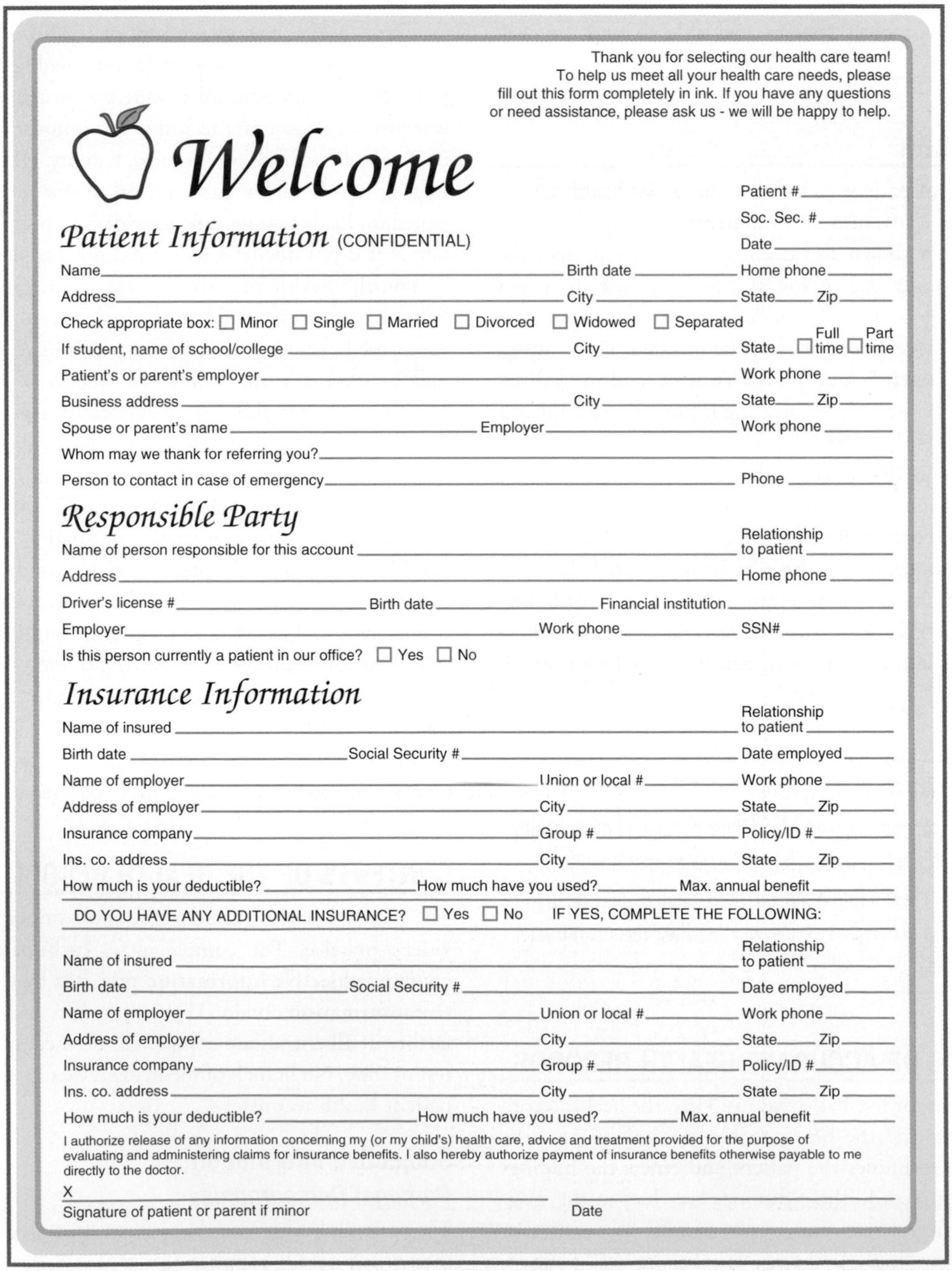

Thank you for selecting our health care team!
To help us meet all your health care needs, please fill out this form completely in ink. If you have any questions or need assistance, please ask us - we will be happy to help.

Welcome

Patient Information (CONFIDENTIAL)

Patient #_____
Soc. Sec. #_____
Date _____

Name_____ Birth date _____ Home phone_____
Address_____ City _____ State_____ Zip_____
Check appropriate box: ☐ Minor ☐ Single ☐ Married ☐ Divorced ☐ Widowed ☐ Separated   ☐ Full time ☐ Part time
If student, name of school/college _____ City_____ State_____
Patient's or parent's employer_____ Work phone _____
Business address _____ City_____ State_____ Zip_____
Spouse or parent's name _____ Employer_____ Work phone _____
Whom may we thank for referring you?_____
Person to contact in case of emergency_____ Phone _____

Responsible Party

Name of person responsible for this account _____   Relationship to patient _____
Address _____ Home phone _____
Driver's license #_____ Birth date _____ Financial institution_____
Employer_____ Work phone_____ SSN#_____
Is this person currently a patient in our office? ☐ Yes ☐ No

Insurance Information

Name of insured _____   Relationship to patient _____
Birth date _____ Social Security #_____ Date employed _____
Name of employer_____ Union or local #_____ Work phone _____
Address of employer_____ City_____ State_____ Zip_____
Insurance company_____ Group #_____ Policy/ID #_____
Ins. co. address_____ City_____ State_____ Zip_____
How much is your deductible? _____ How much have you used?_____ Max. annual benefit _____

DO YOU HAVE ANY ADDITIONAL INSURANCE? ☐ Yes ☐ No   IF YES, COMPLETE THE FOLLOWING:

Name of insured _____   Relationship to patient _____
Birth date _____ Social Security #_____ Date employed _____
Name of employer_____ Union or local #_____ Work phone _____
Address of employer_____ City_____ State_____ Zip_____
Insurance company_____ Group #_____ Policy/ID #_____
Ins. co. address_____ City_____ State_____ Zip_____
How much is your deductible? _____ How much have you used?_____ Max. annual benefit _____

I authorize release of any information concerning my (or my child's) health care, advice and treatment provided for the purpose of evaluating and administering claims for insurance benefits. I also hereby authorize payment of insurance benefits otherwise payable to me directly to the doctor.

X_____   _____
Signature of patient or parent if minor   Date

FIGURE 11-1 The patient information form provides all the information the medical assistant needs to construct the patient's record.

surgeries the patient has had (Figure 11-2). It also includes information about the patient's daily health habits. Stickers can be used on the front of paper health records to indicate allergies, advance directives, and other information (Figure 11-3). In an EHR there will be alerts that may appear as a pop-up window when the record is accessed that will indicate that the patient has allergies, that immunizations are due, or that there is no advance directive on file. These are useful for helping the health professional keep important facts about the patient in the forefront of the mind while treating the individual.

Past Health History. The past health history will include information about previous illnesses/injuries (including childhood illnesses such as chickenpox or measles), previous hospitalizations, and previous surgeries. The dates that these occurred will need to be documented, as well as any complications. The provider needs to be aware

of this information because it could affect the patient's current condition.

Patient's Family History. The family history comprises the physical condition of the various members of the patient's family, any illnesses or diseases individual members may have had, and a record of the causes of death. This information is important because certain diseases may have a hereditary pattern. Most providers are interested in the immediate family: parents, grandparents, siblings, and children.

Patient's Social History. The social history includes information about the patient's lifestyle. If the patient drinks alcohol, how many drinks per day or per week are consumed? If the patient uses nicotine, how much is used in a day, and what type (i.e., cigarettes or smokeless tobacco)? Drug use, living situation, exercise, and nutrition information can be considered part of the social history.

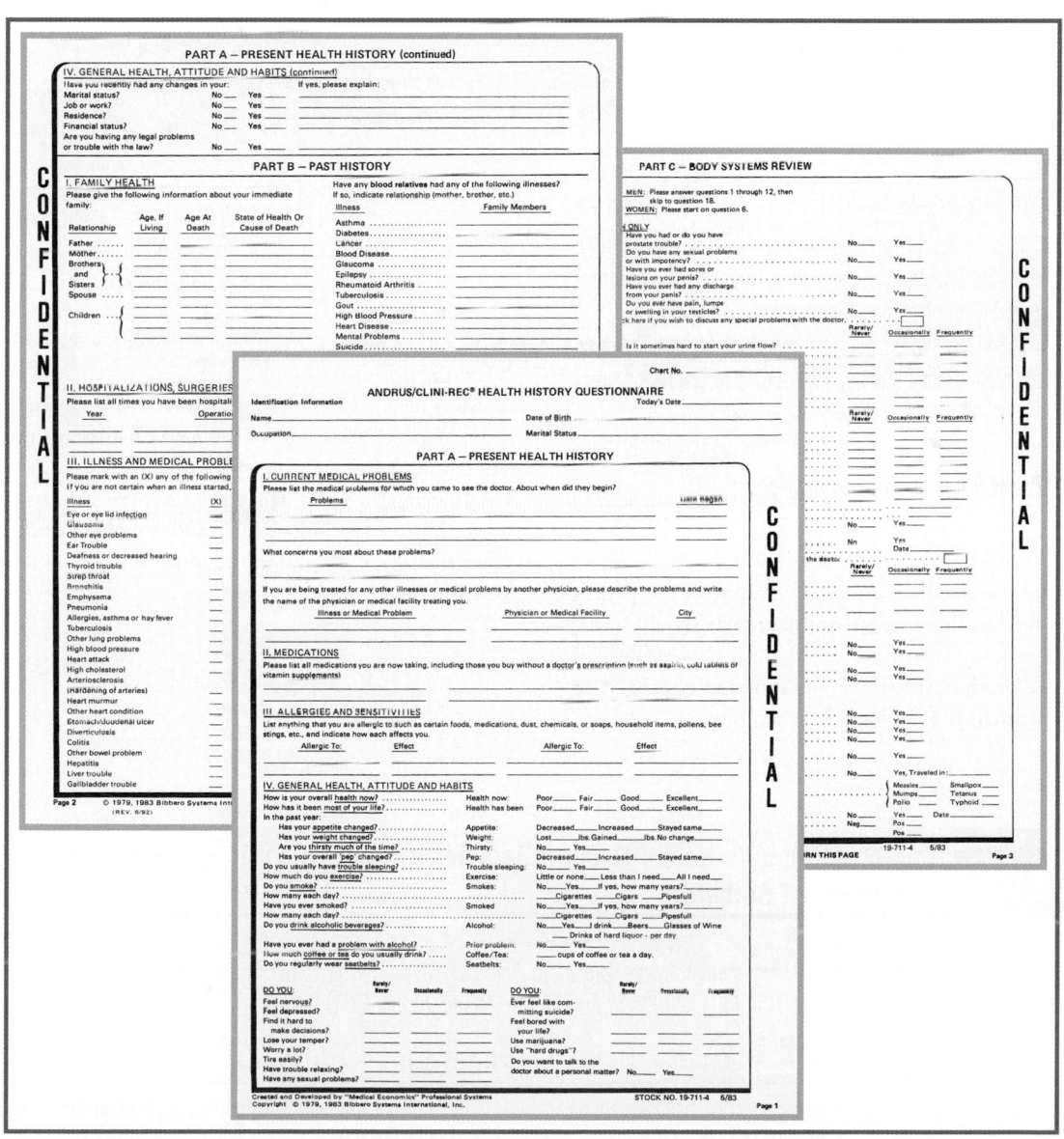

FIGURE 11-2 Database self-administered general health history questionnaire: Lengthy questionnaires should be completed by the patient before the individual is seen by the provider. Either mail the questionnaire to the patient in advance or ask the patient to come in early to complete the paperwork. (Courtesy Bibbero Systems, Petaluma, California.)

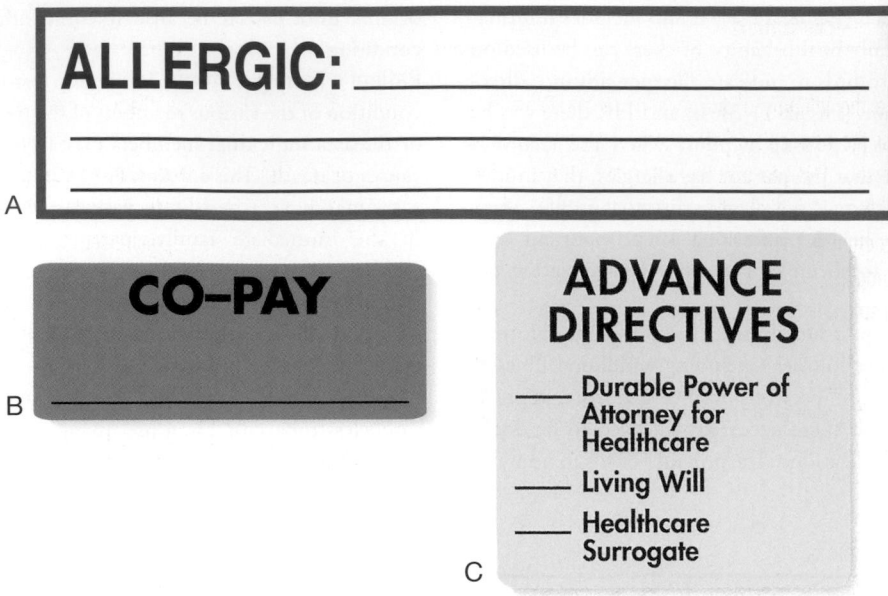

FIGURE 11-3 Record stickers: Information on stickers on the outside of the record allows the provider and medical staff to see important information about the patient quickly. (Courtesy Bibbero Systems, Petaluma, California.)

CRITICAL THINKING APPLICATION   **11-2**

While taking a patient's medical history, Susan asks about his social history. She asks whether he drinks alcohol. The patient immediately becomes defensive and accuses Susan of getting too personal about his affairs.

- How might Susan explain her reasons for asking these questions? What options are available if the patient refuses to discuss his social history with Susan?
- Could this opposition to questions about the social history raise suspicion in Susan's mind? What might she suspect?

Patient's Chief Complaint

The patient's chief complaint is a concise account of the patient's symptoms, explained in the patient's own words. It should include the following:

- The nature, location, frequency, and duration of pain, if any
- When the patient first noticed the symptoms

- Treatments the patient may have tried before seeing the provider and whether they have helped with the symptoms or not; when the last dose was taken
- Whether the patient has had the same or a similar condition in the past
- Other medical treatment received for the same condition in the past

Most medical facilities use a pain scale to determine the severity of the patient's discomfort. The medical assistant might ask, "How bad is your pain on a scale of 1 to 10, with 1 being almost no pain, and 10 being the worst pain you've ever experienced?" The pain scale or wording used in individual facilities should be documented in the office policy and procedures manual and followed by the medical assistant.

| PROCEDURE 11-1 | Create a Patient's Health Record: Register a New Patient in the Practice Management Software |

Goal: *Register a new patient in the practice management software, prepare a Notice of Privacy Practices (NPP) form and a Disclosure Authorization form for the new patient, and document this in the electronic health record (EHR).*

EQUIPMENT and SUPPLIES

- Computer with SimChart for the Medical Office or practice management and EHR software
- Completed patient registration form
- Scanner

PROCEDURAL STEPS

1. Obtain the new patient's completed registration form. Log into the practice management software.
2. Using the patient's last and first names and date of birth, search the database for the patient.

PROCEDURE 11-1 *—continued*

PURPOSE: To help ensure the integrity of the practice management and EHR systems, a search for the new patient's name must always be done before registering that person. This prevents a double record from being created if the patient had been entered into the database at an earlier time.

3. If the database does not contain the patient's name, add a new patient and enter the patient's demographics from the completed registration form.

4. Verify that the information entered is correct and that all fields are completed before saving the data.

PURPOSE: Errors during the registration process can affect the communication with the patient (e.g., if a wrong address or e-mail is entered) or can affect billing (e.g., if the incorrect insurance information is added). Accuracy is extremely important when entering the patient's information.

NOTE: The software will generate a health record number for the patient.

5. Using the EHR software, prepare and print a copy of the NPP and a Disclosure Authorization form for the new patient. The Disclosure Authorization form should indicate the disclosure will be to the patient's insurance company.

PURPOSE: Before the medical office can release patient information to the insurance company, the patient has to give consent in writing.

SCENARIO UPDATE: The patient received both documents and signed the Disclosure Authorization form.

6. Using the EHR, document that the patient received a copy of the NPP and signed the Disclosure Authorization form. Scan the Disclosure Authorization form and upload it into the EHR.

PURPOSE: Documentation in the health record provides a legal record of what was done or communicated to the patient.

7. Log out of the software upon completion of the procedure.

PURPOSE: Logging into and out of the software helps to protect the integrity of the data saved in the software and prevents unauthorized people from viewing the information.

Objective Information

Objective findings, sometimes referred to as *signs,* are findings that can be observed and measured. They can include vital signs, measurements, and observations made by the medical assistant and findings from the provider's examination of the patient.

Vital Signs and Anthropometric Measurements

The medical assistant's responsibilities include taking the patient's vital signs (i.e., temperature, pulse, respirations, blood pressure, pulse oximetry) and height and weight. These measurements are documented in the patient's health record and are used by the provider in his or her assessment. If the medical assistant observes other signs such as a rash, this would also be documented in the patient's health record and brought to the provider's attention.

Findings and Laboratory and Radiology Reports

After the provider has examined the patient, the physical findings are documented in the health record. The results of other tests or requests for these tests are then documented or, if they appear on separate sheets, are attached to the health record. When an EHR is being used the separate sheet may be scanned so that it is in an electronic format and can be added to the patient's EHR.

Diagnosis

Based on all the evidence provided in the patient's past history, the provider's examination, and any supplementary tests, the provider notes his or her diagnosis of the patient's condition in the health record. If some doubt remains, this may be labeled a **provisional diagnosis**. A *differential diagnosis* is the process of weighing the probability of one disease causing the patient's illness against the probability that other diseases are causative. For example, the differential diagnosis of rhinitis, or a runny nose, could indicate allergic rhinitis (i.e., hay fever), the common cold, or even abuse of drugs or nasal decongestants.

Treatment Prescribed and Progress Notes

The provider's suggested treatment is listed after the diagnosis. Generally, instructions to the patient to return for follow-up treatment within a specific period also are noted here. If surgery or other treatment is going to be performed during the current visit, the patient must sign a consent form.

On each subsequent visit, when using a paper record, the date must be entered on the record; information about the patient's condition and the results of treatment, based on the provider's observations, must be added to the health record. Notations of all medications prescribed or instructions given, and the patient's own report of how they are doing, should be documented in the health record. If the patient is hospitalized, the name of the hospital, the reason for admission, and the dates of admission and discharge are documented. Much of this information can be obtained from the hospital discharge summary.

Condition at the Time of Termination of Treatment

When the treatment is terminated, the provider documents that information. For example: *August 18, 2016. Wound completely healed. Problem resolved.*

The Medical Assistant's Role

When the medical assistant is responsible for documenting the patient's history, care must be taken to ensure that the patient's answers are not heard by others. If privacy is not possible, the patient should be given a form to fill out, and the information should be transferred to the permanent record later. When privacy is available, the medical assistant may ask the patient questions and document the answers directly into the health record. This method offers an opportunity to become better acquainted with the patient while completing the necessary records and also ensures the patient understands what all the questions mean. If new patients must complete a lengthy questionnaire, the questionnaire may be mailed to the patient with a request that it be completed and returned to the provider before the appointment. If the record is electronic the patient may access his or her record through a **patient portal** and document the information directly into the EHR system. It would then be reviewed by the medical assistant and provider during the office visit. Another option with an EHR is for the patient to complete a paper form and the medical assistant to enter the information into the EHR while reviewing the form with the patient.

The medical assistant may document the patient's chief complaint, but the provider will question the patient in more detail. Many practitioners write their own entries on the record in longhand if a paper record is used. Some may document the findings directly into the computer if an electronic record is used. Others may dictate the material, either directly to the medical assistant or by using a recording device. If the material is dictated and transcribed, the provider should verify each entry and then initial the entry to verify its accuracy before it is entered into the patient's record. For a record to be admissible as evidence in court, the person dictating or writing the entries must be able to attest that they were true and correct at the time they were written. The best indication of this is the provider's signature or initials on the typed entry. In an EHR the provider's electronic signature is proof of the accuracy of the entries.

OWNERSHIP OF THE HEALTH RECORD

Who owns the health record? Patients often assume that because the information in the health record is about them, ownership of the record rightfully is theirs. However, the owner of the physical health record is the provider or medical facility, often called the "maker," that initiated and developed the record. The patient has the right of access to the information within the record but does not own the physical record or other documents pertaining to the record. The patient has a **vested** interest and therefore has the right to demand confidentiality of all information placed in the record.

The actual paper health record should never leave the medical facility where it originated. Even the provider should refrain from taking the record from the office to the hospital or nursing facility. If information from the record is needed, copies can be placed in a file, and progress notes can be written on site and inserted into the original record later. This is not an issue with an EHR because the record can be accessed by multiple users at the same time. Patients' paper records should be kept in a locked room or locked filing cabinets when the office is closed. EHRs must be protected from unauthorized access. Health Insurance Portability and Accountability Act (HIPAA) regulations state that each user must have a unique user name and password; individual access is determined by the system administrator.

Written health records must be legible. Each record should be written as if the provider and staff expect it to eventually be involved in a lawsuit; therefore every word must be legible to an average reader years after it is written. The record can help the provider prove that he or she treated a patient in a competent manner, or it can prove that the patient was not given competent care. Every person on staff at the provider's office is responsible for writing legibly in every health record.

EHRs eliminate the issue of legibility in the record, but it is just as important to be sure that all patient care is documented in the electronic record. If care is not documented, this will leave the healthcare facility open to potential lawsuits and can affect patient care. If services are not documented, they cannot be billed for either.

CRITICAL THINKING APPLICATION   **11-3**

On Susan's third day at work, a man comes into the office and demands to see his mother's health record. Susan accesses the record and sees that the mother has not granted permission for information to be given to her son. What should Susan do in this situation? Are there any viable reasons the son should have access to his mother's medical information?

TECHNOLOGIC TERMS IN HEALTH INFORMATION

Some confusion has arisen regarding the acronyms *EMR* and *EHR*. These acronyms have been used interchangeably for many years. To **alleviate** the confusion, the Office of the National Coordinator for Health Information Technology (ONC) has established definitions for EMR and EHR that are easy to understand. The EHR is an electronic record of health-related information about a patient that conforms to nationally recognized **interoperability** standards and that can be created, managed, and consulted by authorized clinicians and staff from *more than one healthcare organization.* The **electronic medical record (EMR)** is an electronic record of health-related information about an individual that can be created, gathered, managed, and consulted by authorized clinicians and staff *within a single healthcare organization.* An EMR is an electronic version of a paper record.

EMR is being used less and less as the federal regulations regarding electronic records have been established. There is a significant push toward having all electronic records meet the definition of an EHR. There are many advantages to having an electronic record system that can be accessed from more than one healthcare organization. The continuity of patient care is much more easily established when all providers have access to the same records regardless of what organization they are working for. There should be less running of duplicate tests and procedures, which will help reduce the cost of providing healthcare.

A **personal health record (PHR)** is defined by the ONC as an electronic record of health-related information about an individual that conforms to nationally recognized interoperability standards and that can be drawn from multiple sources, but that is managed, shared, and controlled by the individual. There are several ways that a PHR can be created. Some health insurance companies offer PHRs for those who they insure; some employers offer it as a service for their employees; and some healthcare facilities offer it to their patients. It is important to remember that the patient maintains a PHR. The information from an EHR does not automatically transfer to a PHR.

Another way for patients to access their healthcare information is through a patient portal. Patient portals allow patients to access their actual EHRs. At any time a patient can view progress notes, laboratory results, medications, or immunizations. Many patient portal systems also allow for communication between the patient and provider, completion of forms online, and ability to request prescription refills and schedule appointments. By establishing effective patient portals, healthcare facilities can meet some of the meaningful use requirements.

HIPAA uses the term *protected health information* (PHI), which is any information about health status, the provision of healthcare, or payment for healthcare that can be linked to an individual patient. HIPAA requires that all PHI be protected; this applies to EHRs, EMRs, PHRs, and patient portals.

AMERICAN RECOVERY AND REINVESTMENT ACT

The American Recovery and Reinvestment Act of 2009 (ARRA), commonly known as the Economic Stimulus Package, was passed to promote economic recovery. This legislation was signed into law by President Barack Obama on February 17, 2009. The health information technology aspects of the bill provide slightly more than $31 billion for healthcare infrastructure and EHR investment. The sections of the ARRA that pertain to healthcare are collectively known as the Health Information Technology for Economic and Clinical Health Act, or HITECH Act.

THE HEALTH INFORMATION TECHNOLOGY FOR ECONOMIC AND CLINICAL HEALTH ACT AND MEANINGFUL USE

The HITECH Act provides financial incentives for the meaningful use of certified EHR technology to achieve health and efficiency goals. It was incorporated into the ARRA to promote the adoption and meaningful use of health information technology. Remember, HIPAA was created in large part to simplify administrative processes using electronic devices. *Meaningful use,* defined simply, means that providers must show that they are using EHR technology in ways that can be measured significantly in quality and quantity. If providers meet the meaningful use requirements, they will qualify for incentive payments. Three main components of meaningful use can be identified, including:

- Use of certified EHR in a meaningful manner, such as **e-prescribing**
- Use of certified EHR technology for electronic exchange of health information to improve the quality of healthcare
- Use of certified EHR technology to submit clinical quality reports, procedure and diagnosis codes, surveys, and other measures

Criteria for meaningful use were designed to be implemented in three stages:

- Stage 1 (2011 and 2012): Electronic data capture and sharing
- Stage 2 (2014): Advanced clinical processes
- Stage 3 (expected to be implemented in 2016): Improved outcomes

In Subtitle D of the HITECH Act, privacy and security concerns related to the electronic submission of health information are addressed. Several provisions strengthen the civil and criminal penalties of the HIPAA rules, most of which became effective in February 2009. More of the provisions will become effective over the next few years, subject to future lawmaking.

Included in the February 2009 modifications of HIPAA were:

- Establishment of categories of violations that reflect increasing levels of **culpability**

TABLE 11-1 Categories of Health Insurance Portability and Accountability Act Violations and Associated Penalties

CATEGORY: SECTION 1176(A)(1)	EACH VIOLATION	ALL SUCH VIOLATIONS OF AN IDENTICAL PROVISION IN A CALENDAR YEAR
(A) Did not know	$100 to $50,000	$1.5 million
(B) Reasonable cause	$1,000 to $50,000	$1.5 million
(C) (i) Willful neglect—corrected	$10,000 to $50,000	$1.5 million
(C) (ii) Willful neglect—not corrected	$50,000	$1.5 million

- Requirements that penalties be determined based on the nature and extent of the violation and the nature and extent of the harm resulting from the violation
- Establishment of tiers of increasing penalty amounts that determine the range of and authority to impose civil monetary penalties (Table 11-1)

As indicated in Table 11-1, minimum and maximum penalty amounts are established and can be assessed by the Department of Health and Human Services (HHS), depending on the nature of the violation. The HHS determines the penalties on a case-by-case basis and may provide or continue to provide a waiver for violations that arise from a **reasonable cause** and are not **willful neglect** incidents that are not corrected in a timely manner. The DHHS will also consider whether the covered entity has provided **reasonable diligence** in its attempts to bring the facility into compliance with the law. Providers can expect reductions in the amounts they are paid from Medicare and Medicaid if they are not in compliance. Remember, the computer system in the medical office must be more than a tool for data recall to be considered an EHR system; the provider must use the system for tasks, at a minimum, such as e-prescribing and **computerized provider/provider order entry (CPOE)**.

ADVANTAGES AND DISADVANTAGES OF THE EHR

According to a 2014 survey done by the National Ambulatory Medical Care Survey (NAMCS), 82.8% of providers in office-based practices use full or partial EMR systems. This is up from 18% in 2001.

The EHR has several advantages over a paper health record. Most experts agree that the EHR can reduce medical errors by keeping prescriptions, allergies, and other information organized; it also can reduce costs by preventing duplicate tests. Staffing needs also may be reduced, because fewer personnel are needed to manage an EHR system. Because a computer keyboard is used to enter information into the record, the record is not nearly as likely to be illegible as a written record. Typed copy certainly is easier to read than handwriting, even if the record is several years old. EHR systems require individual user names and passwords, which secure the system from unauthorized users.

Compared with walls and file cabinets full of paper health records, the EHR requires less storage space. One or two external hard drives with a terabyte of disk space each conceivably could hold all the health records of all patients throughout the life of a provider's practice. This would eliminate the need to purge inactive files, and the resulting space requirement for the external hard drive may be no bigger than a large shoebox. The files may be duplicated regularly and placed off site as a backup. Using thumb drives as backup would meet HIPAA requirements as long as they were stored somewhere other than the healthcare facility. More facilities are using cloud storage to protect the EHR content.

Information can be accessed in a variety of locations, and more than one person can see the record at any given time. The patient database usually allows various types of statistical information to be recalled, which is a valuable tool. Patient information is available quickly in an emergency, even when the patient is not in his or her hometown. The provider and medical assistants can access progress notes, test results, and any other information about the patient, including patient education and appointment no-shows. The provider and medical assistants can access patient information using a smart phone or tablet.

Once the provider and staff become familiar with the system, they may find that they are able to see more patients in the course of a day than when paper records were used. All of these advantages lead to cost savings and more efficient patient care.

However, the EHR system is not without disadvantages. Studies show that lack of capital is the most significant obstacle to adoption of the system; another stumbling block is the reluctance of employees in providers' offices to make such substantial changes and to learn a new computer system. Employees who are not very familiar with computers may fear that they will not be able to learn the system or that an EHR may mean that they no longer will have a job. Providers may have the same fears of learning a new system and wonder about how much more time it will take them to do their job. Employees may not be the only individuals resistant to a changeover to electronic records; patients often are fearful that their private health information will be available to unauthorized individuals, and they often assume that their records will be posted on the Internet.

The startup costs of conversion to an EHR system usually are quite high, although most providers realize that the system eventually will be worth the cost. "The Financial and Nonfinancial Costs of Implementing Electronic Health Records in Primary Care Practices," an article in the online journal *Health Affairs,* suggests that the startup cost for a five-provider practice is approximately $162,000, with $85,500 going toward maintenance costs during the first year (Fleming et al., 2011). The study also suggested that the implementation team would need an average of 611 hours to prepare for the implementation, and end-users, such as the providers, medical assistants, and other staff members, would need about 134 hours of training to use the system. Both the provider and staff require extensive training in the EHR system and must be receptive to even more training to use the system to its full capacity. Training

is time-consuming and takes the provider and staff away from treating patients for certain periods. Because not all computer systems are user friendly, care must be taken to choose a system that has technologic support, both live and online, that is available during the hours the healthcare facility is operating. Space for the equipment can be an issue, although usually less space is required than for a paper record system. Finally, security and confidentiality are major concerns of both the healthcare professionals and the patients.

Reassuring Patients About the Security and Confidentiality of the Electronic Health Record

- Explain the conversion before the office changes and during the conversion.
- Never display a negative attitude about the change to an electronic health record (EHR) system; patients tend to reflect the attitude you show them.
- Prepare a pamphlet explaining the processes that will change in your particular office with use of the EHR.
- Take a moment to show the patient a little about the software once it has been implemented (using only their record). Most patients are interested in what the EHR can accomplish. Show the individual the log-in process (without revealing passwords) to reassure him or her that access to records is private and secure.
- Explain the records backup process to help alleviate patients' fears that their health information may be lost.
- Explain the office access policy regarding who can access and view patients' records.

Successful Conversion to an Electronic Health Record System

- Get the entire facility "on board" with the change.
- Provide leadership to the staff.
- Encourage and praise the staff's hard work in making the conversion successful.
- As a medical assistant, be loyal and promote loyalty to the facility during the change.
- Use good people management skills, especially with those who are against the conversion. Many people who were initially averse to conversions later say they do not know how they ever worked without the EHR.
- Always provide patients, visitors, and co-workers excellent customer service.
- Work as a team with other staff members.
- Use every employee's strengths where they are needed.
- Be willing to venture into a new system and keep a positive attitude.
- Remember that if healthcare is anything, it is constant change.

Some of the patients who visit Dr. Adkins and Dr. Brooks have expressed concern that electronic health records (EHRs) may not be private enough and that their health information will be "floating around on the Internet." They are worried that unauthorized individuals could somehow access their information on the computer and do them harm.

- How might Susan alleviate the patients' fears about their records being available on the Internet?
- What disadvantages with regard to confidentiality are associated with the EHR?

Capabilities of Electronic Health Record Systems

The EHR system can perform a multitude of tasks, saving time and money in the provider's office (Figure 11-4). The following are some of the features of a typical EHR system.

- **Specialty software.** Patient data are captured and processed into a system that is specialty specific, so that the terminology and patient care treatments are compatible with the provider's specialty. However, additional features can allow the provider to include terminology from other specialties.
- **Appointment scheduler.** The appointment scheduler allows the staff to track and schedule appointments, matrix the schedule, and account for recurring time blocks (Figure 11-5). The appointments can be merged into specific types with default times so that lengthy procedures are not scheduled in short appointment blocks. The scheduler features also allow various search **parameters**; if a patient calls because he or she

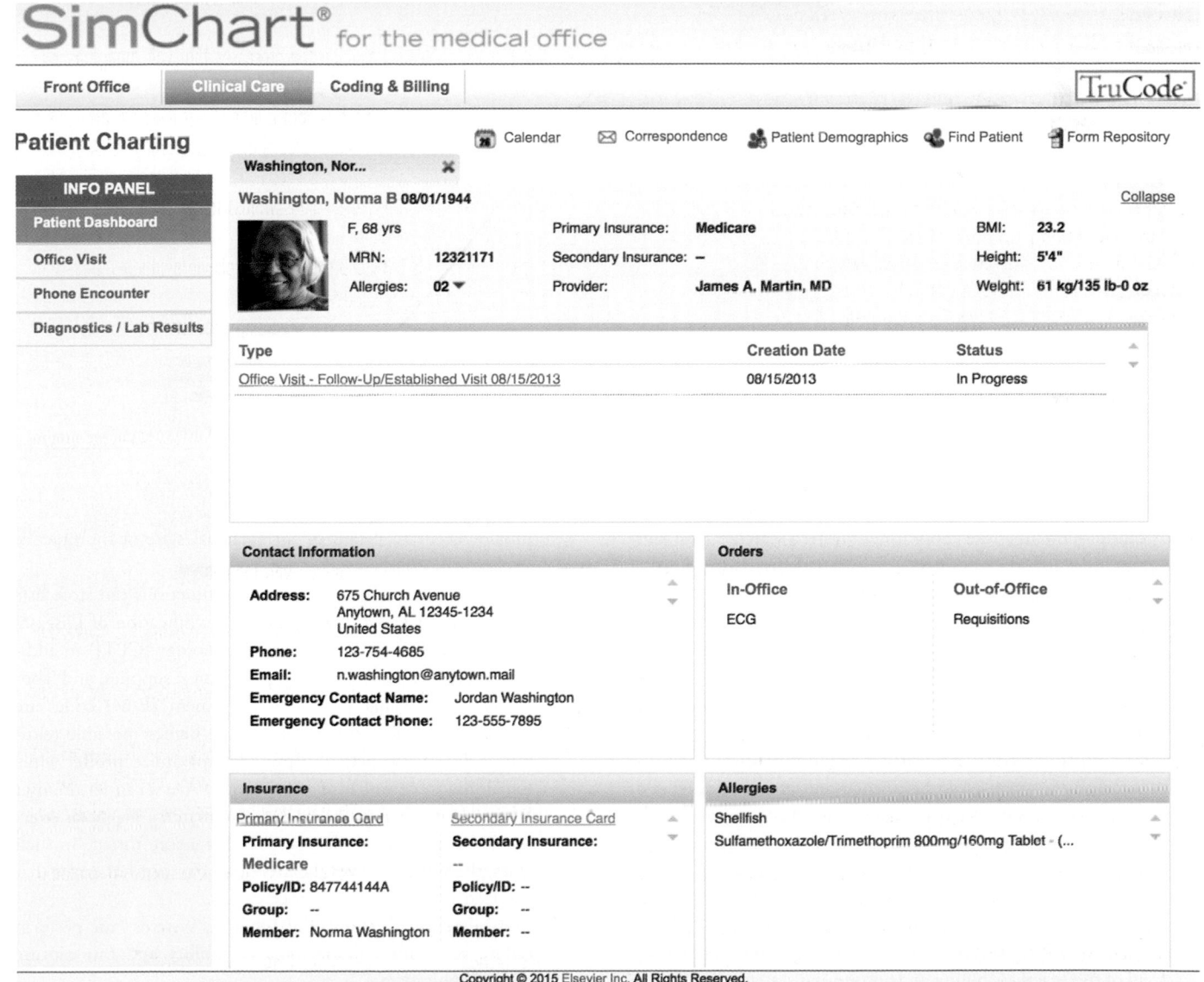

FIGURE 11-4 The electronic health record (EHR) can perform numerous tasks in addition to displaying personal information about the patient. This allows the provider and medical assistants to interact with patients and provide better service.

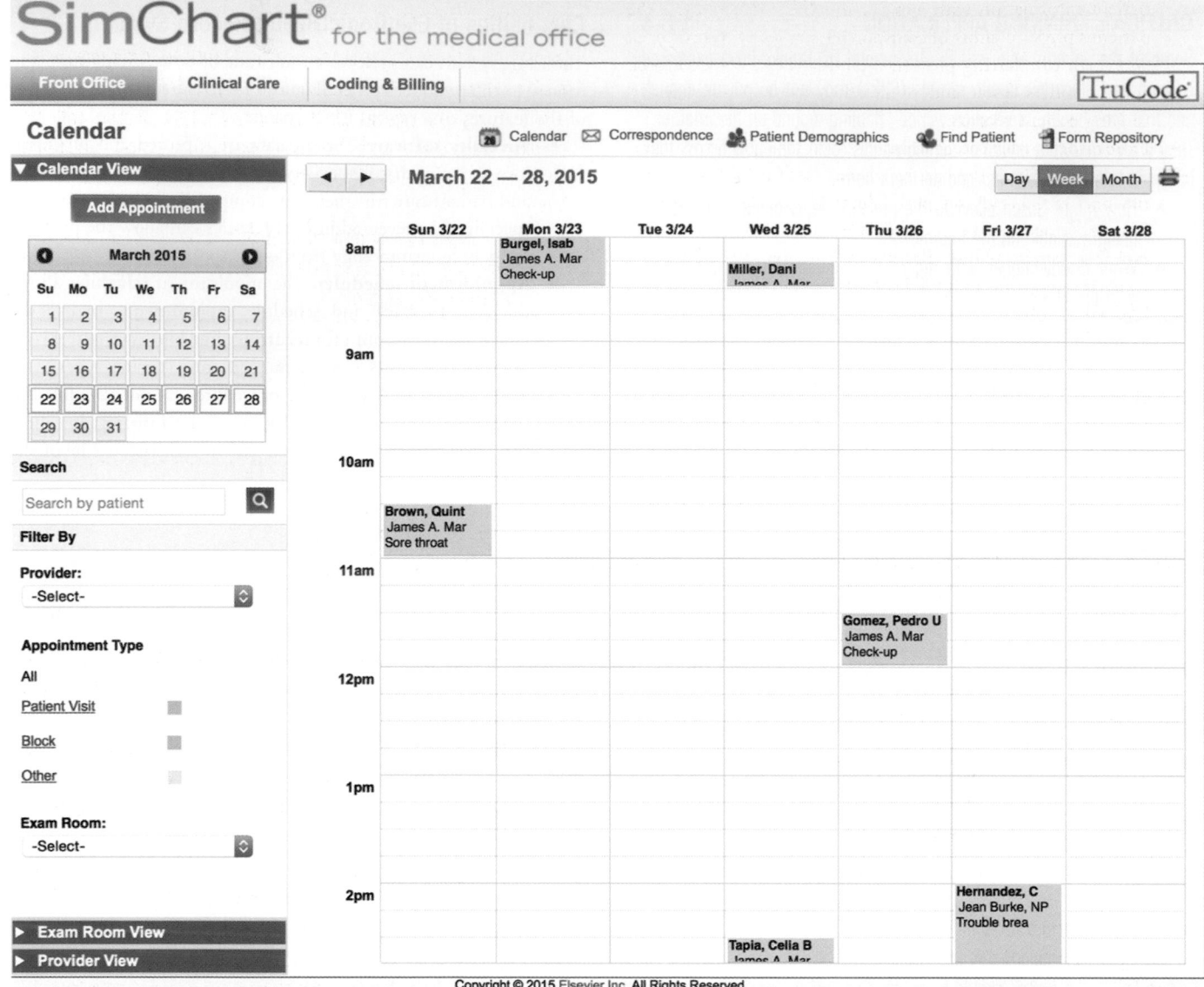

FIGURE 11-5 The EHR usually has a scheduling system that can be changed to manage the needs of the provider and office staff.

cannot remember the appointment time, a search can be initiated using the date, provider's name, patient's name, or other search keywords.

- **Appointment reminder and confirmation.** The system can be programmed to initiate automatic reminder or confirmation calls to patients. The staff can record the reminders, and patients are prompted to choose options, such as "Press one" to confirm or reschedule appointments.
- **Prescription writer.** The EHR system can produce electronic prescriptions, which can be printed and given to patients or automatically submitted to a pharmacy. Lists can be created with the provider's most common drug choices and dosages. A patient allergies function can block the prescription of drugs the patient cannot take, and the system can generate a patient information sheet on new prescriptions.
- **Medical billing system.** The EHR billing system can manage all of the practice's billing and accounting systems. The system also can interface with clearinghouses for electronic claims submission and tracking. Reports can be generated that

provide accurate details of the financial state of the practice at certain intervals or whenever requested.

- **Charge capture.** The charge capture functions can store lists of billing codes (e.g., International Classification of Diseases [ICD] and Current Procedural Terminology [CPT]) in addition to charges associated with procedures, supplies, and laboratory tests. Evaluation and Management (E/M) codes are used during office visits to obtain the highest possible reimbursement; these help the provider maximize profits while remaining in compliance with the law. Alerts can let the user know when a certain charge does not match a diagnosis code; for instance, a blood glucose done for a sore throat. In such cases, the software alerts the user and helps prevent errors that can lead to denial of insurance claims.
- **Eligibility verification.** EHR billing systems can perform online verification of insurance eligibility and can capture demographic data.
- **Referral management.** Current and referring providers can be coordinated and automated, allowing the provider to share

patient information with another provider. This reduces the patient's physical effort of transporting copies of records back and forth to referring providers, eliminates the costs of such copies, and is faster and more efficient than copying and mailing patient records.

- **Laboratory order integration.** The laboratory order integration feature allows the user to interact with outside laboratories and to receive and post laboratory results to patients' records. Tests can be ordered from the provider's laptop, tablet, or smart phone. Results can be transmitted by fax, scan, or e-mail and uploaded directly into the patient's record (Procedure 11-2).

PROCEDURE 11-2 **Organize a Patient's Health Record: Upload Documents to the Electronic Health Record**

Goal: *Scan paper records and upload digital files to the EHR.*

Scenario: A new patient brings in a laboratory report and a radiology report that he would like to be added to his EHR. You need to scan in the original documents and upload them to the EHR.

EQUIPMENT and SUPPLIES

- Scanner
- Computer with SimChart for the Medical Office or EHR software
- Patient's laboratory and radiology reports

PROCEDURAL STEPS

1. Obtain the patient's name and date of birth if not on the reports.
   PURPOSE: You will need the patient's name and date of birth to find the patient's EHR.
2. Using a scanner that is connected to the computer, scan each document, creating an individual digital image for each.
   PURPOSE: The reports should be scanned separately and not combined to create one file. Each type of report must be uploaded separately to the correct location in the EHR.
3. Locate the file of the two scanned images in the computer drive. Open the files to ensure the images are clear.

PURPOSE: When scanning and uploading documents to the EHR, it is crucial that the image of the document is clear and can be easily read by the provider. If the image is blurred, rescan the document.

4. In the EHR, search for the patient, using the patient's last and first name. Verify the patient's date of birth.
   PURPOSE: Before uploading to or documenting in the EHR, it is critical to verify that the correct record is opened.
5. Locate the window to upload diagnostic/laboratory results and add a new result. Enter the date of the test. Select the correct type of result. Browse for the image file of the laboratory file and attach it. Save the information. Select the option to add a new result and repeat the steps to upload the second report. Verify that both documents were uploaded correctly.
   PURPOSE: Errors during the upload may affect the ability to see the files. Verifying at the time of the upload will help ensure providers can see the results in the future.

NONVERBAL COMMUNICATION WITH THE PATIENT WHEN USING THE ELECTRONIC HEALTH RECORD

Although many patients are covered under a type of insurance that requires them to choose a primary care provider (PCP) and to have a referral to a specialist, remember that the patient has the option of changing that PCP or specialist. The patient may decide to change providers simply because he or she does not feel comfortable with that particular provider.

Because the change process is relatively easy, the provider wants to keep his or her patients (in most cases), because losing patients means loss of income. If the care begins to seem impersonal, patients may feel a strong desire to change providers. Remember, patients are consumers of healthcare services, and they expect quality healthcare.

When using the EHR, the medical assistant must make sure his or her nonverbal communication sends the right message to the patient. Eye contact is absolutely essential (Figure 11-6). If the medical assistant constantly looks at the electronic device, the patient feels largely alienated from the information exchange process. Make eye contact with the patient while asking questions, looking at the screen only when needed to enter information. Do not insinuate by physical action that the EHR is a "hidden entity"; for example, do not necessarily shield the device from the patient's view when entering information. Although patients may not understand anything they see on the screen, they will feel more at ease if their information is not hidden from them. Also, modify your stance so that the patient feels like a part of the information process. Just as sitting in a chair

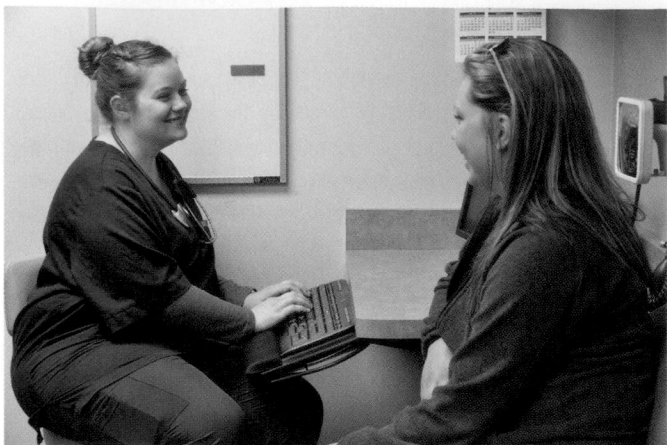

FIGURE 11-6 The medical assistant must make eye contact with the patient when using an EHR.

across from a supervisor's desk can be intimidating, the patient may feel the same emotions sitting across from a medical assistant entering information into the EHR. Take an open stance; sit next to or at an angle to the patient to support the impression that those in the healthcare facility and the patient are partners in the healthcare plan.

Remember that patients have the right to make decisions in most aspects of their healthcare plans; therefore offer choices wherever possible. Never expect patients to make quick decisions about their care. They may want to consult family members or give some thought to important medical decisions. The medical assistant needs to promote time to think unless the patient is faced with a critical, time-sensitive decision. Providers often assume that patients will automatically follow their instructions or orders; however, some patients prefer some time to think. Always follow up and make note of any wait time the patient requests, notify the provider, and enter that information into the EHR. Make sure timely communication is done with the patient and that any additional orders that need to be put in place are completed. The many features of the EHR allow the medical assistant to be efficient and highly competent if he or she is willing to make an extra effort to master the EHR system.

Also make sure patients understand all instructions given to them regarding test procedures or preparation for procedures. Most EHRs can print an instruction sheet, which the medical assistant can review with the patient. The customer service aspect of patient care is even more important when the facility uses an EHR system.

CRITICAL THINKING APPLICATION   **11-6**

Jennifer walks behind Susan's desk and notices that she is looking at the progress notes on a patient who was recently arrested and indicted for child abuse. The case has been in the newspaper and on television consistently for several weeks. Jennifer asks Susan why she has accessed that record. Susan hesitates and then says she must have entered the wrong patient ID number.

- Does Susan's explanation sound convincing?
- Why is Jennifer concerned about Susan looking at the patient's record?
- Just because the individual is a patient at the clinic, does that mean any employee has the right to look at the patient's EHR?

BACKUP SYSTEMS FOR THE ELECTRONIC HEALTH RECORD

Even the best or most expensive EHR system cannot function without power. If a natural disaster occurs and the provider's office is without electricity for several days or weeks, the provider must have a backup system for the EHR so that the office can function. HIPAA requires that the facility adopt a backup and recovery plan that includes daily off-site software backup for the EHR system. Several alternatives can be used for data preservation and backup.

- *External hard drive.* An external hard drive connects to the main computer, and with fairly simple programming can copy the information in the EHR daily. Seven electronic folders, one for each day of the week, can hold the information from the previous day; these folders are replaced with new, updated information at designated periods. CDs and DVDs can hold daily data, and some thumb drives have enough capacity to perform this task. Once a habit of a daily backup to the external hard drive has been established, the method is relatively simple and reliable.

- *Full server backup.* The provider may want to back up the EHR system on a dedicated server, which is a large-capacity computer set aside specifically for the EHR system. With these servers, a full backup should be performed monthly. Many large medical facilities and hospitals have one or more dedicated servers for the EHR system.

- *Online backup system.* An online backup system can be used, usually for a subscription fee. Although the cost may be higher than for some other methods, online systems are easy to use because there is no external drive to carry and no CD or thumb drive to put through the process of downloading data. However, a time investment is involved, because the process of contacting the company that offers the service and then downloading all the data takes several hours. Also, the initial download can take quite a while. Even so, an online system is very stable and reliable.

All these backup methods require an alternative power source in case of a disaster that interrupts electrical service. Remember that backup systems are not effective if the data are stored at the medical facility, and the disaster happens at or affects that physical address. Information technology professionals usually recommend using two of these three methods for the best protection. The system must be protected from theft and unauthorized use, just as is the on-site system.

Medical assistants should keep their paper health records skills sharp in case the EHR system is down for an extended period. Always have a supply of the most commonly used forms in a paper format available for alternative use in such instances. When the EHR system comes back up these paper forms can be scanned into the patients' EHRs.

Transfer, Destruction, and Retention of Electronic Health Records

In most medical offices, records are classified in three ways:

- *Active,* which are the records of patients currently receiving treatment.
- *Inactive,* which generally are the records of patients whom the provider has not seen for 6 months or longer.

- *Closed,* which are the records of patients who have died, moved away, or otherwise terminated their relationship with the provider.

The process of moving a file from active to inactive status is called **purging**. An EHR system can be set up to automatically move the inactive records to another server so that processing time will not be slowed down, but the records are still readily accessible if the patient returns to the healthcare facility. Closed EHRs are also separated from the active records and are typically stored elsewhere. They may be placed on CDs, computer hard drives, or maintained in inactive cloud space by the EHR vendor.

Retention and Destruction

Providers have an obligation to retain patient records, whether they are paper or electronic, that may reasonably be of value to a patient, according to the American Medical Association (AMA) Council on Ethical and Judicial Affairs. Currently, no nationwide standard rule exists for establishing a records **retention schedule**.

Medical considerations are the primary basis for deciding how long to retain health records. For example, operative notes and chemotherapy records should always be part of the patient's health record. The laws regarding the retention of health records vary from state to state, and many governmental programs have their own guidelines for specific records retention. When no rules specify the retention of health records, the best course is to keep the records for 10 years. However, for minors, the facility should keep the records until the minor reaches the **age of majority** plus the statute of limitations.

If a particular record no longer needs to be kept for medical reasons, the provider should check the state law for any requirement that records be kept for a minimum time (most states do not have such a provision). The time is measured from the last professional contact with the patient. In all cases, health records should be kept for at least the period of the statute of limitations for medical malpractice claims, which may be 3 years or longer, depending on state law. In the case of a minor, the statute of limitations may not apply until the patient reaches the age of majority. In summary, know the state requirements related to health records retention and follow those guidelines; the office policy manual should address records retention pertaining to the state where the practice exists.

The records of any patient covered by Medicare or Medicaid must be kept at least 10 years. The HIPAA privacy rule does not include requirements for the retention of health records. However, the privacy rule does require that appropriate administrative, technical, and physical safeguards be applied so that the privacy of health records is maintained.

Some providers refuse to destroy or discard old records. Storage is less of an issue with EHRs as they take up much less physical space. Always refer to state laws when discarding health records.

Before old records are discarded, patients should be given an opportunity to claim a copy of the records or have them sent to another provider. The medical facility should keep a master list of all records that have been destroyed. To legally destroy an EHR, the record, including the backup record, has to be overwritten using utility software.

RELEASING HEALTH RECORD INFORMATION

The healthcare facility must be extremely careful when releasing any type of medical information. The patient must sign a release for information to be given to any third party.

Requests for medical information should be made in writing (Figure 11-7). Electronic signatures may be accepted as long as they are obtained with proper process controls. HIPAA has designated that very specific information must be included on the Release of Information form, including specifically who the information is being released to, what specific information is to be released, and an expiration date for the release. Accepting a faxed request for medical information or a faxed release of information from a patient is unwise. Even requests from the patient's attorney or third-party payers must be cleared by the patient for them to obtain information.

If a provider is involved in a liability suit there will be a required exchange of information. As both parties to a lawsuit begin to prepare their cases, they enter the discovery process. Each side must disclose the pertinent facts of the case that may influence the final outcome of that case. On each occasion that information is needed from the provider, a separate request must be sent. Because this request form is signed by the patient, it serves as a release.

Most offices charge a fee to print or copy health records, whether it is a per-page charge or a per-record fee. If the records are sent electronically there is no fee charged. Follow the steps in the policy and procedures manual for the release of records. Some providers designate the office manager to handle requests for records releases.

Pay particular attention to records release requests involving a minor. In most cases, the parent or legal guardian is entitled to read through the patient's health records; however, according to the HHS, there are three situations in which the parent may not be legally entitled to review the records of his or her minor child:

- When the minor is the one who consents to care and the parent is not required to also consent to care under state law
- When the minor obtains medical care at the direction of a court or a person authorized by the court
- When the minor, parent, and provider all agree that the doctor and minor patient can have a private, confidential relationship

If the provider believes that the minor might be in an abuse situation or that the parent or legal guardian may be harming the patient, the provider is required, both legally and ethically, to report the abuse.

Sometimes patients want to look at their own records. They certainly have a right to see this information, but some patients may not understand the terminology used in the record. A staff member should always remain with a patient who is looking at his or her health record. Remember, the original health record should never leave the medical facility. Always follow office policy when releasing health records.

When a release is presented to the office, copy only the records requested in the release. Do not provide additional information that is not requested. The patient must specify that substance abuse, mental health, and/or human immunodeficiency virus (HIV) records are to be released. Remember that the patient ultimately decides

Central Texas Dermatology Clinic   •   102 Westlake Drive   •   Austin, Texas 78746

AUTHORIZATION TO DISCLOSE HEALTH INFORMATION

I hereby authorize the use or disclosure of information from the medical record of:

Patient Name: _____   Date of Birth: _____

Social Security# _____   Daytime Phone: _____

I authorize the following individual or organization to disclose the above named individual's health information:

_____   Address: _____

This information may be disclosed TO and used by the following individual or organization:

_____   Address: _____

Please release the following:

____ Progress Notes   ____ Pathology Reports   ____ Lab Reports   ____ Any and all Records

____ Other Diagnostic reports (specify _____

____ Other (specify) _____

       Including Information (if applicable) pertaining to:

       ____ Mental Health   ____ Drug/Alcohol   ____ HIV/AIDS   ____ Communicable Treatment

Purpose or Need for Disclosure:

____ Continued Patient Care   ____ Personal Use

____ Attorney/Legal   ____ Insurance Claim/Application

____ Disability Determination   ____ Other(specify) _____

I understand that the information in my health record may include information relating to sexually transmitted disease, acquired immunodeficiency syndrome (AIDS), or human immunodeficiency virus (HIV). It may also include information about behavioral or mental health services, and treatment for alcohol and drug abuse.

I understand that the information released is for the specific purpose stated above. Any other use of this information without the written consent of the patient is prohibited.

I understand that I have the right to revoke this authorization at any time. I understand that if I revoke this authorization I must do so in writing and present my written revocation to the individual or organization releasing information. I understand that the revocation will not apply to information already released in response to this authorization. I understand that the revocation will not apply to my insurance company when the law provides my insurer the right to contest a claim under my policy. Unless otherwise revoked, this authorization will expire on following date, event or condition: _____

_____

If I fail to specify an expiration date, event or condition, this authorization will expire in six months.

I understand that authorizing the disclosure of this health information is voluntary. I can refuse to sign the authorization. I need not sign this form in order to ensure treatment. I understand that I may inspect or copy the information to be used or disclosed, as provided in CFR 164.524. I understand that any disclosure of information carries with it the potential for an unauthorized re-disclosure and the information may not be protected by federal confidentiality rules. If I have questions about disclosure of my health information, I can contact Theresa Farren at 512-327-7779.

_____   _____

Signature of Patient or Legal Representative   Date

_____   _____

Relationship to Patient (If Legal Representative)   Witness

COMPLETE ONLY IF INFORMATION IS TO BE RELEASED DIRECTLY TO PATIENT:

I understand that my medical record may contain reports, test results, and notes that only a physician can interpret. I understand and have been advised that I should contact my physician regarding the entries made in my medical record to prevent my misunderstanding of the information contained in these entries. I will not hold Central Texas Dermatology liable for any misinterpretation of the information in my medical record as a result of not contacting my physician for the correct interpretation.

_____   _____

Signature of Patient or Legal Representative   Date

_____   _____

Relationship to Patient (If Legal Representative)   Witness

Dr. review/signature/date _____

Date request completed _____   # of pages copied _____

Staff Signature _____

PHI Log completed _____

FIGURE 11-7 Authorization to release health records: All requests for health records should be made in writing, and the request should be kept in the patient's record.

whether a record can be released. If any question arises about what is to be released, consult the office manager or the provider.

Health Information Exchanges

The demand for electronic health information exchange (HIE) from one healthcare facility to another, together with nationwide efforts to improve the efficiency and quality of healthcare, is creating a demand for HIEs. As more and more providers move to EHRs it only makes sense to have a system in place that will facilitate the exchange of that information electronically to improve the timeliness of that exchange. Patient care can be improved because all providers will have access to the information needed to treat the patient.

The ONC states, "There are currently three forms of HIE:

- Directed Exchange—ability to send and receive secure information electronically between care providers to support coordinated care
- Query-Based Exchange—ability for providers to find and/or request information on a patient from other providers, often used for unplanned care
- Consumer-Mediated Exchange—ability for patient to aggregate and control the use of their health information among providers"

The implementation of HIE varies from state to state. There is some federal funding for the implementation of HIE that is being administered by the ONC.

CREATING AN EFFICIENT PAPER HEALTH RECORDS MANAGEMENT SYSTEM

The paper health records management system should provide an easy method of retrieving information. The files should be organized in an orderly fashion, the information must be documented accurately, and corrections should be made and documented properly. The wording in the record should be easily understood and grammatically correct. An efficient method of adding documents to the record must be established so that the provider always has the most up-to-date information.

Above all, the health records management system must work for the individual facility.

Organization of the Health Record

Source-Oriented Medical Records

The traditional patient record is a source-oriented medical record (SOMR); that is, observations and data are cataloged according to their source—provider (progress notes), laboratory, radiology, hospital, or consultant. Forms and progress notes are filed in **reverse chronologic order** (i.e., most recent on top) and in separate sections of the record according to the type of form or service rendered (e.g., all laboratory reports together, all x-ray reports together, and so on). Reverse chronologic order is used so that the provider and staff members do not have to search to the bottom of the record to find a recent laboratory report or a test.

Problem-Oriented Medical Records

The problem-oriented medical record (POMR) is a departure from the traditional system of keeping patient records. The POMR is a record of clinical practice that divides medical action into four categories:

- The *database,* which includes the chief complaint, present illness, patient profile, review of systems, physical examination, and laboratory reports.
- The *problem list,* a numbered, titled list of every problem the patient has that requires management or workup. This may include social and demographic troubles in addition to strictly medical or surgical ones.
- The *treatment plan* includes management, additional workups needed, and therapy. Each plan is titled and numbered with respect to the problem.
- The *progress notes* include structured notes that are numbered to correspond with each problem number.

Several companies have developed file folders for organizing patient data according to the POMR. The problem list (Figure 11-8) is placed at the front of the record. Special sections are provided for current major and chronic diagnoses/health problems and for inactive major or chronic diagnosis/health problems. Progress notes usually follow the SOAP approach. SOAP is an acronym for the following:

- *S*ubjective impressions or patient reports
- *O*bjective clinical evidence or observations
- *A*ssessment or diagnosis
- *P*lans for further studies, treatment, or management

Some medical offices also use an *E* in the record to represent evaluation; others include *E* for education and *R* for response. The education notation shows that the patient was educated about his or her condition or given a patient information sheet. The response section is used to record an assessment of the patient's understanding of and possible compliance with the treatment plan.

The POMR has the advantage of imposing order and organization on the information added to a patient's health record. The records are more easily reviewed, and the likelihood of overlooking a problem is greatly reduced. The SOAP method forces a rational approach to the patient's problems and assists the formulation of a logical, orderly plan of patient care (Figure 11-9). The POMR is especially advantageous in clinics, group practices, and hospitals, where more than one person must be able to find essential information in the record.

DOCUMENTING IN AN ELECTRONIC HEALTH RECORD

Documentation in an EHR involves using radio buttons, drop-down menus, and free-text boxes. The radio buttons and drop-down menus allow for standardization of the content in the EHR and the free-text boxes allow for the documentation of the unique circumstance found with each patient (Figure 11-10). It is important to carefully review the choices made with the radio buttons and drop-down menus. Information documented using the free-text boxes should be proofread before submitting.

DOCUMENTING IN A PAPER HEALTH RECORD

When documenting in a paper health record the entry will always start with the date in the MM/DD/YYYY format. The date will be followed by the time. This may be written in standard or military

MASTER PROBLEM LIST

For use of this form, see AR 40-66; the proponent agency is the Office of The Surgeon General

MAJOR PROBLEMS

PROBLEM NUMBER	DATE ONSET	DATE ENTERED	PROBLEM	DATE RESOLVED
1.				
2.				
3.				
4.				
5.				
6.				
7.				
8.				
9.				
10.				
11.				
12.				

TEMPORARY (MINOR) PROBLEMS

PROBLEM LETTER	PROBLEM	DATES OF OCCURRENCES				
A.						
B.						
C.						
D.						
E.						
F.						
G.						
H.						

PATIENT'S IDENTIFICATION (Use mechanical imprint if available; for typed or written entries give: Name, SSN, Unit, Sex, Birthdate, and Duty Phone)

SUMMARY OF PROBLEMS, ALLERGIES, MEDICATIONS, SURGERIES AND TRAUMAS:

NOTE: DO NOT DISCARD FROM CHART

FIGURE 11-8 A problem list designed for a problem-oriented health record (POMR).

FIGURE 11-9 SOAP progress notes: The SOAP method keeps information organized and in a logical sequence. An actual progress note would include the provider's or medical assistant's signature or initials after this entry. (Courtesy Bibbero Systems, Petaluma, California.)

time. If standard time is used it must be followed by AM or PM (e.g., 2:00 PM). If military time is used it is in a four-digit format without a colon (e.g., 1400). All entries must be written in black or blue ink following the format designated by the healthcare facility. Documentation should be in the order in which the steps were completed. If temperature, pulse, and respiration (TPR) measurement is done it would be documented in the "O" or Objective section of the SOAP note starting with temperature, then pulse, and lastly respirations.

MAKING CORRECTIONS AND ALTERATIONS TO HEALTH RECORDS

Corrections sometimes must be made to health records. The first step is to verify the proper procedure for making corrections in the facility's policy and procedures manual. Some providers prefer a specific method for correcting errors in the health record. Erasing, using correction fluid, or any other type of **obliteration** is never acceptable. To correct a handwritten entry:

1. Draw a line through the error.
2. Insert the correction above or immediately after the error in a spot where it can be read clearly.
3. If indicated by the policy and procedures manual, write "Error" or "Err." in the margin.

4. The person making the correction should write his or her initials or signature below the correction and the date. Follow the format indicated in the policy and procedures manual (Figure 11-11).

Errors made while using the computer are corrected in the usual way. However, an error discovered in an entry at a later date is corrected in the same manner as for a handwritten entry. This is sometimes called an *addendum*. Never attempt to alter health records without using this specific correction procedure, because this alteration of records may indicate a fraudulent attempt to cover up a mistake made by a staff member or the provider. Do not hide errors. If the error could in any way affect the patient's health and well-being, it must be brought to the provider's attention immediately. An EHR system will track the changes made within the record.

DICTATION AND TRANSCRIPTION

With the increased use of EHRs and voice recognition software, there is decreased need for **transcription.** If **dictation** is still done in the healthcare facility the administrative medical assistant may find that transcribing the dictation is a job they perform periodically. Transcription can be done from handwritten notes, or more likely from machine dictation. Smooth operation of the facility may depend on the timely, accurate performance of assigned responsibilities, such as record documentation and preparation of special reports. Accuracy and speed are primary **requisites,** as is a strong grasp of medical terminology and principles, especially anatomy and physiology.

Dictation may be done using a machine transcription unit or a portable transcription unit. Many healthcare facilities now use a system that is accessed by telephone; the provider calls the system using passwords or access codes and records the information for the health record while speaking into the telephone. Later, employees transcribe the information into the health record. The provider must acknowledge and initial all transcription before it is placed in the health record.

Voice Recognition Software

Some healthcare facilities use voice recognition software for transcription. When first installed, the software requires the user to say several sentences into the unit so that it "learns" to recognize the user's voice. The system can be used to dictate progress notes, letters, e-mails, and virtually any document in the healthcare facility that needs to be created. These documents will need to be approved by the provider before they are permanently attached to the patient's record. Some systems have an authentication component that allows a type of electronic signature, such as those needed for hospital record dictation.

Transfer, Destruction, and Retention of Paper Health Records

As with EHRs, paper health records are also classified as active, inactive, and closed. A paper record system must have a system established for regular transfer of files from active to inactive status or possibly destruction. The expansion of records and the file space available can influence the transfer period. Records for patients currently hospitalized may be kept in a special section for quick

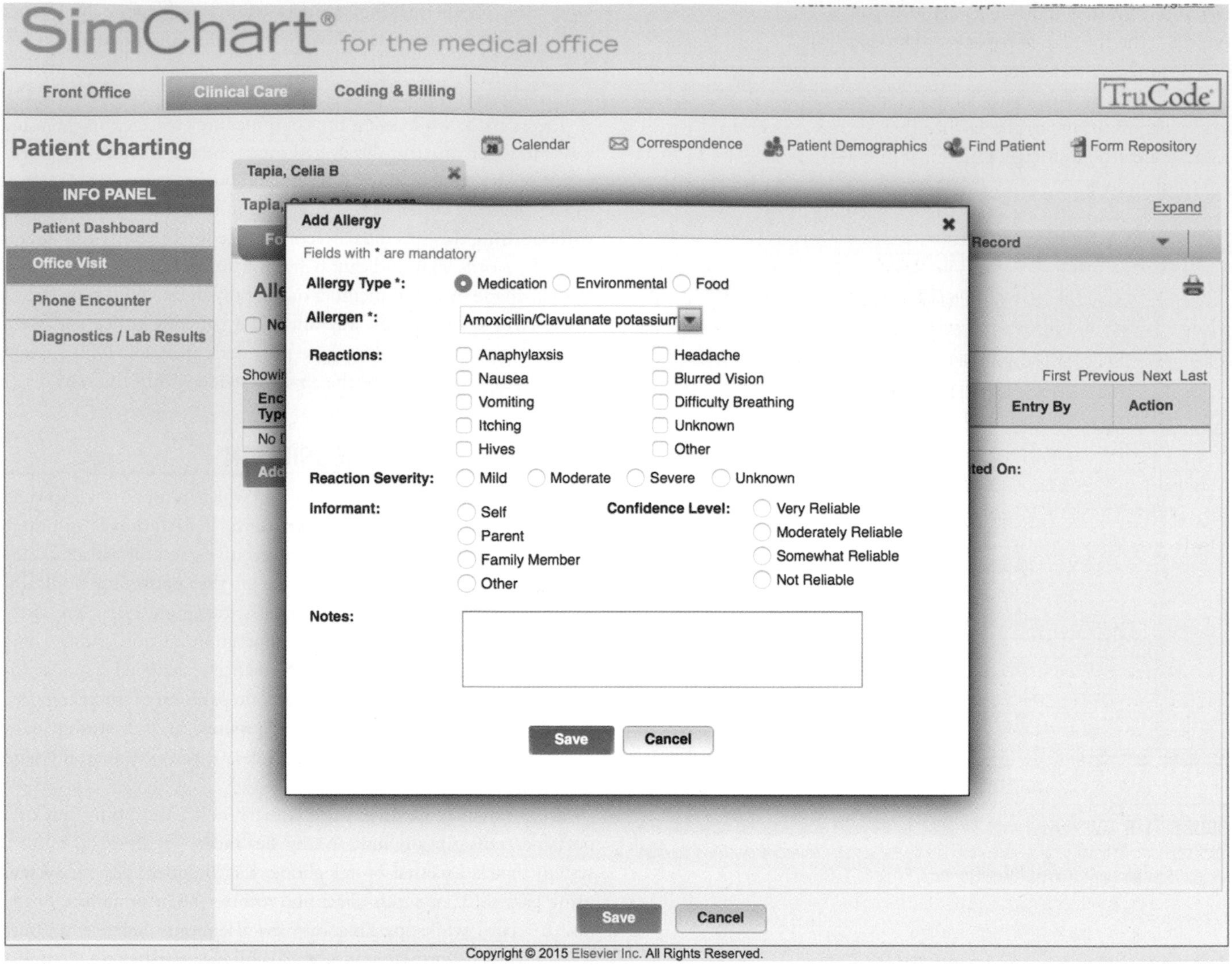

SimChart for the medical office

| Front Office | Clinical Care | Coding & Billing | | TruCode |

Patient Charting   📅 Calendar   ✉ Correspondence   👥 Patient Demographics   🔍 Find Patient   📄 Form Repository

INFO PANEL
Patient Dashboard
Office Visit
Phone Encounter
Diagnostics / Lab Results

Tapia, Celia B   ✕

Tapia, Celia B   Expand

Add Allergy   ✕

Fields with * are mandatory

Allergy Type *:   ◉ Medication   ○ Environmental   ○ Food

Allergen *:   Amoxicillin/Clavulanate potassium ▾

Reactions: ☐ Anaphylaxsis   ☐ Headache
                 ☐ Nausea   ☐ Blurred Vision
                 ☐ Vomiting   ☐ Difficulty Breathing
                 ☐ Itching   ☐ Unknown
                 ☐ Hives   ☐ Other

Reaction Severity: ○ Mild   ○ Moderate   ○ Severe   ○ Unknown

Informant: ○ Self   **Confidence Level:**   ○ Very Reliable
                 ○ Parent   ○ Moderately Reliable
                 ○ Family Member   ○ Somewhat Reliable
                 ○ Other   ○ Not Reliable

Notes: [   ]

        Save   **Cancel**

        Save   **Cancel**

FIGURE 11-10 Documentation in an EHR is done using radio buttons, drop-down menus, and free-text boxes.

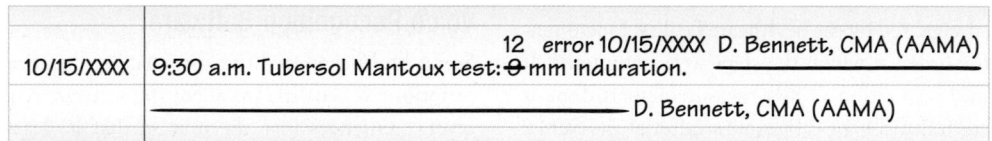

| 10/15/XXXX | 9:30 a.m. Tubersol Mantoux test: ~~0~~ mm induration. | 12 error 10/15/XXXX D. Bennett, CMA (AAMA) |
| | | ——————————————— D. Bennett, CMA (AAMA) |

FIGURE 11-11 Corrections to health records must be done in a legible manner and must be clearly understood. Always initial and date corrections to health records. (From Bonewit-West K: *Today's medical assistant,* ed 2, St. Louis, Saunders, 2013.)

reference and then placed in the regular active file when the patient is discharged from the hospital. In a surgical practice, the record frequently includes the specific date on which the patient is discharged from the provider's care, and the notation is made on the record, "Return prn" (from the Latin *pro re nata,* "as the occasion arises" or "when needed"). This record may safely be placed in the inactive file.

Most medical facilities use a year sticker on the file folder that indicates the last year the patient visited the clinic. If the file has a sticker showing that the patient's last visit was in 2014, and he or she presents to the clinic on January 5, 2016, a *2016* sticker should be placed over the one that indicates *2014.* These stickers often are

included with color-coded filing systems. The medical assistant can easily look at a group of files and see which ones need to be changed to inactive or closed status.

Retention and Destruction

Retention and destruction guidelines are the same for paper health records as for EHRs.

Long-Term Storage

Large healthcare facilities may find it advisable to convert their paper health records to **microfilm** for storage if the facility has not yet begun to scan documents into an EHR. If documents are stored electronically, they must be regularly backed up for storage. Another option is the transfer of paper records onto optical disks. Microfilm and optical disk technology are both expensive and probably are not practical for any but a very large group practice or health maintenance organization, so the facility should be moving toward some form of electronic storage. Using that method, health records can be kept indefinitely.

CRITICAL THINKING APPLICATION   **11-7**

Susan learned about SOAP documentation in school and is eager to use it in her new job. Dr. Thomas is seeing a patient that reports to Susan that she has had nausea and vomiting for the past 3 days. Susan obtains a weight of 132.5 pounds, temperature (T): 101.2° F tympanically, pulse (P): 94 beats/min, respiration (R): 14 breaths/min, and blood pressure (BP) 122/84 mm Hg in the right arm. What information would be documented in the Subjective field? What information would be documented in the Objective field? Who would document information in the Assessment field?

FILING EQUIPMENT

The vertical, four-drawer steel filing cabinet, used with manila folders with the patient's name on the tab, was the traditional system of choice for years. The most popular system today is color-coding on open horizontal shelves. Rotary, lateral, compactable, and automated files also are available. Some records are kept in card or tray files. Some factors that should be considered when selecting filing equipment are:

- Office space availability
- Structural considerations
- Cost of space and equipment
- Size, type, and volume of records
- Confidentiality requirements
- Retrieval speed
- Fire protection
- Cost

Drawer Files

Drawer files should be full suspension; they should roll easily, close securely, and be equipped with a locking device. The best cabinets have a center trough at the bottom of each drawer with a rod for holding divider guides. A drawback of the vertical four-drawer files is that only one person can use a file cabinet at a time. Filing also is slower, because the drawer must be opened and closed each time a file is pulled or filed.

File cabinets are heavy and can tip over, causing serious damage or injury unless reasonable care is taken. Open only one file drawer at a time, and close it when the filing has been completed. A drawer left even slightly open can injure a passerby.

Horizontal Shelf Files

Shelf files should have doors that lock to protect the contents. A popular type of shelf file has doors that slide back into the cabinet; the door from a lower shelf may be pulled out and used for work space. Open shelf units hold files sideways and can go higher on the

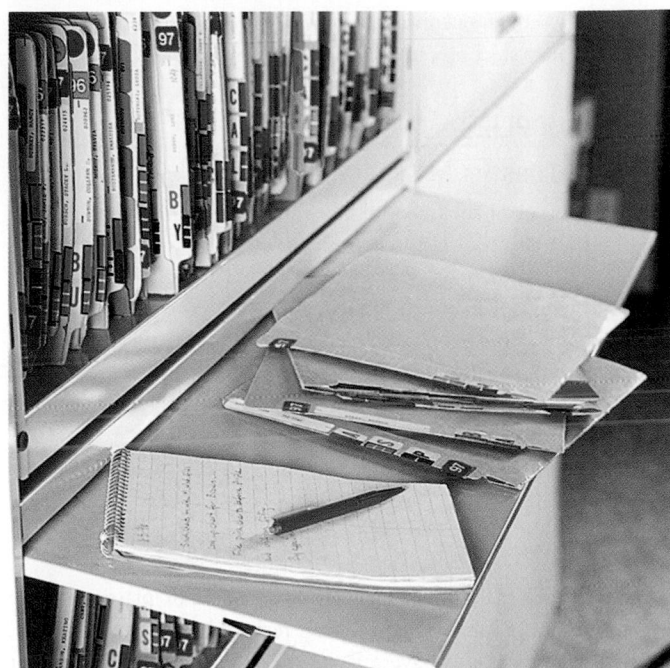

FIGURE 11-12 Open shelf filing is an efficient method, especially for color-coded filing systems. The shelf doors often can be used as workspace.

wall because no drawers need to be pulled out (Figure 11-12). File retrieval is faster, because several individuals can work simultaneously.

Rotary Circular Files

Rotary circular files can hold a large volume of records. They save space and clerical motion. The files revolve easily; some have push-button controls. Several people can work at one rotary file and use records at the same time. One disadvantage is that they afford less privacy and protection than files that can be closed and locked.

Compactable Files

An office with little space and a great volume of records might use compactable files, which are a variation of open shelf files. The files are mounted on tracks in the floor, and the units slide along the tracks so that access is gained to the needed records. One drawback is that not all records are available at the same time.

Automated Files

Automated files are very expensive initially and require more maintenance than other types of filing equipment. They are likely to be found only in very large facilities, such as clinics or hospitals. These files bring the record to the operator instead of the operator going to the record. When the operator presses a button indicating the appropriate shelf, the shelf automatically moves into position in front of the operator for record retrieval. The automated or power file is fast and can store large numbers of records in a small amount of space. However, only one person can use the unit at one time.

Card Files

Almost every office has some occasion to use a card file. This may be for patient ledgers, a patient index, a library index, an index of surgical tray setups, telephone numbers, or numerous other records. A good-quality steel box or tray is a sound investment.

FILING SUPPLIES

Divider Guides

Each file drawer or shelf should be equipped with plenty of dividers or guides. Some authorities recommend one guide for approximately each $1\frac{1}{2}''$ of material, or every eight to 10 folders. Guides should be of good-quality **pressboard** or strong plastic. Less-well-constructed guides soon become bent and frayed and have to be replaced. Divider guides have a protruding tab, which may be an integral part of the card or may be made of metal or plastic. The guides reduce the area of search and serve as supports for the folders. They are available in single, third, or fifth cut (i.e., one, three, or five different positions).

Outguides

Outguides are made of heavyweight cardboard or plastic and are used to replace a folder that has been removed temporarily (Figure 11-13). They may also have a large pocket to hold any filing that may come in while the folder is out. They should be of a distinctive color for quick detection. This makes refiling simpler and alerts the file clerk that a file is missing. Several colors may be used, each color designating the temporary location of the file. The outguide may have lines for recording information, or it may have a plastic pocket for inserting an information card.

File Folders

Most records to be filed are placed in covers or tabbed folders. The most commonly used is a general purpose, third-cut manila folder that may be expanded to $\frac{3}{4}''$. These are available with a double-thickness, reinforced tab, which greatly extends the life of the folder. Folders kept in drawers have tabs at the top; those kept on shelves have tabs at the side. Many folder styles are available for special purposes.

The vertical pocket, which is of heavier weight than the general purpose folder, has a front that folds down for easy access to contents and is available with up to a $3\frac{1}{2}''$ expansion. These are used for bulky histories or correspondence.

Hanging, or suspension, folders are made of heavy stock and hang on metal rods from side to side in a drawer. They can be used only with files equipped with suspension equipment.

Binder folders have fasteners that are used to bind papers in the folder. These offer some security for the papers, but filing the materials is time-consuming.

The number of papers that will fit in one folder depends on the thickness of the papers and the capacity of the folder. Near the bottom edge of most folders are one or more score marks, which should be used as the contents of the folders expand. Papers should never protrude from the folder edges, and they should always be inserted with their tops to the left. When papers start to ride up in any folder, the folder is overloaded.

Labels

The label is a necessary filing and finding device. Use labels to identify each shelf, drawer, divider guide, and folder. A label on the drawer or shelf identifies the nature of its contents. It should also indicate the range (i.e., alphabetic, numeric, or chronologic) of the material filed in that space.

The label on the divider guide identifies the range of folder headings following that divider guide up to the next divider (e.g., BaBo).

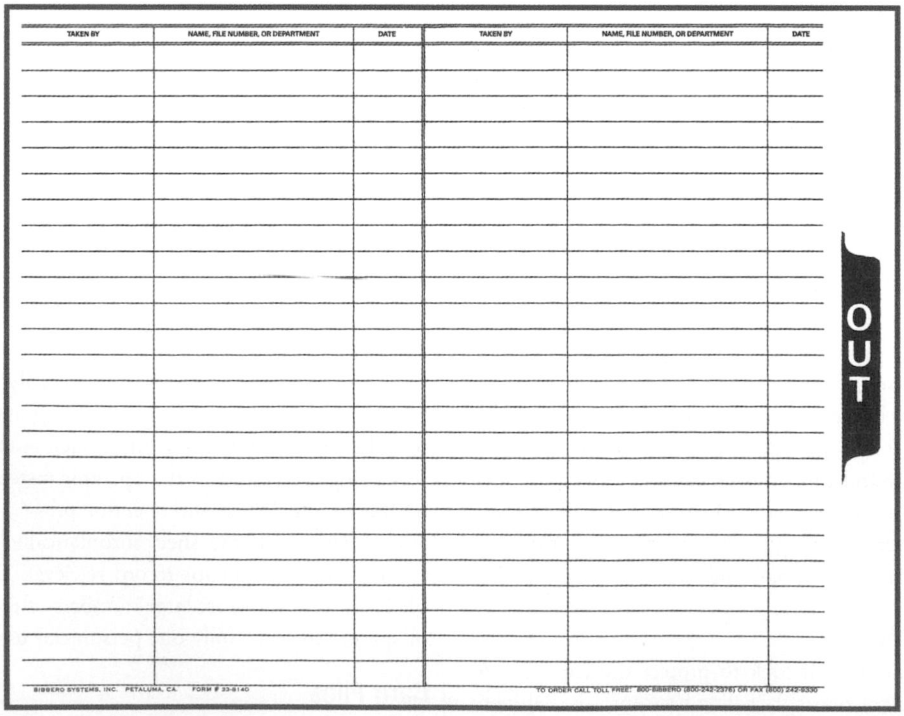

TAKEN BY	NAME, FILE NUMBER, OR DEPARTMENT	DATE	TAKEN BY	NAME, FILE NUMBER, OR DEPARTMENT	DATE

OUT

BIBBERO SYSTEMS, INC. PETALUMA, CA. FORM # 33-8140

TO ORDER CALL TOLL FREE: 800-BIBBERO (800-242-2376) OR FAX (800) 242-9330

FIGURE 11-13 Outguides allow tracking of a file not in its proper location by providing information on the location of the file. (Courtesy Bibbero Systems, Petaluma, California.)

The label on the folder identifies the contents of that folder only. This may be the name of the patient, subject matter of correspondence, a business topic, or anything at all that needs to be filed. Label a folder when a new patient is seen, existing folders are full, or materials need to be transferred within the filing system.

Labels are available in almost any size, shape, or color to meet the individual needs of any facility. Visit an office supply Web site and review the catalogs to find the best product to meet the needs of the facility.

A narrow label applied to the front of the folder tab is the easiest to use and satisfactory for folders kept in a drawer file. Labels for shelf filing should be identifiable from both front and back. Always type the label before separating it from the roll or protective sheet. Type the **caption** on the label in indexing order (Procedure 11-3).

Indexing Rules

Indexing rules (Table 11-2) are standardized and based on current business practices. The Association of Records Managers and Administrators takes an active part in updating these rules. Some establishments adopt variations of these basic rules to accommodate their needs. In any case, the practices need to be consistent within the system.

1. Last names are considered first in filing; then the given name (first name), second; and the middle name or initial, third. Compare the names beginning with the first letter of the name. When a letter is different in the two names, that letter determines the order of filing.
2. Initials precede a name beginning with the same letter. This illustrates the librarian's rule, "Nothing comes before something."
3. With hyphenated personal names, the hyphenated elements, whether first name, middle name, or surname, are considered to be one unit.
4. The apostrophe is disregarded in filing.
5. When indexing a foreign name in which you cannot distinguish between the first and last names, index each part of the name in the order in which it is written. If you can make the distinction, use the last name as the first indexing unit.
6. Names with prefixes are filed in the usual alphabetic order, with the prefix considered part of the name.

TABLE 11-2 Applying Indexing Rules

INDEXING RULE	NAME	UNIT 1	UNIT 2	UNIT 3
1	Robert F. Grinch	Grinch	Robert	F.
	R. Frank Grumman	Grumman	R.	Frank
2	J. Orville Smith	Smith	J.	Orville
	Jason O. Smith	Smith	Jason	O.
3	M. L. Saint-Vickery	Saint-Vickery	M.	L.
	Marie-Louise Taylor	Taylor	Marielouise	
4	Charles S. Anderson	Anderson	Charles	S.
	Anderson's Surgical Supply	Andersons	Surgical	Supply
5	Ah Hop Akee	Akee	Ah	Hop
6	Alice Delaney	Delaney	Alice	
	Chester K. DeLong	Delong	Chester	K.
7	Michael St. John	Stjohn	Michael	
8	Helen M. Maag	Maag	Helen	M.
	Frederick Mabry	Mabry	Frederick	
	James E. MacDonald	Macdonald	James	E.
9	Mrs. John L. Doe (Mary Jones)	Doe	Mary	Jones (Mrs. John L.)
10	Prof. John J. Brock	Brock	John	J. (Prof.)
	Madame Sylvia	Madame	Sylvia	
	Sister Mary Catherine	Sister	Mary	Catherine
	Theodore Wilson, MD	Wilson	Theodore (MD)	
11	Lawrence W. Jones, Jr.	Jones	Lawrence	W. (Jr.)
	Lawrence W. Jones, Sr.	Jones	Lawrence	W. (Sr.)
12	The Moore Clinic	Moore	Clinic (The)	

7. Abbreviated parts of a name are indexed as written if that form generally is used by that person.

8. Mac and Mc are filed in their regular place in the alphabet. If the files have a great many names beginning with Mac or Mc, some offices file them as a separate letter of the alphabet for convenience.

9. The name of a married woman, who has taken her husband's last name, is indexed by her legal name (her husband's surname, her given name, and her middle name or maiden surname). There should be a cross-reference, such as an outguide placed where her maiden name falls directing you to her new name.

10. When followed by a complete name, titles may be used as the last filing unit if needed to distinguish the name from another, identical name. Titles without complete names are considered the first indexing unit.

11. Terms of seniority or professional or academic degrees are used only to distinguish the name from an identical name.

12. Articles (e.g., the, a) are disregarded in indexing.

PROCEDURE 11-3   Create and Organize a Patient's Paper Health Record

Goal: *Create a paper health record for a new patient. Organize health record documents in a paper health record.*

EQUIPMENT and SUPPLIES

- End tab file folder
- Completed patient registration form
- Divider sheets with different color labels (4)
- Progress note sheet (1)
- Name label
- Color-coding labels (first two letters of last name and first letter of first name)
- Year label
- Allergy label
- Black pen or computer with word processing software to process labels
- Health record documents (i.e., prior records, laboratory reports)
- Hole puncher

PROCEDURAL STEPS

1. Obtain the patient's first and last name.
   PURPOSE: To customize the record for the patient, the first and last name will be required.

2. Neatly write or word process the patient's name on the name label. Left-justify the last name, followed by a comma, the first name, middle initial and a period (e.g., Smith, Mary J.).
   PURPOSE: The label should be easy to read. The last name always comes before the first name.

3. Adhere the name label to the bottom left side of the record tab. When the record is held by the main fold in your left hand, the writing should be easy to read. (For directional purposes, assume the record main fold is on the left and the tab is at the bottom.)

4. Put the color-coding labels on the bottom right edge of the folder. Start by placing the first letter of the last name at the farthest right edge. Working left, place the second letter of the last name, then the first letter of the first name, and lastly the year label. The year label should be close to the name label.
   PURPOSE: When the folders are in the file cabinet, the folders are sorted by the colored labels, starting with the top label (first letter of the last name), followed by the second and remaining labels.

5. Place the allergy label on the front of the record. If allergies are known, clearly write the allergy on the label in red ink.

6. Place the divider labels on the record divider sheets, if they come separately. Ensure the labels on the divider sheets are staggered so they do not overlap. Print the name of the section on the front and back of the label. The print should be easy to read when the record is held by the main fold. (Suggested names for dividers: Progress Notes, Laboratory, Correspondence, and Miscellaneous.)
   PURPOSE: Placing divider labels on the divider sheets in a staggered pattern allows the provider to easily see all sections of the health record.

7. Using the prongs on the left-hand side of the record, secure the registration form.
   PURPOSE: The registration form should be in an easy-to-find location in the record.

8. Using the prongs on the right-hand side of the record, secure the index dividers with a progress note sheet under the progress note tab.
   PURPOSE: The provider will need the progress note sheet to document data regarding the visit.

Scenario: The patient authorized his/her prior provider to send health records to your agency. You need to organize these records within the paper health record.

9. Verify the name and the date of birth on the health records and ensure they match the information on the health record.
   PURPOSE: Before organizing and filing documents in a patient's health record, it is critical to ensure the health record is for the correct patient.

10. Open the prongs on the right side of the record and carefully remove the record to the point of where the documents need to be inserted. For the documents being inserted, punch holes in the proper location. Insert the papers into the record and then reassemble the remaining part of the record. Continue to do this until all the documents are filed within the health record.
    PURPOSE: Documents need to be placed in the correct location in the record so the provider can easily find information.

FILING METHODS

The three basic filing methods used in healthcare facilities are:

- Alphabetic by name
- Numeric
- Subject

Patients' records are filed either alphabetically by name or by one of several numeric methods. Subject filing is used for business records, correspondence, and topical materials.

Alphabetic Filing

Alphabetic filing by name is the oldest, simplest, and most commonly used system. It is the system of choice for filing patients' records in most small providers' offices.

The alphabetic system of filing is traditional and simple to set up, requiring only a file cabinet or shelf, folders, and some divider guides (Procedure 11-4). It is a **direct filing system** in that the person filing needs to know only the name to find the desired file. Alphabetic filing does have some drawbacks:

- The correct spelling of the name must be known.
- As the number of files increases, more space is needed for each section of the alphabet. This results in periodic shifting of folders to allow for expansion.
- As the files expand, more time is required for filing or retrieving each folder because of the greater number of folders involved in the search. The time can be greatly reduced by color-coding.

Numeric Filing

Some form of **numeric filing** combined with color and shelf filing is used by practically every large clinic or hospital. Management consultants differ in their recommendations; some recommend numeric filing only if more than 5,000 to 10,000 records are involved. Others recommend nothing but numeric filing. Numeric filing is an **indirect filing system**, or one that requires use of an alphabetic cross-reference to find a given file. Some object to this added step and overlook the advantages of numeric filing, which are:

- It allows unlimited expansion without periodic shifting of folders, and shelves usually are filled evenly.
- It provides additional confidentiality to the record.
- It saves time in retrieving and filing records quickly. One knows immediately that the number 978 falls between 977 and 979. By contrast, an alphabetic system, even with color-coding, requires a longer search for the exact spot.

Several types of numeric filing systems can be used. In the straight, or consecutive, numeric system, patients are given consecutive numbers as they first start using the practice. This is the simplest numeric system and works well for files of up to 10,000 records. It is time-consuming, and the chance for error is greater, when documents with five or more digits are filed. Filing activity is greatest at the end of the numeric series.

In the terminal digit system, patients also are assigned consecutive numbers, but the digits in the number usually are separated into groups of twos or threes and are read in groups from right to left instead of from left to right. The records are filed backward in groups. For example, all files ending in 00 are grouped together first, then those ending in 01, and so on. Next the files are grouped by their middle digits so that the 00 22s come before the 01 22s. Finally, the files are arranged by their first digits, so that 01 00 22 precedes 02 00 22.

Middle-digit filing begins with the middle digits, followed by the first digit, and finally by the terminal digits. Numeric filing requires more training, but once the system has been mastered, fewer errors occur than with alphabetic filing.

CRITICAL THINKING APPLICATION   **11-8**

Susan is unsure whether alphabetic or numeric filing is best in the healthcare facility. What are some advantages and disadvantages of each method?

PROCEDURE 11-4   File Patient Health Records

Goal: *File patient health records using two different filing systems: the alphabetic system and the numeric system.*

Scenario: The agency utilizes the alphabetic system. You need to file health records in the correct location.

EQUIPMENT and SUPPLIES

- Paper health records using the alphabetic filing system
- Paper health records using the numeric filing system
- File box(es) or file cabinet

PROCEDURAL STEPS

1. Using alphabetic guidelines, place the records to be filed in alphabetic order.
   PURPOSE: Placing the records in alphabetic order before filing in the box or cabinet will make the filing process more efficient.

2. Using the file box or file cabinet, locate the correct spot for the first file.
3. Place the health record in the correct location. Continue these filing steps until all the health records are filed.
4. Using numeric guidelines, place the records to be filed in numeric order.
   PURPOSE: Placing the records in numeric order before filing in the box or cabinet will make the filing process more efficient.
5. Using the file box or file cabinet, locate the correct spot for the first file.
6. Place the health record in the correct location. Continue these filing steps until all the health records are filed.

Subject Filing

Subject filing can be either alphabetic or **alphanumeric** (e.g., A 1-3, B 1-1, B 1-2, and so on) and is used for general correspondence. The main difficulty with subject filing is indexing, or classifying; that is, deciding where to file a document. Many papers require cross-referencing. An example would be if you had a subject folder for Laboratory Supplies and the same organization provides you with your General Medical Supplies; there should be a notation in the Laboratory Supplies folder stating to See Also General Medical Supplies and vice versa. All correspondence dealing with a particular subject is filed together. The papers in the folders are filed chronologically with the most recent on top. The subject headings are placed on the tabs of the folders and filed alphabetically.

Color-Coding

When a color-coding system is used, both filing and finding files is easier, and misfiling of folders is kept to a minimum. The use of color visually restricts the area of search for a specific record. A misfiled record is easily spotted even from a distance of several feet. In color-coding, a specific color is selected to identify each letter of the alphabet. Any selection of colors may be used, and the division of the alphabet is determined by one's own needs. However, studies have shown that the frequency with which different letters occur varies widely.

Alphabetic Color-Coding

As medicine continues to consolidate into larger facilities with more patients in one system, the filing of patients' records becomes more complicated, and color-coding becomes more useful. Several color-coding systems use two sets of 13 colors: one set for letters A to M, and a second set of the same colors on a different background for letters N to Z.

Many ready-made systems are available for use. Self-adhesive, colored letter blocks with either two or three letters in the specific colors are supplied in rolls. The color blocks with the appropriate letter are placed on the index tab of the folder, along with the patient's full name. The letters are in pairs so that they can be seen from either side of the record. Strong, easily differentiated colors are used, creating a band of color in the files that makes spotting out-of-place folders easy (Figure 11-14).

Numeric Color-Coding

Color-coding is also used in numeric filing. Numbers 0 through 9 are each assigned a different color. In a terminal digit filing system, the colors for the last two numbers are affixed to the tab. If the number 1 is red and 5 is yellow, all files with numbers ending in 15 have a red and yellow band. Usually a predetermined section of the number is color-coded.

Other Color-Coding Applications

Color can work in many other ways for the efficient healthcare facility. Small tabs in a variety of colors can be used to identify certain types of insured patients and other specific information. For example, a red tab over the edge of the folder may identify a patient on Medicare; a blue tab may identify a Medicaid patient; a green tab may identify a workers' compensation patient; matching tabs may be attached to the insured's ledger card; research cases may be identified

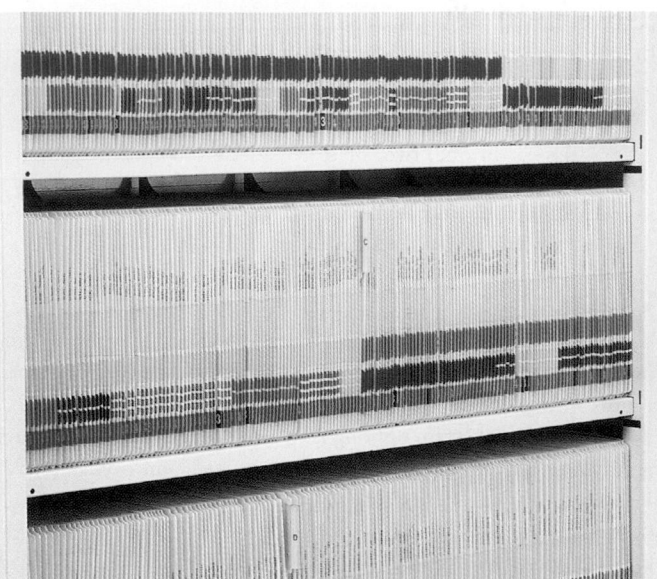

FIGURE 11-14 With color-coding of patients' records, a misplaced file is easily spotted. (Courtesy Bibbero Systems, Petaluma, California.)

by a special color tab; and brightly colored labels on the outside of a patient's record can indicate certain health conditions, such as drug allergies. In a partnership practice, a different color folder or label may identify each provider's patients. Color also can be used to differentiate dates: one color for each month or year.

The use of color in filing is limited only by the imagination. One word of caution: Every person in the facility who uses the files must know the key to the coding, and the key should also be written in the facility's policy and procedures manual.

ORGANIZATION OF FILES

Providers find studying a disorganized patient record very difficult. Some systematic method must be followed in placing items in the patient folder. From the filing standpoint, it should be emphasized that when a patient record is not in actual use, it should be in only one place—the filing cabinet or on the shelf. Many precious hours can be lost searching for misplaced or lost records carelessly left unfiled.

The patient's full name, in indexing order, should be typed on a label and the label attached to the folder tab. A strip of transparent tape can be placed on the label to prevent smudging. The patient's full name should also be typed on each sheet in the folder. Some of the types of records common to the healthcare setting, other than patient records, include health-related correspondence, general correspondence, practice management files, miscellaneous files, and tickler or follow-up files.

Health-Related Correspondence

Correspondence pertaining to patients' health should be filed in the patient's health record. Other medical correspondence should be filed in a subject file.

General Correspondence

The provider's office operates as both a business and a professional service. Correspondence of a general nature pertaining to the operation of the office is part of the business side of the practice. Usually, a special drawer or shelf is set aside for the general correspondence. The correspondence is indexed according to subject matter or the names of the correspondents. The guides in a subject file may appear in one, two, or three positions, depending on the number of headings, subheadings, and subdivisions.

Practice Management Files

Of course, the most active financial record is the patient ledger. In facilities that still use a manual system, this is a card or vertical tray file, and the accounts are arranged alphabetically by name. At least two divisions are used: active accounts and paid accounts.

Miscellaneous Files

Papers that do not warrant an individual folder are placed in a miscellaneous folder. In that folder, all papers relating to one subject or with one correspondent are kept together in chronologic order, with the most recent on top, and then filed alphabetically with other miscellaneous material. Related materials may be stapled together. Never use paper clips for this purpose. When as many as five papers accumulate with one correspondent or subject, a separate folder should be prepared. Other business files include records of income and expenses, financial statements, income and payroll tax records, canceled checks, and insurance policies. These papers may be filed chronologically.

Tickler or Follow-Up Files

The most frequently used follow-up method is a **tickler file**, so called because it tickles the memory that something needs to be done or followed up on a particular date. The tickler file is always a chronologic arrangement. In its simplest form, it consists of notations on the daily calendar. If information, such as an x-ray report or laboratory report, is expected about a patient with an appointment to come in, the medical assistant might make a note on the calendar or tickler file a day ahead to check on whether the report has arrived.

The tickler file can be a part of a computerized health record system or could be as simple as an e-mail sent to oneself. Many people put reminders on their cell phones using an application (app) specially designed for memos and reminders. The tickler file could also be a card file; 12 guides, one for each month, are placed at the front of the cabinet, container, or other object used to hold the folders. Notations of actions to be taken are placed behind the guides for specific days of the current month. Notations for future months are placed behind the guide for that month. To be effective, the tickler file must be checked first thing each day.

The tickler file can be used in many ways. It is a useful reminder of recurring events, such as payments, meetings, and so forth. On the last day of each month, all the notations from behind the next month's guide are distributed among the daily numbered guides, and the guide for the month just completed is placed at the back of the file.

CRITICAL THINKING APPLICATION   11-9

Susan is responsible for checking the tickler file daily. What types of documents and duties might she find inside these files?

Transitory or Temporary File

Many papers are kept longer than necessary because no provision is made for segregating those with a limited usefulness. This situation can be prevented by having a transitory or temporary file. For example, if a medical assistant writes a letter requesting a reprint of the new patient brochure, the file copy is placed in the transitory folder until the reprint is received. When the reprint is received, the file copy is destroyed. The transitory file is used for materials with no permanent value. The paper may be marked with a T and destroyed when the action is completed.

CLOSING COMMENTS

Just as in every aspect of the medical profession, advances in health records management are occurring rapidly, allowing providers and other caregivers to perform their duties more efficiently and accurately. A medical assistant must constantly be willing to learn and to adapt to changes arising from legislation and technologic advances. Computers have become generally accepted as a means of recording health information.

A primary goal of all healthcare facilities is to provide efficient, high-quality patient care. The EHR system can help the staff reach that goal. In the future, every provider's office, hospital, pharmacy, and healthcare facility may be able to access information in minutes, which will improve patient care and save lives. Stay abreast of news and articles related to EHR systems. Remember, the healthcare industry is one of constant growth and learning, and today's information technology provides the medical assistant with endless opportunities to make that growth rewarding and applicable to your current position.

Patient Education

Patients worry about the security of their information, particularly about who can access it. Lawsuits often are filed when patients discover that an unauthorized person has accessed their PHI. The medical assistant should listen to a patient's concerns and explain the safety procedures that apply to the EHR in language the patient can understand. Some facilities prepare a brochure to explain the conversion process to the patient and the advantages of the EHR system.

The medical assistant should expect hesitation and even reluctance from patients who are concerned about the privacy of their health information. Patients are concerned about lack of control over who views their records. Be prepared to answer their questions about the safety of their records as related to the EHR. The medical assistant must know how the EHR is protected and what security measures are in place to be able to reassure the patients that their records are protected at all times.

Legal and Ethical Issues

The authority to release information from the health record lies solely with the patient unless such a release is required by law through a **subpoena duces tecum**. Ownership of the record often is a subject of controversy. The record belongs to the provider; the information belongs to the patient.

Remember that the EHR system contains information that is confidential at all times. The patient must authorize the release of health information in electronic form, just as if it were a piece of paper. EHR systems must:

- Maintain the security and confidentiality of data
- Be easily retrievable
- Have safeguards against the loss of information
- Protect patients' rights to confidentiality and privacy
- Require identification and authentication for access

By supporting these requirements, the medical facility remains in compliance with applicable laws and gains the trust of patients, who are reassured that their health information is secure and safe.

Professional Behaviors

Once the medical assistant has been trained on the EHR system and has had the opportunity to use it for a time, daily use should become second nature. In fact, it may be difficult to imagine a workday without the system! By being open to change and willing to learn, the medical assistant can set a good example for all employees and will be more receptive to the process of change. Be encouraging to other staff members while training on the system, and if technology comes easily to you, share your knowledge with others and assist wherever possible. Do not expect to master the system in a week; instead, realize that a new system has a learning curve and be patient with and receptive to the educational process. Keep technical support phone numbers handy and feel free to use them whenever a new or complicated issue arises. Work as a team, and if possible, help others who might find learning the system more of a struggle. Above all, while getting used to the new technology, make sure your attitude is one of enthusiasm, interest, and curiosity.

SUMMARY OF SCENARIO

Susan looks forward to attending her medical assisting classes each day and works diligently to perform to the best of her ability in the classroom. She strives to do well on each procedure check-off and each examination she completes. Her instructors provide excellent feedback and appreciate her contributions to the class.

Susan has the attitude that everything she is allowed to do in the healthcare facility is a learning tool. She regularly asks for additional responsibilities and is always ready to assist a co-worker. Dr. Thomas has recognized that she has the desire to learn, and he gives her many opportunities to glean more knowledge through the everyday activities in the office.

Although she is new to the medical profession, Susan learns quickly and thinks logically. She knows the rules and regulations on patient confidentiality and is always careful about the information she provides to those who request it. She is never hesitant about asking her office manager for guidance if she is unsure about any aspect of her duties. Susan is understanding and respectful when patients are concerned about their privacy. Her confidence and warm personality play a role in the trust she earns from the patients at the clinic.

Susan is willing to admit when she has made an error and has sought advice from Dr. Thomas and her office manager when an error needed correction. Although filing is not one of her favorite duties, she can be counted on to do her best while completing this important task. She realizes that filing is critical because the documents in the patient's health record direct the care provided to the patient. An abnormal laboratory report that is missing can make a crucial difference in the patient's care. She takes pride in her work and is efficient and accurate where health records are concerned. When she is faced with a task new to her, she considers it a learning experience and asks for help if she is not completely sure about the way to handle a situation.

Susan's co-workers are supportive and always willing to assist her as she learns to be the best medical assistant she can be. Her future as a professional medical assistant certainly holds opportunity and chances for advancement. Just as important, patients trust her. She has alleviated patients' concerns about EHRs by taking the time to explain privacy policies and exactly what information will be accessible to third parties. This trust also gives patients the confidence to reveal personal information and to know that it will be held in the strictest confidence, not just by Susan, but by each employee in the provider's office.

SUMMARY OF LEARNING OBJECTIVES

1. Define, spell, and pronounce the terms listed in the vocabulary.
   Spelling and pronouncing terms correctly bolster the medical assistant's credibility. Knowing the definition of these terms promotes confidence in communication with patients and co-workers.

2. Name and discuss the two types of patient records.
   The two major types of patient records are the paper health record and the electronic health record (EHR). The EHR is much more efficient than the paper record and most healthcare facilities have switched to EHRs for a number of reasons.

3. State several reasons that accurate health records are important.
   Health records must be accurate primarily so that the correct care can be given to the patient. The record also helps ensure continuity of care between providers so that no lapse in treatment occurs. The record serves as indication and proof in court that certain treatments and procedures were performed on the patient; therefore, it can be excellent legal support if it is well maintained and accurate. Health records also aid researchers with statistical information.

SUMMARY OF LEARNING OBJECTIVES—*continued*

4. **Differentiate between subjective and objective information in creating a patient's health record.**

   Subjective information is provided by the patient, whereas objective information is provided by the provider. Examples of subjective information include the patient's address, Social Security number, insurance information, and description of what he or she is experiencing. Objective information is obtained through the provider's questions and observations made during the examination.

   Refer to Procedure 11-1 to see how to create a patient's health record and register a new patient in practice management software.

5. **Explain who owns the health record.**

   The provider owns the physical health record, but the patient controls the information contained in it.

6. **Distinguish between an electronic health record (EHR) and an electronic medical record (EMR).**

   The EHR is an electronic record of health-related information about an individual that conforms to nationally recognized interoperability standards and that can be created, managed, and consulted by authorized clinicians and staff from more than one healthcare organization. The EMR is an electronic record of health-related information about an individual that can be created, gathered, managed, and consulted by authorized clinicians and staff within one healthcare organization.

7. **Do the following related to healthcare legislation and EHRs:**

   - Explain how the American Recovery and Reinvestment Act (ARRA) of 2009 applies to the healthcare industry.

     ARRA, commonly known as the Economic Stimulus Package, was meant to promote economic recovery. The health information technology aspects of the bill provide slightly more than $31 billion for healthcare infrastructure and EHR investment. The sections of the ARRA that pertain to healthcare are collectively known as the Health Information Technology for Economic and Clinical Health (HITECH) Act.

   - Define meaningful use and relate it to the healthcare industry.

     Meaningful use, defined simply, means that providers must show that they are using EHR technology in ways that can be measured significantly in quality and quantity. If providers meet the meaningful use requirements, they will qualify for incentive payments.

   - List the three main components of meaningful use legislation.

     The three main components of meaningful use are (1) use of certified EHR in a meaningful manner, such as e-prescribing; (2) use of certified EHR technology for electronic exchange of health information to improve quality of health care; and (3) use of certified EHR technology to submit clinical quality reports, procedure and diagnosis codes, surveys, and other measures.

8. **Explore the advantages, disadvantages, and capabilities of an EHR system, and explain how to organize a patient's health record.**

   Advantages of the EHR include: reduction of errors, reduction of costs, reduction of staffing needs, legible documentation, easy accessibility, and less physical storage space than paper records. Disadvantages of the EHR include: lack of capital, fear of something new, startup costs, and space for equipment. Some capabilities of an EHR system include specialty practice components, appointment scheduling features, prescription writers, medical billing systems, charge capture, eligibility verification, referral management, laboratory order integration, patient portals, and many other features that vary from system to system.

   Refer to Procedure 11-2 for instructions on how to organize a patient's health record and upload documents to the EHR.

9. **Discuss the importance of nonverbal communication with patients when an EHR system is used.**

   Eye contact is critical when an EHR system is used with patients. Body language must indicate that the medical assistant is open to and listening to the patient's concerns, not just concentrating on data entry. Providers and medical assistants alike may have to relearn how to interact with patients in a natural way while using the laptop or tablet in the examination room. Realize that during the implementation period, processing and serving patients may take longer because the staff is using new technology. Most patients are understanding about this if the medical assistant explains that a new system is in place and asks for patience. Because patients are not always technologically savvy, most will be supportive and interested in the EHR system.

10. **Discuss backup systems for the EHR, as well as the transfer, destruction, and retention of health records as related to the EHR.**

    The provider must have a backup system for the EHR in case a medical office is without power for a significant amount of time. The EHR systems can be set to automatically back up the information at specified times during the day. This means that a minimum amount of data would be lost if the power went out. Options include external hard drive, full server backup, and online backup systems. In most medical offices, records are classified in three ways: active, inactive, and closed. The process of moving a file from active to inactive is called purging. Providers have an obligation to retain patient records. The records of any patient covered by Medicare or Medicaid must be kept at least 10 years.

11. **Describe how and when to release health record information; discuss health information exchanges (HIEs).**

    The healthcare facility must be extremely careful when releasing any type of medical information; the patient must sign a release for information to be given to any third party. Requests for medical information should be made in writing. Pay particular attention to records release requests involving a minor.

    There are currently three kinds of HIE—directed exchange, query-based exchange, and consumer-mediated exchange—and the implementation of HIE varies from state to state.

12. **Identify and discuss the two methods of organizing a patient's paper medical record.**

    The source-oriented medical record (SOMR) categorizes the content by its source, such as provider, laboratory, radiology, hospital, and consultation. Within each source category the content is arranged in reverse chronologic order so that the most recent content is viewed first.

Continued

SUMMARY OF LEARNING OBJECTIVES—*continued*

The problem-oriented medical record (POMR) categorizes each of the patient's problems and elaborates on the findings and treatment plans for all concerns. Detailed progress notes are kept for each individual problem. This method addresses each of the patient's concerns separately, whereas a source-oriented record may address all problems and concerns at one time, usually covering one to three patient concerns per office visit. The POMR helps ensure that individual problems are all addressed.

13. **Discuss how to document information in an EHR and a paper health record, and how to make corrections/alterations to health records.**

Documenting information in an EHR involves using radio buttons, drop-down menus, and free-text boxes. When documenting in a paper health record, the entry will always start with the date in the MM/DD/YYYY format. All entries must be written in black or blue ink and follow the format designated by the healthcare facility.

To create a handwritten correction to a health record, a line should be drawn through the error, the correction inserted above or immediately after, and the person making the correction should write his or her initials or signature and the date below the correction. Errors made while using an EHR are corrected in the usual way; however, an error discovered in an entry at a later date is corrected in the same manner as for a handwritten entry.

14. **Discuss dictation and transcription, and discuss transfer, destruction, and retention of medical records as related to paper records.**

With the increased use of EHRs and voice recognition software, there is decreased need for transcription. Transcription can be done from handwritten notes, or more likely from machine dictation. Accuracy and speed are important. Some healthcare offices use voice recognition software for transcription.

As with EHRs, paper health records are also classified as active, inactive, and closed. Large healthcare facilities may find it advisable to convert their paper health records to microfilm.

15. **Identify filing equipment and filing supplies needed to create, store, and maintain medical records.**

Several types of equipment and supplies are needed to manage patients' records. Office space availability; structural considerations; cost of space and equipment; size, type, and volume of medical records; confidentiality requirements; retrieval speed; fire protection; and cost should all be considered when choosing filing equipment. Filing equipment includes: drawer files, horizontal shelf files, rotary circular files, compactable files, automated files, and card files. Filing supplies include divider guides, outguides, file folders, and labels.

16. **Describe indexing rules, and how to create and organize a patient's health record.**

Five basic steps are involved in document filing. (1) The papers are conditioned, which is the preparatory stage for filing. (2) The documents are released, which means they are ready to be filed because they have been reviewed or read and some type of mark has been placed on the document to indicate this. (3) The documents are indexed, which involves deciding where each document should be filed and coding it with some type of mark on the paper indicating that decision. (4) Sorting involves placing the files in filing sequence. (5) The actual filing and storing of the documents is the last step. Refer to Table 11-2 for indexing rules. Refer to Procedure 11-3 for information on creating and organizing a paper health record.

17. **Discuss the pros and cons of various filing methods, as well as how to file patient health records.**

Both the alphabetic and numeric filing systems have advantages and disadvantages. Perhaps most important is the staff's preference. Some find it easier to retrieve files that are in standard alphabetic order, whereas others prefer a numeric system. The numeric system is more confidential than an alphabetic system. Some staff members prefer a combination of the two, called the alphanumeric system. Both effectively keep health records in good order and allow the medical assistant to spot a misfiled record quickly.

Refer to Procedure 11-4 to see how to file patient health records.

18. **Discuss organization of files, as well as health-related correspondence.**

When a patient record is not in actual use, it should only be in the filing cabinet or on the shelf. Health-related correspondence, including general correspondence, should be filed appropriately. Practice management files are usually divided into active and paid accounts. Papers that do not warrant an individual folder are placed in the miscellaneous folder. Follow-up files are frequently called "tickler files." Transitory (i.e., temporary) files can be helpful for material with no permanent value.

19. **Discuss patient education, as well as legal and ethical issues, related to the health record.**

The primary goal of all healthcare facilities is to provide efficient, high-quality patient care. Patients worry about the security of their information and lawsuits can be filed when patients discover that an unauthorized person has accessed their protected health information (PHI). The authority to release information from the health record lies solely with the patient unless such a release is required by law through a *subpoena duces tecum*.

CONNECTIONS

📖 Study Guide Connection: Go to the Chapter 11 Study Guide. Read and complete the activities.

evolve Evolve Connection: Go to the Chapter 11 link at *evolve.elsevier.com/kinn* to complete the Chapter Review Quiz. Check out the other resources listed for this chapter to make the most of what you have learned from The Health Record.

BASICS OF DIAGNOSTIC CODING

12

SCENARIO

Mike Simeone, a recent medical assistant graduate, excelled in his diagnostic coding course. Recently he found an entry-level coding position in a gastroenterology practice managed by Dr. Marcia Buckner and Dr. Kevin Walker.

Mike is a little nervous but also excited about starting ICD-10-CM coding. He has studied the similarities and differences between the previous edition (ICD-9-CM) and the ICD-10-CM, and he knows that they share a similar foundation. Mike has used encoder software in some of his classes, which helped him determine the most specific and accurate code. Mike noticed that the new software update in the medical office has an ICD-10-CM module, which he is eager to try.

Mike has had some previous experience working in health records, which gives him a strong understanding of the importance of accurate, quality documentation. He knows where to look to find diagnostic statements in providers' orders, treatment plans, progress notes, surgical reports, and other medical reports.

While studying this chapter, think about the following questions:

- How do the format, layout, and conventions of the ICD-10-CM manual help the medical assistant search for the most accurate and specific diagnostic code?

- Why is the quality of health record documentation critical to diagnostic coding?
- Why does the medical assistant need to know the steps for performing diagnostic coding?

LEARNING OBJECTIVES

1. Define, spell, and pronounce the terms listed in the vocabulary.
2. Describe the historical use of the *International Classification of Disease* (ICD) in the United States.
3. Describe the transition from ICD-9-CM diagnostic coding to ICD-10-CM diagnostic coding.
4. Identify the structure and format of the ICD-10-CM.
5. Describe how to use the Alphabetic Index to select main terms, essential modifiers, and the appropriate code (or codes) and code ranges.
6. Do the following related to the Tabular List:
   - Explain how to use the Tabular List to select main terms, essential modifiers, and the appropriate code (or codes) and code ranges.
   - Summarize coding conventions as defined in the ICD-10-CM coding manual.

7. Review coding guidelines to assign the most accurate ICD-10-CM diagnostic code.
8. Explain how to abstract the diagnostic statement from a patient's health record.
9. Describe how to use the most current diagnostic codes and perform diagnostic coding.
10. Identify how encoder software can help the coder assign the most accurate diagnostic codes.
11. Explain the importance of coding guidelines for accuracy, and discuss special rules and considerations that apply to the code selection process.
12. Use tactful communication skills with medical providers to ensure accurate code selection.
13. Review medical coding ethical standards.

VOCABULARY

abstract A summary of the diagnostic statement and/or procedures and services performed.

acute The initial assessment and treatment of the disease, condition, or injury.

chronic A disease that manifests over a long period because medical treatment has not resolved it.

Coding Clinic An industry journal that provides insight into the coding of complex medical cases. The journal is sponsored by

the American Hospital Association (AHA), which also supports a website (*www.codingclinicadvisor.com*) that can accept questions from coders on specific cases.

diagnostic statement Information about a patient's diagnosis or diagnoses that has been extracted from the medical documentation, such as the history and physical finding, operative reports, and encounter form.

encounter Every meeting between a patient and a healthcare provider. The patient's history and chief complaint, in addition to the medical services provided, are documented in the patient's health record.

etiology The cause of a disorder; a claim may be classified according to the etiology.

histologic The microscopic composition of tissue.

impending A term used in the diagnosis of a condition that can be imminently threatening. For example, a patient showing signs of prediabetes may in the near future develop diabetes; therefore, in this case, diabetes is an impending condition.

manifestation An indication of the existence, reality, or presence of something, especially an illness; a secondary process.

neoplasm A growth of uncontrolled, abnormal tissue; a tumor. The ICD-10-CM assigns diagnostic codes for neoplasms based on six criteria, which can be found in a table that follows the Alphabetic Index.

notations Instructions or guides for assigning classifications, defining category content, or using subdivision codes. Notations are found in both the Alphabetic Index and the Tabular List.

reimbursement The process by which the medical office submits a claim to the insurance company, which then pays the provider for services rendered. All insurance claims must submit diagnoses and procedures as codes, not as descriptions.

THE HISTORY OF MEDICAL CODING

Medical coding began as medical classification in seventeenth century England. John Graunt, a statistician, wanted to study causes of mortality in children under age 6, so he developed a medical classification system. In the mid-1800s, William Farr, a medical statistician, established a more organized disease classification to widen the system to patients of all ages. The principles of Farr's classification method, and those of Jacques Bertillon, chief of statistics for the city of Paris, developed into the *International List of Causes of Death,* which was published in Chicago in 1893 by the International Statistics Institute. This list was revised every 10 years. After the League of Nations was established in 1920, its members saw the need for use of the classification system by a variety of stakeholders, including insurers, health administrators, hospitals, and military medical providers. The name of the list was changed to the *International List of Diseases.*

In 1946 the International Commission of the World Health Organization (WHO) established codes to define specific infectious diseases, parasites, symptoms, and causes of death. This code set was called the *Manual of the International Statistical Classification of Diseases, Injuries, and Causes of Death* (ICD).

(*Note:* It is important to understand the difference between the ICD and the *Clinical Modification* versions (i.e., ICD-9-CM and ICD-10-CM). The ICD is the international version, copyrighted and published by WHO. WHO authorized an adaptation for use in the United States, although all modifications had to conform to WHO conventions.* The adaptation currently used in the United States is the ICD-10-CM. [Other countries also may apply for adaptations.] The *Clinical Modification* version provides much more detail and sometimes has separate sections for procedures.)

The *Clinical Modification* version previously used in the United States (ICD-9-CM) was approved and put into use in 1975. This code set had 3-character categories, 4-character subcategories, and 5-character subdivisions.

In 1995 WHO approved the development of the *International Classification of Diseases, Tenth Revision, Clinical Modification* (ICD-10-CM) code set. This code set has a different format from that of the ICD-9-CM.

Medical Coding in the United States

As history dictates, the original purpose of medical coding was to collect statistical data. The United States is the only country in the world that uses coding for health insurance **reimbursement** purposes. Providers are responsible for billing the insurance company for any services rendered during the *encounter* (i.e., any meeting between a patient and a healthcare provider), and the provider must use approved medical codes for these procedures and services to obtain reimbursement. This means that the provider must supply diagnostic information that demonstrates the need for the rendered procedures and/or services. A *diagnosis* is the determination of the nature of a condition, illness, disease, injury, or congenital defect; the provider assigns a diagnosis through *assessment* of the patient.

All components of the encounter (i.e., diagnostic findings, procedures, and services) are used to determine the charges and to generate an insurance claim. This chapter focuses on the ways the medical assistant should gather diagnostic information and translate it into a diagnostic code. The ICD-10-CM coding manual is used for this purpose.

GETTING TO KNOW THE ICD-10-CM

What Is Diagnostic Coding?

Diagnostic coding is the translation of written descriptions of diseases, illnesses, or injuries into alphanumeric codes. The ICD-10-CM code set identifies the disease or injury for which a patient was treated as a code consisting of up to 7 characters, with a period after the 3rd character (Figure 12-1). Using the ICD-10-CM can help ensure accurate health record documentation and efficient claims processing.

The ICD-10-CM code set is available as online documents from the Centers for Medicare and Medicaid Services (*cms.gov*),

---

*Conventions are abbreviations, punctuation, symbols, instructional notations, and related entities that help the coder select an accurate, specific code.

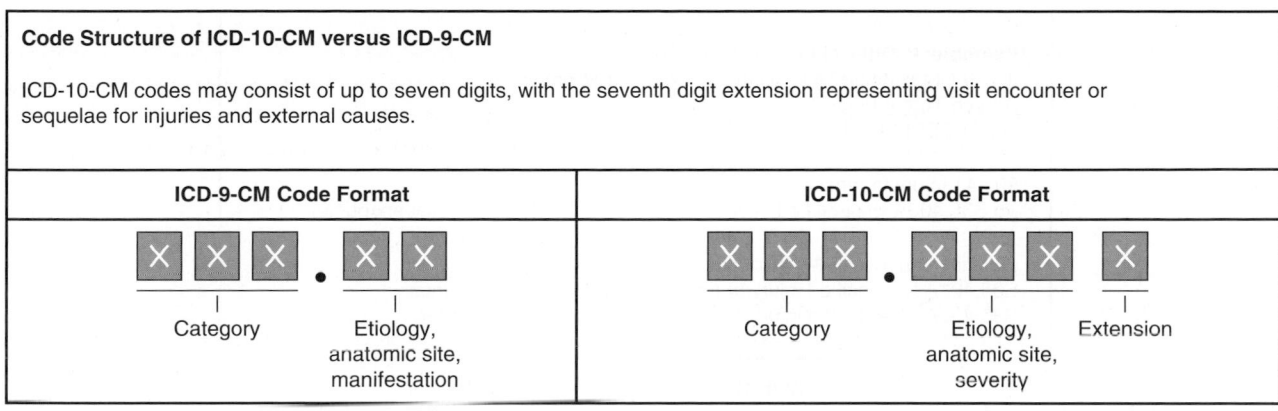

Code Structure of ICD-10-CM versus ICD-9-CM

ICD-10-CM codes may consist of up to seven digits, with the seventh digit extension representing visit encounter or sequelae for injuries and external causes.

ICD-9-CM Code Format	ICD-10-CM Code Format
X X X . X X	X X X . X X X X
Category — Etiology, anatomic site, manifestation	Category — Etiology, anatomic site, severity — Extension

FIGURE 12-1 Code structure and format in the ICD-9-CM and ICD-10-CM.

and as a manual, which is produced by several publishers. Different publishers may use different layouts, symbols, color coding, and some other features. For the coding manual, however, the format, conventions, tables, appendixes, content, and basic structure are the same.

When you use the ICD-10-CM, you will choose a standardized alphanumeric code for the **diagnostic statement** assigned by the provider. Diagnostic statements are found in operative reports, discharge summaries, history and physical exam (H&P) reports, and reports on *ancillary diagnostic services* (e.g., radiology, pathology, and laboratory reports); all of these should support the patient's diagnosis or diagnoses. These reports are used by healthcare providers to code and report clinical information; this coding is required for participation in Medicare and Medicaid insurance programs and by most third-party payers and insurance carriers. The ICD-10-CM also keeps track of various healthcare statistics related to disease and injury. Practice management software, clearinghouses, and third-party payers recognize these codes, which simplifies the coding process and speeds reimbursement to healthcare providers.

Transitioning from ICD-9-CM to ICD-10-CM

As of the publication of this textbook, ICD-10-CM diagnostic coding will be a fairly new process, so it is important to be familiar with the differences between the ICD-9-CM and the ICD-10-CM.

The ICD-9-CM code set (see Figure 12-1) is made up of three volumes. Volumes 1 and 2 are used for diagnostic coding.

- Volume 1 contains the ICD-9-CM Tabular List of Diseases and Injuries (commonly called the *Tabular List*). It contains all the diagnostic codes for disease and injury, grouped into 17 chapters.
- Volume 2 contains the ICD-9-CM Index to Diseases and Injuries (also known as the *Alphabetic Index*). This is an alphabetic list of the *main terms* (discussed later) from the Tabular List and their associated codes. Volume 2 also contains *V codes* (Classification of Factors Influencing Health Status and Contact with Health Service) and *E codes* (Supplementation Classification of External Causes of Injury and Poisoning).

TABLE 12-1   Comparison of the ICD-9-CM and ICD-10-CM Code Sets

The ICD-10-CM differs from the ICD-9-CM in its organization and structure, code composition, and level of detail.

ICD-9-CM CODES	ICD-10-CM CODES
• Consist of 3 to 5 characters	• Consists of 3 to 7 characters
• Character 1: Numeric or alpha (E or V)	• Character 1: Alpha
• Characters 2, 3, 4, 5: Numeric	• Characters 2, 3: Numeric
• Always have at least 3 characters	• Characters 4, 5, 6, 7: May be alpha or numeric
• Decimal placed after character 3	• Decimal placed after character 3
	• Use all letters used except U

- Volume 3 is used by hospitals to code inpatient procedures and services performed in the hospital environment. Most medical offices do not use Volume 3 codes.

The ICD-10-CM follows the same hierarchal structure as the ICD-9-CM in that the first 3 characters represent the code category. Table 12-1 lists some of the significant differences between the ICD-9-CM and ICD-10-CM code sets.

General Equivalence Mappings

To assist with the changeover from the ICD-9-CM to the ICD-10-CM, the Centers for Medicare and Medicaid Services (CMS) has developed code maps, or general equivalence mappings (GEMs) (Figure 12-2). GEMs are used to accurately report ICD-10-CM codes that most closely match ICD-9-CM codes. The translation from ICD-9-CM codes to ICD-10-CM codes through GEMs is based on the description and meaning of the code. According to the CMS, "The purpose of GEMs is to create a useful, practical, code-to-code translation reference dictionary for both code sets, and to offer acceptable translation alternatives wherever possible."

As a medical assistant coder, you must still learn how to assign ICD-10-CM codes. However, GEMs can be helpful and can increase your efficiency in ICD-10-CM coding. A complete list of GEMs is available on the CMS website (*cms.gov*).

Example: ICD-9-CM to ICD-10-CM GEM
ICD-9-CM code 902.41 has the following GEM entry:
<u>Source Target Flags</u>
90241 S35403A 10000

902.41 Injury to renal artery
To S35.403A Unspecified injury of unspecified renal artery, initial encounter

Not included in ICD-9-CM to ICD-10-CM GEM
S35.401A Unspecified injury of right renal artery, initial encounter
S35.402A Unspecified injury of left renal artery, initial encounter

FIGURE 12-2 General equivalence mappings (GEMs).

CRITICAL THINKING APPLICATION   **12-1**

Mike is currently updating the electronic encounter form for the gastroenterology group. However, he is unsure of the accuracy of converting the ICD-9-CM codes to ICD-10-CM codes. What resource can he use to obtain accurate ICD-10-CM codes?

Structure and Format of the ICD-10-CM

The ICD-10-CM also has a Tabular List (officially, the ICD-10-CM Tabular List of Diseases and Injuries) and an Alphabetic Index (the ICD-10-CM Index to Diseases and Injuries). Every ICD-10-CM code begins with an alphabetic letter that indicates the chapter in the Tabular List from which the code originates (Table 12-2). (All the letters of the English alphabet are used except U, which WHO has reserved to assign to new diseases of uncertain **etiology**.) Some conditions use more than one alphabetic letter in their code ranges. For example, the codes in Chapter 1, Certain Infectious and Parasitic Diseases (A00–B99), begin with the letter A or B.

Every year the CMS reviews the ICD-10-CM coding manual, and the update is published on October 1. Additions, revisions, and deletions are made to many of the diagnostic codes, code descriptions, and guidelines. As mentioned previously, *you must always use the current year's coding manual to ensure accurate coding and to comply with regulatory guidelines.*

The CMS prepares Official Guidelines for Coding and Reporting to be used with the ICD-10-CM codes, in addition to instructions on how to report the codes on insurance claim forms. The guidelines are a set of rules that have been developed to accompany and complement the official conventions and instructions provided in the ICD-10-CM proper.

The Alphabetic Index

The Alphabetic Index consists of an alphabetic list of diagnostic terms and related codes. This index includes main terms, nonessential modifiers, essential modifiers, and subterms.

- **Main terms:** These terms appear in bold type.
- **Nonessential modifiers:** These terms follow the main term and are enclosed in parentheses. They are supplementary words or explanatory information; therefore, they do not affect the code assignment.

- **Essential modifiers:** These terms are indented one space to the right under the main term. They change the description of the diagnosis in bold type.
- **Subterms:** These terms are indented one space to the right under an essential modifier (two spaces to the right under the main term). These diagnoses are used when all conditions exist.

Figure 12-3 provides an example of the main term **Colitis**. Follow the list to the modifying term Ischemic, which is indented once. The subterm **acute** is indented once more, twice from the main term. The nonessential modifiers included with the subterm "acute" (i.e., catarrhal, chronic, noninfective, hemorrhagic) do not affect the code assignment.

Colitis (acute) (catarrhal) (chronic (noninfective)
          (hemorrhagic)—*see also* Enteritis K52.9
    allergic K52.2
    amebic (acute) (*see also* Amebiasis) A06.0
        nondysenteric A06.2
    anthrax A22.2
    bacillary—*see* Infection, Shigella
    balantidial A07.0
    Clostridium difficile A04.7
    coccidial A07.3
    collagenous K52.89
    cystica superficialis K52.89
    dietary counseling and surveillance (for) Z71.3
    dietetic K52.2
    due to radiation K52.0
    eosinophilic K52.82
    food hypersensitivity K52.2
    giardial A07.1
    granulomatous—*see* Enteritis, regional, large
        intestine
    infectious—*see* Enteritis, infectious
    ischemic K55.9
        acute (fulminant) (subacute) K55.0
        chronic K55.1
        due to mesenteric artery insufficiency K55.1
        fulminant (acute) K55.0
    left sided K51.50
        with
            complication K51.519

continued

FIGURE 12-3 The main term **Colitis** in the Alphabetic Index.

TABLE 12-2   ICD-1Ø-CM Tabular List of Diseases and Injuries

CHAPTER	TITLE	CODE RANGE	POSSIBLE DIAGNOSIS*	ICD-1Ø-CM CODE
1	Certain Infectious and Parasitic Diseases	AØØ–B99	Measles	BØ5.9
2	Neoplasms	CØØ–D49	Colon cancer	C18.9
3	Diseases of the Blood and Blood-Forming Organs and Certain Disorders Involving the Immune Mechanism	D5Ø–D89	Iron-deficiency anemia	D5Ø.9
4	Endocrine, Nutritional, and Metabolic Diseases	EØØ–E89	Type I diabetes	E1Ø
5	Mental, Behavioral, and Neurodevelopmental Disorders	FØ1–F99	Dementia	FØ3
6	Diseases of the Nervous System	GØØ–G99	Parkinson's disease	G2Ø
7	Diseases of the Eye and Adnexa	HØØ–H59	Glaucoma	H4Ø.9
8	Diseases of the Ear and Mastoid Process	H6Ø–H95	Otitis media, left ear	H6Ø.92
9	Diseases of the Circulatory System	IØØ–I99	Hypertensive heart disease	I11.9
1Ø	Diseases of the Respiratory System	JØØ–J99	Acute sinusitis	JØ1.91
11	Diseases of the Digestive System	KØØ–K95	Inguinal hernia	K4Ø
12	Diseases of the Skin and Subcutaneous Tissue	LØØ–L99	Pressure ulcer of right heel	L89.619
13	Diseases of the Musculoskeletal System and Connective Tissue	MØØ–M99	Rheumatoid arthritis	MØ5
14	Diseases of the Genitourinary System	NØØ–N99	Endometriosis	N8Ø.9
15	Pregnancy, Childbirth, and the Puerperium	OØØ–O94	Ectopic pregnancy	OØØ.9
16	Certain Conditions Originating in the Perinatal Period	PØØ–P96	Neonatal jaundice	P59.9
17	Congenital Malformations, Deformations and Chromosomal Abnormalities	QØØ–Q99	Cleft lip	Q37.9
18	Symptoms, Signs and Abnormal Clinical and Laboratory Findings, Not Elsewhere Classified	RØØ–R99	Abdominal pain	R1Ø.9
19	Injury, Poisoning and Certain Other Consequences of External Causes	SØØ–T88	Left ankle fracture	S82.92xA
2Ø	External Causes of Morbidity	VØØ–Y99	Snowboard accident Fall from cliff Exposure to excessive natural cold	VØØ.318A W15 X31
21	Factors Influencing Health Status and Contact With Health Services	ZØØ–Z99	Pregnancy state	Z33.1

*All diagnoses presented are NOS (not otherwise specified).

CRITICAL THINKING APPLICATION   12-2

Mike sometimes is confused as to which term is the main term and which are modifying terms. What documents or references can help him determine the main term? Whom can he consult in the practice to make sure he understands the main term? What can happen if he selects a modifier or subterm instead of a main term?

Supplementary Sections of the Alphabetic Index

The Alphabetic Index section includes two important tables.

- *Table of Neoplasms:* This table lists neoplasms by anatomic location. For coding purposes, neoplasms are further classified into six categories: Malignant Primary; Malignant Secondary; Ca [cancer] in situ; Benign; Uncertain Behavior; and Unspecified Behavior.
- *Table of Drugs and Chemicals:* This table presents a classification of drugs and other chemical substances; it is used to identify poisonings and external causes of adverse effects.

The six coding classifications are: Poisoning, Accidental (Unintentional); Poisoning, Intentional Self-Harm; Poisoning, Assault; Poisoning, Undetermined, Adverse Effect; and Underdosing.

The Tabular List

The Tabular List is divided into 21 chapters. Most chapter titles specify a particular group of diseases and injuries, and all titles are followed by a code range in parentheses; for example, Chapter 1, Certain Infectious and Parasitic Diseases (A00–B99) (see Table 12-2). Some chapters use a body part or an organ system to group the codes; for example: Chapter 7, Diseases of the Eye and Adnexa (H00–H59); and Chapter 9, Diseases of the Circulatory System (I00–I99). Other chapters group conditions by etiology or the nature of the disease process; for example, Chapter 2, Neoplasms (C00–D49). Chapter 15, Pregnancy, Childbirth, and the Puerperium (O00–O94) groups codes related to the prenatal and postnatal periods. Chapter 20, External Causes of Morbidity (V00–Y99), replaces the V and E codes used in the ICD-9-CM. Chapter 20 also groups codes related to external causes of injury and poisoning. Chapter 21 is Factors Influencing Health Status and Contact With Health Services (Z00–Z99).

Each chapter is subdivided into subchapters, or *blocks,* and each subchapter has a designated 3-character code; these subchapter codes and code ranges form the foundation of the ICD-10-CM code set.

In each chapter, all the 3-character block codes begin with the alphabetic letter assigned to that chapter; for example, in Chapter 6, Diseases of the Nervous System (G00–G99), all the block codes (and their versions) begin with G. If a chapter's code range includes two letters [e.g., Chapter 1, Certain Infectious and Parasitic Diseases (A00–B99)] each 3-character block code begins with one of those two letters. The letter character is followed by a 2-character number.

A summary of the blocks (Figure 12-4) at the beginning of each chapter provides an overview of the chapter.

As mentioned, the ICD-10-CM manual is produced by a variety of publishers, but many of the optional features are similar (remember, the important elements are always the same, regardless of the publisher). For instance, to enable the coder to better maneuver through the Alphabetic Index, each page has *guide words,* which are the first and last words on that page (this is the same arrangement used for the pages of a dictionary). Each chapter of the Tabular List has a different-colored border strip; in some manuals this strip shows the chapter title and the range of codes found on that specific page. In the chapters in the Tabular List, the codes for each category/block are arranged alphabetically (by the initial alpha character) and then numerically. Familiarizing yourself with these tools can help you improve your proficiency as you work through the manual to find the most accurate code.

It is important to note that some codes do not need to be extended beyond the 3-character code, and these are considered valid codes as is; for example, code **I10 {Essential (primary) hypertension}**. If a code has only three characters, do not add a decimal after the 3rd character. If a code has more than three characters, add a decimal point after the 3rd character; for example, **K11.7 {Disturbances of salivary secretion}**. Most ICD-10-CM codes have 4 to 7 characters.

CRITICAL THINKING APPLICATION   **12-3**

Mike is reviewing the Tabular List of the ICD-10-CM coding manual. He notices that each chapter begins with a list of diagnostic categories with a corresponding range of codes. What is this called? How can this feature be used as a tool for accurate ICD-10-CM code assignment?

EXCLUDES 2	
	certain conditions originating in the perinatal period (P04-P96)
	certain infectious and parasitic diseases (A00-B99)
	complications of pregnancy, childbirth and the puerperium (O00-O99)
	congenital malformations, deformations and chromosomal abnormalities (000-Q99)
	endocrine, nutritional and metabolic diseases (E00-E90)
	injury, poisoning and certain other consequences of external causes (S00-T98)
	neoplasms (C00-D49)
	symptoms, signs and abnormal clinical and laboratory findings, not elsewhere classified (R00-R94)

This chapter contains the following blocks:
N00-N08	Glomerular diseases
N10-N16	Renal tubulo-interstitial diseases
N17-N19	Acute kidney failure and chronic kidney disease
N20-N23	Urolithiasis
N25-N29	Other disorders of kidney and ureter
N30-N39	Other disorders of the urinary system
N40-N51	Diseases of male genital organs
N60-N65	Disorders of male genital organs
N70-N77	Inflammatory diseases of female pelvic organs
N80-N98	Noninflammatory disorders of female genital tract
N99	Intraoperative and postprocedural complications and disorders of the genitourinary system, not elsewhere classified

FIGURE 12-4 Chapter blocks in the Tabular List.

Reporting NEC and NOS Codes

In some cases, because of limited documentation in the patient's health record, the medical assistant coder can find it difficult to assign an ICD-10-CM code with a higher specificity. The ICD-10-CM code set accommodates these coding circumstances by establishing "not elsewhere classified" (NEC) and "not otherwise specified" (NOS) guidelines.

- NEC means that the diagnostic statement contains specific wording, but no specific classification exists to match the wording. For example, an NEC code would be assigned if a patient seeks medical attention for **chronic** postoperative pain. The ICD-10-CM code would be **G89.28** {Other chronic postprocedural pain}. For all NEC codes, the last character is always 8.
- NOS codes are used more often than NEC codes. For example, sinusitis with no documentation of the specific sinus site is assigned the NOS code **J32.9** {Chronic sinusitis, unspecified}. The coder should keep in mind that the lack of documentation does not mean that all the patient's sinuses are inflamed; the provider must document the exact site of the sinusitis for a non-NOS code to be assigned. For all NOS codes, the last character is always 9.

Conventions Used in the Tabular List

As mentioned, *conventions* are abbreviations, punctuation, symbols, instructional **notations**, and related entities that help the coder select an accurate, specific code. Conventions are found in the Tabular List, but not in the Alphabetic Index. Understanding their meaning and using them as guides are crucial to accurate coding. The following are the most common conventions.

Placeholder Character. The ICD-10-CM uses the dummy placeholder X in two different ways. The dummy placeholder can be used as the 5th character in certain six-character codes; this allows for future expansion of the code set without interruption of the six-character structure.

Example 12-1—Using the Dummy Placeholder for the 5th Character. T43.4X1A Poisoning by butyrophenone and thiothixene neuroleptics, accidental, initial encounter (unintentional)

Specific categories have a 7th character, but may not use the 4th, 5th, or 6th characters. In these cases, the dummy placeholder X is used to fill the empty character spaces. Note that a dummy placeholder would not be needed for codes with less than 7 characters.

Example 12-2—Using the Dummy Placeholder in 7-Character Codes. S50.01XA Contusion of right elbow

In this case, the 7th character indicates "initial encounter" (see the following section).

The appropriate 7th character is to be added to each code from category S03.
A   initial encounter
D   subsequent encounter
S   sequela

FIGURE 12-5 A 7th character box below the main term.

Codes with 7 Characters. In the ICD-10-CM, the 7th character typically provides specificity about the coded condition. This extension may be a number or letter, and it is always assigned to the 7th character position. A list of possible 7th character codes can be found under the main term in the Tabular List (Figure 12-5).

When Additional Characters Are Required

Every ICD-10-CM code has at least 3 characters: an alphabetic letter followed by two digits. When additional characters are required for accurate coding, the ICD-10-CM coding manual includes symbols indicating how many characters are required. An additional symbol indicates that the 7th character code should follow placeholder X. These symbols are considered a coding convention and provide guidance to ensure coding accuracy.

CRITICAL THINKING APPLICATION   12-4

Mike is looking for the ICD-10-CM code for morbid obesity. From the Alphabetic Index, Mike looked up the code E66 in the Tabular List. The main term, **Overweight and obesity**, has a symbol that indicates a 4th character is needed. What is Mike's next step to assign the most accurate code? Can Mike just use E66? Why or why not?

Punctuation. Four basic forms of punctuation are used in the Tabular List: brackets, parentheses, colons, and braces (Figure 12-6). Each form serves a different purpose to help you read and understand the code descriptions.

Instructional Notations. Instructional notations, which are found in both the Alphabetic Index and the Tabular List, are critical to correct coding practices. They are located directly under the main term.

- **Includes** notes: The word "includes" is used in the Tabular List to clarify the conditions included within the particular chapter, section, category, subcategory, or code. Includes notes begin with the word "includes" when they appear at the beginning of a chapter, section, or category. At the code level, the word "includes" is not present; only a list of terms included in the code is

[ ]	Brackets enclose synonyms, alternative wording, or explanatory phrases.
( )	Parentheses are used to enclose supplementary words, which may be present or absent in the statement of a disease or procedure. These supplementary words do not usually affect the code number selected, but instead provide further definition or specificity to the code description.
:	Colons are used in the Tabular Index after an incomplete term that needs one or more of the modifiers or adjectives that follow to make it assignable to a given category.
{ }	Braces enclose a series of terms, each of which is modified by the statement appearing to the right of the brace.

FIGURE 12-6 Punctuation used in the ICD-10-CM.

provided. For example, to code the diagnostic statement "inflammation due to an infection" correctly, you must include the code for the infectious agent.

- **Excludes** notes: The ICD-10-CM uses two types of exclusion notes, Excludes1 and Excludes2. Either or both statements may be present under a category, subcategory, or code.
  - Excludes1: This is a clear "NOT CODED HERE!" message. It means that the excluded code should never be used with the code above the Excludes1 note. For example, code **G14 {Postpolio syndrome}**, has this Excludes1 note: sequelae of poliomyelitis (B91). As another example, consider that a defect cannot be coded as both a congenital defect and an acquired defect.
  - Excludes2: This means "not included here." The excluded condition is not part of the condition represented by the code; however, a patient may have both conditions concurrently. Excludes2 notes have a corresponding code for the excluded condition. When an Excludes2 note is present, the coder may code both conditions if the patient presents with both. For example, code **F02 {Dementia in other diseases classified elsewhere}** has the following Excludes2 note: vascular dementia (F01.5). This means that vascular dementia is not part of the condition coded as F02; therefore, you can code both dementia (F02) and vascular dementia (F01.5) if the patient has both.
- **Code first/Use additional code** notes: *Code first* notes (Figure 12-7) appear under *manifestation* codes. Manifestation codes specify the way in which an underlying condition appears, or manifests, as a result of an underlying etiology; the main terms of most manifestation codes include the words "in diseases classified elsewhere." A *Code first* note indicates that the underlying condition must be sequenced first, before that manifestation code. For these etiology/manifestation combination codes, a *Use additional code* note is found with the etiology code. The *Code first* and *Use additional code* notes indicate the order in which the codes are arranged: etiology code first, followed by the manifestation code.

  For example, when you code for pain, the code sequence depends on the reason for the encounter. If the reason is that the patient wants a pain management procedure, code for the site of the pain, such as lumbar region pain (**M54.5- Low back pain**) or shoulder pain (**M25.51- Pain in shoulder**). If the patient seeks treatment for an ailment such as an ankle fracture, but is also suffering from limb pain (**M79.6- Pain in limb, hand, foot, fingers and toes**), code the ankle fracture first and the limb pain second.

Cross Reference Notes. Cross reference notes in the Alphabetic Index instruct the coder to check elsewhere in the Index before assigning a code. The ICD-10-CM uses the following three types of cross reference notes:

- *See:* The *see* note (preceded by a long dash) follows a main term. It directs the coder to another main term. The correct code will be found with the main term indicated by the *see* note. For example, **Acidopenia**—*see* Agranulocytosis.
- *See also:* The *see also* note (preceded by a long dash) follows a main term. It indicates that another main term may be checked that may provide additional useful Index entries. For example, **Adiposis**—*see also* Obesity. However, if the original main term provides the necessary code, it is not necessary to follow the *see also* note.
- *See* category: The *see* category note directs the coder to a specific category (which is given as the category's 3-character code). For example: *[main term]* **Intoxication**, *[essential modifier]* meaning, *[subterm]* inebriation—*see* category F10. The *see* category instruction must *always* be followed.

Relational Terms. These terms are used in both the Alphabetic Index and the Tabular List to clarify the context of the disease or injury.

- *And:* In the Tabular List code titles, *and* should be interpreted as meaning "and/or."
- *With:* The term *with* should be interpreted as meaning "associated with" or "due to" when it appears in the Alphabetic Index, or in an instructional note or code title in the Tabular List. In the Alphabetic Index, the word *with* follows immediately after the main term, not in alphabetical order.
- *Due to:* In both the Tabular List and the Alphabetic Index, the term *due to* signifies relationship between two conditions. This assumption can be made when both conditions are present or when the diagnostic statement indicates this relationship.

Coding Guidelines

The coding manual begins with the ICD-10-CM Official Guidelines for Coding and Reporting every coding guideline for the entire ICD-10-CM code set is included in this section. The guidelines are a set of rules that have been developed to complement the official conventions and instructions provided in the ICD-10-CM proper. The guidelines are organized into four sections.

Section I. Conventions, General Coding Guidelines and Chapter Specific Guidelines: This section covers the structure and conventions of the ICD-10-CM classification system, in addition to the general guidelines that apply to the entire system. It also contains chapter-specific guidelines for each of the Tabular List's 21 chapters.

Section II. Selection of Principal Diagnosis: This section includes guidelines for selection of a principal diagnosis for non-outpatient settings.

G30	**Alzheimer's disease**
	Use additional code to identify:
	dementia with behavioral disturbance (F02.81)
	dementia with behavioral disturbance (F02.80)
F02	**Dementia in other diseases classified elsewhere**
	Code first the underlying physiological condition, such as:
	Alzheimer's (G30.-)
	F02.80 Dementia in other diseases classified elsewhere, without behavioral disturbance
	F02.81 Dementia in other diseases classified elsewhere, with behavioral disturbance

FIGURE 12-7 *Code first note.*

Section III. Reporting Additional Diagnoses: This section includes guidelines for reporting additional diagnoses in non-outpatient settings.

Section IV. Diagnostic Coding and Reporting Guidelines for Outpatient Services: As the title indicates, this section includes diagnostic coding and reporting guidelines for outpatient services.

The coding guidelines start with a table of contents for each of the four sections, including the related chapters of disease and injury. After the table of contents, the coding guidelines are presented in section order (i.e., Sections I through IV). For the purposes of outpatient medical office billing, you are most likely to need Sections I and IV.

PREPARING FOR MEDICAL CODING
Extracting Diagnostic Statements
To prepare for medical coding, you must analyze the patient's health record and **abstract** the diagnostic statement documented in the various reports. Sources of diagnostic statements include the encounter form, treatment notes, discharge summary, operative report, and radiology, pathology, and laboratory reports.

Encounter Form
The encounter form (also known as a *superbill*) can be viewed in the electronic health record (EHR). This form is most commonly used to obtain the list of medical services rendered and the treating diagnosis when the total charges are calculated. Although it is a convenient coding reference for the provider and medical staff, possible outdated codes can reduce or delay reimbursement. It is vital that the form used by the medical practice be reviewed annually to ensure that all codes on it have been updated, revised, or deleted according to the latest information from all current coding manuals. Medical practices should ensure that their current encounter form uses ICD-10-CM codes, not ICD-9-CM codes; otherwise, problems with reimbursement will result.

History and Physical Exam
The history and physical exam (H&P) are the starting point of the patient's narrative medical evaluation, which includes the reason the person sought medical attention. The H&P begins with a statement in the patient's own words that describes the reason for seeking medical attention. This statement, called the *chief complaint,* is often abbreviated in the history documentation in the health record. After the chief complaint, the provider documents any other pertinent history about medical, behavioral, and social factors, such as smoking, drinking, drug use, family history, previous surgeries, and hospitalizations.

After recording the patient's history, the provider performs a physical examination. This includes both objective and subjective assessments of the patient's physical status. The final sections of an H&P include an assessment and a plan. The assessment is the provider's evaluation of the findings from the H&P, and it includes a diagnostic statement. The plan is the treatment plan for the conditions noted in the assessment; it may include x-ray studies, laboratory tests, surgery, administration of medications, or other treatments.

Treatment or Progress Notes
Treatment notes are the second most common medical document from which diagnostic statements can be extracted. The format healthcare providers most commonly use for their notes is *SOAP notes,* a system of charting in which information is divided into subjective findings, objective findings, assessment, and plan for treatment. Just as in the H&P, the diagnostic statement can most often be found in the assessment section of the SOAP notes.

Discharge Summary
The discharge summary is used primarily for extracting diagnostic information for patients who were hospitalized, rather than those seen in a provider's office. The main elements of a discharge summary are the patient's admission date, date of discharge, H&P findings, clinical course during hospitalization, health condition on discharge, discharge diagnosis, and aftercare plan. Diagnostic statements are abstracted from the discharge diagnosis section. The medical office can use a discharge summary as an overview of the patient's condition, especially if the discharge was recent.

Operative Report
For patients who underwent surgery as an outpatient or inpatient, the operative report also is used to extract diagnostic statements. An operative report includes the preliminary diagnosis, the final diagnosis, and a detailed description of the operative procedure from start to finish. The medical assistant uses the final diagnosis when searching for and selecting a diagnosis code.

Radiology, Laboratory, and Pathology Reports
Radiology, laboratory, and pathology reports are used to support and/or establish the diagnostic statement. Any findings from these reports must be documented in the treatment notes in the health record so that they can be used for diagnostic coding, charge entry, or insurance billing purposes.

STEPS IN ICD-10-CM CODING
Accurate ICD-10-CM coding requires 8 basic steps (Table 12-3). The first step involves abstracting the diagnostic statement from the health record and determining the main and modifying terms from the various medical reports. The next steps are performed using the Alphabetic Index to search for the code, or code ranges that best fit the diagnostic statement. The remaining steps are performed using the Tabular List to verify and confirm that the code or codes located in the Alphabetic Index fully match the diagnostic statement and are the most specific and accurate diagnostic codes. Procedure 12-1 details the basic coding steps using the ICD-10-CM manual and also encoder software (i.e., TruCode).

CRITICAL THINKING APPLICATION 12-5
In reviewing an encounter form, Mike noticed that the diagnostic statement indicated that the patient needed to be treated for a left inguinal hernia. However, Mike also noted that the surgical report indicated that the left inguinal hernia was obstructed. What should Mike use as the final diagnostic statement? Should he ask the provider which diagnostic statement to use?

TABLE 12-3   Diagnostic Coding Step-by-Step: Parkinson's Disease

Step 1	• *Determine the correct diagnosis from the diagnostic statement.* Parkinson's Disease
Step 2	• *Use the main term to look up the diagnosis in the Alphabetic Index.* **Parkinson's disease, syndrome or tremor** — *see* Parkinsonism
Step 3	• *Look up the "see" term in the Alphabetic Index.* **Parkinsonism** (idiopathic) (primary) G20

Step 4	• *Review the essential modifiers under the main term.*
	Parkinsonism
	  with neurogenic orthostatic hypotension (symptomatic) G90.3
	  arteriosclerotic G21.4
	  dementia G31.83 *[F02.80]*
	    with behavioral disturbance G31.83 *[F02.81]*
	  due to
	    drugs NEC G21.19
	      neuroleptic G21.11
	  neuroleptic induced G21.11
	  postencephalitic G21.3
	  secondary G21.9
	    due to
	      arteriosclerosis G21.4
	      drugs NEC G21.19
	        neuroleptic G21.11
	      encephalitis G21.3
	      external agents NEC G21.2
	      syphilis A52.19
	    specified NEC G21.8
	  syphilitic A52.19
	  treatment-induced NEC G21.19
	  vascular G21.4

Step 5	• *Choose the correct essential modifier based on the diagnostic statement.* Because the diagnostic statement only indicates Parkinson's Disease, code G20 should be chosen.
Step 6	• *Look up code G20 in the Tabular List.* **G20 Parkinson's disease**

Step 7	• *Check for any coding guidelines, conventions, inclusion or exclusion notes, or an additional character symbol.*
	Includes Hemiparkinson's
	                    Idiopathic Parkinsonism or Parkinson's disease
	                    Paralysis agitans
	                    Parkinsonism or Parkinson's disease NOS
	                    Primary Parkinsonism or Parkinson's disease dementia with
	Excludes 1 Parkinsonism (G31.83)

Step 8	• *Assign the final ICD-10-CM code.* **G20 Parkinson's disease**

PROCEDURE 12-1 | Perform Coding Using the Current ICD-10-CM Manual

Goal: *To perform accurate diagnosis coding using the ICD-10-CM manual.*

EQUIPMENT and SUPPLIES

- ICD-10-CM manual (current year)
- Encounter form and other relevant health records

PROCEDURAL STEPS

Preparation

1. Abstract the diagnostic statement from the patient's encounter form and/or other health records:
   (1) Determine the main terms in the diagnostic statement that describe the patient's condition.
   (2) Determine what essential modifiers describe the main term in the diagnostic statement.
   PURPOSE: To extract all diagnoses or diagnostic statements from the health record and to ensure that all parts of the diagnostic statement are included in the encounter form or health record, with nothing missing or added. Then, to identify the main term, essential modifiers, and subterms to be used to search the Alphabetic Index.

Alphabetic Index

1. Locate the main terms from the diagnostic statement in the Alphabetic Index.
   PURPOSE: To provide a starting point for searching the Alphabetic Index.
2. Locate the essential modifiers listed under the main term in the Alphabetic Index.
   PURPOSE: To ensure further specificity of the codes found in the Alphabetic Index.
3. Review the conventions, punctuation, and notes in the Alphabetic Index.
   PURPOSE: To ensure that no additional searches, exclusions, or similar terms are needed to complete the search in the Alphabetic Index.
4. Choose a tentative code, codes, or code range from the Alphabetic Index that matches the diagnostic statement as closely as possible.

PURPOSE: To prevent backtracking and repeated searches in the Alphabetic Index.

Tabular List

1. Look up the codes chosen from the Alphabetic Index in the Tabular List.
   PURPOSE: To begin the process of determining whether the codes selected from the Alphabetic Index are appropriate and accurate.
2. Review notes, conventions, and the Official Coding Guidelines associated with the code and code description in the Tabular List.
   1. Review conventions and punctuation.
   2. Review instructional notations:
      - *Includes* and *excludes* notes
      - *Code first, code also,* and *code additional* notes
      - *and, or,* and *with* statements
   PURPOSE: To ensure that the code or codes selected are appropriate for use and to determine whether they require additional codes or further specificity, or are excluded from use.
3. Verify the accuracy of the tentative code in the Tabular List.
   1. Make sure all elements of the diagnostic statement are included in the codes selected.
   2. Make sure the code description does not include anything not documented in the diagnostic statement.
   PURPOSE: To ensure that the most accurate and specific code is selected and that no contraindication exists to use of the code or codes selected.
4. Extend the codes to their highest level of specificity (up to the 7th character, if required). If a 7th character is required and no codes are present for the 4th, 5th, or 6th characters, it is appropriate to use the dummy placeholder X for these positions.
5. Assign the code (or codes) selected from the Tabular List as the appropriate code for the patient's condition by documenting it in the patient's health record.
   PURPOSE: To ensure that the health record and/or electronic encounter form contain documentation of the code or codes assigned.

PROCEDURE 12-1 *—continued*

Using the TruCode Encoder Software

1. Type in the diagnosis from the diagnostic statement in the search box as in Figure 1.

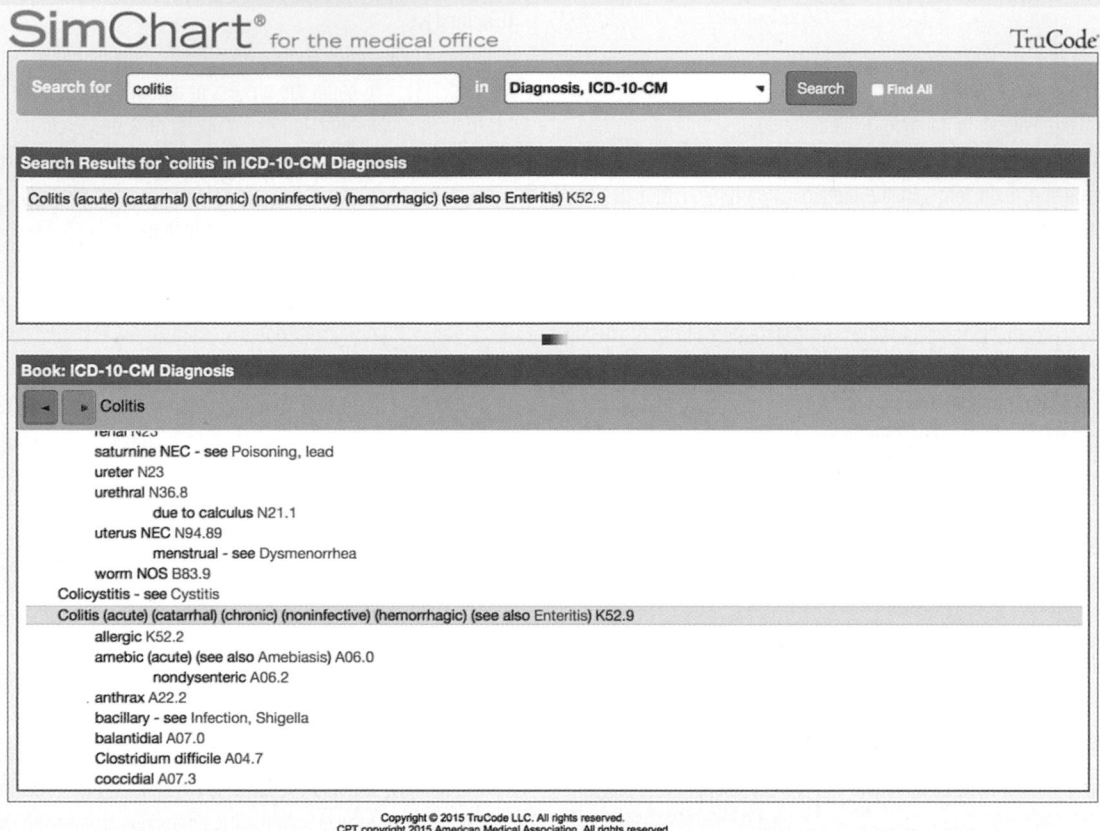

1

2. The software will provide a list of main terms that could be related to the diagnosis typed in the search box. The coder chooses the main term that represents the diagnostic statement.

3. Based on the main term chosen, a list of essential modifiers is presented (Figure 2). The coder must review the diagnostic statement to ensure that all documented modifying terms are identified. If the provider does not document a modifying term, the coder should not assume that a modifying term was implied.

PROCEDURE 12-1   *—continued*

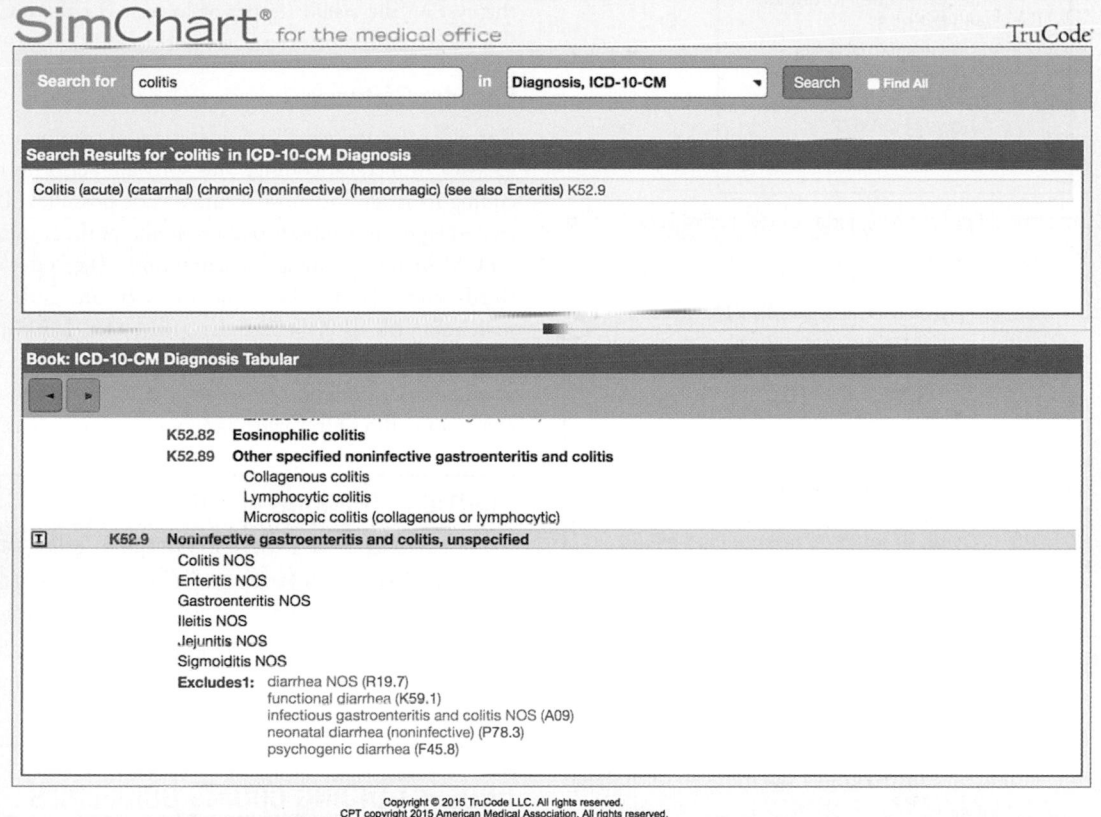

SimChart® for the medical office   TruCode®

Search for [colitis]   in [Diagnosis, ICD-10-CM ▾]   [Search] ☑ Find All

Search Results for `colitis` in ICD-10-CM Diagnosis

Colitis (acute) (catarrhal) (chronic) (noninfective) (hemorrhagic) (see also Enteritis) K52.9

Book: ICD-10-CM Diagnosis Tabular

[◄] [►]

	K52.82	**Eosinophilic colitis**
	K52.89	**Other specified noninfective gastroenteritis and colitis**
		Collagenous colitis
		Lymphocytic colitis
		Microscopic colitis (collagenous or lymphocytic)
Ⓣ	K52.9	**Noninfective gastroenteritis and colitis, unspecified**
		Colitis NOS
		Enteritis NOS
		Gastroenteritis NOS
		Ileitis NOS
		Jejunitis NOS
		Sigmoiditis NOS
		Excludes1: diarrhea NOS (R19.7)
		functional diarrhea (K59.1)
		infectious gastroenteritis and colitis NOS (A09)
		neonatal diarrhea (noninfective) (P78.3)
		psychogenic diarrhea (F45.8)

2

4. In the preceding figure, note the yellow on the left of the chosen diagnosis. In the TruCode program, click on the yellow area, and an instructional notes textbox, which includes coding guidelines, will appear as in Figure 3. To determine the most accurate code, follow these coding guidelines.

5. Once all the menus of essential modifiers and subterms have been presented, choose the most accurate and specific code based on the diagnostic statement.

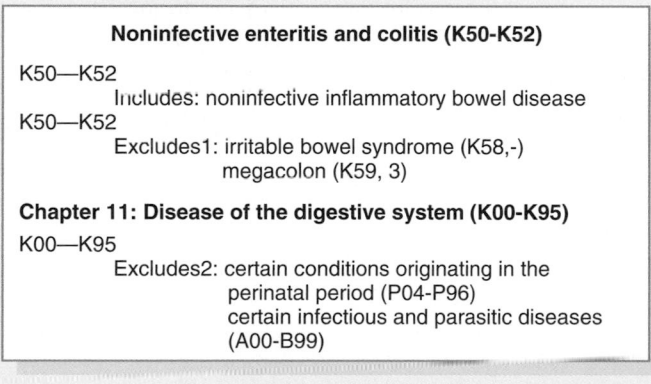

Noninfective enteritis and colitis (K50-K52)

K50—K52
        Includes: noninfective inflammatory bowel disease
K50—K52
        Excludes1: irritable bowel syndrome (K58,-)
                megacolon (K59, 3)

Chapter 11: Disease of the digestive system (K00-K95)

K00—K95
        Excludes2: certain conditions originating in the
                perinatal period (P04-P96)
                certain infectious and parasitic diseases
                (A00-B99)

3

Using the Alphabetic Index

After has been abstracted from the diagnostic statement from the health record have been identified the main terms, start searching for the best code, or code range, in the Alphabetic Index. It is important to note that the Alphabetic Index should be used only as a tool to locate the appropriate code or code range. The Tabular List, with its conventions, punctuation, notes, and guidelines, must always be used to confirm that the code or codes selected are accurate and specific and that no contraindications exist to the use of the code found in the Alphabetic Index. For this reason, never assign a code directly from the Alphabetic Index. Even if only one code is

```
Cyst—continued
    eyelid (sebaceous) H02.829
        infected—see Hordeolum
        left H02.826
            lower H02.825
            upper H02.824
        right H02.823
            lower H02.822
            upper H02.821
```

FIGURE 12-8 Cross section of Cyst (main term); eyelid (essential modifier) in the Alphabetic Index.

```
H02.82    Cysts of eyelid
          Sebaceous cyst of eyelid
    H02.821    Cysts of right upper eyelid
    H02.822    Cysts of right lower eyelid
    H02.823    Cysts of right eye, unspecified eyelid
    H02.824    Cysts of left upper eyelid
    H02.825    Cysts of left lower eyelid
    H02.826    Cysts of left eye, unspecified eyelid
    H02.829    Cysts of unspecified eye, unspecified
               eyelid
```

FIGURE 12-9 Tabular List main term: **Cysts of eyelid**.

found in the Alphabetic Index, it may be used only if a thorough review of the conventions and instructional notations in the Tabular List does not contraindicate it.

Figure 12-8 presents an excerpt from the Alphabetic Index for the main term **Cyst.** The first essential modifier, which is indented one space under **Cyst**, is eyelid. Note the nonessential modifier—sebaceous—in parentheses after eyelid. (Remember, nonessential modifiers add detail, but they do not have to be present in the diagnostic statement for the code to be acceptable for use.) Directly below the essential modifier eyelid, and indented one space under it, are the subterms. Note that there are separate subterms for the left eye and for the right eye. In addition, the diagnostic codes for each eye are further modified by the location of the cyst (upper or lower).

Using the Tabular List

Once are identified at least the first three characters of the code in the Alphabetic Index, turn to the Tabular List. The chapters in the Tabular List are arranged alphabetically according to the initial letter of the 3-character code or codes assigned to each chapter. For example, Chapter 1 has code range A00–B99; Chapter 2 has code range C00–D49; Chapter 3 has code range D50–D89, and so on.

You've determined that the code you probably need is in the H02 code range, turn to the chapter that includes that range (Chapter 7). Figure 12-9, an excerpt from the Tabular List, shows **Cysts of eyelid** as a main term, with the code H02.82. (Note that the nonessential modifier, sebaceous, is not shown in parentheses; rather, it appears under the main term in the nonbold phrase "Sebaceous cyst of eyelid.")

In the coding manual, note the "additional character" symbol, which indicates that code H02.82 requires one more character. All possible diagnoses with six-character codes are indented below the main term. A closer look at the disorders and their codes shows that the 6th character specifies the right or left eye and the location of the cyst on the eyelid (upper or lower). For the not specified code, 9 is placed in the 6th character position.

Encoder Software

Encoder software (e.g., TruCode) is a tool commonly used by coders to assist in medical coding. This software performs computer-aided coding to assign the most accurate code possible. (TruCode is especially helpful to students because it allows them to search the ICD-10-CM manual using a few key terms.) The coder types a few key words into a Search box, and the software finds the most likely matches in the Alphabetic Index. The coder then clicks on a specific code, and the software searches the Tabular List to assign the most accurate code. Encoder software can increase the speed and efficiency of coding for a wide variety of medical cases.

CRITICAL THINKING APPLICATION   12-6

Mike has determined a diagnostic statement to be "Perforation of the tympanic membrane in the left ear." What keyword should be used for the TruCode software search box? To what main term will the encoder go in the Alphabetic Index? What should Mike click to get to the Tabular List? At what point can Mike be sure that he has assigned the most accurate and specific code?

UNDERSTANDING CODING GUIDELINES

Remember that all ICD-10-CM coding manuals, regardless of the publisher, have comprehensive instructional notations and conventions to help the coder select the most accurate diagnostic code or codes. When any discrepancy occurs between reference sources (including this text), the current year's ICD-10-CM coding manual is the final authority; this fact cannot be overemphasized. When coding, you must always refer to and thoroughly review the conventions, instructional notations, code definitions, and other guidelines in the Alphabetic Index and Tabular List in the current year's version of the ICD-10-CM.

The following instructions are designed to provide some additional guidance in selecting diagnostic codes from various chapters in the ICD-10-CM; however, they are not to be considered a replacement for the ICD-10-CM manual, nor do they provide all the coding information, definitions, or explanations found in the manual. The steps for diagnostic coding (see Procedure 12-1) are the same for all chapters of the ICD-10-CM; however, special rules and considerations apply to some chapters that affect the code selection process.

Coding of Signs and Symptoms

Signs and symptoms are coded only if the provider has not yet reached a determination of the final diagnosis. For example, if the provider's notes contain terminology such as "rule out" or "suspected," the coder should use the patient's documented signs and symptoms, including subjective and objective findings. Subjective findings include the patient's chief complaint or statements about why the patient is seeking medical care. Objective findings

---

- Use only if there is no final or determining diagnosis
- Use if "rule out" or "suspected" are included in the assessment or diagnostic statement.
- Signs and symptoms can be subjective and/or objective findings
  - Subjective: Chief complaint or patient's verbal statements
  - Objective: Any measurable indicators found during the physical examination

---

FIGURE 12-10 Rules for coding signs and symptoms.

are any measurable indicators found during the physical examination.

In the Tabular List, ill-defined conditions, signs, and symptoms are found in Chapter 18, Symptoms, Signs, and Abnormal Clinical and Laboratory Findings, Not Elsewhere Classified (R00-R99). Figure 12-10 shows the signs and symptoms section of Chapter 18.

Conditions, signs, and symptoms included in Chapter 18 include the following:

- Not elsewhere classified (NEC) cases, even after all the facts of the medical case have been examined
- Signs or symptoms that existed on the first encounter but were temporary and for which causes could not be determined
- Conditional diagnosis for a patient who failed to return for further care and the cause of whose condition had not yet been determined
- Medical cases referred elsewhere for treatment before a diagnosis could be made
- Not otherwise specified (NOS) cases in which a more precise diagnosis was not available for any reason
- Certain symptoms, for which supplementary information is provided, that represent important problems in the medical care provided

Coding the Etiology and Manifestation

Etiology refers to the underlying cause or origin of a disease. *Manifestation* describes the signs and symptoms of the disease. In the Alphabetic Index, the etiology and manifestation codes are listed together. The etiology code is always listed first, and the manifestation code is listed beside it in italics and enclosed within brackets.

Multiple Coding

In addition to the signs and symptoms that require two codes to fully describe a single condition affecting multiple body systems, other single conditions may require more than one code. In the Tabular List, *Use additional code* notes appear with codes that are not part of an etiology/manifestation pair, but in which a secondary code is useful to fully describe a condition. The sequencing rule is the same as for the etiology/manifestation pair: *use additional code* indicates that a secondary code should be added after the condition code.

For example, consider a bacterial infection that is not included in Chapter 1, Certain Infectious and Parasitic Diseases (A00–B99). A secondary code may be required to identify the organism causing the infection. This secondary code may come from category **B95** {*Streptococcus, Staphylococcus,* and *Enterococcus* as the cause of diseases classified elsewhere} or from category **B96** {Other

bacterial agents as the cause of diseases classified elsewhere}. A *use additional code* note normally is found at the infectious disease code, indicating that the organism code must be added as a secondary code.

As mentioned, *code first* notes are used for certain conditions that involve both an underlying etiology and multiple body system manifestations caused by that etiology. In such cases, the underlying condition should be sequenced first, before the manifestations.

A *code, if applicable, any causal condition first* note indicates that this code may be assigned as a principal diagnosis when the causal condition is unknown or not applicable. If the causal condition is known, the code for that condition should be sequenced as the principal, or first-listed, diagnosis.

Multiple codes may be needed for sequelae, and complication codes and obstetric codes may be needed to more fully describe a condition. See the specific guidelines for these conditions.

Sequela (Late Effects) Codes

Sequelae are the lingering effects produced by a health condition after the acute phase of an illness or injury has ended. The acute phase is considered the first 30 days of a condition with no improvement. There is no time limit on when a sequela code can be used. The residual effect may be apparent early (e.g., another stroke), or it may occur months or years later (e.g., the consequences of a previous injury). Coding of sequelae generally requires two codes sequenced in the following order: the original condition or nature of the sequela is sequenced first; the sequela code is sequenced second.

An exception to the above guidelines are instances in which the code for the sequela is followed by a manifestation code identified in the Tabular List; or, the sequela code has been expanded (at the 4th, 5th, or 6th character) to include the manifestation or manifestations. The code for the acute phase of an illness or injury that led to the sequela is never used with a code for the late effect. The following box presents the rules for coding **impending**, or threatened, conditions.

Rules for Coding Impending or Threatened Conditions

Code any condition described at the time of discharge as "impending" or "threatened."
1. If it did occur, code as a confirmed diagnosis.
2. If it did not occur, consult the Alphabetic Index to determine whether the condition has a subterm for impending or threatened; also check main term entries for Impending and Threatened.
3. If the subterms are listed, assign the given code.
4. If the subterms are not found, code the existing underlying condition or conditions, signs, or symptoms and not the condition described as "threatened" or "impending."

Coding Complications of Care

A complication from medical care generally requires additional procedures or services for a patient, but often the complication is not mentioned as part of the diagnostic statement; this can result in reduced reimbursement. It is important to review the medical documentation to determine whether a complication exists and to code the complication in addition to the diagnostic statement. Keep in mind, not all conditions that occur during or after medical care or surgery are classified as complications. Two criteria must be met: a cause-and-effect relationship must be established between the care provided and the condition; and the documentation must indicate that the condition is a complication.

Coding Infectious and Parasitic Diseases

Multiple diagnostic codes are needed to code infectious or parasitic diseases. The first code identifies the disease or condition (e.g., throat infection), and the second code identifies the organism causing the disease (e.g., enterovirus). The second code can be found in the Tabular List in Chapter 1. The basic coding principles for the use of either combination or multiple codes apply throughout this section of the ICD-10-CM.

Coding Organism-Caused Diseases

The two-step process of coding organism-caused diseases begins with the affected anatomical site. In the case of a throat infection caused by enterovirus, you should first assign the diagnostic code for throat infection, or pharyngitis. In the Tabular List, code **J02.8** {**Acute pharyngitis due to other specified organism**} is accompanied by the following *Use additional code* note: "Use additional code (B95–B97) to identify infectious agent." In the Tabular List, the B95–B97 category/block (found in Chapter 1) is titled Bacterial and Viral Infectious Agents. Starting with code B95, search for the code that specifies enterovirus; this happens to be code **B97.1** {**Enterovirus as the cause of diseases classified elsewhere**}. Note that code B97.1 requires a 5th character; however, no other information is provided by the medical record. Therefore, you can assign code B97.19 {**Other enterovirus as the cause of diseases classified elsewhere**} as the final organism code.

Human Immunodeficiency Virus (HIV) Infection and Acquired Immunodeficiency Syndrome (AIDS)

To code HIV infection and AIDS correctly, it is essential first to understand the descriptions of the codes available. The key is whether the patient has symptoms.

- Human immunodeficiency virus (HIV): This indicates only that the virus is present.
- Acquired immunodeficiency syndrome (AIDS): AIDS is a syndrome; a syndrome is defined as a "group of symptoms occurring together." AIDS is the manifestation of signs and/or symptoms that can occur as a result of HIV infection.

Never code a patient as having HIV unless it is clearly documented as confirmed. Probable and suspected cases are never coded; instead, the signs and symptoms present should be coded. Remember that stringent restrictions are placed on the disclosure of medical information about patients with HIV infection and/or AIDS. Make sure the patient has signed the appropriate release of medical information form before any disclosures are made to third parties.

Selection and Sequencing of HIV Codes

(a) Patient Admitted for HIV-Related Condition. If a patient is admitted for an HIV-related condition, the principal diagnosis should be **B20** {**Human immunodeficiency virus [HIV] disease**}, followed by additional diagnostic codes for all reported HIV-related conditions.

(b) Patient with HIV Disease Admitted for Unrelated Condition. If a patient with HIV disease is admitted for an unrelated condition (e.g., a traumatic injury), the code for the unrelated condition (e.g., the nature of injury code) should be the principal diagnosis. Other diagnoses would be B20, followed by additional diagnostic codes for all reported HIV-related conditions.

(c) HIV Infection in Pregnancy, Childbirth, and the Puerperium. During pregnancy, childbirth, or the puerperium, a patient admitted (or presenting for a healthcare encounter) because of an HIV-related illness should receive a principal diagnostic code **O98.7-** {**Human immunodeficiency [HIV] disease complicating pregnancy, childbirth, and the puerperium**}, followed by B20 and the code for the HIV-related illness. Codes from Chapter 15, Pregnancy, Childbirth, and the Puerperium (O00–O9A), always take sequencing priority.

Patients with asymptomatic HIV infection status who are admitted (or presenting for a healthcare encounter) during pregnancy, childbirth, or the puerperium should receive codes of O98.7- and **Z21** {**Asymptomatic human immunodeficiency virus [HIV] infection status**}.

(d) Encounters for Testing for HIV. If a patient is being seen to determine his or her HIV status, use code **Z11.4** {**Encounter for screening for human immunodeficiency virus [HIV]**}. Use additional codes for any associated high-risk behavior.

If a patient with signs or symptoms is being seen for HIV testing, code the signs and symptoms. An additional counseling code—**Z71.7** {**Human immunodeficiency virus [HIV] counseling**} may be used if counseling is provided during the encounter for the test.

When a patient returns to be informed of his or her HIV test results and the test result is negative, use code Z71.7. If the results are positive, see previous guidelines and assign codes as appropriate.

Coding Neoplasms

A **neoplasm**, or new growth, is coded by the site or location of the neoplasm and its behavior. The Table of Neoplasms (Figure 12-11) is located just after the Alphabetic Index in the coding manual. This table lists the ICD-10-CM codes for neoplasms by anatomic site in alphabetic order. Six possible code numbers exist for each anatomic site, depending on whether the neoplasm is malignant or benign, exhibits uncertain behavior, or is of an unspecified nature. In the Table of Neoplasms, malignant neoplasms are categorized into three separate subclassifications: Malignant Primary, Malignant Secondary, and Ca in situ (carcinoma in situ).

Terms Defining Malignant Neoplasm Sites

- *Primary:* Identifies the originating anatomic site of the neoplasm. A primary malignancy is defined as the original site or sites of the cancer.
- *Secondary:* Identifies sites to which the primary neoplasm has metastasized (spread). A secondary malignancy is defined as a second location to which the cancer has spread from the primary location.
- *Ca in situ:* Carcinoma in situ is defined as the absence of invasion of surrounding tissues. Tumor cells are undergoing

	Malignant Primary	Malignant Secondary	Ca in situ	Benign	Uncertain Behavior	Unspecified Nature		Malignant Primary
bladder (urinary)	C67.9	C79.11	D09Ø	D30.3	D41.4	D49.4	marrow NEC	C96.9
dome	C67.1	C79.11	D09Ø	D30.3	D41.4	D49.4	unspecified side	C40.1Ø
neck	C67.5	C79.11	D09Ø	D30.3	D41.4	D49.4	marrow NEC	C96.9
orifice	C67.9	C79.11	D09Ø	D30.3	D41.4	D49.4	cartilage NEC	C41.9
ureteric	C67.6	C79.11	D09Ø	D30.3	D41.4	D49.4	clavicle	C41.3
urethral	C67.5	C79.11	D09Ø	D30.3	D41.4	D49.4	marrow NEC	C96.9
overlapping lesion	C67.8	—	—	—	—	—	clivus	C41.Ø
sphincter	C67.8	C79.11	D09Ø	D30.3	D41.4	D49.4	marrow NEC	C96.9
trigone	C67.Ø	C79.11	D09Ø	D30.3	D41.4	D49.4	coccygeal vertebra	C41.4
urachus	C67.7	—	D09Ø	D30.3	D41.4	D49.4	marrow NEC	C96.9
wall	C67.9	C79.11	D09Ø	D30.3	D41.4	D49.4	coccyx	C41.4
anterior	C67.3	C79.11	D09Ø	D30.3	D41.4	D49.4	marrow NEC	C96.9
lateral	C67.2	C79.11	D09Ø	D30.3	D41.4	D49.4	costal cartilage	C41.3
posterior	C67.4	C79.11	D09Ø	D30.3	D41.4	D49.4	costovertebral joint	C41.3
blood vessel—*see* Neoplasm, connective tissue							marrow NEC	C96.9
							cranial	C41.Ø

FIGURE 12-11 Table of neoplasms.

malignant changes but are still confined to the point of origin, without invasion of surrounding normal tissue. The *Ca in situ* column is used only if the provider documents that precise terminology.

Definitions of Benign, Uncertain Behavior, and Unspecified Nature Neoplasms

- *Benign:* The growth is noncancerous, nonmalignant, and has not invaded adjacent structures or spread to distant sites.
- *Uncertain Behavior:* The pathologist is unable to determine whether the neoplasm is benign or malignant.
- *Unspecified Nature:* Neither the behavior nor the **histologic** type of neoplasm is specified in the diagnostic statement.

The ICD-9-CM instructional notes state that the behavior of the neoplasm should be determined first for coding.

Most coding decisions on malignant neoplasms are between the primary and secondary classifications. Other terms are used in the following cases:

- *In situ* is used only when the diagnostic statement contains that exact phrase.
- *Unspecified* is used only when no pathologic study has been done, and the neoplasm is still described with a term such as "tumor" or "growth."
- *Uncertain* is used by the provider when it has not been determined whether malignant or benign.

Six Steps for Coding Neoplasms

The following steps can help determine the most specific and accurate diagnostic code for a neoplasm. These steps can be used in addition to the basic diagnostic steps.

1. Using the Table of Neoplasms, determine the site (anatomic location) of the neoplasm and select the row in the table in which it appears.
2. Determine whether the neoplasm is malignant or benign.

3. If the neoplasm is benign, select the column in the table by reviewing the diagnostic statement.
4. If the neoplasm is malignant, determine the table column that best fits its behavior: Malignant Primary, Malignant Secondary, or Ca in situ.
5. Link the appropriate column to the appropriate row.
6. Check the code in the Tabular List to make sure it complies with the guidelines, conventions, and instructional notations in the Tabular List.

The ICD-10-CM manual always provides additional information, definitions, and guidelines for coding neoplasms in the tabular list, just as it does for all other diseases, illnesses, and injuries.

Coding for Diabetes Mellitus

Diabetes mellitus (DM) is classified as type 1 or type 2. Patients with DM type 1 develop the disease because the pancreas is unable to produce insulin. In individuals with DM type 2, the pancreas becomes unable to maintain the level of insulin the body needs to function, or the person has developed target cell resistance to insulin.

The diabetes mellitus codes are combination codes; they include the type of diabetes mellitus, the body system affected, and the complications affecting that body system. Use as many codes within a particular category/block as necessary to describe all the complications of the disease. These codes should be sequenced according to the reason for a particular encounter. Assign as many codes from category/block E08 to E13 (Diabetes Mellitus) as needed to identify all the patient's associated conditions.

Diabetes Mellitus and the Use of Insulin

In the ICD-10-CM, the primary codes for diabetes mellitus (E08–E13) do not include whether the individual is using insulin. Therefore, if insulin use is documented in the health record, a second code is required: **Z79.4 {Long term (current) use of insulin}**. Code Z79.4 should not be assigned if insulin is given temporarily during an encounter to bring the blood glucose level under control in a patient with DM type 2.

Gestational Diabetes

Gestational, or pregnancy induced, diabetes can occur during the second and third trimesters of pregnancy in women who were not diabetic before pregnancy. Gestational diabetes can cause complications in the pregnancy similar to those of pre-existing diabetes mellitus. It also puts the woman at greater risk of developing diabetes after the pregnancy. Codes for gestational diabetes are in subcategory **O24.4** {**Gestational diabetes mellitus**}. No other code from category O24 {**Diabetes mellitus in pregnancy, childbirth, and the puerperium**} should be used with a code from subcategory O24.4. The codes under subcategory O24.4 include diet controlled (O24.410) and insulin controlled (024.414). If a patient with gestational diabetes is treated with both diet and insulin, only the code for insulin controlled is required.

Code **Z79.4** {**Long-term (current) use of insulin**} should also be assigned with codes from subcategory O24.4 if the patient is being treated with insulin.

An abnormal glucose tolerance level in pregnancy is assigned a code from subcategory **O99.81** {**Abnormal glucose complicating pregnancy, childbirth, and the puerperium**}.

Coding for the Circulatory System

Providers use a wide variety of terms and phrases to identify components of the circulatory system. To code disorders of the circulatory system accurately, the coder must carefully review all inclusions, exclusions, conventions, guidelines, and instructional notations associated with each potential code selected.

Myocardial Infarction

A myocardial infarction (MI) is coded as follows:

- As *acute* if it is documented as such in the diagnostic statement or has a stated duration of 8 weeks or less.

- As *chronic* if it is so stated in the diagnostic statement or if symptoms persist after 8 weeks.

Other MI coding considerations include the following:

- If an MI is specified as "old" or "healed" without any current or presenting symptoms, it should be coded using category **I21** {**ST elevation (STEMI) and non-ST elevation (NSTEMI) myocardial infarction**}.

- A history of an MI uses code **I25.2** {**Old myocardial infarction**}. This code is used only if the patient has no symptoms and only if the old MI was diagnosed by means of an electrocardiogram.

- If the patient is symptomatic, code the underlying condition or symptoms only if the underlying condition is not known: **I21.3** {**ST elevation (STEMI) myocardial infarction of unspecified site**}.

Hypertensive Disease

A distinction is made in the ICD-10-CM between "elevated" and "high" blood pressure. High blood pressure is defined as hypertension [**I10 Essential (primary) hypertension**]. If a diagnostic statement does not contain the word "hypertension" or the phrase "high blood pressure," the condition is coded as elevated blood pressure [**R03.0 Elevated blood-pressure reading, without diagnosis of hypertension**], not hypertension.

Hypertension frequently is the cause of various forms of heart and vascular disease; however, the mention of hypertension in the diagnostic statement does not mean that a combination code for hypertensive heart disease should be used. If a cause-and-effect relationship exists between the hypertension and the heart disease, it should be clearly documented in the clinical record or diagnostic statement.

The hypertension table in the ICD-9-CM was not included in the ICD-10-CM. Review Figure 12-12 for a comparison between ICD-9-CM and ICD-10-CM for hypertension coding.

Heart conditions classified to category **I50** {**Heart failure**} or subcategories I51.4–I51.9 are assigned to a code from category **I11**

Hypertension	Malignant	Benign	Unspecified	Hypertension
Hypertension, hypertensive	401.0	401.1	401.9	I10 Essential (primary) hypertension
with CKD stage I-IV, or unspecified	403.00	403.10	403.90	I12.9 Hypertensive chronic kidney disease with stage 1-4 CKD, or unspecified chronic kidney disease
with CKD stage V, or ESRD	403.01	403.11	403.91	I12.0 Hypertensive chronic kidney disease with stage 5 CKD or end stage renal disease
Hypertensive heart	402.00	402.10	402.90	I11.9 Hypertensive heart disease without heart failure
Cardiorenal (disease)	404.00	404.10	404.90	I13.10 Hypertensive heart and chronic kidney disease without heart failure, with stage 1- 4 CKD, or unspecified CKD

FIGURE 12-12 Coding for hypertension in the ICD-9-CM and ICD-10-CM code sets. (Data from *www.ihs.gov/businessoffice/documents/2013pres/ICD-10CM-DiseasesOfTheCirculatorySystem.pdf*.)

{**Hypertensive heart disease**} when a causal relationship is stated in the health record ("as a result of hypertension") or implied ("hypertensive"). Use an additional code from category I50 to identify the *type* of heart failure in patients with heart failure.

The same heart conditions (category I50 or subcategories I51.4–I51.9) with hypertension, but without a stated causal relationship, are coded separately. The codes should sequence according to the circumstances of the admission or encounter.

Coding for Chronic Kidney Disease

Assign codes from category **I12** {**Hypertensive chronic kidney disease**} when both hypertension and a condition classifiable to category **N18** {**Chronic kidney disease (CKD)**} are present. Unlike for hypertension with heart disease, the ICD-10-CM presumes a cause-and-effect relationship and classifies chronic kidney disease with hypertension as hypertensive chronic kidney disease.

The appropriate code from category N18 should be used as a secondary code with a code from category I12 to identify the stage of chronic kidney disease.

If a patient has hypertensive chronic kidney disease and acute renal failure, an additional code for the acute renal failure is required.

Coding for Atherosclerotic Cardiovascular Disease

The ICD-10-CM has combination codes for atherosclerotic heart disease with angina pectoris. The subcategories for these codes are **I25.11** {**Atherosclerotic heart disease of native coronary artery with angina pectoris**} and **I25.7** {**Atherosclerosis of coronary artery bypass graft(s) and coronary artery of transplanted heart with angina pectoris**}.

When you use one of these combination codes, you do not need to use an additional code for angina pectoris. A causal relationship can be assumed in a patient with both atherosclerosis and angina pectoris, unless the documentation indicates that the angina is due to something other than the atherosclerosis.

If a patient with coronary artery disease is admitted because of an acute myocardial infarction (AMI), the AMI should be sequenced before the coronary artery disease.

Coding for Skin Ulcers

Codes from category **L89** {**Pressure ulcer**} are combination codes that identify the site of the pressure ulcer and the stage of the ulcer. The ICD-10-CM classifies pressure ulcer stages based on severity, which is designated by stages 1 to 4; unspecified stage; or unstageable. Unspecified and unstageable codes are used for pressure ulcers in which the stage cannot be clinically determined (e.g., the ulcer has been treated with a skin or muscle graft). These codes also are used for pressure ulcers documented as a deep tissue injury, but not documented as being due to trauma. The modifying term defines each stage, depending on the location of the ulcer (Figure 12-13).

L89.21 Pressure ulcer of right hip
- **L89.210 Pressure ulcer of right hip, unstageable**
- **L89.211 Pressure ulcer of right hip, stage I**
  - Healing pressure ulcer of right hip back, stage I
  - Pressure pre-ulcer skin changes limited to persistent focal edema, right hip
- **L89.212 Pressure ulcer of right hip, stage II**
  - Healing pressure ulcer of right hip, stage II
  - Pressure ulcer with abrasion, blister, partial thickness skin loss involving epidermis and/or dermis, right hip
- **L89.213 Pressure ulcer of right hip, stage III**
  - Healing pressure ulcer of right hip, stage III
  - Pressure ulcer with full thickness skin loss involving damage or necrosis of subcutaneous tissue, right hip
- **L89.214 Pressure ulcer of right hip, stage IV**
  - Healing pressure ulcer of right hip, stage IV
  - Pressure ulcer with necrosis of soft tissues through to underlying muscle, tendon, or bone, right hip
- **L89.219 Pressure ulcer of right hip, unspecified stage**
  - Healing pressure ulcer of right hip NOS
  - Healing pressure ulcer of right hip, unspecified stage

FIGURE 12-13 Coding Example: Pressure Ulcer, Left hip.

Coding for Complications of Pregnancy, Childbirth, and the Puerperium

Coding for the obstetric patient is like using a specialty codebook within the ICD-10-CM coding manual. This is challenging for coders who do not code obstetrics often. Some important clinical terms regarding pregnancy are:

- *Antepartum:* Meaning pregnancy (applies as soon as a pregnancy test result is positive)
- *Childbirth:* Meaning delivery
- *Postpartum:* The puerperium (the first 6 weeks after delivery)
- *Peripartum:* The period from the last month of pregnancy to 5 months' postpartum

Obstetrics cases use codes from Chapter 15, Pregnancy, Childbirth and the Puerperium (O00-O9A). These codes have sequencing priority over codes from other chapters.

Additional codes from other chapters may be used in conjunction with Chapter 15 codes to further specify conditions. If the provider documents that the pregnancy is incidental to the encounter, **Z33.1** {**Pregnant state, incidental**} should be used instead of any Chapter 15 codes. It is the provider's responsibility to state that the condition being treated is not affecting the pregnancy. Codes from Chapter 15 are documented only in the maternal health record; they are never used in the health record of the newborn.

Most of the codes in Chapter 15 have a sixth character indicating the trimester of pregnancy. Assignment of the final character for trimester should be based on the provider's documentation of the trimester (or number of weeks) for the current admission or encounter. This applies to the assignment of trimester for pre-existing conditions, in addition to those that develop during or are due to the pregnancy. The provider's documentation of the number of weeks may be used to assign the appropriate code identifying the trimester.

When a patient is admitted to a hospital for complications in pregnancy during a specific trimester and remains in the hospital into a subsequent trimester, the trimester character for the antepartum complication code should be assigned on the basis of the trimester when the complication developed, not the trimester of the discharge. If the condition developed before the current admission or encounter, or represents a pre-existing condition, the trimester character for the trimester at the time of the admission or encounter should be assigned.

7th Character for Fetus Identification

Where applicable, a 7th character is assigned for certain categories to identify the fetus for which the complication code applies. Assign the 7th character "0":

- For single gestations
- When the documentation in the record is insufficient to determine whether the fetus is affected and it is not possible to obtain clarification
- With more than one fetus, when it is not possible to determine clinically which fetus is affected

Outcome of Delivery and Liveborn Infant Codes

When a delivery occurs, the principal diagnosis should correspond to the main circumstances or complication of the delivery. In cases of cesarean delivery, the selection of the principal diagnosis should be the condition assigned after the encounter that was responsible for the patient's admission. If the patient was admitted with a condition that resulted in the performance of a cesarean procedure, that condition should be selected as the principal diagnosis. If the reason for the admission was unrelated to the condition resulting in the cesarean delivery, the condition related to the reason for the admission/encounter should be selected as the principal diagnosis.

For example, a maternity patient was admitted to the hospital for pneumonia, but because of complications, a cesarean section was performed. In this case, the pneumonia would be the primary diagnosis. A code from category **Z37** {**Outcome of delivery**} should always be included in the maternal health record when a delivery has occurred. Codes from category Z37 are not to be used in subsequent records or in the newborn's health record.

Code **O80** {**Encounter for full-term uncomplicated delivery**} should be assigned when a woman is admitted for a full-term vaginal delivery and delivers a single, healthy infant without any complications antepartum, during the delivery, or postpartum during the delivery episode. Code O80 is always a principal diagnosis.

Newborn Coding

Chapter 16, Certain Conditions Originating in the Perinatal Period (P00–P96), also is used for coding and reporting purposes. The perinatal period extends from just before the birth through day 28 after the birth. When you code the birth episode in a newborn's health record, assign a code from category **Z38** {**Liveborn infants according to place of birth and type of delivery**} as the principal diagnosis. A code from category Z38 is assigned only once, to a newborn at the time of birth. If a newborn is transferred to another institution, a code from category Z38 should not be used at the receiving hospital. When a newborn is admitted to another hospital, the newborn's admitting diagnosis is the health condition that required the hospital transfer.

Coding for Injuries

When you code injuries, assign separate codes for each injury unless a combination code is provided, in which case the combination code is assigned. Code **T07** {**Unspecified multiple injuries**} should not be assigned in the inpatient setting unless documentation for a more specific code is not available. Traumatic injury codes (**S00–T14.9**) are not to be used for normal, healing surgical wounds or to identify complications of surgical wounds.

The code for the most serious injury, as determined by the provider and the focus of treatment, is sequenced first.

Superficial Injuries

Superficial injuries, such as abrasions and contusions, are not coded when they are associated with more severe injuries at the same site.

Primary Injury With Damage to Nerves and/or Blood Vessels

When a primary injury results in minor damage to peripheral nerves or blood vessels, the primary injury is sequenced first. Any additional code or codes for injuries to nerves and the spinal cord and/or injury to vessels or nerves are coded as secondary.

Coding for Traumatic Fractures

The principles of multiple coding of injuries should be followed in the coding of fractures. Fractures of specified sites are coded individually by site in accordance with the level of detail furnished by the health record. The traumatic fracture categories include the following: A02, S12, S22, S32, S42, S49, S52, S59, S62, S72, S82, S89, and S92. A fracture not indicated as open or closed should be coded as closed. A fracture not indicated as displaced or not displaced should be coded as displaced.

Coding for Burns and Corrosions

The same principles for multiple coding apply to burns. Code each burn separately unless specific combination codes are given in the Tabular List. There are many combination codes. Most burn codes are found in Chapter 19 (Injury, Poisoning, and Certain Other Consequences of External Origin); the applicable codes are T20–T32. Because burns are coded by site and degree and by the extent of body surface involvement, all burn cases should have at least two codes and a third if the wound is infected. Other types of wounds, lacerations, punctures, and so on use a different 5th character to show that they are infected and therefore complicated. However, burn codes use the 5th character for other information; therefore, these diagnoses require an additional code to indicate infection.

The ICD-10-CM makes a distinction between burns and corrosions. The burn codes are used for the following: thermal burns (except sunburns) caused by a heat source, such as a fire or hot appliance; burns resulting from electricity; and burns resulting from radiation. Corrosions, on the other hand, are burns caused by chemicals. The guidelines are the same for burns and corrosions.

Current burns (T20–T25) are classified by depth, extent, and burn agent (X code). Depth is categorized as first degree (erythema), second degree (blistering), and third degree (full-thickness involvement). Burns of the eye and internal organs (T26–T28) are classified by site but not by degree.

Coding for Drug Toxicity

Chapter 19 also includes coding for the following drug toxicity classifications:

- *Poisoning* (T36–T50): A reaction to the improper use of a medication, which can be the result of an error made by the prescribing provider, intentional overdose, interaction with drugs or alcohol, or a reaction caused when a nonprescribed medication interacts with a prescribed and properly administered medication.
- *Adverse effect:* An unfavorable side effect that occurs even though a medication is correctly prescribed and properly administered.
- *Underdosing:* Patient takes less of a medication than is prescribed by the provider or by the manufacturer's instructions.
- *Toxic effect:* Patient ingests or comes in contact with a toxic substance.

Codes in categories T36–T65 are combination codes that include the substance taken and the intent. No additional external cause code is required for poisonings, toxic effects, adverse effects, and underdosing codes. When you are coding, do not code directly from the Table of Drugs and Chemicals. Always refer back to the Tabular List.

Coding for External Causes of Morbidity

In the ICD-9-CM, external causes of morbidity were coded with E codes (e.g., a fall from a ladder was coded E881.0). E codes were used to identify an accident or injury. However, E codes are not included in the ICD-10-CM code set.

Instead of using E codes, the ICD-10-CM has added Chapter 20, External Causes of Morbidity (V00-Y99). External cause codes are intended to provide data for research on injuries and for evaluation of injury prevention strategies. These codes capture how the injury or health condition happened (cause); the intent (unintentional or accidental; or intentional, such as suicide or assault), the place where the event occurred; the activity of the patient at the time of the event; and the person's status (e.g., civilian, military).

Place of Occurrence Guideline

Codes from category **Y92** {**Place of occurrence of the external cause**} are secondary codes; they are used after other external cause codes to identify the location of the patient at the time of the injury or other condition.

A place of occurrence code is used only once, at the initial encounter for treatment. No 7th character is used in Y92 codes. Only one code from category Y92 should be recorded on the patient's health record. Do not use place of occurrence code **Y92.9** {**Unspecified place or not applicable**} if the place is not stated or if it is not applicable.

Activity Codes

Activity codes **Y93** {**Activity codes**} are used to define the activity the patient was involved in at the time of injury or when the health condition developed. Only one code from category Y93 should be recorded in the patient's health record. An activity code should be used in conjunction with a place of occurrence code (Y92). The activity codes are not applicable to poisonings, adverse effects, misadventures. or sequelae.

Do not assign code **Y93.9** {**Unspecified activity**} if the activity is not stated.

A code from category Y93 can be used with external cause (Y99) and external cause codes if identifying the activity provides additional information about the event.

For example, you are coding a closed ankle fracture that occurred while the patient was playing soccer in a public park. First, you must identify what should be coded first. In this case, the ankle fracture is coded first: **S92.111A** {**Displaced fracture of neck of right talus**} (remember, "A" indicates initial encounter). The second code is the activity code; the patient was playing soccer, so the code for this activity is **Y93.66** {**Activity, soccer**}. Remember, if the report did not state an activity, do not add **Y93.9** {**Unspecified activity**}. Finally, when an activity code is used, a place of occurrence code should also be used. In this scenario, the patient was playing in a public park; therefore, the place of occurrence code is **Y92.830** {**Public park**}.

Coding for Health Status and Contact With Health Services

In the ICD-10-CM, Chapter 21, Factors Influencing Health Status and Contact with Health Services (Z00-Z99), replaces the V codes used in the ICD-9-CM to describe circumstances or encounters with a healthcare provider when no current illness or injury exists. The 16 categories of Z codes include contact/exposure, inoculations and vaccinations, health status, history of screening, observation, aftercare, follow-up, donor counseling, encounters for obstetric and reproductive services, newborns and infants, routine and administrative examinations, and other health encounters that do not fall into any one of the mentioned categories.

Maximizing Third-Party Reimbursement

The most important thing to remember in using the ICD-10-CM is to code the diagnosis to the highest level of specificity. Obtaining the correct reimbursement is important to the practice's cash flow, and it depends on proper coding and billing techniques. Some other crucial points to remember when submitting diagnostic codes for claims include:

- Use the current year ICD-10-CM manual and stay informed of all changes, revisions, and additions published for that year to both the codes and the official coding guidelines.
- Code accurately from documented information, making sure the appropriate code or codes are assigned for all parts of the diagnostic statement, with no additions or omissions.
- Be sure the diagnosis corresponds to the symptoms and treatment. Many codes are specific to age and gender.
- Review data entry to make sure no digits have been transposed.
- Know the insurance carrier's rules and requirements for completion and submission of claims.
- Incomplete or inaccurate codes may result in delay a possible or denial of reimbursement. An inaccurate diagnosis may have a lifelong negative effect on the patient.

Providers and Accurate Coding

Detailed documentation in the patient's health record can help coders to code to the highest specificity. Therefore, providers should be trained in how to document patient health records appropriately. Respectfully discuss with providers that diagnostic codes cannot be assigned unless clear documentation is found in the patient's health record. Some providers may feel that because they care for the same type of cases, specialized diagnostic statements should be implied. However, the medical assistant should stress to providers the high value of detailed documentation and how developing this practice not only improves ICD-10-CM code assignment, but also may result in higher health insurance reimbursements.

Staff meetings to review third-party requirements should be held regularly by the medical billing supervisor (Figure 12-14). Medical assistants should be respectful to the healthcare provider when third-party requirements compel more effort on their part. An understanding and patient attitude toward the healthcare provider goes a long way in building a trusting relationship.

Ethical Standards of Medical Coding

At times coders can feel pressured by decreasing insurance reimbursements and their employers to use fraudulent coding practices. However, if a medical practice is convicted of fraudulent billing, the coders may lose their coding license and face federal fines. A number of ethical standards have been established for medical coding, and most of these can help coders identify unethical coding behaviors. The following tips explain how to proceed in scenarios that may pose ethical dilemmas.

1. **Understand what ethical coding standards mean.** Coders face stress from all sides: financial issues, providers, and other coders. However, stress cannot be a compelling reason coders intentionally report diagnoses and/or higher specificity codes without sufficient documentation.
2. **Stand your ground.** When coding, be true to yourself, even though it can be hard in a stressful environment. When you know a chart needs additional documentation to justify reporting certain codes, don't be afraid to speak up to the provider. Conduct research ahead of time to strengthen your case. For example, search through and print out applicable issues of *Coding Clinic* from the American Hospital Association website: *ahacentraloffice.org*. The more backup documentation you have, the more likely it is that management will support your ethical coding decision.
3. **Say something.** Other coders may not follow the same ethical coding standards as you. If you observe unethical coding practices, bring it to the attention of the coder and allow him or her to make the needed adjustments. Broaching this issue with a colleague can be challenging, but encourage the other coder to reflect on the ethics of his or her actions. If the unethical coding practices continue, be sure to inform the next person in command.
4. **Keep in communication with the office manager.** Some coding situations require more management involvement than others. For example, if your conversation with a colleague does nothing to dissuade unethical behavior, bring your manager into the loop. Or,

if you know you need to query a provider about a health record that might yield a higher reimbursement, but that provider is on vacation for 7 days, enlist your office manager's help in flagging the health record until the provider returns to clarify it.
5. **Review notes from other health providers.** In most scenarios, coders are not allowed to code from documentation by anyone other than a provider; however, notes from ancillary staff members may encourage a coder to ask the provider whether the diagnosis does exist. For example, if a consultation with a dietitian suggests that a patient is malnourished, but the provider does not document this anywhere, you may be able to use the dietitian's clinical information as the basis for querying the provider. The diagnosis cannot be coded based solely on the dietitian's clinical information; the code can be assigned only after the provider confirms the diagnosis.

DeVault K. Know your ethical obligations regarding coding and documentation. www.hcpro.com/HOM-236942-5728/Know-your-ethical-obligations-regarding-coding-and-documentation.html. Accessed May 8, 2015.

CRITICAL THINKING APPLICATION   12-7

Mike used the GEMs to map the out-of-date ICD-9-CM codes to current ICD-10-CM codes, and then he updated the encounter form electronically. After a few days, Dr. Walker comes into Mike's office to ask that the old encounter form be printed out for him because he is not comfortable using the new electronic encounter form with the updated ICD-10-CM codes. What approach should Mike take in discussing Dr. Walker's concerns with him? How can Mike help Dr. Walker appreciate the need for the ICD-10-CM code updates?

CLOSING COMMENTS

Diagnostic coding using the ICD-10-CM, and its almost 70,000 codes, can seem overwhelming. Successful medical coders follow specific steps very closely to assign the most accurate ICD-10-CM code. Encoder software (e.g., TruCode) can search the ICD-10-CM electronically to facilitate faster coding. Detailed documentation in the patient's health record and accurate coding work hand in hand to maximize reimbursement for services rendered. The medical

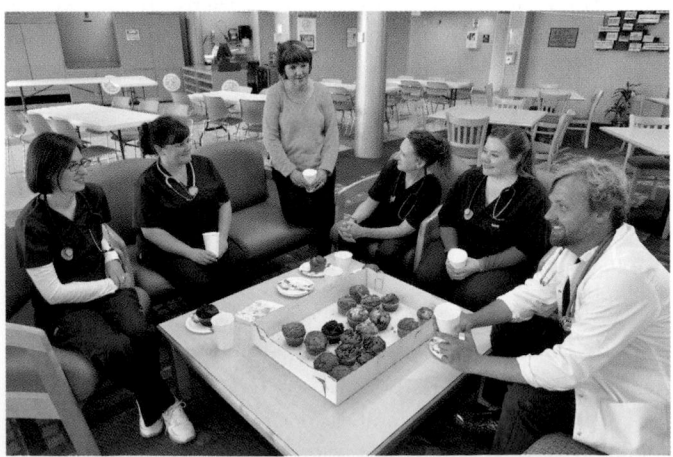

FIGURE 12-14 Regular staff meetings encourage accurate coding.

assistant can best communicate with healthcare professionals about accurate coding by showing them respect and patience. Medical assistants are expected to adhere to ethical standards, assigning and reporting only codes clearly supported by concise documentation in the patient's chart. When in doubt, a medical assistant should consult the attending healthcare provider for clarification. A coding professional is responsible for maintaining and continually enhancing his or her coding skills and for keeping informed of changes in the codes, guidelines, and regulations.

Patient Education

Most patients know very little about medical coding, so they may not understand how the codes on their encounter forms relate to their diagnosis. If the patient has questions, explain that the codes represent his or her diagnosis to the most specific and accurate level. Because the coding system is much like a foreign language to patients, be patient when explaining this process and answering questions, so that the patient is able to understand the insurance billing process.

Legal and Ethical Issues

Using the medical coding system allows providers to express the simplicity or complexity of a medical treatment or procedure. This specificity leads to the maximum reimbursement to the provider. The medical assistant must perform coding procedures accurately so that they reflect exactly what happened during the treatment. Codes must not be exaggerated to increase reimbursement to the provider.

Professional Behaviors

Although providers may be overly concerned about the need to maximize insurance reimbursements, coders should never feel coerced into fraudulent coding practices. Successful coders rely solely on medical documentation as the source of diagnostic statements. Coders should never assume that additional complications or conditions exist if they are not documented. In these cases, strong communication between the coder and the provider is necessary to clarify the appropriate diagnoses.

SUMMARY OF SCENARIO

Mike's experience using the ICD-10-CM coding manual and encoder software on actual medical office cases has made him even more enthusiastic about his new responsibilities, and he enjoys the coding process more. He knows that as he gains experience in ICD-10-CM coding, he will be able to set a positive example for the staff. As Mike progresses with diagnostic coding, he also will be able to help the providers and medical assistant staff be attentive to details when documenting in a health record.

Although the electronic encounter form for entering billing codes is an easy tool, Mike has learned that knowing how to use the ICD-10-CM Alphabetic Index and Tabular List is a necessary asset to ensure accurate coding. He also knows

it is important when coding a diagnosis to make sure the medical documentation matches the encounter form and that all elements of the diagnostic statement are included. Furthermore, he must ensure that the diagnosis listed on the encounter form is fully documented in the patient's health record. Mike is feeling more comfortable about referring to coding guidelines to ensure the most accurate code and ensuring that every character for the ICD-10-CM code is present. Every feature of the manual provides guidance in choosing and confirming a diagnostic code that matches the diagnostic statement on the encounter form and in the health record. Searching for codes in the encoder also has helped Mike develop his coding skills more quickly.

SUMMARY OF LEARNING OBJECTIVES

1. **Define, spell, and pronounce the terms listed in the vocabulary.**
   Spelling and pronouncing medical terms correctly reinforce the credibility of the medical assistant. Knowing the definition of these terms promotes confidence in communication with patients and co-workers. Also, understanding the medical terms found in the diagnostic statement is essential for identifying and selecting the most accurate and appropriate diagnostic code or codes.

2. **Describe the historical use of the *International Classification of Disease* (ICD) in the United States.**
   In 1946, the International Commission of the World Health Organization (WHO) established a code set called the *Manual of the International Statistical Classification of Diseases, Injuries, and Causes of Death* (ICD). Eventually, WHO approved an adaptation of this code set for use in the United States; the ninth edition, the *International Classification of*

Diseases, Ninth Revision, Clinical Modification (ICD-9-CM), was approved and put into use in 1975. The United States adopted ICD-10-CM diagnostic coding on October 1, 2015.

3. **Describe the transition from ICD-9-CM diagnostic coding to ICD-10-CM diagnostic coding.**
   As of the publication of this textbook, ICD-10-CM diagnostic coding will be a somewhat new process, so it is important to familiarize yourself with the differences between the ICD-9-CM and the ICD-10-CM. The ICD-10-CM follows the same hierarchal structure as the ICD-9-CM, in which the first three characters represent the category of the code. (Review Table 12-1 to compare the differences in the ICD-9-CM and ICD-10-CM code sets.) To aid the transition, the CMS has provided General Equivalence Mappings (GEMs), which help convert ICD-9-CM codes to the appropriate ICD-10-CM codes.

Continued

4. **Identify the structure and format of the ICD-10-CM.**

Depending on the publisher, the ICD-10-CM coding manual will vary somewhat in layout, symbols, color coding, and some other features. However, the format, conventions, tables, appendixes, content, and basic structure are always the same.

Every ICD-10-CM code begins with an alphabetic letter that indicates the chapter of disease and injury in which the code is listed. (All the letters in the English alphabet are used except U, which WHO has reserved to assign to new diseases with uncertain etiologies.) Codes contain up to 7 alphanumeric characters; the first 3 characters are followed by a period. Codes that require a 7th character may use an X as a placeholder for the 4th, 5th, and 6th characters if no other code can be used for those characters.

5. **Describe how to use the Alphabetic Index to select main terms, essential modifiers, and the appropriate code (or codes) or code ranges.**

The ICD-10-CM Index to Diseases and Injuries (commonly called the *Alphabetic Index*) consists of an alphabetic list of diagnostic terms and related codes. This index includes main terms, nonessential modifiers, essential modifiers, and subterms. Figure 12-3 provides an example of the *main term* **Colitis**; which is followed by the *nonessential modifiers* (acute), (catarrhal), (chronic), (noninfective), and (hemorrhagic). The second *essential modifier* listed under the main term is "amebic (acute)," and the *subterm* listed under amebic is "nondysenteric." The *main term* is bold face; the *nonessential modifiers* that follow it are enclosed in parentheses; the *essential modifier* is indented one space under the main term; and the *subterm* is indented one space under the essential modifier (two spaces under the main term). The nonessential modifiers (i.e., acute, catarrhal, chronic, noninfective, and hemorrhagic) do not affect the code assignment. The hyphen (-) at the end of the code indicates that additional characters are required to complete the code.

6. **Do the following related to the Tabular List:**

- *Explain how to use the Tabular List to select main terms, essential modifiers, and the appropriate code (or codes) or code ranges.*

The ICD-10-CM Tabular List of Diseases and Injuries (commonly called simply the *Tabular List*) is divided into 21 chapters. Each chapter is divided into categories, or *blocks,* that have been assigned 3-character codes. These codes form the foundation of the ICD-10-CM code set.

In most of the chapters, the title is composed of a group of diseases and injuries, followed by a code range in parentheses. For example, Chapter 1 is: Certain Infectious and Parasitic Diseases (A00–B99). However, some chapter titles use a part of the body or an organ system to group the codes; for example: Chapter 9, Diseases of the Circulatory System (I00–I99). Still other chapters group conditions together by etiology or the nature of the disease process, as in Chapter 2, Neoplasms (C00–D49). Chapter 15, Pregnancy, Childbirth, and the Puerperium (O00–O9A), groups codes related to the prenatal and postnatal periods. Chapter 20, External Causes of Morbidity (V00–Y99), replaces the V and E codes used in the ICD-9-CM.

Chapter 20 also groups codes related to external causes of injury and poisoning. Chapter 21 is Factors Influencing Health Status and Contact with Health Services (Z00–Z99).

- *Summarize coding conventions as defined in the ICD-10-CM coding manual.*

Conventions are abbreviations, punctuation, symbols, instructional notations, and related elements that help the coder select an accurate, specific code. Conventions are found in the Tabular List, but not in the Alphabetic Index. Understanding their meaning and using them as guides are crucial to accurate coding.

7. **Review the Official Coding Guidelines to assign the most accurate ICD-10-CM diagnostic code.**

An important section of the coding manual is the ICD-10-CM Official Guidelines for Coding and Reporting. Every coding guideline for the entire ICD-10-CM code set is included in this Coding Guidelines section at the beginning of the manual. These guidelines are a set of rules developed to accompany and complement the official conventions and instructions provided in the ICD-10-CM proper.

8. **Explain how to abstract the diagnostic statement from a patient's health record.**

To prepare for medical coding, the medical assistant must analyze and abstract the diagnostic statements documented in the various reports in the patient's health record. Sources of diagnostic statements include the encounter form; treatment notes; discharge summary; operative report; and radiology, pathology, and laboratory reports.

9. **Describe how to use the most current diagnostic codes and perform diagnostic coding.**

Ten basic steps are required for accurate ICD-10-CM coding (see Table 12-3). The first step involves abstracting the diagnostic statement from the health record and determining the main and essential modifiers from the various medical reports. The next steps are performed using the Alphabetic Index to search for the code, codes, or code ranges that best fit the diagnostic statement. The remaining steps are performed using the Tabular List to verify and confirm that the code or codes located in the Alphabetic Index fully match the diagnostic statement and are the most specific and accurate diagnostic codes.

The medical assistant's knowledge of accurate diagnostic coding contributes to the legal and financial health of the practice. In most cases, ICD-10-CM codes are found on the encounter form. However, with literally thousands of current diagnostic codes, it may be necessary to code from the ICD-10-CM manual. The process for diagnostic coding is outlined in Procedure 12-1.

10. **Identify how encoder software can help the coder assign the most accurate diagnostic code.**

Encoder software is computer-aided coding, which helps determine the most accurate code possible. The coder types a few key words into a Search box, and the software matches the entry with main terms in the Alphabetic Index. The coder then clicks on a specific code to hyperlink to the Tabular List.

SUMMARY OF LEARNING OBJECTIVES—*continued*

11. **Explain the importance of coding guidelines for accuracy, and discuss special rules and considerations that apply to the code selection process.**

    All ICD-10-CM coding manuals, regardless of the publisher, have comprehensive instructional notes and conventions to help the coder select the most accurate diagnostic code or codes. When a discrepancy occurs between reference sources, including this text, the current year's ICD-10-CM coding manual is the final authority. When coding, the medical assistant must always refer to and thoroughly review the conventions, instructional notations, code definitions, and other guidelines in the Alphabetic Index and Tabular List.

12. **Use tactful communication skills with medical providers to ensure accurate code selection.**

    The medical assistant coder must speak respectfully with providers about the importance of accurate health record documentation in maximizing reimbursements. Providers must understand that diagnostic codes cannot be assigned unless clear documentation is found in the patient's health record, even though some providers may feel that because they care for the same type of cases, specialized diagnostic statements should be implied.

13. **Review medical coding ethical standards.**

    At times medical coders can feel pressure from decreasing insurance reimbursements and their employers that they justify fraudulent coding practices. If a medical practice is convicted of fraudulent billing, it will lose its coding license, and it and the coder also may face federal fines. A number of standards have been established for ethical coding, and most of these can help coders recognize unethical coding behaviors.

CONNECTIONS

Study Guide Connection: Go to the Chapter 12 Study Guide. Read and complete the activities.

evolve Evolve Connection: Go to the Chapter 12 link at *evolve.elsevier.com/kinn* to complete the Chapter Review Quiz. Check out the other resources listed for this chapter to make the most of what you have learned from Basics of Diagnostic Coding.

13 BASICS OF PROCEDURAL CODING

SCENARIO

Sherald Vogt, a medical assisting student, works in an ambulatory surgery center run by Dr. John Caddell. Sherald really enjoyed learning about diagnostic coding in the *International Classification of Diseases, Tenth Revision, Clinical Modification* (ICD-10-CM), and now she looks forward to learning about procedural coding. Sherald recognized that a strong understanding of anatomy and pathophysiology was vital to correct diagnostic coding, and she believes the knowledge she has gained will help her in procedural coding. Sherald will be using the *Current Procedural Terminology* (CPT) coding system for most procedures and services provided in the medical office. In addition, she will use the *Healthcare Common Procedure Coding System* (HCPCS; pronounced "hic-pix") for auxiliary medical products and services.

As she did with the ICD-10-CM, Sherald will learn that accurate coding begins with the proper analysis of the clinical diagnosis (or diagnoses) and supporting documentation, from which she will abstract the correct data to assign an accurate procedure code. Just as does the ICD-10-CM, the CPT has coding guidelines, symbols, and formal steps specific to procedural coding, which Sherald will learn to use. However, unlike with ICD-10-CM diagnostic coding, in CPT and HCPCS coding, Sherald must determine how and when to use modifiers. Dr. Caddell wants to give Sherald some experience so he allows her to review some healthcare records so she can practice coding.

While studying this chapter, think about the following questions:

- What code set will be used for outpatient procedural coding?
- What will Sherald find similar to what she learned with the ICD-10-CM as she performs procedural coding?
- What will help Sherald select the most specific and accurate CPT code?
- What are the differences between CPT coding and HCPCS coding?
- How will Sherald use and apply modifiers in CPT and HCPCS coding?
- What will Sherald learn about the legal implications of inaccurate coding?

LEARNING OBJECTIVES

1. Define, spell, and pronounce the terms listed in the vocabulary.
2. Describe the organization of the *Current Procedural Terminology* (CPT) manual.
3. Report the history of procedural coding.
4. Distinguish between the Alphabetic Index and the Tabular List in the CPT code set.
5. Classify the six different sections of the CPT code set.
6. Discuss special reports, and explain the importance of modifiers in assigning CPT codes.
7. Review various conventions in the CPT code set.
8. Identify the required medical documentation for accurate procedural coding.
9. Describe how to use the most current procedural coding system and perform procedural coding for surgery.
10. Discuss how to use the Alphabetic Index.
11. Identify common CPT coding guidelines for evaluation and management (E/M) procedures.
12. Identify common CPT coding guidelines for anesthesia procedures.
13. Identify common CPT coding guidelines for surgical procedures.
14. Discuss coding factors for the integumentary system and muscular system, and for maternity care and delivery.
15. Identify common CPT coding guidelines for the Radiology, Pathology and Laboratory, and Medicine sections.
16. Do the following related to the HCPCS code set and manual:
    - Identify procedures and services that require HCPCS codes.
    - Describe how to use the most current HCPCS level II coding system.
17. Perform procedural coding of an office visit and an immunization.
18. Summarize common HCPCS coding guidelines.

VOCABULARY

Certified Registered Nurse Anesthetist (CRNA) A nursing healthcare professional who is certified to administer anesthesia.

CPT Assistant An online CPT coding journal, supported by the American Medical Association (AMA), that addresses subjects such as appealing insurance denials, validating coding to auditors, training staff members, and answering day-to-day coding questions.

debridement The surgical removal of dead, damaged, or infected tissue to improve the function of healthy tissue.

eponym In medical terms, a name of a medical diagnosis or procedure derived from the name of the person who discovered it.

global services For purposes of CPT coding, medical services and procedures performed for the patient before, during, and after a surgical procedure that is included with the assigned CPT code.

procedural statement The statement in the health record that specifically describes the procedures and services provided during the encounter.

special report Additional medical documentation required to confirm the need for the use of unlisted, unusual, or newly adopted medical procedures.

Procedural coding is the method of assigning a defined code for each specific medical procedure or service delivered by a qualified healthcare professional. Three types of procedure codes are used for medical coding for reimbursement: ICD-10-PCS, CPT, and HCPCS (Table 13-1). Because the medical assistant most likely will work in the outpatient setting, this chapter focuses on the CPT and HCPCS code sets. The medical biller is responsible for maintaining accurate medical recordkeeping and for processing insurance claims efficiently by using the CPT and HCPCS codes, which identify appropriate procedures and services common to the physician's office.

INTRODUCTION TO THE CPT MANUAL

The Current Procedural Terminology (CPT) system was developed and is maintained by the American Medical Association (AMA). It is updated each year and released on October 1. The CPT coding manual consists of descriptive terms and identifying codes for reporting professional and technical services. CPT codes convert free text procedural data into discrete data; that is, they establish a standard language that accurately describes medical and surgical services.

THE ORGANIZATION OF THE CPT MANUAL

Category I Codes

Category I codes are located in the Tabular List of the CPT manual and arranged by sections. For example, codes beginning with 7 (e.g., 70100—radiologic examination of the mandible, partial, with less than four views) are located in the Radiology section of the manual. Each code has a description of the service or procedure performed. Some CPT codes (e.g., Category II and Category III codes, discussed later) are alphanumeric.

Category II Codes

Category II codes are a set of supplemental tracking codes that providers use for performance measurement. Category II codes are optional; they cannot be used as a substitute for Category I codes, and they are not reported as part of the insurance billing process. These codes describe clinical components that may be typically included in Evaluation and Management services or clinical services. In a Category II code, the 5th digit is the letter F.

Category II codes are described and listed in Appendix H of the CPT manual. They are listed in alphabetic order by condition. Category II codes are reviewed by the Performance Measures Advisory Group, which is composed of members from various medical organizations and government agencies. In some publishers' editions of the CPT manual, Category II codes are also listed in their own section, after the Medicine section and before the appendices.

Category III Codes

Category III codes are temporary codes assigned for emerging and new technology, services, and procedures that have not been officially added to the Tabular List of the CPT manual. Category III codes are intended to be used for data collection purposes, to substantiate widespread use, or as part of the approval process of the U.S. Food and Drug Administration (FDA). In a Category III code,

TABLE 13-1   Comparison of Procedural Code Sets

CODE SET	USED FOR	CODE FEATURES	EXAMPLE	DESCRIPTION	DEVELOPER	UPDATED
ICD-10-PCS	Inpatient hospital procedures	7-digit alphanumeric code	0TTJ0ZZ	Appendectomy	National Center for Health Statistics	Annually, October 1
CPT	Outpatient procedures; professional and technical services	5-digit numeric code; a 2-digit modifier can be added	44970	Laparoscopic appendectomy	American Medical Association (AMA)	Annually, January 1
HCPCS	Auxiliary medical treatment, including vaccines, medical transport, drugs, durable medical equipment	5-digit alphanumeric code; a 2-digit modifier can be added	A0428	Ambulance service, basic life support, nonemergency transport	Centers for Medicare and Medicaid Services (CMS)	Annually, October 1

the 5th digit is the letter T. Category III codes may be used in billing and reporting if no code in the Tabular List accurately describes the technology, service, or procedure performed and no Category I code matches the medical documentation. Category III codes have no reimbursement value. In most publishers' editions of the CPT manual, Category III codes are also listed in their own section, after the Medicine section and before the appendices.

THE EVOLUTION OF CPT CODING

The AMA first published the CPT coding manual in 1966. The first edition contained only surgical codes, and the codes had only 4 digits.

The second edition of the CPT, published in 1970, presented an expanded system of five-digit codes to designate diagnostic and therapeutic procedures in surgery, medicine, radiology, laboratory, pathology, and medical specialties. At that time, the four-digit classification was replaced with the current five-digit coding system. The fourth edition, published in 1977, included significant updates in medical technology. At the same time, a system of periodic annual updating was introduced to keep pace with the rapidly changing environment.

Format of the CPT Coding Manual

- Comprehensive instructions for using the manual, including the steps for coding
- The Alphabetic Index
- Tabular List includes the following six sections:
    Evaluation and Management
    Anesthesia
    Surgery
    Radiology
    Pathology and Laboratory
    Medicine
- Coding Guidelines, Conventions, and Notes
- Appendices (15; A-O)

THE ALPHABETIC INDEX

The CPT coding manual is separated into the Alphabetic Index and the Tabular List. The Alphabetic Index is organized by main terms; these terms represent the type of surgery, the anatomic site, or **eponym** (Figure 13-1).

THE TABULAR LIST

The Tabular List is divided into six sections, with codes listed in numeric order in each section. As in the ICD-10-CM, the codes in the Tabular List include definitions, guidelines, and notes, which enable the coder to select the most specific code based on the procedural statement and service descriptions documented in the health record. The six sections of the Tabular List and their CPT code ranges are:

- Evaluation and Management (99201-99499)
- Anesthesia (00100-01999, 99100-99140)

Fracture

Acetabulum	
Closed Treatment	27220-27222
Open Treatment	27226-27228
with Manipulation	27222
without Manipulation	27220
Alveolar Ridge	
Closed Treatment	21440
Open Treatment	21445
Ankle	
Bimalleolar	27808, 27810, 27814
Lateral	27786, 27788, 27792, 27808, 27810, 27814
Medial	27760, 27762, 27766, 27808, 27810, 27814
Posterior	27767-27769, 27808, 27810, 27814
Trimalleolar	27816, 27818, 27822-27823
Ankle Bone	
Medial	27760-27762
Bennett's	
See Thumb, Fracture	
Blow-Out Fracture	
Orbital Floor	21385-21387, 21390, 21395
Bronchi	
Reduction	31630
Calcaneus	
Closed Treatment	28400-28405
Open Treatment	28415-28420
Percutaneous Fixation	28406
with Manipulation	28405-28406
without Manipulation	28400

FIGURE 13-1 Alphabetic Index: Fractures.

- Surgery (10021-69990)
- Radiology, including nuclear medicine and diagnostic ultrasound (70010-79999)
- Pathology and Laboratory (80047-89398)
- Medicine (90281-99199, 99500-99607)

Sections are subdivided into *subsections*; *subsections* are subdivided into *categories*; and *categories* can be subdivided into *subcategories*. Each level of a section provides more specificity about the procedure or service performed and the anatomic site or organ system involved. Each section and subsection provides coding guidelines and, if needed, a reference to the **CPT Assistant**. In most instances, all four levels are found, although this is not a hard-and-fast rule.

In the CPT manual, the subsection is listed below the section and indented two spaces. The subsection usually describes an anatomic site or an organ system, as in the following examples:

- Anatomic site: heart, femur, or skull
- Organ system: digestive, integumentary, or cardiovascular

A category is listed below the subsection and indented two spaces. It generally refers to a specific procedure or service, but it can also indicate a more specific anatomic site:

- Procedures: esophagoscopy, incision and drainage, or cardiac catheterization
- Specific anatomic site: mitral valve, distal femur, or occipital bone

Subcategory is the lowest level of code description. The subcategory is listed below the category and indented two spaces. It provides even more specificity about an anatomic site or the procedure or service performed.

CRITICAL THINKING APPLICATION **13-1**

To practice her coding skills, Sherald is reviewing a surgical report for a gallbladder removal. Will she be able to find the main term "gallbladder" in the Alphabetic index? Why or why not? What main term should she be looking for? Once she finds the range of codes in the Alphabetic Index, what is her next step?

Evaluation and Management Section

The Evaluation and Management (E/M) section contains codes for the different types of encounters or patient visits. The code range in the E/M section is 99201 to 99499. The E/M section is further divided into subsections that include different types of services (e.g., office visits, hospital visits, consultations, skilled nursing facility, or nursing home visits). Each of these subsections is divided into codes that specify whether the patient is new or established. The subcategories of E/M services are further classified into levels of E/M services that are identified by specific codes. This classification is important because the nature of a provider's work varies by type of service, place of service, and the patient's status.

Anesthesia Section

The Anesthesia section includes CPT-4 codes for services by anesthesiologists and anesthetists. The code ranges in the Anesthesia section are 00100 to 01999 and 99100 to 99140. The CPT-4 codes include any type of anesthesia administered (e.g., general, local, and sedation anesthesia) for the surgery performed on the specified area of the body. Other support services, including the anesthesiologist's preoperative and postoperative encounters with the patient; evaluation of the patient's physical status; administration of anesthesia, fluids, and/or blood; and monitoring services, such as blood pressure, temperature, and electrocardiography, are also included in this code. Figure 13-2 presents examples of CPT-4 Anesthesia codes.

Surgery Section

The Surgery section, the largest section of the CPT Tabular List, includes standardized codes for all *invasive surgical procedures* performed by providers or other qualified professionals. An invasive procedure is any medical procedure in which a body orifice or the skin must be penetrated by cutting or puncture (Figure 13-3 shows the Surgery section for procedures of the larynx). In most instances, each subsection is further divided into categories and subcategories, which describe procedures and services unique to that anatomic subsection. This section is divided into subsections that typically identify specific body systems, beginning with the integumentary system (skin) and ending with the ophthalmologic (eye) and otologic (ear) systems.

Radiology Section

The Radiology section includes codes for diagnostic imaging, including x-ray studies, body scans, and for therapy used in the treatment of cancer. The code range in the Radiology section is 70000 to 79999. Radiology codes are designed for use by radiologists and other medical professionals by simply adding or changing a modifier. Radiology codes are differentiated by the number of views taken (Figure 13-4).

Forearm, Wrist, and Hand

01810	Anesthesia for all procedures on nerves, muscles, tendons, fascia, and bursae of forearm, wrist, and hand
	CPT Assistant Mar 06:15, Nov 07:8, Oct 11:3, Jul 12:13
01820	Anesthesia for all closed procedures on radius, ulna, wrist, or hand bones
01829	Anesthesia for diagnostic arthroscopic procedures on the wrist
	CPT Changes: An Insider's View 2003
01830	Anesthesia for open or surgical arthroscopic/endoscopic procedures on distal radius, distal ulna, wrist, or hand joints; not otherwise specified
	CPT Changes: An Insider's View 2003
01832	total wrist replacement
01840	Anesthesia for procedures on arteries of forearm, wrist, and hand; not otherwise specified
01842	embolectomy
01844	Anesthesia for vascular shunt, or shunt revision, any type (eg, dialysis)
01850	Anesthesia for procedures on veins of forearm, wrist, and hand; not otherwise specified
01852	phleborrhaphy
01860	Anesthesia for forearm, wrist, or hand cast application, removal, or repair
	CPT Assistant Nov 07:8, Jul 12:13

FIGURE 13-2 CPT-4 Anesthesia Codes.

Larynx
Excision

31300	Laryngotomy (thyrotomy, laryngofissure); with removal of tumor or laryngocele, cordectomy
31320	diagnostic
31360	Laryngectomy; total, without radical neck dissection
	CPT Assistant Aug 10:4
31365	total, with radical neck dissection
	CPT Assistant Oct 01:10, Aug 10:4
31367	subtotal supraglottic, without radical neck dissection
	CPT Assistant Aug 10:4
31368	subtotal supraglottic, with radial neck dissection
31370	Partial laryngectomy (hemilaryngectomy); horizontal
31375	laterovertical
31380	anterovertical
31382	antero-latero-vertical
31390	Pharyngolaryngectomy, with radical neck dissection; without reconstruction
31395	with reconstruction
31400	Arytenoidectomy or arytenoidopexy, external approach (For endoscopic arytenoidectomy, use 31560)
31420	Epiglottidectomy

FIGURE 13-3 Surgery Section and Subsection: Larynx Excision.

Pathology and Laboratory Section

Codes are included for all diagnostic tests performed on bodily fluids and tissues (including urine, blood, sputum, and feces); for those performed on excised or biopsied cells, tissue, or body organs; and for evaluation of those fluids and tissues to identify any pathology or disease present. The code ranges for the Pathology and Laboratory section are 80047 to 80076 for Organ or Disease-Oriented Panels and 80100 to 89999 for all other tests. Organ or Disease-Oriented Panel CPT codes are *bundled* into one specific code,

CRITICAL THINKING APPLICATION   **13-2**

Sherald reviewed a coded medical record for a Basic Metabolic Panel with total Calcium that had listed specific CPT codes for each panel test. Is this the correct way of coding for the organ panel? According to Figure 13-5, how should this organ panel be coded?

Spine and Pelvis

72010   Radiologic examination, spine, entire, survey study, anteroposterior and lateral
➲ *CPT Assistant* May 02:18, Jan 07:29
➲ *Clinical Examples in Radiology* Fall 09:10, Spring 13:9

72020   Radiologic examination, spine, single view, specify level
➲ *CPT Assistant* Jul 13:10
➲ *Clinical Examples in Radiology* Spring 13:8, 9

72040   Radiologic examination, spine, cervical; 2 or 3 views
➲ *CPT Assistant* Sep 01:7, Jul 13:10; *CPT Changes: An Insider's View* 2001, 2013, 2014
➲ *Clinical Examples in Radiology* Fall 09:10, Summer 11:8, Fall 11:9, Spring 13:8, 9

72050   4 or 5 views
➲ *CPT Changes: An Insider's View* 2013
➲ *Clinical Examples in Radiology* Summer 11:8, Fall 11:9, Spring 13:9

72052   6 or more views
➲ *CPT Changes: An Insider's View* 2013
➲ *Clinical Examples in Radiology* Summer 11:8, Fall 11:9, Spring 13:9

FIGURE 13-4 Radiology Section: Spine and Pelvis.

80047   Basic metabolic panel (Calcium, ionized)
This panel must include the following:
Calcium, ionized (82330)
Carbon dioxide (bicarbonate)(82374)
Chloride (82435)
Creatinine (82565)
Glucose (82947)
Potassium (84132)
Sodium (84295)
Urea Nitrogen (BUN)(84520)
➲ *CPT Assistant* Apr 08:5, Apr 13:10; *CPT Changes: An Insider's View* 2008

80048   Basic metabolic panel (Calcium, total)
This panel must include the following:
Calcium, total (82310)
Carbon dioxide (bicarbonate)(82374)
Chloride (82435)
Creatinine (82565)
Glucose (82947)
Potassium (84132)
Sodium (84295)
Urea Nitrogen (BUN)(84520)
➲ *CPT Assistant* Jan 98:6, Sep 99:11, Nov 99:44, Jan 00:7, Aug 05:9; *CPT Changes: An Insider's View* 2000, 2008, 2009

FIGURE 13-5 Laboratory Section: Organ Panel.

which lists the included tests, along with their specific CPT code (Figure 13-5).

Medicine Section

The codes for the Medicine section range from 90281 to 99199 and 99500 to 99607 (excluding the anesthesia code ranges described in

---

A View of the Outer Cochlear Implant
92601-92604

An example of the elements that are addressed in the diagnostic analysis and reprogramming of the cochlear implant.

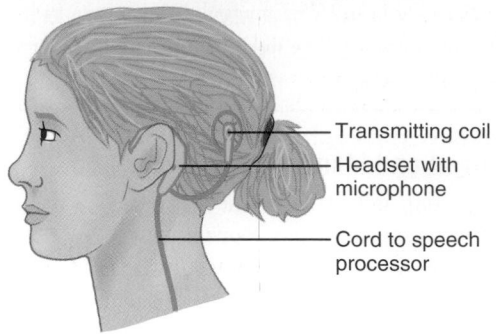

— Transmitting coil
— Headset with microphone
— Cord to speech processor

92601   Diagnotic analysis of cochlear implant, patient younger than 7 years of age; with programming
➲ *CPT Assistant* Mar 03:1, Jan 06:7, Jul 11:17, Oct 13:7, Jul 14:4; *CPT Changes: An Insider's View* 2003

92602   subsequent reprogramming
➲ *CPT Assistant* Mar 03:1, Jan 06:7, Oct 13:7; *CPT Changes: An Insider's View* 2003
(Do not report 92602 in addition to 92601)
(For aural rehabilitation services following cochlear implant, including evaluation of rehabilitation status, see 92626-92627, 92630-92633)

92603   Diagnostic analysis of cochlear implant, age 7 years or older; with programming
➲ *CPT Assistant* Mar 03:2, 4, Jan 06:7, Jul 11:17, Oct 13:7; *CPT Changes: An Insider's View* 2003

92604   subsequent reprogramming
➲ *CPT Assistant* Mar 03:2, 21, Jan 06:7, Jul 11:17, Oct 13:7, Jul 14:4; *CPT Changes: An Insider's View* 2003
(Do not report 92604 in addition to 92603)

92605   Evaluation for prescription of non-speech-generating augmentative and alternative communication device, face-to-face with the patient; first hour
➲ *CPT Assistant* Mar 03:2, 4, Oct 13:7; *CPT Changes: An Insider's View* 2003, 2012

#✚92618   each additional 30 minutes (List separately in addition to code for primary procedure)
➲ *CPT Changes: An Insider's View* 2012
(Use 92618 in conjunction with 92605)

92606   Therapeutic service(s) for the use of non-speech-generating device, including programming and modification
➲ *CPT Assistant* Mar 03:2, 4; *CPT Changes: An Insider's View* 2003

FIGURE 13-6 Medicine Section: Analysis of Cochlear Implant.

the Anesthesia section). The Medicine section includes many and varied subsections, categories, and subcategories. This section can be considered a catchall section in that it includes codes for services and procedures that do not fit into any of the other sections of the CPT manual. Medical specialties, such as ophthalmology, otolaryngology, and allergy, which involve procedures and services that vary greatly from the traditional office encounter, are grouped in the Medicine section rather than the E/M section. Noninvasive diagnostic tests such as diagnostic analysis of cochlear implants, ECGs, and allergy testing, are included in the Medicine section rather than in the Surgery section (Figure 13-6).

UNLISTED PROCEDURE OR SERVICE CODE

Occasionally, even with the best, detailed documentation, an accurate, specific code to match the procedure or service performed cannot be found in the CPT manual. In each section (and sometimes in subsections, categories, and/or subcategories), nonspecific codes have been provided. These codes are known as Unlisted Procedures and Services. For example, code 29999 is found in the Surgery section, Musculoskeletal subsection. It describes an "unlisted procedure, arthroscopy." Unlisted codes can be used only when no Category I or Category III code exactly matches the medical documentation. When an unlisted code is used, a **Special Report** must be sent with the insurance claim that describes the procedure or service in detail.

CPT CODING GUIDELINES

Coding guidelines, which are found at the beginning of each section and some subsections of the Tabular List, add definitions and descriptions necessary to appropriately interpret and report the procedures and services in that section or subsection. Coding guidelines enhance the coder's understanding of when and under what circumstances specific codes may be used. Therefore, it is important to thoroughly read and apply the coding guidelines provided in the Tabular List. Because coding guidelines are updated every year on October 1, it is also important to reread the guidelines after every new edition is released. Selecting a code without reading the guidelines usually leads to selection of the wrong code. Not only will this result in possibly delayed or denied reimbursement, but also, continued inappropriate code selection can be considered fraud or abuse and can result in serious civil or criminal penalties.

Modifiers

Modifiers are two-digit, alphanumeric codes that report or indicate specific criteria, a specific condition, or a special circumstance. They are used with CPT codes to indicate that a service or procedure performed was altered by specific circumstances (Table 13-2). Modifiers are included with the five-digit CPT code to supply additional information or to describe extenuating circumstances that affected the rendered procedure or service. For instance, modifier -50 adds the detail that a procedure was performed bilaterally, or on both sides of the body. To describe a situation in which an assistant surgeon is needed for a surgical procedure, modifier -80 can be used to allow the assistant surgeon to submit charges for his or her time and services. Modifiers can also determine which side of the body a medical procedure was performed. The code 19100 RT indicates that the right breast was biopsied. A list of modifiers can be found in the CPT coding manual in Appendix A.

CPT CONVENTIONS

Conventions, or special symbols (Figure 13-7), are used to provide additional information about specific codes. For example, one of the codes in the Surgery section, Integumentary subsection, is +15401. Code 15401 describes "each additional 100 sq. cm ..." Just above code 15401 is code 15400, which describes a "xenograft of the

TABLE 13-2 Commonly Used CPT Code Modifiers

MODIFIER	DESCRIPTION
-50	Bilateral procedure. If the procedure was performed on both sides of the body (e.g., both knees, both eyes) and the code description does not indicate that the procedure or service was performed bilaterally, modifier -50 is used.
-62	Two surgeons. When two surgeons work together as primary surgeons performing distinct parts of a procedure, each surgeon should report the procedure he or she performed to the insurance carrier using modifier -62. This prevents the insurance carrier from possibly rejecting a surgical charge as a duplicate.
-26	Professional component. This modifier is used when a technician performs the service to provide his professional opinion.
-RT, -LT	Indicates the side of the body on which the procedure took place. (e.g., 19100-LT — Breast biopsy, left side)

Symbols
- ▲ Revised code
- ● New code
- ►◄ New or revised text
- ➲ Reference to *CPT Assistant, Clinical Examples in Radiology,* and *CPT Changes*
- + Add-on code
- ⊘ Exemptions to modifier 51
- ⊙ Moderate sedation
- ⁄ Product pending FDA approval
- ○ Reinstated or recycled code
- # Out-of-numerical sequence code

FIGURE 13-7 CPT conventions.

skin ... the first 100 sq. cm. or less ..." If the medical documentation states that a "200 sq. cm. xenograft of the skin" was performed, the medical assistant would code the first 100 sq. cm. using code 15400, and the second 100 sq. cm. by using add-on code 15401 (+15401).

Another example of a symbol convention is a circle with a small round dot in the center. This symbol indicates that conscious sedation, rather than a general anesthetic, was used during a surgical procedure.

In the Tabular List in most CPT manuals, the legend explaining the meanings of the convention symbols is found at the bottom of each page of the Tabular List.

APPENDICES

The CPT coding manual uses appendices to organize changes to the original code set. There are 15 appendices. A list of appendices and the codes they contain can be found in Table 13-3.

TABLE 13-3   Appendices of the CPT Manual

APPENDIX	TITLE	DESCRIPTION
A	Modifiers	All modifiers applicable to CPT codes
B	Summary of Additions, Deletions, and Revisions	Shows the actual changes made to the annual CPT manual
C	Clinical Examples	Provides helpful narrative examples to aid selection of the correct and most specific level of Evaluation and Management (E/M) codes
D	Summary of CPT Add-on Codes	A list of CPT add-on codes
E	Summary of CPT Codes Exempt from Modifier 51	CPT codes that cannot use modifier 51, which indicates multiple procedures
F	Summary of CPT Codes Exempt from Modifier 63	CPT codes that cannot use modifier 51, which indicates procedures done on infants weighing < 4 kg
G	Summary of CPT Codes That Include Moderate (Conscious) Sedation	A list of CPT codes that do not use an additional code for conscious sedation
H	Alphabetic Listing of Performance Measures	Contains an alphabetic index of performance measures by clinical condition or topic
I	Genetic Testing Modifiers	Contains genetic testing modifiers
J	Electrodiagnostic Medicine Listing of Sensory, Motor, and Mixed Nerves	A list in which each sensory, motor, and mixed nerve is assigned its appropriate nerve conduction study code, to enhance accurate reporting of codes 95907 to 95913
K	Product Pending FDA Approval	Vaccine products that have been assigned a CPT code in anticipation of approval from the Food and Drug Administration (FDA)
L	Vascular Families	A diagram of veins to the first, second, and third order. assuming that the starting point is catheterization of the aorta
M	Renumbered CPT Codes— Citations Crosswalk	A summary of crosswalked, deleted, and renumbered codes, in addition to descriptors with the associated *CPT Assistant* references for the deleted codes
N	Summary of Resequenced CPT Codes	A list of CPT codes that do not appear in numeric sequence, which allows existing codes to be relocated to an appropriate location
O	Multianalyte Assays with Algorithmic Analysis	A list of CPT codes that includes a set of administrative codes for Multianalyte Assays with Algorithmic Analyses procedures; these typically are unique to a single clinical laboratory or manufacturer

CRITICAL THINKING APPLICATION   **13-3**

Sherald is trying to look up the CPT code for a left arm cyst biopsy. She has found the code, but how can she show that the procedure took place on the left side? Sherald also came across CPT code 32491 (removal of lung, pneumonectomy), but she needs to also code for the repair of a portion of the bronchus. The code has a (+) in front of it; what does this mean?

MEDICAL DOCUMENTATION FOR CPT CODING

Medical records used for procedural coding can include any or all of the following:

- Encounter form (Figure 13-8)
- History and physical report (H&P)
- Progress notes
- Discharge summary
- Operative report
- Pathology report
- Anesthesia record
- Radiology report

When comparing the medical documentation to the code, all of the elements of the description must match substantially, with nothing added or missing. For example, review CPT codes 21325 and 21320. Both codes describe the closed treatment of a nasal bone fracture. However, 21325 indicates that there is no stabilization and 21320 indicates that there is stabilization. The coder abstracts the procedural statement and then assigns the CPT code with the description that most closely resembles the medical document.

John Porter, MD   Daniel Berg, MD
Roman Jagla, MD   Katherine Olson, PNP
Ann Johnson, MD   Emily Luther, FNP

YOUR NAME CLINIC
1234 College Avenue
Saint Paul, Minnesota 55316
Phone: (555) 555-2133   Fax: (555) 555-2134

TELEPHONE:
FAX:

PATIENT'S NAME		CHART #		DATE	

☐ MEDI-MEDI   ☐ MEDICAL
☐ MEDICARE   ☐ PRIVATE
☐ SELF PAY   ☐ HMO _____

✔	CPT/Md	DESCRIPTION	FEE	✔	CPT/Md	DESCRIPTION	FEE	✔	CPT/Md	DESCRIPTION	FEE	✔	CPT/Md	DESCRIPTION	FEE
	OFFICE VISIT—NEW PATIENT					LAB STUDIES				PROCEDURES (continued)				INJECTIONS	
	99202	Focused Ex.			36415	Venipucture			93235	Holter, 24 Hour			90724	Influenza	
	99203	Detailed Ex.			81000	Urinalysis			10061	I & D Abscess Comp.			90732	Pneumococcal	
	99204	Comprehensive Ex.			81003	–w/o Micro			10060	I & D Abscess Simple			J0295	Ampicillin, 1 gr	
	99205	Complex Ex.			84703	HCG (Urine, Pregnancy)			94761	Oximetry w/Exercise			J0696	Rocephine	
	OFFICE VISIT—ESTABLISHED PATIENT				82948	Glucose			93720	Plethysmography			J1030	Depomedrol 40 mg	
	99212	Focused Ex.			82270	Hemoccult			94760	Pulse Oximetry			J2000	Lidocaine 50 cc	
	99213	Expanded Ex.			85023	CBC-diff.			10003	Rem. Sebaceous Cyst			J2175	Demerol	
	99214	Detailed Ex.			85024	CBC w/part diff			11100	Skin Bx			J3360	Valium 5 mg	
	99215	Complex Ex.			85018	Hemoglobin			94010	Spirometry			J1885	Toradol 30 mg IV	
	PREVENTATIVE MEDICINE—NEW PATIENT				88155	Pap Smear			92801	Visual Acuity			J1885	Toradol 60 mg IM	
	99381	< 1 year old			87210	KOH/Saline Wet Mount			17100	Wart Removal			90720	DTP–HIB	
	99382	1–4 year old			87430	Strep Antigen			17101	Wart Removal, 2nd			90746	HEP B—HIB	
	99383	5–11 year old			87060	Throat Culture			17102	Wart Removal, 3–15			90707	MMR	
	99384	12–17 year old			80009	Chem profile			11042	Wound Debrid.			86580	PPD	
	99385	18–39 year old			80061	Lipid profile			X-RAY				86580	PPD w/control	
	99386	40–64 year old			82465	Cholesterol			70210	Sinuses			90732	Pneumovax	
	99387	65+ year old			99000	Handling fee			70360	Neck Soft Tissue			90716	Varicella	
	PREVENTATIVE MEDICINE—ESTABLISHED PATIENT				PROCEDURES				71010	CXR (PA only)			82607	Vitamin B12 Inj.	
	99391	< 1 year old			92551	Audiometry			71020	Chest 2V			90712	Polio	
	99392	1–4 year old			29705	Cast Removal			72040	C-Spine 2V			90788	TD Adult	
	99393	5–11 year old			2900_	Casting (by location)			72100	Lumbrosacral			95115	Allergy inj., single	
	99394	12–17 year old			92567	Ear Check			73030	Shoulder 2V			95117	Allergry inj., multiple	
	99395	18–39 year old			69210	Ear Wax Rem. 1 2			73070	Elbow 2V					
	99396	40–64 year old			93000	EKG			73120	Hand 2V					
	99397	65+ year old			93005	EKG tracing only			73560	Knee 2V					
					93010	EKG. Int. and Rep			73620	Foot 2V					
					11750	Excision Nail			74000	KUB					
					94375	Flow Volume									

DESCRIPTION   **ICD-10-CM**

____ Abdominal pain/unspec...... R10.9	
____ Abscess.......................... L02._	
____ Allergic reaction................ T78.40_	
____ Alzheimer's disease.......... G30	
____ Anemia/unspec................. D64.9	
____ Angina/unspec.................. I20.9	
____ Anorexla........................ R63.0	
____ Anxiety/unspec................. F41.9	
____ Apnea, sleep.................... G47.30	
____ Arrhythmia, cardiac........... I49.9	
____ Arthritis, rheumatoid........... M06.9	
____ Asthma/unspec.................. J45.909	
____ Atrial fibrillation................ I48.0	
____ B-12 deficiency................. E53.8	
____ Back pain, low.................. M54.5	
____ BPH.............................. N40	
____ Bradycardia/unspec........... R00.1	
____ Broncitis, acute................ J20._	
____ Bronchitis, chronic............ J42	
____ Bursitis/unspec................ M71.9	
____ CA, breast...................... C50._	
____ CA, lung........................ C34._	
____ CA, prostate.................... C61	
____ Cellulitis........................ L03._	
____ Chest pain/unspec............. R07.9	
____ Cirrhosis, liver/unspec....... K74.60	
____ Cold, common.................. J00	
____ Colitis/unspec.................. K51.90	
____ Confusion....................... R41.0	
____ CHF.............................. I50.9	
____ Constipation.................... K59.00	
____ COPD............................ J44.9	
____ Cough............................ R05	
____ Crohn's disease/unspec...... K50.90	
____ CVA.............................. I63.9	
____ Decubitus ulcer................ L89._	
____ Dehydration..................... E86.0	

____ Dementia/unspec............... F03	
____ Depression, major/unsp...... F32.9	
____ Diab I, no complications...... E10.0	
____ Diab II, no complications..... E11.9	
____ w/kidney complic........ E11.2_	
____ w/ophthalmic compl..... E11.3_	
____ w/neurolog compl........ E11.4_	
____ w/circularltory compl... E11.5_	
____ Insulin use...................... Z79.4	
____ Diarrhea/unspec............... R19.7	
____ Diverticulitis.................... K57.92	
____ Diverticulosis.................. K57.90	
____ Dizziness....................... R42	
____ Dysuria.......................... R30.0	
____ Edema/unspec.................. R60.9	
____ Endocarditis.................... I38	
____ Esophageal reflux............. K21.0	
____ Fatigue (lethargy)............. R53.83	
____ FUO.............................. R50.9	
____ Gastritis......................... K29.70	
____ Gastroenteritis (colitis)....... K52.9	
____ G.I. bleed....................... K92.2	
____ Gout/unspec.................... M10.9	
____ Headache....................... R51	
____ Health exam.................... 200._	
____ Hematuria/unspec............. R31.9	
____ Herpes simplex................ B00.9	
____ Herpes zoster.................. B02.9	
____ Hiatal hernia................... K44.9	
____ HTN (HBP)...................... I10	
____ Hyperlipidemia/unspec....... E78.5	
____ Hypothyroidism/unspec...... E03.9	
____ Impotence....................... N52._	
____ Influenza, respiratory......... J10.1	
____ Insomnia........................ G47.0	
____ IBS, diarrhea................... K58.	
____ Lupus, systemic erythm...... M32.9	

____ MI, acute....................... I21._	
____ MI, old.......................... I25.2	
____ Migraine........................ G43.9	
____ Myalgia......................... M79.1	
____ Neck pain...................... M54.2	
____ Neuropathy.................... G62.9	
____ Nausea......................... R11.1	
____ Nausea/vomitting............. R11.0	
____ Obesity/unspec................ E66.9	
____ Osteoarthritis (site).......... M19._	
____ Otitis media.................... H66.9_	
____ Parkinson's disease......... G20	
____ Pharyngitis, acute............ J02.9	
____ Pleurisy......................... R09.1	
____ Pneumonia..................... J18.9	
____ Pneumonia, viral.............. J12.9	
____ Prostatitis/unspec............ N41.9	
____ PVD............................. I73.9	
____ Radiculopathyp............... M54.1_	
____ Rectal bleeding............... K62.5	
____ Renal failure................... N19	
____ Sciatica........................ M54.3_	
____ Shortness of breath.......... R03.02	
____ Sinusitis, chr./unspec........ J32.9	
____ Syncope........................ R55	
____ Tachycardia/unspec.......... R00.0	
____ Tachy., supraventric.......... I47.1	
____ Tedinitix/unspec............... M77.9	
____ TIA.............................. G45.9	
____ Ulcer, duodenal/unspec..... K26.9	
____ Ulcer, gastric/unspec........ K25.9	
____ Ulcer, peptic/unspec......... K27.9	
____ URI/unspec.................... J06.9	
____ UTI.............................. N39.0	
____ Vertigo......................... R42	
____ Weight gain................... R63.5	
____ Weight loss.................... R63.4	

DIAGNOSIS: (IF NOT CHECKED ABOVE)

PROCEDURES: (IF NOT CHECKED ABOVE)

TODAY'S FEE

AMT. REC'D.

RETURN APPOINTMENT INFORMATION:

(____ DAYS)(____ WKS.)(____ MOS.)(____ PRN)

REC'D BY:
☐ CASH
☐ CR. CARD
☐ CHECK
_____

BALANCE

FIGURE 13-8 Encounter form.

Some providers have CPT and ICD-10-CM codes printed on their encounter forms; however, these codes should be treated only as a reference. Medical coders must also review the health record carefully and an abstract of all the procedures and services rendered during an encounter, regardless of all codes highlighted on the encounter form. For example, a provider may circle the procedure for a preventive health visit for a 4-year-old on the encounter form, but forgets to record the injections provided during the encounter. When the medical assistant reviews the patient's electronic health record (EHR), he or she discovers that the provider's notes state routine injections were indeed administered. If the medical assistant had not reviewed the EHR, the clinic would have lost reimbursement because the claim would not have included all the CPT codes applicable to the visit. Encounter forms should be updated annually to ensure that code additions, changes, and revisions are current.

STEPS FOR EFFICIENT CPT PROCEDURAL CODING

The CPT coding process, which includes use of the Alphabetic Index and the Tabular List, applies to all sections of the CPT manual, except for the E/M and Anesthesia sections.

To start the procedural coding process, you must first determine the procedures or services that were provided. This is accomplished with two basic steps:

1. Analyze and abstract the procedural statement documented in the health record.
2. Compare it with the encounter form, operative report, or other documentation to ensure that all services and procedures have been recorded.

For practice on CPT surgery coding, refer to Procedure 13-1.

Abstracting

The term *abstract*, used as a verb in this context, is the process of collecting pertinent medical information needed to assign the correct code.

Abstracting ensures that all medical procedures and services are identified and none are omitted. The abstracted data are then broken down into main terms and modifying terms. A main term is usually the primary procedure or service performed, and a modifying term further defines or adds information to the main term. Next, the main and modifying terms are used to find the code or code ranges in the Alphabetic Index. Last, the code selected is confirmed by reviewing the guidelines, notes, and conventions in the Tabular List to verify that the most accurate code has been chosen.

PROCEDURE 13-1   Perform Procedural Coding: Surgery

Goal: *To use the steps for CPT procedural coding to find the most accurate and specific CPT surgery code.*

EQUIPMENT and SUPPLIES

- CPT coding manual (current year)
- Surgery report (Figure 1)
- TruCode encoder software

PROCEDURAL STEPS

Using the CPT Coding Manual

1. Abstract the procedures and/or services from the procedural statement in the surgical report.
2. Select the most appropriate main term to begin the search in the Alphabetic Index.
3. Once the main term has been located in the Alphabetic Index, review and select the modifying term or terms if required.
   PURPOSE: For additional specificity and to narrow the search for the most accurate CPT code or code range in the Alphabetic Index.
4. If the main term cannot be found in the Alphabetic Index, repeat steps 2 and 3 using a different main term possibly based on the procedural statement.
5. Once the CPT code or code range is identified in the Alphabetic Index, disregard any code or code range containing additional descriptions or modifying terms not found in the health record.
6. Record the code or code ranges that best match the procedural statements in the surgical report.
   PURPOSE: To prevent repeated reference to the Alphabetic Index by recording all possible matches to the code or code range sought. This saves time and prevents redundant effort.

7. Turn to the Tabular List and find the first code or code range from your search of the Alphabetic Index.
   PURPOSE: To begin the process of finding the most specific and accurate code.
8. Compare the description of the code with the procedural statement in the surgical report. Verify that all or most of the health record documentation matches the code description and that there is no additional information in the code description that is not found in the documentation.
9. Review the coding guidelines and notes for the section, subsection, and code to ensure that there are no contraindications to use of the code. Review the coding conventions and add-on codes, if any.
   PURPOSE: To ensure there are no instructions that would prevent the use of the code selected.
10. Determine whether a modifier is needed.
    PURPOSE: To select any appropriate modifiers that provide additional information for the chosen code to explain certain circumstances or provide additional detail.
11. Determine whether a Special Report is required.
    PURPOSE: To clarify and add additional detail when an unusual or extenuating circumstance exists or if a Category III or unlisted procedure Category I code is used.
12. Record the CPT code selected in the health record documentation next to the procedure or service performed and in the appropriate block of the insurance claim form.
    PURPOSE: To complete the documentation and recording requirements.

PROCEDURE 13-1   *—continued*

Operative Report

PATIENT NAME: Sonia Sample
ROOM NUMBER: 222 West
MR NUMBER: 12-34-56

DATE OF PROCEDURE: 04/22/00
PREOPERATIVE DIAGNOSIS: Acute cholecystitis
POSTOPERATIVE DIAGNOSIS: Acute cholecystitis
NAME OF PROCEDURE: 1. Laparoscopic cholecystectomy
                           2. Intraoperative cystic duct cholangiogram
SURGEON: Claude St. John, M.D.
ASSISTANT: Mark Weiss, D.O.
ANESTHESIOLOGIST: Angela Adams, M.D.
ANESTHESIA: General

DESCRIPTION OF THE OPERATION:
    The patient was placed in the supine position under general anesthesia. The oral gastric tube was placed. The Foley catheter was placed. The patient received appropriate antibiotics. The abdomen was prepped with iodine and draped in the usual fashion. Using a midline subumbilical incision, we entered the subcutaneous fat to find the aponeurosis of the rectus abdominis. Two stay sutures were placed 0.5 cm from the midline bilaterally and we left on these sutures, creating an opening in the linea alba.
    Under direct vision, the catheter was placed. The Hasson cannula was placed in the abdominal cavity and all was normal except an acute necrotizing and probably gangrenous gallbladder. There were multiple omental adhesions. Three other trocars were placed in the right subcostal plane in the midline, midclavicular line, and midaxillary line using a #10, #5, and #5 mm trocar, respectively. The gallbladder was punctured and emptied of clear white bile indicating a hydrops of the gallbladder. It was grasped at its fundus and at Hartmann's pouch retracted cephalad and to the right, respectively. We found the cystic duct and the cystic artery after circumferential dissection and isolated the cystic duct completely.
    When we were sure that this structure was a deep cystic duct, the clip was placed at the most distal aspect to make an opening immediately proximally and we placed a Reddick cholangiocatheter into it via #14 gauge percutaneous catheter. The cholangiogram showed normal arborization of the liver radicals. Normal bifurcation of the common hepatic duct. Normal common hepatic duct. Long large cystic duct. The common bile duct had numerous stones within it. They could not be emptied from the common bile duct. There was good flow into the duodenum.
    The impression was choledocholithiasis. This was corroborated by the radiologist. The decision was made to prepare the patient most probably for endoscopic retrograde cholangiopancreatography postoperatively, and no further intervention of the common bile duct was done in this setting.
    The cholangiocatheter was removed. An attempt was made to milk the bile out, but no stones came out. Three clips were placed on the proximal aspect of the cystic duct and the duct was then cut distally. The artery was isolated and double clipped proximally and single clipped distally and cut in the intervening section. We then peeled the gallbladder off the gallbladder bed with some difficulty because of the intense edema and inflammation. It was then removed from the liver bed completely. Cautery, suctioning and irrigation were used copiously to create a bloodless field. A last check was made and there was no bleeding and no bile leaking. A #15 Jackson-Pratt type drain was placed into Morrison's pouch and brought out through the lateral most port. We then removed, with great difficulty, the gallbladder from the umbilicus. Because of its enormous size and a 3 cm stone within it that was very difficult to macerate, the opening of the umbilicus had to be enlarged.
    As this was done, we removed the gallbladder completely and sent it for pathologic section. Two separate figure-of-eight 0 PDS were used to close the abdominal fascia. The Jackson-Pratt drain was then sutured in place with 2.0 nylon. The skin was closed throughout with subcuticular 3-0 PDS after copious irrigation of the subcutaneous plane. Mastisol and Steri-Strips were placed on the wound. The patient remained stable although she did have bigeminy during surgery and was on a Lidocaine drip. She will be going to the intensive care unit but as she left, she was extubated in the recovery room and was fully alert. She is moving all limbs.
    I will discuss with the gastroenterologist postoperative endoscopic retrograde cholangiopancreatography.
    SPECIMEN: Gallbladder.

Claude St. John, M.D.
CSJ/ld:
D. 04/22/00
T: 04/22/00 9:21 am
CC: Maria Acosta, M.D.

1

PROCEDURE 13-1   *—continued*

Using the TruCode Software

1. Abstract the procedures and/or services from the procedural statement in the surgical report.
2. Type the main term into the encoder Search box and select the CPT. Then click on Show All Results.
3. If the main term cannot be found through the search, repeat steps 2 and 3 using a different main term based on the procedural statement.
4. Choose the procedure description that is closest to the procedural statement in the surgical report as shown in Figure 2.

PURPOSE: To prevent upcoding or downcoding errors or other possible fraud and/or abuse circumstances.

5. Record the CPT code that best matches the procedural statements in the surgical report in the patient's health record.

PURPOSE: To prevent repeated reference to the Alphabetic Index by recording all possible matches to the code or code range being sought. This saves time and prevents redundant effort.

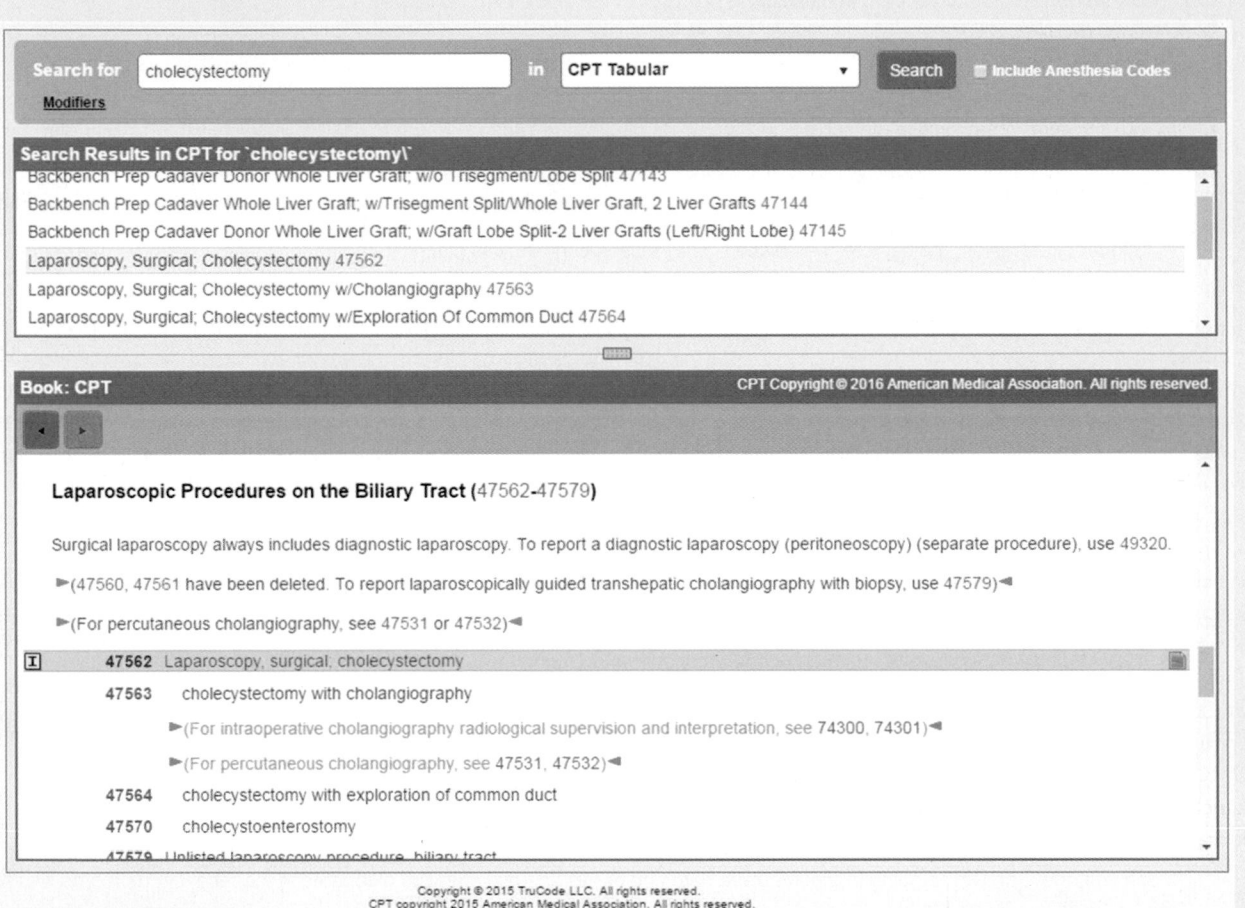

2

USING THE ALPHABETIC INDEX

Although the Alphabetic Index is a comprehensive, alphabetic listing of all main terms, there are no code descriptions. Therefore, it would not be effective to assign a CPT code simply by finding it through the Alphabetic Index. The Alphabetic Index is not a substitute for the Tabular List. Even if an individual is only looking for one code, the Tabular List must be used to ensure the code is accurate.

The Alphabetic Index is used as a guide to search for one or more codes or code ranges. The index is similar to that found in the back of any textbook; it is an alphabetic list of main and modifying terms found in the Tabular List of the coding manual. In a typical index,

the term or concept listed in the index is followed by a reference page or pages, where detailed information is presented in the body of the book. The Alphabetic Index in the CPT coding manual is used in the same way, except that it references codes or code ranges rather than pages. As discussed earlier, the Tabular List is divided into sections, and the procedures and services are listed in numeric order by the Category I code.

The Alphabetic Index is organized by main terms, and modifying terms are indented two spaces below the main term. Modifying terms further describe and add information needed to narrow the search for an appropriate procedure or service code. A main term can be a procedure, such as an excision, and each modifying term could provide further information about the anatomic location or the organ excised, the type of instrument used, a special technique, or whether other procedures were performed at the same time as the excision, such as obtaining biopsy tissue for examination. *Modifying terms affect the selection of appropriate codes; therefore, it is important to review the list of modifying terms when selecting a code or code range.*

Searching the Alphabetic Index

Begin the search of the Alphabetic Index by using one of the four primary classifications (or types) of main and modifying term entries:
- Procedure or service (e.g., examination, excision, scope, revision, repair, drainage)
- Organ or anatomic site (e.g., clavicle, mandible, humerus, liver, colon, uterus)
- Condition, illness, or injury (e.g., cholelithiasis, ulcer, fracture, pregnancy, fever)
- Eponym, synonym, abbreviation, or acronym (e.g., Naffziger operation, MRI [magnetic resonance imaging], TURP [transurethral resection of the prostate]).

When searching the Alphabetic Index, use the name of the performed procedure or service (anastomosis, splint, repair, stress test, therapy, vaccination); the organ or other anatomic site of the procedure (tibia, colon, salivary gland, aorta); the condition, illness, or injury (abscess, fracture, cholelithiasis, strabismus); or, if applicable, synonyms, eponyms, or abbreviations (ECG [electrocardiography], Stookey-Scarff procedure, Mohs' micrographic surgery).

Sometimes searching for a Main Term may not yield any results. When a Main Term cannot be found, search by another primary classification in the Alphabetic Index. Let's search the following procedural statement: Removal of Skin Tags on Neck. Begin by identifying the Main Terms that closely match the four primary classifications in the Alphabetic Index.
1. Procedure of Service: Removal
2. Organ or Anatomic Site: Neck Skin
3. Condition, Illness, or Injury: Skin Tag
4. Eponym: none in this case

Once all possible Main Terms have been abstracted, the coder can quickly search through the Alphabetic Index for the code or code range that matches the procedural statement.

Using *See* and *See Also* in the Alphabetic Index

The *see* statement in the Alphabetic Index points to another location in the Alphabetic Index to find the code or code range. The *see also* statement points to additional codes or code ranges in the Alphabetic Index that may be useful to the code found in the original search.

Use of the Semicolon

A semicolon (;) at the end of a main description indicates that modifying terms and descriptions follow. Every indented description below a stand-alone code is related to that stand-alone code. If a main term has no additional modifying terms, the next entry is a stand-alone description of a different procedure, which is positioned flush left, without indentation. As shown in Figure 13-9, the highlighted CPT code 61314 uses the semicolon and provides two locations.

61314	Craniectomy or craniotomy for evacuation of hematoma, infratentorial; extradural or subdural

FIGURE 13-9 Use of semicolon.

Stand-Alone Codes and Code Ranges

In the Alphabetic Index, a procedure or service may list a single code or a range of possible codes that may match the medical documentation. Remember that the Alphabetic Index is an index; it is designed as a guide to the most suitable codes that match the documentation. At this point, the search is only for the closest match or matches to the procedural statement.

Because some medical procedures and diagnostic tests can be quite complex, there may be a single (stand-alone) code or a code range that may include one main term but has several modifying terms from the Main Term. For example, the code for *Craterization, phalanges, toe* is 28124, a stand-alone code. However, using the same main term, *Craterization,* but adding *any of the phalanges* yields a range of codes: 26235-29236. The code range is shown with a hyphen to indicate that all codes within that range could be appropriate.

In some cases a stand-alone code and a range of codes are listed for the same service or procedure. For example, *Craterization, femur,* lists both the stand-alone code 27360 and the code range 27070-27071. Once a stand-alone code or code range has been found in the Alphabetic Index, the next step is to look up each of those in the Tabular List and select the code or codes that most closely match the medical documentation.

Steps for Using the CPT Alphabetic Index

1. Abstract the procedural statement from the medical documentation and determine the Main and/or Modifying Terms.
2. Select the most appropriate main term to begin searching in the Alphabetic Index.
3. Once the main term has been located, select one or more modifying terms, if needed, to narrow the search.
4. If no main or modifying term produces an appropriate code or code range, repeat steps 2 and 3 using a different main term.
5. Find the code or code ranges that include all or most of the description of the procedure or service found in the medical record.

CRITICAL THINKING APPLICATION 13-4
Sherald is having trouble finding a removal of a cataract procedure code in the Alphabetic Index. What are some options and/or alternative ways she can perform an Alphabetic Index search?

USING THE TABULAR LIST

Once the code or code ranges have been selected from the Alphabetic Index, the next stop is the Tabular List, where the procedural coding decision takes place. In the Tabular List, the conventions, symbols, guidelines, notes, and even the punctuation all play a part in choosing the most accurate code possible.

In the Tabular List, look up each code or code range found in the Alphabetic Index numerically. Read the description of each code thoroughly to ensure that the main terms abstracted from the procedural statement in the medical documentation are all included in the code description, with nothing substantial omitted or added. Read the section guidelines and notes to determine whether additional codes should be used, add-on codes or modifiers are required, or use of the code is contraindicated.

> 5. Determine whether any special circumstances require the use of a modifier or whether a Special Report is required.
> 6. Record the CPT code selected in the health record documentation next to the procedure or service performed and in the appropriate block of the insurance claim form.

Steps for Using the CPT Tabular List

Except for the special considerations required for coding from the Evaluation and Management (E/M) and Anesthesia sections, the following steps apply to all sections of the CPT manual.

1. Look up the code or code range from the Alphabetic Index Search in the Tabular List numerically.
2. Compare the description of the code with the procedural statement from the medical documentation. Verify that all or most of the health record documentation matches the code description and that there is no additional element or information in the code description that is not found in the documentation.
3. Read the guidelines and notes for the section, subsection, and code to ensure that there are no contraindications to use of the code.
4. Evaluate the conventions, especially add-on codes (+) and exemption from modifier -51.

SECTION-SPECIFIC CPT CODING GUIDELINES

Common CPT Coding Guidelines: Evaluation and Management Section

To properly code E/M services, the medical assistant must apply different code lookup techniques from the basic steps outlined earlier. Assigning the correct E/M code includes identifying the section, subsection, category, and subcategory of the procedure or service; reviewing the reporting instructions and guidelines for the code chosen; reviewing the level of E/M service; determining the extent of history obtained and examination performed; and determining the complexity of medical decision making.

The E/M section is divided into broad subsections, such as *office visit, emergency room visit, hospital visit,* and *consultation.* These subsections are further divided into subcategories, which include the place where the services were rendered (e.g., the provider's office, a hospital emergency department, a skilled nursing facility, or the patient's home) and the patient status (i.e., whether the patient is new or established). Procedure 13-2, part A, explains how to perform CPT coding for an office visit.

The first two steps in choosing an E/M code are:
1. Identify the place of service (POS)
2. Identify the patient status (new or established)

PROCEDURE 13-2   Perform Procedural Coding: Office Visit and Immunizations

Goal: *To use the steps for CPT Evaluation and Management coding and HCPCS coding to find the most accurate and specific CPT E/M and HCPCS codes using the coding manuals and the TruCode encoder.*

EQUIPMENT and SUPPLIES

- CPT coding manual (current year)
- HCPCS coding manual (current year)
- Progress Note (see Study Guide Chapter 13) (Figure 1)
- TruCode encoder software

Part A: CPT E/M Coding

1. Determine the place of service from the encounter form.
   To determine the most accurate CPT E/M code, the place of service needs to be identified.
2. Determine the patient's status.
   PURPOSE: To determine the most accurate CPT E/M code, the patient should be identified as new or established.
3. Identify the subsection, category, or subcategory of service in the E/M section.

PURPOSE: To ensure that the correct place of service and patient status are used and the appropriate level of service is selected.
4. Determine the level of service:
   - Determine the extent of the history obtained.
   - Determine the extent of the examination performed.
   - Determine the complexity of medical decision making.
   PURPOSE: To ensure that the correct level is chosen for the history, examination, and medical decision making.
5. If necessary, compare the medical documentation against examples in Appendix C, Clinical Examples, of the CPT manual.
   PURPOSE: To help the coder select the appropriate level of service.
6. Select the appropriate level of E/M service code, and document it in the patient's health record.
   PURPOSE: To complete the documentation and reporting requirements.

PROCEDURE 13-2 *—continued*

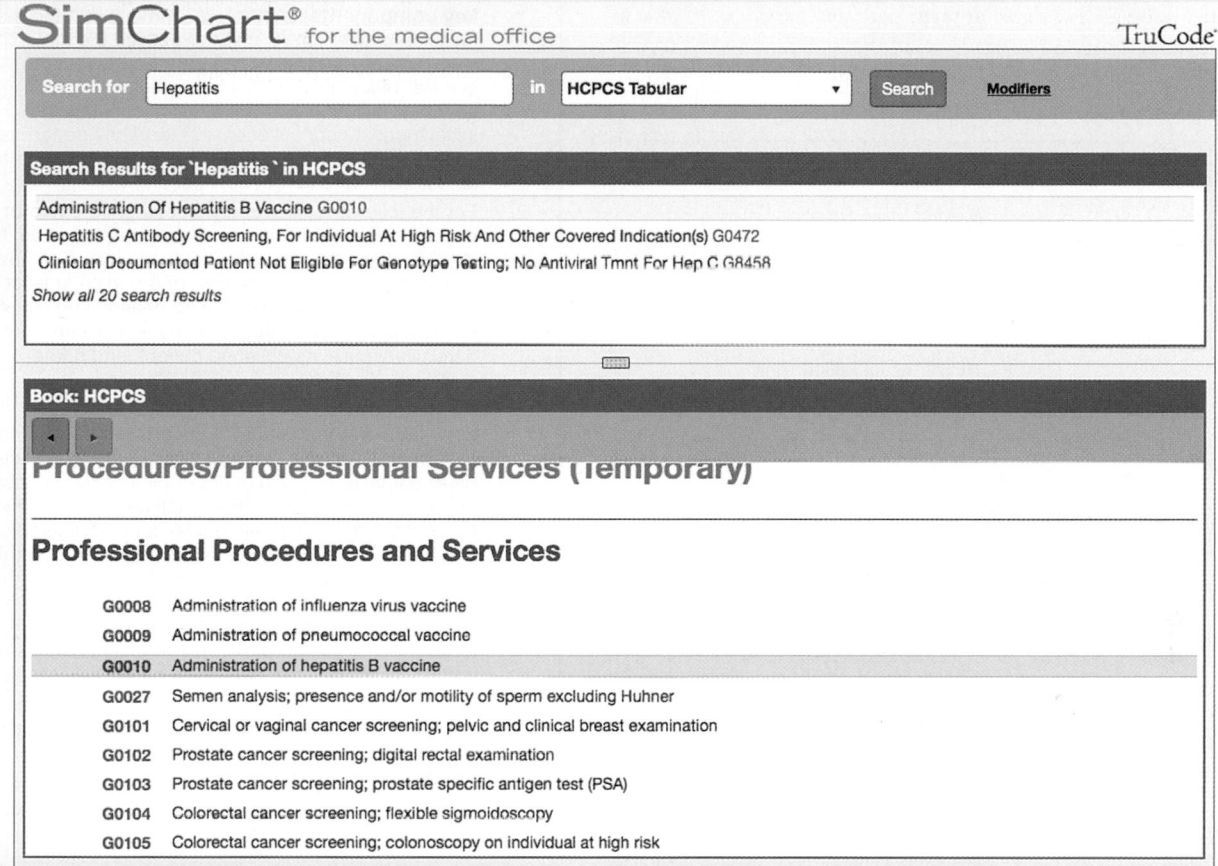

SimChart® for the medical office   TruCode·

| Search for | Hepatitis | in | HCPCS Tabular ▾ | Search | **Modifiers** |

Search Results for `Hepatitis` in HCPCS

Administration Of Hepatitis B Vaccine G0010
Hepatitis C Antibody Screening, For Individual At High Risk And Other Covered Indication(s) G0472
Clinician Documented Patient Not Eligible For Genotype Testing; No Antiviral Tmnt For Hep C G8458
Show all 20 search results

Book: HCPCS

◄   ►

Procedures/Professional Services (Temporary)

Professional Procedures and Services

G0008	Administration of influenza virus vaccine
G0009	Administration of pneumococcal vaccine
G0010	Administration of hepatitis B vaccine
G0027	Semen analysis; presence and/or motility of sperm excluding Huhner
G0101	Cervical or vaginal cancer screening; pelvic and clinical breast examination
G0102	Prostate cancer screening; digital rectal examination
G0103	Prostate cancer screening; prostate specific antigen test (PSA)
G0104	Colorectal cancer screening; flexible sigmoidoscopy
G0105	Colorectal cancer screening; colonoscopy on individual at high risk

1

Part B: HCPCS Coding with TruCode Encoder Software

1. Review the provider documentation.
   PURPOSE: To ensure that all procedures and/or services are listed on the encounter form; that all procedures and services on the encounter form match the health record; and that nothing documented in the health record is missing from the encounter form.
2. Type the main term into the Search box of the encoder and choose the HCPCS Tabular code set for accurate coding.
3. If no modifying term produces an appropriate code or code range, repeat steps 2 and 3 using a different main term.

PURPOSE: To help find the most appropriate code or code range by using alternative methods of searching the Alphabetic Index.
4. Compare the description of the code with the medical documentation.
   PURPOSE: To avoid upcoding and downcoding errors and to ensure there are no contraindications to use of the code selected.
5. Select the appropriate HCPCS immunization code, and document it in the patient's health record.
   PURPOSE: To complete the documentation and reporting requirements.

Identifying the Place of Service

The place of service (POS) is the healthcare facility where the encounter between the patient and the provider occurred and where the medical service was delivered. The two most common places of service are "office" and "hospital." Table 13-4 presents a list of common POS locations and their two-digit identifying numbers, or POS codes.

Identifying the Patient Status

The patient status choices are "new" or "established" patient. A new patient (NP) is one who has not received any professional services from the provider, or from another provider of the exact same specialty and subspecialty who belongs to the same group practice, within the past 3 years. An established patient (EP) is one who has received professional services from the provider, or from another

TABLE 13-4 Commonly Used Codes for Place of Service

CODE	NAME
01	Pharmacy
11	Office
12	Home
13	Assisted Living Facility
14	Group Home
15	Mobile Unit
17	Walk-In Retail Health Clinic
20	Urgent Care Facility
21	Inpatient Hospital
22	Outpatient Hospital
23	Emergency Room—Hospital
24	Ambulatory Surgery Center
31	Skilled Nursing Facility
34	Hospice
51	Inpatient Psychiatric Facility
60	Mass Immunization Center
65	End-Stage Renal Disease Treatment Facility
71	Public Health Clinic
72	Rural Health Clinic
81	Independent Laboratory

Select the Appropriate Level of E/M Services Based on the Following

1. For the following categories/subcategories, **all of the key components**, ie, history, examination, and medical decision making, must meet or exceed the stated requirements to qualify for a particular level of E/M service: office, new patient; hospital observation services; initial hospital care; office consultations, initial inpatient consultations; emergency department services; initial nursing facility care; domiciliary care, new patient; and home, new patient.

2. For the following categories/subcategories, **two of the three key components** (ie, history, examination, and medical decision making) must meet or exceed the stated requirements to qualify for a particular level of E/M services: office, established patient; subsequent hospital care; subsequent nursing facility care; domiciliary care, established patient; and home, established patient.

3. When counseling and/or coordination of care dominates (more than 50%) the encounter with the patient and/or family (face-to-face time in the office or other outpatient setting or floor/unit time in the hospital or nursing facility), then **time** shall be considered the key or controlling factor to qualify for a particular level of E/M services. This includes time spent with parties who have assumed responsibility for the care of the patient or decision making whether or not they are family members (eg, foster parents, person acting in loco parentis, legal guardian). The extent of counseling and/or coordination of care must be documented in the medical record.

FIGURE 13-10 Appropriate assignment of E/M codes.

provider of the exact same specialty and subspecialty who belongs to the same group practice, within the past 3 years.

Once the POS and patient status have been established, the next step in selection of an E/M code is to determine the level of service provided.

Determining the Level of Service Provided

Key Components and Contributing Factors. The three key components for determining the level of service for E/M coding are the history, examination, and medical decision making. The four contributing factors are counseling, the nature of the presenting problem, coordination of care, and time. The history, examination, and medical decision-making components are considered primary key; that is, they are typically the three most important components for deciding the level of service. Counseling, the nature of the presenting problem, coordination of care, and time are secondary considerations. Figure 13-10 presents criteria for choosing the appropriate E/M code.

History. To understand the levels of the history, it is important to know the definition and components of the patient history. The history relates to the patient's clinical picture and depends on the patient for answers to specific questions.

Levels of History. The following are the four levels of history taking.

Problem-focused history: A problem-focused history concentrates on the chief complaint; it looks at the symptoms, severity, and duration of the problem. It usually does not include a review of systems (ROS) or the family and social histories.

Expanded problem-focused history: The provider proceeds as in the problem-focused history but includes a review of systems that relate to the chief complaint. Usually the past, family, and social histories are not included.

Detailed history: The detailed history consists of the chief complaint; extended history of present illness; problem-pertinent system review extended to include a review of a limited number of additional systems; and the pertinent past, family, and/or social histories directly related to the patient's problems.

Comprehensive history: A comprehensive history includes the chief complaint; extended history of present illness; an ROS that is directly related to the problem or problems identified in the history of the present illness plus a review of all additional body systems; and complete past, family, and social histories.

Examination. The examination is the objective part of the patient's visit. The provider examines the patient, obtains measurable findings, and makes notes referring to body areas and/or organ systems as follows:

- *Body areas:* Head, including face and neck; chest, including breasts and axillae; abdomen; genitalia, groin, and buttocks; and back, including spine and extremities
- *Organs and organ systems:* Constitution (e.g., vital signs, general appearance); eyes; ears, nose, throat, and mouth; cardiovascular; respiratory; gastrointestinal (GI); genitourinary; musculoskeletal; skin; neurologic; psychiatric; and hematologic, lymphatic, and immunologic

Levels of Examination. The examination is divided into the following levels:

- *Problem-focused examination:* The examination is limited to the single body area or single system mentioned in the chief complaint.
- *Expanded problem-focused examination:* In addition to the limited body area or system, related body areas or organ systems are examined.
- *Detailed examination:* An extended examination is performed on the related body areas or organ systems.
- *Comprehensive examination:* A complete multisystem examination is performed or a complete examination of a single organ system.

Medical Decision Making. When a provider makes medical decisions, the decisions are based on many years of education and experience. Three elements comprise the medical decision-making process:

1. The number of diagnoses and/or management options
2. The amount and/or complexity of data obtained, reviewed, and analyzed
3. The risk of significant complications and/or morbidity and/or mortality

Number of Diagnoses and Management Options. The provider's notes during the history and examination should help identify whether the patient's problem is minor, acute, stable, or worsening. The medical documentation should also identify whether a new problem exists or whether the provider plans to order any diagnostic tests to further investigate the patient's illness or injury.

Amount and Complexity of Data Reviewed. The medical documentation should also identify what laboratory tests, x-ray diagnostic procedures, and other tests have been ordered or reviewed.

Risk of Complications and Morbidity or Mortality. Risk is often involved in medical care, either from the treatment given to the patient or from the lack of treatment and professional care. *Morbidity,* the relative incidence of disease, and *mortality,* which relates to the number of deaths from a given disease, are integral parts of the provider's assessment of risks.

Complexity Levels in Medical Decision Making. The complexity of medical decision making is categorized into four levels: straightforward, low complexity, moderate complexity, and high complexity. Table 13-5 presents descriptions of the different levels of complexity of medical decision making.

Factors That Contribute to E/M Complexity

Counseling. Counseling is a discussion with a patient and/or family members about the diagnostic results, impressions, recommended diagnostic studies, prognosis, risks and benefits of management or treatment options, and instructions for management, treatment, and/or follow-up. Almost all E/M services involve a degree of counseling with the patient and/or family. This is factored into the E/M code, and as long as this factor does not exceed 50% of the time spent with the patient, it is included in the E/M code. It can be considered a contributing factor when the counseling exceeds 50% of the encounter.

Nature of the Presenting Problem. The presenting problem is usually explained in the chief complaint. It can range from something as simple as a cold in an otherwise healthy patient to a life-threatening problem. Unless dealing with the nature of the presenting problem exceeds half of the patient encounter, it is included in the E/M code description and is not a factor in selecting the level of service.

Coordination of Care. Some patients need assistance in arranging for care beyond the visit or hospitalization. Some will need care in a skilled nursing facility or home health care. Others will need hospice care. The primary provider usually coordinates this care. Coordination of care is also factored into the E/M code and is a consideration for determining the level of service only when it exceeds 50% of the patient encounter.

Time. Time is included in the E/M code descriptions only to assist providers in selecting the most appropriate level of E/M service. The times expressed in the code descriptions are averages, and time is not a determining factor in code selection unless counseling exceeds more than 50% of the encounter. Only then can time be used as a determining component to code level selection.

TABLE 13-5 Complexity of Medical Decision Making			
NUMBER OF DIAGNOSES OR MANAGEMENT OPTIONS	**AMOUNT AND/OR COMPLEXITY OF DATA TO BE REVIEWED**	**RISK OF COMPLICATIONS AND/OR MORBIDITY OR MORTALITY**	**TYPE OF MEDICAL DECISION MAKING**
Minimal	Minimal or none	Minimal	Straightforward
Limited	Limited	Low	Low complexity
Multiple	Moderate	Moderate	Moderate complexity
Extensive	Extensive	High	High complexity

At first, E/M coding can be difficult to understand and put into practice. The E/M coding process provided here can serve as a guide to medical assistants in determining the place of service, patient status, and level of care provided, so that they can select the most accurate E/M code. Using the clinical examples in Appendix C of the CPT manual and comparing them to the medical documentation also can help medical assistants acquire a better understanding of E/M coding.

CRITICAL THINKING APPLICATION   13-5

Dr. Caddell performed a colonoscopy at the ambulatory surgery center on Cecil Matthews, who has been Dr. Caddell's patient for several years. Mr. Matthews came to the office with left lower quadrant pain and a history of colon cancer. What other factors or information would Sherald need to know to properly code Mr. Matthews' office visit? What medical documentation would Sherald need to properly code Mr. Matthews' colonoscopy?

Common CPT Coding Guidelines: Anesthesia

Anesthesiologists and **Certified Registered Nurse Anesthetists (CRNAs)** use codes in the Anesthesia section, which are also known as CPT-4 codes. These codes always start with a zero (0) and identify the anatomic location of the surgery performed. CPT-4 codes are used for unconscious sedation, or for putting patients to sleep during the medical procedure; codes for conscious sedation are found in the Medicine section.

Anesthesia coding differs from any other form of coding in the way anesthesia services are billed. These professionals are paid a standard amount per unit compared to surgeons, who are paid by the procedure. A standard formula has been established to determine the number of units they can bill for each procedure for which they provide anesthesia.

$$\text{Basic unit values} + \text{Time units} + \text{Modifying units } (B + T + M)$$

Anesthesia Formula

All healthcare providers who can administer anesthesia, including anesthesiologists and CRNAs, use CPT-4 codes for anesthesia services based on the anatomic region of the body where the surgery was performed.

Basic Unit Value (B)

The Anesthesia Society of America (ASA) publishes a Relative Value Guide (RVG) that lists the codes for anesthesia services. The RVG compares anesthesia services and assigns a numeric value to each service based on the level of complexity; this numeric value is called the *basic unit value.*

Time Units (T)

Anesthesia services are provided based on the time during which the anesthesia was administered, in hours and minutes. Typically 15 minutes equals 1 time unit, although this can vary because insurance carriers make that determination independently. The time starts when the anesthesiology provider begins preparing the patient to receive anesthesia, continues through the procedure, and ends when

the patient is no longer under the professional care of the anesthesiology provider. The hours and minutes during which anesthesia was administered are recorded in the patient's anesthesia record (Figure 13-11).

Modifying Units (M)

Modifying units reflect circumstances or conditions that change or modify the environment in which the anesthesia service was provided. The two modifying characteristics for anesthesia services are qualifying circumstances and physical status modifiers.

Qualifying Circumstances (QC). Sometimes anesthesia is provided in situations that make administration more difficult. These types of cases include provision of anesthesia in emergency situations, to patients of extreme age, during the use of controlled hypotension, and with hypothermia. There are four qualifying circumstances (QC) codes. Each of the five-digit codes is preceded by a plus sign symbol (+), indicating that it is an add-on code; these codes are used in addition to the Category I anesthesia code.

Physical Status Modifiers. Physical status modifiers are used to indicate the patient's physical condition at the time anesthesia was provided. There are five physical status modifiers, each composed of two characters: first the letter P, followed by a ranking of 1 to 6 (e.g., P1, P2, P3, and so on). P1 represents a normal, healthy patient, and P6 represents a brain-dead patient whose organs are being harvested. Table 13-6 presents a list of physical status modifiers and their

TABLE 13-6 Anesthesia Physical Status and Qualifying Circumstances Modifiers

MODIFIER	DESCRIPTION
Physical Status Modifiers*	
P1	A normal healthy patient
P2	A patient with mild systemic disease
P3	A patient with severe systemic disease
P4	A person with severe systemic disease that is a constant threat to life
P5	A moribund patient who is not expected to survive without the procedure
P6	A declared brain-dead patient whose organs are being removed for donor purposes
Qualifying Circumstances CPT Codes†	
99100	Anesthesia for a patient of extreme age (i.e., <1 yr or >70 yr)
99116	Anesthesia complicated by utilization of total body hypothermia
99135	Anesthesia complicated by utilization of controlled hypothermia

*A physical status modifier is required for performing anesthesia calculations.
†Use a qualifying circumstances modifier code, if appropriate, in addition to the primary CPT Category I Anesthesia code.

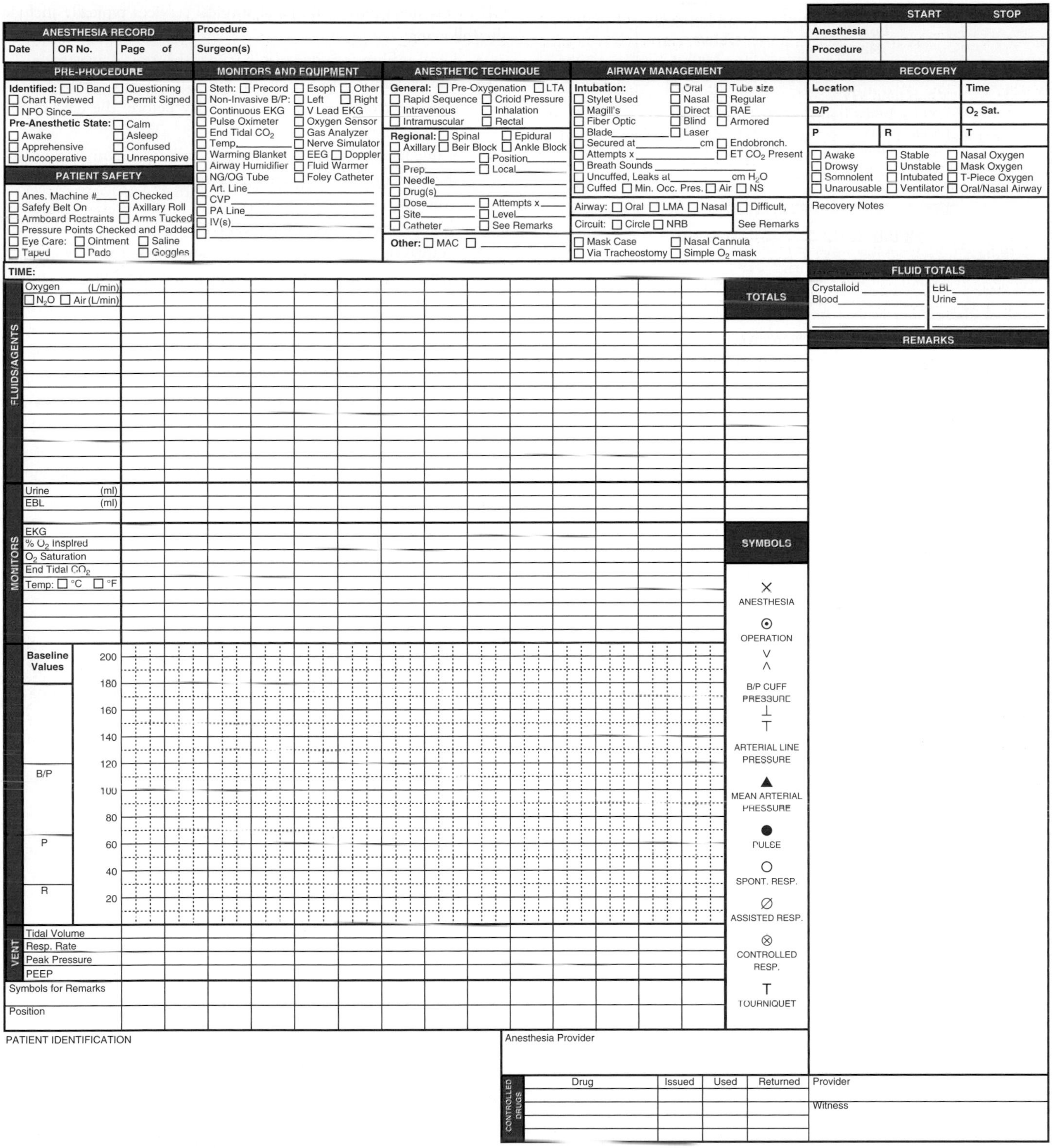

ANESTHESIA RECORD | Procedure | START | STOP
Date | OR No. | Page of | Surgeon(s)
Anesthesia | Procedure

PRE-PROCEDURE
Identified: ☐ ID Band ☐ Questioning ☐ Chart Reviewed ☐ Permit Signed ☐ NPO Since____
Pre-Anesthetic State: ☐ Calm ☐ Awake ☐ Asleep ☐ Apprehensive ☐ Confused ☐ Uncooperative ☐ Unresponsive

PATIENT SAFETY
☐ Anes. Machine #____ ☐ Checked ☐ Safety Belt On ☐ Axillary Roll ☐ Armboard Restraints ☐ Arms Tucked ☐ Pressure Points Checked and Padded ☐ Eye Care: ☐ Ointment ☐ Saline ☐ Taped ☐ Pads ☐ Goggles

MONITORS AND EQUIPMENT
☐ Steth: ☐ Precord ☐ Esoph ☐ Other ☐ Non-Invasive B/P: ☐ Left ☐ Right ☐ Continuous EKG ☐ V Lead EKG ☐ Pulse Oximeter ☐ Oxygen Sensor ☐ End Tidal CO_2 ☐ Gas Analyzer ☐ Temp.____ ☐ Nerve Simulator ☐ Warming Blanket ☐ EEG ☐ Doppler ☐ Airway Humidifier ☐ Fluid Warmer ☐ NG/OG Tube ☐ Foley Catheter ☐ Art. Line____ ☐ CVP____ ☐ PA Line____ ☐ IV(s)____ ☐

ANESTHETIC TECHNIQUE
General: ☐ Pre-Oxygenation ☐ LTA ☐ Rapid Sequence ☐ Crioid Pressure ☐ Intravenous ☐ Inhalation ☐ Intramuscular ☐ Rectal
Regional: ☐ Spinal ☐ Epidural ☐ Axillary ☐ Beir Block ☐ Ankle Block ☐ ____ ☐ Position____ ☐ Prep____ ☐ Local____ ☐ Needle____ ☐ Drug(s)____ ☐ Dose____ ☐ Attempts x____ ☐ Site____ ☐ Level____ ☐ Catheter____ ☐ See Remarks
Other: ☐ MAC ☐

AIRWAY MANAGEMENT
Intubation: ☐ Oral ☐ Tube size ☐ Stylet Used ☐ Nasal ☐ Regular ☐ Magill's ☐ Direct ☐ RAE ☐ Fiber Optic ☐ Blind ☐ Armored ☐ Blade____ ☐ Laser ☐ Secured at____cm ☐ Endobronch. ☐ Attempts x____ ☐ ET CO_2 Present ☐ Breath Sounds____ ☐ Uncuffed, Leaks at____cm H_2O ☐ Cuffed ☐ Min. Occ. Pres. ☐ Air ☐ NS
Airway: ☐ Oral ☐ LMA ☐ Nasal ☐ Difficult, See Remarks
Circuit: ☐ Circle ☐ NRB
☐ Mask Case ☐ Nasal Cannula ☐ Via Tracheostomy ☐ Simple O_2 mask

RECOVERY
Location | Time
B/P | O_2 Sat.
P | R | T
☐ Awake ☐ Stable ☐ Nasal Oxygen ☐ Drowsy ☐ Unstable ☐ Mask Oxygen ☐ Somnolent ☐ Intubated ☐ T-Piece Oxygen ☐ Unarousable ☐ Ventilator ☐ Oral/Nasal Airway
Recovery Notes

TIME:
Oxygen (L/min) ☐ N_2O ☐ Air (L/min)
FLUIDS/AGENTS
Urine (ml) EBL (ml)
TOTALS
FLUID TOTALS: Crystalloid____ EBL____ Blood____ Urine____
REMARKS
MONITORS: EKG, % O_2 Inspired, O_2 Saturation, End Tidal CO_2, Temp: ☐ °C ☐ °F
Baseline Values: B/P, P, R — 200, 180, 160, 140, 120, 100, 80, 60, 40, 20
SYMBOLS: × ANESTHESIA; ⊙ OPERATION; V Λ B/P CUFF PRESSURE; ⊥ T ARTERIAL LINE PRESSURE; ▲ MEAN ARTERIAL PRESSURE; ● PULSE; ○ SPONT. RESP.; Ø ASSISTED RESP.; ⊗ CONTROLLED RESP.; T TOURNIQUET
VENT: Tidal Volume, Resp. Rate, Peak Pressure, PEEP
Symbols for Remarks
Position
PATIENT IDENTIFICATION
Anesthesia Provider
CONTROLLED DRUGS: Drug | Issued | Used | Returned | Provider | Witness

FIGURE 13-11 Anesthesia record.

descriptions; a list also can be found in the Anesthesia section of the CPT manual.

Conversion Factors

A *conversion factor* is the dollar value of each basic unit value. Each third-party payer issues a list of conversion factors. The conversion factor for any given geographic location is multiplied by the number of basic unit values assigned to each procedure (Figure 13-12).

Calculating Anesthesia Services

Using the basic unit value (B), modifying unit (M), time unit (T), physical status (PS) modifier, if applicable, and the conversion factor

Locality Name	Anesthesia Conversion Factor
Manhattan, NY	22.65
NYC suburbs/Long I., NY	22.74
Queens, NY	22.28
Rest of New York	19.91
North Carolina	20.23
North Dakota	19.70

FIGURE 13-12 Anesthesia conversion factors.

Medical Narrative

A 25-year-old female patient in good physical condition has anesthesia services while undergoing laparoscopy (CPT-4 Code 00840). The time for the anesthesia administration was 2 hours. For the purposes of this example the RBV basic unit value will be 4.

Basic Unit Value	= 4
+ Modifying Units: PS	= 0
+ QC	= 0
+ Time Units	= 8
= 12 Total Units	

The total units value of 12 is then multiplied by the conversion factor for the geographic location of the anesthesiologist's office. For the purposes of this exercise, the conversion factor for Manhattan, NY, will be \$20.48, and for North Carolina, \$15.77. For the office located in Manhattan, NY, multiply \$20.48 by 12. The fee for the anesthesia services would be \$245.76. For the office located in North Carolina, multiply 12 times \$15.77, for a fee of \$189.24.

FIGURE 13-13 Anesthesia formula and calculation.

(Figure 13-13), the fee for anesthesia services is calculated according to the anesthesia billing formula:

$$(B + M + T + PS) \times \text{Conversion factor}$$

Common CPT Coding Guidelines: Surgical Section

Specific guidelines and notes related to surgery coding must be considered when a CPT code is assigned. Always review the current year's guidelines for the Surgery section for the most up-to-date information. The following sections discuss a few of the more common guidelines. When coding procedures and services, be sure to read the guidelines and notes thoroughly for accurate coding assignment.

Surgical Package Definition

The CPT code set is designed to include patient prep, surgical care, and postsurgical care in a single code; these are considered **global services** because they are already built into the surgical package cost of the assigned CPT code. Medical coders that include any of these global services as a separate CPT code are acting fraudulently. The

CPT code descriptions of global surgical services typically include the following:
- Local infiltration, digital block, and/or topical anesthesia
- Subsequent to the decision for surgery, one related E/M encounter on the day of, or the day before, the date of the procedure
- Immediate postoperative care, including documentation in the patient's health record and talking with family and/or other physicians
- Writing orders for postsurgical care
- Evaluating the patient in the postanesthesia recovery area
- Typical postoperative follow-up care (includes care for approximately 6 to 8 weeks after surgery and is usually done at the provider's office)

NCCI Edits and Unbundled Codes

In 1996, in an effort to prevent fraudulent medical coding, the Centers for Medicare and Medicaid Services (CMS) established the National Corrective Coding Initiative (NCCI) edit list. This list contains two columns of codes, and the codes in the two columns are mutually exclusive. Submitted claims that contain mutually exclusive codes are automatically rejected. Figure 13-14 presents instructions on how to use the NCCI edits.

When a CPT procedure is billed, this code includes services related to prepping the patient for the procedure, performing the procedure, and suturing to complete the procedure; the single code for the procedure is called a *bundled code* because it represents all of the stages of surgery. When each step of the procedure is listed separately, these are called *unbundled codes*. Unbundled codes are used when the components of a major procedure are separated and reported separately. When these codes are separated and used individually, a special report should be used to describe the circumstances that made the unbundling necessary because unbundled CPT codes have higher reimbursements because each code is paid separately. Medical billers that regularly unbundle CPT codes may be cited for fraud and/or abuse.

Integumentary System

Excision of Lesions—Benign or Malignant

Excision of benign lesions includes a simple closure and anesthesia. If an incision, excision, or traumatic lesion requires intermediate or complex closure, the repair by intermediate or complex closure is coded and reported separately.

Levels of Closure (Repair)
- *Simple repair:* Performed when the wound is superficial (epidermis, dermis, or subcutaneous) without significant involvement of deeper structures. This includes local anesthesia and chemical or electrocauterization of wounds not closed.
- *Intermediate repair:* Includes simple repair with a need for a layered closure of one or more of the deeper layers of subcutaneous tissue and superficial fascia in addition to the skin closure. Single-layer closure of heavily contaminated wounds that required extensive cleaning or removal of particulate matter also constitutes intermediate repair.
- *Complex repair:* Includes wounds that require more than layered closure (e.g., scar revision, extensive undermining, or stents or retention sutures). Necessary preparation includes creation of a

A	B	C	D	E	F
Column 1/Column 2 Edits					
① Column 1	② Column 2	③ * = In existence prior to 1996	④ Effective Date	⑤ Deletion Date * = no data	Modifier ⑥ 0 = not allowed 1 = allowed 9 = not applicable
99215	G0101		19980401	19980401	9
99215	G0102		20000605	*	0
99215	G0104		19980401	19980401	9

① Column 1 indicates the payable code.
② Column 2 contains the code that is not payable with this particular Column 1 code, unless a modifier is permitted and submitted.
③ This third column indicates if the edit was in existence prior to 1996.
④ The fourth column indicates the effective date of the edit (year, month, date).
⑤ The fifth column indicates the deletion date of the edit (year, month, date).
⑥ The sixth column indicates if use of a modifier is permitted. This number is the modifier indicator for the edit. (The Modifier Indicator Table, shown on page 7 of this booklet, provides further explanation.)

FIGURE 13-14 Example of use of NCCI edits.

limited defect for repairs or **débridement** of complicated lacerations. Complex repair does not include excision of benign or malignant lesions, excisional preparation of a wound bed, or débridement, or the removal of damaged tissue or foreign objects from a wound, an open fracture, or an open dislocation.

Listing Services for Wound Repair

- The repaired wound or wounds should be measured and recorded in centimeters; it also should be indicated whether the wound was curved, angular, or in a starlike pattern.
- When multiple wounds are repaired, add together the lengths of those in the same classification (simple, intermediate, or complex) and from all anatomic sites that are grouped together into the same code descriptor. Do not add lengths of repairs from different groupings of anatomic sites (e.g., face and extremities) or from different classifications (intermediate and complex).
- When wounds of more than one classification are repaired, list the more complicated repair as the primary procedure and the less complicated repair as the secondary procedure, using modifier -59.
- Débridement is considered a separate procedure only when gross contamination requires prolonged cleansing, when large amounts of dead or contaminated tissue must be removed, or when débridement is carried out separately without immediate primary closure.
- Wound repair that involves nerves, blood vessels, and/or tendons should be reported under the appropriate system for repair of those structures. The repair of these associated wounds is included in the primary procedure unless it qualifies as a complex repair, in which case modifier -59 applies.

Musculoskeletal System

Fractures

- *Closed fracture:* The fractured bone does not protrude through the dermis or epidermis.
- *Open fracture:* The fractured bone cuts through the skin layers and can be directly visualized.

- *Closed treatment:* The fracture site is not surgically opened (exposed to the external environment and directly visualized). The three methods of closed treatment of fractures are (1) without manipulation, (2) with manipulation, and (3) with or without traction.
- *Manipulation:* Attempted reduction or restoration of a fracture or dislocated joint into its normal anatomic alignment by manually applied forces.
- *Open treatment:* Used when (1) the fractured bone is surgically opened or (2) an opening is made remote from the fracture site to insert an intramedullary nail across the fracture site.
- *Percutaneous skeletal fixation:* Fracture treatment that is neither open nor closed. The fracture fragments are not visualized, but a fixation device (e.g., pins) is placed across the fracture site, usually under x-ray imaging.

Maternity Care and Delivery

The services normally provided in uncomplicated maternity cases include antepartum care, delivery, and postpartum care.

- *Antepartum* care includes the initial and subsequent history; physical examinations; recording of weight, blood pressure, and fetal heart tones; routine chemical urinalysis; monthly visits up to 28 weeks' gestation; biweekly visits to 36 weeks' gestation; and weekly visits until delivery. Any other visits or services provided within this period should be coded separately, including any routine tests (e.g., sonography, routine laboratory tests).
- *Delivery* includes admission to the hospital, the admission history and physical examination, management of uncomplicated labor, vaginal delivery (with or without forceps or episiotomy), or cesarean delivery. Medical problems complicating labor and delivery should be identified by using the codes in the Medicine and E/M sections in addition to codes for maternity care.
- *Postpartum care* includes hospital and office visits after vaginal or cesarean section delivery.

Common CPT Coding Guidelines: Radiology Section

Assigning CPT codes for the Radiology section is the same procedure as the Surgery section. The Radiology section contains all diagnostic imaging codes, including x-ray studies, ultrasound, MRI, and nuclear medicine procedures, in addition to radiation oncology and several other types of diagnostic imaging procedures, services, and therapies. The Radiology section is divided into subsections: head and neck; chest, spine, and pelvis; upper and lower extremities; abdomen, gastrointestinal and urinary tracts; and gynecologic, obstetric, heart, and vascular procedures. The next subdivision, categories, defines the types or functions of various procedures (e.g., diagnostic ultrasound, radiation oncology, and so on) unique to the anatomic site subsection. In addition to the radiology procedure codes, codes are included for physician supervision and interpretation of diagnostic imaging data and for clinical and radiation treatment planning and administration of contrast materials during radiologic procedures.

Common CPT Coding Guidelines: Pathology and Laboratory Section

Assigning CPT codes for the Pathology section is the same procedure as the Surgery section. The subcategories for the Pathology and Laboratory section include organ panels and disease panels, drug testing, therapeutic drug assays, evocative or suppression testing, consultations, urinalysis, chemistry, molecular diagnostics, infectious agents, microbiology, anatomic pathology, cytopathology, cytogenetic studies, and surgical pathology.

For purposes of coding from the Laboratory section, organ or disease panels are groupings of numerous tests performed to diagnose the health or disease status of specific organ systems. A panel code can be used only if all the tests listed under the code selected were performed. Otherwise, the individual tests should be billed using a separate code for each. There are two types of drug testing, qualitative and quantitative. The codes for drug testing are *qualitative;* that is, they are based on the type of drug found. *Quantitative* assays, on the other hand, are performed to determine the amount of drug present.

Common CPT Coding Guidelines: Medicine Section

The Medicine section of the CPT contains codes for a variety of therapeutic procedures and diagnostic testing. This section also contains codes for dialysis, ophthalmology, acupuncture, chiropractic manipulation, and conscious sedation. The steps for determining Medicine codes are similar to those for choosing Surgery codes.

Immune Globulins

When you code administration of **immune globulins**, identify the immune globulin product administered and the method of administration using the codes in the hydration, therapeutic, prophylactic, and diagnostic injections and infusions subsection.

Hydration codes are intended to report a hydration intravenous (IV) infusion consisting of prepackaged fluid and electrolytes; they are not used to report the infusion of drugs or other substances. When multiple drugs are administered, report the service or services and the specific materials or drugs for each (Figure 13-15).

Medicine
Immune Globulins

▶Codes 90281-90399 identify the immune globulin product only and must be reported in addition to the administration codes 90765-90768, 90772, 90774, 90775 as appropriate. Immune globulin products listed here include broad-spectrum and anti-infective immune globulins, antitoxins, and various isoantibodies.◀

- ⊘ 90281 Immune globulin (Ig), human, for intramuscular use
- ⊘ 90283 Immune globulin (IgIV), human, for intravenous use
- ⊘ 90287 Botulinum antitoxin, equine, any route
- ⊘ 90288 Botulism immuno globulin, human, for intravenous use
- ⊘ 90291 Cytomegalovirus immune globulin (CMV-IgIV), human, for intravenous use
- ⊘ 90296 Diphtheria antitoxin, equine, any route
- ⊘ 90371 Hepatitis B immune globulin (HBIg), human, for intramuscular use
- ⊘ 90375 Rabies immune globulin (RIg), human, for intramuscular and/or subcutaneous use
- ⊘ 90376 Rabies immune globulin, heat-treated (RIg-HT), human, for intramuscular and/or subcutaneous use

FIGURE 13-15 Relationship of immune globulins and infusions in CPT.

Immunization Administration for Vaccines/Toxoids

Codes 90465-90474 must be reported in addition to the vaccine and toxoid code(s) 90476-90749.
Report codes 90465-90468 only when the physician provides face-to-face counseling of the patient and family, during the administration of the vaccine. For immunization administration of any vaccine that is not accompanied by face-to-face physician counseling to the patient/family, report codes 90471-90474.
In a significant separately identifiable Evaluation and Management service (e.g., office or other outpatient services, preventive medicine services) is performed, the appropriate E/M service code should be reported in addition to the vaccine and toxoid administration codes.
        (For allergy testing, see 95004 et seq)
        (For skin testing of bacterial, viral, fungal extracts, see 86485-86586)
▶(For therapeutic or diagnostic injections, see 90772-90779)◀

90465   Immunization administration under 8 years of age (includes percutaneous, intradermal, subcutaneous, or intramuscular injections) when the physician counsels the patient/family; first injection (single or combination vaccine/toxoid), per day
        (Do not report 90465 in conjunction with 90467)

+90466   each additional injection (single or combination vaccine/toxoid), per day (List separately in addition to code for primary procedure)
        (Use 90466 in conjunction with 90465 or 90467)

FIGURE 13-16 Relationship of immune vaccines/toxoids and administration codes in CPT.

Immunization for Vaccines or Toxoids

The immunization for vaccines or toxoids codes are for the administration of vaccines and toxoids only and should be reported in conjunction with the appropriate codes in the immunization administration for vaccine/toxoids subsection (Figure 13-16).

Vaccines/Toxoids Codes. These codes identify the vaccine product only. Codes in the immunization administration for vaccines/toxoids subsection must be used in addition to the vaccine or toxoid product codes. To meet the reporting requirements of immunization registries, vaccine distribution programs, and reporting systems, the exact vaccine product administered must be reported on the insurance claim.

Home Health Procedures and Services

The home health procedures and services codes are used by non-physician healthcare professionals only. They are used to report services provided in a patient's residence, including assisted-living apartments, group homes, nontraditional private homes, custodial care facilities, and schools.

HCPCS CODE SET AND MANUAL

Healthcare Common Procedure Coding System (Level II) codes have five alphanumeric digits, beginning with one letter followed by four numerals. HCPCS uses five coding conventions for special instructions relating to specific codes (Figure 13-17). The modifiers for HCPCS are codes composed of two alphanumeric characters. Like the modifiers for CPT Category I codes, the HCPCS modifiers do not change the description of the code, but rather provide additional information or describe extenuating circumstances. Like the CPT manual, the HCPCS manual is divided into two parts: the Alphabetic Index and the Tabular List. As with the CPT, procedures and services can be looked up in the Alphabetic Index and then confirmed as the most accurate and appropriate code by using the Tabular List. The HCPCS manual has no subsections, categories, or subcategories; it has only sections. An appendix contains all the HCPCS modifiers and their descriptions.

The coding steps for HCPCS are almost identical to those for CPT Category I codes. Clinical documentation is the starting point for HCPCS coding, and the final code selected should add nothing to or omit anything from the description in the medical documentation. The final step is determining whether the code selected can stand alone or requires a modifier to further define or add needed information.

Sometimes HCPCS codes are used along with CPT codes, especially in the medical office setting. For example, a well-baby visit would include the E/M code for the patient visit and also HCPCS codes for the administration of immunizations. Procedure 13-2, part B, explains how to code an office visit involving immunizations.

Healthcare Common Procedure Coding System (HCPCS)

HCPCS is a collection of codes and descriptions for procedures, supplies, products, and services not covered by or included in the CPT coding system (Figure 13-18). As are CPT codes, HCPCS codes are updated annually by the Centers for Medicare and Medicaid Services (CMS). These codes are designed to promote standardized reporting and collection of statistical data on medical supplies, products, services, and procedures.

COMMON HCPCS CODING GUIDELINES

Ambulance Transport

HCPCS codes for ambulance transport range from A0021 to A0999. These codes require specific modifiers (Table 13-7) to be added to ensure code specificity. This section provides codes for a variety of medical transport, including ambulance services, nonemergency transportation, and medical supplies used during the transport. A waiting time calculation table also is available, if needed.

Medical and Surgical Supplies

HCPCS codes for medical and surgical supplies range from A4000 to A8999. The HCPCS manual provides some figures that offer guidance as to what the medical and surgical supplies look like, so they can be billed properly. Medical assistants can code only for surgical supplies purchased by the medical office. For example, pharmaceutical and medical equipment representatives can provide the medical office with some supplies that can be used for patient care. However, it is unethical to bill the patient's insurance company for supplies that were provided to the provider for free. All medical and

Special coverage instructions.
Indicates that there are instructions provided regarding circumstances in which the code might be included for reimbursment.
Not covered by or valid for Medicare.
These codes might result in reimbursement by private health insurance payors but not by Medicare. Their value may be only for statistical data collection but not for reimbursement.
Carrier discretion.
These codes may or may not be paid by health insurance carrier including Medicare.
New.
Revised.
The revised symbol is placed in front of codes with any data, payment, or miscellaneous change from the prior year.

FIGURE 13-17 HCPCS conventions.

Humidifiers/Compressors/Nebulizers for Use with Oxygen IPPB Equipment

E0550	Humidifier, durable for extensive supplemental humidification during IPPB treatments or oxygen delivery
E0555	Humidifier, durable, glass or autoclavable plastic bottle type, for use with regulator or flowmeter
E0560	Humidifier, durable for supplemental humidification during IPPB treatment or oxygen delivery
E0561	Humidifier, nonheated, used with positive airway pressure device
E0562	Humidifier, heated, used with positive airway pressure device
E0565	Compressor, air power source for equipment which is not self-contained or cylinder driven
E0570	Nebulizer, with compressor
E0571	Aerosol compressor, battery powered, for use with small volume nebulizer
E0572	Aerosol compressor, adjustable pressure, light duty for intermittent use
E0574	Ultrasonic/electronic aerosol generator with small volume nebulizer
E0575	Nebulizer, ultrasonic, large volume
E0580	Nebulizer, durable, glass or autoclavable plastic, bottle type, for use with regulator or flowmeter
E0585	Nebulizer, with compressor and heater

FIGURE 13-18 *Healthcare Common Procedure Coding System* (HCPCS) Tabular List.

TABLE 13-7   Modifiers Used for HCPCS Ambulance Transport Codes

TRANSPORTATION SERVICES MODIFIERS*	DESCRIPTION
D	Diagnostic or therapeutic site other than P or H when those are used as origin codes
E	Residential, domiciliary, custodial facility
G	Hospital-based end-stage renal disease (ESRD) facility
H	Site of transfer (e.g., airport or helicopter pad) between modes of ambulance transport
I	Free-standing ESRD facility
J	Skilled nursing facility
N	Physician's office
P	Residence
R	Scene of accident or acute event
S	Intermediate stop at physician's office on the way to hospital

*Includes ambulance HCPCS origin modifiers.

surgical supplies used during patient care should be documented on the encounter form in the patient's EHR.

Durable Medical Equipment

HCPCS codes for durable medical equipment range from E0100 to E9999. Examples of durable medical equipment include crutches, wheelchairs, walkers, and other products that assist patients with mobility. Some equipment is kept in the medical office inventory. If the practice purchases the medical equipment wholesale, it is allowed to bill patients and/or their insurance company for the retail value of the equipment. Just as with medical and surgical supplies, it is important for the provider to document the dispensing of the durable medical equipment on the encounter form or medical record.

CLOSING COMMENTS

The CPT and HCPCS coding manuals are updated and published every year, so the updated manuals should be ordered in the early fall so that they arrive in enough time for the medical assistant to review them. Always use the current year's manuals so that the codes are accurate. The Introduction in each manual discusses and highlights changes and/or new coding guidelines. Annual updates should be uploaded to reflect any coding changes in the encoder to ensure that all codes are up to date for the current year.

Legal and Ethical Issues

Medical assistants are responsible for keeping up to date on CPT coding to ensure that no fraud takes place in the coding and claims submission process. Medical assistants should also ensure that proper precautions are taken to avoid incorrect coding, data entry errors, and false claims submissions because these activities can be considered fraud.

Medical coders should be familiar with the NCCI edits, which are published every year by the Centers for Medicare and Medicaid Services (CMS). Medicare can cite a healthcare facility for fraud or abuse (or both) if claims submitted by the facility regularly show unbundled codes. Not only is unbundling an unethical practice, it incurs very stiff monetary penalties. According to the Civil Monetary Penalties Law, medical practices can be cited for penalties of up to $50,000 per violation, and assessments of up to three times the amount claimed for each item or service, or up to three times the amount of remuneration offered, paid, solicited, or received.

Professional Behaviors

Two rules should be followed when you code any procedure or service:
1. Be as specific as possible in code selection, and use all pertinent words in the description given in your documentation.
2. Never add or delete any words, modifying terms, or descriptors to the procedure or service code description that change the definition of the procedure or service or that are not documented.

SUMMARY OF SCENARIO

Sherald has learned that procedural coding using the CPT is similar in many ways to ICD-10-CM diagnostic coding. The two coding manuals have unique but also similar steps, conventions, and guidelines. She also has learned that proper abstraction of procedural data from the health record is equally important for ICD-10-CM and the CPT coding. Sherald also has learned that HCPCS codes are used to describe procedures and services not found in the CPT, such as vaccinations, ambulance services, and durable medical equipment.

Sherald uses documentation by the provider in the encounter form, in a patient's electronic health record, to identify the procedures performed. However, she realizes that she also must know how to use the CPT manual because some notes must be coded from procedures or services delivered. As with diagnostic coding, Sherald reviews the patient's EHR for research and documentation if any questions arise about a claim. She knows that coding to the highest level of specificity helps to ensure accuracy and also enables the practice to obtain the maximum reimbursement allowed. Sherald also uses the Internet to network and research. She realizes the importance of keeping up to date with the CPT and HCPCS codes, so she plans to order the updated CPT manual every year. As Sherald continues to learn procedural coding, she envisions herself becoming well rounded in her knowledge of the practice's administrative operations.

SUMMARY OF LEARNING OBJECTIVES

1. **Define, spell, and pronounce the terms listed in the vocabulary.**
   Spelling and pronouncing medical terms correctly reinforce the medical assistant's credibility. Knowing the definitions of these terms promotes confidence in communication with patients and co-workers.

2. **Describe the organization of the *Current Procedural Terminology* (CPT) manual.**
   The CPT manual comprises three category codes: Category I, Category II, and Category III codes. Category I codes are 5-digit codes that are listed in the Tabular List. Category II codes are used for performance measurement, and their use is optional. Category III codes are temporary codes for emerging medical technologies.

3. **Report the history of procedural coding.**
   The second edition of the CPT, published in 1970, presented an expanded system of codes to designate diagnostic and therapeutic procedures in surgery, medicine, radiology, laboratory, pathology, and medical specialties. At that time, the 4-digit classification was replaced with the current 5-digit coding system. The fourth edition was published in 1977 and included significant updates in medical technology. At the same time, a system of periodic annual updating was introduced to keep pace with the rapidly changing environment.

4. **Distinguish between the Alphabetic Index and the Tabular List in the CPT code set.**
   The CPT has two primary divisions, the Alphabetic Index and the Tabular List. The Alphabetic Index is like any other index in a textbook; it is simply a guide to finding data in the body of the textbook. The Tabular List is divided into six sections, and codes are listed in numeric order in each section.

5. **Classify the six different sections in the Tabular List of the CPT code set.**
   The six sections of the Tabular List are Evaluation and Management, Anesthesia, Surgery, Radiology, Pathology and Laboratory, and Medicine. Sections are divided into subsections; subsections are further divided into categories; and categories can be subdivided into subcategories.

6. **Discuss special reports, and explain the importance of modifiers in assigning CPT codes.**
   When a bill is submitted for a service that is unlisted, unusual, or newly adopted, the third-party carrier requires a special consultation report. Modifiers are used in CPT codes to indicate that a service or procedure performed was altered by specific circumstances. Two-digit alphanumeric modifiers, included with the 5-digit CPT code, can be used to supply additional information or to describe extenuating circumstances that affected the rendered procedure or service.

7. **Review various conventions in the CPT code set.**
   Conventions are used to provide additional information about certain codes. Examples of conventions include triangular and round symbols, which indicate that a code or description was revised, removed, or added.

8. **Identify the required medical documentation for accurate procedural coding.**
   Medical records used for procedural coding can include any or all of the following: encounter form, history and physical report (H&P), progress notes, discharge summary, operative report, pathology report, anesthesia record, and/or radiology report. When the medical documentation is compared against any code description, all the elements of that code must substantially match, with nothing added or missing.

9. **Describe how to use the most current procedural coding system and perform procedural coding for surgery.**
   The basic steps in procedural coding are: (1) read, analyze, and abstract the procedure or service documented in the health record and (2) compare it with the encounter form, operative report, or other documentation to ensure that all services and procedures have been recorded. After searching the Alphabetic Index, the medical assistant should turn to the appropriate codes in the Tabular List to perform the final coding steps. Read the section thoroughly to determine the most accurate code to assign to the procedure or service, and then code the procedure or service. The process for procedural coding for surgery with the CPT code set is detailed in Procedure 13-1.

10. **Discuss how to use the Alphabetic Index.**
    The Alphabetic Index is a comprehensive, alphabetic listing of all main terms used in procedural coding. However, it is not a substitute for the Tabular List. It is organized by main terms, and modifying terms are indented two spaces below that term. Begin the search of the Alphabetic Index by using one of the four primary classifications of main and modifying term entries. In the Tabular List, look up each code or code range found in the Alphabetic Index.

11. **Identify common CPT coding guidelines for Evaluation and Management (E/M) procedures.**
    To properly code E/M services, the medical assistant must understand important differences, or variations, from the basic steps. Assigning the correct E/M code includes identifying the section, subsection, category, and subcategory of the procedure or service; reviewing the reporting instructions and guidelines for the code chosen; reviewing the level of E/M service; determining the extent of the history obtained and examination performed; and determining the complexity of medical decision making.

12. **Identify common CPT coding guidelines for Anesthesia procedures.**
    Anesthesia coding differs from any other form of coding in the way anesthesia services are billed. A standard formula has been established for payment of anesthesia services: Basic unit values (B) + Time units (T) + Modifying units (M) + Physical Status (PS): B + T + M + PS. The total number of units is then multiplied by the conversion factor.

13. **Identify common CPT coding guidelines for surgical procedures.**
    Specific guidelines and notes related to surgery coding must be considered when assigning a CPT code. Always review the current year's guidelines in the Surgery section for the most up-to-date information.

14. **Discuss coding factors for the integumentary system and muscular system, and for maternity care and delivery.**
    Excision of benign lesions includes a simple closure and anesthesia. Different instructions are provided for each type of wound repair. Fractures are handled according to the type. The services normally provided

Continued

in uncomplicated maternity cases include antepartum care, delivery, and postpartum care.

15. **Identify common CPT coding guidelines for Radiology, Pathology and Laboratory, and Medicine sections.**

Assigning accurate CPT codes for the Radiology section is similar to the process for the Surgery section. The Radiology section contains all diagnostic imaging codes, including x-ray studies, ultrasound, magnetic resonance imaging (MRI), and nuclear medicine procedures, in addition to radiation oncology and several other types of diagnostic imaging procedures, services, and therapies.

Assigning accurate CPT codes for the Pathology and Laboratory section also is similar to the process for the Surgery section. The subcategories for the Pathology section include organ panels and disease panels, drug testing, therapeutic drug assays, evocative or suppression testing, consultations, urinalysis, chemistry, molecular diagnostics, infectious agents, microbiology, anatomic pathology, cytopathology, cytogenetic studies, and surgical pathology. In the Laboratory section, organ or disease panels are groupings of numerous tests performed to diagnose the health or disease status of specific organ systems.

The Medicine section contains codes for a variety of therapeutic procedures and diagnostic testing. This section also contains codes for Dialysis, Ophthalmology, Acupuncture, Chiropractic Manipulation, and Conscious Sedation. The steps for determining codes in the Medicine section are similar to those for determining codes in the Surgery section.

16. **Do the following related to the HCPCS code set and manual:**
    - *Identify procedures and services that require HCPCS codes.*
    HCPCS is a collection of codes and descriptions that represent procedures, supplies, products, and services not covered by or included in the CPT coding system. HCPCS codes, like CPT codes, are updated annually by the Centers for Medicare and Medicaid Services (CMS). These codes are designed to promote standardized reporting and collection of statistical data on medical supplies, products, services, and procedures.

- *Describe how to use the most current HCPCS level II coding system.*
Like the CPT manual, the HCPCS manual is divided into two parts: the Alphabetic Index and the Tabular List. As with the CPT, procedures and services are looked up in the Alphabetic Index, and the Tabular List then is used to confirm that the code is the most accurate and appropriate one. The HCPCS manual has no subsections, categories, or subcategories; it has only sections. An appendix contains all the HCPCS modifiers and their descriptions. The coding steps for HCPCS are almost identical to those for CPT Category I codes.

17. **Perform procedural coding for an office visit and an immunization.**

To code an office visit, the coder first must determine the level of all key components, which include the history, examination, and medical decision making. (See Procedure 13-2, part A.)

An immunization procedure is coded using the HCPCS code set. Coding for HCPCS is almost identical to coding for CPT because both manuals have an Alphabetical Index and a Tabular List. After searching the Alphabetic Index, the coder turns to the appropriate codes in the Tabular List to perform the final coding steps. The coder reads the section thoroughly to determine the most accurate code to assign to the procedure or service, and then codes the procedure or service. (See Procedure 13-2, part B.)

18. **Summarize common HCPCS coding guidelines.**

Ambulance Transport codes require specific modifiers to ensure code specificity. The HCPCS manual provides some figures that offer guidance as to what the medical and surgical supplies look like so they can be billed properly. Medical assistants can only bill for surgical supplies that were purchased by the medical office. The medical office can purchase the medical equipment wholesale but still bill patients and/or their insurance companies for the retail value of the equipment. When the insurance company is billed, it is vital that the medical assistant fill in the "Number of Units" box on the health insurance claim form for equipment provided to the patient.

CONNECTIONS

📖 Study Guide Connection: Go to the Chapter 13 Study Guide. Read and complete the activities.

evolve Evolve Connection: Go to the Chapter 13 link at *evolve.elsevier.com/ kinn* to complete the Chapter Review Quiz. Check out the other resources listed for this chapter to make the most of what you have learned from the Basics of Procedural Coding.

BASICS OF HEALTH INSURANCE

14

SCENARIO

Jodie Rimmell, a registered medical assistant (RMA), has worked for Dr. Ted Crawford, an endocrinologist, for 3 years. Jodie started with Dr. Crawford as a receptionist; Dr. Crawford recognized that Judy was very detail-oriented, so he promoted her to take charge of the health insurance policies and procedures manual for the practice 2 years ago. Jodie trains all new medical assistants on how to verify patient health insurance coverage and eligibility. Because Jodie has learned quite a bit about health insurance, she can answer most of the patients' questions about their coverage, benefits, and/or exclusions of their policies. She knows where to direct patients who have more complicated questions and how to follow up—one of the most important duties of a professional medical assistant. She has a great attitude about assisting patients with insurance questions and does not hesitate to call the third-party payer on the patient's behalf. She provides patients with exceptional customer service. When patients call her for assistance, she responds within 24 hours (often within 1 hour) with answers to their questions or a resource to help them. Jodie is willing to help any staff member with other duties when necessary and prides herself on being a patient advocate. She is an enthusiastic team player who puts patients first.

While studying this chapter, think about the following questions:

- How important is the verification of services and benefits for reimbursement?
- How are privately sponsored health insurance plans and government-sponsored health insurance plans different?
- What is the Affordable Care Act and how does this legislation affect healthcare facilities?

- Why is it important to verify eligibility and preauthorize services before the patient appointment is scheduled?
- Is preauthorization necessary for patients who have a managed care health plan? Why or why not?
- Why is it important to educate patients on their health insurance benefits?

LEARNING OBJECTIVES

1. Define, spell, and pronounce the terms listed in the vocabulary.
2. Discuss the purpose of health insurance and explain the health insurance contract between the patient and the health plan.
3. Identify types of third-party plans.
4. Discuss the Affordable Care Act's effect on patient healthcare access.
5. Summarize the different health insurance benefits available and interpret information on a health insurance identification (ID) card.
6. Explain the importance of verifying eligibility and be able to verify eligibility of services, including documentation.
7. Explain the health insurance contract between the healthcare provider and the health insurance company.

8. Explain how insurance reimbursements are determined and discuss the effect health insurance has on provider reimbursements.
9. Summarize privately sponsored health insurance plans.
10. Differentiate among the different types of managed care models.
11. Outline managed care requirements for patient referral and obtain a referral with documentation.
12. Describe the process for preauthorization and how to obtain preauthorization including documentation.
13. List and discuss various government-sponsored plans.
14. Review employer-established self-funded plans.

VOCABULARY

beneficiary A recipient of health insurance benefits.

capitation A contract between the health insurance plan and the provider for which the health insurance plan will pay an agreed-upon monthly fee per patient and the provider agrees to provide medical services on a regular basis.

explanation of benefits (EOB) A document sent by the insurance company to the provider and the patient explaining the allowed charge amount, the amount reimbursed for services, and the patient's financial responsibilities.

fee-for-service A reimbursement model in which the health plan pays the provider's fee for every health insurance claim.

gatekeeper The primary care provider, who can approve or deny when the patient seeks additional care via a referral to a specialist or further medical tests.

government-sponsored health insurance Health insurance programs that are sponsored by the government and offer coverage for the elderly, disabled, military, and indigent.

online provider insurance Web portal An online service provided by various insurance companies for providers to look up patient insurance benefits, eligibility, claims status, and explanation of benefits.

privately sponsored health insurance Health insurance companies that operate for profit and use managed care plans to reduce the costs of healthcare.

qualified Medicare beneficiaries (QMB) Low-income Medicare patients who qualify for Medicaid for their secondary insurance.

third-party administrator (TPA) The intermediary and administrator who coordinates patients and providers, as well as processes claims, for self-funded plans.

subscriber The person who is the signer on the health insurance policy.

utilization management A process of managing healthcare costs by influencing patient care decision making through case-by-case assessments of the appropriateness of care.

waiting period The amount of time a patient waits for disability insurance to pay after the date of injury.

PURPOSE OF HEALTH INSURANCE

Health insurance is a third-party payer system that reimburses a provider when services are rendered for an insured patient. A monthly *premium,* or payment, is paid for a list of health insurance benefits detailed in the contract; the premium can be paid by the employer if the **subscriber** is employed with benefits, or it is paid by the patient for individual coverage. The patient provides evidence of the health insurance contract to the healthcare provider in the form of an insurance identification (ID) card. The provider then submits a claim to the health insurance company for services rendered. The third party then *reimburses,* or pays, the claim to the healthcare provider for services already rendered.

To understand the specifics of the insurance plan, it is vital to review the terms of the health insurance contract with the patient and the healthcare provider.

CONTRACT WITH PATIENTS

To obtain health insurance coverage, applicants need to apply either through their employer or privately. There are two types of health insurance plans in the United States: **privately sponsored health insurance plans** and **government-sponsored health insurance plans**. Health insurance plans typically cover health services and procedures that are deemed *medically necessary,* or health services that are necessary to improve the patient's current health condition. Most insurance policies do not cover *elective procedures,* or medical procedures that are not deemed medical necessary, or needed to improve the patient's current health, such as a facelift. Most of today's health insurance policies cover *preventive care,* which includes services provided to help prevent certain illnesses or that lead to an early diagnosis. Some preventative care services include yearly routine vaccinations, blood tests, urine analysis, and hearing and vision testing; preventative coverage depends on the insurance policy.

HEALTH INSURANCE PLANS

Government-Sponsored Health Insurance Plans

Government-sponsored health insurance plans are federal- or state-sponsored plans that require patients to pay minimal to no monthly premiums. In order to qualify, patients must meet the program requirements such as age, disability, income level, or occupation. However, these health insurance plans offer benefits and healthcare access is limited to healthcare providers that are contracted with them.

Employer-Sponsored Group Policies

In the recent past, businesses have offered their eligible full-time employees health insurance as a *group policy,* a privately sponsored health insurance plan purchased by an employer for a group of employees. The employer exercises the right to establish how much their employees pay for health insurance coverage for themselves, their spouse (i.e., domestic partner), and children. Employers usually sponsor a percentage of the monthly premium, thus making health insurance coverage more affordable for their employees. Employers also determine the health insurance benefits under the group policy. Health insurance monthly premiums and benefits can vary from employer to employer. For example, the health insurance plan for Employer A covers chiropractic care but the health insurance plan for Employer B does not. Group policies usually provide greater benefits at lower premiums because of the large pool of employees. Often the employee shares the cost of the monthly premium through payroll deductions.

Individual Health Insurance Plans

Not so long ago it was very difficult for individuals who did not work full time to obtain affordable health insurance coverage if they did not qualify for a government-sponsored health insurance plan. Although there were individual insurance health plans, health insurance not sponsored by an employer, these were very difficult to qualify for. If an applicant had a preexisting condition, which is a health condition that existed before the application that needed ongoing medical care, the health insurance plan exercised the right to deny coverage or charged exorbitant monthly premiums.

The Affordable Care Act

In the early 2000s it became clear that a large number of Americans lacked basic health insurance. *Preexisting conditions* made it difficult for Americans who did not work full time or were self-employed to obtain health insurance. In addition, the health insurance market was discriminating against young adults of 18+ years that may not have been qualified to receive health benefits because they could not find full-time employment.

In 2010 the Patient Protection and Affordable Care Act, which is also known as the *Affordable Care Act* and also Obamacare, was enacted. It increased the quality, availability, and affordability of private and public health insurance for more than 44 million uninsured Americans. The legislation includes new qualifying regulations, taxes, mandates, and subsidies. The federal mandate not only opens opportunities for more Americans to obtain affordable health insurance, but also works to reduce overall healthcare spending in the long run. Other patient protections and provisions under the Affordable Care Act include:

- Insurance companies are prohibited from dropping patient health coverage if the individual gets sick or makes an unintentional mistake on the health insurance application
- Eliminates preexisting conditions and gender discrimination so patients cannot be charged more based on their health status or gender
- Young adults can remain on their parent's or guardian's insurance policy until age 26
- Creates *Health Insurance Marketplaces* where low-to-middle-income Americans can compare plans and lower their costs on healthcare coverage
- States will expand Medicaid coverage to 15.9 million Americans to include those who qualify for cost assistance through the marketplace
- Requires all Americans to obtain and maintain minimum essential insurance coverage through the year or there will be a monthly tax penalty imposed. For those who cannot afford health insurance based on their household income, tax deductions and payment subsidies are available
- Individuals seeking health insurance can only apply during the open enrollment period, which is established by each state

With more Americans having health insurance, the number of office visits to providers across the country is expected to increase. Refer to Box 14-1 for the Affordable Care Act essential health benefits. Thus efficient health insurance management policies should be instituted to meet the new demand for services.

Box 14-1   Essential Health Benefits Outlined by the Affordable Care Act

Ambulatory patient services
Emergency services
Hospitalization
Maternity and newborn care
Mental health and substance abuse disorder services, including behavior health services
Prescription drugs
Rehabilitative and habilitative services and devices
Laboratory services
Preventive services and wellness services; chronic disease management
Pediatric services, including oral and vision care

Affordable Care Act Navigators Program

Affordable Care Act Navigators are certified enrollment counselors who assist consumers through a variety of outreach, education, enrollment, postenrollment, and renewal support services including, but not limited to, the following:

- Inform eligible consumers of the availability and benefits of obtaining healthcare coverage
- Promote the value of purchasing healthcare coverage
- Motivate consumers to act
- Help consumers to shop and compare plans
- Facilitate enrollment into respective health insurance marketplaces
- Assist consumers with the eligible renewal process
- Provide postenrollment outreach and support to eligible consumers

The Navigators Program is federally mandated for all state health exchanges. The navigators help consumers, small businesses, and employees as they look for health coverage options through the marketplace, including completing eligibility and enrollment forms. These individuals and organizations are required to be unbiased. Their services are free to consumers.

BENEFITS

Every health insurance contract is tailored to the needs of each individual or group policy, and the combinations of benefits are limitless. Benefits cover the *amount loss,* or the amount that should be paid to the healthcare provider for services rendered. Employers can pick and choose the benefits they want for their employees; this is also called "cafeteria style." A policy may contain one or any combination of the benefits found in Table 14-1. Medical assistants should be familiar with how to look up patient benefit information to inform patients of their financial responsibilities before scheduling an appointment.

Hospitalization

Hospital coverage pays the cost of all or part of the patient's hospital room and board including specific hospital services, such as the hospital surgical room fee or a hospital stay of less than 30 days. Hospital insurance policies frequently set a maximum amount payable per day and a maximum number of days of hospital care; these policies and procedures are established by the health insurance plan.

Surgical

Surgical coverage pays all or part of a surgeon's fee; some plans also pay for an assistant surgeon. Surgery may be performed in a hospital, provider's office, or outpatient surgery center. The insurance company frequently provides the guarantor with a surgical fee schedule that establishes the amount they will pay for commonly performed procedures.

Basic Medical

Basic medical coverage pays all or part of a healthcare provider's fee for nonsurgical services, including hospital, home, and office visits and consultations. Payments are made for many different types of

TABLE 14-1   Types of Health Insurance and Plan Benefits

BENEFIT	COVERED	PAYS	BENEFIT	COVERED	PAYS
Hospitalization	Cost of all or part of the hospital room and board; and specific hospital services (i.e., costs involved in having surgery in a hospital)	Maximum amount per day and maximum number of days	Dental care	Preventive care; treatment and repair of teeth and gums	Typically pays 100% for preventive care, 50% for repair and treatment
Surgical	Any surgical procedure, including but not limited to incision or excision; removal of foreign bodies; aspiration; suturing; reduction of fractures	Surgeon's fee Assistant surgeon's fee	Vision care	Eye examination and glasses or contacts	Set benefit amount, depending on vision care policy for examination and glasses
Basic medical	Outpatient and provider office procedures and services	Provider's fees; diagnostic, radiologic, laboratory, and pathology fees	Medicare supplement	Deductible and co-insurance amounts unpaid by Medicare	Deductible and co-insurance amounts unpaid by Medicare
Major medical	Catastrophic or prolonged illness or injury	Takes over when basic medical, hospitalization, and surgical benefits end	Life insurance	Loss of life	Usually a lump sum payment of the life insurance benefit
Disability	Accident or illness resulting in an inability for patient to work; can be paid whether work-related or not	Cash benefits paid in lieu of salary while patient is unable to earn an income	Long-term care	Long-term skilled nursing or rehabilitation care	Set amount determined by policy benefits

healthcare professional's visits including nurses, physical therapists, and occupational therapists. The insurance plan may include a provision for diagnostic laboratory, radiology, and pathology expenses. Basic medical covers a percent of the fee schedule's allowed cost; it is common for the insurance plan to cover 80%, with the additional 20% being the patient's financial responsibility.

Disability (Loss of Income) Protection

Disability insurance is a form of insurance that insures the beneficiary's earned income against the risk that a disability will make working uncomfortable (e.g., psychological disorders), painful (e.g., back pain), or impossible (e.g., coma). It encompasses paid sick leave, short-term disability benefits, and long-term disability benefits.

Weekly or monthly cash benefits are provided to employed policyholders who become unable to work as a result of an accident or illness. Many disability policies have a **waiting period** until benefits can be paid. Payments are made directly to the **beneficiary** and are intended to replace lost income resulting from an illness or other disability. It is not intended for payment of specific medical bills, and it should not be confused with a regular health insurance plan.

Dental Care

Dental benefits offer a variety of options in the form of either fee-for-service or managed care plans that reimburse or discount a portion of a patient's dental expenses.

Most dental plans have preventive dental care (e.g., cleaning and x-ray films) covered 100% twice a year, with most other services covered at a discount.

Vision Care

Vision care insurance usually provides coverage of a yearly eye examination and a discount on frames, lenses, and contact lenses. Some vision plans also pay for corrective procedures, such as laser eye surgery.

Medicare Supplement

Basic medical coverage for Medicare Part B is 80% after the deductible; this means that all Medicare patients are financially responsible for 20%. So some Medicare beneficiaries choose to purchase a privately sponsored supplemental health insurance policy to help cover the 20% medical cost incurred; these supplemental health insurance plans are known as *Medigap* policies. Medigap policies cover the difference between Medicare reimbursement and patient financial responsibilities. Federal regulations now require Medicare supplement policy benefits to be uniform to avoid confusion for the purchaser.

Liability Insurance

Liability insurance covers losses to a third party caused by the insured. There are many types of liability insurance, including automobile, business, and homeowners' policies. Liability policies often include benefits for medical expenses resulting from traumatic injuries, lost wages, and sometimes pain and suffering payable to victims injured by the insured person's home or car, without regard to the insured person's actual legal liability for the accident.

Life Insurance

Life insurance provides payment of a specified amount upon the insured's death, either to his or her estate or to a designated beneficiary. A subtype of life insurance, an *endowment policy*, allows the policyholder to build up funds to be dispersed on a specified schedule during his or her lifetime. Annuity life insurance policies provide monthly cash benefits if the policyholder becomes permanently and totally disabled. Sometimes the proceeds from life insurance are used to meet the expenses of the insured person's last illness.

Long-Term Care Insurance

Long-term care insurance is a relatively new type of insurance that covers a broad range of maintenance and health services for chronically ill, disabled, or developmentally delayed individuals. Medical services may be provided on an inpatient basis (e.g., at a rehabilitation facility, nursing home, or mental hospital), on an outpatient basis, or at home.

CRITICAL THINKING APPLICATION   **14-1**

Michael Sherman, an elderly patient, called to make an appointment, but was unsure what his benefits were. How can Jodie find out what benefits he qualifies for? Is it appropriate for Jodie to educate Michael on his health insurance benefits? Why or why not?

Premiums

Patients covered by an *employer-sponsored group health insurance plan*, or health insurance offered by their employer, typically share the cost for the monthly premium. Individual health insurance plans offered through federal- and state-sponsored health insurance marketplaces make monthly premium payments. Indigent, elderly, federally employed, or military patients who seek healthcare from the government have little or no monthly premiums.

Health Insurance Identification Card

As proof of health insurance coverage, patients are issued a health insurance ID card with the health insurance company, health plan name, health plan type, patient's name, subscriber ID, and health plan contact phone numbers. Review Figure 14-1 for a sampling of different insurance ID cards for common third-party payers. Refer to Procedure 14-1 on how to interpret information on the health insurance ID card.

PROCEDURE 14-1   Interpret Information on an Insurance Card

Goal: *To identify essential information on the health insurance identification (ID) card to confirm co-payment obligations and send accurate health insurance claims for reimbursement.*

EQUIPMENT and SUPPLIES

- Scanned copy of patient's health insurance ID, both sides
- Scanned copy of patient's state-issued ID card

PROCEDURAL STEPS

1. Review the scanned copy of the patient's health insurance ID card and state-issued ID card in the electronic health record (EHR). If the patient is a minor, then scan a copy of the insured's state-issued ID card.
   <u>PURPOSE:</u> To confirm the patient's identity is the name on the health insurance ID card.
2. Identify the subscriber on the health insurance ID card with the patient's name. If the patient is different than the insured name on the card, then obtain the relationship with the insured and the insured's date of birth and gender.
   <u>PURPOSE:</u> To submit an accurate health insurance claim, the insured's date of birth and gender is required.
3. Identify the insurance plan and health maintenance organization (HMO) network, if present.

<u>PURPOSE:</u> To confirm that the provider is a participating provider for the insurance plan or the HMO network. If the provider is out of network, the patient should be informed that they would either have to pay more out of pocket or the medical services rendered will not be covered by the insurance plan.

4. Identify the insured's policy number and group number.
   <u>PURPOSE:</u> To accurately submit the health insurance claim under the correct insurance policy number and group number.
5. Identify the patient's co-payment, which is due before the appointment. Collect the correct amount. For example, if the provider is a general practitioner, then collect the co-payment for the primary care provider (PCP).
   <u>PURPOSE:</u> To ensure the proper co-payment is paid by the patient.
6. On the back of the health insurance ID card, ensure that a customer service phone number and medical claims address is present.
   <u>PURPOSE:</u> To ensure that the provider can contact customer service and has the correct mailing address.

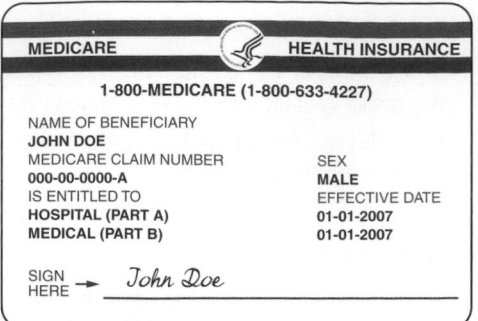

Medicare: The Medicare card uses the patient's social security number as the ID number. The card also details the plan coverages, in this case Part A and Part B.

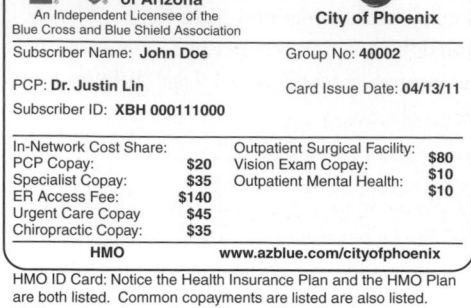

HMO ID Card: Notice the Health Insurance Plan and the HMO Plan are both listed. Common copayments are listed are also listed. HMO members are required to choose PCP which is designated on their health ID card.

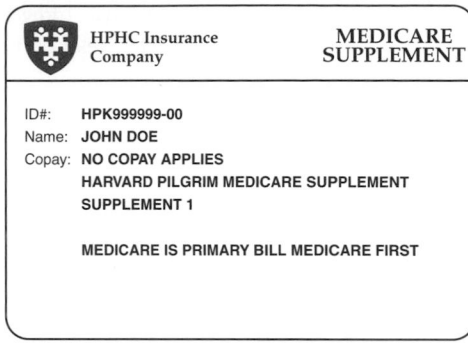

Medicare Secondary Insurance: The ID card states that it is a supplement to Medicare, thus Medicare should be billed as the primary. The ID number does not match the Medicare card.

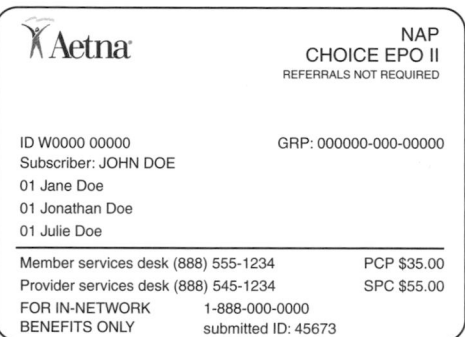

EPO Plan ID Card: Members are not required to choose a PCP, but can only use their benefits for in-network providers and facilities. Notice the ID number stays the same for the insured and all family members listed.

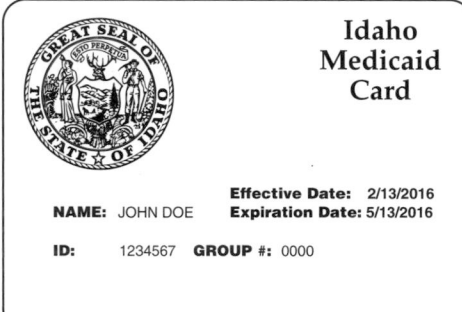

Medicaid: Medicaid cards have the state seal printed on them indicating that services can only be performed by the sponsoring state. These cards contain a effective and expiring date. If a patient presents a card with an expired date, contact Medicaid to confirm their benefits have been extended.

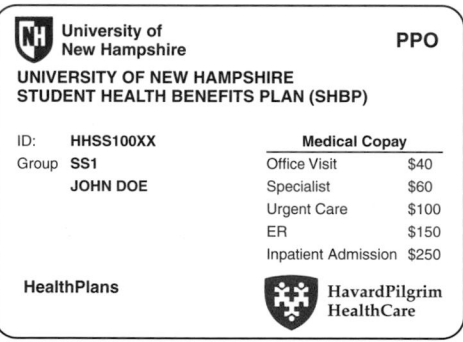

PPO plan ID card: PPO patients have the most flexibility to visit whichever provider, primary care of specialist they choose. Notice the medical copays are slightly higher than HMO copayments.

FIGURE 14-1 A variety of different health insurance identification cards.

VERIFYING ELIGIBILITY OF SERVICES

Verification of eligibility is the process of confirming health insurance coverage for the patient for the medical service on the date of service. It is vital for the healthcare facility to ensure that the patient who is seeking healthcare is in the provider's network of contracted health insurance plans. Before scheduling the appointment, health insurance information should be collected over the phone (unless it is an emergency situation). The medical assistant should verify the *effective date,* or date the insurance coverage began, and confirm that the patient is covered on the date the medical services will be rendered. The medical assistant should make it a practice to review the **online insurance Web portal**, which can verify insurance eligibility, benefits, and exclusions prior to the patient's appointment. If the online insurance provider portal is not available, the medical assistant should contact the provider services desk; the phone number should be listed on the back side of the patient's health insurance ID card. Refer to Procedure 14-2 on how to verify eligibility of services, including documentation.

Online Insurance Provider Portals

In the recent past, the medical assistant would have to call the health insurance company to verify eligibility for each and every patient. Each call to the health insurance company automated system would take at least 5 minutes and the medical assistant would not have access to all of the patient's benefit information unless he or she spoke to a member services agent, which would take even more time. Today, most privately sponsored health insurance plans have offered online insurance provider portals, which allows for quick and easy verification of eligibility (Figure 14-2). The healthcare facility will have to apply for access to the online insurance provider portal. Once approved, patient benefits can be looked up in their entirety in seconds instead of minutes. Patient benefit plan information can be uploaded to the electronic health record (EHR) very quickly; this process reduces the use of paper in the healthcare facility.

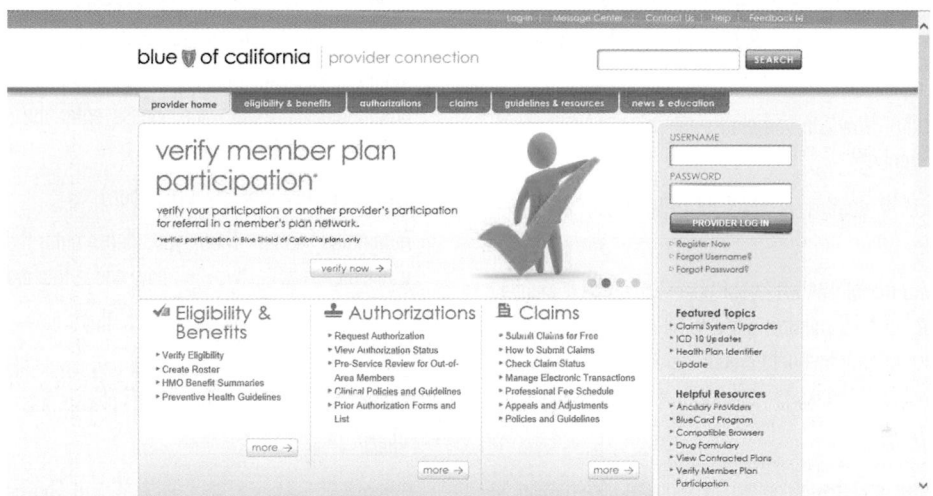

FIGURE 14-2 Online health insurance provider web portal. (From Fordney MT: *Insurance handbook for the medical office,* ed 14, St. Louis, 2017, Elsevier.)

PROCEDURE 14-2   Verify Eligibility of Services, Including Documentation

Goal: *To confirm that the patient's insurance is in effect; to determine the benefits covered, exclusions, and noncovered procedures and services; and to determine whether preauthorizations are included or required.*

EQUIPMENT and SUPPLIES

- Patient health record
- Patient's health insurance identification (ID) card

PROCEDURAL STEPS

1. When a patient calls for an appointment, identify the patient's insurance plan. Ask for information on the patient's ID card including the subscriber number, the group number, and the phone number for provider services. Choose a partner and read the following scripted scenario between Shelly the medical assistant and Amy the patient.

   Shelly: Hello, you've reached Dr. Crawford's office, how can I help you?

   Amy: Yes, I would like to make an appointment to see Dr. Crawford.

   Shelly: Have you been seen by us before?

   Amy: No, this is the first time.

   Shelly: Well, welcome to our office! The first available appointment we have for new patients is next Monday at 9 AM; does that work for you?

   Amy: Sure.

   Shelly: Ok, please tell me your full name, last name first.

   Amy: Palmer, Amy.

   Shelly: Great, and now your date of birth.

   Amy: 11/12/1964.

   Shelly: Can I have your home address?

   Amy: 3434 Homestead Place, Wichita, Kansas, 39493.

   Shelly: And phone number?

   Amy: 585 896-5632.

   Shelly: Great! Now will you be using your health insurance?

   Amy: Yes, I have Blue Shield.

   Shelly: Amy, do you know if it is a PPO or an HMO plan?

   Amy: It is an HMO plan.

Shelly: Ok, if you have the card in front of you, can you please tell me the HMO plan name?

Amy: It is the Wichita Community IPA.

Shelly: Great, we are contracted with them. Are you the insured? Or are you a dependent?

Amy: This is my husband's insurance.

Shelly: Ok, can I get his full name and his date of birth?

Amy: Yes, his name is David Christopher Palmer and his date of birth is 8/1/1962.

Shelly: Thanks for that info. Now can you please tell me the insurance ID number and the group number?

Amy: Yes, the insurance ID number is XEA900000900 and the group number is X0009000.

Shelly: Thanks! Amy, you are all set with your appointment next Monday at 9 AM. Please come at least 15 minutes early to fill out any paperwork. I will verify your insurance information before your appointment and contact you if there are any problems. Thanks for calling, have a great day!

Amy: Thanks, see you Monday.

<u>PURPOSE</u>: To prepare for and begin gathering required information to perform both insurance verification and insurance claim completion procedures.

2. At the time of the appointment, obtain and photocopy both sides of the patient's health insurance ID card(s) and a state-issued ID card.
<u>PURPOSE</u>: To ensure that the correct ID, group, and policy numbers are obtained, in addition to the name, address, and phone number of the insurance carrier or carriers. The state-issued ID card is used to confirm the patient's identity.

3. Call the health insurance company with the contact number listed on the back of the patient's health insurance ID card or you can log into the online

provider insurance Web portal when you have access. Use the following script to initiate a verification of eligibility encounter with the health insurance plan's automated phone system.

Automated System: Thank you for calling Anthem Blue Cross of California. Please choose from one of the following options: Press 1 for verification of eligibility; press 2 to request a referral; press 3 to request an authorization of a medical service; press 5 to request an authorization of a formulary drug; and press 0 to speak to a representative.

Shelly: (Presses 1 to verify patient eligibility.)

Automated System: Thank you for using the Anthem Blue Cross of California automated verification line. Please enter the subscriber's ID number and press the # key.

Shelly: (Enters patient's ID number.)

Automated System: Thank you. Please enter the patient's date of birth with a two-digit month, two-digit day, and a four-digit year.

Shelly: (Enters patient's date of birth.)

Automated System: Thank you. If you would like to hear eligibility information for the patient "Miriam Cho" please press 1.

Shelly: (Presses 1.)

Automated System: Thank you. Miriam Cho has a PPO and is eligible for benefits for (today's date). Would you like to hear the co-payment and deductible amount? Press 1 for yes; hang up if you are finished.

Shelly: (Presses 1.)

Automated System: Thank you. The patient has a co-pay of $30 for the PCP, $50 for the specialist, and $60 for urgent care. The plan has a $4000 deductible, of which $2200 has been met as of (today's date). If you are done, please hang up. If you would like more benefit information, please press 0 for a customer service representative.

Shelly: (Records benefit information and hangs up the phone.)

ACCESSING HEALTHCARE

When the insured patient seeks medical care, a healthcare provider renders medical services at any *in-network* healthcare facility, which are locations that are contracted in the patient's health insurance plan, including medical offices, urgent care centers, and hospitals. In-network healthcare providers and facilities are contracted with the health insurance plan and have agreed to provide health services at a reduced fee. Many health insurance plans do not reimburse for healthcare services provided at *out-of-network* facilities; so prior to the appointment scheduled, the medical assistant should verify that the provider and the healthcare facility are in-network of the patient's insurance plan.

Participating Provider Contracts

With all government-sponsored health plans and most privately sponsored health plans, healthcare providers must become *participating providers* (PARs): These providers are contracted with the insurance plan and have agreed to accept the contracted fee schedule. Healthcare providers can apply to become PARs through a process called *credentialing*. Credentialing is the process of confirming the healthcare provider's qualifications, including the healthcare provider's license to practice medicine, affiliated organizations, and his or her education and professional background.

Once the healthcare provider is credentialed, the health insurance plan issues a contract to become an in-network PAR. The contract includes a fee schedule that the health insurance company will use to reimburse the provider for health services rendered; by signing the contract, the provider agrees to accept the health insurance plan's fee schedule, even if it is lower than their fee schedule.

Contracted Fee Schedules

In the United States payment for services is typically made after the health services are rendered. In other words, healthcare providers are paid weeks, sometimes months, after medical services have been provided to the patient. Once the service is provided to the patient, the healthcare provider must submit a health insurance claim, which includes the diagnosis and procedure codes and total charges. Although the healthcare provider establishes their own fee schedule, or list of charges associated with various medical services provided, health insurance plans maintain their own rates at which they reimburse.

A healthcare provider has three commodities to sell: time, expertise, and services. In every case, healthcare providers must place an estimate on the value of these services. Fees for medical procedures and services differ from office to office based on the type of practice and the needs of the facility. Providers establishing the practice normally set the fees for procedures and services. In the past, most providers worked on a **fee-for-service** basis; that is, patients were charged for the provider's service based on each individual service performed.

In recent years, health insurance plans, particularly government-sponsored and managed healthcare organizations, have greatly influenced what healthcare providers can be reimbursed by establishing the allowable charge. The *allowable charge* is the maximum that third-party payers will pay for a procedure or service. The patient cannot be charged for the amount above the allowable charge if the provider and/or the healthcare facility are contracted in-network.

How Reimbursements Are Determined

Insurance benefits may be determined and paid in one of several ways:

- Determination of the usual, customary, and reasonable (UCR) fees
- Indemnity schedules
- Service benefit plans
- Resource-based relative value scale (RBRVS)

Usual, Customary, and Reasonable Fees

Some insurance companies agree to pay on the basis of all or a percentage of a UCR fee. Charges for a specific service are compared with a database showing (1) charges to other patients for the same service by the same type of provider and (2) charges to patients by other providers performing the same or similar services in the same geographic area. The insurance company determines whether the provider's charge is UCR, and sets the allowed charges.

Indemnity Schedules

Indemnity plans are traditional health insurance plans that pay for all or a share of the cost of covered services, regardless of which provider, hospital, or other licensed healthcare provider is used. Because providers and other providers are paid for each office visit, test, procedure, or other service they deliver, indemnity plans are often called fee-for-service plans.

An indemnity health insurance plan, also known as *major medical,* is a more flexible yet more costly option. Many people refer to this as a traditional plan because it preceded the advent of managed care (e.g., health maintenance organizations [HMOs], preferred provider organizations [PPOs], and point of service [POS] plans).

Policyholders of indemnity plans and their dependents choose when and where to get healthcare services. When the policy is purchased, the subscriber is often given a schedule of indemnities (i.e., a fee schedule), which explains the benefit payment amounts. Indemnity benefits are usually paid to the person insured unless that person has authorized payment directly to the provider, which is a common practice.

Service Benefit Plans

In *service benefit plans,* the health insurance company agrees to pay for certain surgical or medical services without additional cost to the person insured. There is no set fee schedule. In a service benefit plan, surgery with complications would warrant a higher fee than an uncomplicated procedure. Premiums are sometimes higher for this type of coverage, but reimbursements are also larger. Benefit payments are sent directly to the provider and are considered full payment for services rendered. Consider this example: the service benefit plan states that it will pay $900 for a cholecystectomy. If Dr. Jones charges $1500 for this procedure, he must accept the $900 as payment in full and write off the difference.

Resource-Based Relative Value Scale

The *RBRVS* is one of the outcomes of the Medicare Physician Payment Reform that was enacted in the Omnibus Budget Reconciliation Act of 1989 (*OBRA '89*). Originally, Medicare Part B had paid providers using a fee for-service system based on UCR charges. However, implementation of the RBRVS in 1992 changed this system to a fee scale consisting of three parts:

- Provider work
- Charge-based professional liability expenses
- Charge-based overhead

The provider work component includes the degree of effort invested by a provider in a particular service or procedure and the time it consumed. The professional liability and overhead components are computed by the Centers for Medicare and Medicaid Services (CMS).

The RBRVS fee schedule is designed to provide nationally uniform payments after adjustment to reflect the differences in practice costs across geographic areas. The fee schedule includes a conversion factor, which is a single national number applied to all services paid under the fee schedule. Conversion factors are changed by Congress, usually annually, at the request of the CMS.

Depending on the contract between the provider and the insurance carrier (especially Medicare, Medicaid, and other government programs), the provider either writes off the difference between the RBRVS schedule and his or her fee.

Contracts between the provider of service and the insurance payer vary greatly, depending on the insurance or third-party payer. It is important for the medical assistant to know the contract terms for each third-party payer and, upon receipt of payment, to examine the **explanation of benefits (EOB)** from the insurance carrier closely to ensure that all benefits have been reimbursed appropriately and correctly.

PRIVATELY SPONSORED HEALTH INSURANCE PLANS

Privately sponsored health insurance plans, also known as commercial insurance plans, are for-profit organizations. As such, health insurance companies make annual changes to the participating provider contract to negotiate lower reimbursements. Most privately sponsored plans use managed care to reduce the costs of delivering quality healthcare.

Blue Cross/Blue Shield

Blue Cross and Blue Shield (BC/BS) are America's oldest and largest system of privately sponsored insurers. BS began in 1900 from the lumber and mining camps of the Pacific Northwest. BC began in 1929 when an executive at Baylor University came up with a plan for teachers to budget for their future hospital bills. Both BC and BS set the precedent for monthly prepaid healthcare.

BC/BS offers incentive contracts to healthcare providers. PARs agree to write off the difference or balance between the amount charged by the provider and the approved fee established by the insurance plan. They also agree to bill the patient only for the deductible and co-pay/co-insurance amounts that are based on BC/BS allowed rates, and the full charge for any uncovered services.

Other Commercial Insurances

Most Americans seeking health insurance from the Health Insurance Marketplace are covered by health insurance sponsored by private insurance companies (e.g., Aetna, BC, BS, CIGNA, Kaiser Permanente, Metropolitan, and Prudential). Private insurance companies operate to make a profit, and therefore have established protocols to reduce healthcare costs. To control how patients receive medical care, private insurance companies have established *managed care organizations* (MCOs).

MANAGED CARE ORGANIZATIONS

MCOs are a type of healthcare organization which contracts with various healthcare providers and medical facilities at a reduced payment schedule for their insurance members. Patient care is coordinated through a diverse network of providers and hospitals. There are different types of managed care plans such as *health maintenance organizations* (HMOs) and *preferred provider organizations* (PPOs) that provide healthcare in return for scheduled payments and that coordinate healthcare through a defined network of primary care providers (PCPs), hospitals, and other providers.

The goal of MCOs is to reduce the cost of delivering quality care to patient members. MCOs negotiate reduced rates with contracted providers; in return, the managed care plan increases the provider's patient care load. Managed care plans also require *referrals* for their patients to be treated with a specialist provider, thus limiting patient access to more expensive care. The *preauthorization* process can further control patient care costs; medical care, testing, and medication therapy is only provided when it is justified to the health insurance plan. It is important that medical assistants be well versed in the various models of managed care to fully understand their effects on healthcare costs (Table 14-2).

TABLE 14-2   Advantages and Disadvantages of Managed Care

ADVANTAGES	DISADVANTAGES
Healthcare costs are usually controlled	Access to specialized care and referrals can be denied or limited
Contracted and agreed-upon fee schedule	Providers' choices in the treatment of patients can focus more on cost effectiveness instead of necessity of treatment
Authorized services are usually paid for	More paperwork may be required
Most preventive medical treatment is covered	Treatment may be delayed because of preauthorization requirements
Patients' out-of-pocket expenses tend to be less than with traditional insurance	Reimbursement historically is less than with traditional insurance

Models of Managed Care Plans

Health Maintenance Organization

The passage of the Health Maintenance Organization Act in 1973 provided for federal aid to health insurance prepayment plans that met certain criteria, this legislation brought about a rapid growth in HMOs. HMOs are state-licensed health plans that are regulated by HMO laws that require them to include preventive care, such as routine physical examinations and other services, as part of their benefits package. The goal of the HMO health insurance plan is to reduce the cost of healthcare. HMO plans typically have the lowest monthly premiums among other health insurance plans, with lower patient financial responsibility. Patients are required to select a *primary care physician* (PCP), a general practitioner who acts as the **gatekeeper** to more specialized care. The insurance plan will not pay for services that are not in their provider network; patients are 100% financially responsible for medical expenses incurred outside the HMO network of providers. For example, patients wanting to visit the dermatologist for eczema must visit their PCPs first; they would be fully financially responsible if they made an appointment with a dermatologist directly. The PCP can either offer the patient a medication therapy or refer them to the specialist.

PCPs receive financial incentives when they reduce the cost of patient care. In the earlier example, prescribing medicine to the patient is more cost effective than referring the patient to the specialist. HMOs always require referrals from the PCP to specialists, for precertification and preauthorization, for hospital admissions, outpatient procedures, and treatments. There are several different types of HMO models.

Independent Physician Association

An independent physician association (IPA) is an independent group of providers and other healthcare professionals who are under contract to provide services to members of different HMOs, in addition to other insurance plans, usually at a fixed fee per patient. The providers in the IPA, who usually have separately owned practices, formally organize a physician association and continue to practice in their own offices. A healthcare provider may be contracted with several IPAs. Payments to providers by an IPA can be structured either as **capitation** or fee-for-service fee schedule.

Staff Model

A staff model HMO hires salaried healthcare providers. Rather than contracting with providers to create a network, the HMO owns the network. Medical care is authorized by the patient's PCP. No capitation or fee-for-service payment structure is used with the staff model; however, the providers may receive bonuses biannually or annually based on the number of patients treated or the cost savings.

Group Model

A group model HMO contracts with a multispecialty medical group to deliver care to its members. The HMO reimburses the providers' group, which is responsible for reimbursing provider members and contracted healthcare facilities. This arrangement is similar to an IPA in that the multispecialty group may organize a physician association; however, the group members typically practice together in one facility. The payment structure to the providers can be either capitation or fee-for-service. Refer to Table 14-3 to compare the different types of HMOs.

CRITICAL THINKING APPLICATION   **14-2**

Stephanie Hudson is a patient who called to make an appointment with the endocrinologist because she was having trouble managing her diabetes. She told Jodie over the phone when she was making the appointment that she has Aetna HMO. Will Jodie be able to schedule Miss Hudson's appointment with the endocrinologist? Why or why not? What would she need to make an appointment?

TABLE 14-3 Health Maintenance Organization Models

MODEL	STRUCTURE	CONTRACT TYPE
IPA	General or family practice provider or provider group that practices independently and may contract with several IPAs	Capitation or fee-for-service
Staff	One or more providers hired by an HMO	Salaried
Group	Multispecialty group with or without a PCP (i.e., gatekeeper); may contract with several IPAs	Capitation or fee-for-service

Preferred Provider Organization

A PPO is a managed care network that contracts with a group of providers; the providers agree on a predetermined list of charges for all services, including those for both normal and complex procedures. The PPO model of managed healthcare preserves the fee-for-service concept that many providers prefer. Typically, the patient's financial responsibilities represent on average 20% to 25% of the allowed charge, but this depends on the patient's health insurance benefits. A provider who joins a PPO does not need to alter the manner of providing care and continues to treat and bill the patients on a fee-for-service basis. When a patient covered under a PPO plan comes for treatment, the provider treats the patient and bills the PPO. Patients do not need to visit their PCP to obtain a referral to a specialist for more specialized care and they have more control over healthcare choices.

PPOs furnish their subscribers with a list of participating providers and healthcare facilities from which they can access in-network healthcare at PPO reduced rates. Rates are quite often lower than those charged to non-PPO patients.

Although patients have the option to visit a specialist when they feel the need, they are still required to obtain preauthorization for referrals for more expensive medical therapy such as formulary medication and some medical testing.

CRITICAL THINKING APPLICATION   **14-3**

Henry Hudson called Jodie; he was upset because he received a patient statement balance. He told Jodie that he has full coverage insurance through his employer and did not know why he had a balance. What information can Jodie share with Henry to explain his financial responsibility?

Exclusive Provider Organization

An EPO combines features of an HMO (e.g., an enrolled group or population, PCPs, and an authorization system) and a PPO (e.g., flexible benefit design and fee-for-service payments). Patients with EPO coverage will not be covered for services outside the designated network of providers (unless there is an emergency), but may not need to obtain a referral for specialized care. EPO plan members are not required to choose a PCP as HMO members are.

Professional Courtesy

Professional courtesy occurs when the health provider decides to reduce or eliminate the patient's financial obligations for healthcare provided. Providers used professional courtesy to eliminate the patient's financial responsibility because they either had a personal relationship with or had made financial arrangements before the service. However, the onset of strict managed care policies and procedures have all but eliminated professional courtesy. Managed care plans want to ensure that patients meet their financial responsibility to prevent fraud and to ensure quality care is delivered. Managed care contractors may request financial records, including patient account balance statements, confirming that healthcare providers are making an effort to collect payments from their patients.

Referrals

Patients seeking specialized care must first visit their assigned PCP to obtain a referral to a specialist or for more specialized therapy or care. Patients with HMO plans can only obtain a referral to the specialist by visiting their assigned PCP. HMOs will measure how many patients are referred to specialists by individual PCPs. Approval or denial of a referral can take anywhere from a few minutes to a few days. The three types of referrals are as follows:

- A *regular referral* usually takes 3 to 10 working days for review and approval. This type of referral is used when the provider believes that the patient must see a specialist to continue treatment.
- An *urgent referral* usually takes about 24 hours for approval. This type of referral is used when an urgent but not life-threatening situation occurs.
- A *STAT referral* can be approved online when it is submitted to the utilization review department through the provider's

Web portal. A STAT referral is used in an emergency situation as indicated by the provider.

A *regular referral* is the most common type and can be inconvenient for the patient. With most managed care plans, preauthorization needs to be obtained for a referral (Procedure 14-3). Remember this cardinal rule: never tell the patient the referral has been approved unless you have a hard copy of the authorization. A referral is authorized after the approval has been received. When a referral is approved the PCP's office and the patient should receive a copy of the authorization. Always review the authorization thoroughly and confirm details such as approved diagnosis and procedure codes and the exact period of time the authorization lasts. The patient will receive a letter with an authorization number and details regarding the approved services. The patient must bring the authorization to the specialist's office on the date of their appointment.

PROCEDURE 14-3   Obtain a Referral with Documentation

Goal: *To obtain a referral from a health plan's provider services desk phone number listed on the back of the patient's health insurance ID card.*

EQUIPMENT and SUPPLIES

- Patient health record
- Preauthorization form (Figure 14-3)
- Patient's insurance identification (ID) card

PROCEDURAL STEPS

1. Assemble the necessary documentation such as the patient ID card, the verification of eligibility, and the online insurance provider Web portal log-in information.
   PURPOSE: To avoid wasting time searching for information needed to perform the task.
2. Examine the patient's health record and determine the service or procedure for which preauthorization is being requested, including, if applicable, the specialist's name and phone number and the reason for the request.
   PURPOSE: To correctly complete the required form for gaining authorization from the patient's insurance carrier for the specified treatment.
3. Fill out the preauthorization form providing all information requested, which may include the following:
   - The patient's demographic and insurance information

- If the patient is a dependent: Information about the guarantor, such as name, date of birth, and gender.
- The provider's identification information, including the National Provider Identifier (NPI) and group ID number(s)
- The diagnosis and planned procedure or treatment, or the name and contact information of the provider to whom the patient is being referred.
NOTE: This can also be completed through the online insurance provider Web portal.
4. Proofread the completed form.
   PURPOSE: To ensure the accuracy of the information.
5. Attach a copy of the preauthorization submission confirmation to the patient's health record. This information should include the following:
   - A letter that preauthorizes the specified treatment
   - An authorization number
   - Confirmation of the specific number of procedures, services, or treatment sessions allowed; authorization for referral of the patient to a specialist

Preauthorization for Surgical Procedures

Many insurance companies require preauthorization, usually within 24 hours, if a patient is to be hospitalized or undergo certain medical procedures. Insurance claims for payment will be denied if proper preauthorization is not obtained. Refer to Procedure 14-4 on how to perform a preauthorization for surgery.

All managed care plans, including HMOs, PPOs, and EPOs, require preauthorization for medical services such as surgery,

expensive medical tests, and medication therapy. Preauthorization may be requested by calling the health insurance plan provider desk services number listed on the patient's health insurance ID card and by submitting a completed request for a preauthorization form (Figure 14-3). A preauthorization provides the following information:

- An authorization code, which may be alphabetic, numeric, or alphanumeric

- The date on which the referral request was received by the utilization review department
- The date on which the referral was approved and its expiration date
- The exact time period the authorization is valid.
- Authorized diagnosis and procedural codes
- The name, address, and telephone number of the contracted specialist where the authorized services will be provided
- The comments section: This is the most critical area of a referral because this area designates the services that have been approved.
- The specified number of authorized visits to the specialist
- An authorization may be issued for (1) evaluation only, (2) evaluation and treatment plan, (3) evaluation and biopsy, (4) evaluation and one injection, and so on.

Notes about the authorization process:

- If the authorization expires and services have not been provided, an extension may be requested. **Utilization manage-** **ment** will need to extend the expiration date and this will generate a new authorization with a new number. Be sure to update the authorization number for dates of services beyond the original authorization time window.
- If services are provided after the preauthorization's expiration date, the claim will be denied. If this happens, contact utilization management to request approval. Sometimes the patient, the specialist's office, or both must be involved in this process.
- Always ensure that any specialist to whom the provider refers a patient is contracted with the same managed care plan as the PCP.
- The medical assistant should explain to the patient specifically which services were approved.
- The PCP's office and/or the patient are notified if a referral is denied because of insufficient information or lack of medical necessity. When the PCP's office provides the utilization management committee with the necessary information, the referral can be reviewed again (Figure 14-3).

Preauthorization Request Form

TO BE COMPLETED BY PRIMARY CARE PHYSICIAN OR OUTSIDE PROVIDER

☐ Medicare ☑ Blue Cross/Blue Shield ☐ Tricare ☐ Health Net
☐ Medicaid ☐ Aetna ☐ Cigna ☐ Other
Group No.: 54098XX

Name: (First, Middle Initial, Last) Louann Campbell   Date: 7-14-20XX
☐ Male ☑ Female   Birthdate: 4-7-1952   Home Telephone Number: (555) 450-1666
Address: 2516 Encina Avenue, Woodland Hills, XY 12345-0439
Primary Care Physician: Gerald Practon, MD
Referring Physician: Gerald Practon, MD
Referred to: Raymond Skeleton, MD   Office Telephone number: (555) 486-9002
Address: 4567 Broad Avenue, Woodland Hills, XY 12345
Diagnosis Code: M54.5   Diagnosis: Low back pain
Diagnosis Code: M51.27   Diagnosis: Sciatica
Treatment Plan: Orthopedic consultation and evaluation of lumbar spine; R/O herniated disc L4-5
Authorization requested for: ☐ Consult only ☐ Treatment Only ☐ Consult/Treatment
☑ Consult/Procedure/Surgery ☐ Diagnostic Tests
Procedure Code: 99244   Description: New patient consultation
Procedure Code: Description:
Place of service: ☑ Office ☐ Outpatient ☑ Inpatient ☐ Other   Number of visits: 1
Facility: Length of stay:
List of potential future consultants (i.e., anesthetists, surgical assistants, or medical/surgical):
Physician's Signature: Gerald Practon, MD

TO BE COMPLETED BY PRIMARY CARE PHYSICIAN
PCP Recommendations: See above   PCP Initials: GP
Date eligibility checked: 7-14-20XX   Effective Date: 1-15-20XX

TO BE COMPLETED BY UTILIZATION MANAGEMENT
Authorized: Auth. No.   Not Authorized:
Deferred: Modified:
Effective Date: Expiration Date:

FIGURE 14-3 Preauthorization Request Form.

Utilization Management/Utilization Review

Utilization management is a form of patient care review by healthcare professionals who do not provide the care but are sponsored by health insurance companies. It is a necessary component of managed care to control costs. A *utilization review committee* reviews individual cases to make certain that medical care services are medically necessary (the specificity of diagnosis coding is critical) to ensure that providers are using their resources efficiently. This committee also reviews all provider referrals and cases of emergency department visits and urgent care. For referrals, the committee reviews the referral and either approves or denies it, so it is important to submit accurate documentation. The medical assistant should contact the utilization review department directly; it should never be left to the patient to contact this department.

PROCEDURE 14-4   Obtain Preauthorization for a Surgical Procedure with Documentation

Goal: *To obtain preauthorization from a patient's managed care organization (MCO) for requested services or procedures with documentation.*

EQUIPMENT and SUPPLIES

- Patient health record
- Preauthorization form (Figure 14-3)
- Patient's insurance identification (ID) card

PROCEDURAL STEPS

1. Assemble the necessary information such as the patient ID card, the verification of eligibility, and the health plan's provider services desk phone number listed on the back of the patient's health insurance ID card.
   <u>PURPOSE</u>: To avoid wasting time searching for information needed to perform the task.

2. Examine the patient's health record to determine the procedure for which preauthorization is being requested and assign the appropriate diagnosis and procedural codes for the surgical procedure.

3. Fill out the preauthorization form, providing all information requested, which may include the following:
   - The patient's demographic and insurance information

- If the patient is a dependent: Information about the guarantor, such as name, date of birth, and gender
- The provider's identification information, including the National Provider Identifier (NPI) and group ID number(s)
- The facility, including the NPI number and address

NOTE: This can also be completed through the online insurance provider Web portal.

4. Proofread the completed form.
   <u>PURPOSE</u>: To ensure the accuracy of the information.

5. Attach a copy of the preauthorization submission confirmation to the patient's health record. This information should include the following:
   - A letter that preauthorizes the surgery
   - An authorization number
   - Confirmation of the authorization to schedule the surgery
   <u>PURPOSE</u>: To document in the patient's health record the authorization for the procedure.

6. Call the patient to schedule the surgery.

GOVERNMENT-SPONSORED PLANS

Government-sponsored health insurance plans provide health insurance coverage with reduced or no monthly premiums for the indigent, the elderly, the military, and government employees. There are a variety of different insurance plans, but patients need to qualify either by age, income, government occupation, or health condition. A patient who is age 65 or older can qualify for *Medicare* insurance coverage. A low-income patient may be eligible for *Medicaid*. Dependents of military personnel are covered by *TRICARE*; and surviving spouses and dependent children of veterans who died in the line of duty are covered by the *Civilian Health and Medical Program of the Veterans Administration* (CHAMPVA). Some wage earners are protected against the loss of wages and the cost of medical care resulting from an occupational accident, disease, or disability through *workers' compensation insurance*.

Medicare

Established in 1966, Medicare is a federal health insurance program that provides healthcare coverage for individuals age 65 and older, the disabled, and patients with diagnosed end stage renal disease (ESRD). Today Medicare is the world's largest insurance program. In 2015 there were more than 55 million beneficiaries. The Medicare program was developed by the Healthcare Financing Administration (HCFA) as part of Title XVIII of the Social Security Act. HCFA now is known as the Centers for Medicare and Medicaid Services (CMS), a division of the Department of Health and Human Services (DHHS). Laws enacted by Congress regulate the Medicare program.

The Medicare plan is divided into four parts: Part A, Part B, Part C, and Part D (Table 14-4). Part A is hospital insurance for qualified Medicare participants and is financed with special contributions deducted from employed individuals' salaries, with matching contributions from their employers. These sums are collected, along with regular Social Security contributions, from wages and self-employment income earned during a person's working years, so there is no monthly premium paid. Part B is medical insurance for ambulatory care, including primary care and specialists for which patients are required to pay a monthly premium; Part B functions similar to a PPO in that patients can visit any specialist without a referral. Part C is an option for Medicare-qualified patients to turn their Part A and Part B benefits into a privately sponsored plan that can offer some additional benefits. Part D is a prescription drug program offered to Medicare-qualified individuals that requires an additional monthly premium. Optional Medigap policies pay the deductible and the 20% co-payment for those who choose to pay for the additional coverage.

TABLE 14-4   Comparing Medicare Plans

	COVERED SERVICES	MONTHLY PREMIUM	DEDUCTIBLE
Part A	Inpatient hospital care, skilled nursing facilities, home healthcare, and hospice services	$0	$1288 deductible for each benefit period; Days 1-60: $0 co-insurance for each benefit period; Days 61-90: $315 co-insurance per day of each benefit period; Day 91 and beyond: $630 co-insurance per each "lifetime reserve day" after day 90 for each benefit period (up to 60 days over a lifetime)
Part B	Outpatient hospital care, durable medical equipment, provider's services, and other medical services	$104.90	$166, plus 20% co-insurance for all medical services
Part C	Expanded inpatient hospital and outpatient hospital care benefits	Varies by plan	Varies by plan
Part D	Prescription drugs	Varies by income	Varies by plan

CRITICAL THINKING APPLICATION   14-4

Beatrice Hampton is a Medicare patient who has Part A and Part B coverage. Will Medicare cover her office visit with the endocrinologist? What percent of the bill will she be financially responsible for?

Medicaid

In 1965 the federal government provided for the medically indigent through a program known as Medicaid. Title XIX of Public Law 89 to 97, under the Social Security Amendments of 1965, provided for agreements involving cost sharing between federal and state governments to provide medical care for people meeting specific eligibility criteria. All states and the District of Columbia have Medicaid programs, but these programs vary by state. A person eligible for Medicaid in one state may not be eligible in another state, and covered medical services may differ.

The federal government provides funding to the state for Medicaid programs and the states individually decide whether to provide funds for extension of benefits. The state determines the type and extent of medical benefits that will be covered within the minimum standards established by the federal government; the Affordable Care Act has amended these standards.

A medical office has the right to limit the number of Medicaid patients they accept to their practice for financial reasons. The Medicaid Fee Schedule is the lowest of all insurance companies and it may not be in the medical office's financial interest to accept Medicaid patients. The provider who does accept Medicaid patients automatically agrees to accept Medicaid payments as payment in full for covered services. The patient cannot be billed for the difference between the Medicaid payment and the amount the provider charged. Eligibility for benefits is determined by the respective states, but most Medicaid recipients also are some or all of the following:

- Individuals who are medically needy
- Recipients of Aid to Families with Dependent Children (AFDC)

- Individuals who receive Supplemental Security Income (SSI)
- Individuals who receive certain types of federal and state aid
- Individuals who are **qualified Medicare beneficiaries (QMBs)**—Medicaid pays for Medicare Part B premiums, deductibles, and co-insurance for qualified low-income elderly individuals
- Individuals in institutions or receiving long-term care in nursing facilities and intermediate-care facilities

Government-Sponsored Health Maintenance Organization Plans

In an effort to reduce costs and increase the delivery of care efficiently, many Medicare and Medicaid state programs have provided their members options to join a health maintenance organization (HMO) plan. Medicare or Medicaid may sponsor these patients, but they may have a privately sponsored insurance card. These insurance identification (ID) cards state that they are government sponsored, which means that they may not cover all medical services as privately sponsored insurances do. Medical assistants should be diligent about patient verification to ensure what medical services will be covered and share this information with the patient before services are provided.

Children's Health Insurance Program

Children's Health Insurance Program (CHIP) is a state-funded program for children whose family income is above the Medicaid qualifying income limits. CHIP premiums are typically 5% of the family monthly income. State CHIP programs cover routine checkups, immunizations, doctor visits, prescriptions, dental care, vision care, inpatient and outpatient hospital care, laboratory tests, x-rays, and emergency services. CHIP programs are similar to HMO plans in that care is only covered through the designated network of providers. There are smaller co-payments for medical services for CHIP patients.

TRICARE

After World War II and the Korean War, there were a large number of military veterans who did not have access to effective healthcare during peacetime. To address this problem, Congress passed the Dependents Medical Care Act of 1956 and the Military Medical Benefits Amendments of 1966, which allowed the Secretary of Defense to contract with civilian healthcare providers. This civilian healthcare program became known as the Civilian Health and Medical Program of the Uniformed Services (CHAMPUS) in 1966. The program administering these benefits became CHAMPUS, which today is known as TRICARE. TRICARE is now the comprehensive healthcare program for all seven uniformed services: the Army, Navy, Marine Corps, Air Force, Coast Guard, Public Health Service, and the National Oceanic and Atmospheric Administration. TRICARE also covers family members of active duty personnel, military retirees and their eligible family members under the age of 65, and the survivors of all uniformed services.

The TRICARE program is managed by the military in partnership with civilian hospitals and clinics. It is designed to expand access to healthcare, ensure high-quality care, and promote medical readiness. All military hospitals and clinics are part of the TRICARE program and offer high-quality healthcare at low cost to plan users. TRICARE offers three types of plans: TRICARE Prime, TRICARE Extra, and TRICARE Standard. Review Table 14-5 for a comparison of the different TRICARE plans.

TABLE 14-5   Comparing TRICARE Plans

ACTIVE FAMILY DUTY MEMBERS		
	TRICARE PRIME	**TRICARE EXTRA**	**TRICARE STANDARD**
Annual deductible	None	$150/individual or $300/family for E-5 & above; $50/$100 for E-4 & below	$150/individual or $300/family for E-5 & above; $50/$100 E-4 & below
Annual enrollment fee	None	None	None
Civilian outpatient visit	No cost	15% of negotiated fee	20% of allowed charges for covered service
Civilian inpatient admission	No cost	Greater of $25 or $13.90 a day	Greater of $25 or $13.90 a day
Civilian inpatient mental health	No cost	$20/day	$20/day
Civilian inpatient skilled nursing facility care	$0 per diem charge per admission; no separate co-payment/cost-share for separately billed professional charges	$11/day ($25 minimum) charge per admission	$11/day ($25 minimum) charge per admission
RETIREES (UNDER 65), THEIR FAMILY MEMBERS, AND OTHERS		
	TRICARE PRIME	**TRICARE EXTRA**	**TRICARE STANDARD**
Annual deductible	None	$150/individual or $300/family	$150/individual or $300/family
Annual enrollment fee	$260/individual or $520/family	None	None
Civilian co-pays		20% of negotiated fee	25% of allowed charges for covered service
Outpatient emergency care mental health visit	$12 $30 $25 $17 (group visit)		
Civilian inpatient cost share	$11/day ($25 minimum) charge per admission	Lesser of $250/day or 25% of negotiated charges plus 20% of negotiated professional fees	Lesser of $512/day or 25% of billed charges plus 25% of allowed professional fees
Civilian inpatient skilled nursing facility care	$11/day ($25 minimum) charge per admission	$250 per diem co-payment or 20% cost-share of total charges for institutional care, whichever is less, plus 20% cost-share of separately billed professional charges	25% cost-share of allowed charges for institutional services plus 25% cost-share of allowable separately billed professional charges

Civilian Health and Medical Program of the Veterans Administration

CHAMPVA, a health benefits program similar to TRICARE, was established in 1973 for the spouses and dependent children of veterans suffering total, permanent, service-connected disabilities and for surviving spouses and dependent children of veterans who died as a result of service-related disabilities. The Department of Veterans Affairs (VA) shares with eligible beneficiaries the cost of certain healthcare services and supplies.

Workers' Compensation

Workers' compensation is an insurance plan for individuals who are injured on the job either by accident or an acquired illness. An example of an acquired illness would be mesothelioma from inhaling asbestos while on the job. The insurance plan covers all healthcare expenses related to the injury or illness and also includes monetary compensation for loss of income. Compensation benefits include medical care and rehabilitation benefits, weekly income replacement benefits for temporary disability, permanent disability settlements, and survivor benefits when applicable. The provider accepts the workers' compensation reimbursements as payment in full and does not bill the patient. Time limitations are set for the prompt reporting of workers' compensation cases. The employee is obligated to promptly notify the employer; the employer, in turn, must notify the insurance company and must refer the employee to a source of medical care.

State legislatures in all 50 states have passed workers' compensation laws to protect workers against the loss of wages and the cost of medical care resulting from an occupational accident or disease, as long as the employee was not proven negligent. State laws differ as to the classes of employees included and the benefits provided by workers' compensation insurance. Federal and state legislatures require employers to maintain workers' compensation coverage to meet minimum standards, covering a majority of employees, for work-related illnesses and injuries. The purpose of workers' compensation laws is to provide prompt medical care to an injured or ill worker so that the person may be restored to health and return to full earning capacity in as short a time as possible.

EMPLOYER-ESTABLISHED SELF-FUNDED PLANS

Many large companies or organizations have enough employees that they can fund their own insurance program. This is called a *self-funded plan*. Technically, a self-funded plan is not insurance by true definition. The employer pays employee healthcare costs from the funds collected from employee monthly premiums. Usually the costs of benefits and premiums for self-funded plans are similar to those for group plans. Self-funded plans tend to work best for companies that are large enough to offer good benefit coverage and reasonable premium rates and are able to pay large claims for expensive medical services. Often a **third-party administrator (TPA)** handles paperwork and claim payments for a self-insured group.

Self-funded healthcare is an arrangement in which an employer provides health or disability benefits to employees with its own funds.

This is different from fully insured plans, in which the employer contracts an insurance company to cover the employees and dependents. In self-funded healthcare, the employer assumes the direct risk for payment of the claims for benefits. The terms of eligibility and coverage are set forth in the insurance plan document, which includes provisions similar to those found in a typical group health insurance policy.

CLOSING COMMENTS

Health insurance and benefits coverage can be confusing to the patient, so medical assistants should educate themselves on the specific details of all plans accepted at the healthcare facility. The Affordable Care Act allows health insurance to be accessible to more Americans than any other time in history, so the demands on the current healthcare system will greatly increase over the next few years. Managed care has often been criticized in the media for its cost-saving practices; however, extra efforts made by medical assistants to overcome these challenges and educate their patients on how to use their health insurance plans will improve the quality of care delivered to their patients. Providers and healthcare facilities need to evaluate their ability to accept the fee schedule of insurance plans they are contracted with, especially since Medicaid's fee schedule is the lowest in the industry.

Patient Education

It is important for patients to understand how their insurance works. Many people, especially elderly individuals, believe that if they have health insurance, all charges for their healthcare will be covered. The responsibilities of a medical assistant include keeping the patient informed of his or her financial responsibilities and answering questions about their benefits and exclusions. Often healthcare facilities provide their patients with informational brochures that explain how health insurance and reimbursement work and provide definitions of some of the more common terms used in the insurance claims process. If patients are well advised and comfortable with insurance facts before treatment begins, the medical experience will go more smoothly, and collection of their financial responsibilities will be easier. The medical assistant must practice good communication skills, patience, and tact when discussing reimbursement and financial responsibilities issues with patients.

Legal and Ethical Issues

Verification of eligibility is a process that is important not only to ensure the insurance plan is valid at the time of service, but to ensure patient identity. Falsifying one's identity to use someone else's health insurance benefits is a common fraudulent practice. The only way to prevent this type of health insurance fraud is to diligently verify all patients when they schedule appointments with the healthcare facility. A state issued ID should be presented with the patient's health insurance ID to verify identity. If the medical assistant suspects fraud, he or she should report it to the health insurance plan immediately and the patient should be informed that they cannot be seen by the medical professional until issues relating to the health insurance are resolved.

Professional Behaviors

Patients can be confused or angered when insurance companies deny authorization of services or referrals. Although these decisions are made by insurance companies, many times the blame is put on the medical front office assistants. In situations like these, it is important for medical assistants to stay calm and listen to the patient's concerns. In most cases, the patient will come to realize that there is nothing the medical assistant can do, but the patient may need to express frustration. Once the patient has calmed down, the medical assistant can then recommend options such as paying cash, making payment arrangements, or bringing attention to the patient's insurance member services hotline. Compassionately assure patients that their health is most important and that you will do what you can so they can receive the appropriate medical treatment.

If the patient continues to escalate the situation and/or becomes belligerent, excuse yourself from the discussion and ask either an office manager or another medical assistant to step in. A medical assistant should never return anger and/or frustration to the patient. Remember, the patient may be mentally compromised and frustrated from extensive health care problems, so don't exacerbate the situation by releasing your own anger. If the patient's health is made the primary concern, the healthcare facility can work with the insurance company so the patient can receive appropriate medical care.

SUMMARY OF SCENARIO

Although she initially was nervous about explaining fees to patients and asking for payment, Jodie has become more comfortable in doing this aspect of her job because she understands the business aspect of the practice. The provider is operating the practice to make a profit and support his family, and the practice also is a source of support for the employees' families. Patients understand that providers must charge for their services, and have become accustomed to co-payments and co-insurance amounts. Many times, these fees are collected in advance, before the patient sees Dr. Crawford. This practice saves time on checkout, and most patients believe that the co-pay is a small cost compared with the entire fee that providers charge to manage their care in one office visit.

Jodie has noticed that the usual, customary, and reasonable fees that Dr. Crawford charges his patients directly affect the reimbursements that are paid by various insurance and managed care companies. Jodie has attended several health insurance billing seminars sponsored by Medicare and Blue Cross/Blue Shield and has noticed a drop in health insurance claim rejections. Dr. Crawford commented that he uses professional courtesy much less frequently than in the past because of the many rules and regulations placed on providers by managed care companies. He still offers the occasional patient a professional discount when it does not violate the managed care contract that he holds with the insurer or managed care company.

SUMMARY OF LEARNING OBJECTIVES

1. **Define, spell, and pronounce the terms listed in the vocabulary.**
   Spelling and pronouncing medical terms correctly bolster the medical assistant's credibility. Knowing the definitions of these terms promotes confidence in communication with patients and co-workers.

2. **Discuss the purpose of health insurance and explain the health insurance contract between the patient and the health plan.**
   Health insurance is a third-party payer system that reimburses a healthcare provider when services are rendered for an insured patient. A monthly premium is paid for a list of health insurance benefits detailed in the contract. The patient then provides evidence of the health insurance contract to the healthcare provider. The provider then submits a claim to the health insurance company for services rendered. The third party then reimburses the healthcare provider.

   Health insurance is a contract between a guarantor and a third-party payer. The guarantor agrees to pay a monthly premium to the health insurance company for health services coverage. When the guarantor or any of their dependents seeks health services, the health insurance will pay for all medically necessary services on the guarantor's behalf as detailed in the health insurance contract.

3. **Identify types of third-party plans.**
   There are two types of health insurance plans in the United States: privately sponsored health insurance plans and government-sponsored health insurance plans. Health insurance plans typically cover health services and procedures that are deemed medically necessary, or health services that are required to improve the patient's current health condition. Most insurance policies do not cover elective procedures, or medical procedures that will not improve the patient's current health, such as a facelift. Most of today's health insurance policies cover preventive care, which includes services provided to help prevent certain illnesses or that lead to an early diagnosis.

4. **Discuss the Affordable Care Act's effect on patient healthcare access.**
   In 2010, the Patient Protection and Affordable Care Act was enacted, which is also known as the *Affordable Care Act* or Obamacare. It increased the quality, availability, and affordability of private and public health insurance for more than 44 million uninsured Americans. The legislation includes new qualifying regulations, taxes, mandates, and subsidies. The federal mandate not only opens opportunities for more Americans to obtain affordable health insurance, but also works to reduce overall healthcare spending in the long run.

5. **Summarize the different health insurance benefits available and interpret information on a health insurance identification (ID) card.**
   Insurance packages are often tailored to the needs of each individual or group, and the ways to combine benefits are limitless. Health insurance policies normally contain a combination of the different benefits, such as surgical, medical, hospitalization, and major medical.

   As proof of health insurance coverage, patients are issued a health insurance ID card with the health plan name, patient's name, subscriber ID, and health plan contact information (Figure 14-1). Refer to Procedure 14-1 on how to interpret information on the health insurance ID card.

SUMMARY OF LEARNING OBJECTIVES—*continued*

6. Explain the importance of verifying eligibility and be able to verify eligibility of services, including documentation.

It is important to verify insurance benefits before providing services to patients. Verifying benefits is necessary to ensure that the patient is covered by insurance and to determine what benefits will be paid for routine and special procedures and services. Verification protects the provider and the patient against unexpected medical care costs.

Many problems for both the patient and the medical office can be prevented if the medical assistant develops and follows a procedure for verifying insurance benefits before services are rendered. This procedure includes gathering as much information as possible about the demographics of the patient and his or her insurance coverage. A pragmatic and tactful discussion with all new patients to explain the facility's established policy on insurance claims processing and the collection of fees not covered by the patient's policy will pay off. Refer to Procedure 14-2 on how to verify eligibility with documentation.

7. Explain the health insurance contract between the healthcare provider and the health insurance company.

In the United States payment for services is typically after the health services are rendered. In other words, healthcare providers are paid weeks, sometimes months, after medical services have been provided to the patient. Once the service is provided to the patient, the healthcare provider must submit a health insurance claim, which includes the diagnosis, the procedure, and total charges. Although the healthcare provider establishes their own fee schedule, or list of charges associated with various medical services provided, health insurance plans maintain their own rates at which they reimburse.

8. Explain how insurance reimbursements are determined and discuss the effect health insurance has on provider reimbursements.

Benefits are determined and paid in one of several ways: indemnity schedules; service benefit plans; usual, customary, and reasonable (UCR) fees; and the resource-based relative value scale (RBRVS). Medical assistants should become familiar with each of these methods and be able to differentiate the types of schedules, fees, and scales to determine which insurance payer uses them and how they affect reimbursement to the provider.

Healthcare providers have three commodities to sell: time, judgment (i.e., expertise), and services. In every case healthcare providers must place an estimate on the value of these services. However, in recent years health insurance plans, particularly government and managed healthcare organizations, have greatly influenced what healthcare providers can charge by establishing the allowable charge. The allowable amount is the maximum that third-party payers will pay for a particular procedure or service.

9. Summarize privately sponsored health insurance plans.

Privately sponsored health insurance plans, also known as commercial insurance plans, are for-profit organizations. As such, health insurance companies make annual changes to the participating provider contract to negotiate lower payments. Most privately sponsored plans use managed care to reduce the costs of delivering quality healthcare.

10. Differentiate among the different types of managed care models.

Managed care is a broad term used to describe a variety of healthcare plans developed to provide healthcare services at lower costs. It is important for the medical assistant to be familiar with various plan types such as the health maintenance organization (HMO), preferred provider organization (PPO), and exclusive provider organization (EPO) and to understand the policies of each one.

11. Outline managed care requirements for patient referral and obtain a referral with documentation.

Obtaining preauthorization for making referrals must be done according to the guidelines of the individual insurance companies. If the medical assistant is uncertain about the procedure, he or she should always refer to the insurance plan's policies and procedures manual.

The medical assistant should refer to the insurance plan's policies and procedures to accurately obtain preauthorization for a referral. Refer to Procedure 14-3 on how to obtain a referral with documentation.

12. Describe the process for preauthorization and how to obtain preauthorization with documentation.

Managed care plans, including HMOs, PPOs, and EPOs, require preauthorization for medical services such as surgery, expensive medical tests, and medication therapy. Preauthorization may be requested by calling the health insurance plan, which should be documented in the patient's electronic health record (EHR).

Many insurance companies require preauthorization, usually within 24 hours, if a patient is to be hospitalized or undergo certain medical procedures. Insurance claims for payment will be denied if proper preauthorization is not obtained. Refer to Procedure 14-4 on how to perform a preauthorization for surgery.

13. List and discuss various government-sponsored plans.

Government-sponsored health insurance programs include Medicare, Medicaid, TRICARE, CHAMPVA, CHIPS, and worker's compensation. The elderly, disabled, military, indigent, and those injured at work may qualify for one of these programs. Because these programs are sponsored by the government, participating providers (PARs) must accept a lower fee schedule for reimbursements.

14. Review employer-established self-funded plans.

Self-funded healthcare or self-insurance is an arrangement in which an employer provides health or disability benefits to employees with its own funds. This is different from fully insured plans, in which the employer contracts with an insurance company to cover the employees and dependents. In self-funded healthcare, the employer assumes the direct risk for payment of the claims for benefits.

CONNECTIONS

Study Guide Connection: Go to Chapter 14 Study Guide. Read the Case Study and Workplace Applications and complete the assignments. Do online research for answers to the questions in the Internet Activities associated with the basics of health insurance.

evolve Evolve Connection: Go to the Chapter 14 link at *evolve.elsevier.com/kinn* to complete the Chapter Review Quiz. Check out the other resources listed for this chapter to make the most of what you have learned from Basics of Health Insurance.

15

MEDICAL BILLING AND REIMBURSEMENT

SCENARIO

The instructor in Ann Snyder's administrative medical assistant class, Grant Wilson, knows that working with health insurance can be quite rewarding. Mr. Wilson works with Ann and her classmates, answering their questions and helping them to see that medical insurance is not as complicated as it may seem.

A medical assistant who is detailed oriented enjoys billing and coding activities. The individual who performs these duties in the provider's office is a critical staff member because tasks related to billing have a significant effect on the provider's income. That income is used to pay the clinic's expenses, including payroll, so the facility staff indirectly counts on accurate and timely billing. Medical assistants who continually develop their coding skills are assets to the practice and can look forward to a long and rewarding career.

Mr. Wilson is sure to show the students several different Explanation of Benefits (EOBs) from a variety of insurance companies so that the students can learn how the reimbursement process works for a variety of health insurance plans. Ann will learn about the importance of verifying patient billing information and the steps for obtaining precertification for medical procedures; she also will learn how to discuss the patient's billing record professionally.

While studying this chapter, think about the following questions:

- Why is it important for Ann to obtain accurate patient billing information?
- Why is it important to verify insurance eligibility and process precertification before the patient receives medical services?
- How can Ann complete a CMS-1500 Health Insurance Claim Form?
- Will Ann be able to read an EOB to determine the patient's financial responsibility?
- How can Ann successfully inform patients of the financial responsibilities they face as a result of third-party requirements?

LEARNING OBJECTIVES

1. Define, spell, and pronounce the terms listed in the vocabulary.
2. Identify steps for filing a third-party claim
3. Identify the types of information contained in the patient's billing record.
4. Apply managed care policies and procedures, describe processes for precertification, and obtain precertification, including documentation.
5. Explain how to submit health insurance claims, including electronic claims, to various third-party payers.
6. Review the guidelines for completing the CMS-1500 Health Insurance Claim Form, and complete an insurance claim form.
7. Differentiate between fraud and abuse.
8. Discuss the effects of upcoding and downcoding.
9. Discuss methods of preventing the rejection of claims, and display tactful behavior when speaking with medical providers about third-party requirements.
10. Describe ways of checking a claim's status.
11. Review and read an Explanation of Benefits.
12. Discuss reasons for denied claims.
13. Define "medical necessity" as it applies to diagnostic and procedural coding; also, apply medical necessity guidelines.
14. Explain a patient's financial obligations for services rendered, and inform a patient of these obligations.
15. Show sensitivity when speaking with patients about third-party requirements.

VOCABULARY

audit A process done before claims submission to examine claims for accuracy and completeness.

capitation agreement A contract between a provider and an insurance company in which the health plan pays a monthly fee per patient, while the provider accepts the patient's copay as payment in full for office visits.

claims clearinghouse An intermediary that accepts the electronic claim from the provider, reformats the claim to the specifications outlined by the insurance plan, and submits the claim.

CMS-1500 Health Insurance Claim Form (CMS-1500) Form used by most health insurance payers for claims submitted by providers and suppliers.

coinsurance A policy provision in which the policyholder and the insurance company share the cost of covered medical services in a specified ratio.

copayment A patient financial responsibility, which is due at the time of the office visit.

deductible A patient financial responsibility that the subscriber for the policy is contracted per year to pay toward his or her health care before the insurance policy reimburses the provider.

downcoding When a lower specificity level, or more generalized code, is assigned.

explanation of benefits (EOB) A form that is sent by the insurance company to the provider who submitted the insurance claim, which accompanies a check or a document indicating that funds were electronically transferred.

intentional Determining whether fraudulent medical billing practices were done with purpose or by accident.

medical necessity A health insurance carrier's decision that the CPT and HCPCS codes (services or supplies) used to treat the patient's diagnosis (indicated by the ICD code) meet the accepted standard of medical practice.

National Provider Identifier An identifier assigned by the Centers for Medicare and Medicaid Services (CMS) that classifies the healthcare provider by license and medical specialties.

participating provider A healthcare provider who has signed a contract with a health insurance plan to accept lower reimbursements for services in return for patient referrals.

precertification The process of obtaining the dollar amount approved for a medical procedure or service before the procedure or service is scheduled.

release of information A form completed by the patient that authorizes the medical office to release medical records to the insurance company for health insurance reimbursement.

remark codes The area on the EOB where the payer indicates the conditions under which the claim was paid or denied.

upcoding When the provider may be inclined to code to a higher specificity level than the service provided actually involved.

Medical billing and reimbursement represent the financial lifeline of the healthcare facility. Collecting accurate patient health insurance information is essential to submit accurate health insurance claims. Each health insurance company has its own claims submission policies and procedures for timely reimbursement. A successful medical assistant in insurance billing learns the various insurance company requirements and submits accurate claims. Many health insurance companies have setup online provider webportals, and this has made the process of checking the status of a claim quick and easy. The medical assistant also needs to interpret the **explanation of benefits (EOB)** to determine the patient's **coinsurance** and/or **deductible**. Clear communication with the patient about his or her financial responsibilities takes patience and sensitivity.

STEPS IN MEDICAL BILLING

Medical billing tasks begin when the patient seeks medical services from the provider, usually when an appointment is made. If you plan to work in this area in the healthcare facility, you typically would follow these steps in performing insurance billing tasks.

- Collect patient information when the patient calls to schedule an appointment. This includes information about the insured, his or her employer, demographic information, and health insurance data. When the patient arrives for the appointment, you should inform the patient of his or her **copayment** responsibility and collect it before medical services are provided.
- At the time of the appointment, make a copy or scan of both sides of the patient's insurance card and also of a government-issued picture ID.
- Verify the patient's eligibility, confirming that the patient's contract with the insurance company is valid for the date of service. Patient eligibility can be confirmed by calling the provider services desk phone number on the back of the health insurance ID card, or by using the provider Web portal sponsored by the patient's health insurance company. Review patient benefits and exclusions for certain medical procedures and services.

- If **precertification** is needed, contact the health insurance company's representative to request it.
- After services have been rendered to the patient, code the diagnosis and procedures and review the encounter form/superbill for completeness. The charges for the procedure or procedures should be provided automatically by the medical billing software.
- Complete the **CMS-1500 Health Insurance Claim Form (CMS-1500)** (see Figure 15-8) or an electronic claim form. Submit the form to the insurance company or **data clearinghouse**.
- Review the electronic claims submission report to ensure that the claim was submitted accurately. Correct any discrepancies through the claims clearinghouse and resubmit denied claims.
- Meet the timely filing requirements of each of the different health insurance carriers. Health insurance companies do not pay claims submitted after the established filing period, and this balance cannot be billed to the patient.
- Post payments in the patient's account using the EOB to identify the line items that were paid, reduced, or denied. Patient account statements for their financial responsibility should be mailed out. Health insurance claims for patient accounts with secondary insurance should be submitted.
- Each payment for a procedure line item must be posted correctly in the patient's account. Patient accounts should reflect that the amount above the contracted allowed amount needs to be adjusted per line item.

CRITICAL THINKING APPLICATION   **15-1**

The medical billing manager informs Ann that she has noticed an increase in the number of insurance claim rejections that state the patient cannot be identified. Which step of the medical billing process might be addressed to resolve this problem?

TYPES OF INFORMATION FOUND IN THE PATIENT'S BILLING RECORD

The claim submission process begins after the patient receives services from the provider. When the first appointment is made for a patient, it is routine to ask the patient for all pertinent insurance billing information. Much of this information is collected on the patient registration/intake form, which is completed when the patient comes to the medical office for the initial visit (Figure 15-1). This information should always be collected from every new patient seen by the provider. Returning or established patients should be asked before every visit whether any changes have been made to their health insurance plan and whether their insurance information is complete and up-to-date.

Obtaining accurate patient information for submitting a health insurance claim is important, but a medical release of information form, signed by the patient, also should be kept in the person's health record. The release form allows the authorized release of medical information to the health care insurer. Even though the patient expects the insurance form to be filled out and submitted for

---

Patient Registration Form

PATIENT INFORMATION (Please print clearly)   Social Security# 123-45-6789

Please check one: ☐ Married   ☑ Single   ☐ Divorced   ☐ Separated   ☐ Widowed

Patient's Full Name   Rose Dawson   Age 81 DOB 02/17/XX   Sex F

Address 123 Titanic Place

City New York   State NY   Zipcode 10001

Home Phone (212) 545-1212   Driver's License # N/A

Occupation Retired

Patient's Employer None   Phone Number

Address

City   State   Zipcode

Spouse None   Social Security #

Address

City   State   Zipcode

Occupation   Driver's License Number

Family Physician Robert Wilson, MD   Referred by

In case of emergency, contact Marie Dawson   Relationship daughter

Address 123 Titanic Place

City New York   State NY   Zipcode 10001

INSURANCE INFORMATION

Primary Coverage, Name of Carrier: Medicare

    Identification # 123-45-6789A

    Group #

    Subscriber   Rose Dawson

    Effective Date 2/17/20XX

Secondary Coverage Name of Carrier: AARP Secondary Policy

    Identification # 123-45-6789A

    Group #

    Subscriber   Rose Dawson

    Effective Date 2/17/20XX

PAYMENT AUTHORIZATION

Although covered by insurance, I am aware that I am personally responsible for all charges. An electronic copy of this authorization will be as valid as the original.

Rose Dawson   12/15/20XX

Signature of Patient   Date

FIGURE 15-1 Completed patient registration/intake form.

payment, this cannot be done without a signature in the patient's health record granting permission.

MANAGED CARE POLICIES AND PROCEDURES

Medical billers should familiarize themselves with procedures commonly used by managed care organization (MCO) health plans, such as precertification. Medical assistants must keep in mind that services provided to patients who are sponsored by an MCO plan may not be reimbursed if the policies and procedures specific to the insurance plan are not followed. For example, pain management services typically require a preauthorization. If a pain management facility were to provide these services to the patient without preauthorization, the MCO would deny all insurance claims. To submit accurate health insurance claims, medical assistants should establish office procedures for applying MCO policies and procedures (Procedure 15-1). To find out more about training offered by MCOs for medical billing purposes, review the following box.

Health Plan–Sponsored Training in Medical Billing

Some major health plans offer annual training in newly implemented medical billing policies and procedures. These sessions usually are held in a metropolitan area, and training can range from 1 day to a week of informative seminars. Although these training sessions can be expensive, the knowledge gained from them ensures that the most accurate health insurance claims are submitted for reimbursement. The experts conducting the seminars also can answer questions about specific medical billing situations, which can prove valuable for future claims submissions. Medical billers should visit the insurance company's website to see whether any training sessions are scheduled that they can attend. It is wise for an office representative to attend a workshop at least once a year for most of the insurance companies to which the practice submits claims.

PROCEDURE 15-1   Show Sensitivity When Communicating With Patients Regarding Third-Party Requirements

Goal: To demonstrate sensitivity through verbal and nonverbal communication when discussing third-party requirements with patients.

Scenario: Ken Thomas saw Jean Burke N.P. for his asthma today. He was prescribed a fluticasone inhaler 220 mcg and a refill on his Albuterol inhaler. When Ken stops at the check-out desk, to make a follow-up appointment, he looks concerned. You inquire how you can help him and he states that he is wondering if his new insurance will pick up the fluticasone inhaler. He further explains that he has used it in the past with great results, but he recently switched insurance plans and he is finding it doesn't have the same coverage as his old plan.

Role play #1: You call the insurance company and discuss the coverage with the insurance carrier's representative. The representative tells you that the fluticasone inhaler is not covered. The representative gave you names of two other inhalers that would be covered.

Role play #2: You must explain to Ken, who is upset with his insurance coverage, that he would have to cover the $250 inhaler.

EQUIPMENT and SUPPLIES

- Copy of patient's health insurance ID card
- Prescription for new medication

PROCEDURAL STEPS

1. Gather a copy of the patient's health insurance ID card and the prescription for the new medication.
   PURPOSE: Having the required documents will help you to be more efficient as you perform the task.
2. Review the insurance card for coverage information and the phone number for providers.
   PURPOSE: You will need the phone number from the ID card to call the insurance carrier. You will also need to provide the insurance representative the patient's information.
3. Call (use role play #1) the insurance company and clearly state the patient's information, the patient's question, and the new medication.

PURPOSE: The insurance representative will need the patient's information and the question to assist you. Speaking clearly as you provide the information will help the listener understand what you are asking.
4. Demonstrate professionalism through verbal communication skills, by stating a respectful, clear, organized message while pronouncing medical terminology and medications correctly.
5. Explain to the patient (use role play #2) the message from the insurance representative using language that can be understood by the patient.
   PURPOSE: For the patient to understand your message, you need to use language that he can understand.
6. Demonstrate sensitivity to the patient by paying attention to and responding appropriately to the patient's nonverbal body language and verbal message.
   PURPOSE: Demonstrating sensitivity can come from verbal messages and body language. Paying attention to the patient and responding appropriately to the patient's message and nonverbal communication is important.

PROCEDURE 15-1   *—continued*

7. Demonstrate sensitivity to the patient by showing empathy and clarifying that you understand what the patient is stating. Give the patient your full attention during the conversation and reserve judgment.

8. Demonstrate sensitivity to the patient by using a pleasant, courteous tone of voice. Use body language to communicate respect (e.g., eye contact if culturally appropriate, keep arms uncrossed and relaxed).
   PURPOSE: As the person's frustration and anger increase, it is important to use a pleasant, courteous, and normal tone of voice. Keeping your body appearance relaxed (e.g., arms uncrossed, hands relaxed) will help to show the patient you are calm.

9. Provide the patient with options if appropriate.
   PURPOSE: Providing the patient with choices also shows the patient that you care.

Precertification

In an effort to control costs, many MCOs require precertification for specialized medical services. Precertification is the process of obtaining the dollar amount approved for a medical procedure or service before the procedure or service is scheduled. To obtain precertification, the medical assistant typically calls the provider services desk phone number on the back of the patient's health insurance ID card. Precertification does not guarantee payment of services after submission of the health insurance claim; however, the process ensures that both the healthcare provider and the patient are informed of the amount that will be reimbursed and the amount the patient will have to pay.

The policies and procedures for each individual health plan determine whether precertification is required before a procedure is scheduled. Almost every health maintenance organization (HMO) insurance plan requires precertification, but medical assistants must confirm the requirement by contacting provider services. Successful medical billers are diligent in obtaining precertification.

The precertification process (Procedure 15-2) is very similar to the preauthorization process in that the health insurance plan is contacted after the primary care provider (PCP) recommends the specialized medical procedure or service. In fact, many health insurance companies use the terms <u>precertification</u> and <u>preauthorization</u> interchangeably. However, precertification specifically determines the dollar amount approved for the medical procedure, whereas preauthorization gives the provider approval to render the medical service.

Using a Health Insurance Company's Online Web Portal to Apply for Precertification

Typically in modern healthcare facilities, the medical assistant can request precertification online through the health insurance company's online Web portal. Consider this case, which is laid out in stepwise fashion to make it easier for you to follow the events:

1. Dr. Thomas Shea is the primary care provider (PCP) for Mary Tolbert, who has heartburn that has not improved with medication.

2. Because Ms. Tolbert's condition is not improving, Dr. Shea requests preauthorization for her to see Dr. Eduard Hamilton, a gastrointestinal (GI) specialist. Ms. Tolbert is insured by a health management organization (HMO).

3. The HMO plan authorizes Ms. Tolbert to see Dr. Hamilton; this authorization is sent to Ms. Tolbert, Dr. Shea, and Dr. Hamilton. When Ms. Tolbert receives the authorization, she schedules an appointment with Dr. Hamilton.

4. After evaluating Ms. Tolbert, Dr. Hamilton orders a colonoscopy. However, Ms. Tolbert is concerned about her financial responsibility. Therefore, Dr. Hamilton's office requests precertification for the colonoscopy on Ms. Tolbert's behalf.

5. The HMO plan notifies Dr. Hamilton that the plan would reimburse a total of $1,500, and Ms. Tolbert would be financially responsible for $400. The precertification is sent both to Dr. Hamilton and Ms. Tolbert, who agree to its financial terms and schedule the procedure.

PROCEDURE 15-2   **Perform Precertification with Documentation**

Goal: *To obtain precertification from a patient's insurance carrier for requested services or procedures.*

EQUIPMENT and SUPPLIES

- Paper method: Patient's health record, Prior Authorization (Precertification) Request form, copy of patient's health insurance ID card, a pen
- Electronic method: SimChart for the Medical Office (SCMO)

PROCEDURAL STEPS

1. For the paper method, gather the health record, precertification/prior authorization request form, copy of the health insurance ID card, and a pen. For the electronic method, access the Simulation Playground in SCMO.

PROCEDURE 15-2   *—continued*

2. Using the health record, determine the service or procedure that requires precertification/preauthorization.
3. For the paper method, complete the Precertification/Prior Authorization Request form using a pen. For the electronic method, click on the Form Repository icon in SCMO. Select Prior Authorization Request from the left INFO PANEL. Use the Patient Search button at the bottom to find the patient. Complete the remaining fields of the form.
   PURPOSE: This provides information on the ordered procedure or service to the insurance carrier, who will then notify the provider's representative if it will be covered under the plan.

4. Proofread the completed form and make any revisions needed.
   PURPOSE: To ensure the accuracy of the information.
5. Paper method: File the document in the health record after it is faxed to the insurance carrier. Electronic method: Print and fax or electronically send the form to the insurance carrier and save the form to the patient's record.
   PURPOSE: Copies of all forms completed for the patient need to be maintained in the health record.

SUBMITTING CLAIMS TO DIFFERENT THIRD-PARTY PAYERS

All health insurance companies accept the CMS-1500 as the standard for submitting professional and technical claims for a variety of healthcare facilities. However, each health insurance plan has its own policies and procedures for the submission of claims.

Visit Medicare and Medicaid administrator websites for specific guidelines on submitting accurate claims in the provider's state. The MCO-sponsored insurance plans associated with **capitation agreements** have specific guidelines on the types of medical services that are billable. Privately sponsored health insurance plans have their own policies and procedures for submitting claims, and the medical assistant should research those of the health plans commonly seen in the practice.

The medical assistant can successfully manage the requirements of the different insurance plans by keeping a medical billing manual. The manual should contain the billing policies and procedures for most common third-party payers for the healthcare facility. The individual in charge of the manual should make sure that every medical biller has a copy and that the policies and procedures are up-to-date. For example, the date for Medicare's annual billing procedures and policies is October 1. Whenver an update is released, the medical billing manual also should be updated.

GENERATING ELECTRONIC CLAIMS

Since 2006 Medicare has required that all health insurance claims be sent electronically, and most health insurance plans have followed the same practice. If more than 90% of health insurance claims are submitted electronically, why is it important to learn the different fields of the CMS-1500 paper form? Electronic claims are submitted as a collection of data, and the data fields are identical to those on the CMS-1500. Therefore, a medical assistant who is familiar with a paper CMS-1500 will have no problem collecting data for an electronic health insurance claim.

Electronic claims are insurance claims that are transmitted over the Internet from the provider to the health insurance company through *electronic data interchange*. Electronic data interchange is the electronic transfer of data between two or more entities. When submitting electronic health insurance claims, a healthcare facility transmits the data for the claim, and the health insurance company accepts it. A *transmitter ID*, which is found on the patient's health insurance ID card, is needed to identify the specific health plan to which the claim should be submitted. Most medical billing software is designed to generate electronic claims.

Just as for paper claims, when electronic claims are submitted, accurate data are essential. When the medical assistant reviews the claim for accuracy, the claim is prepared for submission.

Electronic Claims Submission

Electronic claims are submitted in the HIPAA 5010 format and can be transmitted directly to the insurance carrier or to a claims clearinghouse.

Direct Billing

Direct billing is the process by which an insurance carrier allows a provider to submit insurance claims directly to the carrier electronically. Most major insurance carriers, including Medicare and Medicaid, provide software packages to providers that are used to enter patient and insured information, charges, and provider details. Many carrier-direct systems are supplied free of charge to the provider, but the direct system can transmit only to specific carriers. A transmitter ID is not needed when electronic claims are submitted through direct billing.

Clearinghouse Submissions

A claims clearinghouse is a healthcare entity that acts as an intermediary between the healthcare facility and the health insurance company. The clearinghouse accepts electronically submitted claims from healthcare agencies, **audits** the claims for completeness, and reformats them to meet the insurance companies' specifications. The claims are sorted by insurance plans and then sent in batches electronically to the appropriate insurance carriers. The insurance companies then send a report through the data clearinghouse to confirm the receipt of claims, claim status on previously submitted claims, and claim payment notification. A clearinghouse charges the healthcare facility a small fee for the service of sending and receiving claims transmissions, checking and preparing the claims for processing, consolidating claims so that one transmission can be sent to each carrier, and submitting claims in correct data format to the appropriate insurance payer. A typical fee is 25¢ per submitted claim. Other services that clearinghouses typically provide include:

- Reporting the number of claims submitted, and the number of errors and their specifics
- Forwarding claims to insurance carriers that accept electronic claims (e.g., Medicare, Medicaid, Blue Cross/Blue Shield, and others) or to another clearinghouse that may hold the contracts with specific payers
- Keeping provider offices updated as new carriers are added to the database
- Generating informative statistical reports

Medical Documentation with Electronic Claims

The electronic submission process sends only health insurance claim information; no other medical documentation can be sent at this time. If a health insurance company requires additional documentation, it notifies the medical office to provide specific documentation. Reimbursement is suspended until the documentation has been received and reviewed by the health insurance plan. Medical assistants should look through mail for documentation requests from insurance companies to facilitate faster reimbursements.

COMPLETING THE CMS-1500 HEALTH INSURANCE CLAIM FORM

The CMS-1500 Health Insurance Claim Form is used by most health insurance payers for claims submitted by providers and suppliers. The form has 33 blocks. These blocks are divided into three sections:

- *Section 1: Carrier.* The first section indicates the type of insurance plan to which the claim is being submitted; this section includes only Block 1.
- *Section 2: Patient and Insured Information.* The second section contains information about the patient and the insured; it includes Blocks 1a through 13.
- *Section 3: Physician or Supplier Information.* The third section contains information about the provider or supplier; it includes Blocks 14 through 33.

Table 15-1 presents a summary of the information needed to complete the CMS-1500 accurately.

Section 1: Carrier—Block 1 (Figure 15-2)

This block shows the type of insurance the patient has. Indicate the type of health insurance coverage applicable to this claim by putting an **X** in the appropriate box, marking only one box. This information directs the claim to the correct payer.

Section 2: Patient and Insured Information—Blocks 1a to 13 (Figure 15-3)

The CMS-1500 distinguishes between the patient and the insured. The insured is the individual who is directly contracted with the insurance company. For example, if an insurance claim for Sabrina Rudman is submitted and Blue Cross covers her through her employer, she is both the patient and the insured. However, if the insurance claim is for Chris Rudman, her son, Sabrina Rudman is the insured, and Chris Rudman, her dependent, is the patient. Every CMS-1500 requires the name, gender, and birth date of both the insured and the patient, even if they are different individuals. The blocks in Figure 15-3 highlighted in yellow are for the patient's information, and the blocks highlighted in blue are for the insured's information.

Blocks 1a, 4, 7, and 11(a-d)

Information required for the insured individual includes the person's health plan ID number, name, address, policy group number, birth date, gender, employer's name (if applicable), the name of the insurance plan, and whether the insured has another health benefit plan.

Blocks 2, 3, 5, 6, and 10 a-c

Required information for the patient includes the person's name, birth date, gender, address, relationship to the insured, patient status, and whether the patient's condition is related to his or her job, an automobile accident, or some other accident.

CRITICAL THINKING APPLICATION   15-2

Ann is preparing an insurance claim to bill to Blue Cross. She notes that the patient is the dependent of the insured, so she reviews the patient registration intake form and finds that the date of birth for the insured is not present. Can Ann accurately complete the CMS-1500?

Block 9

Block 9 is for recording information about any secondary insurance plan that may be applicable. The data required include the other insured person's name, policy or group number, birth date, gender, and employer (if applicable), and the name of the other insurance plan.

HEALTH INSURANCE CLAIM FORM

APPROVED BY NATIONAL UNIFORM CLAIM COMMITTEE (NUCC) 02/12

| PICA | | | | | | | PICA |

1. MEDICARE	MEDICAID	TRICARE CHAMPUS	CHAMPVA	GROUP HEALTH PLAN	FECA BLK LUNG	OTHER
☐ (Medicare #)	☐ (Medicaid #)	☐ (Sponsor's SSN)	☐ (Member ID#)	☐ (SSN or ID)	☐ (SSN)	☐ (ID)

CARRIER →

FIGURE 15-2 Section 1: Carrier (Block 1).

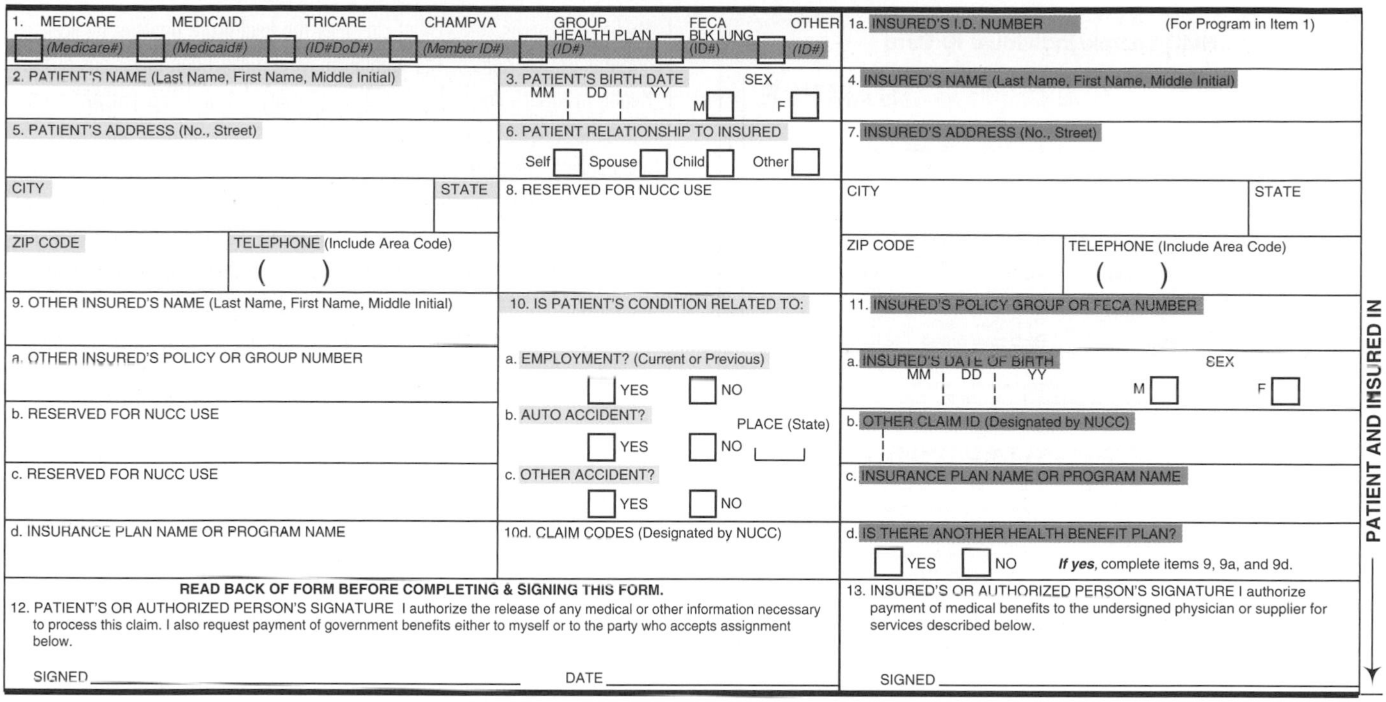

1. MEDICARE MEDICAID TRICARE CHAMPVA GROUP HEALTH PLAN FECA BLK LUNG OTHER		1a. INSURED'S I.D. NUMBER (For Program in Item 1)	

(Medicare#)   (Medicaid#)   (ID#DoD#)   (Member ID#)   (ID#)   (ID#)   (ID#)

2. PATIENT'S NAME (Last Name, First Name, Middle Initial)	3. PATIENT'S BIRTH DATE SEX	4. INSURED'S NAME (Last Name, First Name, Middle Initial)
	MM DD YY M □ F □	
5. PATIENT'S ADDRESS (No., Street)	6. PATIENT RELATIONSHIP TO INSURED	7. INSURED'S ADDRESS (No., Street)
	Self □ Spouse □ Child □ Other □	
CITY STATE	8. RESERVED FOR NUCC USE	CITY STATE
ZIP CODE TELEPHONE (Include Area Code) ( )		ZIP CODE TELEPHONE (Include Area Code) ( )
9. OTHER INSURED'S NAME (Last Name, First Name, Middle Initial)	10. IS PATIENT'S CONDITION RELATED TO:	11. INSURED'S POLICY GROUP OR FECA NUMBER
a. OTHER INSURED'S POLICY OR GROUP NUMBER	a. EMPLOYMENT? (Current or Previous) □ YES □ NO	a. INSURED'S DATE OF BIRTH SEX MM DD YY M □ F □
b. RESERVED FOR NUCC USE	b. AUTO ACCIDENT? PLACE (State) □ YES □ NO	b. OTHER CLAIM ID (Designated by NUCC)
c. RESERVED FOR NUCC USE	c. OTHER ACCIDENT? □ YES □ NO	c. INSURANCE PLAN NAME OR PROGRAM NAME
d. INSURANCE PLAN NAME OR PROGRAM NAME	10d. CLAIM CODES (Designated by NUCC)	d. IS THERE ANOTHER HEALTH BENEFIT PLAN? □ YES □ NO *If yes*, complete items 9, 9a, and 9d.
READ BACK OF FORM BEFORE COMPLETING & SIGNING THIS FORM. 12. PATIENT'S OR AUTHORIZED PERSON'S SIGNATURE I authorize the release of any medical or other information necessary to process this claim. I also request payment of government benefits either to myself or to the party who accepts assignment below. SIGNED_____ DATE_____		13. INSURED'S OR AUTHORIZED PERSON'S SIGNATURE I authorize payment of medical benefits to the undersigned physician or supplier for services described below. SIGNED_____

PATIENT AND INSURED IN

FIGURE 15-3 Section 2: Patient and Insured Information (Blocks 1a to 13).

Primary and Secondary Insurance Determination

In most cases, Medicare is usually the primary insurance, and there is a secondary policy to cover the 20% financial responsibility. In some cases, however, Medicare can be the patient's secondary insurance. This typically happens when a Medicare patient is still covered under an employer-sponsored group policy because the patient works full time. In other cases, a patient may have two insurance coverages, such as when both the patient and his or her spouse have employer-sponsored group insurance.

In the case of a child whose mother and father both carry the child as a dependent on their employer-sponsored health insurance plans, primary and secondary insurance status is determined by the birthday rule: whichever parent's birth date falls first in a calendar year is considered to have the primary insurance. The year of the parent's birth is not used. Therefore, if the mother's birth date is February 20 and the father's birth date is May 1, the mother's insurance is the primary insurance and the father's insurance is the secondary insurance.

Billing for HMO Health Plans

Health insurance ID cards for members of health maintenance organizations (HMOs) show two names: the name of a sponsoring health insurance company, and a separate name for the HMO health insurance plan (Figure 15-4). This can make it confusing for a medical assistant to identify where the claim should be submitted. The first step is to call the HMO plan and ask where the medical claim should be sent. Some HMOs require that insurance claims for medical office procedures be sent to the address for the HMO insurance plan, whereas claims for hospital procedures are sent to the sponsoring health insurance. Because medical billing policies and procedures change with every HMO plan, it is wise to keep this process up-to-date in the office billing manual.

Assignment of Benefits

In the health insurance contract between the third-party payer and the patient, the patient receives the benefit when a claim is submitted. For the medical practice to receive the benefit reimbursement directly from the insurance company, the patient must sign an *assignment of benefits* (Figure 15-5). The assignment of benefits transfers the patient's legal right to collect benefits for medical expenses to the provider of those services, authorizing the payment to be sent directly to the provider. In other words, the assignment of benefits authorizes the provider to not only submit the insurance claim on behalf of the patient, but also to be reimbursed directly by the third-party payer. When the patient has signed the assignment of benefits, the medical assistant completes Blocks 12 and 13 on the CMS-1500 with the statement "Signature on File" and the claim filing date.

Blocks 12 and 13

Block 12 requires the signature of the *patient* or an authorized person, and Block 13 requires the signature of the *insured* or an authorized person. In Block 12, the signature authorizes the release of any medical or other information necessary to process or adjudicate the claim. In block 13, the signature affirms that the insured has a signature on file authorizing payment of medical benefits directly to the provider (whose name appears in Block 31). The phrase "Signature on File" may be entered in these fields.

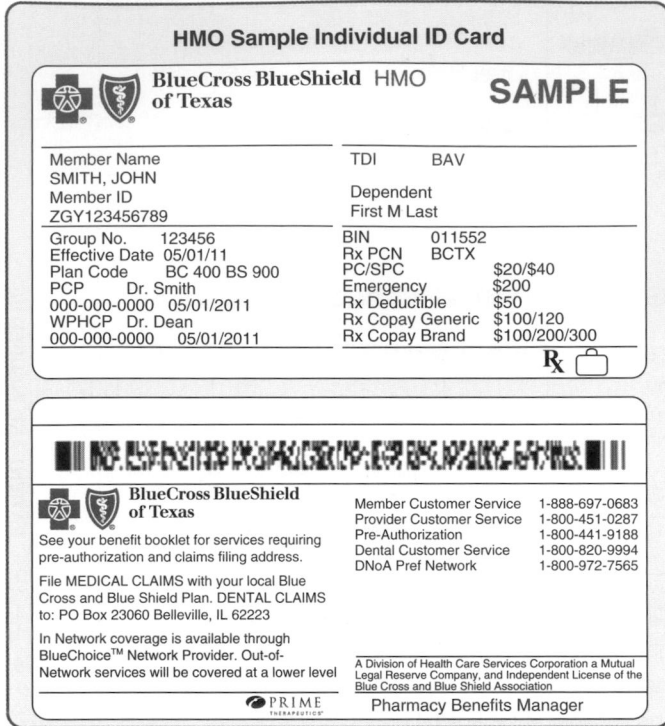

HMO Sample Individual ID Card

BlueCross BlueShield HMO of Texas   **SAMPLE**

Member Name SMITH, JOHN Member ID ZGY123456789	TDI BAV Dependent First M Last

Group No.   123456
Effective Date 05/01/11
Plan Code   BC 400 BS 900
PCP   Dr. Smith
000-000-0000   05/01/2011
WPHCP   Dr. Dean
000-000-0000   05/01/2011

BIN   011552
Rx PCN   BCTX
PC/SPC $20/$40
Emergency $200
Rx Deductible $50
Rx Copay Generic $100/120
Rx Copay Brand $100/200/300

℞

BlueCross BlueShield of Texas

See your benefit booklet for services requiring pre-authorization and claims filing address.

File MEDICAL CLAIMS with your local Blue Cross and Blue Shield Plan. DENTAL CLAIMS to: PO Box 23060 Belleville, IL 62223

In Network coverage is available through BlueChoice™ Network Provider. Out-of-Network services will be covered at a lower level

Member Customer Service   1-888-697-0683
Provider Customer Service   1-800-451-0287
Pre-Authorization   1-800-441-9188
Dental Customer Service   1-800-820-9994
DNoA Pref Network   1-800-972-7565

A Division of Health Care Services Corporation a Mutual Legal Reserve Company, and Independent License of the Blue Cross and Blue Shield Association

PRIME THERAPEUTICS®

Pharmacy Benefits Manager

FIGURE 15-4 *Patient HMO Health Insurance ID Card.* (From Fordney MT: *Insurance handbook for the medical office*, ed 14, St Louis, 2017, Saunders.)

Section 3a: Physician or Supplier Information—Blocks 14 to 23 (Figure 15-6)

Block 14

Date of Current Illness, Injury, or Pregnancy (LMP). Block 14 requires the date of the current illness, injury, or pregnancy. The date should be the date on which the current illness or condition began; the date an injury occurred; or, in the case of pregnancy, the date of the last menstrual period (LMP).

Block 15

Other Date. If the patient had the same or a similar illness or condition before the current one, enter the date of onset of the earlier condition.

Block 16

Dates Patient Unable to Work in Current Occupation. These dates are used to help determine an employee's long- or short-term disability payments.

Block 17 and 17b

Name of Referring Provider or Other Source. If the patient was referred by another provider, that provider's name goes in Block 17 and his or her **National Provider Identification (NPI)** number is entered in Block 17b.

National Provider Identification

Most government-sponsored insurance claims require that the National Provider Identifiers (NPIs) for the referring and rendering providers be printed in Blocks 17b and 24J, respectively. Every healthcare entity is required to have an NPI. The NPI is an identifier assigned by the Centers for Medicare and

Medicaid Services (CMS) that classifies the healthcare provider by license and medical specialties. The Administrative Simplification provisions of the Health Insurance Portability and Accountability Act of 1996 (HIPAA) mandated the adoption of standard unique identifiers for healthcare providers and health plans. The purpose of these provisions is to improve the efficiency and effectiveness of the electronic transmission of health information.

Some privately sponsored insurance companies may require claims to be submitted with the NPI. However, each privately sponsored insurance plan in each state has its own policies and procedures, so medical assistants will find that some third-party payers require NPIs, whereas others do not.

Block 18

Hospitalization Dates Related to Current Services. Block 18 is not used for claims from an ambulatory care practice.

Block 19

Additional Claim Information (Designated by NUCC). Some insurance plans ask for specific identifiers in Block 19. The medical assistant should check the instructions from the applicable third-party payer.

Block 20

Outside Lab?/$Charges. Applies to diagnostic laboratory services provided by an independent or a separate provider (who is listed in Block 32). Put an X in the YES box to indicate that the diagnostic test was performed by an entity other than the provider billing for the service (i.e., the provider listed in Block 33), and that the provider in Block 33 paid the laboratory directly. Include the amount the provider was charged by the diagnostic laboratory.

Block 21

Diagnosis or Nature of Illness or Injury. The ICD-10-CM diagnosis code or codes are entered. Enter one code for each of the 12 fields; the primary diagnosis should be recorded in the first field.

Block 22

Resubmission Code/Optional Reference Number. Both the resubmission code and the original reference number assigned by the insurance payer must be entered in this block.

Block 23

Prior Authorization Number. The preauthorization number obtained from the insurance company is entered.

Section 3b: Physician or Supplier Information—Blocks 24 to 33 (Figure 15-7)

Procedure codes, such as the Current Procedural Terminology (CPT) codes and/or the Healthcare Common Procedure Coding System (HCPCS) codes, are listed in Block 24. Each procedure code is considered a line item; the line numbers are found to the left of Block 24. The insurance claim form is read horizontally; therefore, all data in one line belongs to the coordinated CPT/HCPCS code. For claims that require more than six line items, a second CMS-1500 should be generated. Check with the insurance company to confirm how to indicate that the claim has multiple pages; some insurance

Assignment of Benefits

IMPORTANT: Please Fill-Out This Form Completely and Legibly (Do not leave anything blank)

Patient Name: _Rose Dawson_ DOB _02/17/XX_

Insurance Policy # _123-45-6789A_ Group # _____

Insured Name (if other than patient): _____ Insured DOB _____

Insured's Social Security# _123-45-6789_ Insured's Employer _None_

Your relationship to the Insured: (Self) Parent Spouse Other: _____

I hereby instruct and direct my health insurance policy to pay by check made out and mailed to:

Feel Better Family Practice, 101 Jack Place, New York, NY 10001

If my current health insurance policy prohibits direct payment to the clinic, please sign over the insurance check directly to the Feel Better Family Practice or Robert Wilson, MD and **mail it to the above address** as payment toward the total charges for the professional services rendered.
   This is a direct Assignment of my rights and benefits under this insurance policy.

(Check each box and sign at the bottom)
- ☑ A copy of this Assignment that has been signed shall be considered as effective and valid as the original.
- ☑ I authorize the release of any health information related to the claim for my insurance company, payment adjuster, or attorney involved for the purpose of processing claims and reimbursements for services rendered.
- ☑ I authorize the use of my signature on all insurance submissions.
- ☑ I understand that I am financially responsible for all charges whether or not paid by insurance.

Dated this _15_ day of _December_, 20_XX_.

Rose Dawson
Signature of Insured   Witness

_____
Signature of Patient, If other than Policyholder

FIGURE 15-5 Completed Assignment of Benefits form.

14. DATE OF CURRENT ILLNESS, INJURY, or PREGNANCY(LMP) MM DD YY QUAL.	15. OTHER DATE QUAL. MM DD YY	16. DATES PATIENT UNABLE TO WORK IN CURRENT OCCUPATION MM DD YY MM DD YY FROM TO
17. NAME OF REFERRING PROVIDER OR OTHER SOURCE	1/a. 17b. NPI	18. HOSPITALIZATION DATES RELATED TO CURRENT SERVICES MM DD YY MM DD YY FROM TO
19. ADDITIONAL CLAIM INFORMATION (Designated by NUCC)		20. OUTSIDE LAB? $ CHARGES ☐ YES ☐ NO
21. DIAGNOSIS OR NATURE OF ILLNESS OR INJURY Relate A-L to service line below (24E) ICD Ind. A. |____ B. |____ C. |____ D. |____ E. |____ F. |____ G. |____ H. |____ I. |____ J. |____ K. |____ L. |____		22. RESUBMISSION CODE ORIGINAL REF. NO. 23. PRIOR AUTHORIZATION NUMBER

FIGURE 15-6 Section 3a: Physician or Supplier Information (Blocks 14 to 23).

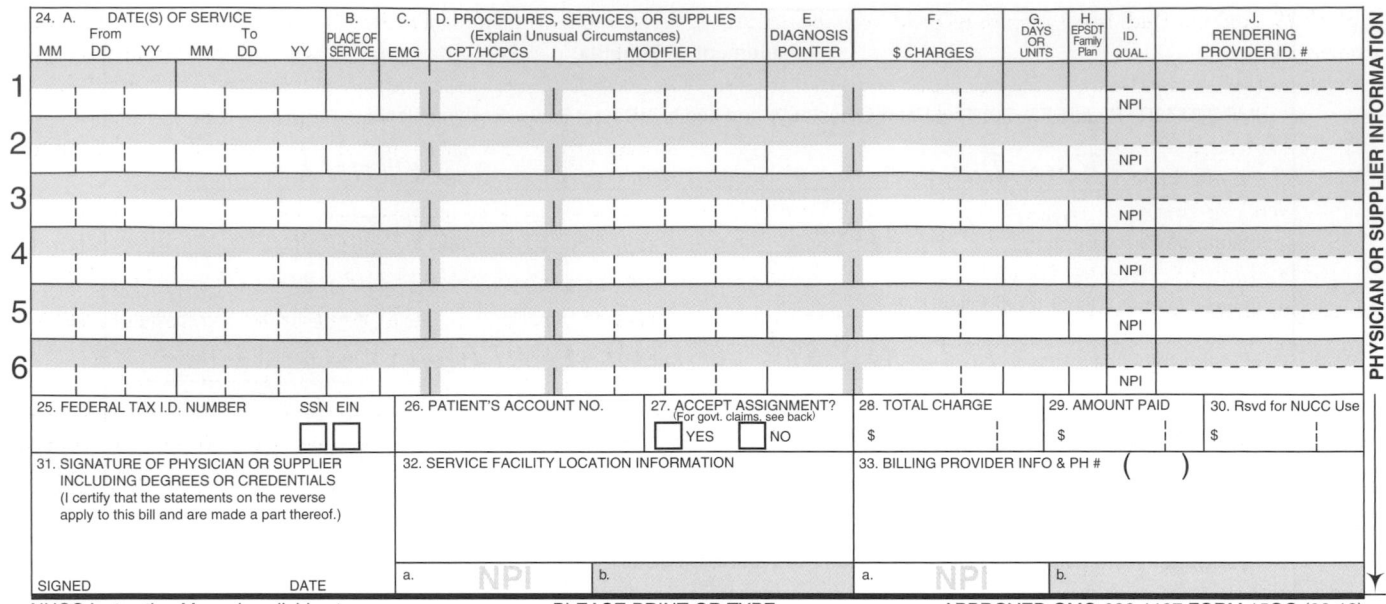

FIGURE 15-7 Section 3: Physician or Supplier Information (Blocks 24 to 33).

companies require the statement "Continued" or "Page 1 of 2" in Box 28, Total Charges.

Block 24

Procedures and Charges. Look at Block 24, line 1, in Figure 15-7. Note that the date of service (Block 24A) is the same for both From and To. This indicates that the patient was discharged after the procedure, so there was no inpatient stay. If the patient had had a hospital stay, the dates would be different.

The place of service (POS) code is entered in Block 24B. For services provided in an ambulatory care setting, the POS code is 24. As shown in Table 15-2, this two-digit code indicates that the procedure took place in an Ambulatory surgical center.

If Block 24C (EMG [emergency]) does not contain a Y, the procedure most likely was scheduled.

Block 24D (CPT/HCPCS and Modifier) provides room for a single five-digit code and up to four separate two-digit modifiers. Turning again to Figure 15-7, note that the CPT code is 19100. According to the CPT code set, the description for code 19100 is "biopsy of breast; percutaneous, needle core, not using imaging guidance." Modifier -50 indicates a bilateral procedure, so we can assume that both breasts were biopsied. The medical assistant should always check with the insurance company to determine whether the plan's medical billing policies and procedures require additional modifiers. No space is provided for a written description of the code; only the code is required. As Block 24D indicates, any unusual circumstances that affected the ability to choose an accurate CPT or HCPCS code should be explained beyond the CMS-1500.

The diagnosis pointer (Block 24E) indicates which diagnosis is used for each line item. Figure 15-7 shows only one diagnosis (N63 Unspecified lump in breast), so the diagnosis pointer is A. If more than one diagnosis is required, the pointer block separates the numbers with a comma.

In Block 24F ($ Charges), the dollar amount of the provider's fee for the service is entered. This fee is calculated in the office based on

work, expertise, and time. If a series of services was performed on any one line, multiply the number of days or units (Block 24G) by the charge for one procedure or service and enter the total amount for all days or units. This field is most commonly used for multiple visits, units of supplies, or anesthesia units.

Block 24H (EPSDT/Family Plan) identifies specific services covered under state health insurance plans. Refer to the appropriate insurance payer's guidelines (typically Medicaid or the Medicaid intermediary) for instructions on completing this block. Leave this block blank for Medicare; TRICARE and CHAMPVA (military insurance plans); group health plans; Federal Employees Compensation Act (FECA)/Black Lung; and most other types of insurance. (EPSDT stands for Early and Periodic Screening, Diagnosis, and Treatment, the child health program under Medicaid).

In Block 24I (Rendering Provider ID Qualifier) and Block 24J (Rendering Provider ID Number), enter the NPI of the provider who rendered the service, as identification.

Block 25 to 33

Facility Information. The Federal Tax ID Number (Block 25) of the provider filing the claim can be listed as a Social Security number (SSN) or an Employer Identification Number (EIN); mark the appropriate box with an **X**.

In Block 26 (Patient's Account No.), enter the account number or medical record number assigned to the patient by the provider of the service.

In Block 27 (Accept Assignment?), put an **X** in the YES box if the provider will accept assignment; this means that he or she is a **participating provider** and agrees to abide by the terms of the agreement with the insurance company to accept what the plan pays on the contracted fee schedule.

Block 28 (Total Charge) shows the amount billed on the claim form for all services rendered. To arrive at this amount, add up the charges reported in Block 24F for all the lines of service on the claim form.

Block 29 (Amount Paid) is the amount received from the patient or other payers.

Block 30 (Reserved for NUCC Use). Some secondary insurance claims use this box for the claim amount due after the primary insurance has paid.

Block 31 (Signature of Physician or Supplier) is the provider's signature, verifying that he or she provided the services listed, and they have been checked for accuracy.

In Block 32 (Service Facility Location Information), enter the name, address, city, state, and ZIP code for the site where the services listed in the claim were rendered. Enter the facility's NPI in Block 32a.

In Block 33 (Billing Provider Info & PH #), enter the address and phone number of the provider asking to be paid on this claim. In Block 33a, enter the same NPI number listed in Block 24J.

Procedure 15-3 shows how to complete a health insurance claim form using the information from an insurance card and an encounter form.

CRITICAL THINKING APPLICATION **15-3**

Ann is reviewing an encounter form that has one CPT code and two HCPCS codes with one diagnosis code for the same office visit. How many lines in Box 24 of the CMS-1500 will she need to use? Will all three CPT/HCPCS codes point to the same diagnosis? Why or why not?

TABLE 15-1 Information Required for Completion of the CMS-1500 Health Insurance Claim Form

BLOCK	INFORMATION NEEDED	BLOCK	INFORMATION NEEDED
	Completed patient registration/intake form	10a-c	If patient's condition or illness is related to employment, auto accident, or some other type of accident, make sure information is obtained as outlined in Block 1
	Photocopy of insurance card or cards (front and back)		
	Encounter form	10d	Claim codes as designated by NUCC
	Preauthorization or precertification number (when applicable)	11	Insured's policy, group, or FECA number (primary insurance)
SECTION 1: CARRIER		11a	Primary insured's date of birth and gender
1	Type of insurance	11b	Other claim ID designated by NUCC
SECTION 2: PATIENT AND INSURED INFORMATION		11c	Primary insured's insurance plan or program name
1a	Insured's identification (ID) number (primary insurance)	11d	Determine whether the patient also is covered by a secondary health insurance plan
2	Patient's full name	12	Confirm that the patient's release of information form has been signed dated and is in the patient's record
3	Patient's date of birth and gender		
4	Insured's name (primary insurance)	13	Confirm that the insured's authorization of benefits form has been signed dated and is in the patient's record
5	Patient's address and telephone number • Permanent address (including apartment number if appropriate) • City, state, ZIP code • Telephone number	**SECTION 3: PHYSICIAN OR SUPPLIER INFORMATION**	
		14	Date current illness, injury, or pregnancy began
6	Patient's relationship to insured	15	Determine whether patient has had the same or similar symptoms
7	Insured's address and telephone number • Permanent address (including apartment number if appropriate) • City, state, ZIP code • Telephone number	16	From-To dates if patient was unable to work at current occupation
		17	Name of ordering or referring provider
		17a	Not required
		17b	Ordering or referring provider's NPI
9	Other insured's name (secondary insurance)*	18	From-To dates if patient encounter included an inpatient hospital stay
9a	Policy or group number (secondary insurance)*		
9b	Secondary insured's date of birth and gender*	19	Determine whether insurance carrier in carrier block and Block 1 requires any information to be entered in this field
9c	Secondary insured's employer or school name*		
9d	Secondary insured's insurance plan or program name*	20	Determine whether an outside laboratory was used; if so, enter charges billed to provider for outside lab services

Continued

TABLE 15-1 Information Required for Completion of the CMS-1500 Health Insurance Claim Form—*continued*

BLOCK	INFORMATION NEEDED	BLOCK	INFORMATION NEEDED
21	ICD-10-CM code or codes for patient's condition, illness, or injury (maximum of four per claim)	24I	Qualifier ID code (if no NPI available)
22	Is Medicaid claim being resubmitted? If yes, provide reference number from original Medicaid claim submitted	24J	Rendering (treating) provider's NPI—unshaded field PIN (if no NPI is available)—shaded field
		25	Rendering provider's federal tax ID number (EIN or SSN)
23	If prior authorization and/or referral is required, provide authorization (approval) number from insurance payer (preauthorization or precertification number)	26	Patient's account number with rendering provider
		27	Determine whether contract or agreement between provider and insurance carrier allows provider to accept assignment
24A	From-To dates of service for current encounter	28	Total charges from Block 24F, lines 1-6
24B	Place of service (POS) code	29	Amount paid by patient, insured, or other insurance
24C	If an emergency, put a Y in this box	30	Balance due (if any amount paid is shown in Block 29)
24D	CPT and/or HCPCS code CPT and/or HCPCS modifier(s) (maximum of four per charge line)	31	Signature of provider performing service or procedure
		32	Address of facility where services were rendered
24E	Block 21 field or reference number (1, 2, 3 and/or 4)	32a	NPI number of service facility listed in Block 32
24F	Total charge for CPT- or HCPCS-coded services listed in Block 24D • If more than 1 day or unit is indicated in Block 24G, multiply the charge for the service(s) coded in Block 24D by the number of days/units in Block 24G; enter the result in Block 24F	32b	Qualifier ID number and PIN of facility listed in Block 32 (if no NPI available)
		33	Name, address, and phone number of performing (rendering) provider
		33a	NPI of provider listed in Block 33
24G	Total number of days or units	33b	Qualifier ID number and PIN of provider listed in Block 33 (if no NPI available)
24H	EPSDT or Family Plan code (Medicaid or AFDC)		

*Only required if a secondary insurance exists and is to be submitted to the insurance carrier.
AFDC, Aid to Families with Dependent Children; *CPT,* Current Procedural Terminology coding system; *EIN,* Employer Identification Number; *EPSDT,* Early and Periodic Screening, Diagnosis, and Treatment; *FECA,* Federal Employees Compensation Act; *HCPCS,* Health Care Common Procedural Coding System coding method ; *ICD-10-CM,* International Classification of Diseases, Tenth Revision, Clinical Modification coding method; *NPI,* National Provider Identifier; *PIN,* personal identification number; *POS,* place of service.

TABLE 15-2 Place of Service Codes

CODE	DESCRIPTION	CODE	DESCRIPTION
11	Doctor's office	33	Custodial care facility (domiciliary or rest home services)
12	Patient's home	34	Hospice (domiciliary or rest home services)
21	Inpatient hospital	35	Adult living care facilities (residential care facility)
22	Outpatient hospital	41	Ambulance—land
23	Emergency department—hospital	42	Ambulance—air or water
24	Ambulatory surgical center	50	Federally qualified health center
25	Birthing center	51	Inpatient psychiatry facility
26	Military treatment facility/uniformed service treatment facility	52	Psychiatric facility—partial hospitalization
31	Skilled nursing facility (swing bed visits)	53	Community mental health care (outpatient, 24-hour/day services, admission screening, consultation, and educational services)
32	Nursing facility (intermediate/long-term care facilities)		

TABLE 15-2   Place of Service Codes—*continued*

CODE	DESCRIPTION	CODE	DESCRIPTION
54	Intermediate care facility/mentally retarded	65	End-stage renal disease treatment facility
55	Residential substance abuse treatment facility	71	State or local public health clinic
56	Psychiatric residential treatment center	72	Rural health clinic
60	Mass immunization center	81	Independent laboratory
61	Comprehensive inpatient rehabilitation facility	99	Other unlisted facility
62	Comprehensive outpatient rehabilitation facility		

PROCEDURE 15-3   Complete an Insurance Claim Form

Goal: *To accurately complete a CMS-1500 Health Insurance Claim Form (see Figure 15-8).*

EQUIPMENT and SUPPLIES

- Patient's health record
- Copy of patient's insurance ID card or cards
- Patient registration/intake form
- Encounter form
- Insurance claims processing guidelines
- Blank CMS-1500 Health Insurance Claim Form

PROCEDURAL STEPS

Background: Almost all medical billing is done electronically through a practice management billing software. The paper CMS-1500 Health Insurance Claim Form is provided only to help students practice and develop their medical billing skills.

Complete each block (as appropriate) of the CMS-1500 (see Table 15-2 for block descriptions).

1. Gather the documents required to complete the claim form.
2. Complete the claim form using a pen. Use capital letters. Do not use punctuation (commas or dollar signs) unless indicated in the insurance manual or guidelines. Use a hyphen to hyphenate last names.
3. Using the patient's health insurance ID card, determine the type of insurance, and the insurance ID number. Enter this information into block 1 and 1a.
   PURPOSE: After selecting the appropriate type of health insurance, the medical assistant can refer to the claims processing guidelines for that plan.
4. Using the ID card, the encounter form, and the registration/intake form, determine the patient's information and insured individual's information. Accurately complete blocks 2, 3, 5, 6, 9, and 10 a-c by entering in the patient's information. Complete 4, 7, and 11, a-d with the insured's information.
   PURPOSE: By distinguishing between the patient and the insured, the medical biller can determine whether the insurer requires additional information for submission of an accurate claim.
5. Complete blocks 12 and 13, by entering "signature on file" and the date.

NOTE: The assignment of benefit form should have been signed by the patient and/or the insured at registration. Enter the dates in either the six (6)–digit format (MM/DD/YY) or the eight (8)–digit format (MM/DD/YYYY).
PURPOSE: To submit an insurance claim, the medical practice must be authorized to release the service information on behalf of the patient or the insured.

6. Accurately enter the physician or supplier information by completing blocks 14-23. Use the eight (8)–digit format (MM/DD/YYYY) when needed.
7. Using the encounter form, complete blocks 24 and the appropriate blocks from 24A through 24H.
   NOTE:
   - Block 24A: Enter the dates of service, both From and To. For ambulatory services, enter the same date in the FROM and TO fields. Enter a date for each procedure, service, or supply in eight (8)–digit format (MM/DD/YYYY).
   - Block 24F: Enter the charge for the listed service or procedure. *Do not use commas when reporting dollar amounts.* The cents column is the small column to the right.
   - Block 24G: Enter the number of days or units. This block is usually used for multiple visits, units of supplies, anesthesia units or minutes, or oxygen volume. If only one service is performed, enter 1.
8. Complete blocks 24I through 27 by entering information on the provider's or healthcare facility where the service was provided and the patient's account number. Check the correct box to indicate acceptance of assignment of benefits.
9. Complete blocks 28 – 29 by entering the total charges, total amount paid, and the total amount due. Complete blocks 31-33a by entering in the provider's and facility's information.
10. Review the claim for accuracy and completeness before submitting. Correct any errors or missing information.
    NOTE: Before sending the claim, make a copy of the form and file the copy in the patient's insurance claim file.
    PURPOSE: It is important to double-check the form for accuracy and missing required information.

ACCURATE CODING TO PREVENT FRAUD AND ABUSE

Accurate coding in any healthcare environment is essential to prevent fraud and abuse in reimbursement (Box 15-1). According to the Health Insurance Portability and Accountability Act (HIPAA):

> Fraud is defined as knowingly and willfully executing or attempting to execute a scheme to defraud any healthcare benefit program or to obtain by means of false or fraudulent pretenses, representations, or promises any of the money or property owned by any healthcare benefit program.

Abuse in medical billing can be likened to actions that are contrary to ethical standards in the medical office. Unlike fraud, abuse is an inadvertent action that directly or indirectly results in an overpayment to the healthcare provider. Abuse is similar to fraud, except that it is unclear if the unethical practice was committed deliberately. The term **intentional** is important when determining whether fraudulent medical billing practices were done with purpose or accident.

Violations of the laws governing reimbursement may result in nonpayment of claims, civil monetary penalties (CMPs), exclusion from the payer program, criminal and civil liability, and in extreme cases, jail time. These laws may be changed or updated, so the person who is responsible for coding must pay close attention to detail and act as a sort of "medical detective" to build a case against a provider or clinic. The ICD-10-CM manual is updated annually. The *Federal Register* announces most changes, and new coding manuals often have a few pages dedicated to the updates for that particular year. Accurate use of the ICD-10-CM manual is essential for correct translation of the diagnostic statements in the health record into alphanumeric codes.

UPCODING AND DOWNCODING

Because diagnostic coding is directly related to insurance reimbursements, providers may be inclined to code to a higher specificity level than the service provided actually involved. This practice is called **upcoding,** and when it is performed regularly, it is a type of fraud and abuse. An example of upcoding would be to include a diagnosis of hyperlipidemia for an otherwise healthy person to justify a higher evaluation and management (E/M) procedure code. The medical assistant should respectfully inform the provider that this is a fraudulent practice and that fines and other penalties can be associated with this course of action.

In **downcoding,** a lower specificity level, or more generalized code, is assigned. Downcoding can be done by a variety of different stakeholders, including the coder, the insurance company, and/or a coding auditor. A coder may downcode a diagnosis to a not otherwise specified (NOS) code to avoid taking the time to look up a more accurate code. An insurance carrier may downcode a diagnosis and/or a procedure code after reviewing requested medical documentation, thus lowering the amount reimbursed to the provider. A coding auditor may downcode diagnosis and/or procedure codes when auditing patients' health records. All downcoding results in lower reimbursements to the provider.

Box 15-1   Guidelines for Reviewing Claims before Submission

The following guidelines can help ensure that clean insurance claims are submitted.

- Proofread the form carefully for accuracy and completeness.
- Make certain any necessary attachments are included with the completed form.
- Follow office policies and guidelines for claim review and signatures.
- Forward the original claim to the proper insurance carrier either by mail or electronically.
- When creating a paper claim for a workers' compensation claim, scan a copy of the completed and signed claim form into the patient's health record.
- Make sure the patient's and/or insured's name, address, and ID, group, and/or policy number are identical to the information printed on the insurance card.
- Make sure the patient's birth date and gender are the same as in the medical record.
- Section 2, Patient and Insured Information **(Blocks 1-13)**: Complete these blocks accurately, according to the insurance carrier's guidelines.
  - **Block 11**: Enter the word NONE if Medicare is the primary payer.
  - **Block 12**: Make sure the patient has authorized the **release of information**, and that Block 12 has a handwritten signature, the words "Signature on File," or the acronym SOF.

- **Blocks 17** and **17b**: If applicable, enter the referring, provider's name and National Provider Identifier (NPI) number.
- **Block 27** (Accept Assignment?): Put an X in the YES box if the provider is a participating provider (PAR) or has an agreement with the insurance carrier or payer to accept assignment.
- Make sure the diagnosis is not missing or incomplete.
- Check that the diagnosis has been coded accurately, according to the ICD-10-CM coding manual, and corresponds to the treatment.
- **Blocks 14–24J** (required fields for diagnosis and procedure): Make sure these blocks are completed accurately, according to the guidelines of the third-party payer or insurance company.
- List the fees for each charge individually; or, if more than 1 day or unit is entered in **Block 24G**, they must be computed correctly
- **Block 25**: Double-check the provider's federal Social Security number (SSN) or Employer Identification Number (EIN) to ensure accuracy.
- **Block 31**: Check for the provider's signature, which must be on the form.
- **Block 24J** and **Blocks 33a, 33b**: Make sure the provider's NPI, corresponding to the insurance carrier being billed, has been entered in Block 24J and again in Block 33a. When applicable, enter the provider's personal identification number (PIN) in Block 33b, with the qualifying number, when applicable.

PREVENTING REJECTION OF A CLAIM

It is important for the medical assistant to understand and comply with the specific guidelines for completing a CMS-1500 established by each third-party payer and insurance company; this prevents delays in reimbursement and denial of payment. The guidelines for Medicare, Medicaid, TRICARE, and workers' compensation can be found online at the websites for these healthcare insurers. Most practice management billing systems have built-in "claim scrubbers" (i.e., software that automatically corrects some common billing errors), which help in the process. If claims are sent electronically through a clearinghouse, claims auditing is done before the clearinghouse transmits the claim to the third-party payer. Claims without significant errors of any type are called *clean claims*. Claims with incorrect, missing, or insufficient data are called *dirty claims*.

Communicating with Providers About Third-Party Requirements

It can be challenging for a provider to keep up with the annual changes set forth by Medicare, private health insurance companies, and the ICD-10-CM updates. This is why healthcare practitioners do well to trust their medical office staff to keep well informed on the various changes in the health insurance industry.

Some providers may be so focused on patient care that they feel uncomfortable with change. This may be the case with the encounter form/superbill used in patient care. A provider may feel comfortable using the same form, but over time, some codes may have changed or become obsolete, or new medical services offered may not be listed on the form.

A medical coder should tactfully discuss with the provider the benefits of using an updated encounter form. If the provider is still reluctant to change the form, even though it is outdated, the medical coder may suggest that the form will not be changed, just the codes on it. Adjust the encounter form to include an open text box for the provider to add medical procedures that he performs occasionally.

When communicating with the provider about coding issues, you must always show a respectful attitude, even though you may be the expert on coding and medical billing. The many changes occurring in medical coding and billing can be overwhelming and confusing for some providers; the approach of coding professionals should be to guide them patiently through these changes.

CHECKING THE STATUS OF A CLAIM

The medical biller should keep track of every submitted claim to ensure timely reimbursement. Clearinghouses send a confirmation report right after submission of a claim. The medical biller should always reconcile the claims submitted through the medical billing software with the claims listed on the confirmation report. Medical assistants should maintain this practice to ensure that every claim is submitted correctly.

The claim submission confirmation report also indicates claims that were rejected because they were incomplete. These claims should be corrected and resubmitted electronically immediately. Often these claims are rejected for typographical errors, so the medical biller should compare the patient's account in the practice management software to the information on the patient's registration/intake form, to ensure accuracy.

It takes 10 to 14 business days for insurance companies to process insurance claims electronically, but allow up to 30 days. If no further response is received from the insurance company about the claim after a month, the medical biller can visit the company's provider Web portal or call the provider services number on the back of the patient's health insurance ID card to check the status of a claim. To confirm claim status, you must provide the insured subscriber's member number and birth date; the patient's name and birth date; and the date of service. The state insurance commission has standards that third-party payers must abide by, including claim processing times and payment guidelines. Medical assistants should keep the commission's contact information in the office medical billing manual as a reference in case a claim should be reported.

EXPLANATION OF BENEFITS

An **Explanation of Benefits (EOB)** is sent by the insurance company to the provider who submitted the insurance claim, which accompanies a check or a document indicating that funds were electronically transferred. Medicare sends a remittance advice (RA) with confirmation of electronic funds transfer; although it has a different name, the document is the same as the EOB. The medical practice cannot deposit the check and disregard the EOB, which provides detailed accounting for the submitted insurance claim. The EOB breaks down each line item charge from Block 24 on the CMS-1500 into the charged amount, the amount allowable, and the paid amount as shown in Figure 15-8.

Reading the Explanation of Benefits

The EOB contains essential information about the submitted health insurance claim. To apply payments to a patient's account properly, it is vital that the medical assistant understand all the elements of an EOB. Figure 15-8 shows a completed CMS-1500. When interpreting the EOB, review the following steps.

1. Verify that the EOB applies to the correct patient by comparing the account number and date of service on the EOB with the submitted CMS-1500.

HEALTH INSURANCE CLAIM FORM

APPROVED BY NATIONAL UNIFORM CLAIM COMMITTEE (NUCC) 02/12

| | PICA | | | | | | | | PICA | |

1. MEDICARE	MEDICAID	TRICARE	CHAMPVA	GROUP HEALTH PLAN	FECA BLK LUNG	OTHER	1a. INSURED'S I.D. NUMBER (For Program in Item 1)
✓ (Medicare#)	(Medicaid#)	(ID#/DoD#)	(Member ID#)	(ID#)	(ID#)	(ID#)	123-45-6789A

2. PATIENT'S NAME (Last Name, First Name, Middle Initial)	3. PATIENT'S BIRTH DATE / SEX	4. INSURED'S NAME (Last Name, First Name, Middle Initial)
ROSE DAWSON	MM 02 DD 17 YY XX M ☐ F ✓	ROSE DAWSON

5. PATIENT'S ADDRESS (No., Street)	6. PATIENT RELATIONSHIP TO INSURED	7. INSURED'S ADDRESS (No., Street)
123 TITANIC PLACE	Self ✓ Spouse ☐ Child ☐ Other ☐	123 TITANIC PLACE

CITY	STATE	8. RESERVED FOR NUCC USE	CITY	STATE
NEW YORK	NY		NEW YORK	NY

ZIP CODE	TELEPHONE (Include Area Code)		ZIP CODE	TELEPHONE (Include Area Code)
10001	( )		10001	( )

9. OTHER INSURED'S NAME (Last Name, First Name, Middle Initial)	10. IS PATIENT'S CONDITION RELATED TO:	11. INSURED'S POLICY GROUP OR FECA NUMBER
ROSE DAWSON		123-45-6789A

a. OTHER INSURED'S POLICY OR GROUP NUMBER	a. EMPLOYMENT? (Current or Previous)	a. INSURED'S DATE OF BIRTH / SEX
123-45-6789	☐ YES ✓ NO	MM 02 DD 17 YY XX M ☐ F ✓

b. RESERVED FOR NUCC USE	b. AUTO ACCIDENT? PLACE (State)	b. OTHER CLAIM ID (Designated by NUCC)
	☐ YES ✓ NO	

c. RESERVED FOR NUCC USE	c. OTHER ACCIDENT?	c. INSURANCE PLAN NAME OR PROGRAM NAME
	☐ YES ✓ NO	MEDICARE

d. INSURANCE PLAN NAME OR PROGRAM NAME	10d. CLAIM CODES (Designated by NUCC)	d. IS THERE ANOTHER HEALTH BENEFIT PLAN?
AARP SECONDARY POLICY		✓ YES ☐ NO *If yes*, complete items 9, 9a, and 9d.

READ BACK OF FORM BEFORE COMPLETING & SIGNING THIS FORM.

12. PATIENT'S OR AUTHORIZED PERSON'S SIGNATURE I authorize the release of any medical or other information necessary to process this claim. I also request payment of government benefits either to myself or to the party who accepts assignment below.

SIGNED SIGNATURE ON FILE   DATE 01/14/20XX

13. INSURED'S OR AUTHORIZED PERSON'S SIGNATURE I authorize payment of medical benefits to the undersigned physician or supplier for services described below.

SIGNED SIGNATURE ON FILE

14. DATE OF CURRENT ILLNESS, INJURY, or PREGNANCY (LMP) MM DD YY QUAL.	15. OTHER DATE QUAL. MM DD YY	16. DATES PATIENT UNABLE TO WORK IN CURRENT OCCUPATION FROM MM DD YY TO MM DD YY

17. NAME OF REFERRING PROVIDER OR OTHER SOURCE	17a.	18. HOSPITALIZATION DATES RELATED TO CURRENT SERVICES
ROBERT WILSON, MD	17b. NPI 11122233344	FROM MM DD YY TO MM DD YY

19. ADDITIONAL CLAIM INFORMATION (Designated by NUCC)	20. OUTSIDE LAB? $ CHARGES
	☐ YES ☐ NO

21. DIAGNOSIS OR NATURE OF ILLNESS OR INJURY Relate A-L to service line below (24E) ICD Ind.	22. RESUBMISSION CODE ORIGINAL REF. NO.
A. E11.22 B. C. D.	
E. F. G. H.	23. PRIOR AUTHORIZATION NUMBER
I. J. K.	

24. A. DATE(S) OF SERVICE		B. PLACE OF SERVICE	C. EMG	D. PROCEDURES, SERVICES, OR SUPPLIES (Explain Unusual Circumstances) CPT/HCPCS MODIFIER	E. DIAGNOSIS POINTER	F. $ CHARGES	G. DAYS OR UNITS	H. EPSDT Family Plan	I. ID. QUAL.	J. RENDERING PROVIDER ID. #
From MM DD YY	To MM DD YY									
1 01 14 XX	01 14 XX	11		99213	1	$125 00	1		NPI	11122233344
2									NPI	
3									NPI	
4									NPI	
5									NPI	
6									NPI	

25. FEDERAL TAX I.D. NUMBER SSN EIN	26. PATIENT'S ACCOUNT NO.	27. ACCEPT ASSIGNMENT? (For govt. claims, see back)	28. TOTAL CHARGE	29. AMOUNT PAID	30. Rsvd for NUCC Use
098-76-5432 ☐ ✓	RW125638	✓ YES ☐ NO	$ 125 00	$ 0	

31. SIGNATURE OF PHYSICIAN OR SUPPLIER INCLUDING DEGREES OR CREDENTIALS (I certify that the statements on the reverse apply to this bill and are made a part thereof.) *Robert Wilson, MD* 01/14/XX SIGNED DATE	32. SERVICE FACILITY LOCATION INFORMATION Feel Better Family Practice 101 Jack Place New York, NY, 10001 (212) 555-1212	33. BILLING PROVIDER INFO & PH # ( ) Robert Wilson, MD 101 Jack Place New York, NY, 10001 (212) 555-1212
	a. 22233344455 b.	a. 11122233344 b.

NUCC Instruction Manual available at: www.nucc.org   **PLEASE PRINT OR TYPE**   APPROVED OMB-0938-1197 FORM 1500 (02-12)

FIGURE 15-8 Completed CMS-1500 Health Insurance Claim Form.

CARRIER · *PATIENT AND INSURED INFORMATION* · *PHYSICIAN OR SUPPLIER INFORMATION*

2. Confirm that the EOB shows the same figures as the submitted CMS-1500 for the amount charged per line (Block 24F) and the number of lines (Block 24J); in other words, the line items and charges should match. Sometimes the EOB summarizes the entire claim in one charged amount. In this case, confirm that the total charged is the same as in Block 28.

3. Post the payment and adjusted amount per line item. In the practice management billing software, these are posted on the same line. The patient's responsibility, as determined by the primary insurance EOB, is calculated using the following equation:

Charged amount − Payment amount − Adjusted amount
= Patient's responsibility

4. Once the patient's responsibility has been determined, check the patient's health record to see whether a secondary insurance is listed. If one is, submit a health insurance claim with the balance due determined by the primary insurance EOB. If no secondary insurance is listed, the patient is billed for the balance due.

5. Review the **remarks codes** on the EOB for any additional messages or information about the claim. The remarks codes area is where the payer indicates the conditions under which the claim was paid. For example, code 01 states that the claim amount allowed was established by the contract between the health insurance plan and the provider. Other remarks codes give the reasons a claim was denied or rejected. Some remarks codes indicate that the claim is pending, awaiting specific information.

6. All remarks codes on pending or denied claims should be followed up immediately upon receipt of the EOB, to prevent further delay in payment for other claims.

Rejected Claims

The EOB provides detailed information on rejected claims. Just as payments on the EOB, rejected claims are presented as line items, just as in Block 24 of the CMS-1500. All rejected claims have a code, with a legend toward the bottom the page. Some of the reasons claims are rejected are:

- The interval specified for filing the claim had expired (check the insurance plan's billing policies manual for details).
- Incorrect ICD-10-CM, CPT, and/or HCPCS codes or combinations of codes were entered.

- The insurer claims that the ICD-10-CM code and the CPT/HCPCS codes do not match; that is, the claim lacks **medical necessity**.
- More than one CPT/HCPCS code was filed on the same date of service, and they are mutually exclusive when billed together.
- The claim was submitted to the wrong insurance plan.

Rejected claims should be corrected and resubmitted for payment electronically unless otherwise specified. Use Block 22 on the CMS-1500 according to insurance plan billing guidelines to indicate a resubmitted claim. These claims should be resubmitted as soon as possible to prevent further delay in reimbursement.

DENIED CLAIMS

The two main reasons for denial of payment are technical errors and insurance policy coverage issues. Technical errors include incorrect, incomplete information, typographic and/or mathematical errors. Common reasons for denial include:

- The patient was not covered by the insurance plan on the date of service.
- A listed procedure was not an insurance benefit.
- Preauthorization for the service was not obtained.
- Medical necessity

Medical Necessity

To obtain the correct reimbursement for a provider, the medical biller must submit the correct codes. The diagnosis code is the reason the medical procedure rendered was necessary. For example, if a claim submitted to the insurance company indicated, through coding error, that a bunionectomy was performed for a tonsillitis diagnosis, the insurer will deny the claim based on medical necessity. Therefore, maintaining accurate health records and efficient claims processing are possible only if *each and every* procedure and service provided during an office visit or encounter is justified.

If an insurance claim is denied for medical necessity, and the medical assistant believes that a payment should be made, an appeal letter should be sent to the insurance plan (Procedure 15-4). The appeal letter should not only identify the denied claim, but also include a statement from the provider detailing the medical reasoning for performing the procedure. Additional medical reports (e.g., laboratory reports, operative reports, and history and physical examination findings [H&P]) should be sent if they support the provider's treatment decision.

PROCEDURE 15-4   Utilize Medical Necessity Guidelines: Respond to a "Medical Necessity Denied" Claim

Goal: *To resolve the insurance company's denial of medical necessity by completing an accurate claim.*

Scenario: *You are working at Walden-Martin Family Medical Clinic, 1234 Anystreet, Anytown, AL 12345 (phone: 123-123-1234).*

You receive a letter indicating that Medicare has denied the following claim for not being medically necessary:

Patient: Norma B. Washington   DOB: 08/07/1944   Policy/ID Number: 847744144A
Date of Service: 06/13/20XX   ICD: G43.101 (Migraine) CPT: J3420 (B-12 injection)
Provider: Julie Walden MD

PROCEDURE 15-4   —continued

You did some research and the information above was the only information sent to Medicare for that encounter. The following information was the correct information for the encounter:

Patient: Norma B. Washington   DOB: 08/01/1944   Date of Service: 06/15/20XX
ICD: G43.101 (Migraine)   CPT: J1885 (Toradol 15 mg—$15.50) and 90772 (Injection, Ther/
                                                          Proph/Diag—$25.00)
ICD: D51.0 (Vitamin B12 deficiency anemia)   CPT: J3420 (B-12 injection—$24.00) and 90772 (Injection, Ther/
                                                          Proph/Diag—$25.00)
To be billed to: Medicare, 1234 Insurance Road, Anytown, AL 12345-1234

EQUIPMENT and SUPPLIES

- Paper method: Patient's health record, copy of patient's insurance ID card or cards, patient registration/intake form, encounter form, blank CMS-1500 Health Insurance Claim Form, and a pen
- Electronic method: SimChart for the Medical Office
- Insurance denial letter or scenario (see above)

PROCEDURAL STEPS

1. Review the insurance denial letter (scenario) carefully. Compare the patient's information from the denial letter to the health record, claim, and encounter form. Look for errors in the patient's name and date of birth.
   PURPOSE: Errors in patient information can be a reason for denial.
2. Compare the insurance denial letter (scenario) to the health record, claim, and encounter form. Look for errors in the date of service, the diagnosis, and the procedure codes. The procedure must be medically necessary for the diagnosis indicated.
   PURPOSE: Errors related to the encounter must be matching for the claim to be accepted. The procedure codes must indicate an acceptable standard of treatment for the diagnosis listed. In some cases, the encounter form may contain a diagnosis that did not make it into the original claim form. Review the patient's health record to determine whether the procedure was medically necessary.
3. Complete a claim (either CMS-1500 or an electronic claim using SimChart) by entering in the information about the carrier, patient, and insured.
4. Enter the information regarding the physician, procedures, and diagnosis. Make sure to include all of the information from the encounter.
5. Proofread the claim form for accuracy before submitting the claim.

The Patient's Financial Responsibility

Most MCO health insurance contracts require patients to pay a **copayment,** which is collected at the time of service (Table 15-3). Copayments usually range from $10 to $75 for office visits; they vary, depending on whether the patient is seen by a PCP or a specialist, in urgent care, or in the emergency department. Office visits and prescription copayments do not count toward the yearly contracted deductible. The medical assistant must make sure that the proper copayments are received and credited to patients' accounts.

A **deductible** is an amount that the policyholder for the policy is contracted per year to pay toward his or her healthcare before the insurance company begins to reimburse the healthcare provider. The deductible amount is stated in the insurance contract between the patient and the health insurance company.

Coinsurance is a policy provision in which the policyholder and the insurance company share the cost of covered medical services in a specified ratio. For example, the plan may set an 80/20 ratio; this means that after the yearly deductible has been met, the insurance carrier pays 80% of the cost of services, and the insured pays 20%. The patient's deductible, or coinsurance financial responsibility, is documented on the EOB.

To help patients understand their health insurance benefits, the medical assistant must be confident in defining the terms copayment, coinsurance, and deductible, taking on the role of patient navigator.

The medical office can contact the insurance company on the patient's behalf to determine the amount of the deductible and/or coinsurance the patient has already paid in the calendar year. The process of precertification enables the healthcare provider to inform patients of how much the procedure will cost them.

TABLE 15-3   Comparing Patient Financial Responsibilities

PATIENT FINANCIAL RESPONSIBILITY	WHEN PATIENT PAYS	AMOUNT PATIENT PAYS
Copayment	At the time of medical service	Fixed amount, $10 to $75 per visit
Deductible	After the provider has been paid	Variable amount, up to 30%
Coinsurance	After the provider has been paid	Variable amount, up to 30%, but not to exceed deductible

Allowed Amount

For providers to become participating providers in an insurance network, they must agree to accept the insurance plan fee schedule as payment in full for services rendered. This means that all fees above the plan's allowed amount should be adjusted. The allowed amount may be all or part of a charge for a service or procedure. For example, a provider typically may charge $80 for a Level I office visit; however, the insurance plan's allowable amount may be only $60. If the provider is a participating provider, he or she is obligated to adjust the difference between these two amounts—$20. However, if the provider is not a participating provider, he or she can bill the patient for the $20 balance. Because contracts between third-party payers and providers vary greatly, it is important for the medical assistant to examine the EOB closely and to be knowledgeable about the contract provisions between the provider and all insurance carriers he or she uses to recognize the appropriate contracted amount.

CRITICAL THINKING APPLICATION   15-6

Ann is reviewing a Remittance Advice (RA) for a Medicare patient with no secondary insurance. The charge for the office visit was $100; the insurance company allowed 80%, of which the insurance company paid 50%. What did the insurance company reimburse and what is the patient's responsibility? What amount should be adjusted?

Calculating the Coinsurance and Deductible

Consider this example: Mrs. Anita Jones' health insurance plan has a $500 annual deductible, after which the insurance company pays 95% of all charges. Mrs. Jones, therefore, has a 5% coinsurance expense in addition to the deductible. She also has a $1,000 out-of-pocket expense maximum; this means that once Mrs. Jones has paid $1,000 total (which includes the deductible), the insurance company pays 100% of any balance remaining. Mrs. Jones has incurred a $10,000 charge for cardiac surgery performed by her provider. Now look at Figures 15-9 and 15-10.

- In Figure 15-9, Column A shows that Mrs. Jones' paid the $500 deductible, and 5% of $10,000 (i.e., an additional $500). The insurance company then paid the remaining balance of $9,000.
- In Figure 15-10, Column B shows that Mrs. Jones' cardiac surgery cost $20,000. Mrs. Jones' total out-of-pocket expense remains $1,000; therefore, in this case the insurance company is responsible for payment of the balance of $19,000. Because her maximum out-of-pocket expense, according to the plan, is $1,000, even though the charges were doubled, she still pays only the $1,000 total out-of-pocket expense.

	Column A	Column B
Total charge	$10,000	$20,000
Deductible (paid by Mrs. Jones)	(500)	(500)
5% (Mrs. Jones' portion)	(500)	(500)
Total amount paid by Mrs. Jones	$1000	$1000
Total amount paid by insurance	$9000	$19,000

FIGURE 15-9 Calculation of deductible and coinsurance.

Using the example in Figure 15-9, if the allowable amount for Mrs. Jones' $10,000 cardiac surgery is $8,500, the $1,500 difference between the provider's charge and the allowed amount (i.e. the additional $500 above Mrs. Jones's out-of-pocket expense) would be either written off or passed on to the patient as an out-of-pocket expense. In Column A, a line has been added to show the $8,500 allowable amount and that $1,500 has been billed to the patient. In Column B, the provider adjusts the charged amount above the contracted amount.

Discussing Patients' Financial Responsibility

Patients must understand that the guarantor is the person ultimately responsible for the entire bill. Remember, the insurance policy is a contract between the policyholder and an insurance plan. The provider is not a party to this contract.

Providers and their staff members, therefore, are not responsible for pursuing insurance payment for the patient's benefit. However, it is in the practice's best interest to actively assist patients if problems arise in securing payment. This is true for two reasons. First, the staff is almost always more knowledgeable than the patient about the health insurance business. Many patients do not even read their insurance policies and have no idea what is and is not covered. Some patients expect insurance to pay all costs simply because they are paying a premium. The medical assistant may need to educate these patients about their policies and offer advice on how patients can effectively work with their insurance company to get answers to questions and make sure they are receiving all the benefits to which they are entitled.

The second reason for helping patients understand their health insurance plan is that this helps ensure that the provider is compensated for his or her services. If the medical assistant acts as a patient navigator with the insurance company, his or her efforts usually result in regular reimbursements (Figure 15-11).

Medical assistants gain knowledge about the insurance industry when they actively assist patients with their concerns. The more experience a medical assistant has in working with insurance and third-party payers, the more helpful he or she can be to patients. As mentioned previously, medical assistants should keep a manual of medical billing policies and procedures for most of the insurances plans they handle; this can serve as an excellent source of guidance and suggestions for working with a particular payer.

Always be sure to obtain the guarantor's signature on an agreement to pay for services. Most patient information sheets have a

	Column A	Column B
Total charge	$10,000	$20,000
Deductible (paid by Mrs. Jones)	(500)	(500)
5% (Mrs. Jones' portion)	(500)	(500)
Allowable amount $8500	(1500)	
Allowable amount $8500 with write off		(1500)
Total amount paid by Mrs. Jones	$2500	$1000
Total amount paid by insurance	$7500	$17,500

FIGURE 15-10 Calculation of allowable amount.

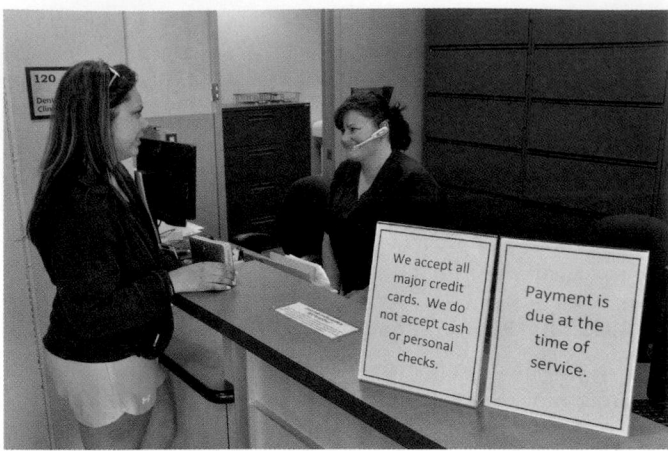

FIGURE 15-11 Medical assistant informing a patient of her financial responsibility.

section referring to the guarantor. A statement may be included, which the guarantor signs, that serves as an agreement to pay the costs of medical care. States have varying statutes that deal with guarantors, so be sure the office's policies comply with those laws. It is especially important to secure a written agreement to pay for services when the care will be long term for costly treatment or surgical procedures. Procedure 15-5 explains how to inform patients of their financial obligations for services rendered.

CRITICAL THINKING APPLICATION   **15-7**

The providers in the practice where Ann works are not in network of a preferred provider organization (PPO) that is often used in their geographic area. Many patients are confused when they have to pay a larger out-of-pocket fee for their medical services. How can Ann explain the reason for these higher fees to patients?

PROCEDURE 15-5   Inform a Patient of Financial Obligations for Services Rendered

Goal: Inform patient of his/her financial obligation and to demonstrate professionalism when discussing the patient's billing record.

Scenario: During this role play, Christi Brown is meeting with you regarding the bill she received in the mail. When she called to make the appointment, she voiced her confusion about the bill, stating she thought her insurance covered everything. You check her record and see that she met her deductible and now needs to pay 20% of the billed amount. She owes $170.

EQUIPMENT and SUPPLIES

- Patient's account record
- Copy of patient's insurance card.

PROCEDURAL STEPS

1. Determine the patient's financial responsibility under the insurance plan by reviewing the copy of the patient's insurance card.
   PURPOSE: Having an understanding of the patient's financial responsibility from the insurance plan will help you to explain the terms to the patient.
2. Determine the amount the patient owes by reviewing the patient's account record.
   PURPOSE: It is important that when working with a patient that you are familiar with the facts of the situation.

3. Discuss the situation with the patient. (Role play the above scenario.)
4. Demonstrate professionalism when discussing the situation with the patient. Verbal and nonverbal communication should demonstrate patience, understanding, and sensitivity. The medical assistant should refrain from inappropriate and unprofessional behavior, including eye rolling, harsh words, disrespectful comments, and similar behaviors.
5. Demonstrate professionalism by respectfully providing the patient with payment options based on the clinic's policies and what the patient can pay on a monthly basis.
   PURPOSE: The medical assist should not force or harass the patient in paying. The medical assistant will be more successful if the communication with the patient is respectful.

Showing Sensitivity When Discussing Patients' Finances

Most patients use health insurance, but they do not always recognize that they will have financial obligations after the insurance plan pays its share. This is common among Medicare patients, who often feel that they should have all their medical expenses paid because they have government insurance. It usually falls to the medical assistant to inform patients of their coinsurance responsibilities.

Patients seeking medical care are not usually feeling like themselves because they may be (or have been) suffering through pain and discomfort. As a result, their behavior may not be typical when the medical assistant suggests discussing their financial responsibilities.

Medical assistants should show patience and sensitivity when discussing a patient's financial obligations (Figure 15-12). Patients should never be harassed to make a payment or forced into payment arrangements. Medical assistants should always be courteous when discussing payments with patients. In addition, the medical practice should offer a variety of payment methods to meet patients' needs, including credit cards, and online payment options.

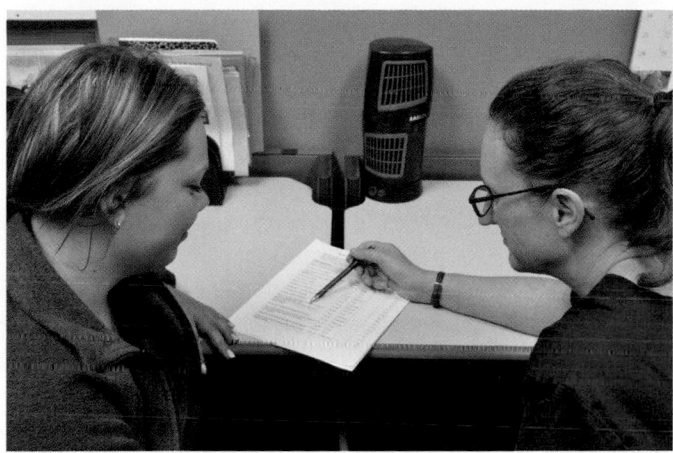

FIGURE 15-12 Medical assistants must show respect and sensitivity when discussing financial issues with patients.

CRITICAL THINKING APPLICATION   15-8

An elderly patient comes to the office and complains that Medicare did not pay her bill in full. "Medicare is supposed to pay 80% of all of my bills, and I have already paid my portion," she insists. What information does Ann need to get to the bottom on this problem? How can she explain situations like this to other patients?

CLOSING COMMENTS

Accurate insurance billing practices are essential for the financial success of every healthcare facility. Medical assistants are strong assets to the healthcare facility when they can submit claims electronically, manage denied and rejected claims, and discuss financial responsibilities with patients professionally. Medical assistants should always maintain a positive attitude toward patients and keep in mind that those who are ill or facing challenges are not always at their best and may not respond in a positive way when discussing their financial responsibilities.

Patient Education

Most patients are unaware of their benefits and coverages through their insurance policies. The medical assistant should encourage patients to read the entire policy to become familiar with its limitations and exclusions. Inform patients that when they call the insurance company with questions, they should always write down the date, the time, and the name of the person with whom they spoke. Using email is helpful because a record of the correspondence can easily be saved or printed. Making sure that patients have a general understanding of their health insurance coverage is well worth the effort.

Often patients do not dispute the decision or question the insurance company when a claim is rejected or not paid in the expected amount. Encourage them to call the company and question rejections if they do not understand why the claim was denied.

Legal and Ethical Issues

From time to time patients may ask for a reduced fee after the insurance has already paid. If the provider is a participating provider with the health insurance plan, he or she is obligated to follow the terms of contract. This includes collecting the patient's financial responsiblitiy detailed in the EOB. The insurance plan can penalize the healthcare facility if a concerted effort is not made to collect the patient's coinsurance and deductible amounts, thus not following the terms of the participating provider health insurance contract.

Professional Behaviors

Medical billers must have strong organizational skills. Not only are they responsible for submitting claims electronically in a timely manner, they also must manage claim denials and rejections. Denied and rejected claims need to be adjusted and rebilled for prompt payment. An organized medical biller ensures that all medical billing activities are worked on daily.

SUMMARY OF SCENARIO

Ann realizes that the best way to keep track of all the carriers is to keep an up-to-date manual that contains the addresses, phone numbers, and medical billing policies and procedures for each insurance plan the healthcare facility accepts. This manual can help prevent the rejection and denial of many claims because they will be submitted accurately the first time.

The medical assistant's understanding of how to calculate deductibles, coinsurance, and allowed amounts for procedures and services benefits both the provider and patient. The provider's productivity, income, and losses can be easily tracked, and the patient can be educated as to the exact amounts he or she is responsible for paying.

Ann also has learned the importance of being courteous to patients when discussing their financial obligations. She has learned how to use the Assignment of Financial Responsibility form to communicate what the patient owes in a clear, straightforward manner.

SUMMARY OF LEARNING OBJECTIVES

1. **Define, spell, and pronounce the terms listed in the vocabulary.**
   Spelling and pronouncing medical terms correctly reinforce the medical assistant's credibility. Knowing the definitions of these terms promotes confidence in communication with patients and co-workers.

2. **Identify steps for filing a third-party claim.**
   The medical assistant's medical billing tasks begin when the patient seeks medical services from the provider, usually when an appointment is made. Insurance billing and coding tasks typically completed by the

Continued

medical assistant include collecting accurate information and submitting a complete insurance claim.

3. Identify the types of information contained in the patient's billing record.

When the first appointment is made for a patient, it is routine to ask the patient for all pertinent insurance billing information. Much of this information is on the patient registration/intake form, which is completed when the patient comes to the medical office for the initial visit.

4. Apply managed care policies and procedures, describe processes for precertification, and obtain precertification, including documentation.

Medical assistants should be aware that services provided to patients who are sponsored by an MCO plan may not be reimbursed if the policies and procedures of the specific insurance plan are not followed. To submit accurate health insurance claims, medical assistants should establish office procedures for applying MCO policies and procedures. (See Procedure 15-1.)

In an effort to control costs, many MCOs require precertification of specialized medical services. The policies and procedures of each insurance plan determine whether precertification is required before a medical procedure is scheduled. Preauthorization helps the medical assistant ensure that the provider will be paid for procedures and services provided to the patient. The process for obtaining preauthorization (precertification) is outlined in Procedure 15-2.

5. Explain how to submit health insurance claims, including electronic claims, to various third-party payers.

Medical billers should familiarize themselves with the claim submission policies and procedures of the health insurance plans commonly seen in their office. A medical assistant can successfully manage the requirements of the different insurance plans commonly seen in the practice by keeping an up-to-date manual containing the billing policies and procedures of these third-party payers. Electronic claims are insurance claims that are transmitted over the Internet from the provider to the health insurance company. Most claims-processing software is designed to generate electronic claims.

6. Review the guidelines for completing the CMS-1500 Health Insurance Claim Form, and complete an insurance claim form.

The medical assistant should follow an established list of guidelines for completing the CMS-1500 Health Insurance Claim Form, including obtaining a signed assignment of benefits. The CMS-1500 has 33 blocks; except for specific blocks that require information about the patient and the insured, the requirements for completing the form vary from payer to payer. Accuracy in completing the CMS-1500 is vital. The process for completing claim forms accurately is outlined in Procedure 15-3.

7. Differentiate between fraud and abuse.

Abuse in coding can be likened to actions that are contrary to ethical standards in the medical office. Unlike fraud, abuse is an inadvertent action that directly or indirectly results in an overpayment to the healthcare provider. Abuse is similar to fraud, except that it is unclear whether the unethical practice was committed deliberately. The term "intentional" is important in defining fraud and abuse and in deciphering whether the coding practices were ethical or not.

8. Discuss the effects of upcoding and downcoding.

Medical coders have an ethical responsibility to prevent fraud and abuse resulting from upcoding. Coders also must be careful not to downcode, or assign codes that are not specific enough. Downcoding can be done by the coder, the insurance company, or even a coding auditor; it always results in lower reimbursements. When providers take the responsibility to assign either diagnostic or procedural codes, they should be guided on the importance of accurate codes and their relation to maximizing reimbursement.

9. Discuss methods of preventing the rejection of claims, and use tactful behavior when speaking with medical providers about third-party requirements.

It can be challenging for a provider to keep up with the annual changes published by Medicare, private health insurance companies, and the ICD-10-CM code set updates. Staff meetings to review third-party requirements should be conducted regularly by the medical billing supervisor. Medical assistants should be respectful to the healthcare provider when discussing third-party requirements that demand more effort on the provider's part. An understanding and patient attitude goes a long way. Rejection and delay of claims cost the medical facility time and money. Proven methods of preventing rejection and delay should be established and followed; these may include reviewing electronic claims submission reports and following up on aging reports.

10. Describe ways of checking a claim's status.

It is important to track health insurance claims once they have been submitted electronically. A regular practice of confirming submission of a claim with the health insurance plan or the clearinghouse is essential for prompt payment. If more than 2 weeks passes after a claim submission without a response from the insurance company, it is wise to follow up either through the online insurance provider Web portal or by phone.

11. Review and read an Explanation of Benefits (EOB).

The EOB is sent by the insurance company to the provider who submitted the insurance claim, along with a check or a document indicating that funds were transferred electronically. The EOB breaks down each line item charge into the amount allowable, how much the insurance plan paid, and how much the patient is contracted to pay to the provider.

12. Discuss reasons for denied claims.

The two main reasons for denial of payment are technical errors and insurance policy coverage issues. Technical errors include incorrect or incomplete information and typographic and/or mathematical errors.

13. Define "medical necessity" as it applies to diagnostic and procedural coding; also, apply medical necessity guidelines.

To ensure correct reimbursement, accurate diagnosis codes must be submitted, and they must be linked to the medical procedure code reported. The diagnosis code is the reason the medical procedure performed was necessary. If an insurance company denies a claim on the

SUMMARY OF LEARNING OBJECTIVES—*continued*

grounds that the medical treatment provided was not medically necessary, an appeal letter should be sent (Procedure 15-4). The appeal letter should not only identify the denied claim in question, but also include a statement from the provider detailing the medical reasoning for providing the billed treatment. Additional medical reports should be sent (e.g., lab reports, operative reports, H&P) if these documents support the provider's decision to treat the patient.

14. **Explain a patient's financial obligations for services rendered, and inform a patient of these obligations.**

Patients must understand that the guarantor is the person ultimately responsible for the entire bill. The insurance policy is a contract between an insurance company or MCO and the policyholder, or a group of people (e.g., through an employer). The provider is not a party to this contract. Therefore, providers and their staff members are not responsible for pursuing insurance payment for the benefit of the patient. However, it is in the best interest of the staff to actively assist the patient if problems occur securing payment.

Always be sure to secure guarantors in writing (see Figure 15-11). Most patient information sheets have a section referring to the guarantor. A statement may be included for the guarantor sign, indicating an agreement to pay the costs of medical care. States have varying statutes that deal with guarantors, so be sure the office's policies reflect compliance with those laws. It is especially important to secure a written agreement to pay for services when the care will be long term or when a costly treatment or surgical procedure must be done. Procedure 15-5 explains how to inform patients of their financial obligations for services rendered.

15. **Show sensitivity when speaking with patients about third-party requirements.**

Medical assistants should show patience and sensitivity when discussing a patient's financial obligations. Patients should never be harassed to make a payment or forced into payment arrangements. Medical assistants should always be courteous when discussing payments with patients.

CONNECTIONS

Study Guide Connection: Go to the Chapter 15 Study Guide. Read and complete the activities.

evolve Evolve Connection: Go to the Chapter 15 link at *evolve.elsevier.com/kinn* to complete the Chapter Review Quiz. To sharpen your test-taking skills, click on the Medical Assisting Exam Review and answer the practice questions. In addition, check out the other resources listed for this chapter to make the most of what you have learned from Medical Billing and Reimbursement.

16 PATIENT ACCOUNTS, COLLECTIONS, AND PRACTICE MANAGEMENT

SCENARIO

Brenda Newman works in patient accounts for Dr. Susan Wilkins, a neurologist. Among her responsibilities are posting all transactions to patient accounts, monitoring accounts receivable, negotiating patient accounts and making payment arrangements, making collection calls for outstanding patient accounts, and some simple bookkeeping for Dr. Wilkins. Dr. Wilkins also works with Grant Schmidt, a certified public accountant (CPA), who assists her with supervising her office bookkeeping, creating financial statements, and overall money management of her practice. Mr. Schmidt is always willing to offer advice to the clinic's staff if any bookkeeping questions arise.

The team effort involving Dr. Wilkins, Brenda, and Mr. Schmidt results in a balanced budget for the clinic, and as a result, staff members are able to enjoy more benefits and perks.

While studying this chapter, think about the following questions:

- Why is a continuous flow of income preferable to a once-a-month influx for a provider's office?
- Why is it important to post charges, payments, and adjustments in a timely manner?
- What should Brenda do when a patient wants to make payments on an outstanding patient account balance?
- What should Brenda do when patient accounts are outstanding for more than 90 days after the date of service?

LEARNING OBJECTIVES

1. Define, spell, and pronounce terms listed in the vocabulary.
2. Define bookkeeping and all the different transactions recorded in patient accounts.
3. Do the following related to patient account records:
   - List the necessary data elements in patient account records.
   - Discuss a pegboard (manual bookkeeping) system.
   - Explain when transactions are recorded in the patient account.
   - Perform accounts receivable procedures for patient accounts, including charges, payments, and adjustments.
4. Describe special bookkeeping procedures for patient account records, including credit balances, third-party payments, and refunds; explain how to interact professionally with third-party representatives.
5. Discuss payment at the time of service, and give an example of displaying sensitivity when requesting payment for services rendered.
6. Describe the impact of the Truth in Lending Act on collections policies for patient accounts.
7. Discuss ways to obtain credit information, and explain patient billing and payment options.
8. Review policies and procedures for collecting outstanding balances on patient accounts.
9. Do the following related to collection procedures:
   - Describe successful collection techniques for patient accounts.
   - Discuss strategies for collecting outstanding balances through personal finance interviews.
   - Describe types of adjustments made to patient accounts, including nonsufficient checks (NSF) and collection agency transactions.
10. Define bookkeeping terms, including *accounts receivable* and *accounts payable*.
11. Discuss patient education, in addition to legal and ethical issues, related to patient accounts, collections, and practice management.

VOCABULARY

accounts payable The management of debt incurred and not yet paid.

accounts receivable Money that is expected but has not yet been received. The amount charged on the encounter form becomes the account receivable for the healthcare facility.

adjustments Credits posted to the patient account record when the provider's fee exceeds the amount allowed stated on the EOB.

anti-kickback statute A criminal law that prohibits the exchange of anything of value to reward the referral of a patient sponsored by a government insurance plan.

bookkeeping The recording of financial transactions in the patient account. records.

cash on hand The amount of money the healthcare facility has in the bank that can be withdrawn as cash.

collections The process of using all legal resources available to collect payment for past due patient account balances.

credit A bookkeeping entry that increases accounts receivable; money owed to the provider.

descendant A family member who takes responsibility for the patient's estate after his or her death.

executor An individual assigned to make financial decisions about the estate of a deceased patient.

guarantor The individual who subscribes to an insurance plan and accepts financial responsibility for the patient.

intangible Something of value that cannot be touched physically.

invoice A list of products or services provided to the healthcare facility for payment.

medically indigent Patients that are in need of medical care, yet cannot pay.

nonsufficient funds check (NSF) When a patient pays a check without having sufficient funds in the bank to cover the payment so it is returned to the provider unpaid.

pegboard system A manual bookkeeping system that uses a day sheet to record all financial transactions for the date of service and maintains patient account balances by using physical cards.

plaintiff The party filing a complaint.

provider's fee schedule Fees established by the provider for services rendered.

refunds Payments returned to insurance companies for overpayments made on patient accounts.

small claims court A last resort option to collect payment from an outstanding patient account; in small claims court, the healthcare facility can sue the patient for the balance.

trustee The coordinator of financial resources assigned by the court during a bankruptcy case.

unsecured debt Debt that is not guaranteed by something of value; credit card debt is the most common type of unsecured debt.

Every patient encounter is a financial transaction for a healthcare facility. Transactions generated by the patient encounter include a variety of charges, payments, and adjustments that need to be accounted for on a daily basis. Financial management is essential if the owner of a healthcare practice is to pay his or her business operating expenses. If the expenses of operating the healthcare facility exceed the fees collected for services rendered, the business will be forced to close.

A *patient account,* a running balance of all financial transactions under the patient's account record, is created when the healthcare provider renders services. Charges are applied to the patient account when an *encounter form* (Figure 16-1) is completed during the office visit; this form lists all the procedures and charges for services rendered.

BOOKKEEPING IN THE HEALTHCARE FACILITY

Bookkeeping is the recording of financial transactions in the patient account records. Most healthcare facilities use practice management software for daily bookkeeping transactions. The charges documented on the encounter form are used to complete the health insurance claim form, which shows the diagnosis, procedures, and associated charges. *Payments* to the healthcare facility come as reimbursement from the insurance company or a patient payment. **Adjustments** are made to a patient's account when it is necessary to add or subtract an amount, which is not a payment, from the balance; for example, the difference between the provider's charged amount and the contracted insurance payment amount.

PATIENT ACCOUNT RECORDS

All charges and payments for professional services are posted to the patient's account record daily. In this way, the record becomes a reliable source of information for answering all inquiries from patients about their financial responsibilities. The patient account record should include all information pertinent to collecting the account, such as:

- Name and address of the **guarantor**
- Insurance identification information
- Home and business telephone numbers
- Name of employer
- Any special instructions for billing
- Emergency or alternative contact information

The patient account statement (Figure 16-2) provides a running balance, the result of all of the different financial transactions performed in the account, including charges, payments, adjustments and **credits**.

Entering and Posting Transactions in Patient Accounts

When a practice management software system is used, charges are entered into the record automatically from the encounter form after the office visit.

When a pegboard system is used (see the Manual Bookkeeping box), transactions are initiated before the patient goes to the exam room. The patient account ledger card is inserted under the first or next available receipt, and the first available writing line of the card is aligned with the carbonized strip on the receipt. Enter the receipt number and the date; enter the account balance in the space labeled *previous balance;* and then enter the patient's name. A copy of the receipt is detached and clipped to the patient's chart to be routed to the provider.

Posting Charges

Whether practice management software or a pegboard system is used, the charges posted to the patient's account should be taken

STATE LIC.# C1503X
SOC. SEC. # 000-11-0000
PIN # _____

College Clinic
4567 Broad Avenue
Woodland Hills, XY 12345-4700

Phone: 555-486-9002

☐ Private ☒ Bluecross ☐ Ind. ☐ Medicare ☐ Medi-cal ☐ Hmo ☐ Ppo

Patient's last name	First		Account #:	Birthdate	Sex ☐ Male	Today's date
Smith	Lydia		13845	09/ 13 / 92	☒ Female	09/ 17 / 20XX

Insurance company	Subscriber		Plan #	Sub. #	Group
Blue Shield of CA	Lydia Smith		0473	186-72-10XX	849-37000

ASSIGNMENT: I hereby assign my insurance benefits to be paid directly to the undersigned physician, I am financially responsible for non-covered services.
SIGNED: Patient, or parent, if minor *Lydia Smith*   Today's date 09 /17 /20XX

RELEASE: I hereby authorize the physician to release to my insurance carriers any information require to process this claim.
SIGNED: Patient, or parent, if minor *Lydia Smith*   Today's date 09 /17 /20XX

✓	DESCRIPTION	CODE	FEE	✓	DESCRIPTION	CODE	FEE	✓	DESCRIPTION	CODE	FEE
	OFFICE VISITS	NEW / EST.			Venipuncture	36415			OFFICE PROCEDURES		
	Blood pressure check	99211			TB skin test	86580			Anoscopy	46600	
	Level II	99202 / 99212			Hematocrit	85013			Ear lavage	69210	
	Level III	99203 / 99213			Glucose finger stick	82948			Spirometry	94010	
X	Level IV	(99204) 99214	$175		IMMUNIZATIONS				Nebulizer Rx	94664	
	Level V	99205 / 99215			Allergy inj. X1	95115			EKG	93000	
	PREVENTIVE EXAMS	NEW / EST.			Allergy inj. X2	95117			SURGERY		
	Age 65 and older	99387 / 99397			Trigger pt. inj.	20552			Mole removal (1st)	17110	
	Age 40 - 64	99386 / 99396			Therapeutic inj.	96372			(2nd to 14th)	17003	
	Age 18 - 39	99385 / 99395			VACCINATION PRODUCTS				Flat warts (1st - 14th)	07110	
	Age 12 - 17	99384 / 99394			DPT	90701			15 or more	17111	
	Age 5 - 11	99383 / 99393			DT	90702			Biopsy, 1 lesion	11100	
	Age 1 - 4	99382 / 99392			Tetanus	90703			Addt'l. lesions	11101	
	Infant	99381 / 99391			MMR	90707			Endometrial Bx	58100	
	Newborn ofc	99432			OPV	90712			Skin tags to 15	11200	
	OB/NEWBORN CARE				Polio inj.	90713			Each addt'l. 10	11201	
	OB package	59400			Flu	90662			I & D abscess	10060	
	Post-partum visit N/C				Hemophilus B	90645			SUPPLIES/MISCELLANEOUS		
	LAB PROCEDURES				Hepatitis B vac.	90746			Surgical tray	99070	
	Urine dip	81000			Pheumovax	90670			Handling charge	99000	
	UA qualitative	81005			VACCINE ADMINISTRATION				Special report	99080	
X	Pregnancy urine	81025	20.00		Age: Through 18 yrs. (1st inj.)	90460			DOCTOR'S NOTES:		
	Wet mount	87210			Age: Through 18 yrs. (ea. addt'l. inj.)	90461					
	kOH prip	87220			Adult (1st inj.)	90471					
	Occult blood	82270			Adult (ea. addt'l. inj.)	90472					

DIAGNOSES ICD-10-CM			
___ Abdominal pain/unspec. . . R10.9	___ Colitis/unspec. K51.90	___ FUO R50.9	___ Osteoarthritis (site). . . . . . M19._
___ Absess . . . . L02._	___ Confusion R41.0	___ Gastritis. K29.70	___ Otitis media . . . . H66.9_
___ Allergic reaction . . . . T78.40_	___ CHF. I50.9	___ Gastroenteritis (colitis) . . K52.9	___ Parkinson's disease G20
___ Alzheimer's disease G30	___ Constipation K59.00	___ G.I. bleed K92.2	___ Pharyngitis, acute. J02.9
___ Anemia/unspec. D64.9	___ COPD J44.9	___ Gout/unspec. M10.9	___ Pleurisy R09.1
___ Angina/unspec. I20.9	___ Cough R05	___ Headache R51	___ Pneumonia. J18.9
___ Anorexia. R63.0	___ Crohn's disease/unspec. . K50.90	___ Health exam . . . . 200.__	___ Pneumonia, viral J12.9
___ Anxiety/unspec. F41.9	___ CVA. I63.9	___ Hematuria/unspec. R31.9	___ Prostatitis/unspec. N41.9
___ Apnea, sleep G47.30	___ Decubitus ulcer. . . . . L89._	___ Herpes simplex. B00.9	___ PVD I73.9
___ Arrhythmia, cardiac I49.9	___ Dehydration. E86.0	___ Herpes zoster. B02.9	___ Radiculopathy . . . . M54.1_
___ Arthritis, rheumatoid. M06.9	___ Dementia/unspec. F03	___ Hiatal hernia K44.9	___ Rectal bleeding K62.5
___ Asthma/unspec. J45.909	___ Depression, major/unsp. . F32.9	___ HTN (HBP) I10	___ Renal failure N19
___ Atrial fibrillation. I48.0	___ Diab I, no complications . . E10.0	___ Hyperlipidemia/unspec. . E78.5	___ Sciatica. . . . . M54.3_
___ B-12 deficiency. E53.8	___ Diab II, no complications. . E11.9	___ Hypothyroidism/unspec. . E03.9	___ Shortness of breath R03.02
___ Back pain, low M54.5	___ w/kidney complic. . . . . . E11.2_	___ Impotentce . . . . N52._	___ Sinusitis, chr./unspec. . . . J32.9
___ BPH N40	___ w/ophthalmic compl. . . E11.3_	___ Influenza, respiratory . . . J10.1	___ Syncope R55
___ Bradycardia/unspec. R00.1	___ w/neurolog.compl. . . . . E11.4_	___ Insomnia. G47.0	___ Tachycardia/unspec. R00.0
___ Broncitis, acute. . . . . J20._	___ w/circulatory cmpl. . . . E11.5_	___ IBS, diarrhea . . . . K58.	___ Tachy., supraventric. I47.1
___ Bronchitis, chronic. J42	___ Insulin use. Z79.4	___ Lupus, systemic erythm. . M32.9	___ Tendinitis/unspec. M77.9
___ Bursitis/unspec. M71.9	___ Diarrhea/unspec. R19.7	___ MI, acute. . . . . I21._	___ TIA G45.9
___ CA, breast . . . . C50._	___ Diverticulitix. K57.92	___ MI, old. I25.2	___ Ulcer, duodenal/unspec. . K26.9
___ CA, lung . . . . C34._	___ Diverticulosis. K57.90	___ Migraine G43.9	___ Ulcer, gastric/unspec. . . . K25.9
___ CA, prostate C61	___ Dizziness. R42	___ Myalgia. M79.1	___ Ulcer, peptic/unspec. K27.9
___ Cellulitis . . . . L03._	___ Dysuria R30.0	___ Neck pain M54.2	___ URI/unspec. J06.9
___ Chest pain/unspec. R07.9	___ Edema/unspec. R60.9	___ Neuropathy G62.9	___ UTI N39.0
___ Cirrhosis, liver/unspec. . . K74.60	___ Endocarditis I38	___ Nausea R11.1	___ Vertigo R42
___ Cold, common J00	___ Esophageal reflux K21.0	X Nausea/vomiting R11.0	___ Weight gain R63.5
	___ Fatigue (lethargy) R53.83	___ Obesity/unspec. E66.9	___ Weight loss R63.4

Diagnosis/additional description: Pregnancy	Doctor's signature/date *Dr. B. Caesar* 09-17-20XX	
Return appointment information: -with whom (Self) other	Rec'd by: ☐ Cash	Total today's fee $195
Days Wks. (Mos.) 1 month	☐ Check	Co-payment $35
PLEASE RMEMBER THAT PAYMENT IS YOUR OBLIGATION, REGARDLESS OF INSURANCE OR OTHER THIRD PARTY INVOLVEMENT.	☐ Credit # _____	Amount rec'd today

FIGURE 16-1 Encounter form with charges. (Courtesy of Bibbero Systems, an InHealth Company, Petaluma, Calif.)

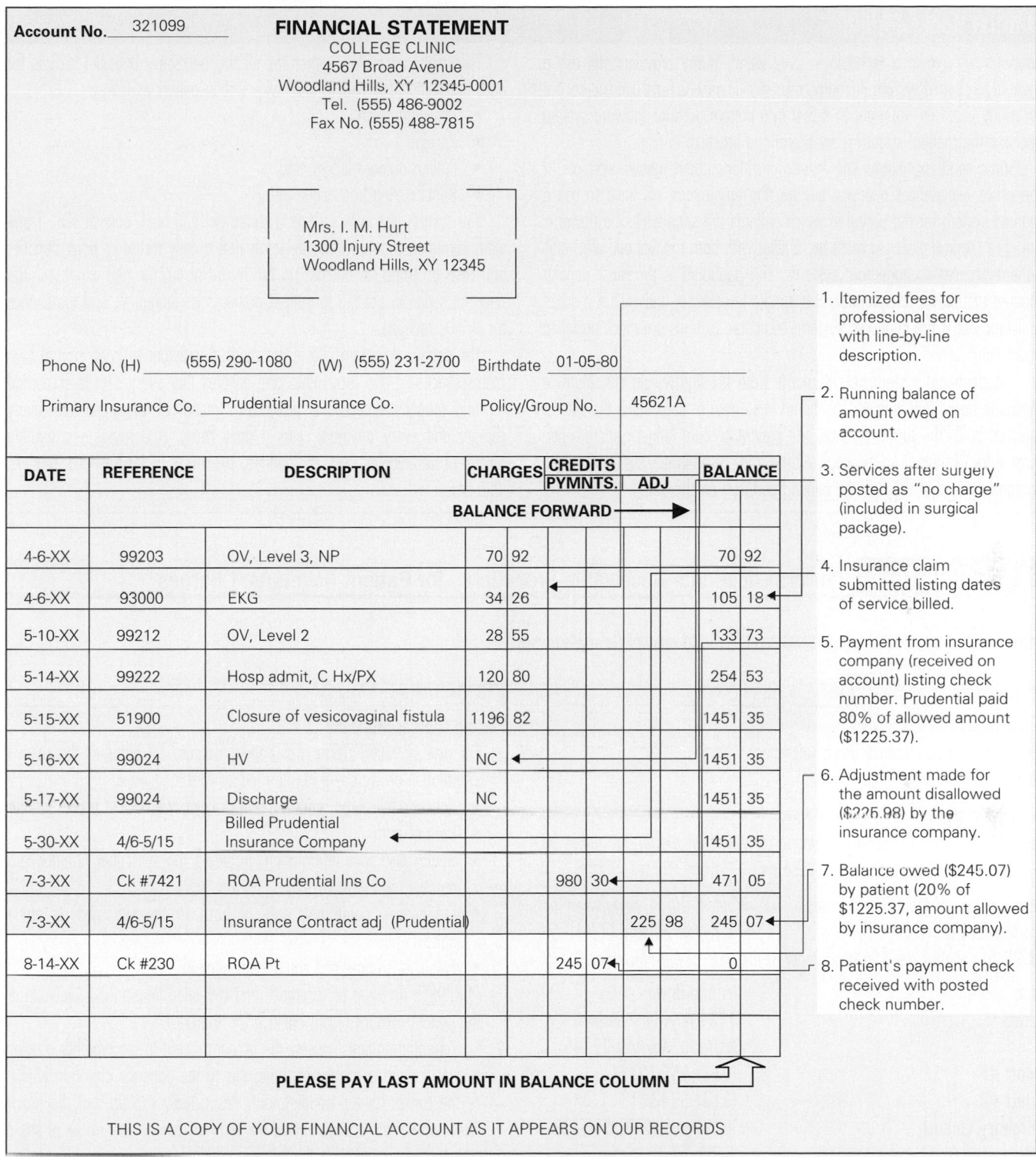

Account No. 321099

FINANCIAL STATEMENT
COLLEGE CLINIC
4567 Broad Avenue
Woodland Hills, XY 12345-0001
Tel. (555) 486-9002
Fax No. (555) 488-7815

Mrs. I. M. Hurt
1300 Injury Street
Woodland Hills, XY 12345

Phone No. (H) (555) 290-1080 (W) (555) 231-2700 Birthdate 01-05-80

Primary Insurance Co. Prudential Insurance Co. Policy/Group No. 45621A

DATE	REFERENCE	DESCRIPTION	CHARGES	CREDITS PYMNTS.	ADJ	BALANCE
		BALANCE FORWARD ➡				
4-6-XX	99203	OV, Level 3, NP	70 92			70 92
4-6-XX	93000	EKG	34 26			105 18
5-10-XX	99212	OV, Level 2	28 55			133 73
5-14-XX	99222	Hosp admit, C Hx/PX	120 80			254 53
5-15-XX	51900	Closure of vesicovaginal fistula	1196 82			1451 35
5-16-XX	99024	HV	NC			1451 35
5-17-XX	99024	Discharge	NC			1451 35
5-30-XX	4/6-5/15	Billed Prudential Insurance Company				1451 35
7-3-XX	Ck #7421	ROA Prudential Ins Co		980 30		471 05
7-3-XX	4/6-5/15	Insurance Contract adj (Prudential)			225 98	245 07
8-14-XX	Ck #230	ROA Pt		245 07		0

PLEASE PAY LAST AMOUNT IN BALANCE COLUMN ⬆

THIS IS A COPY OF YOUR FINANCIAL ACCOUNT AS IT APPEARS ON OUR RECORDS

1. Itemized fees for professional services with line-by-line description.

2. Running balance of amount owed on account.

3. Services after surgery posted as "no charge" (included in surgical package).

4. Insurance claim submitted listing dates of service billed.

5. Payment from insurance company (received on account) listing check number. Prudential paid 80% of allowed amount ($1225.37).

6. Adjustment made for the amount disallowed ($226.98) by the insurance company.

7. Balance owed ($245.07) by patient (20% of $1225.37, amount allowed by insurance company).

8. Patient's payment check received with posted check number.

FIGURE 16-2 Patient account statement. (From Fordney WT: *Insurance handbook for the medical office,* ed 14, St. Louis, 2017, Elsevier.)

from the **provider's fee schedule.** Patient account management software systems automatically put in the correct fees or charges when a CPT/HCPCS* code is entered (Procedure 16-1).

CPT, Current Procedural Terminology; HCPCS, Healthcare Common Procedure Coding System.

When checking out a patient using a pegboard system, the medical assistant should insert the ledger card under the proper receipt and check the number previously entered to make sure the correct card is being used. Record the service by procedure code, post the charge from the fee schedule, enter any payment made, and write in the current balance. If there is no balance, place a zero or a straight line in the balance column.

Manual Bookkeeping

Although we live in a technology-savvy world, many providers still use a manual **pegboard system**. In many cases, providers who have been in practice for many years do not want to invest in a patient account software system because the manual system is so logical and practical to use.

Some certifying exams still include questions about manual systems. If the office experiences a power outage, the employees will have to use a manual system for the period in which patients are seen while the power is out. The medical assistant must be familiar with both manual and electronic patient account management systems. The pegboard is the most popular manual system for this purpose. It is simple to operate, and once a medical assistant learns the pegboard system, computer systems are much easier to understand.

The pegboard system gets its name from the lightweight aluminum or Masonite board that is used. This board has a row of pegs along the side or top that holds the forms in place. The patient account ledger cards are perforated for alignment on the pegs. All the forms used in any system must be compatible so that they can be aligned perfectly on the board.

The pegboard system generates all the necessary financial records for each transaction (by writing once with carbon paper) as follows:
- Encounter form
- Receipt
- Patient account ledger card
- Bookkeeping transaction entry

The system also may include a statement and bank deposit slip. It provides current accounts receivable totals and a daily record of bank deposits and **cash on hand**, in addition to the record of income and expenses. The need for separate posting to patient accounts is eliminated, and the chance for error is reduced.

The pegboard system allows the medical assistant to keep control over cash, collections, and receivables and ensures that every cent is accounted for and properly entered. It provides a record of every patient, every charge, and every payment, plus a daily recap of earnings—a running record of receivables and an audited summary of cash—and requires little time.

PROCEDURE 16-1   Perform Accounts Receivable Procedures for Patient Accounts: Charges

Goal: *To enter charges into the patient account record manually and electronically.*

EQUIPMENT and SUPPLIES

- Patient account ledger card
- SimChart for the Medical Office software
- Encounter form/Superbill
- Provider's fee schedule

Scenario 1: *Ken Thomas is a returning patient of Dr. Martin. He makes his $50 copayment at the time of the office visit.*

Scenario 2: *Martha Bravo is seeing Dr. Walden. He is being seen for hypertension (ICD-10-CM I10) for the first time for hypothyroidism (ICD-10-CM E03.9). She makes the $30 copayment at the time of the office visit.*

Name	Martha Bravo
Address	1234 Anywhere Station
	Anytown, Anystate 12345
Contact #1	(212) 555-1212
Contact #2	(212) 554-1313
Emergency Contact	John Bravo (212) 555-2627
DOB	1/23/56
SSN	111-22-3333
Health Insurance Information	Aetna
	Subscriber: Martha Bravo
	Subscriber DOB: 1/23/56
	ID #: XEK3332328748
	Group #: X1000
	Effective Date: 1/1/20-
Employer Information	Name: Malibu Gardening
	Contact: (212) 555-5151

PROCEDURAL STEPS

Posting Charges Manually

1. For new patients, create the patient account by entering the following information on a patient account ledger card:
   - Patient's full name, address, and at least two contact phone numbers
   - Date of birth
   - Health insurance information, including the subscriber number, group number, and effective date
   - Subscriber's name and date of birth (if the subscriber is not the patient)
   - Employer's name and contact information

   PURPOSE: To keep all insurance and collection information available with the patient account record balance for reference.

2. For returning patients, review the account record to see whether a balance is due. If there is a balance, bring this to the patient's attention when he or she comes for the appointment. Respectfully explain that the provider would appreciate a payment on the previous balance before he or she can care for the patient. Use the following dialogue:

   Brenda: Good morning, Ken. How are you feeling today?

   Ken: Not so good, I really need to see Dr. Martin again because my headaches have been getting worse.

   Brenda: I'm sorry to hear that. Let's get you in to see the doctor right away. I can collect the $50 copayment for today's visit, and here is a statement for your previous balance of $214. How would you like to take care of that today?

   Ken: Oh, I didn't know about the previous balance. Can I just pay the copayment today?

PROCEDURE 16-1 *—continued*

Brenda: Dr. Martin would like at least half of this previous balance paid before seeing you today, please. I know that medical bills can pile up pretty quick, but Dr. Martin would like to continue to provide you with quality care so you can feel back to yourself really soon.

Ken: Yes, I know you're right. I need to keep coming to see Dr. Martin. I can pay half of the $214 today, along with the copayment.

Brenda: Thanks, I know Dr. Martin really appreciates you as a patient. Would that be check or credit card?

Ken: Credit card, please.

Brenda: Okay, here is the credit card receipt and a copy of the updated statement. By the way, I'd like to document on your patient account when you will be able to pay the rest of this statement amount.

Ken: I'll pay the balance next month; is that okay?

Brenda: I'll let Dr. Martin know and put a note in your account. Thanks; you'll be called in shortly.

<u>PURPOSE:</u> To respectfully inform the patient of his or her financial obligations and the provider's intention of having the previous balance paid in full.

3. After seeing the patient, the provider completes the encounter form, which includes all procedures and the associated fee schedule. Using the completed encounter form (see Figure 16-1), enter the charges manually on the ledger

card for the patient's account record. Total all the charges on the encounter form for the services rendered. Then subtract the copayment made from the total charges. The previous balance, if any, is added to this new total. Use the following worksheet to calculate the new balance. The new balance-due amount should be presented to the patient before he or she leaves the healthcare facility.

Total Charges $_____
Amount paid (copayment) $_____
+ Previous balance (if any) $_____
= New Balance Due $_____

PROCEDURAL STEPS

Posting Charges in SimChart for the Medical Office

1. After logging into SimChart, locate the established patient by clicking on Find Patient, enter the patient's name, verify DOB, and click on the radio button. This will bring you to the Clinical Care tab. If there is no encounter shown, create an encounter by clicking on Office Visit under Info Panel on the left, select a visit type, and click on Save. Once an encounter has been created, return to the Patient Dashboard and click on the Superbill link on the right (or click on the Coding and Billing tab).

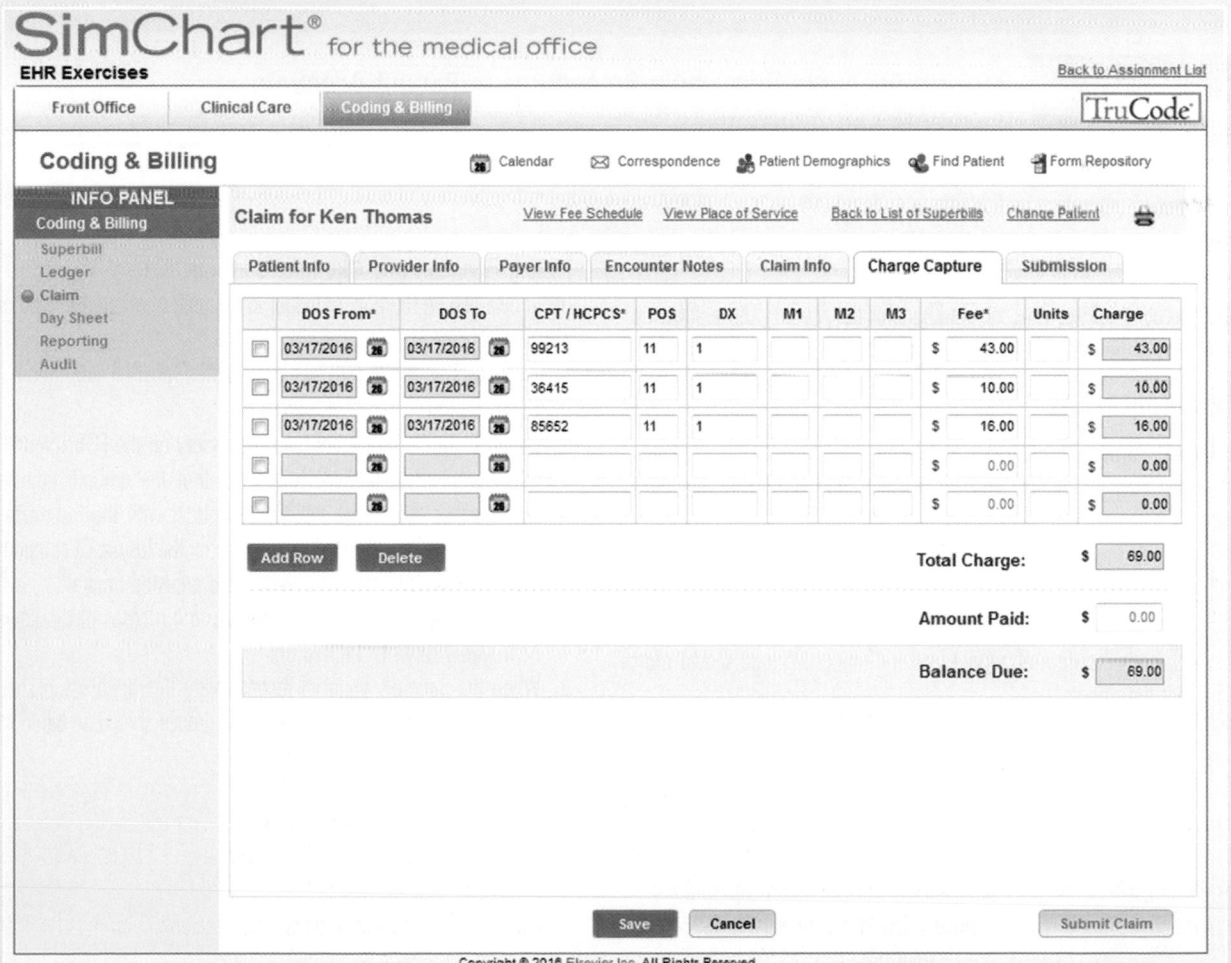

PROCEDURE 16-1 *—continued*

2. From the Superbill area, in the Encounters Not Coded section, click on the encounter (in blue). On page 1 enter the diagnosis in the Diagnosis field and document the services provided (additional services are found on pages 2-3 of the Superbill).
3. Complete the information needed on page 4 of the Superbill and submit.

4. Click on Ledger on the left and search for your patient. Once your patient has been located, click on the arrow across from the name in the ledger.
5. Enter the services provided and the payment received. Click on the Add Row button to continue to add services. The balance will be auto-calculated for you.

Posting Payments

All payments, including those received by mail or electronically, or when the patient pays the copay at the time of the appointment, are entered into the patient's account as a credit.

Payments should be posted by line item corresponding to the submitted health insurance claim (Procedure 16-2). All insurance payment amounts posted should match the total amount paid on the Explanation of Benefits (EOB) (Figure 16-3).

Posting Adjustments

Adjustments are credits posted to the patient account record when the provider's fee exceeds the amount allowed stated on the EOB. Adjustments should always be posted to the patient account record at the same time as the payment. Under the Health Information Technology for Economic and Clinical Health (HITECH) Act of 2009, healthcare providers may not discount the patient's financial responsibility after the health insurance has paid its portion;

PROCEDURE 16-2 **Perform Accounts Receivable Procedures in Patient Accounts: Payments and Adjustments**

Goal: *To process payments and adjustments to patient accounts records accurately.*

EQUIPMENT and SUPPLIES

- Patient account ledgers card, or SimChart for the Medical Office software
- Explanation of Benefits (EOB) (see Figure 16-3)

PROCEDURAL STEPS

Posting Payments and Adjustments Manually

1. Review the EOB for multiple patient accounts received by the healthcare facility.
2. Look up the ledger card for the patient account (or the patient ledger in SimChart) and compare the date of service on the EOB and with the date shown on the ledger card. Also, compare the amount charged for the dates of service; both the date of service and the amount charge should match on the two documents.
   PURPOSE: To confirm that the payment and adjustment posted are shown for the correct patient, date of service, and procedure.
3. Post the payment and adjustment line by line. To confirm the accuracy of the figures, the following formula can be used:

Total charged = Insurance payment amount + Amount adjusted
+ Patient responsibility or Secondary
insurance responsibility

Posting Payments and Adjustments in SimChart

Use a new line on the patient ledger in the patient account to post an insurance payment.

1. After one line on the EOB has been posted, post all subsequent lines on the EOB separately.
2. Confirm that the adjustment was necessary on the EOB (Figure 1). Review the amount paid. If there is concern that the amount adjusted was too much, either review the provider's contract with the insurance company's fee schedule to compare payments, or call the insurance company's provider services to inquire about the applicable adjusted amount.
   PURPOSE: Adjustments may be necessary in cases of disallowed charges, noncovered services, and so on.
3. When the patient's financial responsibility has been established, send the patient a statement. The secondary insurance should be billed if the patient is covered.

PROCEDURE 16-2 *—continued*

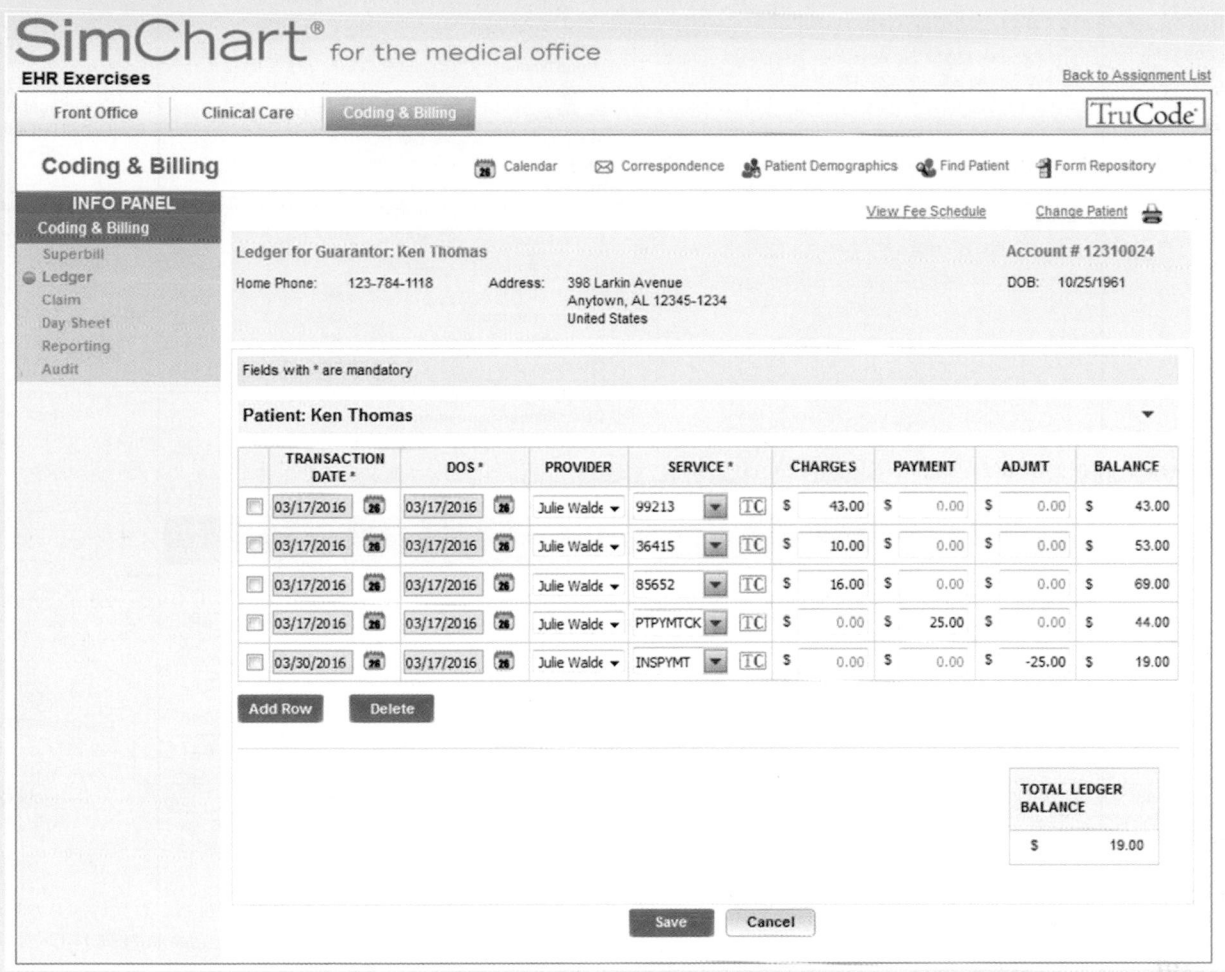

1

Special Bookkeeping Entries for Patient Account Records

The following special bookkeeping entries are sometimes necessary to keep the patient account record in balance. They may be performed either with the practice management software or a pegboard system:

- Credit balances
- Third-party payments
- Refunds

Credit Balances

A *credit balance* occurs when a patient has paid in advance, or an overpayment or duplicate payment is made. For example, an overpayment occurs if the patient makes a partial payment and later the insurance allowance is more than the remaining balance. When this happens, the patient account will show a credit balance, or an amount that the provider owes. The medical assistant should

therefore, providers can adjust only the amount in the patient account approved by the health insurance company. The only other circumstance in which an adjustment can be made is when a patient or guarantor files for bankruptcy; the entire patient account balance then must be adjusted off the books.

The patient account record should have a column for the adjustment to be posted as a credit. Remember, payments and adjustments are both credits; however, payments are money that is received in the healthcare facility, and adjustments simply reduce the balance the patient owes on the account. When the payments and adjustments are subtracted from the charged amount, the balance is either the patient responsibility or the amount billed to the secondary insurance.

Before continuing to post to the next EOB line item, confirm that the payment amount, the adjusted amount, and the patient responsibility/secondary insurance balance match exactly the amounts calculated on the EOB (see Procedure 16-2).

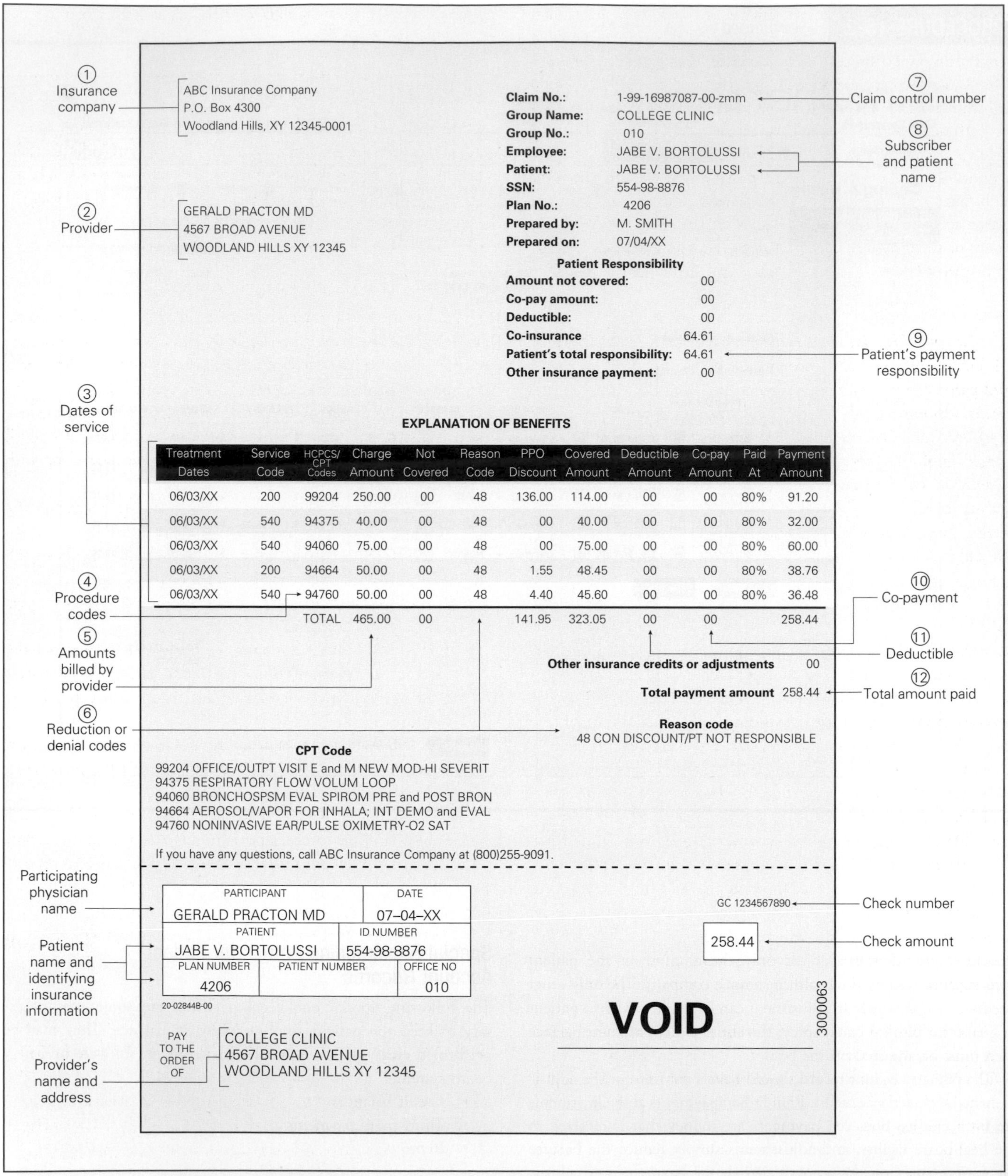

ABC Insurance Company
P.O. Box 4300
Woodland Hills, XY 12345-0001

GERALD PRACTON MD
4567 BROAD AVENUE
WOODLAND HILLS XY 12345

Claim No.: 1-99-16987087-00-zmm
Group Name: COLLEGE CLINIC
Group No.: 010
Employee: JABE V. BORTOLUSSI
Patient: JABE V. BORTOLUSSI
SSN: 554-98-8876
Plan No.: 4206
Prepared by: M. SMITH
Prepared on: 07/04/XX

Patient Responsibility
Amount not covered: 00
Co-pay amount: 00
Deductible: 00
Co-insurance 64.61
Patient's total responsibility: 64.61
Other insurance payment: 00

EXPLANATION OF BENEFITS

Treatment Dates	Service Code	HCPCS/ CPT Codes	Charge Amount	Not Covered	Reason Code	PPO Discount	Covered Amount	Deductible Amount	Co-pay Amount	Paid At	Payment Amount
06/03/XX	200	99204	250.00	00	48	136.00	114.00	00	00	80%	91.20
06/03/XX	540	94375	40.00	00	48	00	40.00	00	00	80%	32.00
06/03/XX	540	94060	75.00	00	48	00	75.00	00	00	80%	60.00
06/03/XX	200	94664	50.00	00	48	1.55	48.45	00	00	80%	38.76
06/03/XX	540	94760	50.00	00	48	4.40	45.60	00	00	80%	36.48
		TOTAL	465.00	00		141.95	323.05	00	00		258.44

Other insurance credits or adjustments 00

Total payment amount 258.44

Reason code
48 CON DISCOUNT/PT NOT RESPONSIBLE

CPT Code
99204 OFFICE/OUTPT VISIT E and M NEW MOD-HI SEVERIT
94375 RESPIRATORY FLOW VOLUM LOOP
94060 BRONCHOSPSM EVAL SPIROM PRE and POST BRON
94664 AEROSOL/VAPOR FOR INHALA; INT DEMO and EVAL
94760 NONINVASIVE EAR/PULSE OXIMETRY-O2 SAT

If you have any questions, call ABC Insurance Company at (800)255-9091.

PARTICIPANT	DATE
GERALD PRACTON MD	07–04–XX

PATIENT	ID NUMBER
JABE V. BORTOLUSSI	554-98-8876

PLAN NUMBER	PATIENT NUMBER	OFFICE NO
4206		010

20-02844B-00

GC 1234567890

258.44

VOID

3000063

PAY TO THE ORDER OF
COLLEGE CLINIC
4567 BROAD AVENUE
WOODLAND HILLS XY 12345

① Insurance company
② Provider
③ Dates of service
④ Procedure codes
⑤ Amounts billed by provider
⑥ Reduction or denial codes
⑦ Claim control number
⑧ Subscriber and patient name
⑨ Patient's payment responsibility
⑩ Co-payment
⑪ Deductible
⑫ Total amount paid
Participating physician name
Patient name and identifying insurance information
Provider's name and address
Check number
Check amount

FIGURE 16-3 Explanation of Benefits (EOB). (From Fordney MT: *Insurance handbook for the medical office*, ed 14, St Louis, 2017, Elsevier.)

investigate to whom the credit balance is owed (i.e., the patient or the insurance company). The first place to investigate is the EOB from the insurance company; this document shows the exact amount of the patient's financial responsibility. The medical assistant should confirm that all the line items match the corresponding amounts on the EOB because many credit balances are created when an error is made in payment posting. If the patient's payment exceeded the amount indicated on the EOB, the provider must send a check for the balance to the patient. A credit balance creates a *debit* in the patient account, or an amount that is due by the provider to the patient or the insurance company, depending on which party made the overpayment.

Third-Party Payments

Third-party payments are reimbursement payments made by an insurance company that provides benefits for the patient. In other words, third-party payers pay the healthcare provider on behalf of the patient. Once the third party pays the insurance claim for the date of service, the total owed to the provider becomes the amount charged minus the payment amount and the amount adjusted by the third party. The remaining balance is still owed to the provider by the patient.

The total charged = insurance payment amount + amount adjusted + patient responsibility or secondary insurance responsibility.

Refunds

Just like credit balances, refunds create a credit in the patient account that needs to be accounted for. **Refunds** are returned payments made to the insurance companies for overpayments made on patient accounts. Sometimes overpayments occur if the health insurance company pays for the same patient, date of service, and procedures more than once by accident. The medical assistant should compare the original EOB to the second EOB to confirm that an overpayment has occurred. If both EOBs show the same payment for the same date of service, refund one payment. If the two EOBs show two different payments, call provider services for the health insurance plan to ensure proper payment to the patient account. The healthcare facility cannot keep the higher payment and return the lower payment. The medical assistant should contact provider services at the health insurance plan to confirm which payment they were supposed to receive and the reasoning behind the payment amount.

Once the amount of the refund has been confirmed, the medical office manager should send the insurance company a check, along with the necessary documentation confirming the refund amount, including a copy of both EOBs and a printout of the patient account ledger.

Most patient account management software can enter charges, payments, and adjustments. As discussed previously, charges increase what is owed to the provider, whereas payments and adjustments reduce what is owed to the provider. However, credit balances and refunds, if not handled properly, can reduce what is owed to the provider erroneously. A credit balance or refund is owed to the patient or to the insurance company; it does not belong to the healthcare facility. A note indicating that there is a refund on the patient account should be recorded, and the healthcare facility office

manager should document all credit balances and refunds in a separate electronic ledger file.

Interacting With Third-Party Representatives

Most health insurance plans sponsor an online provider Web portal for checking on verification of eligibility and claim status. However, in some circumstances medical assistants must interact with third-party representatives. This can be a time-consuming process involving waiting on hold on the telephone for long periods; nevertheless, medical assistants represent their healthcare facility, and they still must interact professionally. Here are some tips for interacting with third-party representatives:

- Before calling provider services, have all documents readily accessible to discuss the patient account
- Use headphones so that the music played while the phone call is on hold does not disturb the rest of the office
- If a long wait time is expected, work on other tasks that do not require phone use
- When the health insurance representative comes on the phone, refrain from telling him or her how long the wait was; representatives usually do not have much control over wait times
- Use the documents set aside for the phone call to confirm the patient's identity quickly so as to get to the purpose of the call
- Document the details of the phone conversation with the health insurance representative in the patient account record, including the representative's name and the date and time of the call
- If the conversation is a follow-up call, share the details collected from the previous call from notes documented in the patient account record

Payment at the Time of Service

Healthcare facilities accept the patient's health insurance card and copayment as good faith that the practice will be paid for the services rendered. For the most part, patients are expected to pay their copayment at the time of service unless previous arrangements have been made (Figure 16-4). Patients without health insurance should pay

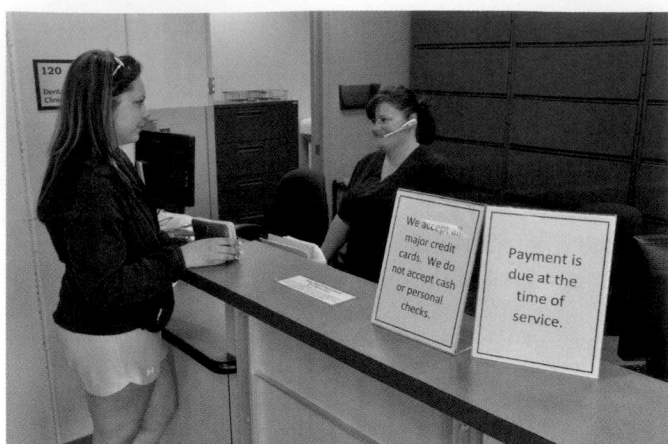

FIGURE 16-4 Most healthcare facilities display a sign informing patients that payments are due at the time of service.

after the charges for the day have been totaled. Patients should be informed when making an appointment that payment is expected at the time of service so that they are not surprised when asked for payment at the healthcare facility. The medical assistant may say, "Your charge for today is $25. Will that be cash, check, credit, or debit card?" If a patient asks to be billed, the medical assistant may say, "Our normal procedure is to pay at the time of service unless other arrangements are made in advance."

Displaying Sensitivity When Requesting Payment

The medical assistant must believe that the provider has a right to charge for the services rendered. Do not be embarrassed to ask for payment for the valuable services that have been provided. Remember that the practice is a business, and the provider must meet the obligations involved in keeping it fiscally healthy, including salary expenses. When tact and good judgment are used in billing and collecting, patients appreciate the service they receive and the help the medical assistant provides. Give each patient individual attention and personal consideration; also, be courteous and show a sincere desire to help the patient with financial problems.

CRITICAL THINKING APPLICATION   **16-3**

Adam Page comes to the front desk to pay his copay with a credit card. His card is declined. How can Brenda handle the situation? What options could be offered to Mr. Page to make a payment at the time of service?

Billing After a Payment Agreement Has Been Made

Most providers prefer payment before or at the time of service. However, if fees for surgery or long-term or expensive therapy are involved, payment arrangements become necessary, and a regular system of billing must be established. The medical assistant therefore must explain to the patient the professional fees, the services the charges cover, and the office credit policies. In most healthcare practices, the appropriate staff member sits down with the patient for a financial consultation before a payment arrangement contract is offered (Figure 16-5). The payment arrangement contract states the

monthly payment; how many months it must be paid; the payment due date; whether interest will be charged; and the penalties of nonpayment.

Using Credit for Medical Services

Some healthcare facilities distribute information about credit cards or loans available specifically for healthcare treatments. This is very popular for cosmetic surgeries, dental procedures, and laser eye surgeries. Offices that offer these types of procedures may want to investigate such alternative financing services. Although these options are valuable when used properly and repaid on time, they do create additional debt for the patient. As an alternative, the healthcare facility may allow the patient to split large healthcare expenses into two or three interest-free lump sum payments so that the patient does not incur credit card interest charges.

TRUTH IN LENDING ACT

When offering credit options for patients, the medical practice should be in compliance with Regulation Z of the Truth in Lending Act (TILA). TILA is enforced by the Federal Trade Commission (FTC) and is part of the Consumer Credit Protection Act. TILA requires that individuals be provided certain information when credit is extended, including the annual percentage rate (APR), the terms of the loan, and the total costs to the borrower. If an agreement exists between provider and patient that the practice will accept full payment in more than four installments, the practice must provide a Federal Truth in Lending Statement (Figure 16-6), even if no finance fees are charged. The statement is signed by the practice's representative and the patient.

Healthcare facilities occasionally allow their patients to pay in installments (although this practice is much less common than in the past). As long as no specific agreement has been made for payment to the provider in more than four installments and no finance charge is assessed, the account is not subject to TILA and does not require a signed Truth in Lending Statement.

OBTAINING CREDIT INFORMATION

Credit information is confidential. It should be guarded as carefully as confidential health information and should never be disclosed to unauthorized individuals. If a call is received about a patient's credit history, follow the healthcare facility's policy, based on regulations established by the Health Insurance Portability and Accountability Act (HIPAA) and legal guidelines in your state. When asking for credit information from patients in the office, do so in a private area where others cannot overhear the conversation. A patient should be able to complete a credit application in an area separate from the reception area, where the patient can sit in total privacy. Never access a credit report on patients unless it is necessary to process an application for credit privileges at the healthcare facility and the patient authorizes it.

MONTHLY PATIENT ACCOUNT STATEMENTS

Healthcare facilities should send monthly statements for all patient account records that have a balance due. These statements should be

---

PATIENT AGREEMENT

Patient's Name_____ James Doland _____ Soc. Sec. # _431-XX-1942_

Address_ 67 Blyth Dr., Woodland Hills, XY 12345 _____Tel. No. _555 372-0101_

WC Insurance Carrier_____ Industrial Indemnity Company _____

Address_____ 30 North Dr., Woodland Hills _____ Telephone No. _555-731-7707_

Date of illness___ 2-13-20XX _____Date of first visit____ 2-13-20XX _____

Emergency Yes ___X___No_____

Is this condition related to employment   Yes_X___ No_____

If accident: Auto_____Other_____

Where did injury occur?____Construction site _____

How did injury happen?____ fell 8 ft from scaffold suffering fractured right tibia __

Employee/employer who verified this information_____ Scott McPherson _____

Employer's name and address__ Willow Construction Company _____

Employer's telephone no.____ 555-526-0611 _____

In the event the claim for workers' compensation is declared
fraudulent for this illness or condition or it is determined by the
Workers' Compensation Board that the illness or injury is not a
compensable workers' compensation case, I_James Doland_ ,
hereby agree to pay the physician's fee for services rendered.

I have been informed that I am responsible to pay any
services rendered by Dr. _Raymond Skeleton_ with regard to the
discovery and treatment of any condition not related to the workers'
compensation injury or illness. I agree to pay for all services not
covered by workers' compensation and all charges for treatment and
personal items unrelated to my workers' compensation illness or
injury.

Signed_____ *James Doland* _____   Date__ 2-13-20XX ____

FIGURE 16-5 Patient payment agreement. (From Fordney MT: *Insurance handbook for the medical office*, ed 14, St Louis, 2017, Elsevier.)

---

computer generated at the beginning of each month for patient accounts that are 90 days past due or less. The patient account statement should make a visual impact, just as a letter does; therefore, the statement heads should be printed on clean, good-quality paper. Payment options such as check, e-check, online payments, and/or credit card should be presented clearly. The font on the statement should be large enough to be read easily and should provide itemized details on the following:
- Charges for the date of service
- Insurance payments and adjustments
- Patient payments, including copayments at the time of service

Envelopes should be imprinted with "Address Service Requested" in the appropriate place to maintain up-to-date mailing lists. A self-addressed return envelope included with the statement is convenient for the patient and encourages prompt payment. The statement should also indicate how old the balance is, such as "Balance now 30 days past due." For accounts that are more than 60 days past due, some offices apply neon-colored stickers to emphasize the need to pay the balance as soon as possible, thus avoiding further collection activity.

Medicare Advance Beneficiary Notices

Medicare does not cover some healthcare services so the *Advanced Beneficiary Notice* (ABN) is presented to patients in these circumstances. The ABN provides an option for patients to pay the provider's fee in full to receive services that Medicare does not cover. The patient decides whether he or she still wants to receive the services from the provider and completes the information on the form (Figure 16-7).

Professional Courtesy

In the past some providers did not charge professional colleagues or their close family members for medical care; this concept is called *professional courtesy*. However, this has led to fraud in the industry because some providers would recommend patients to auxiliary facilities from which the provider would receive compensation for the referral. The Stark law, which was passed to eliminate such fraud, imposes the following restrictions on professional courtesy:
- The professional courtesy must be extended to all members of the healthcare facility, not just a single provider
- The services provided must be routine for the healthcare facility extending the professional courtesy

LEONARD S. TAYLOR, M.D.
2100 West Park Avenue
Champaign, Illinois 61820
———
Telephone 351-5400

FEDERAL TRUTH IN LENDING STATEMENT
For professional services rendered

Patient _____ Joseph Brookhurst _____
Address _____ 353 West Terry Lane _____
_____ Birmingham, Alabama 35209 _____
Parent _____

1. Cash Price (fee for service)	$	1200.00
2. Cash Down Payment	$	200.00
3. Unpaid Balance of Cash Price	$	1000.00
4. Amount Financed	$	1000.00
5. FINANCE CHARGE	$	–0–
6. Finance Charge Expressed As Annual Percentage Rate		–0–
7. Total of Payments (4 plus 5)	$	1000.00
8. Deferred Payment Price (1 plus 5)	$	1200.00

"Total payment due" (7 above) is payable to __Dr. Leonard S. Taylor__ at above office address in __five__ monthly installments of $ __200.00__ . The first installment is payable on __May 1__ 19 __XX__ , and each subsequent payment is due on the same day of each consecutive month until paid in full.

__4-15-2xxx__   *Joseph Brookhurst*
Date   Signature of Patient; Parent if Patient is a Minor

FORM 9402 COLWELL SYSTEMS, INC., CHAMPAIGN, ILLINOIS

FIGURE 16-6 Truth in Lending Statement. (Courtesy Colwell Systems, Champaign, Ill.)

- The professional courtesy must be set forth in writing in advance by the healthcare facility's board of directors
- The professional courtesy cannot be extended to Medicare patients or other federal beneficiaries unless there is documentation of financial need
- The professional courtesy cannot violate any **anti-kickback statute** or state law

CRITICAL THINKING APPLICATION   16-4
Dr. Wilkins has just finished seeing Dr. James Franklin, who came to her as a patient. Dr. Franklin insists to Brenda that Dr. Wilkins always extends him professional courtesy. Brenda is not aware of an approved professional courtesy agreement with Dr. Franklin. However a professional courtesy agreement with Dr. Franklin is not on file. Whom should Brenda talk to?

Billing Minors

According to federal regulations, minors cannot be held financially responsible for their patient account balance unless they are emancipated. Bills for minors are usually addressed to a parent or legal guardian. If a bill is addressed to a minor, parents could take the attitude that they are not responsible because they never received a statement.

If the parents are separated or divorced, the parent who brings the child in for treatment is responsible for payment. Whatever financial agreement exists between the parents is strictly their personal business and should not concern the healthcare practice. The responsible parent should be so informed from the first appointment.

If a minor appears in the office and requests treatment, and you can ascertain that the person is legally emancipated, the minor can assume financial responsiblity. It may be wise to make a determination either with the office manager or with the provider as to whether the office wishes to treat an emancipated minor. Minors can be treated for certain conditions, such as sexually transmitted diseases (STDs), pregnancy, and birth control, without parental consent. In these cases, the medical assistant must determine where the patient account statement should be sent.

Medical Care for Those Who Cannot Pay

The medical profession traditionally has accepted the responsibility of providing medical care occasionally for individuals unable to pay for these services. Despite the increased scope of government-sponsored care for the **medically indigent,** providers still spend thousands of dollars each year providing services before securing some type of payment.

In many instances medical care of the indigent is available through social service agencies. Medical assistants should learn about local organizations and agencies that can aid patients in obtaining the necessary assistance. The provider can provide only medical services. Other agencies provide hospitalization, for example, or arrange for paying the costs of special therapy, rehabilitation, or medications. Unfortunately, another segment of the population consists of uninsured employees who are not eligible for public assistance, are not covered under a group policy, and cannot afford the high premiums for private medical insurance. Give special attention to helping these people arrange payment of their medical bills. If a provider accepts a case in advance for which a fee will not be paid, complete records must still be kept on the patient. The only deviation in procedure is that the financial record indicates no charge in the debit column.

Fees in Hardship Cases

Sometimes a healthcare practice is faced with the problem of deciding whether to reduce or cancel a fee in a hardship case. Before adjusting or canceling a fee, the provider or medical assistant should have a frank discussion with the patient about his or her financial situation. Find out whether the patient is entitled to or qualifies for medical assistance. For instance, if the patient's injuries are the result of a car accident, there may be medical insurance through the automobile policy. Circumstances may qualify the patient for local or state public assistance, such as crime victim assistance. Maintain information about such agencies that are available in the area and direct the patient to the appropriate one.

Discuss the fee in advance and make payment arrangements if the circumstances of hardship are known before services are rendered. The healthcare practice may suggest that a medically indigent patient seek care at a county hospital with public assistance. A provider should be free to choose his or her form of charity and should

A. Notifier: John Doe, MD, College Clinic, 4567 Broad Avenue, Woodland Hills, XY 12345 555-486-9002

B. Patient Name: Mary Judd **C. Identification Number:** 0920XX7291

Advance Beneficiary Notice of Noncoverage (ABN)

NOTE: If Medicare doesn't pay for D. _B12 injections_ below, you may have to pay.
Medicare does not pay for everything, even some care that you or your health care provider have good reason to think you need. We expect Medicare may not pay for the D. _B12 injections_ below.

D.	E. Reason Medicare May Not Pay:	F. Estimated Cost
B12 injections	Medicare does not usually pay for this injection or this many injections	$35.00

WHAT YOU NEED TO DO NOW:
- Read this notice, so you can make an informed decision about your care.
- Ask us any questions that you may have after you finish reading.
- Choose an option below about whether to receive the D. _B12 injections_ listed above.
  Note: If you choose Option 1 or 2, we may help you to use any other insurance that you might have, but Medicare cannot require us to do this.

G. OPTIONS: **Check only one box. We cannot choose a box for you.**

☒ **OPTION 1.** I want the D. _B12 injections_ listed above. You may ask to be paid now, but I also want Medicare billed for an official decision on payment, which is sent to me on a Medicare Summary Notice (MSN). I understand that if Medicare doesn't pay, I am responsible for payment, but **I can appeal to Medicare** by following the directions on the MSN. If Medicare does pay, you will refund any payments I made to you, less co-pays or deductibles.

☐ **OPTION 2.** I want the D. _____ listed above, but do not bill Medicare. You may ask to be paid now as I am responsible for payment. **I cannot appeal if Medicare is not billed.**

☐ **OPTION 3.** I don't want the D. _____ listed above. I understand with this choice I am **not** responsible for payment, and **I cannot appeal to see if Medicare would pay.**

H. Additional Information:

This notice gives our opinion, not an official Medicare decision. If you have other questions on this notice or Medicare billing, call **1-800-MEDICARE** (1-800-633-4227/TTY: 1-877-486-2048).
Signing below means that you have received and understand this notice. You also receive a copy.

| I. Signature: _Mary Judd_ | J. Date: _March 20, 20XX_ |

According to the Paperwork Reduction Act of 1995, no persons are required to respond to a collection of information unless it displays a valid OMB control number. The valid OMB control number for this information collection is 0938-0566. The time required to complete this information collection is estimated to average 7 minutes per response, including the time to review instructions, search existing data resources, gather the data needed, and complete and review the information collection. If you have comments concerning the accuracy of the time estimate or suggestions for improving this form, please write to: CMS, 7500 Security Boulevard, Attn: PRA Reports Clearance Officer, Baltimore, Maryland 21244-1850.

Form CMS-R-131 (03/11)   Form Approved OMB No. 0938-0566

FIGURE 16-7 Advance Beneficiary Notice for Medicare patients. (From Fordney MT: *Insurance handbook for the medical office*, ed 14, St Louis, 2017, Elsevier.)

not feel obligated to substantially reduce or cancel a fee when the circumstances are known in advance.

The provider and the patient may agree on a fee, but special circumstances may subsequently arise that create a hardship. If the provider agrees to reduce the fee, the patient should be told that the reduction will be effective only after the adjusted amount is paid in full. For instance, if a fee of $500 is reduced to $350, the full amount of the $500 charge should appear on the ledger, and when $350 has been received, the remainder can be written off as an adjustment.

Pitfalls of Fee Adjustments

Problems can arise when a provider begins to reduce his or her fees. Patients may begin to expect fees to be reduced in all circumstances. Patients may even doubt the competency of a provider who habitually reduces fees. Make fee reductions the exception rather than the norm.

Take great care in reducing the fee for care of a patient who dies. The provider's sympathy is with the family in such instances, but generosity in reducing a fee could be misinterpreted and result in a suit for malpractice. The family may suspect that the fee was reduced because the provider knows he or she made an error.

If the provider agrees to settle for a reduced fee in a situation in which the patient is disputing the cost, ensure the negotiations are "without prejudice." By taking this precaution, the provider protects his or her right to collect the original sum should the patient refuse to pay the lowered fee. The discount offer, therefore, should be made in writing; should include the words "without prejudice"; and should state a definite time limit for making payment. Prepare two copies of the agreement and have the signatures witnessed by a staff member.

A fee should never be reduced because of poor results or as a means of obtaining payment to avoid the use of a collection agency. A fee reduction for these reasons degrades the provider and the practice of medicine.

COLLECTION PROCEDURES

When to Start Collection Procedures

Collection is the process of using all legal resources available to collect payment for past due patient account balances. Sometimes a patient may have difficulty meeting all of his or her financial obligations. The patient may have lost a job or insurance coverage. An emergency could arise that depletes finances. When patients must choose between paying their medical bills and having electricity, the provider often is forced to wait for payment. Although a few patients absolutely refuse to pay for their medical care, most are honest and willing to pay but may need help with a payment plan. Terms can be arranged for collecting payment in full when the office and the patient cooperate with each other. The medical assistant should attempt to work out a plan that the patient can abide by, and the patient should be expected to make promised payments.

Preparing Patient Accounts for Collection Activity

Sometimes it becomes necessary to aggressively attempt to collect the balances that patients owe the practice. Persuasive collection procedures include telephone calls, collection reminders and letters, and personal interviews.

Before you begin collection action, it is essential to determine which accounts have a balance due and how old the account balance is. Some accounts are grouped together, or "aged," according to the dates of the last payment activity, whereas others are grouped according to the original date of service. Patient account management software programs can create aging patient account reports that are grouped by month, beginning with the month the bill was first charged (Figure 16-8). Common account aging categories are:

- 0-30 days
- 30-60 days
- 60-90 days
- 90-120 days

Most bills with balances less than 30 days old are probably waiting for the health insurance to reimburse, so no collection action is needed. Patient account balances more than 90 or 120 days old require a final demand letter before the account is turned over to a collection agency. Always allow the provider to review and approve the list of patient accounts being sent to a collection agency. Once patient account balances are aged, follow the most appropriate collection activity, according to the practice's policy.

The medical assistant can use a variety of techniques to collect patient accounts, such as collection phone calls, collection letters, and skip tracing. Often more than one technique must be used to obtain payment. Always be courteous and kind when using all collection techniques.

Collection Phone Calls

A telephone call at the right time, in a negotiable demeanor, is more successful than notes, patient account statements, or collection letters. The personal contact call often prompts patients to mail in their payment or to make payments over the phone with a credit card. In the absence of time to make calls, the collection letter is the next best approach, but if collections are a serious problem, it may be worth an extra salary to hire a person to make the phone calls.

Always treat patients with the utmost respect on the telephone. Keep their financial record close by in case they have questions about their bill; also have their insurance company's phone number handy. Remember that some patients may not understand anything about insurance or third-party payers, so guide them to that understanding and be their advocate in getting as much reimbursement as possible so that the patient's share is smaller. Never simply insist that the insurance plan has paid and the patient's balance is due. This puts the patient in a negative mindset. Try using phrases such as the following:

- "Mrs. Diggs, it looks as if your insurance company paid late last month. I believe you have a co-insurance for your surgery which amounts to $450. Is that what you were expecting? Would you like to take care of the whole balance or split that into two payments? Let me review some of your payment options."
- "Mr. Hildebrand, we're showing that you have a balance due from your surgery. Your insurance has paid, and it looks as if you owe $700. We would be happy to help you by splitting that into two or three payments. When can I schedule that first payment for you?"
- "Mrs. Crumley, it seems that you have a balance due of $450 from your surgery, and I called to see whether I could help you budget that. You could pay $50 this week and split the remaining $400 into two payments over the next 2 months?"

Always abide by office policy when making payment arrangements in collection situations. Never be belligerent with a patient.

AETNA									
Patient Name	Acct #	Primary Insurance	Secondary Insurance	Aging Analysis					Total Balance
				0-30	31-60	61-90	91-120	over 120	
Bassett, Eleanor	75846	AETNA		$145.00	$0.00	$0.00	$0.00	$0.00	$145.00
Herron, John	83029	AETNA		$0.00	$42.41	$0.00	$0.00	$0.00	$42.41
Holt, Maxine	64739	AETNA	BLUE SHIELD	$145.00	$0.00	$0.00	$0.00	$0.00	$145.00
Kellog, Keenan	24537	AETNA		$0.00	$0.00	$145.00	$0.00	$0.00	$145.00
Lincoln, Frank	85940	AETNA		$0.00	$15.00	$0.00	$0.00	$0.00	$15.00
Markham, Melanie	14263	AETNA	MEDICARE	$0.00	$0.00	$0.00	$260.00	$0.00	$260.00
McDonald, Lydia	56374	AETNA		$260.00	$0.00	$0.00	$0.00	$0.00	$260.00
McLean, Mary	24395	AETNA		$0.00	$0.00	$0.00	$0.00	$260.00	$260.00
Aetna Aging Total :				**$550.00**	**$57.41**	**$145.00**	**$260.00**	**$260.00**	**$1,272.41**

FIGURE 16-8 Sample aging report. (From Fordney MT: *Insurance handbook for the medical office,* ed 14, St Louis, 2017, Elsevier.)

If he or she becomes irate, simply state that the person can call back when ready to discuss a solution for paying the account, say good-bye, and gently hang up the phone. Never listen to expletives or allow verbal abuse. Respectfully end the phone call by saying thank you and good bye; do not slam the phone.

Written notification is a must before making a final demand for payment indicating that legal or collection proceedings will be started. Each patient account should be handled individually on the basis of the experience with the patient involved.

General Rules for Telephone Collections

What to Do

- Call the patient when it can be done privately.
- Call only between 8 AM and 9 PM.
- Determine the identity of the person with whom you are speaking. If you ask, "Is this Mrs. Noble?" and she answers, "Yes," it could be the patient's mother-in-law or daughter-in-law, who is also "Mrs. Noble." Use the person's full name. Include suffixes, such as "Thomas Melborn, III." This may sound too formal, but it helps to ensure that the correct person is on the phone.
- Be dignified and respectful. One can be friendly and professional at the same time.
- Ask the patient whether it is a convenient time to talk. Unless you have the attention of the called party, there is little to be gained by continuing. If told that it is an inopportune time, ask for a specific time to call back or get a promise that the patient will call the office at a specified time.
- After a brief greeting, state the purpose of the call. Make no apology for calling, but state the reason in a friendly, business-like way. The provider expects payment, and the medical assistant is interested in helping the patient meet the financial obligation. Open the call with a phrase such as, "This is Alice, Dr. Crawford's medical assistant. I'm calling about your account." A well-placed pause at this point in the call sometimes gets an immediate response from the debtor with regard to the nonpayment.
- Assume a positive attitude. For example, convey the impression that the patient intended to pay, and it is only a matter of working out some suitable arrangements.
- Keep the conversation brief and to the point; do not make threats of any kind.
- Try to get a definite commitment—payment of a certain amount by a certain date.
- Follow up on promises made by the patient. This is best accomplished by using a tickler file or a note on the calendar. If the payment does not arrive by the promised date, remind the patient with another call. If the medical assistant fails to do this, the whole effort has been wasted.

What Not to Do

- Do not call between 9 PM and 8 AM. To do so may be considered harassment.
- Do not make repeated telephone calls on the same day.
- Do not call the debtor's place of work if the employer prohibits personal calls.
- If a call is placed to the debtor at work and the person cannot take the call, leave a message asking the debtor to "call Mrs. Black at 951-727-9238" without revealing the nature of the call; that is, do not state that the call is from "Dr. Crawford's office" or "Dr. Crawford's medical assistant."
- Refrain from showing any kind of hostility. An angry patient is a poorly paying patient. Insulted patients often do not pay at all.

Collection Letters

Some consultants believe that a printed collection letter or reminder enclosed with a statement is more effective than a personal letter. Their attitude is that a patient may be embarrassed by a personal letter and feel that he or she has been singled out for attention. An impersonal printed message will probably encourage the debtor to send a payment.

Letters that are friendly requests for an explanation of why payment has not been made are effective in most cases. These letters should indicate that the provider is sincerely interested in the patient's health and well-being and wants to help resolve the financial obligation. Invite the patient to the office to explain the reasons for nonpayment so that payment arrangements can be made. To lessen the patient's embarrassment, these letters can suggest that previous statements may have been overlooked.

When receiving these letters, most patients make some effort to explain their failure to make payment. If a patient really is having financial difficulties, he or she may be able to get public assistance. If it is a temporary financial problem, the provider and the patient may together be able to work out a satisfactory installment plan for payment.

The medical assistant often is given a free hand in designing collection patterns and composing collection letters. Many medical assistants compose a series of collection letters using example letters they have found effective. Such a series usually includes at least five letters in varying degrees of forcefulness.

Sometimes even a person with poor paying habits will pay if treated with respect and consideration. The medical assistant should never go beyond the authority granted by the provider in pursuing collections. If questions arise about special collection problems, always check with the provider before proceeding. This is particularly important with patients you do not know personally (e.g., patients the provider has seen in the hospital or at home and patients with no credit history). It is difficult to say whether the effects of pressing collections too hard (which can result in loss of patient good will) are more detrimental than the effects of not pursuing collections diligently enough (which can result in loss of revenue). The provider and the medical assistant should agree on general collection policies, as outlined earlier in this chapter, and the policies should be followed. In all cases in which an account is to be assigned to a collection agency, make sure the provider is aware of this and approves.

In most healthcare facilities, the medical assistant signs collection letters using his or her title, such as "Medical Assistant" below the typewritten signature. Do not list "Collections" below the name, because the patient may assume that the account has been placed with a collection agency. Some providers want to sign these communications personally, but generally the medical assistant who handles the patient accounts also signs the collection letters.

Personal Finance Interviews

Personal finance interviews with patients sometimes can be more effective than a whole series of collection letters. By speaking with a patient face to face, the medical assistant can come to an understanding of the problem more quickly, and an agreement about future payment plans can be reached (Figure 16-9).

Occasionally a patient may undergo a long course of treatment and yet make no attempt to pay anything on the account. Perhaps such a patient is only waiting for the provider or the medical assistant to suggest that a payment be made. When it is known in advance that the patient requires extensive treatment, the matter of payment should be discussed early in the course of treatment, the credit policy should be explained, and some agreement should be reached on a payment plan.

Because medical services are far more **intangible** than any commercial service, collection efforts must not be delayed too long. Any responsible, sincere patient will call the provider's office after receiving a second statement and explain the delay in payment or ask for a payment plan. This is best accomplished in a private, personal interview.

If the account ultimately must be referred to a collector, find a good agency with a high recovery rate. The value of medical accounts diminishes in direct proportion to the length of time that has elapsed since service was provided. All collection activity is costly. Know when to stop and call on the services of a professional agency.

Special Collection Situations

Tracing "Skips"

When a patient account statement is returned marked "Moved—no forwarding address," you may consider this account a "skip." This generally is accepted as an indication that the patient is attempting to avoid liability for debts, although some skips are innocent errors. The patient may have been careless in not leaving a forwarding address, or the mistake may have occurred in the healthcare facility. However, immediate action should be taken with regard to returned patient account statements. Do not wait until the next billing cycle to attempt to trace the debtor.

The Internet can be a valuable tool in tracing skips. You can use the online white pages to search for the patient's name.

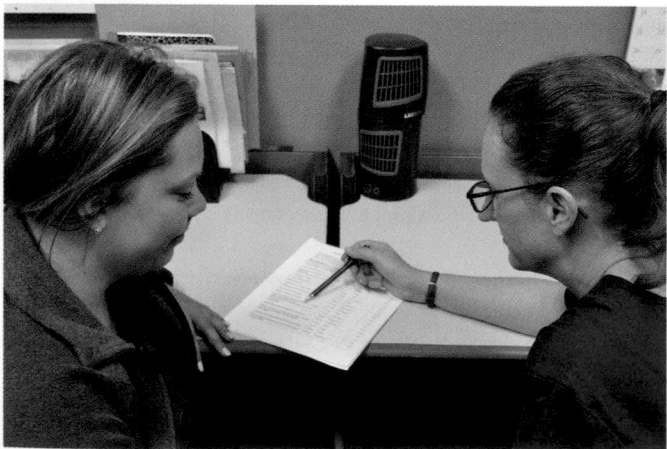

FIGURE 16-9 A face-to-face personal finance interview may motivate patients to take steps to settle their account balances.

Patients might even be found on social networking sites, such as Facebook, and that information may provide clues about the person's whereabouts. Investigate the search results carefully so that collection efforts are directed at the right person. If all attempts fail, turn the account over to a collection agency without delay. Do not keep a skip account too long because as time passes, the trail may become so cold that even collection experts will be unable to follow it.

Suggestions for Tracing Skips

- Examine the patient's original office registration card.
- Call the telephone number listed in the patient account record. Occasionally a patient may move without leaving a forwarding address but will transfer the old telephone number.
- If you are unable to contact the individual by telephone, make a few discreet calls to the references listed on the registration card to get leads.
- Check the Internet to secure the names and telephone numbers of neighbors or the landlord and contact these people to secure information about the debtor's whereabouts.
- Do not inform a third party that the patient owes money. Simply state that you are trying to locate or verify the location of the individual.
- Check the guarantor's place of employment for information. If the person is a specialist in his or her field of work, the local union or similar organizations may be contacted. Although they may not give you the person's current address, they will relay the message that you are seeking to contact him or her. Often people are stirred to pay if they think their employer may learn of their payment failure.
- Do not communicate with a third party more than once. This is specifically forbidden by law (Public Law 95-109, Sec. 804) unless the third party requests the collector to do so.

Claims Against Estates

The patient account record of a deceased patient may be handled a little differently from regular bills. Courtesy dictates that a bill not be sent during the initial period of bereavement, but do not delay longer than 30 days. The **executor** will expect to receive the statements from all healthcare providers. Use the following format to address the statement:

- Estate of (name of patient)
- c/o (spouse or next of kin, if known)
- Patient's last known address

Do not address the statement to a relative unless you have a signed agreement that that person will be financially responsible. If for some reason the statement cannot be addressed as just suggested (e.g., if the patient was in an assisted-living facility or a skilled nursing facility and no relative's name is available), seek information from the county where the estate is being settled.

A will generally is filed within 30 days of a death. The name of the executor usually can be obtained by sending a request to the Probate Department of the Superior Court, County Recorder's Office, in the county where the **decedent** lived. The time limits for filing an estate claim are determined by the state where the decedent resided.

After the name of the administrator or executor of the estate has been obtained, send a duplicate itemized statement of the account to that person by certified mail, return receipt requested. If no response is received in 10 days, contact the executor or the county clerk where the estate is being settled and obtain forms for filing a claim against the estate. This claim against the estate must be made within a certain time, which varies from 2 to 36 months, depending on the state where it is filed.

The executor of the estate either accepts or rejects the claim, and if it is accepted, sends an acknowledgment of the debt. Payment often is delayed because of the legal complications involved in settling an estate, but if the claim has been accepted, the provider eventually receives the payment. If the claim is rejected and there is full justification for claiming the bill, file a claim against the executor according to state laws. The time limit in such cases starts with the date on the letter of rejection sent in response to the original claim.

Because states have different time limits and statutes with regard to these issues, the medical assistant should contact the provider's attorney or the local court for the exact procedure to follow; or, the provider may prefer to turn such matters over to his or her legal counsel immediately.

Bankruptcy

Bankruptcy laws were passed to secure equal distribution of the assets of an individual among the individual's creditors. These are federal laws that apply in all the states. When notified that a patient has declared bankruptcy, do not send statements or make any attempt to collect on the account from the patient.

Chapter 7 bankruptcy usually is a "no asset" situation. Because the provider's charges are considered an **unsecured debt**, there is little purpose in pursuing collection. Chapter 13 is known as *wage earner bankruptcy*, which means that the patient-debtor pays to a **trustee** a fixed amount agreed upon by the court. This money is passed on to the creditors. During this period, none of the creditors can attach the debtor's wages or otherwise attempt to collect the debt. However, the debts are paid in order, secured debts first; consequently, the provider may never receive payment from a debtor who has filed bankruptcy.

Using a Collection Agency

The medical assistant should try every means possible to collect on accounts before they become delinquent. As soon as the account is determined uncollectible through the office (i.e., the patient has failed to respond to the final letter or has failed to fulfill a second promise on payment), the provider should send the account to the collector. Skips should be assigned immediately.

Even though collection by an agency means sacrificing 40% to 60% of the amount owed, further delay only reduces the chances of recovery by the professional collector. If the agency finds that the case deserves special consideration, it will ask the provider's advice before proceeding further.

The collection agency chosen represents the healthcare practice. Therefore, the practice should ensure that its patients are treated with as much respect and dignity as possible through the collection process. There are many different collection agencies, so if one doesn't work out, prepare to switch to another that can better represent the healthcare practice.

CRITICAL THINKING APPLICATION   **16-5**

Brenda has had several complaints about the collection agency used by the office. Patients have called to report that the collectors are threatening and unprofessional. The collection agency's supervisor has been disrespectful to patients and has said that because they owe the money, the collection agency's job is to collect the account in whatever way necessary. How should the healthcare facility approach the collection agency about these complaints?

Working With the Collection Agency

A collection agency needs certain data to enable it to begin collection procedures on overdue accounts:

- Full name of the guarantor
- Name of the spouse
- Last known address
- Full amount of the debt
- Date of the last entry on account
- Occupation of the debtor
- Employer address and phone number

After an account has been released to a collection agency, the healthcare facility can make no further collection attempts. Once the agency has begun its work, a number of guidelines and procedures should be followed:

- Send no more patient account statements.
- The patient account record should be closed for activity because the account was forwarded to a collection agency.
- Refer the patient to the collection agency if he or she contacts the office about the account.
- Promptly report any payments made directly to your office to the collection agency and pay the collection agency's fee.
- Call the agency if any information is obtained that will be of value in tracing or collecting the account.

Making the Decision to Sue

The provider must decide whether he or she will benefit or suffer loss of good will by suing for a balance due rather than writing it off as a loss. Some providers believe it is unwise to resort to the court to collect medical bills unless extraordinary circumstances apply.

An account must be considered a 100% loss to the provider before legal proceedings are started. Remember never to threaten to begin legal proceedings unless the provider is prepared to carry out the threat and has decided to pursue legal action. If the provider decides in favor of a lawsuit, investigate thoroughly and obtain as much information as possible for the proceedings. Litigation to collect a balance due generally is in order when the following are true:

- The patient can afford to pay without hardship.
- The provider can produce office records that support the bill.
- The provider can justify the amount of the bill by comparing it with fee practices in the community.
- The patient's general condition after treatment is satisfactory.
- The persuasive powers of an ethical collection agency have been exhausted, and the agency advises suing.
- The patient can be given ample warning of the provider's intention to sue.

- The defendant (whether a patient or a parent or legal guardian) is legally liable for the services rendered to the patient.
- The statute of limitations has ruled out any possible malpractice action.
- The provider is neither indignant nor in a negative frame of mind.

Small Claims Court

Many healthcare practices find **small claims court** a satisfactory, inexpensive means of collecting delinquent accounts. The state law places a limit on the amount of debt for which relief may be sought in small claims court; this limit should be checked in local courts before recovery is sought in this manner.

Parties to small claims actions are not represented by an attorney at the hearing but may send another person to court on their behalf to produce records supporting the claim. Providers often send their medical assistant with records of unpaid accounts to show the judge.

If the court awards a judgment for the amount owed, the **plaintiff** in small claims court may also recover the costs of the suit. For a very small investment in time and money, the provider who uses this method saves the time of a civil court action and eliminates attorneys' fees.

After being awarded a judgment, the healthcare practice must still collect the money. The only person in a small claims action who has the right of appeal is the defendant. An appeal by the defendant may have the judgment set aside. The plaintiff cannot file an appeal in a small claims action; the decision of the court is final.

The necessary papers for filing action and full instructions on the course to follow may be obtained from the clerk of the local small claims court. It would be wise for a medical assistant who has never appeared in court to attend once as a spectator to preview the procedure; this should allow him or her to feel more at ease when appearing for the provider.

A collection agency to which an account may have been assigned may not file or handle a small claims action. It must either sue in the regular municipal or justice court or attempt to collect the debt in some other manner.

Special Bookkeeping Entries for Collections

Some patient accounts are difficult to collect on; the patient may send a bad check for payment or may lack the desire or ability to pay. These situations call for special bookkeeping entries to keep the patient account in balance. Such entries may be made either with the practice management software or a pegboard system:

- Nonsufficient funds checks (NSF)
- Collection agency transactions

Nonsufficient Funds Checks (NSF)

Nonsufficient funds (NSF) checks occur when a patient pays with a check without having sufficient funds in the bank to cover the payment. The bank will return the check to the healthcare practice marked NSF and will charge the practice's bank account a returned check fee. The payment posted to the patient account must be reversed. It is important to note that the original payment is not deleted; instead, a charge line item is added to the patient account record with the amount of the NSF check. The transaction description should read "NSF Date 02/23/20–". Many medical offices add additional line items for NSF fee charges, but this is up to the discretion of the provider.

Posting Collection Agency Transactions

Collection agencies charge the healthcare practice different percentages of the amount owed to collect delinquent accounts; the agency with the cheapest fee is rarely the most effective. Agencies pay the *net back,* which is the amount of money paid to the practice after the agency has been paid its fee. The net back is the figure that should be considered when a collection agency is used, not simply the fee percentage. If a patient sends a payment after the account has been turned over to a collection agency, the payment must be recorded in the patient account record. Because the agency charges a fee for their collection efforts, the amount sent to the healthcare facility might be less than the actual payment amount. For instance, if the agency charges 25%, a $100 payment results in a $75 payment to the healthcare facility and the agency keeps $25. When posting the payment, the patient account must credit the full amount paid to the collection agency. This would be done by posting a $75 payment and $25 adjustment.

MANAGING FUNDS IN THE HEALTHCARE FACILITY

As mentioned previously, the purpose of financial management is to ensure that the healthcare facility earns enough money to cover its operating expenses. The financial records of the healthcare facility should show the following at all times:

- How much money was earned in a given period
- How much money was collected
- How much money is owed
- The distribution of all operational expenses

An accountant hired by the healthcare facility can prepare monthly and annual financial records from daily bookkeeping records. Periodic analyses of financial resources result in improved business practices, improved time management, elimination of unprofitable services, and more efficient expense budgeting. For the medical assistant, it is crucial to understand the difference between accounts receivable and accounts payable.

Accounts Receivable (A/R)

Accounts receivable is money that is expected but has not yet been received. The amount charged on the encounter form becomes the account receivable for the healthcare facility. When the payment on the patient account record is made, the received payment becomes cash on hand.

To disclose any discrepancies between the balance in all patient accounts and the current account receivable balance, a *trial balance* should be performed monthly, using the following computation:

Accounts receivable at first of month	$ _____
Plus total charges for month	$ _____
Subtotal	$ _____
Less total payments for month	$ _____
Subtotal	$ _____
Less total adjustments for month	$ _____
Accounts receivable at end of month	$ _____

The end of the month accounts receivable figure must agree with the figure arrived at by adding all the patient account balances. The accounts are then said to be *in balance*. If the two totals do not agree, this discrepancy should be brought to the attention of the accountant for resolution.

Accounts Payable (A/P)

Accounts payable is the management of debt incurred and not yet paid. All invoices, statements, and operational expenses are included in accounts payable. When expenses have been paid, they are no longer categorized as accounts payable.

Invoices and Statements

If delivered products are not paid for at the time of purchase, the vendor usually includes an **invoice** for payment with delivery of the merchandise. An invoice describes the products delivered and shows the amount due. Always check to verify that the items listed on the packing slip and invoice are included in the delivery.

Invoices should be placed in a designated accounts payable folder until paid. The healthcare facility may make more than one purchase from the same vendor during the month and send only a single payment at the end of the month for all deliveries.

Paying for Purchases

At the time of payment, compare the statement with the invoice to verify its accuracy. Then, fasten the statement and invoice together, write the date, the amount paid, and the check number on the statement, and place it in the Paid file.

CRITICAL THINKING APPLICATION   16-6

Brenda does not recall ordering a certain item from the office supply company. However, it was included in her last shipment and was shown on the packing list. How can she determine whether the item was ordered?

CLOSING COMMENTS

Patient accounts management and collections are critical responsibilities in the healthcare facility, and a responsible medical assistant is a great asset in this important area. Always maintain a positive attitude with patients when discussing financial matters. Remember that people who are ill or facing challenges are not always cordial, so they may not respond positively to discussion of their patient account balances. Make every attempt to work with each patient to develop a financial plan for settling the account balance. The healthcare facility works hard to collect every dollar, so effective financial management is essential for practice success.

Patient Education

In some cases patients may not fully appreciate all the costs involved in providing high-quality health care. The medical assistant may need to respectfully educate the patient about the basic costs associated with the services provided by the healthcare facility. Patients may not need a lengthy explanation, but they should be informed that the provider does not set his or her fees arbitrarily. The healthcare facility office is a small business, and like thousands of other small businesses, it should collect enough money to cover its operating expenses.

Legal and Ethical Issues

A patient who has filed for bankruptcy cannot be contacted or billed further. Another legal concern is that a threat to send a patient's account into collections should not be made unless this is the provider's intention. Never tell a patient that the provider intends to take action if the provider does not plan to follow through.

Because collection laws vary greatly from state to state, medical assistants should review the statutes pertaining to billing and collecting in the area of the healthcare facility's address. Develop a strong understanding of what is required of small businesses in collecting fees and billing patients for their financial responsibility. Remember that laws change often, so it is important to update the healthcare facility's policies on billing and collecting to reflect current statutes.

Professional Behaviors

The medical assistant is responsible for coordinating communication between the patient and the provider about financial issues. Some patients may act belligerently toward or try to bully the medical assistant in an effort to reduce their financial obligation. Be sure to inform the patient that the provider's decision about the patient's financial responsibility is not based on the medical assistant's discretion. Also, explain that the medical assistant represents the provider in his or her financial decision making. If the patient's behavior is out of control, politely excuse yourself and consult with the office manager. Inform the manager of all the details of the encounter, including the healthcare provider's instructions regarding the patient's account. The more information you give the office manager, the better able he or she will be to represent you in discussing the matter with the patient. During the entire encounter, remember to remain professional and treat the patient with respect, even though that respect may not be reciprocated.

SUMMARY OF SCENARIO

Brenda has learned much about the different types of bookkeeping transactions performed daily in the healthcare facility. She is never hesitant to confer with Mr. Schmidt, the CPA, whenever she has a question about how to post a transaction in the patient account record. As she gains more experience, she appreciates the important role of patient accounts collection in their practice's cash flow and their ability to cover its operating expenses.

Dr. Wilkins follows a conservative philosophy when it comes to accounts payable, which enables her to manage her finances wisely. As a result, Dr. Wilkins can provide job security to her best employees, including Brenda.

SUMMARY OF LEARNING OBJECTIVES

1. **Define, spell, and pronounce the terms listed in the vocabulary.**
   Spelling and pronouncing bookkeeping terms correctly reinforce the medical assistant's credibility. Knowing the definitions of these terms promotes confidence in communication with patients and co-workers.

2. **Define bookkeeping and all of the different transactions recorded in patient accounts.**
   Bookkeeping is the recording of financial transactions in the patient account records. Charges, payments, and adjustments can all be recorded in patient accounts.

3. **Do the following related to patient accounts records:**
   - *List the necessary data elements in patient accounts records.*
     Patient account records should include all information pertinent to collecting the account, such as the name and address of the guarantor, insurance identification, home and business telephone numbers, name of employer, any special instructions for billing, and emergency or alternative contact information.
   - *Discuss a pegboard (manual bookkeeping) system.*
     Although we live in a tech-savvy world, many providers still use a manual pegboard system. There are advantages and disadvantages in using a manual bookkeeping system.
   - *Explain when transactions are recorded in the patient account.*
     Once the provider has entered the procedures into the electronic encounter form, the medical assistant reviews the encounter form and enters the charges into the patient account record.
   - *Perform accounts receivable procedures for patient accounts, including charges, payments, and adjustments.*
     Practice management software systems automatically calculate the correct fees or charges when a CPT/HCPCS code is entered (see Procedure 16-1). All insurance payment amounts posted should also match the total amount paid on the Explanation of Benefits (EOB). The patient account record should have a column for the adjustment to be posted as a credit (Procedure 16-2).

4. **Describe special bookkeeping procedures for patient account records, including credit balances, third-party payments, and refunds; explain how to interact professionally with third-party representatives.**
   A credit balance occurs when a patient has paid in advance or an overpayment or duplicate payment is made. Third-party payments are reimbursement payments made from an insurance company that provides benefits for the patient. Refunds are made to insurance companies for overpayments made on patient accounts.

   Some tips for interacting professionally with third-party representatives include (1) before dialing provider services, have all documents readily accessible to discuss the patient account, and (2) when the health insurance representative comes on the phone, refrain from telling him or her how long the wait was; the representatives usually don't have much control over wait times.

5. **Discuss payment at the time of service, and give an example of displaying sensitivity when requesting payment for services rendered.**
   The medical assistant must believe that the provider and the facility have a right to charge for the services provided. Do not be embarrassed to ask for payment for the valuable services the clinician provides. When tact and good judgment are used in billing and collecting, patients appreciate the service they receive and the help the medical assistant provides. Give each patient individual attention and personal consideration; also, be courteous and show a sincere desire to help the patient with financial problems.

6. **Describe the impact of the Truth in Lending Act on collections policies for patient accounts.**
   If credit options are offered for patients, the healthcare facility should be in compliance with Regulation Z of the Truth in Lending Act (TILA). If an agreement exists between provider and patient that the healthcare facility will accept full payment in more than four installments, the healthcare facility must provide a Federal Truth in Lending Statement, even if no finance fees are charged, and it should be signed by the healthcare facility representative and the patient.

7. **Discuss ways to obtain credit information, and explain patient billing and payment options.**
   Credit information is confidential and should be guarded carefully. Healthcare facilities usually send patient account statements for payment in cycles, which allows a consistent flow of income to the office. A section of patient accounts is billed either weekly or biweekly, and patients send in their payments by mail, bring them in personally, or use an online payment system. Payment is usually requested at the time of service, especially if the patient uses a managed care system that requires a copayment. Medicare Advance Beneficiary Notices provide an option for patients to pay the provider's fee schedule in full to receive services that Medicare does not cover. Minors cannot be held financially responsible for a bill unless they are emancipated, and the medical profession traditionally has accepted the responsibility of providing occasional medical care for those unable to pay for services rendered. Problems can arise when a provider begins to reduce his or her fees.

8. **Review policies and procedures for collecting outstanding balances.**
   Most of today's healthcare facilities use statements from their practice management software to prompt patients to pay overdue bills. Often a message can be added to monthly statements that are increasingly more urgent, depending on the age of the account. Outstanding balances are also collected using telephone calls, e-mails, and personal discussions with the patient or guarantor. More advance collection methods must be used, under the provider's supervision, if the patient account balance goes without payment. Providers may take special circumstances into consideration (e.g., patient financial hardship) in deciding whether to assign a patient account to collection.

SUMMARY OF LEARNING OBJECTIVES—*continued*

9. Do the following related to collection procedures:

- *Describe successful collection techniques for patient accounts.*
  The medical assistant can use a variety of techniques to collect patient accounts, such as collection phone calls, collection letters, and skip tracing. Often more than one technique must be used to obtain payment. Always be courteous and kind when using collection techniques.

- *Discuss strategies for collecting outstanding balances through personal finance interviews.*
  Personal finance interviews with patients sometimes can be more effective than a whole series of collection letters. By speaking with a patient face to face, the medical assistant can come to an understanding of the problem more quickly, and an agreement about future payment plans can be reached.

- *Describe types of adjustments made to patient accounts, including nonsufficient checks (NSF) and collection agency transactions.*
  With a check drawn on an account with insufficient funds, the bank returns the check to the healthcare facility marked "NSF" and charges the healthcare facility bank account a returned check fee. The payment posted to the patient account must be reversed. Note that the originally payment is not deleted; rather, a charge line item is added with the amount of the NSF check; the transaction description should read

"NSF Date 02/23/20-". Many medical offices add additional line items for NSF fee charges, but this is up to the discretion of the provider. Because collection agencies charge a fee for their collection efforts, the amount credited to the patient's account might be less than the actual payment amount.

10. Define bookkeeping terms, including *accounts receivable* and *accounts payable*.
Accounts receivable is money that is expected but has not yet been received. The amount charged on the encounter form becomes the account receivable for the healthcare facility. Accounts payable is the management of debt incurred and not yet paid. All invoices, statements, and operational expenses are included in accounts payable. Once expenses have been paid, they are no longer categorized as accounts payable.

11. Discuss patient education, in addition to legal and ethical issues, related to patient accounts, collections, and practice management.
Patient accounts management and collections are critical responsibilities in the healthcare facility, and a responsible medical assistant is a great asset in this important area. The medical assistant may need to respectfully educate a patient about various things related to payment. Medical assistants should always review their state's statutes pertaining to billing and collecting.

CONNECTIONS

Study Guide Connection: Go to the Chapter 16 Study Guide. Read and complete the activities.

evolve Evolve Connection: Go to the Chapter 16 link at *evolve.elsevier.com/kinn* to complete the Chapter Review Quiz. Check out the other resources listed for this chapter to make the most of what you have learned from Patient Accounts, Collections, and Practice Management.

17

BANKING SERVICES AND PROCEDURES

SCENARIO

Laura has been working at Ambulatory Surgical Care Associates in the back office for the past 3 years. Her primary job has been preparing the daily deposits and visiting the bank every day to make the deposits. A bank representative stopped by the healthcare facility to show Laure some time efficient ways to bank with mobile depositing and online banking. Before she started her medical assisting education, Laura had worked as a part-time teller at City National Bank. She is looking forward to using online banking and managing the healthcare facility's many bank accounts.

Although Laura had some banking experience, working at Ambulatory Surgical Care Associates has helped her realize that she still has much to learn about the daily financial duties in a healthcare facility, including working with the patient account management software, making daily deposits, reconciling bank statements, and many other banking responsibilities.

Laura wants to increase the value of the healthcare facility's bank accounts by looking for bank accounts that pay a higher interest rate and by reducing the office's operational expenses. Laura also wants to encourage patients at the healthcare facility to use debit or credit cards, instead of checks, to pay for services, because she knows that returned patient checks have created problems.

While studying this chapter, think about the following questions:
- How is online banking affecting banking in healthcare facilities?
- How can an office manager determine whether an employee can be trusted with banking procedures?
- What precautions should the healthcare facility take when accepting patient payments?
- Why is making daily deposits a good idea?
- How can the office manager reconcile the bank account, and why is this important?

LEARNING OBJECTIVES

1. Define, spell, and pronounce the terms listed in the vocabulary.
2. Explain the purpose of the Federal Reserve Bank and the types of banks it manages.
3. Identify common types of bank accounts.
4. Do the following related to banking in today's business world:
   - Discuss the importance of signature cards.
   - Explain how online banking has made standard banking processes more efficient.
   - Review the benefits of customer-oriented banking.
5. Do the following related to checks:
   - Compare different types of negotiable instruments.
   - Identify precautions in accepting checks from patients.
   - Explain how checks are processed from one account to another.
   - Review the procedure followed when the healthcare facility receives a nonsufficient funds (NSF) check.
6. Identify precautions in accepting cash.
7. Discuss the use of debit and credit cards, including advantages and precautions.
8. Do the following related to banking procedures in the ambulatory care setting:
   - Describe banking procedures as related to the ambulatory care setting.
   - Explain the importance of depositing checks daily.
   - Prepare a bank deposit.
   - Compare types of check endorsements.
9. Review check-writing procedures used to pay the operational expenses of a healthcare facility.
10. Understand the purpose of bank account reconciliation for auditing purposes.
11. Discuss patient education, as well as legal and ethical issues, related to banking services and procedures.

VOCABULARY

checking account A bank account against which checks can be written and funds can be transferred to the payable party.

discretionary income Money in a bank account that is not assigned to pay for any office expenses.

embezzlement The misuse of a healthcare facility's funds for personal gain.

EMV chip technology Global technology that includes imbedded microchips that store and protect cardholder data; also called *chip and PIN* and *chip and signature*.

endorser The person who signs his or her name on the back of a check for the purpose of transferring all rights in the check to another party.

Federal Reserve Bank The central bank of the United States. The Federal Reserve system consists of a seven-member Board of Governors with headquarters in Washington, D.C., and 12 Federal Reserve banks in major cities throughout the country.

interest A payment the bank makes in exchange for using money.

negotiable instruments A document used to withdraw money from one bank account and deposit it into another.

principal A capital sum of money due as a debt or used as a fund for which interest is either charged or paid.

Financial transactions in the healthcare facility involve the accepting of funds from insurance companies and patients. Most healthcare institutions use bank accounts to deposit their reimbursements to pay their expenses. A medical assistant who works in the front office is responsible for accepting a variety of payments, endorsing and depositing checks, writing checks for office expenses, and regularly reconciling bank and credit card statements. Mobile deposit allows for healthcare facilities to deposit checks on the date payments are received because it is conveniently done in the office. The medical assistant will have to master basic math skills such as addition and subtraction for all banking functions.

BANKING IN TODAY'S BUSINESS WORLD

Banks can be used to centralize all financial transactions for a healthcare facility. The bank account details all deposits, withdrawals, and transfers so that the opening balance exactly matches the closing balance at the end of the previous month. Monthly bank account balances can help healthcare facilities establish and maintain a monthly operational budget. Banks also provide opportunities to earn **interest** and to invest for future financial gain. Overall, banks organize funds for the financial management of the healthcare facility.

Fees for banking services depend on the bank and products used (Table 17-1). The type of bank the medical practice will use is a decision made by the provider and the office manager, depending on the needs of the medical practice.

Although the **Federal Reserve Bank** manages all banks in the United States, healthcare facilities can choose from a number of different types of banks with which to do business:

- *Retail banks:* Offer basic banking services to the public; these banks have hundreds of branches to provide easy consumer access.

TABLE 17-1	Common Banking Fees		
FEE	**DESCRIPTION**	**AVERAGE FEE**	**WAIVABLE?**
Account maintenance fee	Fee for using the bank account	$5 to $25 per month	Some bank accounts waive monthly account maintenance fees if a specific balance is maintained in the account or if direct deposit is used.
Overdraft fee	Fee for the bank paying a check or debit when the balance is not in the account	$25 to $40 per occurrence	Not usually. To avoid the fee in the future, tie the checking account with an overdraft account just in case the balance is low.
Returned deposit fee	Fee charged when a deposited check is returned from the drawer's account	$5 to $10 per occurrence	Not usually. However, the practice can require the check drawer to cover this expense because the check did not clear his or her account.
Hard copy statement fee	Fee for the bank to send paper copies of bank statements	$5 to $10 per statement	This fee can be avoided by downloading all electronic bank statements when they are released.
Nonsufficient funds (NSF) fee	Fee charged when a check is written against an account with not enough funds and the check is returned unpaid	$25 to $40 per occurrence	Not usually. To avoid the fee in the future, tie the checking account with an overdraft account just in case the balance is low.
Transaction fee	Fee charged when too many transactions are made on a bank account	$.50 to $1.00 per transaction	Online banking is usually free, but nowadays banks are charging fees to visit bank branches and to complete transactions with customer service over the phone.

- *Commercial banks:* Offer business banking services to businesses of all sizes; they are equipped to handle large volumes of check deposits and credit card transactions.
- *Credit unions:* Nonprofit banking institutions owned by members; credit unions use the funds deposited to make loans to their members, which enables them to offer loans at lower than market rates.
- *Online banks:* Offer basic banking services at competitive rates because all banking transactions are done online; there are no branch locations to visit.

The medical assistant most likely will manage only the bank accounts set up for the income and operational expenses of the healthcare facility.

The Federal Reserve

In 1913, to provide the nation with a safer, more flexible, and stable monetary and financial system, Congress created the Federal Reserve Banking System, making it the central bank of the United States. The system consists of a seven-member Board of Governors with headquarters in Washington, D.C., and 12 Federal Reserve banks in major cities throughout the country (Figure 17-1).

The Federal Reserve Bank monitors the movement of money in the form of checks from one bank account to another. Each check has a routing number, an account number, and an American Bankers Association (ABA) number; these numbers identify which Federal Reserve Bank jurisdiction, bank location, and specific bank accounts are used in each transaction.

For additional information on the Federal Reserve System and its regional banks, visit the system's website at *www.federalreserve.gov.*

Because of the large volume bookkeeping transactions, many healthcare facilities use accounting management software and most online banking systems can download bank account data. These software systems can be complicated to use, so the medical assistant should be in regular contact with the accountant chosen by the provider who can answer questions when needed.

Common Types of Bank Accounts

Checking Accounts

By placing an amount of money on deposit in a bank, a depositor can set up a **checking account.** Simply stated, a checking account is a bank account against which checks can be written and funds can be transferred to the payable party. Banks typically charge a monthly account maintenance fee. In addition, there may be fees associated with banking services such as transferring funds to other banks or using the checking overdraft.

A provider who also owns a healthcare facility often requires at least three separate bank accounts:

- A personal checking account for depositing income and managing personal expenses
- Another checking account for depositing checks for the healthcare facility and for paying office expenses
- A savings account for monies set aside for paying insurance premiums, property taxes, and other seasonal expenses

Savings Accounts

Money that is not needed for current expenditures can be saved and deposited into a savings account. In most cases, savings accounts earn interest on the amount on deposit; that is, the bank pays the depositor a specified monthly percentage to use the money in the savings account. Interest is a payment the bank makes in exchange for using money. It usually is calculated as a percentage of the **principal**. Simple interest is computed annually. Compound interest is figured on the principal and on any previous interest that has been added to the original sum of money; in addition, compound interest can be computed using a variety of time increments (e.g., daily, monthly, quarterly, and so on). Interest-bearing checking accounts draw a small amount of interest, usually 1% or 2%, on the average daily balance. Savings accounts typically pay a higher rate of interest than checking accounts. Interest rates fluctuate with the financial market.

A standard savings account earns interest at the lowest prevailing rate and has no minimum balance requirement and no check-writing privileges. However, penalties apply for withdrawing funds from a savings account more than four times per month. The provider may deposit a certain percentage of **discretionary income** into a savings account each month to earn interest.

Money Market Savings Account

An insured money market savings account requires a minimum balance, anywhere from $500 to $5,000; it draws interest at money market rates (usually a higher percentage rate than for a regular savings account); and it allows only a specified number of checks (frequently three) to be written per month, which requires most bill payments managed through online banking. Such checks usually are written to transfer funds to a checking account. Some businesses transfer excess funds from the business checking account to a money market account over the weekend or over an extended holiday period to draw interest on the funds.

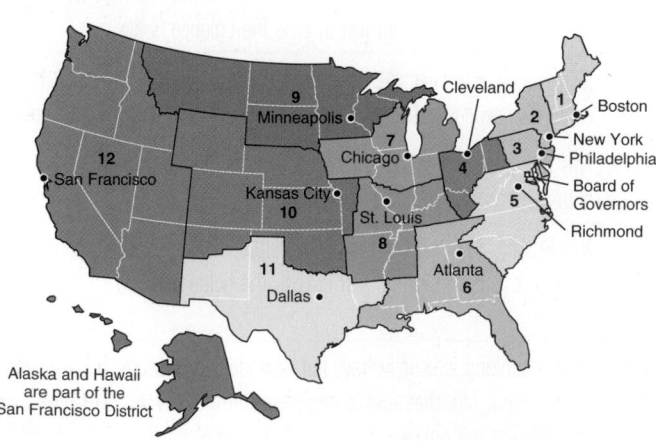

FIGURE 17-1 The 12 Federal Reserve districts.

CRITICAL THINKING APPLICATION 17-1

Dr. Webber knows that Laura worked part-time in a local bank before coming to the clinic. She tells Laura that she is considering changing banks and asks her to research the interest rates on money market accounts at local banks. How does Laura accomplish this task? What type of account would be best for the facility?

Signature Cards

When an account is opened at a bank branch, the account signer is required to provide his or her handwritten signature on a physical or electronic card, which is kept on file with the bank. If a check comes through and some suspicion arises that the depositor's signature has been forged, bank personnel compare the signature on the check with the original on the signature card.

The provider often delegates the task of paying bills to a responsible medical assistant. In this case, any staff member who has been authorized to sign the medical facility's checks must go to the bank and add his or her handwritten signature to the signature card. Only those whose names appear on the signature card are authorized to sign checks, and the bank is responsible for verifying any questionable signatures. The provider is able to designate specific times when the secondary signer is authorized if, for example, the provider is on vacation.

Online Banking

Internet banking has changed the way financial institutions manage money. People once had to fight traffic and wait in line at crowded banks; now, they can bank from their offices any time of day. A healthcare facility's banking transactions, such as paying bills, and transferring funds between accounts, can be done online. In addition, staff members have access to supply companies online and can review costs easily from the office instead of driving to numerous companies to compare prices.

Online banking is a means of performing banking services electronically via the Internet. All banks and credit unions have this capability, and most of them offer both basic and advanced services. With basic services, a customer usually can do the following:

- Check account balances
- Transfer funds between accounts in the same bank
- Pay bills electronically and create checks
- Determine whether a check has cleared the bank
- Download account information
- View images of transactions

A major concern with online banking is fraud. Concern that unauthorized users may gain access to the healthcare facility's account balances are valid. Some experts believe that online banking involves a slightly greater risk of fraud than does conventional banking. Despite the disadvantages, studies show that Internet banking is now mainstream.

Customer-Oriented Banking

Americans want to conduct business and take care of personal concerns on laptops or cell phones on their way to and from work. In addition, the rapid pace of life requires rapid or "instant" solutions; convenience has become a basic expectation of consumers where the banking industry is concerned.

Mobile banking is a customer-oriented innovation that is emerging through the wireless technology. Using wireless devices, such as smart phones and tablets, customers can conduct a variety of financial transactions, set up alerts and notifications when bills are due, and make electronic transfers to pay these bills. Many banks offer banking software applications, which can be downloaded for free on smart phone, tablets, and computers, that allow the user to deposit checks from any location.

A healthcare facility's management personnel should consider the services available through local banks when choosing the best bank for the healthcare facility.

CHECKS

A *check* is a bank draft, or an order to pay a certain sum of money, on demand, to a specified person or entity. When a check is presented for payment, the *drawee* (the bank on which the check is drawn or written) pays the specified sum of money written on the face of the check to the *holder* (the person presenting the check for payment).

A check is considered a *negotiable* instrument. For a check to be negotiable, it must:

- Be written and signed by the drawer
- Contain a promise or order to pay a sum of money
- Be payable on demand or at a fixed future date
- Be payable to order to the drawee

To ensure that the amount is taken from the correct account number, the routing and account numbers are printed with magnetic ink on the bottom of the check. The check should have the amount written as a number and as verbiage to confirm the amount. Finally, the check must be signed and dated by the drawer of the account.

Routing and Account Numbers

A *routing transit number* (RTN) is a nine-digit code printed on the bottom left side of checks. A RTN is assigned to every banking institution under the Federal Reserve Banking System, so it identifies the bank upon which the check was drawn. RTNs also are used for direct deposits and the wiring of funds between banks. The first two digits indicate the Federal Reserve district where the bank is located. The third digit indicates the specific district office. And the rest of the digits represent the individual accounts that belong to the bank.

Bank account numbers are assigned to each individual account. No two accounts in the same financial institution can be the same, even if they belong to the same account holder. *Wire transfers* and *automated clearinghouse (ACH) transfers* use the routing and account numbers to transfer funds between exact accounts. Wire transfers are between two separate banking institutions in which both accounts are verified, so funds are available quickly. ACH transfers also involve two different banking institutions, but because both accounts are not verified, a few extra days are needed for funds to be available.

American Bankers Association Number

The *American Bankers Association number (ABA)* appears in the upper right area of a printed check. The number is used as a simple means of identifying the area location of the bank on which the check is written and the particular bank in that area. The code number is expressed as a fraction (Figure 17-2).

In the top part of the fraction, before the hyphen, the numbers 1 to 49 designate cities in which Federal Reserve banks are located or other key cities; the numbers 50 to 99 refer to states or territories. The part of the number following the hyphen is a number issued to each bank for its own identification purposes. The bottom part of the fraction includes the number of the Federal Reserve district where the bank is located and other identifying information. The ABA number is used to prepare deposit slips and to identify each check.

Types of Negotiable Instruments

The following are different types of **negotiable instruments** are documents used to withdraw money from one bank account and deposit it into another:

- Personal check
- Cashier's check
- Money order
- Business check
- Voucher check

Precautions for Accepting Checks

- Inspect the check carefully for the correct date, amount, and signature.
- Do not accept a check with corrections on it.
- Ask for a state-issued picture ID and compare the signature on the ID to the check signature.
- Do not accept an out-of-town check, government check, payroll check, starter check, unnumbered check, or a non-personalized check.
- Do not accept a third-party check. For example, Mrs. Richards, a patient, receives a check written to her by her neighbor for $30. Mrs. Richards brings the check to her visit with the provider and presents it to the clinic to pay her copayment. If the check is accepted and subsequently returned by the bank, obtaining reimbursement from the patient or the neighbor may be difficult. A check from the patient's health insurance carrier is the only exception.

- When accepting a postal money order for payment, make sure it has only one endorsement. Postal money orders with more than two endorsements will not be honored.
- Do not accept a check marked "Payment in Full" unless it does pay the account in full, up to and including the date on which it is received. If a check so marked is less than the amount due, you will be unable to collect the balance on the account once you have accepted and deposited such a check. It is illegal to cross out the words "Payment in Full."
- Do not accept a check written for more than the amount due; returning cash for the difference between the amount of the check and the amount owed is poor policy. If the check is not honored by the bank, your office suffers the loss not only of the amount of the check, but also of the amount returned in cash.

Personal Check

A personal check is drawn by a bank against funds deposited to a personal account in another bank. Patients typically write these checks for copayments and other financial responsibilities.

Cashier's Check

A cashier's check is a bank's own check, drawn on itself and signed by the bank cashier or other authorized official. A cashier's check is obtained by paying the bank the amount of the check, in cash. Many banks charge a fee for this service. Cashier's checks often are issued to accommodate a savings account customer who does not keep a checking account.

Money Order

Domestic money orders can be purchased at banks, some retail stores, and the U.S. Postal Service. Money orders often are used to pay bills by mail when a person does not have a checking account. The maximum face value varies, depending on the source. Cashier checks are preferable to money orders when larger amounts need to be paid.

Business Checks

Today, most business checks can be prepared through the online banking portal. The checkbook most widely used in the professional office is a ledger-type book with three checks per page and a

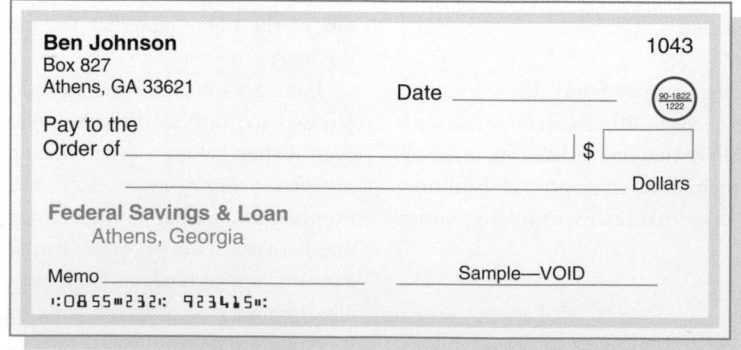

FIGURE 17-2 American Bankers Association (ABA) number.

perforated stub at the left side of the check. Checks may be bound in a soft cover or punched for a ring binder. The checks and matching stubs are numbered in sequence and preprinted with the depositor's name and account number, along with any additional information, such as address and telephone number. Business checks can also be printed through accounting management software programs when vendors submit invoices.

Voucher Check

A voucher check has a detachable voucher form or could be attached to an Explanation of Benefits (EOB). The voucher portion is used to itemize or specify the purpose for which the check was drawn. It shows the amount charged by the provider, the allowable amount, and the amount paid by the insurance company. The voucher portion of the check is removed before the check is presented for deposit; the voucher then is given to the insurance payment poster to post in the patient account record (Figure 17-3).

CRITICAL THINKING APPLICATION 17-2

A new patient wants to pay for his services at the end of the office visit. The charge is $75. The patient writes a check for $100 and asks Laura for $25 in currency in return. How should Laura handle the situation?

How Checks Are Processed from One Bank to Another

Checks received by the drawee's bank are turned over daily to a regional banking clearinghouse, which clears each one. The identifying code numbers, printed on the face of the check with magnetic ink, enable this "clearing" process to be accomplished quickly and efficiently. Checks due from and to all banks outside a specific region are settled by electronic entries. The bank keeps the canceled checks and an electronic copy of the check is returned to the *drawer*, or the writer of the check. When the drawer needs proof of payment, a copy of the check can be requested from the bank, or the drawer can review monthly bank statements for printed copies of cleared checks. Check copies can also be obtained online through the banking portal.

Electronic Checks

In an effort to prevent check fraud, many healthcare facilities accept only electronic checks. When the patient presents a personal check to the healthcare facility, the bottom of the check, which includes the routing and account numbers, is scanned. The funds are then automatically transferred from the patient's checking account and into the healthcare facility's account. Once the transaction has been approved, the paper check is returned to the patient with "VOID" printed across it to show that it has already been used. Electronic checks reduce the time involved in transferring funds from one account to another.

Nonsufficient Funds Check (NSF)

When a check that had been deposited is returned back to the agency, it is called a *nonsufficient funds* (NSF) check ("the check

bounces"). A NSF check is not honored by the bank issuing the check, because there were not sufficient funds in the entity's bank account or the account had been closed. The medical assistant must add the amount of the check plus the NSF fee back to the patient's account balance. Some healthcare facilities will have a set amount that is billed to the patient when a check "bounces."

If the healthcare facility receives an NSF check, call the signer of the check immediately and ask him or her to stop by the office to pay the amount needed to cover the check and the additional fee. Most offices require that such payment be made by another form of payment, preferably credit card. Legal remedies are available for the provider if the check remains unpaid.

Many NSF problems can be cleared up quickly and easily with courtesy and tact, assuming the situation was simply a mistake or an oversight. Bad checks may be reported to several organizations, and once the writer is in their databases, the person will have difficulty writing a check to any business. Credit associations often are a great help when such problems arise. Turn the account over to a qualified collection agency if the practice is unable to collect on the account within a short time. To save time and resources, it may be wise to write off NSF check patient accounts with balances less than $100 if the patient has refused to pay after several requests.

CRITICAL THINKING APPLICATION 17-3

The bank calls Laura to inform her that three of the patient checks deposited last week were NSF. What steps should Laura take to collect the NSF check amounts from the patients? Are there additional charges she can add to the patients' balances to cover the inconvenience?

CASH MANAGEMENT

Some patients may prefer to pay in cash instead of by check or by debit or credit card. Cash transactions can occur with little or no paperwork; therefore, an audit trail is harder to establish.

Patients can request a receipt when they pay cash. However, if there is no canceled check or debit/credit card slip, an employee can easily provide a receipt for payment but then pocket the money for themselves, leaving the balance on the patient's account. To prevent the mismanagement of cash, many healthcare facilities do not allow patients to pay cash for services. Healthcare facilities that have a no-cash payment policy should post a sign in the lobby to inform patients of this in advance. If a patient does not have a bank account, the medical staff can kindly refer the patient to a local money order dealer. Patients may see this as an inconvenience, but the medical assistant should explain that the policy is intended to protect the patient's account.

If the healthcare facility chooses to accept cash payments, keep in mind the following precautions:
- Make sure the cash is not counterfeit; use a marker or tool designed for this purpose to confirm its authenticity. If you suspect that the cash may be counterfeit, do not accept the payment and contact the local FBI office.
- Establish a checks and balance system in which the employee accepting cash must document cash payments on a register and in the patient's account to establish an audit trail.
- Inform patients that change cannot be made for larger bills.

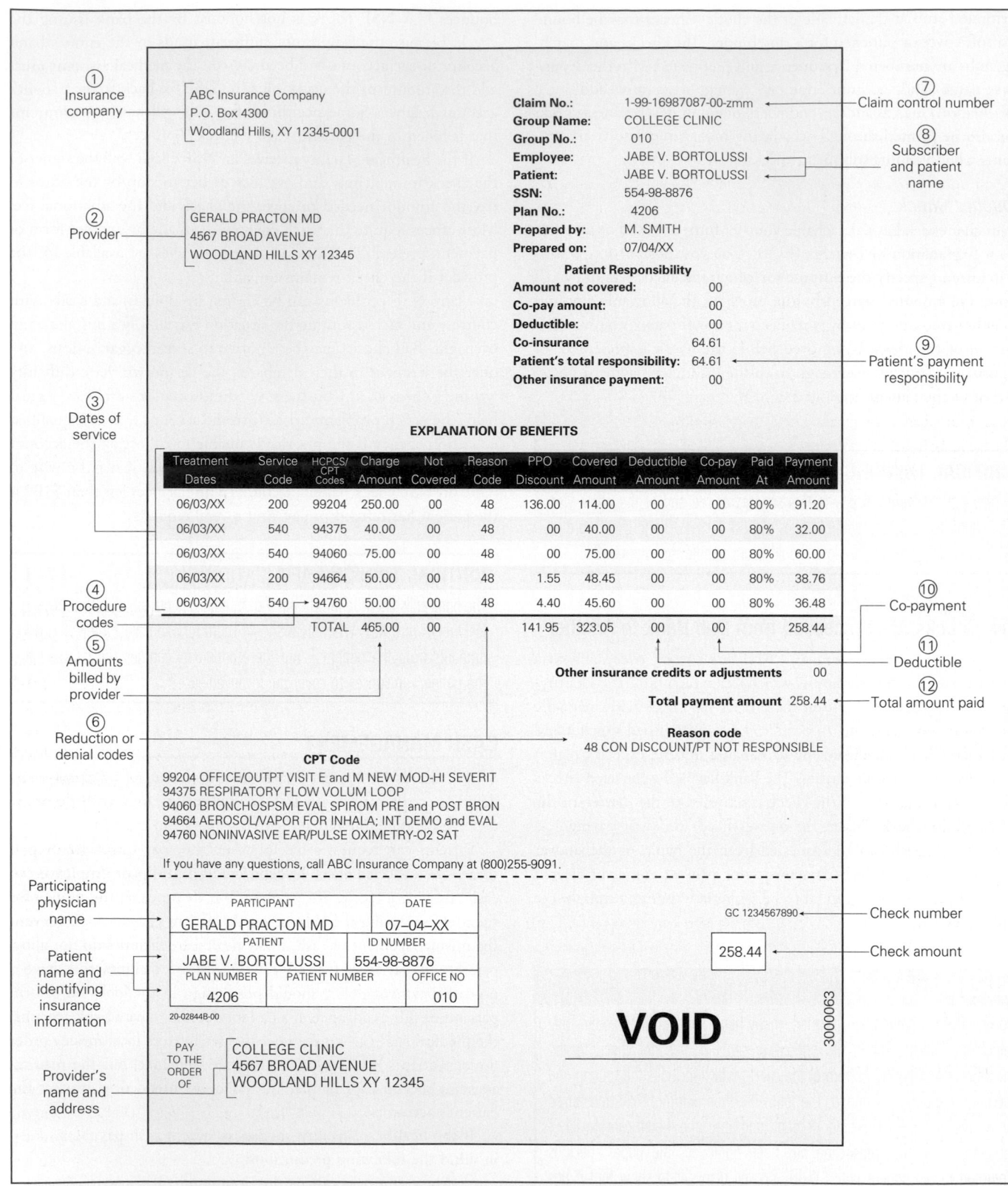

① Insurance company

ABC Insurance Company
P.O. Box 4300
Woodland Hills, XY 12345-0001

② Provider

GERALD PRACTON MD
4567 BROAD AVENUE
WOODLAND HILLS XY 12345

Claim No.:	1-99-16987087-00-zmm
Group Name:	COLLEGE CLINIC
Group No.:	010
Employee:	JABE V. BORTOLUSSI
Patient:	JABE V. BORTOLUSSI
SSN:	554-98-8876
Plan No.:	4206
Prepared by:	M. SMITH
Prepared on:	07/04/XX

⑦ Claim control number

⑧ Subscriber and patient name

Patient Responsibility

Amount not covered:	00
Co-pay amount:	00
Deductible:	00
Co-insurance	64.61
Patient's total responsibility:	64.61
Other insurance payment:	00

⑨ Patient's payment responsibility

EXPLANATION OF BENEFITS

③ Dates of service

Treatment Dates	Service Code	HCPCS/ CPT Codes	Charge Amount	Not Covered	Reason Code	PPO Discount	Covered Amount	Deductible Amount	Co-pay Amount	Paid At	Payment Amount
06/03/XX	200	99204	250.00	00	48	136.00	114.00	00	00	80%	91.20
06/03/XX	540	94375	40.00	00	48	00	40.00	00	00	80%	32.00
06/03/XX	540	94060	75.00	00	48	00	75.00	00	00	80%	60.00
06/03/XX	200	94664	50.00	00	48	1.55	48.45	00	00	80%	38.76
06/03/XX	540	94760	50.00	00	48	4.40	45.60	00	00	80%	36.48
		TOTAL	465.00	00		141.95	323.05	00	00		258.44

④ Procedure codes

⑤ Amounts billed by provider

⑥ Reduction or denial codes

⑩ Co-payment

⑪ Deductible

Other insurance credits or adjustments   00

Total payment amount   258.44 ← Total amount paid

Reason code
48 CON DISCOUNT/PT NOT RESPONSIBLE

CPT Code
99204 OFFICE/OUTPT VISIT E and M NEW MOD-HI SEVERIT
94375 RESPIRATORY FLOW VOLUM LOOP
94060 BRONCHOSPSM EVAL SPIROM PRE and POST BRON
94664 AEROSOL/VAPOR FOR INHALA; INT DEMO and EVAL
94760 NONINVASIVE EAR/PULSE OXIMETRY-O2 SAT

If you have any questions, call ABC Insurance Company at (800)255-9091.

Participating physician name

PARTICIPANT	DATE
GERALD PRACTON MD	07–04–XX

PATIENT	ID NUMBER
JABE V. BORTOLUSSI	554-98-8876

PLAN NUMBER	PATIENT NUMBER	OFFICE NO
4206		010

20-02844B-00

Patient name and identifying insurance information

GC 1234567890 ← Check number

258.44 ← Check amount

VOID

3000063

PAY TO THE ORDER OF	COLLEGE CLINIC 4567 BROAD AVENUE WOODLAND HILLS XY 12345

Provider's name and address

FIGURE 17-3 Sample voucher check. (From Fordney MT: *Insurance handbook for the medical office*, ed 14, St Louis, 2017, Elsevier.)

Debit Cards

The use of debit cards has vastly increased in the United States. Most debit cards are connected to a checking account. When the debit card is used, the amount of the transaction is immediately withdrawn from the available balance in the account. A personal identification number (PIN) is assigned to the card for cash withdrawal and point-of-sale (POS) purchases. The cards usually have a MasterCard or Visa logo and can be used as a credit card wherever they are accepted. The account can still be overdrawn; in most situations, when there are not enough funds in the account to make a purchase, the card is denied unless the account has some type of overdraft protection. Substantial fees may be charged if the bank elects to pay the debit when the account has insufficient funds. Currently, some banks decline debit card charges at the point of sale when an account has insufficient funds, and they do not charge an insufficient funds fee toward the attempted purchase. Stay abreast of recent banking legislation and always follow office policy when accepting debit cards as payment for medical services. The medical assistant may see various types of debit cards in the provider's office. Many states issue a debit card to individuals receiving child support payments or some types of state financial assistance.

Advantages of Using Debit Cards

Using debit cards to transfer funds has many advantages:

1. Debit cards are both safe and convenient, particularly for making payments online.
2. Transactions are completed quickly.
3. The cards can be used either as debit or credit cards. For use as a debit card, the user must have a PIN. For use as a credit card, the user often must provide identification.
4. Specific payments can be easily located online.
5. If stolen or lost, the debit card can be cancelled quickly with minimum liability.
6. Receipts and statements provide a permanent, reliable record of disbursements for tax purposes.
7. The debit card statement provides a summary of receipts.
8. The cards usually can be used anywhere that accepts MasterCard or Visa.

Credit Cards

Credit cards are one of the most common methods of payment from patients. New technology, called *contactless payment systems*, allows payment with a phone or other device that is linked to a credit or debit card. Drawbacks of credit card payments include the small processing fee that is deducted from the amount deposited into the healthcare facility's bank account. There is also an increased risk of fraud when using credit cards.

To help reduce fraud, magnetic strip cards are being replaced with cards imbedded with **EMV chip technology**. These chip cards offer advance security for in-person payments, but the EMV chip cards require a special terminal to read the chips. If a healthcare facility accepts credit or debit cards, it is important to have a terminal that processes the EMV chip cards. Businesses that cannot process the chip cards may be liable for fraud losses to their customers.

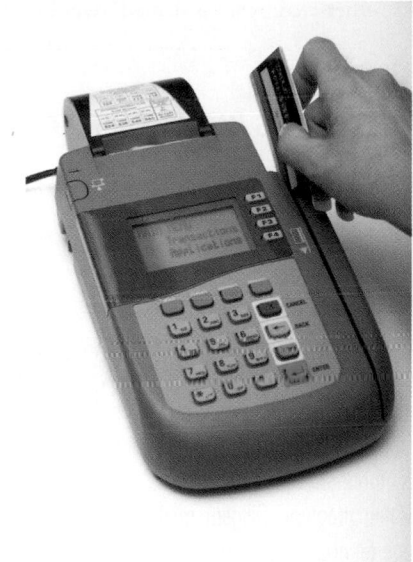

FIGURE 17-4 Example of a magnetic strip card terminal. (From Gaylor LJ: *The administrative dental assistant*, ed 3, St Louis, 2012, Saunders.)

Many credit card processing terminals can accept both credit cards and debit cards (Figure 17-4), and some can also process check payments electronically. Debit card transactions use a PIN but do not need a patient's signature. Credit card transactions do not need a PIN, but patients must sign a credit card slip. Electronic check processing requires patients to submit a signed check in which the routing number and account number are scanned by the credit card terminal. Once these numbers have been scanned, a transfer of funds into the healthcare facility's bank account is initiated. All three types of accounting transactions will transfer the amount charged directly into the healthcare facility's bank account.

Although using the credit card processing terminal incurs per-transaction charges, valuable time is saved because an office employee does not need to visit the bank branch to make the daily deposit. Credit card transactions also can reduce the chances of money mismanagement in the office, such as **embezzlement**.

Precautions for Accepting Credit and Debit Cards

Just as the medical assistant must take precautions when accepting checks, care must be taken when accepting a credit or debit card as payment for medical services. The first precaution should be to make certain the person presenting the card is the person to whom it was issued. Always ask for a state-issued ID, and compare the name and signature to the ones on the credit card. Follow the healthcare facility's policy on verifying identity if the name on the state-issued ID does not match the name on the credit card. Sometimes, a married couple may use each other's cards, but if the office is strict about the card acceptance policy, then the spouse may need to be present in the office for the medical assistant to accept the card. Some patients may use a prepaid credit card, which is purchased with cash and does not have the patient's name printed on it, to make payments on their accounts. These cards, if allowed by office policy, pay just like a normal credit card. If a patient becomes belligerent if his or her credit card is denied, refer him or her to the office manager.

BANKING PROCEDURES IN THE AMBULATORY CARE SETTING

Healthcare facilities use bank accounts to deposit (as cash, checks, or debit or credit card transactions) and to pay their operational expenses by check or credit card (Box 17-4).

BOX 17-4   Accounting Management Software

Accounting management software can simplify the banking transactions of healthcare facilities. This type of software is compatible with many online banking portals; therefore, daily transactions can be downloaded directly into the accounting program. Diligent medical assistants who download daily can manage all account balances on a regular basis. Office expenses and invoices can be entered into the accounting management software as accounts payable, and payments can be scheduled for entered invoices. Checks to vendors can be printed at any time from the accounting software, documenting the transaction—and documented transactions make bank reconciliation a snap!

Making Bank Deposits

The medical assistant should make daily bank deposits, which minimizes the risks of keeping large sums of money on hand, and it also makes the money available for paying expenses. Depositing checks daily is important for these reasons:

- Checks may have a restricted time payment or may be lost, misplaced, or stolen over time.
- A stop-payment order may be placed, or it may be returned for insufficient funds.
- Prompt processing is a courtesy to the payer.

Preparing the Deposit

The medical assistant must prepare a deposit slip (ticket) that accompanies the funds being deposited. The deposit slip can be paper or electronic and itemizes the cash or checks being deposited. It provides the bank account information into which the funds need to be deposited (Figure 17-5). All details of the daily deposit should be recorded in the accounting software program; each check should be entered separately. The check number, payer, and check amount should also be recorded in the accounting software program so that the deposit amount from the software matches the bank deposit record. Many banks require that deposits be made before 3 PM if the deposit is to be credited that business day (Procedure 17-1).

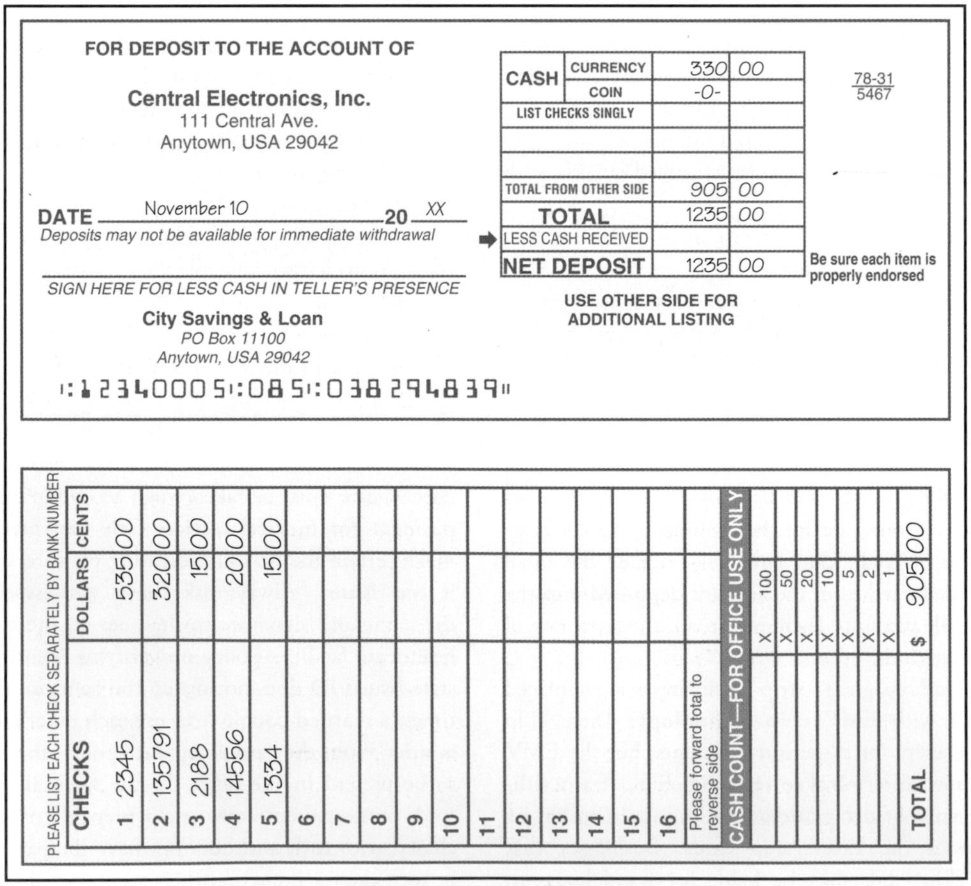

FIGURE 17-5 Front and back of a deposit slip.

Other options to deposit checks include using a credit card terminal that processes checks electronically at the time of payment. Small healthcare facilities can snap a picture of the check and use the bank's app to do a mobile deposit. For facilities receiving a high volume of checks, a mobile check scanner can be used (Figure 17-6). Checks are scanned individually and are documented as a bank transaction on the monthly statement. Mobile deposits can save staff time and do not require a deposit slip since the software (app) is linked to the bank account being used. When using mobile deposits, the daily deposit amount must match the exact daily deposit amount in the accounting management software.

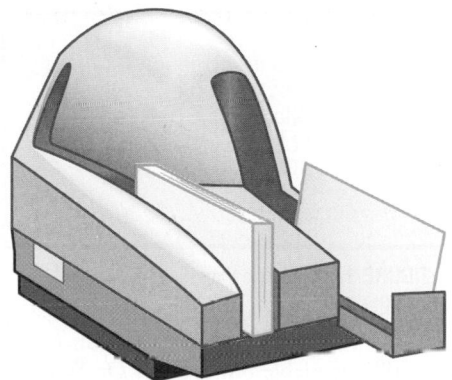

FIGURE 17-6 Mobile check scanner.

PROCEDURE 17-1   Prepare a Bank Deposit

Goal: *To prepare a bank deposit for currency, coins, and checks.*

Scenario: *The following checks need to be deposited: #3456 for $89; #6954 for $136; #9854-10 for $1366.65; #8546 for $653.36; and #9865 for $890.22. The following currency and coins need to be deposited: (19) $20 bills; (10) $10 bills; (46) $5; (73) $1; (43) quarters; and (155) nickels. The healthcare facility's name is Walden-Martin Family Medicine Clinic, account number 123-456-78910, and the bank is Clear Water Bank, Anytown, Anystate.*

EQUIPMENT and SUPPLIES

- Checks, currency, and coins for deposit (see scenario)
- Check for endorsement
- Calculator
- Paper method: bank deposit slip
- Electronic method: SimChart for the Medical Office (SCMO)

PROCEDURAL STEPS

1. Gather the documents to be used. For the electronic method, enter into the Simulation Playground in SCMO. Click on the Form Repository icon. On the INFO PANEL, click on Office Forms and then select Bank Deposit Slip.
2. Add the date on the deposit slip.
3. Using the calculator, calculate the amount of currency to be deposited. Enter the amount in the CURRENCY line, completing the dollar and cent boxes.

4. Calculate the amount of coins to be deposited. Enter the amount in the COIN line, completing the dollar and cent boxes.
5. Add the currency and coins and enter the total amount in the TOTAL CASH line.
6. For each check to be deposited, enter the check number, the dollars, and cents. List each check on a separate line.
   PURPOSE: The bank requires that each check be listed separately, and it also helps when verifying the checks before the deposit.
7. Calculate the total to be deposited and enter the number in the TOTAL FROM ATTACHED LIST box.
8. Enter the number of items deposited in the TOTAL ITEMS box.
9. Before completing the deposit slip, verify the check amounts listed and recalculate the totals. For the electronic method, click on SAVE.
   PURPOSE: It is crucial to verify the accuracy of check amounts and totals.
10. Place a restrictive endorsement on the check(s).
    PURPOSE: To protect checks from loss or theft.

Check Endorsements

An endorsement is a signature plus any other writing on the back of a check by which the **endorser** transfers all rights in the check to another party. Endorsements are made with either a pen or rubber ink stamp. The medical assistant needs to endorse the back of the check in the box indicated. Regardless of how checks are deposited, they all need to be endorsed.

Types of Endorsements

Four principal kinds of endorsements can be used: blank, restrictive, special, and qualified. Blank and restrictive endorsements are most commonly used.

Blank Endorsement. In a blank endorsement, the payee signs only his or her name. This makes the check payable to the bearer. It is the simplest and most common type of endorsement on personal checks but should be used only when the check is to be cashed or deposited immediately.

Restrictive Endorsement A restrictive endorsement specifies the purpose of the endorsement (Figure 17-7). It is used in preparing checks for deposit to the provider's checking account.

Special Endorsement. A special endorsement includes words specifying the person to whom the endorser makes the check payable. For instance, a check written to Helen Barker as the payee may be endorsed to the provider by writing on the back of the check as follows:

Pay to the order of
Theodore F. Wilson, M.D.
Helen Barker

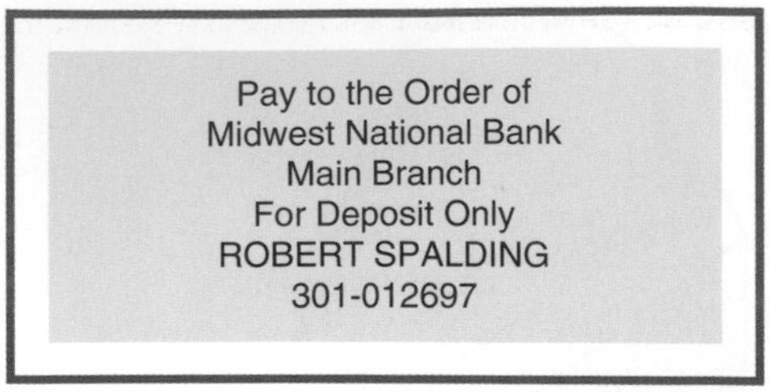

FIGURE 17-7 Example of a restrictive endorsement.

The check is still negotiable but requires Dr. Wilson's signature or endorsement.

Qualified Endorsement. With a qualified endorsement, the effect of the endorsement is qualified by disclaiming or destroying any future liability of the endorser. Usually the words "without recourse" are written above by an attorney who accepts a check on behalf of a client but who has no personal claim in the transaction.

Methods of Endorsement

Any endorsement should match exactly with the name on the pay to line of the check. If the name of the payee is misspelled, the payee usually must endorse the check the way the name is spelled on the face, followed by the correctly spelled signature.

Stamp. As checks from patients and other sources arrive, they should be recorded in the ledger and immediately stamped with the restrictive endorsement "For Deposit Only." This is a safeguard against lost or stolen checks. Most banks accept routine stamp endorsements that are restricted to For Deposit Only if the customer is well known and maintains an established account.

Signature. Some insurance checks or drafts require a personal signature endorsement; a stamped endorsement is not acceptable. This is stated on the back of the check. In such cases ask the payee to endorse the check, then stamp immediately below the signature the restrictive endorsement "For Deposit Only."

USING CHECKS FOR HEALTHCARE FACILITY EXPENSES

How to Write a Check

Checks are written in ink or produced using software. Write or key the check by the following steps:

- Date the check using one of these formats: May 23, 20XX; 05/23/XX; or 5/23/XX.
- On the "Pay to the Order of" line, correctly write or key the person's name or the company's name.
- On the line with the dollar sign, write out the exact amount of the check starting next to the dollar sign (e.g., $135.00, not $135).
- On the line below the recipient's name, write out the amount, making sure to start at the left edge. The cents are written in a fraction. Draw a single line through the rest of the line to prevent any additions (e.g., One hundred thirty-five and 50/100_____).
- On the Memo line, indicate the purpose of the payment (optional).

- The check needs to be signed to be valid. If the provider is signing the check, clip the invoice to the check and place it on the provider's desk for a signature. If you are responsible for signing checks, your name must be on the signature card on file at the bank. For checks over a certain amount, two signatures will be needed.
- If you make a mistake when writing the check, it cannot be altered by crossing out or changing anything that was written. You will need to void the check and rewrite another check. Write "VOID" on the stub and on the check. File the voided check with other accounting documents for auditing purposes. If using accounting software, indicate the check number has been voided in the software.

Preventing Check Fraud in the Healthcare Facility

The National Check Fraud Center suggests the following steps to minimize the chance of check fraud in the healthcare facility:

- Check bank statements immediately after receiving them. If check fraud is not reported within 30 days of receipt of a monthly statement, the bank usualy does not have to reimburse the loss.
- Make sure all extra checks, deposit slips, bank statements, and records are stored securely (e.g., locked file cabinet or secure electronic folder).
- Bank statements and records should be maintained for up to 7 years and then shredded before disposal.

For more information on how to prevent check fraud or what to do if fraud occurs, consult the National Check Fraud Center's website at *ckfraud.org*.

Writing Cash Checks

A check is made payable to Cash and is completely negotiable. Because these checks are easily cashed, it is poor policy to write cash checks until a person is physically at the bank. These checks most often are used to replenish petty cash funds. Some bank personnel may require that the person receiving the cash endorse the check. Many experts in the banking business advise their customers not to endorse a check written for cash often; if a problem arises, the person who endorses the check is liable. To avoid being accused of embezzlement, a medical assistant should never endorse a check written from the facility's account that is written for cash.

Mailing Checks

When checks are sent through the mail, the check should not be visible through the envelope. Either place the check within a letter or fold it into a plain sheet of paper. Checks may be folded at the right end to conceal the amount of money written. Make sure the envelope is sealed before mailing. The medical assistant should personally mail all checks as soon as possible.

Overdraft

When a depositor draws a check for more than the amount on deposit in the account, the account is overdrawn. Issuing a check for more than the amount on deposit in the bank is illegal. Such a check is said to "bounce." Should this happen through error or oversight and a check is written by an established depositor, the bank may honor the check and notify the depositor that the account is overdrawn. If the bank thus pays or covers the check, it issues an overdraft on the depositor's account. Considerable fees ($10 to $35) normally are charged for an overdraft.

Stop-Payments

A depositor or check writer who wants to rescind the check has the right to request that the bank stop payment on it. Stop-payment orders should be used only when absolutely necessary; as with overdrafts, most banks charge a fee for this service. Reasons for stop-payment requests include:

- Loss of a check
- Disagreement about a purchase
- Disagreement about a payment

PAYING BILLS TO MAXIMIZE CASH FLOW

Establish a systematic plan for paying bills. Some offices have incorporated an online bill paying system and pay bills as soon as they are received. In establishing the procedure for accounts payable, a medical assistant should keep in mind that most vendors allow 30 days to pay. When each invoice is received, check the "terms," which usually are located at the top of the document. Sometimes occasions arise when a bill can be discounted if a bill is paid within a specified time, such as 10 days. A few vendors offer a discount (normally 1% to 2%) if bills are paid within a shorter time; such discounts usually are indicated at the bottom of invoices or billing statements. If the terms say "Net 30," this means the total amount of the bill is due within 30 days.

Remember to allow a certain number of days for mailing (2 to 5, depending on where the payment is sent). If the business checking account is an interest-bearing one, do not pay bills before their due date. In this way, the funds in the account continue to draw interest until it is time to write the check. Also, if the practice has a weekly service (e.g., a laundry or cleaning service) that bills several times a month, accumulate the invoices and issue only one check per month.

Online Bill Pay

Online banking is a common practice for personal and business accounts. The bank pays bills by automatically debiting the customer's account and crediting the merchant's account. Many bills can be scheduled through the online banking portal (Figure 17-8). However, not all vendors accept electronic transfers in payment of bills. It will take longer for vendors to receive payment, so schedule payments accordingly. Some routine bills that are due monthly or on a regular billing cycle, such as insurance premiums, rent payments, and utility bills, can be set up to be automatically withdrawn on the online banking portal. All banking transactions can be downloaded into an accounting management program for efficient money management. Online banking also is an excellent way to research the checks that have cleared the bank and to compute accurate bank balances.

Direct Deposit

Direct deposit, also known as *electronic funds transfers* (EFT), is the electronic payment of payroll, money owed to vendors or business establishments, and payments from government agencies. Direct deposit payments are safe, secure, efficient, and less expensive than paper checks. Their greatest advantage is the cost savings: the U.S.

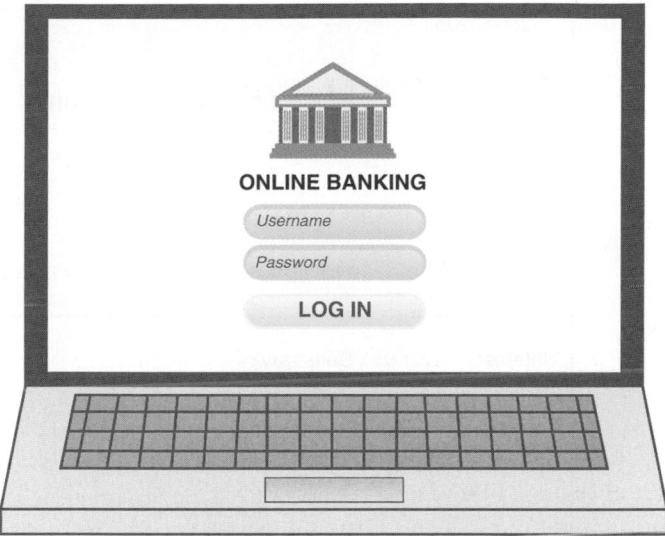

FIGURE 17-8 Online banking portal.

government pays $1.03 to issue each check payment, but only 10.5¢ to issue a direct deposit. Electronic processing becomes more prevalent each day, and business transactions are processed faster and more efficiently through electronic means.

Reward Credit Cards

More and more vendors are accepting credit cards for payment. Many different credit cards offer rewards, such as airline points, hotel rewards, reward points for products, or cash back rewards. If one of these credit cards is used for monthly expenses instead of a checking account, the provider can earn a variety of rewards. To get the greatest advantage from the credit card, be prepared to pay the credit card balance in full at the end of each billing statement to avoid interest charges.

BANK STATEMENTS AND RECONCILIATION

The bank creates a statement at the end of each monthly period, and the medical assistant can download the bank statement directly into the accounting management software, which has a *reconciliation* feature. The purpose of reconciliation is to start with the beginning balance and then add all deposits and subtract all checks and other debit transactions, leaving the ending statement balance. It is extremely important to make sure at the end of reconciliation that the ending balance is achieved. The bank statement reconciliation is used as an audit, or to ensure that the bank is managing the funds in the account accurately. Any errors on the bank statement should be reported to the bank immediately. Bank statements typically contain the following elements (Figures 17-9 and 17-10):

- Beginning balance
- Deposits made
- Checks paid (including images of all cleared checks)
- Transfer transactions
- Online payment transactions
- Bank charges
- Ending balance

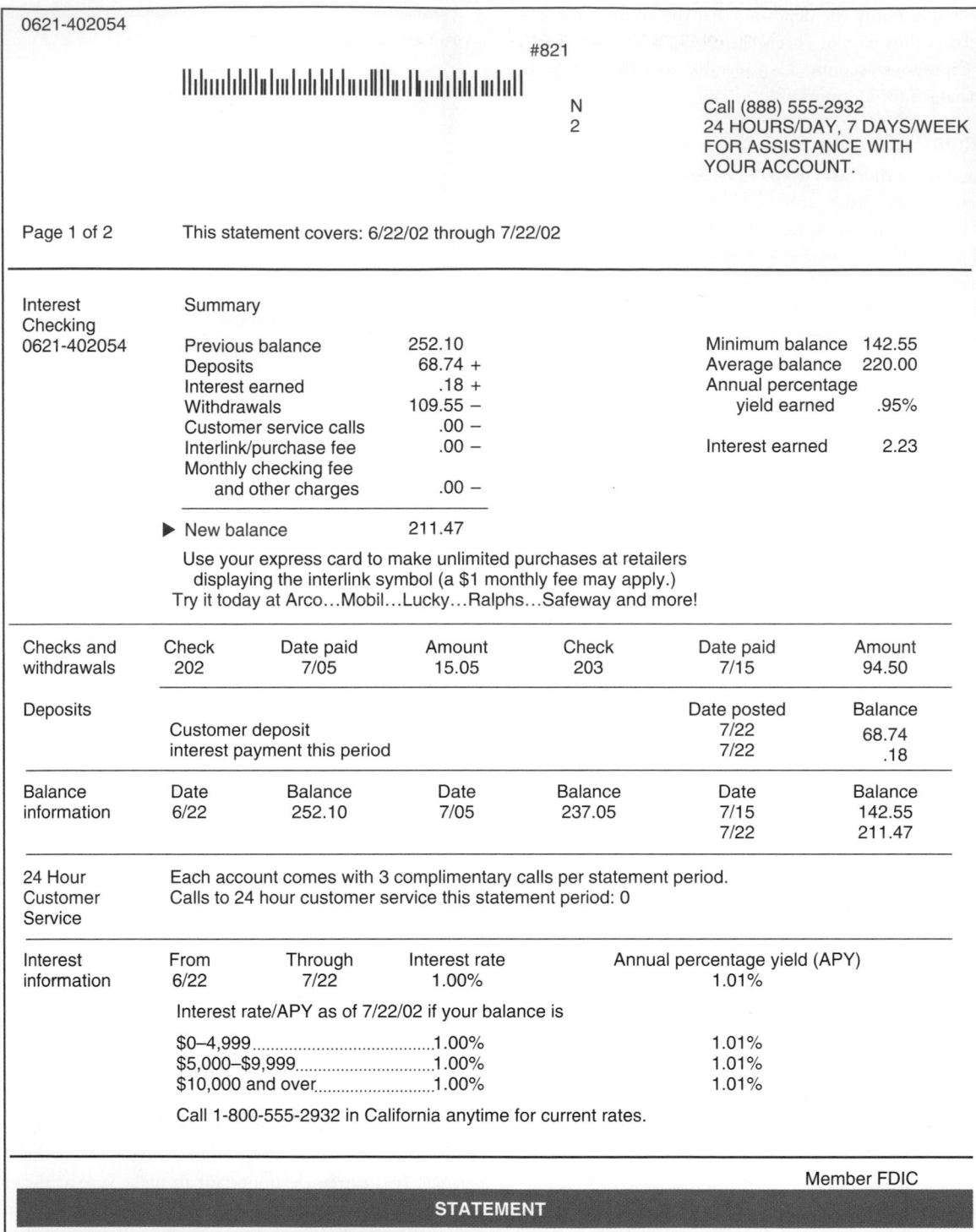

FIGURE 17-9 Example of a regular checking account statement.

This worksheet is provided to help you balance your account

1. Go through your register and mark each check, withdrawal, Express ATM transaction, payment, deposit or other credit listed on this statement. Be sure that your register shows any interest paid into your account, and any service charges, automatic payments, or Express Transfers withdrawn from your account during this statement period.

2. Using the chart below, list any outstanding checks, Express ATM withdrawals, payments or any other withdrawals (including any from previous months) that are listed in your register but are not shown on this statement.

3. Balance your account by filling in the spaces below.

ITEMS OUTSTANDING	
NUMBER	AMOUNT
TOTAL	$

Enter

The new balance shown on
this statement .... $_____

Add

Any deposits listed in your register $_____
or transfers into your account which $_____
are not shown on this statement. $_____
                                       +$_____

Total.................+ $_____

Calculate the subtotal... $_____

Subtract

The total outstanding checks and
withdrawals from the chart at left............................– $_____

Calculate the ending balance

This amount should be the same
as the current balance shown in
your check register.. $_____

If you suspect errors or have questions about electronic transfers

If you believe there is an error on your statement or Express ATM receipt, or if you need more information about a transaction listed on this statement or an Express ATM receipt, please contact us immediately. We are available 24 hours a day, seven days a week to assist you. Please call the telephone number printed on the front of this statement. Or, you may write to us at United Trust Company, P.O. Box 327, Anytown, USA.

1. Tell us your name and account number or Express card number.

2. As clearly as you can, describe the error or the transfer you are unsure about, and explain why you believe there is an error or why you need more information.

3. Tell us the dollar amount of the suspected error.

You must report the suspected error to us no later than 60 days after we sent you the first statement on which the problem appeared. We will investigate your question and will correct any error promptly. If our investigation takes longer than 10 business days (or 20 days in the case of electronic purchases), we will temporarily credit your account for the amount you believe is in error, so that you may have use of the money until the investigation is completed.

FIGURE 17-10 Reverse side of a bank statement, which is used for reconciling a checking account.

What to Do When the Balances Do Not Match

When a medical assistant manages a large number of transactions from check deposits and bill payment activities, it can be challenging to match the closing balance of the bank statement with the closing balance indicated in the accounting management software. Keeping accurate records of deposits and bill payment activities makes the bank reconciliation much smoother. All deposit copies should be maintained with a copy of the calculator tape totaling the day's deposit. Every online bill pay transaction should be recorded accurately in the accounting management system.

If you have diligently recorded every transaction and the balances still do not match, ask yourself the following questions:

- Is your arithmetic correct? Could a deposit, check, or online bill pay amount be transposed?
- Did you forget to include one of the outstanding checks?
- Did you fail to record a deposit or did you record one twice?

Most banks ask to be notified within a reasonable time (e.g., 10 days) of any error found in the statement. The bank statement should be reconciled as soon as it is received. Most banks provide a form for reconciliation on the last page of the bank statement.

Bank Statement Reconciliation Formula

Bank statement balance	$ _____
Minus outstanding checks	$ _____
Plus deposits not shown	$ _____
Corrected bank statement balance	$ _____
Checkbook balance	$ _____
Minus any bank charges	$ _____
Corrected checkbook balance	$ _____

If the two corrected balances agree, stop there. If they do not agree, subtract the lesser figure from the greater figure; the difference usually provides a clue to the error. For instance, if the shortage is $35, examine all the transactions for $35 on the statement and checkbook register and determine whether one of them has a posting error. Check the math and make sure all figures were added and subtracted correctly. Look at each figure and make sure none has been transposed. These tips usually catch the mistake.

CLOSING COMMENTS

Patient Education

It should be emphasized that patients are financially responsible for balances on their accounts; patients should be informed of the healthcare facility's payment policy at the very first appointment. If a patient submits an NSF check, the medical assistant should immediately call the patient and explain the problem, requesting that he or she correct the matter as soon as possible. It is important to remember, however, that most overdrafts are simply the result of mathematic errors or a delay in deposited funds being available for withdrawal. Therefore, the medical assistant should be patient and courteous when discussing NSF issues with patients. However, patients need to know that overdrafts are costly not only to them but also to the medical facility.

Legal and Ethical Issues

If a mistake is made in preparing a check, do not destroy the check. Rather, write "VOID" across the face of the check, make a note on the check stub, and file the check with other important accounting documents available for auditing purposes.

A stop-payment order may be placed with the bank in an emergency, such as when a check is lost or a disagreement occurs with regard to a purchase or payment.

Do not accept a check made payable to another party without the endorsement of the person who gives the check to you. If the check is returned by the bank for any reason, the check will be charged to the last endorser, not the last person to receive the money.

Professional Behaviors

Despite the advances in online banking, the healthcare facility will need a responsible employee to handle money to be deposited or withdrawn from the bank. The healthcare facility manager should be diligent in ensuring that the individual handling the bank deposits or transactions is trustworthy. An employee in this position should undergo a background check, including a credit check, and drug screening. It also is wise for the practice to take out a *fidelity bond,* which is a financial protection against any fraudulent behavior by the bonded employee. Detailed money management policies prevent the misuse of the healthcare facility's funds and/or embezzlement. An effective healthcare facility manager recognizes the power of unaccounted money and protects employees by establishing strict money management rules.

SUMMARY OF SCENARIO

After the visit by the bank representative, Laura has implemented a few changes in bank account management, which has increased productivity in the office. For one, Laura requested that the bank send a mobile deposit machine so this could be done in-house; this has saved Laura a lot of time.

Laura has also set up online bill pay and manages all invoice payments through the banking portal online. She sits down once a month and sets up all payments for the month. In this way she can budget the office expenses for the month and can transfer unused funds to a money market account that pays a higher interest rate.

Laura is working closely with the providers at Ambulatory Surgical Care Associates to make some financial policy changes in the office to streamline banking processes. As of January 1 of the new year, the sign at the healthcare facility's lobby window will explain that cash will no longer be accepted for services and that a $0.25 fee will be charged for the use of a credit or debit card. Laura believes that handling fewer checks will eliminate returned patient checks.

SUMMARY OF LEARNING OBJECTIVES

1. **Define, spell, and pronounce the terms listed in the vocabulary.**
   Spelling and pronouncing terms correctly reinforce the medical assistant's credibility. Knowing the definitions of these terms promotes confidence in communication with patients and co-workers.

2. **Explain the purpose of the Federal Reserve Bank and the types of banks it manages.**
   The Federal Reserve Bank manages all banks in the United States. Healthcare facilities have a choice among different types of banks with which to do business, such as retail and commercial banks, credit unions, and online-only banks.

3. **Identify common types of bank accounts.**
   The bank accounts most commonly used by healthcare facilities are checking, savings, and money market accounts.

4. **Do the following related to banking in today's business world:**
   - *Discuss the importance of signature cards.*
     When an account is opened at a bank branch, the depositor is required to provide a handwritten signature on a physical or electronic card, which is kept on file with the bank. If a check comes through and some suspicion arises that the depositor's signature has been forged, bank personnel compare the signature on the check with the original on the signature card.
   - *Explain how online banking has made standard banking processes more efficient.*
     Online banking allows healthcare facilities to perform mobile deposits, thereby reducing the number of times a staff member visits the bank branch. Online banking also provides up-to-the-minute account balances, online bill pay, and easy account balance transfers so that the healthcare facility's manager can spend less time managing the bank account.
   - *Review the benefits of customer-oriented banking.*
     Customer-oriented banking opens opportunities for customers to perform banking tasks from their office instead of going to the bank regularly. The Federal Reserve Banks are located across the United States. Local branches operate under the assigned Federal Reserve Bank.

5. **Do the following related to checks:**
   - *Compare different types of negotiable instruments.*
     The different types of negotiable instruments used to transfer funds from one bank account and deposit them in another are the personal check, cashier's check, money order, business check, and voucher check.
   - *Identify precautions in accepting checks from patients.*
     When accepting a check, compare the name and address on the check to the name and address in the patient's health record. Scan the check carefully for the correct date, amount, and signature. Do not accept a check with corrections on it. If you do not know the person presenting a personal check, ask for identification and compare signatures.
   - *Explain how checks are processed from one account to another.*
     Local branches are assigned a routing number, which is printed on the bottom left side of the check. The check also has the specific account

number assigned by the branch, which specifies the account from which funds are taken. When a check is presented to the bank, the check is sent to a regional banking clearinghouse, which requests funds from the check-sponsoring financial institution. Then the funds are moved from the payer's account to the payee's account. The endorsement on the back of the check includes the number of the account into which the funds are to be deposited.
   - *Review the procedure followed when the healthcare facility receives a nonsufficient funds (NSF) check.*
     When the healthcare facility is informed that a patient's check has been returned for nonsufficient funds, the patient should be contacted immediately. Inform the patient that the balance plus the overdraft fee is payable by money order or debit or credit card immediately. The patient should also be informed that he or she can no longer pay by check for any future services.

6. **Identify precautions in accepting cash.**
   Many healthcare facilities refuse to accept cash from patients to prevent employees being tempted to embezzle. In addition, cash cannot be deposited by mobile deposit, and maintaining records for accepting cash can be difficult.

7. **Discuss the use of debit and credit cards, including advantages and precautions.**
   The advantages of debit cards include their safety and convenience, in addition to the availability of receipts and statements. The most important precaution in accepting credit cards is to verify the patient's identity by asking to see the person's state-issued ID. Patients must know the debit card's PIN, so this is considered a verification of identity.

8. **Do the following related to banking procedures in the ambulatory care setting:**
   - *Describe banking procedures as related to the ambulatory care setting.*
     Banking procedures include withdrawals, deposits, writing checks, reconciling bank statements, paying bills, and other transactions, most of which can be done conveniently in the healthcare facility through online banking or through accounting management software.
   - *Explain the importance of depositing checks daily.*
     Deposits should be made daily for these reasons: a stop-payment order may be placed; the check may be lost, misplaced, or stolen; delay may cause the check to be returned because of insufficient funds; the check may have a restricted time for cashing; prompt processing is a courtesy to the payer; and the accounts receivable may be inflated because payments have not been deposited daily.
   - *Prepare a bank deposit.*
     Bank deposits should be made daily. The process for preparing a bank deposit is outlined in Procedure 17-1.
   - *Compare types of check endorsements.*
     Endorsements include (1) a blank endorsement, in which the payee simply signs his or her name on the back of the check; (2) a restrictive endorsement, which specifies in which bank and which specific account the funds are to be deposited; (3) a special endorsement,

Continued

SUMMARY OF LEARNING OBJECTIVES—*continued*

which names a specific person on the back of the check as payee; and (4) a qualified endorsement, which disclaims future liability. This type of endorsement is used when the person who accepts the check has no personal claim in the transaction.

9. **Review check-writing procedures used to pay the operational expenses of a healthcare facility.**

Writing checks is a routine and basically simple function; however, certain guidelines should be followed to prevent potential problems. The bank account should have a check signer that is on file with the bank, and correction fluid for errors should not be used on checks.

10. **Understand the purpose of bank account reconciliation for auditing purposes.**

The procedure for reconciliation starts with the beginning balance; then, all deposits are added, and all checks and other debit transactions are subtracted—the ending statement balance should be left. It is extremely important to make sure that the ending balance is achieved at the end of reconciliation. The bank statement reconciliation is used to audit the account; that is, to ensure that the bank is managing the funds in the account accurately. Any errors on the bank statement should be reported to the bank immediately.

11. **Discuss patient education, in addition to legal and ethical issues, related to banking services and procedures.**

Patients are financially responsible for the balance on their accounts, and they should be informed of the healthcare facility's payment policy at the very first appointment. Do not accept a check made payable to another party without the endorsement of the person who gives you the check.

CONNECTIONS

📖 Study Guide Connection: Go to the Chapter 17 Study Guide. Read and complete the activities.

evolve Evolve Connection: Go to the Chapter 17 link at *evolve.elsevier.com/ kinn* to complete the Chapter Review Quiz. Check out the other resources listed for this chapter to make the most of what you have learned from Banking Services and Procedures.

SUPERVISION AND HUMAN RESOURCE MANAGEMENT

18

Katherine Martinson is the office manager for Fair Oaks Pediatrics, a pediatric group practice in a metropolitan area. The office manages a full appointment schedule each day. Katherine encourages the medical office staff to communicate and work as a cohesive team to meet the goal of providing exceptional care to the practice's young patients. Katherine knows that positive motivation will encourage the office team to meet this goal. At weekly staff meetings, employees are free to offer their suggestions on office procedures. Katherine regularly consults her team members and always asks for their thoughts on how the office can function more effectively. She recognizes that employees need to feel that they are part of the team, and by implementing some of the procedures her team members suggest, she creates a forward-thinking and empowered work environment for the office staff.

Katherine has been praised by the pediatricians as a transformational manager because she has implemented new and efficient health information systems and technologies in the pediatrics practice. In addition, when an office position becomes vacant, Katherine is careful about whom she hires. She always checks at least three references per applicant and verifies each previous place of employment. She also always requests a background check, a credit check,

a drug test, and a bond if the applicant will be assigned to manage office money matters.

Katherine trains each new employee herself, using the office's policies and procedures manual. She makes sure the employee knows that this manual also contains a detailed job description, so the employee knows the duties expected of his or her job. Katherine regularly reviews employee performance and keeps checklists that reflect that new employees are trained accurately. All new employees are probationary until they have been evaluated by Katherine at 90 days after hire. She works hard to improve the types of benefits offered to her team, to improve employee satisfaction and retention.

Katherine makes sure each employee has the tools needed to do his or her job effectively. She also trains the team in ways to reduce expenses and waste in the medical office. Major office changes are presented to the entire staff, and although the pediatricians make the final decision, Katherine seeks the suggestions of the employees. The cooperative attitude between the management and employees of the healthcare facility provides a great atmosphere for teamwork, and Katherine and the pediatricians are pleased with the team-building atmosphere they have implemented.

While studying this chapter, think about the following questions:

- How friendly should office managers become with the staff members?
- Why are checking references and a background check important when considering a new staff member?

- How should negative employee evaluations be handled?
- How can the office manager promote a teamwork atmosphere in the medical office?

LEARNING OBJECTIVES

1. Define, spell, and pronounce the terms listed in the vocabulary.
2. Define the qualities and responsibilities of a successful office manager in a healthcare facility.
3. Explain the chain of command in the medical office.
4. Do the following related to the power of motivation:
   - Identify several ways in which employees are motivated.
   - Explain how the abuse of power and authority can negatively affect productivity in a healthcare facility.
5. Do the following related to creating a team atmosphere:
   - Discuss strategies to create a team environment in the healthcare facility.
   - Recognize and overcome communication barriers.
   - Demonstrate respect for individual diversity, including gender, race, religion, age, economic status, and appearance.

6. Summarize strategies to introduce a new office manager.
7. List several ways to prevent burnout.
8. Do the following related to finding the right employee for the job:
   - Identify the need to find the right employee for an opening in the medical office.
   - Review a general job description for medical assistants.
   - Explain how to search through résumés and applications for potential candidates.
   - List and discuss legal and illegal interview questions.
   - Explain how to select the most qualified candidates.
   - Identify follow-up activities the office manager should perform after an interview.

VOCABULARY

diversity The inclusion of every individual, despite age, religion, race, disability, and/or gender, in the medical practice.

affable Pleasant and at ease in talking to others; characterized by ease and friendliness.

blatant Completely obvious, conspicuous, or obtrusive, especially in a crass or offensive manner; brazen.

chain of command A series of executive positions in order of authority.

cohesive Sticking together tightly; exhibiting or producing cohesion.

compliance Ensuring that the healthcare facility meets standards and regulations according to the office's established policies and procedures.

disparaging Slighting; having a negative or degrading tone.

empower To delegate more responsibilities to employees (a management theory).

extern A student working in an ambulatory care environment, who is learning the job and not earning a wage.

Human Resources File (HR File) Contains all documents related to an individual's employment.

incentives Things that incite or spur to action; rewards or reasons for performing a task.

mentor A steady employee whom a new staff member can approach with questions and concerns.

retention A term referring to actions taken by management to keep good employees.

subordinate Submissive to or controlled by authority; placed in or occupying a lower class, rank, or position.

The management of a professional healthcare facility can greatly influence the success of the business. Good management allows the provider to see and treat patients in a functional environment with the confidence that the business side of the facility is operating as it should be. A well-managed office is not something that just happens. Great effort and teamwork are necessary to ensure that the day-to-day activities are carried out efficiently and that the many details needing attention are handled urgently.

Although most medical assistants do not enter medical office management right after graduation, they can look forward to advancing their careers as they gain experience. The information in this chapter can help the medical assistant understand what it takes to become a good manager. Many of these traits can be developed as a new employee after graduation, such as punctuality, respect, and responsibility. Additionally, the medical assistant will learn the employment process from the office manager's point of view. This information also is valuable to a new medical assistant who is applying for a position. By studying office management, the medical assistant prepares for future management positions, but also learns to see both the employee side and the manager side of the operating healthcare facility.

TODAY'S OFFICE MANAGER

The office manager in today's medical facilities must be able to perform many different tasks successfully. The more duties the office manager can perform, the more valuable he or she is to the facility. This is why many medical office managers seek opportunities for continuing education. Office managers should always be

open to learning more management responsibilities because taking on management positions usually results in an increase in salary and benefits. A capable medical assistant who is ready to learn will advance quickly and find a variety of opportunities in the healthcare industry.

Qualities of an Effective Manager

- Uses good judgment
- Organized and manages time well
- Enjoys pursuing continuing education
- Creative and problem solving
- Has leadership ability
- Fair with all employees
- Takes a personal interest in employees
- Remains calm under stress
- Sees the potential of fellow employees
- Can communicate with staff, patients, providers, insurance companies, and upper management
- A good listener
- Approachable
- Comfortable using the computer

Responsibilities of the Medical Office Manager

The responsibilities of medical office managers vary from practice to practice. Some providers take a much more active role in office management than others. The best management plan for the provider is to hire a trustworthy, reliable office manager and then allow the manager to run the daily business aspects of the office. This frees the provider to concentrate on taking care of patients (Figure 18-1).

Some of the tasks performed by the medical office manager include:

- Preparing and updating the policies and procedures manual
- Training and evaluating employees to ensure they follow the healthcare facility's policies and procedures
- Establishing job descriptions for each position in the medical office
- Recruiting future employees
- Conducting performance and salary reviews
- Terminating employees
- Planning staff meetings
- Building strong teams in the office
- Establishing workflow guidelines
- Ensuring human resource compliance with all federal and state regulations
- Improving the office's operational efficiency
- Supervising the purchase and care of equipment
- Educating patients on aftercare, insurance benefits, and their financial responsibility
- Marketing for the practice

Office management is most successful when an office policies and procedures manual is developed and followed.

Variables Affecting Responsibilities in an Ambulatory Healthcare Setting

- Office size
- Number of providers
- Whether medical billing is done in-house or outsourced
- Number of employees
- Amount of provider/owner involvement in daily activities

CHAIN OF COMMAND IN THE MEDICAL OFFICE

If the office has only one medical assistant, that individual must be able to assume many management responsibilities, with cooperation from the provider. When the office has two medical assistants, one administrative and one clinical, the administrative medical assistant often is expected to assume management duties.

A facility with three or more employees should designate one person as supervisor or office manager. This individual needs management skills and experience in personnel supervision. Employees answer to the office manager, and the office manager answers to the provider. A **chain of command** allows the office staff to consult with the provider about administrative or clinical problems, complaints, or grievances; this allows the individuals whom the provider has placed in charge to have the first opportunity to solve problems. It also allows the provider to check on the operation of the office, disseminate information on policy changes, and correct errors or grievances by dealing with one person instead of all employees.

Office management problems often can be prevented by clearly defining areas of authority and the responsibilities of each employee. Many office managers claim that friction among workers is their most common personnel problem. The importance of the chain of command cannot be overemphasized, and the provider must not undermine the office manager's authority by circumvention. When employees know what is expected of them, they can plan both their daily and long-term work more effectively.

THE POWER OF MOTIVATION

Managers have a great deal of influence over the staff they supervise. Successful managers must be interested in people they work with on a daily basis. It is said that if one helps others get what they want in life, the individual usually also gets what he or she wants.

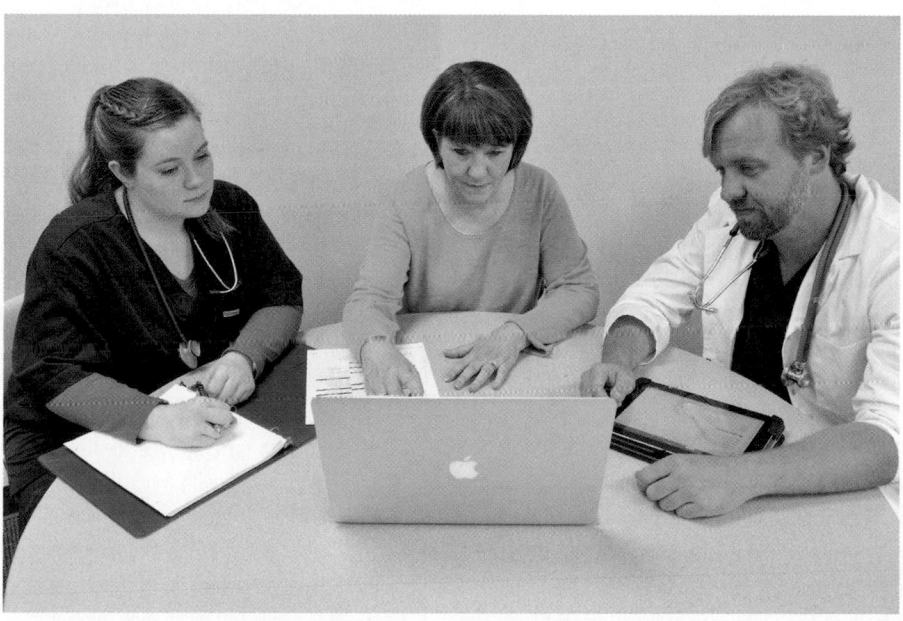

FIGURE 18-1 Staff training is a regular part of an office manager's job.

Successful managers learn that their employees should be encouraged to perform at optimum levels, and managers should be confident enough in their own skills to give credit to employees who develop ideas and concepts for the team. These managers know how to let their employees help them "look good." A manager with a group of outstanding employees usually is looked on as an effective leader.

Frederick Herzberg, known as the Father of Job Enrichment, stated, "Quality work that fosters job satisfaction and health enjoys top priority in industry all over the world." In his book, *The Motivation to Work,* Herzberg stated three points:

1. Jobs must be satisfying and must motivate employees to grow and reach their full capabilities.
2. Employees who show greater ability should be given more responsibility.
3. If the job does not allow the employee to use his or her full ability, a different employee who can grow and find motivation in the work should be placed in that position.

Effective medical office managers, or office team leaders, recognize that employees are more than static workers. Therefore, motivation is a key component to developing successful employees.

The Power of Motivation

A number of factors can motivate a person to reach a goal, including:

- Challenging work
- Money
- Recognition
- Satisfaction
- Freedom
- Fear
- Family
- Insecurity
- Competition
- Fulfillment
- Integrity
- Honor
- Reputation
- Responsibility
- Prestige
- Needs
- Love

Any of these motivators can prompt an employee to action. There are two general types of motivation. *Intrinsic motivation* is internal, or originates within a person. Intrinsic motivation is long term and can be focused toward a lifelong goal. *Extrinsic motivation* is external and more material in nature. Generally, extrinsic motivation is short-lived and less satisfying than intrinsic motivation.

CRITICAL THINKING APPLICATION 18-1

The staff is nervous about the implementation of a new EHR system, and morale has been low because training has been taking a long time. How can Katherine reassure her team of her confidence in their potential?

Keeping the Management Relationship Professional

When people work together for an extended period, they often become **affable**, and sometimes relationships develop into close friendships. This is a normal occurrence, but the office manager must be careful about becoming too close to his or her employees. When the relationship is friendly, reprimanding an employee when needed sometimes is difficult. Some employees take advantage of a good relationship with the office manager and may begin to arrive late or call in sick more than usual. A healthy respect for each other must be maintained. The manager can have a good rapport with employees without becoming overly friendly, and this is the best policy. Some facilities have strict rules about fraternization with subordinates outside the work facility. It is advisable to keep the relationship on a professional level at all times.

Use of Incentives and Employee Recognition

The staff of the provider's office should feel satisfaction with the working conditions and atmosphere in the facility. The office manager plays a part in ensuring that this happens.

CRITICAL THINKING APPLICATION 18-2

The clinical medical assistants at the Fair Oaks Pediatrics office usually celebrate payday by going out to eat after work every other Friday. After about 6 months on the job, they invite Katherine to join them. Should she go with the employees? Why or why not?

Most offices plan parties for Christmas or at other times during the year. Are these good for employee morale, or should they be avoided?

Incentives give employees reasons to perform over and above the level expected of them. An important element to incentive success is that management established clear and attainable goals. If the staff meets or exceeds a goal that has been set, the provider may elect to provide tickets to a sports or entertainment event for the entire staff. Some providers have an incentive program for outstanding patient account collection for a given period. These ideas provide a goal for the employees to work toward and an opportunity to expand their efforts as a team.

Incentives and Employee Recognition

Incentives and employee recognition should reward employees for a job well done; also, they will motivate staff members to keep up the great work! Here are some sensible incentives and employee recognition opportunities:

- After an office accomplishment, take the office out to lunch, order lunch into the office, or schedule a potluck lunch.
- Recognize an employee for his or her exceptional work during a team meeting with a personalized certificate and modest award.
- Set aside a specific time to play office games, trivia, or bingo for modest prizes at the end of a workweek.
- Schedule a weekend activity, such as a company picnic, to which employees can invite their families.

Recognition is a strong method of improving employee morale and encouraging outstanding performance. Certificates for peak performance are a great way to motivate employees. For instance, the office manager may decide to award a certificate each month to the employee who provides the highest rated customer service. Patients could even be involved by allowing them to nominate employees for this honor. When an award is at stake, most employees enjoy participating and striving to accomplish the goals that have been set.

CRITICAL THINKING APPLICATION   **18-3**

Katherine has noticed that the medical coding department has been running behind, more than usual. As a result, health insurance reimbursements have been lagging. What can Katherine do to motivate her employees?

Abuse of Power and Authority

Unfortunately, managers may abuse the power they have. As a result, the patients, the staff, and the overall morale of the office suffer. A manager who puts up barriers and erects emotional walls with employees has difficulty building effective office teams. Some managers use other people as tools to get what they want, and other managers cling to upper management, relating only to the inner circle of decision makers in the facility.

When an organization has no checks and balances, power can be abused. Working with a manager who cannot look inside himself or herself and see mistakes is difficult. Some managers stress rules and conformity, leaving no gray areas where a **subordinate** is concerned. Some show a false humility and pretend to care, but most employees can see right through this half-effort at a relationship. Others only hire "yes" people, who agree with everything the manager says. All these are abuses of power and indications of a poor manager.

These types of managers cannot be successful for an extended time. Eventually their conduct negatively affects the quality of care given to patients. It doesn't take long before upper management grows tired of unresolved office issues, such as high employee turnover and dissatisfied patients. Future candidates for jobs in medical office management should focus on developing the qualities of an effective manager, so that they are ready when ineffective managers must be replaced.

CREATING A TEAM ATMOSPHERE

Teamwork is critical in the medical profession. Communication improves when staff members collaborate as a team in the healthcare workplace, and improved communication can reduce medical errors and increase patient satisfaction. Therefore, the manager must promote an atmosphere in which employees are willing to work together toward common goals. Morale in the office may be low because of recent changes in policies or procedures, changes in staff or management, recent terminations of employees, lack of business, or for any number of other reasons. Some managers try to shield employees from negative information, but this practice can cause rumors to circulate and worsen morale.

One of the most effective ways to improve employee morale is to communicate openly and honestly. Regular staff meetings, e-mails, and memos are critical for good communication and the smooth operation of a medical facility (Figure 18-2). Communicating changes and developments that affect employees helps to improve morale. Morale can also be improved by scheduling activities that involve the families of employees.

Recognize and Overcome Barriers to Communication

Effective communication is important to increase efficiency and improved teamwork. Recognizing barriers to communication in the workplace is critical to the health of the team. The following are five barriers that can occur in a healthcare agency. It is important for the

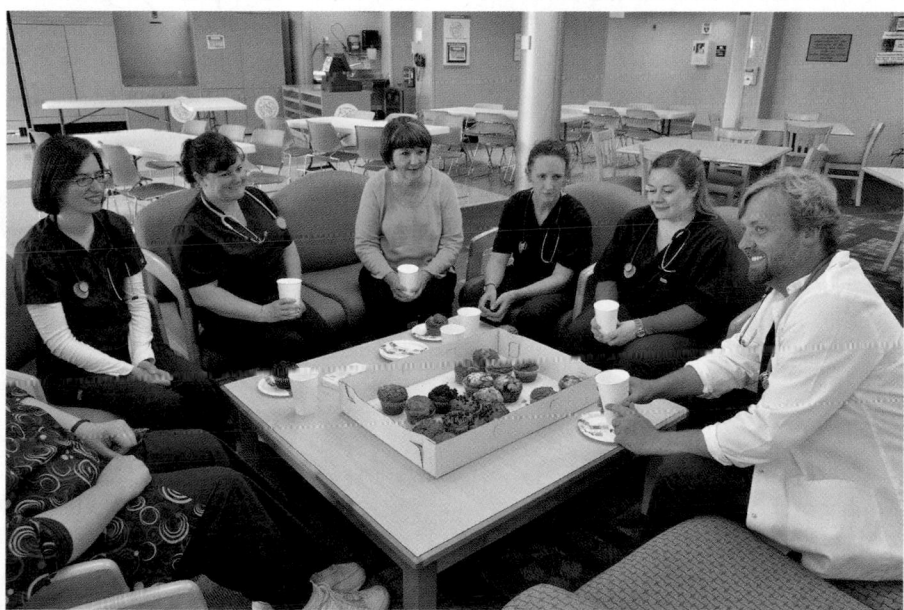

FIGURE 18-2 Communication is vital when building a team. Employees appreciate good communication with management. Sharing good and bad news openly with employees leads to fewer rumors and eases workers' concerns.

medical assistant to recognize the barriers and help the team overcome them.

- **Physical separation barriers** In large healthcare facilities, employees can be separated by departments or even by distance, if they are in different buildings. Communicating via email can be difficult and communication cues can be missed, leading to misinterpretation of the message. Using technology (e.g., videoconferencing and webcams) can help employees interact and strengthen communication.
- **Language barriers** Our workplaces are becoming more diverse. Employees live and train in different areas, learning different communication styles and different words for the same thing. For instance, a surgical instrument may be known by several names, as a result of providers training in different parts of the world. Supervisors who encourage awareness and acceptance of everyone's language and culture differences will strengthen the team's communication.
- **Status barriers** People may perceive that only those in higher ranking positions in a healthcare organization are important. This can lead to communication barriers and malfunctioning teams. It is important for the supervisor to promote awareness and acceptance that everyone counts and every position on the team is important.
- **Gender difference barriers** Males and females communicate differently, with females typically preferring a closer, more personal communication style than males. In some situations, the minority gender in an organization may not be as comfortable in communicating with peers. It is important for the supervisor to ensure that all employees, regardless of gender, feel empowered to communicate openly with others.
- **Cultural diversity barriers** Behaviors, words, and gestures have different meanings from one cultural group to another. How persons of different cultural groups communicate can also be different. For instance, some cultural groups do not believe in eye contact, whereas other groups may perceive a person to be lying or uncomfortable if eye contact is minimal. It is important for the supervisor to help the team embrace the cultural differences among the members, and educating the team on the differences can help promote understanding and cohesion.

INTRODUCING A NEW OFFICE MANAGER

The medical assistant will encounter various reactions when entering a facility as the new office manager. Often, he or she will face negative reactions from employees. They may have felt an intense loyalty to the previous manager and may resent that that person left for another job or was terminated, or they may have settled into a routine with an office manager they had worked with easily for many years. Most individuals resist change, and getting accustomed to a new supervisor can be extremely stressful. A new office manager wants to create a positive work environment; therefore, he or she must find ways to win the support of current employees.

The first thing a new office manager can do to begin gaining support is nothing. Never storm into an office and begin making radical changes in the first few days. Always observe for at least a few weeks and make notes about problem areas. Then, meet with the provider and share the information observed and present a plan

for changes. Ask for the provider's suggestions because he or she may know the history of difficult situations and can provide guidance in moving forward with plans for change.

After discussing these plans with the provider, use strategy to try to move employees toward achieving office goals. Schedule individual meetings with employees and allow them to tell you three things they like about their jobs, three things they dislike, and three things they need to do their jobs more effectively. This information provides a preliminary road map for management because the employees' responses give the new manager an excellent idea about what is important to them and where the problem areas are in the office. Hold staff meetings and move toward eliminating negative aspects and increase positive aspects of employees' jobs. These strategies will help employees realize that the new manager can get things done and that their opinions matter.

Realize that some employees still will resist, which may make the new office manager feel frustrated. At some point staffing changes may be necessary, and this might include terminating employees who do not get on board with the office moving in a positive direction. Although any terminations are stressful for the entire office, realize that this is a common situation when new managers begin their positions. This process is the first step in building a functional team.

PREVENTING BURNOUT

Burnout is defined as exhaustion of physical or emotional strength or motivation, usually as a result of prolonged stress or frustration. Medical professionals are particularly susceptible to burnout because of the intensity of their jobs, in which even small decisions can affect a patient's life.

Some of the causes of burnout include a stressful, disorganized home or work environment; poor human relations skills; a feeling of being out of control of one's life; excessive expectations from supervisors or family members; long work hours or time away from family and friends; and not being able to relax either at home or in the work environment. Management may make efforts to prevent employee burnout, but ultimately the employee must take steps to prevent it.

Personal Tips for Preventing Burnout

- Ask for help.
- Devote specific times to introspection or meditation.
- Understand what can be changed and what cannot be changed.
- Get some exercise.
- Organize and prioritize tasks.
- Understand your personal limitations.
- Take short vacations at least twice a year.
- Identify goals and try to perform only tasks that lead to reaching them.
- Consider options, including changing jobs.
- Personalize your work space with pictures and comforting items.
- Get a good understanding of a position and the stress involved before accepting it.

FINDING THE RIGHT EMPLOYEE FOR THE JOB

The most important asset of any healthcare facility is a staff that genuinely cares for patients. From providers to the receptionist, all play a vital role in the quality of the healthcare delivered. Hiring staff members who can be molded into a **cohesive** team is not an easy task. Care should be taken to choose employees who have the necessary skills and the right personality for the ambulatory care facility.

When the need for a new employee arises, the office manager should discuss with the providers the type of employee needed and the job description for that individual. Ask what qualities the providers desire for the position and the tasks for which the person will be responsible. Once the need has been established and the duties confirmed, the office manager can begin the recruiting process.

One of the most effective methods of finding new employees is allowing medical assistant students to complete their practicum at the healthcare facility. This provides the student the opportunity to learn about the facility and the staff, providers, and supervisor to see how the student interacts with others. Even if no openings exist, supervisors can ask the students for a resume to keep on file until a position opens up. Another effective method for finding new employees is advertising on local job boards. Larger facilities will post the job on their employment website page and link to other job boards. Smaller agencies will usually advertise on local free or low-cost job boards and advertise in local newspapers.

When creating an online ad or a job posting on an employment website, list the basic responsibilities and expectations for the position. Briefly describe the office, location, and the qualifications needed. Some offices also list a few of the benefits offered to attract applicants and also may disclose a salary range.

Job Description for a Medical Assistant

Medical assistants are qualified for a variety of tasks in the ambulatory care site. To fill any open medical assisting positions, the manager must determine which specific experience meets the facility's needs. With experience, professional skills can develop in specific aspects in the medical assisting profession. The website *monster.com* provides the following general job description for medical assistants.

Medical Assistant's Job Responsibilities
Helping patients through information, services, and assistance.

Medical Assistant's Job Duties
- Interviews patient to collect health data; records medical history and confirms purpose of the visit.
- Collects vital patient data by taking blood pressure, weight, and temperature; reports patient history summary.
- Secures patient's private information and preserves patient confidentiality according to HIPAA standards.
- Performs diagnostic and procedural coding, medical billing, and collection procedures for all patient accounts.
- Schedules patient appointments in the medical office and for surgery. Prepares the health record, pre-admit paperwork, and all required consent forms.
- Counsels patients on following provider's orders and answers patients' questions about follow-up care.
- Manages biohazardous waste and infection control to protect patients and medical office staff.
- Works with the medical care team to create a safe, secure, and healthy work environment by following office policies and procedures.
- Maintains inventory for medical supplies in the office by taking stock, placing orders, and verifying receipts.
- Supports healthcare facility equipment maintenance by following operating instructions, troubleshooting equipment failure, conducting preventive maintenance, and calling for repairs.
- Displays exceptional customer service to all patients, regardless of age, race, gender, religion, or socioeconomic background.

Medical Assistant's Skills and Qualifications
Customer service, clinical skills, written and verbal communication, infection control management, time management, scheduling, professionalism, confidentiality, working on a team.

Job Description

The job description is a tool designed to inform job candidates about the duties they would be expected to perform. Well-written and detailed job descriptions list the essential functions of the job and reveal the chain of command the employee should follow when questions or concerns arise. These documents provide a good guideline for potential employees so that they will understand exactly what is expected of them and their responsibilities at work.

Job descriptions are essential in the search for the perfect candidate. They highlight the specific educational background and skill set needed to be successful in the position. A clear job description in the hiring process increases the chance that an applicant with the required skills will apply for the open position. If a job description is too vague, many unqualified applicants may apply, and sorting through all the applications to find the right person for the position will be difficult.

The job description should include a statement that says the employee must perform any additional duties as assigned by the supervisor. With this statement in place, the employee cannot say, "That's not my job." All employees should be willing to pull together and assist with any tasks, but this statement gives added weight to assignments that are not specified in the written job description.

An effective manager understands the phrase "inspect what you expect." When duties are assigned, the manager should ensure that the tasks were completed correctly and in a timely manner. New employees should be monitored to make sure their delegated tasks are being done and done right. Without inspection, the manager cannot know whether the new employee is meeting expectations. Once employees have earned a degree of trust, inspecting their work is not as necessary as in the beginning. Some managers practice a skill called "management by walking around." By strolling through the areas where subordinates work, managers can observe and hear about issues that might be brewing, and at the same time improve morale by offering encouragement and praise.

Reviewing Applications

Depending on the situation, the manager may look at the applications as they come in or at the closing date. With today's technology, many agencies are having applicants submit cover letters, resumes, and applications online, although some still use paper documents. The first step in reviewing resumes includes separating out those that meet the minimal qualifications and those that do not. Typically, the minimal qualification includes successful completion of a medical assistant program and/or a medical assistant credential.

From those that meet the minimal qualifications, divide those into three stacks: those to call for an interview, possible candidates but not the strongest, and those that will not be called for an interview. Usually, the manager makes these decisions after reviewing the resume. Those with related experience, strong related skill sets (e.g., customer service), no unexplained employment gaps, and customized, error-free resumes and cover letters are more apt to be moved to the top of the pile.

Online Job Applications

Many healthcare facilities request job applicants to complete their employment application online. The online job application portal is beneficial for the job applicant and the health facility. The health facility can provide specific details about the open medical assisting positions, including the job responsibilities, a brief description of the benefits package, and a description of the company, including its mission statement. For the healthcare facility employer, online medical assisting applicants can be filtered by each individual professional experience, skills, certifications, and educational background. These portals allow employers to ask for more information specific to the job description; they can reduce the pool of applicants to just a few skilled candidates.

Once the original stack of applications has been reviewed, the office manager can return to the qualifying applications to determine which candidates to interview. Careful judgment and objectivity must be used in the search for an employee suitable for the healthcare facility. The manager should review the final applications with the following questions in mind:

- Does the applicant's grammar meet the office's standards? Can the applicant write a business letter?
- Does the applicant have basic computer skills?
- Has the applicant been employed previously in an ambulatory care facility? What were some of his or her responsibilities? Is this experience in line with the job description of the open position?
- If the applicant was previously employed, how long was he or she in the last position? Why did the applicant leave?
- Does the applicant seem to accept and enjoy responsibility? Does he or she have any professional goals that the medical office can train the individual to achieve?
- What is the applicant's formal education? Is he or she registered or certified?
- Is the applicant a member of a professional organization? Does he or she attend meetings?

Arranging the Personal Interview

In many of the larger healthcare facilities, a human resources representative will conduct a prescreening interview either over the phone or using technology like Skype. At this time, basic questions can be asked by the representative to gauge the interest of the applicant. That information is then forwarded to the office manager. In other agencies, the office manager may conduct the prescreening interview, to evaluate the person's telephone voice, attitude, and communication skills. In addition, the manager may want to ask several questions about the person's education, skills, and professional experience. Because the employee probably will speak with patients on the telephone, a qualified candidate should speak with ease. Those who perform well during the prescreening phone call should be scheduled for an interview.

CRITICAL THINKING APPLICATION   18-4

Katherine was impressed with Carol Limpken's résumé and application, but when scheduling an interview on the telephone, she noticed that Carol's grammar was not as professional as Katherine would like. Should this influence Katherine's decision whether to hire Carol?

Why is speech such an important issue in a healthcare facility?

Should Katherine be concerned about a candidate's grammar and spelling errors on the résumé or application? Why or why not?

Set a time for the personal interview when the applicant can be given undivided attention. An applicant who is being considered for employment should have an opportunity to see the facility during a period of fairly normal activity. The candidate who is interviewed in a peaceful, quiet office may not be prepared for the activity on a normal working day.

Before interviewing any applicant, become thoroughly familiar with the federal, state, and local fair employment practice laws affecting hiring practices. The Equal Employment Opportunity Act of 1972 prohibits inquiries into an applicant's race, color, gender, religion, and national origin. Inquiries about medical history, arrest records, or previous drug use also are illegal. Office managers must research the laws that pertain to employment in their own states or work with the human resources team, who are more familiar with these laws. It is important to develop a list of questions that will be asked to all interviewees. Creating a question list before the interviews helps to ensure no illegal questions are asked and that all interviewees are fairly evaluated (Table 18-1).

Laws Affecting Employment

Numerous laws affect the way employees are treated, from the interview through the end of employment. The office manager should be familiar with these laws and how they affect the practice.

Fair Labor Standards Act
- State standards for minimum wage and overtime pay; employees must be paid minimum wage and time and a half for overtime hours, as they apply
- Prohibits those under age 18 from performing certain kinds of work and restricts the hours of workers under age 16

Occupational Safety and Health Act
- Regulates conditions affecting employees' safety and health in the workplace

Workers' Compensation
- Regulates the benefits of employees who have been injured on the job
- Determines pay for employees who are not working because of an on-the-job injury

Family and Medical Leave Act
- Requires employers of 50 or more employees to offer up to 12 weeks of unpaid, job-protected leave to eligible employees for the birth of a child, an adoption, or a personal or family illness

Pregnancy Discrimination Act
- Forbids employers to refuse to hire a woman based on pregnancy, childbirth, or related medical conditions
- Requires employers to hold open a job for a pregnancy-related absence the same length of time that a job would be held open for employees on sick or disability leave

Americans with Disabilities Act
- Prohibits discrimination against individuals with disabilities

Age Discrimination Act
- Prevents discrimination in hiring on the basis of age
- Prevents discrimination in promoting, discharging, and compensating employees

The Interview

The interview is usually conducted by the office manager or with a panel of employees. If a panel is being used, they should meet before the interview to create a list of interview questions and discuss the flow of the interview. Each interviewee needs to be asked the same questions.

The interview typically starts with an introduction of the interviewers and a review of the job description. Usually, the first question (e.g., "Tell us about yourself") is meant to put the person at ease and get a summary of the person's professional and educational background. As the interview progresses, different types of questions will be asked to explore the person's past experiences and personality. Straightforward questions relate to the position duties. Behavioral questions are given to explore how the person behaved during a difficult past situation to anticipate how he or she might handle

future issues. Situational questions help the interviewers understand how the person would handle a hypothetical situation. The interviewers use the questions to explore the person's personality and past experiences and to judge how the person might fit into the existing team.

After the questions are completed, the manager should give the interviewee an opportunity to ask questions. Some interviews conclude with a discussion of the benefits and pay, but many times this occurs when the job is being offered to the applicant, since the human resources representative is the best resource for this information. Lastly, the office manager should give the interviewee an idea of the next steps in the process and when the decision will be made. If the person hasn't completed an application form, it is important to have that completed before the person leaves. References should also be collected from the interviewee.

Once the applicant leaves, the interviewers should rate or summarize their impressions of the applicant, listing the strengths and weaknesses on the interview question form. Be objective and professional and do not write **disparaging** information. The form will be kept on file in case of discrimination claims in hiring practices.

Usually, discussions of the candidate among the interview team are not encouraged until after all the interviews are completed. After all the interviews are conducted, the interviewers as a group should rank the candidates and finalize the top choices.

Bonding of Employees

To protect their business establishments from embezzlement or other financial loss caused by employees who handle large sums of money, providers often purchase fidelity bonds. Fidelity bonds reimburse the medical practice for any monetary loss caused by employees. Bonding normally requires a personal background investigation. The three types of bonding are:
- *Position-schedule bonding,* which covers a specific position rather than an individual, such as a bookkeeper or receptionist
- *Blanket-position bonding,* which covers all employees
- *Personal bonding,* which covers specific individuals

Follow-Up Activities

Always carefully check all references and follow through on any leads for information. Contact all listed references. When speaking with a candidate's former employer, be sure to "listen between the lines." Note the tone of the replies to the questions. Do not ask questions

TABLE 18-1 Legal and Illegal Interview Questions

LEGAL QUESTIONS	ILLEGAL QUESTIONS
• Why did you leave your last job?	• How long have you been working?
• What are your strengths and weaknesses?	• When was the last time you used drugs?
• What motivates you to succeed?	• Do you have any children?
• What are some of your hobbies?	• What religion do you practice?
• Are you willing to work more than 40 hours a week?	• Are you married?

that might incriminate the person answering them. The following questions are effective as an introduction:

- When did (the applicant) work for you? For how long?
- What were his or her duties and responsibilities? Did the employee assume responsibility well?
- Did the employee work well in a team environment? Did any conflicts arise that we should know about?

Some employers provide information only on the date of hire, job title, and date of termination of the employment. However, if the employer states, "She worked in our office from May, 2011, to July, 2012, and is not eligible for rehire," the reasonable assumption is that the employee did not perform well. The tone of voice and emphasis on the word "not" should be clues that this person is probably not right for the job. Still, if all other references are glowing, call and ask the applicant about the facility that gave the negative response. There could be a reasonable explanation for what might have been a bad experience. Respect the company's policy and do not press for further information.

After the applicant list has been narrowed to two or three candidates whose references have been checked thoroughly, a second interview may be arranged. The providers may want to participate in these interviews.

Selecting the Right Applicant

Once the final interviews have been conducted, it is time to choose the best candidate. Never rely strictly on a "gut instinct" about a potential employee. Base hiring decisions on logical conclusions drawn from all contacts with the applicant, including:

- Grammar and enunciation
- Office manners and customer service skills
- Professional appearance
- Work history
- Match to required job skills
- Friendly, personable attitude

When a decision has been reached to hire someone, either a human resource representative or the office manager will contact the person. This is the most common time to discuss wages and benefits. The applicant may request 2 to 3 days to think over the offer. Make sure you have a firm date when the applicant will make his or her decision.

When the position is filled, the human resources representative or the office manager needs to contact all the applicants and explain the job has been filled. This notification can occur through email, a letter, or a phone call. Be courteous in the notification and thank the individual for applying.

PAPERWORK FOR NEW EMPLOYEES

The office manager should develop a checklist of the paperwork needed for newly hired staff members and all the information that should be covered with the new employee at the start of the job. Basic new employee paperwork often includes:

- HIPAA confidentiality statement
- Computer passwords and agreement statement
- Job application
- Form I-9 (Employment Eligibility Verification)
- W-4 Form (Employee's Withholding Allowance Certificate)

- Notice of Workers' Compensation coverage
- Consent for background check, drug testing, and search (if applicable)
- Acknowledgment of receipt of company handbook or policy manual
- Agreements regarding pay, wage deductions, benefits, schedule, work location, and so on
- Notices of at-will employment status
- Direct deposit application
- Occupational Safety and Health Administration (OSHA) compliance acknowledgement or checklist

All of these forms, once completed and signed, should be kept in the employee's personnel file. Other forms and paperwork may be necessary that vary from state to state and company to company. The Form I-9 (Employment Eligibility Verification) is required by the federal government (Figure 18-3). This form must be completed for all newly hired employees to verify their identification and authorization to work in the United States. The most current form is available at http://www.uscis.gov along with training materials. The newly hired employee should complete the first section of the form and provide it to the human resource representative or office manager on the first day of work. The remaining information is completed by the representative or manager. Specific documents need to be shown to prove the person's identification and authorization to work in this country. A person who cannot provide the required documentation should not be allowed to remain as an employee.

Employees should also understand the *at-will employment* status. Under the at-will employment principle, the employer can terminate the employment at any time, for any reason/cause and without notice. Unless the employer violated labor laws or the employee rights, the employee has little recourse. Only a few states protect employees from termination without good cause. At-will employment also means that the employee can leave the employment at any time, but professionally it is important to give the employer the required notice.

ORIENTATION AND TRAINING: CRITICAL FACTORS FOR SUCCESSFUL EMPLOYEES

The hiring process does not end with hiring a new employee. Orientation and training help new employees understand what is expected and develop to their full potential (Figure 18-4). A critical error made when bringing new staff members aboard is failing to provide them with a fair orientation and training period.

Some managers assign a **mentor** to assist the new employee during the initial probationary period. This type of "buddy" system is a good practice because the new person does not feel isolated and alone during the first few weeks on the job.

Acquaint the new employee with the following:

- Staff members and their names
- Physical environment and layout of the office
- Nature of the practice and specialty
- Types of patients seen in the office
- Office policies and procedures
- Employee benefits
- Short- and long-range expectations
- HIPAA and computer training

Department of Homeland Security
U.S. Citizenship and Immigration Services

**Form I-9, Employment
Eligibility Verification**

Read instructions carefully before completing this form. The instructions must be available during completion of this form.

ANTI-DISCRIMINATION NOTICE: It is illegal to discriminate against work-authorized individuals. Employers CANNOT specify which document(s) they will accept from an employee. The refusal to hire an individual because the documents have a future expiration date may also constitute illegal discrimination.

Section 1. Employee Information and Verification *(To be completed and signed by employee at the time employment begins.)*

Print Name: Last	First	Middle Initial	Maiden Name

Address *(Street Name and Number)*		Apt. #	Date of Birth *(month/day/year)*

City	State	Zip Code	Social Security #

I am aware that federal law provides for imprisonment and/or fines for false statements or use of false documents in connection with the completion of this form.

I attest, under penalty of perjury, that I am (check one of the following):

☐ A citizen of the United States

☐ A noncitizen national of the United States (see instructions)

☐ A lawful permanent resident (Alien #) _____

☐ An alien authorized to work (Alien # or Admission #) _____
until (expiration date, if applicable - *month/day/year*)

Employee's Signature	Date *(month/day/year)*

Preparer and/or Translator Certification *(To be completed and signed if Section 1 is prepared by a person other than the employee.) I attest, under penalty of perjury, that I have assisted in the completion of this form and that to the best of my knowledge the information is true and correct.*

Preparer's/Translator's Signature	Print Name

Address *(Street Name and Number, City, State, Zip Code)*	Date *(month/day/year)*

Section 2. Employer Review and Verification *(To be completed and signed by employer. Examine one document from List A OR examine one document from List B and one from List C, as listed on the reverse of this form, and record the title, number, and expiration date, if any, of the document(s).)*

	List A	OR	List B	AND	List C
Document title:					
Issuing authority:					
Document #:					
Expiration Date *(if any)*:					
Document #:					
Expiration Date *(if any)*:					

CERTIFICATION: I attest, under penalty of perjury, that I have examined the document(s) presented by the above-named employee, that the above-listed document(s) appear to be genuine and to relate to the employee named, that the employee began employment on *(month/day/year)* _____ **and that to the best of my knowledge the employee is authorized to work in the United States. (State employment agencies may omit the date the employee began employment.)**

Signature of Employer or Authorized Representative	Print Name	Title

Business or Organization Name and Address *(Street Name and Number, City, State, Zip Code)*	Date *(month/day/year)*

Section 3. Updating and Reverification *(To be completed and signed by employer.)*

A. New Name *(if applicable)*	B. Date of Rehire *(month/day/year) (if applicable)*

C. If employee's previous grant of work authorization has expired, provide the information below for the document that establishes current employment authorization.

Document Title:	Document #:	Expiration Date *(if any)*:

I attest, under penalty of perjury, that to the best of my knowledge, this employee is authorized to work in the United States, and if the employee presented document(s), the document(s) I have examined appear to be genuine and to relate to the individual.

Signature of Employer or Authorized Representative	Date *(month/day/year)*

Form I-9 (Rev.) Y Page 4

FIGURE 18-3 The I-9 Form (Employment Eligibility Verification) is designed to help the employer gather the documents necessary to prove that an employee is eligible to work in the United States.

Continued

LISTS OF ACCEPTABLE DOCUMENTS

All documents must be unexpired

LIST A		LIST B		LIST C
Documents that Establish Both Identity and Employment Authorization	**OR**	**Documents that Establish Identity**	**AND**	**Documents that Establish Employment Authorization**
1. U.S. Passport or U.S. Passport Card		1. Driver's license or ID card issued by a State or outlying possession of the United States provided it contains a photograph or information such as name, date of birth, gender, height, eye color, and address		1. Social Security Account Number card other than one that specifies on the face that the issuance of the card does not authorize employment in the United States
2. Permanent Resident Card or Alien Registration Receipt Card (Form I-551)				
3. Foreign passport that contains a temporary I-551 stamp or temporary I-551 printed notation on a machine-readable immigrant visa		2. ID card issued by federal, state or local government agencies or entities, provided it contains a photograph or information such as name, date of birth, gender, height, eye color, and address		2. Certification of Birth Abroad issued by the Department of State (Form FS-545)
				3. Certification of Report of Birth issued by the Department of State (Form DS-1350)
4. Employment Authorization Document that contains a photograph (Form I-766)		3. School ID card with a photograph		
		4. Voter's registration card		4. Original or certified copy of birth certificate issued by a State, county, municipal authority, or territory of the United States bearing an official seal
5. In the case of a nonimmigrant alien authorized to work for a specific employer incident to status, a foreign passport with Form I-94 or Form I-94A bearing the same name as the passport and containing an endorsement of the alien's nonimmigrant status, as long as the period of endorsement has not yet expired and the proposed employment is not in conflict with any restrictions or limitations identified on the form		5. U.S. Military card or draft record		
		6. Military dependent's ID card		
		7. U.S. Coast Guard Merchant Mariner Card		5. Native American tribal document
		8. Native American tribal document		
		9. Driver's license issued by a Canadian government authority		6. U.S. Citizen ID Card (Form I-197)
		For persons under age 18 who are unable to present a document listed above:		7. Identification Card for Use of Resident Citizen in the United States (Form I-179)
6. Passport from the Federated States of Micronesia (FSM) or the Republic of the Marshall Islands (RMI) with Form I-94 or Form I-94A indicating nonimmigrant admission under the Compact of Free Association Between the United States and the FSM or RMI		10. School record or report card		8. Employment authorization document issued by the Department of Homeland Security
		11. Clinic, doctor, or hospital record		
		12. Day-care or nursery school record		

Illustrations of many of these documents appear in Part 8 of the Handbook for Employers (M-274)

Form I-9 (Rev.) Y Page 5

FIGURE 18-3, cont'd

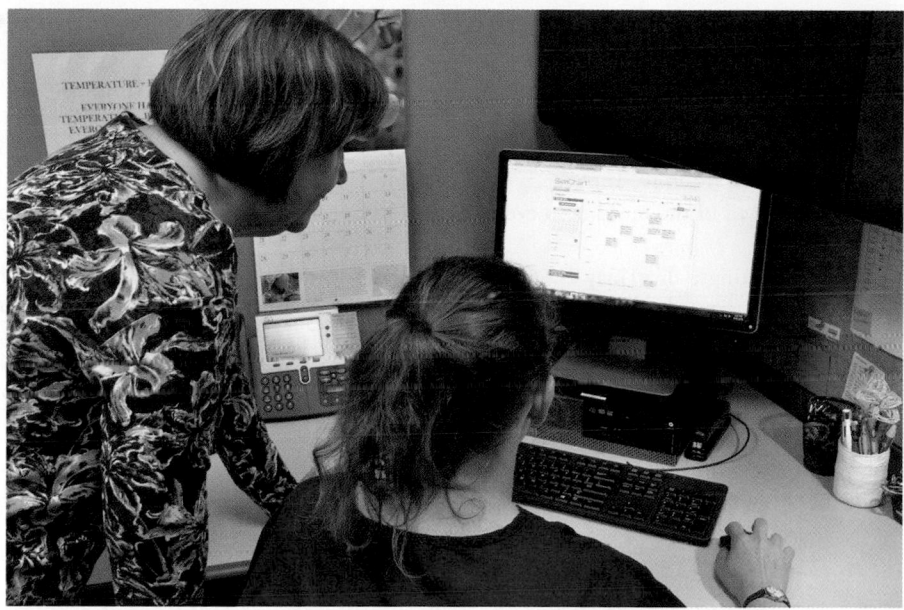

FIGURE 18-4 The training of successful employees begins with the job orientation.

Types of Employee Benefits

- *Employer-sponsored health insurance:* The employer pays a percentage of the employee's health insurance premium.
- *Dental and vision benefits:* The employer may offer dental and vision benefits for employees but may choose not to sponsor any of the premium.
- *Cafeteria plan:* A tax-free account in which employees can invest some of their paycheck and from which they can withdraw amounts for qualified health and/or child day care expenses.
- *401k retirement account matching:* The employer matches the exact amount or a percentage of the investment the employee makes every pay period (2% to 3%), up to a specific amount ($1,500).
- *Life insurance:* The employer pays for a small life insurance policy (usually up to $15,000) for minimal after-death expenses.
- *Disability insurance:* A benefit employees pay for that pays them if they are disabled and unable to work.

All new employees should be required to familiarize themselves with important office policies and procedures by reviewing the manual. It is advisable for the manager to require the employee to sign a statement verifying that the manual has been read.

Make sure the employee's file is complete before allowing the person to work even 1 hour. Also, make sure all federal and state regulations that apply to new employees have been met.

CRITICAL THINKING APPLICATION 18-5

Katherine is hiring a new employee who must begin work on the following Monday because the staff has been short one person for approximately 2 weeks. However, Katherine will be going on vacation the same day. How can she ensure that the new employee is trained properly?

Staff Development and Training

Continuous training and staff development are vital aspects of any medical facility. Technology is always advancing, so all employees must be kept up to date. Meetings should be held at least quarterly to ensure **compliance** in the use of health information technologies and the safety of patient health information. The staff should be trained to use the latest techniques and current regulations when dealing with issues that confront the medical facility. Keep an eye out for e-mails for seminar opportunities that will allow employees to earn continuing education units (CEUs) and develop more skills that will benefit the office. Ask employees to suggest topics about which they'd like to learn more and look for those opportunities. Professional organizations, such as the American Association of Medical Assistants (AAMA) and the American Medical Technologists (AMT), offer CEUs on a regular basis; encourage all staff members to become certified and to join professional organizations. Most hospitals have numerous continuing education classes that they allow employees of affiliated healthcare offices to attend.

Staff Meetings

As discussed, staff meetings are a formal channel used to keep the office manager and other team members current and communicating on a regular basis. One of the most common complaints from office personnel is that they are unable to discuss problems with the providers. The solution to this issue may be to hold regular staff meetings, which may be scheduled as frequently as weekly but should be held no less often than quarterly. Some of the best ideas on improvement come from the office staff; the expression and exchange of good ideas should be encouraged.

Set aside a specific time for regular meetings at an hour when most people can attend with the least disruption (Procedure 18-1). The meetings need not be long or overly formal, but to be effective, they must be planned and organized. There must be a leader, and someone should be appointed to take notes. The effectiveness of the leader, a person who can balance firmness with fairness, is an important aspect of the meeting. This usually is either the provider or the office manager or supervisor. All members of the staff should be encouraged to submit ideas for discussion.

Draw up a simple agenda listing the issues to be discussed and prepare any supporting data needed for the meeting. The agenda can be distributed to the team members ahead of the meeting so everyone can prepare and participate.

There are many kinds of staff meetings; they may be purely informational, problem-solving, or brainstorming meetings. They may be work sessions for updating manuals, training seminars, or whatever is necessary to the individual practice. Meetings also may be scheduled to discuss new ideas and any changes in office procedures. Some meetings are held simply to resolve specific problems. The staff meeting must not be allowed to deteriorate into a gripe session. Individual complaints should be handled privately.

The meeting agenda might be similar to that of any business meeting:
1. Reading of the last meeting's minutes
2. Discussion of any unfinished business
3. Discussion of any problems in the clinical area
4. Discussion of any problems in the administrative area
5. Discussion of any problems in common areas
6. Adjournment

Some providers like to combine the staff meeting with breakfast or lunch. The time or place is not important as long as it meets the needs of the practice. Meetings should be conducted democratically, and without interruption. Meetings should be kept as brief as possible. Always follow up on the items discussed; otherwise, the only result will be frustration and a reluctance to discuss problems at future meetings. The status of action items from the staff meeting should be introduced in the next staff meeting as *minutes*.

PROCEDURE 18-1   Prepare for a Staff Meeting

Goal: *Prepare for the meeting by creating an agenda and notifying the staff.*

Scenario: *You are a medical assistant team leader in a family practice department. Over the last 2 months there has been an increase in patient complaints related to long wait times in the reception area. Your supervisor asks you to prepare for a staff meeting to discuss these complaints and find ways to increase patient satisfaction.*

EQUIPMENT and SUPPLIES

- Computer with word processing software and email
- Paper and pen

PROCEDURAL STEPS

1. Using word processing software, create an agenda. Start by stating the attendees, start and end time, and location of the meeting.
2. Add the purpose and goal of the meeting.
3. Add a list of items to be discussed. The list needs to support or relate to the purpose of the meeting.
   PURPOSE: A well-written agenda provides the reader all the necessary information regarding the meeting.
4. Identify any supplies or materials the attendees should bring to the meeting.
5. Create a professional email to the attendees informing them of the meeting. The email should have an appropriate topic on the subject line. It should include a greeting, appropriate message, and a closing.

NOTE: In some facilities, the email can be sent as an invitation through the scheduling software. When the person accepts the invitation, a notation is then made on the person's schedule.
6. Use correct grammar, spelling, capitalization, and sentence structure in both the agenda and email.
   PURPOSE: Mistakes in the agenda and/or email can impact the reader's understanding of the information.
7. Proofread both the email and the agenda. Attach the agenda to the email and send it.
8. Create a list of items and equipment need for the meeting (e.g., whiteboard, easel pad and easel, projector, and computer).
9. Create a list of activities needed to prepare for the meeting and prepare the room for the meeting (e.g., appoint a person to take notes and order food).

Delegation of Duties

Delegating duties to subordinates allows managers to concentrate on the most critical aspects of their own jobs. Delegation also provides an opportunity to **empower** employees to develop their skills and experiences. Some managers are hesitant to assign duties to employees because they believe the tasks are too important not to be performed by staff employees. This hesitation suggests either a refusal to release control or mistrust of the employees. However, these manager types are typically overrun with tasks and unable to complete them. Managers should place trust in employees who have earned it and allow them to prove their abilities. Mistrust is a symptom of a poor hire. Discover the strengths of individual employees and then assign them tasks that will allow them to use those strengths. For example, if a medical assistant was hired to do administrative duties but is good with phlebotomy, empower the employee to assist with venipunctures whenever needed.

USING PERFORMANCE REVIEWS EFFECTIVELY

A new employee should be granted a probationary period. The traditional period is 60 to 90 days, but many employers believe that 2 weeks is sufficient to determine whether the employee will be able to learn and adapt to the position. Set a specific date for a performance review covering the probationary period when the new employee is hired. This review should not be squeezed in between patient visits or be given a token few minutes at the end of a day. Schedule a time that provides the opportunity to relax and talk. Tell the new employee how well expectations have been met and whether there are any deficiencies; then give the employee an opportunity to ask questions. Sometimes an employee fails to perform because he or she was never told what was expected. Although the probationary period does not always allow time to train an individual fully for a specific position, it is fair to assume that the potential for being a satisfactory employee can be judged at this time. Now is the time to talk about any problems and make suggestions for improvement. Sometimes the employee is released after an unsuccessful probationary period.

The formal performance appraisal usually occurs at the end of the probationary period and then at the hiring date anniversary. A typical appraisal includes feedback on teamwork, punctuality and attendance, motivation, accuracy with skills, customer service, professionalism, and potential continuing education and future goals. In many facilities, the appraisal relates to the pay increase the person will receive. Agencies do performance appraisals differently, yet one of the more common methods is for the supervisor to gather input from peers that work with the employee. The 360-degree evaluation is a process in which the supervisor, peers, and those who interact with the employee outside of the department provide feedback for the performance appraisal. If an employee works well with peers in the department, yet is rude and unprofessional to employees in other areas of the facility, the 360-degree evaluation will provide that information. This evaluation process holds the employee accountable for all his or her interactions in the facility.

When negative information is to be relayed to the employee during a performance appraisal, sandwich the negative comment between two positive ones whenever possible. For instance, tell the employee, "Jewel, you are a pro at greeting patients and making them feel at home. I would like to see you improve your time management skills, however, because I feel you are spending too much time with individual patients. I must confess that they feel a part of the clinic family. Let's work on some time management issues, and keep making them feel so welcome!"

Managers also may use the "feel, felt, found" approach when talking with employees about their performance. For example, "Jewel, I feel the same way you do about patients taking up a lot of our time. I know there are some that want to talk with us for hours, and I have felt the pressure of wanting to make them feel comfortable but having so much to do, too. I have found that if I explain that I have a meeting or another patient to assist, they are very understanding and not offended. Perhaps you can try that approach, too."

No supervisor enjoys giving an evaluation (Figure 18-5) that is not a positive one. It is difficult to know exactly where to begin when the employee has not performed as expected or hoped. Perhaps the best way to open the conversation is to say, "Rebecca, your review today is not going to be a positive one. It seems that we do not have a meeting of the minds about your duties and our expectations of you. Let's talk about your performance and discuss whether this position is a good match for you." Having detailed documentation of performance issues leaves little room for argument and places the manager on the offensive. The employee may be apprehensive or even defensive at this point, but the phrasing will certainly get his or her attention, and the discussion should produce either the motivation to improve or the clarity that termination is in order.

Problem Employees

Occasionally, employees do not perform at the expected level or demonstrate unprofessional behaviors. Counseling these employees

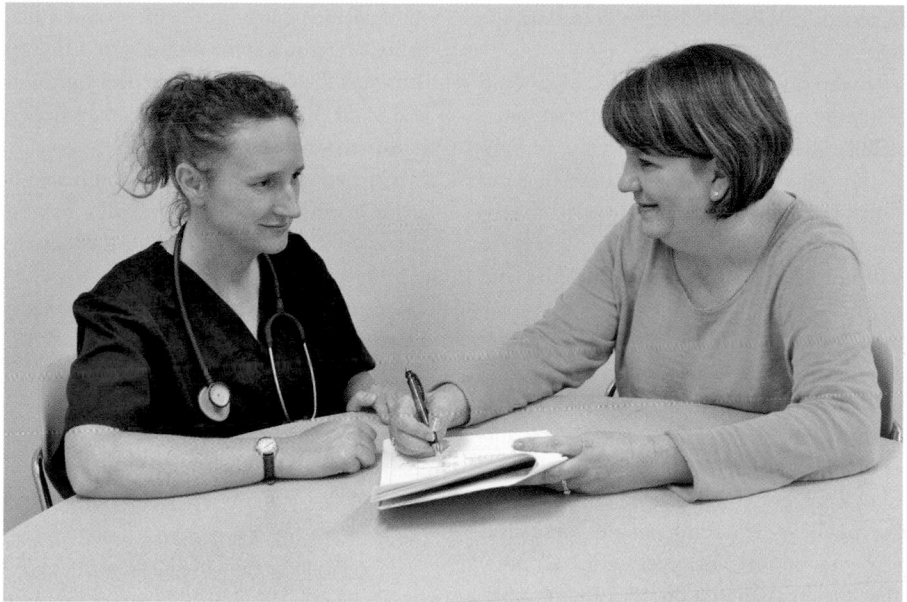

FIGURE 18-5 Performance evaluation and development plan. Performance evaluations should be considered tools that help employees reach their personal goals and the goals of the organization.

to determine the source of their difficulties is the first step toward resolution. Many employees can be redirected to become productive staff members with a little patience and understanding on the manager's part. Employees who display a willingness to improve their attitude are worth the investment the office manager makes to help them succeed.

Many offices allow one verbal warning before written reprimands go into the employee's file. It is important that the manager document the specific times, dates, and descriptions of incidents, even issues like tardiness. If the manager does not make a habit of writing a *formal warning* in the employee's **human resources file (HR file)**, there may be insufficient documentation of problems. The manager should never be in a position in which the termination of an employee cannot be justified through documentation.

CRITICAL THINKING APPLICATION   18-6

Katherine has two employees who have never seemed to get along. One of the employees has a history of being vindictive and manipulative, but never in an obvious enough way for Katherine to have sufficient proof to reprimand her in writing. One day, one of the employees comes to Katherine's office to report that she saw the other employee, who has an exemplary record, taking drugs from the supply cabinet. How does Katherine handle this situation? What steps should Katherine take from here?

Terminating Employees

Terminating an employee is unpleasant at best, but if the ground rules are decided in advance, written into the office policies and procedures manual, and explained to all employees, the problem is partially solved. The policies must be applied equally and impartially to all employees. The providers of the healthcare facility will most probably make the final decision on dismissal, but it may be based on the recommendation of the office manager. Unless there are mitigating factors that suggest otherwise, the person who does the hiring should do the firing.

A probationary employee who does not prove satisfactory should be dismissed at the end of the probationary period, with tact and a full explanation of the reasons for dismissal. In all fairness, an individual should be told why the employment is being ended and not be given weak excuses or untruths that do not help correct deficiencies. If the manager is not straightforward in giving the reason for dismissal, the employee will not have the opportunity to grow and improve his or her performance.

An employee who has been in service for some time and is not performing satisfactorily should be warned and given an explanation of the specific improvements expected. If a second chance does not produce improvement in performance or attitude, dismissal must follow. It should be done privately, with tact and consideration.

Most practice consultants believe that firing should come close to the end of the day and end of the workweek, after all other employees have left, and that the break should be clean and immediate. If the office policy provides for 2 weeks' notice when an employee resigns, the provider may want to offer 2 weeks' pay unless the circumstances that led to the dismissal were extremely **blatant**. A dismissed employee should never be allowed to train or influence a replacement.

The exit meeting should be planned just as carefully as the employment interview. Be honest with the employee. Discuss both the employee's assets and liabilities and give the reasons for the termination. There is no need to dwell on the employee's deficiencies. These should have been thoroughly discussed at the warning interview, and the employee need only be told that the necessary improvements have not been made. Listen to the employee's feedback, unless it becomes lengthy or abusive. This may reveal some important administrative problems that need correction.

After dismissing an employee, do not leave that person in the office unattended. Request the office keys and any other equipment in the employee's possession immediately, before the dismissed employee leaves the building, and block all access to the healthcare facility's electronic health records (EHRs). Most states have strict payday laws that do not allow holding the final paycheck for any reason. Do not offer to give the employee a good reference unless it can be done sincerely. If there is any indication that an employee may become abusive or violent once told about the termination, the supervisor should bring a representative from the human resources department or security to the final interview. It is possible that an employee can "snap" and suddenly become violent; however, more often it is the warning flags raised by an employee's behavior before termination that justify care in the termination interview. This is why supervisors should always document any strange or suspicious employee behavior and any breach of office policy or procedures in the employee's personnel file, according to office policy. Documenting everything creates a clear picture of the employee's actions throughout the time of employment. Of course, the supervisor must be willing to confront an employee about his or her negative actions in the workplace.

Some specific employee behaviors in the workplace, such as embezzlement, insubordination, and violation of patient confidentiality, are grounds for immediate dismissal without warning. These behaviors display a lack of respect for the healthcare facility and can lead to the mistreatment or endangerment of patients if the employee is not terminated immediately.

Occasionally an employee voluntarily leaves a position without giving a valid reason. The provider or office manager may want to follow up with a letter to the former employee to determine whether a problem prompted the resignation. The employee may reveal serious issues with other personnel or with the office that need to be addressed and corrected.

CRITICAL THINKING APPLICATION   18-7

While Katherine is explaining to a particularly poor employee why she plans to terminate her, the employee begins screaming and accusing Katherine of discrimination and harassment. How should Katherine handle this situation? What are Katherine's options if the employee does not stop the inappropriate behavior?

Fair Salaries and Raises

Medical office managers should recruit employees who want to remain with the office for a long time. There are always such situations as a part-time worker returning to college, or a summer worker going back to school. However, good employee **retention** is the goal.

To retain good employees, the practice must pay them a fair salary with regular raises if they perform as expected. The office manager can find information about salary comparisons on the Internet. Periodically review job descriptions and salary analyses online to see whether the salary the medical facility offers is comparable to that for similar jobs in the area.

Merit raises are increases based on an employee's commendable performance. Cost of living increases are given when earned, usually after specific periods or annually, and are based on national statistics and trends. An employee who is promoted should also be awarded a salary increase. When the office pays a fair salary for work done, the facility retains happy employees.

CLOSING COMMENTS

Medical assistants are not likely to go into office management immediately after graduation. The goal of this chapter is to introduce and discuss further professional opportunities in office management and the supervision of the healthcare facility staff. Successful office managers care about their employees and the vision for the healthcare facility. The areas of authority and responsibility must be clearly defined to prevent management problems. A detailed office policies and procedures manual helps the healthcare manager run an efficient facility.

Legal and Ethical Issues

Office managers must stay abreast of current employment laws and regulations for all the different agencies that govern the medical office. Joining a local office managers' association can help the manager keep the office up to date and in compliance. Periodic online checks of the websites of various organizations (e.g., OSHA) are a good way for the office manager to keep up with the most recent changes in policies and rules.

HIPAA compliance training should be required for all healthcare facilities. The facility's office manager should be knowledgable not only about all HIPAA provisions, including those affecting the privacy and security of patient health information, but also about the penalties associated with information breaches.

Professional Behaviors

Managers that encourage their staff create a strong team in the healthcare facility. By focusing on team building, office managers can accomplish more tasks efficiently, delegate some of their workload, and promote high-quality patient care. Office managers can become immersed in their daily office responsibilities; however, they must keep in mind that slacking off on staff training and team development meetings results in lower office productivity. Staff meetings should be scheduled in advance and their attendance should be mandatory for all staff members.

SUMMARY OF SCENARIO

Katherine has had a positive effect on her team at the Fair Oaks Pediatrics office. She treats her employees well and is fair about administering office policies and procedures. Her staff appreciates her flexibility and professionalism as she manages the day-to-day operations of the facility. Katherine treats her employees as team members, never speaking to them as if she were superior to them. She shares vital information with the staff so that they feel a part of the whole team, and she believes that even negative information should be relayed to the staff so that everyone is aware of the challenges the office faces. She makes strong hiring decisions and firmly believes in a good orientation and training program. Dr. Elaine Collins, the senior member of the pediatrician staff, has placed a great deal of trust in Katherine, and she has performed well, proving to be a reliable office manager.

Katherine knows that she should display a friendly attitude toward her staff members when it is appropriate to do so. She is kind and considerate and treats the staff as individuals. She does not fraternize with them but is open to having lunch with the staff at various times and participates in all casual office activities. She maintains a healthy distance so that she can be an effective manager, but she listens to those who are experiencing difficulty and is compassionate about helping whenever possible.

Katherine knows that when hiring for a vacant position, she must be diligent in checking references so that she brings reliable, qualified individuals on board as staff members. Unless she receives acceptable references, she will not hire a medical assistant to become a part of her team. Once she hires someone, she conducts a thorough training program and takes special care to share the experience and skills of the new staff member with the rest of the team.

When Katherine must give a negative employee evaluation, she states that fact at the beginning of the meeting. Although she is compassionate, she is able to point out a staff member's shortcomings in a detailed, fair way. She usually is willing to give an employee time to improve, but if he or she fails to perform, Katherine does not hesitate to end the employment.

Katherine leads a group of cooperative team members who function well together every day, and this results in an efficient office and a pleasant work environment.

SUMMARY OF LEARNING OBJECTIVES

1. **Define, spell, and pronounce the terms listed in the vocabulary.**
   Spelling and pronouncing medical terms correctly reinforce the medical assistant's credibility. Knowing the definitions of these terms promotes confidence in communication with patients and co-workers.

2. **Define the qualities and responsibilities of a successful office manager for a healthcare facility.**
   The provider counts on the office manager to run the business aspects of the office so that he or she can focus on providing good patient care. A high degree of trust is placed in the office manager. A good office manager is fair and flexible. Good communication skills are necessary, as is attention to detail. The manager should care about the employees and have a sense of fairness. The ability to remain calm in a crisis is important, as are the use of good judgment and the ability to multitask. Successful medical office managers work to promote a positive team environment to facilitate cohesion.

3. **Explain the chain of command in the medical office.**
   The provider/owner is ultimately responsible for all activities in the medical office. The provider and the medical office manager work together to handle the day-to-day activities. The provider trusts the medical office manager to handle employee issues. The medical office manager also defines job descriptions so that each member of the team is aware of his or her responsibilities.

4. **Do the following related to the power of motivation:**
   - *Identify several ways in which employees are motivated.*
     Employees are motivated by various factors, including money, praise, insecurity, honor, prestige, needs, love, fear, satisfaction, and many others. An effective manager attempts to discover what motivates an employee to do a good job. Employees can also be motivated by incentives and recognition.
   - *Explain how the abuse of power and authority can negatively affect productivity in a healthcare facility.*
     A manager who berates and insults the staff members because he or she feels superior to them creates a distrusting, stressful, and nonproductive environment. Eventually the conduct of these types of managers negatively affects the quality of the care given to patients.

5. **Do the following related to creating a team atmosphere:**
   - *Discuss strategies to create a team environment in the medical office.*
     Teamwork is critical in the medical profession. In the healthcare facility, the manager must promote an atmosphere in which employees are willing to work together toward common goals. Morale in the facility may be low because of recent changes in policies or procedures, changes in staff or management, recent terminations of employees, lack of business, or any number of other reasons. The wise manager takes steps to improve employee morale continuously, including scheduling frequent meetings and keeping employees abreast of changes and developments that affect them.
   - *Recognize and overcome barriers to communication.*
     It is important for the medical assistant to recognize the barriers and help the team overcome them. Physical separation barriers can be reduced by using technology (e.g., video-conferencing and webcams). Language barriers can be addressed by encouraging awareness and acceptance of everyone's language and cultural differences. Status barriers can be reduced by promoting awareness and acceptance that everyone counts and every position on the team is important. Gender difference barriers can be addressed by helping all employees feel empowered to communicate openly with others. Cultural diversity barriers can be reduced by helping the team embrace the cultural differences among the members and educating the team on the differences.
   - *Demonstrate respect for individual diversity including gender, race, religion, age, economic status, and appearance.*
     Encouraging workplace diversity is part of the method of encouraging strong teams in the healthcare facility. Management should focus on the strengths that each staff member brings to the team. Staff members should be trained to provide the best medical care they can for all patients, without discrimination.

6. **Summarize strategies to introduce a new office manager.**
   As a new office manager, the first thing you can do to begin gaining support is nothing. Never storm into an office and begin making radical changes in the first few days. Work with the providers to determine the office goals. Then, schedule individual meetings with employees; allow them to tell you three things they like about their jobs, three things they dislike, and three things they need to do their jobs more effectively. After discussing your findings with the providers, use strategy to put the helpful suggestions into practice and attempt to move employees toward achieving the office goals.

7. **List several ways to prevent burnout.**
   Some of the causes of burnout include a stressful, disorganized home or work environment; poor human relations skills; a feeling of being out of control of one's life; excessive expectations from supervisors or family members; long work hours or time away from family and friends; and not being able to relax either at home or in the work environment. Although management may make efforts to prevent employee burnout, the employee ultimately must take steps to prevent it.

8. **Do the following related to finding the right employee for the job:**
   - *Identify the need to find the right employee for a job opening in the medical office.*
     From the providers to the receptionist, all play a vital role in the quality of healthcare delivered to patients. Hiring staff members who can be molded into a cohesive team is not an easy task. Care should be taken to choose employees who have the necessary skills and the right personality for the ambulatory care facility. When the need for a new employee arises, the office manager should discuss with the providers the type of employee required and the job description for that individual.
   - *Review a general job description for medical assistants.*
     Medical assistants are qualified for a variety of tasks in the healthcare facility. To fill an open medical assisting position, the manager must

SUMMARY OF LEARNING OBJECTIVES—*continued*

determine the specific experience that meets the facility's needs. Management should summarize the educational and skills sets needed to be successful at the position in the job description.

- *Explain how to search through résumés and applications for potential candidates.*

  Résumés and applications should be reviewed for accuracy and completeness. Gaps in employment dates should be explained fully, and the office manager should verify any references. Documents should be legible, and the information should be consistent and without oversights.

- *List and discuss legal and illegal interview questions.*

  The interviewer should be aware of various federal and state laws protecting the interviewee. Title VII of the Civil Rights Act of 1964, as amended by the Equal Employment Opportunity Act of 1972, prohibits inquiries into an applicant's race, color, gender, religion, and national origin. Inquiries about a person's medical history, arrest record, or previous drug use also are illegal. Most states have laws designed to protect the rights of job applicants, and these laws may impose additional restrictions. Office managers must research the laws that pertain to employment in their own states.

- *Explain how to select the most qualified candidates.*

  The first step in reviewing resumes includes separating out those that meet the minimal qualifications and those that do not. From those that meet the minimal qualifications, divide those into three stacks: those to call for an interview, possible candidates but not the strongest, and those that will not be called for an interview. Those with related experience, strong related skill sets (e.g., customer service), no unexplained employment gaps, and customized, error-free resumes and cover letters are more apt to be moved to the top of the pile.

- *Identify follow-up activities the office manager should perform after the interview.*

  When the interview is over, the office manager or interview team should immediately take a few moments to rate or summarize the applicant's strength and weaknesses. After all the interviews have been conducted, the team then rates the interviewees and identifies the top candidates. References are checked and a second interview may occur before the final person has been selected.

9. **Review new employee orientation, including paperwork, training, and development; also, explain how to conduct a staff meeting with an agenda.**

The office manager should develop a checklist of the paperwork needed for newly hired staff and all the information that should be covered with the new employee at the start of the job. Basic new employee paperwork often includes a job application; Form I-9 (Employment Eligibility Verification); W-4 Form (Employee's Withholding Allowance Certificate); Notice of Workers' Compensation coverage; consent for a background check and drug testing; acknowledgement of receipt of the company handbook or policy manual; agreements regarding pay, wage deductions, benefits, schedule, work location, and so on; notices of at-will employment status; acknowledgement of ethics statement; direct deposit application; and the OSHA compliance acknowledgement or checklist. Orientation and training help new employees to understand what is expected and to develop to their full potential.

The process for arranging a staff meeting is outlined in Procedure 18-1.

10. **Discuss strategies for addressing a problem employee, giving an employee a poor evaluation, terminating an employee, and determining fair salaries and raises.**

When negative information is to be relayed to an employee during a performance appraisal, the office manager should sandwich the negative comment between two positive ones whenever possible. Counseling these employees to find the source of their difficulties is the first step toward resolution. Many employees can be redirected to become productive staff members with a little patience and understanding on the manager's part. The manager should have good documentation of the problems that led to the poor evaluation. An employee who has been in service for some time and is offering unsatisfactory performance should be warned and given an explanation of the specific improvements expected. If a second chance does not produce improvement in performance or attitude, dismissal must follow. It should be done privately, with tact and consideration.

To keep good employees, the practice must pay a fair salary with regular raises if the staff member performs as expected. The office manager can find information about salary comparisons on the Internet. The manager should periodically review job descriptions and salary analyses online to see whether the salary the medical facility offers is comparable to those for similar jobs in the area.

CONNECTIONS

Study Guide Connection: Go to the Chapter 18 Study Guide. Read and complete the activities.

evolve Evolve Connection: Go to the Chapter 18 link at *evolve.elsevier.com/kinn* to complete the Chapter Review Quiz. Check out the other resources listed for this chapter to make the most of what you have learned from Supervision and Human Resource Management.

19 MEDICAL PRACTICE MARKETING AND CUSTOMER SERVICE

Medical assistant Monica Raymond was hired by the Clear Skin Dermatology practice 2 years ago, after she had graduated from a medical assisting program. Dr. Julie Huang regularly praises Monica for her customer service skills. Dr. Huang is aware that effective marketing is essential to grow the practice, so she has asked Monica if she would be willing to assume some marketing responsibilities for the practice. Dr. Huang knows that Monica is comfortable using the Internet and is social media–savvy. Monica is excited about this opportunity. She realizes that she first must determine the type of patients the practice usually serves.

Dr. Huang has suggested a small budget and a few marketing tools that Monica may want to implement. In turn, Monica has suggested some updates to staff members' training, to improve their customer service skills and thus patient retention.

Monica has started designing the practice's website. She plans to incorporate a few features she found on other medical practice websites, including online appointment scheduling, an "ask the provider" e-mail exchange, and uploading of new patient intake forms. Knowing the importance of social networking, Monica intends to establish the dermatology practice on several social media platforms, such as Facebook and YouTube.

While studying this chapter, think about the following questions:

- Why is it important to identify the target market?
- What are some cost-effective marketing tools that a healthcare practice can use?
- Can social media help a healthcare practice stay in closer communication with its patients? If so, how?
- Why is customer service so important when delivering patient care?
- What type of resources can the healthcare practice provide to meet the needs of its patients?

LEARNING OBJECTIVES

1. Define, spell, and pronounce the terms listed in the vocabulary.
2. Do the following related to the marketing needs of a healthcare practice:
   - Explain the need for marketing for a healthcare facility.
   - Identify the target market.
   - Discuss why a SWOT analysis is important to identify the target market.
3. Do the following related to marketing tools:
   - Review ways a healthcare practice or facility can promote their practice through community involvement.
   - Define and discuss automated call distribution.
   - Explain how newsletters and blogs can be effective marketing tools.
   - Discuss marketing through print ads in magazines and newspapers.
   - Determine the value of Internet marketing for a healthcare practice or facility.
4. Distinguish between advertising and public relations.
5. Discuss the value of marketing through social media.
6. Develop website content, organization, and design to attract new patients; also, review strategies to increase website traffic.
7. Explain how to successfully deliver high-quality customer service, including how to identify with patients, and the value of patient surveys.
8. Identify strategies to manage problem patients.
9. Review the importance of the new patient information packet, and develop a current list of community resources related to patients' healthcare needs.
10. In the role of patient navigator, facilitate referrals to community resources.
11. Define a patient-centered medical home (PCMH).
12. Discuss applications of electronic technology (e.g., telemedicine) in professional communication.

VOCABULARY

advocate An individual who represents the patient when healthcare decisions are made.

blog An online journal that providers can use to share their experiences in caring for patients.

cost benefit analysis An assessment that weighs the benefit of attracting patients against the cost required.

liaison An individual assigned to communicate between multiple parties when the financial responsibilities of a deceased patient's estate are settled.

patient centered medical home (PCMH) A model philosophy intended to improve the effectiveness of primary care. This approach is promoted by the National Committee for Quality Assurance (NCQA).

patient navigator A person who identifies patients' needs and barriers and assists by coordinating care and identifying community and healthcare resources to meet the needs.

site map A list of all Web page links on a website.

social media Internet sponsored, two-way communication between individuals, individuals and businesses, or between businesses.

target market The groups of people most likely to need the medical services the practice offers.

telemedicine Video-conferencing technology that enables the delivery of quality healthcare at a distance.

A medical practice is a business; therefore, success lies in bringing in new patients and retaining current patients to maintain cash flow. Marketing and customer service are both essential for a healthcare facility to grow. *Marketing* is the process of informing the local community of the medical procedures and services the healthcare practice provides. Once customers visit the healthcare facility and become patients, customer service can enhance their experience so they want to return.

Marketing can be expensive and ineffective at increasing patient traffic if it is not planned out well. Some healthcare facilities work hard to find patients in the community, but then lose the patients' business through the lack of customer service. Customer loyalty ensures the longevity of a healthcare business. Therefore, following a well-thought-out marketing plan and building loyalty through customer service can ensure the healthcare practice's long-term financial success.

MARKETING NEEDS OF THE HEALTHCARE FACILITY

All healthcare practices must have some sort of marketing plan to attract new patients. There are many ways to market a healthcare practice. A billboard near a freeway is a great way to promote the practice because of the number of potential patients it can reach; however, this type of marketing can be very expensive. A healthcare practice can print business cards for about $20 and then have someone leave a card at all the stores in a retail center. Although relatively inexpensive, this method doesn't ensure that the right patients are being reached (Table 19-1). The most important element of the marketing plan is to identify the right target market.

Identifying the Target Market

Identifying the **target market** is the key to successful marketing. Reaching the target market means that the targeted groups are made aware of the healthcare practice and what it has to offer.

The first step in identifying the target market is to determine who will need the medical procedures and services the healthcare facility offers. For example, the elderly population would most benefit from a long-term care facility. Women who are or who want

TABLE 19-1 Marketing Strategies for the Medical Office	
STRATEGY	**COST**
Maintain a professional website	$$$
Manage an active Facebook, Twitter, Instagram, and/or other social media handle	No cost
Actively participate in community health fairs and events	$
Mail yearly checkup reminders	$$
Purchase billboard or magazine advertisements promoting the medical office	$$$$
Invite the public to an open house	$

to become pregnant would benefit from an obstetrician's office and so on.

To bring more focus to the target market, the healthcare practice can review the demographics of its current patients. It may find, for example, that most of the patients for the long-term care facility come from the 78253 ZIP code. A gynecologist's office may find that most of its patients are between the ages of 20 and 25. In established medical offices, the medical assistant should keep a spreadsheet file for all patients with the following fields:

- Reason for visit
- Patient's age
- ZIP code
- Gender
- Marital status
- Ages of children
- How the patient found out about the healthcare facility

These demographics provide the details of the healthcare facility's specific target market. To identify the target market further, a SWOT analysis should be performed.

SWOT Analysis

The acronym SWOT stands for:

S – Strengths
W – Weaknesses
O – Opportunities
T – Threats

The SWOT analysis provides an evaluation of the business environment (Figure 19-1). This tool evaluates how economic forces affect the healthcare facility internally and externally. The Strengths and Weaknesses categories evaluate internal economic forces, and the Opportunities and Threats categories evaluate external economic forces.

Strengths and Weaknesses. The strengths of a healthcare practice are the advantages it has over its competitors, such as in the following categories:

- Reduced patient wait times
- Advanced medical technique and health information technology
- Flexible appointment hours
- Patient information Web portals
- E-prescribing

Weaknesses are the exact opposite of strengths. In other words, the weaknesses tool evaluates whether the healthcare practice's competitors are better in any of these categories.

No healthcare practice has only strengths. It would be too expensive for the practice to offer every benefit for their patients, but not be able to gain all the patients in their target market. Therefore, the healthcare practice should perform a **cost benefit analysis**, which is an assessment that weighs the benefit of attracting patients against the cost required. For example, a healthcare practice could invest in an in-house magnetic resonance imaging (MRI) machine, which would cost millions of dollars in lease payments over the next 5 years. But how many patients will use the machine in their healthcare facility? How much revenue will having the equipment generate for the medical office? Are there more significant advantages compared to referring patients go to a laboratory facility for an MRI?

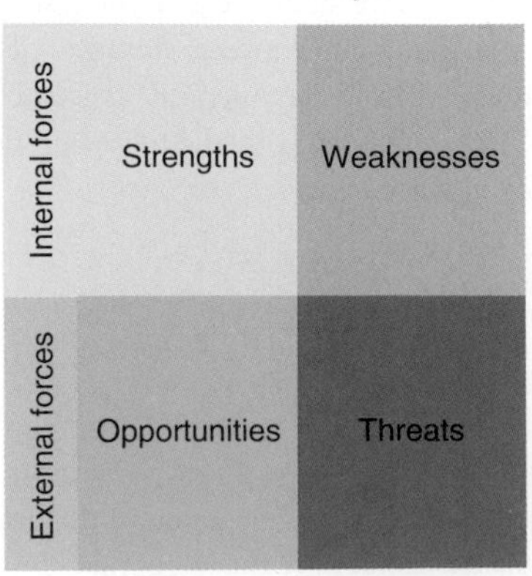

Opportunities and Threats. Opportunities review the prospect of increased business due to external forces. Healthcare practices have little or no control over the external market environment; however, a practice that recognizes opportunities can improve its internal strengths. Likewise, disregarding changes in the market can worsen a practice's weaknesses.

Some examples of opportunities include:

- Medical technology that reduces the cost of healthcare and hospital stays
- The increased number of Americans with health insurance because of the Affordable Care Act
- Electronic management of patient information, which reduces the time needed to care for each patient
- Public health campaigns, which highlight the importance of seeing the provider for specialized care

Threats can damage the long-term viability of a healthcare practice. A key threat is resisting the integration of electronic health record (EHR) systems into the practice. EHR systems facilitate the delivery of quality healthcare to patients and can support the continuity of patient care through collaboration among different healthcare providers. Although the implementation of electronic systems in healthcare facilities can be expensive at first, the long-term market outlook for them is good.

CRITICAL THINKING APPLICATION   **19-1**

Monica reviews the clinic's spreadsheet file of dermatology patients and finds that 40% of the patients come in for treatment of their acne. Would it be a good idea for the dermatology practice to expand its treatments for acne patients?

MARKETING TOOLS

As mentioned, some marketing strategies can be very expensive and also ineffective. Once the target market has been clearly identified, a number of marketing tools can effectively increase patient volume.

Promoting the Practice Through Community Involvement

Patients trust medical offices that participate in the local community. Some healthcare practices have participated in local health fairs offering free screenings, have partnered with farmer's markets to promote healthier eating, or even sponsored a local 5K run/walk to encourage exercise. To increase the healthcare practice's involvement in the community, some staff members can attend public community events and distribute brochures and pamphlets about conditions such as diabetes, heart disease, and hypertension. The practice may also sponsor specific charities annually. Some healthcare practices have volunteer programs in which staff members are recognized for their participation in community activities. Screenings for cholesterol and blood pressure checks are good ways to market a practice and gain new patients. The more the public views the healthcare practice actively participating in the community, the more likely it is that this will increase the number of appointments made at the medical office.

SWOT Analysis

FIGURE 19-1 A SWOT analysis can be done to define the target market.

Automated Phone Calls

Automated appointment reminders are a popular means of communicating with a large number of patients. A computer dials multiple phone numbers at the same time and plays a recorded message. Similar systems can send out text messages because most patients use their cell phones as their primary phone line. For instance, if a healthcare practice is planning to move to another part of the city, a program could be initiated to notify all patients that the office will be moving after a certain date. The message could include the address of the new location and even prompt patients to "Press 1" if they need to schedule an appointment. The same principle could be applied to news about an upcoming health fair or a special seminar about a certain illness.

Newsletters and Blogs

Many providers refer their patients to medical research about a variety of health topics, including ways to be treated. Some providers communicate this medical information as an e-newsletter, which is sent periodically, typically every month. However, providers are careful not to offer medical advice electronically; the intention of the e-newsletter should be to inform patients about health conditions that the provider typically sees in the medical office. For example, as an introduction to outdoor summer activities, an e-newsletter may promote healthy sun habits, such as wearing hats, sunglasses, and sunscreen. Or, in the fall, the provider can publish an e-newsletter to discuss ways to avoid catching the flu and may include a short video on how to properly wash hands to prevent the spread of disease.

A **blog** is an online journal that providers can use to share their experiences in caring for patients. Usually, providers do not follow a schedule for blog posts; they post when they have an experience to share for prevention, for care, and to inform. For example, a provider may document a patient who came in with a second-degree sunburn. To protect the patient's identity, the provider must uphold all privacy and confidentiality rules established by the Health Insurance Portability and Accountability Act (HIPAA), but he or she can post how the patient suffered through an unfortunate incident that could have been prevented. Sometimes blogs can include a v-log, or video log; at times providers post surgery videos online to inform patients of the services they provide.

Print Ads in Magazines and Newspapers

Advertising in magazines, newspapers, or mailers can inform the public of the healthcare practice and the services it offers. However, it is important to ensure that the target market can be reached by advertising this way because it is significantly more expensive and reaches a wider audience. Advertising in local magazines and/or newspapers is a more effective marketing strategy and can establish a business in the community. Magazine and newspaper ads can be effective tools, but finding free sources to promote the practice is less of a strain on the budget and allows expansion in other areas. The effectiveness of a newspaper and magazine marketing strategy can be evaluated by asking new patients how they learned about the practice. If a significant percentage mention the magazine or newspaper ad, the target market was reached.

Mailers are postcards or flyers that are mailed directly to hundreds of homes in a geographic area (Figure 19-2). This practice can be costly, and the target market may be wider than the area covered in the mailing, so the strategy may not be as effective. The more specialized the service the healthcare practice offers, the less likely it is that a mailer campaign could reach the target market and thus would be successful in increasing patient traffic.

Internet Marketing

Nowadays it is common to read many customer reviews on websites before patronizing a business. Businesses with more and better reviews tend to attract new customers. A healthcare practice has many opportunities to build a strong reputation through Internet marketing because patients can post reviews of their experiences on many different popular websites. The key is to ask every patient before he or she leaves to post a review of the services the person received; as the number of reviewers grows, the potential for new patients also will grow. A medical assistant can take responsibility for monitoring customer reviews on websites to confirm that the reviews are mostly positive. Some websites allow businesses to address negative comments, so the medical assistant should be ready to post a reply, such as, "We're sorry that you feel you did not receive the care that you deserve. Please feel free to call our office manager, Grace Townsend, to discuss how we could have improved your experience. Thank you for your feedback."

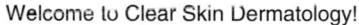
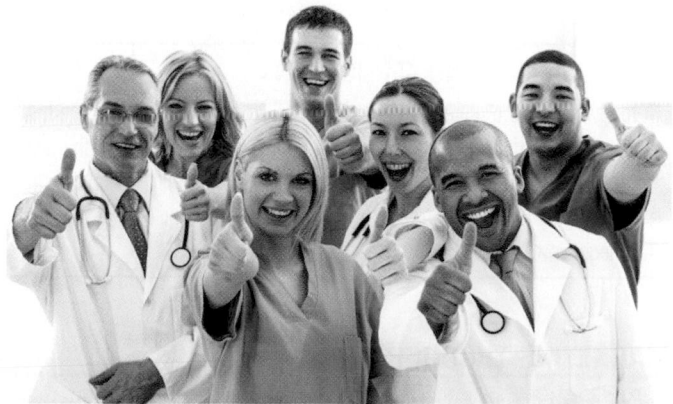

Welcome to Clear Skin Dermatology!

FIGURE 19-2 A mailer promoting the healthcare facility.

ADVERTISING VERSUS PUBLIC RELATIONS

There is a difference between advertising and public relations. Advertising involves creating or changing attitudes, beliefs, and perceptions by influencing people with purchased broadcast time, print space, or other forms of written and visual media. Broadcast time could take the form of television commercials, radio broadcasts, or audiovisual aids. Print could be a newspaper, magazine, or trade journal, and written and visual media may include a flier, brochure, or billboard.

Public relations is a similar field but relies more on news broadcasts or reports, magazine or newspaper articles, and blogs and radio reports to reach the audience. Most public relations efforts are free, but often it is difficult to get others interested enough in the activities the medical practice is planning to warrant coverage.

Addressing Bad Press

Occasionally a healthcare facility will face some cases of medical error, poor healthcare delivery, the leaking of personal health information, and/or mitigating circumstances that have found their way into the national headlines. Because healthcare is a personal issue, negative health news stories can destroy the trust the community has in the provider and the medical office. The first defense is to establish a high standard of customer service in the medical practice. Many patients will overlook small mistakes if the medical staff is apologetic and humble about the error.

If a medical error has been published in any type of media, it is wise for the medical practice to post an official apology statement on its website. This statement should not defend the actions of the provider and/or the medical practice, but rather express concern for any that were negatively affected in any way. The statement should also inform the public of the practice's rededication to delivering quality healthcare to all its current patients. A copy of the statement can also be displayed in the reception area of the medical office.

After the error has been published, the medical practice and the provider must work to overcome the stigma. Greater participation in the local community can help win back patients' trust, but patience and diligence may be needed to rebuild a thriving medical practice. It may be wise for a medical practice to hire a public relations consultant to help it improve its image in the community.

CRITICAL THINKING APPLICATION 19-4

A few weeks ago a patient posted on a public review website that she had had a bad reaction to a chemical peel she received at the clinic; she also complained that the medical office staff had done nothing to rectify the problem. This is the most recent review. What can Monica do to address the negative customer review?

MARKETING THROUGH SOCIAL MEDIA

Social media (e.g., Facebook, Twitter, YouTube) allow for two-way communication between a business and the consumer. Social media outlets promote the business, and customers can respond positively or negatively about the service they received. Traditional media outlets, such as newspapers and magazines, allow only limited ability to respond; a person can write a letter to the editor of a newspaper, but the letter is not an immediate two-way exchange. Social media are considered a blending of technology and social interaction that creates an effective marketing tool.

Many websites now have icons that link to Facebook, Instagram, Twitter, YouTube, Pinterest, and other types of social media to promote interaction, in the hope of creating loyal patient relationships.

Medical offices are taking advantage of social media to promote the services they offer. Just like the "About Us" Web page, social media allow patients to gain insight into the care delivered. Providers can post nutritional counseling videos on YouTube, announce a community event on Twitter, and post the event pictures on Instagram. Patients can use Facebook to refer their friends and family to the medical practice. At-home remedies for some conditions, such as migraines, can be posted on Pinterest. Social media can bring the provider-patient relationship closer without the provider spending more time with the patient.

It is easy to understand how an aggressive, well-planned social media approach can positively affect the financial health of a practice. These outlets put individuals "into" the Web, making the experience more interactive and responsive. A medical assistant who can promote the healthcare practice on social media in a professional way is a valuable asset to the practice.

BUILDING A MEDICAL PRACTICE WEBSITE

One of the most popular and beneficial marketing tools for the healthcare facility is a professional website. An essential part of the marketing budget is the cost of having a Web developer create a website and maintain it on a monthly basis (Figure 19-3).

Five basic steps are involved in building a website for a medical practice:
1. Choosing a website name
2. Creating a site map
3. Designing the pages, including graphics and written content
4. Increasing traffic to the website
5. Using social media to increase public awareness of the website

Choosing a Website Name

Choosing a website name should be part of the healthcare facility's marketing strategy. Patients should commonly associate the website name with the medical office. The ideal website name typically is 7 to 15 letters and is related to the practice's name. The Internet has been around for some time, so many website names have already been taken; therefore, an Internet search should be done to check the availability of the preferred name before it is given to the Web page designer. Most websites begin with *www.*, followed by the name with no spaces, and usually end with *.org*, *.com* or *.net*. Some other website endings (e.g., *.gov* for government sites and *.edu* for educational institutions) would not be appropriate for a healthcare facility.

There is no requirement that the website name reflect the provider's name or the name of the medical office. Some practices identify themselves as the local specialist, as in *www.riversidegastroenterologists.com*.

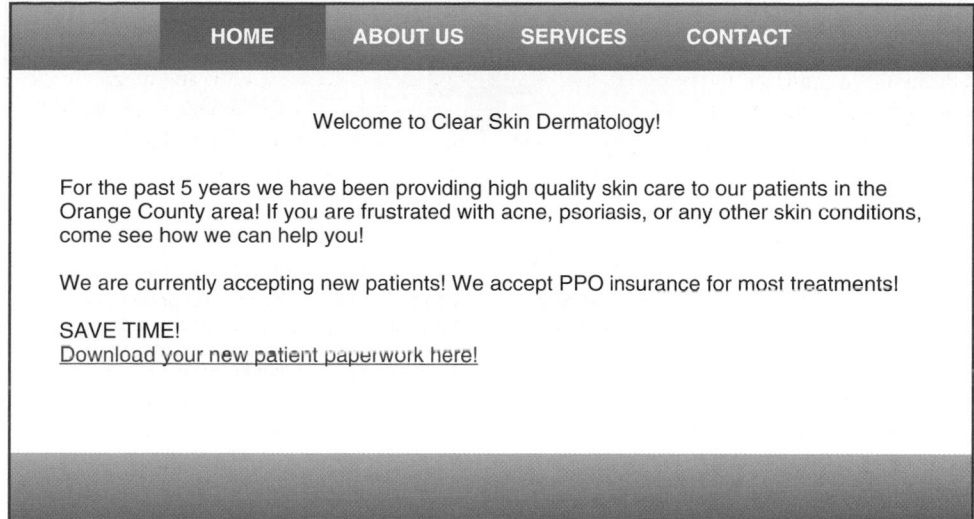

FIGURE 19-3 Common website format, with an introduction to the healthcare facility and site map.

Creating a Site Map

A successful website will attract many patients. An organized **site map** makes the website user friendly. When the website is designed, it is important to identify which informational pages should be included. A standard basic website has a Home page, an About Us page, a Testimonials or Information page, a Specials page, and a Contact Us page.

Home Page

The Home page is the introduction to the entire website. It is the first page viewed when the patient types the website into the address bar. The purpose of the Home page is to introduce the medical practice to the patient. Design is a key element of this page; colors should be appealing to the eye, and there should be a balance of images and content.

The Home page should contain the practice's name, the address, phone number, and any social media handles. The links to other pages, or the navigational menu, on the website should also be presented vertically or horizontally along the Web page. Most medical practices have a link to a patient portal, which provides access to personal health records; the user name and password are assigned by the practice. Typically the link to new patient paperwork also is found on the Home page.

About Us Page

The About Us page offers a unique opportunity to introduce all the healthcare providers in the medical office. Many healthcare facilities include photos of their providers, medical professionals, and/or support staff. These profiles are a marketing tool in that they inform possible patients about the services the medical practice offers. Each profile should include a friendly photograph of the medical practitioner, biographic information about his or her background, the number of years in practice, and a personal note. The personal note should focus on the type of care the patient can expect to receive.

Testimonials or Information Page

The Testimonials or Information page is an opportunity for the practice to customize the website. Some healthcare facilities prefer to include positive patient reviews about the practice; the page could have a link to a public reviewer website with more reviews. Other medical offices use the page for more informational purposes by publishing monthly e-newsletters here. The page can also be used to present any research papers a provider in the practice has published. The content of this page is up to the discretion of the medical staff.

Specials Page

Healthcare facility management decides the content of the Specials page. There may be times in the year when a practice, in an effort to attract more patients, can offer specials for various services. Many patients who still do not have health insurance look for specials for more affordable healthcare. For example, the practice can offer a special for flu vaccination for $20, no appointment necessary. Offering specials shows that the medical practice is invested in the good health of the community in general, not just in those with health insurance.

Contact Us Page

The Contact Us page contains a form that patients can fill out to be contacted for more information. This page also can be used as an "Ask the Provider" e-mail service (Figure 19-4). The patient can send an e-mail to the provider and expect a response within the next 24 hours. This type of provider-patient communication is popular and can increase patient retention.

Once the form has been filled out, the data collected are sent to the medical office e-mail address associated with the Web page. A medical assistant should be assigned to monitor this e-mail to respond to the patient in a timely manner.

Designing Pages

Once the site map has been created, the Web designer can begin brainstorming ideas about what the site will look like on the computer screen. Graphics, color choices, animation, and fonts enhance a website's look, and those four elements should be kept in balance. For example, smaller fonts make the text difficult to read for patients

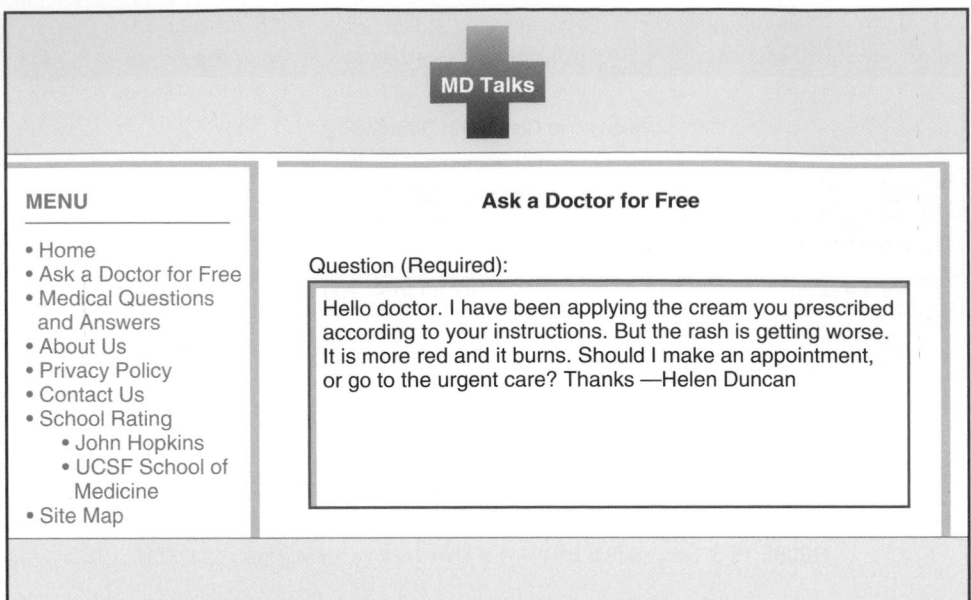

FIGURE 19-4 *"Ask the Provider" e-mail feature in the patient portal.*

with poor vision. Too many graphics crowd out the content of the website. The navigational menus should be designed so that viewers can move easily through the site. Most users appreciate a means to go back to the page previously viewed, and they become frustrated with sites that have an excessive number of pop-up boxes. Consistency is important, so it is a good idea to keep the same design theme on each page of the website.

Photographs, graphics, and video can add fun to the website, but be careful not to overdo them. Larger graphic files can take time to download. Most people will not wait longer than about 10 seconds for a Web page to load before clicking elsewhere. When you design Web page graphics, remember that smaller is better. Graphics can be found by searching for "index of GIF files" or "GIF library." Always respect any copyrights that are designated on any graphic file used. Many websites offer these file for free or charge a small fee.

The most important part of the website is the script, which should be developed by the office manager and the provider. It has been said that every word in a book must add to the story, and this is a good way to look at the text in a website. Avoid too much repetition, and remain clear about what is being communicated on the site. Headings and titles help clarify the theme of each page. Use a spell-checker before uploading the message and making it available for public viewing.

Hyperlinks are words or graphics on a Web page that, when clicked, take the viewer to another page or another website. To add a hyperlink, simply highlight the text field or graphic, select the hyperlink icon, and specify the destination address, or the *uniform resource locator* (URL). Always specify the full URL to ensure that the link directs the user to the desired page.

Increasing Website Traffic

A well-organized website has no value if patients are not aware that it exists. When patients search medical offices in their geographic area on a search engine website, the website should pop up. In order for the search engine to pick up the website, the Web designer includes appropriate key words into the website developer code. All healthcare facility websites should include keywords such as city, state, medical specialty, types of insurances accepted, and so on. These keywords are not viewable on the website but are included in the design code.

Website traffic should be monitored on a regular basis by healthcare facility management. Counters often can be added to the website that indicate how many people have viewed it. This helpful tool allows the medical practice to track how many people are viewing which pages. A sharp decline in website traffic may indicate a technical problem with the website, so it is important to monitor website traffic regularly and ensure that all Web pages are working properly.

HIGH-QUALITY CUSTOMER SERVICE

Once a patient comes to a medical practice, the key is to retain the patient for his or her future care needs. High-quality customer service not only can retain loyal patients, but also prompts them to refer their friends and family to the healthcare facilty. The delivery of high-quality customer service, therefore, is also considered an effective marketing tool.

Loyal Patients

The most effective way to increase the number of patients is word of mouth. When patients are satisfied with the treatment they receive, they refer other patients to the provider. However, if they are dissatisfied, they will tell everyone they know about their negative experience, which may affect the facility's future business.

Because patients often have a choice about who provides their healthcare services, it is important that the healthcare facility become the patient's first choice. Some patients are so loyal to a certain provider that even if their healthcare coverage no longer pays for visits, they continue to see that provider.

A Helpful Attitude

The provider and staff members should project a helpful attitude in every contact with the patient. They should sincerely ask, "How may I help you?" and then take steps to assist the patient in whatever way possible (Figure 19-5). Instead of pointing in the general direction of the radiology department, a staff member should take the patient there and introduce him or her to the receptionist. Instead of telling a patient on the telephone, "Ann handles the insurance billing. I'll transfer you to her," say, "One moment, Mrs. Brown, let me see if Ann is at her desk." Place Mrs. Brown on hold, call Ann, and let her know that she has a call. Then return to Mrs. Brown, tell her that Ann is at her desk, and transfer the call at that time. Be courteous and kind to every patient and visitor to the office. Good customer relations must be one of the primary goals of the medical facility. Patients count on staff members to be reliable and available to help them to the best of their abilities.

Office management should emphasize to all staff members the importance of delivering quality customer service. Staff meetings should be scheduled regularly to discuss customer service failures, review how those situations should have been handled, and recognize staff members who display high-quality customer service.

Identifying with Patients

Patients appreciate staff members who can be empathetic with the problems patients are facing. This is especially effective when a patient is upset or angry. For example, if a patient comes to the office complaining that charges were placed on his account for procedures that were not performed, the medical assistant may respond with a phrase such as, "Mr. Roberts, I understand that you are upset about these additional charges. Let me do some research on your account and let you know what I find. Let me help you by doing this ..."

Identifying with the patient shows understanding on the part of the staff member, no matter how upset the patient may be. Always acknowledge and restate the patient's concern. It proves that the medical assistant was listening and is interested in resolving the problem.

Remember, it costs much more to find new customers than to keep existing customers happy. Providing helpful, personal service impresses even the most difficult patient. To patients and visitors to the clinic, the employees to whom they speak represent the whole practice. Perceptions and opinions likely will be formed based on experiences with only one person. Each individual employee must be aware that to the patient, each employee is the healthcare practice.

CRITICAL THINKING APPLICATION   **19-5**

Monica thinks it would be beneficial for staff members to receive some of the dermatologic treatments so that they can recommend them to patients. Monica takes her idea to the providers as a marketing tool. Could this be a strong marketing tool? Might the staff members relate to patients better after experiencing the same medical treatments?

What Do Patients Expect?

First, patients expect to be treated according to the Golden Rule. They expect their concerns to be met with responsiveness, which means that the medical assistant should have a caring attitude (Figure 19-6). They also expect the professionals in the medical office to be knowledgeable about their field or specialty. An insurance biller should know more than just the basics of insurance filing. The office manager should have a certain degree of authority to handle problems and complaints. Patients also expect confidentiality and trust from the staff of the medical office. They expect an organized office that runs on schedule. They also expect that if a staff member promises to do something, it is as good as done.

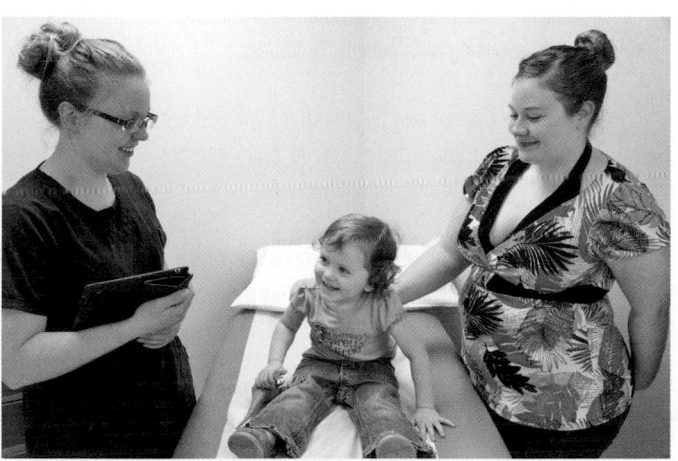

FIGURE 19-5 Helpful staff members provide the best customer service.

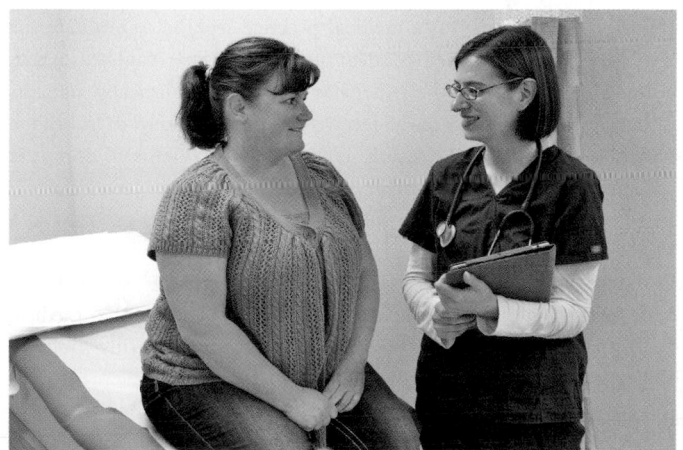

FIGURE 19-6 Friendly staff members are the best marketing tool. A smile is an excellent way to make patients feel welcome in the medical facility.

Thank you so much for visiting Clear Skin Dermatology! We want to ensure your experience with us was excellent! Your experience is important to us, so please share your thoughts by completing this survey. All surveys are confidential and are used to improve our service only. Thank you so much for your time and we look forward to caring for you soon!

		YES	NO
1.	Is the location of our office convenient?	☐	☐
2.	Do you find our reception area comfortable?	☐	☐
3.	Do you feel relaxed in the reception area?	☐	☐
4.	Do you find our front office personnel (Receptionist, etc.)	☐	☐
	Friendly?	☐	☐
	Courteous?	☐	☐
	Rude or indifferent?	☐	☐
5.	Do you find our business personnel (practice manager, billing specialist, etc.)	☐	☐
	Friendly?	☐	☐
	Courteous?	☐	☐
	Rude or indifferent?	☐	☐
6.	Are phone calls handled in a prompt, courteous, competent manner?	☐	☐
7.	Do we provide adequate help with your insurance?	☐	☐
8.	Have you received a copy of our financial policies?	☐	☐
9.	Have our payment and billing policies been explained to your satisfaction?	☐	☐
10.	Do you find our nurses and other clinical allied health workers:	☐	☐
	Friendly?	☐	☐
	Courteous?	☐	☐
	Rude or indifferent?	☐	☐

Comments/complaints: _____
_____
_____
_____

FIGURE 19-7 Sample patient survey.

Patient Surveys

There is no better way to understand the quality of the care delivered than by asking the patients themselves! A patient survey (Figure 19-7) is vital for a medical practice seeking to evaluate the level of quality provided to their patient. Surveys can be mailed, e-mailed, or posted in the patient Web portal. Realistically, patients unhappy with the care they received are more likely to submit a patient survey. Sending friendly reminders for patients to complete the survey would be appropriate. Some medical offices have offered a small reward for completing the survey, such as a $10 gift card to a local coffee shop.

Successful medical practices take these surveys seriously by addressing patients' commendations and concerns. The medical office manager should review some of the responses during monthly staff meetings to discuss any changes that can be implemented to improve customer service. For the most part, surveys are anonymous. However, if a patient identifies himself or herself and addresses a specific concern, the office manager should contact the patient immediately to offer a possible remedy.

Phrases and Body Language That Undermine Successful Customer Service

The following are examples of phrases and body language that should never be used when speaking with patients or visitors.

- "I don't know."
  Say instead: "I'm not exactly sure, but I will find out." Medical assistants will not know the answer to every question, but they must be willing to find out the information.
- "I don't care."
  Say instead: "We care about your concerns and want to help." If the medical assistant cannot honestly make this statement, he or she should consider another profession.
- Body language that implies the staff member can't be bothered with the patient's concern.
  Instead: Look at the patient directly and say, "I truly want to give this matter my full attention. How can I contact you once I have looked into it?"

Some people may expect immediate attention and service, but they may have to be patient and wait their turn to receive assistance.

- "Ask someone else."
  Say instead: "I will be happy to find out who handles that for you." The medical assistant should never project the attitude that the patient's concerns are unimportant.
- "It's not my job."
  Say instead: "I am not one of the employees who files insurance, but I will be happy to ask Amanda, our insurance supervisor, to contact you and answer your questions." Do not ever tell the patient or a supervisor that a certain duty is not your responsibility. Find the right person to help the patient.
- "It's not my fault."
  Say instead: "I was not involved with that decision, but I know that our office manager would be happy to speak with you about it." Although blame should never be placed on another employee, any touchy issue should be referred to the office manager, especially if the medical assistant is not the final decision-making authority.
- "I didn't do it."
  Say instead: "I will see if I can get to the root of this issue." Be willing to assist the patient even if you are not involved in the situation at hand.
- "I know that."
  Say instead: "Yes, I understand. Let me try to help you." Do not use sarcasm, and never make snippy remarks.
- "I'm right, you're wrong."
  Say instead: "Our policy is clear about this matter, but let's see if we can come up with a compromise." Accusatory remarks should never be made to a patient.

All of the preceding alternate phrases give the patient a more positive view of both the office and those who work in it.

PROBLEM PATIENTS

Patients can sometimes be quite challenging for the provider's staff and office manager. Most patients are genuinely concerned about their health and are very cooperative. However, a few patients require extra understanding, which may lead to intervention by the office manager. Types of problem patients may include those who are:

- Complainers
- Angry
- Needy
- Demanding
- Violent
- Nonpaying
- Noncompliant
- Drug seeking
- Reschedulers

The office manager may act as a **liaison** between the patient and the providers when issues arise that are somewhat complicated. Some patients may feel ignored or mistreated by office staff. Others may

have a general lack of trust that makes complying with the provider's orders difficult for them. Cultural differences, social issues, and financial problems all can affect a patient's compliance and attitude.

Both the medical assistant and the office manager should serve as patient **advocates**, but they can never hold back information the provider needs to know. For instance, if a patient tells the medical assistant or office manager that he has been smoking, although he told the provider he quit, the information must be presented to the provider. Information that is shared with the medical assistant must be shared with the provider, even if the patient objects. Medical assistants should inform the patient respectfully that they are ethically obligated to share all information collected with the provider.

"WELCOME TO OUR OFFICE" PACKET

Only a very small percentage of practices have a Welcome to Our Office packet that explains the operational and service aspects of the practice. Yet, the provider and staff can easily compile a patient information booklet cooperatively during a staff meeting. Experience has shown that if such a packet is given to every new patient, the number of patient calls to the office can be reduced by an average of 20% to 30%. It also can reduce misunderstandings and forgotten instructions. The packet should be custom tailored to the specific practice.

Introduction to the Medical Office

The welcome packet should begin with an introduction letter to the practice. The information should be the same or similar to what would be found in the "About Us" Web page on the website. The healthcare facility letterhead should be used, which includes the address, contact numbers, website, and/or any social media user names.

A statement of philosophy frequently is included in the introduction, followed by a description of the practice. Consider this example:

The doctors and staff would like to welcome you to our office. We work as a team with the goal of providing prompt and thorough care to improve your health. We are always working to improve our care and service in any way possible. Our practice is limited exclusively to dermatology and related disorders. Therefore, it is important for each patient to have a primary care provider, such as a pediatrician, a family provider, or an internist, to oversee the patient's primary medical care. Our role is most effective as a consultant to your primary care provider.

List all providers in the practice; state their educational backgrounds, training, and board certifications; and define their specialties. List the names of key clinical and administrative staff members, such as registered nurses and nurse practitioners, medical assistants, the office manager, and the business manager. Provide the practice address, a map of how to get there, and information about the parking facilities.

Missed Appointments and Cancellation Policy

The office policy regarding missed appointments and cancellations, telephone calls, and the function of the answering service should also be mentioned in the welcome packet. For example:

We always strive to answer telephone calls quickly, but at times you may be asked to wait as we finish handling prior patient calls. Your call is important to us, and we appreciate your patience. If you wish to speak to the provider, the receptionist will take your information and the provider will contact you during the next available break or at the end of the office day. Our triage nurse and the provider's medical assistant also would be happy to help you.

If you want to speak to a doctor, your call usually will be returned during the next available break period or at the end of the office day. Therefore, the receptionist usually will take a message, and your call will be returned as soon as possible. Please inform the receptionist if your problem is urgent, and he or she will inform the doctor. Patients can also use the "Ask the Provider" e-mail service located on the "Contact Us" page on the website.

In case of emergency, call 911. If you have a nonemergency concern, one of the doctors in the group is always on call. You may reach him or her by calling our office telephone number (714) 555-2323; the answering service will put you in touch with the doctor on call at that time. Our doctors are on staff at St. Joseph Hospital (714) 555-3333, and for children, Children's Hospital of Orange County (714) 555-4444.

Medical Office's Financial Policy

Spell out the practice's policies on billing and collection procedures, and make it clear that patients are responsible for their financial portion of the fees. If payment is expected at the time of service, add this in the welcome folder. Keep the language simple and straightforward so that the message is clear:

We ask that our services be paid for at the time they are rendered. There is usually a greater charge for the initial visit because this involves more time and evaluation than follow-up visits. If you are referred to an outside office for laboratory testing or special x-ray procedures, you will be billed separately by that office. We will bill your insurance on your behalf; thank you for accepting financial responsibility for the amount the health insurance assigns as your co-insurance and/or deductible.

Patient Information Web Portal

Patients should be granted access to their patient portal through the healthcare facility website. The username and password are assigned at the patient's first office visit. Patients can gain access to laboratory reports, test results, consultation reports, and any other medical encounter records in their personal Web portal.

Patients can also request pharmaceutical refills, update health insurance information, and request an appointment through the patient portal. However, patients should be aware that the patient

Web portal manages records from this specific medical office, not from any other specialists, laboratories, or hospitals.

Patient Instruction Sheets

In most medical offices, some patient procedures are performed over and over again. Instead of attempting to instruct a patient orally each time, the practice can develop instruction sheets (Figure 19-8) that can be reviewed with the patient and then uploaded to the patient portal. The following are some suggested topics for patient instruction sheets:

- Preparation for an x-ray procedure or laboratory tests
- Preoperative and postoperative instructions
- Dietary guidelines
- Performing an enema
- Dressing a wound
- Taking medications
- Using a cane, crutches, walker, or wheelchair
- Care of casts
- Exercise therapy

List of Community Resources

Community organizations can collaborate with the healthcare provider to meet the patient's health needs. As a participant in the health of the local community, the practice should generate a list of community resources to assist patients in their efforts to improve their health (Procedure 19-1). These resources can represent a wide variety of services, such as:

- Meals assistance and food banks
- Adult day care services and centers
- Grief support groups
- Chronic disease support groups
- Medical equipment suppliers
- Home healthcare centers
- Long-term healthcare facilities (e.g., convalescent care, skilled nursing facilities, rehabilitation centers, and psychiatric hospitals)
- Assisted-living information
- Hospice services
- Immunization clinics
- Smoking cessation programs
- Local board of health
- Alcoholics and Narcotics Anonymous meetings

Local communities have many outreach programs with which the healthcare practice should network. For example, the American Cancer Society provides support to cancer patients in the community by providing rides to treatment, lodging near treatment centers, and hair loss and mastectomy products. The healthcare facility should maintain and update the list of resources on a regular basis, but it is not responsible if the services are no longer available.

NIH U.S. National Library of Medicine

MedlinePlus
Trusted Health Information for You

Search MedlinePlus [GO]

About MedlinePlus Site Map FAQs Contact Us

Health Topics   Drugs & Supplements   Videos & Tools   Español

Home → Drugs, Herbs and Supplements → Clindamycin and Benzoyl Peroxide Topical

Clindamycin and Benzoyl Peroxide Topical
pronounced as (klin da mye' sin) (ben' zoe ill) (per ox' ide)

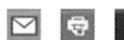

Why is this medication prescribed?

The combination of clindamycin and benzoyl peroxide is used to treat acne. Clindamycin and benzoyl peroxide are in a class of medications called topical antibiotics. The combination of clindamycin and benzoyl peroxide works by killing the bacteria that cause acne.

How should this medicine be used?

The combination of clindamycin and benzoyl peroxide comes as a gel to apply to the skin. It is usually applied twice a day, in the morning and evening. To help you remember to use clindamycin and benzoyl peroxide gel, apply it at around the same times every day. Follow the directions on your prescription label carefully, and ask your doctor or pharmacist to explain any part you do not understand. Use clindamycin and benzoyl peroxide gel exactly as directed. Do not use more or less of it or use it more often than prescribed by your doctor.

To use the gel, follow these steps:

1. Wash the affected area with warm water and gently pat dry with a clean towel.
2. Use you fingertips to spread a thin layer of gel evenly over the affected area. Avoid getting the gel in your eyes, nose, mouth, or other body openings. If you do get the gel in your eyes, wash with warm water.
3. Look in the mirror. If you see a white film on your skin, you have used too much medication.
4. Wash your hands.

Other uses for this medicine

This medication may be prescribed for other uses; ask your doctor or pharmacist for more information.

FIGURE 19-8 Sample patient instruction sheet.

PROCEDURE 19-1	Develop a Current List of Community Resources Related to Patients' Healthcare Needs and Facilitate Referrals

Goal: *Identify community resources related to patients' healthcare needs and to facilitate referrals to community resources in the role of a patient navigator.*

EQUIPMENT and SUPPLIES

- Computer with Internet and/or a telephone book
- Paper and pen
- Community Resource Referral Form or referral form

- **Scenario 1:** Herman Miller is a 72-year-old male who was just diagnosed with dementia. He currently lives with his daughter, Ruby, who works full-time. Ruby is feeling overwhelmed with being his only caregiver and realizes that she needs to find someone to provide care to her father while she is working.

- **Scenario 2:** Leslie Green just tested positive for pregnancy. She is still a teenager and doesn't feel that she has a support system to help her make decisions.

PROCEDURE 19-1 —continued

- **Scenario 3:** Marcia Carrillo's husband of 30 years, died suddenly 1 month ago. Marcia stated that she feels alone and has no one to talk to. Her daughter feels that she needs the support of others who have gone through the same thing.

PROCEDURAL STEPS

1. Identify the possible types of community resources that would assist the patient and/or family.
   PURPOSE: A variety of community resources are available for patients and families dealing with chronic illnesses and death. The resources range from daycare, meals, transportation, medical equipment, assistive living, support groups, and reduced costs for medications.
2. Using the Internet and/or the phone book, identify local resources for the patient. Make a list of resources for the patient and/or family member. Include the name of the organization, the addresses, and the contact information.
   PURPOSE: As an advocate and patient navigator, it is important to provide patients and families with the contact information for various community

resources. Information provided helps the family find the best solution for the situation.
3. Summarize the services provided by the organization.
   PURPOSE: Patients and families may not be familiar with the services that local organizations provide. By providing a summary of the services, you are educating the patient and family, and it may promote them to seek out these services.
4. (Role-play) Provide the patient and/or family member with the list of resources and identify which service(s) they would be interested in.
5. Use professional, tactful verbal and nonverbal communication as you work with the patient and family.
   PURPOSE: Patients and family members are more apt to respond positively to assistance if the medical assistant's communication is professional, empathic, and tactful. Talking down to patients or acting superior are unprofessional behaviors that negatively impact the working relationship with patients.
6. Complete the referral form to help facilitate the referral to community resource(s).

THE PATIENT NAVIGATOR

The **patient navigator** program was established at the Harlem Hospital Center in 1990 to assist cancer patients in accessing quality healthcare. With the assistance of the 2005 Patient Navigator, Outreach and Chronic Disease Prevent Act, many patient navigator positions were funded throughout the U.S. Today, patient navigator positions are found in clinics and hospitals around the country, helping patients find emotional, financial, administrative, or cultural resources within the healthcare community and the local community.

There are many models for patient navigator programs, but the goal is the same—to help patients find the resources they need. Patient navigators are responsible for, but not limited to, the following:

- Interview patients to identify their needs and barriers to wellness and healthcare.
- Provide patients resources based on their needs and barriers.
- Coordinate appointments and care for patients.
- Assist with reducing language barriers, by identifying bilingual providers and translators.
- Discuss special needs patients have with their healthcare team.
- Identify community resources, which may include transportation, medical equipment, adult daycare and assistive living, support groups, low cost medication programs, low-cost preventative screening and immunizations, and adoption services.

A medical assistant can work in the patient navigator role and assist the healthcare team by identifying patients' needs and barriers to wellness and healthcare. The medical assistant then matches the patient to appropriate community resources (e.g., support groups, low cost/free meals, and transportation) and provides the patient

with information on the resources (see Procedure 19-1). For healthcare related resources (e.g., medical equipment, hospice), the medical assistant works with the provider and completes the required insurance and referral forms.

PATIENT-CENTERED MEDICAL HOME

The **patient-centered medical home (PCMH)** is a model philosophy intended to improve the effectiveness of primary care. This approach is promoted by the National Committee for Quality Assurance (NCQA). The PCMH model sets the following standards in the delivery of primary health care:

- Providers and patient care teams should work together to bring care to the patient.
- Patients should be treated with respect, dignity, and compassion by the medical care team.
- Medical care should be coordinated with the patient's needs and wants.
- The use of health information technology should be maximized in the delivery of patient care.
- A chain of command that creates a forum for decision making for the entire patient care team should be established; this helps organize and unify network practices.

The intent of the PCMH model is to improve healthcare in America by transforming how primary care is organized and delivered. The model has five key domains (Table 19-2):

- Comprehensive Care
- Patient-Centered Care
- Coordinated Care
- Accessible Services
- Quality and Safety

TABLE 19-2   Key Domains of the Patient-Centered Medical Home (PCMH)

DOMAIN	DESCRIPTION
Comprehensive Care	The PCMH is designed to meet a majority of a patient's physical and mental health care needs through a team-based approach to care.
Patient-Centered Care	The delivery of primary care oriented toward the whole person. This can be achieved by partnering with patients and families through an understanding of and respect for culture, unique needs, preferences, and values.
Coordinated Care	The PCMH coordinates patient care across all elements of the healthcare system, such as specialty care, hospitals, home healthcare, and community services, with an emphasis on efficient care transitions.
Accessible Services	The PCMH seeks to make primary care accessible through minimizing wait times, enhanced office hours, and after-hours access to providers through alternative methods, such as telephone or e-mail.
Quality and Safety	The PCMH model is committed to providing safe, high-quality care through clinical decision-support tools, evidence-based care, shared decision making, performance measurement, and population health management. Sharing quality data and improvement activities also contribute to a systems level commitment to quality.

From the Agency for Healthcare Research and Quality: pcmh.ahrq.gov.

Health Internet Technology (IT), the workforce, and finance support these key domains. Health IT supports PCMH by collecting and storing relevant data to improve process outcomes. The workforce, which includes the team of providers and other healthcare personnel, provides care based on PCMH principles. Finance calls for the reform of health insurance reimbursement for primary care services.

ELECTRONIC TECHNOLOGY IN PROFESSIONAL COMMUNICATION

Telemedicine

More and more, providers are using technology to improve the care delivered to their patients. Advances in video conferencing technology have enabled providers to evaluate and treat patients who live hundreds of miles away. **Telemedicine** opens health care access to many patients in rural areas where access is limited. Patients in rural areas must drive farther to receive care; because of this inconvenience, many of these patients go without regular medical care. Case studies have shown that providers who use telemedicine improve not only the quality of the patient's health, but also customer service.

Video conferencing through a secured Web portal in which the provider can view the patient for evaluation. Some telemedicine organizations provide 24-hour support for patients all over the country. Providers can allow patients to keep the recording of the consultation so they can remember the provider's recommendations. Telemedicine also has greatly reduced the number of unnecessary emergency and urgent care visits.

CLOSING COMMENTS

Marketing is essential to the future financial success of a medical practice. Once a target market has been identified, many different marketing tools can be used to assist the practice in attracting new patients. A well-organized website is useful for reaching new patients and creating a loyal relationship with current patients. The most inexpensive marketing strategy is delivering exceptional customer service. Providing good customer service is a commitment that must be made by every employee of the healthcare practice, every single day. There will be times when the customer does not act respectfully, but he or she should be treated with dignity and respect at all times. In addition, a skilled customer service provider has a knack for making the customer think he or she was right all along! For medical practices, providing good service results in an excellent reputation for the clinic, built by those who matter most—the patients.

Patient Education

A practice's marketing efforts provide endless opportunities for patient education. Most providers agree that part of the obligation of the medical profession is to educate patients about healthcare issues specific to their needs. Medical assistants should listen carefully to the patient's needs and then make referrals to community resources if these can help the patient meet his or her health needs. For patients who are more private about their personal health struggles, it may be beneficial to post links to different online resources, such as Alcoholics Anonymous meetings and stop smoking seminars.

Legal and Ethical Issues

The provider must take care that patients do not use the information in brochures or on the practice website as medical advice or as a substitute for the provider's medical advice. Before attaching a link to another website, the medical assistant must be sure the site is reputable; government websites are always recommended. The patient may consider information on the practice's website to be an extension of the provider's advice, so make sure everything on the website is accurate.

The provider should carefully review all printed information used to promote the medical facility. Make sure there are no misleading statements. A stated disclaimer should be included to remind patients that the information given in brochures and on websites is for general use only. Patients should be advised to discuss specific issues with the provider or to use the "Ask the Doctor" feature.

Professional Behaviors

Building a successful medical practice starts with effective marketing tools and strong customer service standards. As mentioned, customer service is the key to building a loyal patient base and growing the practice through referrals. Medical assistants, whether just out of school already established in their career must strive to provide patients with good customer service. Patients do not hesitate to tell the provider if the medical assistant is not cordial and helpful. Providing excellent customer service is mandatory for every employee of the practice.

SUMMARY OF SCENARIO

Monica is confident that a simple marketing plan will enable the practice to experience steady, continuous expansion. She has performed a SWOT analysis and reviewed the spreadsheet of patient demographics and determined a specific target market.

A monthly newsletter and the practice's website are some of the marketing tools Monica plans to use to reach the target market. One of her first steps is to develop an annual calendar of special events and community outreach. The newsletter, which will provide health information and details about upcoming events, will be available both in print and online. The patients in the office database who have e-mail addresses will automatically receive a computer-generated e-mail message with a link that takes them directly to the online newsletter. Monica also has planned one special community event for each month of the upcoming year.

Monica plans to track the responses to each event promoted on the healthcare facility website to determine what marketing tools were most effective in promoting the clinic. The website allows her to count the number of visits and to determine which pages are the most popular. She will keep Dr. Huang informed, and be open to their suggestions. Monica also has found that using social media for marketing has increased traffic to the practice's website, which offers patients several options to increase their knowledge about health-related subjects and find opportunities to participate in events that promote good health.

The clinic's staff members understand that no matter what efforts are used to promote the practice and obtain new patients, it is their responsibility to provide exceptional customer service so that patients are happy with their experience. People have choices as to who provides their healthcare, so they must be treated cordially and fairly by medical professionals who truly want to serve their needs.

SUMMARY OF LEARNING OBJECTIVES

1. **Define, spell, and pronounce the terms listed in the vocabulary.**
   Spelling and pronouncing medical terms correctly reinforce the medical assistant's credibility. Knowing the definitions of these terms promotes confidence in communication with patients and co-workers.

2. **Do the following related to the marketing needs of the healthcare practice:**
   - *Explain the need for marketing for a healthcare practice or facility.*
     All healthcare practices and facilities must have a marketing plan in order to attract new patients. There are many ways to market a healthcare practice/facility.
   - *Identify the target market.*
     Identifying the *target market* (i.e., the groups of people most likely to need the medical service provided by the practice) is the key to successful marketing. Reaching the target market means that the targeted groups are made aware of the practice and what it has to offer.
   - *Discuss why a SWOT analysis is important to identify the target market.*
     A SWOT analysis provides an evaluation of the business environment. This tool evaluates how economic forces affect the healthcare practice internally and externally. The strengths and weaknesses categories evaluate internal economic forces, and the opportunities and threats categories evaluate the external economic forces.

3. **Do the following related to marketing tools:**
   - *Review ways a healthcare practice or facility can promote itself through community involvement.*

   Patients trust medical practices that participate in the local community. Some practices participate in local health fairs to provide free screenings and farmers' markets to promote healthier eating. Some even sponsor a local 5K run/walk to encourage vigorous exercise. The more the public views the practice as active in the community, the more likely it is that this will increase the number of appointments made at the medical office.
   - *Define and discuss automated call distribution.*
     Automated call distribution is a popular means of communicating with large numbers of people. A computer dials multiple numbers at the same time and plays a recorded message, which can be the actual provider with news about a new procedure or a new associate joining the practice.
   - *Explain how newsletters and blogs can be effective marketing tools.*
     Many providers refer their patients to the same medical research about a variety of health topics, including ways to be treated. Some providers communicate this medical information as an e-newsletter, which is sent periodically, typically every month. However, providers must be careful not to offer medical advice electronically; the intention of the e-newsletter should be to inform patients about health conditions that the provider typically sees in the medical office.
   - *Discuss marketing through print ads in magazines and newspapers.*
     If the marketing budget allows, advertising in magazines and newspapers or through mailers can inform the public about the practice and the services it offers. However, it is important to ensure that the

SUMMARY OF LEARNING OBJECTIVES—*continued*

target market can be reached by advertising this way because it is significantly more expensive and reaches a wider audience. Advertising in local magazines and/or newspapers is a more effective marketing strategy and can establish the practice in the community.

- *Determine the value of Internet marketing for a healthcare practice or facility.*

On the Internet, businesses that have a greater number of and more favorable reviews tend to attract new business. There are many opportunities for a healthcare practice to build a strong reputation through Internet marketing because there are many different popular websites in which people post reviews of their experiences. The key is to ask every patient before he or she leaves to post a review of the services the person received; as the number of reviewers grows, the potential for new patients also will grow.

4. **Distinguish between advertising and public relations.**

Advertising is a medium that attempts to create or change attitudes, beliefs, and perceptions through printed material, the Internet, or other forms of communication. Public relations is a similar field but relies more on news broadcasts or reports, magazine or newspaper articles, and radio reports to reach the audience.

5. **Discuss the value of marketing through social media.**

A social media outlet promotes a business, and customers can respond positively or negatively about the service they received. Traditional media outlets, such as newspapers and magazines, allow only limited ability to respond; a person can write a letter to the editor of a newspaper, but the letter does not generate an immediate two-way response. Social media is considered a blending of technology and social interaction that creates an effective marketing tool.

6. **Develop website content, organization, and design to attract new patients; also, review strategies to increase website traffic.**

A successful website will be able to attract many patients. An organized site map makes a website user friendly. In the design of a website, it is important to identify which informational pages should be included. A standard basic website has a Home page, an About Us page, testimonials or an informational page, specials, and a Contact Us page.

A well-organized website has no value if patients are not aware that it exists. When patients search for medical offices in their geographic area on a search engine website (e.g., Google), the practice's website should pop up. To enable the search engine to pick up the website, the Web designer must include appropriate key words in the website developer code. All medical office websites should include keywords such as city, state, medical specialty, types of insurances accepted, and so on. These keywords are not viewable on the website but are included in the design code.

7. **Explain how to successfully deliver high-quality customer service, including how to identify with patients, and the value of patient surveys.**

High-quality customer service not only can create a loyal patient, it can prompt that patient to refer his or her friends and family so that they can receive the same quality of care. Therefore, delivering high-quality customer service is considered an effective marketing tool.

For staff members, identifying with the patient means showing understanding, no matter how upset the person may be. Always acknowledge and restate the patient's concerns. This proves that the medical assistant was listening and is interested in resolving the problem.

For a medical practice seeking to evaluate the quality of its customer service, periodic evaluation is vital. Patients' perspectives can provide insight into areas needing improvement that staff members may not be able to perceive from inside the office. Evaluations can be mailed, e-mailed, or posted on the patient Web portal.

8. **Identify strategies to manage problem patients.**

Cultural differences, social issues, and financial problems all can affect a patient's compliance and attitude. The rare patient may have a personality disorder or psychological problem that staff members find frustrating as they provide medical treatment. Some patients may have a general lack of trust that makes complying with the provider's orders difficult for them.

9. **Review the importance of the new-patient information packet.**

Experience has shown that if an information packet is given to every new patient, the number of patient calls to the office can be reduced by an average of 20% to 30%. This also can reduce misunderstandings and instances of forgotten instructions. The packet should be custom tailored to the specific practice.

10. **In the role of patient navigator, facilitate referrals to community resources.**

Patient navigators help identify patients' barriers and needs to wellness and healthcare. The patient navigators then provide patients with referrals or information about community resources. For healthcare related needs, the patient navigator works closely with the patient's healthcare team to resolve the issues.

11. **Define a patient-centered medical home (PCMH).**

The patient-centered medical home (PCMH) is a model philosophy intended to improve the effectiveness of primary care. This approach is promoted by the National Committee for Quality Assurance (NCQA).

12. **Discuss applications of electronic technology (e.g., telemedicine) in professional communication.**

Video conferencing takes place through a secure Web portal in which the provider can view the patient for evaluation. Some telemedicine organizations provide 24-hour support for patients all over the country.

CONNECTIONS

Study Guide Connection: Go to the Chapter 19 Study Guide. Read and complete the activities.

evolve Evolve Connection: Go to the Chapter 19 link at *evolve.elsevier.com/ kinn* to complete the Chapter Review Quiz. Check out the other resources listed for this chapter to make the most of what you have learned from Medical Practice Marketing and Customer Service.

20

INFECTION CONTROL

SCENARIO

Rosa Lucia is a certified medical assistant working in a pediatric practice with several physicians. She is quite concerned about contracting an infectious disease while caring for her patients. Rosa learned about Standard Precautions while enrolled in her medical assisting program and now must implement that knowledge in the workplace. Two important factors in preventing the spread of infection are (1) understanding how to break the chain of infection and (2) recognizing the importance of correct and frequent hand washing.

While studying this chapter, think about the following questions:

- How can Rosa achieve these goals?
- What is the significance of an Exposure Control Plan in Rosa's pediatric office?
- What are the important details of the office's compliance with the guidelines established by the Occupational Safety and Health Administration (OSHA)?
- How can Rosa implement required infection control procedures in the pediatric office?

LEARNING OBJECTIVES

1. Define, spell, and pronounce the terms listed in the vocabulary.
2. Describe the characteristics of pathogenic microorganisms.
3. Do the following related to the chain of infection:
   - Apply the chain of infection process to healthcare practice.
   - Compare viral and bacterial cell invasion.
   - Differentiate between humoral and cell-mediated immunity.
4. Summarize the impact of the inflammatory response on the body's ability to defend itself against infection.
5. Analyze the differences among acute, chronic, latent, and opportunistic infections.
6. Do the following related to OSHA standards for the healthcare setting:
   - Specify potentially infectious body fluids.
   - Integrate OSHA's requirement for a site-based Exposure Control Plan into facility management procedures.
   - Explain the major areas included in the OSHA Compliance Guidelines.
   - Discuss protocols for disposal of biologic chemical materials.
7. Remove contaminated gloves while following Standard Precautions principles.
8. Perform an eye wash procedure to remove contaminated material.
9. Summarize the management of postexposure evaluation and follow-up and participate in blood-borne pathogen training and a mock exposure event.
10. Identify the regulations established by the Centers for Disease Control and Prevention (CDC) that affect healthcare workers.
11. Apply the concepts of medical and surgical asepsis to the healthcare setting.
12. Discuss proper hand washing, and demonstrate the proper hand-washing technique for medical asepsis.
13. Differentiate among sanitization, disinfection, and sterilization procedures and select barrier/personal protective equipment while demonstrating the correct procedure for sanitizing contaminated instruments.
14. Discuss the role of the medical assistant in asepsis.
15. Apply patient education concepts to infection control.
16. Discuss legal and ethical concerns regarding medical asepsis and infection control, and perform compliance reporting based on public health statutes covering reportable communicable diseases.

VOCABULARY

anaphylaxis (an-uh-fuh-lak´-sis) An exaggerated hypersensitivity reaction that in severe cases leads to vascular collapse, bronchospasm, and shock.

antibodies (an´-ti-bah-dees) Immunoglobulins produced by the immune system in response to bacteria, viruses, or other antigenic substances.

antigen (an´-ti-juhn) A foreign substance that causes the production of a specific antibody.

antiseptics (an-ti-sep´-tiks) Substances that inhibit the growth of microorganisms on living tissue (e.g., alcohol and povidone-iodine solution [Betadine]); they are used to cleanse the skin, wounds, and so on.

autoimmune (o-to-im´-yuhn) Pertaining to a disturbance in the immune system in which the body reacts against its own tissue. Examples of autoimmune disorders are multiple sclerosis, rheumatoid arthritis, and systemic lupus erythematosus.

candidiasis (kan-duh-de-uh´-sis) An infection caused by a yeast that typically affects the vaginal mucosa and skin.

coagulate (ko-ag´-yuh-late) To form into clots.

contaminated Soiled with pathogens or infectious material; nonsterile.

disinfectant A liquid chemical that is capable of eliminating many or all pathogens but is not effective against bacterial spores; it cannot be used on the skin.

flora Microorganisms that live on or within the body; they compete with disease-producing microorganisms and provide a natural immunity against certain infections.

fomites Contaminated, nonliving objects (e.g., examination room equipment) that can transmit infectious organisms.

germicides (jur´-muh-sides) Agents that destroy pathogenic organisms.

hereditary (huh-re´-duh-ter-e) Pertaining to a characteristic, condition, or disease transmitted from parent to offspring on the DNA chain.

interferon (in´-tuhr-fir-on) A protein formed when a cell is exposed to a virus; the protein blocks viral action on the cell and protects against viral invasion.

nosocomial infections (nos-uh-koh´-mee-uhl) Infections that are acquired in a healthcare setting.

opportunistic infections Infections caused by a normally nonpathogenic organism in a host whose resistance has been decreased.

palliative (pah-lee-ah-tive) A substance that relieves or alleviates the symptoms of a disease without curing the disease.

parenteral (puh-ren´-tuh-ruhl) The injection or introduction of substances into the body by any route other than the digestive tract (e.g., subcutaneous, intravenous, or intramuscular administration).

pathogenic (path´-o-jen-ik) Pertaining to a disease-causing microorganism.

permeable (pur´-me-uh-buhl) Allowing a substance to pass or soak through.

pyemia (pi-em´-e-uh) The presence of pus-forming organisms in the blood.

relapse The recurrence of the symptoms of a disease after apparent recovery.

remission The partial or complete disappearance of the clinical and subjective characteristics of a chronic or malignant disease.

rhinitis (rin-i´-tis) Inflammation of the mucous membranes of the nose.

spore A thick-walled, dormant form of bacteria that is very resistant to disinfection measures.

sterile (ster´-il) Free of all microorganisms, pathogenic and nonpathogenic.

tinea (tin´-e-uh) Any fungal skin disease that results in scaling, itching, and inflammation.

urticaria (uhr-tuh-kar´-e-uh) A skin eruption that creates inflamed wheals; hives.

vectors Animals or insects (e.g., ticks) that transmit the causative organisms of disease.

The concepts of disease transmission and the body's response to infection form the basis for understanding the importance of the first line of defense in preventing disease. Before we can assist in the prevention of disease, we have to look at methods we can use to minimize the chances of being a carrier of disease. One of the simplest ways to prevent the spread of disease is to wash your hands or use alcohol-based hand rubs. As you continue through the remainder of this textbook, you should refer to the fundamental concepts of this chapter when faced with an infection control issue. Because of the need for infection control and the impact on medical practice of the guidelines established by the Occupational Safety and Health Administration (OSHA), every procedure must begin and end with hand hygiene practices. The guidelines in this chapter are basic to all clinical skills, and following them can reduce the transmission of disease organisms and lessen the severity of disease. They also may save a patient's or co-worker's life, or even your own.

DISEASE

Disease is defined as any sustained, harmful alteration of the normal structure, function, or metabolism of an organism or cell. This pathologic condition presents a group of clinical signs, symptoms, and laboratory findings that set it apart as an abnormal entity, different from other normal and pathologic conditions. We recognize and categorize many types of diseases: **hereditary** (genetic), drug induced, **autoimmune**, degenerative, communicable, and infectious, to name only a few. Sometimes a specific disease may fit two or more categories.

Any disease caused by the growth of **pathogenic** microorganisms in the body falls into the category of *infectious diseases*. The entrance of a living microbe into the body is not disease because until the infected cell or individual shows a harmful alteration in structure, physiology, or biochemistry, disease either is not detected or is not considered present. In fact, a pathogen may be ingested, injected, or inhaled and never cause disease. However, an unaffected person still can transmit the infection to another person. In this case we call the unaffected person a *carrier*.

Microorganisms are almost everywhere. We carry them on our skin, in our bodies, and on our clothing. They can be in ice, boiling water, the soil, and the air. The only places free of microorganisms are certain internal body organs and tissues and sterilized medical equipment and supplies. In the normal state, organs and tissues that do not connect with the outside by means of mucus-lined membranes are free of all living microorganisms.

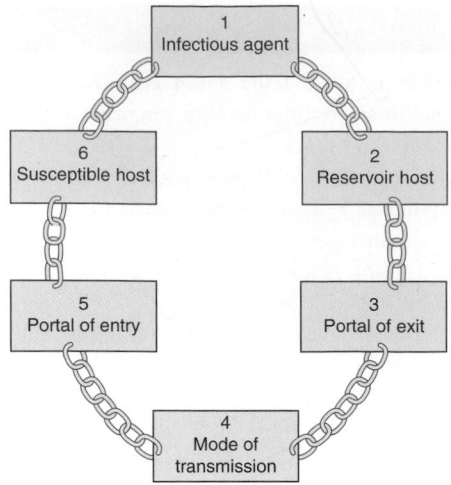

FIGURE 20-1 The chain of infection.

Conditions Required for Microbial Growth

To grow and flourish, microbes require certain conditions. To maintain a healthcare environment as free of pathogenic organisms as possible, the medical assistant must prevent or eliminate as many of these growth requirements as possible.

- *Nutrients:* Pathogens thrive on contaminated surfaces and equipment. Most microbes need the same nutrients we do: carbohydrates, proteins, and fats.
- *Moisture:* Microbes require moisture for cellular activities.
- *Temperature:* Most pathogenic microbes flourish at body temperature (98.6° F [37° C]).
- *Oxygen:* Some microbes, called *aerobes,* require oxygen to grow and multiply; others, called *anaerobes,* thrive in environments without oxygen.
- *Neutral pH:* pH refers to the acid-base level of a solution on a scale of 1 to 14, with 7 being neutral. Most pathogens prefer a neutral pH for optimum growth.

THE CHAIN OF INFECTION

Certain factors are required for an infectious disease to spread. These factors, or links, make up the chain of infection. Break the chain, and you break the infection process (Figure 20-1).

The chain of infection starts with the infectious agent. Five groups make up the potentially pathogenic agents or microorganisms: viruses, bacteria, protozoa and helminths, fungi, and rickettsia. Infection cannot occur without the presence of an infectious microorganism, so the best way for healthcare workers to prevent the spread of disease is to use adequate infection control procedures, such as consistent hand washing and proper use of **antiseptics**, in addition to effective disinfection and sterilization methods.

The smallest of all pathogens, viruses, lead the list of important disease-causing agents. Viral microorganisms are intracellular para-

sites that take over the deoxyribonucleic acid (DNA) or ribonucleic acid (RNA) of the invaded cell. Viral invasion may not cause significant immediate symptoms because host cells infected with viruses can produce a substance called **interferon**, which protects nearby cells. Interferon leaves the infected cell and acts somewhat like a Paul Revere, warning neighboring cells that "a virus is coming!" The neighboring cells then produce antiviral proteins, which prevents the virus from replicating inside the cells, thus slowing and halting the infection.

Antibiotics are unable to destroy viral invaders that enter a normal cell and multiply within the cell. The only way to destroy a viral invader is to destroy the host cell. Therefore, the treatment for viral infections typically focuses on relieving symptoms, or **palliative** treatment, and antiviral medications that slow the rate of viral replication. Interferon and the antiviral agents acyclovir (Zovirax), valacyclovir hydrochloride (Valtrex), adefovir dipivoxil (Hepsera), penciclovir (Denavir), Oseltamivir (Tamiflu), and famciclovir (Famvir) may be prescribed, depending on the specific viral agent. Viral diseases include the common cold, influenza, herpes, infectious hepatitis (e.g., hepatitis B and C), and acquired immunodeficiency syndrome (AIDS), which is caused by the human immunodeficiency virus (HIV).

Bacteria are tiny, simple cells that produce disease in a variety of ways. Pathogenic bacteria can secrete toxic substances that damage human tissues, act as parasites inside human cells, or grow on body surfaces, disrupting normal human functions. Bacteria are classified according to their shape, or *morphology;* they may be spherical (cocci), rod shaped (bacilli), or spiral shaped (spirilla). Some bacteria can produce resistant internal structures, called **spores**, that make treatment difficult. When bacteria invade the body, the patient can be treated in a number of ways. The most common approach is to use antibiotics to destroy the invader or inhibit its growth. We all have nonpathogenic bacteria that reside in various body systems; for example, a harmless form of *Escherichia coli (E. coli)* lives in the large intestine. These bacteria protect against disease by competing for nutrients that pathogenic bacteria require to grow and multiply. Common diseases caused by bacteria include tuberculosis, urinary tract infections, pneumonia, and strep throat.

Antibiotic Resistance

Antibiotic resistance is one of the world's most significant public health problems. Infectious microorganisms that once were easily treated with antibiotics are growing increasingly resistant to the actions of these drugs. The Centers for Disease Control and Prevention (CDC) reports that at least 2 million people in the United States become infected with antibiotic-resistant bacteria, and at least 23,000 people die each year as a direct result of these infections. Resistance occurs when an antibiotic is used inappropriately to treat an infection, resulting in a change or mutation of the pathologic organism that in some way reduces or eliminates the effectiveness of the drug.

If antibiotic medication is prescribed inappropriately (e.g., for a viral infection) or inaccurately (e.g., lower dosage, fewer days than recommended) or perhaps not taken by the patient as prescribed, some of the bacteria that survive the initial antibiotic treatment may mutate, allowing the microorganism to survive even in the presence of the antibiotic. Although mutations are rare, overuse of antibiotics provides more opportunity for them to occur. Antibiotics should be used to treat bacterial infections; however, they are not effective against viral infections, such as the common cold, most sore throats, and the flu. Cautious use of antibiotics is the key to preventing the spread of resistance. The CDC recommends that providers:

- Prescribe antibiotic therapy only when it will benefit the patient.
- Treat the patient with an antibiotic that is specific to the infecting pathogen.
- Prescribe the recommended dose and treatment duration of the medication.

CRITICAL THINKING APPLICATION   20-1

Susie Chen, a 3-year-old patient, is being seen today because of complaints of a cough and nasal congestion. Susie's father does not understand why the pediatrician did not order an antibiotic for his daughter's viral infection. Rosa needs to reinforce the doctor's decision. How can she help the father understand the proper use of antibiotics?

Protozoa are unicellular parasites that can replicate and multiply rapidly once inside the host. Examples of diseases caused by protozoa include giardiasis, which typically is caused by the ingestion of water contaminated by feces, and malaria, in which *Plasmodium* organisms invade the blood system. Protozoal infections frequently are seen in tropical climates, which have large insect populations. These insects serve as **vectors** for many protozoal diseases. For example, the mosquito transmits the organisms that cause malaria. Protozoa and helminths (worms) are usually grouped together as parasites. Helminths include tapeworms and roundworms. Tapeworms live in the intestines of some animals and can be transferred to humans who eat undercooked meat from infected animals. Most parasitic roundworm eggs are found in the soil and enter the human body when a person picks them up on the hands and then transfers them to the mouth. Roundworms eventually end up or live in human intestines and cause infection and disease.

Fungi may be unicellular or multicellular; they include such organisms as mushrooms, molds, and yeasts. Many forms are pathogenic and can cause disease, such as **candidiasis** and **tinea** infections. Fungi grow best in warm, moist environments. Treatment with antifungal agents includes application of topical preparations (e.g., Lotrimin) for tinea infections; vaginal suppositories (e.g., Monistat) for candidiasis; and oral medications, such as fluconazole (Diflucan), ketoconazole (Nizoral), and terbinafine (Lamisil). Fungal infections also are called *mycotic* infections.

Rickettsiae are microorganisms that have characteristics of both bacteria and viruses. Like viruses, they are obligate parasites that must live within a host cell for growth; however, they are larger than viruses, so they can be viewed with a microscope. Vectors such as fleas, ticks, and mites usually transmit pathogenic forms of rickettsiae. Diseases caused by rickettsiae can be treated with antibiotics; they include Rocky Mountain spotted fever, which is transmitted by a tick.

The second link in the chain of infection is the reservoir. Reservoirs may be people, insects, animals, water, food, or **contaminated** instruments and equipment. Most pathogens must gain entrance into a host or else they die. The reservoir host supplies nutrition for the organism, allowing it to multiply. The pathogen either causes infection in the host or, in the case of vector-borne diseases, exits the host in great enough numbers to cause disease in another host.

The chain of infection continues with the means, or portal, of exit; that is, how the pathogen escapes the reservoir host. Exits include the mouth, nose, eyes, ears, intestines, urinary tract, reproductive tract, and open wounds. The use of Standard Precautions (e.g., gloves, masks, proper wound care, correct disposal of contaminated products, hand washing) helps control the ability of infectious material to spread from one host to another.

After exiting the reservoir host, organisms spread by transmission. Transmission either is direct or indirect. Direct transmission occurs from contact with an infected person or with discharges from an infected person, such as feces or urine. Indirect transmission occurs from droplets in the air expelled by coughing, speaking, or sneezing; vectors that harbor pathogens; contaminated food or drink; and/or contact with contaminated objects (called **fomites**). Proper sanitation of water and food; the use of sanitization, disinfection, and sterilization procedures; and the use of **germicides** (e.g., Wavicide and Cidex) help control the transmission of pathogens.

The next link in the chain of infection is the means, or portal, of entry. This is how the transmitted pathogen gains entry into a new host. Like the means of exit, the means of entry may be the mouth, nose, eyes, intestines, urinary tract, reproductive system, or an open wound. The first line of defense against pathogenic invasion is the intact *integumentary* system, or skin, which serves as a mechanical barrier to infection. Anatomic defense mechanisms also include tears, cilia, mucous membranes, and the pH of body fluids. The body's second line of defense includes the inflammatory process and immune system response. The immune system responds by producing **antibodies** specifically designed to combat the presence of a foreign substance, or **antigen**. This process is called *humoral immunity* and is the responsibility of the body's B cells. The immune system also reacts at the cellular level, with T-cell activity in *cell-mediated immunity*, by causing the destruction of pathogenic cells at the site of invasion. An example of cell-mediated immunity is *phagocytosis,* in which specialized immune system cells, called *macrophages,* actually ingest and destroy pathogenic microbes.

The final link in the chain of infection is exposure of the pathogen to a susceptible host. If the host is susceptible (i.e., capable of supporting the growth of the infecting organism), the organism multiplies. Factors that contribute to a host's susceptibility include the location of entry, the dose of organisms, and the individual's state of health. Health is affected by a multitude of factors, including stress, poor nutrition, other illnesses, and contributing lifestyle factors. If conditions are right, the organism reaches infectious levels, and the susceptible host can start the chain of infection all over again.

Individuals who are successfully immunized against a disease (e.g., hepatitis B virus [HBV] infection), are not susceptible to the disease, even if they are exposed to the pathogen, because their immune system has created antibodies to protect them. However, some people do not develop immunity to diseases even after following immunization guidelines. The Centers for Disease Control and Prevention (CDC) estimate that 1% to 5% of the time, depending on the vaccine, individuals do not develop immunity. The provider can check for postimmunization effectiveness by ordering an antibody titer. A *titer* is a laboratory test that measures the level of antibodies in a blood sample. If a vaccine stimulated a person's immune system to create antibodies to a disease, the antibodies will be present in adequate amounts in the titer. If not, the physician decides whether another dose of the vaccine should be given to try to boost the person's immune response.

The Body's Natural Protective Mechanisms

The body has multiple levels of protection against the invasion of pathogenic microorganisms. The following are some of these mechanisms:

- Intact skin serves as a natural barrier to disease.
- Mucous membranes lining the openings of the body help protect underlying tissues and trap foreign substances.
- Tiny, hairlike projections, called *cilia,* line the respiratory tract and move in a coordinated upward motion to expel trapped foreign substances.
- Trapped substances can be expelled with sneezing and coughing before the organisms invade underlying tissue.
- Some body secretions, such as tears, have antimicrobial properties that help destroy invading pathogens.
- The natural pH of many of the body's organs discourages the growth of microbes. The acidic pH of urine, the vaginal mucosa, and the stomach helps prevent pathogenic invasion. The body's resident microbes create and maintain this environment.

CRITICAL THINKING APPLICATION   20-2

Tommy Anderson, a 5-year-old patient, is seen in the office because of an outbreak of impetigo. Rosa must apply the concepts of the chain of infection and infection control methods to teach Tommy and his mother how to prevent the spread of the infection to other members of the family. What procedures should she follow after Tommy's visit to prevent the spread of the infection to other patients, other staff members, and herself?

THE INFLAMMATORY RESPONSE

When the body experiences trauma or is exposed to pathogens, protective mechanisms are alerted, and the body responds in a predictable manner, called the *inflammatory response* (Figure 20-2). To defend itself, the body initiates specific responses to destroy and remove pathogenic organisms and their byproducts; or, if this is not possible, to limit the extent of damage caused by the invading pathogen. This process results in the four classic symptoms of inflammation: *erythema* (redness), *edema* (swelling), pain, and heat.

When the body is exposed to an infectious agent or a foreign substance, cellular damage occurs at the site. Inflammation mediators (i.e., histamine, prostaglandins, and kinins) are released, causing three different responses at the cellular level. All three actions are designed to increase the number of white blood cells (WBCs) at the injury site.

First, blood vessels at the site dilate, causing an increase in local blood flow, which results in redness (inflammation) and heat. Blood vessel walls become more **permeable**, which assists in the movement of WBCs through the vessel wall to the site. The WBCs begin to form a fibrous capsule around the site to protect surrounding cells from damage or infection. Blood plasma also filters out of the more permeable vessel walls, resulting in edema (swelling), which puts pressure on the nerves and causes pain. Finally, chemotaxis, or the release of chemical agents, occurs, attracting even more WBCs to the site. The increased number of WBCs at the site results in phagocytosis, or the engulfing and destruction of microorganisms and damaged cells. Destroyed pathogens, cells, and WBCs collect in the area and form a thick, white substance called *pus.* If the pathogenic invasion is too great for localized control, the infection may collect in the body's lymph nodes, where more WBCs are present to help fight the battle. This causes swollen glands, or *lymphadenopathy.* If the body is too weak or the number of pathogens is too great, the infection may spread to the bloodstream. A systemic infection, called *septicemia* or *blood poisoning,* may occur, which ultimately could affect the entire body. Another term for septicemia is **pyemia.** Without appropriate medical intervention, death can occur from a systemic infection.

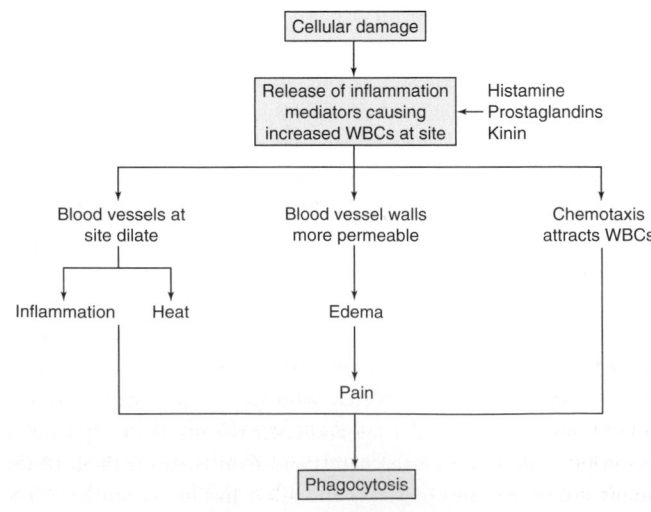

FIGURE 20-2 The inflammatory response.

TYPES OF INFECTIONS

Acute Infection

An acute infection has a rapid onset of symptoms but lasts a relatively short time. The *prodromal period* of an acute infection is that time when the patient first shows vague, nonspecific symptoms of disease. For example, the person is not vomiting nor does he or she have a fever, but the individual just doesn't feel well. In an acute viral infection, the host cell typically dies within hours or days. Symptoms appear after the tissue damage begins. In most acute infections, such as the common cold, the body's defense mechanisms eliminate the virus within 2 to 3 weeks.

Chronic Infection

An infection that persists for a long period, sometimes for life, is called a *chronic* infection. In the case of chronic viral hepatitis B infection, patients are *asymptomatic*, or without symptoms, but the virus is detectable with blood tests and remains transmissible throughout the person's life. Hepatitis B infection, or serum hepatitis, is transmitted by blood or blood products and by all body fluids. It is a serious health hazard to medical personnel. All individuals employed in a healthcare setting should be immunized against hepatitis B. OSHA requires all employers to offer hepatitis B vaccination to their employees.

Latent Infection

A *latent infection* is a persistent infection in which the symptoms cycle through periods of **relapse** and **remission**. Cold sores and genital herpes are latent viral infections caused by the herpes simplex virus (HSV) types 1 and 2, respectively. The virus enters the body and causes the original lesion. It then lies dormant, in nerve cells away from the surface, until a certain trigger (illness with fever, sunburn, or stress) causes it to leave the nerve cell and seek the surface again. Once the virus reaches the superficial tissues, it becomes detectable for a short time and causes a new outbreak at the site. Another herpes virus, varicella-zoster virus, causes chickenpox (varicella). This virus may lie dormant along a nerve pathway for years and later erupt as the painful disease shingles (herpes zoster).

Opportunistic Infections

Opportunistic infections are caused by organisms that are not typically pathogenic but that occur in hosts with an impaired immune system response, such as individuals infected with HIV. Over time, the person's immune system becomes weakened, and diseases result that are not typically seen in patients with a healthy immune system, such as *Pneumocystis carinii* pneumonia and oral candidiasis.

Ebola Virus

The Ebola virus causes a type of viral hemorrhagic fever, Ebola hemorrhagic fever (EHF). Depending on the strain and the individual infected with the disease, EHF may be fatal in 50% to 90% of cases. Workers performing tasks involving close contact with symptomatic individuals with EHF are at risk of exposure. These include healthcare workers, those in mortuary and death care, and travel service employees.

Individuals with EHF have symptoms typical of viral illnesses, including fever, fatigue, muscle pain, headache, and sore throat. The illness progresses to nausea, vomiting, diarrhea, impaired organ function, rash, and internal and/or external bleeding. Symptoms typically appear abruptly, within 2 to 20 days after exposure to the virus (8 to 10 days is most common). EHF is believed to be contagious only when symptoms appear, and the illness runs its course within 14 to 20 days of symptom onset.

In areas of Africa where Ebola viruses are common, suspected reservoirs include primate and bat populations. Naturally occurring EHF outbreaks are believed to start from contact with infected wildlife (alive or dead) and then spread from person to person through direct contact with body fluids, such as blood, urine, sweat, semen, breast milk, vomit, and feces. The infection is spread when body surfaces that can easily absorb blood-borne pathogens (e.g., open cuts, scrapes, or mucous membranes such as the lining of the mouth, eyes, or nose) come into direct contact with infectious blood or body fluids. There is currently no treatment, antiviral therapy, or approved vaccine for EHF or Ebola virus.

The risk of infection with Ebola virus is minimal if a person has not been in close contact with the body fluids of someone sick with or recently deceased from EHF. Although there are no known animal reservoirs of the disease in the United States, the possible spread of EHF is a concern because of the availability and reach of global travel. Under certain conditions, exposure to just one viral particle can result in the development of EHF.

Ambulatory care facilities may develop policies and procedures to manage patients who report that they have recently travelled to areas where Ebola infections have occurred. The CDC recommends the following measures:

- Staff members should be ready to take three steps: Identify, Isolate, and Inform.
- Ask every patient if, in the last 20 days, he or she has traveled to a country with widespread transmission (Guinea, Liberia, or Sierra Leone) or has had contact with a person with confirmed EHF.
- If a patient appears to be at risk for EHF, isolate the patient immediately, avoid unnecessary direct contact, determine the PPE needed, and notify the health department. Refer to the CDC website (www.cdc.gov/vhf/ebola/healthcare-us/ppe/guidance.html) for detailed information on how to put on and take off appropriate PPE.
- Do not transfer the patient without first notifying the health department; these patients should be transferred only to a facility approved by public health authorities.

Modified from www.osha.gov/SLTC/ebola/index.html and www.cdc.gov/vhf/ebola/healthcare-us/outpatient-settings/index.html. Accessed March 11, 2015.

OSHA STANDARDS FOR THE HEALTHCARE SETTING

In 1987, in response to concern about the increasing prevalence of HIV and HBV, the CDC recommended a new approach to potentially infectious materials called *Universal Precautions*. The underlying concept of Universal Precautions is that because healthcare workers cannot know whether a patient has an infectious disorder, all blood and certain body fluids must be treated as if known to be infectious for blood-borne pathogens. Therefore, precautions must be implemented for all patients, regardless of the information available about the person's individual health history. In turn, Universal Precautions protect patients from any blood-borne infection the healthcare worker may carry.

In 2001 OSHA developed the Bloodborne Pathogens Standard (Standard Precautions) to safeguard all healthcare employees and their patients who are at risk of exposure from blood and other body fluids.

Potentially Infectious Fluids
Items contaminated with any of the following potentially infectious materials require special handling: • Cerebrospinal fluid (CSF); mucus; and synovial, pleural, pericardial, peritoneal, and amniotic fluids* • Liquid or semiliquid blood • Vaginal and seminal secretions • Saliva in dental procedures • Body fluid visibly contaminated with blood • Unknown body fluid • Wound drainage • Human tissue, including tissue culture, cells, or exudates

*The human immunodeficiency virus (HIV) has been isolated from CSF, synovial, and amniotic fluids; hepatitis antigens have been detected in synovial, amniotic, and peritoneal fluids.

Exposure Control Plan

OSHA recognizes that healthcare employees face significant health risks as the result of occupational exposure to blood or other potentially infectious materials that may contain HBV, the hepatitis C virus (HCV), or HIV. In July, 1992, OSHA began enforcing work practice controls to reduce or eliminate occupational exposure to blood-borne pathogens. Employers whose workers are at risk for occupational exposure to blood or other infectious materials must implement an Exposure Control Plan that details employee protection procedures. The Exposure Control Plan must identify job classifications and/or specific work-related tasks in which an employee may be exposed to blood and/or body fluids. The plan must describe how an employer will use a combination of controls, including personal protective equipment (PPE), training, medical surveillance, HBV immunizations, record keeping of occupational injuries, post-exposure follow-up, and labeling of hazardous materials. Engineering controls, such as safer medical equipment, puncture-proof sharps containers, and shielded needle devices, in addition to PPE (e.g., gloves, gowns, and face shields), are recommended as the primary ways to reduce or eliminate employee exposure.

The Exposure Control Plan must be reviewed and updated at least annually to incorporate the use of safer medical devices designed to eliminate or minimize occupational exposure to contaminated waste. In addition, the plan must be readily available to all employees for review and training. It does not have to be a separate document and may be included as part of the facility's policies and procedures manual, or in the health and safety manual developed by the site.

CRITICAL THINKING APPLICATION   **20-4**

Based on what you have learned about OSHA requirements for environmental safety in a healthcare facility, evaluate your clinical laboratory at school. Does it meet all of OSHA's standards? Is an environmental safety plan in place? Develop an Exposure Control Plan for your facility and share it with your peers.

The Bloodborne Pathogens Standard

In response to the CDC's concern about employee risk, Congress passed the Needlestick Safety and Prevention Act, which took effect in April, 2001. Employers are required to keep a confidential sharps injury log that describes the device involved in the incident and the details of how and where the incident occurred. Employers also must make available to employees effective sharps management devices, such as syringes with self-sheathing needles, needles that retract after use, and needleless intravenous (IV) systems that do not require sharps for **parenteral** administration. Parenteral exposure includes accidental needlesticks, occupation-related human bites, and exposure of nonintact skin (e.g., cuts and abrasions on the employee's hands) to potentially infectious material. An employer who fails to comply with OSHA's Bloodborne Pathogens Standard could face a maximum penalty of $7,000 for the first violation and up to $70,000 for repeated violations.

The Bloodborne Pathogens Standard also clarifies the use of washing or flushing of any exposed body area or mucous membrane immediately or as soon as possible after exposure to potentially infectious materials. This includes hand washing after the removal of gloves or other PPE.

Although the hands should be washed with antimicrobial soap and warm, running water when available, studies have shown that correct use of alcohol-based hand rubs significantly reduces the number of microorganisms on the skin, takes less time than traditional hand washing, and causes less irritation to the skin, especially if the solution is mixed with emollients (Figure 20-3). Allergic contact dermatitis from alcohol hand rubs is uncommon.

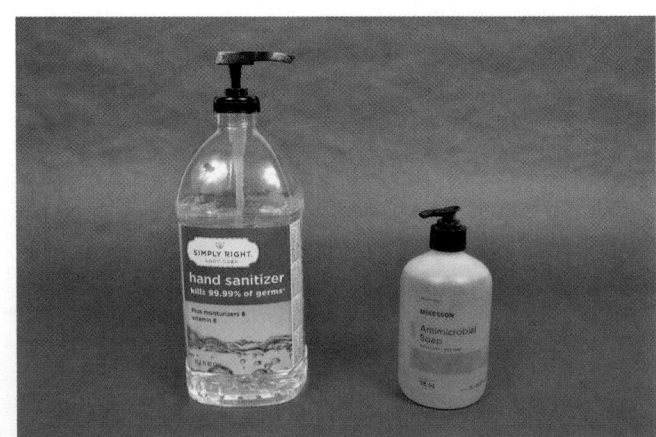

FIGURE 20-3 Antimicrobial soap and alcohol-based hand rubs.

The CDC's recommendations for adequate hand hygiene are as follows:

- Visibly soiled hands should be washed for a minimum of 15 seconds with antimicrobial soap and warm, running water.
- Alcohol hand rubs should be used before and after contact with each patient, and also after removing gloves, to prevent cross-contamination among patients and healthcare workers.
- To use an alcohol hand rub properly, apply the label-recommended amount to the palm of one hand and rub the hands together, covering all surfaces until the hands are dry.

- Artificial nails should not be worn; studies show that even after careful hand hygiene, healthcare workers with artificial nails have more pathogenic microbes under their nails and on their fingertips than workers with natural nails. Artificial nails also cause nail changes that contribute to the transmission of microbes.
- Natural nail tips should be no longer than $\frac{1}{4}$ inch to prevent microbial growth in the nail bed.

The best way to reduce the occupational risk of infection is to follow the Bloodborne Pathogens Standard. Healthcare workers must take adequate and consistent precautions to protect themselves and their patients. Figure 20-4 summarizes the Bloodborne

---

Requirements of Employers: OSHA Bloodborne Pathogens Standard

EXPOSURE CONTROL PLAN

Each medical office must develop a written exposure control plan (ECP). The purpose of an ECP is to identify tasks where there is the potential for exposure to blood and other potentially infectious materials.

- A timetable must be published indicating when and how communication of potential hazards will occur.
- The employer must offer employees the hepatitis B vaccine within 10 working days of employment (at no cost to the employee). If employees sign a form to refuse the vaccine, they can change their mind at no cost to the employee.
- The employer must document the steps that should be taken in case of an exposure incident, including a postexposure evaluation and follow-up, strict record keeping, implementation of engineering controls, provision for personal protective equipment, and general housekeeping standards. This plan must be posted in the medical office.
- There must also be written procedures for evaluating the circumstances of an exposure incident.
- Training records must be kept for 3 years.

ENGINEERING CONTROLS AND WORK PRACTICES

The employer must provide engineering controls, or equipment and facilities that minimize the possibility of exposure. Examples of engineering controls include the following:

- Providing puncture-resistant containers for used sharps.
- Providing handwashing facilities that are readily accessible.
- Equipment for sanitizing, decontaminating, and sterilizing.

The employer must also enforce work practice controls. Work practice controls also minimize the possibility of exposure by making sure employees are using the proper techniques while working. Examples include the following:

- Enforcing proper handwashing or sanitizing procedures.
- Enforcing proper technique for using and handling needles to prevent needle sticks.
- Enforcing proper techniques to minimize the splashing of blood.

PERSONAL PROTECTIVE EQUIPMENT

Employers must provide, and employees must use, personal protective equipment (PPE) when the possibility exists of exposure to blood or contaminated body fluids. This equipment must not allow blood or potentially infectious material to pass through to the employee's clothes, skin, eyes, or mouth. Examples of PPE include the following:

- Gowns
- Face shields
- Goggles
- Gloves

If an employee has an allergy to powder or latex, the employer must provide hypoallergenic or powderless gloves. The employee cannot be charged for PPEs.

EXPOSURE INCIDENT MANAGEMENT

An exposure incident is contact with blood or biohazard infectious material that occurs when doing one's job. When an exposure incident is reported, the employer must arrange for an immediate and confidential medical evaluation. The information and actions required are as follows:

- Documenting how the exposure occurred.
- Identifying and testing the "source" individual, if possible.
- Testing the employee's blood, if consent is granted.
- Providing counseling.
- Evaluating, treating, and following up on any reported illness.

Medical records must be kept for each employee with occupational exposure for the duration of employment plus 30 years.

COMMUNICATION OF POTENTIAL HAZARDS TO EMPLOYEES

A medical assistant will be exposed to hazardous chemicals on the job. Most chemicals handled by assistants are not any more dangerous than those used in the home. In the workplace, however, exposure is likely to be greater, concentrations higher, and exposure time longer.

The "right to-know" law, OSHA's hazard communication standard, states that each employee has a right to know what chemicals he or she is working with in the workplace. The right-to-know law is intended to make the workplace safer by making certain that all information regarding chemical hazards is known to the employee. This information is supplied in the material safety data sheet (MSDS), a fact sheet about a chemical that includes the following information:

- Identification of the chemical
- Listing of the physical and health hazards
- Precautions for handling
- Identification of the chemical as a carcinogen
- First-aid procedures
- Name, address, and telephone number of manufacturer

Many SDS information sheets can be obtained in repositories on the Internet. An SDS should be updated at least every 3 years. Employers must ensure that all products have an up-to-date SDS when they enter the workplace.

Potential hazards are also communicated with labels and color. Any containers with biohazard waste must be orange (or reddish orange) and must display the biohazard symbol. These labels and colors alert employees to the risk of possible exposure.

FIGURE 20-4 Requirements of employers: OSHA's Bloodborne Pathogens Standard. (www.osha.gov. Accessed 8/13/2015)

Pathogens Standard. Healthcare facilities must establish specific policies and procedures for the management of an exposure incident (e.g., accidental needlestick) and the exposed employee.

Compliance Guidelines

Because the Bloodborne Pathogens Standard is written to cover employees working in all health fields, only some of the regulations apply to the ambulatory care setting. Safety and infection control fundamentals go beyond hand washing and knowledge of the disease cycle. The information is presented here as it applies to the medical assisting profession.

Barrier Protection

Medical assistants routinely should use appropriate barrier precautions when contact with blood or other body fluids is expected. Barrier protection, or PPE, includes specialized clothing or equipment that prevents the healthcare worker from coming in contact with blood or other potentially infectious material, thereby preventing or minimizing the entry of infectious material into the body. Barrier devices include disposable gloves, face masks, face shields, protective glasses, shoe covers, laboratory coats, barrier gowns, mouthpieces, and resuscitation bags (Figure 20-5).

Since the implementation of Standard Precautions, the use of disposable examination gloves is required in healthcare facilities. Because of the frequent allergic reactions associated with latex products, facilities now use nonlatex gloves. If the facility where you work still uses latex gloves, signs of an allergic reaction include localized **urticaria**, dermatitis, conjunctivitis, and **rhinitis**. Hypersensitive reactions can be systemic, producing asthma symptoms or **anaphylaxis**. If a healthcare worker or a patient shows signs of sensitivity to latex, the healthcare provider is required to provide products made of nonallergenic materials. Gloves must be worn if the medical assistant is at all likely to be involved in any of the following activities (Procedure 20-1):

- Touching a patient's blood, body fluids, mucous membranes, or skin that is not intact.

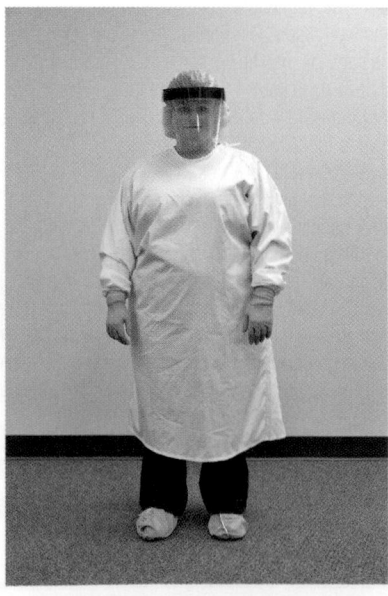

FIGURE 20-5 Personal protective equipment.

- Handling items and surfaces contaminated with blood and body fluids.
- Performing venipuncture, finger sticks, injections, and other vascular procedures.
- Assisting with any surgical procedure. If a glove is torn during the procedure, the glove should be removed, the hands washed carefully, and a new glove put on as soon as possible.
- Handling, processing, and disposing of all specimens of blood and body fluids.
- Cleaning and decontaminating spills of blood or other body fluids.

The same pair of gloves cannot be worn for the care of more than one patient; new disposable gloves must be used for each individual patient.

Safety Alert

Protective equipment contaminated with body fluids of any kind must be removed and placed in a designated area or biohazard container. The hands or any other exposed areas must be washed or flushed as soon as possible. Face shields that cover the mouth, nose, and eyes must be worn whenever splashes, sprays, or droplets are possible. Utility gloves may be reused if they are intact (i.e., have no cracks, tears, or punctures). All PPE must be removed before the medical assistant leaves the medical facility (Figure 20-6).

CRITICAL THINKING APPLICATION   20-5
Rosa is caring for an injured 3-year-old child with an open wound on his right knee. She puts on disposable gloves to clean the wound, and the mother demands to know why. How can she explain her actions?

Environmental Protection

Environmental protection refers to minimizing the risk of occupational injury by isolating or removing any physical or mechanical health hazard in the medical workplace. Every medical assistant must adhere to these safety rules.
- Read warning labels on biohazard containers and equipment.
- Minimize splashing or spraying of potentially infectious materials. Blood that splatters onto open areas of the skin or mucous membranes is a proven mode of HBV transmission.
- Bandage any breaks or lesions on your hands before gloving.
- If any body surface is exposed to potentially infectious material, scrub the area with antimicrobial soap and warm, running water as soon as possible after the exposure.
- If your eyes come in contact with body fluids, continuously flush them with water as soon as possible for a minimum of 15 minutes using an eye wash unit. A stationary unit connected to warm, running water is the best method for properly flushing potentially infectious material out of the eyes (Figure 20-7 and Procedure 20-2).
- Contaminated needles and other sharps should never be recapped, bent, broken, or resheathed; needle units must have protective safety devices to cover the contaminated needle after injection.

PROCEDURE 20-1

Participate in Bloodborne Pathogen Training: Use Standard Precautions to Remove Contaminated Gloves and Discard Biohazardous Material

Goal: *To minimize exposure to pathogens by aseptically removing and discarding contaminated gloves.*

EQUIPMENT and SUPPLIES

- Disposable examination gloves
- Biohazard waste container with labeled red biohazard bag

PROCEDURAL STEPS

1. With the dominant hand, grasp the glove of the opposite hand near the palm and begin removing the first glove (Figure 1). The arms should be held away from the body with the hands pointed down.
   PURPOSE: Holding the hands down and away from the body helps prevent possible contamination.

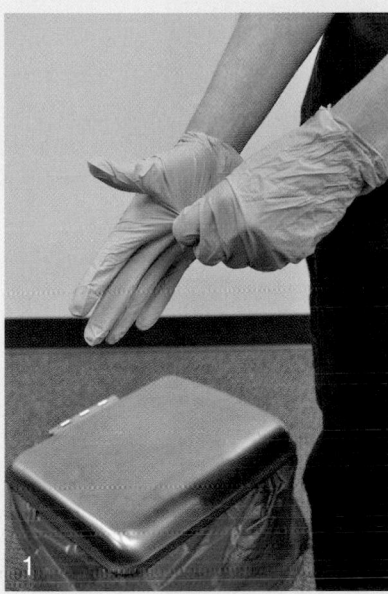

2. Pull the glove inside out (Figure 2). After removal, ball it into the palm of the remaining gloved hand.
   PURPOSE: Taking off the glove inside out prevents transmission of pathogens to another surface.

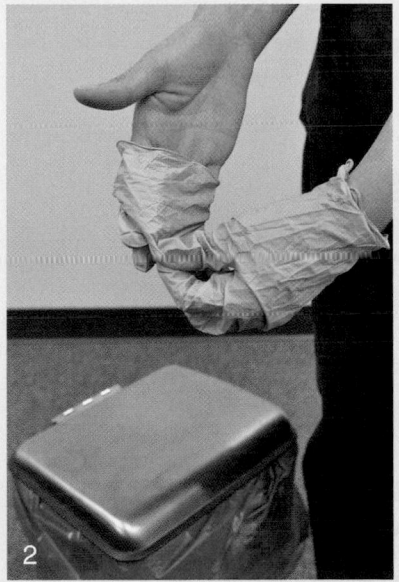

3. Insert two fingers of the ungloved hand between the edge of the cuff of the other contaminated glove and the hand (Figure 3).

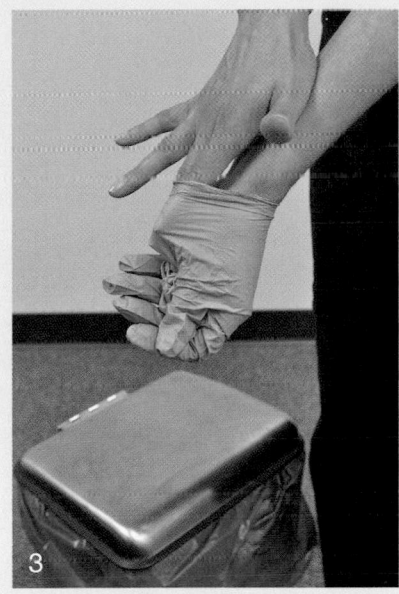

4. Push the glove down the hand, inside out, over the contaminated glove being held, leaving the contaminated side of both gloves on the inside.
   PURPOSE: This technique protects the wearer from the contaminated surfaces of both gloves.

5. Properly dispose of the inside-out, contaminated gloves in a biohazard waste container (Figure 4).
   PURPOSE: To prevent the spread of infection.

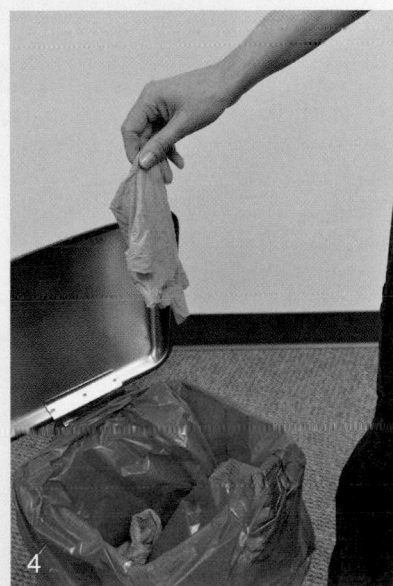

6. Perform a medical aseptic hand wash as described in Procedure 20-4 or sanitize the hands with an alcohol-based rub.
   PURPOSE: To minimize the number of pathogens on the hands, thereby reducing the number of transient flora and the risk of transmission of pathogens.

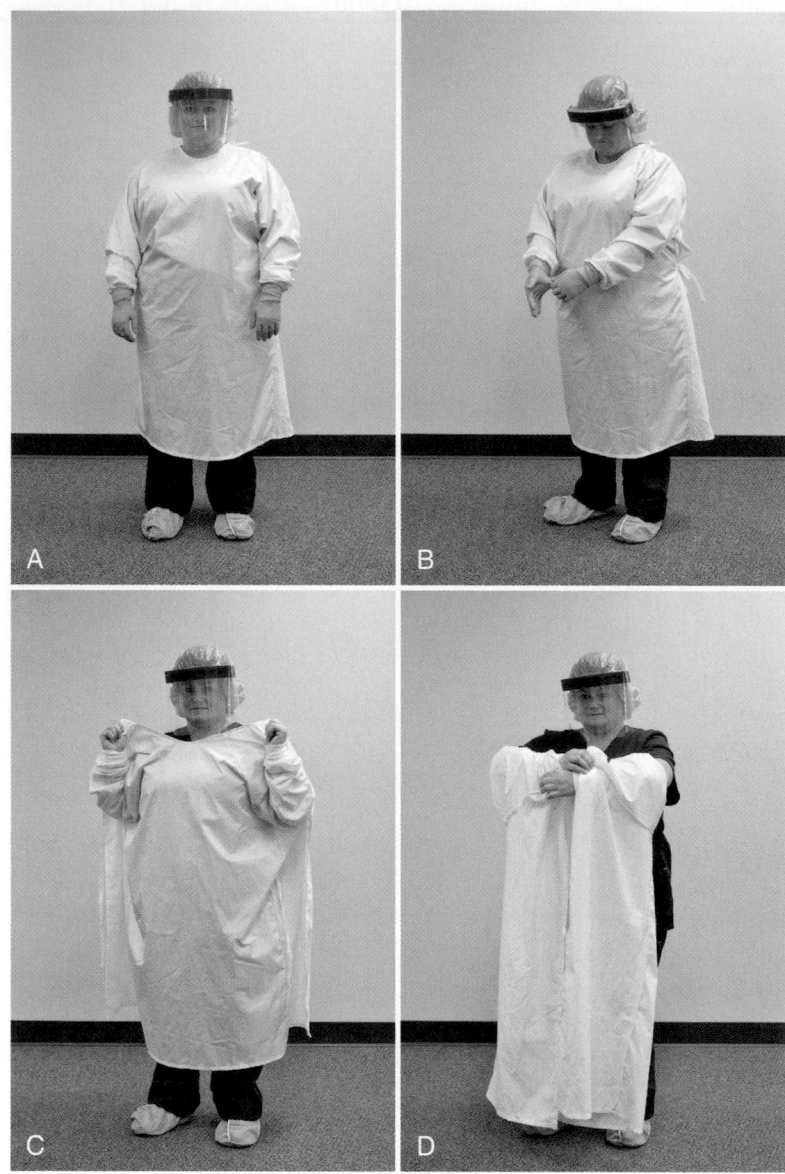

FIGURE 20-6 Removing a contaminated gown.

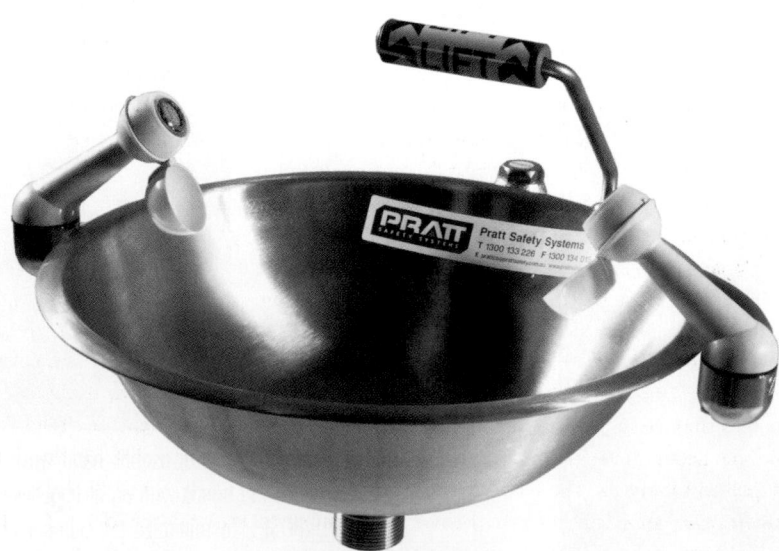

FIGURE 20-7 Eye washing unit.

PROCEDURE 20-2   Demonstrate the Proper Use of Eye Wash Equipment: Perform an Emergency Eye Wash

Goal: *To minimize the risk of occupational exposure to pathogens if body fluids come in contact with the eyes.*

EQUIPMENT and SUPPLIES

- Plumbed or self-contained eye wash unit
- Disposable gloves

PROCEDURAL STEPS

1. Put on gloves and remove contact lenses or glasses.
   <u>PURPOSE:</u> To ensure flushing of all material in the eyes.
2. Following the manufacturer's directions, turn on the eye wash unit. If it is a plumbed unit, the control valve should remain on until the unit is manually shut off.
   <u>PURPOSE:</u> The unit must be plumbed so that it can remain on until manually turned off.
3. Hold the eyelids open with the thumb and index finger to ensure adequate rinsing of the entire eye and eyelid surface (Figure 1).
   <u>PURPOSE:</u> The normal reflex is to close the eyes tightly, which prevents removal of all the contaminated material.
4. Avoid aiming the water stream directly onto the eyeball.
   <u>PURPOSE:</u> A direct water stream may cause discomfort and/or damage the eye.
5. Flush the eyes and eyelids for a minimum of 15 minutes, rolling the eyes periodically to ensure complete removal of the foreign material.
   <u>PURPOSE:</u> To completely remove the potentially dangerous substance from the eyes.
6. Remove gloves using Procedure 20-1, dispose of them in a properly labeled biohazard bag, and sanitize your hands.
   <u>PURPOSE:</u> To prevent cross-contamination.

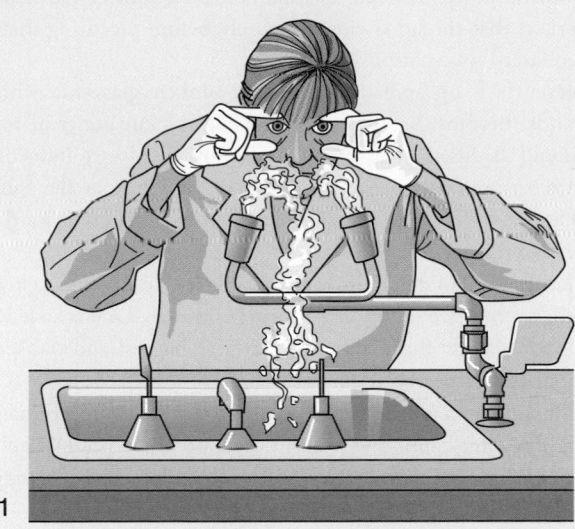

1

7. After completion of the eye wash, follow postexposure follow-up procedures.
   <u>PURPOSE:</u> Depending on the type of exposure, the facility's policies may include provider completion of an exposure incident form and provider follow-up.

- Contaminated sharp instruments, such as biopsy scissors, should not be processed in a way that requires employees to reach into containers to grasp them.
- Immediately after use, dispose of syringes and needles, scalpel blades, and other disposable sharp items in a labeled, leakproof, puncture-resistant biohazard container. The container must be located as close as possible to the area where the item is used.
- All specimens must be placed in a container that prevents leakage during collection, handling, processing, storage, transport, and shipping. Avoid contaminating the outside of the container or the label with the specimen substance. The container must have a biohazard label to alert others that it holds potentially infectious material. Gloves should be worn throughout this procedure.
- Equipment requiring repair that has been contaminated with blood or body fluids should be decontaminated before being repaired in the office or transported for repair. There is no documented evidence of HIV transmission from contaminated environmental surfaces, but surface contamination is a proven mode of transmission of HBV.

- Smoking, eating, drinking, applying cosmetics or lip balm, and handling contact lenses are prohibited in work areas where there is a reasonable likelihood of contamination by pathogens.
- Food and beverages cannot be kept in refrigerators, freezers, or cabinets or on countertops where infectious materials could be present.

Housekeeping Controls

The Bloodborne Pathogens Standard requires certain housekeeping measures to ensure a sanitary work area. Facilities must post a schedule for cleaning and decontaminating each work area where exposures could occur. This documentation must include information about the surface cleaned, the type of waste encountered, and procedures performed in the designated area.

- After accidental spills of blood or body fluids, at the end of each procedure, and at the end of each shift, work surfaces must be immediately cleaned and then disinfected with a **disinfectant** registered with the Environmental Protection Agency (EPA).

- All reusable containers must be disinfected and decontaminated on a routine basis.
- Sharps containers must be kept as close as possible to the work area. Never attempt to reach inside a sharps container, and do not overfill them. Replace containers on a routine basis, and be certain that the lid is closed securely before preparing them for biohazard waste disposal.
- Never pick up spilled material or broken glassware with the hands. Brooms, brushes, dustpans, and pickup tongs or forceps should be used. The material should be placed immediately into an impervious biohazard bag or container at the spill site (Figure 20-8). Use an absorbent, professional biohazard spill preparation as directed to decontaminate the site.
- Handle soiled linen as little as possible and always wear gloves or other protective equipment during disposal. Linens soiled with blood or body fluids should be double-bagged and transported in labeled, leakproof biohazard bags.
- Contaminated materials and/or infectious waste must be handled with extreme caution to prevent exposure. Biohazard waste must be collected in impermeable, red polyethylene or polypropylene biohazard-labeled bags or containers and sealed (Figure 20-9). This waste must be disposed of in accordance with all federal, state, and local regulations. Disposal methods include treatment by heat, incineration, steam sterilization, chemical treatment, or other equivalent methods that renders the waste inactive before it is placed in a landfill.

CRITICAL THINKING APPLICATION   20-6

Your office manager asks you to prepare a fact sheet for your co-workers that summarizes the details of OSHA's Bloodborne Pathogens Standard. What should you include?

Protocols for Disposal of Biologic Chemical Materials

The Medical Waste Tracking Act set the standards for governmental regulation of medical waste; however, that law expired in 1991. The states were then given responsibility for regulating the disposal of medical waste. The

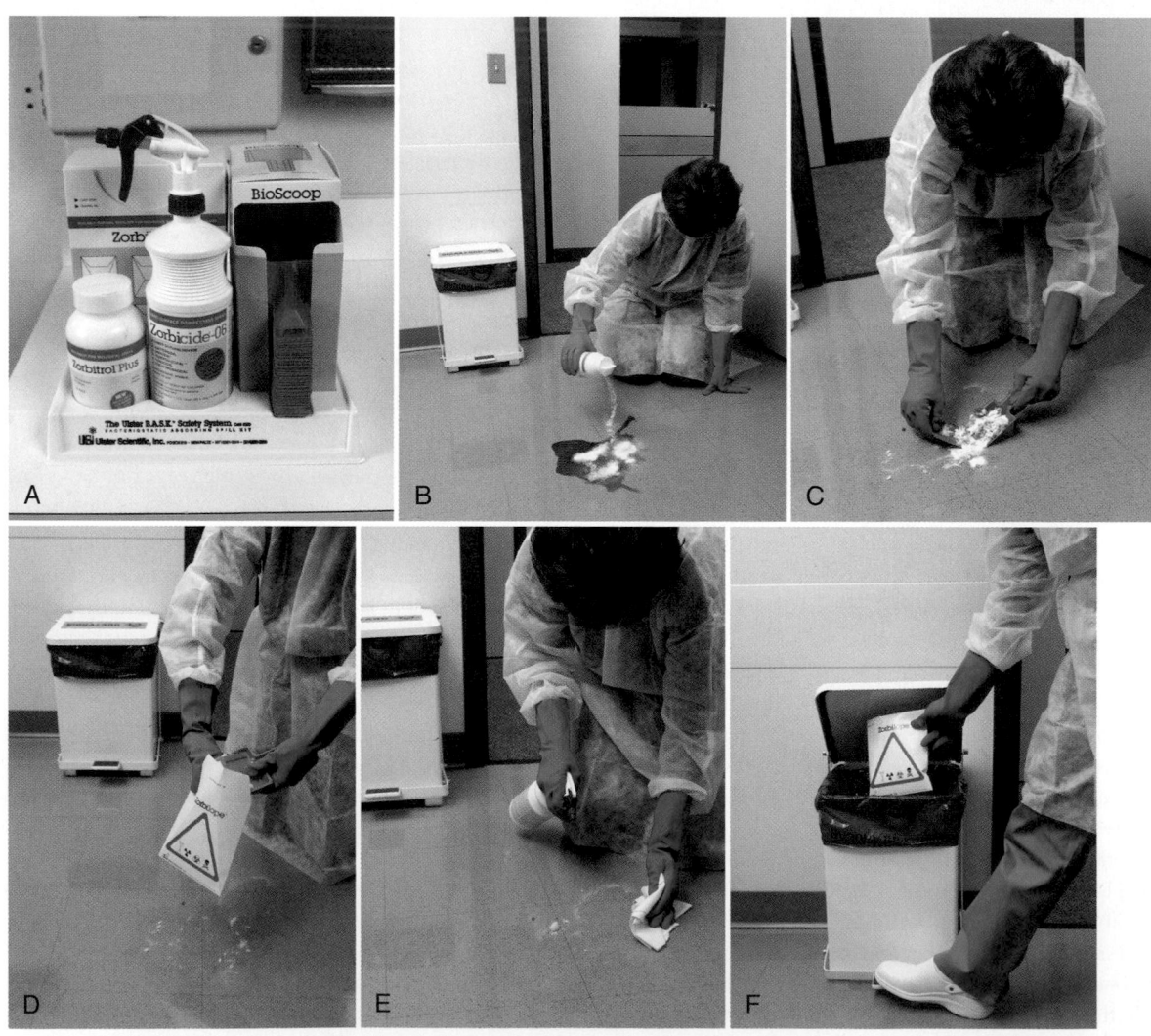

FIGURE 20-8 Cleaning up spilled material. **A,** Clean-up kit with printed instructions. **B,** Sprinkle congealing powder over the spill. **C,** Scoop up the spill. **D,** Place the contents in a biohazard bag. **E,** Wipe the area thoroughly with a germicide. **F,** Place all contaminated material in a biohazard bag or container.

50 states vary in their degree of regulation, ranging from no regulation to very strict rules. The following are some examples of regulations covering the disposal of hazardous materials.

- Biomedical waste should be collected in containers that are leakproof and strong enough to prevent breakage during handling; the containers must be labeled with the biohazard symbol.
- Workers who handle biomedical waste should observe Standard Precautions.
- Biologic waste containers and boxes should not be held in the healthcare facility for longer than 30 days.
- Sharps are instruments intended to cut or penetrate the skin; they include lancets, scalpel blades, needles, and syringe/needle combinations. Sharps must be placed in red, hard plastic sharps boxes after use; sharps boxes should be closed when three-fourths full.
- Boxes for disposal of chemicals should be labeled with the chemicals' names and any other pertinent data; they must be adequately sealed to prevent breakage or leakage.
- Each healthcare facility must hire a biomedical waste disposal service whose employees are trained to collect and haul away biomedical waste in special containers (usually cardboard boxes or reusable plastic bins) for treatment at a facility designed to handle biomedical waste.
- The cost to the healthcare facility for biomedical waste disposal is typically based on the weight of the contaminated items collected (i.e., the weight of filled sharps containers, biohazard boxes, and bags).

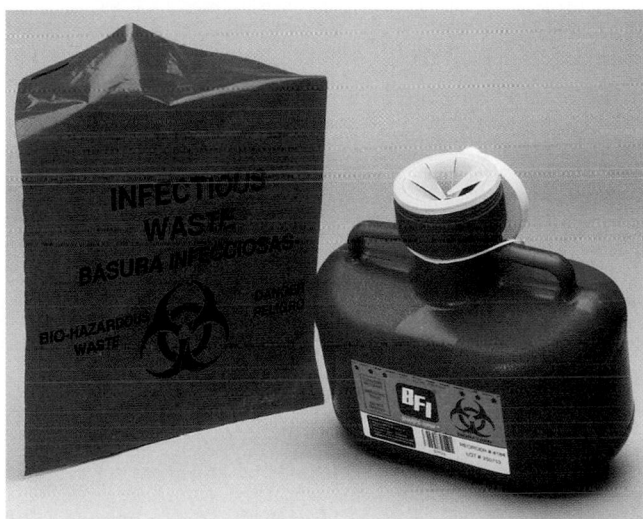

FIGURE 20-9 Biohazard bag and biohazard sharps container.

Hepatitis B Vaccination

HBV vaccination must be available free of charge to all employees at risk for occupational exposure to blood-borne pathogens, whether they are full-time or part-time workers, within 10 days of starting employment. The vaccine is administered by intramuscular injection in three doses. The second injection is administered 4 weeks after the first, and the third injection 6 months after the first. The U.S. Public Health Service does not currently recommend routine boosters for hepatitis B immunization. However, if they are recommended in the future, boosters must be made available to eligible employees without cost.

FIGURE 20-10 Sample hepatitis B declination form. (https://www.osha.gov/SLTC/etools/hospital/hazards/bbp/declination.html. Accessed 10/7/2015.)

After three intramuscular doses of hepatitis B vaccine, more than 90% of healthy adults and more than 95% of infants, children, and adolescents (from birth to 19 years of age) develop adequate antibody responses. Despite this, healthcare workers with a high risk of exposure should have a blood titer drawn after completion of the injection cycle to determine whether they have created antibodies against the disease. Postvaccination antibody testing should be done 1 to 2 months after completion of the vaccine series. If the employee did not respond to the first series or if the series was not completed, revaccination with a second three-dose series is recommended. If antibodies still do not develop, no further vaccination is given.

Employees have the right to decline hepatitis B immunization, but they are required to sign a declination form (Figure 20-10) that is kept on file as a record of their refusal. The statement can be signed only after the employee has received training about hepatitis B, hepatitis B vaccination, and the safety, route of administration, and benefits of vaccination, in addition to being informed that the vaccine will be administered free of charge. Employees who change their mind may receive the vaccine at a future date free of charge.

Postexposure Follow-Up

If a worker is exposed through an accidental needlestick, a human bite, exposure to broken skin, or from a splash or splatter onto mucous membranes, such as the eyes, certain procedures must be followed. Procedure 20-3 presents the specific steps to be taken after exposure to contaminated waste.

- Immediately, or as soon as possible after exposure, the worker should wash or flush the exposed area.
- The exposure incident must be immediately reported to the supervisor.
- The employee must immediately receive a confidential medical evaluation. The provider caring for the exposed employee must receive written details of the exposure incident, including the route and circumstances surrounding the incident. All documentation related to the exposure must remain confidential, may not be disclosed to any individual without the employee's express written permission, and must be kept for at least the duration of the worker's employment plus 30 years.

PROCEDURE 20-3	Participate in Bloodborne Pathogen Training and a Mock Environmental Exposure Event with Documentation of Steps

Goal: *To manage an exposure incident according to OSHA standards.*

Scenario: *As Rosa administers a hepatitis B injection intramuscularly (IM), the patient jumps back. The needle becomes dislodged from the patient's arm, and Rosa is accidentally jabbed in the hand by the contaminated needle. The patient is receiving ongoing treatment for hepatitis C but is not HIV positive. After Rosa notifies her site supervisor, what procedural steps must she take to comply with OSHA standards?*

EQUIPMENT and SUPPLIES

- Antibacterial soap and warm running water
- Exposure incident report form

Sample Blood and Body Fluid Exposure Report Form from the Centers for Disease Control (CDC) can be found at *http://www.cdc.gov/sharpssafety/pdf/AppendixA-7.pdf*

PROCEDURAL STEPS

1. Remove gloves and immediately wash the exposed site with antibacterial soap and warm running water.
   <u>PURPOSE:</u> To sanitize and disinfect the exposure site as quickly and thoroughly as possible.

2. Immediately report the exposure incident to the site supervisor.
   <u>PURPOSE:</u> The facility supervisor (e.g., office manager, practice manager, provider) is responsible for following through with the facility's Exposure Control Plan.

3. Complete an exposure incident report that details the type of injury, the details surrounding the incident, the equipment involved, and any other pertinent details.
   <u>PURPOSE:</u> The facility must report exposure incidents to OSHA. OSHA evaluates the incident based on required standards, including employee training, availability of current protective devices (e.g., needle safety covers and location of sharps containers), and the extent of employee injury. The incident report also serves as a written record of the incident, which establishes the need for employee healthcare.

- An incident report must be filed that documents the details surrounding the exposure incident, the route or type of exposure, and the identity, if known, of the source individual. The source individual is the person, living or dead, whose blood or potentially infectious material was the source of the occupational exposure.
- The source individual is screened for HBV, HCV, and HIV. Depending on state regulations, consent may or may not be required from the source individual to perform the screening. If consent is required but not given, the employer must document that consent was not received from the source individual. If screening is done, OSHA requires that the employee be informed of the results of the source individual's tests.
- The exposed worker is tested for HBV, HCV, and HIV if consent is given to determine whether the employee already has one of these infectious diseases. If the employee refuses the tests but blood is drawn, the sample must be stored 90 days for the worker to decide whether screening is wanted.
- If the employee has not been vaccinated against HBV, vaccination is offered.
- The injured employee must receive a copy of the healthcare provider's written opinion within 15 days of completion of the evaluation.
- The exposed worker must receive health counseling about the risk of illness or other adverse outcomes of exposure and the potential for and consequences of transmission of the disease to family, patients, and others.

Healthcare students are at risk for blood-borne pathogen exposure and should follow all OSHA guidelines designed to protect individuals from exposure. A complete, unabridged copy of OSHA's Bloodborne Pathogens Standard may be obtained at the OSHA website *(www.osha.gov)*.

The CDC has developed a checklist that ambulatory care facilities can use to systematically assess employee adherence to infection prevention and to ensure that the facility has policies and procedures

---

Risk of Infection After an Occupational Exposure

Hepatitis B Virus (HBV)
Healthcare workers who have received hepatitis B vaccine and have developed immunity to the virus are at virtually no risk for infection. For an unvaccinated person, the risk from a single needlestick or a cut exposure to HBV-infected blood ranges from 6% to 30%.

Hepatitis C Virus (HCV)
The estimated risk for infection after a needlestick or cut exposure to HCV-infected blood is approximately 1.8%. The risk after a blood splash is unknown but is believed to be very small.

Human Immunodeficiency Virus (HIV)
The average risk for HIV infection after a needlestick or cut exposure to HIV-infected blood is about 1 in 300; the risk after exposure of the eye, nose, or mouth is 1 in 1,000; the risk after exposure of the skin to HIV-infected blood is estimated to be less than 0.1%.

www.cdc.gov/OralHealth/infectioncontrol/faq/bloodborne_exposures.htm. Accessed March 10, 2015.

in place and adequate supplies available to prevent infections at the site. If the answer to any of the questions is "No," the facility must do all it can to correct the problems with either staff or supplies (Table 20-1).

Postexposure Management

- *Hepatitis B virus (HBV):* Hepatitis B vaccine series started in any unvaccinated person; postexposure prophylaxis (PEP) with hepatitis B immune globulin and/or hepatitis B vaccine series if the post-vaccination antibody test is negative.
- *Hepatitis C virus (HCV):* Immune globulin and antiviral agents (e.g., interferon with or without ribavirin) are not recommended for PEP of hepatitis C; determine the HCV status of the source and the exposed person; provide follow-up HCV testing for the employee if the source is HCV positive.
- *Human immunodeficiency virus (HIV):* Four-week PEP regimen of two drugs (zidovudine [ZDV] and lamivudine [3TC]; 3TC and stavudine [d4T]; or didanosine [ddI] and d4T) for most HIV exposures and a third drug for HIV exposures that pose an increased risk for transmission; employees should receive follow-up counseling, postexposure testing, and medical evaluation, regardless of whether they receive PEP. After baseline testing at the time of exposure, follow-up testing could be performed at 6 weeks, 12 weeks, and 6 months after exposure.

CRITICAL THINKING APPLICATION 20-7

Rosa's office has been especially busy today. While administering an injection to a frightened 6-year-old child, a co-worker accidentally sticks herself with the needle. She tells Rosa about the incident, but she doesn't know what to do next. What steps should be taken to manage the situation?

ASEPTIC TECHNIQUES: PREVENTING DISEASE TRANSMISSION

Asepsis means freedom from infection or infectious material. *Medical asepsis* is defined as the destruction of disease-causing organisms after they leave the body. When we practice the principles of medical asepsis, we are working to prevent reinfection of the patient or the cross-infection of other patients or ourselves. The goal is to eliminate or minimize pathogens by following OSHA's Bloodborne Pathogens Standard and disinfecting objects as soon as possible after contamination. This creates a healthcare environment as free of pathogens as possible.

Surgical asepsis is the destruction of organisms before they enter the body. This technique is used for any procedure that invades the body's skin or tissues, such as surgery or injections. Anytime the skin or a mucous membrane is punctured, pierced, or incised (or will be during a procedure), surgical aseptic techniques are practiced. Everything that comes in contact with the patient should be **sterile**, including gowns, drapes, instruments, and the gloved hands of the surgical team. Minor surgery, urinary catheterization, injections, and some specimen collections, such as blood collection and biopsies, are performed using surgical aseptic technique.

Because the hands themselves cannot be sterilized, the goal of hand washing is to reduce the amount of skin **flora** through the use of mechanical friction, antimicrobial soaps, and warm, running water. Normally, two types of flora are found on the skin: normal resident flora and transient flora that are associated with infection. Normal resident flora lives harmlessly on the skin; transient flora includes bacteria, viruses, and other organisms picked up on the hands. The goal of thorough hand washing is to remove or reduce the number of transient flora on the surface of the skin, thus preventing their transfer to patients.

The most effective barrier against infection is the unbroken skin. If the skin and mucous membranes are intact, medical asepsis can be practiced for most noninvasive procedures (i.e., those that do not penetrate human tissues), such as pelvic and proctologic examinations. Instruments and objects used in medical aseptic procedures must be sanitized and disinfected or sterilized before use on another patient. Medical aseptic procedures may include the use of gowns and masks, but these are not sterile and are worn to protect the healthcare worker more than the patient.

Another practical application of aseptic technique is to set up work areas in the medical office's laboratory so that one side of the laboratory is the "clean" side, where only noninfectious procedures are performed, and the other is the "dirty" side, where potentially infectious materials are processed or cleaned.

Hand Washing

The hands must be washed, using the correct technique, before and after each patient is examined or treated and also when stipulated by the Bloodborne Pathogens Guidelines. A lengthy scrub is not necessary each time, but the first scrub in the morning should be extensive, lasting 2 to 4 minutes. Subsequent hand washing may be brief unless the hands are excessively contaminated. A good antimicrobial soap with chlorhexidine (e.g., Hibiclens), which has antiseptic residual action that lasts several hours, should be used. Each office sink should be equipped with a liquid soap dispenser. A water-soluble lotion may be rubbed into the hands after they have been washed and dried. Dry, cracked, chapped skin is no longer intact and can result in the transmission of disease.

Proper hand washing depends on two factors: running water and friction. The water should be warm, because water that is too hot or too cold causes the skin to become chapped. Friction is the firm rubbing of all surfaces of the hands and wrists. Remember that your fingers have four sides, and fingernails have two sides. For medical hand washing, all jewelry except a plain wedding band is removed. A wristwatch may be left on if it can be moved up on the forearm away from the wrist area. The hands are washed under running water with the fingertips pointing downward. Soap and friction are applied to the hands and wrists. The water is allowed to wash debris away from the wrists and down toward the fingertips (Procedure 20-4).

Remember, the goal of aseptic hand washing is to protect you from infection and prevent cross-contamination from one patient to another. Use this procedure after you finish with one patient and before you attend to another patient; after you finish handling one specimen and before you handle another specimen; before and after you use toilet facilities; whenever you touch something that causes

TABLE 20-1 Modified CDC Infection Prevention Checklist*			
FACILITY POLICIES	**PRACTICE PERFORMED**		**IF ANSWER IS NO, DOCUMENT PLAN FOR REMEDIATION**
1. Administrative Policies and Facility Practices			
a. Written infection prevention policies and procedures are available and reflective of current research.	Yes	No	
b. At least one individual trained in infection prevention is employed by or regularly available to the facility.	Yes	No	
c. Supplies necessary for adherence to Standard Precautions are readily available.	Yes	No	
d. Healthcare personnel receive job-specific training on infection prevention policies and procedures and OSHA Bloodborne Pathogens Standard and are observed for compliance when hired and at least annually.	Yes	No	
e. The facility maintains a log of needlesticks, sharps injuries, and other employee exposure events.	Yes	No	
f. Following an exposure event, post-exposure evaluation and follow-up, including prophylaxis as appropriate, are available at no cost to employee.	Yes	No	
g. Hepatitis B vaccination is available at no cost to all employees at risk of occupational exposure.	Yes	No	
h. Post-vaccination screening for hepatitis B surface antibodies is conducted.	Yes	No	
i. All personnel are offered annual influenza vaccination at no cost.	Yes	No	
j. All personnel with potential exposure to tuberculosis (TB) are screened for TB upon hire and annually (if negative).	Yes	No	
2. Surveillance and Disease Reporting			
a. Updated list of reportable diseases is readily available to all personnel.	Yes	No	
3. Hand Hygiene			
a. Facility provides training and supplies necessary for adherence to hand hygiene.	Yes	No	
4. Personal Protective Equipment (PPE)			
a. Facility provides training and supplies for appropriate PPE.	Yes	No	
b. Impermeable gowns are worn during procedures where contact with blood or body fluids is anticipated.	Yes	No	
c. PPE is removed and discarded prior to leaving the exam room.	Yes	No	
d. Hand hygiene is performed immediately after removal of PPE.	Yes	No	
5. Environmental Cleaning			
a. Policies and procedures exist for routine cleaning and disinfection of environmental surfaces.	Yes	No	
b. Cleaning procedures are periodically monitored and assessed to ensure that they are consistently and correctly performed.	Yes	No	
c. The facility has a policy/procedure for decontamination of spills of blood or other body fluids.	Yes	No	

Modified from www.cdc.gov/HAI/settings/outpatient/checklist/outpatient-care-checklist.html. Accessed March 5, 2015.
*The complete checklist is available at the CDC website for Infection Prevention in Outpatient Settings: www.cdc.gov/HAI/settings/outpatient/checklist/outpatient-care-checklist.html.

your hands to become contaminated; when you arrive at work and before you leave the facility; before and after eating; and at the end of the day.

As stated earlier, alcohol-based hand rubs may substitute for hand washing unless the hands are visibly contaminated. Evidence suggests that hand antisepsis with an alcohol-based hand rub is more effective at reducing **nosocomial infections** than plain hand washing. Using antimicrobial-impregnated wipes (e.g., towelettes) is not a substitute for using an alcohol-based hand rub or antimicrobial soap.

According to the CDC, proper hand hygiene must be performed in the following instances even if disposable gloves are worn:
- Before and after contact with the patient or his or her immediate care environment
- Before performing an aseptic task (e.g., giving an injection, drawing blood)
- After contact with blood, body fluids, or contaminated surfaces
- When hands move from a contaminated body site to a clean body site during patient care

---

PROCEDURE 20-4   Participate in Bloodborne Pathogen Training: Perform Medical Aseptic Hand Washing

Goal: *To minimize the number of pathogens on the hands, thus reducing the risk of transmission of pathogens.*

EQUIPMENT and SUPPLIES

- Sink with warm running water
- Antimicrobial liquid soap in a dispenser (bar soap is not acceptable)
- Disposable nail brush or orange stick
- Paper towels in a dispenser
- Water-based antimicrobial lotion
- Covered waste container with foot pedal

PROCEDURAL STEPS

1. Remove all jewelry except your wristwatch, if it can be pulled up above your wrist, and a plain wedding ring.
   PURPOSE: Jewelry can harbor microorganisms.
2. Turn on the faucet with a paper towel and regulate the water temperature to lukewarm.
   PURPOSE: Use a paper towel to prevent touching of contaminated surfaces; water that is too hot can cause skin to become dry and chapped.
3. Wet your hands, apply soap, and lather using a circular motion with friction while holding your fingertips downward (Figure 1). Rub well between your fingers. If this is the first hand wash of the day, use a nail brush or an orange stick and clean under every fingernail. Inspect your nails thoroughly.
   PURPOSE: Friction removes soil and contaminants from the hands and wrists.

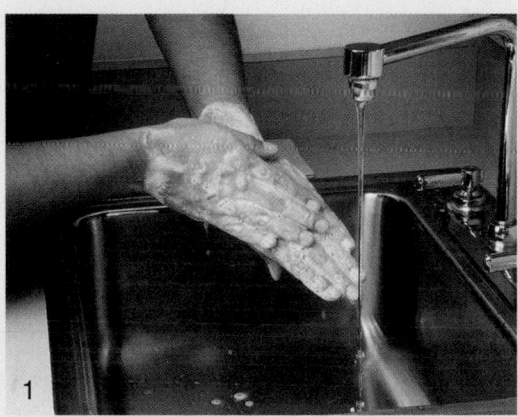

4. Rinse well, holding your hands so that the water flows from your wrists downward to your fingertips (Figure 2).
   PURPOSE: Soil and contaminants will wash off the skin and down the drain.

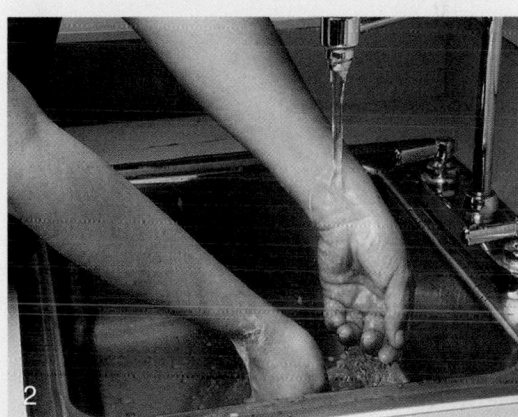

5. If this is the first hand wash of the day or if your hands are obviously contaminated, wet your hands again and repeat the scrubbing procedure using a vigorous, circular motion over the wrists and hands for at least 1 to 2 minutes.
   PURPOSE: Time is required for friction and motion to eliminate all possible soil and contaminants.
6. Rinse your hands a second time, keeping the fingers lower than your wrists.
   PURPOSE: To ensure removal of all transient flora.
7. Dry your hands with paper towels. Do not touch the paper towel dispenser as you are obtaining towels (Figure 3).
   PURPOSE: Touching the dispenser contaminates your hands, and you will need to start over.

PROCEDURE 20-4 —*continued*

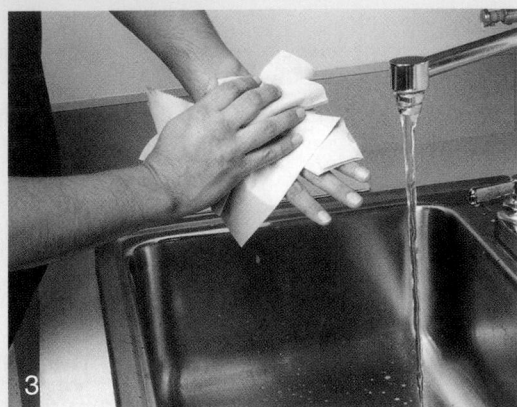

3

8. If the faucets are not foot operated, turn them off with a paper towel (Figure 4).
<u>PURPOSE</u>: The faucet is dirty and will contaminate your clean hands.

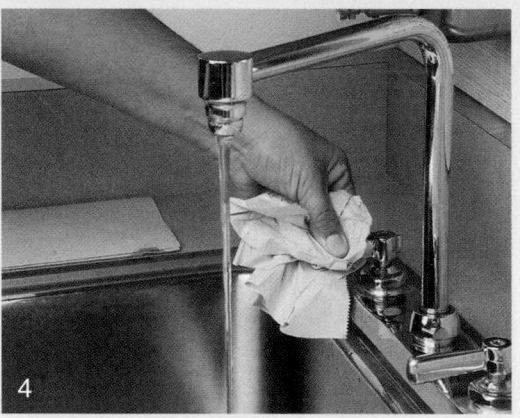

4

9. After you finish drying your hands and turning off the faucets, place used towels into a covered waste container.
<u>PURPOSE</u>: Always discard contaminated waste in a covered waste container immediately to eliminate the source of infection.

10. If needed, apply a water-based antibacterial hand lotion to prevent chapped or dry skin.
<u>PURPOSE</u>: Chapped skin eliminates the first line of defense against infectious organisms.

11. Repeat the procedure as indicated throughout the day.
<u>PURPOSE</u>: To eliminate contaminants and prevent the transmission of pathogens to yourself and others.

Sanitization

Instruments and other items used in office surgery, examination, or treatment must be carefully cleaned before proceeding with the steps of disinfection or sterilization. Sanitization is the cleansing process that reduces the number of microorganisms to a safe level, as dictated in public health guidelines. This cleansing process removes debris such as blood and other body fluids from instruments or equipment. Blood and debris must be removed so that later disinfection with chemicals or sterilization with steam, heat, or gases can penetrate to all the instrument's surfaces (Procedure 20-5).

The medical assistant should always wear gloves (thick utility gloves if the instruments have sharp or pointed edges) while performing sanitization to prevent possible personal contamination with potentially infectious body fluids that may be present on the articles being cleaned. The procedure should be completed immediately after use of the instruments in a separate workroom or on the "dirty" side of the utility room to prevent cross-contamination of clean instruments and equipment. If this is not possible, rinse the used items under cold water immediately after the procedure and place them in a low-sudsing, rust-inhibiting, enzyme-containing detergent solution. Never allow blood or other substances that can **coagulate** to dry on an instrument.

When you are ready to sanitize instruments, drain off the soaking solution and rinse each instrument in cold running water. Separate the sharp instruments from the others because metal instruments may damage the cutting edges, and sharp instruments may damage other instruments or injure you. Clean all sharp instruments at one time, when you can concentrate on preventing injury to yourself. Open all hinges and scrub serrations and ratchets with a small scrub brush or toothbrush. Rinse the instruments in hot water and then check carefully that they are in proper working order before they are disinfected or sterilized. The items should be hand dried with a towel to prevent spotting.

Sanitization is a very important step, and it cannot be overlooked or done carelessly. The use of disposable instruments minimizes the need for sanitization, disinfection, and sterilization.

Ultrasonic Sanitization

Sound waves can be used to sanitize instruments. The instruments are placed in an ultrasonic bath of cleaner and water. Sound waves cause the solution to vibrate, which loosens the materials attached to the instruments. Ultrasonic cleaners are beneficial because they do not damage even the most delicate instruments, and workers do not run the risk of an accidental sharps injury.

| PROCEDURE 20-5 | Select Appropriate Barrier/Personal Protective Equipment and Demonstrate Proper Disposal of Biohazardous Material: Use Standard Precautions for Sanitizing Instruments and Discarding Biohazardous Material |

Goal: *To follow Standard Precautions in removing all contaminated matter from instruments in preparation for disinfection or sterilization while wearing appropriate personal protective equipment (PPE).*

EQUIPMENT and SUPPLIES

- Sink with cold and hot running water
- Sanitizing agent or low-sudsing soap with enzymatic action
- Decontaminated utility gloves that show no signs of deterioration
- Chin-length face shield or goggles and face mask if contamination with blood-borne pathogens is possible
- Impermeable gown
- Disposable brush
- Disposable paper towels
- Disposable gloves
- Disinfectant cleaner prepared according to manufacturer's directions
- Covered waste container with foot pedal
- Biohazard waste container with labeled red biohazard bag

PROCEDURAL STEPS

1. Put on an impermeable gown and face shield or goggles and mask if potential for splashing of infectious material exists (Figure 1).
   PURPOSE: To provide personal protection against potentially infectious matter.

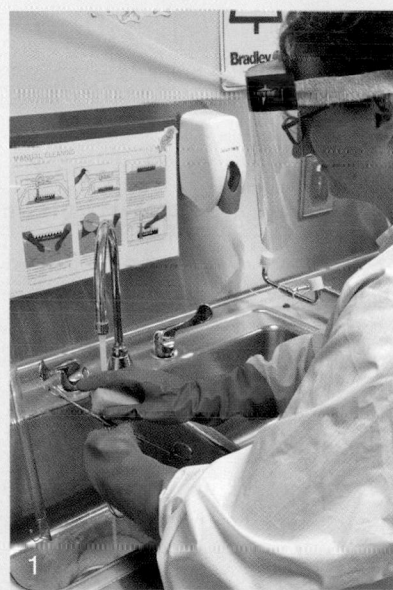

2. Put on utility gloves.
   PURPOSE: To provide personal protection against potentially infectious matter and sharp instruments.
3. Separate the sharp instruments from other instruments to be sanitized.
   PURPOSE: To prevent possible self-injury and exposure to infectious matter.
4. Rinse the instruments under cold running water.
   PURPOSE: To help remove debris and prevent coagulation of body fluids.

5. Open hinged instruments and scrub all grooves, crevices, and serrations with a disposable brush (Figure 2).
   PURPOSE: Microorganisms can hide under contaminants and may not be destroyed by the disinfection process.

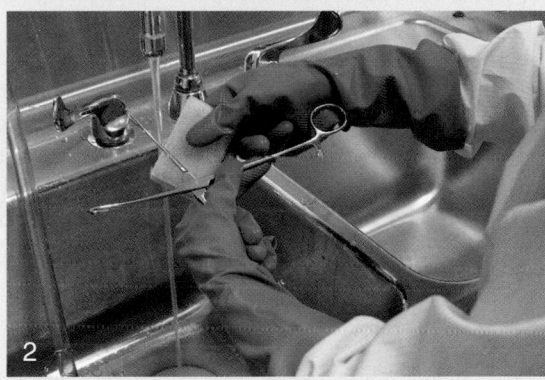

6. Rinse well with hot water.
   PURPOSE: Hot water removes all soap and contaminant residue.
7. Towel-dry all instruments thoroughly and dispose of contaminated towels and disposable brush in a biohazard waste container. Do not touch the paper towel dispenser as you are obtaining towels.
   PURPOSE: All contaminated material must be discarded in a labeled biohazard container and/or a labeled red biohazard bag. Touching the dispenser with the utility gloves contaminates the dispenser. Wet instruments can rust or become dull and also dilute disinfectant or sterilizing chemicals.
8. Remove the utility gloves and wash your hands according to Procedure 20-4.
   PURPOSE: To remove any possible contaminants.
9. Towel-dry your hands and put on disposable gloves. Decontaminate the utility gloves and work surfaces using disinfectant cleaner.
   PURPOSE: To prevent personal exposure to contaminants. All equipment and working surfaces should be cleaned and decontaminated with a disinfectant to prevent transmission of infectious organisms.
10. Dispose of the contaminated towels in a covered waste container.
    PURPOSE: All contaminated material must be disposed of in a labeled biohazard container and/or a labeled red biohazard bag.
11. Place sanitized instruments in a designated area for disinfection or sterilization.
    PURPOSE: Sanitized instruments must be removed from the cleaning area to prevent possible cross-contamination.
12. Remove the disposable gloves according to Procedure 20-1. Dispose of the gloves in a biohazard waste container. Sanitize the hands.
    PURPOSE: To prevent the spread of infectious organisms and to remove any possible contaminants.

Disinfection

Disinfection is the process of killing pathogenic organisms or of rendering them inactive. It is not always effective against spores, tuberculosis bacilli, and certain viruses. Disinfectant chemicals may kill microbes within a short time, but they usually are very hard on instruments. Some chemicals, such as Cidex, are effective enough to kill all organisms, but the usual immersion time for these sterilants is 10 hours or longer. For equipment and countertop surfaces, the cheapest and most reliable method of disinfection is to use a 1:10 bleach solution. This is an effective and noncaustic disinfectant that can be used to wipe laboratory countertops where human blood and other body fluid samples are handled. It also can be used for soaking reusable rubber goods before sanitization. In addition, bleach solution is an effective disinfectant for surfaces that have come in contact with viruses, including HIV.

Many types of disinfecting agents are available and have varying degrees of effectiveness. It is important to follow the manufacturer's guidelines on how to use each product properly and to understand its advantages and disadvantages and the possible sources of error.

Disinfection is very difficult to verify, because no convenient indicators ensure destruction of organisms. Even when the manufacturer's directions for chemical strength and immersion times are followed, common errors can cause chemicals to lose their effectiveness:

- Instruments are not thoroughly sanitized, and attached organic matter inhibits or prevents the action of the disinfectant. No chemical can kill unless it reaches all instrument surfaces; therefore, complete sanitization is absolutely necessary.
- Sanitized instruments are not dried, and the moisture on the instruments dilutes the disinfectant solution beyond effective concentration levels.
- The disinfectant solution is left in an open container, and evaporation changes its concentration.
- Solutions are not changed after the recommended period for use has expired.
- Solutions are not prepared properly or are not mixed properly before use.
- The manufacturer's recommended temperature for use and storage is not maintained.

Chemical disinfectants cannot be used on skin or tissues because they can damage them. Therefore, antiseptics, such as alcohol, are used on the skin to reduce the number of pathogens. Alcohol is the most widely used antiseptic, but recent studies indicate that it is not as effective as other products in inhibiting the growth and reproduction of microorganisms on the skin's surface. Other antiseptic chemicals, such as povidone-iodine solution (Betadine), are effective antimicrobial agents that are safe to use on a patient's skin.

Sterilization

Sterilization, or the destruction of all microorganisms, is essential for surgical asepsis. Sterilization can be achieved by moist heat in an autoclave, dry heat, ultraviolet or ionizing radiation, gas, or with chemicals. Medical facilities typically use the autoclave method. Steam under pressure in the autoclave is an excellent method of sterilization because it kills all pathogens and spores.

Guidelines for Disinfection of Endoscopes

Because typical sterilization procedures can damage endoscopes, high-level disinfection of these instruments is crucial to prevent the spread of nosocomial infections. Disinfection must follow the manufacturer's guidelines for the instrument. This process has five steps:

1. *Leak test*: Pressurize the endoscope with air and submerge it in water to check for damage or leaks.
2. *Clean*: Wipe and/or brush internal and external surfaces; brush internal channels and flush each internal channel with water and a detergent or enzymatic cleaner.
3. *Disinfect*: Immerse the endoscope in a high-level disinfectant or chemical sterilant (e.g., Cidex). Aspirate and flush all channels with the chemical for the length of time recommended by the manufacturer.
4. *Rinse*: Rinse the endoscope and all channels with water to remove the chemical disinfectant.
5. *Dry*: Rinse the insertion tube and inner channels with alcohol, and dry with forced air before storage. Scopes should be hung vertically to store.

CRITICAL THINKING APPLICATION   20-8
Rosa is responsible for the orientation of the new medical assistant in the office's sanitization and disinfection procedures. Outline the important concepts and methods of each.

You will learn more about surgical asepsis and the sterilization process in the Surgical Asepsis and Assisting with Surgical Procedures chapter.

ROLE OF THE MEDICAL ASSISTANT IN ASEPSIS

Asepsis is one of the few procedures that directly affect the health of the patient, the provider, and the staff. The spread of pathogens in the ambulatory care setting can be controlled only through effective, consistent application of the Bloodborne Pathogens Standard and by proper sanitization, disinfection, and sterilization of supplies, equipment, and work surfaces.

The medical assistant must develop an inner sense for performing aseptic procedures properly. It is important that these techniques be done on such a routine basis that they become an unbreakable habit. The use of disposable items is highly recommended for infection control purposes. However, when disposable equipment is used, the assistant must follow recommended disposal guidelines to ensure infection control.

CLOSING COMMENTS
Patient Education

The medical assistant should take every opportunity to educate patients about the infection process and ways to prevent the transmission of disease. The best time to instruct a patient in aseptic techniques that can be used at home is while performing the aseptic procedure. For example:

- While washing your hands, explain to the patient that this routine is particularly important for patients who are very young or old or who seem to get sick frequently. Instruct the patient that the hands should be washed before and after meals; after sneezing, coughing, or blowing the nose; after using the restroom; before and after changing a dressing; and after changing an infant's diaper.
- Advise the patient to carry an alcohol-based hand rub and to use it as indicated throughout the day.
- Explain to the patient that coughing or sneezing into a bent elbow is an effective method for preventing the spread of disease.
- Instruct the patient in the differences between sterile and clean dressings and bandages. Demonstrate each step in changing a dressing properly and explain how to dispose of contaminated items.

A medical assistant can help patients live healthier lives in many ways. For example, here are a few more suggestions for teaching the patient about asepsis and infection control:

- Set up an information table in the waiting room with take-home pamphlets and literature.
- Mail, e-mail, or post on the healthcare facility's website a periodic newsletter to patients about infection control, especially during flu season.
- Demonstrate and explain aseptic procedures to patients and family members, inviting them to participate.

Legal and Ethical Issues

Medical asepsis and infection control in ambulatory care practices give rise to numerous legal and ethical concerns. Personal discipline is the primary concern in medical asepsis. Typically, the medical assistant is alone when performing an aseptic procedure; therefore, if contamination occurs, he or she is the only one who knows. If contamination should occur, the medical assistant must start over again with clean supplies.

A primary reason for performing aseptic procedures completely and effectively is to prevent the development of nosocomial infections in susceptible patients. These infections, which are acquired in the healthcare environment, can be especially dangerous for elderly or debilitated patients. Ignorance of the various aseptic techniques or carelessness can be dangerous and is inexcusable before the law.

Professional Behaviors

One of the medical assistant's main responsibilities is to perform sanitization, disinfection, and sterilization procedures with precision and total effectiveness. There is no room for compromise. Patients should have absolute assurance that they are being treated in an aseptic atmosphere and under aseptic conditions. This assurance is just as important for the protection of the provider and staff as it is for the patient. Allowing the provider to assume that the correct aseptic techniques were used when preparing a procedure and allowing him or her to use contaminated equipment on a patient may result in a malpractice lawsuit. Honesty on the part of the medical assistant builds self-respect and contributes to professional achievement.

Partial List of CDC National Notifiable Infectious Conditions*

Each state has laws requiring that certain diseases be reported to state health authorities when they are identified by healthcare providers, nurses, laboratory directors, infection control practitioners, healthcare facilities, state institutions, schools, or day care workers (see Procedure 20-6). However, it is voluntary for states to provide this information to the CDC. The list of reportable diseases varies among states and over time.

The procedure for reporting public health threats varies among the states, but the general rules are as follows:

- Some infectious diseases, such as anthrax, measles, polio, and tuberculosis, must be reported immediately by phone to the local health department and followed up with submission of a confidential case report form.
- In addition to the diseases identified by the state as reportable, any unusual disease (e.g., severe food poisoning) that could possibly be caused by an infectious agent or toxin is reportable.
- If there is a cluster of cases of any communicable disease (e.g., head lice, scabies, streptococcal sore throat), this outbreak should be reported.
- States may require that cases of HIV infection, HIV-related illness, and AIDS be reported on special forms.

Examples of some of the infectious diseases that may be reported by individual states include:

Anthrax	Mumps
Botulism	Pertussis
Chlamydia trachomatis infection	Poliovirus infection
Cholera	Rabies, animal and human
Diphtheria	Rubella
Giardiasis	Salmonellosis
Gonorrhea	Smallpox
Hepatitis A, B, C	Spotted fever rickettsiosis
HIV infection	Syphilis
Influenza-associated pediatric mortality	Tetanus
Lyme disease	Tuberculosis
Malaria	Typhoid fever
Measles	Varicella
Meningococcal disease	Viral hemorrhagic fever

Modified from wwwn.cdc.gov/NNDSS/script/ConditionList.aspx?Type=0&Yr=2013. Accessed March 11, 2015.
*For the entire list, refer to the CDC website: wwwn.cdc.gov/NNDSS/script/ConditionList.aspx?Type=0&Yr=2013

| PROCEDURE 20-6 | Perform Compliance Reporting Based on Public Health Statutes |

Goal: *To report suspected or confirmed communicable diseases as mandated by state law.*

Scenario: *The provider is reviewing laboratory results on a new patient and notes that the patient is hepatitis C positive. Hepatitis C is a reportable infectious disease, so the case must be reported to the local health department. The provider asks Rosa to file the report. How should she perform this procedure?*

EQUIPMENT and SUPPLIES

- Website, mailing address, phone number of the local health department where the patient resides
- CDC website:
  - To find state health departments: *www.cdc.gov/mmwr/international/relres.html*
  - To determine individual state reportable diseases: *wwwn.cdc.gov/NNDSS/script/ConditionList.aspx?Type=0&Yr=2013*

PROCEDURAL STEPS

1. Search online for procedures for filing reportable diseases to the local health department. New cases of hepatitis C must be reported within 24 hours, but this can be done either online or by mail.
2. Complete the online form that requests details for new hepatitis C cases and submit it to the local health department.
3. Electronically save the submitted form and/or print a copy for the provider's review.

SUMMARY OF SCENARIO

Implementing Standard Precautions throughout daily practice is crucial to the welfare and protection both of the patient and the healthcare worker. Rosa must be sure to wash her hands routinely and/or to use an alcohol hand rub. She also must familiarize herself with the office's Exposure Control Plan; follow OSHA's Bloodborne Pathogens Standard; use PPE when needed; follow environmental protection guidelines; use appropriate procedures for cleaning up contaminated spills and other housekeeping controls; and understand postexposure follow-up if an accidental exposure occurs. In addition, Rosa must follow guidelines for sanitization, disinfection, and sterilization of appropriate instruments and equipment.

SUMMARY OF LEARNING OBJECTIVES

1. **Define, spell, and pronounce the terms listed in the vocabulary.**
   Spelling and pronouncing medical terms correctly reinforce the medical assistant's credibility. Knowing the definitions of these terms promotes confidence in communication with patients and co-workers.

2. **Describe the characteristics of pathogenic microorganisms.**
   Pathogenic microorganisms include viruses, bacteria, protozoa, fungi, and rickettsiae. Viral microorganisms are intracellular parasites that take over the deoxyribonucleic acid (DNA) or ribonucleic acid (RNA) of the invaded cell. Bacteria are tiny, simple cells that produce disease by secreting toxins, act as parasites inside human cells, or grow on body surfaces, disrupting normal human functions. Bacteria are classified according to their shape. Protozoa are unicellular parasites that can replicate and multiply rapidly once inside the host. They are frequently carried by insects that serve as vectors for the disease. Fungi may be unicellular or multicellular; they include molds and yeasts and cause tinea infections. Rickettsia are microorganisms that have characteristics of both bacteria and viruses; they are obligate parasites that must live within a host cell for growth but are larger than viruses so can be viewed with a microscope.

3. **Do the following related to the chain of infection:**
   - *Apply the chain-of-infection process to healthcare practice.*
     The chain of infection is the way infectious disease is spread. It begins with the infectious agent and moves to the host, the means or portal of exit from the host, the mode of transmission, and the means or portal of entry into a new host. It ends with the presence of the infection in a susceptible host. At least one of these links must be broken to stop the spread of infection.
   - *Compare viral and bacterial cell invasion.*
     Bacterial infections can be treated with antibiotics, but viral infections, which involve viral takeover of cellular DNA or RNA material, cannot be treated with antibiotics because viruses are not cells but parasites within a cell.
   - *Differentiate between humoral and cell-mediated immunity.*
     Humoral immunity creates specific antibodies to combat antigens through the action of B cells. The immune system also reacts at the cellular level with T-cell activity in cell-mediated immunity by causing the destruction of pathogenic cells at the site of invasion.

4. **Summarize the impact of the inflammatory response on the body's ability to defend itself against infection.**
   The inflammatory response is one aspect of the body's ability to defend itself against infection. It involves the body's reaction to the introduction of a foreign substance or antigen, an increase in blood flow to the site, and the release of inflammatory mediators that attract white blood cells to the site. WBCs isolate and destroy the source of inflammation.

5. **Analyze the differences among acute, chronic, latent, and opportunistic infections.**

Acute diseases have a rapid onset and short duration. Chronic diseases are present over a long period, perhaps a lifetime. Latent diseases cycle through relapse and remission phases. Opportunistic infections are caused by organisms that are not typically pathogenic but that occur in hosts with an impaired or weakened immune system response, such as individuals with HIV.

6. **Do the following related to OSHA standards for the healthcare setting:**

- *Specify potentially infectious body fluids.*
Potentially infectious body fluids include CSF; mucus; synovial, pleural, pericardial, peritoneal, and amniotic fluids; blood; vaginal and seminal secretions; saliva; and human tissue.

- *Integrate OSHA's requirement for a site-based Exposure Control Plan into facility management procedures.*
OSHA requires incorporation of a site-based Exposure Control Plan into facility management procedures. The plan must be revised annually and must be available for employees to review. It must reflect current safety technology, identify employees at risk for exposure, and contain specifics about protection from blood-borne pathogens, including PPE, training, hepatitis B immunization, exposure, follow-up, record keeping, and the labeling and disposal of all biohazard waste.

- *Explain the major areas included in the OSHA Compliance Guidelines.*
The OSHA Compliance Guidelines include barrier protection devices, environmental protection, housekeeping controls, hepatitis B immunization, and postexposure follow-up.

- *Discuss protocols for disposal of biologic chemical materials.*
States vary in their degree of regulation of disposal of hazardous waste, ranging from no regulation to very strict rules. Typical regulations include specific hazardous waste containers; the use of standard precautions; the length of time that the containers should be kept on site; the management of contaminated sharps; labeling and properly packing chemicals for disposal; and hiring a biomedical waste disposal service

7. **Remove contaminated gloves while following Standard Precautions principles.**
Refer to Procedure 20-1.

8. **Perform an eyewash procedure to remove contaminated material.**
Refer to Procedure 20-2.

9. **Summarize the management of postexposure evaluation and follow-up and participate in blood-borne pathogen training and a mock exposure event.**
Postexposure evaluation and follow-up are as follows: The site is cleaned and the exposed individual reports to his or her supervisor immediately.

Medical assessment is performed immediately. Testing of the source individual's and the worker's blood is performed if possible and if consent is given. Health counseling is provided. Strict confidentiality of all medical records is maintained. Procedure 20-3 summarizes the steps required for the management of a postexposure needlestick.

10. **Identify the regulations established by the Centers for Disease Control and Prevention (CDC) that affect healthcare workers.**
Table 20-1 summarizes the main points of the CDCs' Infection Prevention Checklist that is to be used by facilities to systematically assess employee adherence to infection prevention and to ensure that the facility has policies and procedures in place and adequate supplies available to prevent infections at the site. The CDC has also developed specific hand hygiene guidelines and guidelines for disinfection of endoscopes.

11. **Apply the concepts of medical and surgical asepsis to the healthcare setting.**
Medical asepsis is the removal or destruction of pathogens. Medical aseptic techniques are used to reduce the number of microorganisms as much as possible. Surgical asepsis is destruction of all microorganisms. Surgical asepsis is used when the patient's skin or mucous membranes are disrupted.

12. **Discuss proper hand washing, and demonstrate the proper hand-washing technique for medical asepsis.**
Refer to Procedure 20-4.

13. **Differentiate among sanitization, disinfection, and sterilization procedures and select appropriate barrier/personal protective equipment while demonstrating the correct procedure for sanitizing contaminated instruments.**
Sanitization is cleaning of contaminated articles or surfaces to reduce the number of microorganisms (refer to Procedure 20-5). Disinfection involves the use of physical or chemical means to destroy pathogens or their components on inanimate surfaces or objects. Sterilization removes all living microorganisms.

14. **Discuss the role of the medical assistant in asepsis.**
Asepsis affects the health of the patient, the provider, and the staff. The medical assistant must develop the necessary skills as well as a firm grasp of the principles involved for performing aseptic procedures properly.

15. **Apply patient education concepts to infection control.**
Take every opportunity to demonstrate aseptic techniques, to educate patients about proper management of infectious materials at home, and to emphasize the importance of frequent and consistent hand washing.

16. **Discuss legal and ethical concerns regarding medical asepsis and infection control and perform compliance reporting based on public health statutes regarding reportable communicable diseases.**
The medical assistant is responsible for applying infection control procedures in all situations at all times to prevent cross-contamination and the development of nosocomial infections in patients (refer to Procedure 20-6).

CONNECTIONS

Study Guide Connection: Go to the Chapter 20 Study Guide. Read and complete the activities.

evolve Evolve Connection: Go to the Chapter 20 link at *evolve.elsevier.com/kinn* to complete the Chapter Review Quiz. Check out the other resources listed for this chapter to make the most of what you have learned from Infection Control.

21

PATIENT ASSESSMENT

SCENARIO

Chris Isaacson, CMA (AAMA), works in an ambulatory care clinic at the community hospital. He is responsible for initial patient interviews, taking medical histories, and documentation. Chris is having difficulty gathering the information needed from some of the patients. They do not always respond openly and honestly to him, and the attending physician is not satisfied with his work. His supervisor is responsible for helping him improve his interviewing skills.

While studying this chapter, think about the following questions:

- How can Chris learn to develop helping relationships so that the patient's medical history is as comprehensive as possible?
- Would it help if Chris displayed greater sensitivity to diverse populations?
- Would using active listening techniques and attending to the patient's nonverbal behaviors better enable Chris to develop therapeutic communications skills?
- How can Chris's supervisor help him become a better communicator and demonstrate comprehensive and accurate documentation in patients' health records?

LEARNING OBJECTIVES

1. Define, spell, and pronounce the terms listed in the vocabulary.
2. Employ the concept of holistic care in the patient assessment process.
3. Describe the components of the patient's medical history and how to collect the history information.
4. Discuss how to successfully understand and communicate with patients and display sensitivity to diverse populations.
5. Demonstrate therapeutic communication feedback techniques to obtain information when gathering a patient history.
6. Respond to nonverbal communication when interacting with patients.
7. Identify barriers to communication and their impact on patient assessment; also, compare open-ended and closed-ended questions.
8. Do the following related to the patient interview:
   - Discuss the patient interview.
   - Identify barriers to communication and their impact on the patient assessment.
   - Detect a patient's use of defense mechanisms and the resultant barriers to therapeutic communication.
   - Demonstrate professional patient interviewing techniques.
9. Discuss the use of therapeutic communication techniques with patients across the lifespan.
10. Compare and contrast signs and symptoms.
11. Document patient care accurately in the medical record.
12. Identify and define medical terms and abbreviations related to body systems; also, use medical terminology correctly and accurately to communicate information to providers and patients.
13. Differentiate the documentation systems used in ambulatory care practices.
14. Explain "meaningful use" as it applies to the electronic health record (EHR).
15. Describe the role of patient education, in addition to legal and ethical issues, in the patient assessment process.

VOCABULARY

biophysical (bi-o-fi'-zi-kuhl) The science of applying physical laws and theories to biologic problems.

cognitive (kog'-nuh-tiv) Pertaining to the operation of the mind; referring to the process by which we become aware of perceiving, thinking, and remembering.

congruence (kon-groo'-ents) Agreement; the state that occurs when the verbal expression of the message matches the sender's nonverbal body language.

familial Occurring in or affecting members of a family more than would be expected by chance.

holistic Considering the patient as a whole including the physical, emotional, social, economic, and spiritual needs of the person.

patient portal A secure online website that gives patients convenient 24-hour access to personal health information;

patients have a secure user name and password to view their health information.

present illness The chief complaint, written in chronologic sequence, with dates of onset.

psychosocial Pertaining to a combination of psychological and social factors.

rapport (ra-por') A relationship of harmony and accord between the patient and the healthcare professional.

signs Objective findings determined by a clinician, such as a fever, hypertension, or rash.

symptoms Subjective complaints reported by the patient, such as pain or visual disturbances.

As medical professionals directly involved in gathering information from patients about their health status, medical assistants must remember that a healthy state is more than the absence of disease. The assessment process should be a reflection of the entire patient, not just a report about signs and symptoms. Individual lifestyles and environmental factors can create disease and therefore should be considered when we gather information about the patient's chief complaint. For example, if a patient smokes or works in a stressful occupation, he or she may be more prone to hypertension. As health professionals, we should consider all patient factors, including **cognitive**, **psychosocial**, and behavioral data, when gathering information about the patient's health status. Consider this: do you think a patient who has limited insurance coverage for prescription drugs can always afford his medication? The method of analyzing all factors that may contribute to the development of disease is based on a **holistic** perspective. Holistic patient care recognizes that illness is the result of many factors, not just physical ones.

Assessment factors are a list of **biophysical** signs and symptoms. As the first step in treating a disease process, the provider must determine the patient's medical diagnosis. A *differential diagnosis* considers which one of several diseases may be producing patient symptoms. The possible causes for a set of symptoms are considered in order to arrive at a diagnosis. For example, if a patient presents with moderate to severe knee pain the provider might consider causes like an injury or arthritis. A differential diagnosis is based on information gathered from the patient about symptoms; contributing family, personal, and social histories; and a complete physical examination. Multiple causes are not ruled out in a differential diagnosis because it is possible for patients to be sick with more than one thing at once. Once the provider has considered all the possible factors, he or she comes up with a working diagnosis and begins treatment. A working diagnosis is also called a *clinical diagnosis*. The

clinical diagnosis is arrived at after taking a detailed history and doing a comprehensive physical examination, but before any laboratory tests or x-rays, diagnostic testing is done. For the patient with knee pain, after gathering detailed patient information and conducting a comprehensive physical examination, the provider decides that the clinical diagnosis is arthritic changes in the joint. The provider orders x-rays and an MRI of the knee to confirm the clinical diagnosis. The final diagnosis is determined after all of the diagnostic studies are completed.

However, patient care does not start with the physical examination; it begins when the patient first makes contact with the office. Even before the examination, the medical assistant has the opportunity to interact with the patient to ensure that he or she feels comfortable during the process and that all the necessary information is obtained.

Interviewing patients, assisting with examinations, and documentation are important responsibilities for a medical assistant. You must know the components of a medical history and the techniques for interviewing patients because these will help the provider diagnose and treat the patient. The more complete the medical history, the better able the provider will be to treat the patient.

MEDICAL HISTORY

Collecting the History Information

When a new patient calls or comes in for an appointment, the person is asked to complete a health history form. Besides being useful for diagnosing and treating the patient, the self-history allows the patient more participation in the process. The form may be mailed to the patient's home before the appointment or may be completed in the office during the first visit. Some practices now use electronic forms; these can be e-mailed to the patient before the first appointment and incorporated into the patient's electronic health record

(EHR) when the completed form is e-mailed back. The patient may also be able to complete the form online through a **patient portal**. If a paper form is used, it can be scanned into the patient's EHR after it is completed.

If you are responsible for taking a portion of the medical history, conduct the interview in a private area free of outside interference and beyond the hearing range of other patients. Patients will not talk freely where they may be overheard or interrupted. Legally and ethically, the patient has the right to privacy, and access to the patient's health record is permitted only for healthcare workers directly involved in the patient's care or individuals the patient has specified on his or her Health Insurance Portability and Accountability Act (HIPAA) release form.

Listen to the patient. Do not express surprise or displeasure at any of the patient's statements. Remember, you are there not to pass judgment, but to gather medical data. Documentation of information gathered while taking the medical history is included in the progress notes section of the medical record. The medical assistant records the information in an organized manner, exactly as given by the patient, without opinion or interpretation. The progress notes should include the purpose of the patient's visit, written as the chief complaint (CC), and the patient's vital signs (VS), including height and weight, if preferred by the provider. In addition, if the patient reports pain, it should be documented using a scale of 1 to 10, with 1 being the least amount of pain and 10 being the greatest amount.

In some facilities the provider takes the medical history during the patient's initial visit. The provider correlates the physical findings in the examination with the information in the history. The complete medical history and the physical examination are the starting point and foundation of all patient-physician contacts. EHR systems incorporate the patient's history and physical examination data directly into the health record (Figure 21-1).

Components of the Medical History

Medical history forms vary, depending on the provider's preference, the practice specialty, and the EHR system used in the facility (Figure 21-2). The most commonly used medical history forms include these components:

- *Database:* The record of the patient's name, address, date of birth, insurance information, personal data, history, physical examination, and initial laboratory findings. As new information is added, it becomes part of this database.
- *Chief complaint (CC)* or **present illness** (history of present illness [HPI]): The purpose of the patient's visit. The medical assistant should gather as much information about the health problem as possible and record it concisely, using the patient's own words as often as possible.
- *Past history (PH)* or *past medical history (PMH):* A summary of the patient's previous health. It includes dates and details of the patient's usual childhood diseases (UCD or UCHD), major illnesses, surgeries, allergies, accidents, and immunization record. Each medical practice has a policy on how to document a patient's allergies; they typically are written in red ink or identified by a colored sticker so that all healthcare workers can easily take note of potential allergic reactions.

EHR systems have methods for including allergy information on all pertinent screens in the patient's record. Included in the patient's medication history should be a record of frequently used over-the-counter (OTC) medications, including supplements and currently prescribed drugs.

- *Family history (FH):* Details about the patient's parents and siblings and their health; if they are deceased, the age and cause of death. This information is important because certain diseases and disorders have **familial** and/or hereditary tendencies.
- *Social history (SH):* This section includes information about the patient's lifestyle including whether he or she feels safe at home; use of tobacco, alcohol, or recreational drugs; sleeping and exercise habits; typical diet; education and occupation; dental care history; and for female patients their last menstrual period (LMP), pregnancy history, and method of birth control if sexually active. It may be important to note the patient's cultural and religious background, because these could influence certain lifestyle and dietary choices. This information helps the physician to plan treatment for the patient or to determine causative factors for disease. It also provides a holistic picture of the patient's health.
- *Systems review (SR)* or *review of systems (ROS):* These questions provide a guide to the patient's general health and help detect conditions other than those covered under the present illness. Often a patient may think certain health problems irrelevant and may fail to mention them. However, these problems may help the provider determine the cause of the disorder currently being explored. A systems review is obtained through a logical sequence of questions about the state of health of body systems, beginning with the head and proceeding downward (Figure 21-3). The provider typically completes this section of the medical history while conducting the physical examination.

UNDERSTANDING AND COMMUNICATING WITH PATIENTS

To provide high-quality patient care, we must communicate effectively with the patient and provide a warm, caring environment. Positive reactions and interactions with the patient are vital. Because medical care by nature is extremely personal, a medical assistant must always remember that each patient is an individual with certain anxieties. These anxieties often cause people to act and react in different ways; therefore, effective verbal and nonverbal communication with each patient is absolutely essential.

Healthcare professionals accept the responsibility of developing helping relationships with their patients. The interpersonal nature of the patient–medical assistant relationship carries with it a certain amount of responsibility to forget one's self-interest and focus on the patient's needs. A medical assistant can elicit either a positive or a negative response to patient care simply by the way he or she treats and interacts with patients. You usually are the first person with whom the patient communicates; therefore, you play a vital role in initiating therapeutic patient interactions (Procedure 21-1).

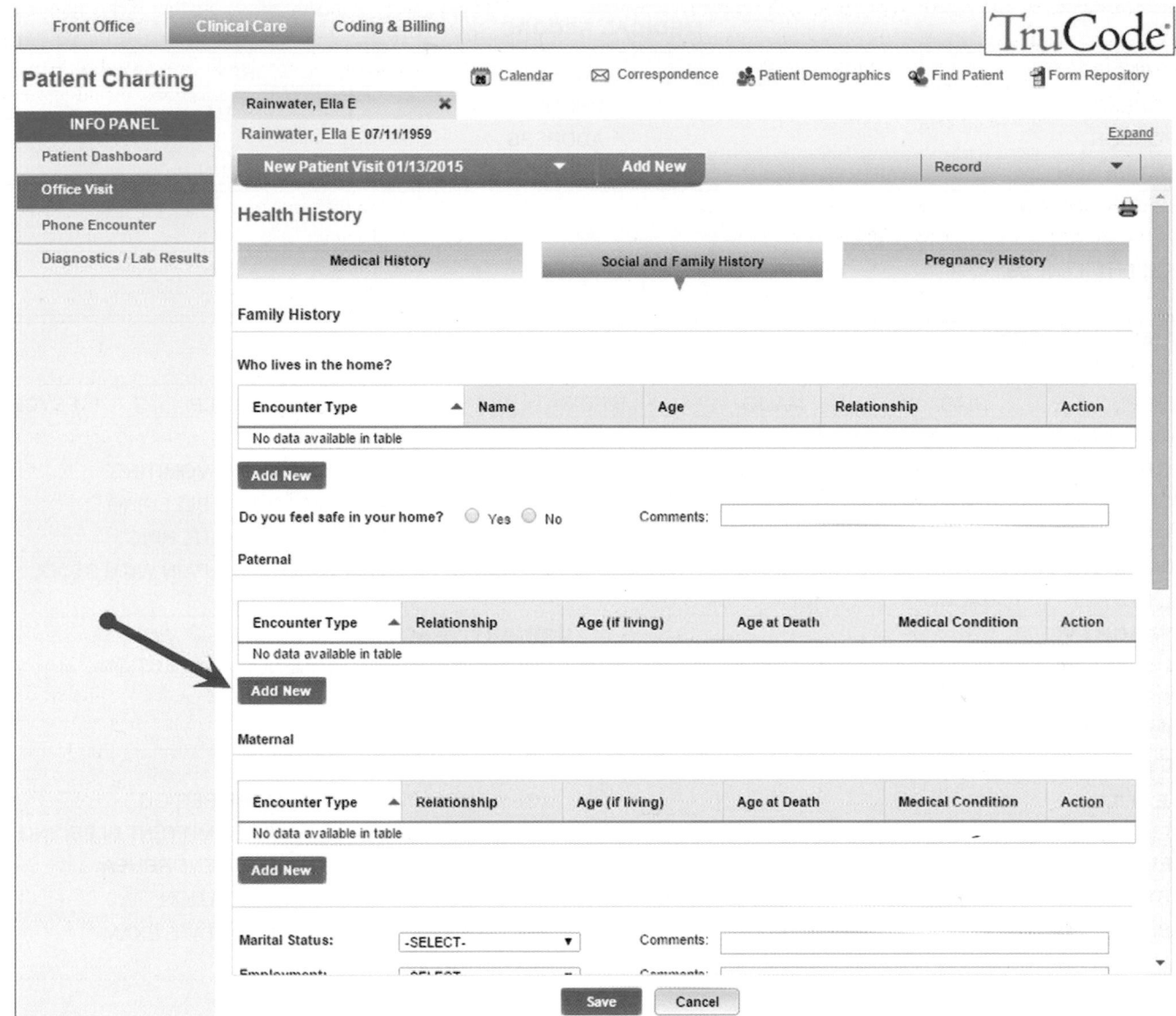

FIGURE 21-1 Example of an electronic health record (EHR) system.

Sensitivity to Diverse Patient Groups

Practicing respectful patient care is extremely important when working with a diverse patient population. Empathy is the key to creating a caring, therapeutic environment. Empathy goes beyond sympathy. A medical assistant who is empathetic respects the individuality of the patient and attempts to see the person's health problem through his or her eyes, recognizing the effect of all holistic factors on the patient's well-being. Empathetic sensitivity to diversity first requires those interested in healthcare to examine their own values, beliefs, and actions; you cannot treat all patients with care and respect until you first recognize and evaluate personal biases. We think and act a certain way for many reasons. The first step in understanding the process is to evaluate your individual value system. Why do you have certain attitudes or beliefs about the worth of individuals or things?

> **CRITICAL THINKING** APPLICATION   **21-1**
>
> What do you value most in life? What is important to you? What influences you to act in a certain way? Make a list of five things you value the most and share them with the class. Try to determine why you feel so strongly about those particular things.

Many different factors influence the development of a value system. Value systems begin as learned beliefs and behaviors. Families and cultural influences shape the way we respond to a diverse society. Other factors that influence reactions include socioeconomic and educational backgrounds. To develop therapeutic relationships, you must recognize your own value system to determine whether it could affect your method of interaction. Preconceived ideas about

MEDICAL RECORD

NAME	AGE	SEX	S / M / D / W
ADDRESS	PHONE	DATE	
SPONSOR	ADDRESS		
OCCUPATION	REF BY	ACKN	

CHIEF COMPLAINT

PRESENT ILLNESS

FAMILY HISTORY

MOTHER	FATHER	SIBLING(S)

TB	DIAB	MALIG	HT DIS	NEPH	EPILEP	PSYCH

PAST HISTORY — GENERAL HEALTH

CHILDHOOD DISEASES

SC FEV   RHEUM FEV   ASTHMA

OTHER

SOCIAL HISTORY

COFFEE   TOBACCO   ALCOHOL   DRUG USE

WEIGHT

USUAL WEIGHT

RECENT WEIGHT FLUCTUATIONS

HX OF EATING DISORDER

REVIEW OF SYSTEMS

E E N T

EYES   EARS   NOSE   THROAT   NECK

NEUROMUSCULAR

STRENGTH   ANXIETY

SLEEP   DEPRESSION

MUSCULAR PAIN   PERIPHERAL NEUROPATHY

JOINT PAIN

CARDIOVASCULAR

HEART DISEASE   MI

CONGENITAL HEART DEFECTS   TIAS

HYPERTENSION   STROKE

EDEMA

LUNGS

PAIN   DYSPNEA

COUGHING UP BLOOD   COUGH

IRREG BREATHING

GASTROINTESTINAL

APPETITE	BOWEL HABITS	VOMITING
INDIGESTION	HEMORRHOIDS	BLEEDING
NAUSEA	DIET	ITCHING
JAUNDICE	PAIN	PAIN WITH STOOL
OTHER		

URINARY TRACT

NOCTURIA	INCONTINENCE	INFECTION
PAIN	FREQUENCY	
BLEEDING	BURNING	

GENITAL TRACT

AGE AT MENST	TYPE PERIOD
PAINFUL PERIOD	INTERMITTENT BLEEDING
AMENORRHEA	DYSMENORRHEA
VAG DISCH	IRRITATION
BREAST EXAM	PROSTATE EXAM
TESTICULAR EXAM	

L M P

AGES OF CHILDREN	CONTRACEPTION TYPE
LMP DATE	NO. OF PREGNANCIES
NO. OF LIVE BIRTHS	AGES OF CHILDREN

OTHER

ACCIDENTS

OPERATIONS

CURRENT MEDICATIONS AND TREATMENTS

COMMENTS

FIGURE 21-2 A general medical history form.

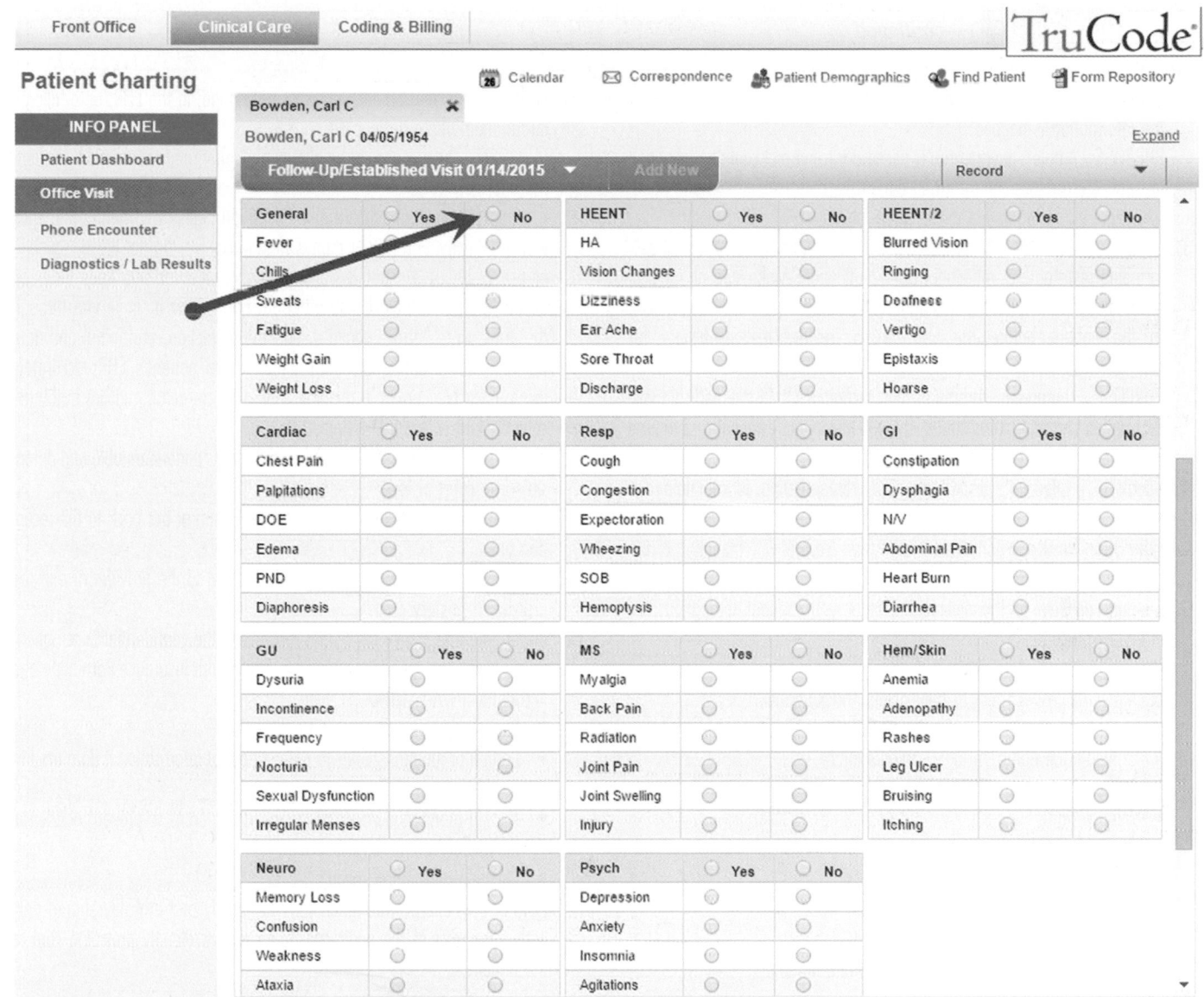

FIGURE 21-3 Example of review of systems (ROS) questions in an EHR.

PROCEDURE 21-1	Demonstrate Therapeutic Communication Feedback Techniques to Obtain Patient Information and Document Patient Care Accurately in the Medical Record

Complete this procedure with another student playing the role of the patient. To make the experience more realistic, choose a student about whom you know very little. To maintain the student's privacy, he or she does not have to share any confidential information.

Goal: *To use restatement, reflection, and clarification to obtain patient information and document patient care accurately.*

EQUIPMENT and SUPPLIES

- History form or EHR system with the patient history window opened
- If using a paper form—a red pen for recording the patient's allergies, and a black pen to meet legal documentation guidelines
- Quiet, private area

PROCEDURAL STEPS

1. Greet and identify the patient in a pleasant manner. Introduce yourself and explain your role.
   <u>PURPOSE</u>: To make the patient feel comfortable and at ease.

PROCEDURE 21-1 —continued

2. Take the patient to a quiet, private area for the interview and explain why the information is needed.
   PURPOSE: A quiet, private area is necessary to protect confidentiality and prevent interruptions. An informed patient is more cooperative and therefore more likely to provide useful information.

3. Complete the history form by using therapeutic communication techniques, including restatement, reflection, and clarification. Make sure all medical terminology is adequately explained. A self-history may have been mailed to the patient before the visit. If so, review the self-history for completeness.
   PURPOSE: Therapeutic communication techniques help the medical assistant gather complete information; the self-history is designed to save time and to involve the patient in the process.

4. Speak in a pleasant, distinct manner, remembering to maintain eye contact with your patient.
   PURPOSE: Positive nonverbal behaviors create a friendly, caring atmosphere.

5. Remain sensitive to the diverse needs of your patient throughout the interview process.
   PURPOSE: Incorporate awareness of your personal biases into treating all patients with respect despite their diverse backgrounds.

6. Record the following statistical information:
   - Patient's full name, including middle initial
   - Address, including apartment number and ZIP code
   - Marital status
   - Sex (gender)
   - Age and date of birth
   - Telephone numbers for home, cell, and work
   - Insurance information if not already available
   - Employer's name, address, and telephone number

7. Record the following medical history:
   - Chief complaint
   - Present illness
   - Past history
   - Family history
   - Social history
   PURPOSE: The provider needs this information to make an accurate assessment and diagnosis. The provider usually completes the review of systems (ROS) during the pre-examination interview.

8. Ask about allergies to drugs and any other substances and record any allergies in red ink on every page of the history form, on the front of the patient record, and on each progress note page; in the EHR, enter allergy information where designated.
   PURPOSE: The presence of an allergy may alter medication and treatment procedures.

9. If using a paper form, record all information legibly and neatly and spell words correctly. Print rather than writing in cursive. Do not erase, scribble, or use whiteout. Do not leave any blank spaces or skip lines between documentation entries. If you make an error, draw a single line through the error, write "error" above it, add the correction, and initial and date the entry. If recording the information in the patient's EHR, accurately locate each box; errors in the EHR should be corrected and are automatically tracked within the system.
   PURPOSE: To maintain a medical record that is understandable and defensible in a court of law.

10. Thank the patient for cooperating and direct him or her back to the reception area.

11. Review the record for errors before you pass it to the provider or exit the EHR health history area.

12. Protect the integrity of the health record and the confidentiality of patient information. Safeguards mandated by the Health Insurance Portability and Accountability Act (HIPAA) include:
    - Passwords to secure access to all EHRs.
    - Computer monitor shields to protect patient information if data are left on the screen.
    - Turning monitors away from patient traffic areas to prevent accidental release of information.
    - Securing all medical records
    PURPOSE: Patient information may be legally and ethically shared only with a member of the healthcare team who is directly providing care to the patient.

DOCUMENTATION PRACTICE

Mr. Bonski is a new patient being seen today for the first time. His CC is dizziness for 2 weeks. He denies having headaches and has no previous Hx of ear infections or hypertension. He does not take any prescribed medications but uses Tylenol as needed for a headache. T 97.6, P 88, R 21, BP 172/94. Document pertinent patient findings using the SOAP method.

S _____

O _____

A _____

P _____

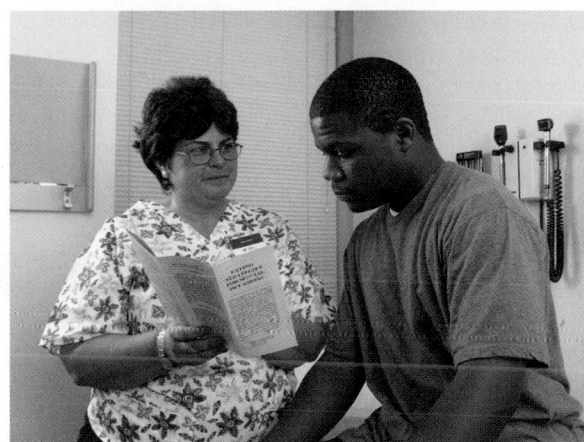

FIGURE 21-4 Respectful patient care.

people because of their race, religion, income level, ethnic origin, sexual orientation, or gender can act as barriers to the development of a therapeutic relationship. You cannot treat your patients empathetically unless you can connect with them in some way. Personal biases or prejudices are monumental barriers to the development of therapeutic relationships (Figure 21-4).

CRITICAL THINKING APPLICATION   **21-2**

Honestly evaluate your personal biases. What do you find unacceptable in people? Do you prejudge an individual based on his or her affiliation with a particular group or because of a certain lifestyle decision? Do these biases create barriers to the development of therapeutic relationships? If so, how can you get beyond these barriers?

Consider the following scenarios and discuss them with your classmates:

- While you are conducting a patient interview, the patient informs you that he has tested positive for the human immunodeficiency virus (HIV). Do you think this will affect your therapeutic relationship?
- You are responsible for recording an in-depth interview on a homeless person with very poor hygiene. Will this cause a problem with your professional manner?
- You are told by your office manager that an inmate of the county prison is being brought in this afternoon for an examination. Do you think his status will affect your interaction with the patient?
- You are attempting to interview a 20-year-old patient who brought her two young children with her to the office today. She is a single mother who is pregnant with her third child and receives public assistance. What do you think? Will you have difficulty being empathetic?

Therapeutic Techniques

The linear communication model describes communication as an interactive process involving the sender of the message, the receiver, and the crucial component of feedback to confirm reception of the message. The message can be sent by a number of different methods, such as face-to-face communication, telephone, e-mail, and letter; however, there is no way to confirm the message was actually received unless the patient provides feedback about what he or she interpreted from the message. Feedback completes the communication cycle by providing a means for us to know exactly what message the patient received and therefore whether it requires clarification.

For example, as a medical assistant, one of your responsibilities will be to provide patient education on how to prepare for diagnostic studies. Let's say you have to explain to an elderly patient how to prepare for a colonoscopy. Even though you provide a detailed explanation of the preparation procedure, in addition to a handout explaining the step-by-step process, how do you really know whether the patient understands? You ask the patient to provide feedback by explaining the process back to you. As a member of the healthcare team, you must become an effective communicator. You will play a vital role in collecting and documenting patient information. If your methods of collection or recording are faulty, the quality of patient care may be seriously impaired.

Active Listening Techniques

Active listeners go beyond hearing the patient's message to concentrating, understanding, and listening to the main points in the discussion. Active listening techniques encourage patients to expand on and clarify the content and meaning of their messages. These techniques are very useful communication tools when a patient is agitated or upset because they help the medical assistant clarify the important details of the patient's chief complaint.

Three processes are involved in active listening: restatement, reflection, and clarification. Restatement is simply paraphrasing or repeating the patient's statements with phrases such as, "My understanding of what you are sayin ..." or "You are telling me the problem is ..."

Reflection involves repeating the main idea of the conversation while also identifying the sender's *feelings*. For example, if the mother of a young patient is expressing frustration about her child's behavior, a reflective statement identifies that feeling with the response, "It sounds like you are frustrated about ..." Or, if a patient who has been newly diagnosed with insulin-dependent diabetes shows anxiety about administering injections, an appropriate reflective statement recognizes the patient's feelings: "You appear anxious about ..." Reflective statements clearly demonstrate to patients that you are not only listening to their words; you also are concerned and are attending to their feelings.

Clarification seeks to summarize or simplify the sender's thoughts and feelings and to resolve any confusion in the message. Questions or statements that begin with "Give me an example of ..." or "Explain to me about ..." or "So what you're saying is ..." help patients focus on the chief complaint and give you the opportunity to clear up any misconceptions before documenting patient information.

Listening is not a passive role in the communication process; it is active and demanding. You cannot be preoccupied with your own needs, or you will miss something important. For the duration of the patient interview, no one is more important than this particular patient. Listen to the way things are said, the tone of the patient's voice, and even to what the patient may not be saying out loud but is saying very clearly with body language.

Nonverbal Communication

Much of what we communicate to our patients is conveyed through the use of conscious or unconscious body language. Our nonverbal actions, such as gestures, facial expressions, and mannerisms, are learned behaviors that are greatly influenced by our family and cultural backgrounds. The body naturally expresses our true feelings; in fact, experts say that more than 90% of communication is nonverbal.

Most of the negative messages communicated through body language are unintentional; therefore, it is important to remember while conducting patient interviews that nonverbal communication can seriously affect the therapeutic process.

The verbal messages you send are only part of the communication process. You have a specific context in mind when you send your words, but the receiver puts his or her own interpretations on them. The receiver attaches meaning determined by his or her past experiences, culture, self-concept, and current physical and emotional states. Sometimes these messages and interpretations do not coincide. Feedback from the patient is crucial in determining whether the patient understood the message. Successful communication requires mutual understanding by the interviewer and the person being interviewed.

Observing your patient during the interview fosters mutual understanding. The purpose of observing nonverbal communication is to become sensitive to or aware of the feelings of others as conveyed by small bits of behavior rather than words. This sensitivity enables you to adapt your behavior to these feelings; to deliberately select your response, either verbal or nonverbal; and thereby to have

a favorable effect on others. The favorable effect may consist of providing emotional support, conveying that you care, defusing the patient's fear or anger, or providing an invitation to release pent-up feelings by talking about the situation that aroused the feelings. Table 21-1 lists some nonverbal behaviors by patients that may indicate anxiety, frustration, or fear.

Helpful Listening Guidelines

- Listen to the main points in the discussion.
- Attend to both verbal and nonverbal messages.
- Be patient and nonjudgmental.
- Do not interrupt.
- Never intimidate your patient.
- Use active listening techniques: restatement, reflection, and clarification.

You can do much to put a patient at ease by the tone of your voice. Your facial expression and the ease and confidence of your movements demonstrate a sincere interest to the patient. Therapeutic use of space and touch also are important ways of sending nonverbal messages to your patients. You should establish eye contact, sit in a relaxed but attentive position, and avoid using furniture as a barrier between you and the patient. Give the patient your undivided attention and let your body language inform each patient that you are interested in his or her medical problems (Figure 21-5 and Procedure 21-2).

The key to successful patient interaction is **congruence** between verbal and nonverbal messages. Although choosing the correct words is very important, less than 10% of the message received is verbal; therefore, to be seen as honest and sensitive to the needs of your patients, you must be aware of your nonverbal behavior patterns. The nonverbal message the patient receives from the medical assistant's listening behavior should be, "You are a person of worth, and I am interested in you as a unique individual."

TABLE 21-1   Observation of Nonverbal Communication in Patients

AREA	OBSERVATION	INDICATION
Breathing patterns	Rapid respirations, sighing, shallow thoracic breathing	Anxiety, boredom, pain
Eye patterns	No eye contact, side-to-side movement, looking down at the hands	Anxiety, distrust, embarrassment
Hands	Tapping fingers, cracking knuckles, continuous movement, sweaty palms	Anxiety, worry, fear
Arm placement	Folded across chest, wrapped around abdomen	Anxiety, worry, fear, pain
Leg placement	Tension, crossed and/or tucked under, tapping foot, continuous movement	Frustration, anger

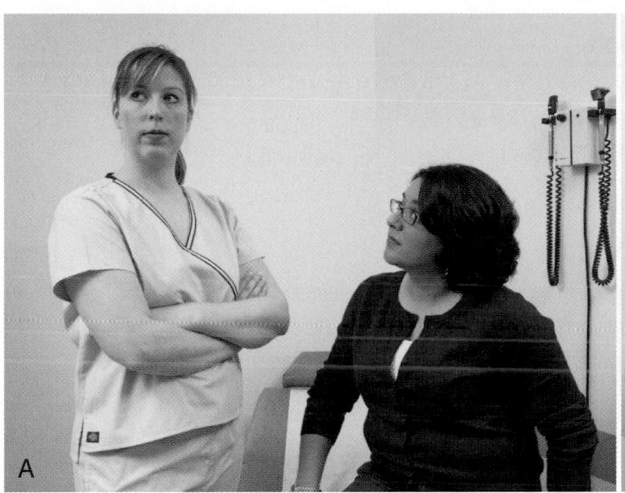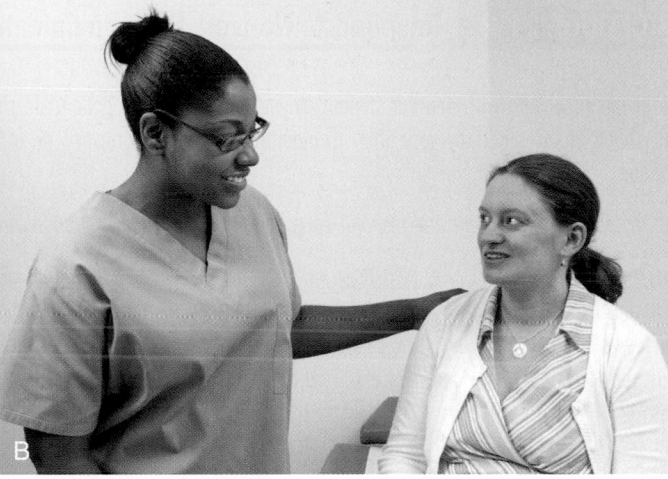

FIGURE 21-5 A, Ineffective nonverbal language. **B,** Therapeutic nonverbal language.

Nonverbal Language Behaviors

Nonverbal behavior—your body language—can have either a positive or negative effect on patient interactions. Positive nonverbal behaviors enhance the patient's experience in the healthcare setting. Communication experts recommend the following:

- When gathering a health history, lean toward the patient to show interest.
- Face the patient squarely and at eye level to help make the process more comfortable and to demonstrate sensitivity and empathy.
- Eye contact is essential for therapeutic communication unless the patient is from a culture that discourages this.
- A closed posture (crossed arms or legs) may indicate disinterest.
- Be sensitive to the patient's personal space when possible. Maintain a comfortable distance from the patient, at least an arm's length, when conducting the interview.
- Be careful with body gestures, such as hand and arm movements. Gestures, such as nodding your head when the patient talks, can display interest, but too much body movement can be distracting.
- Your tone of voice should reflect your interest in the patient. Speaking too quietly or too loudly can detract from therapeutic communication.
- Continually observe the patient's body language during the interview; watch for signs of confusion, boredom, worry, and so on so that you can respond appropriately.
- Documenting in an EHR can be distracting to both the medical assistant and the patient. Remind yourself to frequently look at the patient and use encouraging body language to maintain a personal interaction with the patient.

Environmental Factors

Before you meet with the patient, prepare the physical setting, which may be an examination room or an office. In any location, optimum conditions are important to achieving a smooth, productive interview.

Open-Ended Questions or Statements

An open-ended question or statement asks for general information or states the topic to be discussed, but only in general terms. Use this communication tool to begin the interview, to introduce a new section of questions, or whenever the person introduces a new topic. It is a very effective method of gathering more details from the patient about the chief complaint or health history. Examples include:

"What brings you to the doctor?"

"How have you been getting along?"

"You mentioned having dizzy spells. Tell me more about that."

This type of question or statement encourages patients to respond in a manner they find comfortable. It allows patients to express themselves fully and provide comprehensive information about their chief complaint.

Closed Questions

Direct, or closed, questions ask for specific information. This form of questioning limits the answer to one or two words, in many cases yes or no. Use this form of question when you need confirmation of specific facts, such as when asking about past health problems. For example:

"Do you have a headache?"

"What is your birth date?"

"Have you ever broken a bone?"

PROCEDURE 21-2   Respond to Nonverbal Communication

Complete this procedure with another student playing the role of the patient. To make the experience more realistic, choose a student about whom you know very little. To maintain the student's privacy, he or she does not have to share any confidential information.

Goal: *To observe the patient and respond appropriately to nonverbal communication.*

Scenario: *Jessica Simpert, 39, is a new patient with the CC of intermittent abdominal pain with alternating diarrhea and constipation. Ms. Simpert has experienced this discomfort for several months and appears very frustrated. She is sitting on the end of the exam table with her arms wrapped around her abdomen. She sighs frequently and refuses to maintain eye contact. What is her nonverbal behavior telling you, and how can you establish therapeutic communication with this patient?*

EQUIPMENT and SUPPLIES

- Patient's record

PROCEDURAL STEPS

1. Greet and identify the patient in a pleasant manner. Introduce yourself and explain your role.
   PURPOSE: To make the patient feel comfortable and at ease.
2. Ask the patient the purpose of her visit and the onset, duration, and frequency of her symptoms. Pay close attention to her body language to determine whether what she is telling you is congruent with her body language.
   PURPOSE: Nonverbal language naturally expresses the patient's true feelings. Closely observing body language will help you reach more accurate conclusions about the patient's information.
3. Use restatement, reflection, and clarification to gather as much information as possible about the patient's CC. Make sure all medical terminology is adequately explained.

PURPOSE: Therapeutic communication techniques help the medical assistant gather complete information; using feedback techniques and making sure the patient understands medical terms helps relieve anxiety.
4. Speak in a pleasant, distinct manner, remembering to maintain eye contact with your patient.
   PURPOSE: Positive nonverbal behaviors create a friendly, caring atmosphere. Remain sensitive to the diverse needs of your patient throughout the interview process.
5. Continue to observe nonverbal patient behaviors and select the appropriate verbal response to demonstrate your sensitivity to her discomfort, frustration, and anxiety.
   PURPOSE: Displaying sensitivity and awareness to the patient's nonverbal body language demonstrates your concern for the patient and can help defuse the patient's concerns.

INTERVIEWING THE PATIENT

The interview, or gathering the patient's medical history, is the first and most important part of data collection. The medical history identifies the patient's health strengths and problems and is a bridge to the next step in data collection, the physical examination performed by the provider. At this point, the patient knows everything about his or her own health status and you know nothing. Your skill in interviewing helps glean the necessary information and builds **rapport** for a successful working relationship.

Consider the interview a type of contract between you and your patient. The contract consists of spoken and unspoken language and addresses what the patient needs and expects from the healthcare visit. The patient interview consists of three stages: the initiation or introduction, the body, and the closing.

The initiation of the interview is the time to introduce yourself, to identify the patient, and to determine the purpose of the interview (Figure 21-6). If you are nervous about how to begin, remember to keep it short. The patient probably is nervous, too, and is anxious

to get started. Address the patient by his or her last name and give the reason for the interview. For example: "Mr. Coleman, my name is Stacey, and I am a certified medical assistant who works with Dr. Yang. I have some questions to ask you about your health history."

After the brief introduction, move on to the body of the interview. This is when you use various therapeutic communication techniques to determine the reason the patient is seeking healthcare, the patient's perception of the problem, the characteristics of the problem, and the patient's expectations of care. During this time, use active listening skills, meaningful silence, congruent verbal and nonverbal communication, and a combination of open-ended and closed statements and questions to gather the details of the patient's history and current health problem (Table 21-2).

Conclude the interview by summarizing the results of your interaction. The closing of the interview should clarify the patient's chief complaint, the purpose of the health visit, and the patient's expectations of care. This is the patient's opportunity to add any additional details or to explain further the characteristics of the health problem.

Preparing the Appropriate Environment

- **Ensure privacy:** Make sure the room you use is unoccupied for the entire time allowed for the interview. The patient needs to feel sure that no one can overhear the conversation or interrupt.
- **Prevent interruptions:** Inform your co-workers of the interview, and ask them not to interrupt you during this time. You need to concentrate on the patient and establish rapport. An interruption can destroy in seconds what you have spent many minutes building up.
- **Prepare comfortable surroundings:** Conducting the interview in comfortable surroundings reduces the patient's anxiety. Keep the distance between you and the patient at arm's length. Arrange chairs so that you and the patient are comfortably seated at eye level, and the desk or table does not act as a barrier between you.
- **Take judicious notes:** Note taking should be kept to a minimum while you try to focus your attention on the person. Note taking during the interview has disadvantages, such as breaking eye contact and shifting your attention away from the patient, which diminishes the patient's sense of importance. However, it is important to write down pertinent details as you are interviewing, because you may forget important facts if you do not note them at the time of the discussion. With experience you will develop a personal type of shorthand that you can use during the interview process. If using an EHR medical history template, efficiently open boxes and choose the appropriate data, maintaining eye contact and using active listening techniques periodically throughout the interview.

TABLE 21-2   Therapeutic Communication Techniques

TECHNIQUE	VALUE
Open-ended questions and statements	Encourage the patient to respond in more detail
Direct or closed questions	Ask for specific information; usual reply is yes or no
Active listening	Nonverbally communicates your interest in the patient
Silence	Nonverbally communicates your acceptance of the patient and willingness to wait until the patient is ready to answer
Establishing guidelines	Informs the patient of what to expect during the interview
Acknowledgment	Shows the importance of the patient's role and respect for autonomy
Restating	Checks your interpretation of the patient's message for validation
Reflecting	Shows the patient your acknowledgment of his or her feelings
Summarizing	Helps the patient separate relevant from irrelevant material; provides clarity to the interview

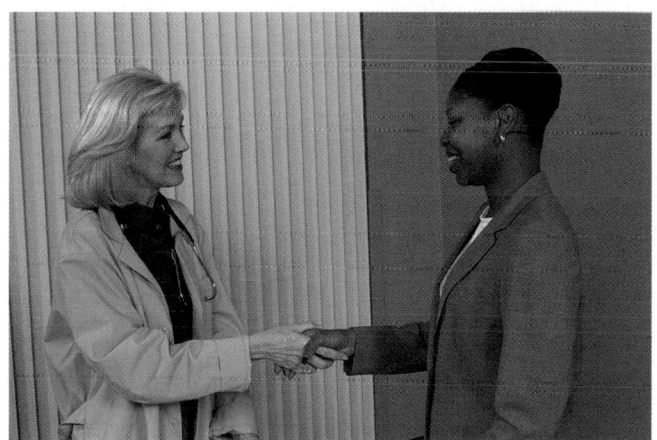

FIGURE 21-6 Greeting the patient.

Interview Barriers

Providing Unwarranted Assurance

Mrs. Miller says to you, "I know this lump is going to turn out to be cancer." The typical reply is almost automatic: "Don't worry, I'm sure everything will be fine." This type of answer indicates that her anxiety is insignificant and denies her the opportunity to discuss her fears further. A reflective response, such as, "You sound really worried about ..." acknowledges her feelings and demonstrates empathy and a willingness to listen to her concerns.

Giving Advice

Mrs. Thompson has just finished talking to the doctor. She looks at you and says, "Dr. Rowe says I need surgery to get rid of these gallstones. I just don't know. What would you do?" If you tell her how you would handle the situation, you may have shifted the accountability for decision making from her to you, and she has not worked out her own solution. Does this woman really want to know what you would do? Probably not. You could respond to her question with, "Based on what the doctor told you, what do you think you should do?" or "Do you need further information to make your decision?" If the patient continues to question the provider's recommendations, the medical assistant should encourage further discussion with the provider.

Using Medical Terminology

You must adjust your vocabulary to fit the patient. The more the patient understands about what is happening and the management of the problem, the better the outcome. Misinterpreted communication is the most common error in patient care. One of the biggest problems for the patient is understanding medical terminology. Closely observe the patient's body language while he or she receives instructions or patient education. If the patient shows signs of not understanding the procedure, ask the patient to repeat back to you the information or instructions. This demonstration–return demonstration form of providing feedback ensures that the patient completely understands what is happening. It also gives the medical assistant the opportunity to clarify any misconceptions.

Leading Questions

During the interview, you ask the patient, "You don't smoke, do you?" By asking questions in this manner, you indicate the preferred answer. Telling you that he or she does smoke would surely meet with your disapproval. Keep your questions positive. A better way of asking would be, "Have you ever smoked?" or "Do you use tobacco?"

Talking Too Much

Some medical assistants associate helpfulness with verbal overload. The patient may let the interviewer talk at the expense of his or her own need to explain what is wrong. Always remember that when interviewing a patient, you should listen more than you talk. Pay close attention to the patient's body language to make sure you are giving the patient ample opportunity to discuss the health problem.

Defense Mechanisms

Many individuals respond to anxiety-provoking situations by automatically relying on defense mechanisms. Because defense mechanisms are used consciously or unconsciously to block an emotionally painful experience, it is understandable that patients facing a traumatic diagnosis or a difficult treatment feel the need to protect themselves from the reality of the situation. The problem is, how can we ensure compliance with treatment if the patient is in denial, projecting feelings onto the healthcare worker, or repressing the need for treatment or diagnostic follow-up? The medical assistant must be sensitive to patients' use of defense mechanisms and must consistently apply therapeutic communication techniques to interactions with patients.

Defense Mechanisms

Patients may use defense mechanisms to protect themselves from a situation or medical information they cannot manage psychologically. Defense mechanisms may hide any of a variety of thoughts or feelings: anger, fear, sadness, despair, or helplessness. A patient who uses defense mechanisms can be very difficult to deal with; however, if the medical assistant is aware of the patient's need for psychological protection, he or she may be able to find a way to provide care for the patient while maintaining a therapeutic relationship. For example, Mrs. Alicia Simone, a 48-year-old patient, has just been told she has breast cancer. The following are defense mechanisms she might display to protect herself from the psychological reality of her disease.

- **Denial:** The patient completely rejects the information. *Example:* "I couldn't possibly have breast cancer. You must be mistaken."
- **Suppression:** The patient is consciously aware of the information or feeling but refuses to admit it. *Example:* "I don't think the test is accurate. My mammograms are always normal."
- **Reaction formation:** The patient expresses her feelings as the opposite of what she really feels. *Example:* If she is angry at the medical assistant for insisting that a biopsy be scheduled, she may express the opposite emotion: "I appreciate your trying to help me, but I just can't come to the hospital that day."
- **Projection:** The patient accuses someone else of having the feelings that she has. *Example:* If the patient is angry about the diagnosis,

she may say to the medical assistant, "You don't have to lose your temper about this," even though the medical assistant's demeanor is completely professional.

- **Rationalization:** The patient comes up with various explanations to justify her response. *Example:* "I think the results are wrong. I didn't follow the directions for the tests like I should have, and besides, there's no history of breast cancer in my family."
- **Undoing:** The patient tries to reverse a negative feeling by doing something that indicates the opposite feeling. *Example:* If the patient feels angry and violated about the diagnosis but she finds those feelings unacceptable, she may say, "Don't worry, dear, I'm not upset with you for telling me about this."
- **Regression:** The patient reverts to an old, usually immature behavior to ventilate her feelings. *Example:* Perhaps instead of discussing the diagnosis and the need for treatment, she just storms out of the office. Or she may say, "I can't possibly schedule a procedure without discussing this with my mother."
- **Sublimation:** The patient redirects her negative feelings into a socially productive activity. *Example:* Mrs. Simone eventually becomes an active member of a local support group for women recovering from breast cancer.

CRITICAL THINKING APPLICATION   **21-3**

Mr. Gonzales, a 48-year-old patient recently diagnosed with hypertension, did not show up today for his follow-up appointment. Chris calls to find out why he failed to keep the appointment, and the patient tells Chris he forgot to come, even though an appointment reminder call was made yesterday. He also tells Chris he has not been taking his medicine and does not understand why it is so important for him and his wife to meet with the dietitian. Is this patient using defense mechanisms? How should Chris respond to the patient? What communications skills might be helpful to promote a therapeutic relationship?

Communication Across the Lifespan

The key to communicating effectively with patients is using an age-specific approach. Given the age and developmental level of your patient, how can you best interact with the person and with significant family members?

For example, Tasha, a 2-year-old patient, is scheduled for a physical examination. How can you best interact with her and her father to ensure that the history phase of the visit is complete and accurate? Therapeutic use of nonverbal language is essential to interacting with children of all ages. Getting down on the child's level, establishing eye contact, and using a gentle but firm voice are ways of gaining

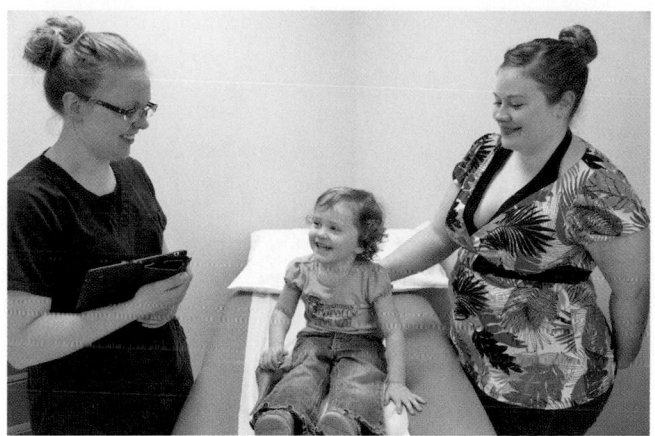

FIGURE 21-7 Interacting with a parent and child.

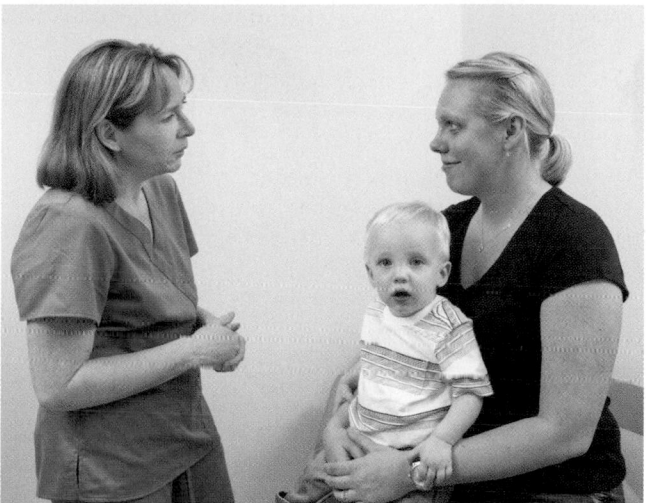

FIGURE 21-8 Responding to parental concerns.

the child's confidence and cooperation. Children fear the unknown, so explaining all procedures with language the child understands is important. At the same time, the medical assistant must communicate with the child's caregiver so that he or she can contribute to the intake process (Figure 21-7). The following are some important guidelines for obtaining the health history of a child.

- Make sure the environment is safe and attractive.
- Do not keep children and their caregivers waiting any longer than necessary because children become anxious and distracted quickly.
- Do not offer a choice unless the child can truly make one. If part of the treatment requires an injection, asking the child whether she'd like her shot now is most likely to get an automatic "No!" However, giving her a choice of stickers after the injection is appropriate.
- Praising the child during the examination helps reduce anxiety and boosts self-esteem. When possible, direct questions to the child so that he or she feels like part of the process.
- Involving the child in the examination by permitting him or her to manipulate the equipment may help relieve anxiety. If possible, use your imagination and make a game of the assessment or the procedure.
- A typical defense mechanism seen in sick or anxious children is regression. The child may refuse to leave the mother's lap or may want to hold a favorite toy during the procedure as a comfort measure. Look for signs of anxiety, such as thumb-sucking or rocking during the assessment, and encourage caregivers to be involved in the process to help make the child feel as safe as possible.
- Listen to parents' concerns and respond truthfully to questions (Figure 21-8).

Older children may also have difficulty during the health visit (Figure 21-9). To help school-aged children gain a sense of control, give them the opportunity to make certain decisions about treatment. For example, Heather, a 13-year-old patient with diabetes, could be given the choice of having her father present during the visit. Or, if she requires an insulin injection, she could choose the site of the injection or perhaps administer the medication herself. This gives the medical assistant an opportunity to observe her technique and allows Heather to exert her independence.

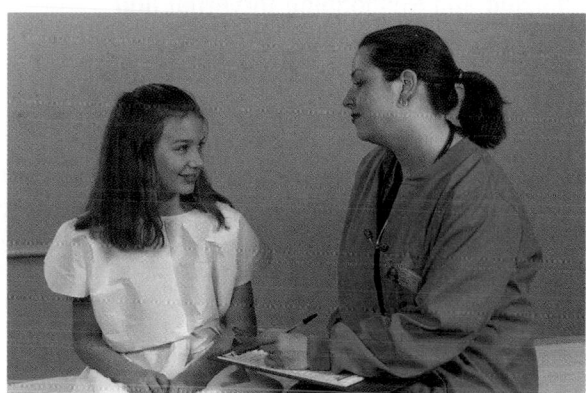

FIGURE 21-9 Interacting with a school-aged child.

Privacy is an important issue to consider with older children, especially adolescents. During the physical examination, respect privacy by keeping body exposure to a minimum and adequately preparing the child for procedures and positions. In addition, older children want to know what is going on during the examination, what to expect, and what the findings mean; therefore, keeping them informed in a language they can understand is important. Teen patients should always be encouraged to ask questions, which should be answered as completely and clearly as possible. Take every opportunity to teach your patients, regardless of their age, about their disease and to share information about significant wellness factors (Figure 21-10).

Patient education is extremely important when interacting with adult patients. Using language the adult patient understands and involving the patient in treatment decisions as much as possible are essential to developing a helping relationship with your older patients. Adults are bombarded by multiple responsibilities, which means that stress-related health problems are not unusual in these patients. Get to know your adult patients, and emphasize preventive healthcare when possible (Figure 21-11).

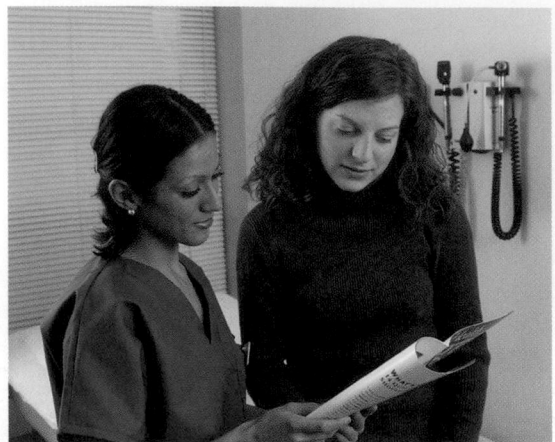

FIGURE 21-10 Interacting with an adolescent.

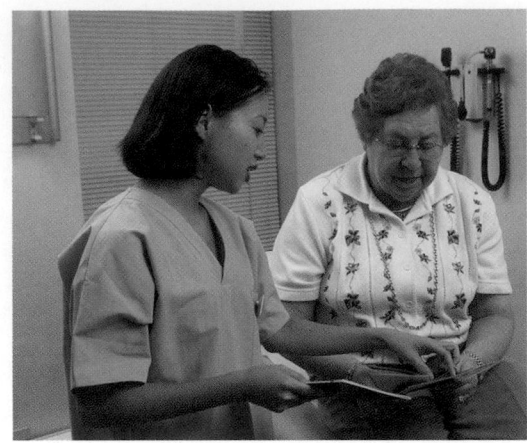

FIGURE 21-11 Adult patient education.

Recognizing and Responding to Verbal and Nonverbal Communications

The medical assistant not only must implement therapeutic communication skills, but also must observe the patient to interpret the person's message and level of understanding. In the following critical thinking exercise, Chris, the medical assistant from the opening scenario, conducts a patient interview using the therapeutic communication skills discussed in this chapter, including active listening techniques, open-ended and closed questions and statements, positive nonverbal interview skills, and effective observation of the patient's body language.

CRITICAL THINKING APPLICATION   **21-4**

Toby Anderson, a 52-year-old patient, was recently diagnosed with hypertension and prescribed Lotensin bid for treatment. He is being seen today for follow-up measurement of his blood pressure. Mr. Anderson is 45 pounds overweight and was given information about a reduced-calorie, low-sodium diet 1 month ago, but he has not lost any weight. He tells Chris that he has been having side effects from the medication. He is sitting with his arms across his chest, tapping his foot and occasionally cracking his knuckles.

Communication factors Chris should consider include the following:

- What nonverbal language is Mr. Anderson using, and how should Chris interpret it?
- Mr. Anderson tells Chris he is not following that crazy diet and never will. What therapeutic communication skills can Chris use to get more information out of Mr. Anderson and to reinforce the provider's recommendations?
- During the discussion, Mr. Anderson tells Chris he stopped taking the Lotensin because of the side effects. What communication techniques and therapeutic body language can Chris use to emphasize the need for Mr. Anderson to take his medicine as prescribed?

ASSESSING THE PATIENT

After the interview is complete, the patient is escorted to an examination room and prepared for the physical examination, which is performed by the physician or a qualified healthcare professional, such as a physician assistant (PA) or nurse practitioner. During the examination, the healthcare provider methodically checks all the body's systems. As this examination proceeds, the provider mentally compares the system with established norms. If something deviates from the accepted normal range, it is documented in the patient's health record. The physical examination typically starts with the head and progresses downward to the feet. However, the order may vary, depending on the provider's specialty.

Signs and Symptoms

After completing the examination, the provider documents all the signs and symptoms gathered during the physical assessment process. To better understand the examination procedure, the medical assistant must know the difference between a sign and a symptom.

Subjective findings, or **symptoms**, are perceptible only to the patient; they are what the patient feels and can be interpreted only by the patient. For example, only the patient experiences and can define the quality of his or her discomfort, pain, nausea, or dizziness. Symptoms of the greatest significance in identifying a disease are called *cardinal symptoms*. For example, crushing chest pain and difficulty breathing are cardinal symptoms of a possible heart attack.

Objective findings, or **signs**, can be observed and/or measured by the provider or medical assistant. They are the indicators of health or disease that a provider detects when examining a patient. The provider feels, sees, hears, or measures the signs that often are associated with a certain disease or abnormal condition. For example, a mass that a provider palpates, or feels, in the patient's abdomen is an objective finding and a sign of an abnormal condition. In addition, objective data can be measured and recorded, and repeat measurements can be taken to confirm the presence of or changes in the sign. The patient's temperature, pulse, respirations, and blood pressure are objective signs the medical assistant measures and records regularly.

The medical assistant also needs to know the difference between a functional disorder and an organic (physical) disorder. When a condition or disease is *functional,* it is without an organic cause; that is, when inspected, the organ appears normal, without any evidence of disease, even though the patient's signs or symptoms indicate a problem. An example of a functional problem would be a patient who has repeated bouts of elevated urinary albumin, but all tests on the kidneys show normal, healthy organs. Or a patient is diagnosed with irritable bowel syndrome even though diagnostic studies have failed to show any evidence of intestinal disease. A functional disorder can be difficult for the patient and provider to deal with because even though the patient is suffering from certain health problems, all diagnostic tests fail to show that anything is wrong with the affected system.

An *organic* disease or condition is one in which the abnormality can be seen or felt or clinically proven through laboratory or other diagnostic tests. For example, an electrocardiogram (ECG) can confirm that a patient with chest pain is having a heart attack. A colonoscopy performed on a patient who complains of bloody stools can reveal evidence of ulcers in the colon.

Assessing Pain

Pain is difficult to assess. We typically rely on the patient's report of symptoms to determine his or her level of pain. Some questions you can ask to evaluate the patient's perception of pain are:

- Where is the pain located? Is it associated with any particular movement?
- Can you describe how it feels? Is it constant or intermittent? Does anything relieve the pain?
- When was the onset of the pain? Did something cause the pain to start?
- Are you taking any medication to relieve the pain? What is it, and how often are you taking it? Is it effective? When was your last dose?
- Does pain affect your daily activities?
- On a scale of 1 to 10, with 10 being the highest level of pain, where would you rate your pain?

DOCUMENTATION

Various methods can be used for documentation, depending on the healthcare provider's preference and/or the facility's EHR system. However, certain charting procedures have been standardized to meet the legal requirements for maintaining medical records accurately and concisely. Complete, accurate documentation is one of the primary responsibilities of a medical assistant (Figure 21-12).

Documentation Guidelines

- Check the name on the record and make sure the information being documented is recorded on the correct form in the correct patient's health record or, with an EHR system, that the correct information is recorded using the correct system prompts. Confirm the patient's identity by checking his or her birth date.
- The month, day, and year must precede the entry; many facilities also require the time of the documentation.
- All unusual complaints, symptoms, or reactions must be noted in detail. Include complete information about the onset (when the problem started), duration (how long episodes last), and frequency (how often episodes occur) of each reported sign and symptom.
  Example: Pt reports night cough, which started 2 days ago, lasts approximately 10 minutes, and occurs 3-4 times per night.
- Describe objective data, such as the presence of a wound, using correct anatomic medical terminology.
  Example: Observed wound on left distal anterior leg approximately 2 cm long and 1 cm wide.
- If the patient reports pain, record the quality and intensity of the pain using a pain scale of 1 to 10.
  Example: Pt c/o dull pain at wound site, a 4 on a scale of 1-10.
- If the patient's comments are entered in the patient's own words, enclose them in quotation marks.
  Example: Pt states, "I fell against a stone foundation while cutting the grass and slashed my leg."

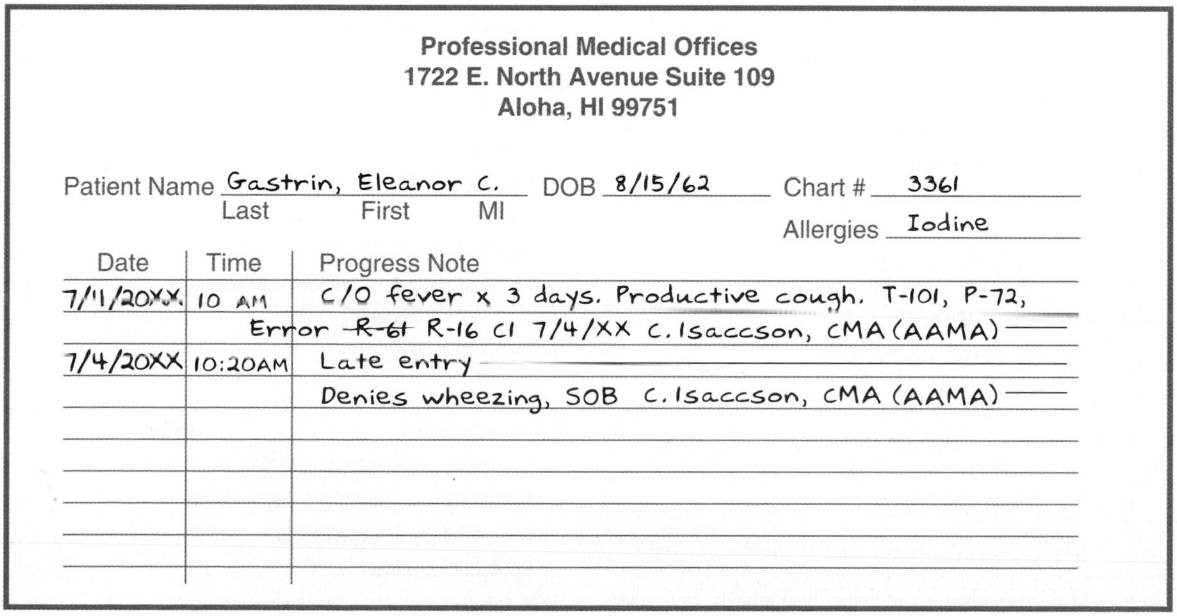

Professional Medical Offices
1722 E. North Avenue Suite 109
Aloha, HI 99751

Patient Name Gastrin, Eleanor C.   DOB 8/15/62   Chart # 3361
              Last   First   MI   Allergies Iodine

Date	Time	Progress Note
7/1/20XX	10 AM	C/O fever x 3 days. Productive cough. T-101, P-72,
		Error ~~R-6~~ R-16 CI 7/4/XX C. Isaccson, CMA (AAMA)
7/4/20XX	10:20AM	Late entry
		Denies wheezing, SOB C. Isaccson, CMA (AAMA)

FIGURE 21-12 Documentation correction.

Physician's Assessment of Body Systems

Appearance
Body build, posture, and gait
Height and weight fluctuation
Nutritional status
Hygiene and grooming
Emotional state and mood

Head and Neck
Size, shape, and contour of head
Hair and scalp
Palpation of neck, thyroid, and trachea
Difficulty swallowing
Change in voice, hoarseness

Eyes
Visual acuity and field
Inspection of eyelids and eyeballs
Pupillary reaction and eye movement
Inspection of internal eye structures
Measurement of ocular pressure

Nose
Size, shape, and symmetry
Deviated septum, nasal congestion
Sense of smell

Ears
Hearing deficits
Inspection of size, symmetry, placement
Discharge, ringing in the ears, infection

Mouth and Throat
Inspection of gums, teeth, tongue, pharynx
Bad breath, changes in salivation
Sense of taste

Respiratory
Size and shape of chest
Breath sounds
Phlegm, cough, sneezing, wheezing
Coughing of blood, asthma, emphysema
Upper or lower respiratory tract infections

Cardiovascular
Shortness of breath, chest pain
Reflected pain in the jaw, arms, upper back
Heart murmur, palpitations, night sweats
Cold or bluish hands, leg cramps, varicose veins
Hypertension, valvular disease

Gastrointestinal
Symmetry, tenderness, pain
Changes in appetite, nausea, vomiting
Jaundice, ulcers, gallstones
Bowel sounds
Change in bowel habits: diarrhea, constipation, hemorrhoids, stool color

Urinary
Changes in urinary habits: hesitancy, urgency, frequency, night voiding, pain when voiding, loss of stream force
Kidney stones, urinary tract infections
Dribbling, incontinence
Indicators of infections

Genitalia (Male)
Infertility, sterility, impotence
Testicular pain or mass
Penile discharge or discomfort
Erections, hernias
Prostate or testicular enlargement

Genitalia (Female)
Menses regularity, flow, pain, duration
Premenstrual symptoms, menopause
Obstetric history, birth control method
Breast symmetry, discharge, masses
Estrogen therapy, reproductive surgeries
Pain during intercourse, sterility

Lymph Glands
Enlargement, tenderness

Neurologic
Level of consciousness, headaches
Reflex reactions, general weakness
Speech changes, memory loss, seizures
Changes in balance, lack of coordination

Endocrine
Weight change, fatigue, bulging eyes
Increased thirst or hunger, neck swelling
Excessive sweating, heat or cold intolerance

Skin
Color, turgor, and tone
Lesions or scars
Temperature, rashes, itching
Moles, sores, acne

Arms and Legs
General appearance and symmetry
Palpation of arm muscles
Range of motion, limitation of movement
Inspection of fingernails
Deformities, joint stiffness
Gait

Legs and Feet
Symmetry, scars, bruises, swelling, open areas
Broken bones, deformity, sprains, strains
Gout, arthritis, osteoporosis
Inspection of toenails

- Document the complete medication history, including both prescription and OTC medications taken on a regular basis, the last dose taken of the medication, its effectiveness, and any other pertinent details.

  Example: Pt reports taking 2 ibuprofen tablets for pain with moderate relief; last dose taken 45 minutes ago.
- Record details about the previous history of the current CC.

  Example: Pt reports having a similar cough 3 weeks ago.
- When entering information in the medical record, sign the entry, including the appropriate initials after your name (e.g., CMA).
- Learn to be observant and to note anything that seems pertinent.
- Use accurate abbreviations, symbols, and terminology (Table 21-3).
- Review your documentation immediately after completion so that you can detect errors while the information is fresh in your mind.
- The electronic record system will automatically track any corrections made to the original documentation entry.
- If documenting in a paper record:
  - Do all charting in black ink except for noting allergies in red ink; never use pencil.
  - Write in a clear, legible manner.
  - Do not leave any blank spaces on the paper record and do not skip lines between documentation entries.
  - Never scribble, erase, or use whiteout on an error. For legal purposes, it is crucial that the corrected error be readable.
  - Correct the error by drawing one line through it. Write "error" above the corrected word or words and date and initial the correction. Then write in the correction.

- If details are omitted, add information by documenting after the last entry. Record "late entry," include date and time of note, and document the omitted information (see Figure 21-13).

Medical Terminology

Medical terminology is a language system based on Latin. It addresses processes that occur in specific body systems, procedures, diagnostics, and diseases. The system depends on the use of a suffix, which is defined first, a root word, and many times a prefix. The parts of the word are connected using a combining form "o," except in terms with a suffix that begins with a vowel. For example, *osteitis* is defined as inflammation (the suffix "-itis") of the bone (root word "oste"). The combining form "o" is not needed to connect the suffix and root word because the suffix begins with an "i." In the term *osteopathic*, the suffix "-ic" means pertaining to, and the two root words "path" (disease condition of) and "oste" (bone) are connected with the combining form "o."

If a word is unfamiliar to you, it is important to learn the meaning, correct spelling, pronunciation, and proper use of the term. Consistent use of a good medical dictionary is essential. To aid your learning, some frequently used medical word parts and their definitions are presented in Table 21-4. In addition, a terminology glossary is included in the back of this textbook, a vocabulary section appears at the beginning of each chapter, and an audio glossary of medical terms can be found on the Evolve website *(evolve.elsevier.com/kinn)*. Because the provider communicates using medical terminology and the medical assistant should use medical terms when documenting in the patient record, it is essential that you become comfortable and familiar with the medical language system and its correct use (Procedure 21-3).

TABLE 21-3 Medical Abbreviations

ABBREVIATION	DEFINITION	ABBREVIATION	DEFINITION
abd	abdomen	BOM	bilateral otitis media
ABG	arterial blood gases	BP	blood pressure
ac	before eating	BUN	blood urea nitrogen
ACLS	advanced cardiac life support	bx	biopsy
ad lib	as desired	c̄	with
AFP	alpha-fetoprotein	C&S	culture and sensitivity
AKA	above the knee amputation	CA	cancer
ASAP	as soon as possible	CABG	coronary artery bypass graft
ASHD	atherosclerotic heart disease	CAD	coronary artery disease
BE	barium enema	CBC	complete blood count
bid	twice a day	CC	chief complaint
BM	bowel movement	CHF	congestive heart failure
BMR	basal metabolic rate	CHO	carbohydrate

Continued

TABLE 21-3 Medical Abbreviations—*continued*

ABBREVIATION	DEFINITION	ABBREVIATION	DEFINITION
CNS	central nervous system	HTN	hypertension
c/o	complains of	Hx	history
COPD	chronic obstructive pulmonary disease	I&D	incision and drainage
CPK	creatinine phosphokinase	I&O	intake and output
CPR	cardiopulmonary resuscitation	IG	immunoglobulin
CSF	cerebrospinal fluid	lytes	electrolytes
CT	computed tomography	MI	myocardial infarction
CVA	cerebrovascular accident	NG	nasogastric
CXR	chest x-ray	NKA	no known allergies
DAT	diet as tolerated	NPO	nothing by mouth
dc	discontinue	N/V	nausea and vomiting
D&C	dilation and curettage	p	after
DDx	differential diagnosis	PE	pulmonary embolism
DM	diabetes mellitus	prn	as needed
DNR	do not resuscitate	pt	patient
DVT	deep vein thrombosis	PE	physical examination
Dx	diagnosis	PT	physical therapy
ECG	electrocardiogram	q	every
ENT	ears, nose, throat	RBC	red blood cells
FBS	fasting blood sugar	R/O	rule out
f/u	follow up	ROM	range of motion
FUO	fever of unknown origin	Rx	treatment
fx	fracture	$\overline{s}$	without
GC	gonorrhea	SOB	shortness of breath
GI	gastrointestinal	STD	sexually transmitted disease
GTT	glucose tolerance test	STAT	immediately
GU	genitourinary	Sx	symptoms
HCT	hematocrit	Tx	treatment
Hgb	hemoglobin	UA	urinalysis
HIV	human immunodeficiency virus	URI	upper respiratory infection
HPI	history of present illness	UTI	urinary tract infection
hs	at bedtime or hour of sleep	VS	vital signs

TABLE 21-4   Medical Word Parts

WORD PART	MEANING	WORD PART	MEANING	WORD PART	MEANING
a-	without	-cele	hernia	gastr/o	stomach
-ac	pertaining to	cephal/o	head	-genesis	forming
aden/o	gland	-cide	killing	gest/o	pregnancy
adip/o	fat	-clast	to break	-globin	protein
-al	pertaining to	colp/o	vagina	gloss/o	tongue
-algesia	sensitivity to pain	contra-	against	gluc/o	glucose, sugar
-algia	pain	crani/o	skull	-gram	recording
angi/o	blood vessel	-crit	to separate	hem/o	blood
ankyl/o	stiff	cyan/o	blue	hemi-	half
ante-	before	cyst/o	urinary bladder	hepat/o	liver
anter/o	front	cyt/o	cell	hist/o	tissue
anti-	against	-derma	skin	hydr/o	water
arter/o	artery	dipl/o	double	hyper-	above; excessive
arthro	joint	dors/o	back	hyp/o	deficient
articulo	joint	-dynia	pain	hyster/o	uterus
-ase	enzyme	dys-	painful, abnormal	-iasis	abnormal condition
ather/o	fatty plaque	-ectasia	dilation, stretching	infra-	below
aur/o	ear	-ectomy	excision	inter-	between
auto-	self	-emesis	vomiting	intra-	within
axill/o	armpit	-emia	blood condition	jaund/o	yellow
bi-	two	encephal/o	brain	kines/o	movement
bi/o	life	endo-	within	lact/o	milk
-blast	immature	enter/o	small intestine	-lapse	to sag
blephar/o	eyelid	eosin/o	red	later/o	side
brady-	slow	epi-	above	leuk/o	white
bucc/o	cheek	erythem/o	flushed; red	lip/o	fat
carcin/o	cancerous	-esis	condition	lith/o	stone
cardi/o	heart	eu-	good; normal	-lithiasis	condition of stones

Continued

TABLE 21-4   Medical Word Parts—*continued*

WORD PART	MEANING	WORD PART	MEANING	WORD PART	MEANING
-logy	study of	path/o	disease	-rrhea	flow
-lysis	to break down	-penia	deficiency	-sclerosis	hardening
macro-	large	-pepsia	digestion	-scope	instrument to visualize
mal-	bad	per-	through	semi-	half
-malacia	softening	peri-	surrounding	somat/o	body
mast/o	breast	-pexy	fixation	spl/o	spleen
medi/o	middle	-phagia	eating	-stasis	to stop
mega-	large	-phasia	speech	-stenosis	tightening
-megaly	enlargement	phleb/o	vein	stomat/o	mouth
morph/o	shape	-plasty	repair	-stomy	new opening
my/o	muscle	-plegia	paralysis	sub-	under
necr/o	death	-pnea	breathing	supra-	above
neo-	new	-poiesis	formation	tachy-	fast
nephr/o	kidney	poly-	many	thorac/o	chest
neur/o	nerve	post-	after	thromb/o	clot
odyn/o	pain	-prandial	meal	-tomy	cutting
olig/o	scanty	pre-	before	tox/o	poison
-oma	tumor; mass	proxim/o	near	trans-	across; through
onych/o	nail	prurit/o	itching	-tresia	opening
oophor/o	ovary	pseudo/o	false	tri-	three
ophthalm/o	eye	-ptosis	drooping; sagging	-tripsy	to crush
orch/o	testis	py/o	pus	ur/o	urine
orth/o	straight	pyel/o	renal pelvis	varic/o	varicose veins
oste/o	bone	pyr/o	fever	vascul/o	vascular
ot/o	ear	quadri-	four	ventr/o	front
pan-	all	ren/o	kidney	viscer/o	internal organs
para	near; beside	-rrhage	bursting forth	vit/o	life

PROCEDURE 21-3	Use Medical Terminology Correctly and Pronounce Accurately to Communicate Information to Providers and Patients

Goal: *To use medical terminology correctly so that you can effectively communicate with providers and explain terminology to patients.*

Scenario: *The physician has just examined Antonio Markus, age 19, and documents in the patient's record that he has bilateral otitis media, an URI, SOB and bronchitis. After the physician leaves the room, Antonio tells you he doesn't understand what the physician told him. Using your knowledge of medical terminology, review the physician's documentation and explain the medical terms to the patient.*

EQUIPMENT and SUPPLIES

- Patient's record
- Medical terminology dictionary or online reference site if needed
- Related educational materials

PROCEDURAL STEPS

1. Greet and identify the patient in a pleasant manner. Introduce yourself and explain your role.
   PURPOSE: To make the patient feel comfortable and at ease.
2. Review the physician's documentation. Look up the terminology if you are not sure of its meaning.
   PURPOSE: Medical terminology can be complicated for patients to understand. Healthcare workers should be cautious about using medical terms to explain a diagnosis.
3. Explain the physician's documentation in lay terms. Use restatement and clarification to make sure the patient understands the diagnosis and treatment plan. Make sure all medical terminology is adequately explained.
   PURPOSE: Therapeutic communication techniques help the medical assistant determine whether the patient understands the terminology; using feedback methods and making sure the patient understands medical terms helps relieve anxiety.
4. After you have explained the medical terms, make sure all the patient's questions have been answered.
5. Provide the patient with education materials that cover the details of his diagnosis and treatment plan.
   PURPOSE: To reinforce the diagnosis and verify treatment so that the patient understands; promotes compliance with the treatment plan.
6. Document the patient education intervention in the patient's health record.
   PURPOSE: Documentation verifies that the patient's questions were answered and educational materials were provided.

Documentation Methods

Problem-Oriented Medical Record

The problem-oriented medical record (POMR) is a form of documentation that introduces a logical sequence to recording the information obtained from the patient. It is based on the scientific method and was designed to present the patient's health problem efficiently and record systematically how it was managed. The medical history and physical examination fit into a special format that clarifies the patient's health problems. Each patient problem, or diagnosis, is defined and documented on a problem list sheet at the beginning of the medical record. Each time the patient is diagnosed with a new health problem, that diagnosis is added to the problem list in numeric order. If the patient is successfully treated for the health problem and cured, the provider documents next to that diagnosis on the problem list "Problem resolved" and dates it accordingly. Typically EHR systems have a section of the medical record that contains a current list of patient problems. Because the patient's diagnoses are identified and numbered at the beginning of the medical record, the POMR is very helpful for record audits. In addition, the format is designed for and easily adapted to EHR systems. The POMR system has four basic parts:

1. *Database:* This includes the patient's health history, the physical examination findings, and the results of baseline laboratory and diagnostic procedures. This information allows the provider to compile a health problem list for the patient.
2. *Problem list:* This list of the identified patient problems is kept in the front of the patient's record. It serves as a table of contents or index for the record and defines the patient's health concerns, including diagnoses, treatments, and educational needs. The problem list takes a holistic approach by including both psychosocial and physical needs. Each problem entered is listed numerically and dated and is supported by the database. The problems then are identified and referred to throughout progress note documentation by their assigned number. If over time an additional problem is identified, it is added to the problem list. If the problem is resolved, the date of problem resolution is entered next to the problem. For example, if Mr. Xu is diagnosed with hypertension and that particular health problem is listed as diagnosis #3, every time Mr. Xu comes to the office for follow-up of his blood pressure, the documentation piece begins by identifying the diagnosis by its number (#3). This system makes it very easy for the provider or medical assistant to scan the progress notes, review all documentation relating to diagnosis #3 (hypertension), and obtain a relatively quick and comprehensive history of how the patient's blood pressure is being managed and controlled.

PATIENT RECORD

Name: Fiddleman, Fred D.

Number:

Blood Type: A+

ALLERGIES/SENSITIVITY
Penicillin

Prob. No.	Date	PROBLEM DESCRIPTION	Date Resolved	Index	Prob. No.	Date	PROBLEM DESCRIPTION	Date Resolved	Index
1	10/2014	Hypertension - essential		✓					
2	10/2014	Diabetes mellitus (mild)		✓					
3	1/2014	Bilat. Grade II Retinopathy							
4	5/3/2015	L lower lobe pneumonia	5/2015						

Prob. No.	CONTINUING MEDICATIONS	Start	Stop	Prob. No.	CONTINUING MEDICATIONS	Start	Stop
1	Sinoserp 1 mg. b.i.d.	10/14	11/14				
2	Orinase 0.5 gm. daily	10/15	11/15				
1	Hydrodiuril 50 mg. A.M.	10/14					
2	1500 cal. diet low Na hi K	2/15					

Periodic Health Examination	Dates	1/13	3/14	3/14	6/15						

FIGURE 21-13 Initial plan for POMR progress notes.

3. *Plan:* This is a documented plan for each problem identified on the problem list. It outlines further studies, treatments, and patient education (Figure 21-13).

4. *Progress notes:* Using the first letter of each part of the progress notes spells the acronym SOAP; therefore, this portion of the POMR system is called the *SOAP notes* (or *SOAPE notes* when evaluation is included) (Figure 21-14). Each progress note uses the following format:

- **S** for *subjective* data: This information includes the purpose of the visit, with the patient's words in quotation marks, or a summary of the patient's statement about the chief complaint. For example, the subjective note may record exactly what the patient says, such as "I feel horrible, exhausted, coughing all night long." If the patient's exact words are not documented in quotation marks, the subjective entry typically starts with "Patient states ..., " "Patient c/o ...," or "Caregiver reports ..." The medical assistant documents this information based on details gained from the patient interview.

- **O** for *objective* data: This is anything that is observed or measurable, including vital signs, the exact anatomic location of an injury, difficulty with gait, and so on. Objective data can be measured repeatedly, which means that regardless of how many different healthcare workers observe the patient or document the sign, the same or very similar numbers or explanations would be given. The medical assistant is responsible for documenting complete and accurate objective data about all of the patient's signs. This information should be in such specific detail that even an individual who has not seen the patient can visualize the person's state of health. Typically the medical assistant documents only the subjective and objective data, leaving the remainder of the documentation to the provider.

- **A** for *assessment* of the problem: Usually this is the provider's preliminary diagnosis of the cause of the patient's chief complaint. The provider makes a judgment about what is wrong with the patient and documents it in this section; the medical assistant is not involved in this piece.

PROBLEM-ORIENTED PROGRESS NOTES

Name		DOB	Doctor
Jessica Michaels		9/20/2009	Frank Edwards, MD

DATE	TIME	PROBLEM NUMBER	FORMAT: Problem Number and TITLE: S = Subjective O = Objective A = Assessment P = Plan
10/15/15	9:30 AM	1	S: Mother states child has runny nose
			and sore throat x 2d. Taking Tylenol prn.
			O: Vital signs: T 98.8 (TA) P 96 R 24; Wt 42 lb.
			C. Isaccson, CMA (AAMA)
			A: Upper respiratory tract infection.
			P: 1. Prescribe Rondec DM, 1/2 tsp q6h prn
			cough and congestion.
			2. Mother to contact office if child does
			not improve. F. Edwards MD

FIGURE 21-14 Structured notes for the POMR system. (Courtesy Bibbero Systems, Petaluma, Calif.)

This is also the section where the medical assistant would go to abstract the diagnosis for billing purposes.

- **P** for the *plan* of care: This is the provider's documentation of how the health problem will be managed, including diagnostic studies, treatments, and patient education.
- **E** for *evaluation:* This is the assessment of the patient's understanding of the treatment or of the person's ability to comply with the treatment plan. It also may be used to document a follow-up on medication or treatments administered in the physician's office. For example, if a patient with asthma receives a breathing treatment during the office visit, a note is made regarding the effectiveness of the treatment.

CRITICAL THINKING APPLICATION **21-5**

Document the following scenario using the POMR method:

The patient c/o a sore throat with pain of 5 on a 1-10 scale and fever for 2 days. He has been taking OTCs for relief of symptoms. His VS are T 100.4, P 88, R 20. He also has an erythemic, papular rash across his chest.

S: ______________________________

O: ______________________________

Source-Oriented Medical Record

The source-oriented medical record (SOMR) is the most common form of record keeping used by physicians practicing in medical offices. The data in the patient record are organized in divided sections, which include the History and Physical (H&P), Progress Notes, Laboratory Results, Consultations, and so on. All information is filed in reverse chronologic order, with the most recent report or progress note placed on top. Progress notes are made each time the patient is seen or contacted by telephone. Documentation in the Progress Notes section is based on details surrounding the patient's chief complaint or the treatment protocol. For example, if a patient is being seen today for the flu, the note may read, "CC flulike symptoms, fever × 3 days, general discomfort, yellow nasal drainage, productive cough." The primary disadvantage of the SOMR system is that it can be very time-consuming to find a back entry about a particular problem or treatment.

Electronic Health Records

EHR systems are used in virtually every ambulatory care setting to collect and maintain patient information and to link healthcare information across healthcare facilities. EHR systems usually are designed for the particular needs of the practice. They are set up so that information is entered directly as the patient is interviewed or

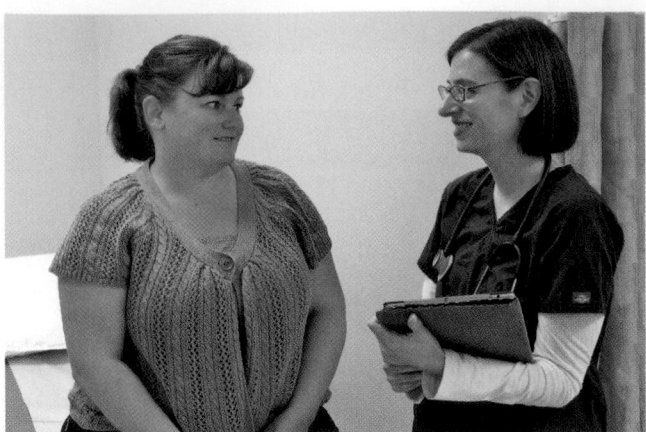

FIGURE 21-15 A medical assistant uses a tablet to conduct the patient interview.

assessed. This is done using tablets, laptop computers, or computer stations located throughout the facility (Figure 21-15).

Proponents of the EHR believe this type of record keeping reduces practice overhead and improves staff efficiency, cuts the cost of running the practice, and improves patient care. The EHR system can cut costs by reducing the physical resources needed to operate the practice (e.g., paper, chart material, copiers, and so on) and by drastically reducing the amount of space needed to store medical records. With the EHR, health records are on computerized files and therefore easily accessible, which saves time for the staff, and all documentation pieces are easily legible. In addition, the clinic's office system can be linked to the hospital or laboratory so that diagnostic tests can be downloaded into a patient's file and be readily available for the provider to review and share with the patient. The provider can also send electronic prescriptions to pharmacies, increasing the efficiency and accuracy of prescribing medication.

The most significant problem with EHR systems is that if a major electrical or computer malfunction occurs, patient information cannot be accessed. Backup files must be maintained, and special attention must be paid to patient confidentiality to prevent accidental sharing of private information.

"Meaningful Use" and Electronic Health Records

According to the EHR Incentive Programs established by the Centers for Medicare and Medicaid Services (CMS), "meaningful use" is the use of certified electronic health record (EHR) technology to:

- Improve the quality, safety, and efficiency of patient care
- Engage and empower patients and their families
- Improve the coordination of care across specialties and between ambulatory and inpatient care facilities
- Maintain the privacy and security of patient health information
- Improve the health of the general population and that of individual patients
- Increase the transparency of patient health information
- Enable the collection of health research data

Medicare and Medicaid EHR Incentive Programs provide financial incentives for the "meaningful use" of certified EHR technology. To receive an EHR incentive payment, eligible professionals and hospitals must show that they are "meaningfully using" their certified EHR technology by meeting certain established objectives. The incentive programs have three stages, each with increasing requirements for participation. All providers were to start meeting stage 1 requirements in 2011-2012 and stage 2 requirements in 2014 for 2 full years; in stage 3, which starts in 2016, providers are expected to show improved patient outcomes.

Some of the requirements for stage 1 included using an EHR system to track patient drug allergies and drug-to-drug interactions; transmit e-prescriptions; maintain current patient medication lists; record pertinent patient demographics (e.g., gender, race, ethnicity, smoking status); document changes in patients' vital signs; provide patients with electronic copies of their health information and clinical summaries for each office visit; protect EHR information with current technology; include lab test results in patient EHRs; use drug formularies; create lists of patients by specific conditions to compare and identify outcomes and possible outreach needs; communicate with patients about disease prevention, education, and follow-up care; evaluate current medication lists on new or referred patients; and provide a summary of care for patients transferring to another provider.

In addition to the core requirements listed for stage 1, in stage 2 providers must show they are using an EHR system to give patients online access to their health information and demonstrate that the system is capable of electronically submitting patient data to registries or immunization information systems as allowed by law; they also must show that they use secure electronic messaging to communicate with patients on relevant health information.

CLOSING COMMENTS

Patient Education

Finding time to conduct patient education in a busy healthcare practice can be challenging. Every opportunity to interact with patients should be considered a potential teaching moment. The perfect time to begin the education process is during the initial patient interview, when you first become aware of lifestyle factors or financial, social, or psychological problems that may affect the patient's wellness. Your interactions with patients and your use of therapeutic communications skills and interview techniques are crucial to the quality of care patients receive in your practice. One of the advantages of EHR systems is ready access to educational materials that can be downloaded and printed for patients to take home or e-mailed to patients upon request. This electronic tool makes it possible for healthcare workers to quickly provide educational materials that meet the patient's current needs.

Legal and Ethical Issues

The medical history is a confidential record that can be shared only with healthcare personnel directly involved in the patient's care. Data provided to you by the patient or that you read in the patient's health record are confidential; you must not share any of this information with anyone. The consequences for disclosing private information to individuals not involved in the patient's care can be very serious and can result in the loss of your job, court-imposed fines, and even imprisonment.

In addition to maintaining patient confidentiality, consistently implementing correct documentation procedures is crucial for medical practices. The medical record is considered a legal document, and court cases can be won or lost based on the clarity and completeness of staff documentation. It is essential that medical assistants document all patient information in a factual, nonjudgmental manner. Risk management practices focus on these problems as a way of reducing the chances of professional liability claims.

Elements of Sound Risk Management Practices

- Periodic review or audit of patients' records
- Consistent documentation of accurate and complete clinical facts and test results
- Adequate office procedures for informing patients of test results and for documenting this communication
- If paper records are used, appropriate use of abbreviations and legible recording in the patient's file; also, corrections made in the legally required manner
- Documentation that shows diagnostic test results were received and reviewed by the provider
- Documented evidence of appropriate discharge and continuing care instructions

Important Provisions of the Health Insurance Portability and Accountability Act (HIPAA)

- The patient has the right to request that the healthcare facility limit the disclosure of protected health information (PHI) for treatment, payment, and healthcare operations (TPO). For example, if the patient had an abortion 5 years ago, she may request that this information not be shared unless absolutely necessary.
- The healthcare facility is not required to comply with this request, but if agreement is reached, the restriction on sharing the information must be documented, and all employees must comply with the agreement. Therefore, if a provider referral includes sending the patient's record to a consulting physician, the medical assistant must make sure the restricted information is not included in the material sent or e-mailed.
- The patient has the right to request that confidential information be sent in a manner that the patient decides is best. For example, some patients may request that all phone calls from the office be made to a work number rather than to home, whereas others may give approval for messages to be left on the home answering machine or voice mail. Patients also can give approval that e-mail be used to send test results or confirm appointments. Whatever the patient's preference, this information must be documented and followed each time the patient is contacted.
- The healthcare facility owns the patient's record, but the patient owns the information in the record. Patient confidentiality must be secured regardless of the type of documentation or record system used in the healthcare setting. Safeguards mandated by HIPAA include:
  - Passwords to secure access to all electronic health records
  - Computer monitor shields to protect patient information if data are left on the screen
  - Turning monitors away from patient traffic areas to prevent accidental release of information
  - Securing all medical records

Professional Behaviors

The ability to communicate effectively is crucial to the role of the professional medical assistant. Effective communication includes the use of all of the therapeutic tools discussed in this chapter. The professional medical assistant should:

- Attend to nonverbal behaviors to verify congruence between what the patient states verbally and demonstrates via body language.
- Modify communication methods as needed to meet the needs of a diverse patient population.
- Use restatement, reflection and clarification to gather pertinent and comprehensive patient information.
- Utilize electronic communication appropriately and effectively.

SUMMARY OF SCENARIO

The office supervisor met with Chris and reviewed essential techniques for gathering patient information. Therapeutic communication includes demonstrating respectful patient care, using active listening skills, observing nonverbal behaviors, and using a combination of both open-ended and closed questions to gather the best possible detail about the patient's chief complaint. The supervisor gave Chris a variety of information on meeting the needs of a diverse patient population and also gave him suggestions on how to develop empathetic, helping relationships with patients. One suggestion she made was that Chris develop a community resource file, to which he can refer if a patient needs assistance outside the healthcare setting. Chris learned to identify the parts of the patient interview and became familiar with typical barriers to patient communication so that interviews would run more smoothly and he could gather more specific information from patients. Chris's workplace uses POMR documentation methods, so he reviewed the specifics of this type of record keeping with his supervisor. The significance of patient confidentiality was emphasized, and Chris agreed to work at implementing the techniques for therapeutic communication.

SUMMARY OF LEARNING OBJECTIVES

1. **Define, spell, and pronounce the terms listed in the vocabulary.**
   Spelling and pronouncing medical terms correctly reinforce the medical assistant's credibility. Knowing the definitions of these terms promotes confidence in communication with patients and co-workers.

2. **Use the concept of holistic care in the patient assessment process.**
   Holistic care involves assessing the patient's health status through the collection of physical, cognitive, psychosocial, and behavioral data. The medical assistant should consider all these factors when collecting data on the patient's health problems.

3. **Describe the components of the patient's medical history and how to collect the history information.**
   The medical history consists of the patient's database, past medical history, and family and social histories, in addition to the review of systems. A new patient should fill out a health history form, either online through a patient portal, electronically, or on paper.

4. **Discuss how to successfully understand and communicate with patients and display sensitivity to diverse populations.**
   Developing a professional helping relationship with patients is the responsibility of all healthcare workers. The helping relationship involves consistent application of respectful patient care that recognizes the impact of a patient's anxieties on interactions and responses to treatment. (See Procedure 21-1.)

   Sensitivity to diverse populations includes the use of empathetic communications and an awareness of the impact of individual value systems and personal prejudices on patient interactions.

5. **Demonstrate therapeutic communication feedback techniques to obtain information when gathering a patient history.**
   The linear communication model illustrates communication as an interactive process between the sender and the receiver of the message, with feedback as a crucial part of the process. Active listening techniques, which include restatement, reflection, and clarification, help the medical assistant go beyond hearing the message to actually listening and appropriately responding to the patient's main point. (Refer to Procedure 21-1.)

6. **Respond to nonverbal communication when interacting with patients.**
   Approximately 90% of patient interactions occur through nonverbal language. The key to successful patient interaction is congruence between verbal and nonverbal messages. (Refer to Procedure 21-2 and Table 21-1.)

7. **Identify barriers to communication and their impact on patient assessment; also, compare open-ended and closed-ended questions.**
   Optimum environmental conditions are important to a productive interview. Open-ended questions ask for general information and should be used to begin the interview, to introduce a new section of questions, or wherever the person introduces a new topic. Closed-ended questions are more direct and limit the answer to one or two words, typically yes or no.

8. **Do the following related to the patient interview:**
   - *Discuss the patient interview.*
     The interview should be considered a contract between you and your patient. Ask a variety of open-ended and closed-ended questions, and conclude the interview by summarizing the results of your interactions.
   - *Identify barriers to communication and their impact on patient assessment.*
     Certain communication styles can be misleading or can restrict the patient's response. The medical assistant must be careful to avoid using such faulty techniques as inappropriately providing reassurance, giving advice, using medical terminology without clarification, asking leading questions, and talking too much. These behaviors interfere with the process of gathering complete data during the interview and are obstacles to developing rapport with the patient.
   - *Detect a patient's use of defense mechanisms and the resultant barriers to therapeutic communication.*
     Patients use defense mechanisms to protect themselves in emotionally challenging situations. A medical assistant must consistently apply nonjudgmental therapeutic communication skills to maintain professional relationships.
   - *Demonstrate professional patient interviewing techniques.*
     The patient interview is divided into the introduction, the body, and the summary, or closing. Throughout the interview, the medical assistant should use professional interviewing techniques, such as empathetic patient care, sensitivity to patient diversity, active listening skills, appropriate nonverbal communication, attention to the interview environment, avoidance of communication barriers, and the framing of questions and statements in an open or closed manner, depending on the information needed and the patient's communication behaviors.

9. **Discuss the use of therapeutic communication techniques with patients across the lifespan.**
   Therapeutic communication techniques vary according to the patient's age and developmental level. A medical assistant should be aware of how to interact most effectively with various age groups, including young children, adolescents, adults, elderly patients, and family members. Age-specific application of interview styles enables clear communication between the health professional and the patient.

10. **Compare and contrast signs and symptoms.**
    Subjective findings are symptoms; they are perceptible only to the patient. *Objective findings* are *signs;* they can be observed and/or measured by the provider or medical assistant.

11. **Document patient care accurately in the medical record.**
    The ability to document accurately and completely is an essential skill for all medical assistants. Documentation should describe the patient's chief complaint, identify all pertinent signs and symptoms, and demonstrate correct use of medical terminology, with appropriate abbreviations. Any error in the health record must be corrected according to legally approved methods.

12. **Identify and define medical terms and abbreviations related to body systems; also, use medical terminology correctly and accurately to communicate information to providers and patients.**
    Medical terminology is a language that addresses processes that occur in specific body systems, procedures, diagnostics, and diseases. The

SUMMARY OF LEARNING OBJECTIVES—*continued*

system depends on the use of a suffix, which is defined first, a root word, and often a prefix. The parts of the word are connected using a combining form "o" except in terms with a suffix that begins with a vowel. (Refer to Tables 21-3 and 21-4 and Procedure 21-3.)

13. **Differentiate the documentation systems used in ambulatory care practices.**
    The POMR method uses SOAPE documentation to define the patient's health problems; the SOMR method organizes patient data into specific sections.

14. **Explain "meaningful use" as it applies to the electronic health record (EHR).**
    Eligible professionals and hospitals must achieve specific objectives to qualify for Medicare and Medicaid EHR Incentive Programs, which provide financial incentives for the "meaningful use" of certified EHR technology.
    "Meaningful use" includes using EHRs to:
    - Improve the quality, safety, and efficiency of patient care
    - Engage and empower patients and their families
    - Improve the coordination of care across specialties and between ambulatory and inpatient care facilities
    - Maintain the privacy and security of patient health information
    - Improve the health of the general population and that of individual patients
    - Increase the transparency of patient health information
    - Enable the collection of health research data

15. **Describe the role of patient education, in addition to legal and ethical issues, In the patient assessment process.**
    The perfect time to initiate patient education is during the initial patient interview. A medical assistant should take advantage of every teaching moment to get to know his or her patients and promote patient wellness. Risk management practices focus on reducing the chances of professional liability claims and maintaining compliance with HIPAA standards. Accurate, complete documentation in the patient's health record is crucial for successful risk management. In addition, maintaining strict confidentiality of patient information and factual, nonjudgmental recording of patient data are essential to professional patient care.

CONNECTIONS

Study Guide Connection: Go to the Chapter 21 Study Guide. Read and complete the activities.

evolve Evolve Connection: Go to the Chapter 21 link at *evolve.elsevier.com/kinn* to complete the Chapter Review Quiz. Check out the other resources listed for this chapter to make the most of what you have learned from Patient Assessment.

22

PATIENT EDUCATION

SCENARIO

Taylor DiSalvo is a medical assistant in a busy family practice. He currently is working with a patient, Sam Ignatio, who is 62 years old and has been married for 30 years. Mr. Ignatio has just been diagnosed with diabetes mellitus (DM) type 2. Although his mother and sister developed DM type 2 in their 60s, he knows very little about the disease and nothing about the strides that have been made in its treatment. In addition, his diet is high in saturated fat and carbohydrates (especially simple sugars because he loves sweet treats), and he does not exercise regularly. Mr. Ignatio is 50 pounds overweight, has functional deafness in his left ear and decreased sound quality in his right ear, and shows early signs of diabetic-related vision loss. Taylor is responsible for assisting with Mr. Ignatio's patient teaching plan.

Mr. Ignatio is faced with a serious illness, and his future health depends on compliance with a wide range of lifestyle changes. The methods Taylor chooses to coach this patient in managing his disease can have a significant effect on his eventual health outcome.

While studying this chapter, think about the following questions:

- How should Taylor begin Mr. Ignatio's patient education?
- What are some of Mr. Ignatio's individual characteristics that may affect his ability to learn all the information required to manage his disease?
- How can Taylor coach Mr. Ignatio so that he understands the importance of following treatment and disease-monitoring guidelines?
- What teaching approaches and materials would best meet the needs of this patient?
- Are any community resources available that could help Mr. Ignatio learn how to manage his disease?

LEARNING OBJECTIVES

1. Discuss the holistic model of patient education related to health and illness; also, instruct patients according to their needs to promote health maintenance and disease prevention.
2. Summarize the stages of grief and suggest therapeutic interactions for grieving patients.
3. List at least five guidelines for patient education that can affect the patient's overall wellness.
4. Do the following related to patient factors that affect learning:
   - Define six patient factors that have an impact on learning.
   - Display respect for individual diversity.
   - Summarize educational approaches for patients with language barriers.
5. Do the following related to the teaching plan:
   - Determine possible barriers to patient learning.
   - Assess the patient's needs.
   - Determine the teaching priorities.
   - Decide on the appropriate teaching materials.
   - Develop a list of community resources related to patients' healthcare needs and facilitate referrals to community resources in the role of patient navigator.
   - Decide on the appropriate teaching methods.
   - Implement the teaching plan.
   - Demonstrate the ability to develop an appropriate and effective patient teaching plan.
6. Describe the role of the medical assistant in patient education.
7. Integrate the legal and ethical elements of patient teaching into the ambulatory care setting; also, discuss applications of the Health Insurance Portability and Accountability Act (HIPAA).

This chapter focuses on helping students recognize the individual learning needs of patients. It also provides guidelines for developing effective teaching approaches. The key to patient compliance with prescribed treatments is empowerment; that is, providing the patient with information and support that enable the person to take charge of his or her health problem. The concepts in this chapter are basic to all patient education interventions. Putting them into practice, as a medical assistant, can help you improve both a patient's understanding of the disease process and his or her willingness to comply with the disease management steps recommended by the provider.

PATIENT EDUCATION AND MODELS OF HEALTH AND ILLNESS

Patient education should begin with the first contact between the patient and the healthcare team. A well-informed patient is more likely to comply with treatment and adopt a healthy lifestyle. However, informing a patient about his or her disease is only part of the health teaching process. The key to successful health teaching is to empower the patient to accept the responsibility of his or her disease process and to become willing to implement teaching guidelines.

As a result of reductions in hospital admissions and shorter hospital stays, patients and families have had to assume responsibility for care that once was provided by the hospital staff. This means that those who work in ambulatory care settings have an even greater responsibility to meet the educational needs of their patients. To develop an effective teaching approach, we must implement a holistic model that considers not only the patient's physical state, but also his or her psychological, sociocultural, intellectual, and economic needs (Figure 22-1). The holistic model suggests that we look at patients and determine their needs based on a complete view of their lives rather than just as an analysis of their specific diseases. It is our responsibility not only to teach patients about disease processes, but also to help them implement related skills and changes in lifestyle to promote recovery and improve function. In the case of Mr. Ignatio, diabetes mellitus is a complicated disease that requires an in-depth understanding of the disease process, in addition to making significant lifestyle changes. When considering the impact of this diagnosis on the patient (in this case, Mr. Ignatio), the medical assistant should keep in mind the following factors, because they will affect the patient's response.

- *Psychological effect of the disease:* Is Mr. Ignatio in shock and denial? Is he angry or depressed? How will his emotional reaction to the diagnosis affect his response to patient education and coaching efforts?
- *Sociocultural impact:* How will his family and employer respond to the demands of the diagnosis? Does he have a support system that will assist him in making healthy lifestyle choices?

- *Intellectual impact:* Is Mr. Ignatio able to understand the complexities of the disease and treatment recommendations?
- *Economic impact:* Can he afford the treatment for diabetes? Does he have health insurance to cover the cost, or will he need assistance in paying for ongoing diagnostic and treatment recommendations?
- *Spiritual impact:* What is Mr. Ignatio's spiritual response to his diagnosis? How might his spiritual beliefs affect his compliance with treatment?

The health belief model may help you understand why some people do not follow recommended guidelines to maintain their health and prevent the development of disease.

The model focuses on individuals' attitudes toward and beliefs about themselves and their health. The model suggests that we first consider how the patient perceives his or her risk of developing a disease and the possible severity of the condition. For example, even though Mr. Ignatio's mother and sister developed diabetes type 2, he may believe he is not going to have the same problem. Therefore, even though wellness information recommends that he lose weight, exercise, and eat a healthy diet, he may not believe he is in danger of developing diabetes; consequently, he doesn't believe he needs to follow disease prevention recommendations. He may also believe that even if he does develop diabetes, the consequences of the disease are not that serious, so why bother altering his lifestyle to prevent it?

Another factor considered in the health belief model is the patient's perceived benefits of action; that is, whether the patient believes altering his or her health behaviors will prevent the person from developing the disease or from suffering serious complications. In this case, because Mr. Ignatio has a strong family history of the disease, he may have decided he was going to get diabetes anyway, so why should he bother exercising and watching his diet? Until the patient believes that teaching and health promotion guidelines affect him and are worth pursuing, he will not follow suggested health promotion tips or comply with treatment protocols.

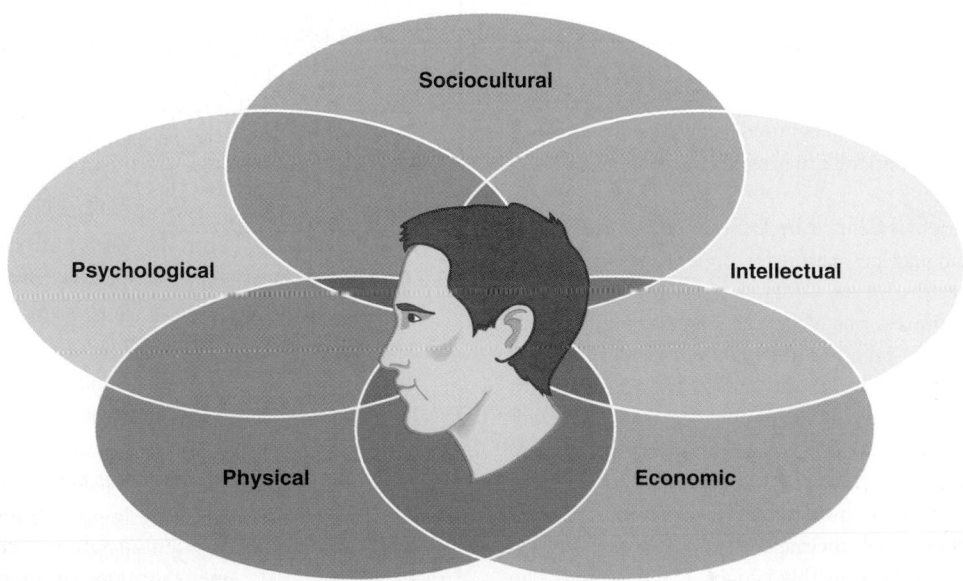

FIGURE 22-1 The holistic approach.

TABLE 22-1	Health Belief Model	
PRINCIPLES	**DEFINITION**	**PATIENT EDUCATION**
Perceived susceptibility	Patient's opinion on the chances of developing a disorder	Supply information on the risk level; individual risk is based on the patient's health habits and family history.
Perceived severity	Patient's opinion on the seriousness of the condition and its health risks	Outline the potential complications of the disease.
Perceived benefits	Patient's belief in the value of altering lifestyle factors and complying with treatment	Emphasize the positive results that can be achieved if the patient complies with healthcare recommendations.
Perceived barriers	Patient's opinion on the financial and psychological costs of compliance	Identify patient barriers and work to reduce them through patient education, family outreach, and use of community resources.
Cues to action	Methods developed to activate patient compliance	Provide one-on-one education interventions; detailed handouts; family involvement in education efforts; follow-up at subsequent office visits; referral to community resources.
Self-efficacy	Patient has the confidence to take action to achieve a healthier state	Provide ongoing education and support.

Table 22-1 outlines the health belief model and suggests methods for applying the model in patient teaching and coaching efforts in the ambulatory care setting.

The five stages of grief, as defined by Dr. Elisabeth Kübler-Ross, are another model that may be helpful for understanding the way patients respond to health threats. When a patient faces a serious health threat, the grief process may delay the person in adjusting to the disease and starting to take control of his or her health. For example, Mr. Ignatio may respond to the news of his diagnosis with what is commonly the first stage of the grief process—denial. Both his father and sister suffered serious complications from diabetes, including blindness and leg amputation, and he may be using denial to deal psychologically with the burden of the diagnosis.

Each individual goes through the stages of grief in his or her own way and at his or her own pace. This process can take weeks to months; however, until the patient reaches the point of accepting the diagnosis and the possible ramifications of the disease, compliance with patient education will be very difficult to achieve.

The five stages of grief are:

- *Denial and isolation.* The patient denies the existence of the disease, may be unwilling to accept the reality of the situation, and refuses to discuss the health problem or remember health teaching interventions. For example, Mr. Ignatio refuses to meet with the dietitian because he says his diet is fine and there is no need to change it.
- *Anger.* The patient may be very angry and hostile when forced to discuss the condition. Mr. Ignatio may say, "Why did this happen to me? I am a good person, why did I get diabetes?"
- *Bargaining.* The patient tries to bargain for privileges or time. Mr. Ignatio may say, "Look, I know I'm supposed to start this new diet, but Christmas is coming. I'll meet with the dietitian after the holidays."
- *Depression.* The patient grieves the loss of health. Mr. Ignatio may be very sad about the diagnosis. He doesn't want to have to deal with the complexities of the disease, he just wants it to go away so he can live his life without the fear of diabetic complications.
- *Acceptance.* The patient finally gets to the point where he or she accepts the diagnosis and is ready to make the best of it. At this point, Mr. Ignatio may be willing to use community resources for education and support.

Therapeutic Interactions for Grieving Patients

Denial and isolation: Reinforce each education intervention with handouts that explain the disease and treatment. Encourage the patient's family to attend visits to the provider's office and to become involved in the patient's care. For example, if a patient has been diagnosed with diabetes, provide a list of approved online resources or YouTube videos so that the patient and/or family can learn more about diabetes privately at home.

Anger: Use therapeutic communication techniques, especially reflection, to acknowledge the patient's feelings about the diagnosis. Recognize the patient's need to use defense mechanisms as protection from the reality of the disease (these topics are addressed in more detail in the Patient Assessment chapter). Remember, the patient is not angry at you or the provider; he or she is angry about the diagnosis and its accompanying challenges.

Bargaining: Rely on the provider's recommendations regarding postponing certain treatments. Discuss the patient's bargaining requests with the provider and other staff members to work out a solution that promotes patient compliance with healthcare recommendations.

Depression: Use available community resources to provide support for the patient and family. The provider may recommend that the patient attend a support group, meet with a dietitian, or use professional counseling services to deal with depression.

Acceptance: Take advantage of this time to renew education efforts by providing multiple methods for learning about the disease, such as DVDs, professional websites, YouTube videos, and community support services.

Patient Factors That Affect Learning

Many factors or characteristics may affect the patient's ability to learn. Medical assistants must be aware of these factors to develop a coaching approach that best meets the needs of each patient.

Guidelines for Patient Education

- Provide knowledge and skills to promote recovery and health.
- Encourage patient ownership and participation in the teaching process.
- With the patient's approval, include the family and significant others in education interventions.
- Promote safe, appropriate use of medications and treatments.
- Encourage patient adaptation to healthy behaviors.
- Provide information about accessing community resources.

Perception of Disease Versus Actual State of Disease

Patients respond to a particular diagnosis in many different ways. One predictor of how a patient will respond, and therefore how he or she will react to health education, is the patient's perception of the disease. Previous life experiences may greatly influence the patient's knowledge base and/or desire to learn about the disease. Does the patient recognize and accept the seriousness of the diagnosis? Or, perhaps, does the patient overreact to potential disease risks? Both of these responses affect the patient's willingness to learn about the disease and his or her compliance with treatment recommendations.

How do you think Taylor's patient education efforts will be affected if Mr. Ignatio does not consider diabetes a serious disease?

Patient's Need for Information

The patient's perception of the impact of the disease on his or her general health also determines the need for information about the disease. Does the patient express a desire to learn all he or she can about the disease, or does the patient resist or act indifferent to teaching efforts? A vital part of patient education is encouraging patient ownership of the learning process. To accomplish this, you first may have to persuade the patient that he or she needs to understand the disease before an improvement in overall wellness can be achieved.

Mr. Ignatio tells Taylor that his father had diabetes and had to have both legs amputated; eventually he died of the disease. Mr. Ignatio says it doesn't matter whether he controls his blood sugar; he'll still have major health complications. What is the appropriate response?

Patient's Age and Developmental Level

Depending on the patient's age and ability to understand information about the disease, you may have to adapt the teaching plan to meet specific learning needs. For example, educating a 9-year-old patient with DM type 1 about disease management requires a different approach from one that would be used for Mr. Ignatio. You should be flexible and creative in providing learning opportunities that support the provider's attempt to educate the patient about

disease prevention and health maintenance. Often the key to patient understanding and compliance is the involvement of family members.

During his assessment of Mr. Ignatio's diet, Taylor learns that his wife cooks all his meals and packs his lunch daily. He loves bread and desserts, and he tells Taylor he's too old to change his diet now. What should Taylor do to make sure Mr. Ignatio's diet complies with diabetic recommendations?

Patient's Mental and Emotional State

Even a well-planned teaching intervention can be ineffective if the patient is unable to pay attention because of anxiety, stress, anger, or denial (Figure 22-2). Frequently patients use defense mechanisms to protect themselves from the reality of a serious illness. It is important that the medical assistant be sensitive to the patient's mental state and adapt teaching interventions as needed. If a patient is overwhelmed by the diagnosis and his body language cues are defensive, limit the amount of information at this time to what he must know immediately about his disease, rather than trying to teach him detailed facts.

Mr. Ignatio has just been diagnosed with diabetes. He has already shared that his father died of diabetes. Do you think he is able to pay attention to coaching efforts about a diabetic diet? What should Taylor do to manage this problem?

Influence of Multicultural and Diversity Factors on Patient Education

Culture, family background, and religious beliefs influence patients' actions. Working with patients from diverse backgrounds is an exciting challenge; however, for your patient education to be successful, it is essential that you recognize and are sensitive to the impact of these factors on patient learning (Figure 22-3). Some questions you should consider when teaching a patient from another background include:

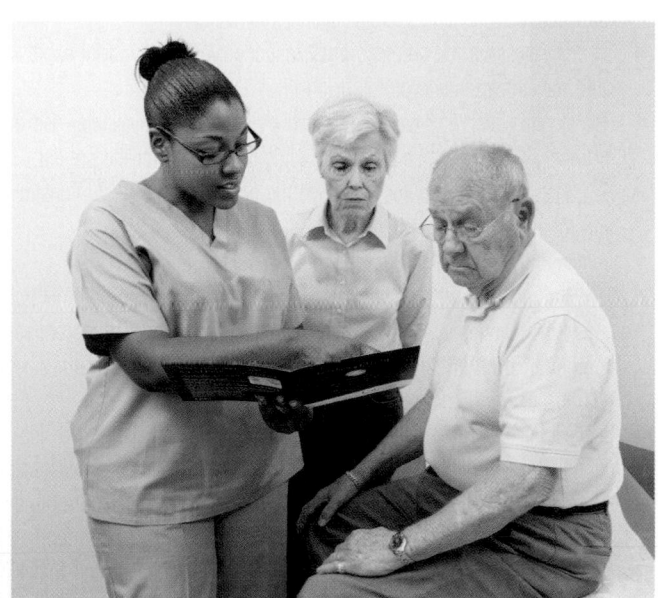

FIGURE 22-2 Demonstrating sensitivity to the patient's needs.

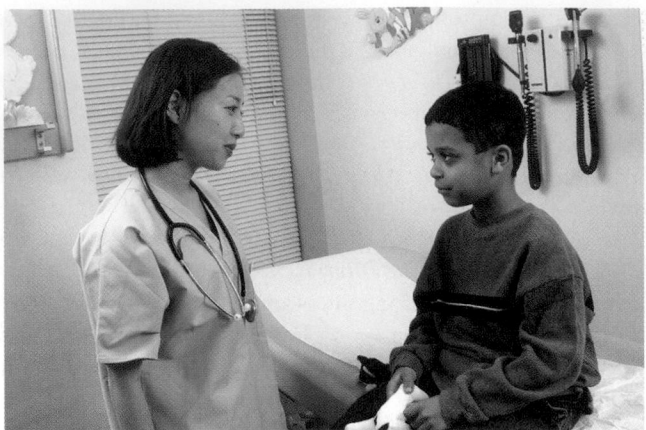

FIGURE 22-3 Considering diversity.

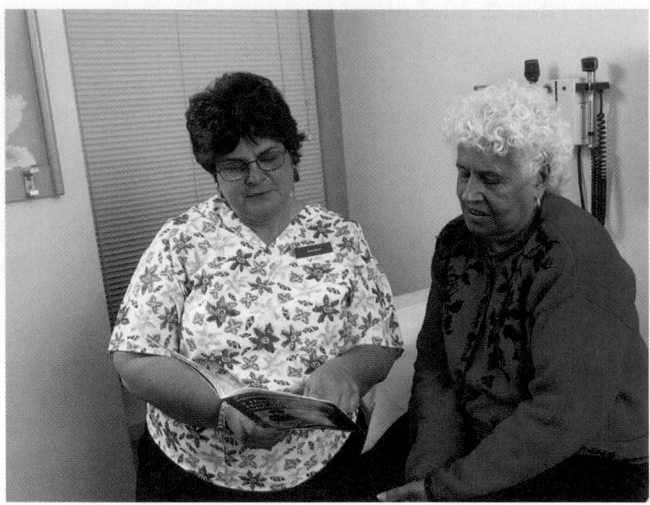

FIGURE 22-4 Using language-appropriate educational booklets.

- Is language an issue with your patient (Figure 22-4)? If the patient is unable to understand spoken English or to read it correctly, do you have an alternative method for getting the information across?
- Do the patient's culture, ethnic background, or religious beliefs influence the way he or she perceives disease and the role of healthcare workers?

Approaches for Language Barriers

- Determine whether the patient can read and/or understand English.
- Address the patient by his or her last name (e.g., Mrs. Martinez, Mr. Nugyen).
- Be courteous and use a formal approach to communication.
- Use gestures, tone of voice, facial expressions, and eye contact to emphasize appropriate parts of the discussion.
- Integrate pictures, handouts, models, and other aids that visually depict the material.
- Carefully observe the patient's body language, especially facial expression, for understanding or confusion.
- Use simple, everyday words as much as possible. If available, use a dictionary that translates as many words as possible for the patient.
- Demonstrate all procedures and have the patient return the demonstration to check for understanding.
- Implement the teaching plan in small, manageable steps.
- Give the patient written instructions for all procedures and treatments.
- If possible, have an interpreter present or have access to an online interpreter; if an interpreter is not available, a family member may be able to help with communication.
- If available, provide educational materials in the patient's native language. For example, vaccine information sheets (VIS) are available online in multiple languages from the Centers for Disease Control and Prevention (CDC); send materials home in English if a family member can interpret the material for the patient; refer the patient and family to online sources of educational materials in their native language.

- What strategies or techniques might minimize patient education problems?
- Are community resources available that could facilitate patient learning?

Patient Learning Style

All of us have a preferred way of learning; that is, methods that work best for us to learn new material. Patients also have a learning preference that reflects their individual learning style. Some patients learn best from discussion or lecture, whereas others must take time to think about the material before they understand it. Some patients can learn from observing; others must act or do something with the material to learn it. Start your teaching intervention by asking your patient how he or she prefers to learn new material, and pattern your teaching interventions along those lines.

Mr. Ignatio tells Taylor that he could never learn things by listening to someone tell him what to do. What approach to learning might best meet his needs?

Impact of Physical Disabilities

The patient first must be assessed to determine whether he or she can adequately hear instructions, see written material, and manipulate any required treatment equipment. All teaching efforts are lost if disabilities interfere with a patient's capacity to understand information or to handle equipment properly. A hearing or speech impairment may require the use of sign language with supplemental written instructions. If the patient is unable to manipulate equipment because of a physical disability or vision problem, family or adaptive equipment may be necessary for the patient to manage his or her care.

Mr. Ignatio's physical assessment revealed hearing and vision problems. Is he able to understand verbal instructions clearly? What can be done to adapt the teaching intervention to meet his needs?

Therapeutic Communication With Patients With Special Needs

Patients With Vision Loss

- Alert the patient that you are in the room and identify yourself; do not touch the patient without warning.
- The patient is unable to pick up on your body language; use clear, concise language and a normal tone of voice.
- Provide all written material in a large font or print size; large-print educational materials often can be ordered
- Supply reliable Internet sources for information and provide audio material if possible.

Patients With Hearing Loss

- Stand in front of the patient or within the person's field of vision before you begin speaking; the patient may be able to lip-read.
- You may need to touch the patient lightly to get her or his attention.
- Use *expanded speech*; lower the tone of your voice and pronounce each syllable. Do not raise your voice or shout to be heard. The louder your voice, the higher the tone, and aging ears find high-pitched sounds the most difficult to interpret.
- Carefully observe the patient's body language for understanding or confusion.
- Use gestures or demonstration as needed to get the message across.
- Clearly print any information needed to clarify the patient teaching.
- If a patient is wearing a hearing aid, ask him or her whether it is on and working before starting the conversation; the patient may turn a hearing aid off to prevent annoying background noise.
- Provide written handouts that review the material being taught.
- Request family assistance in verifying that the patient received and understood the material.
- Refer patients and families to appropriate online resources

---

CRITICAL THINKING APPLICATION 22-1

Implement the holistic education model and the health belief model to determine and respond to Mr. Ignatio's individual learning needs.

THE TEACHING PLAN

What is it that patients need to know to manage a disease effectively? What is it about an individual patient that needs to be addressed for a teaching intervention to work? What are the immediate and long-term goals of patient education? What teaching materials or strategies should be used to meet the patient's learning needs and also effectively relay the information? How can the teaching plan be implemented successfully? How do you, as a medical assistant, manage the limited time available for patient coaching? How do you know the patient is learning and actually converting this knowledge into disease management? A vital aspect of patient teaching is to be flexible and to provide information about what patients want to know when patients want to know it. These and other guidelines for developing an appropriate and effective teaching plan follow.

Assess the Patient's Learning Needs

Developing a teaching plan that works for a particular individual first requires an assessment of the patient as a learner and consideration of any characteristics that might affect the learning process. Many of these factors already have been addressed, such as the patient's learning preference, perception of the illness, age, background, multicultural influences, language barriers, and disabilities. The medical assistant also must consider what the patient already knows about the diagnosis and whether that knowledge includes misconceptions about the disease.

The goal of the assessment process is to create a teaching plan that meets the patient's needs for understanding and managing his or her illness. Therefore, in the learning assessment, the medical assistant should consider what the patient needs to know, what the patient wants to know, and what can be done in the time available for learning.

Before developing a specific approach to patient education, you must consider potential barriers to learning other than those already presented, such as the presence of pain. A patient in acute distress is unable to concentrate on the information. In this case, the amount of material must be adjusted to meet the patient's immediate needs, and time should be planned in the future for a more in-depth teaching session.

Does Mr. Ignatio exhibit any potential barriers to learning about his disease?

Possible Barriers to Patient Learning

- Individual learning style
- Age and developmental level
- Use of defense mechanisms
- Language
- Motivation to learn
- Physical limitations or disabilities
- Emotional or mental state
- Cultural or ethnic background
- Pain
- Time limitations

Determine the Teaching Priorities

Once you have done an adequate assessment of your patient as a learner and you understand your patient's learning needs, the next question is, "Where do I start?" A patient such as Mr. Ignatio has a significant amount of information to learn before he can manage his disease completely. The volume of information might seem overwhelming unless priorities are established. How do you figure out what material should be first? The first question to ask is, "What is the patient's immediate versus long-term needs?" What must this patient learn today to be able to take care of himself, and what does he need to know overall about his illness to promote healthy behaviors?

Because the patient learning assessment told you what your patient knows about his or her disease, that is a good place to start. Confirm what the patient knows about the problem and attempt to correct any potential misconceptions. If you start with something the patient knows and understands, he or she will feel more competent and capable of managing new material. You then should go on to the new material that is causing the patient the most anxiety. If the patient is nervous or afraid about a particular aspect, he or she will be unable to pay attention to any other new material until that anxiety has been addressed.

For example, if Mr. Ignatio is most concerned about pricking his finger for a glucometer reading, that is the first skill he should learn. Once he is confident about that particular part of treatment, he will be able to pay attention to diet and exercise recommendations. You should always begin with the basic details about the disease and add more information during each patient visit.

Every interaction with the patient is an opportunity for health education. A major problem with delivering high-quality patient education in an ambulatory healthcare setting is the lack of time you have to spend with each patient. Therefore, you must take advantage of every "teaching moment"; that is, every time you interact with a patient, use it as an opportunity to assess the patient's current education needs and provide as much information or guidance about that specific learning need as possible during the time available.

Use the waiting room as a place for learning by providing up-to-date educational materials on a wide variety of health issues. Many facilities have DVD equipment in the waiting room for patient education while the patient is waiting to be seen. These can be specific to the type of practice or can provide general health information. Another good location for educational materials is in the examination rooms. The patient may be more likely to pick up brochures on sensitive topics such as types of contraceptives, the procedures for performing testicular or breast exams, or information about sexually transmitted infections in the privacy of a closed exam room.

Decide on the Appropriate Teaching Materials

What teaching materials would best meet the needs of your patient? A wide variety of patient education materials is available, and deciding which materials best meet your patient's needs depends on the patient's learning preference, individual characteristics, and lifestyle factors. Individualized instruction is the key to understanding and patient compliance; however, additional materials can help reinforce the information.

When possible, all patient instruction should include a handout or online reference that reinforces information and that the patient can use as a resource. Patient factors such as the use of defense mechanisms, emotional state, and language barriers can limit the patient's ability to comprehend and remember information. Printed information is needed to help the patient and the patient's family understand what is happening and what needs to be done to improve the patient's health (Figure 22-5). Informational flyers can be ordered from medical office suppliers, pharmaceutical company representatives, and health education companies. In addition, most electronic health record (EHR) systems include a package for printing out or e-mailing diagnose-specific educational materials. Many hospitals also offer free educational materials about diagnostic procedures, immunizations, and other disease-related topics. The ambulatory

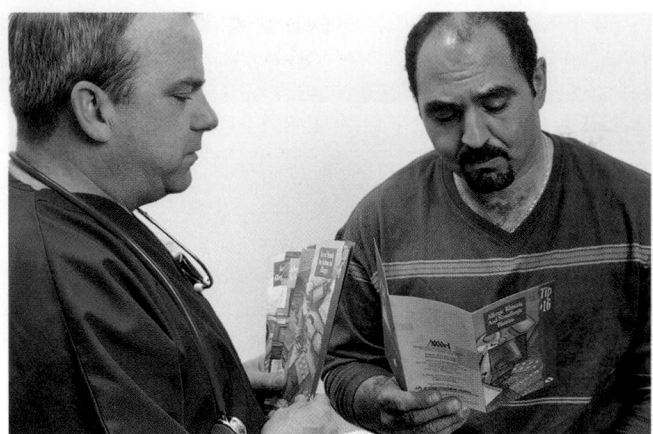

FIGURE 22-5 Reviewing printed information.

care setting where you are employed may develop its own educational materials.

Some guidelines to follow if you are responsible for developing or ordering educational supplies include the following:

- The material should be written in lay language at about a sixth grade level to promote general patient understanding.
- Information should be well organized and clearly described.
- All material should be checked for accuracy.
- Handouts should be attractive and professional.
- Copies should be available in other languages when possible and in large print for visually impaired clients.

Identifying Community Resources

One role of the medical assistant in ambulatory care settings is to assist patients and their families in finding and using community education and support services. The healthcare facility should keep an up-to-date file of area resources. The information should include the name of the group and the services provided; the contact person; a telephone number and address; meeting times and location if applicable; and a related website if available (see Procedure 22-1). This information can be found in a number of locations, such as the blue pages of the local phone book, through the community outreach or speakers bureau of area hospitals, or online by searching for area educational institutions at *.edu* sites or local chapters of national organizations at *.org* sites. For example, the American Cancer Society operates local branches throughout the United States, and information on local services can be found on the national home page (*www.cancer.org*).

An excellent comprehensive Internet site operated by the U.S. National Library of Medicine and the National Institutes of Health is MedlinePlus. Both health professionals and consumers can depend on it for accurate information that is updated frequently. The site provides a variety of information about health issues, an extensive list of diseases and conditions, a medical encyclopedia and dictionary, health information in Spanish, extensive details on prescription and nonprescription drugs, health information from the media, and links to thousands of clinical trials. It can be bookmarked at *medlineplus.gov*. Another excellent source of current information on diseases is the Centers for Disease Control and Prevention (CDC) website at *www.cdc.gov/*.

Other teaching materials include DVDs, approved YouTube links, and health-related applications that can be accessed by smart phone or computer to help patients learn about their disease and track their progress. These learning aids promote self-directed and self-paced learning. They also permit the patient to access material in a nonstressful environment, which improves the patient's learning potential. Depending on the patient's age or access to the appropriate technology, using media resources or referring the patient to provider-approved healthcare sites on the Internet can help develop patient ownership of the learning process and provide excellent resources for patient referral. However, using the Internet as a resource for patient education information has its drawbacks. It is important that the patient understand that there is no oversight or control over information posted on the Web; therefore, some sites may offer information that is erroneous, out of date, or misleading. Provide patients with accurate, well-researched sites and/or keep informed about what sites patients are accessing to make sure online recommendations support the provider's treatment protocol. The following website, posted by the National Institutes of Health, can help you learn how to assess Internet health information: *www.nlm.nih.gov/medlineplus/webeval/*

The Medical Assistant as a Patient Navigator

According to the American Medical Association, a patient navigator is a person who helps patients and families with insurance problems, explains treatment and care, communicates with the healthcare team, assists caregivers, and manages medical paperwork. This definition describes the role of the medical assistant as a patient advocate in ambulatory care settings.

The concept of patient navigation was pioneered in 1990 by Dr. Harold P. Freeman, a surgical oncologist at Harlem Hospital, for the purpose of eliminating barriers to timely cancer care for the indigent and underserved. In response to this need, the Patient Navigator Outreach and Chronic Disease Prevention Act of 2005 was passed to make grants available for the development of patient navigator programs. The original goal of patient navigation was to help people overcome barriers such as poverty, low literacy, or lack of health insurance that were preventing patients from gaining access to medical care. However, the care for illnesses such as cancer can be so complicated that patients, regardless of income or education level, can benefit from expert assistance. In fact, under a new requirement for accreditation by the American College of Surgeons Commission on Cancer, cancer centers must have started providing patient navigation services by 2015. Most recently, the Affordable Care Act required that "insurance navigators" be available to help consumers research and enroll in health insurance through the law's health insurance marketplace.

Because medical assistants are cross-trained in both administrative and clinical skills, they are in a unique position to serve as patient navigators in ambulatory care settings.

PROCEDURE 22-1 | **Develop a List of Community Resources for Patients' Healthcare Needs; also, Facilitate Referrals in the Role of Patient Navigator**

As a medical assistant, one of your roles will be to help patients who need community health education or support services. To prepare for this role, you should collect a minimum of 25 community resources available in your area (e.g., support groups, educational workshops, dietary assistance, national organizations, medical equipment suppliers). In your directory, include the following information: name of the group; services provided; contact person; telephone number; address; meeting times and locations (if applicable); and a related website. As a patient navigator, apply what you have learned about community resources to assist the patient in the following scenario.

Goal: *To develop a list of community resources and perform the role of patient navigator by referring patients to resources.*

Scenario: Role-play the following scenario with your partner.

Mr. Tomás Garcia was admitted to the hospital last week for an acute myocardial infarction (MI). Mr. Garcia is 54 years old, overweight, smokes two packs of cigarettes a day, eats fast food almost daily, has a family history of heart disease, and works as a carpenter. The provider recommends that he lose weight; follow a diet high in fiber and low in saturated fat; and quit smoking. What community resources might help educate and support Mr. Garcia in making these complex lifestyle changes?

EQUIPMENT and SUPPLIES

- Patient's health record
- Educational handouts
- Computer with Internet connection and printer
- Quiet, private area

PROCEDURAL STEPS

1. Greet and identify the patient in a pleasant manner. Introduce yourself and explain your role.
   <u>PURPOSE</u>: To make the patient feel comfortable and at ease.

PROCEDURE 22-1 —continued

2. Take the patient to a quiet, private area that has computer access.
   PURPOSE: A quiet, private area is necessary to protect confidentiality and prevent interruptions.

3. Assess Mr. Garcia's needs, and identify factors that may limit his ability to learn and implement lifestyle changes. Use restatement, reflection, and clarification to verify the information.
   PURPOSE: Therapeutic communication techniques help you gather complete information and address the patient's immediate needs; it also improves the likelihood of success.

4. Speak in a pleasant, distinct manner, remembering to maintain eye contact with your patient.
   PURPOSE: Positive nonverbal behaviors create a friendly, caring atmosphere.

5. Remain sensitive to the individual needs of your patient throughout the interview process.

PURPOSE: Be aware of your personal biases, but do not let them affect the way you treat your patients; make sure to respect patients' diverse backgrounds.

6. Provide Mr. Garcia with appropriate handouts and a list of community resources that might be helpful. Print out this information or e-mail it to the patient for future use. One of the handouts could include a list of provider-approved websites the patient can consult.
   PURPOSE: Make sure the patient has all the handouts with him before he leaves the office; also make sure he has a list of appropriate online sites he can check out later for additional information and support.

7. Answer any questions the patient may have; use clarification and feedback methods to make sure all his questions have been addressed.

8. Document the patient education intervention in the health record.

Decide on the Appropriate Teaching Methods

A variety of methods may be used to get the message across to your patients. One of the best ways to manage a large amount of information within a short time is to use community resources to reinforce the message. Your local area provides a wide range of education services for your patients to help them better understand and manage their health problems, to promote wellness, and to provide support for treatment compliance. Hospitals and many community agencies and organizations provide patient education opportunities, support groups for specific problems or diseases, and learning materials. These same groups may help the patient by providing professional consultation for many topics, including diet, exercise, and emotional support. It is important that the medical assistant be aware of the various resources available in the community for patient education and referral.

Based on your evaluation of Mr. Ignatio's learning needs, what community resources would help him and his family better understand and manage his disease?

Teaching patients specific skills also is an important component of health education. The best way to coach a patient through the process of manipulating and operating medical equipment accurately is to use demonstration and return demonstration of the skill (Figure 22-6). Using the exact piece of equipment the patient will be using at home, you first should demonstrate to the patient how to perform the skill, ask for questions and explain further as needed, and then have the patient return the demonstration before leaving the facility. This gives you the opportunity to observe the patient performing the task and correct any mistakes or clarify any misconceptions before the patient has to use the equipment at home alone.

For some patients, an effective method of monitoring health education is to have the patient keep a journal of his or her activities and response to treatment. For example, a patient trying to adapt to a new diet could record daily intake to get a better idea of whether he or she is following through with dietary recommendations. Some excellent online applications (apps) are available, such as the *MyPlate.gov* site,

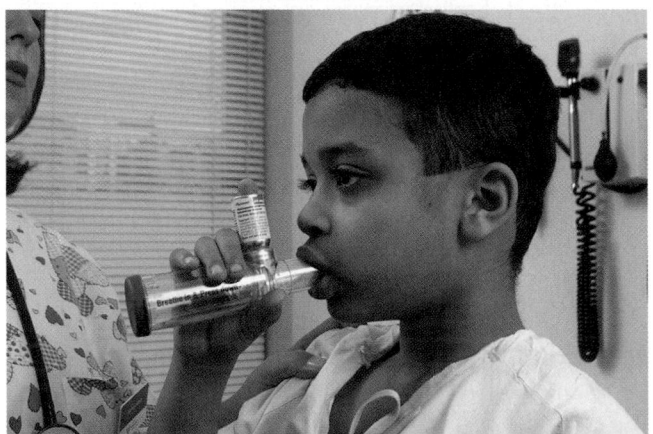

FIGURE 22-6 Demonstration and return demonstration.

that can help patients perform this task. In the case of Mr. Ignatio, referring to the memory log on his glucometer or tracking blood glucose levels with an app on his phone or computer could reinforce the results of his compliance with medication and diet therapies.

Another vital link to the success of patient education is family involvement. If the patient is being treated holistically, the family plays an integral role in patient wellness. Involving family members in patient education efforts provides support and understanding for the patient and manages family concerns about the patient's welfare. An educated family member can be an excellent resource for patient concerns and a vigilant reinforcer of healthy behaviors.

CRITICAL THINKING APPLICATION   **22-2**

The provider recommends that Mr. Ignatio start a 1,200-calorie diabetic diet for weight reduction and blood glucose control and that he take glucometer readings three times a day. After you consider various teaching methods, which strategies do you think would be most useful in helping Mr. Ignatio learn about his disease and follow the provider's recommendations?

Implement the Teaching Plan

After you have completed the patient assessment, decided on teaching materials and methods that match your patient's characteristics and learning needs, and adapted the material and your approach for any potential barriers to learning, it is time to implement the plan. Conduct the lesson in a quiet area away from distractions. Assemble the equipment the patient will need to follow through with treatment. The patient should learn to handle and practice on the same type of equipment that will be used at home so that no problem occurs in transferring the skill. Time is always an issue in the ambulatory care setting, so it is important to present only the material or skill it is possible for the patient to master before the end of the appointment. Throughout the lesson, remember to maintain an adequate pace for learning—not too fast and not too slow—to optimize the patient's understanding.

A crucial aspect of successful patient teaching is to consistently ask for feedback about the process (Figure 22-7). It also helps to restate, repeat, or rephrase the material to make sure the patient understands the process. As patients provide correct feedback about what they are learning or demonstrate skills correctly, it is important to be positive about their progress. It also helps to summarize the material learned or the skills mastered at the end of each teaching intervention, as a way of reviewing the material and clarifying important concepts.

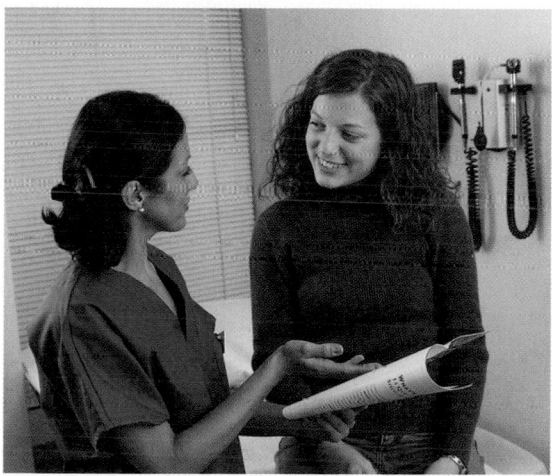

FIGURE 22-7 Patient feedback.

CRITICAL THINKING APPLICATION 22-3

Taylor has just completed the initial patient education session with Mr. Ignatio and his wife. He used demonstration–return demonstration to teach Mr. Ignatio how to check his blood glucose levels properly with the glucometer he will be using at home. Taylor answered Mrs. Ignatio's questions about diabetic diets, but the provider has also referred the couple to the dietitian at the hospital for further information on that topic. Taylor plans to review the skills practiced today at Mr. Ignatio's next appointment and to continue the teaching intervention, emphasizing the importance of Mr. Ignatio checking his feet daily for open areas or any signs of infection.

Accurately and completely document Taylor's initial coaching session with Mr. Ignatio.

The medical assistant should continue to evaluate the teaching plan throughout the process to make sure the time was adequate for learning and that the patient understood the information needed to follow through with care at home. In addition, plans should be made for the education intervention during the patient's next visit. All of this information needs to be included in the progress note about the lesson. Finally, the medical assistant must document details about the material covered, the patient's competency or level of skill in learning treatment techniques, and any referrals made for community and hospital experts or education groups (Procedure 22-2).

Summary of the Patient Teaching Plan

1. Perform an assessment.
   - Consider pertinent patient factors.
   - Identify barriers to learning.
   - Prioritize patient information.
2. Determine the patient's immediate and long-term needs.
   - Decide on the appropriate teaching materials and methods; prepare the teaching area; and assemble the necessary equipment and materials.
   - Demonstrate techniques and procedures using the supplies the patient will use at home.
   - Provide positive feedback when the patient performs skills correctly.
3. Maintain an adequate pace while teaching (not too fast).
4. Repeatedly ask for patient feedback to confirm understanding.
   - Barriers to learning are eliminated.
   - Immediate learning needs can be addressed.
   - Repetition and rephrasing promote understanding.
5. Summarize the material learned or skill mastered at the end of each teaching interaction.
6. Outline a plan for the next meeting.
7. Evaluate the teaching plan.
   - Was there enough time to complete the lesson?
   - Was the patient physically and psychologically ready for the information?
   - Were the goals for the session reached?
8. Document the teaching intervention in the patient's health record.
   - Material covered
   - Patient response or level of skill performance
   - Plans for next session
   - Community referrals

Role of the Medical Assistant as Patient Coach
- Reinforce provider instructions and information
- Encourage patients to take an active role in their health
- Use each patient interaction as an opportunity for health teaching
- Keep information relevant to the patient's needs
- Establish and maintain rapport with the patient
- Communicate clearly
- Be sensitive to the patient's learning factors
- Modify the teaching plan as needed to best meet the patient's needs

PROCEDURE 22-2	Coach Patients in Health Maintenance, Disease Prevention, and Following the Treatment Plan

Goal: *To consider patient factors, such as cultural diversity, developmental life stage, and communication barriers, when coaching patients in health maintenance, disease prevention, and following the treatment plan.*

Scenario: Role-play the following scenario with your partner.

Samuel Wu is a 74-year-old patient who was recently diagnosed with hypertension. The provider has designed a treatment plan for health maintenance and disease prevention that includes a low sodium diet, weight loss, and hypertensive medication. What patient education approaches should the medical assistant use that are age- and culturally appropriate? Should the medical assistant provide an educational brochure for Mr. Wu that he can take home for reinforcement of patient education? Include in your discussion the importance of following the provider's instructions for diet and weight loss.

EQUIPMENT and SUPPLIES

- Patient's health record
- Educational handouts and/or access to online resources that can be printed
- Quiet, private area

PROCEDURAL STEPS

1. Greet and identify the patient in a pleasant manner. Introduce yourself and explain your role.
   PURPOSE: To make the patient feel comfortable and at ease.
2. Take the patient to a quiet, private area. If this room has a computer with Internet access, you can help Mr. Wu research appropriate sites and print educational materials for his use at home.
   PURPOSE: A quiet, private area is necessary to protect confidentiality and prevent interruptions.
3. Identify factors that may limit the patient's ability to learn and implement lifestyle changes. Mr. Wu is of Chinese descent and is 74 years old. Will these patient factors affect learning?
   PURPOSE: You can promote patient learning if you identify and address the patient's primary concern and are sensitive to possible barriers to patient education, such as cultural influences, developmental stage, and possible communication barriers.
4. Prioritize the patient information and determine the patient's immediate and long-term needs. What does Mr. Wu need to know to maintain his health, prevent complications related to hypertension, and to follow the provider's treatment plan?
5. Prepare the teaching area and assemble necessary equipment and materials, making sure to use the same supplies and equipment the patient will use at home. Mr. Wu has a wrist blood pressure machine that he will use at home to monitor his blood pressure. Monitoring his blood pressure at home will help Mr. Wu determine if he is following diet restrictions and taking his medication as ordered.
   PURPOSE: Using the same equipment that the patient uses at home reinforces learning and limits the need to apply newly learned skills to a different type of equipment. Taking his blood pressure routinely will help reinforce diet restrictions, and the need for taking his medication as ordered.
6. Use restatement, reflection, and clarification to promote understanding.
   PURPOSE: Therapeutic communication techniques help you gather complete information.
7. Remain sensitive to the individual needs of your patient throughout the interview process.
   PURPOSE: Consistently keep in mind the patient's cultural background, developmental stage, and possible communication barriers as you progress through the teaching intervention. Treat all patients with respect.
8. Summarize the material learned or the skill mastered at the end of each teaching interaction and outline a plan for the next meeting. Emphasize the importance of following the treatment plan to maintain health and prevent disease complications.
   PURPOSE: Summarizing the material covered helps clarify the information for the patient and also helps you determine where to start or what to review at the next appointment.
9. Give the patient appropriate handouts and/or conduct an online search of community resources that might be of benefit. Print out this information or e-mail it to the patient for future use.
   PURPOSE: Make sure the patient takes the handouts when leaving the office; include a list of online sites that can be checked for additional information and support.
10. Document the teaching intervention, including the material covered; the patient's response or level of skill performance; plans for the next session; and any community referrals.
    PURPOSE: Documentation in the health record of the teaching intervention and the patient's comprehension helps ensure consistency and appropriate follow-up for subsequent visits.

CLOSING COMMENTS

Legal and Ethical Issues

Providing adequate, correct, understandable information to patients is integral to the informed consent mandate in the Patients' Bill of Rights. All patients have the right to information before they agree to receive care. An extension of this concept is the right of patients to understand their disease process and to manage their health. Another consideration arising from the Patients' Bill of Rights is the issue of patient confidentiality as it relates to patient education. When developing and implementing the teaching plan, designing teaching interventions and strategies, and referring patients for community assistance, the medical assistant must protect the patient's confidentiality.

Essential factors in risk management for the ambulatory care setting include conducting adequate patient education and follow-up. Also integral to risk management is the importance of documenting each patient education intervention completely and accurately. The patient's health record should clearly describe the education intervention, methods and materials used, the patient's response to the intervention, the date of each session, and the individual who conducted each intervention. Each documentation entry should completely describe the material covered and the patient's feedback about the information so that no doubt exists that the patient understood the information and was able to perform any related skills properly and adequately.

Teaching interventions should demonstrate sensitivity to multicultural factors and diverse populations. Meeting the needs of all patients without evidence of prejudice is a key risk management step.

HIPAA Applications

- The patient has the right to restrict who can receive protected health information (PHI). At the first office visit, the patient should complete a release of information form, if he or she wants to do so. This form identifies a particular family member, close friend, or any other individual who the patient states can receive disclosures of health information.
- Only the person or persons identified on the HIPAA release form completed by the patient have the right to the patient's personal information. Therefore, if an individual requests information about the patient, the medical assistant first must check the release form to determine whether the individual was approved by the patient before discussing the patient's condition. This holds true regardless of the individual's relationship to the patient.
- If the provider believes that it is in the patient's best interest that family members be involved in patient health education, the medical assistant can contact the family only if the patient has given approval. This permission should be included in the patient's HIPAA information and should be documented in the medical record so that all employees can read evidence of the patient's approval.

Professional Behaviors

Medical assistants are members of a profession in which information about disease, treatment, diagnostics, and management of health problems is constantly changing. Keeping up with current medical information requires a commitment to lifelong learning from all members of the healthcare team. To be effective patient educators, we first must be sure to have adequate knowledge ourselves. Medical assistants are perfectly placed in the healthcare team to represent the patient; that is, to perform the duties of a patient navigator. Who else in the ambulatory care setting is better able to understand the complex administrative and clinical skills needed for patients to navigate their care? From understanding treatment protocols to helping patients with insurance issues, medical assistants can serve as intermediaries who represent and support the patient throughout the healthcare environment.

SUMMARY OF SCENARIO

After working with Mr. Ignatio, Taylor realizes the significance and complexity of educating patients in the ambulatory care setting. Despite the time constraints typical in this particular healthcare setting, patients still must learn how to manage their disease and follow treatment guidelines. Approaching each patient as an individual learner with particular needs and characteristics is crucial to the ultimate success of the teaching plan. By using a holistic approach and taking into account the health belief model, Taylor has considered the ramifications of diabetes mellitus for Mr. Ignatio's life and has made efforts to include family and community resources in the management of his disease.

SUMMARY OF LEARNING OBJECTIVES

1. **Discuss the holistic model of patient education related to health and illness; also, instruct patients according to their needs to promote health maintenance and disease prevention.**

   The holistic model suggests that patient education should consider all aspects of the patient's life, including physical, sociocultural, intellectual, economic, and psychological needs. (See Table 22-1 and Figure 22-1.) The health belief model analyzes what people believe to be true about themselves and their health. This model suggests that healthcare practitioners consider how the patient perceives the risk of developing the disease and whether he or she believes that altering health behaviors will prevent the disease. Dr. Elisabeth Kübler-Ross's stages of grief may also help explain a patient's reaction to a particular diagnosis, especially if the disease requires a drastic change in lifestyle. Grief is an ongoing process, with patients moving through denial, anger, bargaining, depression, and finally resolution, at their own pace and in their own way.

   Many factors or patient characteristics may affect the patient's ability to learn. Medical assistants must be aware of these factors to develop a patient education approach that best meets the needs of each patient.

2. **Summarize the stages of grief and suggest therapeutic interactions for grieving patients.**
   - *Denial and isolation:* Reinforce each education intervention and encourage family members to attend visits.
   - *Anger:* Use therapeutic communication techniques to acknowledge the patient's feelings about the diagnosis.
   - *Bargaining:* Discuss the patient's bargaining requests with the provider to work out a solution.
   - *Depression:* Use available community resources to provide support for the patient and family.
   - *Acceptance:* Renew education efforts by providing multiple methods for learning about the disease.

3. **List at least five guidelines for patient education that can affect the patient's overall wellness.**

   The guidelines for patient education include providing knowledge and skills that promote recovery and health; including family in education interventions; encouraging patient ownership of the education process; promoting safe use of medications and treatments; encouraging healthy behaviors; and providing information on how to access community resources.

4. **Do the following related to patient factors that affect learning:**
   - *Define six patient factors that have an impact on learning.*
     Patient factors that have an impact on learning include the patient's perception of disease versus the actual state of disease; the need for information; age and developmental level; mental and emotional state; the influence of multicultural and diversity factors; individual learning style; and the impact of physical disabilities on the education process.
   - *Display respect for individual diversity.*
     Culture, family background, and religious beliefs influence a patient's actions. For patient education to be successful, it is essential that the medical assistant be aware of and sensitive to the impact of these

   factors on patient learning. Consider the patient's language, ability to understand English verbally or read it correctly, and cultural relationships to healthcare workers. Develop techniques to minimize the patient's education problems.
   - *Summarize educational approaches for patients with language barriers.*
     Educational approaches for patients with language barriers include addressing the patient formally and courteously; using nonverbal language to promote understanding; integrating pictures or models that illustrate the material; observing the patient for understanding or confusion; using simple lay language; demonstrating procedures; implementing teaching in small, manageable steps; providing written instructions; and using an interpreter when available.

5. **Do the following related to the teaching plan:**
   - *Determine possible barriers to patient learning.*
     Possible barriers to patient education include the patient's learning style, physical limitations, age, and developmental level; any emotional or mental state that interferes with learning; use of defense mechanisms; cultural or ethnic factors; language; the presence of pain; a patient's lack of motivation to learn; and limited time for teaching.
   - *Assess the patient's needs.*
     The goal of the assessment process is to create a teaching plan that meets the patient's needs for understanding and managing his or her illness.
   - *Determine the teaching priorities.*
     Every interaction with the patient is an opportunity for health education. Use the waiting room as a place for learning by providing up-to-date educational materials on a variety of issues.
   - *Decide on the appropriate teaching materials.*
     When possible, all patient information should include a handout or online reference that reinforces information and that can be used as a resource. Other teaching materials include DVDs, approved YouTube links, and health-related applications that can be accessed by smart phone or computer.
   - *Develop a list of community resources related to patients' healthcare needs and facilitate referrals to community resources in the role of a patient navigator.*
     The medical assistant should assist patients and their families in finding and using community education and support services when needed. The healthcare facility should maintain a current file of area resources that give the name of the group and the services provided; the contact person; a telephone number and address; meeting times and location if applicable; and a related website if available. Patients should be provided with accurate, well-researched sites to make sure that online recommendations support the provider's treatment protocol. A patient navigator is a person who helps patients and families with insurance problems, explains treatment and care, communicates with the healthcare team, assists caregivers, and manages medical paperwork. This definition describes the role of the medical assistant as an advocate for

SUMMARY OF LEARNING OBJECTIVES—*continued*

the patient in the ambulatory care setting. (Refer to Procedure 22-1.)

• *Decide on the appropriate teaching methods.*

A variety of methods may be used to get the message across to patients. Some excellent apps are available that can help patients keep track of their progress. Family involvement is also important.

• *Implement the teaching plan.*

The medical assistant should consistently ask for feedback about the process. It also helps to restate, repeat, or rephrase the material to make sure the patient understands.

• *Demonstrate the ability to develop an appropriate and effective patient teaching plan.*

The parts of the teaching plan include assessing learning needs; eliminating learning barriers; determining teaching priorities; using appropriate teaching materials and methods; gathering feedback repeatedly to ensure that the patient understands; summarizing the material at the end of each education session; planning for the next meeting; evaluating the effectiveness of the session; and completely and accurately

documenting the details of the teaching intervention. (Refer to Procedure 22-2.)

6. **Describe the role of the medical assistant in patient education.**

The role of the medical assistant in patient education is to reinforce the provider's instructions and information by encouraging patients to take an active part in their health; using teaching moments effectively; keeping information relevant to the patient; establishing and maintaining patient rapport; communicating clearly; remaining aware of learning factors; being flexible with the teaching plan; and using community resources for learning and support.

7. **Integrate the legal and ethical elements of patient teaching into the ambulatory care setting; also, discuss HIPAA applications.**

Appropriate patient education reflects the emphasis of the Patients' Bill of Rights on patient confidentiality and informed consent. Risk management practices related to patient education include accurate and complete documentation of patient education sessions, sensitivity to the needs of the individual patient, and application of HIPAA rules.

CONNECTIONS

Study Guide Connection: Go to the Chapter 22 Study Guide. Read and complete the activities.

evolve Evolve Connection: Go to the Chapter 22 link at *evolve.elsevier.com/kinn* to complete the Chapter Review Quiz. Check out the other resources listed for this chapter to make the most of what you have learned from Patient Education.

23

NUTRITION AND HEALTH PROMOTION

Marcia Schwartz, CMA (AAMA), is employed by an internal medicine practice in her hometown. She recognizes that many of the patients seen in the practice have diseases that are influenced by diet and lifestyle factors. She learned about the importance of good nutrition and wellness in her medical assisting program.

In addition, Marcia has continued to attend workshops and read about current trends in nutrition, so she is prepared to provide assistance to her patients as directed by the provider.

While studying this chapter, think about the following questions:
- How can Marcia help her patients understand the importance of and suggested requirements for the primary nutrients?
- What should Marcia know about the dietary guidelines for carbohydrates, proteins, and fats?
- What is the importance of vitamins and minerals and in what foods can they be found?
- How can Marcia educate patients using the Choose My Plate website?
- Is Marcia able to teach patients the significance of the body mass index (BMI)?
- What are the general guidelines for therapeutic nutrition?
- Is it important that Marcia be able to coach patients about understanding food labels?
- What factors contribute to a healthy lifestyle?

LEARNING OBJECTIVES

1. Define, spell, and pronounce the terms listed in the vocabulary.
2. Analyze the relationship between poor nutrition and lifestyle factors and the risk of developing diet-related diseases.
3. Recognize the reasons for people's food choices and the effects of cultural eating patterns.
4. Describe digestion and classify the types and functions of dietary nutrients.
5. Describe the roles of various nutrient components, including carbohydrates, fats, and proteins, in the daily diet.
6. Explain the function of appropriate amounts of vitamins, minerals, and water in the diet.
7. Apply the Dietary Guidelines for Americans using the Choose My Plate website developed by the U.S. Department of Agriculture (USDA).
8. Implement nutritional assessment techniques by measuring a patient's body fat and correlating a patient's calculated body mass index (BMI) with the risk for diet-related diseases.
9. Do the following related to therapeutic nutrition:
   - Compare the concepts of therapeutic nutrition.
   - Instruct a patient according to the patient's dietary needs; coach a patient with diabetes about the Glycemic Index of foods.
10. Interpret food labels, explain their application to a healthy diet, and demonstrate to the patient how to understand nutrition labels on food products.
11. Discuss food-borne diseases and food contaminants.
12. Summarize the causes of eating disorders and obesity and their impact on a patient's health.
13. Define the concepts of health promotion.
14. Describe the role of the medical assistant in patient education; also, explain the legal and ethical issues related to nutrition and health promotion.

VOCABULARY

amino acids The organic compounds that form the chief constituents of protein; they are used by the body to build and repair tissues.

cholesterol (kuh-les'-tuh-rol) A substance produced by the liver and found in animal fats; it can produce fatty deposits or atherosclerotic plaques in blood vessels.

deficiencies (di-fi'-shun-sees) Conditions that result with below-normal intake of particular substances.

diabetes mellitus type 1 A disease in which the beta cells in the pancreas no longer produce insulin. The individual must rely on daily insulin administration to use glucose for energy and prevent complications.

diabetes mellitus type 2 A disease in which the body is unable to use glucose for energy as a result either of inadequate insulin production in the pancreas or resistance to insulin on the cellular level.

digestion The process of converting food into chemical substances that can be absorbed and used by the body.

diverticulosis (di-vuhr-ti-kyuh-lo'-sis) The presence of pouchlike herniations through the muscular layer of the colon.

free radicals Compounds with at least one unpaired electron, which makes the compound unstable and highly reactive. Free radicals are believed to damage cell components, ultimately leading to cancer, heart disease, or other diseases.

hydrogenated (hi-drah'-juh-na-ted) Combined with, treated with, or exposed to hydrogen.

macular degeneration A progressive deterioration of the macula of the eye that causes loss of central vision.

neural tube defect Any of a group of congenital anomalies involving the brain and spinal column that are caused by failure of the neural tube to close during embryonic development.

obesity An excessive accumulation of body fat; defined as a body mass index (BMI) of 30 or higher.

osteoporosis (ah-ste-o-puh-ro'-sis) Loss of bone density; lack of calcium intake is a major factor in its development.

psyllium (si'-le-um) A grain found in some cereal products, in certain dietary supplements, and in certain bulk fiber laxatives; a water-soluble fiber.

registered dietitian (RD) An individual with a minimum of a bachelor's degree in food and nutrition who is concerned with the maintenance and promotion of health and the treatment of diseases through diet; to become an RD, the individual must pass a national examination.

statins A class of drugs that lowers the level of cholesterol in the blood by reducing the production of cholesterol by the liver; statins block the enzyme in the liver that is responsible for making cholesterol.

triglyceride (tri-gli'-suh-ride) A fatty acid and glycerol compound that combines with a protein molecule to form high-density or low-density lipoprotein.

turgor A term referring to normal skin tension; the resistance of the skin to being grasped between the fingers and released. Turgor is decreased with dehydration and increased with edema.

vertigo Dizziness; a sensation of spinning or an inability to maintain normal balance.

Good health is a state of emotional and physical well-being that is determined to a large extent by diet and lifestyle factors. Health promotion and disease prevention practices focus on sound nutrition, regular exercise, avoidance of smoking and tobacco, limited alcohol intake, management of stress, and avoidance of environmental contaminants. We are what we eat because the food we consume is used to build and repair every part of our bodies. A well-nourished person is also better able to ward off infections. Consequently, a poor diet and risky lifestyle behaviors are directly related to multiple health problems.

The provider, the medical assistant, and the **registered dietitian (RD)** are all closely involved in the nutritive care of a patient. The provider prescribes the diet, and ideally the dietitian instructs the patient in how to follow it. If professional aid is not available, the medical assistant may be asked to discuss the diet with the patient, answer questions, and explain certain aspects of the modifications involved. The patient may hesitate to ask the provider about details of a recommended diet, or he or she may call with questions on how to implement the diet after leaving the office. Therefore, you frequently are the person to whom the patient turns for answers. You should be able to answer basic questions on healthy nutrition, and you should have a fundamental knowledge of the diets most often prescribed.

Health Problems Related to Poor Nutrition and Lifestyle Factors

- *Anemia:* Low iron or folate intake
- *Cancers:* High-fat, low-fiber, low–complex carbohydrate diet; high alcohol and sodium intake; sedentary lifestyle; tobacco use
- *Constipation:* Low fiber, inadequate fluids; high-fat diet; sedentary lifestyle
- *Diabetes mellitus type 2:* High-calorie, high-fat, low–complex carbohydrate diet; obesity; sedentary lifestyle
- *Hypercholesterolemia* and *atherosclerosis:* High-fat, low-fiber diet; high sugar and alcohol intake; tobacco use; sedentary lifestyle
- *Hypertension:* High-calorie, high-fat diet; high alcohol and sodium intake; tobacco use; sedentary lifestyle; obesity; stress
- *Osteoporosis:* Low calcium intake; inadequate vitamin D intake or lack of sun exposure; high alcohol intake; sedentary lifestyle; tobacco use
- *Stroke:* High-fat, low-fiber, low–complex carbohydrate diet; high alcohol intake; tobacco use; stress

People eat the way they do for many reasons. When encouraging patients to make significant changes in their diets, the medical assistant must be sensitive to these reasons. The choices people make about what they eat are greatly influenced by their background and relationships. Every culture, religion, and ethnic group has its own beliefs and practices with regard to food. For example, according to the Hindu religion, eating beef is forbidden. Certain Jewish practices govern the types of foods that are eaten and how they are prepared. Food is more than sustenance; it represents family and celebrations and has an entire psychological component that you must recognize to care for the individual patient most effectively.

Reasons for People's Food Choices

- *Convenience:* People choose what is easiest and quickest, including eating out and take-home meals.
- *Cost:* What a person can afford.
- *Emotional comfort:* "Feel good" foods are chosen based on cultural and psychological influences.
- *Routine:* People eat what they always eat out of habit, personal preference, and availability.
- *Positive experiences:* A food is associated with a fond memory, eaten by someone the person admires, or chosen because of the influence of marketing and advertising.
- *Ethnic or regional influences:* The person grew up with the food; it is associated with the individual's cultural background; or it is part of the regional diet where the person lives.
- *Health and weight:* People think a particular food is good for them or will help them maintain or lose weight.

Cultural Eating Patterns

- *Asian diets* emphasize whole grains in the form of millet, rice, and noodles, in addition to fruits, vegetables, legumes, nuts and seeds; fats are derived largely from vegetable oils, such as peanut or sesame oils. Dairy products are not traditionally eaten. Protein sources typically are broiled or stir-fried fish and seafood, egg whites, tofu, and nuts.
- *Latin American diets* emphasize food from plant sources at each meal, especially maize (corn) and potatoes, in addition to fruits, vegetables, whole grains, beans, and nuts. Poultry, fish, and dairy typically are consumed daily and meat and eggs weekly.
- *Mediterranean diets* emphasize whole grains, fresh fruits and vegetables, and all types of legumes, such as beans, lentils, and peas daily; olive oil replaces other fats and oils; fish, poultry, and eggs are consumed weekly and meat monthly.
- *Mexican diets* emphasize corn or flour tortillas, cabbage, legumes, squash, tomatoes, corn, and potatoes daily. Dairy is used in the form of cheeses, but milk is not regularly consumed. Protein sources typically are fish, beef, poultry, lamb, and many types of beans.

NUTRITION AND DIETETICS

The term *nutrition* refers to all the processes involved in the intake and use of nutrients. *Nutrients* are the organic and inorganic chemicals in food that supply the energy and raw materials for cellular activities. Nutrients include carbohydrate, fat, protein, vitamins, minerals, and water.

Metabolism is the process in which nutrients are used at the cellular level for growth and energy production and excretion of waste. Metabolism occurs in two phases, anabolism and catabolism. *Anabolism* is the building phase, in which smaller molecules, such as **amino acids**, are combined to form larger molecules, such as proteins. An example of anabolism is the liver's creation of *glycogen,* a stored form of glucose. In this process, many units of glucose are combined to form a more complex glycogen molecule. *Catabolism* is the breaking-down phase, in which larger molecules are broken down and converted into smaller units, such as when stored glycogen is broken down into glucose molecules for energy.

Digestion is a combination of mechanical and chemical processes that occur in the mouth, stomach, and small intestine. These processes result in the breakdown of nutrients into absorbable forms, including amino acids, fatty acids, glycerol, and glucose. Most nutrients are absorbed in the small intestine and then carried by the bloodstream to all parts of the body.

The term *nutrition* also is used to indicate nutritional status, or the condition of the body resulting from the use of nutrients. *Dietetics* is the practical application of nutritional science to individuals; it is the combined science and art of feeding individuals or groups, given a wide range of economic factors and/or health conditions, according to the principles of nutrition and dietary management. A registered dietitian's role is the promotion of good health through proper diet and the therapeutic use of diet in the treatment of disease.

Nutrients

To nurture life, the nutrients in food must perform one or more of three basic functions in the body: (1) provide a source of fuel or energy, (2) supply material to build and repair tissues, and (3) regulate metabolic processes. Because no one food supplies all the nutrients required, a combination of different foods is necessary to promote health. With a little planning, all the body's needs can be met by a well-balanced diet. Dietary **deficiencies** result in undernourishment or malnourishment and may lead to a variety of diseases. Good nutrition is an important part of health promotion for all individuals but especially for pregnant women, young children, and the elderly.

The role of diet in supplying energy is crucial to body functions. Every action of the body, whether voluntary or involuntary, requires energy. Even when a person is asleep, the body needs a source of energy to keep vital organs functioning. *Basal metabolism* is the amount of energy needed to maintain essential body functions. The *basal metabolic rate* (BMR) is the amount of energy used by a fasting, resting individual to maintain vital functions. The rate is determined by the amount of oxygen used and is defined in units of heat energy, called *calories* (cal). Because this unit represents a relatively small amount of energy and because metabolism involves much larger amounts of energy, the large calorie (Cal), or kilocalorie (kcal), is commonly used. A kilocalorie is defined as the amount of heat required to raise the temperature of 1 kg of water 1°C.

Of the seven food constituents (carbohydrates, proteins, fats, water, minerals, vitamins, and fiber), only carbohydrates, proteins, and fats are capable of furnishing the body with energy. The amount of energy, or kilocalories, a person needs varies according to the individual's activity level and basal metabolic requirements, and whether disease is present. Most adults age 20 to 40 require 1,800 to 2,200 kcal/day. A patient generally is said to be overweight or underweight depending on how his or her current weight compares with nutritional assessment standards. **Obesity** is likely to result when more calories are consumed than are expended or because of certain endocrine imbalances.

Nutrients can be categorized as those that are a required part of the diet and those that can be anabolized in the body. An *essential* nutrient cannot be manufactured by the body and therefore must be included in the diet or a deficiency disease occurs. Certain amino acids are examples of essential nutrients. A *nonessential* nutrient can be created in the body and therefore does not need to be included in the diet; for example, both **cholesterol**, which is manufactured in the liver, and vitamin D, which is synthesized from exposure to the sun, are nonessential nutrients.

Nutrient Components

Carbohydrates

Carbohydrates (CHO) are chemical organic compounds composed of carbon, hydrogen, and oxygen that are primarily plant products. They are divided into three groups based on the complexity of their molecules: simple sugars (e.g., table sugar, molasses, syrup, honey, candy, baked goods, and milk); complex carbohydrates (starch) (e.g., whole-grain products, cereal, pasta, rice, potatoes, legumes, fruits, vegetables, and seeds); and dietary fiber, which is found in bran, oatmeal, whole-grain breads, beans, fruits, vegetables, seeds, and dried fruits. Each has a function in health and consists of many variations. With the exception of fiber, carbohydrates are easily digested and absorbed into the body. Simple sugars are quickly absorbed, whereas complex carbohydrates must be processed before they can be absorbed in the intestinal tract. Dietary fiber is indigestible and passes through the gastrointestinal tract unchanged.

How Many Terms Can Apply to Bread?

Grains are divided into two groups, whole grains and refined grains. Whole grains contain the entire grain kernel: the bran, germ, and endosperm. Examples of whole grains include whole-wheat flour, bulgur (cracked wheat), oatmeal, whole cornmeal, and brown rice. Refined grains have been processed to remove the bran and germ. This is done to give grains a finer texture and improve their shelf life, but it also removes dietary fiber, iron, and many B vitamins. Some examples of refined grain products are white flour, white bread, and white rice. Most refined grains are *enriched*, which means certain B vitamins (thiamin, riboflavin, niacin, folic acid) and iron are added back after processing. Fiber is not added back to enriched grains.

Dietary guidelines recommend that at least half of the grains consumed each day come from a whole-grain source. People who eat whole grains

---

as part of a healthy diet have a reduced risk of some chronic diseases. However, labels can be confusing. How do you know which is a healthy choice? Understanding the following definitions associated with grain foods can help. Review the definitions and see what you think about the healthiest grain choices.

- *Bran:* The tough, fibrous covering of a grain that is the primary source of fiber in grain products.
- *Enriched* or *fortified bread:* Since 1942, and with legislation amended in 1996 to include folate, the U.S. government has required that thiamin, riboflavin, niacin, folate, and iron be added to refined grain products because the process of creating white flour destroys these nutrients.
- *Refined* or *white flour bread:* Bread produced through a process that removes the coarse parts of the grain (the fiber and nutrients); the flour is bleached to create the white color.
- *Stone-ground flour:* A process used to grind the grain; it may include white flour.
- *Unbleached flour:* Similar to white flour in nutritional value and nutrient content.
- *Wheat bread* or *brown bread:* Bread made from wheat (white bread also is made of wheat) or any other type of flour that contains molasses or another product to color the bread brown.
- *Whole-grain* or *whole-wheat flour:* Flour from which the entire grain kernel is ground; unrefined flour. This is the healthiest bread choice.

The main function of carbohydrates is to supply fuel for energy and for all basic cellular activities. To meet energy needs, carbohydrate is metabolized at a rate of 4 cal/g. When digested, carbohydrate is converted into glucose, which is carried by the bloodstream to cells that need energy. A small amount of concentrated glucose is stored in the liver and muscles as glycogen. This stored glucose is available to supplement dietary supplies of carbohydrate. As with all nutrients, excess amounts of carbohydrate are converted into fat and stored in the body as *adipose* tissue. In addition to serving as the body's primary energy source, carbohydrate also is needed to regulate protein and fat metabolism. As long as sufficient amounts of dietary carbohydrate are available to meet the body's energy needs, protein and fat are not needed to supply energy. This *protein-sparing* effect allows protein to be used for its intended purpose: the repair and growth of tissues.

Carbohydrate is used for energy with limited production of waste materials, whereas protein and fat metabolism creates byproducts that are challenging for the body to process and excrete. For example, the metabolism of fat for energy results in the production of ketone bodies, which can cause an increase in the acidity of the blood and possibly kidney damage from the excretion of ketones. In addition, the central nervous system (CNS) requires a constant minute-to-minute supply of glucose to function properly. Neurons find it difficult to use fat or protein for energy.

Dietary fiber, commonly called *roughage*, is the portion of a plant that cannot be digested or absorbed. However, fiber's inability to be digested makes it an important dietary asset. Fiber adds bulk to the intestinal tract that stimulates peristalsis and promotes regular bowel movements. In addition, *soluble fiber*, which is found in oat bran, peas, beans, certain fruits, and **psyllium**, lowers blood cholesterol levels, reducing the risk of heart disease. Soluble fiber combines with cholesterol in the intestine and is excreted through the bowel, which prevents the absorption of cholesterol into the bloodstream. *Insoluble fiber*, which is found in whole grains and beans, promotes regular bowel movements, which prevents constipation and hemorrhoids. It also prevents **diverticulosis** by stimulating and toning the muscles lining the large intestine, and it is thought to help prevent colon cancer. The recommended daily fiber intake is 20 to 35 g, and 5 to 10 g of this should be soluble fiber. Table 23-1 identifies food sources of both soluble and insoluble fiber. Eating unpeeled fruit and raw vegetables can greatly increase the fiber content of the diet.

Recommendations for Carbohydrate Consumption

- Carbohydrates should account for 45 to 65 percent of the total calories consumed each day (i.e., 225 to 358 g of carbohydrates a day for a 2,000 to 2,200-calorie diet).
- Fiber-rich fruits, vegetables, and whole grains should be eaten as often as possible.
- People should consume 14 g of fiber for every 1,000 calories.

- The intake of simple sugars, especially sugar-sweetened drinks, should be reduced, and snacking on foods high in sugars and starches should be limited.
- Fruits and vegetables: Based on the typical 2,000-calorie diet, 2 cups of fruit and 2½ cups of vegetables should be eaten daily; a variety of dark green, orange, and starchy vegetables and legumes should be consumed.
- Whole grains: At least three 1-ounce servings should be eaten each day. Whole grains should make up at least half of the daily grain consumption. One ounce is equal to one slice of bread, 1 cup of dry cereal, or ½ cup of cooked rice, pasta, or cereal.
- Dairy: Includes milk, yogurt, cheese, and fortified soymilk. These provide calcium, vitamin D, potassium, protein, and other nutrients. Choose low-fat or fat-free products to limit calories and saturated fat. Recommended amounts are 3 cups per day of fat-free or low-fat milk and milk products for adults and children and adolescents ages 9 to 18 years; 2½ cups per day for children ages 4 to 8 years; and 2 cups for children ages 2 to 3 years. Toddlers should have 2 cups of whole milk from age 1 through age 2. One cup is equal to 1 cup of yogurt, 1½ ounces of natural cheese, or 2 ounces of processed cheese.

TABLE 23-1   Food Sources of Fiber

FOOD	SERVING SIZE	TOTAL FIBER (g)	SOLUBLE FIBER (g)	INSOLUBLE FIBER (g)
Spaghetti, cooked	1 cup	2	0.5	1.5
Whole-wheat bread	1 slice	2.5	0.5	2
White rice, cooked	½ cup	0.5	0	0.5
Bran flake cereal	¾ cup	5.5	0.5	5
Corn flake cereal	1 cup	1	0	1
Oatmeal, cooked	¾ cup	3	1	2
Banana	1 medium	2	0.5	1.5
Apple, with skin	1 medium	3	0.5	2.5
Orange	1 medium	2	0.5	1.5
Pear, with skin	1 medium	4.5	0.5	4
Strawberries	½ cup	1	0	1
Broccoli	½ cup	2	0	2
Corn	½ cup	1.5	0	1.5
Potato, baked, with skin	1 medium	4	1	3
Spinach	½ cup	2	0.5	1.5
Kidney beans	½ cup	4.5	1	3.5
Popcorn	1 cup	1	0	1

A patient, George Hawthorne, recently was diagnosed with hypertension and hypercholesterolemia. He has a family history of colon cancer. The provider recommends a high-fiber diet. Describe how Marcia could reinforce the provider's information by explaining the purpose of dietary fiber, the difference between soluble and insoluble fibers, and the types of foods Mr. Hawthorne should include in his diet.

Fats

Fats are the storage form of fuel used to back up carbohydrates as an available energy source. Fat is a much more concentrated form of fuel, producing 9 cal of energy per gram when metabolized. Dietary fats, or *lipids,* provide essential fatty acids and are needed for the absorption of the fat-soluble vitamins, A, D, E, and K. Fat gives food flavor and creates a feeling of *satiety,* or satisfaction, after eating. *Adipose* tissue, the stored form of fat in the body, supports and protects vital organs, insulates the body to help in the regulation of body temperature, and plays an important role in protecting nerve fibers and relaying nerve impulses. Lipids are also crucial to cell membrane development.

Saturated and Unsaturated Fatty Acids. When digested, fats are broken down into fatty acids and glycerol. The main building blocks of fat are *fatty acids,* which can be either saturated or unsaturated. *Unsaturated* fatty acids can take on more hydrogen under the proper conditions and therefore are less heavy and less dense. If fatty acids have one unfilled hydrogen bond, the fat is called *monounsaturated.* Olives and olive oil, peanuts and peanut oil, canola oil, pecans, and avocados contain monounsaturated fats. *Polyunsaturated* fats, such as safflower, corn, cottonseed, and soy oils, have two or more unfilled hydrogen bonds. Unsaturated fats are found in plants and are usually liquid at room temperature. Monounsaturated fat should be used as frequently as possible to replace saturated fat in the diet. Research on olive oil indicates it may offer some protection against heart disease and breast cancer; canola oil is another rich source of monounsaturated fatty acids.

The chemical structure of a *saturated* fatty acid contains all the hydrogen possible; these fats, therefore, are denser, heavier, and solid at room temperature. Saturated fats are found in whole milk dairy products, eggs, lard, meat, and **hydrogenated** fats, such as margarine. Some saturated fats, such as those in soft margarines, are partially hydrogenated. These fats usually are soft at room temperature. Most saturated fats come from animal sources. The main exceptions are coconut and palm oils, which are of plant origin but are exceptionally high in saturated fat. The primary dietary factor associated with high blood cholesterol levels is a high intake of foods high in saturated fat.

What Is a Trans Fat?

Trans-fatty acids are byproducts created when polyunsaturated oils are solidified by the addition of hydrogen. Manufacturers use this process to preserve food products because the foods are much more resistant to rancidity after hydrogenation. This lengthens the shelf life of the processed food, and the product tastes better. Trans fats are found naturally in meat and dairy products, but Americans consume most of their trans fats in processed foods, such as margarine, crackers, cookies, doughnuts, biscuits, chips, frozen meals, french fries, and other items containing or fried in partially hydrogenated oils.

Trans fats raise the level of low-density lipoprotein (LDL), the so-called bad cholesterol, and lower the level of high-density lipoprotein (HDL), or "good" cholesterol, in the blood. Scientific evidence indicates that saturated fat and trans fat combine to raise the LDL level, resulting in an increased risk of coronary heart disease (CHD). According to the National Institutes of Health, more than 12.5 million Americans have CHD, and more than 375,000 die from its complications each year. Food labels must list the amounts of saturated fat, dietary cholesterol, and trans fats if the amount exceeds 0.5 g per serving. Label readers should be cautious, however, because eating more than the designated serving size can drastically increase the amount of trans fats consumed.

Benefits of Omega-3 Fatty Acids

The omega-3 fatty acids have a number of beneficial effects in the body:
- They are present in large amounts in the cerebral cortex.
- They help form the retina.
- They have antiinflammatory effects, including improving the immune response, protecting blood vessels (e.g., the coronary arteries), and inhibiting the formation of blood clots.

Omega-3 fatty acids are found in cold-water fish, including mackerel, salmon, tuna, and trout; in certain oils, including canola, flaxseed, soybean, and wheat germ oil; and in walnuts, soybeans, and soybean kernels. The benefits of omega-3 fatty acids can be obtained by consuming two servings of cold-water fish weekly.

Foods High in Saturated Fat. Even a fat-free food can become high in saturated fat, depending on how it is prepared (e.g., a fat-free potato cooked as french fries). Therefore, we not only need to lower our intake of foods with saturated fat, we also need to be cautious about how foods are prepared. Foods should be grilled, roasted, broiled, baked, or cooked in the microwave rather than fried. Only lean meats should be used, and visible fat should be cut off before eating. Low-fat or fat-free products should be substituted when possible. Some foods high in saturated fat include the following:

Whole-milk dairy products	Oil-packed fish
Whole-milk cheeses	Salad dressing
Butter	Mayonnaise
Cream	Meat (especially red meat)
Ice cream	Palm oil

A **triglyceride** molecule is created when three fatty acids attach to a molecule of glycerol. This structure is the main storage form of lipids. Triglyceride molecules are transported throughout the body via the bloodstream as lipoproteins. Recent research indicates that a diet high in added sugars, especially in the form of sugar-sweetened drinks, simple carbohydrates (such as desserts and white bread), and saturated fat increases serum triglyceride levels and blood pressure. The total amount of triglycerides in the blood is used as a diagnostic tool for determining a patient's risk for hypertension and heart disease. A desirable triglyceride level is less than 150 mg/dL.

Cholesterol. Cholesterol is a nonessential nutrient that plays a vital role in metabolic activities. It is synthesized only in animal tissue, so it is not found in plant foods. Research now indicates that cholesterol in our diet may not be as directly linked to heart disease as has been thought. All animal sources of food contain cholesterol, but because cholesterol is a nonessential nutrient (it is manufactured in the liver), dietary sources of cholesterol may not increase blood cholesterol levels as much as once was believed. However, that doesn't mean it is healthy to eat a high-fat diet. High fat means high in calories, which can lead to obesity, and high cholesterol in the blood still contributes to the development of heart disease. Just because food isn't a major direct contributor doesn't mean people can ignore cholesterol blood levels. What the data show us is that people tend to replace cholesterol in their diets with foods high in added sugars, rather than with healthier choices such as fruits and vegetables. Diet aside, risks that elevate cholesterol in the body include obesity, smoking, lack of exercise, and diabetes.

The confusion over "good" and "bad" fat stems from the distinction between the fat in food and the fat in our bodies. The good fats in our diet are monounsaturated and polyunsaturated fats. The bad dietary fats are trans fats and saturated fats. As mentioned, the fat in our bodies is divided into two lipoprotein categories. The good fats, or high-density lipoproteins (HDLs), carry cholesterol from body tissues or the bloodstream to the liver for metabolism and excretion. The bad fats, or low-density lipoproteins (LDLs), carry cholesterol to the cells. LDL forms atherosclerotic plaques on arterial walls, and these plaques frequently result in heart disease, hypertension, and strokes. However, serum LDL levels often can be lowered through diet and exercise. Using polyunsaturated and monounsaturated fat products reduces total serum cholesterol levels. In addition, using monounsaturated fats (olive, peanut, and canola oils) reduces LDL levels.

Aerobic exercise is an important tool for lowering total serum cholesterol levels, increasing HDL levels, and reducing triglycerides. The higher the serum HDL level, the greater the protection against cardiovascular disease. The best HDL level is 60 mg/dL or higher. A level below 40 mg/dL is considered a major risk for heart disease. A low LDL cholesterol level is considered good for heart health. The recommended level varies, based on individual heart disease risk. For those not at risk, an LDL level of 100 to 129 mg/dL is recommended; for those at very high risk, the LDL level should be below 70 mg/dL. Recent research recommends that individuals with a high risk of heart disease (e.g., LDL level of 190 mg/dL or higher and DM type 2) should be treated with **statins** (Table 23-2).

Another potential health risk from a high-fat diet is obesity. Too much fat in the diet is deposited in the body as stored adipose tissue. Currently fats make up 35% to 40% of the total calories in the American diet. Nutritionists and epidemiologists believe that reducing dietary fat to 30%, with saturated fat and trans fat making up no more than 10% of calories, would reduce the risks of cancer, atherosclerosis, hypertension, and heart disease.

Recommendations for Fat Consumption

- Keep total fat intake to 20% to 35%, or approximately 17 g of fat per day for a 2,000-calorie diet.
- No more than 10% of daily calories should come from saturated or trans fats.
- Use only lean cuts and smaller portions of meat; trim visible fat.
- Substitute poultry and fish for red meat; remove poultry skin before eating.
- Avoid adding fat during cooking.
- Limit intake of organ meats.
- Use low-fat or fat-free products, including milk and milk products.
- Choose liquid monounsaturated oils, such as canola or olive oil.

CRITICAL THINKING APPLICATION   **23-2**

Mr. Hawthorne is attempting to control his hypercholesterolemia with diet and exercise. What recommendations about fat intake can Marcia make that will help him lower his total cholesterol and LDL levels and raise his HDL level?

Antioxidants. High blood cholesterol levels contribute to the development of atherosclerotic plaque and coronary artery disease. Studies indicate that the problem may lie not with the cholesterol itself, but with the way it reacts with oxygen, or the process of oxidation, in the bloodstream. The normal body process of using oxygen for energy, combined with environmental factors, such as pollution and tobacco smoke, creates **free radicals**, which can cause cellular damage. Our bodies have developed mechanisms to protect us against oxidizing free radicals through the use of antioxidant vitamins C, E, and beta carotene, but their amounts are not always sufficient. When enough antioxidants are circulating in the blood, cholesterol is prevented from oxidizing. If the level of antioxidants is insufficient, the opposite is true, and damage to arteries begins. Therefore, in addition to lowering saturated fat and trans fat intake, increasing dietary intake of antioxidants may prove beneficial in preventing cardiovascular disease. Research indicates that a diet rich in antioxidant vitamins also may be linked to protection against some cancers and **macular degeneration**. Naturally occurring antioxidants are found in many fruits and vegetables and certain seasonings.

TABLE 23-2	Recommendations for Total and Low-Density Lipoprotein (LDL) Cholesterol Levels					
	TOTAL CHOLESTEROL (mg/dL)			**LDL CHOLESTEROL (mg/dL)**		
AGE (yr)	**ACCEPTABLE**	**BORDERLINE**	**HIGH**	**ACCEPTABLE**	**BORDERLINE**	**HIGH**
2-20	<170	170-199	>200	<110	110-129	>130
>20	<200 (<180 is optimal)	200-239	>240	<130	130-159	>160

Foods Containing Antioxidants

Vitamin C	Beta Carotene
Broccoli	Apricots
Cabbage	Broccoli
Cauliflower	Cantaloupe
Grapefruit	Carrots
Lemons	Kale and spinach
Oranges	Mustard greens
Peppers	Pumpkin
Strawberries	Sweet potatoes
Tangerines	Winter squash
Vitamin E	**Mixed Antioxidants**
Almonds	Cloves
Chickpeas	Green tea
Oatmeal	Oregano
Soybeans	Rice
Sunflower seeds	Rosemary
Wheat germ	Sesame
	Thyme
	Wheat bran
	Red wine

Functions of Protein

- Builds and repairs body tissue, including new tissue, blood, enzymes, and hormones
- Aids the body's defense mechanisms against disease by creating antibodies
- Regulates the fluid and electrolyte balance
- Provides energy when carbohydrate and fat stores are depleted

Food Sources of Protein

Complete proteins: Meat, fish, poultry, eggs, and dairy products
Incomplete proteins: Whole grains (e.g., barley, bulgur, cornmeal, oats, rice, whole-grain breads), cashews, sesame seeds, sunflower seeds, walnuts; soy products, dried legumes, peanuts; broccoli; dark green, leafy vegetables

Proteins

Proteins are very large, complex molecules. They are composed of units known as *amino acids,* which are the materials the body uses to build and repair tissues. Twenty amino acids are necessary for normal growth and maintenance of tissues. Of these, eight are essential amino acids that must be included in the diet because humans do not have the enzymes necessary for their formation.

Proteins are classified according to whether they contain all essential amino acids in good proportion. *Complete proteins* come from animal sources and have a mixture of all eight essential amino acids. *Incomplete proteins* do not supply the body with all the essential amino acids. These are the vegetable proteins, which must be used in specific combinations because each is missing or extremely low in one or more of the essential amino acids.

To prevent the wasting of protein for energy and to permit the creation of needed amino acid compounds, dietary protein must be adequate, the diet must supply essential amino acids, and enough carbohydrate and fat must be consumed to prevent the burning of protein for energy. Fortunately, most foods have a mixture of proteins that supplement one another. Because little, if any, storage of amino acids occurs in the body, it is important that a source of protein be included at each meal. Patients with extensive burns or those with wound healing problems often are prescribed high-protein diets to encourage tissue regeneration. The recommended dietary allowance for adults over the age of 18 is 0.8 grams per kilogram of body weight per day. Each pound is equal to 2.2 kg so a person who weighs 150 pounds should consume about 68 g of protein per day. The average North American diet contains close to twice that amount. Excess protein is metabolized and either converted to glucose, burned as fuel, or stored as fat in adipose tissue.

Recommendations for Protein Consumption

- Consume no more than 18% of daily calories from protein.
- The U.S. Department of Agriculture (USDA) recommends eating 5½ to 6 ounces of cooked lean meat, poultry, or fish each day.
- One ounce of meat equals 1 egg, ¼ cup of dry beans, 1 tablespoon of peanut butter, ½ cup of cooked beans, or ½ cup of tofu.

If incomplete proteins are the only source of protein in the diet, a food that is protein deficient in one amino acid should be eaten with one that is high in the same amino acid to get the needed mix of essential amino acids. Vegetarianism has become increasingly popular, and there are many different forms. Some vegetarians consume no red meat but eat fish and poultry. Lacto-ovo vegetarians eat primarily vegetable foods but include eggs and/or dairy products in their diets. Lacto-vegetarians consume milk and milk products in addition to vegetables but no other animal sources of food. Vegans consume no animal proteins at all, relying solely on vegetable foods for protein.

Those who eat some animal protein in the form of fish, eggs, and milk generally are not at risk nutritionally. However, vegans must include a variety of vegetable foods to ensure the nutritional adequacy of their diets. To supply sufficient protein, vegetables that complement each other must be eaten together to get the correct proportion of amino acids. This is customarily done in the diets of different cultures. For example, in Mexico, beans are combined with rice, and in Middle Eastern countries, wheat bread is combined with cheese.

Tips for vegetarians from the USDA website (*http://www.choosemyplate.gov/tips-vegetarians*) include the following:

- Build meals around protein sources that are naturally low in fat, such as beans, lentils, and rice, rather than high-fat cheeses.

- Try calcium-fortified, soy-based beverages in place of milk.
- Try vegetarian products such as soy-based sausage patties or links and veggie burgers made from soybeans, vegetables, and/or rice.
- Add meat substitutes, such as tempeh (cultured soybeans with a chewy texture), tofu, or wheat gluten (seitan), to soups and stews to boost protein without adding saturated fat or cholesterol.

Examples of Nutritionally Balanced Incomplete Protein Combinations

Combining two or more sources of incomplete amino acids provides a complete protein. For example:

- Black beans and rice
- Peanut butter sandwich on whole-grain bread
- Split-pea soup with whole-grain bread
- Lentil soup and cornbread
- Walnuts, peanuts, and rice
- Whole-wheat pasta, broccoli, and spinach
- Sunflower seeds and navy bean soup

Vitamins (Micronutrients)

Vitamins are organic substances that occur in minute quantities in plant and animal tissues; they are needed for specific metabolic processes to proceed normally. Vitamins function as catalysts and help or allow metabolic reactions to proceed. Originally they were lettered or numbered as they were discovered. However, as they have been identified chemically, they have been given more specific names. In many cases their chemical names are as well known as their letter designations.

Vitamins are divided into two groups: *fat soluble* (A, D, E, and K) and *water soluble* (B complex and C). Some vitamins are nonessential, meaning they can be manufactured in the body. Vitamin A is produced from beta carotene food sources, such as carrots, pumpkin, and sweet potatoes. Ultraviolet light from the sun initiates the production of vitamin D in the skin. Vitamin K is created from intestinal bacteria.

Functions of Vitamins

- Regulate the synthesis of bone, skin, glands, nerves, brain, and blood
- Aid in the metabolism of protein, carbohydrates, and fats
- Prevent nutritional deficiency diseases
- Support good health at all ages

Vitamins do not cure an illness other than a health problem that is caused by the lack of a specific vitamin. For example, adding vitamin C to a patient's diet does not cure bleeding gums unless the condition is specifically caused by a lack of ascorbic acid (the chemical name for vitamin C). It should also be noted that toxic symptoms from excessive ingestion of fat-soluble vitamins can occur because these vitamins can be stored in adipose tissue. Water-soluble vitamins typically are excreted in the urine. However, a large intake of some water-soluble vitamins may cause adverse effects (Table 23-3). Nutrition experts agree that vitamins provide the greatest benefit when they are obtained through food as part of the diet rather than in supplement form. However, supplements may be needed in the following cases:

- Patients showing signs and symptoms of a vitamin or mineral deficiency
- Folate for women planning to become pregnant or in their childbearing years
- Iron and folate for pregnant and lactating women
- Calcium for lactose-intolerant individuals
- Daily vitamins for the elderly, who may have difficulty chewing, have malabsorption problems, live alone, or make poor food choices
- Postsurgical or burn patients, who require more protein and nutrients to grow and repair tissue
- Strict vegetarians, who may need vitamins B_{12} and D, along with iron and zinc
- Patients who have had gastric bypass surgery, who may require multiple nutrients, including vitamin B_{12}, protein, and iron

Extensive research is under way studying the role vitamins play in disease prevention and treatment. Research indicates that antioxidant vitamins (C, E, and A) may prevent cell membrane damage that leads to cancer and heart disease. Vitamins C and E also appear to protect against the development of cataracts. Vitamin E is recommended to help prevent blood clot formation and coronary heart disease (CHD). The B vitamins may help lower LDL levels, and folic acid is recommended for women planning a pregnancy to prevent **neural tube defects**.

A diet that includes certain vitamins can affect the action of prescribed medications. For example, vitamin K can interfere with the action of warfarin anticoagulants. Therefore, a sudden dietary increase or decrease in vitamin K–rich foods can alter how long it takes a clot to form in patients undergoing anticoagulant therapy. High levels of vitamin K are found in dark green, leafy vegetables such as kale, collards, Swiss chard, broccoli, and spinach; green tea; and lentils and soybeans. For stable anticoagulant treatment, patients should not increase or reduce their intake of vitamin K–rich foods without consulting their provider. They also should inform the provider if they are taking vitamin supplements that contain vitamin K.

Because vitamins and dietary supplements are categorized as food and not as drugs, no standards or regulatory mechanisms apply to their production. Therefore, various brands differ in the amount of substance available, its quality, and its level of absorption. The U.S. Pharmacopoeia (USP), an independent organization that sets standards for drugs, recently developed standards for vitamins. Consumers should look for the USP label for products that adhere to these standards.

TABLE 23-3 Vitamin Facts

VITAMIN	U.S. RDA*	BEST SOURCES	FUNCTIONS	DEFICIENCY SYMPTOMS†	TOXIC?	PROCESSING TIPS	DID YOU KNOW?
A (carotene)	500-700 mcg/day	Yellow or orange fruits and vegetables; green, leafy vegetables; fortified oatmeal; liver; dairy products	Formation and maintenance of skin, hair, and mucous membranes; aids vision in dim light; bone and tooth growth	Night blindness; dry, scaly skin; frequent fatigue	Yes, in high doses, but beta carotene is nontoxic	Serve fruits and vegetables raw and keep covered and refrigerated; steam vegetables; broil, bake, or braise meats.	Low-fat and skim milk often are fortified with vitamin A, which is removed with the fat.
B_1 (thiamine)	1.2 mg/day	Fortified cereals and oatmeal, meat, rice, pasta, whole grains, liver	Helps the body release energy from carbohydrates during metabolism; growth and muscle tone	Heart irregularity, fatigue, nerve disorders, mental confusion	No, high doses are excreted by the kidneys	Do not rinse rice or pasta before and after cooking; cook in minimal water.	Pasta and breads made of refined flours have B_1 added because it is lost in the milling process.
B_2 (riboflavin)	1.1 to 1.3 mg/day	Whole grains; green, leafy vegetables; organ meats; milk; eggs	Helps the body release energy from protein, fat, and carbohydrates during metabolism	Cracks in the corners of the mouth, rash, anemia	No toxic effects reported	Store food in containers that light cannot penetrate; cook vegetables in minimal water; roast or broil meats.	Most ready-to-eat cereals are fortified with 25% of the U.S. RDA for vitamin B_2.
B_6 (pyridoxine)	1.3 mg/day	Fish, poultry, lean meats, bananas, prunes, dried beans, whole grains, avocados	Helps build body tissue and aids metabolism of protein	Convulsions, dermatitis, muscular weakness, skin cracks, anemia	Long-term megadoses may cause nerve damage in hands and feet	Serve fruits raw or cook for shortest time in little water; roast or broil meats.	Because vitamin B_6 aids in the use of protein in the body, the need for it increases with protein intake.
B_{12} (cobalamin)	2.4 mcg/day	Meats, milk products, seafood	Aids cell development, functioning of the nervous system, and metabolism of protein and fat	Anemia, nervousness, fatigue, and in some cases neuritis and brain degeneration	No toxic effects reported	Roast or broil meat and fish.	Vegetarians who do not eat any animal products may need a supplement.
Biotin	30 mcg/day	Cereal/grain products, yeast, legumes, liver	Involved in the metabolism of protein, fats, and carbohydrates	Nausea; vomiting; depression; hair loss; dry, scaly skin	No toxic effects reported	Storage, processing, and cooking do not appear to affect this vitamin.	Biotin deficiency is extremely rare in the United States.
Folate (folacin, folic acid)	400 mcg/day	Green, leafy vegetables; organ meats; dried peas, beans, and lentils	Aids in genetic material development and is involved in red blood cell production	Gastrointestinal (GI) disorders, anemia, cracks on the lips	Some evidence of toxicity in large doses	Store vegetables in refrigerator and steam, boil, or simmer in minimal water.	Deficiencies can occur in premature infants and pregnant women.

Continued

TABLE 23-3   Vitamin Facts—*continued*

VITAMIN	U.S. RDA*	BEST SOURCES	FUNCTIONS	DEFICIENCY SYMPTOMS†	TOXIC?	PROCESSING TIPS	DID YOU KNOW?
Niacin	14-16 mg/day	Meat, poultry, fish, enriched cereals, peanuts, potatoes, dairy products, eggs	Involved in carbohydrate, protein, and fat metabolism	Skin disorders, diarrhea, indigestion, general fatigue	Nicotinic acid form should be taken only under provider's care	Roast or broil beef, veal, lamb, and poultry; cook potatoes in minimal water.	Niacin is formed in the body by converting an amino acid found in proteins.
Pantothenic acid	5 mg/day	Lean meats, whole grains, legumes, vegetables, fruits	Helps in the release of energy from fats and carbohydrates	Fatigue, vomiting, stomach stress, infections, muscle cramps	No toxic effects reported	Serve fruits and vegetables raw.	It is believed that some pantothenic acid is produced in the GI tract.
C (ascorbic acid)	75-90 mg/day	Citrus fruits, berries, and vegetables, especially peppers	Essential for structure of bones, cartilage, muscle, and blood vessels; also helps maintain capillaries and gums and aids in absorption of iron	Swollen or bleeding gums, slow wound healing, fatigue/depression, poor digestion	Intake of 1 g or more can cause nausea, cramps, and diarrhea	Do not store or soak fruits and vegetables in water; refrigerate juices and store only 2 to 3 days.	Smokers may benefit from an increased intake of vitamin C.
D	15 mcg/day	Fortified milk, sunlight, fish, eggs, butter, fortified margarine	Aids bone and tooth formation; helps maintain heart action and nervous system	In children: Rickets and other bone deformities In adults: Calcium loss from bones	High intakes may cause diarrhea and weight loss	Storage, processing, and cooking do not appear to affect this vitamin.	Sunlight starts vitamin D production in the skin.
E	15 mg/day	Fortified and multigrain cereals; nuts; wheat germ; vegetable oils; green, leafy vegetables	Protects blood cells, body tissue, and essential fatty acids from harmful destruction in the body	Muscular wasting, nerve damage, anemia, reproductive failure	Relatively nontoxic	Store in airtight containers away from light.	Most fortified cereals have 40% of RDA.
K	90-120 mcg/day	Green, leafy vegetables; fruit; dairy and grain products	Essential for blood clotting functions	Bleeding disorders in newborns and those on blood-thinning medications	Not toxic as found in food	Store in containers away from light.	Vitamin K is also formed by bacteria in the colon.

Information for this chart was obtained from the U.S. Food and Drug Administration at http://fnic.nal.usda.gov/dietary-guidance/dietary-reference-intakes/dri-tables-and-application-reports. Accessed November 4, 2015.

mg, Milligrams; *mcg,* micrograms; *RDA,* recommended dietary allowance.

*For adults and for children over 4 years of age.

†Many of these symptoms also can be attributed to conditions other than vitamin deficiency. If they persist, the patient should see the healthcare provider.

Tips for Buying Dietary Supplements

Dietary supplements may contain a combination of vitamins, minerals, herbs, plants, amino acids, and enzymes. Individuals who have been prescribed other medications should check with their healthcare providers before taking dietary supplements.

Consider the following tips before buying a dietary supplement:

- Be cautious about chasing the latest headline; watch out for "quick fix" claims that do not follow well-researched dietary guidelines.
- More may not be better; some products can be harmful when consumed in high amounts or for a long period.
- Learn to spot false claims in advertising and on supplement labels; if something sounds too good to be true, it probably is.
- Beware of claims about limited availability and requirements for advance payment.
- Supplements can be quite expensive; ask yourself if the product is worth the money.

US Food and Drug Administration: www.fda.gov/ForConsumers/ConsumerUpdates/ucm118079.htm#why. Accessed March 23, 2015.

Minerals (Electrolytes)

The human body requires minerals in relatively small amounts; nevertheless, they are absolutely essential for life (Table 23-4). Of the 19 or more minerals that form the mineral composition of the body, at least 13 are needed to maintain a healthy state. Minerals must be supplied by the diet or by supplements. Recommended daily intakes have been established for 12 minerals. Minerals contribute to the body's water-electrolyte balance and acid-base balance and are essential components of enzymes. Minerals also help regulate muscular and nervous activities, blood clotting, and normal heart rhythm.

Dietary recommendations for the daily intake of minerals, based on a 2,000-calorie diet, are:

- Potassium: 4,000 mg
- Sodium: 1,800 mg
- Calcium: 1,300 mg
- Magnesium: 400 mg
- Copper: 2 mg
- Iron: 18 mg (8 mg for those older than 51)
- Phosphorus: 1,800 mg
- Zinc: 14 mg

Minerals recommended in the largest amounts include sodium, potassium, calcium, chlorine, phosphorus, and magnesium. Those present in very small amounts, the trace elements, include iron, zinc, copper, selenium, chromium, manganese, iodine, and fluorine. The minerals needed only in trace amounts seem either to behave as part of a hormone or enzyme system or to work with vitamins in various metabolic reactions throughout the body. For example, iodine is part of the thyroid hormone thyroxine, and zinc is part of the hormone insulin. Cobalt is an essential part of vitamin B_{12}.

Calcium, iodine, and iron are the minerals most frequently missing in the American diet. One of the leading mineral deficiencies is **osteoporosis** from lack of vitamin D and/or calcium and iron-deficiency anemia. High sodium levels are associated with hypertension. Current

dietary guidelines recommend that everyone, even children, reduce their sodium intake to less than 2,300 mg/day, which is about 1 teaspoon of salt per day. Adults age 51 or older, African-Americans of any age, and individuals with high blood pressure, diabetes, or chronic kidney disease should consume less than 1,500 mg of sodium a day.

Sodium, Blood Pressure, and the DASH Diet

Thirty percent of U.S. adults have high blood pressure; it is especially common among African-Americans, who tend to develop it at an earlier age, and among older Americans. Research has proven that individuals with a sodium intake of more than 2,400 mg a day have a high risk of developing hypertension. On average, adults in the United States are estimated to consume almost 4,000 mg of sodium per day. A healthy body excretes excess sodium through the kidneys, but sodium's attraction for fluid can cause hypertension to develop.

How can you cut down on salt intake? You should avoid pickles, olives, and sauerkraut; all processed meats (lunch meat) and processed fish, but especially those that are smoked; salty snacks; fast and processed foods; canned soups; and cheese, especially processed.

The Dietary Approaches to Stop Hypertension (DASH) diet is recommended to help lower blood pressure. Daily guidelines for the DASH diet include the following:

- Four to five servings of both fruits and vegetables
- Seven to eight servings of whole grains
- 6 ounces or less of meat, fish, and poultry
- Four to five servings per week of nuts, seeds, and dry beans
- 2 to 3 cups of low-fat or fat-free milk
- 2 to 3 teaspoons of oils
- 5 tablespoons of added sugar per week
- 1,500 to 2,000 mg of sodium per day
- Total fat should not exceed 22% of calories

Water

Water is all too often overlooked when nutritional status is evaluated. The body is approximately 80% water and can survive longer without food than it can without water. Water is part of almost every vital body process.

Water is lost daily from the body in urine, feces, sweat, and expiration. Extensive water losses from diarrhea, vomiting, burns, or perspiration can lead to electrolyte losses that result in life-threatening imbalances. Water is contained in almost all foods; however, a healthy diet should include about eight 8-ounce glasses of water a day.

Functions of Water

- Plays a key role in the maintenance of body temperature
- Acts as a solvent and the medium for most biochemical reactions
- Acts as the vehicle for transport of substances such as nutrients, hormones, antibodies, and metabolic waste
- Acts as a lubricant for joints and mucous membranes

TABLE 23-4 Functions of Minerals in the Body

FUNCTIONS	SOURCES	DEFICIENCY SYMPTOMS	TOXICITY SYMPTOMS
Calcium (Ca^{2+})			
• Helps muscles contract and relax, thereby helping to regulate the heartbeat • Plays a role in normal functioning of the nervous system • Aids blood coagulation and functioning of some enzymes • Helps build strong bones and teeth • May help prevent hypertension	Primarily found in milk and milk products; also found in dark green, leafy vegetables; tofu and other soy products; sardines; salmon with bones; and hard water	Poor bone growth and tooth development, leading to stunted growth and increased risk of dental caries, rickets (bowing of the legs) in children, osteomalacia (soft bones) and osteoporosis (brittle bones) in adults, poor blood clotting, and possible hypertension	Kidney stones
Chloride (Cl$^-$)			
• Involved in the maintenance of fluid and acid-base balance • Provides an acid medium, in the form of hydrochloric acid, for activation of gastric enzymes	Major source is table salt (sodium chloride); also found in fish and vegetables	Disturbances in acid-base balance, with possible growth retardation, psychomotor defects, and memory loss	Disturbances in acid-base balance
Magnesium (Mg^{2+})			
• Helps build strong bones and teeth • Activates many enzymes • Participates in protein synthesis and lipid metabolism • Helps regulate heartbeat	Raw, dark green vegetables; nuts and soybeans; whole grains and wheat bran; bananas and apricots; seafood; coffee, tea, and cocoa; and hard water	Rare but in disease states may lead to central nervous system (CNS) problems (confusion, apathy, hallucinations, poor memory) and neuromuscular problems (muscle weakness, cramps, tremor, cardiac arrhythmia)	Drowsiness, weakness, and lethargy Severe toxicity: skeletal paralysis, CNS depression, respiratory depression, and ultimately coma and death
Phosphorus (P)			
• Helps build strong bones and teeth • Present in the nuclei of all cells • Aids the oxidation of fats and carbohydrates (energy metabolism) • Helps maintain acid-base balance	Milk and milk products, eggs, meats, legumes, whole grains, soft drinks (used to make the "fizz")	Rare but with malabsorption can cause anorexia, weakness, stiff joints, and fragile bones	Hypocalcemic tetany (muscle spasms)
Potassium (K$^+$)			
• Plays a key role in fluid and acid-base balance • Transmits nerve impulses, helps control muscle contractions, and promotes regular heartbeat • Needed for enzyme reactions	Apricots, bananas, oranges, grapefruit, raisins, green beans, broccoli, carrots, greens, potatoes, meats, milk and milk products, peanut butter and legumes, molasses, coffee, tea, cocoa	Possibly impaired growth, hypertension, bone fragility, CNS changes, renal hypertrophy, diminished heart rate, and death	Hyperkalemia (excess potassium in the blood) with cardiac function disturbances
Sodium (Na$^+$)			
• Plays a key role in the maintenance of acid-base balance • Transmits nerve impulses and helps control muscle contractions • Regulates cell membrane permeability	Salt (sodium chloride) is the major dietary source; minor sources are foods such as milk and milk products and several vegetables	Hyponatremia (too little sodium in the blood)	May cause hypertension, which can lead to cardiovascular diseases and renal (kidney) disease; salt tablets can cause gastric irritation

TABLE 23-4   Functions of Minerals in the Body—*continued*

FUNCTIONS	SOURCES	DEFICIENCY SYMPTOMS	TOXICITY SYMPTOMS
Chromium (Cr^{3+})			
• Activates several enzymes • Enhances the removal of glucose from the blood	Liver and other meats, whole grains, cheese, legumes, and brewer's yeast	Weight loss, abnormalities of the CNS, and possible aggravation of diabetes mellitus	Inhibited insulin activity
Copper (Cu^{2+})			
• Aids in the production and survival of red blood cells • A component of many enzymes involved in respiration • Plays a role in normal lipid metabolism	Shellfish (especially oysters), liver, nuts and seeds, raisins, whole grains, and chocolate	Anemia, CNS problems, abnormal electrocardiograms, bone fragility, impaired immune response; may be a factor in failure to thrive in premature infants	In Wilson's disease and Huntington's chorea (both hereditary diseases), copper accumulation causes neuron and liver cell damage
Fluorine (Fl$^-$)			
• Aids the formation of solid bones and teeth, thereby reducing the incidence of dental caries, and may help prevent osteoporosis	Fluoridated water (and foods cooked in fluoridated water), fish, tea, gelatin	Increased susceptibility to dental caries	Fluorosis and mottling of teeth
Iodine (I$^-$)			
• Helps regulate energy metabolism as part of thyroid hormones • Essential for normal cell functioning, helps to keep skin, hair, and nails healthy	Primarily from iodized salt, also found in saltwater fish, seaweed products, and vegetables grown in iodine-rich soils	Goiter, cretinism in infants born to iodine-deficient mothers, with accompanying mental retardation and diffuse CNS abnormalities	Little toxic effect in individuals with normal thyroid gland functioning
Iron (Fe^{3+})			
• Essential to the formation of hemoglobin, which is important for tissue respiration and ultimately growth and development • A component of several enzymes and proteins in the body	Heme sources: Organ meats, especially liver, red meats, and other meats. Nonheme sources: Iron-fortified cereals; dark green, leafy vegetables; legumes; whole grains; blackstrap molasses; dried fruit; and foods cooked in iron pans	Iron-deficiency anemia and possible alterations that impair behavior	Idiopathic hemochromatosis, which can lead to cirrhosis, diabetes mellitus, skin pigmentation, arthralgias (joint pain), and cardiomyopathy
Manganese (Mn^{2+})			
• Needed for normal bone structure, reproduction, and normal functioning of cells and the CNS • A component of some enzymes	Nuts, whole grains, vegetables and fruits, coffee, tea, cocoa, and egg yolks	None observed in humans	Iron-deficiency anemia through inhibiting effect on iron absorption; pulmonary changes, anorexia, apathy, impotence, headaches, leg cramps, and speech impairment; in advanced stages of toxicity resembles Parkinson's disease

Continued

TABLE 23-4   Functions of Minerals in the Body—*continued*

FUNCTIONS	SOURCES	DEFICIENCY SYMPTOMS	TOXICITY SYMPTOMS
Selenium (Se)			
• Acts as an antioxidant with vitamin E to protect cells from oxidative damage • A component of an enzyme system	Protein-rich foods (meat, eggs; milk), whole grains, seafood, liver and other meats, egg yolks, and garlic	Keshan's disease (a human cardiomyopathy) and Kashin-Bek disease (an endemic human osteoarthropathy)	Physical defects of the fingernails and toenails; also hair loss
Zinc (Zn^{2+})			
• Plays a role in protein synthesis • Essential for normal growth and sexual development, wound healing, immune function, cell division and differentiation, and smell acuity	Whole grains, wheat germ, crabmeat, oyster, liver and other meats, brewer's yeast	Depressed immune function, poor growth, dwarfism, impaired skeletal growth and delayed sexual maturation, acrodermatitis	Severe anemia, nausea, vomiting, abdominal cramps, diarrhea, fever, hypocupremia (low blood serum copper), malaise, fatigue

From Poleman CM, Peckenpaugh NJ: *Nutrition essentials and diet therapy,* ed 6, Philadelphia, 1991, Saunders; Garrison RH, Somer E: *The nutrition desk reference,* New Canaan, Conn., 1985, Keats Publishing; and Griffeth HW: *Complete guide to vitamins, minerals and supplements,* Tucson, 1988, Fisher Books.

CHOOSE MY PLATE

In 1992, to reflect dietary guidelines that called for more consumption of grains and less consumption of meat, sweets, and fats, the USDA introduced the Food Guide Pyramid. In 2011 the Pyramid design was changed to a dinner plate icon that represents how to build a healthy plate at mealtime. The plate includes choices from the five basic food groups, with recommendations based on the Dietary Guidelines for Americans (Figure 23-1). At the Choose My Plate website (*www.choosemyplate.gov*), consumers can determine individual dietary needs that match their particular age, health status, exercise level, and food preferences. Students should use the website to take advantage of the many learning opportunities it offers. It is also an excellent source for patient education information on dietary guidelines.

The Dietary Guidelines for Americans encourages daily dietary choices that are low in saturated fat, added sugars, and sodium. Sodium, saturated fat, and added sugars should be reduced and replaced with healthier options. The guidelines include the following recommendations:

1. *Balance calorie intake*: Use the Choose My Plate website to determine how many calories are needed each day to manage your weight; include exercise to help balance calories; enjoy food but eat less; avoid oversized portions. Use a smaller plate, bowl, and glass. When eating out, choose a smaller size option, share a dish, or take home part of your meal.

2. *Foods to eat more often*: Increase your daily intake of vegetables, fruits, whole grains, legumes, nuts, and fat-free or 1% milk and dairy products. Make half your plate fruits and vegetables. Make half your grains whole grains.

3. *Foods to eat less often*: Cut back on foods high in solid fats, added sugars, and salt. Use food labels to compare sodium content and choose lower sodium versions.

4. *Drink water instead of sugary drinks.*

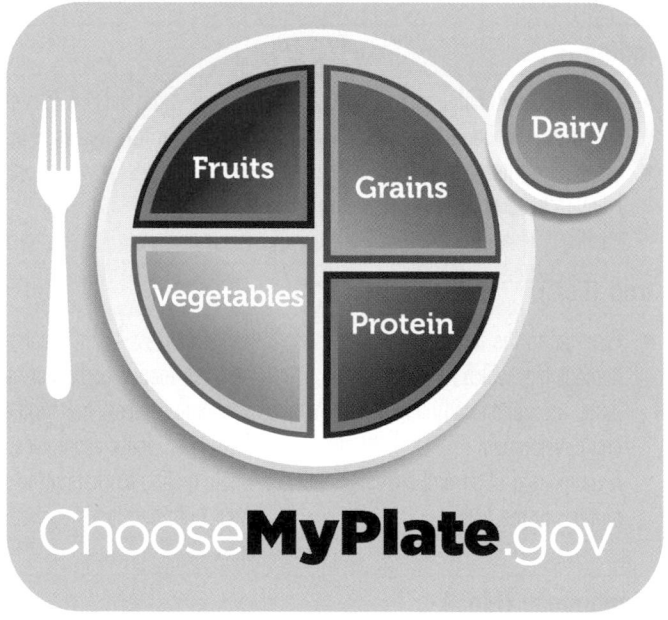

FIGURE 23-1   Choose My Plate. (From the US Department of Agriculture. www.choosemyplate.gov. Accessed March 22, 2015).

Many patients have never been educated in nutrition and do not know how to plan a healthy diet for themselves or their families. Good nutrition is a balance of carbohydrates, protein, vitamins, minerals, fiber, and water, with limited amounts of fat, sodium, sugar, and alcohol. Calorie intake must be balanced with energy output to maintain a healthy body weight.

Highlights of the U.S. Department of Agriculture's Dietary Recommendations

Adequate Nutrients Within Caloric Needs
- Consume a variety of nutrient-dense foods while limiting saturated and trans fats, cholesterol, added sugars and salts, and alcohol.
- Meet dietary recommendations by adopting a balanced eating pattern.
- Added sugars should be reduced in the diet and not replaced with low-calorie sweeteners, but rather with healthy options, such as water in place of sugar-sweetened beverages.
- Most Americans need to increase consumption of vitamin E, calcium, potassium, and fiber.
- Childbearing women should increase their intake of iron-rich and folic acid–containing foods or take supplements.
- Individuals over age 50 should consume vitamin B_{12}–fortified foods.
- Aging individuals, those with dark skin, and people who are not exposed to sunlight should eat vitamin D–fortified foods or take a supplement.

Weight Management
- Balance the intake of calories with those expended.
- With aging, calories should be decreased and physical activity increased to prevent gradual weight gain over time.
- Those who need to lose weight should do so slowly.
- Reducing the caloric intake by 50 to 100 calories per day prevents weight gain; reducing it by 500 calories a day promotes weight loss.
- Control portion sizes and reduce the intake of saturated fats, added sugars, and alcohol.

Carbohydrates
- Choose fiber-rich fruits, vegetables, and whole grains.
- Limit the use of added sugar and sweeteners; added sugars should account for no more than 10% of total calories per day.
- Practice good dental hygiene and limit sugary snacks to reduce dental caries.

Sodium and Potassium
- Consume less than 2,300 mg of sodium per day (approximately 1 teaspoon of salt).
- Consume potassium-rich foods.

Alcoholic Beverages
- Practice moderate consumption: one drink per day for women and two for men.
- Avoid alcohol if you are or may become pregnant or if lactating.

Food Safety
- Clean all fruits, vegetables, and cooking surfaces.
- Keep raw, cooked, and ready to eat foods separate.
- Cook foods to the recommended temperature to kill microbes.
- Chill perishable foods and defrost foods properly.
- Avoid unpasteurized milk products, raw eggs, and raw or undercooked meats.

Physical Activity
- Engage in 30 to 60 minutes of moderate physical activity per day to prevent weight gain; 60 to 90 minutes for weight loss.
- Children and adolescents should be physically active 60 minutes a day.
- Aging people should participate in regular exercise to maintain function.
- Include aerobic activity, stretching, and weight training.

Food Groups to Encourage
- For a 2,000-calorie diet, consume 2 cups of fruit and $2\frac{1}{2}$ cups of vegetables a day.
- Eat dark green and orange vegetables, legumes, and starches several times a week.
- At least half of the grains consumed should be whole grains.
- Consume 3 cups of fat-free or low-fat milk or milk products a day; children age 2 to 8 years should consume 2 cups a day.

Fats
- Less than 10% of calories should come from saturated fats; keep trans fats as low as possible.
- Consume less than 35% of calories from fat.
- Choose low-fat or fat-free milk products and lean meats.

Modified from the Dietary Guidelines Advisory Committee. http://health.gov/dietaryguidelines/2015-scientific-report/. Accessed November 4, 2015.

NUTRITIONAL STATUS ASSESSMENT

During the provider's examination, he or she will assess the patient's nutritional status. The provider considers the patient's age; height and weight; body mass index (BMI); overall health status; any recent changes in weight; diet and exercise habits; and lifestyle, culture, and educational background. In addition to this information, the provider may check the patient's skin **turgor** to determine the level of hydration and perform various techniques to assess the percentage of body fat.

Body Fat Measurement

The location of body fat may be related to an increased risk of developing diabetes, stroke, hypertension, and coronary artery disease. Studies indicate that the body has two places to store fat: at the hips and in the abdomen. Fat at the hips is more common in women and is used to store energy for special purposes, such as during pregnancy and breastfeeding. Abdominal fat, or central obesity, seems to be more dangerous to overall health. Health risks related to weight range from no increased risk with normal weight to severe risk from central obesity, with the risk from other types of obesity falling somewhere in between.

To determine the patient's status, the waist and hips are measured and correlated with the waist-to-hip ratio (the bigger the belly, the higher the ratio). Normal ratios are less than 0.75 in women and 0.90 to 0.95 in men. Waist measurements also can predict the risk of developing a weight-related disease. Men at increased risk for disease have a waist measurement greater than 40 inches (102 cm); for women, the risk is increased with a waist measurement greater than 35 inches (88 cm).

At the provider's request, the medical assistant may perform body fat measurements on a patient. The percentage of body fat may be an indicator of overall health and of risk for cardiovascular disease. Body fat can be measured by several methods. A reliable method of measuring body fat uses a specially designed caliper to measure the thickness of a fold of tissue in three areas: the triceps, the subscapular, and the suprailiac regions (Figure 23-2). However, an increasing number of patients have fat folds that are too large for calipers to measure. The provider may also order a dual energy x-ray absorptiometry (DEXA) scan, in which two x-ray beams are used to give accurate feedback on the body fat percentage, where the fat is distributed, and bone density.

Body Mass Index

To determine how healthy an adult patient's weight level is, the provider may ask the medical assistant to calculate the patient's BMI. The BMI is the relationship of weight to height that mathematically correlates the patient's measurements with health risks. It is a more accurate predictor of weight-related diseases than traditional height-weight charts because it provides a good estimate of the degree of body fat.

A patient's BMI can be calculated by dividing the weight in kilograms by the square of the height in meters: BMI = Weight (kg) ÷ Height (m²)]. However, to determine the BMI, clinics can use a wheel device that compares the patient's height to weight, or an online BMI calculator, or can refer to a BMI chart (Table 23-5). This is not necessary with EHR systems because the program automatically calculates the BMI after the patient's height and weight have been documented. Table 23-6 shows the correlation between a patient's BMI and the risks for disease.

Individuals with a BMI of 19 to 22 are thought to live the longest. Death rates are significantly higher for people with a BMI of 25 or above. If the risk is anything other than acceptable, dietary modifications may be needed. The provider makes this decision after evaluating all the patient's data.

CRITICAL THINKING APPLICATION   **23-3**

The provider encourages Mr. Hawthorne to lose weight to lower his BMI of 29. Explain how Marcia could coach Mr. Hawthorne about the importance of his BMI and how he can monitor his BMI at home. What educational materials might be helpful?

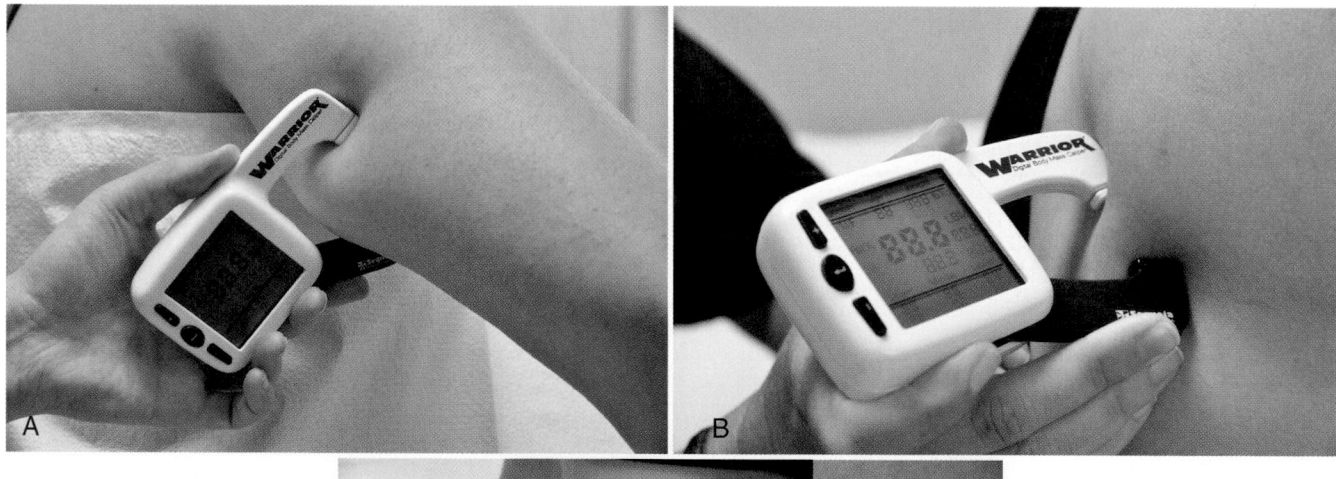

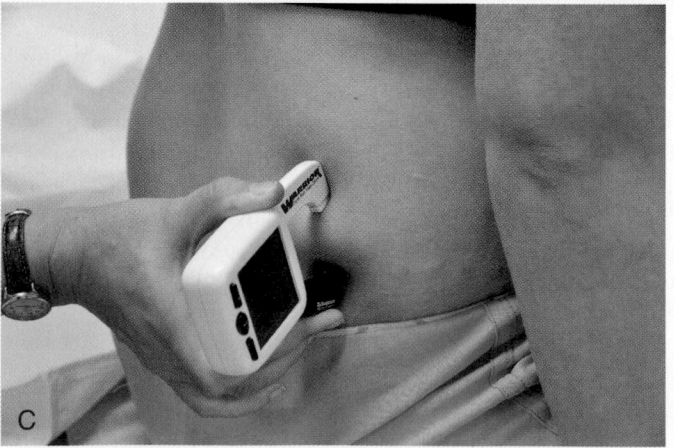

FIGURE 23-2 Determining fat fold measurements. **A,** Triceps. **B,** Subscapular. **C,** Suprailiac.

TABLE 23-5   Body Mass Index Chart*

	BODY WEIGHT (lb)																
HEIGHT (in)	19	20	21	22	23	24	25	26	27	28	29	30	31	32	33	34	35
58	91	96	100	105	110	115	119	124	129	134	138	143	148	153	158	162	167
59	94	99	104	109	114	119	124	128	133	138	143	148	153	158	163	168	173
60	97	102	107	112	118	123	128	133	138	143	148	153	158	163	168	174	179
61	100	106	111	116	122	127	132	137	143	148	153	158	164	169	174	180	185
62	104	109	115	120	126	131	136	142	147	153	158	164	169	175	180	186	191
63	107	113	118	124	130	135	141	146	152	158	163	169	175	180	186	191	197
64	110	116	122	128	134	140	145	151	157	163	169	174	180	186	192	197	204
65	114	120	126	132	138	144	150	156	162	168	174	180	186	192	198	204	210
66	118	124	130	136	142	148	155	161	167	173	179	186	192	198	204	210	216
67	121	127	134	140	146	153	159	166	172	178	185	191	198	204	211	217	223
68	125	131	138	144	151	158	164	171	177	184	190	197	203	210	216	223	230
69	128	135	142	149	155	162	169	176	182	189	196	203	209	216	223	230	236
70	132	139	146	153	160	167	174	181	188	195	202	209	216	222	229	236	243
71	136	143	150	157	165	172	179	186	193	200	208	215	222	229	236	243	250
72	140	147	154	162	169	177	184	191	199	206	213	221	228	235	242	250	258
73	144	151	159	166	174	182	189	197	204	212	219	227	235	242	250	257	265
74	148	155	163	171	179	186	194	202	210	218	225	233	241	249	256	264	272
75	152	160	168	176	184	192	200	208	216	224	232	240	248	256	264	272	279
76	156	164	172	180	189	197	205	213	221	230	238	246	254	263	271	279	287

National Institutes of Health/National Heart, Lung, and Blood Institute: *Clinical guidelines on the identification, evaluation, and treatment of overweight and obesity in adults: the evidence report,* June 1998. www.nhlbi.nih.gov/guidelines/obesity/bmi_tbl.htm. Accessed March 22, 2015.

*To use the table, find the appropriate height in the left-hand column. Move across to a given weight. The number at the top of the column is the BMI at that height and weight. Pounds have been rounded off.

TABLE 23-6   Body Mass Index and Disease Risk

BODY MASS INDEX	CLASSIFICATION	DISEASE RISK
≤18.5	Underweight	Low
18.5-24.9	Normal weight	Low
25-29.9	Overweight	Increased
30-34.9	Obese	High
35-39.9	Obese	Very high
≥40	Extremely obese	Extremely high

THERAPEUTIC NUTRITION

Although most patients are treated medically without a therapeutic diet, patient treatment may include the use of special diets. For example, patients with hypertension, hypercholesterolemia, certain gastrointestinal diseases, and **diabetes mellitus type 1** and **diabetes mellitus type 2** all benefit from a therapeutically planned diet. It is important to take into consideration the patient's lifestyle, cultural influences, and background to ensure cooperation.

Modifying a Diet

The following features of a normal diet (or combinations of them) can be modified to create a therapeutic diet:

- Consistency
- Calorie level
- Amounts of one or more nutrients

- Degree of bulk or fiber
- Spiciness
- Levels of specific foods

In general, a normal diet is modified by restricting or increasing the foods that are sources of the nutrient involved in the disease process. Except for the nutrient in question, the recommended daily allowances usually can be met. However, if several restrictions are ordered for the same patient, a nutrient supplement may be necessary.

Liquid Diet

Two types of liquid diets are used. A clear liquid diet includes only transparent or translucent liquids, such as broth soups, tea, and gelatin. In some cases, apple juice and cranberry juice may be allowed. A full liquid diet includes all foods allowed on a clear liquid diet plus milk, custards, strained cream soups, refined cereals, eggnog, milkshakes, and all juices. This diet may be indicated as part of preparation for certain diagnostic tests (e.g., colonoscopy) or for the first several days after major surgery.

Soft or Light Diet

When a soft or light diet is prescribed, foods with roughage are eliminated (no raw fruits or vegetables). No strongly flavored or gas-forming vegetables are allowed (e.g., onions, beans, broccoli, and cauliflower), and spices also may be limited. This diet often is used after surgery to place less strain on the gastrointestinal system or for patients with certain gastrointestinal disorders.

Mechanical Soft Diet

A mechanical soft diet is a regular diet in which the food is chopped, ground, or pureed, depending on the degree of texture change required. No foods or spices are restricted. This diet may be used after dental or oral surgery or for patients who have difficulty chewing or swallowing.

Bland Diet

A bland diet restricts dietary components classified as gastrointestinal irritants. Such a diet limits any foods that are chemically irritating (e.g., caffeine, pepper, chili, nutmeg, and alcohol) or mechanically irritating (e.g., high-fiber foods). No fried foods or highly concentrated sweets are allowed. Gas-forming vegetables belonging to the onion and cabbage family also are eliminated. A bland diet commonly is used for problems of the gastrointestinal tract. Such a diet should supply sufficient nutrients for the individual to meet the recommended daily allowances unless fruits and vegetables are eliminated.

Lactose Sensitivity and Intolerance

Lactose is a sugar found in milk and milk products. Lactase is an enzyme produced in the small intestine to break down lactose into two simpler forms of sugar, glucose and galactose. The body absorbs these simpler sugars into the bloodstream. Patients with lactose sensitivity or intolerance have either a lactase deficiency or a problem absorbing lactose. They experience a number of gastrointestinal (GI) symptoms, including bloating, diarrhea, and gas after drinking milk or eating dairy products.

Lactose intolerance is sometimes confused with a milk allergy, but an allergy is an immune system response that may even be life-threatening, whereas lactose intolerance is a GI disorder that results in uncomfortable symptoms. A cow's milk allergy typically occurs in the first year of life, whereas lactose intolerance occurs more often during adolescence or adulthood.

Lactose intolerance is more likely to occur in certain racial and ethnic groups, including African-Americans, Hispanics/Latinos, Native Americans, and Asian-Americans.

The most important health concern with this condition is its effect on calcium and vitamin D intake. Individuals with lactose sensitivity or intolerance can manage the condition by using lactose-free and lactose-reduced milk and milk products and by taking lactase tablets or drops when eating or drinking milk products. The lactase enzyme digests the lactose in the food and decreases the chances of developing GI symptoms.

Elimination Diet

Elimination diets involve removing specific foods or ingredients from the diet to help diagnose food allergies. Common allergy-causing foods include milk, eggs, fish, crustacean shellfish, wheat, soy, peanuts, and tree nuts. An elimination diet can vary slightly but generally involves elimination of certain foods from the diet and then a gradual reintroduction phase. During the elimination phase, which should last 4 to 8 weeks, all potentially problematic foods must be avoided and replaced with safer alternatives. If the elimination phase results in significant health improvements, the reintroduction phase begins with systematically reintroducing eliminated foods into the diet one at a time and every few days to assess tolerance. Any foods that trigger previous symptoms should be avoided. Foods that don't appear to cause any reaction are considered safe and can become part of the regular diet again. Gluten-free and lactose-free diets are types of elimination diets. Elimination diets may be helpful for individuals with irritable bowel syndrome (IBS), migraine headaches, and other inflammatory diseases, such as rheumatoid arthritis.

Gluten-Free Diets

Gluten is found in grains such as wheat, barley, and rye. A gluten-free diet is primarily used to treat celiac disease, which is an inherited allergy to the gluten protein. There is no treatment for celiac disease other than avoiding gluten in the diet. Gluten causes inflammation in the small intestines of people with celiac disease, and eating a gluten-free diet helps control signs and symptoms and prevents destruction of the small intestine wall. People with celiac disease must eat a strictly gluten-free diet and must remain on the diet for the remainder of their lives. People who don't have celiac disease but have symptoms when they eat gluten are diagnosed with nonceliac gluten sensitivity. People with nonceliac gluten sensitivity may benefit from a gluten-free diet, but there is still some controversy over whether it is actually gluten that is causing their symptoms. Further research is needed in this area.

High- or Low-Fiber Diet

The amount of bulk or fiber in the diet is either increased or decreased, depending on the specific disorder of the colon or large bowel. In either case, foods high in cellulose are considered high in fiber because the body does not digest this carbohydrate well, and a residue is left in the colon. In some instances, a low-residue diet is distinguished from a low-fiber diet. In this case, a low-fiber diet eliminates foods with a high cellulose content, and a low-residue diet restricts milk in addition to fiber content. Either diet should supply all the nutrients needed; however, if milk is restricted drastically, the calcium level must be watched carefully. Low-fiber diets are prescribed for patients with certain gastrointestinal disorders, such as diverticulitis. High-fiber diets are recommended for patients with hypercholesterolemia or diabetes mellitus and to prevent certain forms of cancer.

Diabetic Diet

The specific diet for a patient with diabetes is determined by the individual's health needs. The basic goal of managing the disease is to maintain consistent control of blood glucose levels. When developing a diabetic diet plan, the provider or dietitian must consider additional factors, such as the need for weight control, individual patient preferences, exercise patterns, and lifestyle factors. General guidelines for a healthy diabetic diet include the following:

- Five servings of dark-colored fruits and vegetables and six of whole grains each day
- Two weekly servings of fatty fish (salmon, cod, mackerel)
- Complex carbohydrates that are high in fiber (e.g., whole grains)
- Monounsaturated fats (olive and canola oil)
- Daily serving of nuts, seeds, or legumes
- Fish or soy over poultry or other meat
- Avoidance of fad diets, especially those with high-protein, low-carbohydrate foods
- Reduced salt intake
- Avoidance of saturated fats and trans fats

Traditionally, the diabetic diet has been based on exchange lists, which group foods according to similar calorie, carbohydrate, protein, and fat content. The objective of exchange lists is to achieve the proper balance of carbohydrates, proteins, and fats while maintaining healthy weight and blood glucose levels. Menus are developed based on the food groupings and the optimum number of daily calories needed to meet the patient's needs. Foods can be substituted for one another within an exchange list but not among lists. Table 23-7 lists the number of exchanges per day allowed within certain calorie-restricted diabetic diets.

Cancer and Nutrition

Good nutrition is important when one is diagnosed with cancer and during cancer treatment. Although the nutrient needs of people with cancer vary, listed below are some general guidelines.

Extra protein is usually needed to heal tissues and help fight infection. Choose monounsaturated and polyunsaturated fats to help create stored energy, insulate body tissues, and transport fat-soluble vitamins.

Carbohydrates are needed for energy and proper organ function; fruits, vegetables, and whole grains provide vitamins, minerals, and fiber.

If there is vomiting or diarrhea, extra fluid intake may be required. Drink at least 1 cup of liquid after each loose bowel movement to prevent dehydration.

When undergoing cancer treatment, it is common to have a poor appetite; try eating frequent small meals, avoiding liquids with meals, and keeping high-calorie, high-protein snacks on hand.

Try bland, soft, easy-to-digest foods if nauseated.

The provider or dietitian may suggest a daily multivitamin and mineral supplement.

Do not take large amounts of vitamins or any herbs unless the provider is aware of it and approves.

Nutrition for People With Cancer. The American Cancer Society http://www.cancer.org/treatment/survivorshipduringandaftertreatment/nutritionforpeoplewithcancer/index?sitearea=M. Accessed February 10, 2016.

TABLE 23-7 Diabetic Diet Exchanges per Day

EXCHANGE GROUPS AND SERVING SIZES	NUMBER OF EXCHANGES OR SERVINGS IN EACH GROUP				
	1,200*	1,500*	1,800*	2,000*	2,200*
Starch or bread: One exchange equals 1 ounce bread and ½ cup cooked cereal, grain, or pasta	5	8	10	11	13
Meat and cheese: One exchange equals 1 ounce; high-fat exchanges should be used no more than three times per week	4	5	7	8	8
Vegetables: One exchange equals ½ cup cooked, 1 cup raw, and ½ cup juice	2	3	3	4	4
Fruits and sugar: No more than 10% of total daily carbohydrates; each exchange equals 15 g carbohydrate	3	3	3	3	3
Milk products: One exchange equals 1 cup (8 ounces); skim and very low fat milk products are recommended	2	2	2	2	2
Fats: One exchange equals 1 teaspoon of fat	3	3	3	4	5

*Number of calories in the prescribed diabetic diet.

Diabetes educators agree that the simplest way to teach patients about the relationship between diet and blood glucose levels is to focus on the total number of carbohydrate grams a patient can consume daily (carb counting) while maintaining the recommended blood glucose level. In this way, patients can decide how they want to distribute their carbohydrate intake throughout the day. The number of carbohydrate grams a patient with diabetes can eat each day is determined by a combination of factors: the patient's weight and whether weight loss or maintenance is part of the treatment plan; the level of exercise because physical activity lowers the blood glucose level; prescribed diabetic medications, including insulin; and other factors, such as age and blood lipid levels.

Therefore, people with diabetes can eat sugary foods as long as they restrict themselves to the total number of carbohydrates allowed for that snack or meal, and the decision to eat that food adheres to the rules of healthy nutrition. In other words, a patient with diabetes can have a whole-wheat raisin bagel for breakfast as long as the total carbohydrate grams for the bagel do not exceed the number of carbohydrate grams that should be eaten for that particular meal. Table 23-8 presents breakfast choices for a patient with diabetes restricted to a total of 50 g of carbohydrate per day.

All carbohydrates raise the blood glucose level to a similar degree. In general, 1 g of carbohydrate raises the blood sugar level of a person who weighs 150 pounds by 4 points; for a person who weighs 200 pounds, it raises the level by 3 points. However, not all carbohydrates raise the blood glucose level at the same rate. Choosing a carbohydrate that takes longer to affect the blood glucose level helps control hyperglycemic peaks, which are associated with the complications of diabetes mellitus. A rating system known as the Glycemic Index (GI) may help solve this problem. The GI rates carbohydrate foods on a scale from slowest to fastest effects on blood glucose levels. The lower the GI value of the food, the longer it takes to raise the patient's blood glucose level. The GI scale is based on 100 glycemic units, which is equivalent to the number of units in a glucose tablet. The Glycemic Index of foods helps people with diabetes understand the impact of different carbohydrates on the blood glucose level, but it can be a complicated tool to understand, and it must be used in conjunction with a dietary plan that considers the nutritional guidelines for all foods (Procedure 23-1). For further information about the Glycemic Index, refer to the American Diabetes Association website (*www.diabetes.org/*).

TABLE 23-8 Carbohydrate (CHO) Content of Breakfast Foods

FOOD TYPE	SERVING SIZE	CHO (g)
1% Reduced fat milk	1 cup	12
Bran Chex	2/3 cup	23
Frosted Flakes	3/4 cup	26
Apples and cinnamon instant oatmeal	1 packet	27
Low-fat granola	1/2 cup	30
Toast	1 slice	15
White table sugar	1 teaspoon	4
Pancakes	2	15
Pancake syrup	2 tablespoons	30
Light pancake syrup	2 tablespoons	4
Fruit yogurt	1 cup	40
Fruit yogurt with NutraSweet	1 cup	19
Fruit juice	1/2 cup	15
Banana	1/2	15

Glycemic Index (GI) Values of Some Foods

FOOD	GI VALUE (0-100 SCALE)
Honey	91
Puffed rice	90
White potato	87
Corn chips	72
White rice	72
Whole-wheat bread	72
Shredded wheat	70
Brown rice	66
Refined sugar	64
Rye bread	64
Oatmeal cookies	57
Potato chips	56
Oatmeal	53
Sweet potato	50
Spaghetti	38
Yogurt	38
Milk	34
Kidney beans	33
Fructose	22
Soybeans	14

CRITICAL THINKING APPLICATION   23-4
Samantha Rashad recently was diagnosed with diabetes mellitus type 2. She has met with the dietitian, but she has some questions about her 1,200-calorie diabetic diet. The goals of her dietary management are to maintain blood glucose levels within normal range while encouraging weight loss. Based on Marcia's knowledge of the components of a healthy diet, what recommendations can she make to Ms. Rashad?

Heart-Healthy Diet

The goals for a heart-healthy diet are to encourage the patient to eat foods that reduce overall cholesterol levels and LDL, increase HDL, and keep blood pressure within normal limits. Other factors that must be considered for patients at risk for heart disease are obesity

PROCEDURE 23-1	Instruct a Patient According to the Patient's Dietary Needs: Coach the Patient on the Basics of the Glycemic Index

The Glycemic Index (GI) rates carbohydrate foods on a scale from slowest to fastest effects on blood glucose levels. The lower the GI value of the food, the longer it takes to raise the patient's blood glucose level. With your partner, role-play how to teach the following patient about the GI index. The patient was recently diagnosed with diabetes type 2, is of Italian descent, and has a family history of diabetes type 2 and a body mass index (BMI) of 30.*

Goal: *To coach the patient the basic principles of a diabetic diet using the Glycemic Index of foods.*

EQUIPMENT and SUPPLIES

- Patient's health record
- Handouts and a list of professional websites that discuss a diabetic diet and the Glycemic Index of foods
- Table of the Glycemic Index of foods
- Pencil and paper

PROCEDURAL STEPS

1. Using the patient's health and family histories, assess the individual to determine cultural influences that may affect dietary choices.
   PURPOSE: Cultural factors may influence the patient's dietary choices.
2. Introduce yourself and explain to the patient that you are going to teach him or her about the Glycemic Index of foods. Be sure to include reasons the patient should use a food's GI value to help plan carbohydrate food choices.
   PURPOSE: Explaining the rationale for consistently referring to the GI value of a carbohydrate food encourages the patient to participate in the education process.
3. Using the GI table, point out the Glycemic Index value of common carbohydrate foods.
   PURPOSE: Using the index when looking up types of carbohydrate foods that the patient typically eats assists learning and reinforces practical applications.

4. Give the patient the pencil and paper to write down the GI value of five favorite carbohydrate foods.
   PURPOSE: Writing down information aids memory retention.
5. Compare the numbers and ask the patient to determine which would be a healthy choice and explain why.
   PURPOSE: Comparing the results reinforces learning.
6. Together, analyze the patient's choices of foods with a low GI value.
   PURPOSE: To gather feedback about the learning experience so that the patient's learning needs are clarified.
7. Ask the patient whether he or she will use this information when shopping and making carbohydrate food choices.
   PURPOSE: Role-play implementation of the information to determine the patient's level of learning.
8. Document the education intervention, including the feedback received from the patient about his or her understanding of how to use the GI.
   PURPOSE: Documentation in the health record provides proof of patient education and an assessment of the patient's ability to apply the knowledge to daily practice.

---

*For further information about the Glycemic Index, refer to the American Diabetes Association website at www.diabetes.org/.

American Heart Association's Diet and Lifestyle Recommendations

- Eat at least 4 ½ cups a day of a variety of fruits and vegetables.
- Eat six or more servings a day of a variety of grain products, with at least three servings a day of fiber-rich whole grains.
- Eat fish at least twice a week; research indicates that eating oily fish containing omega-3 fatty acids (salmon, trout, and herring) may help lower the risk of death from coronary artery disease.
- Include fat-free and low-fat milk products, legumes, skinless poultry, and lean meats.
- Choose fats and oils with 2 g or less of saturated fat per tablespoon (e.g., canola or olive oil).
- Limit the intake of foods high in calories or low in nutrition.
- Limit foods high in saturated fat and trans fat.

- Eat less than 1,500 mg of sodium a day.
- Cut back on beverages and foods with added sugars.
- Eat at least four servings a week of nuts, legumes, and seeds.
- Quit smoking and avoid secondhand smoke.
- Women should limit their alcohol intake to one drink a day; men to two drinks a day.
- Balance calorie intake with the number of calories burned each day. If overweight or obese, multiply your ideal body weight by 15 (active) or 13 (not active) to find the number of calories you should eat to gradually achieve your ideal body weight.
- Get enough physical activity to keep fit. Exercise at least 30 minutes every day.

American Heart Association. www.heart.org/HEARTORG/. Accessed March 23, 2015.

and the patient's typical exercise patterns. Obesity is associated with elevated lipid levels; therefore, weight management must be part of the patient's dietary plan. In addition, researchers report that an aerobic exercise program must be included to maintain cholesterol at a healthy level.

Cross-Cultural Tips for Reducing Sodium and Fat

- Limit the use of soy or teriyaki sauce, even the low-sodium type.
- Eat fresh or frozen fruits and vegetables; rinse fresh produce before eating, or choose canned products low in sodium.
- Bake or broil meats rather than frying; limit beef products; remove skin from chicken before cooking; increase the intake of unprocessed fish.
- Cook with olive or canola oil.
- Limit servings of cured foods, such as ham and bacon; avoid pickles and other foods prepared in brine; limit condiments such as mustard and ketchup.
- Cook rice and pasta without added salt; do not use instant versions, which are higher in sodium.
- Do not add salt to food; use substitute spices, such as lemon, lime, and herbs.

CRITICAL THINKING APPLICATION   23-5

Ms. Rashad's blood pressure at this visit was 182/94. She is concerned about the risks of heart disease and wants to lower her blood pressure. What facts about a heart-healthy diet should Marcia share with her to help her understand the importance of nutrition in overall wellness?

READING FOOD LABELS

The USDA requires that all food products carry a nutrition facts label. Food labels are a source of information about the nutrients in the product. When a designated diet is planned or implemented, the food label can be used as a valuable source of nutritional information (Procedure 23-2).

The U.S. Food and Drug Administration (FDA) is proposing to update the Nutrition Facts label on food packages by 2016-2017 to reflect new public health and scientific information. One major change will be to update the serving size so that it reflects the amount of food people actually eat and drink. In addition, the format of the label will be changed so that the key parts (calories, serving sizes, and percent daily value) are displayed more prominently (Figure 23-3). The following will be some of the requirements for the new label.

- The Dietary Guidelines for Americans recommend reducing the intake of calories from added sugars. Americans on average eat 16% of their total calories from added sugars, the major sources being soda, energy and sports drinks, grain-based desserts, sugar-sweetened fruit drinks, dairy-based desserts, and candy. The new label must include an "Added Sugars" category, indented under "Sugars," so that both are listed.
- "Calories from fat" will no longer be shown because research shows that the total fat calories in the diet are less important than the type of fat consumed. The categories "Total Fat," "Saturated Fat," and "Trans Fat" must still be listed.
- The new label must show the amount of calcium, vitamin D, potassium, and iron because studies show that Americans are consuming inadequate amounts of these nutrients, and their lack

A

Nutrition Facts

Serving size 2/3 cup (55g)
Servings Per Container About 8

Amount Per Serving
Calories 230   Calories from Fat 72

	% Daily Value*
Total Fat 8g	**12%**
Saturated Fat 1g	**5%**
Trans Fat 0g	
Cholesterol 0mg	**0%**
Sodium 160mg	**7%**
Total Carbohydrate 37g	**12%**
Dietary Fiber 4g	**16%**
Sugars 1g	
Protein 3g	
Vitamin A	10%
Vitamin C	8%
Calcium	20%
Iron	45%

*Percent Daily Values are based on a 2,000 calorie diet. Your daily value may be higher or lower depending on your calorie needs.

		Calories: 2,000	2,500
Total Fat	Less than	65g	80g
Sat Fat	Less than	20g	25g
Cholesterol	Less than	300mg	300mg
Sodium	Less than	2,400mg	2,400mg
Total Carbohydrate		300g	375g
Dietary Fiber		25g	30g

B

Nutrition Facts

8 servings per container
Serving size   2/3 cup (55g)

Amount per 2/3 cup
Calories   230

% DV*	
12%	**Total Fat** 8g
5%	Saturated Fat 1g
	Trans Fat 0g
0%	**Cholesterol** 0mg
7%	**Sodium** 160mg
12%	**Total Carbs** 37g
14%	Dietary Fiber 4g
	Sugars 1g
	Added Sugars 0g
	Protein 3g
10%	**Vitamin D** 2mcg
20%	**Calcium** 260mg
45%	**Iron** 8mg
5%	**Potassium** 235mg

• Footnote on Daily Values (DV) and calories reference to be inserted here.

FIGURE 23-3 Nutrition Facts label. (From the US Food and Drug Administration. www.fda.gov/food/ingredientspackaginglabeling/labelingnutrition/ucm114155.htm. Accessed March 22, 2015.)

is associated with the risk of chronic disease. The actual amount of vitamins and minerals in the food must be included.

- The amount per serving must be given in common household measures, such as 1 cup.
- If a claim is made about any of the optional components or if a food is fortified or enriched with any of them, nutrition information for these components must be provided.

How to Use Label Information

When evaluating the nutritional value of a food product, begin with the serving size information, which is listed in household measurements. The amount of each nutrient in the food is expressed in terms of weight per serving. If you eat more or less than the serving size on the label, you will need to adjust the amounts of nutrients and number of calories accordingly. The goal is to choose foods that total 100% of your daily nutrition needs.

The ingredient list on the label also can help you learn more about the foods you eat. Ingredients are listed in descending order of weight; that is, the ingredient with the largest amount in the food is listed first. This helps you get an idea of the proportion of an ingredient in a food (Figure 23-4). Artificial colors must be named in the ingredient list; this is important information for individuals with food allergies and those on specialized diets. In addition, the total percentage of juice in juice drinks must be declared so that you can see exactly how much juice is in the product.

INGREDIENT LABEL

INGREDIENTS: COOKED WHITE RICE, WATER, COOKED CHICKEN TENDERLOINS, GREEN BEANS, CARROTS, RED PEPPERS, BROWN SUGAR. CONTAINS LESS THAN 2% OF MODIFIED FOOD STARCH, MUSTARD (VINEGAR, MUSTARD SEED, SALT, SPICES, TURMERIC), DIJON MUSTARD (WATER, MUSTARD SEED, DISTILLED VINEGAR, SALT, WHITE WINE, CITRIC ACID, TARTARIC ACID, SPICES), HONEY, MALTODEXTRIN (FROM CORN), SALT, EGG YOLK SOLIDS, SODIUM PHOSPHATE, VINEGAR POWDER (MALTODEXTRIN, MODIFIED FOOD STARCH, VINEGAR SOLIDS), XANTHAN GUM FLAVORS, SPICES, LEMON JUICE CONCENTRATE

FIGURE 23-4 Ingredient label.

The front package label is where manufacturers often place statements describing the nutritional qualities of their product. The government has set strict conditions under which statements such as "low fat," "cholesterol free," and "good source of fiber" can be used as part of the front label. The FDA permits claims linking a nutrient or food to the risk of a disease or health-related condition, but only claims supported by scientific evidence are allowed.

PROCEDURE 23-2 Coach a Patient About How to Understand Food Labels

Goal: *To help the patient understand food labels.*

EQUIPMENT and SUPPLIES

- Patient's health record
- Food labels from a protein bar, a granola bar, and a pop tart package
- Pencil and paper

PROCEDURAL STEPS

Role-play the following steps with your partner.

1. Using the patient's health and family histories, assess the individual to determine cultural influences that may affect dietary choices.
   PURPOSE: Cultural factors may influence the patient's dietary choices.
2. Introduce yourself and explain to the patient that you are going to teach him or her how to read a food label. Be sure to include reasons food labels are a valuable source of nutritional information in meal planning.
   PURPOSE: Explaining the rationale for consistently reading food labels encourages the patient to participate in the education process.
3. Using the labels on each product, point out the nutritional information according to the guidelines in the text.
   PURPOSE: Using actual labels assists learning and reinforces practical applications.
4. Give the patient the pencil and paper to write down the serving size of each type of bar.
   PURPOSE: Writing down information aids memory retention.
5. Compare the similarities and differences among the products.
   PURPOSE: Comparing the results reinforces learning.
6. Have the patient write down the total number of calories for a single serving of each food product.
   PURPOSE: To reinforce the significant effect of high-calorie snacks on overall nutritional health.
7. Write down the amount of total, saturated, and trans fats in each product.
   PURPOSE: To review the role of saturated and trans fats in disease.
8. Record the total number of added sugars and sodium in each product.
9. Together, analyze the nutritional level of each.
10. Discuss any new information learned.
    PURPOSE: To gather feedback about the learning experience so that the patient's learning needs are clarified.
11. Ask the patient whether he or she will use this information when shopping and how it will be implemented in menu planning.
    PURPOSE: Role-play implementation of the information to determine the patient's level of learning.
12. Document the education intervention, including the feedback received from the patient about his or her understanding of how to read food labels.
    PURPOSE: Documentation in the health record provides proof of patient education and an assessment of the patient's ability to apply the knowledge to daily practice.

Regulated Nutritional Claims for Food Labels

Calorie-free	Less than 5 calories per serving
Extra lean	Cooked meat or poultry with less than 4.9 g of fat per serving, of which less than 1.8 g is saturated fat
Fat-free	Less than 0.5 g of fat per serving
Fresh	Raw; never frozen, processed, or preserved
High	Provides more than 20% of the recommended daily consumption (per serving) of the nutrient (e.g., high-fiber)
Lean	Cooked meat or poultry with less than 10.5 g of fat per serving, of which less than 3.5 g is saturated fat
Light	One-third fewer calories than the regular product
Low-calorie	Less than 40 calories per serving
Low-fat	3 g or less of fat per serving
Low saturated fat	1 g or less of saturated fat per serving, and not more than 15% of calories from saturated fat
Low-sodium	Less than 140 mg of sodium per serving
Saturated fat–free	Less than 2 g of saturated fat per serving
Sodium-free	Less than 5 mg of sodium per serving
Sugar-free	Less than 0.5 g of sugar per serving

Organic Foods Production Act

In 1990 the USDA initiated regulations for organically grown food, and in 2002 the agency revised the regulations for the production and labeling of organic foods. Until then, organizations from state governments to trade and consumer groups contributed to the regulation of organic products, resulting in often-conflicting standards about which products could be labeled organic. Current government regulations require that foods labeled organic must have been produced without exposure to pesticides, chemical fertilizers, or sewage sludge. The food cannot have been irradiated to extend shelf life, nor can it contain any genetically modified ingredients. In addition, animals raised for organic meat, eggs, and milk cannot be given antibiotics or growth hormones; must be fed organic feed; and must have had access to the outdoors.

Products with a "100 percent organic" label are limited to strictly organic ingredients. Products simply labeled "organic" identify the food as being made up of 95% organic materials. Products that fall into these two categories can display a "USDA Organic" seal. Foods containing at least 70% organic ingredients may be labeled "made with organic ingredients" and may list up to three of them on the package. Any product containing less than 70% organic ingredients may not be marketed as an organic food.

FOOD-BORNE DISEASES

Eating or drinking contaminated food can result in a food-borne disease. Each year, 1 in 6 Americans gets sick by consuming contaminated foods or beverages. Many different types of bacteria, viruses, and parasites can contaminate food, but the most common are *Escherichia coli* and *Salmonella* and *Campylobacter* organisms. Patients may experience a variety of symptoms, but the first typically are

gastrointestinal: nausea, vomiting, stomach pain, and/or diarrhea. Usually a delay of several hours to days occurs after ingestion of the contaminated substance before symptoms begin. This is the *incubation period*, when the microbes are attaching to the intestinal wall and beginning to multiply. The diagnosis is confirmed with laboratory tests, of which the most common is a stool sample. However, more sophisticated tests may be needed to diagnose viral pathogens.

Prevention is the most effective way to limit food-borne disease. Essential to prevention efforts are clean drinking water; inspection of restaurants and meat production facilities; temperature monitoring of food; adequate sewage treatment; and public education on proper hygiene. All patients with a suspected food-borne illness should perform frequent handwashing to prevent the spread of the disease.

Treatment of a food-borne disease depends on the microorganism causing the illness and the patient's symptoms; if diarrhea and vomiting are severe, dehydration is a major concern, especially in young children and older adults. In such cases, replacing fluid and electrolytes is the most important aspect of care. Other treatments include the use of antidiarrheal medications (e.g., Imodium) and drugs that coat the gastrointestinal tract (e.g., Pepto-Bismol). Antibiotics may shorten the duration of the disease but are only prescribed if the organism causing the infection can be identified and will respond to antibiotic therapy.

When you are screening phone calls from patients experiencing gastrointestinal symptoms, complaints that indicate a food-borne illness include:

- Fever of 101.5° F (38.6° C) or higher
- Diarrhea lasting longer than 3 days
- Prolonged vomiting
- Blood in the stool
- Signs of dehydration (reduced urination, dry mouth, **vertigo**, and altered skin turgor)

ENVIRONMENTAL CONTAMINATION OF FOOD

Environmental contamination of food can be a serious problem. The FDA regularly monitors the presence of contaminants in the food chain and issues warnings as needed to protect consumers from possible danger. Mercury is the most common heavy metal found in food, primarily fish. Other environmental contaminants include cadmium from industrial processing; lead found in old paint and old plumbing; and polychlorinated biphenyls (PCBs), which are part of discarded electrical equipment. Each of these can have serious toxic effects on humans. For example, mercury at toxic levels can poison the nervous system, especially that of a developing fetus. The FDA therefore recommends that pregnant women, women of childbearing age, nursing mothers, and young children not eat any fish known to have high mercury levels. These include king mackerel, swordfish, shark, and any fresh water fish from lakes or rivers known to be contaminated with mercury.

EATING DISORDERS

An eating disorder is any eating behavior pattern that can lead to a health problem. These disorders can damage all the body systems and can cause death. Although 90% of reported cases occur in adolescent and young adult women, the incidence in males and middle-aged women is rising.

Anorexia nervosa is characterized by self-induced starvation. Anorexic individuals typically are adolescents when first diagnosed and tend to be perfectionists who are extremely sensitive to failure and any criticism. They use avoidance of food as a way of controlling their feelings and fear of becoming grossly overweight if they allow themselves to eat. As a result, they lose an excessive amount of weight, usually 15% to 60% of their normal body weight, resulting in extreme malnourishment. They can die without medical intervention. If necessary, patients are fed intravenously or by nasogastric tube feedings to establish an immediate level of nourishment to the body systems. Patients with anorexia nervosa have a significantly distorted body image and require psychotherapy to alleviate depression, to deal with their emotional issues, and for assistance in forming a positive self-image.

Bulimia is more common than anorexia and is characterized by cycles of bingeing and purging. This behavior pattern usually begins in adolescence when an individual who is slightly overweight diets but fails to achieve the expected results. Psychologically the person believes that self-worth is related to being thin. Usually the pattern begins with some form of stress that upsets the individual, who then turns to food for consolation. Intake during a binge period can reach as high as 20,000 calories. The eating binge is followed by self-induced punishment in the form of vomiting, using laxatives and enemas, excessive exercise, and food abstinence. Most individuals with bulimia have a normal or an above-normal body weight, but their weight can vary as much as 10 pounds during bingeing and purging cycles. Treatment programs involve a combination of medication, psychotherapy, and nutritional counseling. The goal is to help the patient establish healthy eating patterns and develop an improved self-image.

Binge-eating disorder is similar to bulimia; however, people with binge-eating disorder do not purge themselves of the extra calories or exercise excessively. As a result, people with binge-eating disorder often are overweight or obese. With obesity comes a higher risk of cardiovascular disease and hypertension. These individuals often experience guilt, shame, and anxiety about binge eating, which leads to more binge eating. They have a compulsion to gorge themselves that they cannot control. Typically, people with binge-eating disorder have no obvious physical signs or symptoms. Binge eating is a complicated psychological disorder in which patients express a combination of shame, poor self-image, and self-disgust. Treatment works to address these issues through psychotherapy, although antidepressants and topiramate (Topamax) may help reduce the episodes of bingeing. Complementary and alternative therapies, such as massage, therapeutic touch, and mind-body therapies (meditation, yoga, and hypnosis) may help reduce anxiety and promote an awareness of the body's cues for hunger and fullness.

CRITICAL THINKING APPLICATION   **23-6**

A 22-year-old patient is being seen for the first time for a work-related physical examination. While you are gathering her patient history, she mentions that she takes a laxative after every meal and exercises about 3 hours every night. The young woman is 5 feet, 6 inches tall and is determined to weigh 100 pounds by spring. How should you handle this situation?

OBESITY

Approximately 70% of Americans are overweight or obese. Obese individuals are at risk for a wide range of health problems, including hypertension, DM type 2, coronary artery disease, stroke, gallbladder disease, osteoarthritis, sleep apnea, and certain types of cancer. Assessment of weight-related health risks uses three key measures: the patient's BMI, waist circumference, and the presence of health problems associated with obesity. As the BMI rises, so do the risks for cardiovascular disease, hypertension, diabetes type 2, hypercholesterolemia, and death. According to the National Cancer Institute, obesity is associated with an increased risk of multiple cancers including:

- Esophageal
- Pancreatic
- Colon and rectum
- Breast (after menopause)
- Endometrial (lining of the uterus)
- Kidney
- Thyroid
- Gallbladder

http://www.cancer.gov/about-cancer/causes-prevention/risk/obesity/obesity-fact-sheet. Accessed February 5, 2016.

Medications for Obesity

Weight-loss medications fall into two categories: appetite suppressants and lipase inhibitors. Appetite-suppressant medications, such as phentermine (Adipex-P, Obenix, Suprenza) promote weight loss by reducing the appetite or increasing the feeling of being full. Orlistat (Xenical), blocks the release of the enzyme lipase, which metabolizes fat for absorption. If fat is not broken down, it cannot be absorbed, which results in a decrease in dietary fat absorption by about one third. The FDA also has approved Alli, an over-the-counter weight-loss aid for adults that is a lower dose form of orlistat.

Two new medicines for chronic weight management, lorcaserin hydrochloride (Belviq) and a combination medication made up of phentermine hydrochloride and topiramate (Qsymia), have been approved for adults who have a BMI of 30 or higher, or a BMI of 27 or higher (overweight) if the patient has at least one weight-related health problem.

The response to medications for weight loss varies among patients, but the average weight loss is 5 to 22 pounds, which is more than might have been lost without medication. Most of the weight is lost in the first 6 months of treatment, after which the patient's weight stabilizes or may even increase. The use of weight-loss medications must be combined with improvement in overall nutrition and exercise to have long-lasting effects and reduce weight-related health risks.

Bariatric Surgery for Obesity

Gastrointestinal surgery, or *bariatric* surgery, may be an option for people who are severely obese, have attempted unsuccessfully to lose weight by traditional means, and have been diagnosed with obesity-related health problems. The operation promotes weight loss by reducing the size of the stomach to the point that food intake is restricted and/or by interrupting the digestive process by surgically bypassing part of the small intestine. Two common weight-loss surgeries are banded gastroplasty and Roux-en-Y gastric bypass. With a gastroplasty the surgeon places a band around the stomach, or staples are used to create a small pouch at the top of the stomach. This procedure limits the amount of food and liquids the stomach can hold. The Roux-en-Y gastric bypass surgery creates a small stomach pouch with a bypass around part of the small intestine where most calories are absorbed. This surgery both limits food intake and reduces the amount of nutrients absorbed through the small intestine.

Weight-loss surgery can improve health and weight, but it can be risky. Gastroplasty has fewer long-term side effects, but the patient must limit food intake dramatically. Gastric bypass side effects include nausea, bloating, diarrhea, and faintness. After gastric bypass, the patient typically needs vitamin and mineral supplements because absorption of nutrients is drastically affected.

Patients seeking bariatric surgery must meet certain criteria, including a BMI of 40 or greater, or a BMI of 35 to 40 along with a diagnosed obesity-related health problem, such as DM type 2 or severe sleep apnea. The patient also must undergo counseling and psychiatric evaluation because bariatric surgery requires a lifelong commitment to dietary change. The procedure is successful for long-term weight loss only if the individual is willing to commit to making drastic behavioral changes and undergoing regular medical checkups for the rest of his or her life. In addition, the cost of the procedure ($20,000 to $35,000) may be prohibitive, and insurance coverage varies by state and insurance provider.

HEALTH PROMOTION

The concept of health promotion includes such aspects as adequate nutrition, a healthy environment, ongoing health education, and an overall attempt to prevent disease and maintain optimum wellness. Wellness goes beyond the absence of disease to a state of moving toward fitness, managing stress, and maximizing individual potential. Health promotion uses immunizations, appropriate personal hygiene, environmental sanitation standards, protection against occupational hazards, nutritious diets, and periodic health screenings and examinations to diagnose health problems early and promote wellness.

As a medical assistant, you will play a key role in assisting the provider in many of these areas. In addition, you can serve as a patient navigator by interacting with local social service agencies or insurance companies on the patient's behalf. You also will play an important role in scheduling and assisting the provider with health screenings, physical examinations, and health teaching. Components of wellness that all medical assistants should promote include exercise, stress management, and routine health screenings.

Exercise

Exercise is defined as physical exertion for the maintenance or improvement of health or for the correction of a physical handicap. Exercise improves cardiorespiratory endurance; maintains musculoskeletal health by improving or maintaining strength, flexibility, and bone integrity; and relieves stress. Although most Americans say they know about the benefits of exercise, only 20% to 25% of adults exercise enough to gain significant health benefits. Twenty-five percent are not active at all, and more than half of all American youths 12 to 21 years of age are not vigorously active on a regular basis.

A well-balanced diet is only part of the fitness equation; adequate exercise and sufficient rest are the other elements that help achieve good health. As with special diets, exercise programs must be approved for each individual by the provider. It is the provider who determines the patient's exercise needs and tolerance levels to safeguard the patient from overexertion and possible injury.

Many forms of exercise are available. Some patients may find it best to go to a gym and develop a formal program of physical fitness. Others may purchase home exercise equipment so they can exercise in privacy. Many feel that just getting out in the fresh air and walking is the best form of exercise. Each individual should find the outlet that brings enjoyment and enrichment to his or her own life. It is not the form of exercise, but rather the participation in physical activity, that promotes wellness.

CRITICAL THINKING APPLICATION   23-7

The provider tells Mr. Hawthorne that he must exercise to maintain a healthy lifestyle. What can Marcia tell him about the benefits of exercise and possible methods that might help him follow through with the provider's recommendation?

Stress Management

Stress stimulates the fight-or-flight response that physically prepares us to either fight off a stressor or run away from it. Unfortunately, most of the stress we experience on a daily basis is not something we can either physically battle or effectively run away from. Therefore, the stress response can lead to multiple health problems if it is not managed therapeutically. The stress response results in the release of epinephrine (adrenaline), which increases the heart and respiratory rates, slows peristalsis, increases blood supply to the skeletal muscles while reducing blood to the periphery, causes overall muscular tension, and raises the blood pressure. If stress is permitted to build without release, multiple health problems can occur, some of which can lead to chronic disorders. One of the best methods for reducing stress is by developing adaptive coping mechanisms.

Coping mechanisms are thoughts and actions we use to relieve stressful circumstances over which we have little control. Many factors shape how we respond to stress, such as cultural and family influences; financial status; our perception of the seriousness of the situation; and previous experiences with crisis. Adaptive coping mechanisms—those considered positive—help us regain control over the situation and manage stressful situations. These might include exercise, organizational skills, relaxation techniques, talking over the situation with a trusted person, or using humor to relieve stress. Nonadaptive coping mechanisms often make the stressful situation worse. These negative actions might include anger, denial, isolation, overeating or undereating, or substance abuse. Regardless of how we typically respond to a stressful situation, coping mechanisms are learned behaviors, so it is possible to identify those that do not work well and replace them with more adaptive responses.

Reflect on your stress management style. Make a list of the adaptive and nonadaptive coping mechanisms you typically use when faced with a stressful situation. Share your list with the class and discuss alternatives to your adaptive techniques.

Preventive Services and Health Screening

Routine physical examinations and health screenings are important components of health promotion. The Affordable Care Act requires every health plan to cover all costs associated with preventive services, meaning there is no co-payment or deductible for preventive services. The patient scheduled for a physical examination should have a health history completed or updated and should be weighed; his or her blood pressure, temperature, pulse, and respirations should be recorded; and any complaints should be documented in the health record.

Preventive Services for Women

- Starting at age 21 or approximately 3 years after having sex for the first time, a Papanicolaou (Pap) test at least every 3 years to screen for cervical cancer.
- Women age 65 or older should be tested for osteoporosis; women younger than age 65 who are at risk should also be tested.
- Mammograms should be done every 2 years between the ages of 50 and 74; women with risk factors for breast cancer may need to have mammograms more often or start having them sooner.
- Begin colorectal cancer screening at age 50 and continue until age 75; the patient may need to continue testing until age 85.
- Maintain a current immunization schedule.

Preventive Services for Men

- Check cholesterol levels regularly starting at age 35.
- Start colorectal cancer screening at age 50 and continue until age 75; the patient may need to continue testing until age 85.
- Maintain a current immunization schedule.

CLOSING COMMENTS

Patient Education

Because medical assistants may be asked to discuss a diet plan with a patient, it is extremely important that they have a thorough knowledge of diet therapy. The patient must understand the prescribed diet and the rationale for following it. If the patient feels uneasy or has questions that go unanswered, he or she may be less motivated to follow a diet plan. You can be a valuable asset to the provider, the dietitian, and the patient in the implementation of a specific diet.

The medical assistant may find the following suggestions helpful when talking to patients about a diet:

- Use charts and diagrams to illustrate diets.
- Consider the patient's dietary likes and dislikes.
- Remember that ethnic and cultural foods are important.
- Encourage the patient to play an active role in the learning process.
- Suggest local support groups, other community resources, and online resources that can help in diet maintenance.

Legal and Ethical Issues

Always remember that you are not a provider, nor are you a dietitian; follow the provider's instructions. If you are not sure of the answer to a question, always ask the provider. If your workplace employs a registered dietitian, refer questions about meal patterns and food selection changes to that individual. Direct patients seeking advice in the field of nutrition and exercise programs to a qualified expert. Use community resources as needed.

Professional Behaviors

The medical assistant plays a vital role in health promotion by making sure patients are scheduled for annual examinations and that they follow up with the provider's recommendations for dietary changes, exercise programs, stress management approaches, and health screening procedures. In the role of patient navigator, the medical assistant is the link between the patient and the provider, and between the patient and community resources.

SUMMARY OF SCENARIO

As a certified medical assistant working in an internal medicine practice, Marcia must be familiar with the types and functions of dietary nutrients, the USDA dietary recommendations, including the *choosemyplate.gov* website, how nutritional assessments are conducted, the concepts of therapeutic nutrition, how to apply the interpretation of food labels to patient practice, and the concepts of health promotion. Recommendations for nutrition are constantly changing as research continues on the dietary needs of healthy people. Marcia can refer her patients to the USDA website (*www.usda.gov/dietaryguidelines*) or the MyPlate website (*www.choosemyplate.gov*) for

updated information on dietary recommendations and for educational material on nutrition.

Providers rely on the BMI to determine a patient's risk for diet-related diseases, and medical assistants should be familiar with various therapeutic diets so that they can answer patients' questions about foods that should be included or avoided.

As a certified medical assistant, Marcia must make a commitment to lifelong learning so that she can provide her patients with up-to-date information on nutrition-related topics and can use community resources to support patient care.

SUMMARY OF LEARNING OBJECTIVES

1. **Define, spell, and pronounce the terms listed in the vocabulary.**

   Spelling and pronouncing medical terms correctly reinforce the medical assistant's credibility. Knowing the definitions of these terms promotes confidence in communication with patients and co-workers.

2. **Analyze the relationship between poor nutrition and lifestyle factors and the risk of developing diet-related diseases.**

   Research has found that lifestyle and dietary habits directly correlate with the development of certain diseases and disorders. These include certain types of anemia, constipation, diabetes mellitus type 2, hypercholesterolemia, atherosclerosis, hypertension, osteoporosis, and cerebrovascular accidents.

3. **Recognize the reasons for people's food choices and the effects of cultural eating patterns.**

   People eat the way they do for many reasons. Encouraging patients to make significant lifestyle changes with regard to their diets requires sensitivity to these reasons. The choices people make about what they eat are greatly influenced by their background and relationships. Every culture, religion, and ethnic group has its own beliefs and practices with regard to food.

4. **Describe digestion and classify the types and functions of dietary nutrients.**

   Digestion is a combination of mechanical and chemical processes that occur in the mouth, stomach, and small intestine. Nutrients consist of carbohydrates, fats, proteins, vitamins, minerals, and water. Their primary functions are to provide the body with energy, protection, and insulation; build and repair tissues; and regulate metabolic processes.

5. **Describe the roles of various nutrient components, including carbohydrates, fats, and proteins, in the daily diet.**

   The primary function of carbohydrates is to provide the body with a ready source of energy. Dietary fat provides essential fatty acids and is needed for the absorption of fat-soluble vitamins. Adipose tissue helps protect the organs of the body, insulates, and serves as a concentrated form of stored energy. Protein builds and repairs tissue and assists with metabolic functions.

6. **Explain the function of appropriate amounts of vitamins, minerals, and water in the diet.**

   Vitamins are essential for metabolic functions and are classified as either fat soluble or water soluble. They regulate the synthesis of body tissues and aid the metabolism of nutrients. Vitamins also play a vital role in disease prevention. Minerals help to maintain electrolytes and acid-base balance and to regulate muscular action and nervous activities throughout the body. Water is part of almost every vital body process.

7. **Apply the Dietary Guidelines for Americans using the Choose My Plate website developed by the U.S. Department of Agriculture (USDA).**

   In 2011 the Pyramid design was changed to a dinner plate icon that represents how to build a healthy plate at mealtime. The plate includes choices from the five basic food groups, with recommendations based on the 2010 Dietary Guidelines for Americans. At the Choose My Plate website (*www.choosemyplate.gov*), consumers can determine individual dietary needs that match their particular age, health status, exercise level, and food preferences. (See Figure 23-1.)

8. **Implement nutritional assessment techniques by measuring a patient's body fat and correlating a patient's calculated body mass index (BMI) with the risk for diet-related diseases.**

   The provider's assessment of the patient's nutritional status includes an evaluation of the patient's current health and lifestyle habits and also body fat measurements. Body fat can be measured by using the waist-to-hip ratio, by using calipers to measure fat folds, or by calculating the BMI. (See Figure 23-2.) The BMI is the relationship of weight to height, which correlates with health risks. The BMI is a more accurate predictor of weight-related diseases than traditional height-weight charts because it provides a good estimate of the degree of body fat. Individuals with a BMI of 19 to 22 are thought to live longest. The incidence of diet-related disorders and the mortality rate are significantly higher for people with a BMI of 25 or higher.

9. **Do the following related to therapeutic nutrition:**

   - *Compare the concepts of therapeutic nutrition.*

     Therapeutic nutrition uses various diets to help treat or prevent disease. Diets can be modified in many ways, including changes in consistency and taste, monitoring of caloric levels, altering the amounts and types of specific nutrients, and managing the fiber content of foods. Two examples of diet therapies are the diabetic diet and the heart-healthy diet, both of which can have a significant impact on a patient's wellness.

   - *Instruct a patient according to the patient's dietary needs; coach a patient with diabetes about the Glycemic Index of foods.*

     The GI rates carbohydrate foods on a scale from slowest to fastest effects on blood glucose levels. The lower the GI value of the food, the longer it takes to raise the patient's blood glucose level. (See Procedure 23-1.)

10. **Interpret food labels, explain their application to a healthy diet, and demonstrate to the patient how to understand nutrition labels on food products.**

    The federal government requires all food manufacturers to follow certain guidelines when labeling packages. Labels provide facts on the nutritional value of foods. The food label can be a valuable tool in patient compliance with specialized diets (see Figures 23-3 and 23-4). (See Procedure 23-2 to see how to coach a patient about food labels.)

11. **Discuss food-borne diseases and food contaminants.**

    Many different types of bacteria, viruses, and parasites can contaminate food. The first symptoms of a food-borne disease are usually gastrointestinal. The FDA regularly monitors the presence of contaminants in the food chain and issues warnings as needed to protect consumers from possible danger.

12. **Summarize the causes of eating disorders and obesity and their impact on a patient's health.**

    An eating disorder is defined as any eating behavior pattern that can lead to a health problem. In anorexia nervosa, profound malnutrition occurs because of an individual's attempt to control his or her life by not eating. Bulimia is characterized by bingeing and purging episodes. Obesity has become a national health emergency. Obese individuals have a higher risk of a wide range of health problems, including hypertension, diabetes mellitus type 2, coronary artery disease, stroke, gallbladder disease, osteoarthritis, sleep apnea, and certain types of cancer. Bariatric surgery may be an option for people who are severely obese.

13. **Define the concepts of health promotion.**

    Health promotion considers all aspects of patient care, including the concepts of general wellness, adequate nutrition, environmental health and safety, health education needs, and disease prevention. The components of health promotion include exercise, stress management, regular physical examinations, and preventive services and health screening.

14. **Describe the role of the medical assistant in patient education; also, explain the legal and ethical issues related to nutrition and health promotion.**

    The medical assistant plays a key role in promoting nutrition and health. He or she serves as a patient navigator and as a liaison between the patient and community resources. It is important that medical assistants understand the various implications of nutrition and specific diets, so that they can answer patients' questions, which promotes compliance with treatment.

CONNECTIONS

Study Guide Connection: Go to the Chapter 23 Study Guide. Read and complete the activities.

evolve Evolve Connection: Go to the Chapter 23 link at *evolve.elsevier.com/kinn* to complete the Chapter Review Quiz. Check out the other resources listed for this chapter to make the most of what you have learned from Nutrition and Health Promotion.

SCENARIO

Dr. Susan Xu is a member of a primary care practice with several providers. Each provider has a medical assistant who works directly with him or her. Carlos Ricci, CMA (AAMA), is Dr. Xu's assistant. Carlos graduated from a medical assistant program 3 years ago and enjoys the variety of patients seen in Dr. Xu's practice. One of Carlos' primary responsibilities is to accurately measure and record each patient's vital signs before the patient is seen by Dr. Xu.

While studying this chapter, think about the following questions:

- What factors might alter a patient's vital signs?
- What methods can Carlos use to gather and record a patient's temperature, pulse, respirations, blood pressure, height, weight, and body mass index (BMI)?
- What are the current guidelines for diagnosing and treating hypertension?

LEARNING OBJECTIVES

1. Define, spell, and pronounce the terms listed in the vocabulary.
2. Do the following related to temperature:
   - Cite the average body temperature for various age groups.
   - Describe emotional and physical factors that can cause body temperature to rise and fall.
   - Convert temperature readings between Fahrenheit and Celsius scales.
   - Obtain and record an accurate patient temperature using three different types of thermometers.
3. Do the following related to pulse:
   - Cite the average pulse rate for various age groups.
   - Describe pulse rate, volume, and rhythm.
   - Locate and record pulse at multiple sites.
4. Do the following related to respiration:
   - Cite the average respiratory rate for various age groups.
   - Demonstrate the best way to obtain an accurate respiratory count.
5. Do the following related to blood pressure:
   - Cite the approximate blood pressure range for various age groups.
   - Specify physiologic factors that affect blood pressure.
   - Differentiate between essential and secondary hypertension.
   - Interpret current hypertension guidelines and treatment.
   - Describe how to determine the correct cuff size for individual patients.
   - Identify the different Korotkoff phases.
   - Accurately measure and document blood pressure.
6. Accurately measure and document height and weight.
7. Convert kilograms to pounds and pounds to kilograms.
8. Identify patient education opportunities when measuring vital signs.
9. Determine the medical assistant's legal and ethical responsibilities in obtaining vital signs.

VOCABULARY

apnea (ap'-nee-uh) Absence or cessation of breathing.

arrhythmia An abnormality or irregularity in the heart rhythm.

arteriosclerosis (ar-ter'-ee-o-scler-o-sis) Thickening, decreased elasticity, and calcification of arterial walls.

bounding A term used to describe a pulse that feels full because of increased power of cardiac contraction or as a result of increased blood volume.

bradycardia (brad-i-kahr'-dee-uh) A slow heartbeat; a pulse below 60 beats per minute.

bradypnea (brad-ip-nee'-uh) Respirations that are regular in rhythm but slower than normal in rate.

cerumen (see-room'-men) A waxy secretion in the ear canal; commonly called *ear wax.*

Cheyne-Stokes respirations A breathing pattern characterized by rhythmic changes in the depth of respiration. The patient breathes deeply for a short time and then breathes very slightly or stops breathing altogether; the pattern occurs over and over, every 45 seconds to 3 minutes. The Cheyne-Stokes breathing pattern is seen in patients with heart failure or brain damage, but also in healthy individuals who hyperventilate, at high altitudes, and with hypnotic drug or narcotic overdose and sleep apnea.

VOCABULARY—continued

chronic obstructive pulmonary disease (COPD) A progressive, irreversible lung condition that results in diminished lung capacity.

diurnal rhythm (die-ur'-nl) A pattern of activity or behavior that follows a day-night cycle.

dyspnea (disp-nee'-uh) Difficult or painful breathing.

essential hypertension Elevated blood pressure of unknown cause that develops for no apparent reason; sometimes called *primary hypertension.*

febrile (feb'-ril) Pertaining to an elevated body temperature.

homeostasis Internal adaptation and change in response to environmental factors; multiple functions that attempt to keep the body's functions in balance.

hyperpnea (hahy-per-nee'-uh) An increase in the depth of breathing.

hyperventilation Abnormally prolonged and deep breathing, usually associated with acute anxiety or emotional tension.

hypotension Blood pressure that is below normal (systolic pressure below 90 mm Hg and diastolic pressure below 50 mm Hg).

intermittent pulse A pulse in which beats occasionally are skipped.

orthopnea (or-thop'-nee-uh) A condition in which an individual must sit or stand to breathe comfortably.

orthostatic (postural) hypotension A temporary fall in blood pressure when a person rapidly changes from a recumbent position to a standing position.

otitis externa Inflammation or infection of the external auditory canal; commonly called *swimmer's ear.*

peripheral (puh-rif'-er-uhl) A term that refers to an area outside of or away from an organ or structure.

pulse deficit A condition in which the radial pulse is less than the apical pulse; it may indicate a peripheral vascular abnormality.

pulse pressure The difference between the systolic and diastolic blood pressures (30 to 50 mm Hg is considered normal).

pyrexia (pi rek'-see-uh) A febrile condition or fever.

rales Abnormal or crackling breath sounds during inspiration.

rhonchi (ron'-ki) Abnormal rumbling sounds on expiration that indicate airway obstruction by thick secretions or spasms.

secondary hypertension Elevated blood pressure resulting from another condition, typically kidney disease.

sinus arrhythmia An irregular heartbeat that originates in the sinoatrial node (pacemaker).

spirometer An instrument that measures the volume of air inhaled and exhaled.

stertorous (stuh-tuh'-rus) A term that describes a strenuous respiratory effort marked by a snoring sound.

syncope (sing'-kuh-pee) Fainting; a brief lapse in consciousness.

tachycardia (tak-i-kahr'-dee-uh) A rapid but regular heart rate; one that exceeds 100 beats per minute.

tachypnea (tak-ip-nee'-uh) A condition marked by rapid, shallow respirations.

thready A term describing a pulse that is scarcely perceptible.

wheezing A high-pitched sound heard on expiration; it indicates obstruction or narrowing of respiratory passages.

Measurement of vital signs is an important aspect of almost every patient visit to the medical office. These signs are the human body's indicators of internal **homeostasis** and the patient's general state of health. Because medical assistants are chiefly responsible for obtaining these measurements, it is imperative that they have confidence in the theoretic and practical applications of vital sign measurement. A medical assistant who understands the principles of and the reasons for these measurements becomes a valuable asset to any medical office.

Accuracy is essential. A change in one or more of the patient's vital signs may indicate a change in general health. Variations may suggest the presence or disappearance of a disease process and therefore may lead to alteration of the treatment plan. Although the medical assistant obtains vital signs routinely, it is a task that requires consistent attention to accuracy and detail. These findings are crucial to a correct diagnosis, and vital signs should never be measured with indifference or casualness. In addition to performing accurate measurement, care must be taken when charting the findings in the patient's health record.

The *vital signs* are the patient's temperature, pulse, respiration, and blood pressure. These four signs are abbreviated *TPR* and *BP* and may be referred to as *cardinal signs.* The medical assistant must understand the significance of the vital signs and must measure and record them accurately. *Anthropometric measurements* are not considered vital signs but usually are obtained at the same time as vital signs. These measurements include height, weight, body mass index (BMI), and other body measurements, such as fat composition and an infant's head circumference.

FACTORS THAT MAY INFLUENCE VITAL SIGNS

Vital signs are influenced by many factors, both physical and emotional. A patient may have had a hot or cold beverage just before the examination or may be anxious or fearful about what the provider may find. For example, consider that a patient has been asked to return to have a repeat Papanicolaou (Pap) test because the first one showed the presence of suspicious cells. The medical assistant measures the patient's blood pressure and finds it significantly elevated compared with previous readings. The patient may be anxious and apprehensive about the test results, and the elevated blood pressure readings reflect her anxiety.

What temperature reading might be expected in a patient who could not find a parking place and had to walk four blocks to the office, knowing he would be late for his appointment? If you said it would be elevated, you are right. Certainly, this patient's metabolism would increase because of the physical exercise, and as a result, his temperature would be elevated, along with his pulse, respirations, and blood pressure.

Vital signs are often altered if the patient is in pain. Pay attention to nonverbal signs that might indicate discomfort or pain, especially if the patient's blood pressure, pulse, and respirations are elevated. In addition, many patients are apprehensive about being seen by the provider. These emotions may alter vital signs, and the medical assistant must help the patient relax before taking any readings. Measurements sometimes must be obtained a second time, after the patient is calmer or more comfortable. For a better picture of the patient's vital signs, the medical assistant may be asked to record the vital signs twice: at the beginning of the visit and just before the patient leaves the examination room.

TEMPERATURE

Physiology

Body temperature is defined as the balance between heat lost and heat produced by the body. It is measured in degrees Fahrenheit (F) or degrees Celsius (C). The process of chemical and physical change in the body that produces heat is called *metabolism.* Body temperature is a result of this process. The core body temperature is maintained within a normal range by the thermoregulatory center in the hypothalamus. The average body temperature varies from person to person and is different in each person at different times throughout the day. In a healthy adult, this **diurnal rhythm** varies from 97.6° to 99°F (36.4° to 37.2°C); the average daily temperature is 98.6°F (37°C). Body temperature is lowest in the morning and highest in the late afternoon. Factors that may affect body temperature include the following:

- *Age:* The body temperature of infants and young children fluctuates more rapidly in response to external environmental temperatures. Teething may cause a slight elevation in temperature but should not be the cause of a fever. Aging adults lose their ability to respond therapeutically to environmental temperature extremes, making them more susceptible to hypothermic or hyperthermic reactions.
- *Stress and physical activity:* Both exercise and emotional stress can increase the metabolic rate, causing an elevation in temperature.
- *Gender:* Hormone secretions result in fluctuations of the core body temperature in women throughout the menstrual cycle.
- *External factors:* Smoking, drinking hot fluids, and chewing gum can temporarily elevate an oral temperature.

In illness, an individual's metabolic activity is increased; this causes an increase in internal heat production, which in turn raises the body temperature. The increase in body temperature is thought to be the body's defensive reaction because heat inhibits the growth of some bacteria and viruses.

When a fever is present, superficial blood vessels (those near the surface of the skin) constrict. The small papillary muscles at the base of hair follicles also constrict, creating goose bumps. Chills and shivering may follow, producing internal heat. As this process repeats itself, more heat is produced, and the body temperature becomes elevated or rises above the normal range. When more heat is lost than is produced, the opposite effect occurs, and body temperature drops below normal range.

Fever

Infection, either bacterial or viral, is the most common cause of fever in both children and adults.

Infants do not usually develop **febrile** illnesses during the first 3 months of life; if one is present, it usually is very serious. However, fever, or **pyrexia,** is very common in young children and accounts for an estimated 26% of office visits. Fevers are classified according to the 24-hour pattern they follow. The three most common patterns are:

- *Continuous fever,* which rises and falls only slightly during a 24-hour period. The temperature consistently remains above the patient's average normal temperature range and fluctuates less than 3 degrees.
- *Intermittent fever,* which comes and goes, alternating between elevated and normal levels.
- *Remittent fever,* which fluctuates considerably (i.e., by more than 3 degrees) and never returns to the normal range.

Variation from the patient's average body temperature range may be the first warning of an illness or a change in the patient's current condition. Patients with fever usually have loss of appetite *(anorexia),* headache, thirst, flushed face, hot skin, and general malaise. Some patients experience an acute onset of chills and shivering, followed by an increase in body temperature. A serious possible complication in young children with high fevers is a febrile seizure. Medication to reduce the fever, or *antipyretic* drugs (e.g., acetaminophen or ibuprofen), should be taken as instructed to prevent dangerous spikes in temperature. Age-related normal values for temperature readings are shown in Table 24-1.

Temperatures Considered Febrile

- Rectal, temporal, or aural (ear) temperature over 100.4°F (38°C)
- Oral temperature over 99.5°F (37.5°C)
- Axillary temperature over 98.6°F (37°C)
- Fever of unknown origin (FUO): a temperature over 100.9°F (38.3°C) that lasts 3 weeks in adults and 1 week in children without a known related diagnosis

---

TABLE 24-1	Age-Related Temperature Norms	
AGE	**FAHRENHEIT**	**CELSIUS**
Newborn (temporal)	98.2°	36.8°
1 year	99.7°	37.6°
6 years to adult (oral)	98.6°	37°
Elderly over age 70 (oral)	96.8°	36°

Temperature Readings

A clinical thermometer is used to measure body temperature. It is calibrated in the Fahrenheit or Celsius scale. The Fahrenheit scale is used most often in the United States, but hospitals and many ambulatory care settings use the Celsius scale. Although you can use an online conversion scale or a program in an electronic health record (EHR) system, the mathematical formulas for conversion from one system to the other are:

$$°C = (°F - 32) \times \frac{5}{9}$$

$$°F = \left(°C \times \frac{9}{5}\right) + 32$$

For example, if an infant's temperature is measured at 101°F, the Celsius conversion would be as follows (remember, always complete the equation in parentheses first):

$$°C = (101°F - 32) \times \frac{5}{9}$$

$$= 69 \times \frac{5}{9}$$

$$= 345 \div 9$$

$$= 38.3°C$$

Another formula that can be used is:

$$°C = (°F - 32) \div 1.8$$

$$°C = (101 - 32) \div 1.8$$

$$= 69 \div 1.8$$

$$= 38.3°C$$

If the ambulatory care setting where you work uses a Celsius thermometer, patients may ask you what the temperature is in Fahrenheit degrees because that is the scale they understand. If the facility does not have a conversion chart available, you can convert the temperature mathematically. For example, if an infant's temperature is 39°C, what is the Fahrenheit reading?

$$°F = \left(°C \times \frac{9}{5}\right) + 32$$

$$= \left(39°C \times \frac{9}{5}\right) + 32$$

$$= (351 \div 5) + 32$$

$$= 70.2 + 32$$

$$= 102.2°F$$

Another formula that can be used is:

$$°F = (°C \times 1.8) + 32$$

$$= (39 \times 1.8) + 32$$

$$= 70.2 + 32$$

$$= 102.2°F$$

CRITICAL THINKING APPLICATION   **24-1**

Using the correct formula, convert the following temperatures from one system to the other.

99°F = _____ °C   102°F = _____ °C

38°C = _____ °F   39.5°C = _____ °F

TABLE 24-2	Average Adult Temperatures	
SITE	**FAHRENHEIT**	**CELSIUS**
Oral	98.6°	37°
Axillary	97.6°	36.4°
Tympanic	98.6°	37°
Temporal artery	98.6°	37°

Several types of thermometers and several different methods can be used to take temperature readings. A digital thermometer is placed under the tongue, in the armpit, or rectally; a tympanic thermometer is inserted into the ear; and a temporal artery scanner is moved across the forehead. Average temperature values for adults at the four most common sites are shown in Table 24-2.

Axillary temperatures (A) are approximately 1°F (0.6°C) lower than accurate oral readings because axillary readings are not taken in an enclosed body cavity. When taken correctly, the tympanic (ear) temperature (T) is an accurate measure because it records the temperature of the blood closest to the hypothalamus. However, research on the temporal artery (TA) thermometer indicates that this method is more accurate than tympanic measurement for identifying elevated temperatures in infants. Pediatricians, therefore, may prefer TA temperatures in infants suspected of having a fever. The TA thermometer also records accurate temperature readings in all age groups of patients. The tympanic method still is considered a fast, accurate, and noninvasive way of recording temperatures for older children and adults.

When obtaining an oral temperature, you do not have to indicate the site when documenting the reading in the patient's health record. However, if you use an alternative site, you should write (or put in the correct window in the EHR) the following identifiers after recording the temperature: (T) for tympanic, (A) for axillary, or (TA) for temporal artery; this clarifies that an alternative site was used. The oral temperature cannot be measured accurately in young children because the technique requires the patient to hold the thermometer under the tongue and keep the mouth closed. To take an infant's temperature rectally, lubricate the probe tip (most facilities use a lubricating product such as K-Y Jelly), hold the baby securely with the legs elevated, and insert the probe approximately ½ inch; hold the probe carefully and continue to secure the infant's legs throughout the procedure to prevent rectal damage. The red probe must be used when taking a rectal temperature with an electronic digital thermometer. However, most pediatricians prefer that infants' temperatures be taken with a temporal thermometer because it is more comfortable for the baby, less invasive, and eliminates the possible complication of a perforated rectum.

For patients older than 3 years and for those unable to hold a thermometer properly in their mouth during the procedure, a tympanic or temporal thermometer can be used; if not, a less accurate axillary temperature can be obtained.

CRITICAL THINKING APPLICATION   **24-2**

The mother of a 3-year-old calls the office to report that her child had an axillary temperature of 101° F at 9 o'clock this morning. The schedule is very full today, so Carlos has to decide whether the child should be seen today or first thing tomorrow. When should Carlos schedule the appointment? What is the significance of the axillary temperature reading?

Types of Thermometers and Their Uses

Digital Thermometer

Digital thermometers are battery operated and available in both Fahrenheit and Celsius scales. Disposable covers fit snugly over the probes and are easily and quickly removed by pushing in the colored end of the probe. The instrument sounds a beep when the process is complete (10 to 60 seconds), and the reading appears on a light-emitting diode (LED) screen on the face of the instrument (Procedure 24-1). Because the only part of the instrument that comes in contact with the patient is the probe, which is sheathed, the risk of cross-infection is greatly reduced (Figure 24-1). These thermometers have a digital screen on which the temperature is read, and they should always be covered by a disposable sheath and wiped with an alcohol swab after use.

A temperature should not be taken orally if the patient recently has had something hot or cold to eat or drink or has just smoked because these factors may artificially alter the patient's temperature. In addition, the patient must be able to hold the thermometer under the tongue with the lips tightly sealed around the probe if an accurate oral reading is to be obtained. The digital unit or individual digital thermometers should be routinely cleaned with disinfectant. When ejecting the probe shield or removing the sheath, be careful not to

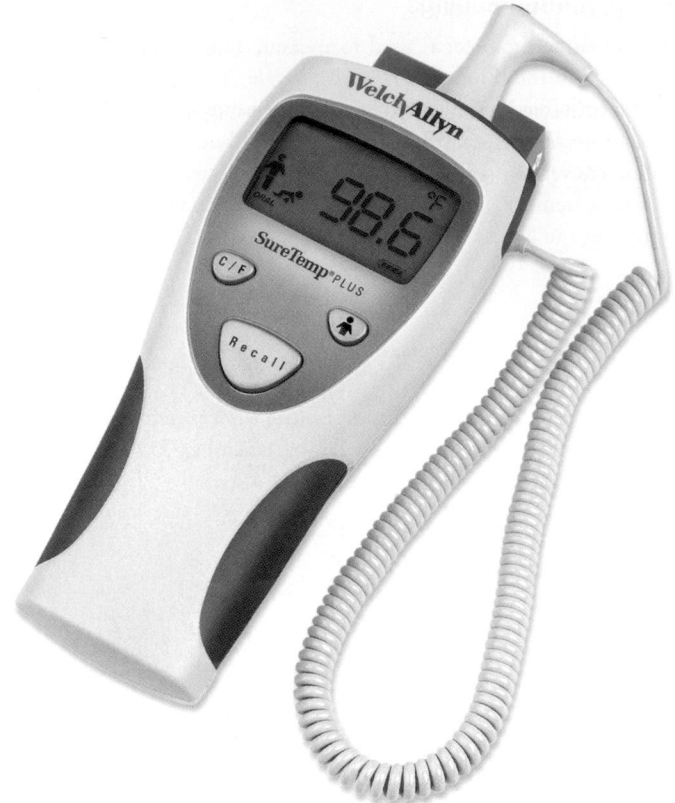

FIGURE 24-1 Digital thermometer. (Courtesy Welch Allyn.)

contaminate the probe or the processing unit. Both the probe shield and the thermometer sheath should be deposited directly into a biohazard waste container. If a chance exists that a patient's body fluids touched the unit, wipe it with disinfectant before returning it to the storage area.

PROCEDURE 24-1   **Obtain Vital Signs: Obtain an Oral Temperature Using a Digital Thermometer**

Goal: *To accurately determine and record a patient's temperature using a digital thermometer.*

EQUIPMENT and SUPPLIES

- Patient's record
- Digital thermometer
- Probe covers
- Disposable gloves as appropriate
- Biohazard waste container

PROCEDURAL STEPS

1. Sanitize your hands.
   <u>PURPOSE</u>: To ensure infection control.

2. Assemble the needed equipment and supplies.

3. Identify your patient and explain the procedure. Make sure the patient has not eaten, consumed any hot or cold fluids, smoked, or exercised during the 30 minutes before the temperature is measured.
   <u>PURPOSE</u>: Identification of the patient prevents errors, and explanations are a means of gaining implied consent and patient cooperation. The temperature will be inaccurate if hot or cold food or fluids have been consumed or if the patient has exercised within 30 minutes.

PROCEDURE 24-1 —continued

4. Prepare the probe for use as described in the package directions (Figure 1). Make sure probe covers are always used.
   PURPOSE: To ensure infection control.

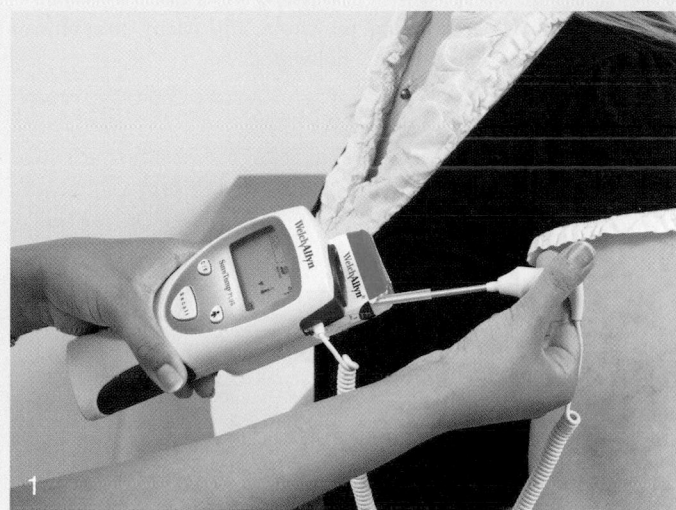

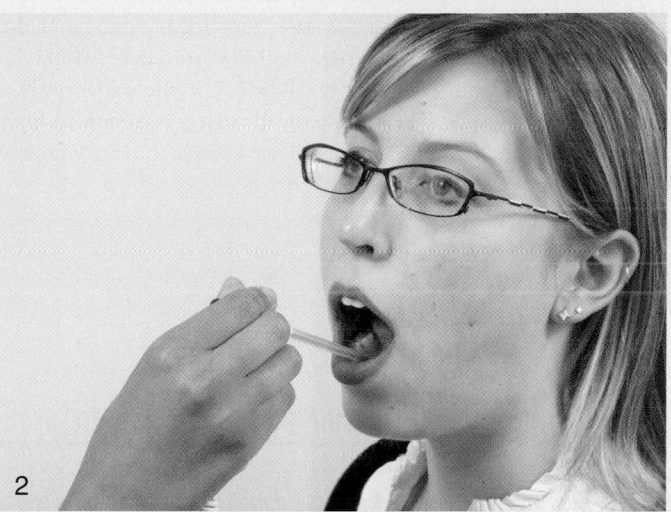

5. Place the probe under the patient's tongue (Figure 2) and instruct the patient to close the mouth tightly without biting down on the thermometer. Help the patient by holding the probe end, or the patient can hold the probe end if that is more comfortable.
   PURPOSE: Air seeping into the mouth interferes with an accurate body temperature reading.

6. When a beep is heard, remove the probe from the patient's mouth and immediately eject the probe cover into an appropriate biohazard waste container.
   PURPOSE: The probe cover is contaminated and must be discarded in a biohazard waste container.

7. Note the reading in the LED window of the processing unit.

8. Record the reading in the patient's medical record (e.g., T - 97.7° F).
   PURPOSE: Procedures that are not recorded are considered not done.

9. Sanitize your hands and disinfect the equipment as indicated.
   PURPOSE: To observe infection control measures and Standard Precautions.

3/27/20— 10:05 AM: T-97.7° F. C. Ricci, CMA (AAMA)

Tympanic Thermometer

The tympanic membrane of the ear can be used for quick, accurate, and safe assessment of a patient's temperature. It shares the blood supply that reaches the hypothalamus, which is the brain's temperature regulator. The ear canal is a protected cavity, so aural temperature is not affected by factors such as an open mouth, hot or cold drinks, or even a stuffy nose, which would prevent a patient from keeping the mouth closed during the procedure. In addition, the covered probe is designed to bounce an infrared signal off the eardrum without touching it, so the risk of spreading communicable diseases during temperature measurement is greatly reduced.

The tympanic measurement system consists of a handheld processor unit equipped with a tympanic probe, which is covered with a disposable speculum for use (Figure 24-2). When the probe is placed into the ear canal, it gently seals the external opening of the canal, and the infrared energy emitted by the tympanic membrane is gathered. This signal is digitized by the processor unit and shown on the display screen. Accurate readings are obtained in less than 2 seconds

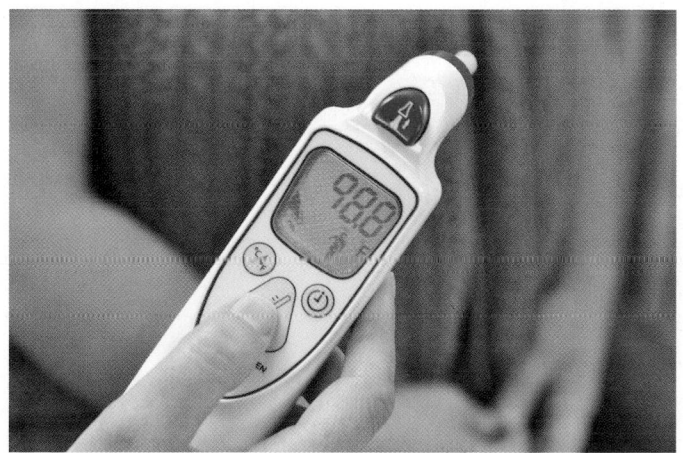

FIGURE 24-2 Tympanic thermometer.

(Procedure 24-2). Both the speed of the tympanic thermometer and the comfort it affords the patient have greatly influenced its popularity. However, this unit should not be used if the patient is complaining of pain in both ears when the ear is touched because he or she may have bilateral **otitis externa**, and the procedure would be uncomfortable for the patient. In addition, if the patient has a history of or has been diagnosed with impacted **cerumen** in both ears, do not use a tympanic thermometer because the reading may be inaccurate.

Insert the probe into the ear canal far enough to seal the opening without applying pressure. To expose the tympanic membrane in children younger than age 3, gently pull the earlobe down and back; for patients older than age 3, gently pull the pinna (top of the ear) up and back. When using a tympanic thermometer on a small child, be conscious of what the child touches. If the processing unit is touched, be sure to wipe it with disinfectant after use. See the manufacturer's manual for cleaning the probe tip. Many recommend cleaning the probe lens with alcohol wipes.

PROCEDURE 24-2 Obtain Vital Signs: Obtain an Aural Temperature Using the Tympanic Thermometer

Goal: *To accurately determine and record a patient's temperature using a tympanic thermometer.*

EQUIPMENT and SUPPLIES

- Patient's record
- Tympanic thermometer
- Disposable probe covers
- Disposable gloves as appropriate
- Alcohol wipes
- Biohazard waste container

PROCEDURAL STEPS

1. Sanitize your hands.
   PURPOSE: To ensure infection control.
2. Gather the necessary equipment and supplies.
3. Identify the patient and explain the procedure.
   PURPOSE: Identification of the patient prevents errors, and explanations are a means of gaining implied consent and patient cooperation.
4. Clean the probe with an alcohol wipe if indicated. Place a disposable cover on the probe (Figure 1).
   PURPOSE: To ensure a clean surface and prevent cross-contamination.

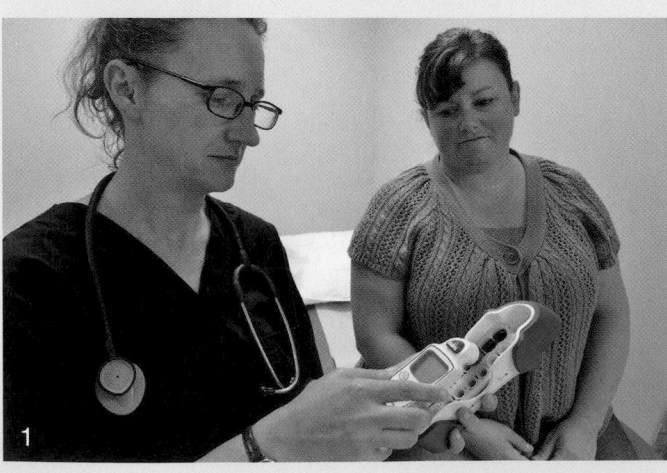

5. Follow the package directions to start the thermometer.

6. Insert the probe into the ear canal far enough to seal the opening. Do not apply pressure. For children younger than age 3, gently pull the earlobe down and back (Figure 2); for patients older than age 3, gently pull the top of the ear (pinna) up and back (Figure 3).
   PURPOSE: The external ear must be pulled gently to open the external auditory canal and expose the tympanic membrane for an accurate reading.

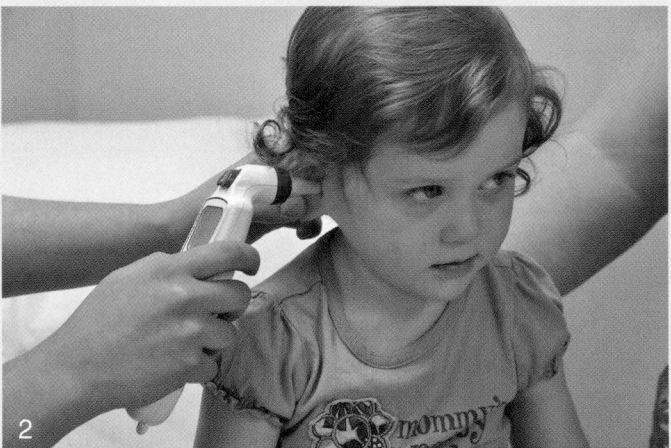

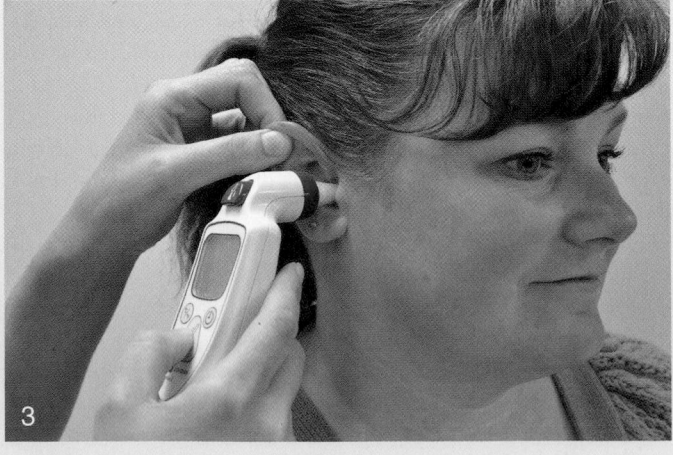

PROCEDURE 24-2   —continued

7. Press the button on the probe as directed. The temperature will appear on the display screen in 1 to 2 seconds.
8. Remove the probe, note the reading, and discard the probe cover into a biohazard waste container without touching it.
   PURPOSE: The probe cover is contaminated and must be discarded in a biohazard waste container.
9. Sanitize your hands and disinfect the equipment if indicated. See the manufacturer's manual for cleaning the probe tip. Many recommend cleaning the probe lens with alcohol wipes.
   PURPOSE: To ensure infection control.

10. Record the temperature results (e.g., T-98.6° F [T]) in the patient's health record.
    PURPOSE: Procedures that are not recorded are considered not done.

3/30/20– 2:20 PM: T-101.2° F (T). C. Ricci, CMA (AAMA)

Temporal Artery Scanner

The temporal artery scanner uses an infrared beam to assess the temperature of the blood flowing through the temporal artery of the lateral forehead, where the artery lies about 1 mm below the skin (Figure 24-3). Because the artery is so close to the skin, it provides good surface heat conduction, allowing the thermometer to obtain a fast, accurate, and noninvasive measurement of body temperature. To perform the procedure, place the probe in the center of the forehead, halfway between the eyebrows and the hairline. Bangs should be pushed back off the forehead (this method cannot be used if bandages cover the area). Depress the button on the scanner and gently stroke the probe across the forehead toward the hairline (at the temples), keeping the probe flat on the patient's skin. As the scanner moves across the forehead, repeated temperature measurements are taken and the highest measurement is recorded; keeping the button depressed, lift the scanner from the temporal area and lightly place the probe behind the earlobe. Release the button and remove the probe. Recording an accurate temperature takes about 3 seconds (Procedure 24-3). Depending on the facility's infection control procedures, disposable covers can be used on the scanner or it can be cleaned between patients with an alcohol wipe.

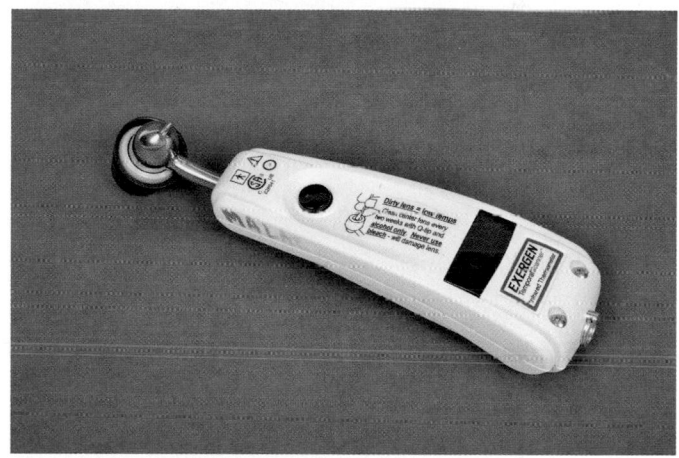

FIGURE 24-3 Professional temporal artery scanner.

PROCEDURE 24-3   Obtain Vital Signs: Obtain a Temporal Artery Temperature

Goal: To accurately determine and record a patient's temperature using a temporal artery scanner.

EQUIPMENT and SUPPLIES

- Patient's record
- Professional temporal artery thermometer with probe covers
- Alcohol swabs
- Biohazard waste container

PROCEDURAL STEPS

1. Sanitize your hands.
   PURPOSE: To ensure infection control.
2. Gather the necessary equipment and supplies.

3. Introduce yourself, identify your patient, and explain the procedure.
   PURPOSE: Identification of the patient prevents errors, and explanations are a means of gaining implied consent and patient cooperation.
4. Remove the protective cap on the probe. Depending on the facility's infection control procedures, disposable covers can be used on the scanner, or it can be cleaned by lightly wiping the surface with an alcohol swab.
   PURPOSE: To ensure infection control.
5. Push the patient's hair up off the forehead to expose the site. Gently place the probe on the patient's forehead, halfway between the edge of the eyebrows and the hairline.
   PURPOSE: This places the probe directly over the temporal artery.

PROCEDURE 24-3   *—continued*

6. Depress and hold the SCAN button and lightly glide the probe sideways across the patient's forehead to the hairline just above the ear (Figure 1). As you move the sensor across the forehead, you will hear a beep, and a red light will flash.
   <u>PURPOSE</u>: This verifies that the scanner is recording temperatures as it moves across the surface of the temporal artery.

7. Keeping the button depressed, lift the thermometer, and place the probe behind the ear lobe (Figure 2). The thermometer may continue to beep, indicating that the temperature is rising.
   <u>PURPOSE</u>: To continue scanning of the temporal artery until the highest temperature is recorded on the thermometer.

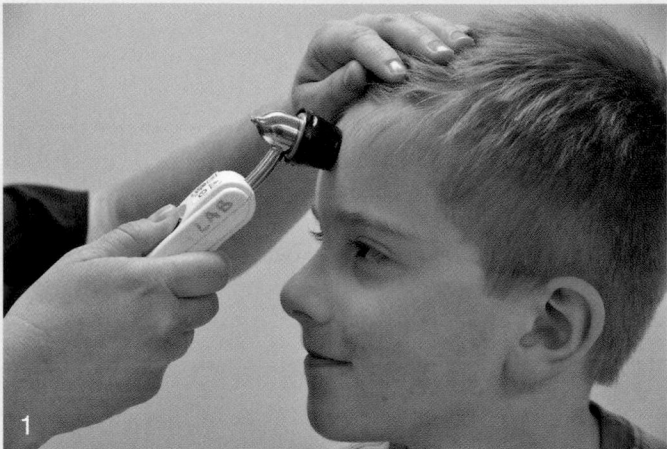

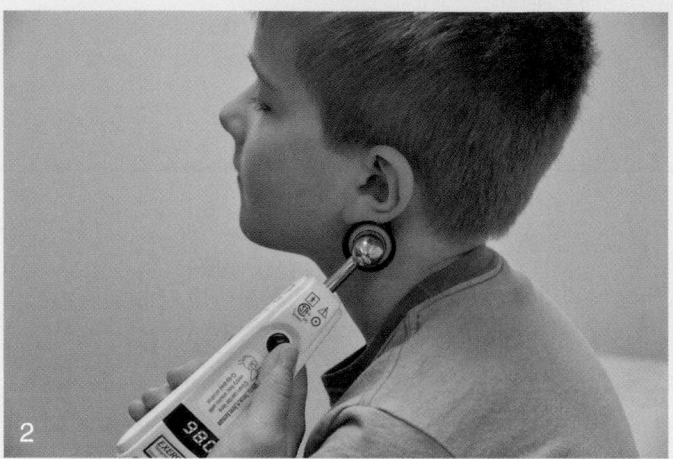

8. When scanning is complete, release the button and lift the probe. Note the temperature recorded on the digital display. The scanner automatically turns off 15 to 30 seconds after release of the button.

9. If a probe cover was used, eject it directly into a biohazard waste container. Disinfect the thermometer if indicated and replace the protective cap.
   <u>PURPOSE</u>: To ensure infection control. Depending on the facility's infection control procedures, disposable covers can be used on the scanner, or it can be cleaned between patients with a disinfectant wipe.

10. Sanitize your hands.

11. Record the temperature results (e.g., T - 101.6°F [TA]) in the patient's health record.
    <u>PURPOSE</u>: Procedures that are not recorded are considered not done.

Axillary Thermometer

Studies indicate that axillary temperatures are accurate when performed correctly. Axillary temperatures take more time to register the correct body temperature, but the method is safe, simple, and easy to perform (Procedure 24-4). Axillary temperatures are taken with a digital thermometer, which is placed into the axillary fold. If the digital thermometer has more than one probe, the oral (blue) probe with a disposable probe cover should be used. Because tympanic and temporal thermometers are relatively expensive, the axillary method may be a viable way for parents of young children to get accurate temperature readings at home. However, parents should be aware that the axillary temperature may be as much as 1° less than the child's actual core temperature.

PROCEDURE 24-4   Obtain Vital Signs: Obtain an Axillary Temperature

Goal: *To accurately determine and record a patient's temperature using the axillary method.*

EQUIPMENT and SUPPLIES

- Patient's record
- Digital unit
- Thermometer sheath or probe cover
- Supply of tissues
- Disposable gloves as appropriate
- Patient gown as needed
- Biohazard waste container

PROCEDURAL STEPS

1. Sanitize your hands.
   PURPOSE: To ensure infection control.
2. Gather the needed equipment and supplies.
3. Introduce yourself, identify your patient, and explain the procedure.
   PURPOSE: Identification of the patient prevents errors, and explanations are a means of gaining implied consent and patient cooperation.
4. Prepare the thermometer or digital unit in the same manner as for oral use.
5. Expose the axillary region. If necessary provide the patient with a gown for privacy.
6. Pat the patient's axillary area dry with tissues if needed.
   PURPOSE: To ensure an accurate reading. Do not rub the area because this may cause an elevated reading.
7. Cover the thermometer or probe and place the tip into the center of the armpit, pointing the stem toward the upper chest, and making sure the thermometer is touching only skin, not clothing.
   PURPOSE: To obtain the most accurate axillary reading; contact with clothing alters the reading.

8. Instruct the patient to hold the arm snugly across the chest or abdomen until the thermometer beeps (Figure 1).
   PURPOSE: To prevent air from leaking in and interfering with the temperature reading.

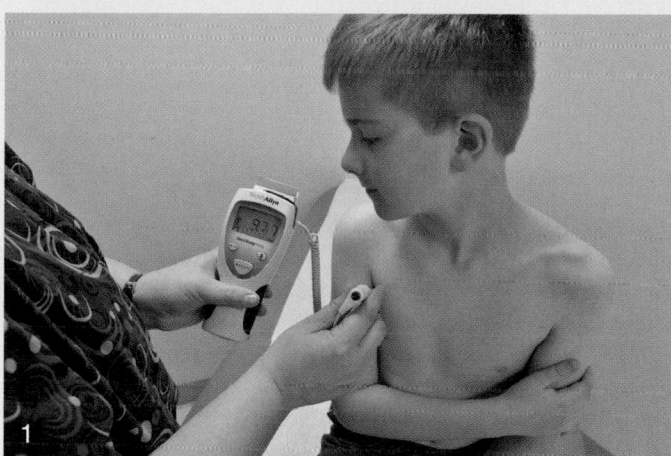

9. Remove the thermometer, note the digital reading, and dispose of the cover in the biohazard waste container.
10. Disinfect the thermometer if indicated.
    PURPOSE: To ensure infection control.
11. Sanitize your hands.
12. Record the axillary temperature in the patient's health record (e.g., T-97.6° F [A]).
    PURPOSE: Procedures that are not recorded are considered not done.

4/2/20– 9:30 AM: T-98.2° F (A). C. Ricci, CMA (AAMA)

Disposable Thermometer

Disposable thermometers (those that are used only once) may be used on small children in the home. The reading is obtained by a heat-sensitive material that changes color according to the elevation of body temperature. Two types of disposable thermometers frequently are used by parents of young children. One type is placed under the child's tongue (Figure 24-4); the other is placed on the forehead. Although both types are fairly reliable, the temperature-sensing materials have expiration dates, which often are overlooked, and specific storage requirements may apply. Disposable thermometers are considered to be good screening devices but are not as accurate as other methods. If you are instructing a parent in the use of a disposable thermometer at home, be sure to emphasize that it should be discarded immediately in a childproof container.

PULSE

A patient's pulse rate reflects the palpable beat of the arteries throughout the body as they expand in response to contraction of the heart.

CRITICAL THINKING APPLICATION   24-3

How should the medical assistant adapt temperature-taking techniques in the following scenarios?
- Patient who talks continuously with the thermometer in his mouth
- 7-year-old patient with bilateral otitis externa
- 3-month-old patient when a temporal artery thermometer is available
- 46-year-old patient with a severe asthma attack
- 72-year-old patient with bilateral impacted cerumen
- 28-year-old patient who has just smoked a cigarette

With every beat, the heart pumps an amount of blood, known as the *stroke volume,* into the aorta. Arteries branch off the aorta as it travels down through the center of the abdomen, transferring the pulse beat throughout the body. To measure the pulse, an artery is used that is close to the body surface and can be pushed against a bone. Palpating a **peripheral** pulse gives the rate and rhythm of the heartbeat and local information about the condition of the artery used.

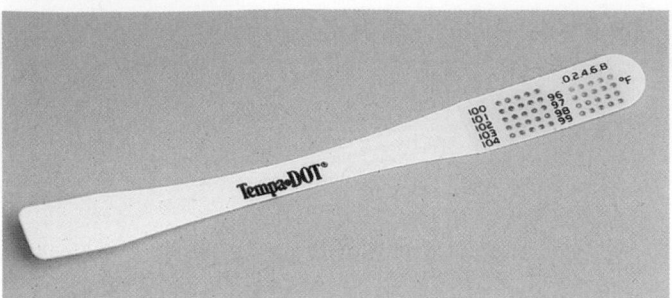

FIGURE 24-4 Tempa-Dot disposable oral strip thermometer. (Courtesy Tempa-Dot, Somerville, NJ.)

Pulse Sites

A pulse rate may be counted anyplace an artery is near the surface of the body and the vessel can be pressed against a bone. The most common pulse sites are the temporal, carotid, apical, brachial, radial, femoral, popliteal, and dorsalis pedis arteries (Figure 24-5).

The *temporal* pulse is located in the temple area of the skull, parallel and lateral to the eyes (Figure 24-6). It is seldom used as a pulse site but may be used as a pressure point to help control bleeding from a head injury.

The *carotid* artery is located between the larynx and the sternocleidomastoid muscle in the front and to the side of the neck (Figure 24-7). It most frequently is used in emergencies and to check the pulse during cardiopulmonary resuscitation (CPR). It can be felt by pushing the muscle to the side and pressing against the larynx.

The *apical* heart rate, or the heartbeat at the apex of the heart, is heard with a stethoscope. It is used for infants and young children because the radial pulse is difficult to palpate in young patients. Apical rates are also recorded on adult patients who have irregular or difficult to feel radial pulses just to make sure you are recording an accurate heart rate. An apical count may be requested if the patient is taking cardiac drugs or has **bradycardia** or **tachycardia**. To determine the presence of a **pulse deficit**, the provider may listen to the apical beat while the medical assistant counts the pulse at another site (usually the radial pulse). The stethoscope is placed at the apex of the heart which is located in the left fifth intercostal space on the midclavicular line, that is, between the fifth and sixth ribs on a line with the midpoint of the left clavicle. The pulse should be counted for 1 full minute and should be documented with (AP) beside the recorded count (Procedure 24-5).

The *brachial* pulse is felt at the inner *(antecubital)* aspect of the elbow. This is the artery that is felt and heard when blood pressure is measured (Figure 24-8). It also can be felt in the groove between the biceps and triceps muscles on the inner surface of the middle upper arm. This is the pulse that is checked on infants and young children receiving CPR.

The *radial* artery is the most frequently used site for counting the pulse rate. It is best found on the thumb side of the wrist, 1 inch below the base of the thumb (Figure 24-9).

The *femoral* pulse is located at the site where the femoral artery passes through the groin. The examiner must press deeply below the inguinal ligament to palpate this pulse.

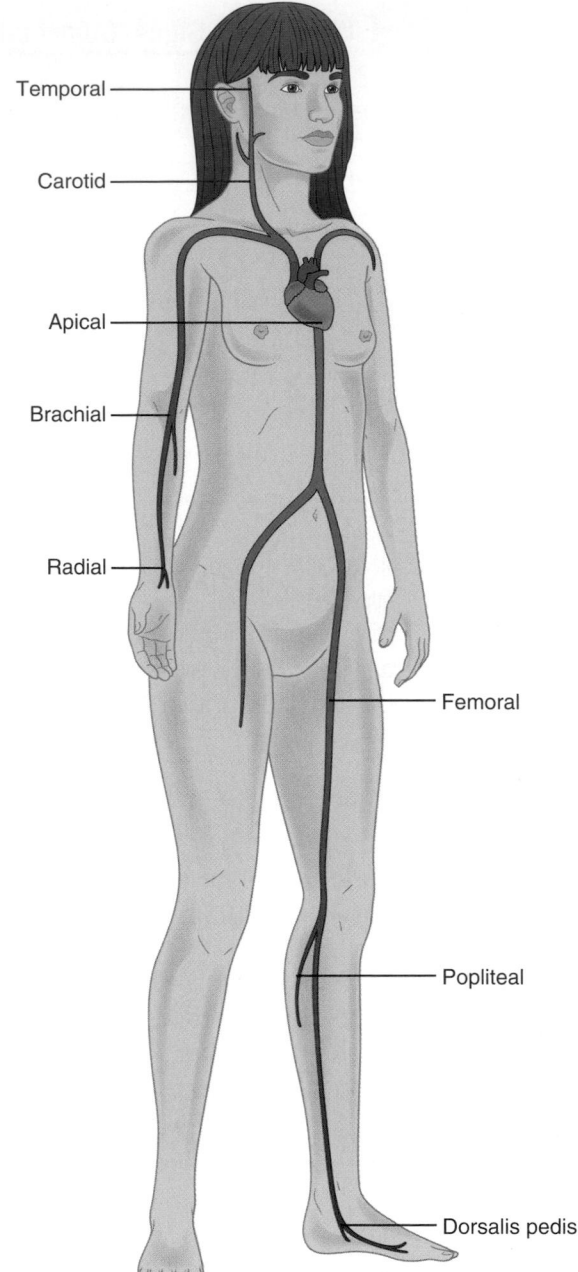

FIGURE 24-5 Pulse sites.

The *popliteal* pulse is found at the back of the leg behind the knee. Palpation of this pulse requires the patient to be in a recumbent position with the knee slightly flexed. The popliteal artery is deep and difficult to feel. It is palpated and also monitored with a stethoscope when a leg blood pressure reading is necessary. The provider checks blood flow through the popliteal artery if a circulatory system problem, such as a blood clot, is suspected in the lower leg.

The *dorsalis pedis* (pedal) artery is felt across the arch of the foot, just slightly lateral to the midline, beside the extensor tendon of the great toe. This pulse may be congenitally absent in some patients. Because a good pulse rate at this site is an indicator of normal lower limb circulation and arterial sufficiency, the provider checks the pedal pulses in patients with peripheral vascular problems, such as patients with diabetes mellitus.

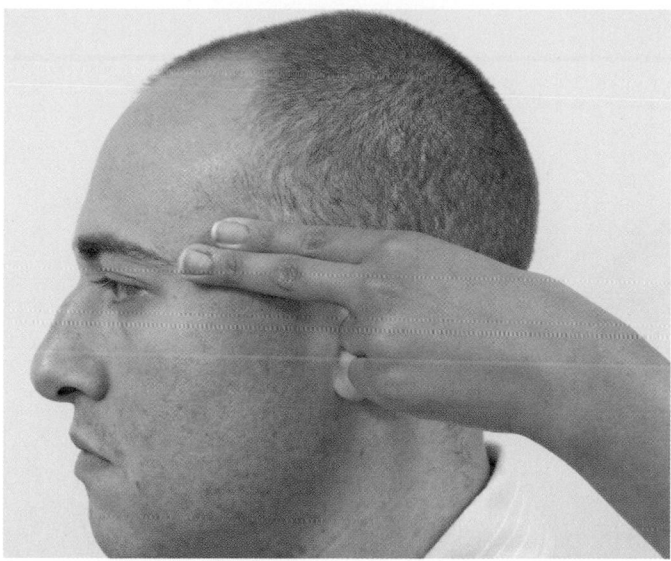

FIGURE 24-6 Temporal pulse.

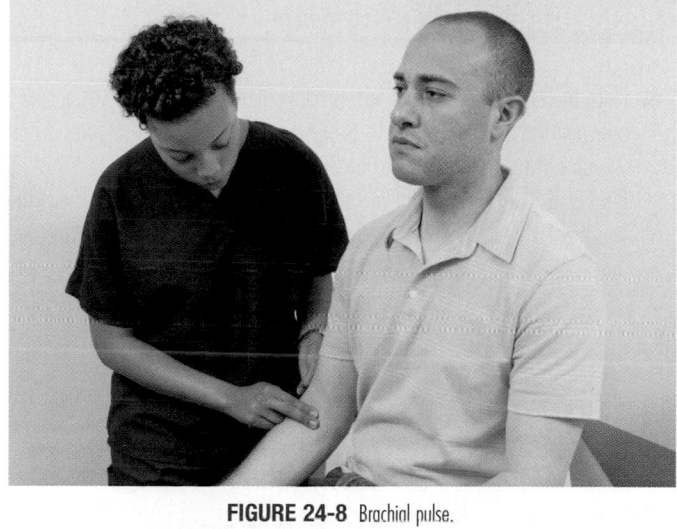

FIGURE 24-8 Brachial pulse.

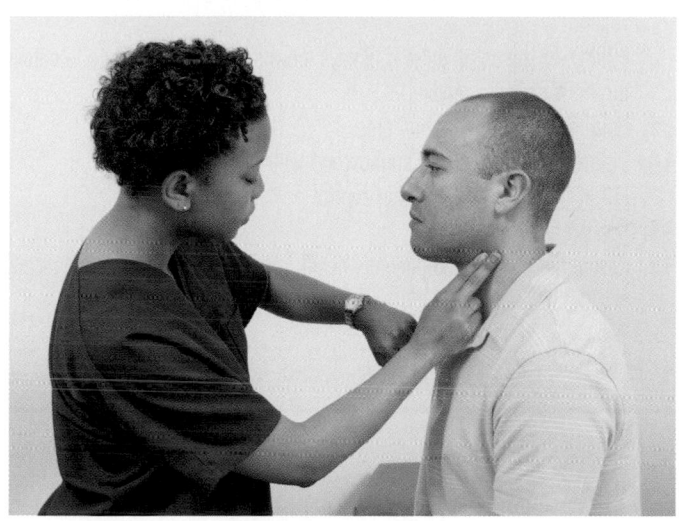

FIGURE 24-7 Carotid pulse.

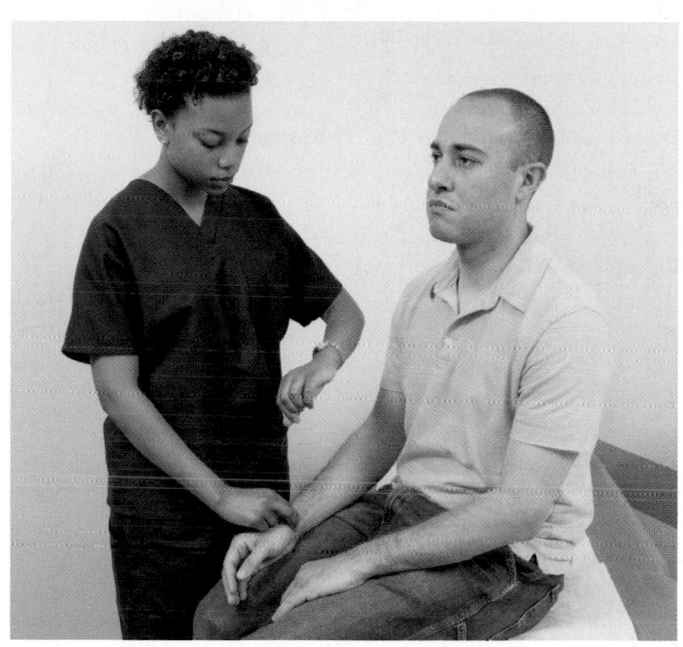

FIGURE 24-9 Radial pulse.

PROCEDURE 24-5   Obtain Vital Signs: Obtain an Apical Pulse

Goal: *To accurately determine and record the patient's apical heart rate.*

EQUIPMENT and SUPPLIES

- Patient's record
- Watch with a second hand
- Patient gown as needed
- Stethoscope
- Alcohol wipes

PROCEDURAL STEPS

1. Sanitize your hands and clean the stethoscope earpieces and diaphragm with alcohol swabs.
   <u>PURPOSE</u>: To ensure infection control and to follow Standard Precautions.

2. Introduce yourself, identify your patient, and explain the procedure.
   <u>PURPOSE</u>: Identification of the patient prevents errors, and explanations are a means of gaining implied consent and patient cooperation.

3. If necessary, assist the patient in disrobing from the waist up and provide the patient with a gown that opens in the front.
   <u>PURPOSE</u>: To expose the chest and provide privacy and warmth.

4. Assist the patient into the sitting or supine position.
   <u>PURPOSE</u>: To allow easier access to the apical site at the apex of the heart.

5. Hold the stethoscope's diaphragm against the palm of your hand for a few seconds.
   <u>PURPOSE</u>: To warm the diaphragm, promoting patient comfort.

PROCEDURE 24-5 —*continued*

6. Place the stethoscope at the left midclavicular line in the intercostal space between the fifth and sixth ribs over the apex of the heart (Figures 1 and 2). Do not touch the bell end of the stethoscope.
   <u>PURPOSE</u>: This is the point of maximum contractile strength, where the heartbeat can be heard best. Touching the bell end of the stethoscope may interfere with the sound.

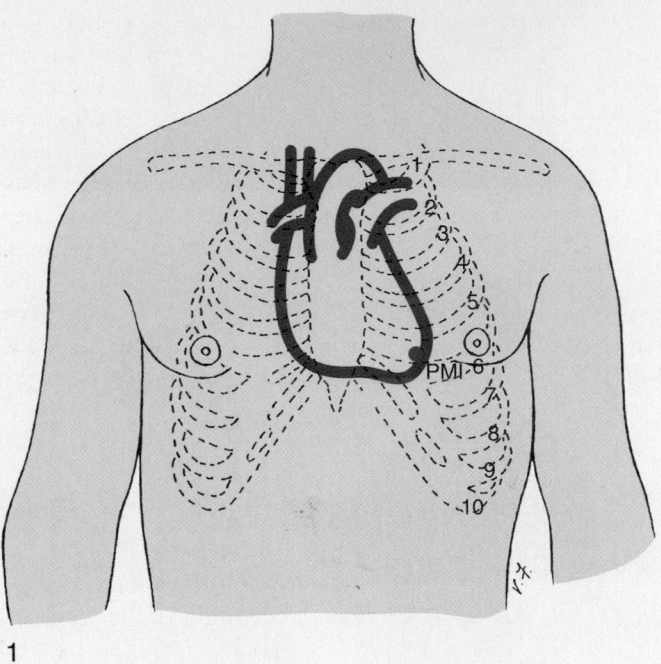

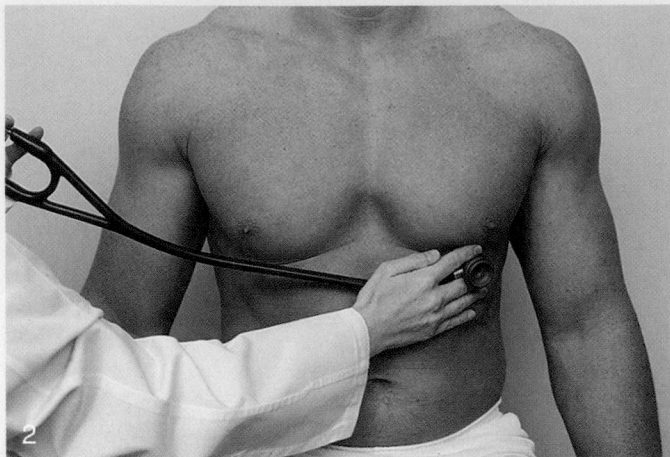

7. Listen carefully for the heartbeat.
8. Count the pulse for 1 full minute. Note any irregularities in rhythm and volume.
   <u>PURPOSE</u>: The apical pulse is always measured for 1 full minute to obtain the most accurate reading.
9. Help the patient sit up and dress.
10. Disinfect the head of the stethoscope with an alcohol wipe.
    <u>PURPOSE</u>: To ensure infection control.
11. Sanitize your hands.
12. Record the pulse in the patient's health record (e.g., AP - 96) and record any arrhythmias.

4/22/20— 4:10 PM: AP-92 irregular. C. Ricci, CMA (AAMA)

Characteristics of a Pulse

When measuring a pulse, you must note three important characteristics: rate, rhythm, and volume. These characteristics vary with the size and elasticity of the artery and the strength and regularity of the heart's contractions. A patient's pulse may reveal valuable information about the cardiovascular system.

Rate

The pulse rate is a measure of the number of heartbeats felt from the movement of blood through an artery. When the heart contracts, pressure throughout the arteries is increased, and the arteries expand. When the heart relaxes, arterial pressure is decreased, and the arteries relax. Each contraction and relaxation of the heart muscle is a heartbeat, and each resulting expansion and relaxation of the arteries is the pulse rate. Normally, the heartbeat (rate) and the pulse rate are the same. The rate of the pulse is the number of heartbeats (pulsations) that occur in 1 minute. Because the body must balance heat loss by increasing circulation (a faster heart rate), the pulse rate is proportionate to the size of the heart. The smaller the body, the greater the heat loss and the faster the heart must pump to compensate. Therefore, infants and children normally have a faster pulse than adults; as aging progresses, the pulse rate declines.

Pulse rates normally vary as a result of a person's age, body size, gender, and health status. The rate is affected by an individual's activities and psychological state, and by certain medications. It usually is faster in women (70 to 80 beats per minute) than in men (60 to 70 beats per minute). Children tend to have more rapid pulse rates than adults. The rate is more rapid when a person is sitting than when he or she is lying down, and it increases when an individual stands, walks, or runs. During sleep or rest, the pulse rate may drop to as low as 45 to 50 beats per minute. Well-conditioned athletes tend to have pulse rates of 50 to 60 beats per minute because consistent aerobic exercise strengthens the heart muscle (the myocardium) so that each heart contraction ejects an increased volume of blood into the arterial system. Table 24-3 lists the normal pulse ranges for various age groups of patients.

Rhythm

The pulse rhythm is the time between pulse beats. A normal rhythm pattern has an even tempo, which indicates that the intervals between the beats are of equal duration. An abnormal rhythm, or **arrhythmia**, is described according to the rhythm pattern detected. An **intermittent pulse** may occur in healthy individuals during exercise or after drinking a beverage containing caffeine. A common

TABLE 24-3 Approximate Age-Related Pulse Ranges

AGE	RANGE (beats/min)	AVERAGE
Newborn	120-160	140
1-2 years	80-140	120
3-6 years	75-120	100
7-11 years	75-110	95
Adolescence to adulthood	60-100	80

irregularity found in children and young adults is **sinus arrhythmia**, in which the heart rate varies with the respiratory cycle, speeding up at the peak of inspiration and slowing to normal with expiration. If beats are frequently skipped or if the beats are markedly irregular, the provider should be advised, because this may indicate heart disease. If an irregular rhythm is detected, the apical pulse should be measured for a full minute to ensure accuracy, and the rate should be recorded for the provider's review. A note also should be made that the patient's pulse was irregular. For example: P-86 irregular.

Volume

The volume (pulse amplitude) reflects the strength of the heart when it contracts. Volume can be assessed by feeling the strength of the pulse as blood flows through the vessel. The force of each pulse beat is described as **bounding**, or full; strong, or normal; or **thready**, or weak. The force of the heartbeat and the condition of the arterial wall (whether hard or soft) influence the volume. The pulse may vary only in intensity and otherwise may be perfectly regular. This condition also can indicate heart disease. The pulse volume is recorded using a three-point scale.

Three-Point Scale for Measuring Pulse Volume

3+	Full, bounding pulse	Pulsation is very strong and does not disappear with moderate pressure.
2+	Normal pulse	Pulsation is easily felt but disappears with moderate pressure.
1+	Weak, thready pulse	Pulsation is not easily felt and disappears with slight pressure.

Determining the Pulse Rate

Radial and Apical Pulse Rates

To record an accurate radial pulse, you must have the patient in a comfortable position with the artery to be used at the same level as or lower than the heart (Procedure 24-6). The limb should be well supported and relaxed. The patient may be lying down or sitting. As with all pulse readings, the pads of the first two or three fingers are placed over the artery. Never use your thumb to determine the pulse

rate; the thumb has its own pulse, and your pulse rate may be confused with the patient's rate. Push the radial artery against the bone until the strongest pulsation is felt. The pulse should be counted for 1 full minute. A 15- or 30-second interval may be used once you become proficient at performing the skill.

Variations from normal quality should be noted, such as an arrhythmia or a pulse that is thready or bounding. Some pulses are more difficult to feel than others, and finding the correct pressure to be used for each patient and site requires repeated practice and experience.

Both you and the patient should be in a relaxed position. Too much pressure obliterates the patient's pulse, and too little pressure prevents detection of irregularities or of all the beats. Record the number of beats in 1 minute. Assess the pulse, including rate, rhythm, and volume. If the pulse rate is counted at any site other than the radial artery, the rate should be recorded along with a notation of the site used. The apical pulse should always be auscultated for a full minute to detect any irregularities in rate and rhythm. Remember, one reason you would decide to take an apical pulse on an adult patient is that you noted irregularities in the heart rate when palpating the radial pulse. Therefore, you should listen to an apical pulse for a full minute to make sure you are accurately counting the number of heartbeats per minute.

CRITICAL THINKING APPLICATION   24-4

Mrs. Arnez has a documented thready pulse. What site should Carlos use to measure the pulse? Why should he listen to the pulse for a full minute?

Femoral, Popliteal, and Pedal Pulses

Pulses in the lower extremities may be difficult to find and equally difficult to hear. A Doppler unit, which is an ultrasound unit that magnifies the pulsation, may be used to locate and count these pulses accurately (Figure 24-10). A Doppler unit is battery operated and can be attached to a stethoscope so that only the provider can hear the beat, or it can be set so that both the provider and the patient can hear the pulsations.

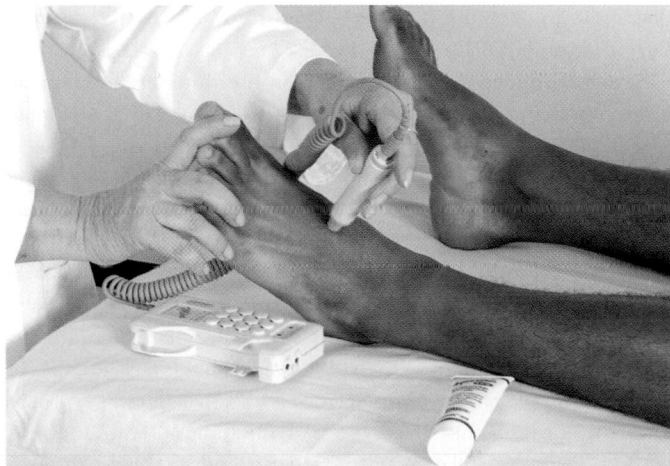

FIGURE 24-10 Doppler ultrasound unit measuring the pedal pulse. (From Jarvis C: *Physical examination and health assessment,* ed 7, St Louis, 2016, Saunders.)

RESPIRATION

Physiology

The purpose of respiration is to provide for the exchange of oxygen and carbon dioxide among the atmosphere, the blood, and the body cells. Oxygen is taken into the body to be used for life-sustaining body processes, and carbon dioxide is released as a waste product.

One complete inspiration and expiration is called a *respiration*. During the inspiratory phase, the diaphragm contracts and drops down and the intercostal muscles pull the ribs up and outward; this causes the lungs to expand and fill with air. During the expiratory phase, the diaphragm returns to its normal elevated position and the intercostal muscles relax; this causes the lungs to expel the waste air back into the atmosphere.

Respiration is both internal and external. *External respiration* is the exchange of oxygen and carbon dioxide in the lungs. *Internal respiration* occurs at the cellular level, when oxygen in the bloodstream is transferred into the cells for energy, and carbon dioxide is released as a waste product and transported back to the lungs for exhalation.

The respiratory center in the medulla oblongata, located in the brain between the top of the spine and the brainstem, is sensitive to changes in blood oxygen and carbon dioxide levels. When blood carbon dioxide levels become elevated, the respiratory control center sends a message to the respiratory system that triggers breathing. Respiration, therefore, is controlled by the involuntary nervous system; this means that we breathe automatically. Because a person can control respiration to a certain extent, it also is a voluntary body function. However, breathing ultimately is under the control of the medulla oblongata, which is why we can hold our breath only for a given length of time. Once the blood's carbon dioxide level rises to the point where cells become oxygen starved, a stimulus is sent to the respiratory muscles (the diaphragm and intercostal muscles) and breathing begins involuntarily.

Characteristics of Respirations

Normally, a person's breathing is relaxed, automatic, and silent. However, respiratory disease or chronic conditions can influence the characteristics of an individual's respirations. **Dyspnea** occurs in patients with pneumonia, asthma, or **chronic obstructive pulmonary disease (COPD)**. It also occurs after physical exertion or at very high altitudes. Other alterations in breathing are **bradypnea**, **apnea**, **tachypnea**, and **hyperpnea**. Hyperpnea usually is accompanied by **hyperventilation** and often occurs when the patient is extremely anxious or in pain. **Orthopnea** frequently occurs in patients with congestive heart failure (CHF) and COPD. **Wheezing** signals difficulty breathing in patients with asthma.

When assessing a patient's respirations, you must note three important characteristics: rate, rhythm, and depth.

- *Rate:* The rate of respiration is the number of respirations per minute and is described as normal, rapid, or slow. Figure 24-11 shows sample rate patterns recorded with a **spirometer**. Typically, a ratio of four pulse beats to one respiration is seen. As a rule, both the pulse and respiratory rates respond to exercise or emotional upset. Table 24-4 lists normal respiratory ranges for patients in various age groups.

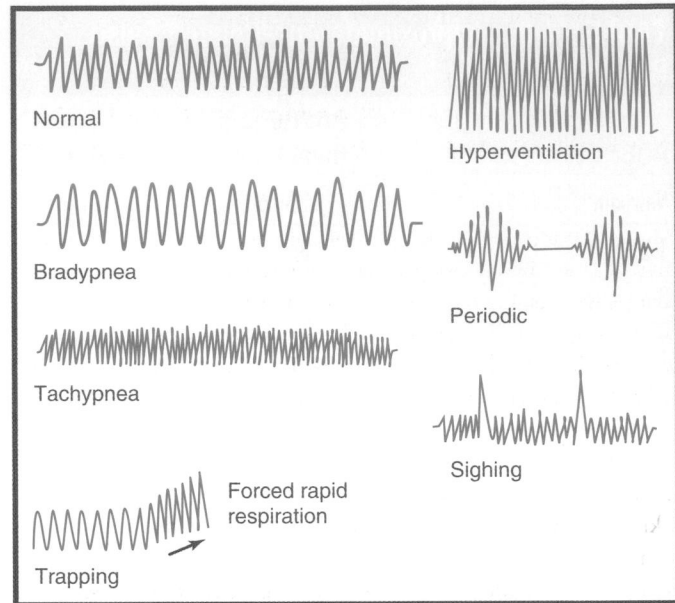

FIGURE 24-11 Respiratory rate patterns, called *spirograms*, are recorded using a spirometer.

TABLE 24-4 Approximate Age-Related Respiration Ranges		
AGE	RANGE (breaths/min)	AVERAGE
Newborn	30-50	40
1-3 years	20-30	25
4-6 years	18-26	22
7-11 years	16-22	19
Adolescence to adulthood	12-20	16

- *Rhythm:* *Rhythm* refers to the breathing pattern. A regular breathing pattern is normal in adults; however, the breathing pattern for infants varies. Automatic interruptions, such as sighing, are also considered normal.
- *Depth:* The *depth* of respiration is the amount of air inhaled and exhaled. When a patient is at rest, normal respirations have a consistent depth, which can be noted as you watch the rise and fall of the chest. Rapid, shallow breathing at rest occurs with some diseases, such as asthma and emphysema. An alteration in the depth and sometimes the rate of breathing is also seen in **Cheyne-Stokes respirations**.

Normally, no noticeable breath sounds occur during the breathing process, except during snoring. Noticeable breath sounds are a sign of certain diseases, such as pneumonia, asthma, and pulmonary edema. After auscultating breath sounds with a stethoscope, the provider can describe the characteristics of breath sounds by using specific terminology (e.g., **rales**, **rhonchi**, **stertorous** breathing).

When an individual cannot inspire enough oxygen to supply all body cells with oxygenated blood, normal skin coloring, particularly around the mouth and the nail beds, changes to a bluish, dusky color. This coloration, which indicates an increased level of carbon dioxide in the blood, is called *cyanosis*. The patient also may have other signs and symptoms, such as vertigo, chest pain *(angina),* and numbness in the fingers and toes.

Counting Respirations

Because most people are unaware of their breathing, do not mention that you will be counting the person's respirations (see Procedure 24-6). The respiratory rate is easily controlled, and patients self-consciously alter their breathing rate when they know they are being watched. Therefore, count the respirations while appearing to count the radial pulse. Keep your eyes alternately on the patient's chest and your watch while you count the pulse rate; then, without removing your fingers from the pulse site, determine the respiratory rate (Figure 24-12). If the patient is supine, the arm on which you are taking the radial pulse may be crossed over the chest so that respirations can be felt with the rise and fall of the chest. Another way of observing respirations is to watch the movement of the patient's shoulders with each inspiration. Count the respirations for 30 seconds and multiply the number by 2. Do not use the 15-second interval because this count can vary by a factor of ±4, which is significant when dealing with such a small number. Note any variation or irregularity in the rate. Record the respiratory count in the health record.

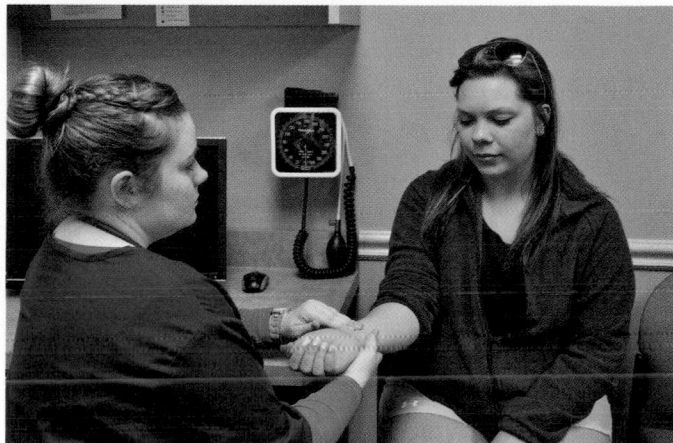

FIGURE 24-12 Hand position when counting respirations. The hands should be left in place as if still counting the patient's pulse.

CRITICAL THINKING APPLICATION **24-5**

Tina Anderson, a 36-year-old patient who is obese, is wearing a heavy knit sweater, and Carlos needs to obtain a respiratory count. What could he do to obtain an accurate measurement of Tina's respiratory rate?

PROCEDURE 24-6 | **Obtain Vital Signs: Assess the Patient's Radial Pulse and Respiratory Rate**

Goal: *To accurately determine and record a patient's radial pulse rate and rhythm and respiratory rate.*

Note: Respirations should be assessed immediately after the radial pulse while the medical assistant is appearing to take the pulse so the patient does not artificially alter breathing patterns.

EQUIPMENT and SUPPLIES

- Patient's record
- Watch with a second hand

PROCEDURAL STEPS

1. Sanitize your hands.
   PURPOSE: To ensure infection control.
2. Introduce yourself, identify your patient, and explain the procedure.
   PURPOSE: Identification of the patient prevents errors, and explanations are a means of gaining implied consent and patient cooperation.
3. Place the patient's arm in a relaxed position, palm at or below the level of the heart.
   PURPOSE: The patient's radial artery is more easily palpated when the patient is relaxed and in this position.
4. Gently grasp the palm side of the patient's wrist with your first two or three fingertips approximately 1 inch below the base of the thumb (Figure 1).
   PURPOSE: This position puts your fingertips directly over the radial artery. Press firmly (but do not press too hard, or you will occlude the artery and feel nothing).

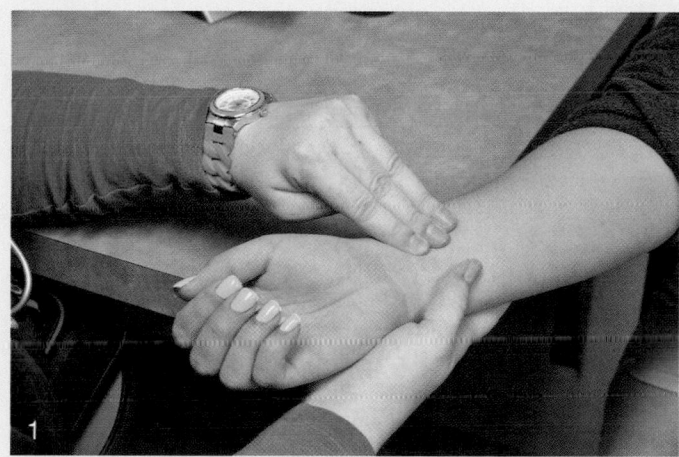

5. Count the beats for 1 full minute using a watch with a second hand.
   PURPOSE: Counting for 1 full minute allows you to obtain an accurate count, including any irregularities in rhythm and volume. Once you become more adept at taking a pulse, you can reduce this to 30 seconds and multiply that number by 2 to record the patient's heart rate.

6. While continuing to hold the patient's arm in the same position used to count the radial pulse, observe the rise and fall of the patient's chest (see Figure 24-12). If you have difficulty noticing the patient's breathing, place the arm across the chest to detect movement.
   PURPOSE: The respiratory count may be altered if the patient is aware that you are counting his or her breaths; placing the arm across the chest allows you to feel or see the rise and fall of the chest wall.

7. Inspiration and expiration make up one complete breathing cycle or respiration. Count the respirations for 30 seconds and multiply by 2.
   PURPOSE: Counting for 30 seconds allows you to obtain an accurate count and determine any irregularities in rhythm or depth or unusual breathing patterns. If respirations are abnormal in any way, count for 1 full minute.

8. Release the patient's wrist.

9. Sanitize your hands.
   PURPOSE: To ensure infection control.

10. Record both the radial pulse and respiration counts with any irregularities on the patient's health record. In a paper record the pulse is recorded immediately after the temperature and respirations after the pulse recording (e.g., P - 72, R - 18).
    PURPOSE: Procedures that are not recorded are considered not done.

5/6/20– 8:35 AM: P-72 reg, R-18. C. Ricci, CMA (AAMA)

BLOOD PRESSURE

The blood pressure reading reflects the pressure of the blood against the walls of the arteries. Each time the ventricles contract, blood is pushed out of the heart and into the aorta, exerting pressure on the walls of the arteries. There are actually two blood pressure readings: the *systolic* pressure is the highest pressure level that occurs when the heart is contracting and the first pulse beat heard; the *diastolic* pressure is the lowest pressure level when the heart is relaxed and is the last sound heard. Systole (heart contraction) and diastole (heart relaxation) together make up the cardiac cycle. The difference between systolic and diastolic pressures is the **pulse pressure**.

Blood pressure is read in millimeters of mercury, abbreviated *mm Hg*. However, you need not include the abbreviation when documenting the reading in the patient's health record. Blood pressure is recorded as a fraction, with the systolic reading the numerator (top) and the diastolic reading the denominator (bottom) (e.g., 130/80). Table 24-5 lists normal blood pressure ranges for patients of various age groups.

Factors Affecting Blood Pressure

Physiologic factors that determine blood pressure include blood volume, peripheral resistance created by blood viscosity (the thickness of the blood), vessel elasticity, and the condition of the heart muscle and arterial walls.

Volume is the amount of blood in the arteries. An increased blood volume raises blood pressure, and a decreased blood volume lowers blood pressure. Therefore, with extensive bleeding or hemorrhage, the blood volume drops, and so does the blood pressure.

The *peripheral resistance* of blood vessels refers to the relationship of the lumen (the diameter of the vessel) to the amount of blood flowing through it. The smaller the lumen, the greater the resistance to blood flow. Blood pressure is higher with a small or reduced-size lumen and lower with a large lumen. Vessels affected by fatty cholesterol deposits (*atherosclerotic plaques*) become narrower over time, resulting in smaller vessel lumens and therefore higher blood pressure.

Vessel elasticity is the ability of an artery to expand and contract to supply the body with a steady flow of blood. With advancing age, certain lifestyle factors, or the presence of **arteriosclerosis**, vessel elasticity may decrease, causing the arterial walls to become firm and resistant; as a result, the blood pressure is increased.

The condition of the myocardium is a primary determinant of the volume of blood flowing through the body. A strong, forceful contraction empties the heart and tends to keep the blood pressure within normal limits. If the myocardium becomes weak, pressure in the vessels begins to increase in an attempt to maintain an adequate level of circulating blood to meet the oxygen and nutrient needs of the body.

Evaluating the Blood Pressure

When a patient's blood pressure is being tracked, frequent readings should be taken at about the same time of day and by the same person using the same-sized cuff and the same arm. **Secondary hypertension** is caused by another underlying pathologic condition, such as renal disease, complications of pregnancy, endocrine

TABLE 24-5   Approximate Age-Related Blood Pressure Ranges

AGE	RANGE SYSTOLIC	DIASTOLIC
Newborn	60-96	30-62
1-3 years	78-112	48-78
4-6 years	78-112	50-79
7-11 years	85-114	52-79
Adolescent	94-119	58-79
Adult	100-119	60-79

imbalance, and brain injury. Temporary hypertension may occur with stress, pain, exercise, and exhaustion. Many patients experience "white coat hypertension"; that is, their blood pressure becomes elevated in the medical environment, although it is normal when they are away from the healthcare facility.

An adult is diagnosed with **essential hypertension** (stage 1 primary hypertension) if the systolic pressure is 140 to 159 or higher and/or the diastolic pressure is 90 to 99 or higher. Essential hypertension is the most common type of hypertension. It is *idiopathic* (no known cause) but is associated with obesity, a high blood level of sodium, elevated cholesterol levels, family history, and race. African-Americans, Mexican Americans, Native Americans, native Hawaiians, and some Asian-Americans are at greater risk of developing hypertension.

Primary, or essential, hypertension is diagnosed if the patient's blood pressure is persistently higher than 119 mm Hg systolic and/or 79 mm Hg diastolic (the criteria for prehypertension) at two or more office visits over several weeks or months. If the medical assistant first notes that a patient's blood pressure is elevated, the pressure should be checked again after the patient has been allowed to sit comfortably for at least 2 minutes. Check the blood pressure in both arms with a cuff that is the proper size for the patient's arm. If the pressure readings are different, the provider uses the higher value for diagnostic purposes. All of these readings must be documented in the patient's record.

The American Heart Association (AHA) guidelines for the diagnosis and management of hypertension include three categories for diagnostic and treatment purposes: prehypertension, stage 1 hypertension, and stage 2 hypertension. The goal of the AHA recommendations is to reduce the number of people who die each year from hypertension-related illnesses, such as coronary artery disease, heart attack, heart failure, kidney disease, and stroke. Hypertension can occur in children or adults, but individuals of African-American descent, middle-aged and elderly people, patients with diabetes mellitus, and those with kidney disease are at greatest risk. Hypertension has been called *the silent killer* because it frequently has no symptoms, and individuals may go for long periods without knowing they have a problem. Hypertension often is discovered during medical treatment for another problem. Signs and symptoms may include blurred vision, angina, vertigo, dyspnea, fatigue, headache, flushing, nosebleeds *(epistaxis)*, and palpitations. Table 24-6 summarizes the stages and recommended treatment for the different levels of elevated blood pressure.

Treatment guidelines for hypertension have four basic aspects:

1. Individuals with prehypertension should be diagnosed and encouraged to make lifestyle changes before they require medical treatment and/or move into the hypertensive category. The AHA recommends limiting intake of salt and eating a diet rich in potassium, calcium, magnesium, and protein while reducing total fat intake, especially saturated fat. Individuals with prehypertension also should restrict their alcohol intake, engage in regular physical activity, and lose weight if necessary to maintain a healthy BMI range. Many times, just losing 10% of a person's weight lowers the blood pressure.
2. In people older than 50 years of age, the systolic reading is more important than the diastolic reading. Individuals over

TABLE 24-6 Stages and Treatment of Hypertension

BLOOD PRESSURE	TREATMENT
Prehypertension 120-139 systolic OR 80-89 diastolic	• Lifestyle modification (reduced sodium, low saturated and trans fat diet; regular aerobic activity; moderate alcohol intake; smoking cessation; weight loss; stress reduction) • Drug therapy for patients with diabetes mellitus or chronic kidney disease
Stage 1 hypertension 140-159 systolic OR 90-99 diastolic	• Consider coexisting conditions • Thiazide-type diuretics (e.g., furosemide [Lasix] or hydrochlorothiazide plus triamterene [Dyazide]) for most patients
Stage 2 hypertension ≥160 systolic OR ≥100 diastolic	• Consider coexisting conditions • Two-drug combination for most patients

From the Seventh Report of the Joint National Committee on Prevention, Detection, Evaluation, and Treatment of High Blood Pressure at http://www.nhlbi.nih.gov/health-pro/guidelines/current/hypertension-jnc-7/. Accessed November 4, 2015.

50 should be treated if they have a systolic pressure of 140 mm Hg or higher, regardless of their diastolic blood pressure. Medical treatment at this age can reduce the development of cardiac and kidney disease later in life.

3. Most patients with hypertension require two or more medications to achieve desired blood pressure levels. The goal of treatment is to maintain blood pressure below 140/90 mm Hg, or below 130/80 mm Hg in patients with diabetes or kidney disease. Patients should be treated with both a diuretic, to help the body excrete excess amounts of fluid and sodium, and an antihypertensive medication.
4. A patient-centered treatment approach should be implemented to motivate patients and to maintain compliance with hypertension management. The medical assistant can play an active role in establishing a therapeutic relationship with the patient by providing ongoing education and support to ensure compliance with provider-recommended treatment. Using community resources, such as local dietitian referrals, may also help patients comply with treatment.

CRITICAL THINKING APPLICATION 24-6

Mr. Samuel Long, a 43-year-old patient, recently was diagnosed with essential hypertension. What should Carlos discuss with Mr. Long to emphasize the dangers of his disease and to teach him about possible lifestyle modifications that he must make to improve his health? Are any community resources available that might help Mr. Long and his family effectively manage his disease?

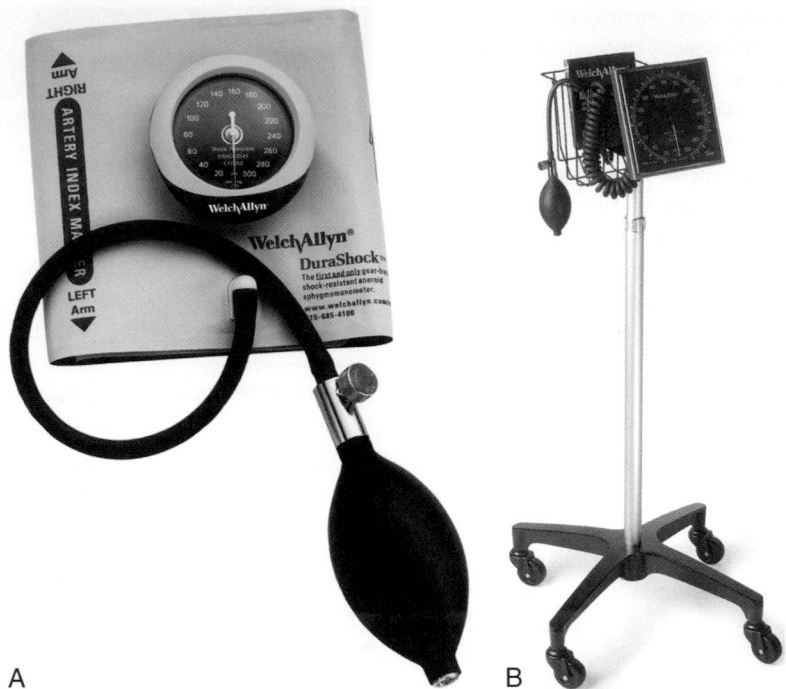

FIGURE 24-13 A, Aneroid dial system with an inflatable cuff. **B,** Aneroid floor model with a large, slanted face.

Hypotension is an abnormally low blood pressure, which may be caused by emotional or traumatic shock; hemorrhage; central nervous system (CNS) disorders; and chronic wasting diseases. Persistent readings of 90/60 mm Hg or lower usually are considered hypotensive. **Orthostatic (postural) hypotension** can cause patients to experience vertigo or **syncope**. Some medications can cause orthostatic hypotension.

Measuring Blood Pressure

The instrument used to measure blood pressure is called a *sphygmomanometer*. The term *manometer* refers to an instrument used to measure the pressure of a liquid or a gas. *Sphygmo-* means pulse. Therefore, *sphygmomanometer* means an instrument used to measure blood pressure in the arteries. The instrument consists of an inflatable cuff, an inflation bulb with a control valve, and a pressure gauge. The blood pressure mechanism consists of an aneroid dial attached to an inflatable cuff (Figure 24-13, *A*); the device may be wall mounted or a floor model (Figure 24-13, *B*). Some systems have a trigger-style air release valve; these can be pumped up and then the air slowly released simply by pushing the trigger (Figure 24-14). With the more traditional sphygmomanometers, the valve must be unscrewed.

Sphygmomanometers are delicately calibrated instruments that must be handled carefully. They should be recalibrated regularly and checked for accuracy by you or by a medical supply dealer. The needle on the aneroid dial sphygmomanometer should rest within the small square or circle at the bottom of the dial. The dial can be calibrated by connecting it to a calibrated manometer. Pump both manometers to 250 mm Hg and record the readings on both machines at least four different times as the pressure is released. A correctly calibrated mechanism shows a difference of no more than

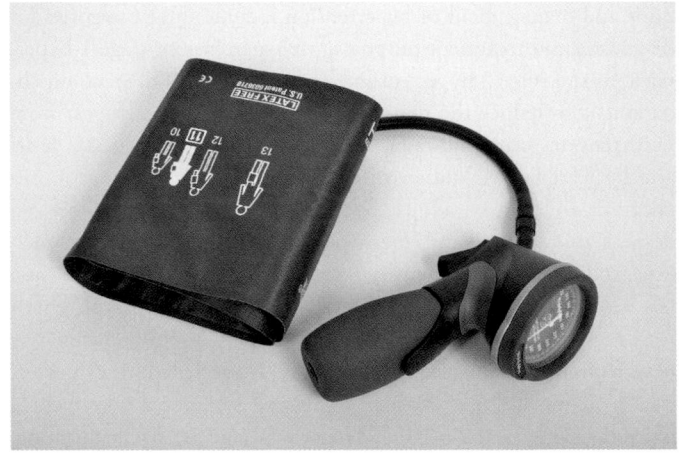

FIGURE 24-14 Trigger-release aneroid blood pressure valve.

3 mm Hg between the two readings at any time during the deflation period. If the sphygmomanometer is not correctly calibrated, the patient's blood pressure reading will be inaccurate.

The sphygmomanometer must be used with a stethoscope. The objective of the procedure is to use the inflatable cuff to obliterate (cause to disappear) circulation through an artery. The stethoscope is placed over the artery just below the cuff, and the cuff is slowly deflated to allow the blood to flow again. As blood flow resumes, cardiac cycle sounds are heard through the stethoscope, and gauge readings are taken when the first (systolic) and last (diastolic) sounds are heard (Procedure 24-7).

To obtain a correct blood pressure reading, the proper-sized cuff must be used. The systolic and diastolic blood pressures can be lowered by as much as 5 mm Hg if the cuff is one size larger than appropriate; the blood pressure can be elevated by up to 6 mm Hg if the cuff is one size smaller. To make sure you are using the correct size, the inflatable part (the bladder) should cover about 80 percent of the circumference of the upper arm. To help with this, most blood pressure cuffs have predetermined markings on the internal side of the cuff (the side placed on the patient's arm); as long as the cuff is secured within these lines it should be the accurate size (Figure 24-15). Table 24-7 presents the various sizes of blood pressure cuffs available.

When placed on the patient's arm, the cuff should cover two thirds of the distance from the elbow to the shoulder. The lower end of the cuff should be 2 to 3 cm (about 2 finger widths, or 1 inch) above the elbow or antecubital space to allow plenty of room to place the stethoscope without touching the cuff. If the stethoscope touches the cuff during the blood pressure reading, the sound of the deflating cuff may interfere with your ability to hear the correct reading. The patient's sleeve must be above the antecubital space; if the sleeve is tight, ask the patient to remove the arm from the sleeve. This is done for two reasons: tight clothing can restrict normal blood flow in the

brachial artery, thus altering the blood pressure, and placing the stethoscope over clothing makes it difficult to hear blood pressure sounds. Provide a patient gown if needed to maintain the patient's privacy.

Blood pressure cuffs and stethoscopes are available in drug and retail stores for patients to use to measure their own blood pressure at home. These units can be aneroid, electronic, or computerized sphygmomanometers (Figure 24-16). If you have patients who are monitoring their pressure at home, be sure they understand the mechanics of obtaining a reading accurately. It is best to have the patient bring his or her equipment to the office and demonstrate its use. While the patient is showing you the home equipment, you will have an ideal opportunity to check technique and calibration and to answer any questions the patient may have about use of the equipment. This is also a good opportunity to reinforce treatment plans, such as medication, diet, and exercise. It is helpful for a patient who is monitoring blood pressure readings at home to keep a log and review it with the provider during visits to help detect blood pressure variations during normal daily activities.

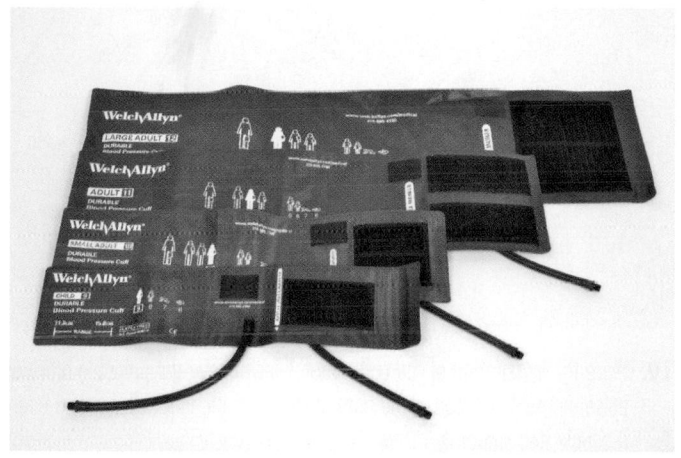

FIGURE 24-15 Variety of blood pressure cuff sizes.

TABLE 24-7	Blood Pressure Cuff Sizes	
	ARM CIRCUMFERENCE	
CUFF	CENTIMETERS	INCHES
Small adult	22-26	9
Adult	27-34	Up to 13
Large adult	35-44	14-17
Adult thigh	45-52	18-20

Data from Pickering TG, Hall JE, Appel LJ et al: Recommendations for blood pressure measurement in humans and experimental animals: Part 1. Blood pressure measurement in humans: a statement for professionals from the Subcommittee of Professional and Public Education of the American Heart Association Council on High Blood Pressure Research, *Hypertension* 45(1):142-161, 2005.

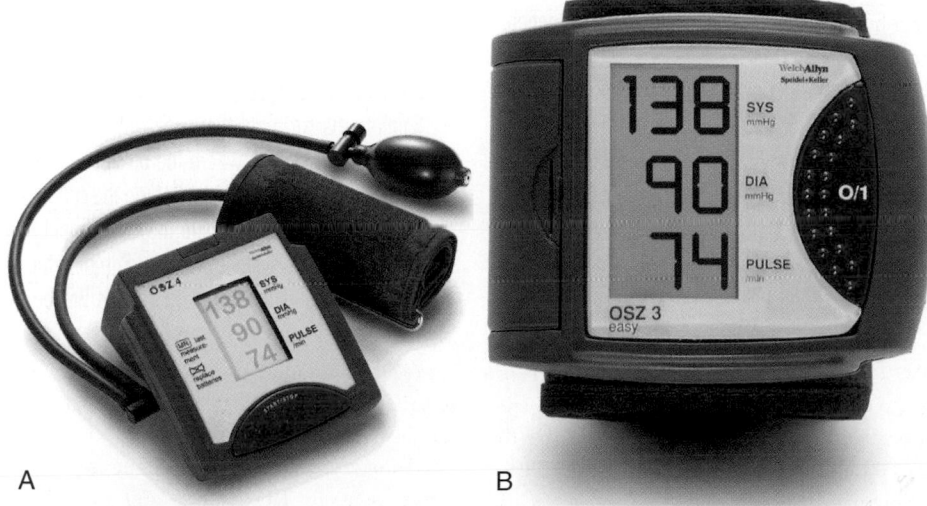

FIGURE 24-16 Personal blood pressure systems. **A,** Digital arm cuff. **B,** Digital wrist cuff.

PROCEDURE 24-7   Obtain Vital Signs: Determine a Patient's Blood Pressure

Goal: *To perform a blood pressure measurement that is correct in technique, accurate, and comfortable for the patient.*

EQUIPMENT and SUPPLIES

- Patient's record
- Sphygmomanometer
- Stethoscope
- Antiseptic wipes/alcohol swabs

PROCEDURAL STEPS

1. Sanitize your hands.
   PURPOSE: To ensure infection control.
2. Assemble the equipment and supplies needed. Clean the earpieces and diaphragm of the stethoscope with alcohol swabs.
   PURPOSE: To follow Standard Precautions.
3. Introduce yourself, identify the patient, and explain the procedure.
   PURPOSE: Identification of the patient prevents errors, and explanations are a means of gaining implied consent and patient cooperation.
4. Select the appropriate arm for application of the cuff (no mastectomy on that side, no injury or disease). If the patient has had a bilateral mastectomy, the blood pressure should be taken using a large thigh cuff with the stethoscope over the popliteal artery.
   PURPOSE: The pressure of the cuff temporarily interferes with circulation to the limb.
   CAUTION: If a female patient has had a mastectomy, the blood pressure should never be taken on the affected side. Compressing the arm may cause complications. If she has had a bilateral mastectomy, another site such as the popliteal artery must be used, which requires use of a thigh cuff.
5. Seat the patient in a comfortable position with the legs uncrossed and the arm resting, palm up, at heart level on the arm of a chair or a table next to where the patient is seated.
   PURPOSE: To expose the brachial artery; also, to promote patient relaxation and ensure a true reading. Crossed legs may increase the blood pressure, and positioning of the arm above heart level may cause an inaccurate reading.
6. Roll up the sleeve to about 5 inches above the elbow or have the patient remove the arm from the sleeve.
   PURPOSE: Tight clothing prevents an accurate reading.
7. Determine the correct cuff size.
   PURPOSE: An incorrect cuff size prevents accurate measurement of blood pressure. The cuff should fit comfortably around the patient's arm, and the bladder should be located over the brachial artery between the lines designated on the cuff. Pediatric, normal adult, and large adult cuff sizes should be available. Thigh cuffs may be needed for obese patients.

8. Palpate the brachial artery at the antecubital space in both arms. If one arm has a stronger pulse, use that arm. If the pulses are equal, select the right arm.
   PURPOSE: A stronger pulse is easier to measure; the right arm is the universal arm of choice.
9. Center the cuff bladder over the brachial artery with the connecting tube away from the patient's body and the tube to the bulb close to the body (Figure 1).
   PURPOSE: Pressure must be applied directly over the artery for an accurate reading. The cuff and its tubing should not touch the stethoscope. Noise from the tubing can interfere with a correct reading.

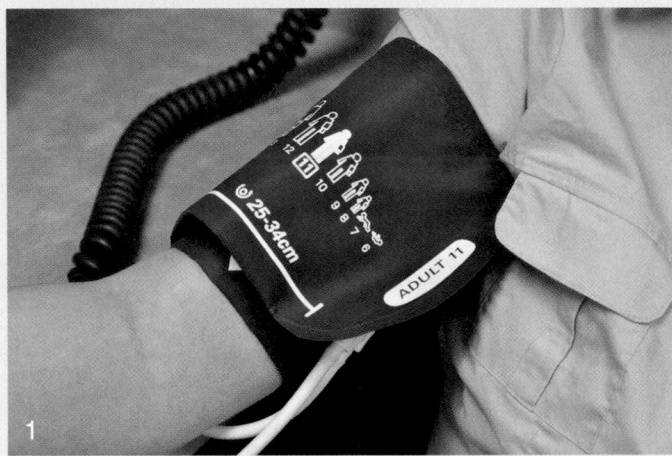

10. Place the lower edge of the cuff about 1 inch above the palpable brachial pulse, normally located in the natural crease of the inner elbow, and wrap it snugly and smoothly.
    PURPOSE: To help ensure an accurate reading. The cuff should be high enough on the arm that the stethoscope does not touch it, so that cuff sounds do not interfere with listening to the blood pressure sounds. A loose cuff results in an inaccurate reading.
11. Position the gauge of the sphygmomanometer so that it is easily seen.
    PURPOSE: An aneroid gauge should show the needle within the zero mark.
12. Palpate the brachial pulse, tighten the screw valve on the air pump, and inflate the cuff until the pulse can no longer be felt. Make a note at the point on the gauge where the pulse could no longer be felt. Mentally add 30 mm Hg to the reading. Deflate the cuff and wait 15 seconds (Figure 2).
    PURPOSE: The point where the brachial pulse is no longer felt provides an estimate of the systolic pressure. Pumping the cuff above that level ensures that phase I of the Korotkoff sounds will be heard.

PROCEDURE 24-7 —continued

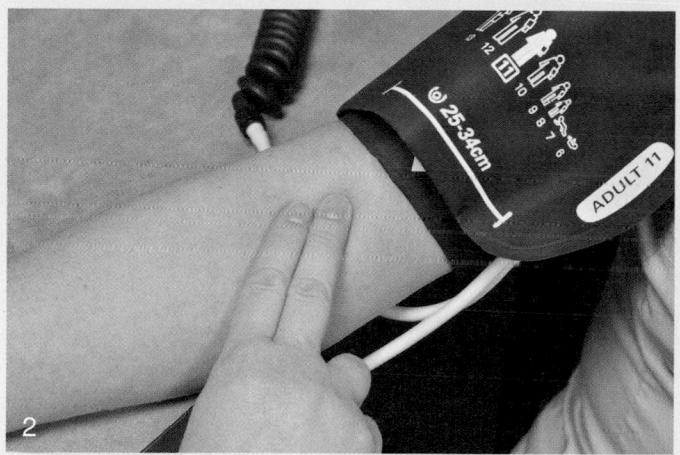

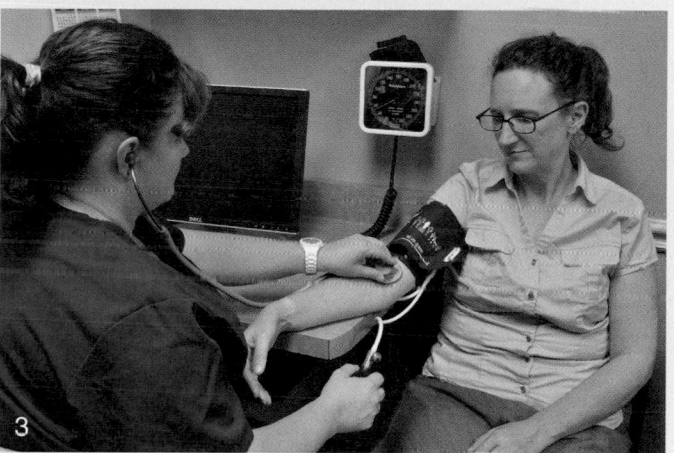

13. Insert the earpieces of the stethoscope turned forward into the ear canals.
    PURPOSE: With the earpieces in this position, the openings follow the anatomic line of the ear canal and the blood pressure will be accurately heard.

14. Place the stethoscope's diaphragm over the palpated brachial artery for an adult patient or the bell for a pediatric patient. Press firmly enough to obtain a seal but not so tightly that the artery is constricted. Only touch the edges of the stethoscope head.
    PURPOSE: Forming a seal around the head of the stethoscope aids listening for blood pressure sounds. Placing your fingers directly over the stethoscope head will cause interference with the sound.

15. Close the valve and squeeze the bulb to inflate the cuff, rapidly but smoothly, to 30 mm above the palpated pulse level, which was previously determined (Figure 3).

16. Open the valve slightly and deflate the cuff at a constant rate of 2 to 3 mm Hg per heartbeat.
    PURPOSE: Careful, slow release allows you to listen to all sounds.

17. Listen throughout the entire deflation; note the point on the gauge at which you hear the first sound (systolic) and the last sound (diastolic) until the sounds have stopped for at least 10 mm Hg.

18. Do not reinflate the cuff once the air has been released. Wait 30 to 60 seconds to repeat the procedure if needed.
    PURPOSE: Not allowing the blood to refill in the brachial artery results in inaccurate readings.

19. Remove the cuff from the patient's arm.

20. Remove the stethoscope from your ears and record the arm used and the systolic and diastolic readings as BP systolic/diastolic (e.g., BP 120/80).
    NOTE: It is recommended that the blood pressure be checked and recorded in each arm during the initial assessment of the patient and then bilaterally periodically after that for patients with hypertension.

21. Clean the earpieces and the head of the stethoscope with alcohol and return both the cuff and the stethoscope to storage.

22. Sanitize your hands.
    PURPOSE: To ensure infection control.
    ADDENDUM: The provider may direct the medical assistant to record the blood pressure with the patient in two different positions to determine whether orthostatic hypotension is a factor. To perform this skill:

    1. Measure and record the patient's blood pressure (as detailed earlier) while the patient is either supine or sitting.
    2. Leave the cuff in place.
    3. Have the patient stand, and immediately measure the blood pressure again.
    4. Record the second blood pressure and any patient symptoms, such as complaints of (c/o) vertigo or lightheadedness.

5/19/20– 11 AM: BP 120/80 ℗ arm. C. Ricci, CMA (AAMA)

Effects of Body Position on Blood Pressure Measurement

Blood pressures are usually taken with the patient in either the sitting or the supine position. However, the diastolic pressure can be as much as 5 mm Hg higher when patients are sitting than when they are supine. In addition, if the patient's back is not supported and there is some muscle tension in the body (as occurs when the patient is seated on an examination table rather than in a chair), the diastolic pressure may be increased by 6 mm Hg; if patients cross their legs during the reading, the systolic pressure may be raised by 2 to 8 mm Hg. The position of the patient's arm can also have a major influence when the blood pressure is measured. If the upper arm is below the level of the right atrium (e.g., dangling at the patient's side), the reading is artificially elevated; if the arm is above the heart level, the reading is lowered. Or, if the arm is held up by the patient, muscular tension will raise the pressure. The arm should be placed at the level of the heart on a table next to an exam room chair or resting on the arm of the chair to avoid these issues (Figure 24-17).

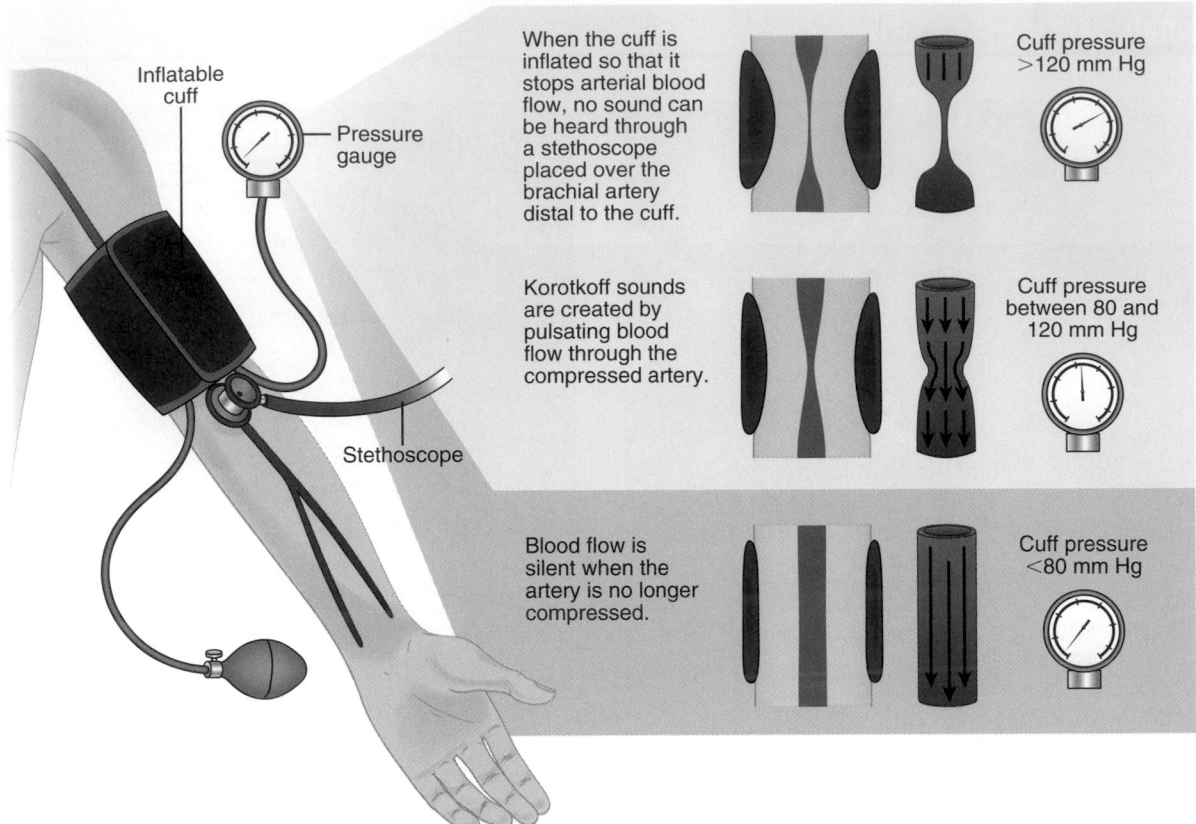

FIGURE 24-17 The science of taking a blood pressure.

Common Causes of Error in Blood Pressure Readings

- The limb used for measurement is above the level of the heart.
- The rubber bladder in the cuff is not completely deflated before a reading is started or retaken.
- The pressure in the cuff is released too rapidly.
- The patient is nervous, uncomfortable, or anxious (may cause a reading higher than the patient's actual blood pressure).
- The patient drank coffee or smoked cigarettes within 30 minutes of the blood pressure measurement.
- The cuff was applied improperly.
- The cuff is too large, too small, too loose, or too tight.
- The cuff was not placed around the arm smoothly.
- The bladder is not centered over the artery, or the bladder bulges out from the cover.
- The practitioner fails to wait 1 to 2 minutes between measurements.
- Instruments are defective:
  - Air leaks in the valve
  - Air leaks in the bladder
  - Aneroid needle not calibrated to zero

Korotkoff Sounds

Two basic heart sounds are produced by the functioning of the heart during the cardiac cycle. The first sound, produced at systole (contraction), is dull, firm, and prolonged and is heard as a *lubb* sound. The second sound, produced at diastole (relaxation), is shorter and sharper and is heard as a *dupp* sound. Therefore, *lubb-dupp* is the sound of one heartbeat.

Korotkoff sounds are the sounds heard during auscultation of blood pressure. These sounds are produced by vibrations of the arterial wall when the blood surges back into the vessel after it has been compressed by the blood pressure cuff. The sounds were first discovered and classified into five distinct phases by Russian neurologist Nikolai Korotkoff.

Phase I

Phase I is the first sound heard as the cuff deflates. The blood is resurging into the patient's artery and can be heard quite clearly as a sharp, tapping sound. Note the gauge reading when this first sound is heard. Record this as the systolic blood pressure.

Phase II

As the cuff deflates, even more blood flows through the artery. The movement of the blood makes a swishing sound. If you did not follow proper procedure in inflating the cuff, you may not hear these sounds because of their soft quality. Occasionally blood pressure sounds completely disappear during this phase. Loss of the sounds, followed by their reappearance later, is called the *auscultatory gap*. The silence may continue as the needle falls another 30 mm Hg. Auscultatory gaps occur particularly in hypertension and certain types of heart disease, so if you notice such a gap, make sure to report it to the provider.

Phase III

In phase III, a great deal of blood is pushing down into the artery. The distinct, sharp tapping sounds return and continue rhythmically. If you do not inflate the cuff enough, you will miss the first two phases completely and you will incorrectly interpret the beginning of phase III as the systolic blood pressure (phase I).

Phase IV

At this point, the blood is flowing easily. The sound changes to a soft tapping, which becomes muffled and begins to grow fainter. Occasionally these sounds continue to zero. This may occur in children, in patients of any age after exercise or with a fever, or in a pregnant patient with anemia. The AHA recommends that the beginning of phase IV be recorded as the diastolic reading for a child. Some providers call the change at phase IV the *fading sound* and want it recorded between systolic and diastolic recordings (e.g., 120/84/70, with 84 representing the gauge reading when the sounds of phase III have ended and those of phase IV are beginning). Other providers consider phase IV the true diastolic pressure.

Phase V

All sounds disappear in this phase. Note the gauge reading when the last sound is heard. Record this as the diastolic pressure.

Palpatory Method

The systolic pressure may be checked by feeling the radial pulse rather than hearing it with the stethoscope. Place the cuff in the usual position and palpate the radial pulse, noting rate and rhythm. Inflate the cuff until the pulse disappears, then add 30 mm Hg more of inflation to get above the systolic pressure. Do not remove your fingers from the pulse or change the pressure of your fingers. Carefully watch the gauge while slowly releasing the pressure in the cuff and wait until you feel the first pulse beat. Note the reading on the gauge, and record the first pulse felt as the systolic pressure. For example, if you first felt the radial pulse at 52 mm Hg, the palpated blood pressure is recorded as 52/P, with P indicating that the systolic reading was palpated. The diastolic and Korotkoff phases cannot be determined by this method. This method can be very useful in times of a medical emergency, such as shock, when the patient's blood pressure cannot be auscultated. If you are having difficulty hearing the systolic blood pressure, you can use the palpatory method first to determine how far you need to pump the cuff to hear that first beat.

CRITICAL THINKING APPLICATION   **24-7**

Vital signs are documented in a paper record in this order: temperature (T), pulse (P), and respirations (R). Blood pressure is recorded after TPR. Depending on the EHR system, they may be ordered differently. Correctly document the following vital signs:

1. Oral temperature 101.2°; apical pulse 90; respirations 22; and orthostatic blood pressure in the right arm is 138/88 supine and 110/70 standing
2. Tympanic temperature 36.8°; radial pulse 66; respirations 18; and bilateral blood pressure 128/76 in the left arm and 132/80 in the right arm
3. Temporal temperature 102.4°; apical pulse 102; and respirations 27
4. Axillary temperature 97.7°; carotid pulse 58; respirations 24; and palpated blood pressure 62

OSHA Guidelines for Measuring Vital Signs

Guidelines established by the Occupational Safety and Health Administration (OSHA) for the measurement of vital signs include the following:

- Wash hands before and after each procedure.
- Always use protective disposable sheaths on all forms of thermometers.
- Immediately disinfect any equipment that becomes contaminated during the procedure.
- Wear gloves if the potential exists for contacting any open areas or body fluids.
- When caring for a patient with a known respiratory infectious disorder (e.g., tuberculosis), use protective clothing, including a face shield or mask as indicated.
- Dispose of all contaminated material, including thermometer covers, gloves, and disinfectant swabs, in the proper biohazard waste containers.

ANTHROPOMETRIC MEASUREMENTS

Anthropometry is the science that deals with measurement of the size, weight, and proportions of the human body. These measurements often are included in the initial recording of vital signs and before the provider performs a physical examination or a well-baby check. Because they are indicators of the patient's state of health and well-being, height and weight measurements and the associated BMI are discussed as aspects of the vital signs. Other measurements are discussed when pertinent in the specialty chapters.

Measuring Weight and Height

A patient's weight and height can be helpful in diagnosis, and the medical assistant must obtain these readings with accuracy and empathy (Procedure 24-8). In many medical settings, weight and height are measured routinely as the patient is escorted to the examination room. To safeguard patient confidentiality, the scale should be located in a private area where other individuals are unable to observe the patient's weight. However, regardless of where the scale is located in the healthcare facility, be sure to safeguard the patient's confidentiality by not repeating the measurement out loud so others nearby can hear this private patient information. If this is the patient's first visit, anthropometric measurements are recorded in the history database and are used as reference information during future visits as needed. EHR systems automatically record vital signs data so that they can be seen on the majority of screens viewed.

Many providers use the BMI to determine the risk for certain diseases, so the medical assistant may have to use the accurately measured height and weight to determine and record the patient's BMI. This is typically done using a BMI chart that converts the patient's height and weight ratio into a BMI number, or with a wheeled device that calibrates the BMI when the height and weight intersect. BMI numbers also can be determined using an online conversion calculator. EHR systems automatically calculate and record the patient's BMI after the height and weight measurements are entered.

Certain medical specialties and specific medical problems may require continuous monitoring of weight. Hormone disorders (e.g., diabetes), growth patterns (seen in children), and eating disorders (e.g., obesity, bulimia) require accurate weight checks as part of every medical visit. In addition, maternity patients must have their weight monitored to make sure they are gaining weight, but also as a precaution against too much weight gain, which may indicate fluid retention. Patients with cardiovascular disorders who tend to retain fluid should have their weight checked each time they are seen in the office. Some scales are calibrated in kilograms, others in pounds. When weight must be converted from one to the other, use the formulas shown later in this chapter or an online conversion calculator. EHR systems do the conversion automatically (Figure 24-18).

Accurate height or length measurements are particularly important for children (see the Pediatrics chapter). The provider also may request routine height screening for patients diagnosed with osteoporosis because these patients may lose height over time.

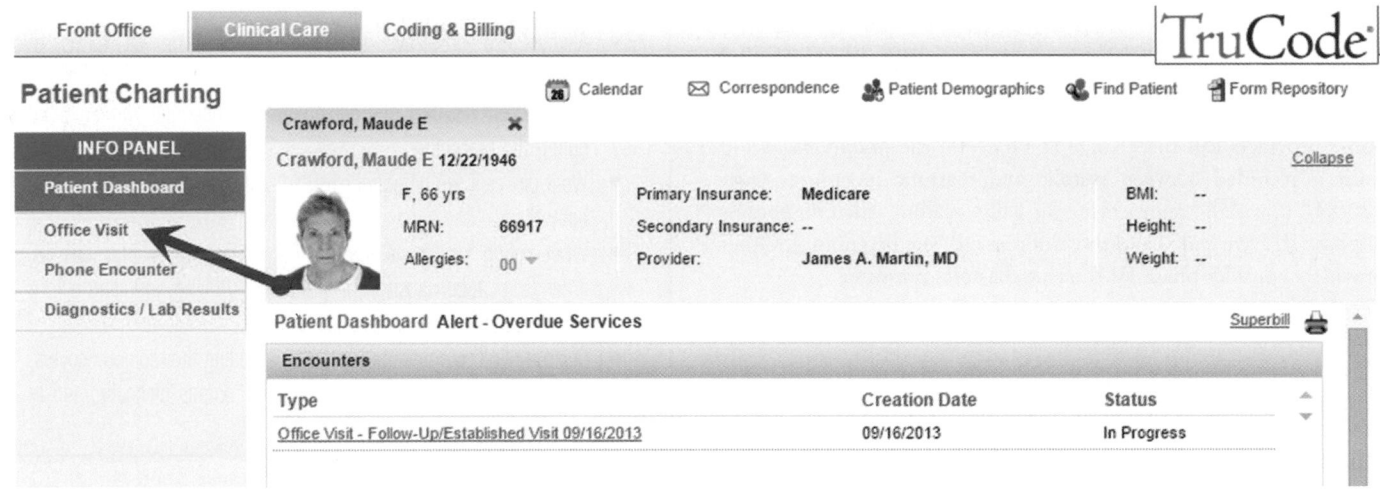

FIGURE 24-18 Electronic health record (EHR) documentation of height, weight, and body mass index (BMI).

PROCEDURE 24-8   Obtain Vital Signs: Measure a Patient's Weight and Height

Goal: *To accurately weigh and measure a patient as part of the physical assessment procedure.*

Note: Make sure the scale is located in an area away from traffic to maintain the patient's privacy.

EQUIPMENT and SUPPLIES

- Patient's record
- Balance scale with a measuring bar
- Paper towel

PROCEDURAL STEPS

1. Sanitize your hands.
   PURPOSE: To ensure infection control.
2. Introduce yourself, identify your patient, and explain the procedure.
   PURPOSE: Identification of the patient prevents errors, and explanations are a means of gaining implied consent and patient cooperation.
3. If the patient is to remove his or her shoes for weighing, place a paper towel on the scale platform. Check to see that the balance bar pointer floats in the middle of the balance frame when all weights are at zero.
   PURPOSE: A floating pointer indicates that the scale is properly adjusted and in balance.

4. Help the patient onto the scale. Make sure a female patient is not holding a purse and that a male or female patient has removed any heavy objects from pockets.
5. Move the large weight into the groove closest to the patient's estimated weight. The grooves are calibrated in 50-lb increments. If you choose a groove that is more than the patient's weight, the pointer will immediately tilt to the bottom of the balance frame. You then must move it back one groove (Figure 1).
6. While the patient is standing still, slide the small upper weight to the right along the pound markers until the pointer balances in the middle of the balance frame.
   PURPOSE: The pointer floats between the bottom and the top of the frame when both lower and upper weights together balance the scale with the patient's weight.
7. Leave the weights in place.
8. Ask the patient to stand up straight and to look straight ahead. On some scales, the patient may need to turn with the back to the scale.

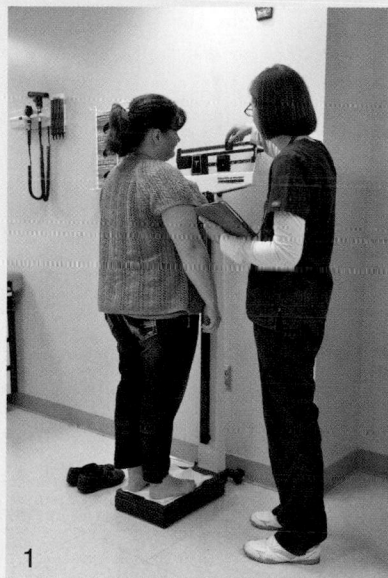

1

9. Adjust the height bar so that it just touches the top of the patient's head (Figure 2).

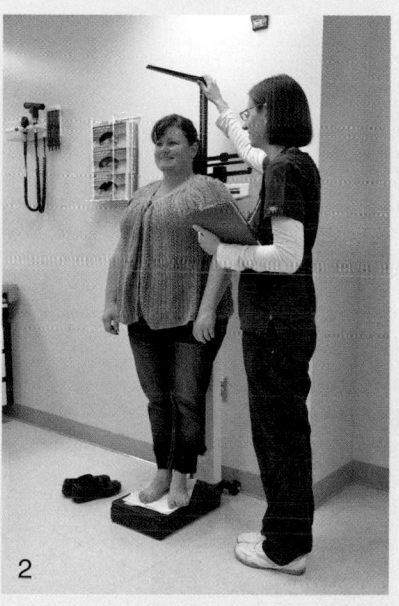

2

10. Leave the elevation bar set.
<u>PURPOSE</u>: To maintain the height recording while protecting the patient from possible injury.

11. Assist the patient off the scale. Make sure all items that were removed for weighing are given back to the patient.

12. Read the weight scale. Add the numbers at the markers of the large and small weights and record the total to the nearest $\frac{1}{4}$ lb in the patient's health record (e.g., Wt-176 $\frac{1}{2}$ lb).

13. Record the height. Read the marker at the movable point of the ruler and record the measurement to the nearest $\frac{1}{4}$ inch on the patient's medical record (e.g., Ht: 66 $\frac{1}{2}$ in) (Figure 3).

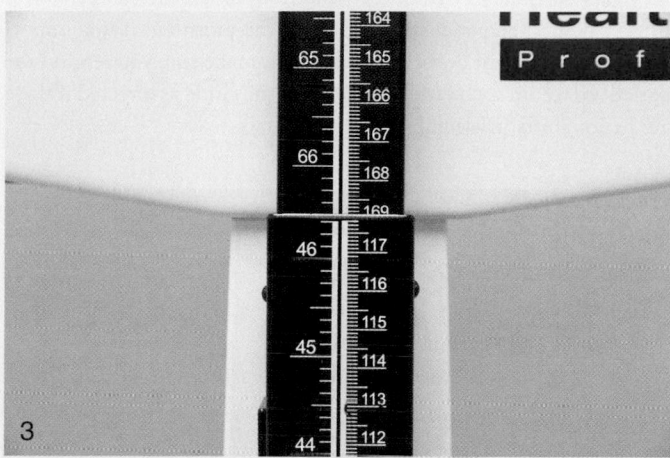

3

14. Use the patient's weight and height to record the BMI if it is not automatically done by the EHR program.

15. Return the weights and the measuring bar to zero.

16. Sanitize your hands.

17. Record the results in the patient's health record.

5/26/20— 11:07 AM: Wt 176 $\frac{1}{2}$ lb, Ht 66 $\frac{1}{2}$ in, BMI 28.5. C. Ricci, CMA (AAMA)

Weight

Your manner and approach are very important in keeping patients from feeling embarrassed or shy when being weighed. Make sure heavy items are removed from pockets and that the patient is not holding a purse. If patients have difficulty with balance or stability, assist them onto the scale and help them balance themselves. If the patient is unable to maintain his or her balance while the scale is calibrating, the ideal equipment to have on hand is a scale with built-in handrails. If the facility does not have this type of scale, a walker can be placed over the scale for the patient to use as hand support when getting on or off, or to maintain balance while on the scale (Figure 24-19).

If the provider prescribes weight measurement at home, make sure the patient understands the importance of getting weighed at the same time each day in clothing of similar weight. Body weight may vary considerably from early morning to late afternoon, so it is usually best if the patient is weighed in the morning. If it is important that the patient be weighed each day, make sure you remind the patient to record each weight and notify the clinic as directed if there are major shifts in weight.

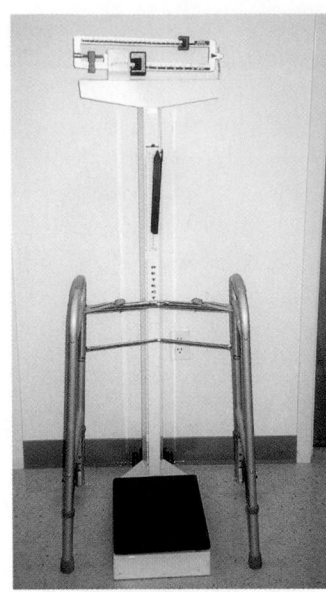

FIGURE 24-19 A walker is placed over the scale to aid the patient's balance.

Weight Conversion Formulas

To Convert Kilograms to Pounds
1 kg = 2.2 lb
  Multiply the number of kilograms by 2.2.
  Example: A patient weighs 68 kg: 68 × 2.2 = 149.6 lb

To Convert Pounds to Kilograms
1 lb = 0.45 kg
  Multiply the number of pounds by 0.45, or divide the number of pounds by 2.2 kg.
  Example: A patient weighs 120 lb: 120 × 0.45 = 54 kg, or 120 ÷ 2.2 = 54.5 kg

---

CRITICAL THINKING APPLICATION   24-8

1. A patient weighs 87 kg; how many pounds does he weigh?
2. A patient weighs 148 lb; how many kilograms does she weigh?

Height

Height can be measured in inches or centimeters. Measurement is easily accomplished by moving the parallel bar attached to a wall ruler or on the scale. Length measurements used in pediatrics and pediatric BMIs are discussed in the Pediatrics chapter.

CRITICAL THINKING APPLICATION   24-9

Mrs. Johnson is being seen for the first time by Dr. Xu. In what order should Carlos take her vital signs and her anthropometric measurements? Should her blood pressure be measured in both arms, with the patient both sitting and standing? If so, what is the rationale?

CLOSING COMMENTS

Patient Education

All patients should know how to use a thermometer safely and accurately, in addition to the preferred site based on age and other patient factors. Because many types of temperature-reading equipment are available, ask the patient what type of equipment he or she uses at home to obtain temperature readings. Inexpensive digital models have greatly simplified home temperature taking.

In teaching a patient how to assess the pulse rate, familiarize him or her with counting the beats and explain how to determine the rate and regularity of the beat. Use diagrams to teach pulse points, and have the patient measure your pulse to assess the person's accuracy and to provide any needed assistance.

Monitoring blood pressure at home has become very common. Suggest that the patient bring his or her equipment to the office and practice with it. In this way, you can make sure the patient is using the equipment correctly and is recording the results accurately in a record book. Computerized home measuring devices typically store a series of recent blood pressure readings in the device's memory. If the patient brings the home device for clinic visits, you can easily check the history of blood pressure recordings taken at home.

Weight management can be a trying and emotional experience for a patient. Explaining to the patient how weight is affected by the time of day, a particular activity, or the type of scale used can help him or her maintain a positive attitude. Have an assortment of weight management literature available for the patient to take home, and use community resources when indicated to help the patient with weight-related issues.

Responsibilities of the Medical Assistant in Obtaining Vital Signs

- Monitoring vital signs is a key responsibility of the medical assistant.
- It is crucial to measure and describe all facets of each vital sign correctly.
- The information must be accurately and clearly documented.
- The medical assistant should take advantage of all opportunities to answer questions and to help the patient understand the significance of healthy vital signs.
- The patient's privacy must be maintained throughout all procedures.
- Family members or caregivers should be included in patient care and education as indicated.
- Community resources should be used to promote holistic patient care.
- The medical assistant should be sensitive to cultural and socioeconomic factors that may affect the patient's compliance with the provider's recommendations, such as diet, exercise, weight control, and the use of medication.

Legal and Ethical Issues

The medical assistant must remember that as the provider's agent, he or she plays an important role in preventing legal claims against the provider and the medical office. The medical assistant must always function within the legal boundaries of the profession. When obtaining vital signs, carefully select your response to a patient who asks about the results. Remember, medical assistants are not qualified to diagnose a patient's problem; that is, never evaluate or give an opinion of what the results may mean. For example, if a patient asks, "Is my blood pressure better?" you might reply, "The reading is 160/90 today." You have not said that it is worse, the same, or better, but you have informed the patient of the current blood pressure reading.

Always be accurate in transcribing results into the patient's health record. If results are incorrectly recorded, the patient may be incorrectly diagnosed or treated; this can result in legal action that may implicate you. A careless attitude toward assessment of vital signs and documentation can lead to possible legal entanglement. Every procedure in this chapter is accompanied by a reminder to record the test results. If no entry has been made, the assumption is that the procedure was not done.

Professional Behaviors

Measuring and recording vital signs are a crucial part of the medical assistant's responsibilities. These procedures can become so routine that we no longer consider that the results can cause the patient anxiety and concern. For example, if you have a patient who is struggling to maintain a healthy blood pressure, it is important that you are sensitive to his concerns. Or if you have a patient who is having difficulty maintaining or losing weight, she can be quite apprehensive, embarrassed, or even depressed about weight results. Demonstrating awareness of the patient's concerns about the measuring and recording of vital signs and showing sensitivity to his or her needs are part of performing as a professional medical assistant.

SUMMARY OF SCENARIO

Carlos recognizes the significance of measuring and recording each patient's vital signs and anthropometric measurements. Dr. Xu relies on Carlos to provide this information accurately. Carlos has never let these procedures become routine and has never done them without focusing on the task because vital signs are an important reflection of a person's health status.

Carlos knows that a number of factors can alter a patient's vital signs, including the external environment, smoking, drinking hot beverages, exercise, and anxiety and pain. Carlos evaluates patient factors such as age, gender, level of compliance, and the presence of disease to determine the best method of accurately measuring vital signs. In addition, Carlos is sensitive to the need for safeguarding the patient's privacy. When he was first hired by Dr. Xu, he was concerned about privacy and confidentiality when he discovered that the patient scale was in the hall next to the waiting room. After he discussed this with the office manager, the scale was moved to an examination room so that patients could be weighed in privacy.

Carlos attended a workshop last year on the AHA guidelines for the diagnosis and treatment of hypertension, and he is prepared to explain those recommendations to patients. He recognizes his role in motivating patients diagnosed with prehypertension to stick with recommended lifestyle changes and follow the provider's treatment protocol. Carlos continues to care for patients while providing valuable assistance to Dr. Xu in her busy primary care practice.

SUMMARY OF LEARNING OBJECTIVES

1. Define, spell, and pronounce the terms listed in the vocabulary.

Spelling and pronouncing medical terms correctly reinforce the medical assistant's credibility. Knowing the definitions of these terms promotes confidence in communication with patients and co-workers.

2. Do the following related to temperature:
- *Cite the average body temperature for various age groups.*

The average body temperature varies from person to person; in a healthy adult, it is typically between 97.6° and 99° F (36.4° and 37.2° C). (See Tables 24-1 and 24-2.)
- *Describe emotional and physical factors that can cause body temperature to rise and fall.*

Multiple factors can affect body temperature, including the external environment, age, stress, physical exercise, gender, and illness.
- *Convert temperature readings between Fahrenheit and Celsius scales.*

Using the formulas presented in this chapter, perform correct calculations to convert temperatures between Fahrenheit and Celsius scales.
- *Obtain and record an accurate patient temperature using three different types of thermometers.*

The patient's temperature can be measured orally and in the axillary region with a digital thermometer, in the ear using an aural thermometer, and at the temporal artery using a temporal artery scanner. The axillary temperature is approximately 1° F (0.6° C) lower than an accurate oral reading because the reading is not taken in an enclosed body cavity. The tympanic temperature is accurate because it records the temperature of the blood closest to the hypothalamus. The temporal artery scanner is considered most accurate for infants. After the temperature reading is documented, (T) is recorded for a tympanic reading; (A) for an axillary reading; and (TA) for a temporal artery reading, to clarify the site. Procedures 24-1 thru 24-4 explain how to take and record patient temperatures using a variety of thermometers.

3. Do the following related to pulse:
- *Cite the average pulse rate for various age groups.*

Infants and children typically have a faster pulse than adults; as aging progresses, the pulse rate declines. As a rule, both the pulse and respiratory rates respond to exercise or emotional upset. (See Table 24-3 for approximate age-related pulse ranges.)
- *Describe pulse rate, volume, and rhythm.*

The pulse *rate* reflects the number of times the heart contracts in 1 minute. The pulse *volume* is the amount of force placed on the arterial walls when the heart beats; the *rhythm* of the pulse is the length of time between beats. Monitor and record the pulse rate, noting whether the rhythm is regular or arrhythmic, and the volume is bounding, normal, or thready.
- *Locate and record the pulse at multiple sites.*

The most common sites used to feel the pulse are the temporal, carotid, apical, brachial, radial, femoral, popliteal, and dorsalis pedis arteries. (Procedures 24-5 and 24-6 present the specifics on recording apical and radial pulses.)

4. Do the following related to respiration:
- *Cite the average respiratory rate for various age groups.*

As a rule, both the pulse and the respiratory rate respond to exercise and emotional upset. Table 24-4 presents a list of normal respiratory rates for patients in various age groups.
- *Demonstrate the best way to obtain an accurate respiratory count.*

Count the number of respirations for 30 seconds and then multiply by 2. This should be done immediately after taking the patient's pulse, while still holding the pulse point and without warning the patient, because the patient may inadvertently alter the respiratory rate if he or she is aware that breaths are being counted. (See Procedure 24-6.)

5. Do the following related to blood pressure:
- *Cite the approximate blood pressure range for various age groups.*

Table 24-5 lists the normal blood pressure ranges for patients of various age groups.
- *Specify physiologic factors that affect blood pressure.*

Physiologic factors that affect blood pressure include the amount or volume of blood in circulation; the condition of the blood vessels, including the presence of atherosclerosis and arteriosclerosis; the degree of blood viscosity; and the strength of the myocardium.
- *Differentiate between essential and secondary hypertension.*

The cause of essential hypertension is unknown; it is diagnosed when a patient has a systolic reading higher than 140 mm Hg and/or a diastolic reading higher than 90 mm Hg. Secondary hypertension is caused by an underlying condition, such as renal disease, pregnancy, or a congenital heart defect.
- *Interpret current hypertension guidelines and treatment.*

AHA guidelines for the diagnosis and management of hypertension include a prehypertension category. Table 24-6 identifies the categories of prehypertension, stage 1 hypertension, and stage 2 hypertension, with suggested treatments. The goal of the AHA recommendations is to reduce the number of people who die each year from hypertension-related illness. Treatment includes a combination of weight management, sodium reduction, lifestyle changes, and the use of two or more antihypertensive and diuretic medications.
- *Describe how to determine the correct cuff size for individual patients.*

The proper size cuff must be used to obtain a correct blood pressure reading. To make sure the size is correct, the inflatable part (bladder) should cover about 80 percent of the circumference of the upper arm. (Table 24-7 presents the various sizes of blood pressure cuffs available.)
- *Identify the different Korotkoff phases.*

The Korotkoff phases are the categories of sounds heard during blood pressure measurement. These sounds are produced by vibrations of the arterial wall when the blood surges back into the vessel after it has been compressed by the blood pressure cuff. Phase I is the first sound heard as the cuff deflates and is the systolic reading; phase II is the swishing sound made by the movement of blood through the artery, although an

SUMMARY OF LEARNING OBJECTIVES—*continued*

auscultatory gap may occur in which sounds completely disappear; phase III involves distinct, sharp tapping sounds made as the blood rushes through the artery; in phase IV, the sound changes to a soft tapping, which becomes muffled and begins to grow fainter; and in phase V, sound completely disappears. The last sound heard is the diastolic reading.
- *Accurately measure and document blood pressure.*

A sphygmomanometer is used with a stethoscope to hear the systolic over diastolic sounds. (Procedure 24-7 outlines the method for performing this skill.)

6. **Accurately measure and document height and weight.**

A patient's height and weight are anthropometric measurements that are recorded during the initial patient visit and periodically after that, depending on the patient's needs and the provider's preference. The scale should be kept in a private location. Variations in weight may indicate physical or emotional disorders, including diabetes, congestive heart failure, hormone abnormalities, depression, and eating disorders. (Procedure 24-8 describes the techniques for weighing a patient; the BMI is determined as indicated.)

7. **Convert kilograms to pounds and pounds to kilograms.**

To convert kilograms (kg) to pounds (lb), multiply the number of kilograms by 2.2. To convert pounds to kilograms, divide the number of pounds by 2.2 kg, or multiply the number of pounds by 0.45 kg.

8. **Identify patient education opportunities when measuring vital signs.**

Patient education about vital signs includes confirming the patient's ability to monitor vital signs at home as needed; providing assistance in helping the patient learn how to use home equipment systems; and confirming the patient's understanding of the need to comply with the provider's recommendations.

9. **Determine the medical assistant's legal and ethical responsibilities in obtaining vital signs.**

Legal and ethical implications for the medical assistant include following the provider's guidelines regarding patient disclosure, monitoring and recording vital signs accurately, and being consistently alert for inaccurate readings or possible carelessness.

CONNECTIONS

Study Guide Connection: Go to the Chapter 24 Study Guide. Read and complete the activities.

evolve Evolve Connection: Go to the Chapter 24 link at *evolve.elsevier.com/kinn* to complete the Chapter Review Quiz. Check out the other resources listed for this chapter to make the most of what you have learned from Vital Signs.

Felicia Grand, a newly hired certified medical assistant (CMA, AAMA), works for Dr. Anna Kosto, a member of a busy primary care practice with several providers. One of Felicia's chief responsibilities will be to assist Dr. Kosto with physical examinations. Her duties include preparing and maintaining the examination room and equipment; getting the patient ready for specific physical examinations; and gowning, draping, and positioning the patient as needed. Because Felicia will be assisting with examinations, she must become familiar with the physical examination procedure and the order in which the provider needs various pieces of medical equipment. It also is important that Felicia protect herself from possible injury by using appropriate body mechanics throughout her day in the office.

While studying this chapter, think about the following questions:

- What equipment does Felicia need to gather before the provider enters the examination room, to make sure the examination goes smoothly and without interruption?
- What examination and treatment positions should Felicia be familiar with, and when should the various positions be used?
- What measures can Felicia take to protect herself from injury when lifting heavy items or assisting with the transfer of patients?

LEARNING OBJECTIVES

1. Define, spell, and pronounce the terms listed in the vocabulary.
2. Describe the structural organization of the human body and the body cavities.
3. Identify the functions of the body systems and the major organs and structures of each system.
4. Discuss the concept of a primary care provider and the role of a medical assistant in a primary care practice.
5. Outline the medical assistant's role in preparing for the physical examination.
6. Summarize the instruments and equipment the provider typically uses during a physical examination.
7. Identify the principles of body mechanics and demonstrate proper body mechanics.
8. Outline the basic principles of gowning, positioning, and draping a patient for examination; also, position and drape a patient in six different examining positions while remaining mindful of the patient's privacy and comfort.
9. Describe the methods of examination, and give an example of each.
10. Outline the sequence of a routine physical examination.
11. Prepare for and assist in the physical examination of a patient, correctly completing each step of the procedure in the proper sequence.
12. Discuss the role of patient education during the physical examination, in addition to the legal and ethical implications and Health Insurance Portability and Accountability Act (HIPAA) applications.

VOCABULARY

auscultation The act of listening to body sounds, typically with a stethoscope, to assess various organs throughout the body.
bruit (broo′-it) An abnormal sound or murmur heard on auscultation of an organ, vessel (e.g., carotid artery), or gland.
clubbing Abnormal enlargement of the distal phalanges (fingers and toes) associated with cyanotic heart disease or advanced chronic pulmonary disease.
colonoscopy A procedure in which a fiberoptic scope is used to examine the large intestine.

electrocardiogram (i-lek-tro-kar′-de-uh-gram) A graphic record of electrical conduction through the heart.
emphysema (em-fuh-ze′-muh) The pathologic accumulation of air in the alveoli, which results in alveolar destruction and overall oxygen deprivation; in the lungs, the bronchioles become plugged with mucus and lose elasticity.
gait The manner or style of walking.
hematopoiesis (hi-ma-tuh-poi-e′-suhs) The formation and development of blood cells in the red bone marrow.

intercellular A term referring to the area between cells.

intracellular A term referring to the area within the cell membrane.

manipulation Movement or exercise of a body part by means of an externally applied force.

mastication (mas-tuh-ka'-shun) Chewing.

murmur An abnormal sound heard during auscultation of the heart that may or may not have a pathologic origin; it is associated with valve disease or a congenital heart defect.

nodules (nah'-juhls) Small lumps, lesions, or swellings that are felt when the skin is palpated.

palpation The use of touch during the physical examination to assess the size, consistency, and location of certain body parts.

peripheral neuropathy A problem with the function of the nerves outside the spinal cord; symptoms include weakness, burning pain, and loss of reflexes; a frequent complication of diabetes mellitus.

peristalsis (per-uh-stahl'-suhs) Rhythmic contraction of involuntary muscles lining the gastrointestinal tract.

sclera The white part of the eye that forms the orbit.

transillumination Inspection of a cavity or organ by passing light through its walls.

trauma A physical injury or wound caused by external force or violence.

vasoconstriction (va-zo-kuhn-strik'-shun) Contraction of the muscles lining blood vessels, which narrows the lumen.

To promote health maintenance, healthcare professionals must understand the anatomy and physiology of the body, the role each part plays, how each component functions, and what happens to the body when disease occurs in body systems.

ANATOMY AND PHYSIOLOGY

Anatomy is the study of how the body is shaped and structured. It encompasses a wide range of subjects, including structural development, levels of organization, relationships among microscopic parts, and the interrelationship of structure and function.

Physiology is the study of body functions. This field is subdivided into areas of study; some physiologists spend their entire lives studying only one function, such as how cells work or how a single organ, such as the small intestine, is interrelated in function with the stomach and the large intestine.

Separating these two sciences is almost impossible because one continuously influences the other. Function affects structure, and structure affects function; for example, an infant can suck effortlessly because of the lack of teeth in the mouth. Once teeth appear, sucking becomes more tiresome, and the child begins to chew and bite. Phenomena in structure and function affect the interrelationships of all body systems.

Structural Development

Cells

The basic unit of life is the cell. Cells determine the functional and structural characteristics of the entire body. Cells are microscopic in size, have a variety of shapes, and perform a vast array of functions. It is estimated that the human body is composed of approximately 100 trillion living, functioning cells. A cell is made up of three primary parts: the plasma membrane that surrounds the cell, creating an outer covering; the **intracellular** environment, which includes the cytoplasm that contains the living material that carries on the

cell's function; and the nucleus of the cell, which contains the genetic code of the cell that determines the cell's function.

Tissues

When cells with similar structure and function are placed together, they form tissues. The study of tissues is known as *histology*. All of the body tissues are grouped into four types. The types of tissues distributed throughout the body and where they are located are as follows:

- *Epithelial tissue:* This type of tissue makes up the skin, glands, and linings of body cavities and organs. It is packed closely together with little or no **intercellular** material, and it is classified according to shape as *squamous* (flat), *cuboidal* (square), *columnar* (long and narrow), or *transitional* (varying shapes that can stretch). Epithelial cells may be arranged in a single layer of cells of the same shape, called *simple epithelium,* or in many layers of cells named according to the shape of the cells in the outer layer; this is called *stratified epithelium.*

- *Connective tissue:* This tissue supports and binds other body tissues. Types of connective tissue include collagen, bone, cartilage, adipose, ligaments, tendons, blood, and lymph. Connective tissue is the most frequently occurring tissue in the body and has the widest distribution.

- *Muscle tissue:* This tissue produces movement. It is classified as skeletal muscle (striated, voluntary), which is attached to bones and produces voluntary body movements when contracted; cardiac muscle (striated and involuntary), which forms the heart muscle wall; or smooth muscle (nonstriated and involuntary), which lines the walls of blood vessels and hollow organs and causes such actions as **peristalsis** and **vasoconstriction**.

- *Nervous tissue:* This type of tissue conducts nerve impulses between the periphery and the central nervous system (CNS). It also effects rapid communication between body structures

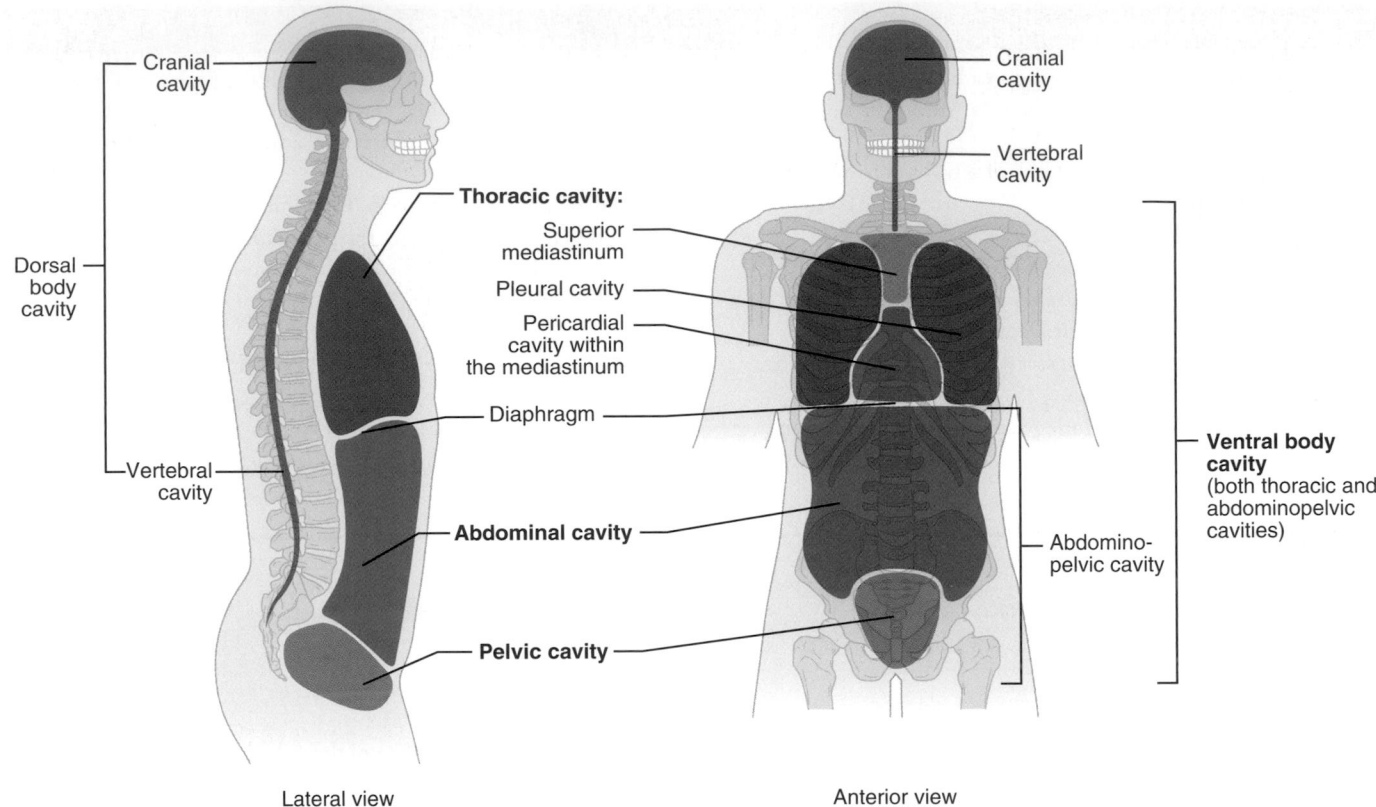

FIGURE 25-1 The body cavities.

and controls the body's functions to maintain homeostasis. Nervous tissue is made up of neurons and supportive structures called *neuroglial* cells.

Organs

An *organ* is composed of two or more types of tissue bound together to form a more complex structure for a common purpose or function. An organ may have one or many functions; for example, the pancreas has an endocrine function because it produces the hormone insulin, and a digestive function because it produces digestive enzymes. Organs also may be part of one or several systems. For example, in the male system, the urethra is part of both the urinary and the reproductive system.

Body Cavities

The body is separated into two main cavities called the *dorsal* (posterior) and *ventral* (anterior) body cavities. The dorsal body cavity protects organs of the nervous system and has two primary areas: the cranial cavity within the skull, which encloses the brain; and the spinal (vertebral) cavity, which surrounds the vertebral column and spinal cord. The ventral cavity is separated into two general areas: the thoracic cavity, which is surrounded by the ribs and muscles in the chest and includes the pleural cavities (each lung is surrounded by its own pleural cavity) and the mediastinum; and the pericardial cavity, which surrounds the heart and is located in the mediastinum. The diaphragm separates the thoracic cavity from the abdominopelvic cavity. The abdominal cavity contains gastrointestinal organs,

including the stomach, spleen, liver, and intestines. The pelvic cavity is not physically separated from the abdominal cavity; it contains the urinary bladder, rectum, and reproductive organs (Figure 25-1).

Systems

A *body system* is composed of several organs and their associated structures. These structures work together to perform a specific function in the body. Each system has specific units, and each performs specific functions. Table 25-1 summarizes the body systems; their primary cells, organs, and structures; and the major functions of each.

PRIMARY CARE PROVIDER

A primary care provider (PCP) is a healthcare practitioner who sees people of all ages for a broad range of diseases and complaints. The PCP treats common medical problems and serves as the main healthcare provider in nonemergency situations. He or she evaluates the patient's total healthcare needs, provides personal medical care in one or more fields of medicine, and refers the patient to a specialist when an advanced or serious condition warrants additional expertise. Primary care usually is provided in an ambulatory care setting; however, the PCP may assist in or direct hospitalized care. PCP professionals include:

- *Family practitioners:* Physicians whose scope of practice includes children and adults of all ages and may include obstetrics and minor surgery.

TABLE 25-1	Organization of Body Systems	
BODY SYSTEM	**CELLS, ORGANS, AND STRUCTURES**	**FUNCTIONS**
Blood	Arteries, arterioles, veins, venules, white blood cells, red blood cells, platelets, plasma	Transports materials and collects wastes throughout the body; white blood cells fight infection; red blood cells carry oxygen; platelets help form clots; plasma carries dissolved nutrients and other materials
Cardiovascular	Heart, valves, arteries, arterioles, veins, venules	Circulatory system transports materials in the blood throughout the body; veins return deoxygenated blood to the heart, which pumps it into the lungs; oxygenated blood is pumped into the aorta and branching arteries to cells throughout the body
Endocrine	Pituitary, pineal gland, hypothalamus, thyroid, pancreas, adrenal cortex and medulla, parathyroid, thymus, ovaries, testes	Produces hormones that circulate in the blood to target tissue that stimulates a particular action
Integumentary	Skin, subcutaneous tissue, sweat and sebaceous glands, hair, nails, sense receptors	Protection, temperature regulation; senses organ activity
Gastrointestinal	Mouth, tongue, teeth, pharynx, esophagus, stomach, small intestine, large intestine, liver, gallbladder, pancreas, appendix	**Mastication**, swallowing, digestion, absorption of nutrients, excretion of waste materials
Lymphatic and immune	Lymph, lymph vessels, lymph nodes, thymus, tonsils, spleen, lymphocytes, antibodies	Maintains fluid balance; protects internal environment; defends against foreign cells and disease; provides immunity to some diseases
Musculoskeletal	Bones, joints, muscles, tendons, ligaments, cartilage	Movement, posture, heat production, support, protection, mineral storage, **hematopoiesis**
Nervous	Brain, spinal cord, neurons, neuroglial cells, peripheral nerves, autonomic nerves	Controls body structures to maintain homeostasis; higher order thinking and reflex centers that control autonomic processes; carries sensory stimulus to the brain and motor impulses to the periphery
Reproductive	*Female:* Estrogen and progesterone, ovum, ovaries, fallopian tubes, uterus, vagina, vulva, mammary glands *Male:* Testosterone, sperm, epididymis, vas deferens, prostate gland, testes, scrotum, penis, urethra	Produces hormones; reproduction
Respiratory	Nose, sinuses, pharynx, larynx, trachea, bronchi, lungs, bronchioles, alveoli	Responsible for inhalation of oxygen and exhalation of carbon dioxide externally and exchange of oxygen and carbon dioxide internally at the cellular level; acid-base regulation
Sensory	Eyes, ears, taste buds, olfactory receptors, sensory receptors	Helps sense changes in the external and internal environments through vision, hearing, balance, taste, and smell
Urinary	Nephron unit, bilateral kidneys, ureters, urinary bladder, urethra	Filters waste material from the blood; reabsorbs fluid and electrolytes as needed; excretes waste in the urine; maintains electrolyte, water, and acid-base balances; regulates blood pressure; activates red blood cells

- *Pediatricians:* Physicians who care for newborns, infants, children, and adolescents.
- *Internists:* Physicians who care for adults of all ages with many different medical problems, such as diabetes mellitus.
- *Obstetricians/gynecologists:* Physicians who serve as PCPs for women, particularly those of childbearing age.
- *Nurse practitioners (NPs)* and *physician assistants (PAs):* Practitioners who have earned advanced degrees and licensure and

who can work in primary or specialty medical practices and clinics.

The medical assistant's clinical responsibilities in a primary care practice include assisting with patients who may have problems in any of the body systems and with procedures in all age groups. With such a diversified scope of practice, the provider and medical assistant must work as a team to use their time efficiently and still provide quality, patient-centered healthcare.

PHYSICAL EXAMINATION

The purpose of a physical examination is to determine the patient's overall state of well-being. All major organs and body systems are checked during a physical examination. As the provider examines the entire body, he or she interprets the findings, and by the time the examination has been completed, the provider has formed an initial diagnosis of the patient's condition. Often laboratory and other diagnostic tests are ordered to supplement the provider's clinical diagnosis. The results of these tests are used to refine the patient's diagnosis, to help the provider plan or revise treatment for the patient, to evaluate and maintain current drug therapy, and/or to determine the patient's progress.

Preparing for the Physical Examination

Role of the Medical Assistant in the Physical Examination

Assessment of the patient begins with the first contact in the office. The administrative medical assistant is responsible for verifying the accuracy of the patient's insurance information according to office policy. In most facilities, the policy is to make a copy of the patient's insurance card when the patient first enters the office or, if the patient has been to the office recently, to ask whether any of the insurance information has changed. Before the examination, the medical assistant has the opportunity to make sure the patient feels comfortable during the examination process and that all the necessary medical information has been obtained. The medical assistant's duties include preparing and maintaining the examination room and equipment, preparing the patient, and assisting the provider during the physical examination.

Preparing the Examination Room. The medical assistant is responsible for making sure the examination room is ready for any procedure that might be performed during the physical examination. The area should be as comfortable as possible for the patient and free of any potential dangers, such as contaminated equipment or unlocked drug cabinets. You should prepare the examination room as follows:

- Check the area at the beginning of each day and between patients to make sure it is completely stocked with equipment and supplies and that all equipment is functioning properly. You must understand how to take care of and operate all equipment and instruments, and you should refer to operation manuals supplied by manufacturers as needed.
- Regularly check expiration dates on all packages and supplies; discard expired materials.
- Make sure the room is private, well lit, and at a comfortable temperature for the patient during the physical examination.
- Clean and disinfect the area daily and between patients to prevent the spread of infection and to ensure patients' comfort. When the patient leaves the room, discard the used exam table paper. Using disinfectant wipes, clean the table and any other potentially contaminated surface. When the table dries, replace the exam table paper.
- Arrange drapes, gowns, and all other patient supplies before the patient enters the room so that they are ready for use.
- To save time, prepare the instruments and equipment needed for the examination, arranging them for easy access, before the provider enters the room.

- Make sure the examination room has all materials required for observing Standard Precautions, including disposable gloves, a sink with an antibacterial hand-washing agent, paper towels, biohazard waste containers, sharps containers, and impervious gowns and face guards. Sharps containers are replaced when they are two-thirds full, as indicated by Standard Precautions.

Assisting the Patient. Getting the patient ready for the examination includes taking care of paperwork before the patient enters the examination room and performing related clinical skills.

- Make sure the health record is complete and that any needed consent forms have been signed; document current medications and allergies; identify any medications that need refills. The medical assistant is not responsible for obtaining informed consent, but he or she should review the paperwork to make sure that informed consent forms were reviewed by the provider and that the patient signed the forms.
- Introduce yourself, verify the patient's identity, and address the patient by his or her preferred name, making sure to show respect at all times. Pay close attention to the patient's nonverbal language to make sure he or she understands what to expect.
- Obtain specimens (e.g., urine, blood) if they have been preordered by the provider or if this practice is part of the office policy.
- Measure and record the patient's height, weight, body mass index (BMI), and vital signs.
- Conduct the initial investigation into the reason for the visit and explain the examination procedure to the patient. Be prepared to answer the patient's questions and allay any fears. If needed, refer the patient's questions to the provider.
- Ask the patient whether he or she needs to empty the bladder before the examination because a full bladder may interfere with the examination and may be uncomfortable for the patient.
- Help the patient physically prepare for the examination. Explain to the patient what clothing should be removed and in what direction to put on the gown (open to the front or to the back, depending on the type of examination); provide a drape to ensure the patient's privacy, and offer assistance as needed.
- Assist the patient into and out of various examination positions as needed.
- Throughout this entire sequence of events, explain what is happening, and consistently maintain the patient's privacy and confidentiality.
- Help the patient with dressing as needed after the examination.

Assisting the Provider. The medical assistant should be prepared to help the provider complete the physical examination as comprehensively and efficiently as possible. During the examination, the provider may expect the medical assistant to do the following:

- Hand him or her instruments and equipment as requested and provide supplies as needed.
- Alter the position of the light source to better illuminate the area being examined and turn lights off and on during specific phases of the examination.

- Position and drape the patient during different phases of the examination.
- Assist in collecting and properly labeling specimens such as urine, Pap test specimens, and throat cultures.
- Conduct any diagnostic tests preordered by the provider, including hearing and visual screenings.
- Conduct follow-up diagnostic procedures as ordered, including an **electrocardiogram** (ECG), urinalysis, and phlebotomy.
- Document patient data in the health record, completing all forms required.
- Schedule postexamination diagnostic procedures, such as mammography, x-ray examination, or **colonoscopy**.

CRITICAL THINKING APPLICATION   25-1

Felicia's first patient for the day is Harry Garcia, a 51-year-old truck driver who is scheduled for a complete physical examination. The provider ordered an ECG and a complete blood panel to be drawn before the physical. What does Felicia need to complete before Dr. Kosto sees the patient?

Supplies and Instruments Needed for the Physical Examination

The instruments typically used during the physical examination are shown in Figure 25-2. They enable the provider to see, feel, inspect, and listen to parts of the body. All equipment must be in good working order, properly disinfected, and readily available for the provider's use during the examination. The instruments most fre-quently used for a physical examination are described in the following paragraphs. Physical examinations typically are performed from the head to the feet; the instruments are listed in the order in which the provider typically would request them.

Ophthalmoscope. An ophthalmoscope is used to inspect the inner structures of the eye. It consists of a stainless steel handle containing batteries and an attached head, which has a light, magnifying lenses, and an opening through which the eye is viewed. Examination rooms usually are equipped with wall-mounted electrical units for the ophthalmoscope and otoscope, a dispenser for disposable specu-lums, and a wall-mounted sphygmomanometer.

Tongue Depressor. A tongue depressor is a flat, wooden blade used to hold down the tongue when the throat is examined.

Otoscope. An otoscope is used to examine the external auditory canal and tympanic membrane. It has a stainless steel handle con-taining batteries or is part of a wall-mounted electrical unit. The head of the otoscope has a light that is focused through a magnifying lens; it should be covered with a disposable ear speculum. The light also may be used to illuminate the nasal passages and throat.

Tuning Fork. Tuning forks are aluminum, fork-shaped instruments that consist of a handle and two prongs (Figure 25-3, A). The prongs produce a humming sound when the provider strikes them against his or her hand. Tuning forks are available in different sizes, and each size produces a different pitch level. A tuning fork is used to check the patient's auditory acuity (Figure 25-3, B) and to test bone vibra-tion (Figure 25-3, C). A tuning fork can also be used to test for diabetic **peripheral neuropathy**.

Tape Measure. A tape measure is a flexible ribbon ruler that is usually printed in inches and feet on one side and in centimeters and meters on the reverse side. Measurements may be used to assess length and head circumference in infants, wound size, and so on.

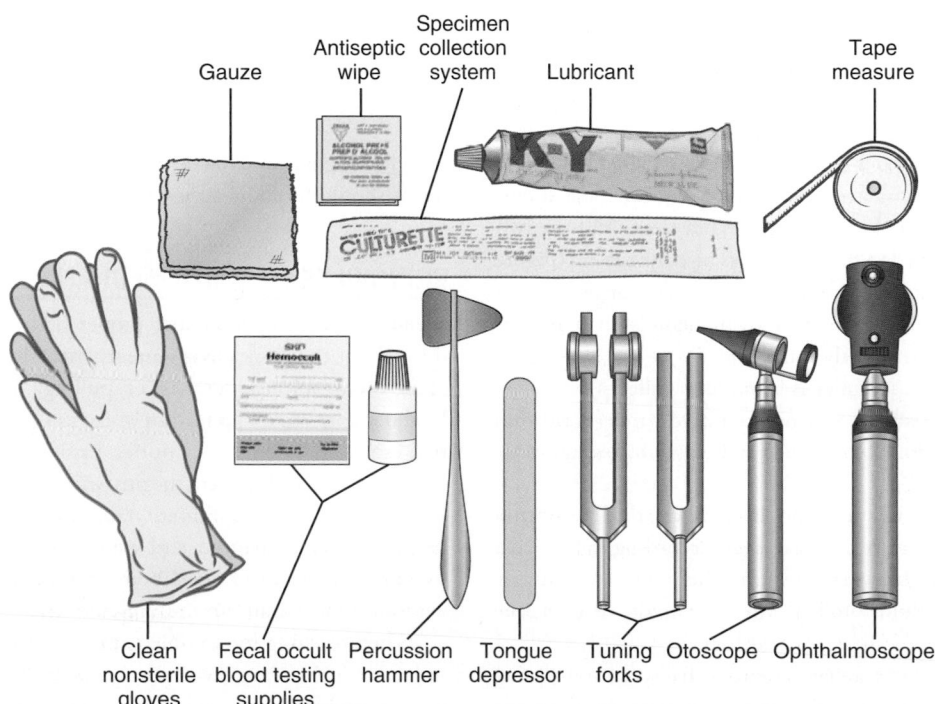

FIGURE 25-2 Instruments for the physical examination.

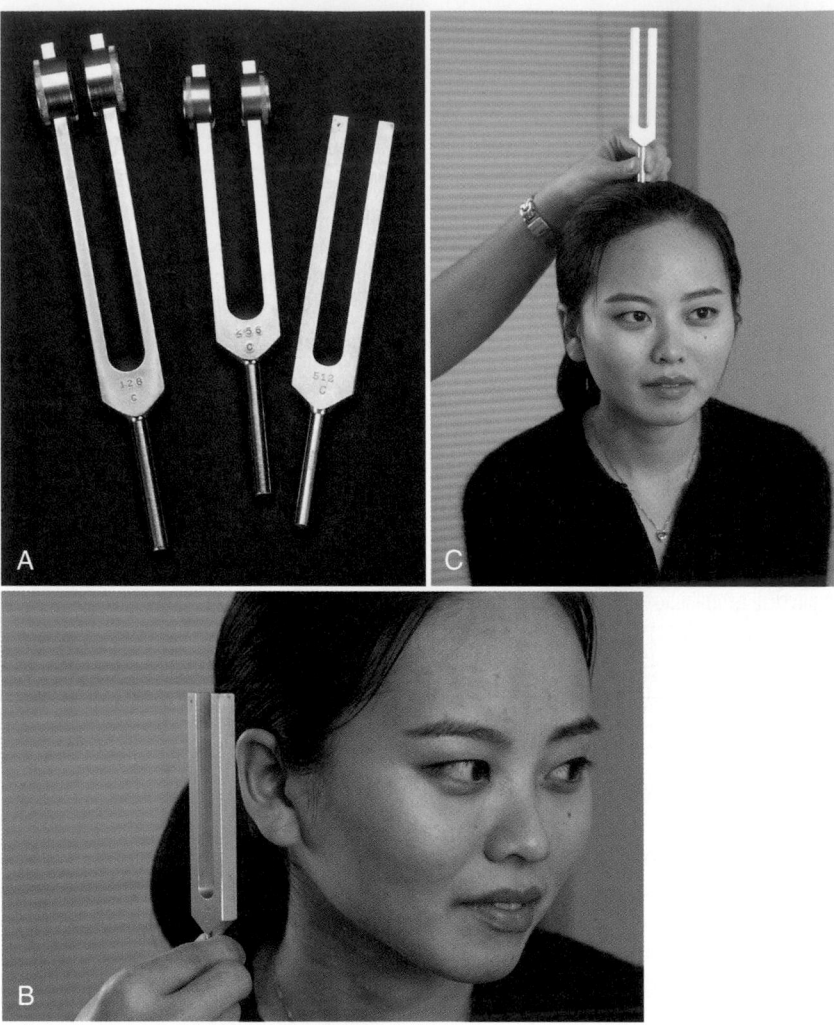

FIGURE 25-3 A, Tuning forks. **B,** Sound vibration test. **C,** Bone vibration test.

Stethoscope. A stethoscope is a listening device used when certain areas of the body are auscultated, particularly the heart and lungs. This instrument is available in many shapes and sizes. All have two earpieces that are connected to flexible rubber or vinyl tubing (Figure 25-4). At the distal end of the tubing is a diaphragm or bell (many have both); when it is placed securely on the patient's skin, it enables the provider to hear internal body sounds.

Reflex Hammer. A reflex hammer is sometimes called a *percussion hammer.* This stainless steel instrument has a hard rubber head that is used to strike the tendons of the knee and elbow to test the neurologic reflexes.

Gloves. Disposable examination gloves protect the healthcare worker and the patient from microorganisms. According to Standard Precautions, gloves must be worn whenever the potential exists for contact with any body fluid, broken skin or wounds, or contaminated items.

Additional Supplies. Gauze squares, cotton balls, cotton-tipped applicators, disposable tissues, specimen containers, fecal occult blood test cards, Pap test supplies for female patients, lubricating jelly for vaginal and rectal examinations, and laboratory request forms should be easily accessible during the examination.

PRINCIPLES OF BODY MECHANICS

Medical assistants should use proper body mechanics consistently throughout the work environment when sitting or standing, lifting or carrying objects, pushing or pulling, or transferring patients. Without consistent application of correct anatomic alignment, injuries, especially lower back injuries, easily occur.

Proper body alignment begins with good posture. Maintaining posture requires a combination of muscle efforts. Good posture keeps the spine balanced and aligned while a person is sitting or standing. A person in good body alignment can maintain balance without undue strain on the musculoskeletal system.

When reaching for an object, avoid twisting or turning; instead, move the feet to face the object needed; this prevents undue strain on the lumbar region. Do not cross the legs while sitting because this interferes with circulation to the legs and feet. When sitting, keep the popliteal area (behind the knees) free of the edge of the chair. Pressure in this area interferes with circulation and may damage nerves behind the knees. Do a mental check of your posture regularly. Hold the head erect, the face forward and the chin slightly up, the abdominal muscles contracted up and in, the shoulders relaxed and back, the feet pointed forward and slightly apart, and the weight evenly distributed to both legs, with the knees slightly bent. Always be on the alert for poor body mechanics that may cause injury (Figures 25-5 and 25-6).

Safe Lifting Techniques

- Always get help if the load is too heavy.
- Maintain correct body alignment, with the legs spread apart for a broad base of support.
- Do not reach for items; clear barriers out of the way and get as close as possible to what needs to be lifted.
- Bend at the knees with the feet shoulder width apart and keep the back straight. Use the major muscle groups of the arms and legs rather than the weaker ones of the back to help lift a heavy item (see Figure 25-5).
- When carrying a heavy item, keep the weight as close to the body as possible (see Figure 25-6).
- Move the feet in the direction of the lift. Do not twist or turn on fixed feet.
- Bend the knees while keeping the back straight when lowering an item at the completion of a lift.
- If possible, slide, roll, or push a heavy item rather than lifting or pulling it.

Transferring a Patient

Patients may need assistance in moving from a chair to the examination table or back again. Patients can be transferred in multiple ways, but all should focus on correct body mechanics. If the patient is in a wheelchair, move the chair at a 45-degree angle toward the foot

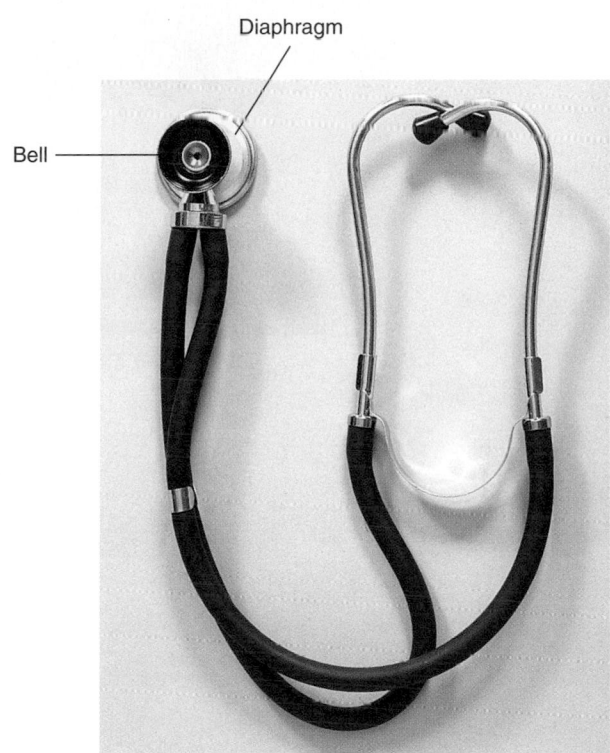

FIGURE 25-4 Stethoscope. (Modified from Ball JW, et al: *Seidel's guide to physical examination,* ed 8, St Louis, 2015, Mosby.)

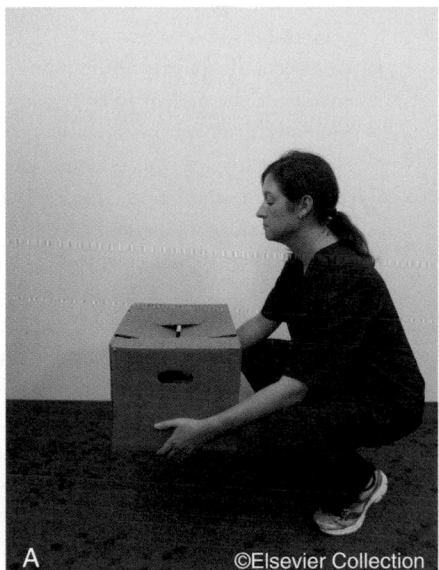 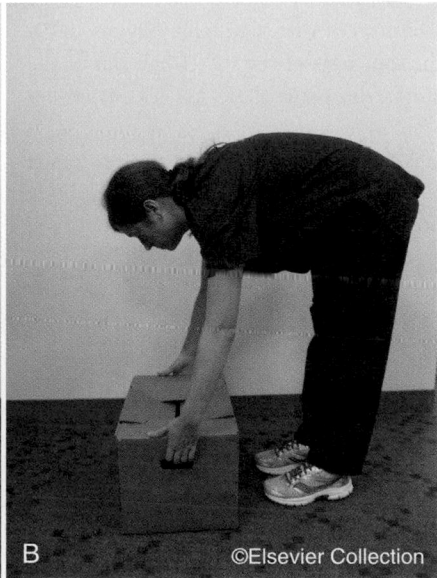

FIGURE 25-5 A, Proper lifting technique. **B,** Improper lifting technique.

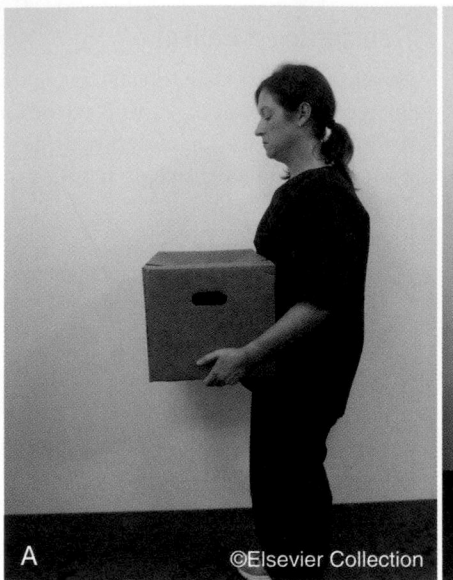 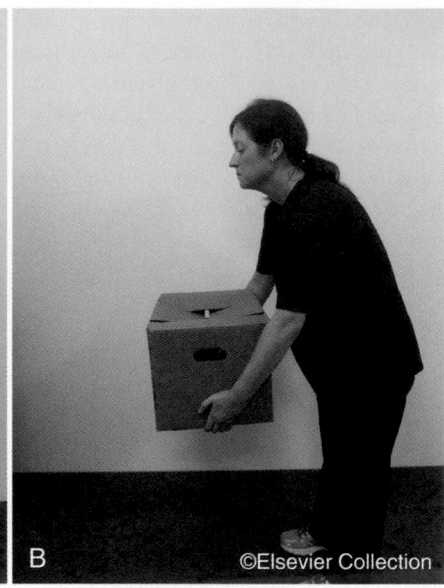

FIGURE 25-6 A, Carrying an item close to the body. **B,** Improper carrying technique.

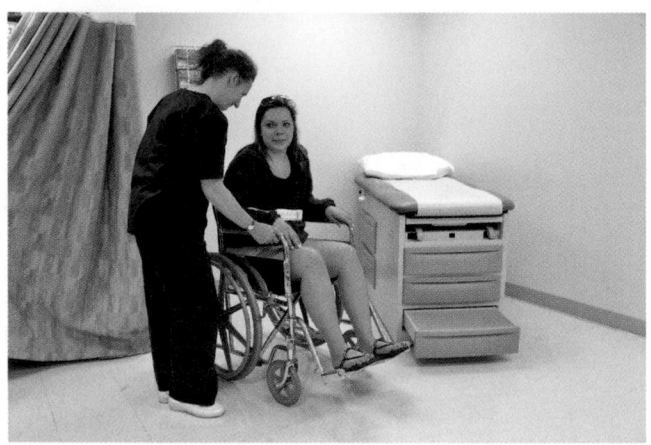

FIGURE 25-7 Wheelchair at a 45-degree angle at the end of the exam table.

rest that extends from the bottom of the exam table (Figure 25-7), lock the wheels, and lift the foot rests of the wheelchair out of the way. Explain the procedure to the patient and ask for his or her assistance.

If one side of the patient is stronger than the other, always provide support on the strong side. Support the patient close to your body on the strong side, with one hand under the axillary region and the other either grasping the patient's hand or holding the forearm. When bending, always bend at the knees and maintain the back's three natural curves, allowing the leg muscles to help in lifting. Give the patient a signal and lift as the patient assists. Help the patient step up onto the foot rest with the strong leg first, then pivot. Ease the patient down onto the table, bending your knees while keeping your back aligned. Make sure the patient is comfortable and safely positioned on the table.

Use a gait belt as needed to help transfer patients to prevent injury to yourself and to safeguard patients from falling. A gait belt is a safety device that is used to help transfer a patient from a wheelchair to the exam table or to help a patient ambulate. The gait belt helps you support the patient while keeping your body in proper alignment, to prevent back injuries. A gait belt should be used if the patient is weak and at risk of falling. To use a gait belt:

- Place the belt around the individual's waist over clothing with the buckle in front.
- Insert the belt through the teeth of the buckle and pull it tight to lock it.
- The belt should be tight, with just enough room to place your fingers under it.
- Grip the belt tightly, bend your knees, and keep your back straight.
- Ask the patient to assist you; then lift, using your arm and leg muscles.
- Avoid twisting or turning as you help the patient stand.
- Keep your body close to the patient's with your knees in front of his or hers at all times to stabilize the patient and prevent falls.
- Complete the transfer without bending or twisting your body; encourage the patient to bear as much weight as possible and to gently sit down on the table.
- After transferring the patient, remove the gait belt for the provider's examination and replace it to help transfer the patient back to the wheelchair after the provider is finished.
- If the patient should start to fall during a transfer, do not try to stop the fall because you may be injured; use the gait belt to help guide the patient to the floor as gently as possible.

You may need to remain with the patient until the examination has been completed to ensure his or her safety. If the provider prefers that the patient be in a supine position, place one arm across the patient's shoulders and the other under the knees, and smoothly lower the patient's upper body to the table while raising the legs. Use the same pivoting techniques with proper body mechanics to help transfer the patient from the examination table back to the locked wheelchair. If the patient must hold onto you, have the person hold your waist or shoulders, not your neck (Procedure 25-1).

PROCEDURE 25-1   Use Proper Body Mechanics

Goal: *To safely transfer a patient from a wheelchair to an examination table using proper body mechanics.*

EQUIPMENT and SUPPLIES

- Patient's record
- Wheelchair
- Examination table with pull-out foot rest
- Gait belt

PROCEDURAL STEPS

1. Sanitize your hands.
   PURPOSE: To ensure infection control.
2. Greet and identify the patient, introduce yourself, and determine how much assistance the patient will need to transfer from the wheelchair to the examination table. Do not proceed if you think you will need additional help.
   PURPOSE: To promote the patient's cooperation during the transfer and prevent personal injury.
3. Place the wheelchair at a 45-degree angle toward the foot rest at the base of the examination table (see Figure 25-7).
4. Lock the brakes on the wheelchair and move the foot rests of the wheelchair out of the way (Figure 1).
   PURPOSE: Never transfer a patient into or out of a wheelchair until the brakes are locked on both sides of the chair.

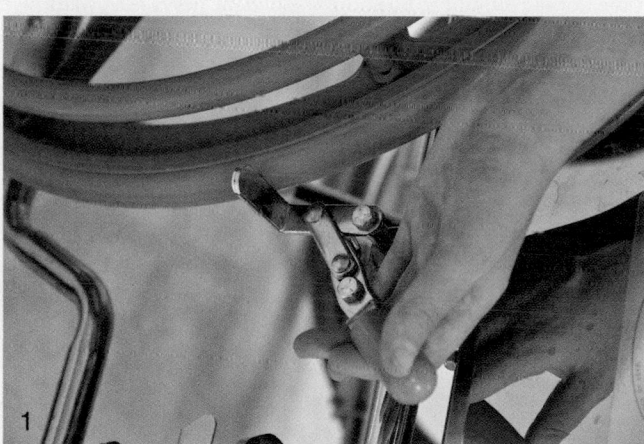

5. Place the gait belt around the patient's waist over clothing with the buckle in front. Insert the belt through the teeth of the buckle and pull it tight to lock it. The belt should be tight with just enough room to place your fingers under it.
6. Request that the patient place both feet flat on the floor with the hands on the armrests.
   PURPOSE: This position helps you grasp the gait belt, the patient can use the wheelchair armrests to help push her into an upright position, and feet flat on the floor help with patient stability.
7. Stand directly in front of the patient with your feet apart, back straight, and knees bent (Figure 2).

PURPOSE: This position helps you maintain good body mechanics during the transfer.

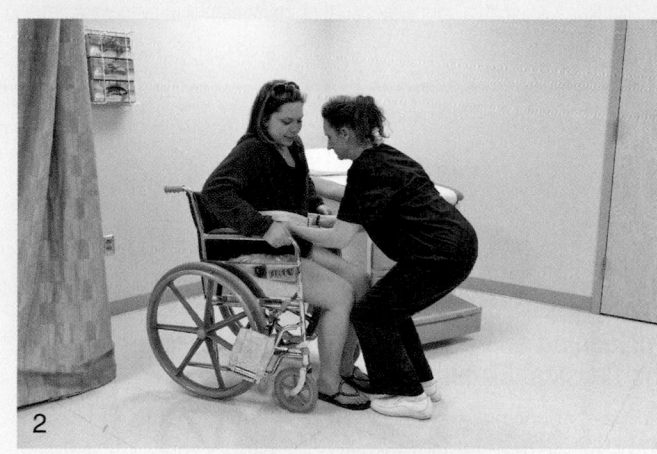

8. Slide your fingers under the gait belt on opposite sides of the patient's waist.
9. Instruct the patient at the count of 3 to push off from the armrests while you at the same time grasp the gait belt and, using your leg muscles, straighten your knees so that the patient is in a standing position.
   PURPOSE: This position allows the patient to assist as much as possible while you are using the large muscles of your legs to help lift her.
10. Ask the patient to step up onto the foot rest at the bottom of the exam table, and assist the person in pivoting and sitting down on the examination table. Remove the gait belt until the provider has completed the examination (Figure 3).

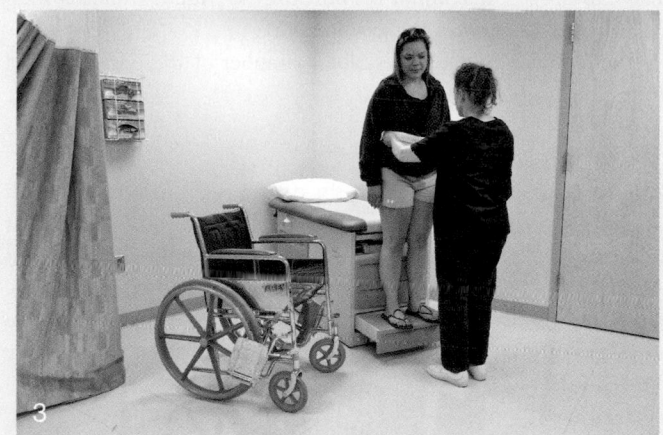

11. After the examination is complete, place the wheelchair at an angle next to the exam table and lock the wheels. Replace the gait belt. Make sure the patient is positioned at the bottom edge of the table.
    PURPOSE: To prepare for transfer back to the wheelchair.

12. Place yourself directly in front of the patient with your back straight and your knees bent. Slide your fingers under the gait belt on opposite sides of the patient's waist.

13. Grasp the gait belt on both sides at the waist. Instruct the patient at the count of 3 to push off from the examination table and, using your leg muscles, straighten your knees so that the patient is in a standing position on the foot rest.

14. Maintaining your hold on the gait belt, ask the patient to step down. Pivot the person so that she can slowly sit in the wheelchair; at the same time, bend your knees but keep your back straight.

15. Remove the gait belt. Replace the wheelchair foot rests and unlock the brakes on the wheelchair.

ASSISTING WITH THE PHYSICAL EXAMINATION

Positioning and Draping the Patient for the Physical Examination

Various patient positions are used to facilitate a physical examination. The medical assistant instructs the patient about and assists the patient into these positions, ensuring as much ease and modesty as possible, and helps the patient maintain the position during the examination with as little discomfort as possible. Do not place a patient into a position that is uncomfortable or that compromises the patient's privacy until it is necessary to complete that part of the examination. Never leave the patient's side if he or she is in a position that could result in a fall.

Draping the patient with an examination sheet protects the individual from embarrassment and keeps the patient warm. However, the sheet must be positioned so that it allows complete visibility for the examiner and does not interfere with the examination. During the general examination, each part of the body is exposed one portion at a time. For gynecologic and rectal examinations, the sheet is positioned on the diagonal across the patient, or in a diamond shape, to provide maximum comfort for the patient while allowing the provider to perform the examination.

The following sections describe a number of the positions used during medical examinations.

Fowler's Position

In Fowler's position, the patient sits on the examination table with the head of the table elevated 90 degrees. This position is useful for examinations and treatments of the head, neck, and chest, and for patients with orthopnea who have difficulty breathing while lying down. Drape placement varies, depending on the type of physical examination done and the need to maintain the patient's privacy (Procedure 25-2).

Semi-Fowler's Position

Semi-Fowler's position is a modification of Fowler's position. The head of the table is positioned at a 45-degree angle instead of at a full 90-degree angle. This position is useful for postoperative examination, for patients with breathing disorders, and for patients suffering from head **trauma** or pain (see Procedure 25-2). The drape and/or gown should cover the entire patient from the nipple line down.

Supine (Horizontal Recumbent) Position

In the supine position, the patient lies flat with the face upward and the lower legs supported by the table extension (Procedure 25-3). This position is used for examination of the front of the body, including the heart, breasts, and abdominal organs. The patient's gown should open down the front, and the drape should be placed over any exposed area that is not being examined.

Dorsal Recumbent Position

In the dorsal recumbent position, the patient lies face upward, with the weight distributed primarily to the surface of the back. This is accomplished by flexing the knees so that the feet are flat on the table. This position relieves muscle tension in the abdomen and may be used for examination and/or inspection of the rectal, vaginal, and perineal areas; or, it may be used if the patient experiences back discomfort when lying supine. This position can be used for digital examination of the vagina and rectum, but it is not used if an instrument such as a speculum is needed. To ensure the patient's privacy, it is important to keep the patient completely draped, with the drape in a diamond shape, until the provider is present (see Procedure 25-3).

Lithotomy Position

The patient should not be placed in the lithotomy position until the provider is in the examination room and is ready for this part of the examination. Place the patient on his or her back with the knees sharply flexed and the arms at the sides or folded over the chest; have the patient slide the buttocks down to the bottom edge of the table. Support the feet in stirrups placed wide apart and somewhat away from the table, with the stirrup arms extended to match the length of the patient's legs. If the heels are too close to the buttocks, the possibility of leg cramps increases, and it is more difficult for the patient to relax the abdominal muscles. Make sure the stirrups are locked in place. Place a drape diagonally over the patient's abdomen and knees. The drape must be long enough to cover the knees and touch the ankles and wide enough to prevent the sides of the thighs from being exposed. The provider lifts the drape away from the pubic area when the examination begins (Procedure 25-4). The lithotomy position is used primarily for vaginal examinations that require the use of a speculum and for Pap tests.

Sims Position

Sims position is sometimes called the *lateral position.* The patient is placed on the left side; the left arm and shoulder are drawn back behind the body so that the body's weight is predominantly on the chest. The right arm is flexed upward for support. The left leg is slightly flexed, and the buttocks are pulled to the edge of the table. The right leg is sharply flexed upward. The drape extends diagonally from under the arms to below the knees. The provider can raise a small portion of the sheet from the back of the patient to expose the rectum sufficiently. The remaining portion of the sheet covers the patient's chest area and thighs. This position is used for rectal examinations, for instillation of rectal medication, and for some perineal and pelvic examinations (Procedure 25-5).

Prone Position

In the prone position, the patient lies face down on the table on the ventral surface of the body. This is the opposite of the supine position and is another of the recumbent positions. The drape should cover from the middle of the back to below the knees, with the gown opening in the back (Procedure 25-6). This position is used for examination of the back and for certain surgical procedures.

Knee-Chest Position

For the knee-chest position, the patient rests on the knees and the chest with the head turned to one side. The arms can be placed under the head for support and comfort, or they can be bent and placed at the sides of the table near the head. The thighs are perpendicular to the table and slightly separated. The buttocks extend up into the air, and the back should be straight. The patient will need assistance to assume the knee-chest position correctly. Most patients have difficulty maintaining this position, so they should not be placed into it until it is required. The medical assistant must remain next to the patient for assistance and support the entire time the knee-chest position is needed. If the correct knee-chest position cannot be obtained, the patient may have to be placed in a knee-elbow position. This position puts less strain on the patient and is easier to

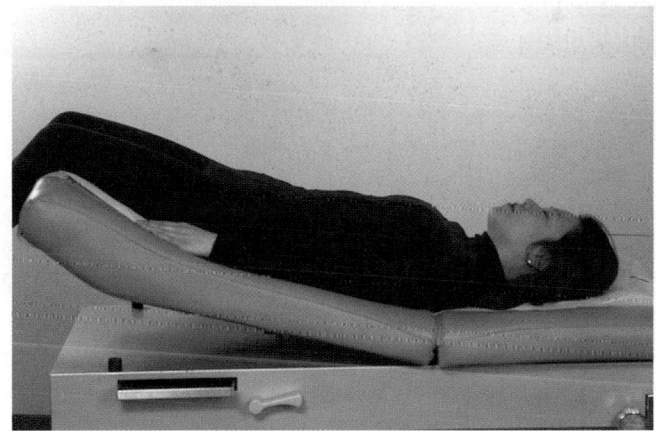

FIGURE 25-8 Trendelenburg position.

maintain. These positions are used for proctologic examination and for sigmoid, rectal, and occasionally vaginal examinations. The patient's gown should open in the back, and a fenestrated (opening) drape or a single sheet should be draped diagonally over the patient's back at the sacral area (Procedure 25-7).

Trendelenburg Position

Trendelenburg position is rarely used in the ambulatory care setting, but it may be needed if a patient has severe hypotension or is going into shock. This position can be achieved only if the examination table separates so that the legs can be elevated higher than the head (Figure 25-8).

CRITICAL THINKING APPLICATION   **25-2**

Determine the correct patient position and method of gowning and draping for the following examinations:
- Insertion of a rectal suppository
- Annual Papanicolaou (Pap) test
- Examination of the back
- Patient with dyspnea
- Breast examination

Text continued on p. 521

PROCEDURE 25-2   Assist Provider with a Patient Exam: Fowler's and Semi-Fowler's Positions

Goal: *To position and drape the patient for examinations of the head, neck, and chest, or patients who have difficulty breathing when lying flat.*

EQUIPMENT and SUPPLIES

- Patient's record
- Examination table
- Table paper
- Patient gown
- Drape
- Disinfectant wipes
- Disposable gloves

PROCEDURAL STEPS

1. Sanitize your hands.
   <u>PURPOSE</u>: To ensure infection control.
2. Greet and identify the patient, introduce yourself, and determine whether the patient understands the procedure. If the patient does not, explain what to expect.
   <u>PURPOSE</u>: To promote the patient's understanding and cooperation during the examination.

PROCEDURE 25-2   *—continued*

3. Give the patient a gown. Explain what clothing must be removed for the particular examination being done and whether the gown should open in the front or the back. Provide assistance as needed. Give the patient privacy while changing. Knock on the examination room door before re-entering to make sure the patient has completed undressing and gowning.

4. For Fowler's position, elevate the head of the bed 90 degrees. If the patient feels more comfortable, she can sit at the end of the table (Figure 1). Extend the foot rest as needed for patient comfort. The patient may be more comfortable in semi-Fowler's position. In this modification of Fowler's position, the head of the table is elevated 45 degrees. Semi-Fowler's position may be used for postoperative follow-up or for patients with a fever, head injury, or pain. It also is a comfortable, supportive position for patients with breathing disorders (Figure 2).

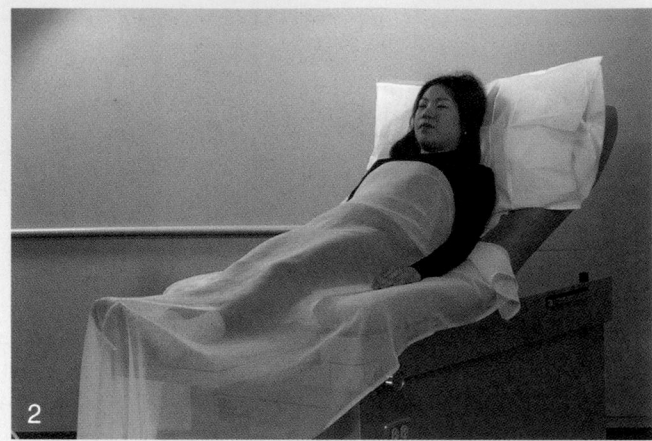

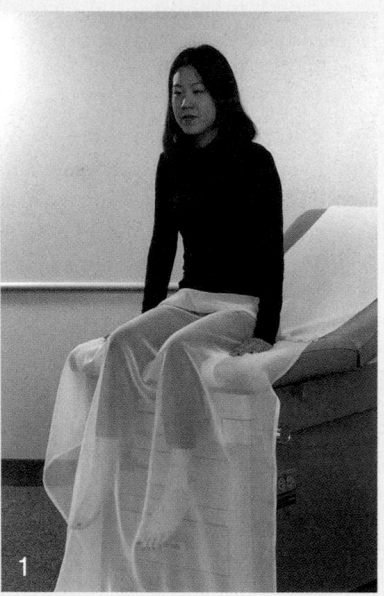

5. Drape the patient according to the type of examination and the required patient exposure.
   PURPOSE: Draping the patient provides warmth and privacy while giving the provider access to the examination site.

6. After the examination has been completed, assist the patient as needed to get off the table and get dressed.

7. Put on gloves and use disinfectant wipes to clean the exam table and all potentially contaminated surfaces. Dispose of used gloves and examination table paper according to facility policies. Pull clean paper over the table.
   PURPOSE: To ensure infection control and to prevent the transmission of pathogens from one patient to another.

8. Sanitize your hands.

9. Follow up with the provider's orders regarding scheduling of diagnostic studies, collection of specimens, and/or scheduling of future appointments.

PROCEDURE 25-3   **Assist Provider with a Patient Exam: Horizontal Recumbent and Dorsal Recumbent Positions**

Goal: *To position and drape the patient for examinations of the abdomen, heart, and breasts in the horizontal recumbent (supine) position, and exams of the rectal, vaginal, and perineal areas in the dorsal recumbent position.*

EQUIPMENT and SUPPLIES

- Patient's record
- Examination table
- Table paper
- Patient gown
- Drape
- Disinfectant wipes
- Disposable gloves

PROCEDURAL STEPS

1. Sanitize your hands.
   PURPOSE: To ensure infection control.

2. Greet and identify the patient, introduce yourself, and determine whether the patient understands the procedure. If the patient does not, explain what to expect.
   PURPOSE: To promote the patient's understanding and cooperation during the examination.

PROCEDURE 25-3   —continued

3. Give the patient a gown. Explain the clothing that must be removed for the particular examination being done and whether the gown should open in the front or in the back. Provide assistance as needed. For the horizontal recumbent position, the gown should be open in the front. Give the patient privacy while changing. Knock on the examination room door before re-entering to make sure the patient has completed undressing and gowning.

4. Do not place the patient in the necessary positions until the provider is ready for that part of the examination.
   PURPOSE: To ensure the patient's privacy, comfort, and modesty.

5. Pull out the table extension that supports the patient's legs. For the horizontal recumbent (supine) position, help the patient lie flat on the table with the face upward (Figure 1). For the dorsal recumbent position, have the patient lie flat on the back and flex the knees so the feet are flat on the table (Figure 2). If needed, help the patient move down toward the foot of the table for the examination.

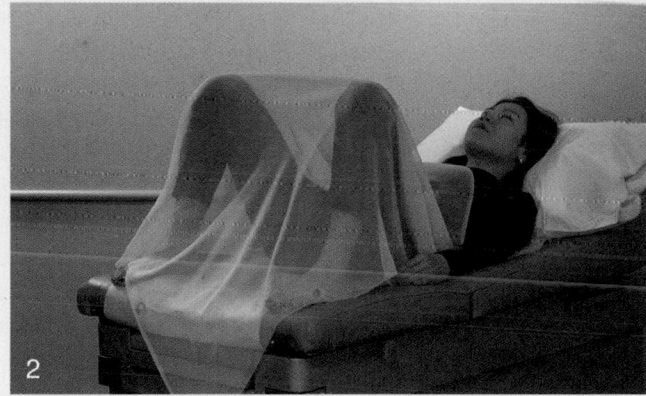

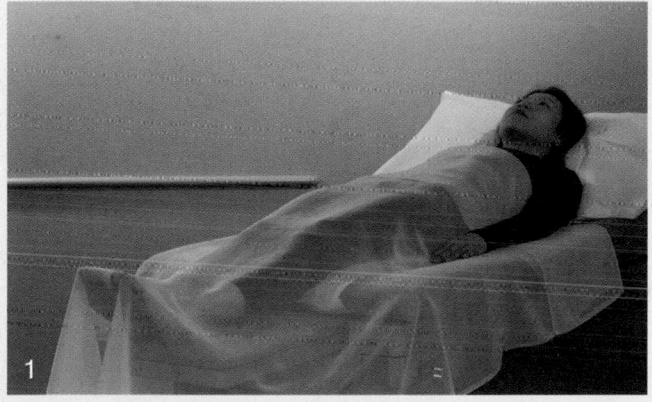

6. Drape the patient from nipple line to feet in the supine position, and diagonally with the point of the drape between the feet for the dorsal recumbent position.
   PURPOSE: Draping the patient provides warmth and privacy while giving the provider access to the examination site.

7. After the examination has been completed, assist the patient as needed to get off the table and get dressed.

8. Put on gloves and use disinfectant wipes to clean the exam table and all potentially contaminated surfaces. Dispose of used gloves and examination table paper according to facility policies. Pull clean paper over the table.
   PURPOSE: To ensure infection control and to prevent the transmission of pathogens from one patient to another.

9. Sanitize your hands.

10. Follow up with the provider's orders regarding scheduling of diagnostic studies, collection of specimens, and/or scheduling of future appointments.

PROCEDURE 25-4   Assist Provider with a Patient Exam: Lithotomy Position

Goal: *To position and drape the patient primarily for vaginal and pelvic examinations and Pap tests.*

EQUIPMENT and SUPPLIES

- Patient's record
- Examination table
- Table paper
- Patient gown
- Drape
- Disinfectant wipes
- Disposable gloves

PROCEDURAL STEPS

1. Sanitize your hands.
   PURPOSE: To ensure infection control.

2. Greet and identify the patient, introduce yourself, and determine whether the patient understands the procedure. If the patient does not, explain what to expect.
   PURPOSE: To promote the patient's understanding and cooperation during the examination.

3. Give the patient a gown. Instruct the patient to undress from the waist down with the gown open in the back. If the provider also will be doing a breast examination, the patient should undress completely and put on the gown so that it opens in the front. Provide assistance as needed. Give the patient privacy while changing. Knock on the examination room door before re-entering to make sure the patient has completed undressing and gowning.

PROCEDURE 25-4   —*continued*

4. Do not place the patient in the lithotomy position until the provider is ready for that part of the examination.
   PURPOSE: To promote the patient's privacy, comfort, and safety.
5. Pull out the table extension that supports the patient's legs and help the patient lie face upward on the table. Pull out the stirrups, adjust their extension length for the patient's comfort, and lock them in place.
6. Reinsert the table extension and have the patient move toward the foot of the table with her buttocks on the bottom table edge. Gently place the patient's legs in the stirrups, checking for comfort. Some offices may stock cloth or paper stirrup covers to protect the patient and make the position more comfortable. The patient's arms can be placed alongside the body or across the chest (Figure 1).

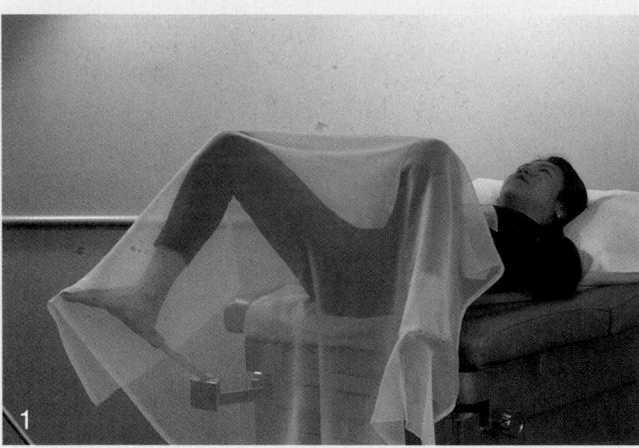

7. Drape the patient diagonally, with the point of the drape between the feet. The drape should be large enough to cover the patient from the nipple line to the ankles and wide enough so the patient's thighs are not exposed.
   PURPOSE: To provide warmth and privacy for the patient while giving the provider access to the examination site.
8. After the examination has been completed, assist the patient as needed to get off the table and get dressed.
9. Put on gloves and use disinfectant wipes to clean the exam table and all potentially contaminated surfaces. Dispose of used gloves and examination table paper according to facility policies. Pull clean paper over the table.
   PURPOSE: To ensure infection control and to prevent the transmission of pathogens from one patient to another.
10. Sanitize your hands.
11. Follow up with the provider's orders regarding scheduling of diagnostic studies, collection of specimens, and/or scheduling of future appointments.

PROCEDURE 25-5   Assist Provider with a Patient Exam: Sims Position

Goal: *To position and drape the patient for examination of the rectum, instillation of rectal medication, perineal examination, and some pelvic examinations.*

EQUIPMENT and SUPPLIES

- Patient's record
- Examination table
- Patient gown
- Table paper
- Drape
- Disinfectant wipes
- Disposable gloves

PROCEDURAL STEPS

1. Sanitize your hands.
   PURPOSE: To ensure infection control.
2. Greet and identify the patient, introduce yourself, and determine whether the patient understands the procedure. If the patient does not, explain what to expect.

PURPOSE: To promote the patient's understanding and cooperation during the examination.

3. Give the patient a gown and explain what clothing must be removed for the particular examination being done. Tell the patient that the gown should open in the back. Provide assistance as needed. Give the patient privacy while changing. Knock on the examination room door before re-entering to make sure the patient has completed undressing and gowning.
4. Do not place the patient in the Sims position until the provider is ready for that part of the examination.
   PURPOSE: To promote the patient's privacy, comfort, and safety.
5. Help the patient turn onto the left side; the left arm and shoulder should be drawn back behind the body so that the patient is tilted onto the chest. Flex the right arm upward for support, slightly flex the left leg, and sharply flex the right leg upward. Help the patient move the buttocks to the side edge of the table (Figure 1).

PROCEDURE 25-5   —continued

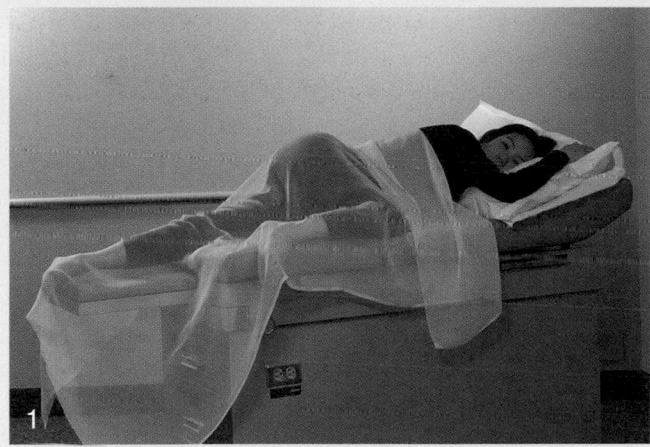

6. Drape the patient diagonally in a diamond shape, with the point of the diamond dropping below the buttocks. Make sure the drape is large enough to prevent exposure of the patient.

PURPOSE: Draping the patient provides warmth and privacy while giving the provider access to the examination site.

7. After the examination has been completed, assist the patient as needed to get off the table and get dressed.

8. Put on gloves and use disinfectant wipes to clean the exam table and all potentially contaminated surfaces. Dispose of used gloves and examination table paper according to facility policies. Pull clean paper over the table.
   PURPOSE: To ensure infection control and prevent the transmission of pathogens from one patient to another.

9. Sanitize your hands.

10. Follow up with the provider's orders regarding scheduling of diagnostic studies, collection of specimens, and/or scheduling of future appointments.

PROCEDURE 25-6   Assist Provider with a Patient Exam: Prone Position

Goal: *To position and drape the patient for examination of the back and certain surgical procedures.*

EQUIPMENT and SUPPLIES

- Patient's record
- Examination table
- Patient gown
- Table paper
- Drape
- Disinfectant wipes
- Disposable gloves

PROCEDURAL STEPS

1. Sanitize your hands.
   PURPOSE: To ensure infection control.

2. Greet and identify the patient, introduce yourself, and determine whether the patient understands the procedure. If the patient does not, explain what to expect.
   PURPOSE: To promote the patient's understanding and cooperation during the examination.

3. Give the patient a gown and explain what clothing must be removed for the particular examination being done. Tell the patient that the gown should open in the back. Provide assistance as needed. Give the patient privacy while changing. Knock on the examination room door before re-entering to make sure the patient has completed undressing and gowning.

4. Do not place the patient in the prone position until the provider is ready for that part of the examination.
   PURPOSE: To promote the patient's privacy, comfort, and safety.

5. Pull out the table extension and help the patient lie down on his or her stomach (Figure 1).

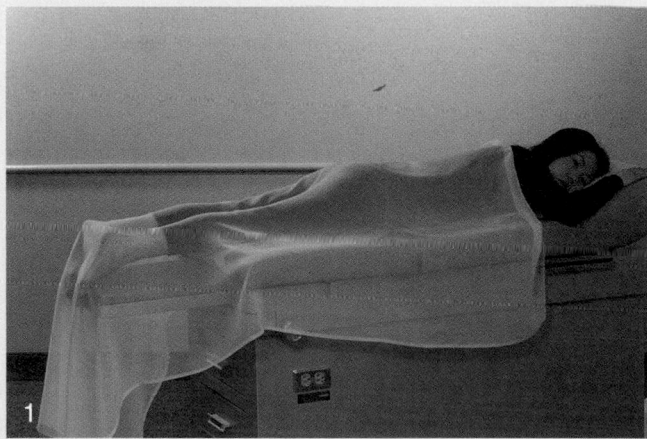

6. Drape the patient over any exposed area that is not included in the examination. For female patients, the drape should be large enough to

PROCEDURE 25-6   *—continued*

cover from the breasts to the feet so that the patient is not exposed accidentally if she is asked to roll over.

PURPOSE: Draping the patient provides warmth and privacy while giving the provider access to the examination site.

7. After the examination has been completed, assist the patient as needed to get off the table and get dressed.

8. Put on gloves and use disinfectant wipes to clean the exam table and all potentially contaminated surfaces. Dispose of used gloves and examina-

tion table paper according to facility policies. Pull clean paper over the table.

PURPOSE: To ensure infection control and to prevent the transmission of pathogens from one patient to another.

9. Sanitize your hands.

10. Follow up with the provider's orders regarding scheduling of diagnostic studies, collection of specimens, and/or scheduling of future appointments.

PROCEDURE 25-7   **Assist Provider with a Patient Exam: Knee-Chest Position**

Goal: *To position and drape the patient for examinations of the back and rectum and for certain surgical procedures.*

EQUIPMENT and SUPPLIES

- Examination table
- Table paper
- Patient gown
- Drape
- Disinfectant wipes
- Disposable gloves

PROCEDURAL STEPS

1. Sanitize your hands.
   PURPOSE: To ensure infection control.

2. Greet and identify the patient, introduce yourself, and determine whether the patient understands the procedure. If the patient does not, explain what to expect.
   PURPOSE: To promote the patient's understanding and cooperation during the examination.

3. Give the patient a gown and explain what clothing must be removed for the particular examination being done. Tell the patient that the gown should open in the back. Provide assistance as needed. Give the patient privacy while changing. Knock on the examination room door before re-entering to make sure the patient has completed undressing and gowning.

4. Do not place the patient in the knee-chest position until the provider is ready for that part of the examination.
   PURPOSE: To promote the patient's privacy, comfort, and safety.

5. Pull out the table extension if necessary. Help the patient lie down on his or her back and then turn over into the prone position. Ask the patient to move up onto the knees, spread the knees apart, and lean forward onto the head so that the buttocks are raised. Tell the patient to keep the back straight and turn the face to either side. The patient should rest his or her weight on the chest and shoulders (Figure 1).

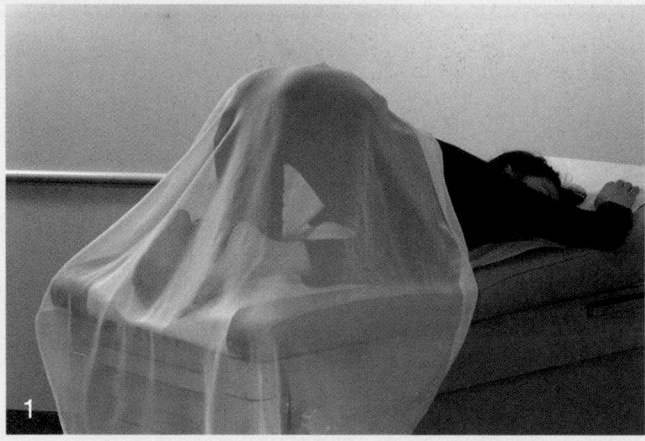

6. If the patient has difficulty maintaining this position, an alternative is to place weight on bent elbows with the head off the table.

7. Drape the patient diagonally so that the point of the drape is on the table between the legs.
   PURPOSE: Draping the patient provides warmth and privacy while giving the provider access to the examination site.

8. After the examination has been completed, assist the patient as needed to get off the table and get dressed.

9. Put on gloves and use disinfectant wipes to clean the exam table and all potentially contaminated surfaces. Dispose of used gloves and examination table paper according to facility policies. Pull clean paper over the table.
   PURPOSE: To ensure infection control and to prevent the transmission of pathogens from one patient to another.

10. Sanitize your hands.

11. Follow up with the provider's orders regarding scheduling of diagnostic studies, collection of specimens, and/or scheduling of future appointments.

Methods of Examination

Examinations are performed as both a routine confirmation of the absence of illness and a means of diagnosing disease. Healthcare providers use six methods to examine the human body: inspection, palpation, percussion, auscultation, mensuration, and manipulation. All six are part of a complete physical examination.

Inspection

During the inspection, the examiner uses observation to detect significant physical features or objective data. This method of examination ranges from focusing on the patient's general appearance (general state of health, including posture, mannerisms, and grooming) to more detailed observations, including body contour, **gait**, symmetry, visible injuries and deformities, tremors, rashes, and color changes.

Palpation

In **palpation**, the examiner uses the sense of touch (Figure 25-9, *A*). A part of the body is felt with the hand to determine its condition or the condition of an underlying organ. Palpation may involve touching the skin or performing a firmer exploration of the abdomen for underlying masses. This technique involves a wide range of perceptions, including temperature, vibration, consistency, form, size, rigidity, elasticity, moisture, texture, position, and contour. Palpation is performed with one hand, both hands (bimanual), one finger

(digital), the fingertips, or the palmar aspect of the hand. A pelvic examination is done bimanually, whereas an anal examination is performed digitally. Do not confuse palpation with *palpitation*, which is a throbbing pulsation felt in the chest.

Percussion

Percussion involves tapping or striking the body, usually with the fingers or a small hammer, to elicit sounds or vibratory sensations. Percussion aids determination of the position, size, and density of an underlying organ or cavity. The effect of percussion is both heard and felt by the examiner; it is helpful in determining the amount of air or solid matter in an underlying organ or cavity. The two basic methods of percussion are direct percussion and indirect percussion. Direct (immediate) percussion is performed by striking the body with a finger or a reflex hammer. With indirect (mediate) percussion, which is used more frequently, the provider places his or her hand on the area and then strikes the placed hand with a finger of the other hand (see Figure 25-9, *B*). Both a sound and a sense of vibration are evident. The examiner quantifies the sound in terms of pitch, quality, duration, and resonance.

Auscultation

For **auscultation**, the provider uses a stethoscope to listen to sounds arising from the body (not the sound produced by the provider, as in percussion, but sounds that originate within the patient's body). Auscultation is a difficult method of examination because the

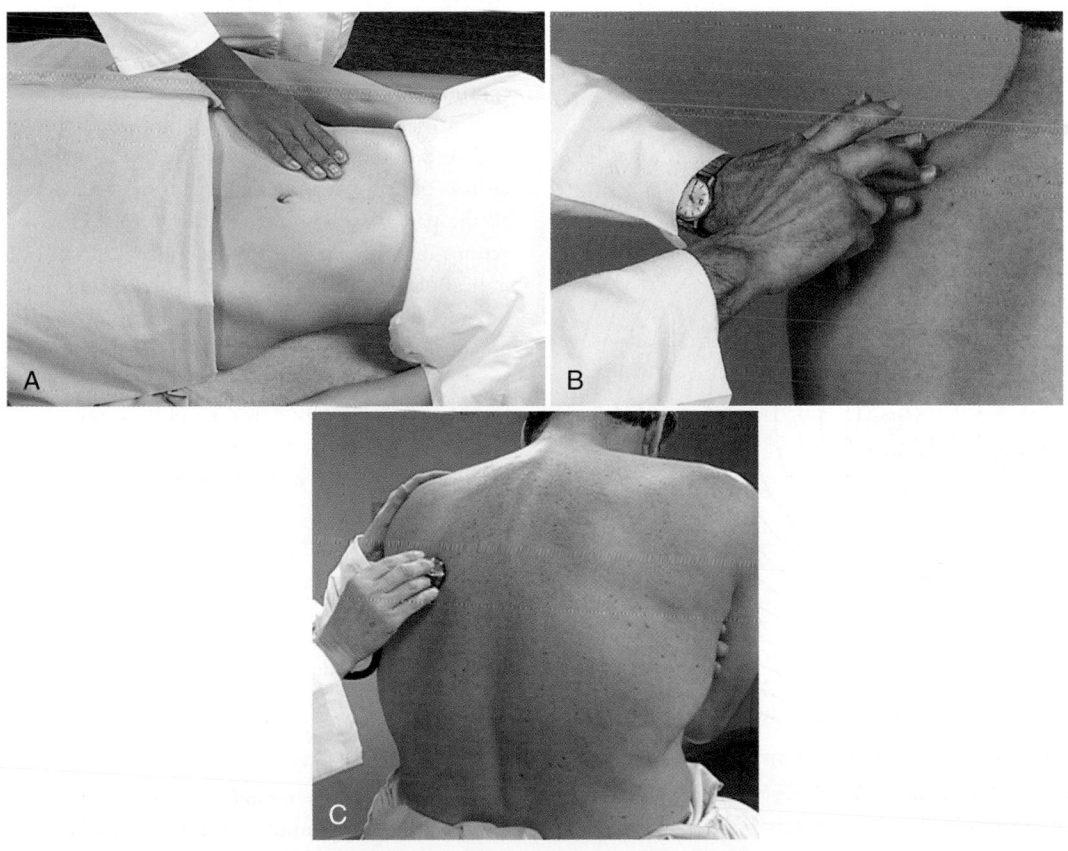

FIGURE 25-9 A, Demonstration of palpation. **B,** Demonstration of percussion. **C,** Demonstration of auscultation. (From Ball JW, et al: *Seidel's guide to physical examination,* ed 8, St Louis, 2015, Mosby.)

provider must distinguish between a normal sound and an abnormal sound (see Figure 25-9, *C*). It is particularly useful for evaluating sounds originating in the lungs, heart, and abdomen, such as a **murmur**, a **bruit**, and bowel sounds.

Mensuration

Mensuration is the process of measuring. Measurements that are recorded include the patient's height and weight, the length and diameter of an extremity, the extent of flexion or extension of an extremity, the size of the uterus during pregnancy, the size and depth of a wound, and the pressure of a grip. Measurements are taken with a flexible tape measure, a circular wound measurement device (Figure 25-10), or a specialized piece of equipment (e.g., a goniometer, which is used to measure joint angles) and usually are recorded in centimeters.

Manipulation

Manipulation is the passive movement of a joint to determine the range of extension or flexion of a part of the body. Manipulation may or may not be grouped with palpation. It usually is considered separate from the four standard methods of examination (inspection, palpation, percussion, and auscultation) and is grouped with mensuration, especially by an orthopedist or a neurologist. Insurance and industrial reports often request this information in detail. For example, a patient involved in a work-related accident that caused joint damage may have to perform assisted range-of-motion (ROM) exercises to the joint, with subsequent measurements of joint flexion and extension to demonstrate improvement or lack thereof.

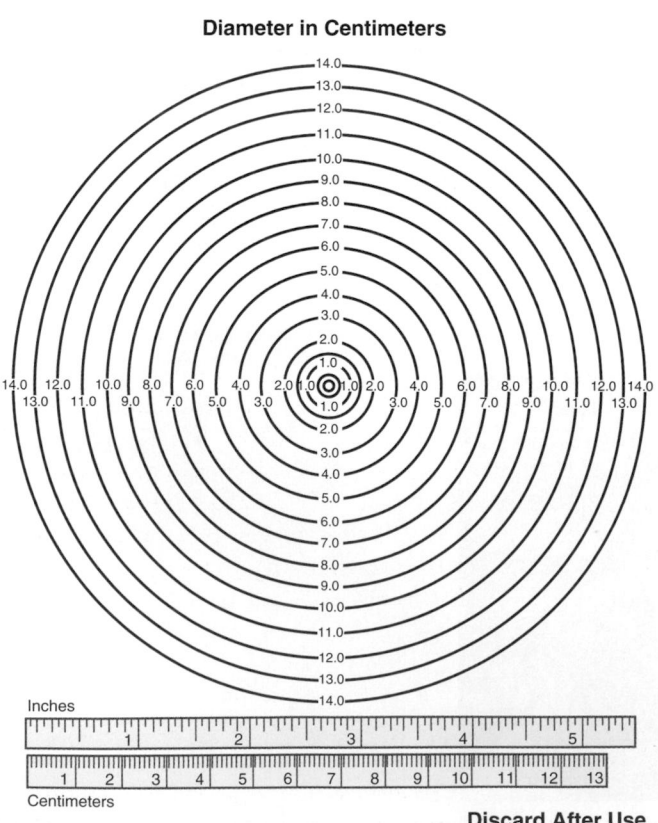

FIGURE 25-10 Circular wound measurement device.

EXAMINATION SEQUENCE

The physical examination sequence is fairly standard; however, variations may occur, depending on the provider's specialty, the medical necessity for the examination, and the provider's preference. Patients are more cooperative and less anxious if they understand what is expected of them; therefore, you should start by giving the patient a brief explanation of the examination process. Assemble all supplies and instruments needed for the examination before the provider enters the room. As the provider proceeds with the examination, make sure the patient remains unexposed by adjusting the drape and gown as needed. In every examination, the medical assistant assists the provider by handing the correct instruments and needed supplies. Having an assistant in the room during the examination can help prevent lawsuits. When the provider begins the examination, the medical assistant should keep conversation to a minimum and remain inconspicuous. The examination usually starts with the patient seated at the end of the exam table or in Fowler's position if the patient needs support. If the provider uses reflected light, the light source should be behind the patient's right shoulder. If illuminated instruments are used, standard overhead lights are sufficient. Take care not to shine a light directly into the patient's eyes; this can be done by turning on lights while they are directed away from the patient and carefully moving the light toward the area.

General Appearance

The provider starts the physical examination by observing the patient's appearance, using an inspection technique. The general appearance explains whether the patient appears well and in good health (e.g., the patient appears disoriented or in distress; well-nourished or undernourished; and answers questions with ease or confusion).

The patient's gait often provides important information. The patient may limp, walk with the feet wide apart, have a shuffle step, or have difficulty maintaining his or her balance. In addition to gait, all the patient's body movements are observed for possible muscle actions that the provider deems unusual. Posture also is checked for indications of pain, stiffness, or difficulty with limb movement. The provider notes body build and proportions. Any gross (immediately obvious) deformities are recorded. Sometimes abnormalities in height or body proportion may be caused by hormonal imbalances. If the medical assistant notes any of these observations or the patient reports any complaints, these should be recorded in the patient's health record, along with the vital signs, before the provider begins the examination.

Speech

Speech may reveal a pathologic condition. Some basic speech defects include *aphonia*, the inability to speak because of loss of the voice, which is commonly seen with severe laryngitis or overuse of the voice; *aphasia*, the loss of expression by speech or writing because of an injury or disease of the brain; and *dysphasia*, lack of coordination and failure to arrange words in proper order, usually caused by a brain lesion. With *motor aphasia*, the patient knows what he or she wants to say but cannot use muscles properly to speak; for example, this may be seen as slurred or incoherent speech that might occur after a cerebrovascular accident (CVA). In *sensory aphasia*, the patient pronounces words easily but uses them inaccurately, as in jumbled speech. Speech is also assessed in well-child checkups. A delay in speech development can indicate an issue (e.g., a neurologic deficit or possible autism spectrum disorder) and the need for a referral.

Breath Odors

Breath odors may or may not be diagnostic, although they often are associated with poor oral hygiene or dental care. Acidosis produces a strong odor of acetone, which is sweet and fruity and may result from diabetes mellitus, starvation, or renal disease. A musty odor usually is associated with liver disease, and the odor of ammonia may be noted in cases of uremia.

Skin

The condition of the skin can be a good reflection of the patient's nutritional status and hydration level. If dehydration is suspected, skin turgor is checked by pinching the skin on the posterior surface of the hands. The tissue is observed to see how quickly it returns to the normal location. A delay indicates a decrease in tissue fluid, confirming the diagnosis of dehydration. Extreme dryness, scaling, extended time for wound healing, or frequent breaks in the skin may indicate systemic disease.

Fingernails and toenails often give some indication of a person's health. Brittle, grooved, or lined nails may indicate local infection or systemic disease. **Clubbing** of the fingertips is associated with some congenital heart or lung diseases. *Spooning* of the nail is seen in some patients with severe iron-deficiency anemia. *Beau's lines* appear after an acute illness but grow out and disappear. The provider may refer a patient with skin disorders to a dermatologist for diagnosis and treatment.

Head

Once the provider makes the overall observations of the patient's general condition, the physical examination typically begins with the head and face and moves downward to the feet. The face reflects the patient's state and tells the provider a great deal about how the patient handles stress and illness. The skull, scalp, and face are palpated for size, shape, and symmetry. The distribution or lack of hair and hair texture may indicate hormonal changes. Excessive hair, especially facial hair in females, indicates a hormonal imbalance. As the head is palpated, the provider assesses possible **nodules**, masses, or signs of trauma.

Eyes

The pupils are checked for reaction by shining a light into one eye at a time. If the pupils constrict equally and smoothly to a light stimulus, the provider documents "PERRLA" (which means the pupils are equal, round, respond to light, and adjust and focus on objects). The **sclera** is checked for color, which ranges from white to pale yellow. If the eye is inflamed, it will be evident in the sclera. A sclera with a yellow tone indicates liver disease. Movements of the eyes are tested by having the patient follow the provider's finger. If eye movement is within average range, "extraocular movement (EOM) intact" is documented. The ophthalmoscope is used to examine the interior of the eye, including the retina and intraocular vessels. Some diseases, such as diabetes mellitus or hypertension, damage the blood vessels of the retina.

Ears

The ears are examined with an otoscope covered with a disposable speculum. The external ear is checked first for inflammation of the external auditory canal or for earwax (cerumen). The tympanic membrane (eardrum) is examined and should appear pearly gray. Scars on the eardrum frequently are the result of earlier, chronic ear infections or perforations. The color of the eardrum is important to the diagnosis because it may indicate fluids such as blood or pus behind the eardrum in the middle ear. The patient may be asked to swallow several times to allow observation of movement of the tympanic membrane, which occurs because of pressure changes in the eustachian tube. The eustachian tube equalizes air pressure between the middle ear and the throat. The ability of the tympanic membrane to move is crucial to the hearing process.

Nose and Sinuses

The mucosa of the nasal cavity is examined for color and texture. The sinuses cannot be seen, but the frontal and maxillary sinuses may be examined by firm palpation over the area and by **transillumination**. When disorders of the eyes, ears, nose, and throat are observed, and the provider believes that the condition warrants the attention of a specialist, the patient is referred to an ophthalmologist or an otorhinolaryngologist (ear, nose, and throat specialist).

Mouth and Throat

The mouth, or oral cavity, usually is thought of in terms of oral hygiene and dental care. Dental hygiene includes the condition of the teeth, how the patient cares for the teeth and gums, and whether the teeth of the upper and lower jaws meet properly (occlude) for chewing. Healthy gums are pale pink, glossy, and smooth and do not bleed when pressure from a tongue depressor is applied. The palatine tonsils usually are visible. The provider may use a tongue depressor and a piece of gauze to grasp the tongue to examine it carefully. The floor of the mouth is examined by both inspection and palpation for enlarged lymph nodes, salivary gland function, and ulcerations. The insides of the cheeks and the gumline are also examined for any abnormal marks or color. The provider may use the otoscope light to help with the examination.

Neck

The neck is examined for ROM by having the patient move the head in various directions. The thyroid gland is given special attention for symmetry, size, and texture. The provider manually palpates the thyroid area while the patient swallows several times because this action elevates the thyroid lobes. The carotid artery is palpated and auscultated for possible bruits. The lymph nodes are palpated. *Lymphadenopathy* (enlargement of the lymph nodes) can occur if the patient has an infection of the face, head, or neck.

Chest

While the patient is still in the sitting position, the chest, heart, and lungs are examined. The chest is examined for symmetric expansion. A tape measure may be used, especially if variation exists between the upper and lower chest expansion. A patient with a history of **emphysema** may have a barrel-shaped chest. The provider may use percussion to determine the density of lung tissues.

Placing a stethoscope on the patient's back, the examiner auscultates lung sounds. The patient is asked to take deep, regular breaths. This may produce slight dizziness, but the patient should be assured that it is only the result of the deep respirations and will rapidly pass. The provider notes the types of respirations and the presence of lung sounds in all lobes.

Because considerable concentration is required to interpret heart sounds, the provider must have complete silence when listening to the patient's heart. In patients with heart disease, the provider may spend an extended time listening to heart sounds. If lung or heart abnormalities are found, the provider typically orders further diagnostic tests, including blood analysis, x-ray evaluation, and an ECG. Once the results of these studies have been analyzed, the provider may refer the patient to a cardiologist for treatment of a heart condition, or a pulmonologist or a respiratory care specialist for treatment of a breathing disorder.

Abdomen

For the abdominal part of the examination, the patient is lowered to the dorsal recumbent or supine position and the drape is lowered to the pubic hair line. The gown is raised to just under the breasts. The patient's arms may be placed at the side, or the hands may be crossed over the chest or under the head. Relaxation of the abdominal muscles is needed for the abdominal examination. To assist in this and to promote patient comfort, a small pillow can be placed under the head and knees. The provider auscultates the abdomen in all quadrants to confirm the presence of complete bowel sounds and palpates the abdomen for any abnormalities. The provider also may use percussion to determine the density, position, and size of underlying abdominal organs.

Reflexes

The patient's reflexes are checked with the patient sitting, in a high Fowler's position, or supine. While the patient is sitting, the biceps are checked with the patient's arm flexed and supported by the examiner. The knee jerk (patellar reflex) and the ankle jerk (Achilles reflex) are checked using tapotement (a tapping or percussing movement) with either the fingers or the reflex hammer. The plantar reflexes (Babinski's reflex and Chaddock's reflex) are tested with the patient in an upright or a supine position.

Breast and Testicles

Careful breast examination is part of the physical examination for every female, regardless of whether she is symptomatic. The breasts are examined both visually and by palpation with the patient in the supine position and the arm on the side that is being examined bent and tucked under the head. Breast cancer is the most common malignancy in women, and early detection is the key to successful treatment. This is a good opportunity to discuss and reinforce the consistent use of monthly breast self-examination (BSE). For male patients who have reached puberty or are 14 years of age or older, the provider performs a testicular examination. The testicular self-examination (TSE) is an important self-examination for all males to perform each month because testicular carcinoma is a major health risk that has a high cure rate if discovered early.

CRITICAL THINKING APPLICATION   25-3
Alice Greenbaum, a 68-year-old patient of Dr. Kosto, is scheduled for an annual physical examination, including a breast check and a Pap test. Mrs. Greenbaum appears anxious about the examination and asks Felicia whether the gynecologic examination is necessary. How should Felicia answer this patient? What might be helpful in easing the patient's fears and preparing her for the examination?

Rectum

The rectal examination usually follows the abdominal examination or may be part of the examination of the male or female genitalia. Preserving the patient's comfort and dignity is vital. For this part of the examination, the provider needs examination gloves and water-soluble lubricating jelly (e.g., K-Y Jelly). The examination light should be directed at the perineal area during the examination.

Fecal occult blood test specimens often are collected at the time of the digital rectal examination. If this is a procedure the provider performs, be sure to include the necessary collection folder with the examination equipment. Patients diagnosed with gastrointestinal (GI) disorders may be referred to a gastroenterologist. Procedure 25-8 presents the steps for assisting with the physical examination.

CRITICAL THINKING APPLICATION   25-4
Dr. Kosto is the provider for residents of group homes for the developmentally delayed. Jimmy Cosgrove, a 38-year-old patient, is being seen today for an annual physical examination. Felicia is responsible for preparing the patient for the examination. Describe how Felicia should prepare the examination room and the patient.

PROCEDURE 25-8   Assist Provider with a Patient Exam

Goal: To aid the provider in the examination of a patient by preparing the patient and the necessary equipment and ensuring the patient's safety and comfort during the examination.

EQUIPMENT and SUPPLIES

- Patient's record
- Stethoscope
- Gauze sponges

- Ophthalmoscope
- Pen light
- Scale with height measurement bar
- Tuning fork

- Tongue depressor
- Biohazard container
- Cotton balls
- Examination light
- Laboratory request forms
- Percussion hammer
- Specimen bottles and laboratory requisitions
- Lubricating gel
- Disposable gloves
- Patient gown
- Sphygmomanometer
- Drapes
- Otoscope with disposable speculum
- Thermometer
- Cotton-tipped applicators
- Tape measure
- Fecal occult blood test supplies
- Disinfectant wipes
- Table paper

PROCEDURAL STEPS

1. Check the examination room at the beginning of each day and between patients to make sure it is completely stocked with equipment and supplies and that the equipment functions properly.
   PURPOSE: The room must be ready for patient services.
2. Check expiration dates on all packages and supplies regularly and discard expired materials.
   PURPOSE: To ensure the patient's safety.
3. Prepare the examining room before and between patients according to acceptable medical rules of asepsis.
   PURPOSE: The room must be aseptically clean to prevent the spread of infection.
4. Sanitize your hands.
   PURPOSE: To ensure infection control.
5. Locate the instruments for the procedure. Set them out in order of use within reach of the provider and cover them until the provider enters the examination room.
   PURPOSE: To promote time management and ensure that all needed equipment and supplies are ready.
6. Greet and identify the patient, introduce yourself, and determine whether the patient understands the procedure. If the patient does not, explain what to expect. Refer any unanswered questions to the provider.
   PURPOSE: To promote the patient's understanding and cooperation during the examination.
7. Review the medical history with the patient and investigate the purpose of the visit. Review current medications, and document any changes or prescription refills needed. Document the interview results.
   PURPOSE: To verify that all information is current and complete.

8. Measure and record the patient's vital signs, height, weight, and body mass index (BMI). Instruct the patient on how to collect a urine specimen, if ordered, and hand the patient a properly labeled specimen container. Obtain blood samples for any tests ordered.
   PURPOSE: To gather data needed before the examination begins.
9. Hand the patient a gown and drape. Explain what clothes should be removed for the examination and whether the gown should open in the front or the back. Help the patient with undressing as needed (most patients prefer to undress in privacy). Knock on the door before re-entering the room to protect the patient's privacy.
   PURPOSE: To assist the patient in preparing for the examination and to safeguard the patient's privacy, comfort, and safety.
10. Assist the patient as needed in sitting at the foot of the examination table; place the drape over the patient's lap and legs. If the patient is elderly, confused, or feeling faint or dizzy, do not leave him or her alone.
    PURPOSE: To provide for the patient's warmth and privacy and to prevent a fall or injury.
11. Place the patient's paper health record in the designated area or make sure the computer is ready for the provider to log in and access the patient's electronic health record (EHR). Be careful to safeguard patient confidentiality during this step of the procedure.
12. Assist during the examination by handing the provider instruments as needed and by positioning and draping the patient.
13. When the provider has completed the examination, allow the patient to rest for a moment, then help the patient from the table. Assist with dressing, if necessary. Use proper body mechanics if assistance in transfer is needed.
    PURPOSE: To ensure the patient's stability and safety and to protect yourself from injury.
14. Return to the patient and ask whether he or she has any questions. Give the patient any final instructions, and schedule tests as ordered by the provider and/or the next appointment.
    PURPOSE: To clarify instructions, eliminate any misunderstandings, and allow the patient to discuss any concerns. If the patient's misunderstandings or concerns are beyond your scope of experience or skill, arrange for the provider to speak with the patient again.
15. Put on gloves and dispose of used supplies and linens in designated biohazard waste containers. Dispose of exam table paper. Use disinfectant wipes to clean the examination table and any other potentially contaminated surface. Disinfect all equipment.
    PURPOSE: To prevent cross-contamination with any potential infectious materials.
16. Remove the gloves, discard them in the biohazard waste container, and sanitize your hands.
    PURPOSE: To ensure infection control.
17. Cover the exam table with fresh paper, replace used supplies, and prepare the room for the next patient.

CLOSING COMMENTS

Patient Education

The physical examination process is an excellent time for the medical assistant to assess the need for patient education. This assessment should be performed to identify the best ways to meet the patient's needs. When identifying these needs, consider the following:

- The information the patient needs to know
- How to convey the information so that the patient understands it
- How the patient will use the information
- Whether any community resources are available that might help the patient understand and learn more about health problems or treatment protocols

Develop a plan to teach the patient. Think about the different modalities available, such as pamphlets, pictures, DVDs, demonstrations, websites, and community resources. The more interesting the information, the more fun it is to teach the patient and the more enjoyment the patient will get out of learning. Many facilities keep patient education files that contain handouts on a wide range of health issues. The medical assistant should always review teaching plans with the provider and follow the provider's direction in patient education.

Legal and Ethical Issues

The medical assistant must recognize that a legal and ethical contract exists between the patient and the provider. As the provider's employee, the medical assistant is part of that contract. Information gained during the physical examination is confidential and must remain that way. The medical assistant must uphold ethical responsibilities as written in the Code of Ethics of the American Association of Medical Assistants (AAMA): to render service, respect confidential information, and uphold the honor and high principles of the profession.

HIPAA Applications

- Remember that conversations in the healthcare facility may be overheard. Guard patient confidentiality when gathering information about the chief complaint, scheduling diagnostic tests, or processing samples. If the front desk has a privacy glass, make sure it remains closed; turn away from the waiting room when talking on the phone; make sure that computer monitors are protected and screened; and avoid any conversations about the patient that may be overheard.
- If paper health records are used in the facility, make sure they are placed on the examination room door with identifying information facing the door to prevent those passing by from recognizing the patient's name. If EHRs are used, safeguard patient information by closing patient files and locking computers when you will be out of the room and by using privacy screen protectors.
- Maintain patient confidentiality during the admissions procedure in the facility. Many facilities no longer use sign-in sheets, but if they are used, the staff must completely block the names of previous patients from sight to maintain confidentiality.

Professional Behaviors

Courteous and respectful care is the hallmark of professional medical assistant behavior. Many times the physical examination process requires patients to expose very private parts of their bodies, which can make them feel quite uncomfortable. Safeguarding the patient's privacy as much as possible with adequate gowning and draping helps prevent undue exposure and embarrassment for patients during the examination process. Treating patients with thoughtful consideration goes a long way in making them feel more comfortable with physical examination procedures.

SUMMARY OF SCENARIO

As a new medical assistant, Felicia has a great deal of responsibility when it comes to assisting with physical examinations. She must prepare the room for the particular examination ordered and must prepare and care for the patient during the procedure. Preparing the room includes making sure appropriate supplies and equipment are readily available for the provider as well as planning how to safeguard the patient's privacy during the examination. Each examination is different, just as each patient has his or her own set of needs. Felicia helps the patient into a variety of positions, depending on the examination, and properly gowns and drapes the patient to safeguard privacy. Felicia is responsible for making sure the examination runs smoothly for the provider and for supporting the patient throughout the process. To protect herself against injury, Felicia uses proper posture and body alignment, remembering to bend at the knees and use her arm and leg muscles, rather than her back, to lift heavy items. She always asks for help if a load is too heavy, and she pushes a heavy item rather than lifting it.

SUMMARY OF LEARNING OBJECTIVES

1. Define, spell, and pronounce the terms listed in the vocabulary.
   Spelling and pronouncing medical terms correctly reinforce the medical assistant's credibility. Knowing the definitions of these terms promotes confidence in communication with patients and co-workers.

2. Describe the structural organization of the human body and the body cavities.
   The human body is made up of trillions of microscopic cells that determine the functional and structural characteristics of the entire body. A cell is

made up of three primary parts: the plasma membrane, the cytoplasm, and the nucleus. When cells with similar structures and functions combine, tissues are formed. The body has four types of tissue: epithelial, connective, muscular, and nervous tissue. A combination of two or more types of tissues creates an organ, and a number of organs joined together form a body system. The body is separated into the dorsal (posterior) and ventral (anterior) body cavities. The dorsal body cavity protects organs of the nervous system and contains the cranial and spinal cavities. The ventral cavity contains the thoracic cavity, which includes the pleural cavities and the mediastinum; the pericardial cavity is in the mediastinum. The diaphragm separates the thoracic cavity from the abdominopelvic cavity. The abdominal cavity contains gastrointestinal organs. The pelvic cavity is not physically separated from the abdominal cavity; it contains the urinary bladder, rectum, and reproductive organs.

3. **Identify the functions of the body systems and the major organs and structures of each system.**

A body system is composed of several organs and their associated structures. These structures work together to perform a specific function in the body. Each of the body's systems has specific units within it, and each performs specific functions. Table 25-1 summarizes the body systems; their primary cells, organs, and structures; and the major functions of each.

4. **Discuss the concept of a primary care provider and the role of a medical assistant in a primary care practice.**

A primary care provider is a healthcare practitioner who sees people of all ages for a broad range of diseases and complaints. The medical assistant's clinical responsibilities in a primary care practice include assisting with patients who may have problems in any of the body systems and assisting with procedures in all age groups.

5. **Outline the medical assistant's role in preparing for the physical examination.**

Before the examination, the medical assistant has the opportunity to interact with the patient to ensure that he or she feels comfortable during the examination process and that all necessary medical information has been obtained. The medical assistant's duties include preparing and maintaining the examination room and equipment; preparing the patient by conducting the initial interview and measuring vital signs; assisting the provider with positioning and draping; and providing instruments and supplies as needed during the physical examination.

6. **Summarize the instruments and equipment the provider typically uses during a physical examination.**

Instruments and supplies typically used in a physical examination include ophthalmoscope, otoscope, tongue depressor, reflex hammer, various tuning forks, stethoscope, sphygmomanometer, thermometer, tape measure, scale, examination light, disposable gloves, biohazard container, specimen bottles, laboratory requisitions, fecal occult blood test supplies, patient gown, drapes, and lubricating gel.

7. **Identify the principles of body mechanics and demonstrate proper body mechanics.**

Proper body alignment begins with good posture. When reaching for an object, avoid twisting or turning; instead, move the feet to face the object needed. Do not cross the legs while sitting, and keep the popliteal area free of the edge of the chair. Hold the head erect, the face forward, and the chin slightly up, the abdominal muscles contracted up and in, the shoulders relaxed and back, the feet pointed forward and slightly apart, and the weight evenly distributed to both legs, with the knees slightly bent.

Good body mechanics principles include maintaining balanced posture, bending the knees while maintaining the back's three natural curves, and using leg muscles to help lift. Move the wheelchair close to the examination table, lock the wheels, and lift the foot rests of the wheelchair out of the way. Provide patient support close to your body on the patient's strong side. Place the wheelchair at a 45-degree angle next to the foot rest at the end of the table, and with one hand under the axillary region and the other grasping the patient, help the patient step up onto the foot rest with the strong leg; then help the patient pivot into a sitting position on the table. Use a gait belt as needed to assist in patient transfer. (Refer to Procedure 25-1.)

8. **Outline the basic principles of gowning, positioning, and draping a patient for examination; also, position and drape a patient in six different examining positions while remaining mindful of the patient's privacy and comfort.**

The patient should be instructed on whether to wear the gown open in the front or the back, depending on the type of examination to be done. The position assumed by the patient during the examination depends on the part of the body to be examined or the procedure to be done. Possible patient positions include *Fowler's position,* in which the patient sits straight up, and *semi-Fowler's position,* in which the patient's torso is elevated 45 degrees; the *dorsal recumbent position,* in which the patient lies on the back with the legs bent; the *supine position,* in which the patient lies flat on the back; the *lithotomy position,* in which the patient's buttocks are at the bottom of the table and the legs are positioned in stirrups; the *prone position,* in which the patient lies on the stomach; *Sims position,* in which the patient lies on the left side with the limbs flexed so that the weight of the body is tilted forward; and the *knee-chest position,* in which the patient is on the knees with the buttocks elevated and the weight of the body tilted downward toward the chest. Trendelenburg position, in which the patient's head is lower than the legs, is not typically used in the ambulatory care setting. Draping requires constant attention to maintaining the patient's privacy throughout the examination while assisting the provider with exposure of the area being examined. The general rule is to cover all exposed body parts until the point in the examination when the provider must evaluate that particular area. Procedures 25-2 through 25-7 outline the steps for positioning and draping patients.

Continued

9. Describe the methods of examination, and give an example of each.

The examiner uses *inspection* to detect significant physical features, such as the patient's general appearance. With *palpation*, the sense of touch is used to feel the brachial pulse before a blood pressure reading is taken. *Percussion* involves tapping or striking the body to elicit sounds or vibratory sensations, as in percussion of the chest to detect fluid in the lungs. A stethoscope is used to *auscultate* or listen to the lungs and heart. *Mensuration* is the process of measuring the patient's height and weight. *Manipulation* is the passive, assisted movement of a joint to determine the range of extension or flexion.

10. Outline the sequence of a routine physical examination.

The examination sequence depends on the type of examination and the provider's preference. The provider typically begins the examination by noting the patient's general health appearance, nutrition status, speech, breath odor, skin condition, and reflexes. The physical examination begins at the head and proceeds down through the body. Any abnormalities are noted and may be further investigated with diagnostic tools after the examination has been completed.

11. Prepare for and assist in the physical examination of a patient, correctly completing each step of the procedure in the proper sequence.

Prepare the examination room and the patient; complete the initial patient interview and measure and record vital signs; gather the needed equipment and place it in the order of use; gown and drape the patient as needed; provide patient instruction and check for understanding throughout the process; assist during the examination by handing the provider instruments, managing changes in lighting, collecting samples as ordered, and conducting diagnostic procedures as ordered; assist the patient when the examination is complete, including helping the patient dress, scheduling further diagnostic tests as ordered, and answering the patient's questions. Complete the documentation, disinfect the examination room and equipment, and restock supplies to ready the room for the next patient. Procedure 25-8 presents the steps for assisting with the physical examination.

12. Discuss the role of patient education during the physical examination, in addition to the legal and ethical implications and HIPAA applications.

Before, during, and after the physical examination are excellent times to provide appropriate patient education. The medical assistant should clarify or reinforce any information given by the provider and should take advantage of "teaching moments" to promote patient well-being.

The medical assistant is part of the legal contract established between the patient and the provider. This contract begins at the time of the first visit to the ambulatory care facility. Maintaining confidentiality and providing respectful service are crucial to the integrity of that patient contract.

CONNECTIONS

Study Guide Connection: Go to the Chapter 25 Study Guide. Read and complete the activities.

evolve Evolve Connection: Go to the Chapter 25 link at *evolve.elsevier.com/kinn* to complete the Chapter Review Quiz. Check out the other resources listed for this chapter to make the most of what you have learned from Assisting with the Primary Physical Examination.

PRINCIPLES OF PHARMACOLOGY

26

SCENARIO

Kathy Augustino, CMA (AAMA), was hired recently to work for a primary care practice in her hometown. Kathy is responsible for managing phone calls and answering patient questions about their medication and prescriptions. Part of her job description is to follow the provider's orders to administer medication to a wide range of patients. To be knowledgeable about the administrative side of medication management, and to give medications to patients accurately and safely, Kathy must understand the basic principles of pharmacology.

While studying this chapter, think about the following questions:

- What should Kathy know about the management of controlled substances in the ambulatory care setting?
- If Kathy is not familiar with a medication, how can she learn about the properties of the drug?
- Is it important that Kathy understand the clinical uses of prescribed drugs and over-the-counter (OTC) drugs?

- The practice uses an electronic prescription program as part of its electronic health record (EHR) package. How does Kathy transmit the provider's drug orders electronically?
- A primary care practice has patients of all ages. What factors related to age might affect the action of medications on Kathy's patients?
- What role does patient education play in drug safety?

LEARNING OBJECTIVES

1. Define, spell, and pronounce the terms listed in the vocabulary.
2. Do the following related to government regulation of medications in the United States:
   - Distinguish among the government agencies that regulate drugs in the United States.
   - Cite the areas covered in the regulations established by the Drug Enforcement Administration (DEA) for the management of controlled or regulated substances.
   - List the DEA regulations for prescription drugs for each of the five schedules of the Controlled Substances Act.
3. Explain the medical assistant's role in preventing drug abuse.
4. Differentiate a drug's chemical, generic, and trade names.
5. Describe the use of drug reference materials, and explain the five pregnancy risk categories for drugs.
6. Discuss tips for studying pharmacology, and define the five medical terms used to describe the clinical use of drugs.

7. Cite safety measures for the use of OTC drugs.
8. Do the following related to prescription drugs:
   - Diagram the parts of a prescription.
   - Demonstrate the ability to transcribe a prescription accurately.
   - Describe e-prescription methods.
9. Relate the principles of pharmacokinetics to drug use.
10. Describe factors that affect the action of a drug, including the physiologic changes associated with aging.
11. Identify the classifications of drug actions.
12. Differentiate among commonly used herbal remedies and alternative therapies.
13. Examine the role of the medical assistant in drug therapy education.
14. Identify the medical assistant's legal responsibilities in medication management in an ambulatory care setting.

VOCABULARY

angina pectoris (an-ji′-nuh/pek′-tuh-ruhs) A spasmlike pain in the chest caused by myocardial anoxia.

bronchodilator (brahn-ko-di′-la-tuhr) A drug that relaxes contractions of the smooth muscle of the bronchioles to improve lung ventilation.

cirrhosis (suh-ro′-suhs) A chronic, degenerative disease of the liver that interferes with normal liver function.

colloidal (kah-loid′-uhl) Pertaining to a gluelike substance.

enteric coated A term describing an oral medication that is coated to protect the drug against the stomach juices; this design is used to ensure that the medicine is absorbed in the small intestine.

formulary A list of drugs compiled by a health insurance company that identifies the drugs the insurance company will cover under benefits.

generic A medication that is not protected by copyright.

hypercholesterolemia (hi-per-kuh-les-tuh-ruh-le′-me-uh) Elevated blood levels of cholesterol.

identity proofing The process by which a credential service provider validates that a person is who he or she claims to be; the provider must complete this verification before being allowed to e-prescribe controlled substances.

lumen An open space, such as within a blood vessel or the intestine, or within a needle or an examining instrument.

metabolic alkalosis A condition characterized by significant loss of acid in the body or an increased amount of bicarbonate; severe metabolic alkalosis can lead to coma and death.

over-the-counter (OTC) drugs Medications sold without a prescription.

spermicide (spuhr′-muh-side) A chemical substance that kills sperm cells.

therapeutic range The blood concentration of a drug that produces the desired effect without toxicity.

tinnitus A noise sensation of ringing heard in one or both ears.

Pharmacology is the broad science of the origin, nature, chemistry, effects, and uses of drugs. *Clinical pharmacology* is the study of the biologic effects of a drug used as a medical treatment and the actions of a drug in the body over time, including the rate at which it is absorbed by body tissues; where it is distributed or localized in the tissues; the route by which it is excreted; and its toxicity, or poisonous effect.

Medical assistants must have a general understanding of the types of drugs available and their uses. For every medication administered, a medical assistant must understand the drug's action, typical side effects, route of administration, and recommended dose, in addition to the individual patient factors that can alter the drug's effects and elimination. Drugs are constantly being developed and released for patient treatment; therefore, medical assistants must continually update their knowledge of specific drugs used in the ambulatory care setting. Correct management of drug administration and patient education are crucial factors in providing safe drug therapy for all patients.

GOVERNMENT REGULATION

Several federal agencies combine forces to regulate, safeguard, and manage the development and use of medications in the United States. The Food and Drug Administration (FDA), a division of the Department of Health and Human Services (HHS), regulates the development and sale of all prescription and **over-the-counter (OTC) drugs**. Pharmaceutical companies developing new medications must gain FDA approval before the drugs can be sold to consumers. The approval process begins with chemical testing in the laboratory and progresses to toxicity testing in laboratory animals, and finally to human clinical trials, which involve volunteers who participate in controlled drug studies. Only 1 of 10 new drugs ever reaches the clinical testing phase. If the drug is found to have an acceptable *benefit-to-risk* ratio (i.e., it is effective without causing an unacceptable degree of harm to the user), the FDA approves the medication for release.

The original manufacturer of the drug is awarded copyright protection on that particular chemical compound. Patents expire 20 years from the date of filing; this means that during the 20-year period, other pharmaceutical companies cannot produce **generic** copies of the drug. However, when patents on brand name drugs are near expiration, manufacturers can apply to the FDA to sell generic versions. Besides approving new drugs for the marketplace, the FDA establishes manufacturing standards for drug purity and strength and ensures that generic brands are effective and safe.

Standards for Generic Drug Manufacturers

On average, the cost of a generic drug is 80 to 85 percent lower than the brand name product. The U.S. Food and Drug Administration (FDA) has found no difference in the rates of reported side effects between brand name and generic drugs. Generic drugs must meet the following standards:

- The generic version must have the same active ingredients, labeled strength, route of administration, and dosage form (tablets, patches, and so on). However, generic drugs do not need to contain the same inactive ingredients or fillers as the brand name product. This difference may alter the absorption rate of a generic product. Because of this, some patients may require continued use of brand name drugs even after a generic becomes available.

- Generics do not have to replicate the human clinical trials of the brand name drugs, but applicants must prove that the product performs exactly as the brand name version does.

- Generic versions must act in the same period of time as the brand name version, delivering the same amount of active ingredient into the bloodstream in the same amount of time.

- The label of the generic drug must contain the same information as the brand name version for patient education.

- The generic manufacturing process must ensure comparable quality and production standards. The FDA continues to monitor the quality of the generic drug and periodically inspects manufacturing facilities to conduct quality control procedures.

www.fda.gov/Drugs/ResourcesForYou/Consumers/BuyingUsingMedicineSafely/. Accessed August 24, 2015.

Controlled Substances

The Drug Enforcement Administration (DEA) was established in 1973 as part of the Department of Justice to enforce federal laws regarding the use of illegal drugs. According to the Controlled Substances Act (CSA) of 1970, a drug or other substance that has the potential for illegal use and abuse must be placed on the controlled substance list. Any new medication with an action similar to a drug already on the controlled substance list also is considered to have the potential for abuse.

Most controlled drugs provide significant assistance to patients in need of their particular actions, such as pain relief or anesthesia for surgery. However, certain guidelines must be followed to comply with the storage of controlled substances, their record keeping, and security requirements. In addition, federal law mandates that all medical personnel, including medical assistants, share the responsibility for managing controlled substances on site. Precautions must be taken to monitor patients' drug use, protect prescription pads and e-prescription programs, maintain the records required by law, and report any known or suspected drug diversion or theft.

According to the guidelines set forth in the CSA, controlled substances are divided into five sections, or *schedules,* depending on their addictive abilities and likely degree of abuse. The classifications range from Schedule I drugs, which are illegal and cannot be prescribed, to Schedule V medications, which have the least potential for addiction and abuse (Table 26-1). A limited number of states also have a Schedule VI category for marijuana (cannabis) and synthetic cannabis products.

Every medical practice that stores and administers medications that fall into any of the schedule categories should have a copy of the controlled substances regulations. This list can be obtained from the regional DEA office or online. It is also important to ensure that the facility is included on the DEA's contact list so that the practice receives updates as drugs are added, deleted, or moved from one schedule to another.

Regulation of Controlled Substances

Specific CSA regulations govern the record keeping, physician registration, and inventory of controlled substances. Complete, accurate records on the purchase and management of scheduled drugs in the ambulatory care setting must be maintained. These records must be kept separate from the patient's medical record for 2 years and must be readily available for inspection by the DEA at all times. Each time

a controlled substance is dispensed and administered in the office, documentation of that process includes the number of doses of the drug on site both before and after the medication is dispensed. Medical practices that dispense and administer controlled substances on site use forms developed for this purpose. Any discrepancy in the count of the medication available must be documented and co-signed by two employees.

Every physician who prescribes or has controlled substances on site must register with the DEA for a Controlled Substance Registration Certificate. The physician receives a specific DEA registration number that must be included on all controlled substance prescriptions. The certificate is renewable every 3 years and is specific to a particular site of practice. Therefore, if the physician dispenses or prescribes scheduled drugs at more than one site, a DEA registration number must be obtained for each site.

All controlled substances must be stored in a safe or immovable double-locked cabinet, and the keys must be kept in a secure location. Prescription forms should be kept out of areas used by patients and preferably secured in an area that prohibits unauthorized or illegal use. All DEA forms used by the facility to order controlled substances also must be kept in a locked area.

Many ambulatory practices no longer keep controlled substances on site. However, if drugs are lost or stolen, the incident must be reported immediately to the regional DEA office and to local law enforcement authorities. If the facility needs to dispose of controlled substances a DEA-authorized collector should be contacted to safely and securely collect and dispose of controlled substances and other prescription drugs. Authorized collection sites may be retail pharmacies, hospital or clinic pharmacies, and law enforcement locations. If these disposal options are not available, the DEA recommends that some medicines, such as Demerol, Dilaudid, and OxyContin

TABLE 26-1   Schedule System of Classification of Controlled Substances

SCHEDULE	GUIDELINES	DRUG EXAMPLES
I	• No accepted medical use • Never prescribed for use • High potential for abuse • Possession of these drugs is illegal	Heroin, lysergic acid diethylamide (LSD), methaqualone (Quaalude), mescaline (peyote), amphetamine variations, phencyclidine (PCP), Ecstasy, gamma hydroxybutyrate (GHB), Acetylcodone, Dipipan. Marijuana is still considered a Schedule I drug by the DEA, even though some U.S. states have legalized marijuana for personal or medical use.
II	• Accepted for medical use but with severe restrictions • High potential for abuse • May cause severe psychological or physical dependence	Opium extracts, morphine, methadone, cocaine precursors, amphetamine, barbiturates, methylphenidate (Ritalin), lisdexamfetamine (Vyvanse); oxycodone (Percocet or OxyContin), hydromorphone HCl (Dilaudid), meperidine HCl (Demerol), codeine, alfentanil (Alfenta), alphaprodine (Nisentil), Burgodin, secobarbital (Seconal), pentobarbital (Nembutal), fentanyl, anileridine (Leritine)
III	• Accepted for medical use • Potential for abuse is less than for Schedule I or II drugs • May cause moderate to low physical dependence or high psychological dependence • Includes combination drugs that contain limited amounts of narcotics or stimulants	Acetaminophen and codeine (Tylenol with codeine), benzphetamine, suppositories with barbiturates, anabolic steroids, testosterone, butabarbital (Butisol), Fiorinal, Empirin, hydrocodone (Vicodin), buprenorphine, Boldione, paregoric, other opium combination products
IV	• Accepted for medical use • Low potential for abuse • May cause limited physical or psychological dependence compared with Schedule III drugs • Includes minor tranquilizers and hypnotics	Chlordiazepoxide (Librium), diazepam (Valium), flurazepam (Dalmane), chloral hydrate, Rohypnol ("date rape" drug), alprazolam (Xanax), triazolam (Halcion), temazepam (Restoril), chlorazepate dipotassium (Tranxene), lorazepam (Ativan), Klonopin, zolpidem tartrate (Ambien), barbital, clonazepam (Klonopin), diethylpropion (Tenuate), Motofen, midazolam (Versed), Donnatal Extentabs, Carisoprodol (Soma), eszopiclone (Lunesta), butorphanol (Stadol), Zaleplon (Sonata)
V	• Accepted for medical use • Low potential for abuse • May cause limited physical or psychological dependence compared with Schedule IV drugs • Includes drug mixtures containing limited amounts of narcotics	Cough medicines containing limited quantity of codeine (Robitussin A-C), alkaloids, kaolin and pectin belladonna (Donnagel), diphenoxylate with atropine (Lomotil), ezogabine (Potiga), lacosamide (Vimpat), pregabalin (Lyrica). May be sold by a pharmacist in some states; buyer must be 18 years old and must show identification

www.dea.gov/druginfo/ds.shtml. Accessed May 26, 2015.

oral doses, be flushed down the sink or toilet as soon as they are no longer needed. A list of medicines recommended for disposal by flushing can be found at http://www.fda.gov/Drugs/Resources ForYou/Consumers/BuyingUsingMedicineSafely/EnsuringSafeUse ofMedicine/SafeDisposalofMedicines/ucm186187.htm#Flush_List.

CRITICAL THINKING APPLICATION   26-1

Kathy is responsible for maintaining the inventory of controlled substances in the office. While checking the supply of meperidine, she notices that the expiration date on the medication is today. She must dispose of the remaining two pills. According to DEA regulations, how should she dispose of the medication?

Individual states also may regulate controlled substances; therefore, it is essential that medical assistants know their state's legal requirements. Specific federal guidelines apply to both written and e-prescriptions for controlled substances:

1. A written, oral, faxed, or DEA-compliant electronic prescription order must include the date the drug is prescribed; the name and address of the patient; and the name, address, and DEA number of the physician.
2. The amount prescribed must be written out ("ten" rather than "10"); the prescription usually is written for small amounts of the drug.
3. The provider must manually sign all paper prescriptions for controlled substances, although the medical assistant can prepare the prescriptions for the provider's signature.
4. Other specific rules may apply, depending on the schedule to which the prescribed controlled substance is assigned. The

symbols C-II, C-III, C-IV, and C-V are used to indicate the specific schedule.

- Schedule II (C-II) prescriptions
  - Must be either a written or an e-prescription; telephone or fax orders are not permitted
  - Cannot be refilled
  - May require specific types of order forms in some states
- Schedules III (C-III) and IV (C-IV) prescriptions
  - May be ordered orally, in writing, or transmitted electronically
  - May be refilled up to five times within 6 months of the original order
- Schedule V (C-V) prescriptions
  - May be ordered orally, in writing, or transmitted electronically
  - May be refilled up to five times within 6 months of the original order
  - Depending on the state, may be dispensed by the pharmacist without a prescription but typically require a photo ID

CRITICAL THINKING APPLICATION   **26-2**

Kathy is responsible for the orientation of a new medical assistant in the practice. Summarize the important points about government regulation of controlled substance prescriptions that she should include in the orientation.

DRUG ABUSE

Any drug, from aspirin to alcohol, can be misused or abused. The use of illegal and legal drugs has increased tremendously. Treatment programs for drug abuse are available throughout the United States for people from all walks of life. Programs include detoxification, rehabilitation, and long-term rehabilitation maintenance.

Medical assistants may encounter patients who are misusing or abusing drugs. It is important to be alert to the symptoms of drug dependence and to notify the provider when you suspect that a patient, or a co-worker, may have a problem with drug or alcohol dependency.

Drug *misuse* is the improper use of common drugs that can lead to dependence or toxicity. Examples of people with chronic dependencies include those who cannot have a bowel movement unless they take a laxative; those who have used nasal decongestants for so long that they cannot breathe without the use of nasal sprays; and those who take so many antacids that they suffer systemic **metabolic alkalosis**.

Drug *abuse* is the continuous or periodic self-administration of a drug that could result in addiction (physical dependence). Drug *dependency* is the inability to function unless under the influence of a substance; it may be psychological or physical. *Psychological dependency* is the compulsive craving for the effects of a substance. *Habituation* is a form of psychological dependency on a substance but without physiologic dependence, such as the need for tobacco. *Physical dependency*, or addiction, is a person's need to use a substance

continuously so that the body can function and also to prevent physical discomfort. This type of dependency occurs when abused substances produce biochemical changes in cells and tissues, most commonly in the nervous system. When a substance that causes physical dependency is discontinued, withdrawal symptoms occur. Withdrawal symptoms may be mild or serious, leading to convulsions and possibly death.

Regardless of the type of drug abused, it will have two effects on the person: acute and chronic. The acute effect is what the person feels when intoxicated, or directly under the influence of a particular substance. Chronic effects include the temporary or permanent physical and mental changes that result from long-term abuse.

Patients may question medical assistants about drug abuse. The medical assistant should read and keep up to date on drug-related issues. Booklets, websites, and agency referral names should be available for patients. In addition, patients' concerns and questions about drug abuse should be conveyed to the provider.

The Medical Assistant's Role in Preventing Drug Abuse

By following these guidelines, the medical assistant can help prevent drug abuse:

- Carefully monitor patients who repeatedly call for prescription refills of controlled substances.
- Request health records from other facilities for patients who report previous prescriptions for scheduled drugs.
- If the facility uses paper prescription pads, keep blank pads in a safe place, away from patient treatment areas, and minimize the number of prescription pads in use at any given time.
- Never use prescription pads for notepads, and never use preprinted or presigned forms.
- Secure computers used for electronic health record (EHR) documentation to prevent patient access to prescription generation.
- Keep only a limited supply of controlled substances on hand.
- Keep accurate, complete records of controlled substances dispensed on site and those prescribed; include specific documentation in the patient's record for all prescribed controlled substances.

DRUG NAMES

A single drug may have up to three names: a chemical name, a generic name, and a trade name. The chemical name represents the drug's exact formula. For example, the chemical name of the analgesic acetaminophen is *N*-(4-hydroxyphenyl); *acetaminophen* is the generic name, and the trade name is *Tylenol*. All drugs are assigned a generic, or nonproprietary (official), name. This name is much simpler than the chemical name, and it is not protected by copyright. The trade (brand) name is assigned by the manufacturer and is protected by copyright. To prevent confusion, the use of generic names rather than trade names is encouraged for medical professionals; however, patients may only recognize the trade names of drugs. Drugs also are classified by their use. For example, Advil is a brand name for the generic drug ibuprofen, which is classified as an analgesic and an antiinflammatory agent.

APPROACHES TO STUDYING PHARMACOLOGY

A pharmaceutical glossary could be a book in itself. Many terms are combinations of the condition to be treated plus the prefix *anti-* (e.g., antianginal, antianxiety, antiarrhythmic, anticoagulant, anticonvulsant, antidiarrheal). Notice how these names emphasize the drug's effect (use) rather than its action in the body. More recent classifications, such as parasympathomimetic and cholinesterase inhibitor, describe the pharmacologic action rather than the therapeutic use. Both viewpoints are necessary for a more complete understanding of drugs and their action in the human body. No one can remember all there is to know about clinical pharmacology. The number of new drugs introduced into use far exceeds the number of older drugs replaced or discontinued. The number of drugs available for clinical use grows beyond the ability to learn all there is to know about each medication. Therefore, it is essential that the medical assistant understand how to use pharmacology resources as references. Several drug index resources are available online that can be used to search for medication information. Examples of these are Rxlist at http://www.rxlist.com/script/main/hp.asp and Drugs.com at http://www.drugs.com/. If the facility promotes online drug research, preferred websites should be posted for staff use.

Drug Reference Materials

Reference books that are updated annually or periodically should be available for easy reference at all medical facilities. Most references list drug information in the following sequence:

1. *Action:* How the drug provides therapeutic results in the body, or the use of the drug.
2. *Indication:* The conditions for which the drug is used.
3. *Contraindications:* Conditions that make administration of the drug improper or undesirable. For example, aspirin is contraindicated in patients with GI bleeding.
4. *Precautions:* Necessary actions that must be taken because of special conditions of the patient, the drug, or the environment; these actions must be considered if the drug is to be successful or not harmful. The drug's pregnancy risk category is included in this section, as are precautions for nursing mothers (Table 26-2).
5. *Adverse reactions:* Commonly observed side effects on a tissue or organ system other than the one targeted by the medication. Adverse reactions include hypersensitivity, which causes an allergic reaction to the drug; idiosyncrasy, or an unexplained, unusual response to the drug; psychological dependence or habituation to the drug; and physical dependence on the compound, causing signs and symptoms of withdrawal in the patient if the medication is removed. For example, patients prescribed certain diuretics (e.g., Lasix) are at risk for potassium depletion, so they must take a potassium supplement or must eat a daily dietary source of potassium (bananas are a common source) to prevent complications.
6. *Dosage and administration:* Usual route, dosage, and timing for administering the drug.

TABLE 26-2   FDA's Pregnancy Risk Drug Categories

CATEGORY	RISK LEVEL/DESCRIPTION
A	Remote risk. Controlled studies in women have failed to demonstrate risk to fetus.
B	Slightly more risk than Category A. Animal studies show no risk, but controlled human studies have not been done; *or* animal studies show risk, but controlled studies in women have shown no risk.
C	Greater risk than Category B. Animal studies have shown risk, but no controlled human studies have been done; *or* no studies have been done in animals or women.
D	Proven risk of fetal harm. Human studies show proof of fetal damage, but the potential benefits of use during pregnancy may make its use acceptable.
X	Proven risk of fetal harm. Studies in women or animals show definite risk of fetal abnormality. Risks outweigh any possible benefit.

FDA, U.S. Food and Drug Administration.

7. *How supplied:* Description of how the medication is packaged and specifics on how it should be administered.

Package Inserts

Every drug package contains an insert describing all the significant aspects of using the drug, including information on the chemical formulation of the drug and clinical studies. The information in the insert is controlled by the FDA and serves as an excellent quick reference on new medications in the ambulatory setting.

Physicians' Desk Reference

The *Physicians' Desk Reference* (PDR) is published annually by Thomson Medical Economics (Oradell, New Jersey). It is supplied free to providers who subscribe to *Medical Economics* magazine. Copies can be purchased through the publisher or in local bookstores. Supplements are published quarterly throughout the year. The PDR contains information on approximately 3,000 drugs and includes product descriptions that are identical to the information provided in package inserts. The drug manufacturers pay for this space, so the PDR could be considered the Yellow Pages of the drug industry. The facility can also purchase an online version of the PDR and smart phone applications that can be used by staff and providers throughout the facility (*www.pdr.net*).

The print version of the PDR contains color-coded sections, which allows for easy cross-reference. The various sections enable you to begin searching for information about a drug from any starting point. You can start with the usage, classification, generic name, manufacturer's name, or trade name of a drug, or what the drug looks like. A special photographic section allows visual identification of products. Once you know which drug you want to study, the product information section lists the actual package insert information alphabetically, first by the manufacturer, then by the brand name. (A separate PDR volume, the *Physicians' Desk Reference for Nonprescription Drugs,* is published annually for OTC drugs and dietary supplements.)

The six sections of the PDR are color coded as follows:

- *Manufacturer's index (white):* Alphabetical listing of pharmaceutical companies; it includes the drugs manufactured by each company and the contact information for each manufacturer
- *Brand and generic section (pink):* Alphabetical listing of all drugs in the PDR volume, with complete information for each
- *Product category index (blue):* Alphabetical listing compiled according to drug category; drugs with similar actions are listed alphabetically in each category
- *Product identification section (gray):* Illustrated section that shows actual-size photographs of the tablets and capsules listed in the PDR
- *General and diagnostic product information area (white):* Alphabetical listing of diagnostic product information and the uses of these products

United States Pharmacopeia/National Formulary

The *United States Pharmacopeia/National Formulary* (USP/NF) is the official source of drug standards for the United States. The *Pharmacopeia* was combined with the *National Formulary,* which lists the chemical formulas for all accepted drugs. This combined reference lists and describes all approved medications in the United States considered useful and therapeutic in the practice of medicine. Single drugs, rather than combined products (compound mixtures), are listed. If a drug name is the same as the official name in this volume, the drug is followed by the initials USP (e.g., digitoxin, USP).

Learning About Drugs

The study of pharmacology is difficult at best. However, the following steps can help make it easier:

1. Take advantage of opportunities to observe the use of drugs in patient care. Studying about atorvastatin calcium (Lipitor) becomes more meaningful when you see how its lipid-lowering action actually affects a patient's blood cholesterol level.
2. Concentrate on the most important drugs in each classification. As you expand your knowledge to other drugs in each category, you will easily understand new drugs by noting the similarities and differences between them and the basic, important drugs you studied first.
3. Learn about a drug's primary action and use, then expand your knowledge to its other actions and uses. Soon you will be able to name the drug that is usually indicated for a particular condition. Knowing a drug's secondary effects will help you understand the side effects that are likely to occur with use of the drug. More important, you will be aware of

contraindications to use of the drug. Knowledge of the drug's actions will enable you to predict what toxic reactions might occur from an overdose.

Terms Describing the Uses of Drugs	
Diagnostic	Helps to determine the cause of a particular health problem (e.g., injecting antigen serum for allergy testing).
Palliative	Indicates that the drug does not cure, but provides relief from pain or symptoms related to the disorder (e.g., the use of an antihistamine for allergy symptoms or narcotics for pain relief).
Prophylactic	Prevents the occurrence of a condition (e.g., vaccines prevent the occurrence of specific infectious diseases or contraceptives prevent pregnancy).
Replacement	Provides the patient with a substance needed to maintain health (e.g., insulin for patients with diabetes, levothyroxine sodium [Synthroid] for patients with hypothyroidism).
Therapeutic	Treats a disorder and cures it (e.g., antibiotics cure bacterial infections).

Dispensing Drugs

Drugs are dispensed in two ways: over the counter and by prescription. OTC drugs are available to the public for self-medication without a prescription. These drugs have been approved by the FDA for general consumer use, but patients taking prescription drugs should keep their healthcare providers informed about their OTC drug use.

A medical assistant directly involved in patient care should have an understanding of some basic facts about OTC drugs and herbal products. Today patients are better informed about their personal healthcare, and many want to be active participants in healthcare decisions. They need facts to make informed choices when using OTC preparations. Most OTC preparations are safe if used as directed on the package; however, patient education contributes greatly to the safe and correct use of OTCs. Patients should be encouraged to do the following when choosing or using an OTC:

- Carefully read the package label and insert for use guidelines.
- Take only the recommended dose.
- Monitor the expiration date and discard the medication when appropriate.
- Never combine an OTC with a prescription drug without the provider's knowledge.
- Recognize that many OTC drugs are contraindicated in pregnancy, for nursing mothers, and for young children, and if certain diseases are present.
- Check with the pharmacist if questions or concerns arise.

The number of prescription drugs that have been granted OTC status is constantly increasing, and as the list of OTC drugs increases, so does the need for consumer education. Many OTC medications influence the safety and effectiveness of prescription drugs; therefore,

TABLE 26-3 Commonly Used OTC Drugs and Possible Complications

DRUG NAME	CLASSIFICATION	INDICATIONS AND DESIRED EFFECTS	SIDE EFFECTS	DRUG INTERACTIONS
Acetylsalicylic acid (ASA), ibuprofen, naproxen	Nonsteroidal antiinflammatory drugs (NSAIDs); analgesics	Inflammation and pain relief	GI bleeding, compromised renal function, tinnitus, diarrhea, and nausea	ACE inhibitors, warfarin
Acetaminophen (Tylenol)	Analgesic, antipyretic	Relief of pain and fever	Liver damage	Warfarin
Pseudoephedrine (Sudafed)	Decongestant	Relief of common cold and allergy symptoms	Hypertension, vasospasm, arrhythmia, CVA	Beta blockers, digoxin
Diphenhydramine (Benadryl and other combination products)	Antihistamines	Cough, cold, allergy, and insomnia	Disrupted sleep, confusion, hallucinations, delirium	Oxybutynin (Ditropan)
Dextromethorphan (Dayquil Cough, Delsym, Robitussin)	Antitussive	Suppression of cough reflex	Dizziness, lethargy, nausea	
Tums, Gaviscon, Pepto-Bismol	Antacids	Treatment of heartburn, GERD symptoms	Diarrhea, constipation, kidney stones	Ibuprofen, tetracycline, isoniazid

ACE, Angiotensin-converting enzyme; *CVA,* cerebrovascular accident; *GERD,* gastroesophageal reflux disease; *GI,* gastrointestinal; *OTC,* over the counter.

gathering information for a complete and accurate pattern of the patient's use of OTC drugs should be part of every healthcare visit. Table 26-3 presents a list of commonly used OTC medications, their side effects, and possible prescription drug interactions.

Prescription Drugs

Federal law makes drugs that are dangerous, powerful, or habit-forming illegal to use except under a licensed provider's order. A prescription is an order written by the provider for the dispensing of a particular medication by the pharmacist and its administration to the patient. As electronic health records (EHRs) have come into use, electronic prescriptions have become commonplace, although some facilities continue to use paper prescription forms (Figure 26-1). The prescription must be signed by the provider, or the order cannot be carried out (Procedure 26-1). If the provider requests that the medical assistant phone or fax a prescription to the pharmacy, all pertinent information for the medication order must be written down and reviewed by the provider for accuracy before the call is made. A note is made in the patient's record that a medication order was phoned or faxed into the pharmacy, with all of the pertinent information about the order included.

Appropriate medical terminology and abbreviations must be used to complete the prescription. The more common terms and abbreviations are listed in Table 26-4. In an attempt to reduce the number of medication errors caused by incorrect use of medical terminology, The Joint Commission has developed a "Do Not Use" list of abbreviations, acronyms, and symbols that should not be used for documentation purposes in accredited institutions. In addition, the commission created an ancillary list of possible future inclusions. Both of these lists are presented in Table 26-5. Besides The Joint Commission lists, facilities have the option of creating their own list of problematic abbreviations that employees should avoid using.

Six Parts of a Prescription

- *Superscription*: Patient's name, address, and date need to be included at the top of the paper prescription; the symbol Rx (for the Latin word *recipe,* meaning "take")
- *Inscription*: Main part of the prescription; name of the drug, dosage form, and strength
- *Subscription*: Directions for the pharmacist; size of each dose, amount to be dispensed, and the form of the drug ordered (tablets, capsules, or some other form)
- *Signature*: Directions for the patient; usually preceded by the symbol Sig (for the Latin word *signa,* meaning "mark"); the place where the provider indicates the instructions to be put on the label to tell the patient how, when, and in what quantities to use the medication
- *Refill information*: May be regulated by federal law if the drug is a controlled substance; the provider must write on the script the number of times a refill is allowed
- *Provider's signature*: Must include the provider's signature (whether it is electronic or manual), in addition to his or her Drug Enforcement Agency (DEA) registration number when indicated

CRITICAL THINKING APPLICATION   26-3

Dr. Simon asks Kathy to prepare the following prescription for his signature: "Take one 20-mg tablet of Lipitor daily at bedtime. Dispense 4 weeks' worth, and the prescription may be refilled two times." How would Kathy write the prescription using the correct format, medical terminology, and abbreviations?

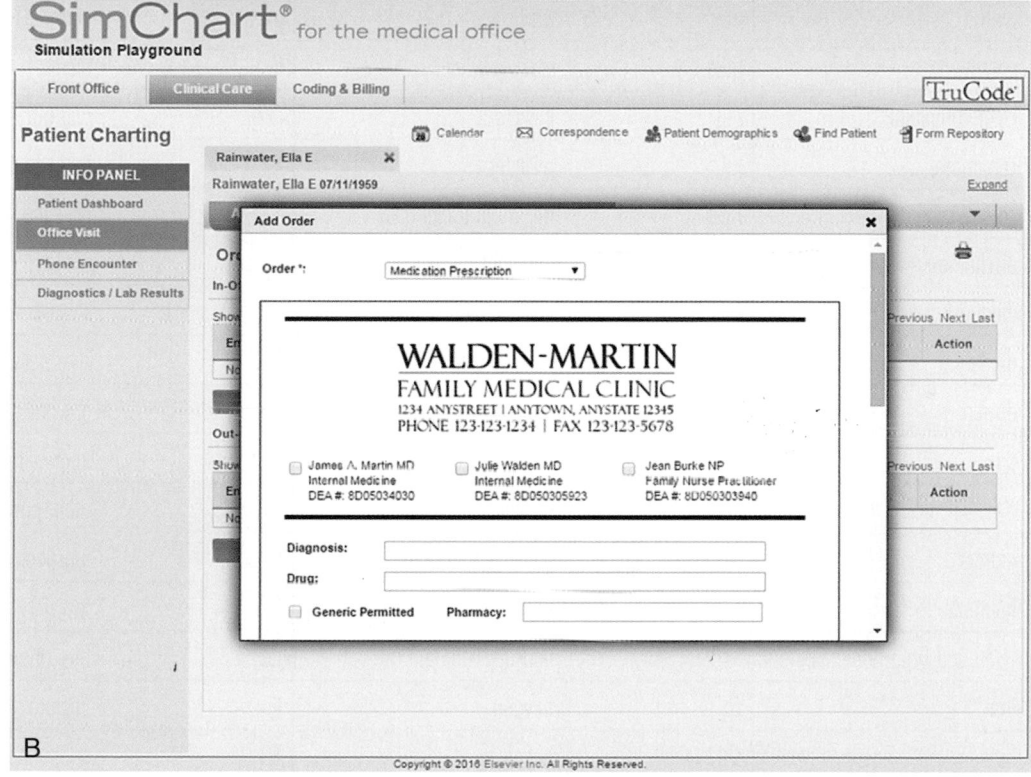

FIGURE 26-1 **A,** Sample paper prescription. **B,** Sample electronic prescription entry. (**B** from Elsevier: *SimChart for the medical office,* St Louis, 2016, Elsevier.)

Electronic Prescriptions

Electronic health record (EHR) systems can create and send prescriptions directly to a pharmacy. EHR programs are designed to automatically check a prescribed drug against the patient's allergies, identify possible drug-drug interactions, access current databases for the patient's medication history, review the patient's insurance drug **formulary** for coverage, and electronically send the script to the patient's pharmacy to be filled. The Department of Health and Human Services (HHS) recognizes the importance of e-prescriptions in quality patient care because they reduce the chances of misinterpretation of a provider's handwriting and promote speed in filling prescriptions through the instant transfer of the script from the ambulatory care facility to the patient's pharmacy. The HHS recommends that an individual, such as a credentialed medical assistant, be designated the practice's expert for e-prescribing so that the process runs smoothly and all regulations for the delivery of prescriptions electronically are followed.

Details on Medicare incentive programs to encourage physicians to adopt e-prescribing programs can be found at the following website: *www.cms.gov/Medicare/E-Health/Eprescribing/index.html?redirect=/Eprescribing.*

TABLE 26-4   Common Prescription Abbreviations

ABBREVIATION	MEANING	ABBREVIATION	MEANING	ABBREVIATION	MEANING
aa	of each	IM	intramuscular	pt	pint
ac	before meals	inj	injection	pulv	powder
ad lib	as desired	IV	intravenous	qh	every hour
agit	shake, stir	K	potassium	q2h	every 2 hours
am	morning	kg	kilogram	q3h	every 3 hours
amp	ampule	KVO	keep vein open	q4h	every 4 hours
ASA	aspirin	L	liter	qid	four times a day
aq	water	lb	pound	qm	every morning
bid	twice a day	LR	lactated Ringer's solution	qn	every night
C	cup, Celsius	mcg	microgram	qs	quantity sufficient
$\overline{c}$	with	med	medicine	qt	quart
cap	capsule	mEq	milliequivalent	R	rectal
CC	chief complaint	mg	milligram	r/o	rule out
cm	centimeter	mL	milliliter	Rx	take, treatment
c/o	complaining of	MLD	minimum lethal dose	S, Sig	give the following directions
D/C	discharge	mn	midnight	$\overline{s}$ or w/o	without
Dx	diagnosis	MO	mineral oil	SC, SQ, subQ	subcutaneous
dil	dilute	MOM	milk of magnesia	SOB	shortness of breath
disp	dispense	MTD	maximum tolerated dose	$\overline{ss}$	one-half
dr	dram	NKA	no known allergies	stat	immediately
EENT	eye, ear, nose, throat	noct	at night	T, tbs	tablespoon
ext	extract	NPO	nothing by mouth	t, tsp	teaspoon
F	Fahrenheit	NS	normal saline	tab	tablet
FDA	Food and Drug Administration	N/V	nausea/vomiting	tid	three times a day
Fe	iron	O₂	oxygen	tinct	tincture
fl	fluid	OD	overdose	TO	telephone order
fx	fracture	OTC	over-the-counter (drugs)	tus	cough
gal	gallon	oz	ounce	ung	ointment
gm, g	gram	pc	after meals	vag	vagina
gr	grain	PL	placebo	ves	bladder
gtt	drops	pm	afternoon	VO	verbal order
h	hour	PMI	patient medication instruction	VS	vital signs
hs	at bedtime	po	by mouth	WNL	within normal limits
HTN	hypertension	pr	per rectum	W/O	water in oil
Hx	history	prn	as needed	x	times
ID	intradermal	pt	patient	y/o	years old

TABLE 26-5 The Joint Commission's Official "Do Not Use" List[1] and Possible Future Inclusions

DO NOT USE	POTENTIAL PROBLEM	USE INSTEAD
U (unit)	Mistaken for "O" (zero), the number "4" (four) or "cc"	Write "unit"
IU (international unit)	Mistaken for IV (intravenous) or the number 10 (ten)	Write "International Unit"
Q.D., QD, q.d., qd (daily) Q.O.D., QOD, q.o.d, qod (every other day)	Mistaken for each other Period after the Q mistaken for "I" and the "O" mistaken for "I"	Write "daily" Write "every other day"
Trailing zero (X.0 mg)* Lack of leading zero (.X mg)	Decimal point is missed	Write X mg Write 0.X mg
MS MSO4 and MgSO4	Can mean morphine sulfate or magnesium sulfate Confused for one another	Write "morphine sulfate" Write "magnesium sulfate"

[1]Applies to all orders and all medication-related documentation that is handwritten (including free-text)

***Exception:** A "trailing zero" may be used only where required to demonstrate the level of precision of the value being reported, such as for laboratory results, imaging studies that report size of lesions, or catheter/tube sizes. It may not be used in medication orders or other medication-related documentation.

Additional Abbreviations, Acronyms and Symbols (for possible future inclusion in the Official "Do Not Use" List)

> (greater than) < (less than)	Misinterpreted us the number "7" (seven) or the letter "L" Confused for one another	Write "greater than" Write "less than"
Abbreviations for drug names	Misinterpreted due to similar abbreviations for multiple drugs	Write drug names in full
Apothecary units	Unfamiliar to many practitioners Confused with metric units	Use metric units
@	Mistaken for the number "2" (two)	Write "at"
cc	Mistaken for U (units) when poorly written	Write "mL" or "ml" or "milliliters" ("mL" is preferred)
μg	Mistaken for mg (milligrams) resulting in one thousand-fold overdose	Write "mcg" or micrograms

www.jointcommission.org. Accessed November 16, 2015.

PROCEDURE 26-1 | **Prepare a Prescription for the Provider's Signature**

Goal: *To accurately prepare a prescription for the provider's signature using the appropriate abbreviations and prescription format.*

EQUIPMENT and SUPPLIES

- Patient's record
- Prescription pad
- Drug reference materials, if needed
- Black pen

PROCEDURAL STEPS

1. Refer to the provider's written order for the prescription. If the provider gives a verbal order to write a prescription, write down the order and review it with the provider for accuracy.
   PURPOSE: To ensure accuracy in writing the ordered medication.
2. If you are unfamiliar with the medication, look it up in a drug reference book (e.g., the *Physicians' Desk Reference* [PDR]).

PURPOSE: The medical assistant should be familiar with the details of the drug, including the correct spelling, form in which it is dispensed, strength, recommended dose, storage guidelines, drug-drug interactions, and possible side effects, to make sure the transcription is correct and to be prepared to answer the patient's questions about the medication.

3. Ask the patient about drug allergies.
   PURPOSE: The patient should be asked about drug allergies each time a medication is prescribed or dispensed because these can change over time.
4. Using a prescription pad that has the provider's name, address, and telephone number, begin to transcribe the provider's order. Add the provider's DEA number if the script is for a controlled substance (see Figure 26-1).

PROCEDURE 26-1 *—continued*

5. Record the patient's name and address and the date on which the prescription is being written.

6. Next to the Rx, write in legible handwriting the name of the drug (correctly spelled), the dosage form (e.g., tablet, capsule, or other, using correct abbreviations), and the strength ordered. This is the inscription. For example, if the provider orders Lipitor, 40-mg tablets, by mouth, one tablet at bedtime, the first line of the prescription should read: Lipitor 40 mg tabs.

7. On the next line, write *Disp*. This is the subscription, which includes directions to the pharmacist on the amount to be dispensed and the form of the drug. For the Lipitor order, the subscription would read: Disp: #30.

8. Next comes the signature. This includes directions for the patient, such as how and when to take the medicine; it usually is preceded by the abbreviation Sig: For the Lipitor order, the signature would read: Sig: T̄ tab PO hs.

9. The provider has told you that the patient can get three refills of the prescription, so this information should be added at the bottom of the prescription on the designated line.

10. The provider must review and sign the prescription before it is given to the patient.

11. Document in the patient's health record the medication order and any pertinent details, including patient education and refill information.
    PURPOSE: All patient education should be documented for future reference. The details about the prescription, in addition to refill information, must be included for future prescriptions and/or refill orders.

Telephoning or Faxing a Prescription Into the Pharmacy or Transmitting an E-Prescription

Using the steps outlined previously, complete the prescription, making sure to include the following elements:

1. Patient's full name and address
2. Provider's full name and address
3. DEA number if the prescription is for a controlled substance (Schedule II drugs must be filled with a written prescription and/or an EHR program authorized to fill scheduled drugs)
4. For the prescribed drug:

- Name
- Strength
- Dosage form
- Quantity prescribed
- Directions for use
- Number of refills (if any) authorized

The provider must review the prescription for accuracy before the medical assistant telephones, faxes, or transmits the prescription to the pharmacy. Document the pharmacy order in the patient's health record as you would for any prescribed drug.

For an e-prescription, access the program for electronic transmission of prescriptions through the patient's record. Complete all the information required, and transmit the prescription to the patient's preferred pharmacy.

DRUG INTERACTIONS WITH THE BODY

Pharmacology is the study of drugs, their desired effects, and what happens to a drug while it is in the body. Different patients may react to the same dose of a drug in very different ways, and the same patient may react to the same dose of a drug differently at various times. Therefore, the management of medication therapy is concerned primarily with the effectiveness of a drug's action and the drug's potential side effects. *Pharmacokinetics* is the study of the movement of drugs throughout the body. Four basic actions occur when a drug is taken: absorption, distribution, metabolism, and excretion. If you know what happens to the drug in the body, you can know the *onset* of a drug's activity (when the drug action starts), when the effects of the drug are likely to peak, the minimum amount of the drug needed to bring about the desired effect (therapeutic dose), and the *duration* of a particular drug's activity. All these factors help the provider determine the appropriate form, amount, route, and frequency of administration of a medication for a particular patient.

Drug Absorption

The rate at which drugs are absorbed from the site of administration into the bloodstream depends on many factors, including the drug's ability to dissolve, the characteristics of the medication, the concentration of the dose, and the route of administration. Liquid oral medications dissolve more rapidly than solid forms because they do not have to be dissolved by GI fluids before they are absorbed. In addition, drugs soluble in fat pass more readily through the cell membrane because cell membranes have a fatty acid layer. More acidic drugs are absorbed well in the stomach, whereas others cannot be absorbed until they reach the small intestine. For some medications, such as antibiotics, the physician may order an initial *loading dose* of the drug, usually twice the typical amount, so that the patient's blood levels reach the **therapeutic range** more quickly.

Oral Route

Oral medications are convenient, safe, and relatively inexpensive. However, drugs that can be destroyed in any way by the digestive tract must be given by injection. Insulin and heparin are examples of drugs that are destroyed by the digestive process and therefore cannot be administered orally. Injection of medications leads to rapid absorption into the bloodstream, but this increases the danger of overdose or infection. Most oral medications are absorbed by the small intestine. After absorption into the bloodstream from the small intestine, drugs are carried to the liver. Much of the drug's potency is inactivated in this organ before the drug circulates to the tissues.

This inactivation by the liver often makes it necessary to administer higher doses orally than those given by injection.

Food slows the absorption of drugs; therefore, many medications are absorbed best when taken either 1 hour before or 2 hours after ingestion of food. Food also may bind with a medication or in some other way inactivate it. For example, tetracycline is destroyed by milk products and antacids containing calcium salts. Therefore, patients taking tetracycline should be advised not to eat dairy products or take liquid or solid forms of antacids. Stomach acid that naturally occurs during digestion may destroy certain drugs. Because some drugs are destroyed by the components of the digestive tract or irritate the empty lining of the stomach, oral drugs may be **enteric coated** to keep them intact for passage into the small intestine or to prevent gastric irritation or vomiting; therefore, enteric-coated medications should not be crushed or chewed.

Some drugs are not affected by digestive processes, but they cannot be absorbed through the intestinal walls into the bloodstream. For example, neomycin has no therapeutic effect when taken orally (unless it is used to sterilize the bowel before bowel surgery). Other drugs may be unable to cross the bowel mucosa because of their poor solubility in lipids (fats), or because they are inactivated by the pH of the GI tract.

It is important to remember these absorption factors when administering medication by the oral route. If a patient has previously responded to a drug but is no longer responding, it may be important to question the patient's food-medication cycle. It could be that the patient is no longer taking the medication on an empty stomach as directed.

Parenteral Route

Parenteral refers to the administration of drugs by injection. The parenteral route results in the fastest action because the medication is administered directly into the bloodstream or into tissues with a rich blood supply. However, several factors determine the effectiveness and rate of absorption of injected medications.

A drug in an aqueous (water) solution is absorbed more quickly in an area with more blood vessels. Therefore, drugs deposited in the muscle are absorbed faster than drugs given subcutaneously. The intramuscular (IM) route is chosen in an emergency for fast action or when larger amounts of the medication must be absorbed. The IM route is also used for oil-based medications (e.g., testosterone), which are typically prepared with oil to extend the absorption rate of the drug. The subcutaneous (SC) route is chosen when a slower, prolonged effect is desired.

Drug absorption also may be controlled physically. Absorption may be quickened by hand massage after injection, but massage should be done only if recommended. Absorption may be slowed by pharmaceutical preparation of the drug in a physical form that slows absorption. These methods include suspending the drug in a solution that prolongs absorption, such as **colloidal** substances, fatty substances (oil), or insoluble salts or esters. Drugs suspended in these substances slowly dissolve in the tissues over a long time, and the patient can be spared costly, frequent, and sometimes painful injections. Local anesthetics sometimes are mixed with epinephrine to keep the medication and its effects in an area longer because epinephrine (adrenalin) constricts blood vessels at the site, reducing circulation and the rate of absorption.

Another parenteral route is the *intravenous* (IV) route, in which the medication is injected directly into the vein. Because of the dangers of IV administration, only members of the medical team who are licensed to do so may inject medication intravenously. Other parenteral routes that are outside the medical assistant's scope of practice include:

- Intrathecal, or intraspinal, injections are used for spinal anesthesia and to administer certain medications into the spinal column.
- Intra-articular injections are used to administer corticosteroids into joints.
- Intralesional medications are injected directly into a lesion, such as an anticancer drug that is administered into a cancerous tumor.

> ### Safety Alert
>
> It is outside the medical assistant's scope of practice to perform IV administration of medications to patients. Because IV administration is so dangerous, medications given intravenously usually are administered in small doses through an IV infusion (IV drip) so that the effects in the body can be monitored.

Another form of parenteral route is an intradermal injection, which is injection of the drug within the dermal layer of the skin and superficial to the subcutaneous tissues. This route is used mostly for allergy testing and skin testing, such as testing for tuberculosis.

Mucous Membrane Absorption

Drugs may be absorbed by the mucous membranes of the mouth, throat, nose, eyes, rectum, vagina, and respiratory tracts. Some applications, such as nasal sprays, eye drops, and rectal suppositories for constipation, have a local effect. Others have a systemic effect, such as a rectal suppository given to control vomiting, or a nitroglycerin tablet dissolved under the tongue *(sublingual)* to dilate coronary arteries and relieve the pain of **angina pectoris**. *Inhalation* is used to concentrate drugs locally in the lower respiratory passages or to produce systemic effects, such as general anesthesia. For example, a **bronchodilator**, such as metaproterenol sulfate (Alupent), is inhaled during an asthma attack to relieve bronchospasms.

Topical Absorption

Topical routes include the application of medications to the skin, eyes, and ears. Drugs in ointments, creams, lotions, and aerosols can be applied for the treatment of skin itching, inflammation, or other discomforts, and for the treatment of skin infections with antibiotics. Nitroglycerin (for angina) can be absorbed through the skin from a dermal patch, which releases it systemically. Hormones such as testosterone and estrogen also can be administered via a dermal patch for systemic purposes.

Drug Distribution

Once a drug has been absorbed, it must be transported by the circulatory system to the area where it will have its effect. In the bloodstream, drugs can attach to plasma proteins and then are freed

Terms Related to Drug Interactions

Antagonism	The action of one drug diminishes the effect or shortens the duration of action of another drug. For example, Naloxone Injection and Evzio (a prefilled naloxone autoinjector) are used to reverse the life-threatening effects of a narcotic overdose.
Synergism	A drug enhances the intensity or prolongs the action of another drug. This can have a positive effect, as when two different antibiotics are used to treat an infection, or a negative effect, as when two drugs lower blood pressure to dangerous levels.
Potentiation	A form of synergism in which the effect of one drug is enhanced by the presence of another drug. In this case, the two drugs have different actions, but one increases the effect of the other. Promethazine, an antihistamine, when given with a painkilling narcotic such as Demerol, intensifies the narcotic's effect, thereby reducing the amount of the narcotic needed.

to pass from the blood into the site of action. Drugs are carried through the fluids into the cells of the tissues and organs. The blood supply to a part affects the speed with which drugs reach certain tissues.

The *blood-brain barrier* is a functional cellular barrier between the brain cells and the capillaries circulating blood through the brain. The barrier is poorly permeable to water-soluble materials, which makes it difficult for dissolved substances in the blood to pass through. For substances that do cross through, the barrier regulates the degree and rate of their absorption into the brain tissue. The general anesthetic thiopental is able to cross the blood-brain barrier immediately and produces sleep within seconds, whereas other sleep-producing drugs, such as the barbiturates, cross slowly and may take as long as 30 minutes to 1 hour to produce the same effect. The blood-brain barrier is a mixed blessing. It provides a physical barrier that protects the brain from potentially dangerous chemicals, but it also makes it very difficult to treat CNS disorders. In contrast, the placenta has no method for blocking substances, so whatever the mother consumes is readily passed through the placenta to the developing fetus. This means that childbearing women must be extremely careful of all chemicals they consume or inhale because they are quickly transferred to the baby's bloodstream.

Drug Action

Regardless of the route of administration, a drug can have one of two actions on the body: local (restricted to one spot or part; not general) or *systemic* (affecting the body as a whole). Most drugs are used for their systemic effects. Even when drugs are used for local purposes, no drug remains completely localized in the body. Any chemical that comes into contact with even the most superficial surface, such as the skin, has the potential to be absorbed into the bloodstream and circulate to other tissues and organs.

Multiple theories explain the actions of drugs. Drugs are believed to combine with body chemicals on the cell surface or within the

cell itself. Pharmaceutical developers create compounds that have an affinity for a specific target cell. The target cell recipient is called a *receptor*, and the drug that has the affinity for it and produces a functional change in the cell is called an *agonist*. Not all drugs that bind to specific cells cause a functional change in the cell. These drugs act as an *antagonist* to the natural process and work by blocking a sequence of biochemical events.

Some drugs are believed to act by affecting the enzyme functions of the body. Drugs attach to enzyme substances and rob the enzymes from cells. As a result, the enzyme products needed for normal cellular function are not supplied, and the cell fails to function properly.

Certain antiinfective drugs have a selected toxicity for pathogens or parasites that have invaded the body. Penicillin and sulfonamides work because they poison or interfere with the life processes of bacteria without affecting the life processes of normal human cells. Research scientists continue to look for differences between cancer cells and normal cells so that they can apply the principle of selected toxicity in cancer treatment. Both drugs that have a selective affinity for cells and those that bind with enzymes may be counteracted by administering large amounts of natural substances with which the drugs compete. This process is known as administering an *antidote* to a drug that may be acting as a poison. For example, an antidote such as naloxone hydrochloride can be administered if a patient receives too much anesthesia or has taken a drug overdose.

Some drugs alter the function of a cell by affecting the physical properties of the cell membrane rather than altering biochemical processes within the cell. This is especially true of drugs that affect nerve cells, such as anesthetics and alcohol. A change in the cell membrane alters the permeability of the membrane, which in turn changes the flow of ions into and out of the cells. This change in ion flow alters the *polarity* (opposite effects at two extremities, the two extremities being inside and outside the cell membrane) on which nerve pulses are conducted, resulting in general sleep or stupor.

Drug Metabolism

After the drug has been absorbed and distributed, it is metabolized for excretion. During metabolism, the drug is converted into harmless byproducts, which are more easily eliminated by the kidneys. Most drugs are broken down by the enzyme activity of the liver. For oral medications that are absorbed in the small intestine, this process begins in the liver before distribution.

The ability to break down the chemical components of a drug varies among individuals. Factors that determine this ability include age, the presence of other drugs, and liver disease. Infants and aging individuals have more difficulty effectively metabolizing medications. Patients taking multiple medications also may be at increased risk for liver-related problems with metabolism because of the sheer number of chemicals the liver is exposed to on a daily basis. Individuals with chronic liver disease, such as **cirrhosis**, may not be able to metabolize even normal doses of medications. A *cumulative effect*, meaning the total amount of the drug present in the body after multiple doses, may result in a toxic condition if the drug is absorbed faster than it is metabolized. Because of these factors, drug therapy must be monitored closely in very young and aging patients, those taking multiple medications, and patients with chronic liver disease.

In contrast, patients receiving long-term drug therapy may develop overstimulation of the enzyme activity of the liver. This results in rapid destruction of the drug, and the patient has to take larger and larger doses for the drug to be effective. This situation is called *tolerance*.

Drug Excretion

After the drug has been metabolized, its byproducts must be excreted from the body. The kidneys are the most important route for the elimination of drugs. Most chemicals are filtered out of the blood, circulated through the kidneys, and excreted in the urine. Because the kidneys are so important in the elimination of chemicals from the body, drug therapy must be carefully monitored in patients with kidney disease or malfunction. Drugs are also eliminated through the sweat glands, saliva, and feces. Exhalation, another mechanism for drug elimination, serves as the basis for measuring alcohol concentrations in the blood by the breathalyzer test. Drugs may be eliminated through the milk glands of a lactating mother, which means that a breastfeeding woman must be extremely careful about taking medications.

The combination of metabolism and excretion reduces the amount of drug in the body at any given time. The *therapeutic dose* of a medication depends on many factors, including the drug's half-life. The *half-life* is the amount of time it takes for half a dose of medication to be metabolized and excreted from the body. Some drugs have extremely short half-lives (only minutes), whereas others can take days to leave the body. The amount of drug lost during one half-life depends on how much drug is present. Providers use the half-life of a drug to determine the timing of medication administration, or the dose intervals. The shorter the half-life of the drug, the closer together are the times when it should be administered. If the next dose of the drug is not given within the half-life, blood levels drop and the patient does not receive adequate therapeutic effects from the treatment.

Pharmacokinetic Terms

Absorption	The movement of a drug into the bloodstream. The rate of absorption depends on many factors, including the route of administration.
Distribution	The transport of a drug from the site of administration to the location in the body where it is meant to act (i.e., the target tissue).
Metabolism	The inactivation of a drug, including the time required for a drug to be detoxified and broken down into byproducts. The liver typically metabolizes medications.
Excretion	The elimination of a drug from the body, including the route of elimination and the time required for this process. The kidneys typically excrete drug metabolites.

FACTORS AFFECTING DRUG ACTION

As was stated earlier, different people react to the same dose of medication in different ways, and the same patient can react to the same dose of the same drug differently on various occasions. A

TABLE 26-6 Physiologic Changes of Age and Effects on Medication Usage

CHANGES WITH AGING	EFFECTS ON MEDICATION
Stomach takes longer to empty, and gastric acidity is reduced.	Increases the risk of stomach irritation and ulceration.
Increased percentage of adipose (fat) tissue in the body.	Increases likelihood of drug storage in fat; may lead to drug toxicity.
Fewer protein-binding sites available in bloodstream.	Reduces drug passage through cell membranes; increases blood level of drug; may lead to toxicity.
Liver function declines.	Slows rate of drug metabolism; increases risk of toxicity.
Kidney function declines.	Slows rate of elimination of drug byproducts; increases risk of toxicity and complications.
Peripheral vascular disease present; venous tone diminished.	Reduces distribution of drug to the periphery.
Fat-soluble medications pass through blood-brain barrier more easily.	May affect central nervous system; increases risk of vertigo and confusion.

number of factors are important in determining the correct medication for a patient.

Body Weight

The effect of a medication is directly related to the person's weight. Basically, the same dose has a lesser effect on a patient who weighs more and a greater effect on a person who weighs less. Manufacturers of adult medications calculate dosages based on a normal adult weight (approximately 150 pounds). Sometimes the provider adjusts the dose to better suit the patient's body size. Pediatric medications are designed for the body weight of the child.

Age

The most significant effect of age on the body's response to a drug occurs in newborns and elderly individuals. This usually is related to immature or deteriorating body systems. In addition, both patient groups are particularly sensitive to drugs that affect the CNS and are at risk of developing toxic drug levels. Consequently, dosage amounts for these two groups must be carefully calculated. The provider may opt to start therapy with very small doses and increase the dose over time based on the presence or absence of side effects. Table 26-6 summarizes the altered effects of medications on aging individuals.

Gender

Drugs may affect men and women differently. As has been mentioned, a pregnant woman must be extremely cautious when taking medications to prevent possible damage to the developing fetus. In addition, the side effects of some drugs can stimulate uterine contractions, causing premature labor and delivery. Intramuscular medications are absorbed faster by men because they generally have higher levels of muscle mass, which is rich in blood vessels. Because women typically have a higher body fat content and less muscle (resulting in fewer blood vessels in peripheral tissues compared with men), intramuscular drugs remain in their tissues longer. In the past, most clinical trials were conducted only on men; therefore, until newer trial results are released that include women, the effect of gender on the action and safety of medications is impossible to predict accurately.

Time of Day

Diurnal refers to during the day or time of light. Diurnal body rhythms play an important part in the effects of some drugs. Sedatives given in the morning are not as effective as those administered before bedtime because the CNS is more alert in the morning, causing increased resistance to the effects of the drug. Corticosteroid administration is preferred in the morning because this best mimics the body's natural pattern of corticosteroid production and elimination.

Pathologic Factors

Patients may adversely respond to drugs if they have liver or kidney disease because the body is unable to metabolize and excrete chemicals properly. Drugs may also produce pathologic conditions of the liver or kidneys, and patients may need to be monitored for potentially serious drug complications. For example, patients taking statin medications (e.g., atorvastatin calcium [Lipitor]) for **hypercholesterolemia** should have liver function studies done routinely because these drugs are very hard on liver cells.

Patients with liver or kidney disease have an increased risk of drug toxicity, which may result in unconsciousness or death. Reactions in patients with other diseases or disorders may be quite different from the expected response. Therefore, a thorough medical history of the patient must always be taken before medications are prescribed and administered.

Immune Responses

The presence of a drug can stimulate a patient's immune response, causing the patient to develop antibodies to a particular chemical. If the same drug is administered again, the patient will have an allergic reaction to the drug, ranging from a mild reaction to anaphylaxis, a serious respiratory and circulatory emergency. Antibiotics are the group of drugs that most commonly cause allergic responses. A typical low-level allergic response to an antibiotic is *urticaria,* or the formation of hives.

Psychological Factors

People may respond differently to a medication because of the way they feel about the drug. If a patient believes in the therapy, even a placebo (a sugar pill or sterile water thought to be a drug) may help or bring about relief. In addition, a patient's personality can affect whether he or she will follow directions for a particular drug; also, a negative mindset or mental attitude can reduce an expected response to a drug.

Tolerance

Tolerance is the phenomenon of reduced responsiveness to a drug. *Acquired tolerance* occurs after a particular drug has been taken for a period of time. *Cross-tolerance* occurs when a patient acquires a tolerance to one drug and becomes resistant to other, similar drugs. *Physical dependence,* such as occurs with narcotic addictions, often accompanies tolerance. The body becomes so adapted to the presence of the drug that it cannot function properly without it. To withdraw the drug is to throw the body out of its equilibrium, causing withdrawal symptoms.

Accumulation

When a drug is taken too frequently to allow for proper elimination, it accumulates in the tissues. The result is a more intense effect and a longer duration. Accumulation can cause overdose and/or toxic effects. An example of a toxic accumulation of medication is *ototoxicity* (a toxic condition affecting the ears), which results in nausea, vomiting, **tinnitus**, and vertigo. Proper dosage and timing of administration are the best methods of preventing drug accumulation.

Idiosyncrasy

Occasionally a person reacts to a drug in a manner that is unexpected and peculiar to that individual. An idiosyncratic response may manifest in many different ways; for example, a hypnotic drug may keep a person awake, acting as a stimulant to this person rather than as a depressant. Usually these reactions cannot be explained.

Drug-Drug Interactions

Special care must be taken with patients who take more than one drug on a regular basis. One medication may increase or decrease the effects of another or may cause unexpected side effects. To safeguard patients from potentially negative drug interactions, it is important at each visit to record a complete list of all drugs the patient is taking, including OTC medications and herbal products. However, because many patients do not know or get confused about the names and dosages of their medications, the best way to maintain an accurate record is to ask that patients bring their medication containers with them to each office visit. This way, you can list information about the medications in the patient's EHR and at the same time ask whether the patient has any questions about his or her treatment. It is also a good idea to advise patients to fill prescriptions at the same pharmacy because the pharmacist can monitor medications for potential drug interactions. One of the positive aspects of EHRs is that the computer program reviews possible drug-drug interactions if a correct list of all a patient's medications is included in the person's electronic record.

An example of a drug interaction is the effect of some antibiotics on oral contraceptives. Certain antibiotics can interact with birth control pills, making the birth control pills less effective and pregnancy more likely. Patients should be told that spotting (midcycle bleeding) may be the first sign that an antibiotic is interfering with the effectiveness of birth control pills. Examples of antibiotics that interact with birth control pills include penicillin (Veetids), amoxicillin (Amoxil), ampicillin (Omnipen), sulfamethoxazole plus trimethoprim (Septra or Bactrim), tetracycline (Sumycin), minocycline (Minocin), metronidazole (Flagyl), and nitrofurantoin (Macrobid or

Macrodantin). If a woman wants to prevent pregnancy while taking an antibiotic, the provider may recommend that she use a condom and **spermicide** as a backup birth control method while taking the medication and for at least 1 week after the completion of treatment.

CRITICAL THINKING APPLICATION   **26-4**

Sylvia Kramer, a 72-year-old patient of Dr. Simon, calls today and asks Kathy how she should be taking her heart medicine, diltiazem HCl (Cardizem). Mrs. Kramer has diabetes, hypertension, and a history of heart disease. She is overweight, has the potential for kidney disease, and takes a number of other prescriptions. What factors may have an impact on the potential effect of Mrs. Kramer's medication?

CLASSIFICATIONS OF DRUG ACTIONS

Clinical pharmacology is a complex subject. To make it easier, drugs are classified into groups according to their actions in the body (e.g., diuretics, emetics); the symptoms they relieve (e.g., antihistamine); or the body system they affect (e.g., drugs that act on the cardiovascular system). The following examples of drug classifications serve as a glossary of terms that describe some basic drug actions. As you read some of the examples, remember that a drug classified as one type of agent may have other uses and actions in other body systems. For example, a drug classified as a diuretic may also be an antihypertensive drug, and a vasodilator may also be a respiratory antispasmodic. It takes time to understand not only the basic classification of a particular drug, but also the many secondary uses and effects the drug has on the human body.

Examples of Drug Classifications

Adrenergics
Desired effects: Cause vasoconstriction (i.e., narrowing of the **lumen** of a blood vessel); dilate pupils and bronchioles; relax muscles of the GI and urinary tracts.
Examples: *Adrenergics used to treat hypotension:* isoproterenol (Isuprel); norepinephrine (Levophed). *Adrenergics used for nasal and ophthalmic decongestion:* naphazoline (Naphcon); phenylephrine (Neo-Synephrine); pseudoephedrine (Sudafed); tetrahydrozoline (Visine).
Indications for use: Stop superficial bleeding; raise and sustain blood pressure; relieve nasal congestion and relieve redness, burning, irritation, and dryness of the eyes.
Side effects and adverse reactions: Chest pain, tachycardia, headache, increased blood glucose levels, nervousness, tremors.

Adrenergic Blockers
Desired effects: Cause vasodilation; reduce blood pressure; increase muscle tone of GI walls.
Examples: valsartan (Diovan); propranolol (Inderal); atenolol (Tenormin); carvedilol (Coreg); tamsulosin (Flomax); metoprolol (Lopressor).
Indications for use: Control hypertension and peripheral vascular disease; treat prostatic hyperplasia.

Side effects and adverse reactions: Confusion, lowering of blood pressure, lowering of blood glucose levels, fatigue, reduced heart rate.

Analgesics
Desired effects: Reduce the sensory function of the brain; block pain receptors.
Examples: *Nonnarcotic OTCs:* aspirin; acetaminophen (Tylenol); ibuprofen (Advil, Motrin). *Narcotic:* hydrocodone w/APAP (Tylenol with codeine); oxycodone (OxyContin); meperidine (Demerol); hydrocodone (Vicodin).
Indications for use: Relieve pain.
Side effects and adverse reactions: *Nonnarcotic:* GI disorders, liver and kidney disorders, tinnitus. *Narcotic:* Suppression of vital signs, agitation, blurred vision, confusion, constipation, oversedation, restlessness.

Anesthetics
Desired effects: Produce insensibility to pain or the sensation of pain; block nerve impulses to the brain, resulting in unconsciousness; dilate pupils; lower blood pressure; reduce respiratory and pulse rates.
Examples: *Local:* benzocaine (Dermoplast, Solarcaine); lidocaine (Xylocaine); bupivacaine (Marcaine); lidocaine topical (Lidoderm); procaine (Novocain). *General:* midazolam (Versed).
Indications for use: Produce local anesthesia (absence of sensation without loss of consciousness) or general anesthesia (loss of consciousness).
Side effects and adverse reactions: Hypotension, cardiopulmonary depression, sedation, nausea, vomiting, headaches.

Antacids/Proton-Pump Inhibitors
Desired effect: Reduce acidity in the stomach.
Examples: omeprazole (Prilosec); esomeprazole (Nexium); rabeprazole (Aciphex); lansoprazole (Prevacid); pantoprazole (Protonix). *OTCs:* magaldrate (Riopan); calcium carbonate (Maalox).
Indications for use: Treat gastric hyperacidity; treatment of gastroesophageal reflux disease (GERD).
Side effects and adverse reactions: Constipation, diarrhea, electrolyte imbalance, flatulence, kidney stones, osteoporosis.

Antianxiety Agents
Desired effects: Reduce anxiety and tension.
Examples: chlordiazepoxide (Librium); clonazepam (Klonopin); chlorazepate (Tranxene); diazepam (Valium); alprazolam (Xanax); temazepam (Restoril); triazolam (Halcion).
Indications for use: Produce calmness and release muscle tension; sedation.
Side effects and adverse reactions: Agitation, amnesia, bizarre behaviors, confusion, reduced white blood cell (WBC) count, depression, drowsiness, lethargy, oversedation, tremors, photosensitivity.

Antibiotics
Desired effects: Kill or inhibit growth of microorganisms.
Examples: azithromycin (Zithromax); levofloxacin (Levaquin); cefaclor (Ceclor); tetracycline (Sumycin); amoxicillin (Amoxil);

amoxicillin/clavulanic acid (Augmentin); cefadroxil (Duricef); ciprofloxacin (Cipro); cephalexin (Keflex); doxycycline (Vibramycin).

Indications for use: Treat bacterial invasions and infections.

Side effects and adverse reactions: Hypersensitivity reaction, nausea, diarrhea, GI distress, light sensitivity, urticaria.

Anticholinergics

Desired effects: Parasympathetic blocking agents; reduce spasms in smooth muscles.

Examples: scopolamine or atropine sulfate; tiotropium inhalation (Spiriva); dicyclomine (Bentyl); ipratropium (Atrovent).

Indications for use: Dry secretions before surgery; prevent bronchospasm.

Side effects and adverse reactions: Blurred vision, confusion, reduced GI and genitourinary motility, dilation of pupils, fever, flushing, headache, increased heart rate.

Anticoagulants

Desired effects: Delay or block clotting of blood.

Examples: rivaroxaban (Xarelto); heparin; enoxaparin sodium (Lovenox); warfarin sodium (Coumadin); tinzaparin (Innohep).

Primary uses: Treat blood clots, thrombophlebitis; prevent clot formation.

Side effects and adverse reactions: Increased bleeding; blood irregularities; GI, liver, and kidney disease.

Anticonvulsants

Desired effects: Prevent seizures; reduce excessive stimulation of the brain.

Examples: clonazepam (Klonopin); gabapentin (Neurontin); phenytoin (Dilantin); phenobarbital; carbamazepine (Tegretol); lamotrigine (Lamictal); pregabalin (Lyrica); topiramate (Topamax); valproic acid (Depakene).

Indications for use: Treat epilepsy and other neurologic disorders (e.g., peripheral neuropathy).

Side effects and adverse reactions: Sedation, vertigo, visual disturbances, GI disturbances, liver complications.

Antidepressants

Desired effect: Treat depression.

Examples: venlafaxine hydrochloride (Effexor); sertraline (Zoloft); escitalopram (Lexapro); duloxetine (Cymbalta); bupropion (Wellbutrin); trazodone HCl (Desyrel); fluoxetine (Prozac); imipramine pamoate (Tofranil); amitriptyline (Elavil); citalopram (Celexa).

Indications for use: Elevate mood; treat other neurologic disorders (e.g., migraines).

Side effects and adverse reactions: Anorexia, anxiety, sexual dysfunction, fatigue, drowsiness, vertigo, weight gain, confusion, blurred vision.

Antiemetics

Desired effect: Act on hypothalamic center in the brain to reduce or prevent nausea and vomiting.

Examples: prochlorperazine (Compazine); trimethobenzamide (Tigan); metoclopramide (Reglan); granisetron (Kytril); ondansetron (Zofran); promethazine (Phenergan).

Indications for use: Prevent and relieve nausea and vomiting; manage motion sickness.

Side effects and adverse reactions: Dry mouth, sedation, drowsiness, diarrhea, blurred vision.

Antifungals

Desired effects: Slow or retard multiplication of fungi.

Examples: miconazole (Monistat); nystatin (Mycostatin); fluconazole (Diflucan); ketoconazole (Nizoral); terbinafine (Lamisil).

Indications for use: Treat systemic or local fungal infections.

Side effects and adverse reactions: Anemia, chills, hypotension, vertigo, fever, kidney and liver damage, malaise, photophobia, muscle and joint pain.

Antihistamines

Desired effects: Counteract the effects of histamine by blocking action in tissues; may be used to inhibit gastric secretions.

Examples: cetirizine (Zyrtec); fexofenadine (Allegra); loratadine (Claritin, Alavert); chlorpheniramine (Chlor-Trimeton); diphenhydramine (Benadryl); promethazine (Phenergan); cimetidine (Tagamet); ranitidine (Zantac).

Indications for use: Relieve allergies; prevent gastric ulcers.

Side effects and adverse reactions: CNS depression, muscle weakness, epigastric distress, dry mouth.

Antihypertensive Agents

Desired effects: Block nerve impulses that cause arteries to constrict; slow the heart rate, reducing its contractility; restrict the hormone aldosterone in the blood.

Examples: amlodipine (Norvasc); atenolol (Tenormin); doxazosin mesylate (Cardura); metoprolol (Lopressor or Toprol); methyldopa (Aldomet); valsartan (Diovan); amlodipine plus benazepril (Lotrel); propranolol (Inderal); diltiazem (Cardizem); nifedipine (Procardia); benazepril (Lotensin); lisinopril (Prinivil, Zestril); losartan (Cozaar).

Indications for use: Reduce and control blood pressure.

Side effects and adverse reactions: Headache, vertigo, GI disturbances, rash, hypotension, nonproductive cough.

Antiinflammatory Agents

Desired effect: Reduce inflammation.

Examples: *Nonsteroidal antiinflammatory drugs (NSAIDs):* ibuprofen (Advil, Motrin); naproxen (Naprosyn); celecoxib (Celebrex); indomethacin (Indocin). *Steroidal antiinflammatory drugs (SAIDs):* dexamethasone (Decadron); prednisone (Cortisone); methylprednisolone (Medrol, Depo-Medrol); montelukast sodium (Singulair); fluticasone propionate (Flonase); mometasone (Nasonex). *Inhalers:* flunisolide (AeroBid); triamcinolone (Azmacort).

Indications for use: Treat arthritis and other inflammatory disorders, including asthma and allergic rhinitis.

Side effects and adverse reactions: GI upset, GI bleeding, hepatitis, drowsiness, tinnitus, irregular heart rate, kidney disorders.

Antimigraine Agents

Desired effect: Alter circulation to the brain.

Examples: topiramate (Topamax); sumatriptan (Imitrex); zolmitriptan (Zomig).

Indications for use: Treatment or prevention of migraine headaches.

Side effects and adverse reactions: Confusion, psychomotor slowing, difficulty concentrating, memory problems, rare but serious cardiac events.

Antineoplastics

Desired effects: Inhibit development of and destroy cancerous cells.

Examples: hydroxyurea (Hydrea); cyclophosphamide (Cytoxan); chlorambucil (Leukeran); raloxifene (Evista).

Indications for use: Cancer chemotherapy and/or prevention.

Side effects and adverse reactions: Nausea, vomiting, bone marrow depression, aplastic anemia, hair loss, GI ulcers.

Antipsychotics

Desired effect: Alter chemical actions in the brain.

Examples: quetiapine (Seroquel); risperidone (Risperdal); aripiprazole (Abilify); olanzapine (Zyprexa); chlorpromazine (Thorazine); haloperidol (Haldol).

Indications for use: Treat the symptoms of schizophrenia and bipolar disorder.

Side effects and adverse reactions: GI distress, hypotension, electrocardiographic (ECG) changes, vertigo, sedation, headache, photosensitivity.

Antipruritics

Desired effect: Relieve itching.

Examples: calamine lotion; hydrocortisone ointment; diphenhydramine (Benadryl).

Indications for use: Treat allergies or topical exposures that cause itching.

Side effects and adverse reactions: Topical agents have no side effects; Benadryl can cause vertigo, sedation, and nervousness.

Antipyretics

Desired effect: Lower body temperature.

Examples: aspirin; acetaminophen; ibuprofen.

Indications for use: Reduce fever.

Side effects and adverse reactions: GI disturbance, liver disease; with aspirin, possibility of Reye's syndrome if given during or after a viral disease.

Antispasmodics

Desired effects: Relieve or prevent spasms from musculoskeletal injury or inflammation.

Examples: methocarbamol (Robaxin); carisoprodol (Soma); cyclobenzaprine (Flexeril).

Indications for use: Treat sports injuries.

Side effects and adverse reactions: CNS suppression, drowsiness, vertigo.

Antitussives

Desired effect: Inhibit the cough center.

Examples: *Narcotic:* codeine sulfate. *Nonnarcotic:* dextromethorphan (Robitussin DM).

Indications for use: Temporarily suppress a nonproductive cough; reduce the thickness of secretions.

Side effects and adverse reactions: Codeine cough suppressants cause CNS depression and constipation.

Antiviral Agents

Desired effects: Inhibit the growth or reduce the spread of viral cells.

Examples: interferon beta-1a (Avonex); sofosbuvir (Sovaldi); dimethyl fumarate (Tecfidera); acyclovir (Zovirax); interferon; valacyclovir (Valtrex); oseltamivir (Tamiflu); famciclovir (Famvir); includes the human immunodeficiency virus (HIV) medications efavirenz, emtricitabine, and tenofovir (Atripla); emtricitabine and tenofovir (Truvada); darunavir (Prezista).

Indications for use: Treat viral infections, including oral and genital herpes, influenza, and HIV.

Side effects and adverse reactions: Confusion, diarrhea, headache, kidney disease, urticaria, vomiting.

Bronchodilators

Desired effect: Relax the smooth muscle of the bronchi.

Examples: theophylline (Theo-Dur); epinephrine (Adrenalin); albuterol (Ventolin HFA, Proventil, ProAir HFA); budesonide and formoterol (Symbicort); isoproterenol (Isuprel).

Indications for use: Treat asthma, bronchospasm; promote bronchodilation.

Side effects and adverse reactions: CNS stimulation, tremors, tachycardia, increased blood glucose level, elevated blood pressure.

Cathartics (Laxatives)

Desired effect: Increase peristaltic activity of the large intestine.

Examples: magnesium hydroxide (Milk of Magnesia); bisacodyl (Dulcolax); casanthranol (Peri-Colace).

Indications for use: Increase and hasten bowel evacuation (defecation).

Side effects and adverse reactions: Nausea, bloating, flatulence, cramping.

Central Nervous System Stimulants

Desired effects: Affect chemicals in the brain that contribute to hyperactivity and impulse control.

Examples: methylphenidate (Concerta, Ritalin); modafinil (Provigil); lisdexamfetamine (Vyvanse).

Indications for use: Treat attention deficit disorder (ADD) and attention deficit/hyperactivity disorder (ADHD).

Side effects and adverse reactions: Irregular heartbeat, rash, sore throat, aggression, hypertension, numbness, fainting.

Contraceptives

Desired effect: Inhibit conception.

Examples: medroxyprogesterone acetate (Depo Provera); Ortho Evra; etonogestrel/ethinyl estradiol (NuvaRing).

Indications for use: Prevent pregnancy.

Side effects and adverse reactions: Breast enlargement and tenderness; cardiovascular risk; GI upset; headache; irregular menstrual bleeding; deep vein thrombosis; pulmonary embolus (PE).

Decongestants

Desired effect: Relieve local congestion in the tissues.

Examples: ephedrine or phenylephrine (Neo-Synephrine); pseudoephedrine (Sudafed); oxymetazoline (Afrin); mometasone (Nasonex).

Indications for use: Relieve nasal and sinus congestion caused by common cold, hay fever, or upper respiratory tract disorders.

Side effects and adverse reactions: Arrhythmias, hypertension, headache, nausea, dry mouth.

Diuretics

Desired effects: Inhibit reabsorption of sodium and chloride in the kidneys; promote excretion of excess fluid in the body.

Examples: hydrochlorothiazide (Dyazide, Esidrix, HydroDiuril); furosemide (Lasix); triamterene (Dyrenium).

Indications for use: Increase urinary output; lower blood pressure.

Side effects and adverse reactions: Dehydration, muscle weakness, fatigue, gout, hyperglycemia.

Erectile Dysfunction Agents

Desired effect: Facilitate an erection.

Examples: sildenafil (Viagra); tadalafil (Cialis).

Indications for use: Facilitates an erection in patients with erectile dysfunction (impotence) and symptoms of benign prostatic hypertrophy (enlarged prostate).

Side effects and adverse reactions: Headache, flushing, nasal congestion, myalgia, prolonged erections, vision and hearing problems, cerebrovascular accident (CVA), myocardial infarction (MI).

Expectorants

Desired effect: Liquefy secretions in the bronchial tubes so that they can be coughed out.

Examples: dextromethorphan (Benylin).

Indications for use: Relieve upper respiratory tract congestion.

Side effects and adverse reactions: Vomiting, diarrhea, abdominal pain.

Hematopoietic Agents

Desired effect: Promote red blood cell production.

Examples: epoetin alfa (Epogen, Procrit); pegfilgrastim (Neulasta).

Primary use: Treat anemia in patients undergoing chemotherapy.

Side effects and adverse reactions: Headache, arthralgia, nausea, hypertension, diarrhea.

Hemostatic Agents

Desired effects: Control bleeding; act as a blood coagulant.

Examples: phytonadione, vitamin K; absorbable hemostatic agents (e.g., Gelfoam, Surgicel) are applied directly to a wound.

Indications for use: Control acute or chronic blood-clotting disorder; promote formation of absorbable, artificial clot.

Side effects and adverse reactions: Hypersensitivity reactions, transient flushing, dizziness; newborn hyperbilirubinemia.

Hormone Replacement Agents

Desired effects: Replace hormones or compensate for hormone deficiency.

Examples: insulin (Levemir, NovoLog, Lantus Solostar, Humalog); levothyroxine sodium (Synthroid or Levoxyl); estrogen (Premarin); vasopressin (Pitressin).

Indications for use: Maintain adequate hormone levels.

Side effects and adverse reactions: *Estrogen replacement therapy:* Hot flashes, decreased sex drive, nausea, vomiting.

Hypnotics (Sedatives)

Desired effects: Induce sleep; lessen the activity of the brain.

Examples: zolpidem tartrate (Ambien); eszopiclone (Lunesta); secobarbital (Seconal); flurazepam (Dalmane); temazepam (Restoril); barbiturates.

Indications for use: Treat insomnia; obtain sedation (lower doses).

Side effects and adverse reactions: Daytime sedation, confusion, dry mouth, vertigo.

Lipid-Lowering Agents

Desired effects: Reduce blood cholesterol levels and/or increase high-density lipoprotein (HDL) level.

Examples: atorvastatin calcium (Lipitor); simvastatin (Zocor); ezetimibe (Vytorin or Zetia); rosuvastatin (Crestor); fenofibrate (Tricor).

Indications for use: Reduce low-density lipoprotein (LDL) and very low density lipoprotein (VLDL) levels and triglycerides; increase HDL.

Side effects and adverse reactions: GI discomfort, muscle pain and weakness, liver complications, hypersensitivity, cataracts, myopathy.

Miotics

Desired effect: Cause the pupil to contract.

Examples: carbachol (Isopto Carbachol); pilocarpine (Isopto Carpine).

Indications for use: Counteract pupil dilation.

Side effects and adverse reactions: Corneal edema, clouding, stinging, tearing, headache.

Monoclonal Antibodies

Desired effect: A class of highly specific antibodies that are produced in a laboratory and used to treat cancer and conditions that cause extreme inflammation, such as rheumatoid arthritis and psoriasis.

Examples: adalimumab (Humira); ustekinumab (Stelara); etanercept (Enbrel); trastuzumab (Herceptin); imatinib (Gleevec); fingolimod hydrochloride (Gilenya); infliximab (Remicade); rituximab (Rituxan); pemetrexed (Alimta); glatiramer (Copaxone); bevacizumab (Avastin).

Indications for use: Cancer treatment; treatment of rheumatoid arthritis, psoriasis, Crohn's disease, ulcerative colitis, multiple sclerosis.

Side effects and adverse reactions: Injection site reactions, headache, rash, sinusitis, hypersensitivity, neurologic complications, respiratory infections.

Mydriatic Agents (Anticholinergic)

Desired effect: Dilate the pupil.

Example: atropine sulfate (Isopto Atropine).

Indications for use: Ophthalmologic examinations.

Side effects and adverse reactions: Stinging, burning, photosensitivity.

Narcotics

Desired effects: Depress the CNS, causing insensibility or stupor.

Examples: *Natural narcotics:* opium group (codeine phosphate, morphine sulfate); buprenorphine and naloxone (Suboxone); oxycodone (OxyContin). *Synthetic narcotics:* meperidine (Demerol), methadone (Dolophine).

Indications for use: Relieve pain.

Side effects and adverse reactions: Suppression of vital signs; agitation, blurred vision, confusion, constipation, oversedation, restlessness.

Oral Hypoglycemic Agents

Desired effects: Reduce blood glucose level by increasing insulin production and/or reducing target cell resistance to insulin, or by delaying glucose absorption.

Examples: liraglutide (Victoza 3-Pak); rosiglitazone (Avandia); sitagliptin (Januvia); metformin HCl (Glucophage); acarbose (Precose); chlorpropamide (Diabinese); glimepiride (Amaryl); glipizide (Glucotrol); glyburide (Micronase).

Indications for use: Manage diabetes mellitus type 2.

Side effects and adverse reactions: GI irritation, fatigue, hypoglycemia, vertigo; possible hypersensitivity reactions.

Osteoporosis Agents

Desired effects: Inhibit bone reabsorption and/or promote use of calcium.

Examples: alendronate (Fosamax); risedronate (Actonel); calcitonin (Miacalcin nasal spray and Calcimar); ibandronate (Boniva); raloxifene hydrochloride (Evista); zoledronic acid (Reclast, Zometa).

Indications for use: Promote bone mineral density and reverse progression of osteoporosis.

Side effects and adverse reactions: GI disorders, esophageal irritation.

Respiratory Corticosteroid Agents

Desired effects: Reduce airway inflammation and bronchial resistance.

Examples: fluticasone and salmeterol (Advair Diskus); fluticasone propionate (Flovent HFA); budesonide and formoterol fumarate dehydrate (Symbicort); tiotropium bromide (Spiriva Handihaler); mometasone furoate monohydrate (Nasonex).

Indications for use: Long-term relief of asthma symptoms; decrease frequency of asthma attacks; manage chronic obstructive pulmonary disease (COPD) and seasonal allergies.

Side effects and adverse reactions: Headache, pharyngitis, myalgia, hypersensitivity, oral candidiasis. Advair Diskus is contraindicated in patients with a milk allergy.

Table 26-7 lists details about the top 50 prescribed drugs in 2014. Review this list to become familiar with some of the most commonly prescribed medications. These are just a few examples of the different classifications of medications. Remember to research and review all medications before administering them.

TABLE 26-7	Top 50 Prescribed Drugs in 2014			
BRAND NAME	**CLASSIFICATION**	**INDICATIONS AND DESIRED EFFECTS**	**SIDE EFFECTS**	**ADVERSE REACTIONS**
Synthroid	Thyroid hormone	Increase BMR; enhance gluconeogenesis; stimulate protein synthesis	Reversible hair loss, dry skin, GI intolerance	Overdosage causes signs of hyperthyroidism, cardiac arrhythmias
Crestor	Cholesterol lowering (antihyperlipidemic)	Decrease LDL, VLDL, triglycerides; increase HDL	Pharyngitis, headache, epigastric distress, myalgia	Hypersensitivity, cataracts, myopathy
Nexium	Proton-pump inhibitor	Increase gastric pH; reduce gastric acid production; esophagitis; GERD; *Helicobacter pylori* ulcers	Headache, diarrhea, abdominal pain	Hepatitis, hypersensitivity, decreased WBC count
Ventolin HFA	Bronchodilator	Relieve bronchospasm, reduce airway resistance; can function as a rescue inhaler to relieve immediate symptoms of an asthma attack	Headache, nausea, restlessness, tremors, dizziness, throat irritation, hypertension	Palpitations, tachycardia, slight increase in BP, chest pain
Advair Diskus	Long-acting respiratory corticosteroid agent	Relieve symptoms of asthma; reduce airway resistance	Headache, pharyngitis, URI, myalgia, nausea	Hypersensitivity, palpitations, chest pain, oral candidiasis
Diovan	Antihypertensive	Cause vasodilation; decrease peripheral vessel resistance; decrease BP	Headache, dizziness, viral infection, fatigue, abdominal pain	Hypotension with overdosage, tachycardia, hypersensitivity
Lantus Solostar	Long-acting insulin	Control glucose levels	Localized reaction at injection site, hypokalemia, allergic reaction	Severe hypoglycemia with insulin overdose, diabetic ketoacidosis

Continued

TABLE 26-7 Top 50 Prescribed Drugs in 2014—*continued*

BRAND NAME	CLASSIFICATION	INDICATIONS AND DESIRED EFFECTS	SIDE EFFECTS	ADVERSE REACTIONS
Cymbalta	Antidepressant	Relieve depression	Nausea, dry mouth, diarrhea, insomnia, headache	Increased heart rate, orthostatic hypotension, skin rashes, GI disorders
Vyvanse	Stimulant	Improve attention span; decrease distractibility and impulsive behavior; treat ADHD	Abdominal discomfort and GI symptoms, decreased appetite, headaches, insomnia, dry mouth, dizziness	Cardiovascular complications in patients with heart problems, hypersensitivity; overdosage may cause arrhythmias, seizures, psychosis
Lyrica	Anticonvulsant	Seizure control; treat fibromyalgia; treat pain caused by nerve damage in diabetic neuropathy, herpes zoster (postherpetic neuralgia)	Muscle pain, weakness, or tenderness; vision problems; easy bruising or bleeding; swelling of hands or feet; rapid weight gain	Mood or behavior changes, anxiety, panic attacks, trouble sleeping, hyperactive, increased depression, suicidal thoughts
Humira	Monoclonal antibody	Reduce inflammation and joint destruction in rheumatoid arthritis	Injection site reactions, headache, rash, sinusitis, nausea	Hypersensitivity, neurologic events, respiratory infections and bronchitis
Enbrel	Antirheumatic, immunomodulator, monoclonal antibody	Relieve symptoms of rheumatoid arthritis, psoriasis, and other inflammatory conditions	Injection site reaction, abdominal pain, URI, headache	Infections, heart failure, hypertension, nervous system disorders
Remicade	Antirheumatic, immunomodulator, monoclonal antibodies	Decrease inflamed areas of intestine, synovitis, and joint erosion	Headache, nausea, fatigue, fever	Hypersensitivity, infusion reactions, lupuslike syndrome
Copaxone	Immunosuppressant	Slow progression of MS	Injection site reactions, arthralgia, vasodilation, anxiety	Infection, lymphadenopathy, hypertension, decreased WBC count
Neulasta	Hematopoietic agent	Increase phagocytosis and decrease incidence of infection during chemotherapy	Bone pain, nausea, fatigue, headache, arthralgia	Allergic reactions, spleen complications
Rituxan	Antineoplastic, monoclonal antibodies	Cytotoxicity, reduce tumor size; reduce joint destruction in RA	Fever, chills, headache, angioedema, nausea, rash	Arrhythmias, acute renal failure, hypersensitivity
Spiriva Handihaler	Bronchodilator	Relieve bronchospasm for patients with COPD	Dry mouth, sinusitis, pharyngitis, dyspepsia, UTI, rhinitis	Chest pain, angioedema, hypersensitivity
Januvia	Antidiabetic agent, oral hypoglycemic	Lower blood glucose and A_{1c} levels over time	Headache, nasopharyngitis, URI, hypoglycemia	Overdose causes severe hypoglycemia, pancreatitis, hypersensitivity
Atripla	HIV antiviral combination drug (three drugs)	Decrease viral load	Lactic acidosis, serious liver problems, serious psychiatric problems, kidney disorder, osteopenia, skin discoloration, diarrhea, dizziness, drowsiness	Serious complications from lactic acidosis and liver disorders
Avastin	Antiangiogenic agent, monoclonal antibody	Treatment of metastatic carcinoma of the colon; glioblastoma, and renal cell cancer	Fainting, anorexia, heartburn, diarrhea, weight loss, dry mouth, sores on the skin or in the mouth, voice changes	Gastric ulcers, bleeding, slow wound healing

TABLE 26-7 Top 50 Prescribed Drugs in 2014—*continued*

BRAND NAME	CLASSIFICATION	INDICATIONS AND DESIRED EFFECTS	SIDE EFFECTS	ADVERSE REACTIONS
OxyContin	Analgesic narcotic; contains codeine and acetaminophen	Relieve pain	Sleepiness, dizziness, hypotension, anorexia, constipation	Overdose causes respiratory failure, hepatotoxicity from overdose of acetaminophen; addiction
Epogen	Hematopoietic agent	Stimulate RBC production; raise H&H; treatment of anemia in chemotherapy patients	Fever, diarrhea, nausea, vomiting, edema	Encephalopathy, thrombosis, CVA, MI, seizures
Celebrex	NSAID, analgesic	Reduce inflammation and relieve pain; treatment of RA and other forms of arthritis	GI disorders, URI, back pain, peripheral edema, rash	Increased risk of CV events and GI bleeding
Truvada	HIV (combination of two antiviral drugs)	Prevent HIV cells from multiplying in the body; reduce risk of HIV infection	New infections, GI disorders, chest pain, dry cough, wheezing, cold sores, tachycardia	Hypersensitivity, lactic acidosis
Gleevec	Antineoplastic, monoclonal antibody	Suppress tumor growth	Nausea, diarrhea, vomiting, headache, fluid retention	Severe fluid retention, decreased WBC and platelet counts; pneumonia
Herceptin	Chemotherapeutic agent; adjunct therapy for cancers of the breast or stomach; monoclonal antibody	Interfere with growth and spread of cancer cells in the body	Nausea, diarrhea, weight loss, fever, headache, sleep problems, cough, trouble breathing, skin rash, bruising, cold symptoms	Cardiomyopathy, infusion reactions, embryo-fetal toxicity, pulmonary toxicity
Lucentis	Ophthalmic injection	Keep new blood vessels from forming under the retina; treat wet age-related macular degeneration and diabetic retinopathy	Itchy or watery eyes, dry eyes, swelling of the eyelids, blurred vision, sinus pain, sore throat, joint pain	Hypersensitivity, exophthalmos from increased intraocular pressure, detached retina, CVA, MI
Namenda	Alzheimer's disease	Reduce deterioration in moderate to severe Alzheimer's disease	Dizziness, headache, confusion, constipation, hypertension, cough	AV block, CNS reactions, hypersensitivity
Zetia	Cholesterol lowering (antihyperlipidemic)	Reduce total cholesterol, LDL, triglycerides; increase HDL	URI, headache, back pain, diarrhea, myalgia	None known
Levemir	Long-acting insulin	Control glucose levels	Localized reaction at injection site, hypokalemia, allergic reaction	Severe hypoglycemia with insulin overdose, diabetic ketoacidosis
Symbicort	Glucocorticoid inhaler, long-term treatment of asthma and COPD	Relieve symptoms of asthma and reduce airway resistance	Headache, URI, sore throat, sinusitis, oral candidiasis	Hypersensitivity, palpitations, ECG changes
Sovaldi	Antiviral	Prevent hepatitis C virus cells from multiplying	Headache, fatigue, mild itching, nausea, insomnia	Hypersensitivity, birth defects or death in unborn baby
Novolog	Combination insulin	Control glucose levels	Localized reaction at injection site, hypokalemia, allergic reaction	Severe hypoglycemia with insulin overdose, diabetic ketoacidosis
Tecfidera	Interferon	Treat relapsing multiple sclerosis	Nausea, diarrhea, stomach pain, flushing	Hypersensitivity, serious viral infection of the brain
Suboxone	Opioid narcotic	Treat narcotic addiction; not used as a pain medication	Tongue pain, redness or numbness inside mouth, constipation, headache, insomnia, swelling of arms or legs	Respiratory arrest, addictive, hypersensitivity

Continued

TABLE 26-7   Top 50 Prescribed Drugs in 2014—*continued*

BRAND NAME	CLASSIFICATION	INDICATIONS AND DESIRED EFFECTS	SIDE EFFECTS	ADVERSE REACTIONS
Humalog	Rapid acting or a combination insulin	Control glucose levels	Localized reaction at injection site, hypokalemia, allergic reaction	Severe hypoglycemia with insulin overdose, diabetic ketoacidosis
Xarelto	Anticoagulant	Prevent new clot formation	Bleeding, pruritus, pain in extremities, muscle spasms	Hemorrhage, hypersensitivity
Seroquel XR	Extended-release antipsychotic	Manage psychotic disorders and schizophrenia; adjunct antidepressant	Headache, sleepiness, dizziness, constipation, orthostatic hypotension	Heart block, hypokalemia, tachycardia
Viagra	Erectile dysfunction (ED) agent	Facilitate an erection	Headache, flushing, nasal congestion, UTI, diarrhea	Severe hypotension, prolonged erections, vision problems, CVA, MI
Alimta	Chemotherapeutic agent	Treatment of lung cancer; interfere with growth and spread of cancer cells in the body	Fatigue, anorexia, weight loss, N/V, diarrhea, rash, hair loss.	Hypersensitivity, kidney and liver damage
Victoza 3-Pak	Antidiabetic agent	Lower blood glucose and A$_{1c}$	Headache, nausea, diarrhea, GERD	Severe hypoglycemia, pancreatitis, hypersensitivity
Avonex	Interferon antiviral	Treatment of relapsing-remitting MS	Headache, flulike symptoms, myalgia, URI, generalized pain, sinusitis	Anemia, rare life-threatening reactions
Nasonex	Corticosteroid allergy agent	Decrease response to seasonal allergens; stabilize asthma	Nasal irritation, sore throat, headache	Hypersensitivity, stimulates wheezing in asthmatics
Cialis	ED agent	Facilitate erection in ED	Headache, myalgia, flushing, nasal congestion	Prolonged erections, vision and hearing problems, CVA, MI
Gilenya	Biologic response modifier, MS agent	Reduce progression of MS	Headache, flulike symptoms, diarrhea, back pain	Increased risk of infections, CVA, hypersensitivity, dyspnea
Stelara	Immunomodulator, antipsoriatic agent, monoclonal antibody	Reduce inflammation, scaling of psoriasis plaques	Headache, fatigue, nasopharyngitis, URI	Hypersensitivity, risk of skin cancer, neurologic complications
Flovent HFA	Corticosteroid inhaler	Prevent or control inflammation and asthma	Throat and nasal irritation, dry mouth, candidiasis	Anaphylaxis, glaucoma, nasal septal perforation
Prezista	Antiretroviral; protease inhibitor	Interrupt HIV replication; slow progression of HIV infection	Diarrhea, abdominal pain, headache, rash, N/V	Immune system reactions, pancreatitis, serious skin rashes, hepatitis
Procrit	Hematopoietic agent, erythropoiesis-stimulating agent (ESA)	Promote production of RBCs to raise H&H; treatment of anemia in chemotherapy patients	Fever, diarrhea, N/V, edema	Encephalopathy, thrombosis, CVA, MI, seizures
Isentress	Antiviral; integrase inhibitor	Prevents HIV cells from multiplying; treatment of HIV strains that are resistant to multiple antiretroviral drugs and for people with drug-sensitive HIV strains	Diarrhea, nausea, headache	Increase in total cholesterol, rash, increased liver enzymes, increased blood glucose, psychiatric disorders

www.medscape.com/viewarticle/825053; and www.webmd.com/news/20140805/top-10-drugs.
ADHD, Attention deficit/hyperactivity disorder; *AV,* atrioventricular; *BMR,* basal metabolic rate; *BP,* blood pressure; *CNS,* central nervous system; *COPD,* chronic obstructive pulmonary disease; *CV,* cardiovascular; *CVA,* cerebrovascular accident; *ECG,* electrocardiogram; *GERD,* gastroesophageal reflux disease; *GI,* gastrointestinal; *HCV,* hepatitis C virus; *HDL,* high-density lipoprotein; *H&H,* hemoglobin and hematocrit; *HIV,* human immunodeficiency virus; *LDL,* low-density lipoprotein; *MI,* myocardial infarction; *MS,* multiple sclerosis; *NSAID,* nonsteroidal antiinflammatory drug; *N/V,* nausea and vomiting; *RA,* rheumatoid arthritis; *RBC,* red blood cells; *URI,* upper respiratory infection; *UTI,* urinary tract infection; *VLDL,* very low density lipoprotein; *WBC,* white blood cells.

HERBAL AND ALTERNATIVE THERAPIES

The use of alternative therapies, often called *complementary* or *holistic medicine,* has become very popular in the United States. According to estimates, more than 42% of adult patients use some form of alternative therapy, such as herbal medicine, acupuncture, massage therapy, chiropractic care, or mind-body therapies. Even though only limited scientific studies prove the effectiveness of herbs, their use to relieve the symptoms of common patient complaints is definitely on the rise. It is estimated that 15 million adults take prescription drugs along with herbal and vitamin supplements. Patients typically are hesitant to discuss their use of herbal products with their provider, which makes it difficult for providers to assess potential drug-herb interactions. Therefore, it is important that medical assistants become familiar with common alternative therapies and that they include questions about the use of these therapies when gathering information about the patient's medication history.

Herbal Products

Regulation of Herbal Products

Herbal medicine uses plant-based products to promote health and treat the symptoms of a wide range of diseases. These remedies typically are marketed by manufacturers and are regulated by the federal government as dietary supplements. The FDA is responsible for regulating dietary supplements under the Dietary Supplement Health and Education Act of 1994 (DSHEA). Under DSHEA, manufacturers are responsible for performing tests and ensuring the safety of dietary supplements before they are sold. However, these products are not registered with the FDA and do not have to go through the rigorous process of FDA approval that new drugs face before they are produced and sold. In addition, there is no federal control over the standardization of herbal dietary supplements. Pharmaceutical companies must prove that each batch of a drug is standardized or consistent with previous batches. Because this is not the case with dietary supplements, there are no guarantees that the amounts of active ingredients in a herbal supplement remain the same over time or are similar to the amounts found in the same supplement produced by a different company.

The FDA has the authority to oversee the manufacture of domestically made and foreign-made supplements. Supplement manufacturers must provide evidence that their products actually contain what the labels claim and that the products are free of contaminants. According to FDA regulations, dietary supplement labels must list the following:

- Product name with the word "supplement" on the label
- Name and location of the manufacturer or distributor
- Structure/function claim: Claims of specific benefits may be made, but the following statement must be included: *This statement has not been evaluated by the Food and Drug Administration. This product is not intended to diagnose, treat, cure, or prevent any disease.*
- Directions for use
- For plant-based herbal preparations: the name of the plant or the part of the plant used
- For blended products created by the manufacturer: the components and the weight of each ingredient

- All nondietary ingredients (e.g., fillers, artificial colors, sweeteners, flavors), listed in descending order of weight
- The label may include warnings about use, but the lack of cautionary statements does not mean that no adverse effects are associated with the supplement.

Commonly Used Herbal Products

Table 26-8 summarizes the most commonly used herbal products. Information about herbal remedies is constantly changing, but the federal government has several websites that can be used as references. These include the National Center for Complementary and Alternative Medicine (*http://nccam.nih.gov/*) and the National Institutes of Health Office of Dietary Supplements (*http://ods.od.nih.gov/index.aspx*).

Alternative Therapies

Acupuncture

Acupuncture treatments are part of traditional Chinese medicine, which is based on the concept that disease is caused by a disruption in the flow of life force and an imbalance between yin and yang. In acupuncture treatments, thin metal needles are inserted through the skin to stimulate specific points in the body to restore and maintain health. Studies indicate that acupuncture may help reduce pain and relieve the nausea associated with chemotherapy treatments. Therapy involves a series of treatments, with the placement of as many as 12 needles in various locations on the body.

During the procedure, the patient is placed supine, prone, or in the Sims position, depending on the needle insertion site. Although the procedure is not painful, the patient may notice a sharp sensation when the needles initially are placed. After the needles have been in place for a time, they may be rotated gently, heated, or electrically stimulated to achieve the benefit sought by the treatment. The needles usually are left in place for 5 to 20 minutes, and after they have been removed, the provider typically discusses the results of treatment with the patient.

Chiropractic Care

Chiropractic providers apply techniques that focus on the body's physical structure (usually the spine) and perform manipulations or anatomic adjustments to correct alignment problems and help the body heal itself. Many patients combine chiropractic therapy with conventional medical treatment to obtain relief of chronic pain in the lower back and neck and to relieve persistent headaches. Chiropractors must earn a Doctor of Chiropractic degree at an accredited college and pass a state licensing examination before they can practice. Besides spinal adjustments, patient treatment plans may include a combination of hot and cold therapies; electrical stimulation; rest and rehabilitation exercises; dietary and lifestyle counseling; and the use of dietary supplements.

Mind-Body Therapy

Mind-body therapy uses biofeedback to teach patients to use their thoughts to control certain body reactions. It is based on the scientific principle that our thoughts can influence the body's involuntary functions. For example, a child experiencing the sudden onset of an asthma attack may become extremely anxious because he or she is having serious difficulty breathing. Panic and anxiety increase the

TABLE 26-8	Commonly Used Herbal Products	
NAME	**USES**	**SIDE EFFECTS AND CAUTIONS**
Acai	Weight loss and antiaging; antioxidant	Little scientific information about the safety of acai; no scientific evidence to support use for any health-related purpose; might affect magnetic resonance imaging (MRI) results.
Black cohosh	Relieve symptoms of menopause; treat menstrual irregularities and premenstrual syndrome; induce labor	Headaches, gastric complaints, heaviness in the legs, weight problems; safety unknown for pregnant women or those with breast cancer.
Echinacea	Treat or prevent colds, flu, and other infections; believed to stimulate the immune system	Most studies indicate echinacea does not appear to prevent colds or other infections; some people experience allergic reactions, including rashes, increased asthma, and anaphylaxis; gastrointestinal (GI) side effects.
Flaxseed	Laxative; treat hot flashes and breast pain; flaxseed oil used to treat arthritis; both flaxseed and flaxseed oil used to treat high cholesterol levels and prevent cancer	Few reported side effects; contains soluble fiber (such as that found in oat bran) and is an effective laxative; should be taken with plenty of water; may diminish body's ability to absorb medications taken by mouth; should not be taken at same time as oral medications.
Garlic	Treat high cholesterol, heart disease, hypertension; prevent certain types of cancer, including stomach and colon cancer	Some evidence indicates garlic can slightly lower blood cholesterol levels and may slow development of atherosclerosis; side effects include breath and body odor, heartburn, GI upset, and allergic reactions; acts as a mild anticoagulant (similar to aspirin); may be a problem during or after surgery—avoid dietary and supplemental garlic for at least 1 week before surgery; interferes with effectiveness of saquinavir, a drug used to treat human immunodeficiency virus (HIV) infection.
Ginger	Treat stomach aches, nausea, diarrhea; ginger extract is a component of many cold and flu dietary supplements; used to alleviate nausea associated with postoperative state, motion sickness, chemotherapy, and pregnancy; used for rheumatoid arthritis, osteoarthritis, and joint and muscle pain	Short-term use can safely relieve pregnancy-related nausea and vomiting; side effects most often reported are gas, bloating, heartburn, and nausea.
Asian ginseng	Support overall health and boost immune system; improve mental and physical performance; treat erectile dysfunction, hepatitis C, and menopause symptoms; lower blood glucose and control blood pressure	Some studies show ginseng may lower blood glucose and possibly boost immune function; when taken by mouth, it usually is well tolerated; most common side effects are headaches, sleep disorders, GI problems, and possible allergic reactions; patients with diabetes using medications for treatment should use ginseng with caution.
Ginkgo biloba	Treat a variety of conditions, including asthma, bronchitis, fatigue, and tinnitus (ringing or roaring sounds in the ears); typically used to improve memory; treat or help prevent Alzheimer's disease and other types of dementia; reduce intermittent claudication (leg pain caused by narrowing arteries); treat sexual dysfunction and multiple sclerosis	Research indicates that ginkgo is ineffective in treating Alzheimer's disease, dementia, and intermittent claudication; side effects may include headache, nausea, GI upset, diarrhea, dizziness, or allergic skin reactions; severe allergic reactions occasionally are reported; can increase bleeding risk, so people who take anticoagulant drugs, have bleeding disorders, or have scheduled surgery or dental procedures should use caution; uncooked ginkgo seeds contain a toxic chemical that can cause seizures.
Glucosamine plus chondroitin sulfate	Natural substances found in and around the cells of cartilage; used to treat arthritis and joint pain	Recent study shows participants with moderate to severe pain had significant relief with the combined supplement. Most common side effect is GI upset.
Green tea	Prevent and treat a variety of cancers and for mental alertness, weight loss, lowering cholesterol levels, and protecting skin from sun damage; laboratory studies suggest may help protect against or slow the growth of certain cancers	Safe in moderate amounts; possible complications include liver problems with concentrated green tea extracts but not when used as a beverage; contains caffeine; contains small amounts of vitamin K, which can make anticoagulant drugs less effective.

TABLE 26-8   Commonly Used Herbal Products—*continued*

NAME	USES	SIDE EFFECTS AND CAUTIONS
Melatonin	Treatment of sleep disorders	May help individuals with normal sleep patterns but has limited or no effect on those with sleep disorders. Most common side effects are nausea and drowsiness.
Milk thistle (silymarin)	Promote liver health, treat cirrhosis, chronic hepatitis, and gallbladder disorders; lower cholesterol; reduce insulin resistance	Studies suggest it may benefit the liver; associated with fewer and milder symptoms of liver disease in patients with hepatitis C; may lower blood glucose levels; can cause allergic reaction.
Saw palmetto	Primarily used to treat urinary symptoms associated with an enlarged prostate gland; also used for chronic pelvic pain, bladder disorders, reduced sex drive, hair loss, and hormone imbalance	Studies suggest it may be effective for treating prostate symptoms, but no evidence indicates that it reduces the size of an enlarged prostate; does not appear to affect readings of prostate-specific antigen (PSA) level, which is used as screening tool for cancer of the prostate; may cause mild GI upset, tender breasts, and decline in sexual desire in male patients.
St. John's wort	Traditionally used to treat mental disorders and nerve pain; may be used as a sedative; treatment for malaria; balm for wounds, burns, and insect bites; currently used for depression, anxiety, and/or sleep disorders	Some scientific evidence shows it helps treat mild to moderate depression; not effective in treating major depression. Side effects include photophobia (increased sensitivity to sunlight), anxiety, dry mouth, dizziness, GI symptoms, fatigue, headache, and sexual dysfunction. Affects the way the body processes or breaks down many drugs; may speed or slow a drug's metabolism. Combined with certain antidepressants, it may increase side effects such as nausea, anxiety, headache, and confusion. Drugs that can be affected include: • Antidepressants • Birth control pills • Cyclosporine (prevents rejection of transplants) • Digoxin (strengthens myocardial contractions) • Indinavir and possibly other drugs used for HIV • Irinotecan and possibly other drugs used to treat cancer • Warfarin and related anticoagulants St. John's wort is not a proven therapy for depression. If depression is not adequately treated, it can become severe.

Modified from the National Center for Complementary and Alternative Medicine. *https://nccih.nih.gov/health/herbsataglance.htm.* Accessed May 26, 2015.

urgency to breathe. If the child can be taught to relax and keep breathing at a normal rate, the asthma attack will not be influenced by the child's anxiety, and medications taken to relieve bronchospasm will be more effective.

Biofeedback specialists use special monitoring equipment to demonstrate the body's reaction to certain stimuli and to help teach patients how to control physical responses to stress. During a biofeedback session, the provider applies electrical sensors to various locations on the body. These sensors monitor and provide feedback about the body's physiologic responses to stress. For example, if a patient is experiencing chronic tension headaches, the sensors demonstrate that the headache is just part of overall muscular tension. Tension that is registering throughout the body may cause a beeping sound or lights flashing from the equipment as a cue for the patient to associate muscular tension with development of the headache. The goal is to help patients recognize that one body action results in another. Once this goal has been achieved, patients are taught

relaxation techniques designed to prevent the stressful response. Biofeedback methods are effective in managing multiple stress-related conditions, including muscle tension, headaches, chronic low back pain, altered heart rates, and hypertension.

Homeopathic Medicine

Homeopathy, or homeopathic medicine, is a medical approach that was developed in Germany over 200 years ago. The primary principle of homeopathic medicine is to administer very dilute substances that are designed to stimulate the body's ability to heal itself. Homeopaths work individually with clients to administer the lowest dose of medication possible, believing that the lower the dose, the more effective the treatment. Remedies are created from plants, minerals, or animals, and include red onion, arnica (mountain herb), and stinging nettle plant.

Homeopaths assess clients holistically and gather details on individual and family health histories, body type, and current physical, emotional, and mental symptoms. Treatments are specifically designed for each client; therefore, it is not unusual for people with the same condition to have different treatment protocols. People seek homeopathic assistance for a wide range of health problems, including allergies, asthma, chronic fatigue syndrome, depression, digestive disorders, ear infections, headaches, and skin rashes.

Homeopathic remedies are regulated in the same manner as OTC drugs. They do not have to comply with the strict testing guidelines required for prescription drugs. However, the FDA does require that homeopathic remedies meet strength, purity, and packaging standards. Labels must identify at least one health condition that the remedy can treat, provide an ingredient list, indicate the dilution of the ingredients, and explain safety instructions.

Homeopathic therapies are not known to interfere with prescription and OTC medications; however, it is important to gather information from patients about the use of homeopathic remedies and to document the details in the patient's record for the provider to review.

CLOSING COMMENTS

Patient Education

It is important for the patient to be aware of the effects a drug may have and should have on his or her system. The medical assistant plays an important role in helping patients understand their medications, promoting compliance with treatment, and preventing complications. Depending on the facility's policies, the administrative medical assistant may be expected to do many of the following tasks when gathering initial information from patients. These points should be considered when gathering a medication history and documenting in the patient's health record.

- Make a comprehensive list of all medications, including OTC agents and alternative therapies that the patient uses regularly.
- Ask female patients whether they are pregnant or breast-feeding.
- Preassess the patient for any adverse effects, such as drug allergies and drug-drug or drug-food interactions.
- Observe the patient for any adverse effects for a minimum of 20 minutes after administration of a medication in the office; also, inform the patient of possible adverse reactions to the medication that may occur at home.
- Discuss with the patient how and when the prescribed drug is to be taken, and whether any special storage precautions are required.
- Reassess that the patient is taking the medication properly.
- Provide comfort, encouragement, and guidance to patients to ensure their understanding, safety, and cooperation while using drug therapy.
- Answer any questions the patient may have. Remember: If you are not sure of the answer, consult the prescribing provider.

Therapeutic Communication with Patients from Diverse Cultures

Health beliefs can affect compliance with medication therapy. Patients from various cultures may be using home remedies or herbal treatments that could interfere with the effectiveness and safety of medications prescribed by the provider. Guidelines that the medical assistant may find helpful include the following:

- Investigate the healing practices of the primary cultures in your area so that you are better equipped to discuss these practices with your patients.
- Encourage cultural sensitivity in your co-workers.
- Provide patients with educational materials in their native language.
- Ask patients if they are using home remedies or are consulting a healer from their culture. If so, get as much detail as possible so that you can share this information with the provider.

Legal and Ethical Issues

The medical assistant plays a key role in the management of controlled substances in the ambulatory care setting. It is important that all rules for record keeping, inventory, prescribing, dispensing, and documenting scheduled drugs are followed according to state and federal regulations. The medical assistant may be responsible for requesting the provider's initial DEA registration and for continuing certification renewal. The area DEA office can provide instructions on this. Each DEA number is specific to a site, so multiple practice locations require a DEA number for each facility.

Accurate, complete documentation is essential for correct management of patient medications. Each time the patient is prescribed or administered a medication, complete details must be included in the patient's record using approved medical terminology and abbreviations. Failure to do this may result in a serious error that could harm the patient and result in litigation.

HIPAA Applications

According to the Health Insurance Portability and Accountability Act (HIPAA), patients have the right to request restrictions on the disclosure of protected health information (PHI) for treatment, payment, and healthcare operations (TPO). For example, if a patient has a history of substance abuse and this information is not pertinent to current TPO circumstances, the patient can request that this information not be disclosed. The facility does not have to agree to the patient's request; however, a process must be established within the practice to review the demand and explain the provider's decision to the patient. If the provider agrees not to release this information, the specific restriction must be documented in the patient's record, and staff members must review and comply with the restrictions each time material is sent out of the facility for TPO purposes.

Professional Behaviors

Participation in drug therapy requires absolute accuracy from the medical assistant. There is no room for error when gathering a medication history, documenting in the patient's health record, and understanding the purpose and effects of prescribed drugs. When a medical assistant performs his or her duties with accuracy, the message is sent that this is a professional who is dedicated to quality care and patient safety. Both the provider and patient rely on the medical assistant to possess accurate information about drug therapy and perform medication-related duties with meticulous care.

Kathy has a great deal of responsibility in managing medications in the primary care practice where she works. She must be familiar with and follow DEA regulations governing the management of controlled substances. In addition, she must be able to use drug reference materials; identify the general clinical uses of prescribed drugs and OTC products; understand the parts of a prescription and use accepted medical terms and abbreviations; recognize the significance of patient education in the safe use of OTC drugs; and understand the factors that affect drug action.

SUMMARY OF LEARNING OBJECTIVES

1. **Define, spell, and pronounce the terms listed in the vocabulary.**
Spelling and pronouncing medical terms correctly reinforce the medical assistant's credibility. Knowing the definitions of these terms promotes confidence in communication with patients and co-workers.

2. **Do the following related to government regulation of medications in the United States:**
- *Distinguish among the government agencies that regulate drugs in the United States.*
Several federal agencies combine forces to regulate drugs in the United States. The FDA regulates the development and sale of all prescription and OTC drugs; the DEA enforces laws designed to prevent drug abuse and educates the public about drug abuse prevention; and the FTC regulates OTC advertisement.
- *Cite the areas covered in the regulations established by the DEA for the management of controlled or regulated substances.*
DEA regulations for the management of controlled substances include specific record-keeping guidelines, in addition to information on physician registration and the inventory, storage, and disposal of controlled substances.
- *List the DEA regulations for prescription drugs for each of the five schedules of the Controlled Substances Act.*
Prescriptions written for controlled substances must comply with both state and federal regulations. The prescription must include details about the patient; information about the physician, including the DEA number; and the amount of the drug, written out ("ten" not "10"). The prescription must be manually or electronically signed by the physician. Orders for Schedule II drugs cannot be phoned in except in an absolute emergency, and these prescriptions cannot be refilled. Schedules III, IV, and V drugs may be prescribed by phone, faxed, or e-prescribed and refilled up to five times in a 6-month period. In some states, Schedule V drugs can be dispensed by the pharmacist without a physician's prescription. (See Table 26-1.)

3. **Explain the medical assistant's role in preventing drug abuse.**
The medical assistant should keep track of patients who repeatedly call for prescription refills of controlled substances; secure computers so there is no access to e prescription programs and keep prescription pads secure; and maintain a small supply of controlled substances in the office and accurately record their administration.

4. **Differentiate a drug's chemical, generic, and trade names.**
The chemical name is the drug's formula. The generic (official) name is assigned to the drug and may reflect the chemical name. The trade (brand) name is given to the compound by the pharmaceutical company that developed it and is protected by law for 20 years.

5. **Describe the use of drug reference materials, and explain the five pregnancy risk categories for drugs.**
The use of drug reference materials is crucial for the safe administration of medications. Most drug references include actions, indications, contraindications, precautions, adverse reactions, dosage, administration guidelines, and method of packaging. The most frequently used drug reference guide is the *Physicians' Desk Reference* (PDR), but package inserts also can be used. A number of websites provide FDA-approved information about medications such as Rxlist at *http://www.rxlist.com/script/main/hp.asp* and *Drugs.com* at *http://www.drugs.com/*. Table 26-2 presents the FDA's five pregnancy risk categories for drugs.

6. **Discuss tips for studying pharmacology, and define the five medical terms used to describe the clinical use of drugs.**
Clinically, drugs are used as therapeutic medications (to cure a condition); palliative medications (to relieve symptoms); prophylactic medications (to prevent the occurrence of a condition); diagnostic medications (to help determine the cause of a disease); and replacement medications (to provide substances that normally occur in the body).

7. **Cite safety measures for the use of OTC drugs.**
OTC drugs may interfere or interact with prescription drugs. Some safety measures for the use of OTC drugs include carefully reading directions, taking only the recommended dose, discarding the drug when it expires, informing the provider of OTC drug use, and being aware of contraindications to OTC drug use in certain conditions. (Refer to Table 26-3.)

8. **Do the following related to prescription drugs:**
- *Diagram the parts of a prescription.*
A prescription consists of the following six parts: (1) superscription, (2) inscription, (3) subscription, (4) signature, (5) refill information, and (6) provider's signature. A prescription also must provide the patient's name and address and the date the drug is prescribed.
- *Demonstrate the ability to transcribe a prescription accurately.*
Procedure 26-1 outlines the method for transcribing a prescription for the physician's signature. It is important that the medical assistant follow a written order; look up information about the medication in a drug reference text or online; ask the patient about drug allergies and record the patient's personal information on the prescription note; and correctly write the name of the drug, form, dosage, strength, route of administration, amount of the drug to be given to the patient, specifics about time of administration if appropriate, and the number

Continued

SUMMARY OF LEARNING OBJECTIVES—*continued*

of refills. The prescription should be reviewed and signed by the provider before it is given to the patient or before the medical assistant transmits an electronic prescription. (Refer to Tables 26-4 and 26-5 to review common prescription abbreviations and The Joint Commission's "Do Not Use" list.)

- *Describe e-prescription methods.*

   EHR systems can be used to create a prescription, print a paper copy of it, and/or send it directly to a pharmacy. EHR programs are designed to automatically check a prescribed drug against the patient's allergies, identify possible drug-drug interactions, access current databases for the patient's medication history, review the patient's insurance drug formulary for coverage, and either print out the prescription for the patient to take to the pharmacy or electronically send the script to the pharmacy.

9. **Relate the principles of pharmacokinetics to drug use.**

   Pharmacokinetics comprises the actions of absorption, which depends on the route of administration (oral, parenteral, mucous membrane, or topical); distribution through the bloodstream; metabolism in the liver; and excretion, primarily by the kidneys.

10. **Describe factors that affect the action of a drug, including the physiologic changes associated with aging.**

   Multiple factors affect a drug's action, including weight, age, gender, diurnal rhythms, pathologic factors, immune responses, psychological factors, tolerance, accumulation, idiosyncrasy, and drug-drug interactions. (Refer to Table 26-6 for the effects of aging on the body's processing of medications.)

11. **Identify the classifications of drug actions.**

   Drugs are classified into groups according to their actions in the body, by the symptoms they relieve, or according to the body system they affect. Drugs may have multiple actions and therefore multiple classifications.

(Refer to Table 26-7 for a summary of the top 50 prescribed drugs in 2014.)

12. **Differentiate among commonly used herbal remedies and alternative therapies.**

   Table 26-8 summarizes common herbal remedies, their uses, and possible side effects. Acupuncture treatments involve the use of thin metal needles inserted through the skin to stimulate specific points in the body to restore and maintain health. Chiropractic providers perform manipulations or anatomic adjustments to correct alignment problems and help the body heal itself. Mind-body therapy uses biofeedback to teach the patient to use his or her thoughts to control certain body reactions. The primary principle of homeopathic medicine is to administer very dilute substances that are designed to stimulate the body's ability to heal itself.

13. **Examine the role of the medical assistant in drug therapy education.**

   The medical assistant plays an important role in helping patients understand their medications, promoting compliance with treatment, and preventing complications. Conducting comprehensive interviews that ask detailed questions about patient use of drugs and documenting this information in the health record provides vital information for the provider. Culturally sensitive interviews with patients help the medical assistant gather details about home remedies and patient belief systems that may affect compliance with drug therapy.

14. **Identify the medical assistant's legal responsibilities in medication management in an ambulatory care setting.**

   The medical assistant's legal responsibilities in medication management include documenting compliance with DEA regulations for controlled substances; maintaining complete and accurate documentation on all medications administered and prescribed for each patient; and following HIPAA regulations on the release of confidential information.

CONNECTIONS

Study Guide Connection: Go to the Chapter 26 Study Guide. Read and complete the activities.

evolve Evolve Connection: Go to the Chapter 26 link at *evolve.elsevier.com/kinn* to complete the Chapter Review Quiz. Check out the other resources listed for this chapter to make the most of what you have learned from Principles of Pharmacology.

PHARMACOLOGY MATH

27

SCENARIO

Heather Izacco, a recent graduate of a medical assistant program in the area, has just been hired by a local family practice physician, Dr. Carlos Angio. One of her responsibilities will be to administer medications under Dr. Angio's supervision. Heather is confident of her ability to administer medications but is unsure of her accuracy in pharmacology math. Heather never did well in math at school and had a difficult time calculating accurate doses and converting between math systems during her medical assisting training. Her supervisor, Mrs. Allison, suggests that Heather review the math section of her textbook at home and be prepared to work out some sample problems next week.

While studying this chapter, think about the following questions:

- How can Heather be sure that she has calculated the correct dosages?
- What are the parts of a drug label, and why are they important?
- Is it critical for Heather to be able to convert dosages from one system to another?
- Are there any differences between calculating an adult dose and calculating a pediatric dose?
- How would Heather go about reconstituting an injectable powder?
- How can Heather's ability to analyze tables prove useful when she is performing pharmacology math?

LEARNING OBJECTIVES

1. Define, spell, and pronounce the terms listed in the vocabulary.
2. Summarize the important parts of a drug label.
3. Demonstrate knowledge of basic math computations.
4. Define basic units of measurement in the metric and household systems.
5. Convert among measurement systems.
6. Do the following when calculating drug dosages for administration:
   - Demonstrate knowledge of basic match computations by calculating the correct dose amount.
- Calculate proper dosages of medication for administration while using mathematical computations.
7. Determine accurate pediatric doses of medication.
8. Summarize how to reconstitute powdered injectable medications.
9. Specify the legal and ethical responsibilities of a medical assistant in calculating drug dosages.

VOCABULARY

dispense To prepare a drug for administration.

unit dose Method used by the pharmacy to prepare individual doses of medication; a dose of medicine prepared in an individual packet for convenience or safety, such as blister packs.

Medical assistants are responsible for being absolutely certain that the medication they prepare and administer to a patient is exactly what the provider ordered. Although drugs often are delivered by the pharmacy or supplied by pharmaceutical representatives in **unit dose** packs, the dosage ordered may differ from the dosage on hand. In this case, the medical assistant must be prepared to calculate the correct dose accurately before dispensing and administering the medication. There is never a margin of error in drug calculations; even a minor mistake may result in serious complications for the patient. The medical assistant, therefore, must take meticulous care in calculating all drug dosages.

DRUG LABELS

The first step in safely calculating a drug dosage is to accurately read the label of the drug on hand to determine whether the provider's order and the packaged drug are in the same system of measurement. Starting at the top, the label shows the drug's name with the brand name capitalized and typically in bold print. The brand name is copyright protected; therefore, it is followed by an ® symbol that indicates the U.S. government has granted a Federal Registration Certificate for the drug. The generic name is printed in lower case letters under the brand name in smaller print. A patent is granted on a drug for 20 years from the date of filing for the patent. Patents are granted at any point in time along the development of a drug. *Exclusivity* is granted by the Food and Drug Administration (FDA) to give exclusive marketing rights to the manufacturers of the drug when it earns FDA approval. This exclusive marketing right can vary from 3 to 5 years. If a medication has been on the market longer than 20 years or after the exclusive rights to the drug have expired, the generic name may be the only one listed (e.g., meperidine instead of Demerol, diazepam rather than Valium). If the medication is ordered from the pharmacy and stocked as a generic drug, only the generic name is printed on the label. In the label examples in Figure 27-1, Cardizem is the brand name of the generic drug diltiazem HCl; on the second label, cephalexin is the generic name for Keflex, and because patent and exclusivity protections have ended, only the generic name is listed on the label.

Under the name of the drug, the dosage strength of the medication is given. Whether listed in milligrams (mg), milliliters (mL), or another unit of measure, the label states how much of the drug is contained in each of the identified units. This is what you must compare with the provider's order to determine whether you must calculate the amount to administer to match the ordered dose of the drug. For example, the provider orders 250 mg of cephalexin, and the label states that the dosage strength is 250 mg per 5 mL; in this case, no calculation is needed—you simply administer 5 mL of the medication. However, if the provider orders 500 mg of the medication for a *loading dose* of the antibiotic, you must make sure you administer the correct amount of the medication to match the order. Sometimes the label helps by providing different but equivalent units of measurement for the dosage strength. For example, if the provider orders 250 mg of cephalexin and asks you to make sure the mother understands how much of the medication she should administer to her sick child, the label may state that 5 mL is equivalent to 1 teaspoon (according to the label, 250 mg of the drug is present in 5 mL of solution); therefore, you can confirm with the parent that the child should receive 1 teaspoon of medication without having to do any calculations.

The label identifies the *route,* or method of administration, for the drug. If the medication is packaged as a tablet or a capsule, it should be given orally; liquid medication is labeled either for oral or for parenteral use. If the drug is powdered *(solute)* and it must be mixed with a liquid *(solvent)* before administration, the label provides instructions on how to prepare the medication. At the bottom of the label is the total amount of the drug contained in the package. For example, the cephalexin label in Figure 27-1 identifies it as a multidose bottle that contains 200 mL of total volume when

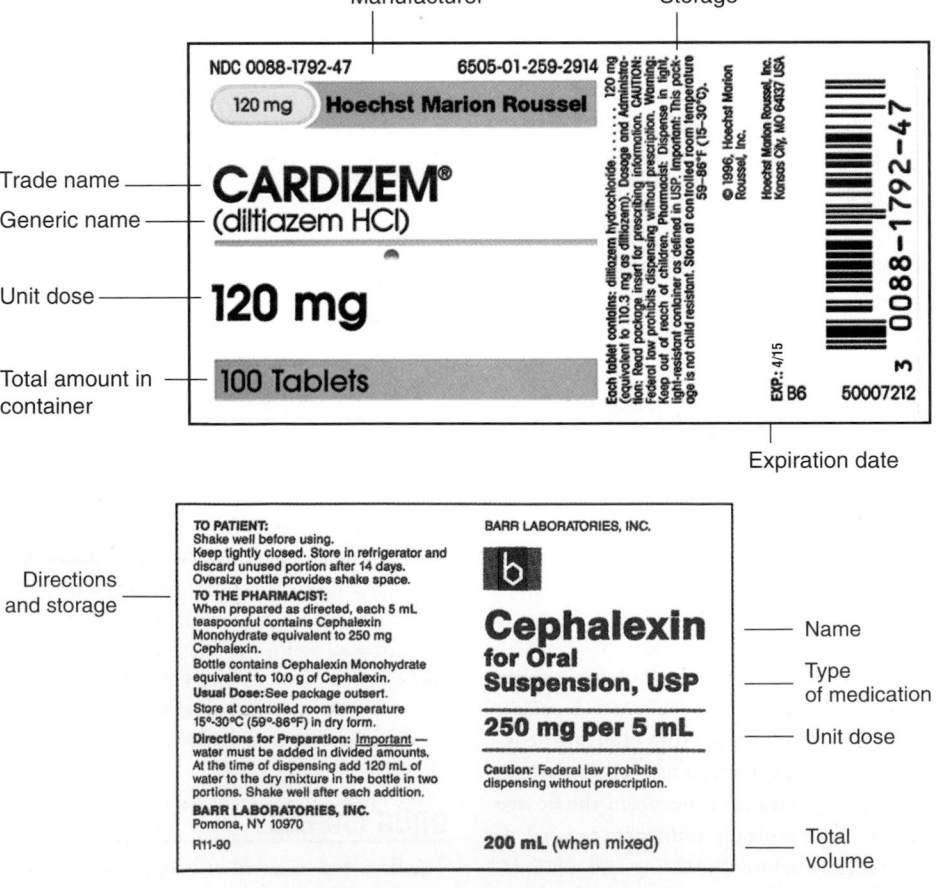

FIGURE 27-1 Drug labels. (From Brown M, Mulholland JM: *Drug calculations: process and problems for clinical practice,* ed 9, St Louis, 2012, Mosby.)

mixed (e.g., 250 mg of cephalexin in each 5 mL of solution). A single-dose bottle would contain one dose of the medication. In the cephalexin example, that would be 250 mg in 5 mL of solution; therefore, a single-dose bottle would contain 5 mL, or 1 teaspoon, of cephalexin. Special storage precautions, such as light or heat sensitivity, are identified on the back or side of the drug container.

The name of the drug's manufacturer appears on the label, as does an expiration date that must be checked each time the medication is dispensed. Dispose of all medications that have reached the label's expiration date. The label also has a lot number stamped on the package so that it can be identified as belonging to a batch of drugs manufactured at the same time. This number becomes important if problems are noted with a particular batch and the medication is recalled. Depending on your employer's preferences, you may need to include the lot number in the documentation of the medication in the patient's record. For example, the lot number of immunization containers must be documented in the facility's vaccination log and the patient's health record for each dose administered. Finally, federal law requires that all labels have a National Drug Code (NDC) number that identifies that particular drug.

Some of the basic information provided on drug labels includes the following:
- *Strength:* The potency of the drug, stated as a percentage of drug in the solution (2% epinephrine); as a solid weight—grams (g), milligrams (mg), micrograms (mcg); or as a milli-equivalent (mEq) or unit.
- *Dose:* The size or amount of the drug available in the drug package. This could be expressed in milliliters, teaspoons, or number of tablets. For example, the label may read "Imitrex, 6 mg/0.5 mL," which means that there is 6 mg of the drug in each 0.5 mL of liquid.
- *Solute:* The pure drug that is dissolved in a liquid to form a solution.
- *Solvent* or *diluent:* The liquid (usually sterile water or sterile saline) that dissolves the solute.

MATH BASICS

You may need to review some basics of arithmetic before you tackle drug calculations. You must thoroughly understand the addition, subtraction, multiplication, and division of fractions and decimals; the relationship of decimals and fractions; and how they are converted from one to the other.

Fractions

A fraction is a part of a whole; that is, fractions are a way of dividing a whole unit into parts. For example, think of dividing a small cherry pie into equal parts for friends after dinner. Four people want dessert, so you can divide the pie into four equal parts; each person receives ¼ of the pie. If only three people want dessert, you can divide the pie into three equal parts; each person receives ⅓ of the pie.

The top number in a fraction is the *numerator,* and the bottom number is the *denominator.* In a *proper fraction,* the numerator is smaller than the denominator. If we go back to the pie example, ¼ and ⅓ of the pie are proper fractions.

In *improper fractions,* the numerator is equal to or greater than the denominator. Another way of looking at improper fractions is

that the numerator is so large it is equal to or greater than 1. For example, the improper fraction ⁵⁄₄ is greater than 1. It is equal to ⁴⁄₄ (the entire pie that was cut into 4 pieces, or 1 whole pie) plus ¼ of another pie. Therefore, if you wanted everyone to have ¼ of a pie for dessert, you would need two pies: one whole pie for four guests (⁴⁄₄) and ¼ of another pie for yourself (1¼ pies). To convert improper fractions into whole numbers, divide the numerator by the denominator. In this case, you need five ¼-pieces of pie, or: 5 ÷ 4 = 1¼ pies.

Review the following examples. Identify the proper and improper fractions. If the fraction is improper, perform the math to get the whole number equivalent.

½ _____   ⅜ _____
⅔ _____   ⁶⁄₄ _____
⁹⁄₁₀ _____   ¹⁴⁄₁₂ _____

Fractions typically are written in their lowest terms. For example, can you reduce the fraction ⁵⁄₁₅ to its lowest term? To reduce a fraction, you must divide the numerator and the denominator by the largest number that goes into each equally. In the case of ⁵⁄₁₅, 5 divides into 5 (numerator) 1 time, and into 15 (denominator) 3 times; this means that ⁵⁄₁₅ can be reduced to ⅓. Other examples include the following:

$$\frac{25}{100} \div \frac{25}{25} = \frac{1}{4} \qquad \frac{9}{45} \div \frac{9}{9} = \frac{1}{5}$$

$$\frac{30}{100} \div \frac{10}{10} = \frac{3}{10} \qquad \frac{6}{8} \div \frac{2}{2} = \frac{3}{4}$$

In some cases, you may have to multiply fractions. For example, let's say you want to multiply ⅓ times ¾. All you have to do is multiply the two numerators (1 × 3) and the two denominators (3 × 4), and then reduce the answer to its lowest terms. After multiplying the numerators and denominators, you have ³⁄₁₂. Now we must reduce that fraction to its lowest terms. Three is the largest number that will divide equally into 3 and 12; therefore, divide the numerator by 3 (3 ÷ 3 = 1) and the denominator by 3 (12 ÷ 3 = 4); the final answer is ¼. The problem can be written in a mathematical "sentence" as follows:

$$\frac{1}{3} \times \frac{3}{4} = \frac{3}{12} = \frac{1}{4}$$

To divide fractions, you must *invert* the divisor (the second fraction) and then multiply the numerators and denominators.

Consider this problem: ⅓ ÷ ¾. The divisor, we know, is ¾, and we also know we must invert it to multiply the numerators and denominators; the problem now is stated: ⅓ × ⁴⁄₃. Next, we multiply the numerators (1 × 4 = 4) and the denominators (3 × 3 = 9) to get the answer: ⁴⁄₉; this fraction cannot be reduced and thus is the final answer.

Decimals

A decimal is similar to a fraction, but it is expressed in units of tenths (0.1), hundredths (0.01), and thousandths (0.001). To perform drug calculations, fractions first must be converted into decimals.

To convert a fraction into a decimal, simply divide the numerator by the denominator.

For example, rather than ordering ¾ of a dose for a patient, the provider orders the decimal equivalent. To perform this math, you may need to add zeroes after the decimal point at the end of the numerator.

$$\frac{3}{4} = 3 \div 4 = 0.75$$

If the answer is less than a whole number, it is crucial to place a zero before the decimal point to prevent a medication error. For example, if you are to administer .5 mL of a medication and the zero is not placed before the decimal point, you may miss the decimal point and think that the correct dose is 5 mL. Also, a zero should never be placed after the decimal point of a whole number. Mathematically, a whole number such as 1 mL is actually 1.0 mL. However, if the decimal point and a zero follow the whole number, the dose may be misinterpreted as 10 mL.

Percent

A percent is a number expressed as part of 100. Decimal numbers can be converted to percentages by dividing the number by 100 *or* by simply moving the decimal point *two spaces to the right*. For example:

$$0.25 = \frac{25}{100} = 25\% \qquad 0.48 = \frac{48}{100} = 48\%$$

$$0.03 = \frac{3}{100} = 3\% \qquad 0.005 = \frac{5}{1,000} = 0.5\%$$

Another way of converting decimals into percentages is simply to move the decimal point two spaces to the right. This works because a percentage is based on an expression of 100.

0.43 (move the decimal point two places to the right) = 43%

0.014 (move the decimal point two places to the right) = 1.4%

0.06 (move the decimal point two places to the right) = 6%

0.5 (move the decimal point two places to the right) = 50%

Ratio and Proportion

A ratio is one way of expressing a fraction or a division problem; it shows the relationship of the numerator to the denominator. The comparison of two ratios is called a *proportion*. A proportion is written as follows:

$$\frac{4}{16} = \frac{1}{4} \text{ or } 4:16 = 1:4$$

This is read as 4 divided by 16 equals 1 divided by 4, or 4 is to 16 as 1 is to 4.

The provider's order for a medication may be a ratio that is different from that of the medication in stock. To determine the correct proportion for administration, the ordered ratio must be compared with the available ratio (what is in stock).

The preceding proportion example has all the answers in it; there is nothing to solve. In calculating dosages, mathematical proportions are used, but with one element unknown. We must solve for that unknown, or *x*. For example:

$$\frac{4}{16} = \frac{1}{x} \text{ or } 4:16 = 1:x$$

This is read as 4 divided by 16 equals 1 divided by x , or 4 is to 16 as 1 is to x.

In a proportion, the problem is always solved by cross-multiplication. Do not confuse this with plain multiplication. An equals sign (=) between two fractions always means that in order to solve for *x*, you must cross-multiply.

Step 1. Set up the equation.

$$\frac{4}{16} = \frac{1}{x}$$

Step 2. Multiply across the equation.

$$4 \times x = 16 \times 1$$

Step 3

$$4x = 16$$

We now know what 4*x* equals, but next we must find what 1*x*, or *x*, equals. To find the value of *x*, we must find a way to leave *x* (or 1*x*) alone on the left side of the equation. We can change 4*x* to 1*x* by dividing the number 4 by itself. However, whatever we do on one side of an equation, we must do on the other side, or the equation will not be equal anymore. Therefore, we also divide 16 by 4:

Step 4

$$4x \div 4 = 1x \quad \text{and} \quad 16 \div 4 = 4$$

$$1x = 4$$

$$\text{Therefore:} \quad x = 4$$

If we go back to our original problem:

$$\frac{4}{16} = \frac{1}{x}, \text{ then } \frac{4}{16} = \frac{1}{4}$$

Another way to make sure your proportion answer is correct is to check your answer by multiplying the *means* (the middle numbers of the equation) and the *extremes* (the outer numbers of the equation). If your answer is correct, multiplication of the means and extremes produces answers that are equal. For example:

$$3:5 = 6:x$$

If the problem is solved by cross-multiplication, the equation looks like this:

$$\frac{3}{5} = \frac{6}{x}$$

After cross-multiplying, we have:

$$3x = 30 \text{ (then divide each side by 3 to find } x)$$

$$x = 10$$

Having found *x*, we can now complete our original equation:

$$3:5 = 6:10$$

TABLE 27-1   Mathematical Equivalents

PERCENT	DECIMAL	FRACTION	RATIO
25	0.25	$^{25}/_{100} = \frac{1}{4}$	1:4
50	0.5	$^{5}/_{10} = \frac{1}{2}$	1:2
60	0.6	$^{6}/_{10} = \frac{3}{5}$	3:5
0.5	0.005	$^{5}/_{1,000} = \frac{1}{200}$	1:200
0.1	0.001	$^{1}/_{1,000}$	1:1,000
85	0.85	$^{85}/_{100} = ^{17}/_{20}$	17:20
1	0.01	$^{1}/_{100}$	1:100

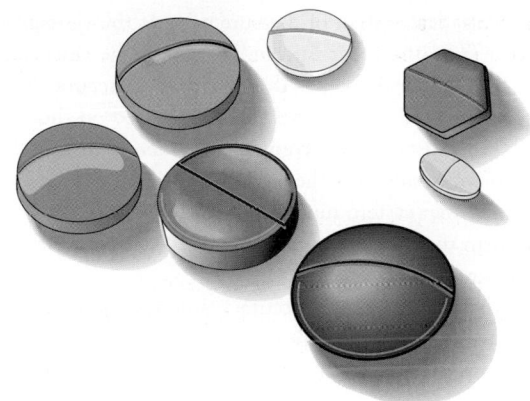

FIGURE 27-2 Examples of scored tablets. (From Fulcher EM, Fulcher RM, Soto CD: *Pharmacology: principles and applications,* ed 3, St Louis, 2012, Saunders.)

To check the accuracy of your equation, multiply the means (5 × 6 = 30) and the extremes (3 × 10 = 30). Because the answers are equal, you know you have the correct proportion. Table 27-1 provides some examples of the relationships between percents, decimals, fractions, and ratios.

Determine the following equivalents:

0.20 = _____ (percent) = _____ (fraction) = _____ (ratio)
37% = _____ (decimal) = _____ (fraction) = _____ (ratio)
$\frac{2}{3}$ = _____ (ratio)   = _____ (percent) = _____ (decimal)
3:4 = _____ (fraction) = _____ (decimal) = _____ (percent)

Rounding Calculations

What should you do if the dose of the supplied drug does not exactly match your calculation? For example, what if you calculate a tablet dose as 1.75 tabs, but you have only whole tablets available? First, check your calculation for accuracy, then check the stocked supply of the drug to make sure no other dosages are available. If the calculation is correct and no other dosages of the drug are available, you will have to round your answer to the nearest amount that matches the dose available. *If the last number in the decimal calculation is 0.5 or greater, round up to the next whole number.* For 1.75 tablets, 0.75 would be rounded up to 1, and the patient should be given two tabs of the medication. However, *make sure you check with the provider before administering a rounded dose of medication.*

Determine the correct doses for the following examples:

1.2 tabs = _____ tablet(s)   1.55 tabs = _____ tablet(s)
1.37 tabs = _____ tablet(s)   0.56 tab = _____ tablet
1.64 tabs = _____ tablet(s)   0.81 tab = _____ tablet

Some tablets are *scored,* which means that the medication was manufactured with an impression or groove down the center of the tablet. This type of tablet can be accurately divided into two equal parts; therefore, calculations can be rounded to the closest half-tab (Figure 27-2). For example, 0.4 tab would be rounded up to one half of a scored tab, and 1.7 tabs would be 2 tabs. *Never* give a partial

dose of a tablet unless the tablet has been scored; if the tablet has been scored, then the dose can be given rounded to the nearest $\frac{1}{2}$.

If a liquid medication is to be administered, it usually is acceptable to round the dose to the *nearest tenth.* Rounding calculations to the nearest tenth is acceptable because most syringes used to administer injected medications are calibrated by 0.1 mL.

For example, say that the correct calculation for an injection of an antibiotic is 1.76 mL. First, note that the 6 is in the hundredths position, and the 7 is in the tenths position. The hundredths number (6) is 5 or greater, so you round up the tenths number (7), which increases by one to 8. Therefore, a 1.76 mL calculation, when rounded to the nearest tenth, equals 1.8 mL of the drug.

There are two important *exceptions* to this rule:

- The injection is to be given to a pediatric patient, and accurate doses for children may be much smaller than adult doses.
- The dose is less than 1 mL and the syringe you are using is calibrated in hundredths (e.g., syringes used for allergy shots or TB tests); in these cases, the medication is rounded to the nearest hundredth.

What are the correct doses of the following medications, rounded to the nearest tenth?

1.47 cc = _____ cc   1.33 mL = _____ mL
2.62 mL = _____ mL   2.15 cc = _____ cc
1.08 mL = _____ mL   1.15 mL = _____ mL

What are the correct doses of the following medications, rounded to the nearest hundredth?

0.078 mL = _____ mL   0.231 mL = _____ mL
0.146 mL = _____ mL   0.937 mL = _____ mL

SYSTEMS OF MEASUREMENT

If the dosage ordered by the provider is different from the dosage on hand, the medical assistant must follow three basic steps to calculate the prescribed dose accurately:

1. Compare the system printed on the drug label with the provider's order to determine whether the order is in the same

mathematical system of measurement. If the systems are different (e.g., the order is in milliliters but the label states that the medication is prepared in teaspoons), accurately convert the order so that it matches the system used on the label. The medical assistant must convert the ordered dose to the measurement system on the drug label (i.e., what is available) because that system must be used to **dispense** the drug.

2. Perform the calculation in equation form using the appropriate formula.

3. Check your answer for accuracy and ask someone you trust to confirm your calculations.

All three steps must be completed before the medication is dispensed and administered. Confirm your calculations with the provider if you have any doubt of their accuracy.

Two different systems of measurement are used for medications: the metric system and the household system. In the ambulatory care setting, the provider orders the drug using the metric system, and drug labels represent the strength of the drug in the metric system; however, the pharmacist will convert the metric dose into a household measurement so that patients can accurately dispense the drug at home. The provider may ask the medical assistant to include the household measurement of the prescribed dose when he or she educates the patient about home administration of the medication. Table 27-2 presents abbreviations and symbols used in the metric and household systems.

Metric System

The metric system of weights and measures is used throughout the world as the primary system for weight (grams), volume (liters), and length (meters). In the United States, the metric system is used for scientific work, including most tasks involving pharmaceuticals.

The metric system of weights and measures is a decimal system based on the number 10, and all calculations are completed by moving decimal points to the right or to the left. Each higher measure is 10 times the measure at hand; each lower measure is 0.1 ($\frac{1}{10}$) the measure. The basic units are multiplied or divided by units of 10. The fraction is always written as a decimal, and the number precedes the letters designating the actual measure. Thus 1½ liters would be written 1.5 L. The cubic centimeter (cc) and the milliliter (mL) are interchangeable; however, The Joint Commission advises against the use of the *cc* abbreviation in documenting medications in the patient's record.

In the metric system, 1 cc is a measurement of area, and an area this size holds exactly 1 mL, or 0.001 ($\frac{1}{1,000}$) of a liter of fluid. The milliliter (mL) measures the *amount* of liquid medication, or the volume, that is to be given orally or by injection. The gram (g) measures the weight, or *strength,* of a solid medication, such as a tablet, powder, or topical preparation. The meter is the measurement for *length* in the metric system. A meter is equal to 39.37 inches, which is slightly longer than a yard, or 3.28 feet. One inch is equal to 2.54 centimeters (cm). The medical assistant may use centimeter measurements when using a wound device to determine the depth and borders of a wound.

The units of measurement in the metric system are based on their prefixes: *kilo-* means 1,000, and *milli-* means 0.001. The prefixes mean the same whether used to measure volume or weight. For example, a kilogram (kg) is 1,000 grams (g), and a kiloliter (kL) is 1,000 liters (L); a milligram (mg) is 0.001($\frac{1}{1,000}$) of a gram, and a milliliter (mL) is 0.001 ($\frac{1}{1,000}$) of a liter.

Conversions within the metric system may be necessary if the provider orders a unit that is different from the one on the drug label. One method of converting units of measurement in the metric system is by moving the decimal point in multiples of 10. For example, when converting grams to milligrams you are converting a large unit (grams) into a smaller unit (milligrams, which are 0.001 or $\frac{1}{1,000}$ of the larger unit). There are 1,000 mg in each gram of the drug. When *larger units of measurement are converted to smaller ones* (in this example, grams to mg) the answer is a larger number, so the *decimal point is moved three places to the right* (0.35 g = 350 mg). When *smaller units of measurement are converted to larger ones* (mg to grams), the answer is a smaller number, so the *decimal point is moved three places to the left* (e.g., 150 mL = 0.15 L). If converting mg to micrograms (mcg) you are converting a larger unit of measurement to a smaller one (1 mg = 1,000 mcg), so move the decimal point three places to the right (0.04 mg = 40 mcg). When converting mcg to mg (a smaller unit to a larger unit of measurement) move the decimal point three places to the left (130 mcg = 0.13 mg).

Another way of converting amounts in the metric system is to multiply or divide the ordered amount by a unit of 10. For example, say you want to convert 0.35 g into milligrams. Think it through: 0.35 is part of a gram; you want to convert it to milligrams (larger unit to a smaller one, therefore the answer will be a larger number); there are 1,000 milligrams in 1 gram. So, to convert 0.35 g into mg, multiply 0.35 by 1,000, which equals 350 mg. Consider these additional examples:

- To convert the smaller unit of milliliters (150 mL) into liters, you divide the number of milliliters by 1,000 (there are 1,000 ml in 1 L); this gives you 0.15 L.

TABLE 27-2 Common Pharmacology Abbreviations and Symbols			
METRIC SYSTEM		**HOUSEHOLD MEASUREMENTS**	
Kg, kg	kilogram	gtt	drop
g	gram	gtt	drops
mg	milligram	t or tsp	teaspoon
mcg	microgram	T or tbsp	tablespoon
m	meter	oz	ounce
mm	millimeter	fl oz	fluid ounce
cm	centimeter	c	cup
cc	cubic centimeter	qt	quart
L	liter	pt	pint
mL	milliliter	gal	gallon
mEq	milliequivalent	lb	pound

- If you need to convert mg to mcg (there are 1,000 mcg in 1 mg), multiply the number of mg by 1,000 (0.18 mg × 1,000 = 180 mcg).
- To convert mcg to mg, you would divide the number of mcg by 1,000 (462 mcg ÷ 1,000 = 0.462 mg).

As you can see, it is much easier to remember the rules about which direction to move decimal points than it is to perform the math calculation.

The following equivalents can be used to make conversions within the metric system:

1 kg − 1,000 g
1 g = 1,000 mg
1 L = 1,000 mL
1 mg = 1,000 micrograms (mcg)
1 mg = 0.001 g or $\frac{1}{1,000}$ of a gram
1 mL = 0.001 L or $\frac{1}{1,000}$ of a liter

CRITICAL THINKING APPLICATION   27-1

The first problems Heather reviewed were conversions within the metric system. Yesterday, Dr. Angio ordered 0.45 L of a drug, but the label gave the contents in milliliters. How many milliliters should Heather have given? To determine the correct dosage you would move the decimal point 3 places to the right (you are converting from a larger unit of measurement to a smaller one, so your answer will be a larger number); or, you could multiply 0.45 by 1,000 (because there are 1,000 mg in 1 gram). Review the examples below. If your answer is less than a whole number, make sure you place a zero before the decimal point so that the number is not mistaken for a whole number.

Examples:

6 g = 6,000 mg	3,200 mL = 3.2 L
0.6 g = 600 mg	320 mL = 0.32 L
0.06 g = 60 mg	32 mL = 0.032 L

Convert the following measurements:

2.5 g = _____ mg	42 g = _____ mg
0.21 g = _____ mg	150 mcg = _____ mg
1.7 g = _____ mg	55 mg = _____ g
3 mg = _____ mcg	74 L = _____ mL
0.28 L = _____ mL	950 mL = _____ L

TABLE 27-3   Approximate Equivalents for Commonly Used Measures

1 kilogram (kg)	=	2.2 pounds (lb)
1 lb	=	454 grams (g)
1 kilogram (kg)	=	1,000 g
1 g	=	1,000 milligrams (mg)
1 mg	=	1,000 micrograms (mcg)
1 inch (in)	=	2.54 centimeters (cm)
1 cup, or 8 ounces (oz), or 16 tablespoons (T or tbsp)	=	240 mL
16 oz or 2 cups = 1 pint (pt)	=	480 mL
2 pt	=	1 quart (qt)
4 qt	=	1 gallon (gal)
1 oz, or 2 Tbsp, or 6 teaspoons (tsp)	=	30 mL
1 tsp	=	5 mL
1 tbsp	=	15 mL
3 tsp	=	1 tbsp
15 gtt	=	1 mL
1 liter (L)	=	1,000 mL

---

directions using the household measurements of volume. Liquid oral medications are taken by the drop, teaspoon, or tablespoon and are supplied in bottles labeled in ounces or pints. Pediatric medications frequently are packaged as liquids, and the label gives instructions for the medication to be given in household measurements (e.g., teaspoon [tsp], tablespoon [Tbsp]). The medical assistant should know that 1 tsp − 5 mL, and 3 tsp = 1 Tbsp = 15 mL. Based on the household equivalents in Table 27-3 convert the following orders:

2 tsp = _____ mL	8 oz = _____ mL
10 mL = _____ tsp	20 mL = _____ Tbsp
3 mL = _____ tsp	4 Tbsp = _____ mL

Household Measurements

The household system is used in most American homes. This system of measurement is important for a patient at home who has no knowledge of the metric system; however, household measurements are not precise, so they should never be used in the medical setting. Nevertheless, a medical assistant must understand the conversions between medical and household measurements so that the patient can be instructed in how to measure the medication most accurately at home.

The basic measure of weight in the household system is the pound (lb); the basic measure of volume is the drop (gt). Medications are not measured in household weights, but many prescriptions contain

Conversions Among Systems of Measurement

Medication orders may have to be converted from one system to another if the order is written in one system and the drug label is in another. Medical assistants can use tables to help convert measurements from metric to household measurements and vice versa. Tables and charts can be helpful tools in many aspects of healthcare, but you must take the time to analyze the information so that it is processed accurately. You can use the conversions in Table 27-3 to directly convert many measurements, or an equivalent can be chosen and the order mathematically converted to the system on the drug label. The conversion is calculated by multiplication or by division. For example, if the provider orders 0.25 ounce (oz) of a liquid medication but the label states that the unit dose of the drug is 5 g/mL, you must convert the order in ounces to milliliters to know how much of the solution to give the patient.

As Table 27-3 shows, 1 oz equals 30 mL; again, the provider has ordered 0.25 oz, and you must determine how much that is of the medication in stock. Therefore, multiply the amount ordered in ounces (0.25) by 30 (the number of mL in 1 oz) to determine how many milliliters to give the patient.

$$0.25 \times 30 = 7.5 \text{ mL}$$

You can also solve the problem by setting up a proportion:

$$0.25 \text{ oz} : x = 1 \text{ oz} : 30 \text{ mL} \quad or \quad \frac{0.25}{x} = \frac{1}{30}$$

$$x = 0.25 \times 30 = 7.5 \text{ mL}$$

Conversions between units of measurement can be done by placing the numbers in an algebraic formula. We know that 1 oz equals 30 mL, and we are looking for the number of milliliters that is equivalent to 0.25 oz. If the amount ordered is placed on the left side of the equation and the conversion factor on the right side, similar units can be cancelled when cross-multiplied, and we can determine the dose.

$$(\text{Ordered amount}) \; 0.25 \text{ oz} \times \frac{30 \text{ mL}}{1 \text{ oz}} \; (\text{Conversion factor})$$

Cross-multiply and the oz unit cancels out:

$$0.25 \times 30 \text{ mL} = 7.5 \text{ mL}$$

To take it one step further, the label states that there are 5 g of the drug per milliliter; therefore, to determine how many grams of the drug the patient will receive, multiply the number of mL to be administered (7.5) by the number of grams per milliliter (5):

$$7.5 \times 5 = 37.5 \text{ g}$$

The patient will receive 37.5 g of the drug.

How would you convert a metric order for a medication into a household unit of measurement that a parent could administer to a sick child? For example, the provider orders 30 mL of an oral antibiotic. What is the equivalent household unit of measurement? As has been stated previously, 1 tablespoon equals 15 mL. You can determine the answer in two ways. Either divide the order by the conversion factor:

$$30 \text{ mL} \div 15 \text{ mL} = 2 \text{ Tbsp}$$

or set up the problem as an equation with the ordered amount on the left side of the equation and the conversion factor on the right side:

$$\frac{30 \text{ mL}}{x} = \frac{15 \text{ mL}}{1 \text{ Tbsp}}$$
$$15x = 30 \text{ Tbsp}$$
$$x = \frac{30 \text{ Tbsp}}{15} = 2 \text{ Tbsp}$$

Or the problem can be set up as a proportion:

$$30 : x = 15 : 1 \text{ Tbsp}$$
$$15x = 30$$
$$x = 2 \text{ Tbsp}$$

Complete the following conversion problems:
1. A patient scheduled for urinary tract diagnostic tests needs to drink a minimum of 2 L of water over the next 12 hours. How many ounces should the patient drink?
2. A pediatric patient is prescribed 8 mL of amoxicillin qid for 10 days. What is the equivalent dose in household measurements?

CALCULATING DRUG DOSAGES FOR ADMINISTRATION

The correct dosage of a medication may depend on the patient's age, weight, and state of health, or on what other drugs the patient is taking. Frequently the provider orders a medication in a dosage that is different from the dosage of the drug in stock. The difference may be in the system of measurement, the strength, or the form. Formulas and mathematical tables of conversion are available online for calculating the correct dosage of medication to be administered. However, because you need to check the answer to make sure you are administering the dose ordered, it is helpful to look at how the correct calculation is performed, one step at a time.

Calculating Dosages

A standard set of formulas is used for calculating dosages (Procedures 27-1 and 27-2). These formulas use the *strength* (potency) and *dose unit* (amount) of the drug. If the drug label reads "5 g/tab," the strength is 5 grams, and the dose unit is 1 tablet. For liquids, the drug strength is an amount of *solute*, which is dissolved in a liquid called the *solvent*. Therefore, if a vial of injectable drug reads "500 mg/mL," 500 mg (strength) of the drug is present in every milliliter (amount) of liquid.

We can use these two examples and the proportion formula to work out two problems: (1) preparing an injectable medication and (2) determining an oral dose.

Problem 1: Preparing an Injectable Dose
Order: Administer 250 mg of cephalexin IM
Available: A vial marked 500 mg/mL
Standard formula:

$$\frac{\text{Available strength}}{\text{Ordered strength}} = \frac{\text{Available amount}}{\text{Amount to give}}$$

When the standard formula is used, the *Available strength* is the strength of the drug that is written on the medication label. In this case, the cephalexin vial states on the label, "500 mg/mL," meaning there is 500 mg (available strength) of cephalexin in each milliliter of the medication. The *Ordered strength* is the dose ordered by the provider (i.e., 250 mg). The *Available amount* is the amount of the drug that must be used to deliver the strength identified on the label. Because the label states "500 mg/mL," we know that the available amount for 500 mg is 1 mL.

Problem: Given the strength of the drug needed (the provider's order of 250 mg), the amount of fluid to be dispensed must be determined.

Step 1. Set up a proportion with the three known quantities: (1) the strength of the drug in the vial, (2) the unit of fluid in which that strength is contained, and (3) the strength of the drug the provider has ordered for administration.

$$\frac{\text{Strength of the drug in the vial}}{\text{Strength the provider ordered}}$$
$$= \frac{\text{Unit of fluid containing that strength}}{\text{(?) Amount to be given}}$$

Step 2. Now, restate the problem in the standard formula, and put in the corresponding numbers. If you get confused about where to place the numbers in the equation, remember that like units of measurement (in this case, mg) must be placed on the same side of the equation.

$$\frac{\text{Available strength (500)}}{\text{Ordered strength (250)}} = \frac{\text{Available amount (1 mL)}}{\text{Amount to give } (x \text{ mL})}$$

Now, with only the numbers:

$$\frac{500 \text{ mg}}{250 \text{ mg}} = \frac{1 \text{ mL}}{x \text{ mL}}$$

The mg units in the numerator and denominator on the left side of the equation cancel each other out. Cross-multiply the equation:

$$500 \times x = 250 \times 1$$
$$500x = 250 \text{ mL}$$

Step 3. To find *x* (the amount to be given), you must divide each side of the equation by 500.

$$\frac{500x}{500} = \frac{250 \text{ mL}}{500}$$
$$x = \frac{1}{2} \text{ mL} = 0.5 \text{ mL}$$

Solution: Administer 0.5 mL of cephalexin

Problem 2: Determining an Oral Dose

Order: Give 10 mg of a drug
Available: A bottle with tablets labeled 5 mg each
Standard formula:

$$\frac{\text{Available strength}}{\text{Ordered strength}} = \frac{\text{Available amount}}{\text{Amount to give}}$$

Problem: Given the strength of the drug needed, the number of tablets to be administered must be determined.
Step 1. Set up a proportion with the three known quantities: (1) the strength of the drug in each tablet, (2) the unit amount in 1

tablet, and (3) the strength of the drug the provider has ordered for administration. Apply the standard formula to the problem:

$$\frac{\text{Available strength}}{\text{Ordered strength}} = \frac{\text{Available amount}}{\text{Amount to give}}$$

with the numbers: $\dfrac{5 \text{ mg}}{10 \text{ mg}} = \dfrac{1 \text{ tab}}{x \text{ (tab)}}$

Step 2. The mg units in the numerator and denominator on the left side of the equation cancel each other out. Cross-multiply:

$$5 \times x = 10 \times 1$$
$$5x = 10$$

Step 3. To find *x* (i.e., the amount to be given), you must divide each side of the equation by 5:

$$\frac{5x}{5} = \frac{10}{5}$$
$$x = 2 \text{ tablets}$$

Solution: Administer 2 tablets

The standard formula can be used for any type of calculation. You may be using strengths that are measured in International Units, as with penicillin, or you may have grams, milligrams, or percentages. The forms in which drugs may be prepared include cc or mL, oz, pints (pt), and gallons (gal) (for making up diluted stock solutions from concentrated solutions, as with alcohol and hydrogen peroxide).

Follow the steps previously shown and, above all, discipline yourself to write down each step with complete calculations. This is the only way to ensure maximum accuracy and the safety of your patients. If you have difficulty with the calculation or the answer does not seem quite right, ask the provider to check your calculation. A double check is always preferred.

Some of your co-workers may use an alternative formula for calculating drug dosages:

$$\frac{D}{H} \times Q$$

D—Desired dose (the provider's order)
H—What is on hand (the dosage strength listed on the medication label)
Q—Quantity in the unit (identified on the label as 1 tablet, 5 mL, and so on)
Regardless of the formula used, the answer will be the same.

More Sample Problems

Problem 1. Dr. Angio orders 500 mg of an antibiotic. The label states that the dosage strength is 250 mg/2 mL. How much should the patient receive?

$$\frac{D}{H} \times Q = \frac{500 \text{ mg (Physician's order)}}{250 \text{ mg (Dosage strength on hand)}} \times 2 \text{ mL (Label quantity)}$$

The mg quantities cancel out:

$$\frac{500}{250} \times 2\ mL = 2 \times 2\ mL$$

$$= 4\ mL\ of\ medication\ should\ be\ given$$

Problem 2. Dr. Angio orders 50 mg of Imitrex to be given to a patient with a severe migraine. The label states, "25 mg/tab."

$$\frac{Dose\ ordered}{Dose\ on\ hand} \times Quantity = Amount\ to\ give$$

$$or\quad \frac{D}{H} \times Q = Amount\ to\ give$$

$$\frac{50\ mg}{25\ mg} \times 1\ tab = 2\ tabs$$

Calculate the following doses.

1. Administer 0.25 mg of Lanoxin. The label reads "0.125 mg/tab." How many tablets should you give?

2. The patient is prescribed 15 mEq of KCl, and the label reads "5 mEq/5 mL." How many milliliters should the patient receive?

3. The phenobarbital label states "15 mg/5 mL." The patient is prescribed 45 mg of the drug. How many milliliters should be administered?

4. The provider orders 25 mg of Compazine IM. The label reads "10 mg/mL." How much medicine should be injected?

CRITICAL THINKING APPLICATION   **27-2**

At work the next day, Dr. Angio asks Heather to administer Acetaminophen Elixir 70 mg to a 6-year-old patient with a fever of 102.6° F (39.2° C). Heather checks the label of the Acetaminophen Elixir in the drug cabinet and discovers that the bottle contains 120 mg per 5 mL in a 100-mL bottle. Using the standard formula presented earlier, how many milliliters should the child receive? If Heather is concerned about her calculation, what should she do?

PROCEDURE 27-1   Demonstrate Knowledge of Basic Math Computations

Goal: *To calculate the correct dose amount and choose the correct equipment to complete the provider's order.*

Order: The provider orders 1 million International Units of penicillin G benzathine (Bicillin).

EQUIPMENT and SUPPLIES

- Patient's record
- Provider's drug order
- Premixed syringes of Bicillin, available as:
  - 0.6 million International Units/syringe in a 1-mL syringe
  - 1.2 million International Units/syringe in a 1-mL syringe
- Pencil and paper

PROCEDURAL STEPS

1. Verify the order with the provider. Read the order in quiet surroundings to make sure you fully understand it.
2. Examine the drug labels to see what strengths and amounts are available. The premixed Bicillin in a 1-mL syringe with a strength of 1.2 million International Units/syringe is the closest to the 1 million International Units ordered by the provider. If you chose the syringe with 0.6 million International Units, you would have to give the patient two injections—a single 0.6 million International Unit syringe plus part of another 0.6 million International Unit syringe—to administer the 1 million International Units ordered.
3. Write down the standard formula.

$$\frac{Available\ strength}{Ordered\ strength} = \frac{Available\ amount}{Amount\ to\ give}$$

<u>PURPOSE</u>: To eliminate the chance of error, orders should never be carried out unless the calculations have been completed in writing.

4. Rewrite the formula, placing the known quantities into the proper place in the formula. The unknown value *(x)* will be the amount of the drug to give.

$$\frac{1.2\ million\ International\ Units}{1\ million\ International\ Units} = \frac{1\ mL}{x}$$

5. Work the proportion problem by cross-multiplying to solve for *x*.

$$x \times 1.2\ million\ International\ Units = 1\ million\ International\ Units$$

6. To solve for *x*, divide each side of the equation by 1.2 million International Units:

$$x \times \frac{1.2\ million\ International\ Units}{1.2\ million\ International\ Units} = \frac{1\ million\ International\ Units}{1.2\ million\ International\ Units}$$

$$x = 0.83\ mL\ of\ the\ 1.2\ million\ International$$

$$Units\ per\ 1\text{-}mL\ syringe$$

PROCEDURE 27-2	Calculate Proper Dosages of Medication for Administration: Convert Among Measurement Systems

Goal: *To choose the correct system of measurement and calculate the correct dose amount per the provider's order.*

Order: The provider orders 4 mL of amoxicillin for a 3-year-old child. She wants the mother to understand the household measurement equivalent of this dose.

EQUIPMENT and SUPPLIES

- Patient's record
- Provider's drug order
- Amoxicillin solution, 50 mg per 1 mL
- Pencil and paper
- Standard mathematical formula:

$$\frac{\text{Available strength}}{\text{Ordered strength}} = \frac{\text{Available amount}}{\text{Amount to give}}$$

- Conversion equivalent: 5 mL = 1 tsp

PROCEDURAL STEPS

1. Verify the order with the provider. Read the order in quiet surroundings to make sure you fully understand it.
2. Write out the order.
3. Examine the drug labels to see what strengths and amounts are available.
4. Convert the ordered system of measurement to the system of measurement on the label.
5. Place the amount ordered on the left side of the equation and the conversion factor on the right side so that similar units (in this problem, mL) can be cancelled.

$$\frac{4\,\text{mL}}{5\,\text{mL}} \times \frac{1\,\text{tsp}}{5} = \frac{20}{5} = 4\,\text{mL} = 0.8\,\text{tsp}$$

6. The label states that there are 50 mg of amoxicillin in every 1 mL of solution. To determine how many mg the child will receive in each dose, use the standard formula:

$$\frac{\text{Available strength}}{\text{Ordered strength}} = \frac{\text{Available amount}}{\text{Amount to give}}$$

PURPOSE: To eliminate the chance of error, orders should never be carried out unless the calculations have been completed in writing.

7. Rewrite the formula, placing the known quantities into the proper place in the formula, and using the system of measurement on the label. The unknown *(x)* will be the amount of the drug to give (amount to give).

$$\frac{1\,\text{mL}}{4\,\text{mL}} = \frac{50\,\text{mg}}{x}$$

8. Work the proportion problem by cross-multiplying to solve for *x*. The mL cancel each other out.

$$x = 200\,\text{mg}$$

The child should receive 0.8 tsp of amoxicillin, measured in a pediatric oral syringe, which contains 200 mg per dose.

PEDIATRIC DOSAGES

Calculating the Dose

Pediatric doses are calculated differently from those for other age groups because of multiple factors, including differences in absorption and drug metabolism. Although formulas have been used in the past that based the dose calculation on age, pediatric doses are much more accurate when based on weight because children of any age can vary greatly in size and body weight. You must be especially careful in calculating dosages for children because even a minor miscalculation can be dangerous. With online calculators available, in addition to tools in EHR programs designed to complete accurate calculations, doses can be determined efficiently and accurately without requiring mathematical calculations. However, it is important that medical assistants be familiar with traditional methods because some providers may continue to use them.

Dosages Based on Body Weight

The most frequently used calculation method relies on the child's accurate weight in kilograms. Kilogram measurements are necessary because most pediatric medication dosages are based on the metric system, with a designated number of milligrams to be administered per kilogram of body weight (mg/kg). Several steps are involved in this type of calculation, but if you follow them closely, you will determine the most accurate amount of medication to administer to a child (Procedure 27-3).

Step 1. Before you begin the dose calculation, carefully weigh the child to make sure you have an accurate weight. If the scale provides a reading in pounds, convert the child's weight to kilograms by dividing the number of pounds by 2.2 (1 kg = 2.2 lb). For example, 36 lb is equal to 16.4 kg (36 ÷ 2.2 = 16.36 = 16.4 kg [rounded up]). If the child's weight is in pounds and ounces, you must convert the ounces to pounds as a decimal and add it to the pounds. For example, if an infant weighs 9 lb 7 oz, first convert 7 oz to the nearest tenth of pounds (1 lb = 16 oz; 7 oz ÷ 16 oz = 0.4 lb [rounded from 0.4375]) and then add it to 9 lb; thus the baby weighs 9.4 lb. Then convert pounds to kilograms by dividing 9.4 by 2.2 (9.4 ÷ 2.2 = 4.3 kg [rounded from 4.2727]).

Step 2. Calculate the total daily dose of the medication by multiplying the child's weight in kilograms by the amount of drug stated on the label that should be administered per kg per day (kg/day). For example, if the label states that the child should receive 4 mg/kg/day, multiply the child's weight in kg by 4 mg to determine the daily dose of the drug.

Step 3. Calculate a single dose of the drug based on how frequently the medication is to be given throughout the day. For example, if the drug is ordered qid, divide the total daily dose by 4; if the medication is ordered for every 8 hours (q8h), divide the total daily dose by 3, because there are three 8-hour periods in a 24-hour day; if the drug is ordered tid, divide the total daily dose by 3; if it is ordered bid, divide the total daily dose by 2.

Step 4. After calculating the amount of a single dose, compare the ordered amount with the drug label. If necessary, apply the standard formula to calculate the amount of medication that should be administered.

Example. An infant who weighs 12 lb 6 oz is prescribed erythromycin q6h. The label states that there is 200 mg of the drug in 5 mL of suspension. The recommended dose of the medication for infants is 30 mg/kg/day. How much should the child receive per dose?

1. Convert 12 lb 6 oz to kg:

$$6 \text{ oz} \div 16 \text{ oz} = 0.375 \text{ lb (0.4 rounded to the nearest tenth)}$$

$$0.4 \text{ lb} + 12 = 12.4 \text{ lb (baby's weight in lb)}$$

$$12.4 \div 2.2 = 5.6 \text{ kg (baby's weight in kg)}$$

2. The total daily recommended dose of the medication is 30 mg times the infant's weight in kilograms:

$$30 \times 5.6 = 168 \text{ mg/day}$$

3. A single dose of the drug is the total daily dose divided by 4 (there are four 6-hour periods in a 24-hour day):

$$168 \text{ mg} \div 4 = 42 \text{ mg/dose}$$

4. The amount of the medication that should be administered in a single dose is determined by the drug label, which states that there are 200 mg in every 5 mL of the suspension. The standard formula can be used as follows to find the answer:

$$\frac{\text{Available strength}}{\text{Ordered strength}} = \frac{\text{Available amount}}{\text{Amount to give}}$$

$$\frac{200 \text{ mg}}{42 \text{ mg}} = \frac{5 \text{ mL}}{x \text{ (mL)}}$$

$$200x = 210$$

$$\frac{200x}{200} = \frac{210}{200}$$

$$x = 1.05, \text{ rounded up to } 1.1 \text{ mL}$$

PROCEDURE 27-3	Calculate Proper Dosages of Medication for Administration: Calculate the Correct Pediatric Dosage Using Body Weight

Goal: *To calculate the correct pediatric dosage by using the body weight method.*

Order: Zithromax suspension 5 mg/kg/day bid for 5 days for a patient who has a diagnosis of otitis media. The patient weighs 22 lb. The suspension is labeled 100 mg/5 mL. Weight conversion: 2.2 lb = 1 kg.

EQUIPMENT and SUPPLIES

- Patient's record
- Provider's drug order
- Suspension labeled 100 mg/5 mL
- Formula for conversion of pounds to kilograms
- Standard math formula:

$$\frac{\text{Available strength}}{\text{Ordered strength}} = \frac{\text{Available amount}}{\text{Amount to give}}$$

- Paper and pencil

PROCEDURAL STEPS

1. Verify the order with the provider. Read the order in quiet surroundings to make sure you fully understand it.
2. Write out the order.
3. Examine the drug label to check the strength and amount available.
4. Convert the patient's weight from pounds to kilograms.

$$22 \text{ lb} \div 2.2 = 10 \text{ kg}$$

PROCEDURE 27-3 *—continued*

5. Calculate the total daily amount of medication by multiplying the weight in kilograms by the mg/kg factor.

$$5\,mg \times 10\,kg = 50\,mg\ of\ Zithromax\ daily\ for\ 5\ days$$

6. Calculate the individual dose of Zithromax; divide the daily dose by 2 (bid is twice a day).

$$50\,mg \div 2 = 25\,mg/dose$$

7. Compare the ordered dose with the dose information on the medication label. The suspension is labeled 100 mg/5 mL (100 mg = 5 mL).

8. Write down the standard formula.
   PURPOSE: To eliminate the chances of error.

$$\frac{Available\ strength}{Ordered\ strength} = \frac{Available\ amount}{Amount\ to\ give}$$

9. Rewrite the formula, placing the known quantities into the proper place in the formula. The unknown x will be the amount of the drug to give.

$$\frac{100\,mg}{25\,mg} = \frac{5\,mL}{x}$$

10. Work the problem by cross-multiplying to solve for x.

$$100x = 125$$
$$x = 1.25\,mL$$

11. State your answer by filling in the blank:
   To administer 5 mg of Zithromax per kilogram of body weight from a suspension labeled 100 mg/5 mL, administer _____ mL.

Reconstituting Powdered Injectable Medications

Some medications are packaged in a vial as crystals or powder (solute) that must be mixed with sterile isotonic saline or sterile distilled water (solvent) to form a solution before it can be injected. In such cases, it is essential to *read the label directions carefully* to determine how much sterile solvent must be added to the solute to create the ordered dosage strength.

Example. The provider orders 500 mg of a drug. The label reads, "Add 5.5 mL of sterile water to make 250 mg/mL; total volume of available solution will be 6 mL."

1. Inject 5.5 mL of sterile water into the vial of medication. Rotate the vial between your hands to mix the solutes and the solvent. The total volume in the vial is now 6 mL.
2. According to the label, every milliliter in the vial contains 250 mg of the drug.
3. On the vial, write the date and time of reconstitution, because the guidelines on the drug label state that once the medication has been mixed, it must be discarded within 7 days.
4. Using the standard formula, calculate the number of milliliters to withdraw from the vial to fulfill the provider's order for 500 mg of the drug.

$$\frac{Available\ strength}{Ordered\ strength} = \frac{Available\ amount}{Amount\ to\ give}$$
$$\frac{250\,mg}{500\,mg} = \frac{1\,mL}{x\,(mL)}$$
$$250x = 500$$
$$\frac{250x}{250} = \frac{500}{250}$$
$$x = 2\,mL$$

Solution: To administer 500 mg from a vial labeled 250 mg/mL, give 2 mL of medication

CLOSING COMMENTS

Legal and Ethical Issues

A medical assistant who is responsible for administering medications must have completely mastered the calculation of dosages, whether the prescribed dose is for a child or for an adult. If the medical assistant is ever in doubt about the accuracy of a calculation, he or she should always have a trusted colleague or the provider check the calculations.

A medical assistant who prepares and administers medications is ethically and legally responsible for his or her own actions. Laws vary from state to state; therefore, it is essential that medical assistants become familiar with the laws in the states where they are employed before they administer medications. In some states, legislation gives physicians broad authority to delegate responsibility for giving medications. In such a case, the medical assistant acts as the "agent" of the physician. However, the assistant is responsible and accountable for the acts performed and may be subject to penalties.

Regardless of the differences in state authorization laws, the courts do not allow the carelessness of healthcare workers to go unpunished, especially when such actions result in harm or death for the patient.

Professional Behaviors

One of the characteristics that mark a true professional is not being afraid to ask for help when it is needed. Calculating drug dosages can be intimidating. The well-being of your patient rests in your hands when you have to calculate a dose of an ordered drug. If you ever have any doubt that your answer may not be correct, do not hesitate to have someone you trust — either your supervisor or a provider in your practice — check your calculations. If you give a patient the wrong dose of a medication, the patient may suffer very serious complications. The best way to prevent this is to seek help when needed with math calculations.

SUMMARY OF SCENARIO

Heather recognizes how important it is to be able to calculate drug dosages correctly. To do so, she must understand the terms involved in dosage preparation, must be able to read a drug label correctly, and must follow the various steps in calculating an accurate dose. The drug label contains a great deal of information, including the brand and generic names; dosage strength; route of administration; instructions on mixing solvents if appropriate; storage guidelines; total amount of drug in the container; name of the drug manufacturer; expiration date; and both the lot number and the NDC identification number.

Heather also must be able to make conversions within and between measuring systems; use the standard formula to determine drug doses; accurately calculate pediatric doses based on the child's weight; and reconstitute powdered drugs for administration by following the label directions regarding the amount of solvent that should be added to the solute. She continues to ask Mrs. Allison or Dr. Angio to check her calculations for accuracy before dispensing and administering any drug for which the order differs from the medication label.

SUMMARY OF LEARNING OBJECTIVES

1. **Define, spell, and pronounce the terms listed in the vocabulary.**
   Spelling and pronouncing medical terms correctly reinforce the medical assistant's credibility. Knowing the definitions of these terms promotes confidence in communication with patients and co-workers.

2. **Summarize the important parts of a drug label.**
   The drug label contains a great deal of information, including the brand and generic names; dosage strength; route of administration; instructions on mixing solvents if appropriate; storage guidelines; total amount of the drug in the container; name of the drug manufacturer; expiration date; and both the lot number and the NDC identification number. Drug label terms must be understood to implement pharmacology math formulas.

3. **Demonstrate knowledge of basic math computations.**
   The medical assistant must thoroughly understand the addition, subtraction, multiplication, and division of fractions and decimals; the relationships of decimals and fractions; and how they are converted from one to the other. Table 27-1 contains examples of mathematical equivalents.

4. **Define basic units of measurement in the metric and household systems.**
   The metric system of weights and measures is a decimal system based on the number 10, and all calculations are completed by moving decimal points to the right or to the left. Each higher measure is 10 times the measure at hand; each lower measure is 0.1 ($\frac{1}{10}$) the measure. The basic units are multiplied or divided by units of 10. The fraction is always written as a decimal, and the number precedes the letters designating the actual measure. The household system is important for a patient at home; however, it is not precise and therefore should never be used in the medical setting. Table 27-2 lists common abbreviations and symbols used in the metric and household systems. Table 27-3 lists approximate equivalents for commonly used metric and household measures.

5. **Convert among measurement systems.**
   Two systems of measurement are used for drugs. The metric system is based on units of 10. The liter is a measure of the liquid volume of a drug, and the gram is a measure of the weight or strength. Units are converted within the metric system by moving the decimal point to the right or to the left. Household measurements are based on pounds and drops. Table 27-3 can be used to convert from one system of measurement to another, or drug measurements can be converted by using the conversion formula.

6. **Do the following when calculating drug dosages for administration:**
   - *Demonstrate knowledge of basic math computations by calculating the correct dose amount.*
     See Procedure 27-1.
   - *Calculate proper dosages of medication for administration while using mathematical computations.*
     The correct dose of an ordered drug can be calculated by using basic arithmetic involving fractions, ratios, and proportions. The standard formula for calculating drug dosage uses information about the drug's strength and amount (found on the label) and the strength of the drug ordered, with the unknown *(x)* being the answer sought. The only way to gain confidence in using the standard formula is to practice dose calculations frequently until you become comfortable with the math. (Refer to Procedure 27-2.)

7. **Determine accurate pediatric doses of medication.**
   The medical assistant must be especially vigilant in calculating pediatric doses, because even a minor error may be dangerous to a child. The most accurate method for determining a pediatric dose is based on the child's weight. Procedure 27-3 describes how to calculate a pediatric dose.

8. **Summarize how to reconstitute powdered injectable medications.**
   In reconstituting powdered injectable medications, the medical assistant must add a particular amount of solvent (as recommended on the drug label) to a vial of powdered or crystalloid medication. Once the solute and the solvent have been combined and mixed in the vial, a solution of medication is formed; the strength is based on equivalents printed on the drug label. After the medication has been mixed, it is important for the medical assistant to read the label carefully to determine how much of the drug must be withdrawn to fulfill the provider's order. This process frequently requires use of the standard conversion formula to determine the accurate dose for administration.

SUMMARY OF LEARNING OBJECTIVES—*continued*

9. **Specify the legal and ethical responsibilities of a medical assistant in calculating drug dosages.**

A medical assistant who prepares, dispenses, and administers medications is ethically and legally responsible for his or her own actions. If any doubt exists about the accuracy of calculations, it is essential that the medical assistant have the provider or another trusted employee review the math before the medication is dispensed and administered. Medical assistants must be aware of state laws that monitor medication administration by allied health workers.

CONNECTIONS

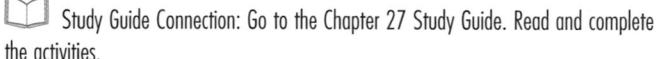 Study Guide Connection: Go to the Chapter 27 Study Guide. Read and complete the activities.

evolve Evolve Connection: Go to the Chapter 27 link at *evolve.elsevier.com/kinn* to complete the Chapter Review Quiz. Check out the other resources listed for this chapter to make the most of what you have learned from Pharmacology Math.

28

ADMINISTERING MEDICATIONS

SCENARIO

Dr. Anna Thau just opened a new primary care office in the community. She is in the process of hiring office staff, and Dorothy Gaston, CMA (AAMA), is being interviewed for a clinical assisting position. One of Dr. Thau's chief requirements is that the medical assistants working in the clinical area be familiar with medications and competent in their administration. Her primary concern is the safety of her patients, so she requires that employees take appropriate safety measures when dispensing and administering oral, topical, and parenteral drugs.

While studying this chapter, think about the following questions:

- What safety guidelines should Dorothy incorporate into her practice each time she receives a drug order from Dr. Thau?
- What information must be included in comprehensive documentation of the administration of medication?
- Are there patient assessment factors that might affect medication administration?
- Why does Dorothy have to understand the details of various drug forms and their administration guidelines?
- What practices mandated by the Occupational Safety and Health Administration (OSHA) must be followed in preparing and administering medications?

- How can Dorothy coach patients about the safe administration of medications while encouraging compliance with the treatment plan and following through with adaptations that are appropriate to meet individual patient needs?
- What does Dorothy need to know about the legal implications of drug administration?

LEARNING OBJECTIVES

1. Define, spell, and pronounce the terms listed in the vocabulary.
2. Do the following related to safety in drug administration:
   - Follow safety precautions in the management of medication administration in the ambulatory healthcare setting.
   - Analyze safety guidelines for specific patient populations.
   - Document the administration of a medication accurately in the health record.
3. Summarize patient assessment factors that can affect medication administration.
4. Identify various drug forms and their administration guidelines, and administer oral medications.
5. Do the following related to parenteral administration of drugs:
   - Specify parenteral administration equipment, including details about needles and syringes.

   - Follow OSHA guidelines in the management of parenteral administration.
   - Describe and demonstrate the types and locations of parenteral administrations with proper use of sharps containers.
6. Recognize the medical assistant's role in coaching patients about the administration of drugs.
7. Assess legal and ethical issues in drug administration in the ambulatory care setting, and complete an incident report related to an error in medication administration.

VOCABULARY

aqueous (ak'-wee-uhs) A waterlike substance; a medication prepared with water.
asymptomatic Without symptoms of a disease process.
bevel (bev'-uhl) The angled tip of a needle.

bronchoconstriction Narrowing of the bronchiole tubes.
edema (i-dee'-muh) An abnormal accumulation of fluid in the interstitial spaces of tissues.

immunosuppressant A substance that suppresses or prevents an immune system response.

immunotherapy Administration of repeated injections of diluted extracts of a substance that causes an allergy; also called *desensitization.*

induration (in-doo-rey'-shuhn) An abnormally hard, inflamed area.

loading dose A large dose administered as the first dose of a medication; it usually is used in antibiotic therapy to quickly achieve therapeutic blood levels of the drug.

meniscus (meh-nis'-kus) The curved surface of liquids in a container.

polyuria (pah-le-yur'-e-uh) Excretion of an unusually large amount of urine.

scored A term referring to a tablet manufactured with an indentation for division through the center.

vasodilation An increase in the diameter of a blood vessel.

viscosity (vis-kos'-uh-te) The quality of being thick and of lacking the capability of easy movement.

wheal (weel) A localized area of edema or a raised lesion.

Previous medication chapters in this text explained general pharmacologic principles and pharmacology math. In this chapter, you will learn about safety factors in drug administration, documentation guidelines, the forms of medications, and how they are administered. It is important to remember that medications can cause serious harm to a patient. Therefore, the process of dispensing and administering medications must always be treated with great care. Each member of the healthcare team involved in medication administration must be constantly vigilant to prevent errors and to deliver high-quality patient care.

No matter the type of medication administered, the order first must come from either the physician or a licensed provider, such as a nurse practitioner or physician assistant. If the provider delegates drug administration to the medical assistant, this must be allowable under state law. Many states have a medical practice act that defines whether a medical assistant can administer drugs under the supervision of a physician. Some states allow medical assistants to administer only certain types of medications; some prohibit medical assistants from giving injections. Contact your state government or medical society for information about the scope of practice for medical assistants in your particular state. You should know what the law states and how your duties fit into that law.

SAFETY IN DRUG ADMINISTRATION

To ensure patient safety in drug administration, the medical assistant must perform certain procedures every time a medication is ordered. First, it is essential that the medical assistant understand the provider's order. Safety starts with a clearly written order that can be easily read and understood. Many times in the clinical setting the provider gives a verbal order for a medication. Patient safety requires that you write down a verbal order and repeat it back to the provider to make sure there are no errors. Ask the provider for clarification if you have any questions about the medication, dose, strength, or route of administration. This step has become much simpler with the use of the electronic health record (EHR). Once the order has been clarified, the medical assistant is responsible for looking up the drug in a pharmacology reference, such as the *Physicians' Desk Reference* (PDR), another drug reference book, or an online drug reference. A medication should never be given until its purpose, possible side effects, precautions, route of administration, and recommended dose are known.

After the medical assistant learns about the drug ordered, the medication is dispensed and administered. To safeguard the patient during this process, use the Seven Rights of proper drug administration. Remember, however, that the patient always has the right to refuse to take a medication. If this occurs, make sure you inform the provider immediately, because he or she may want to follow up with the patient about the importance of the prescribed medication. If a patient refuses to take an ordered medication, be sure to document this refusal in the patient's record. The Seven Rights of drug administration are as follows.

1. *The right patient*	The patient should be identified in two ways: by his or her full name and date of birth (DOB). A patient identification number can also be used, but most patients will not know their medical record number.
2. *The right drug*	This check begins with clarification of the provider's order if needed. *Every* time a drug is dispensed or prepared for administration, and strength. You must be competent in reading and understanding the information on drug labels. The drug's name and strength on the label must exactly match the provider's written order. Compare the provider's written order with the medication label when you: • Take the medication from the storage area • Check the expiration date and dispense the medication from the container • Replace the container to storage or before discarding the used container Remember, each time you are checking for four things—the right (1) drug, (2) dose, (3) route of administration, and (4) strength.

3.	*The right dose*	If the dose ordered does not match the dose available according to the drug label, perform appropriate pharmacology math procedures to determine the accurate dose. *Remember to always recheck your own calculations, and if there is any doubt about the accuracy of the dose, have someone else also check.*
4.	*The right route*	Check the provider's order to clarify the route of administration, whether it is oral, via mucous membrane, or parenteral. Patient assessment includes determining whether this is an appropriate route for that particular patient.
5.	*The right time*	In the ambulatory care setting, most medications are ordered *on a one-time basis.* However, it is important to check the provider's order to clarify the time of administration and to refer to this information when looking up the drug to clarify any questions the patient may have about home administration of the drug.
6.	*The right technique*	A medical assistant must be familiar with the proper techniques for all routes of administration such as the correct method for giving injections. If you have any doubts about your ability to administer a particular drug, always ask for help.
7.	*The right documentation*	Immediately after administering the drug, document the date and time of administration; the drug's name, strength, dose, and route of administration; any reactions the patient has to the medication; and the details of patient education about the drug. Some medications, such as vaccines, also require documentation of the lot number, expiration date, and manufacturer. For parenteral medications, inspect the site of injection before administration for scarring, altered pigmentation, or any other indication of a possible problem with medication absorption. The exact site of administration must be documented. If the patient calls in for a prescription refill, document all pertinent information in the patient's record.

Additional Safety Steps for Medication Administration

- Prepare medications in a quiet, well-lit area.
- Pay close attention to all the steps involved in dispensing drugs.
- Never substitute a drug or drug strength. Consult the provider about any discrepancy between the medication ordered and the medication available.

- Store medications as ordered on the package, and return containers to the proper storage area immediately after dispensing the dose.
- The person who administers the medication is responsible for any drug errors. Never administer a medication that you have not personally prepared.
- If ordered to prepare a medication for the provider to administer, place the container with the dispensed drug so that the provider can verify the seven rights.
- The provider should document every medication order in the patient's electronic health record (EHR) before the medication is administered.
- Routinely check expiration dates when verifying the Seven Rights. Properly discard expired drugs.
- Discard medications with damaged labels to avoid errors caused by inaccurate reading of label information.
- If a medication is not administered after it is dispensed, discard it rather than returning it to the container.
- Before administering any medication, ask the patient about drug allergies; these can change over time.
- Patients should be observed for side effects or adverse reactions for up to 30 minutes after administration of a medication. Any reactions must be reported to the provider and documented in the patient's health record.
- Always provide and document patient education about the medication, time of administration, side effects, and so on, when administering a drug.

CRITICAL THINKING APPLICATION   28-1

Dr. Thau asks Dorothy what safety precautions she would routinely follow when administering a Vitamin B12 injection. Based on the information you have learned about safe drug administration, what steps should Dorothy follow in dispensing and administering the ordered medication?

Patient Assessment Factors

Although medications are given only under the direct order and supervision of the provider, the medical assistant is part of the assessment and problem-solving process. In medicine, assessment never ends, and it is never the responsibility of just one person. A provider gives the order to administer medication to a patient based on a medical assessment, but you must continue to assess the patient and the patient's environment as you follow through with that order. The provider depends on the medical assistant to be alert to patient changes or to new information that could mean that the use of a particular drug should be reconsidered. For example, perhaps the patient denied having any allergies to medications, but right before you administer an injection of penicillin, the patient mentions that she developed a rash after her last penicillin shot. You should stop right then and go back to the provider with this new information. It is vital to continuing patient safety that you assess the patient, the drug, and the environment before giving any medication.

Drug therapy should be based on a holistic approach to patient treatment. The patient is more than a particular disease. Many factors may have an impact on the patient's compliance with drug treatment and on the safety and effectiveness of medication therapy. The first step in holistic medication treatment is collecting a complete and accurate history. This includes gathering details about the patient's health history, current and past use of both prescription and over-the-counter (OTC) drugs and herbal supplements, and any negative responses to medications, especially drug allergies. Every time a patient is seen in the facility, he or she should be asked about drug allergies. Most medical practices and electronic health record (EHR) programs have a specific place on the patient's record to document drug allergies (e.g., in red ink in the upper right corner of each paper documentation sheet) or an alert designed into the EHR template that consistently brings the provider's attention to patient medication allergies. It is crucial that the provider have current and accurate information about drug allergies to prevent serious complications and possibly death.

Patient assessment does not end with the administration of the drug. Observe patients carefully for drug reactions after the administration of all medications, especially those that are injected. Patients receiving penicillin (a drug with a high incidence of allergic response) or **immunotherapy** must remain in the office for 20 to 30 minutes after administration in case of an acute anaphylactic reaction. An acute anaphylactic reaction can result in respiratory failure and circulatory collapse within minutes if not reversed with epinephrine. Lesser allergic reactions that may occur include hives, swelling, and itching. The provider may order an antihistamine, such as diphenhydramine (Benadryl), if these reactions occur.

Because patient factors such as age, weight, and height may be used to determine the correct therapeutic dose, accurate recordings of this information should be documented in the patient's record. Chronic conditions, especially liver and kidney disease, may affect the body's ability to metabolize and excrete medications. Therefore, a complete and accurate medical history is crucial to the patient's safety.

Besides the patient's physical state, other holistic factors play a role in successful drug therapy. The patient must understand the drug regimen, may require family support to follow treatment guidelines, and must be able to afford the prescribed medication. Unless these criteria can be met, the patient may be unable to follow through with the treatment protocol. It is important that the medical assistant investigate these issues and offer appropriate community support, if available, to help the patient maintain proper drug therapy.

Approaches to Special Patient Populations

Pregnant and breast-feeding women must be especially careful when taking OTC and prescription drugs because medications are known to cross the placenta and may affect the developing fetus. A pregnant woman should not take any medication without the knowledge and approval of her provider. The U.S. Food and Drug Administration (FDA) has identified five pregnancy risk categories of drugs. The medical assistant should be familiar with the specific drug category before administering any medication to a pregnant woman. Besides passing through the placenta, medications also are transmitted through breast milk. Therefore, similar precautions must be taken when the provider prescribes medications for a lactating mother.

Special precautions must also be followed in determining the correct dose of medication for children. Pediatric doses are determined primarily by the child's weight; therefore, it is important to measure and record the child's weight accurately at each office visit. A child's body manages drug absorption, distribution, metabolism, and excretion differently from an adult's body, and the provider considers these factors when prescribing pediatric doses.

Aging people also are more sensitive to the effects of medications, so certain factors must be considered when prescribing and administering drugs to this patient population. The metabolic rate typically slows with the aging process, resulting in increased susceptibility to a buildup of chemicals in the body that may lead to toxic conditions. Part of the normal aging process is loss of subcutaneous fat, which may affect the route of administration of some medications, especially parenteral sites. In addition, many elderly people have accompanying chronic diseases, such as circulatory, liver, or kidney disease, that may affect the distribution, metabolism, and excretion of medications. Geriatric patients frequently take multiple medications prescribed by more than one practitioner, which increases the risk of drug contraindications and interactions. In addition, a holistic approach to aging patients should include a nutritional evaluation because a poor diet or restricted fluid intake affects drug actions.

Another very real concern for aging patients is the cost of drug therapy. Many patients on fixed incomes may not be able to afford the ordered drug but hesitate to inform the provider of this problem. It may be up to the medical assistant to ask the patient about his or her ability to pay for the ordered medication and to offer available assistance for prescription drugs. This includes offering drug samples with provider approval and/or investigating drug coverage offered by pharmaceutical companies.

Suggestions for Successful Medication Administration to Children

- Explain why the medication is needed and how it will make the child feel.
- Attempt to gain cooperation by getting down on the child's level and using a soft but firm voice.
- When possible, offer choices of care, such as "Would you like your medicine in your right leg or your left leg?"
- Divert the child to relieve stressful moments.
- If the child refuses to cooperate, get help as needed to restrain the child so the medication can be given safely.
- Encourage parents to participate as much as possible, and make sure that both parents and the child (if of an appropriate age) understand the prescribed drug therapy.
- Offer a "treat," such as a sticker, at the end of the visit.

Guidelines for Administration of Medication to Geriatric Patients

- Educate the patient and family about the purpose of the drug; the time, dose, and route of administration; and common side effects. Instructions should be written clearly for home reference.
- If the patient has difficulty swallowing the medication, crush the medication (if allowed) or mix it into applesauce or pudding.

- Encourage the patient to drink plenty of fluids (at least eight glasses of water per day) while taking the medication.
- Reinforce that the patient should take the medication as prescribed and should not skip or double doses.
- Request that patients bring to every healthcare visit all of the medications they are currently taking in their labeled containers, including over-the-counter (OTC) medications, so a current medication record can be accurately maintained in the patient record.
- If patients are taking multiple medications, suggest the use of daily or weekly medication dispensers. These can be purchased in drugstores and restocked by family members on a weekly basis. It is safest if all prescriptions are filled at the same pharmacy, so the pharmacist can keep track of possible drug interactions or contraindications.
- Encourage patients not to share or "save" medications. All leftover medications should be discarded to avoid use beyond the expiration date.

CRITICAL THINKING APPLICATION   **28-2**

Dr. Thau has both pediatric and geriatric patients. Summarize key items that Dorothy should consider when administering medications to these specialty patient population groups.

Assessment of the Patient's Environment

The patient's surroundings affect the success of medication therapy. The patient may be uncooperative when you attempt to administer a medication (imagine a young child due for immunization updates), or the patient's family may protest the use of the drug. A medical assistant should never administer medication without the presence of a licensed provider. For example, because of the risk of anaphylactic shock, allergy injections should not be given unless a licensed provider is in the facility. In addition, the environment must be safe for drug administration. Make sure the patient is comfortable and protected from accidental injury. If a patient is to receive an injection, take care to place the patient in a position that best exposes the site and protects the person from injury in case he or she faints or has a drug reaction. If the patient is to take an oral medication with water, make sure he or she is seated in a position that prevents choking.

Because any medication is potentially dangerous to a patient, emergency drugs must be readily available to counteract any adverse effects that might occur immediately after the administration of a medication. Emergency drugs should be in injectable form for rapid effect. Emergency carts typically include adrenergics (e.g., epinephrine), anticholinergics (e.g., atropine), bronchodilators, and histamine blockers. Any action to deal with serious adverse effects in a patient or allergic reactions to administered medications must be directed by a licensed provider. It is beyond the medical assistant's scope of practice to make decisions about emergency care for patients.

The following section presents suggested questions that can be asked to obtain as much information as possible from the patient about medication therapy. Any information gathered should be included in your documentation.

Suggested Questions for Gathering Medication Information

- *What provider-prescribed drugs are you currently taking?*
  Record the names, doses, strengths, and routes of administration.
- *Do you take any OTC drugs on a regular basis?*
  Record the purpose, amount, and frequency of use. If appropriate, ask when the last dose was taken. For example, if a mother reports that her child has a fever but the temperature is normal at the time of the visit, perhaps she gave the child a dose of ibuprofen before the visit.
- *What medications, including OTC drugs, have you taken over the past 6 months to 1 year, and why?*
  Ask this question to gather a history of medication use and perhaps to discover health problems that have not been recorded previously.
- *Do you regularly use any alternative or herbal products? What are they? How much do you use and how frequently are they used? For what purpose are they used?*
  Herbal products or alternative methods of treatment may interfere with prescribed medications.
- It is important that patients take their medications as prescribed, so focus a few questions on how currently prescribed drugs are taken.
  - *What time of day do you take your medicine?*
  - *How do you remember to take it?*
  - *Are you having any problems or do you notice side effects from the medication?*
  - *Can you afford to take the medication as prescribed?*
  - *Are you having the desired response to the medication (e.g., pain relief, breathing better, lowered blood pressure)?*
- *Where do you store your medications at home?*
  Review any special storage precautions for prescribed drugs. Most medications should be stored away from any heat source and sunlight, and some must be refrigerated.
- *Have you checked the expiration dates on your containers?*
  Patients often neglect to dispose of unused medication and may take it after the expiration date if not informed of this precaution.
- *Can you tell me why you are taking the prescribed medication?*
  You should periodically check on the need for patient education about drug therapy. Patients are more likely to be compliant with treatment protocols if they understand the importance of taking the medication as prescribed.
- *Do you use the same pharmacy to fill all of your prescriptions?*
  Patients may see more than one provider. An excellent method of keeping track of all prescribed drugs, their contraindications, and possible drug-drug interactions is to strongly suggest that the patient use only one pharmacy. The pharmacist then can monitor overall medication safety.

DRUG FORMS AND ADMINISTRATION

The chosen route of drug administration determines the rate and intensity of the drug's effect. A drug prepared for one route but administered by another route may not have any effect at all and is potentially dangerous. Each route requires different dosage forms.

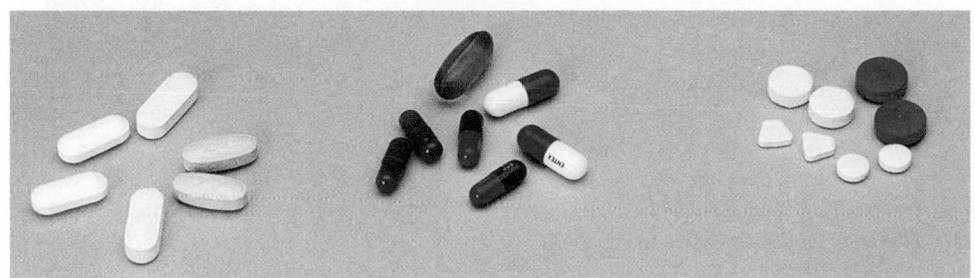

FIGURE 28-1 *Left to right,* Caplets, capsules, and tablets.

Solid Oral Dosage Forms

The basic forms for solid oral dosage are tablets, capsules, and lozenges (troches). Figure 28-1 shows typical caplets, capsules, and tablets. Tablets are compressed powders or granules that, when wet, break apart in the stomach—or in the mouth if they are not swallowed quickly. Tablets may be sugar coated to improve the taste or enteric coated (e.g., erythromycin) to protect the stomach mucosa or to prevent the partial breakdown of the drug in the acidic environment of the stomach. Buffered tablets are also designed to prevent stomach irritation by combining the drug with a buffering agent that reduces the amount of acidity in the compound. Buffered or enteric-coated tablets should never be crushed or dissolved because that would expose the stomach to the irritants in the drug or interfere with the timed-release action of an enteric-coated medication. Only **scored** tablets can be cut in half; this is accomplished with a pill cutter (Figure 28-2).

Some tablets quickly dissolve in the mouth, such as zolmitriptan, which is prescribed to treat the symptoms of migraine headaches. The tablet is placed on the tongue, where it quickly dissolves, rather than being swallowed. This allows for rapid absorption of the medication. Caplets are tablets without a coating; they are solid and oblong, similar in shape to capsules.

Capsules are gelatin coated and dissolve in the stomach, or they may be enteric coated to protect them from stomach acids. Timed- or sustained-release (SR) capsules or spansules are designed to dissolve at different rates over a period of time to reduce the number of times a patient has to take a medication. These drugs should never be crushed or dissolved because this negates their timed-release action and increases the risk that the patient will get an overdose of medication. Another form of oral medication, the lozenge (or troche), is a flattened disk that is dissolved in the mouth to coat the throat, such as a lozenge for a sore throat.

Liquid Oral Dosage Forms

Many liquid forms of medication are available. They differ mainly in the type of substance used to dissolve the drug: water, oils, or alcohol.

A *solution* is a mixture of a liquid, such as normal saline. Liquid forms include the following:

- *Syrups:* A syrup is a solution of sugar and water, usually containing flavoring and medicinal substances. Cough syrups, such as Robitussin, are the most common.
- *Suspensions:* Suspensions are insoluble drug substances contained in a liquid (e.g., amoxicillin solutions for pediatric patients). A solution separates if left standing, so you must

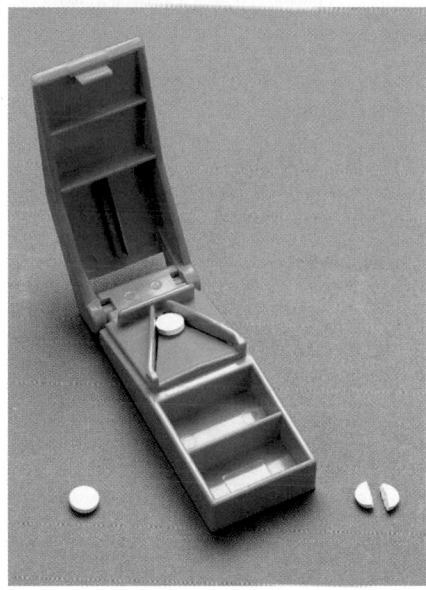

FIGURE 28-2 Pill cutter.

shake the container before administering the medication. Examples of suspensions include:

- *Emulsions:* An emulsion is a mixture of oil and water that improves the taste of otherwise distasteful products (e.g., cod liver oil).
- *Gels* and *magmas:* Gels and magmas consist of minerals suspended in water. Minerals settle; therefore, products containing minerals must be shaken before use. Milk of magnesia is an example.

A drug substance can be mixed with alcohol to enhance the drug's properties. Examples include the following:

- *Fluid extracts:* Fluid extracts are combinations of alcohol and vegetable products that are more potent than tinctures. For example, belladonna fluid extract has a higher percentage of the powdered belladonna leaf than tincture of belladonna.
- *Tinctures:* A tincture is an alcoholic preparation of a soluble drug or chemical substance, usually from plant sources. Examples include tincture of benzoin and tincture of iodine, which are applied externally.
- *Extracts:* Extracts are very concentrated combinations of vegetable products and alcohol or ether that are evaporated until a syrupy liquid, a solid mass, or powder is

formed. Extracts are many times stronger than the crude drug.

- *Elixirs:* An elixir is an aromatic, alcoholic, sweetened preparation. Elixir of phenobarbital is one example. Elixirs differ from tinctures in that they are sweetened. They should be used with caution in patients with diabetes or a history of alcohol abuse. Some pediatric medications retain the name *elixir,* although they no longer contain alcohol.

CRITICAL THINKING APPLICATION   **28-3**

Dorothy is ordered to administer a **loading dose** of cephalexin to a 17-year-old patient with acute bronchitis. Dr Thau's order reads, "Administer cephalexin 500 mg cap PO." The patient is sent home with a prescription for Keflex, 250 mg cap q6h times 7 days. Document the details that should be included in Dorothy's note.

_____

_____

_____

Rectal Administration

The rectal mucosa allows rapid absorption of a drug, even though the surface of the rectum is small. Drugs are absorbed directly into the bloodstream without being altered, as they would be by the digestive processes, and without irritating the patient's gastric mucosa. Rectal medications are useful if the patient is nauseated, vomiting, or unconscious. For example, acetaminophen suppositories may be prescribed for a child who has a fever with nausea and vomiting. Manufacturers supply rectal medications in the form of gelatin- or cocoa butter–based suppositories, which melt in the warmth of the rectum and release the medication (Figure 28-3). Suppositories may also be used to soften the stool or to stimulate evacuation of the bowel; enemas are used to cleanse and evacuate the bowel.

The best time to administer a rectal drug intended for a systemic effect is after a bowel movement or enema. The patient should be cautioned to remain lying down for 20 to 30 minutes to prevent

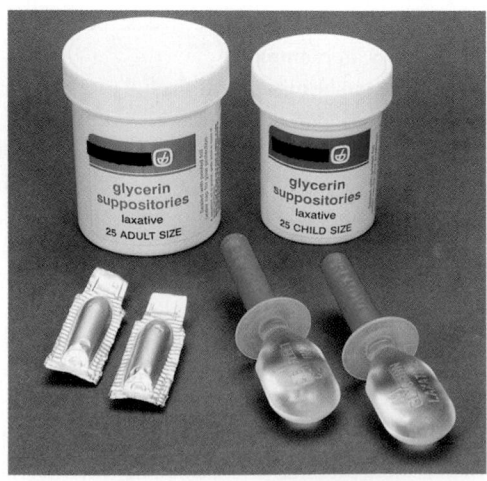

FIGURE 28-3 Sample rectal suppositories.

accidental evacuation of the drug. Of course, suppositories intended to treat constipation are administered to bring about bowel evacuation. The patient should be instructed to remove the outer wrapping and insert the suppository with the pointed end first approximately 2 inches above the rectal sphincter muscles in adults and ½ to 1 inch in children; using a lubricating gel (e.g., K-Y Jelly) can help with insertion. If suppositories are individually wrapped in foil, make sure the patient knows that the foil is the wrapper and is not part of the treatment. Suppositories are typically stored in the refrigerator, but refer to the package insert for storage information.

Vaginal Administration

Vaginal suppositories, tablets, creams, and fluid solutions are used to treat local infections. Cream and foam spermicides are available as local contraceptives. Vaginal instillation is completed with an applicator and most effective if the patient remains lying down after administration to prevent leakage; many preparations, therefore, are intended to be used at bedtime. The patient may need to wear a pad to absorb drainage.

Administration of Medications by Mouth

If the drug is not intended to coat the oral cavity or throat, oral medications should be taken with enough water to transport the drug to the stomach. Make sure the patient is able to swallow the medication. It may be helpful to place the medication on the back part of the tongue. Liquid medications are ideal for children. Solid drugs should not be administered to children until they reach the age at which they can safely swallow a solid drug form without the danger that they will aspirate the drug. Oral syringes are the best way to give liquid medications to children because there is less likelihood the medication will be spilled. Liquid medications, especially those that stain the teeth, can be taken through a straw. If the patient has been vomiting or is nauseated, an alternative route of administration may be necessary. Always remain with the patient until all of the medication has been swallowed. Procedure 28-1 outlines how to dispense and administer oral medications.

Mouth and throat agents come in the form of sprays, swabs, sublingual tablets, and buccal tablets. The mouth and throat membranes may be treated locally with antiseptics for oral hygiene and local infection, with anesthetics for pain relief, and with astringents that form a protective film over the mucous membranes. The patient may have to gargle, or the area may be painted or sprayed. To paint or spray the throat, first look for the area of inflammation to be treated. Otherwise, the part needing treatment may be missed entirely. Avoid touching the posterior pharynx (back of the throat); this causes gagging and possibly vomiting.

Sublingual (SL) tablets are placed under the tongue, where they are rapidly absorbed into the bloodstream by the rich supply of capillaries. Sublingual absorption is systemic and bypasses the acids in the stomach. Nitroglycerin, which is used for treating the chest pains of angina pectoris, may be administered sublingually. Patients should not chew or swallow sublingual medications. Buccal tablets are placed between the cheek and the upper molars and are quickly absorbed by the oral capillaries. The patient should be instructed not to smoke, eat, or drink immediately before or after administration of SL and buccal medications.

PROCEDURE 28-1	Administer Oral Medications

Goal: *To verify the rules of medication administration and safely dispense, administer, and document the administration of an oral medication.*

Order: Administer hydrochlorothiazide (HydroDiuril) 100 mg PO tab STAT for hypertension.

EQUIPMENT and SUPPLIES

- Patient's health record
- Written provider's order, including the drug name, strength, dose, and route of administration
- Container of ordered medication
- Calibrated medication cup
- Water, if appropriate
- PDR, online drug reference, or package insert

PROCEDURAL STEPS

1. Read the order and clarify any questions with the provider.
2. If you are unfamiliar with HydroDiuril, refer to the PDR, online drug reference, or package insert to determine the purpose of the drug, common side effects, typical dose, and any pertinent precautions or contraindications. Be prepared to answer any questions the patient may have about the medication. Use the Seven Rights to prevent errors. This step completes the Right Medication rule of medication administration.
3. Perform calculations needed to match the provider's order. Confirm the answer with the provider if you have any questions.
4. Assemble the equipment and sanitize your hands.
5. Prepare the medication in a well-lit, quiet area.
6. Compare the order with the label on the container of medicine when you remove it from storage. Check the expiration date on the container and dispose of the medication if it has expired.
   PURPOSE: To compare the medication label and the provider's order the first of three times.
7. Compare the order with the label on the container of medicine just before dispensing the ordered dose. Make sure the strength on the label matches the order or that you dispense the correctly calculated dose.
   PURPOSE: To compare the medication label and the provider's order the second of three times. This completes the Right Medication and the Right Dose of the rules of medication administration.

Dispensing Solid Oral Medications (HydroDiuril Tablet)

8. Gently tap the prescribed dose into the lid of the medication container. If too many tablets are dispensed onto the lid, pour the extra tablets back into the container. Do not touch the inside of the lid or the medication (Figure 1).
   PURPOSE: Touching the medication or the inside of the container contaminates the drug.

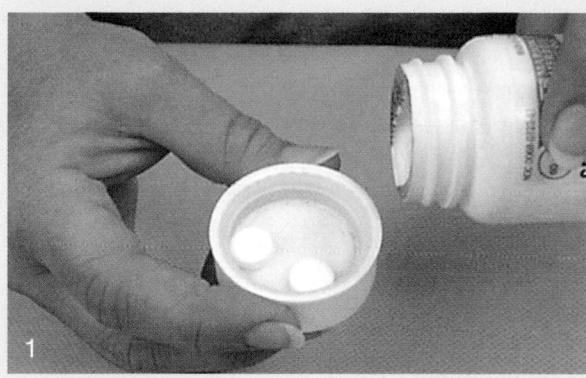

9. Empty the medication in the container lid into a medicine cup.

Dispensing Liquid Oral Preparations (HydroDiuril Solution)

10. Mix medication well if required.
11. When liquid medications are poured, the label should be held in the palm of the hand.
   PURPOSE: To protect the label from medication spills. The medication must be discarded if staff members are unable to read the drug label clearly.
12. Place the medicine cup on a flat surface and, at eye level, pour the medication to the prescribed dose mark on the medicine cup (Figure 2).
   PURPOSE: At eye level, the base of the **meniscus** is where the prescribed dose should be measured.

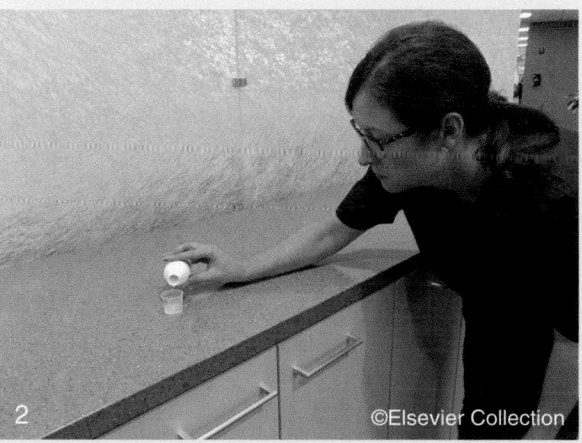

©Elsevier Collection

PROCEDURE 28-1   *—continued*

For Both Solid and Liquid Oral Medications

13. Recap the container and compare the label with the provider's order before replacing the container in storage.
    <u>PURPOSE</u>: To compare the medication label and the provider's order the third of three times.
14. Take the medication to the patient.
15. Greet the patient, and identify him or her by name and date of birth (DOB); compare them to the name and DOB on the order.
    <u>PURPOSE</u>: To make sure you have the right patient. This completes the Right Patient of the rules of medication administration.
16. Mention the name of the drug and the reason it is being given. Ask the patient whether she or he has any allergies to the medication.
    <u>PURPOSE</u>: To educate the patient about drug treatment and to verify that the patient is not allergic to the prescribed medication.
17. If necessary, help the patient into a sitting position.
18. Administer tablets, capsules, or caplets with water. If the patient is receiving liquid medication, offer water after the medication has been taken if appropriate. Make sure the patient swallows the entire dose. This completes the Right Route and the Right Time of the rules of medication administration.

19. Provide patient education about the purpose of the drug, typical side effects, and dosage and storage recommendations. Consult the provider to clarify information if needed.
    <u>PURPOSE</u>: To ensure compliance with home drug therapy and to monitor for side effects.
20. The patient must remain in the office for 20 to 30 minutes after drug administration as a precaution against untoward effects.
21. If the patient experiences any discomfort after taking a medication, the provider should be notified immediately and the incident documented completely and accurately.
22. Sanitize your hands.
23. Document the administration of the drug, including the date and time; the drug name, dose, strength, and route of administration; any patient side effects; and patient education provided about the drug. This completes the Right Documentation of the rules of medication administration.

6/8/20–9:45 AM: HydroDiuril 100 mg tab administered PO per Dr. Thau's order. Pt ed conducted; pt had no questions. Dorothy Gaston, CMA (AAMA)

Nasal Administration

Nose drops and nasal sprays may be used for localized effect; however, like the inhalation drugs, they can spill over into the bloodstream. Some nasal preparations, such as decongestants, can cause an increased heart rate, elevated blood pressure, or central nervous system stimulation. Nasal medications are commonly used for blocked nasal passages (decongestants) and nosebleeds (hemostatics). Nasal decongestant sprays are often misused by patients. Be sure to teach the patient not to exceed the amount or frequency ordered by the provider. If too much is used, these drugs can dry the mucosa and make congestion worse. Nasal inhalants can also be used for their systemic effect, such as the corticosteroid Flonase, which may be prescribed as part of asthmatic treatment.

Topical Forms

Topical drugs are prescribed for both local and systemic effects. Skin medication forms include lotions, liniments, ointments, and transdermal patches. The medical assistant should wear gloves when applying any topical treatment to prevent self-administration of the drug.

Lotions

Often used to control itching, lotions are applied by dabbing with a soft cloth, a cotton ball, or a tongue blade. To prevent contamination, only a sterile item, such as a sterile tongue blade, should be inserted into the lotion container. Calamine is an example. Some lotions are used to relieve inflammation and pain in muscles and joints. After the lotion has been applied, the area may be covered with a thick cloth to retain heat. However, the therapeutic value of these preparations is controversial. The effects of musculoskeletal lotions are limited to the skin surface where the medication is applied.

Liniments

Liniments (emulsions) have a higher portion of oil than lotions, and volatile active ingredients may be added. Liniments are often used to protect dried, cracked, or fissured skin.

Ointments

Ointments, such as bacitracin, are semisolid medications containing bases such as petrolatum and lanolin. An ointment should be removed from a jar or tube with a tongue blade to prevent contamination of the remaining medication.

Transdermal Patches

Certain medications can be absorbed slowly through the skin to create a constant, timed-release systemic effect (Figure 28-4). The

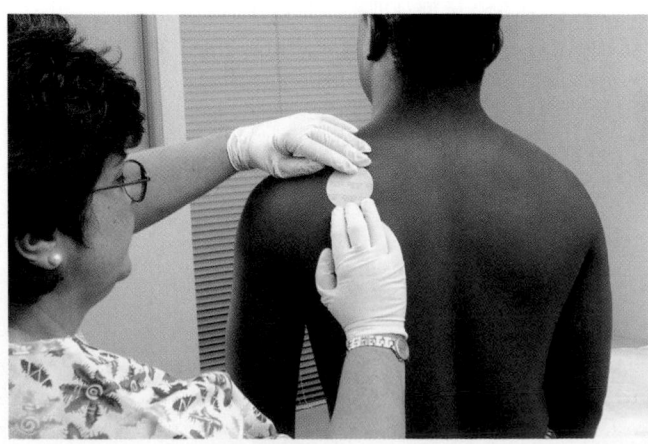

FIGURE 28-4 Transdermal patch.

nitroglycerin patch is particularly useful for patients with frequent attacks of angina. Estrogen and testosterone patches allow the hormones to be absorbed slowly through the skin. With dermal patches, drugs can be administered in a time-released manner for as long as 7 days. The date and time the patch was applied should be written on the patch and documented in the patient's record.

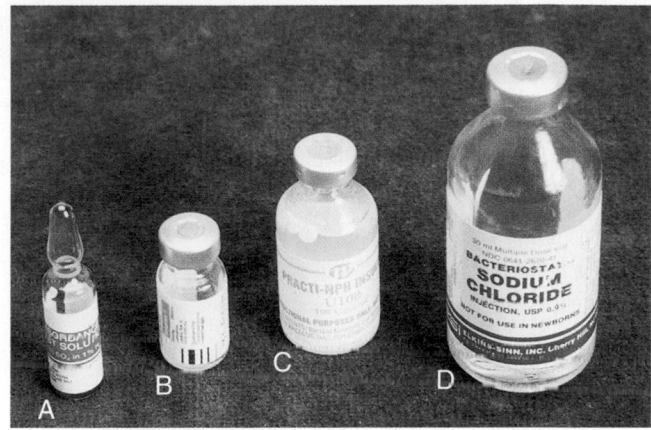

FIGURE 28-5 **A,** Ampule. **B,** Single-dose vial. **C** and **D,** Multidose vials.

Patient Teaching Recommendations for Transdermal Patches

1. Wash your hands.
2. Hold the patch so that the plastic backing is facing you.
3. Peel off one side of the plastic backing.
4. Use the other side of the patch as a handle, and apply the sticky half to your skin in the spot you have chosen.
5. Press the sticky side of the patch against the skin and smooth it down.
6. Fold back the other side of the patch. Hold onto the remaining piece of plastic backing and use it to pull the patch across the skin.
7. Wash your hands again.
8. When you are ready to remove the patch, press down on its center to lift the edges away from the skin.
9. Hold the edge gently and slowly peel the patch away from the skin.

The patient may shower with the patch in place. Rotate sites to prevent skin irritation. Follow package insert directions on where to apply the patch, avoiding scars and areas with a great deal of body hair. If the patch is to remain on for 24 hours or for an extended number of days, apply a new patch at the same time every day. Dispose of used patches by folding them in half with the sticky side together and placing in a garbage can that is out of the reach of children and pets because the old patch may still contain medication.

http://www.nursingcenter.com/journalarticle?Article_ID=789127. Accessed November 16, 2015.

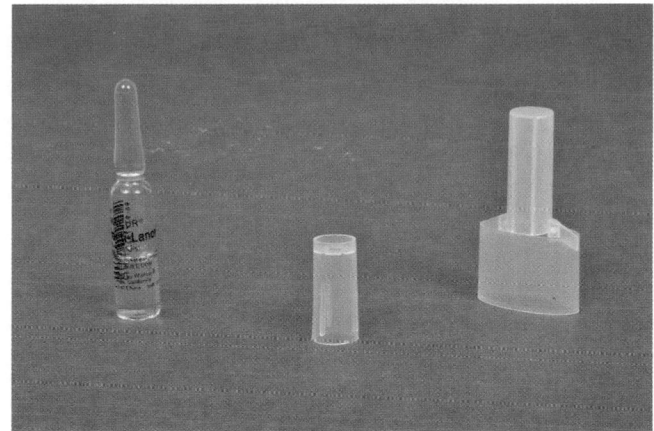

FIGURE 28-6 An ampule opener/breaker.

Parenteral Medication Forms

Injectable medications must be sterile and in liquid form. These medications may be supplied in an ampule, a single-dose vial, or a multidose vial (Figure 28-5). The drug usually is in a solution that is minimally irritating to human tissues (e.g., normal saline solution, sterile water) and may contain a preservative or a small amount of antibiotic to prevent bacterial growth in the vial. All injectable medications are dated. Before use, check the expiration date and examine the solution for possible deterioration. If the medication is discolored or if any sediment has formed at the bottom of the vial, the vial should be discarded. A parenteral medication is administered with a sterile syringe and needle.

Guidelines established by the Occupational Safety and Health Administration (OSHA) must be followed when any sharp instrument is used, including all types of needles, because every needle used on a patient is contaminated with blood and body fluids. The medical assistant must wear disposable gloves when administering parenteral injections, must immediately engage the syringe unit's safety device after use, and must dispose of the unit in a sharps container.

Ampule

An *ampule* is a small glass flask that contains a single dose of medication. Its neck has a scored weak point where the ampule is broken just before use (see Figure 28-5, *A*). Figure 28-6 shows a type of ampule opener/breaker that helps the medical assistant open a glass ampule without the potential for injury. After opening, the top of the ampule must be disposed of in a sharps container. Procedure 28-2 explains the special technique required for opening an ampule of medication and withdrawing medication for administration.

Single-Dose Vial

A single-dose vial is a small bottle with a rubber stopper through which a sterile needle is inserted to withdraw the single dose of medication inside. Before a sterile syringe and needle unit can be introduced into the solution, the rubber stopper must be wiped in a circular motion with alcohol or another suitable disinfectant (Procedure 28-3). The vial is discarded after medication has been withdrawn.

Goal: *To correctly and safely remove medication from a glass ampule for administration.*

EQUIPMENT and SUPPLIES

- Patient's health record
- Written provider's order, including the drug name, strength, dose, and route of administration
- Syringe and needle unit
- Needle of the appropriate length and gauge
- Medication ampule
- Filter needle
- Sterile gauze squares
- Alcohol squares
- Ampule opener/breaker if available
- Sharps container
- PDR, online drug reference, or package insert

PROCEDURAL STEPS

1. Read the order and clarify any questions with the provider.
   PURPOSE: The medical assistant should never dispense or administer a drug without making sure the provider's order is legible and the details of the drug are known.

2. If you are unfamiliar with the medication, refer to the PDR, online drug reference, or package insert to determine the purpose of the drug, common side effects, typical dose, and any pertinent precautions or contraindications. Be prepared to answer any questions the patient may have about the medication. Use the Seven Rights to prevent errors.

3. Perform calculations needed to match the provider's order. Confirm the answer with the provider if you have any questions.

4. Dispense the medication in a well-lit, quiet area.
   PURPOSE: To prevent distractions and possible errors.

5. Assemble the equipment and sanitize your hands.

6. Compare the order with the label on the ampule of medicine when you remove it from storage. Check the expiration date on the container and dispose of the medication if it has expired.
   PURPOSE: To compare the medication label and the provider's order the first of three times.

7. Gently tap the top of the ampule with your fingers to settle all the medication to the bottom portion of the flask (Figure 1).

8. Compare the order with the label on the container of medicine just before dispensing the ordered dose. Make sure the strength on the label matches the order or that you dispense the correctly calculated dose.
   PURPOSE: To compare the medication label and the provider's order the second of three times.

9. Thoroughly disinfect the neck of the ampule with alcohol squares.
   PURPOSE: To prevent possible contamination of the medication.

10. Place the ampule breaker over the top of the ampule and follow the manufacturer's instructions to open/break the ampule (Figure 2). If no ampule breaker is available, wrap the top of the ampule with a gauze square to protect yourself from the glass. Hold the covered ampule between your thumb and finger, in front of you and above waist level (Figure 3).
    PURPOSE: To protect your fingers and maintain eye contact with the medication ampule at all times.

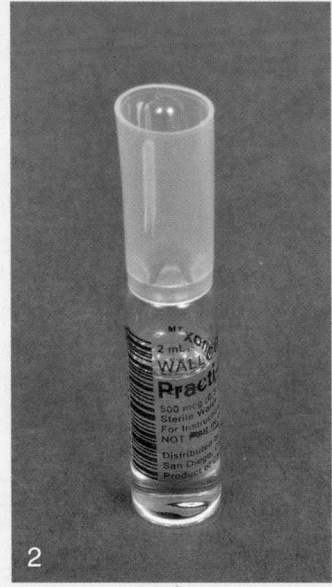

2

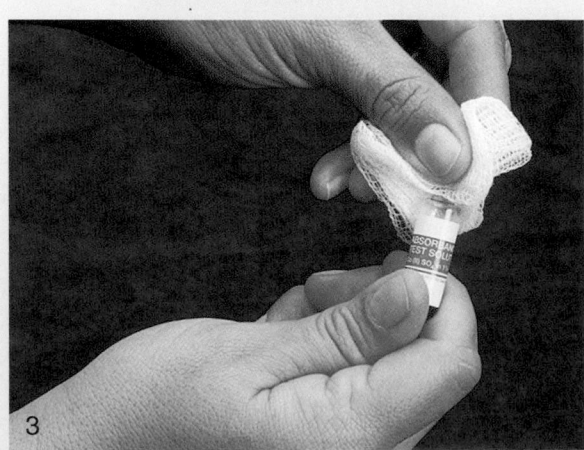

3

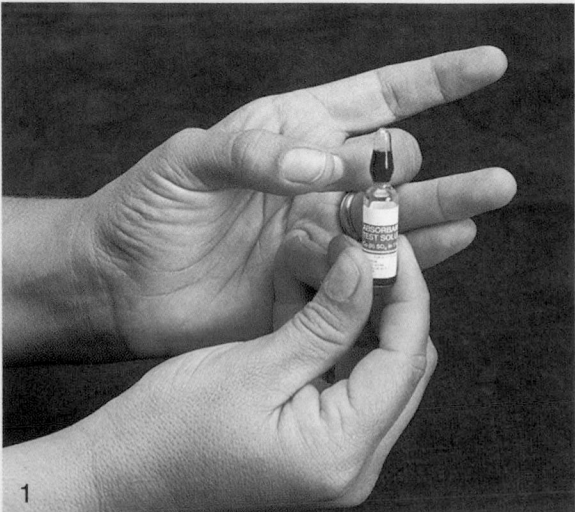

1

PROCEDURE 28-2 —*continued*

11. Follow manufacturer's guidelines for using the ampule opener (Figure 4). If one is not available push the gauze-covered ampule top away from your body to break the neck of the ampule. You will hear a pop because the ampule is vacuum sealed. The glass is designed not to shatter, and the medication will not spill out. Dispose of the ampule opener with the glass ampule top inside (or of the gauze square and the glass top) in the sharps container (Figure 5).

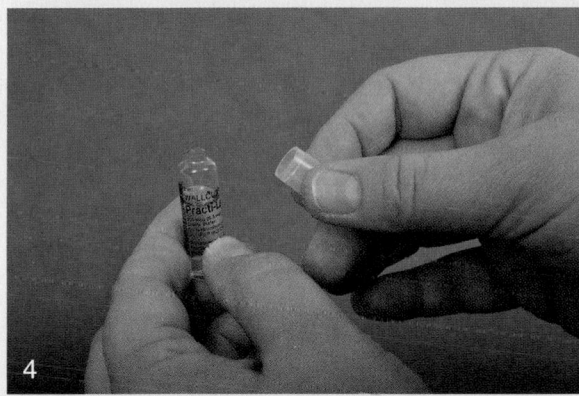

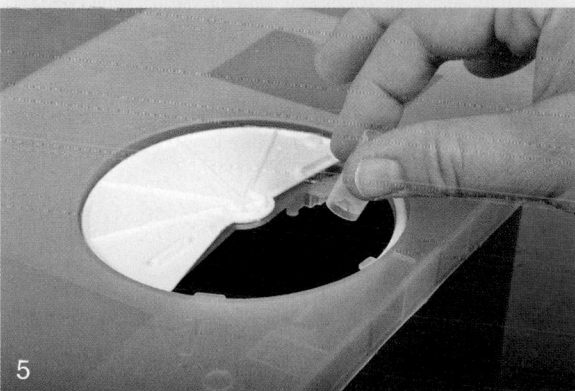

12. Open the sterile syringe and needle unit. Touching the needle covers only, unscrew the needle from the syringe and place it in the sharps container, then attach the sterile filter needle.
    PURPOSE: To maintain the sterility of the unit, only the needle covers are touched. The filter needle is needed to withdraw the medication from the ampule to prevent accidental aspiration of glass fragments into the injection unit.

13. Without touching the outside of the opened ampule, insert the syringe unit with the filter needle attached into the ampule and withdraw the ordered dose. Then place the needle cover back on the filter needle.
    PURPOSE: Touching the needle with anything except the sterile interior of the ampule contaminates the needle. If this happens, start over again with a new filter needle. Recover the filter needle so it can be removed safely.

14. Before discarding the ampule in the sharps container, check the provider's order against the label one more time to complete the three label checks. If you are drawing the medication up for the provider to administer, take the ampule and the syringe unit to the provider for the final safety check.

15. Change the filter needle, safeguarding the sterility of the injection unit, for a needle of the appropriate length and gauge based on the provider's ordered route of administration and patient characteristics. Discard the used filter needle into the sharps container.
    PURPOSE: A new needle is used to prevent the possible injection of glass particles on or inside the filter needle.

16. Dispose of used alcohol and gauze squares.

PROCEDURE 28-3 Fill a Syringe from a Vial

Goal: *To fill a syringe from a multidose vial using sterile technique.*

EQUIPMENT and SUPPLIES

- Patient's health record
- Written provider's order, including the drug name, strength, dose, and route of administration
- Multidose vial containing the medication ordered
- Alcohol wipes
- Sterile needle and syringe unit
- PDR, online drug reference, or package insert

PROCEDURAL STEPS

1. Read the order and clarify any questions with the provider.
   PURPOSE: The medical assistant should never dispense or administer a drug without making sure the provider's order is legible and the details of the drug are known.

2. If you are unfamiliar with the medication, refer to the PDR, online drug reference, or package insert to determine the purpose of the drug, common side effects, typical dose, and any pertinent precautions or

PROCEDURE 28-3   *—continued*

contraindications. Be prepared to answer any questions the patient may have about the medication. Use the Seven Rights to prevent errors.

3. Perform calculations needed to match the provider's order. Confirm the answer with the provider if you have any questions.

4. Dispense the medication in a well-lit, quiet area.
   PURPOSE: To prevent distractions and possible errors.

5. Assemble the equipment and sanitize your hands. Choose the correct syringe and needle unit, depending on the site of administration, patient characteristics, and the amount of medication to be injected (Figure 1).

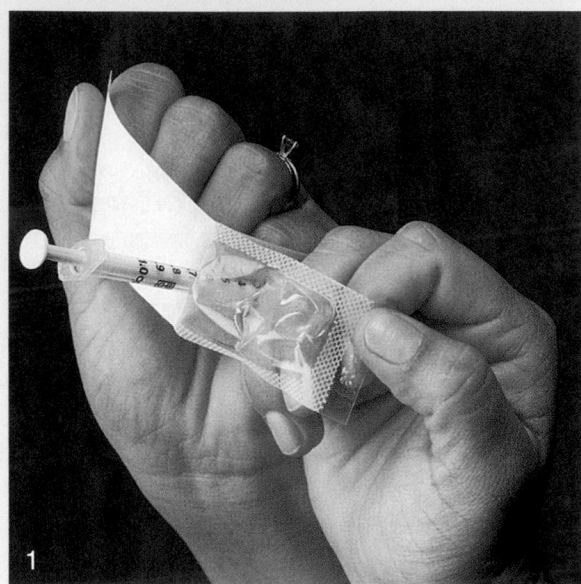

6. Compare the order with the label on the vial of medicine when you remove it from storage. Check the quality of the medication and the expiration date on the container and dispose of the medication if it appears contaminated, contains sediment, or has expired.
   PURPOSE: To compare the medication label and the provider's order the first of three times.

7. Compare the order with the label on the vial of medicine just before dispensing the ordered dose. Make sure the strength on the label matches the order or that you dispense the correctly calculated dose.
   PURPOSE: To compare the medication label and the provider's order the second of three times.

8. Gently agitate the medication by rolling the vial between your palms (Figure 2).
   PURPOSE: To mix any medication that may have settled.

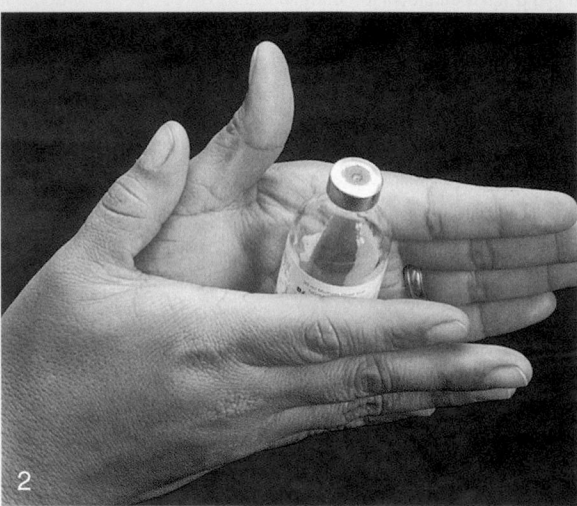

9. Clean the rubber stopper of the vial with the alcohol wipe using a circular motion (Figure 3). Place the vial on a secure, flat surface, leaving the alcohol swab over the rubber stopper.

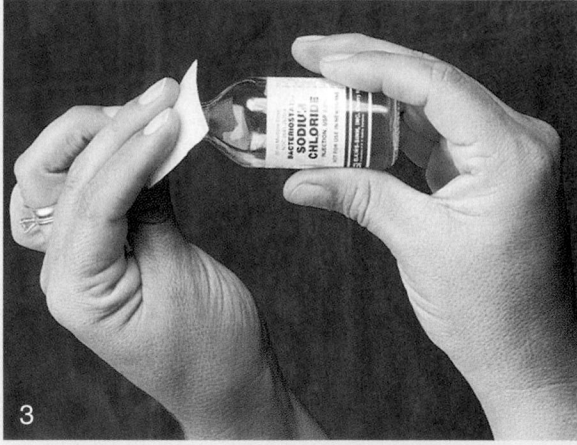

10. With the needle cover in place, grasp the syringe plunger and draw up an amount of air equal to the amount of medication ordered.
    PURPOSE: Not enough replaced air makes it difficult to withdraw the medication; too much replaced air increases the pressure in the vial so that medication is forced into the syringe without the plunger being pulled to withdraw it.

11. Remove the alcohol swab over the rubber stopper and the needle cover and insert the needle into the center of the rubber stopper. Hold the vial firmly against a flat surface and watch carefully that the needle touches only the cleaned rubber area.
    PURPOSE: To maintain the sterility of the needle.

12. Inject the aspirated air in the syringe into the vial.

PROCEDURE 28-3 —continued

13. Keeping the syringe unit in the vial, pick up and invert them (Figure 4). Slowly pull back on the plunger with the unit at eye level and draw up more medication than ordered into the syringe unit.
    PURPOSE: Withdrawing medication rapidly causes air bubbles to form in the syringe. Draw up extra medication so that any bubbles in the syringe can be injected back into the vial while maintaining sterility.

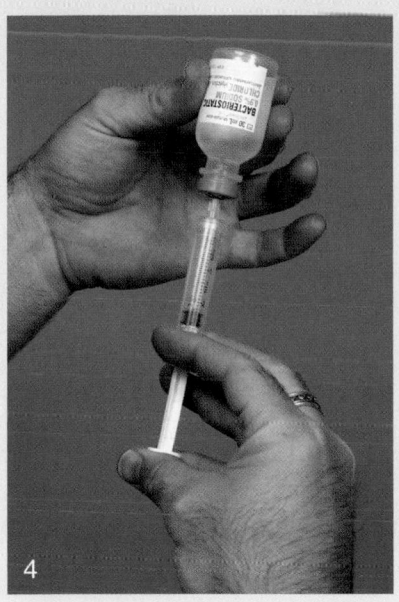

4

14. While the needle is still in the vial, check for air bubbles in the syringe.
    PURPOSE: Air bubbles displace medication, and the patient will not receive the proper amount of medication.
15. If air bubbles are present, slip the fingers holding the vial down to grasp the vial and syringe as a single unit.
    PURPOSE: This frees your dominant hand.
16. With your free hand, tap the syringe until the air bubbles dislodge and float into the tip of the syringe.
17. Inject the air bubbles back into the vial with the extra medication that was withdrawn. At eye level, make sure the accurate amount of medication is in the syringe unit.
18. Withdraw the needle from the vial and carefully replace the needle cover without letting the needle touch the outside of the cover.
19. Return the medication to the shelf or the refrigerator, checking the order against the label one more time to complete the three label checks.
    PURPOSE: This is the third of the three drug label and order checks.
20. Dispose of used alcohol and gauze squares.

Multidose Vial

A multidose vial is a bottle with a rubber stopper that contains enough medication for multiple injections. Multidose vials are labeled as such by the manufacturer and typically contain an antimicrobial preservative to help prevent the growth of bacteria. However, the preservative has no effect on viruses and does not protect against contamination when healthcare personnel fail to follow aseptic practices. The medical assistant should write on the bottle the date the first dose from a multidose vial is administered and should follow the manufacturer's guidelines or the facility's policy on how long the vial can remain on the shelf. The Centers for Disease Control and Prevention (CDC) recommends that if a multidose vial has been punctured with a needle, the vial should be dated and discarded within 28 days unless the manufacturer specifies a different (shorter or longer) date for an opened vial. Because multidose vials are used more than once, extreme caution must be taken every time a needle is inserted into the medication, to protect it from contamination, which could cause a very serious infection in subsequent patients. If at any time you believe an error has been made or you suspect possible contamination, discard the vial. *Never* return unused medication to the vial. If you have more medication than you need in the syringe, eject the excess while the needle remains in the vial. Never inject unneeded medication into the vial once the needle has been removed.

Vials are vacuum sealed. Each time you withdraw medication from a vial, you first must replace the portion of withdrawn medication with the same portion of air. Not enough replaced air makes it difficult to withdraw medication, and too much replaced air increases pressure within the vial, forcing medication into the syringe. See Procedure 28-3 for instructions on how to safely and accurately withdraw medication from a vial.

Prefilled Syringe

A prefilled syringe is a sterile, disposable syringe and needle unit packaged by the manufacturer with a single dose of medication that is ready to administer. Some prefilled syringe units are designed to fit into a reusable cartridge injection system (Figure 28-7). The Carpuject Syringe System is an example of a cartridge system for the injection of prefilled syringes. Most prefilled syringe units are overfilled with medication or may contain more medication than was ordered by the practitioner. Before administration, carefully check the unit and expel any excess medication or air to make sure the patient receives an accurate dose.

Parenteral Medication Equipment

Syringes and needles are manufactured in countless varieties for specific purposes and sometimes for specific medications. For example, a special syringe unit used for insulin is calibrated in units

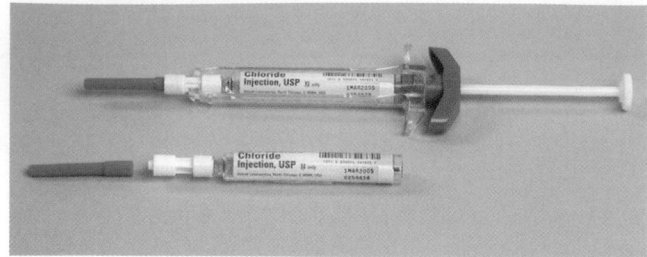

FIGURE 28-7 Carpuject Syringe System with a prefilled syringe and needle with safety device. (From deWit SC, O'Neill PA: *Fundamental concepts and skills for nursing,* ed 4, Philadelphia, 2014, Saunders.)

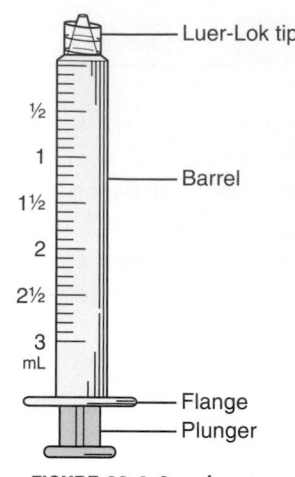

FIGURE 28-9 Parts of a syringe.

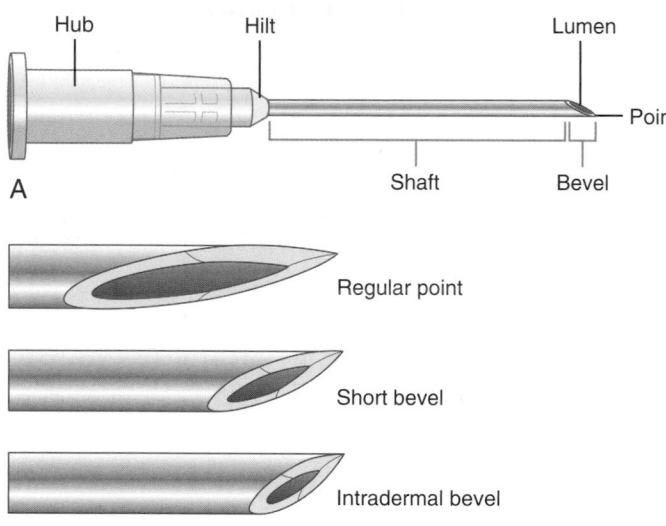

FIGURE 28-8 A, The construction of a hypodermic needle. **B,** Needle points.

of measurement and packaged with a microneedle. Hypodermic needles are manufactured in many lengths and gauges, depending on the depth of the injection, the **viscosity** of the medication to be injected, the ordered route of administration, and patient characteristics. Needles may be purchased separately or as part of a needle-syringe unit. Figure 28-8 shows the parts of a needle and the three common types of **bevel** points. Needles are measured for length from the place where the cannula or shaft joins the hub to the tip of the point.

Needle Gauge

The diameter, or lumen size, of a needle is called its *gauge.* Needle gauges range in size from 14 (the largest) to 31 (the smallest). *The larger the gauge number, the smaller the diameter of the needle.* Gauges 27 and 28 are used for intradermal (ID) injections, as in screening for tuberculosis (TB), when a very small opening is desired. These fine needle widths leave a small amount of medication just below the surface of the skin with a minimum amount of injury. Gauges 25 and 26 are commonly used for subcutaneous (SC) injections. Insulin needles may be as small as 31 gauge.

Medications in an **aqueous** solution and with low viscosity are easily injected through a small opening. In addition, these two gauges cause minimal tissue damage, and the patient experiences

less pain. Larger needles (gauges 20 to 23) usually are necessary for intramuscular (IM) injections when the medication is thick (e.g., penicillin) or when the needle length requires the extra support of a thicker gauge. A patient cannot feel the difference between a 20- and a 22-gauge needle. In fact, the medication is not forced as strongly into the tissues with the larger 20-gauge needle as with the 22-gauge needle, and the patient actually experiences less pain. Needles larger than 20 gauge are not used for drug therapy. They are used mostly for venipuncture, blood donations, and blood transfusions.

Needle Length

Needle lengths range from $\frac{3}{8}$ inch to 4 inches, depending on the area of the body to be injected, the patient's size, and the route (depth) used. ID injections require only the short $\frac{3}{8}$-inch needle. Needles that are $\frac{1}{2}$ or $\frac{5}{8}$ inch long are used for SC injections. Longer needles are needed to deposit drugs intramuscularly. The choice of a 1-inch, $1\frac{1}{2}$-inch, 2-inch, $2\frac{1}{2}$-inch, or 3-inch length depends on both the muscle used and the patient's size.

Syringes

Parts of a syringe include the barrel, a calibrated scale (or scales), the flange, the plunger, and the tip (Figure 28-9). The typical syringe holds up to 3 mL and is calibrated with a milliliter (cubic centimeter) scale, with each calibrated line marked at 0.1 mL. The tuberculin syringe, which is used for small amounts of drug, holds up to 1 mL of injectable material, and each calibrated line is marked at 0.01 mL (Figure 28-10, *A*).

The insulin syringe is calibrated in units specifically for the use of patients with diabetes. Insulin syringes are calibrated to hold 30 units, 50 units, or 100 units of insulin (see Figure 28-10, *B* and *C*). The type of calibration chosen depends on the total amount of insulin to be injected in one dose. When less than 30 units is to be drawn up, the 30-unit syringe should be used; for 30 to 50 units, the 50-unit syringe is used; and for more than 50 units, the 100-unit syringe is used.

The establishment of Standard Precautions and recognition of the danger of needlesticks prompted the development of syringe units with safety needle devices (Figures 28-11 and 28-12); these must be

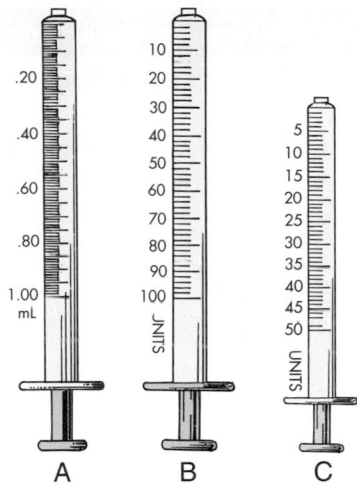

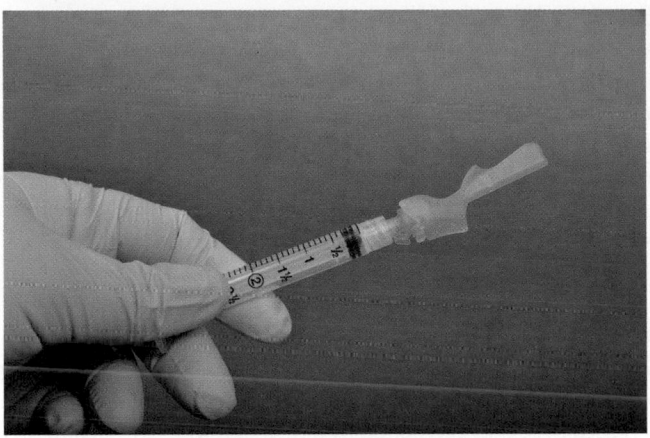

FIGURE 28-11 A safety needle device.

FIGURE 28-10 Types of syringes. **A,** 1-mL syringe. **B,** 100-unit insulin syringe. **C,** 50-unit insulin syringe. (From Perry AG, Potter PA: *Clinical nursing skills and techniques,* ed 8, St Louis, 2014, Mosby.)

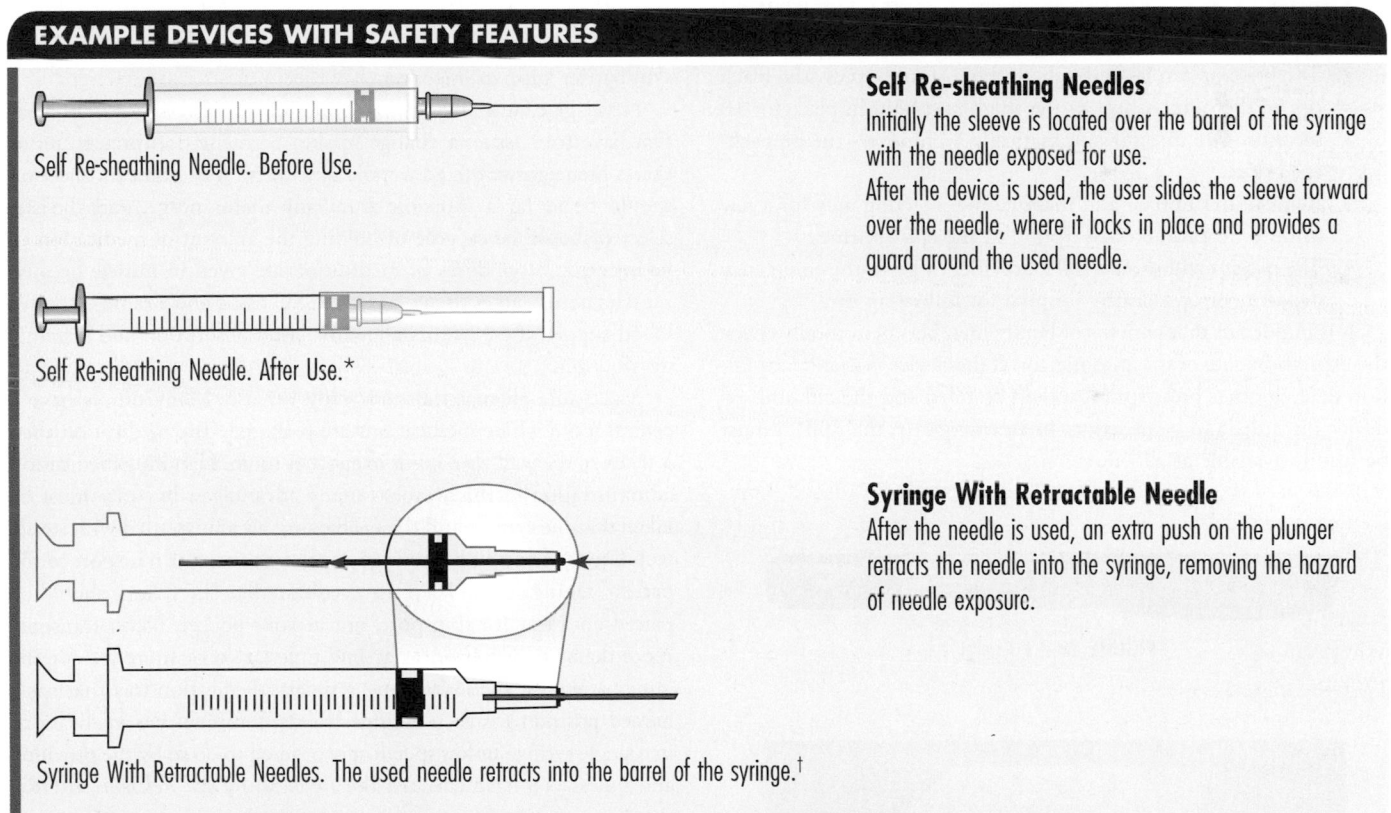

EXAMPLE DEVICES WITH SAFETY FEATURES

Self Re-sheathing Needle. Before Use.

Self Re-sheathing Needle. After Use.*

Syringe With Retractable Needles. The used needle retracts into the barrel of the syringe.†

Self Re-sheathing Needles
Initially the sleeve is located over the barrel of the syringe with the needle exposed for use.
After the device is used, the user slides the sleeve forward over the needle, where it locks in place and provides a guard around the used needle.

Syringe With Retractable Needle
After the needle is used, an extra push on the plunger retracts the needle into the syringe, removing the hazard of needle exposure.

From Occupational Safety and Health Administration, *http://www.osha.gov/SLTC/etools/hospital/hazards/sharps/sharps.html#safer*
*Please note that these safety devices lock in place and do not reset in actual use situations.
†Please note that these safety devices lock in place and do not reset in actual use situations.

FIGURE 28-12 Examples of safety needles.

made available to employees as an OSHA safeguard against accidental needlesticks. A safety needle is an injection device designed with special functions that allow the needle either to be capped after a patient has been injected or to automatically retract back into the barrel after use. Using safety needles is important because it prevents healthcare workers from accidentally being stuck with a needle, thereby reducing the transmission of diseases such as human immunodeficiency virus (HIV) infection and hepatitis.

Disposable syringe and needle units are packaged in sealed, rigid plastic containers or in peel-apart paper wrappers. Both individual needles and syringe-needle units are color coded for easy identification.

Specialty Syringe Units

An example of a specialty syringe unit is an injector pen that can be used by patients who must give themselves injections away from home. Different types are available, depending on the amount of medication to be dispensed per injection and the type of medication used. Administering insulin away from home is easier and more convenient with an insulin pen (Figure 28-13), which contains a predetermined type and amount of insulin that can be injected with minimal preparation.

The EpiPen is an automatic injector system that contains a dose of epinephrine (Figure 28-14). It must be prescribed by a practitioner and comes packaged with the correct dose for an adult (0.3 mg of epinephrine) or for a child (0.15 mg of epinephrine). The EpiPen is carried as a safety precaution by individuals who have anaphylactic reactions to such allergens as bee stings or certain types of foods. Anaphylactic reactions can be fatal if not treated immediately, so patients and their family members should be educated in the signs and symptoms of anaphylaxis and how to manage the EpiPen injection. The steps for EpiPen injection are quite simple:

1. Pull back the gray end of the autoinjector. This sets the device for use.
2. The injector can go through clothing. Firmly press the black tip on the outer aspect of the thigh and hold in place for 10 seconds. The injector automatically administers the prepackaged dose.
3. Remove the EpiPen and massage the injection area for a few minutes to promote absorption of the epinephrine.
4. The patient still should call a provider or go to the emergency department of a nearby hospital for follow-up care.

It is important that patients or family members periodically check the expiration date of the autoinjector. If the device is near its expiration date, another prescription should be filled and the old, unused device discarded. To be of service in an emergency, the EpiPen must be readily available at all times.

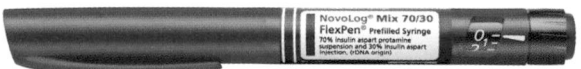

FIGURE 28-13 NovoPen.

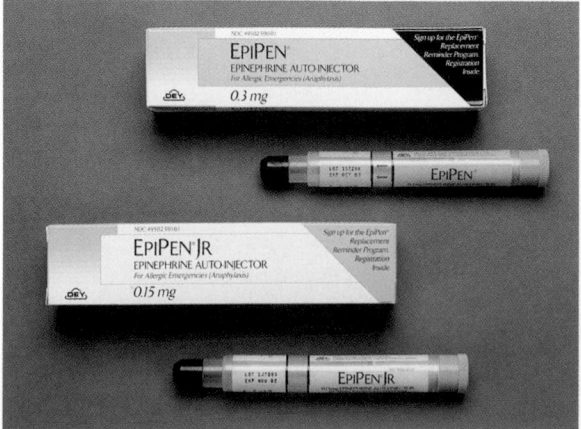

FIGURE 28-14 EpiPen prepackaged autoinjector.

> ### Signs and Symptoms of an Anaphylactic Reaction
>
> - Hypotension resulting from systemic **vasodilation**
> - Hives *(urticaria)*
> - Difficulty breathing *(dyspnea)* resulting from **bronchoconstriction**
> - Difficulty swallowing as a result of **edema**
> - Vomiting and diarrhea

Parenteral Administration

With practice, giving medications by injection becomes easy and even automatic. However, the medical assistant must always follow the provider's orders, perform the three order and label checks while dispensing the medication, and strictly adhere to the Seven Rights throughout the procedure.

Develop and practice techniques that provide maximum safety and comfort for the patient. Injections are least painful when (1) the needle is inserted swiftly; (2) the medication is injected slowly; and (3) the needle is removed quickly, with counterpressure when needed. Remember that the same aseptic conditions necessary for minor surgery are necessary whenever you penetrate the protective skin barrier with an injection.

Never give an injection near bones or blood vessels. Avoid areas that have scar tissue; a change in skin pigmentation or texture; or excess tissue growth (e.g., a mole or a wart). The point of injection should be as far as possible from any major nerve, and the site selected should be capable of holding the amount of medication to be injected. Large doses of medication are given in muscle because muscles have a larger tissue mass than SC tissue and a more extensive blood supply; these factors allow for faster absorption and systemic distribution.

Make sure all materials are ready for use. Many offices have a central room where medications are prepared. The medication then is taken to the waiting patient in another room. Handling medication administration in this way has many advantages, but care must be taken that the syringe and the needle unit are transported with sterile technique. After filling a syringe, replace the cap for transport to the patient, taking care to keep the needle sterile. The syringe should be placed on a tray for transport, not in your pocket. Never transport more than one injection at a time unless two or more are for the same patient or unless you have a special medication tray that has a named position for each syringe. Never combine two medications in a single syringe unless specifically ordered to do so by the provider, and unless you have checked the *Physicians' Desk Reference* (PDR), an online drug resource, or the medication's package insert for contraindications on mixing different types of medications. If you are preparing a medication for the provider to give, place the vial or empty ampule beside the filled syringe. This shows what medication is in the syringe and offers a double check for safety.

Some medications for injection are packaged in vials as sterile powders or crystals that must be mixed with sterile water or saline before they can be administered; the amount of solvent to be added to the dry form of the drug (solute) depends on the provider's order and the label directions. After calculating the correct amount of liquid that must be added to the dry form of the drug to create the dose ordered by the provider, follow the guidelines in Procedure 28-4 to prepare the drug and administer it to the patient.

Guidelines for Parenteral Administration of Medications

1. Use a two-step method to identify the patient, typically asking the patient his or her full name and date of birth (DOB).
2. Use a professional approach, and explain what you are going to do.
3. Sanitize your hands before the procedure—and also afterward.
4. Small talk can keep the patient's mind off the procedure.
5. Never tell a patient that it will not hurt; you may destroy your credibility.
6. Make the patient as comfortable as possible, and allow for privacy.
7. Never allow the patient to stand during the procedure.
8. Keep the syringe unit out of the patient's sight as much as possible.
9. Always wear disposable gloves.
10. Immediately after the injection, activate the needle safety device and dispose of it in a sharps container with the needle inserted first.
11. *Never* recap a contaminated needle.
12. Provide patient education and coaching as needed.
13. Document complete details about the procedure in the patient record.

Intradermal Injections

Intradermal injections are given within the skin layers (Figure 28-15 and Procedure 28-5). The ID site is used for allergy testing and tuberculin screening. The tine test is no longer used to screen for TB because it was found to be unreliable in diagnosing exposures to the TB bacillus. The Mantoux (purified protein derivative [PPD]) ID test now is used routinely to screen for TB exposure. It is the only widely used test for detecting **asymptomatic** TB infection, currently termed *latent tuberculosis infection* (LTBI).

With the Mantoux test, a 0.1-mL tuberculin solution of PPD is injected into the intradermal layers. If the person was infected with the TB bacillus in the past, his or her immune system developed antibodies that recognize and fight the bacteria. When a PPD skin test is performed, these antibodies move to the injection site to try to stop the infection. This immune reaction causes swelling and **induration** in the area approximately 48 hours after administration of the skin test. An induration 5 mm in diameter or larger is considered a positive test result in patients at increased risk of being infected and in individuals who are most likely to develop active disease if infected with TB bacteria. These individuals include those infected with HIV; anyone in close contact with a patient newly diagnosed with TB (e.g., family members); and patients who have undergone recent organ transplantation or are taking **immunosuppressant** medications. A 10-mm or greater induration is read as positive if the person has a moderate likelihood of TB exposure and infection; these individuals include recent immigrants from countries in which TB is prevalent; intravenous (IV) drug users; residents and employees of correctional institutions, homeless shelters, and healthcare facilities (including medical personnel); and children younger than 4 years of age. Regardless of risk factors, anyone with an induration of 15 mm or greater is considered positive.

Patients must return to the office after the specified period so that a staff member can read the results (see Procedure 28-5). Many healthcare facilities now require employees to have a two-step tuberculin skin test (TST) to more accurately diagnose individuals who have been previously exposed to TB. The employee is tested as explained and then 48 to 72 hours later is retested. The first TST may be negative because the immune system did not immediately identify the TB bacillus. However, the second dose helps trigger the immune response and identifies individuals who have been previously exposed to TB.

When an ID injection is administered correctly, a small **wheal** is raised on the skin. A ⅜-inch, 27- or 28-gauge needle is used for ID injections. The angle of insertion is 15 degrees, almost parallel to the skin surface. The best site for injection is the center of the anterior forearm, but the upper chest and back are frequently used for allergy testing (Figure 28-16).

FIGURE 28-15 The intradermal (ID) injection is administered just under the epidermis. Because the drug is dispersed in an area where many nerves are present, it causes momentary burning or stinging. Minute amounts of medication are injected. This method is used to test for allergies, drug sensitivities, and susceptibility to some diseases. Can also be used as an injection technique for influenza vaccines that are pre-packaged with microneedles and are injected into the deltoid region.

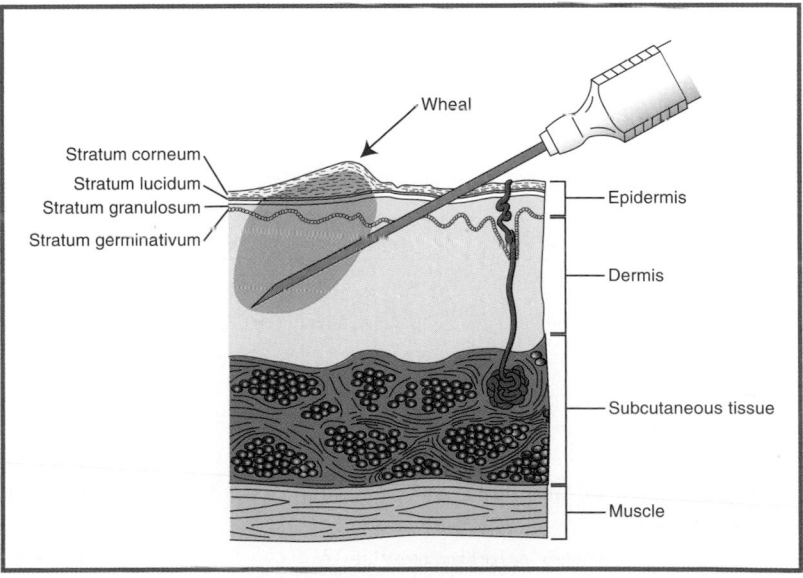

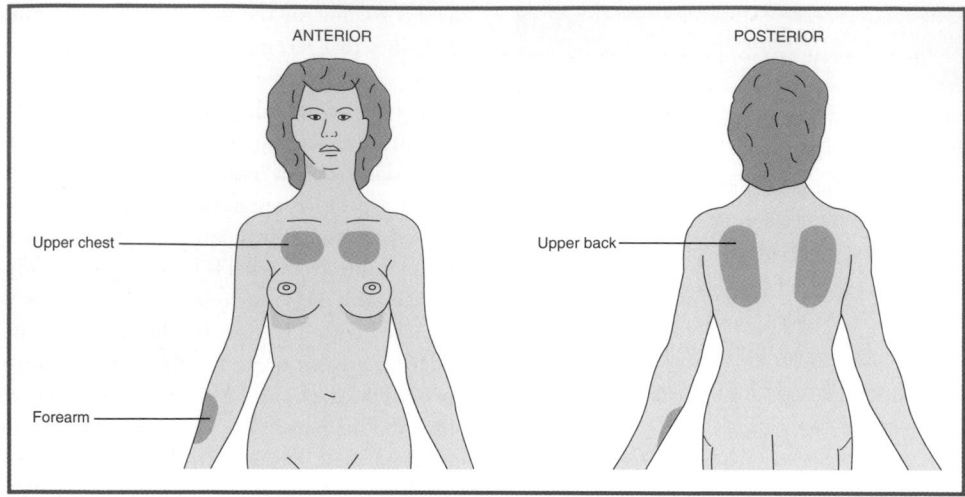

FIGURE 28-16 Sites recommended for intradermal injections.

Fluzone Intradermal Quadrivalent (Influenza Vaccine)

A newly released influenza vaccine is now packaged with a very small needle to enable the delivery of the vaccine into the subcutaneous layer. The technique of administration is similar to an intramuscular injection in the deltoid area but the needle is so small that it only enters the tissue as far as the dermal layer.

- The vaccine is indicated for the prevention of 4 different strains of influenza.
- A single 0.1 mL dose is available for intradermal injection in adults 18 through 64 years of age.
- Packaged as a suspension for injection in a prefilled microinjection system that administers the vaccine into the dermal layer.
- The preferred site of injection is the skin in the region of the deltoid at a 90-degree angle.
- Contraindicated in anyone with a history of a severe allergic reaction to egg protein or to a previous dose of any influenza vaccine.

CRITICAL THINKING APPLICATION   28-4

Dorothy is ordered to give her first Mantoux test since being hired by Dr. Thau. Document the details that Dorothy should include in the patient's health record. She administered 0.1 mL of PPD by ID injection into the patient's right midforearm and instructed the patient on when to return to the office to have the test read.

_____

_____

_____

PROCEDURE 28-4   Reconstitute a Powdered Drug for Administration

Goal: *To reconstitute a powdered drug for intramuscular injection as ordered by the provider.*

EQUIPMENT and SUPPLIES

- Patient's health record
- Written provider's order, including the drug name, strength, dose, and route of administration
- Vial containing the ordered powdered medication
- Diluent: sterile saline
- Alcohol wipes
- Two sterile needle and syringe units
- Sharps container
- PDR, online drug reference, or package insert

PROCEDURAL STEPS

1. Read the order and clarify any questions with the provider.
   <u>PURPOSE</u>: The medical assistant should never dispense or administer a drug without making sure the provider's order is legible and the details of the drug are known.
2. If you are unfamiliar with the medication, refer to the PDR, online drug reference, or package insert to determine the purpose of the drug, common side effects, typical dose, and any pertinent precautions or contraindications. Be prepared to answer any questions the patient may have about the medication. Use the Seven Rights to prevent errors.

PROCEDURE 28-4 *—continued*

3. Perform calculations needed to match the provider's order. Confirm the answer with the provider if you have any questions.
4. Dispense the medication in a well-lit, quiet area.
   PURPOSE: To prevent distractions and possible errors.
5. Assemble the equipment and sanitize your hands. Choose the correct syringe and needle unit, depending on the site of administration, patient characteristics, and the amount of medication to be injected.
6. Select the correct vial of powdered medication from the shelf and the recommended diluent for reconstitution. Compare the order with the label on the vial when you remove it from storage. Check the quality of the medication and the expiration date on the container and dispose of the medication if it appears contaminated, contains sediment, or has expired.
   PURPOSE: To compare the medication label and the provider's order the first of three times.
7. Compare the order with the label on the vial of medicine just before dispensing the ordered dose. Read the label to determine the correct amount of diluent to add to create the dose ordered by the provider. Calculate the correct dose, if necessary.
   PURPOSE: To compare the medication label and the provider's order the second of three times.
8. Remove the tops from each vial and clean each with an alcohol wipe. Leave the wipes in place on top of each vial.
9. Using one of the syringe units with the needle cover in place, grasp the syringe plunger and draw up the amount of air equal to the amount of diluent needed to reconstitute the drug.
   PURPOSE: Not enough replaced air makes it difficult to withdraw the diluent; too much replaced air forces the diluent into the syringe without the plunger being pulled to withdraw it.

10. Remove the alcohol swab over the rubber stopper and the needle cover and insert the needle into the center of the rubber stopper of the diluent. Hold the vial firmly against a flat surface and watch carefully that the needle touches only the cleaned rubber area.
11. Inject the aspirated air in the syringe into the diluent vial.
12. Invert the diluent vial and aspirate the calculated or recommended amount of diluent.
13. Remove the alcohol swab over the rubber stopper of the drug vial. Remove the needle from the diluent vial and inject the diluent into the center of the rubber stopper of the drug vial. Remove the needle from the vial and discard the syringe unit into the sharps container.
   PURPOSE: An unused syringe unit should be used to administer the medication to the patient because the needle on the used unit may not be as sharp as that on a new syringe unit.
14. Roll the vial with the drug and diluent mixture between the palms of your hands to mix it thoroughly. Do not shake the vial unless directed to do so on the drug label. When the medication is completely mixed, no residue or crystals are seen on the bottom of the vial.
15. Aspirate air into the second syringe unit that is equal to the calculated amount of medication to be administered.
16. Inject the air into the mixed drug vial, invert the vial, and withdraw the ordered amount of medication.
17. Check the order against the label one more time to complete the three label checks.
   PURPOSE: This is the third of the three drug label and order checks.

PROCEDURE 28-5 **Administer Parenteral (Excluding IV) Medications: Give an Intradermal Injection**

Goal: *To inject 0.1 mL of purified protein derivative (PPD) intradermally (ID) to perform a Mantoux test as ordered by the provider.*

ORDER:

Administer 0.1 mL PPD ID for a Mantoux test for TB screening.

EQUIPMENT and SUPPLIES

- Patient's health record
- Written provider's order, including the drug name, strength, dose, and route of administration
- Vial of tuberculin PPD
- Alcohol wipes
- 27-gauge, ⅜-inch sterile needle and 1-mL syringe unit with safety needle cover device
- Disposable gloves

- Gauze squares
- Sharps container
- PDR, online drug reference, or the package insert
- Written patient instructions for follow-up

PROCEDURAL STEPS

1. Read the order and clarify any questions with the provider.
   PURPOSE: The medical assistant should never dispense or administer a drug without making sure the provider's order is legible and the details of the drug are known.
2. If you are unfamiliar with the medication, refer to the PDR, online drug reference, or package insert to determine the purpose of the drug,

PROCEDURE 28-5   —continued

common side effects, typical dose, and any pertinent precautions or contraindications. Be prepared to answer any questions the patient may have about the medication. Use the Seven Rights to prevent errors.

3. Perform calculations needed to match the provider's order. Confirm the answer with the provider if you have any questions.

4. Dispense the medication in a well-lit, quiet area.
   PURPOSE: To prevent distractions and possible errors.

5. Assemble the equipment and sanitize your hands. Choose the correct syringe and needle unit, depending on the site of administration, patient characteristics, and the amount of medication to be injected.

6. Compare the order with the label on the vial of medicine when you remove it from storage. Check the quality of the medication and the expiration date on the container and dispose of the medication if it appears contaminated, contains sediment, or has expired.
   PURPOSE: To compare the medication label and the provider's order the first of three times.

7. Compare the order with the label on the vial of medicine just before dispensing the ordered dose. Make sure the strength on the label matches the order or that you dispense the correctly calculated dose.
   PURPOSE: To compare the medication label and the provider's order the second of three times.

8. Warm refrigerated medications by gently rolling the container between your palms.

9. Prepare the syringe and vial as described in Procedure 28-3 and withdraw the correct dose of 0.1 mL.

10. Return the medication to the shelf or the refrigerator, checking the order against the label one more time to complete the three label checks.
    PURPOSE: This is the third of the three drug label and order checks.

11. Take the medication to the patient. Greet the patient, and identify him or her by full name and date of birth; compare them to the name and DOB on the order.
    PURPOSE: To make sure you have the right patient.

12. Ask the patient whether he or she has ever had a positive reaction to a PPD injection (TB test). If yes, report this information to the provider before administering the medication. An individual with a history of a positive PPD test result always has a positive result because of antibody action.

13. Put on gloves and position the patient comfortably.
    PURPOSE: To create a wheal successfully, it is easier if the patient is sitting and the medical assistant is lower than the patient (e.g., on a stool) with the anterior surface of the patient's arm extended straight out and angled downward.

14. Locate the antecubital space, then find a site several fingerwidths down the midanterior aspect of the forearm. Avoid any scarred, discolored, or pigmented areas.

15. Loosen the needle cover so that the needle can be picked up with one hand after the site has been cleansed. Open alcohol wipes so they can be grasped with one hand.

PURPOSE: To be able to remove the needle cover with one hand and prevent contamination of the needle; once the site has been grasped and cleaned, you must keep your hand in place on the patient's arm to avoid injecting the PPD solution into an area that was not cleansed with alcohol; you also will need to grasp alcohol wipes with one hand while the other hand is holding tissue up and away from the injection site.

16. Wrap the thumb and the first two fingers of your nondominant hand around the patient's forearm, pulling downward and apart to stretch the skin of the forearm taut at the location of the injection.
    PURPOSE: Stretching the skin tightens the surface and facilitates insertion of the needle with minimum discomfort to the patient. The skin is not stretched tightly enough if it begins to wrinkle as you start to insert the needle.

17. Cleanse the patient's skin with an alcohol wipe using a circular motion, moving from the center outward (Figure 1).

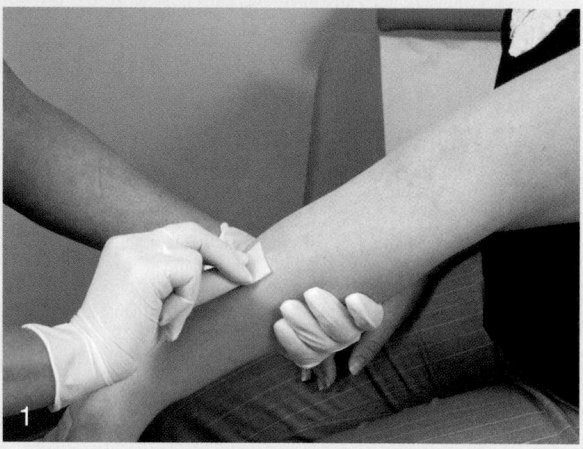

18. Allow the antiseptic to dry while maintaining your grip on the patient's forearm.

19. Pick up the syringe unit, shaking off the already loosened needle cover.

20. Grasp the syringe between the thumb and first two fingers of your dominant hand, palm down, with the needle bevel upward. Hold the syringe close to the plunger end.

21. At a 15-degree angle (Figure 2, A), with the syringe unit parallel to the surface of the skin and the bevel up, carefully insert the needle just until the bevel point is under the skin surface (Figure 2, B).

PROCEDURE 28-5 —continued

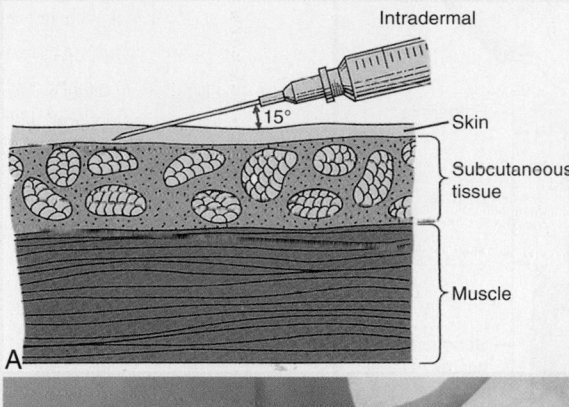

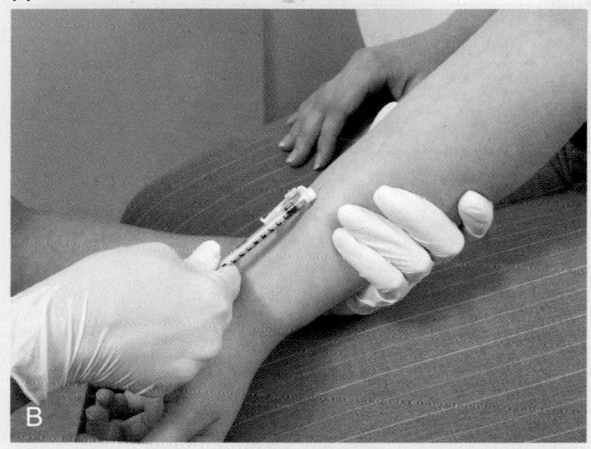

22. Slowly and steadily inject the medication by depressing the plunger with your ring or little finger. Do not aspirate. A wheal should appear.
    PURPOSE: A rapid injection may force the substance through to the surface.
23. After administering all the medication (0.1 mL), withdraw the needle.
24. Immediately cover the contaminated needle with the syringe unit safety device and discard the unit in the sharps container with the needle first.
25. Do not massage the area, but you may blot it with a cotton ball or a gauze square. Do not cover the site with a bandage.
    PURPOSE: Massaging disturbs the wheal and interferes with the intended results.
26. Make sure your patient is comfortable and safe.
27. Observe the patient for any adverse reaction.

28. Dispose of the gloves in the biohazard container and sanitize your hands.
29. In the patient's health record, document the procedure and any reactions that occurred at the site of the injection. Include the exact site of the injection.
    PURPOSE: A procedure is not considered done until it is recorded. The exact site must be known to check for reactions to the PPD in 48 to 72 hours.
30. Help the patient make an appointment to return to the facility for any reaction to be read in 48 to 72 hours.
    PURPOSE: Patient education must be provided to obtain intended results.

Reading the Mantoux Test Results
31. Use the patient's health record to identify the location of the test.
32. Sanitize your hands and put on gloves; using good lighting and with the patient's arm slightly flexed, palpate the injection site with your fingertips and measure the induration. The basis of reading the skin test is the presence or absence of induration, which is a hard, dense, raised area. This is the area that is measured using a disposable millimeter ruler. Do not include any areas of inflammation in the measurement.
    PURPOSE: A positive Mantoux reaction occurs if the induration is inflamed, raised, and 15 mm or larger; an induration of 5 mm or larger is considered positive in patients with human immunodeficiency virus (HIV) infection, those in recent contact with a person who has TB, patients with a positive chest x-ray result, those who have received organ transplants, and anyone who is immunosuppressed. An induration of 10 mm or larger is considered positive in recent immigrants, IV drug users, and children younger than 4 years of age. Further diagnostic tests are ordered to rule out or confirm the diagnosis of tuberculosis.
33. Discard the gloves and measuring device in the biohazard waste container and sanitize your hands.
34. Document in the patient's record the results of the Mantoux test, including a complete description of the size of any induration. Notify the provider.

8/22/20–9:10 AM: Administered Mantoux TB test as ordered by Dr. Thau, 0.1 mL ID, lot #MF4780D, exp date 2/20, to Ⓡ anterior forearm. Pt tolerated procedure well. No questions. Appointment made to return 8/24 for reading. Dorothy Gaston, CMA (AAMA)
    8/24/20–10 AM: Mantoux test site in Ⓡ anterior forearm 3 mm. Dorothy Gaston, CMA (AAMA)

Subcutaneous Injections

Subcutaneous injections are given between the epidermis and the muscle, into the fatty areolar layer called *adipose tissue* (Figure 28-17 and Procedure 28-6). Smaller doses of less irritating drugs (i.e., no more than 2 mL) are given by this method. A ½- to ⅝-inch, 25- or 26-gauge needle is used for SC injections. Insulin microneedles are 31 gauge. The angle of insertion is typically 45 degrees, but the needle length determines the angle of administration. For example, heparin and insulin may be administered at a 90-degree angle when a microneedle (⁵⁄₁₆ inch) is used; or, to reach subcutaneous tissue, the injection may be administered at a 90-degree angle if the patient is obese. The posterior upper arm (about 3 inches above the elbow and 3 inches below the shoulder) is the typical injection site, but the abdomen, the anterior aspect of the thighs, and the upper back also may be used (Figure 28-18). Regardless of the site of the location, subcutaneous injections are administered by pinching up the tissue to create a skinfold before injection to allow for easier access to subcutaneous tissue.

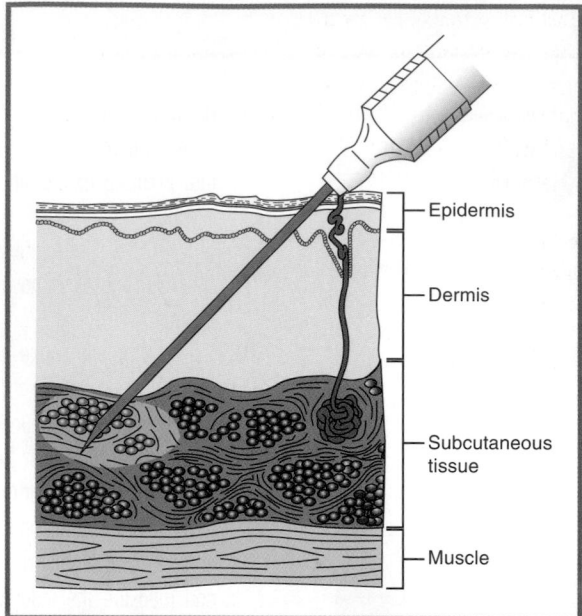

FIGURE 28-17 The subcutaneous (SC) injection is administered with a 25- or 26-gauge, ½- or ⅝-inch needle. This method is used for small amounts of nonirritating medications in aqueous solution. For injection of the medication, the needle is inserted at a 45-degree angle (or, for insulin and heparin, at a 90-degree angle). The most common site is the posterior upper arm.

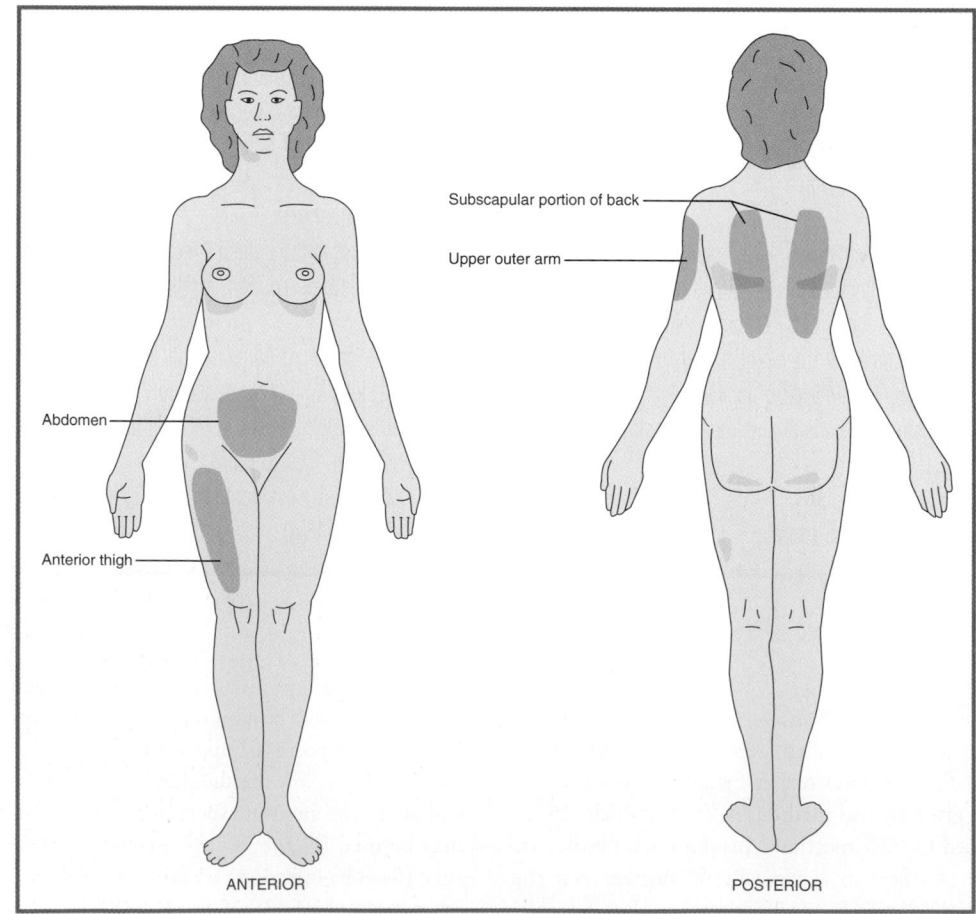

FIGURE 28-18 Areas of the body commonly used for subcutaneous injections.

When multiple or frequent injections are ordered, as with routine insulin administration that requires the patient to receive up to four injections a day, the sites must be rotated to prevent tissue damage and problems with absorption of the medication. Part of patient education for diabetics who rely on insulin for therapy is teaching them how to keep a rotation record (Figure 28-19). It might be helpful for patients to mark the site of the last injection with a spot bandage or a piece of tape. The easiest way to rotate sites is to give subsequent injections in a circular pattern around the site of the first injection in a particular location, such as the right anterior thigh. The goal is to avoid using the same location again for another month. Patients with diabetes typically have to administer two different types of insulin at one time. Many different solutions of insulin are available in premixed, multidose vials; however, you may have to mix two different types of insulin in the ambulatory care setting. Procedure 28-7 explains how to perform this technique.

Insulin Administration Guidelines

- Typically more than one type of insulin is ordered for immediate administration. Check labels carefully, and follow office policy when mixing insulins in the same syringe. Not all insulin products can be mixed.
- Insulin is always ordered in unit amounts. Use the appropriate insulin syringe—30, 50, or 100 units—based on the total amount of insulin ordered.
- Insulin should be stored in the refrigerator and gently rotated between the hands to warm before dispensing.
- Do not massage the site after injection.

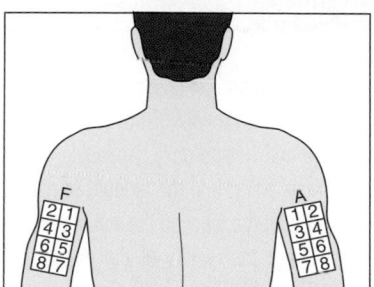

Posterior view

Anterior view

INJECTION LOG

SITE		1	2	3	4	5	6	7	8
Right arm	A								
Right abdomen	B								
Right thigh	C								
Left thigh	D								
Left abdomen	E								
Left arm	F								

FIGURE 28-19 A, Rotation sites for insulin injections. **B,** Rotation log.

PROCEDURE 28-6 | ## Select the Proper Sites for Administering a Parenteral Medication: Administer a Subcutaneous Injection

Goal: To inject 0.5 mL of medication into the subcutaneous tissue using a 25-gauge, ⅝-inch needle and syringe of correct size and type as directed by the provider.

Order: Administer 0.5 mL varicella vaccine SC to Mandy Leno, age 11.

EQUIPMENT and SUPPLIES

- Patient's health record
- Written provider's order, including the drug name, strength, dose, and route of administration
- Vial of ordered medication
- Alcohol wipes
- Gauze squares or cotton balls
- Sterile, 25-gauge, ⅝-inch needle and syringe unit with safety cover device
- Disposable gloves
- Sharps container
- PDR, online drug reference, or package insert
- Vaccine Information Sheet (VIS) for varicella

PROCEDURAL STEPS

1. Read the order and clarify any questions with the provider.
   PURPOSE: The medical assistant should never dispense or administer a drug without making sure the provider's order is legible and the details of the drug are known.
2. If you are unfamiliar with the medication, refer to the PDR, online drug reference, or package insert to determine the purpose of the drug, common side effects, typical dose, and any pertinent precautions or contraindications. Be prepared to answer any questions the patient may have about the medication. Use the Seven Rights to prevent errors.
3. Perform calculations needed to match the provider's order. Confirm the answer with the provider if you have any questions.

PROCEDURE 28-6 *—continued*

4. Assemble the equipment and sanitize your hands. Dispense the medication in a well-lit, quiet area to prevent distractions and possible errors. Choose the correct syringe and needle unit, depending on the site of administration, patient characteristics, and the amount of medication to be injected.

5. Compare the order with the label on the vial of medicine when you remove it from storage. Check the quality of the medication and the expiration date on the container and dispose of the medication if it appears contaminated, contains sediment, or has expired.
   PURPOSE: To compare the medication label and the provider's order the first of three times.

6. Warm refrigerated medications by gently rolling the container between your palms.

7. Compare the order with the label on the vial of medicine just before drawing the ordered dose into the syringe unit. Make sure the strength on the label matches the order or that you dispense the correctly calculated dose.
   PURPOSE: To compare the medication label and the provider's order the second of three times. One medication may be manufactured and prepackaged in different strengths. For instance, a particular drug may be available in vials of 250 mg/mL and 500 mg/mL.

8. Prepare the syringe and withdraw the correct dose, maintaining sterile technique. Compare the order with the label on the vial before disposing of the vial to complete the third label check.

9. Take the medication to the patient.

10. Greet the patient, and identify him or her by full name and date of birth; compare them to the name and DOB on the order. Ask about allergies. Explain the purpose of the immunization, and confirm that the caregiver was given a VIS form to review before administration of the vaccine and that the caregiver has given permission for administration.
    PURPOSE: To make sure you have the right patient, to gain cooperation, and to comply with federal VIS regulations.

11. To administer the injection into the arm, ask the patient to sit upright and help position her comfortably if necessary.

12. Expose the upper posterior arm (back or side of the arm) 3 inches below the shoulder and 3 inches above the elbow. To locate injection sites on the thigh, have the patient sit; then draw an imaginary line above the knee and below the uppermost part of the thigh and down the outer side and the center front of the leg. The area within these imaginary lines is where injections may be given. Another way to think of it is, in the middle third of the lateral aspect of the upper leg. To locate injection sites on the abdomen, draw an imaginary line below the lower ribs as far around as you can pinch up fatty tissue folds. Abdominal injections must avoid a 1-inch area around the navel.

13. Loosen the cap on the needle while keeping the cover over the needle. Open alcohol wipes so that they can be grasped with one hand.
    PURPOSE: To be able to remove the needle cover with one hand and prevent contamination of the needle; you will need to grasp alcohol wipes with one hand while the other hand is holding tissue up and away from the injection site.

14. Put on gloves, and with the thumb and fingers of your nondominant hand, grasp the tissue of the posterior upper arm, pinching up the area to create a tissue fold. Cleanse the patient's skin with the alcohol wipe, using a circular motion and moving outward from the center (Figure 1).

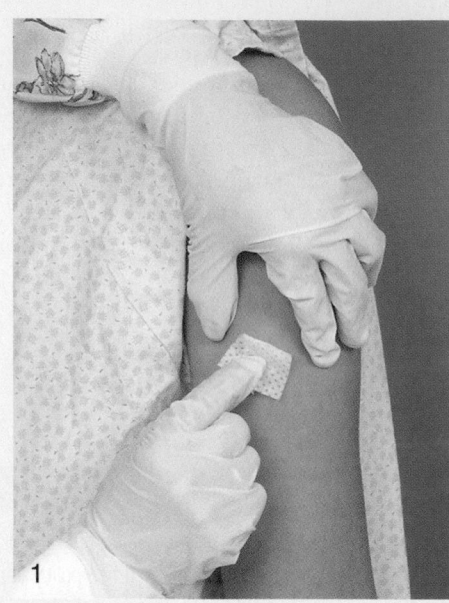

15. Remove the cap from the needle by gently shaking the loosened cover free while maintaining the sterility of the needle unit.

16. Hold the syringe between the thumb and the first two fingers of your dominant hand, and with one swift movement, insert the entire needle up to the hub at a 45-degree angle.
    PURPOSE: The depth of the injection is determined by the choice of needle length, not by how far you insert the needle. Some subcutaneous injections, such as insulin injections with microneedles, are administered at a 90-degree angle.

17. After the needle has been completely inserted into the skin, release the skin that you are grasping. Use your nondominant hand to stabilize the syringe area closest to the skin so that the needle does not move during administration of the drug.
    PURPOSE: To prevent discomfort for the patient, do not move the needle while injecting the medication.

18. Follow the facility's policies and/or the provider's recommendations regarding aspiration before the drug is administered. Push in the plunger slowly and steadily until all medication has been administered.
    PURPOSE: Aspiration before administration of certain medications (e.g., pediatric vaccines, insulin, heparin) is not recommended. A rapid injection may damage the tissues and may be uncomfortable for the patient.

19. As the needle is pulled out of the skin, gently press a gauze square next to the needle insertion site. Immediately cover the contaminated needle with the syringe unit safety device and discard the unit in the sharps container with the needle first.
    PURPOSE: Pressure over the site while removing the needle prevents the skin from pulling back, which may be uncomfortable. The gauze also helps seal the punctured tissue and prevents leakage.

PROCEDURE 28-6 —continued

20. Follow the facility's policy regarding massaging the injection site after drug administration (do not massage the site after insulin or heparin injections). If permitted, press or rub the site for a few seconds.
    PURPOSE: Massage helps increase absorption and reduce pain but is not recommended for certain medications; pressing the site without massage helps control bleeding.
21. Make sure the patient is comfortable and safe.
22. Dispose of gloves in the biohazard waste container and sanitize your hands.
23. Observe the patient for any adverse reaction. You may need to keep the patient under observation for 20 to 30 minutes.
24. Record the drug administration in the patient's medical record, including the exact injection site. Document the vaccine dose in the vaccination log. Each facility has a policy for vaccination documentation.

PURPOSE: The immunization record or vaccination log must be completed each time a vaccine is administered. Information includes the manufacturer; batch and lot numbers, which are stamped on the container; expiration date; dose administered; route of administration; and whether a patient reaction occurred. You must also document that the caregiver received a VIS form and that any questions were answered before the vaccine was administered. (More details about immunization records are presented in the Pediatrics chapter.)

6/14/20–11:35 AM: 0.5 mL varicella virus vaccine administered SQ to ® posterior upper arm as ordered by Dr. Thau, Beck Corp, lot #V5829K, exp date 9/20. VIS form, date 10/20XX, given to mother. She had no questions. Pt tolerated procedure well. Dorothy Gaston, CMA (AAM)

PROCEDURE 28-7   Mix Two Different Types of Insulin in One Syringe

Goal: *To mix two different types of insulin from two different multidose vials in one injection unit for administration.*

Order: Administer 5 units of Lispro and 15 units NPH insulin to Gregor Thomas STAT.

EQUIPMENT and SUPPLIES

- Patient's health record
- Written provider's order, including the drug name, strength, dose, and route of administration
- Multidose vial of Lispro insulin
- Multidose vial of NPH insulin
- Alcohol wipes
- Sterile needle and insulin syringe unit with safety cover device (because the total amount of insulin ordered is 20 units, use a 30-unit insulin syringe)
- PDR, online drug reference, or the package insert

PROCEDURAL STEPS

1. Read the order and clarify any questions with the provider.
   PURPOSE: The medical assistant should never dispense or administer a drug without making sure the provider's order is legible and the details of the drug are known.
2. If you are unfamiliar with the medications, refer to the PDR, online drug reference, or package insert to determine the purpose of the drug, common side effects, typical dose, and any pertinent precautions or contraindications. Be prepared to answer any questions the patient may have about the medication. Use the Seven Rights to prevent errors.
3. Perform calculations needed to match the provider's order. Confirm the answer with the provider if you have any questions.
4. Dispense the medication in a well-lit, quiet area.
   PURPOSE: To prevent distractions and possible errors.
5. Assemble the equipment and sanitize your hands. Choose the correct syringe and needle unit, depending on the site of administration, patient characteristics, and the amount of medication to be injected.
6. Select the correct multidose vials of insulin from the refrigerator. Compare the order with the labels on the vials of insulin when you remove them from the refrigerator. Check the quality of the medication and the expiration date on the containers; dispose of the medication if it appears contaminated, contains sediment, or has expired. Lispro and Regular insulin are clear and colorless. NPH is opaque or cloudy and colorless.
   PURPOSE: To compare the medication label and the provider's order the first of three times; make sure the Lispro vial is not contaminated with NPH; if the Lispro vial is cloudy or if either vial has sediment in the mixture, dispose of the contaminated vial or vials.
7. Mix and warm the insulin vials by gently rolling the vials between your palms.
   PURPOSE: Mixing ensures an equal concentration of medication throughout the vial. Shaking insulin vials can turn the medication frothy, making it difficult to measure the dose accurately.
8. Compare the order with the label on each vial of insulin just before drawing the ordered dose into the syringe unit. Make sure the name on the label matches the order or that you dispense the correctly calculated dose.
   PURPOSE: To compare the medication label and the provider's order the second of three times.
9. Check to make sure the total amount of insulin ordered is less than the insulin syringe chosen.
   PURPOSE: Insulin syringes are available in 30-unit, 50-unit, and 100-unit calibrations. The total amount of insulin ordered in this case is 20 units, so the 30-unit syringe is the most appropriate.

PROCEDURE 28-7   *—continued*

10. Clean the tops of each vial with individual alcohol wipes, leaving the wipe on the top of each vial.
   PURPOSE: To disinfect the top of each vial before drawing up the ordered dose.

11. Remove the alcohol swab and inject 15 units of air into the NPH vial, being careful not to touch the insulin in the vial with the needle, and withdraw the needle (Figure 1).
   PURPOSE: The NPH dose is drawn up last to avoid adding NPH insulin to the Lispro vial. Inject air into the NPH vial before drawing up the Lispro order so that it is ready for dispensing. Touching the NPH insulin with the needle contaminates the Lispro vial.

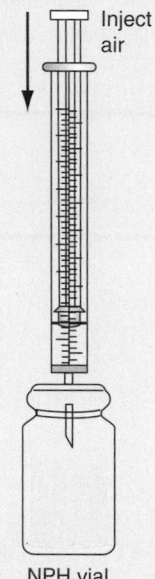

1   NPH vial

12. Remove the alcohol swab and inject 5 units of air into the Lispro vial, keeping the needle in the vial (Figure 2). Invert the vial and withdraw the ordered dose of 5 units (Figure 3).

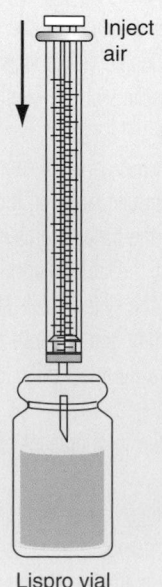

2   Lispro vial

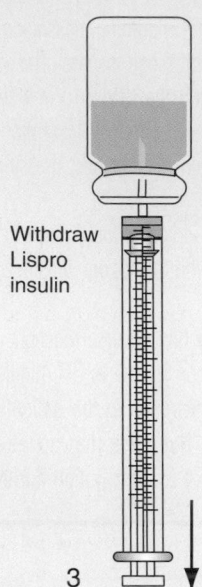

3

13. Reinsert the needle into the NPH vial and carefully withdraw the ordered 15-unit dose. Do not push any insulin back into the vial. If you withdraw more than the ordered dose, discard the syringe unit and restart the procedure (Figure 4).

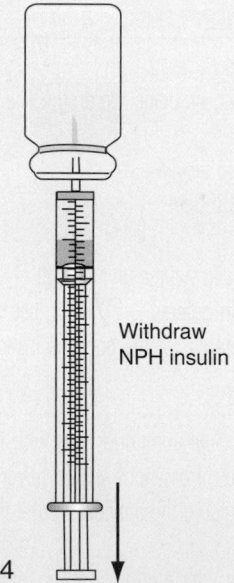

4

14. Complete the third label check by comparing the order with the labels on the insulin vials before returning the multidose vials to the refrigerator.

15. Dispose of used alcohol wipes.

Intramuscular Injections

Injections are given into muscle if the drug would irritate the SC tissues, if more rapid absorption is desired, or if a large volume of medication is to be injected. The angle of insertion is 90 degrees (Figure 28-20), and the preferred sites in an adult are the vastus lateralis, deltoid, ventrogluteal, and gluteus medius muscles (Figure 28-21); in an infant or child, the preferred site is the vastus lateralis. It is important to select a needle that is long enough, especially for obese patients, to ensure that the medication is injected into the muscle and is not deposited in the upper adipose tissue. Fatty tissue does not absorb medication well, and the medication may remain at the site of the injection rather than being distributed systemically as intended. The recommended gauge for an adult is 20 to 23, and the needle length should be 1 to 3 inches, depending on the patient's size.

In adults, the deltoid region can hold up to 2 mL of medication, and the vastus lateralis and gluteal sites can hold up to 3 mL. Infants and children should be given no more than 2 mL in the vastus lateralis or the ventrogluteal site. The most important criterion in choosing an IM site is to use one that is not near large nerves, bones, or blood vessels. If any of these structures are damaged by the injection, the patient may experience nerve injury with lingering pain or may develop an abscess or bone inflammation with infection.

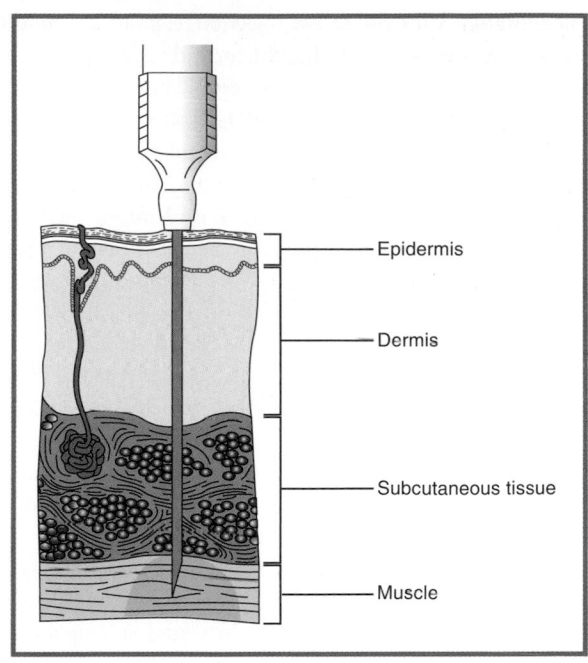

FIGURE 28-20 Anatomic illustration of the intramuscular (IM) injection. Note that the needle is inserted at a 90-degree angle, which deposits the medication into the large central part of the muscle.

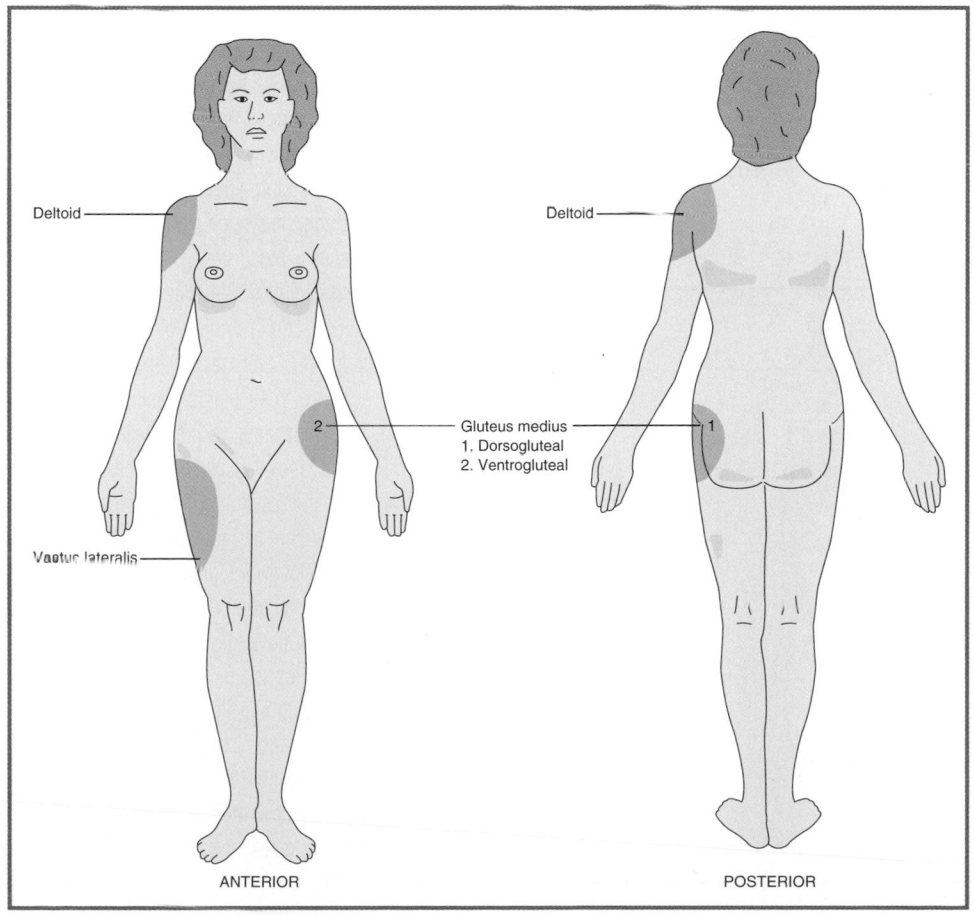

FIGURE 28-21 Muscles commonly used for an intramuscular injection.

When locating a site for an IM injection, expose the site so that you can see and palpate the landmarks correctly. If the patient must receive repeated IM injections, the sites should be rotated to prevent damage to the muscle and to surrounding tissues.

Deltoid Site. The deltoid muscle, the muscular cap of the shoulder, is located at the top of the upper arm. The muscle mass is somewhat limited, so it can hold only 1 to 2 mL of medication. This triangular muscle is located between the acromion and the deltoid tuberosities, and the injection site is approximately 2 fingerbreadths below the acromial process (Figure 28-22). The major nerves and blood vessels, especially the radial nerve and artery, must be avoided. Aqueous medications, such as vitamin B_{12}, are most appropriate here; hepatitis B and flu vaccines are also given in the deltoid.

If frequent injections are ordered, rotate the site and alternate the right and left arms. The deltoid site is acceptable for adults and older children, but it should not be used when the muscle is small or underdeveloped. For a small arm, you may need only a 25-gauge, ⅝-inch needle; the 23-gauge, 1-inch needle most often is used for an arm of average size. The patient may be seated or lying down. To administer the injection, expose the entire shoulder rather than rolling up the sleeve; rest the palm of your hand across the shoulder and grasp the muscle; inject the medication at a 90-degree angle (Procedure 28-8).

Vastus Lateralis (Thigh) Site. The vastus lateralis muscle is part of the quadriceps group of the thigh. It is one of the body's largest muscles, and because it is developed at birth, it is considered the safest IM injection site for infants. Many experts believe that as a site for adult IM injections, the vastus lateralis is better than the deltoid or the dorsogluteal sites because fewer major nerves and blood vessels are in the vastus lateralis. The vastus lateralis muscle fills the midportion of the upper, outer thigh. In an adult, it can be located from 1 handwidth below the proximal end of the greater trochanter to 1 handwidth above the top of the patella (kneecap), or the middle third of the upper outer leg.

Administering injections to infants and small children requires some special considerations. The choice of a site is based on muscular development and the absence of major nerves and blood vessels. As has been mentioned, the most popular site for IM injections in children and infants is the vastus lateralis muscle. Other sites are avoided for the following reasons:

- Infants do not have well-developed deltoid muscles.
- The sciatic nerve, located near the dorsogluteal site, is proportionately larger in the infant.
- The gluteus medius is not well developed until the child is walking.

If you have any doubts, the best policy is to ask the provider to show you exactly where to inject the medication or vaccine. Any site selected for infants and children involves greater risk of error because the muscles are smaller than the muscles of adults.

Infants should be restrained by a co-worker or a parent to prevent injury. If the child is old enough to understand, be honest and explain that the injection may sting for a minute, but that it is important to hold very still. Always get help if giving an injection to an uncooperative child.

The recommended site for vastus lateralis injections in infants and children is below the greater trochanter of the femur but within the upper lateral quadrant of the thigh (Figure 28-23, *A* and *B*).

The Debate Over Needle Aspiration

Traditional procedures for intramuscular (IM) injections of medications and vaccinations have always recommended needle aspiration before administration of a solution into any muscle group. Needle aspiration is the process of pulling back on the syringe plunger before injection to determine whether the needle is in a blood vessel. If blood is aspirated into the syringe, it should be immediately removed and discarded to prevent inadvertent intravenous (IV) administration of a medication that was ordered for IM administration. However, recent analysis of research shows there is no scientific evidence to support this practice.

What does that mean for healthcare workers who administer IM injections? The most recent guidelines published by the American Academy of Pediatrics state that aspiration before intramuscular vaccination may not be necessary. According to the Centers for Disease Control and Prevention (CDC), because there are only two routinely recommended IM sites for administration of vaccines (the vastus lateralis and deltoid muscles) and because there are no large blood vessels in either site, aspiration before injection of vaccines is not necessary. In addition, aspiration may cause more pain during an injection procedure.

However, aspiration should still be part of a dorsogluteal injection because there is danger of needle insertion into the gluteal artery. Because this is a relatively new area of research, medical assistants should follow the procedures established by the facilities where they work, and if there is any question about performing aspiration with IM injections, they should ask a provider in the practice for clarification.

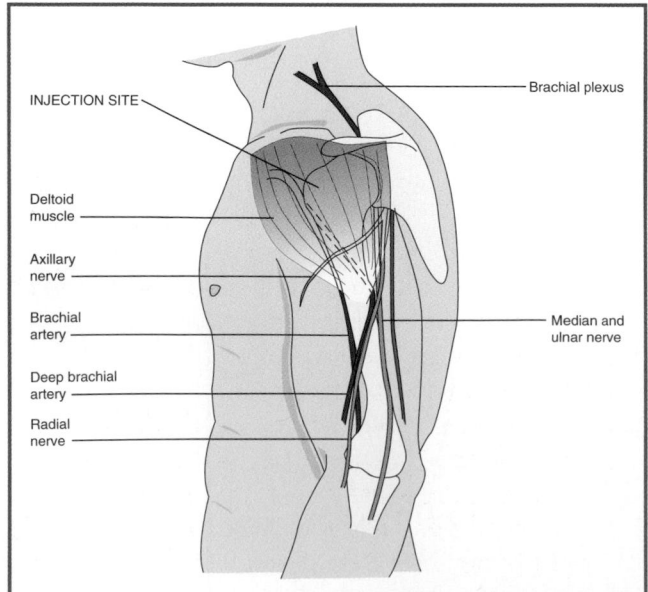

FIGURE 28-22 Deltoid muscle intramuscular site. This site is not recommended for infants because the muscle is not well developed until later in childhood.

When the vastus lateralis site is used, the needle should be inserted at a 90-degree angle. The length of the needle should be adjusted based on the size of the patient. Needle gauges for adults range from 20 to 23, and lengths range from 1 to 1½ inches; the muscle can hold as much as 3 mL of medication. In pediatric patients, the needle gauge should be 22 to 25, and the length should be ⅝ inch; the muscle can hold 0.5 mL in infants and 0.5 to 2 mL in children (Procedure 28-9). An adult patient may sit or lie supine; in pediatric patients, the vastus lateralis is easier to locate with the child lying down.

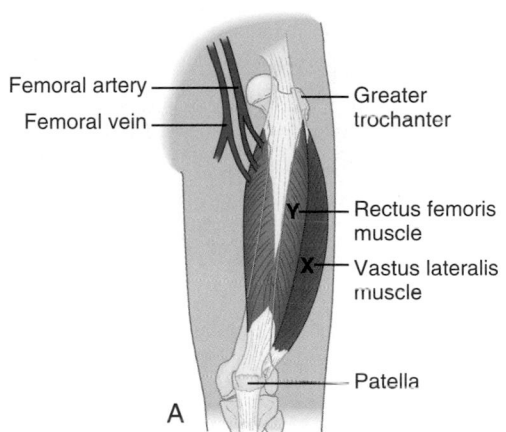
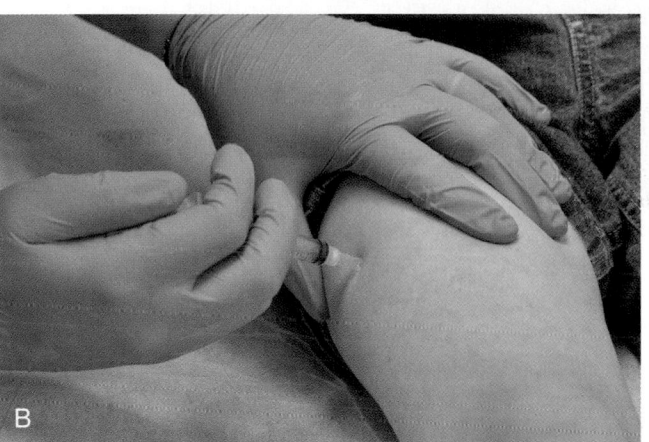

FIGURE 28-23 A, Vastus lateralis intramuscular site. **B,** The recommended site for vastus lateralis injections in infants and children.

PROCEDURE 28-8 | Administer Parenteral (Excluding IV) Medications: Administer an Intramuscular Injection into the Deltoid Muscle

Goal: To inject ordered medication into the muscle using a 22-gauge, 1- to 1½-inch needle and a 3-mL syringe as directed by the provider.

Order: Administer 300,000 units penicillin G IM STAT to Liz Anderson, age 23.

EQUIPMENT and SUPPLIES

- Patient's health record
- Written provider's order, including the drug name, strength, dose, and route of administration
- Vial containing ordered medication
- Alcohol wipes
- Gauze squares
- Sterile needle and syringe unit with safety needle cover
- Disposable gloves
- Sharps container
- PDR, online drug reference, or the package insert

PROCEDURAL STEPS

1. Read the order and clarify any questions with the provider.
   <u>PURPOSE</u>: The medical assistant should never dispense or administer a drug without making sure the provider's order is legible and the details of the drug are known.

2. If you are unfamiliar with the medication, refer to the PDR, online drug reference, or package insert to determine the purpose of the drug, common side effects, typical dose, and any pertinent precautions or contraindications. Be prepared to answer any questions the patient may have about the medication. Use the Seven Rights to prevent errors.

3. Perform calculations needed to match the provider's order. Confirm the answer with the provider if you have any questions.

4. Dispense the medication in a well-lit, quiet area.
   <u>PURPOSE</u>: To prevent distractions and possible errors.

5. Assemble the equipment and sanitize your hands. Choose the correct syringe and needle unit, depending on the site of administration, patient characteristics, and the amount of medication to be injected.

6. Compare the order with the label on the vial when you remove it from storage. Check the quality of the medication and the expiration date on the container; dispose of the medication if it appears contaminated, contains sediment, or has expired.

PROCEDURE 28-8   —*continued*

PURPOSE: To compare the medication label and the provider's order the first of three times; a drug may be manufactured and prepackaged in different strengths; for instance, penicillin G is packaged in vials of 300,000 units/mL and 600,000 units/mL.

7. Mix and warm refrigerated medications by gently rolling the vial between your palms.

    PURPOSE: Mixing ensures an equal concentration of medication throughout the vial. Shaking the vial can turn the medication frothy, making it difficult to measure the dose accurately.

8. Compare the order with the label on the vial just before drawing the ordered dose into the syringe unit. Make sure the name on the label matches the order or that you dispense the correctly calculated dose.

    PURPOSE: To compare the medication label and the provider's order the second of three times.

9. Prepare the syringe and vial as described in Procedure 28-3 and withdraw the correct dose of medication. Compare the order with the label on the vial before disposing of the vial or replacing a multidose vial to storage to complete the third label check.

    PURPOSE: To complete the third of the three label checks.

10. Take the medication to the patient.

11. Greet the patient, and identify her by full name and date of birth; compare them to the name and DOB on the order. Ask the patient whether she is allergic to penicillin or any other antibiotics.

    PURPOSE: To make sure you have the right patient. Antibiotics, especially the penicillin family, are the most likely group of drugs to cause allergies. The patient's response can change over time, so it is important to request allergy information before each administration of an antibiotic.

12. Help the patient into an upright sitting position.

13. Put on gloves and expose the deltoid site. The mid-deltoid site is located approximately 2 to 3 fingerwidths below the acromial process.

14. Loosen the needle cover while keeping the needle within the cover and maintaining the sterility of the unit. Open alcohol wipes so they can be grasped with one hand.

    PURPOSE: To be able to remove the needle cover with one hand and prevent contamination of the needle; you will need to grasp alcohol wipes with one hand while the other hand is holding tissue up and away from the injection site.

15. Clean the patient's skin with the alcohol wipe using a circular motion and moving outward from the center (Figure 1).

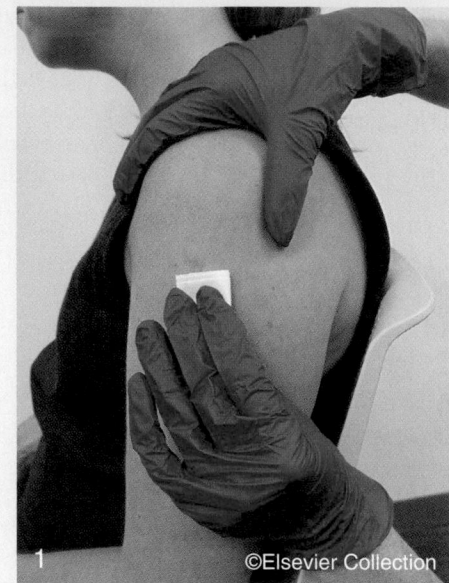
1   ©Elsevier Collection

16. Place your nondominant hand on the patient's shoulder, and with the thumb and first two fingers, spread the skin tightly and grasp the muscle deeply on each side (Figure 2).

    PURPOSE: To compress fat and stabilize the muscle.

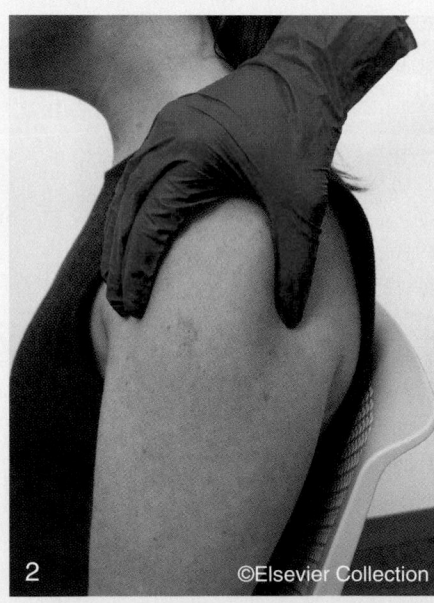
2   ©Elsevier Collection

17. Shake the needle cover off and grasp the syringe as you would a dart and with one swift movement, insert the entire needle up to the hub, at a 90-degree angle, into the muscle.

    PURPOSE: The depth of the injection is determined by the choice of needle length, not by how far you insert the needle. Once the needle is at the tissue layer, release the muscle and stabilize the syringe unit with the nondominant hand so that the needle does not move during aspiration and injection of the medication.

PROCEDURE 28-8 —continued

18. Aspirate; withdraw the plunger slightly to make sure no blood enters the syringe.
    PURPOSE: Blood in the syringe means that the needle is in a blood vessel and is not in the muscle tissue. You may not administer an intramuscular medication by the IV route.
19. If blood appears, immediately withdraw the syringe, cover the contaminated needle with the safety device, discard it in the sharps container with the needle first, and compress the injection site with the cotton ball. Begin again with step 5. If no blood appears in the syringe, push in the plunger slowly and steadily until all medication has been administered.
    PURPOSE: A rapid injection is uncomfortable for the patient.
20. Place the cotton ball next to the needle and apply counterpressure to the area while you withdraw the needle at the same angle used for insertion. Immediately cover the contaminated needle with the syringe unit safety device and discard the syringe unit in the sharps container with the needle first.

21. Gently massage the site with a gauze square.
    PURPOSE: Massage helps promote absorption and reduce pain.
22. Make sure your patient is comfortable and safe.
23. Observe the patient for any adverse reaction. You may need to keep the patient under observation for 20 to 30 minutes.
24. Dispose of the gloves and sanitize your hands.
25. Record the drug administration in the patient's health record and in the required Drug Enforcement Agency (DEA) record if the medication is a controlled substance.
    PURPOSE: A procedure is not considered done until it is recorded.

9/8/20–8:35 AM: 300,000 units penicillin G administered IM to Ⓡ deltoid as ordered by Dr. Thau without complication. Pt observed for allergic reaction and none noted. Pt had no questions. Instructed to call office if she experiences any problems from injection. D. Gaston, CMA (AAMA)

PROCEDURE 28-9   Select the Proper Sites for Administering a Parenteral Medication: Administer a Pediatric Intramuscular Vastus Lateralis Injection

Goal: To inject 0.5 mL of vaccine into the vastus lateralis muscle using a 22-gauge, $\frac{5}{8}$-inch needle.

Order: Administer 0.5 mL of *Haemophilus influenzae* type B (Hib) vaccine IM to Lizzy Dearborne, age 4 months.

EQUIPMENT and SUPPLIES

- Patient's health record
- Written provider's order, including the drug name, strength, dose, and route of administration
- Vial containing Hib vaccine
- Alcohol wipes
- 2 × 2-inch gauze square
- Sterile needle and syringe unit with safety device
- Disposable gloves
- Sharps container
- PDR, online drug reference, or package insert
- Vaccine Information Sheet (VIS) for Hib

PROCEDURAL STEPS

1. Read the order and clarify any questions with the provider.
   PURPOSE: The medical assistant should never dispense or administer a drug without making sure the provider's order is legible and the details of the drug are known.
2. If you are unfamiliar with the medication, refer to the PDR, online drug reference, or package insert to determine the purpose of the drug, common side effects, typical dose, and any pertinent precautions or contraindications. Be prepared to answer any questions the caregiver may have about the medication. Use the Seven Rights to prevent errors.

3. Check the patient's record for a previous allergic reaction to the Hib vaccine. Perform calculations needed to match the provider's order. Confirm the answer with the provider if you have any questions.
4. Dispense the medication in a well-lit, quiet area.
   PURPOSE: To prevent distractions and possible errors.
5. Assemble the equipment and sanitize your hands. Choose the correct syringe and needle unit, depending on the site of administration, patient characteristics, and the amount of medication to be injected.
6. Compare the order with the label on the vial of medicine when you remove it from storage. Check the quality of the medication and the expiration date on the container and dispose of the medication if it appears contaminated, contains sediment, or has expired.
   PURPOSE: To compare the medication label and the provider's order the first of three times.
7. Warm refrigerated medications by gently rolling the vial between your palms.
8. Compare the order with the label on the vial of medicine just before drawing the ordered dose into the syringe unit. Make sure the strength on the label matches the order or that you dispense the correctly calculated dose.
   PURPOSE: To compare the medication label and the provider's order the second of three times.
9. Prepare the syringe and withdraw the correct dose, maintaining sterile technique as shown in Procedure 28-3. Compare the order with the label

PROCEDURE 28-9   —*continued*

on the vial before disposing of the vial or replacing a multidose vial to storage to complete the third label check.

10. Take the medication to the patient.

11. Greet and identify the patient's caregiver, using the child's full name and date of birth; compare the child's name and DOB to those on the order. Check to make sure the caregiver has received the Hib VIS form and that his or her questions have been answered. Confirm that the caregiver has given permission for the child to receive the immunization.
    PURPOSE: To make sure you have the right patient, and to confirm that immunization regulations have been followed.

12. Explain the procedure to the caregiver. Check the baby's temperature and ask the caregiver about recent illnesses. Refer to facility policies if the child has a fever and/or the caregiver reports a recent illness.
    PURPOSE: To promote cooperation; children with a moderate to severe illness should not be vaccinated.

13. Position the infant on her back. Ask the caregiver to remove any clothing necessary to expose the infant's thighs. Choose the right or left thigh for the injection.
    PURPOSE: It is important to expose the entire vastus lateralis muscle to prevent injury to the child.

14. Put on gloves and loosen the needle cover while keeping the needle within the cover and maintaining the sterility of the unit. Open alcohol wipes so that they can be grasped with one hand.
    PURPOSE: To be able to remove the needle cover with one hand and prevent contamination of the needle; you will need to grasp alcohol wipes with one hand while the other hand holds tissue up and away from the injection site.

15. Locate the injection site. The pediatric vastus lateralis site is located below the greater trochanter of the femur but within the upper lateral quadrant (fourth) of the thigh. Grasp the muscle with your nondominant hand, and clean the injection site with the alcohol wipe, using a circular motion and moving outward from the center.

16. Ask for the caregiver's assistance in holding the child still if necessary.

17. Remove the cap from the needle by gently shaking the loosened cover free while maintaining the sterility of the needle unit.

18. With the thumb and first two fingers of the nondominant hand, spread the skin at the site tightly.

19. Grasp the syringe as you would a dart, and with one swift movement, insert the needle at a 90-degree angle into the muscle.

20. After the needle has been completely inserted into the skin, release the muscle that you are grasping. Use your nondominant hand to stabilize the

syringe area closest to the skin so that the needle does not move during administration of the drug. Aspiration is no longer recommended with pediatric vaccination injections, but you should follow the facility's policy.
    PURPOSE: To prevent discomfort for the patient, do not move the needle while injecting the medication.

21. As the needle is pulled out of the skin, gently press a gauze square next to the needle insertion site. Immediately cover the contaminated needle with the syringe unit safety device and discard the unit in the sharps container with the needle first.
    PURPOSE: Pressure over the site while removing the needle prevents the skin from pulling back, which may be uncomfortable. The gauze also helps seal the punctured tissue and prevents leakage.

22. Follow your facility's policy on massaging the injection site after drug administration. If permitted, press or rub the site for a few seconds.
    PURPOSE: Massage helps increase absorption and reduce pain but is not recommended for certain medications; pressing the site without massage helps control bleeding.

23. Make sure the infant is safely held by the caregiver. Observe the patient for 20 to 30 minutes for any adverse reaction.

24. Dispose of your gloves and sanitize your hands.

25. Record the vaccine administration in the patient's health record and complete the vaccination log according to office procedure.
    PURPOSE: A procedure is not considered done until it is recorded. It is important to keep an accurate record of vaccinations performed so that the next dose is timed properly. The immunization record or vaccination log must be completed each time a vaccine is administered. Information includes the manufacturer; batch and lot numbers, which are stamped on the Hib vial; expiration date; dose administered; route of administration; and whether there was a patient reaction. You must also record that the caregiver received a VIS form and that any questions he or she had were answered before the vaccine was administered. (More details about immunization records are presented in the Pediatrics chapter.)

3/27/20–1:30 PM: Hib lot #98525, Beck Corp, exp date 10/20, administered 0.5 mL Hib vaccine IM to Ⓛ vastus lateralis per Dr. Thau order. Caregiver given HIB VIS dated 6/20XX, answered questions regarding follow-up care. No adverse effects noted. Appointment made for next immunizations in 1 month. D. Gaston, CMA (AAMA)

Dorsogluteal (Gluteus Medius) Site. The dorsogluteal region is the traditional site for deep IM injections. However, complications from sciatic nerve injury are common enough that experts have suggested that use of this site be discontinued and that the vastus lateralis and ventrogluteal sites be used instead. Regardless, the dorsogluteal site continues to be popular and is still acceptable for adults if care is taken to locate the exact site. This site should not be used for pediatric patients.

The patient should lie in Sims position with the bottom leg straight and the top leg slightly bent. To locate the site, put the palm of your nondominant hand on the greater trochanter of the femur and point your fingers toward the posterior superior iliac spine. Palpate these bony prominences to make sure you are at the correct site, and draw an imaginary line between these two anatomic markings. The injection is made into the gluteus medius muscle above the imaginary line (Figure 28-24). Needle gauges 20 to 23 and a

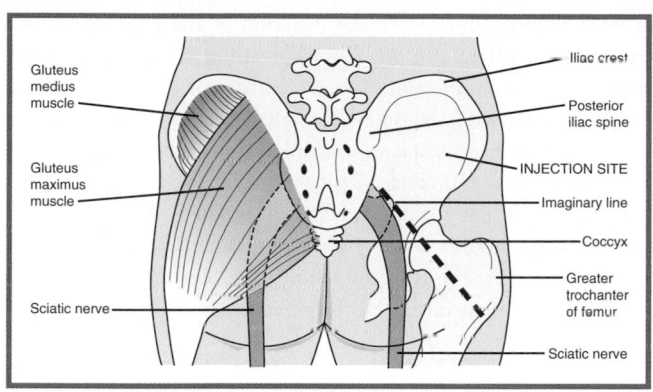

FIGURE 28-24 Many providers still prefer the dorsogluteal (gluteus medius) site.

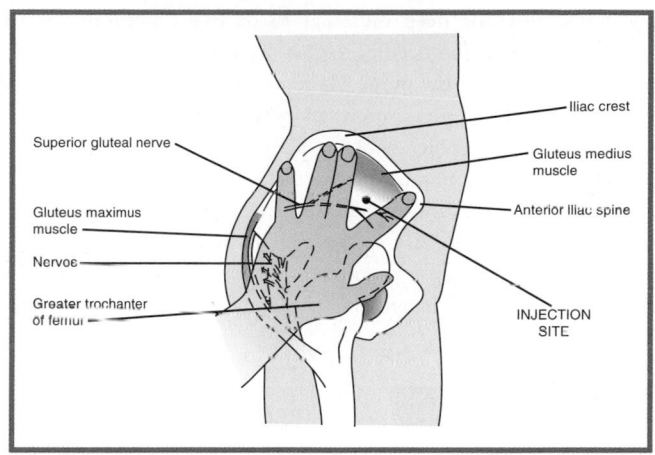

FIGURE 28-25 The ventrogluteal site can be used for most intramuscular injections.

TABLE 28-1	Parenteral Administration of Medications					
ROUTE OF ADMINISTRATION	SITE	NEEDLE GAUGE	NEEDLE LENGTH (in)	SYRINGE	DRUG AMOUNT	EXAMPLE DRUGS
Intradermal	Midanterior forearm	27-28	3/8	1 mL: tuberculin	0.1 mL: allergy tests	Tuberculosis skin test (Mantoux)
Subcutaneous	Posterior upper arm, thigh, abdomen	25-26	1/2, 5/8	3 mL: insulin	Adult: 0.1-2 mL Child: 0.5 mL	Insulin, heparin, vaccines
Intramuscular	Adult deltoid	20-23	1-3	3 mL	1-2 mL	Epinephrine, vitamin B_{12}, antibiotics (e.g., penicillin), meperidine, morphine, vaccines
	Child deltoid	20-23	5/8-1	1-3 mL	0.5-2 mL	
	Adult vastus lateralis, dorsogluteal, ventrogluteal	20-23	1-1½ 1-3 1-3	3 mL	2-3 mL	
	Infant or child vastus lateralis	22-26	5/8	1-3 mL	0.5-2 mL	

needle length of 1 to 3 inches should be used; the site can hold as much as 5 mL of medication. Procedure 28-10 can help you practice finding the dorsogluteal site.

Ventrogluteal (Gluteus Medius) Site. Although considered safe, the ventrogluteal region is not used as frequently as the others previously discussed. This technique uses a larger mass of the gluteus medius muscle than is used for the dorsogluteal site. The area is free of major nerves and blood vessels, and it is considered safe for both infants and adults (Figure 28-25). All types of IM medications can be injected here, including thick, oily preparations. Needle gauges 20 to 23 and needle lengths 1 to 3 inches should be used; the site can hold as much as 3 mL of medication.

To locate the site, place the patient in Sims position and put the palm of your nondominant hand on the greater trochanter of the femur, pointing your fingers toward the patient's head and the index finger toward the anterior superior iliac spine. Spread your middle finger back as far as possible from your index finger to form a triangular injection area. For a child, you will need a 1-inch needle; for an obese adult patient, you may need a 2½- to 3-inch needle to reach the depth of the muscle. Table 28-1 summarizes the details of parenteral administration of medications.

Z-Track Intramuscular Injection

Some IM medications are irritating to the skin and SC tissues; others, such as iron replacement products, leak to the surface and stain surrounding tissues. These medications should be injected in such a way as to prevent any leakage from the deep muscle back into the upper SC layers. The Z-track method displaces the upper tissue laterally before the needle is inserted.

Prepare the medication according to safety guidelines and then put on gloves. Palpate the site using anatomically correct markings, and localize the injection site visually. Push the skin to one side, and clean it as described for IM injections. Insert the needle into the anatomically correct location, aspirate, and slowly release the medication into the deep muscular tissue (see Procedure 28-10). After withdrawing the needle, release the tissue so that the needle tract is to the side of the point where the medication was deposited in the muscle. This process prevents a direct pathway to the surface for the medication, which protects SC and surface tissues from the irritating and/or staining properties of the drug.

The medications for which Z-track injection is appropriate require a large muscle mass, so they should be injected only into the dorsogluteal site. Because the medication is so irritating to tissues, the needle should be changed after the medication has been drawn

up from the vial and before the injection is given. Some facilities require personnel to use the Z-track method when administering abdominal heparin injections because leakage of the drug at the site may cause localized bleeding. Although heparin is administered by SC injection, the technique of pushing the surface tissue to the side before injection is the same.

Medications that require the Z-track method of administration (e.g., heparin) should not be massaged after injection because massaging encourages spread of the medication. Use alternate sides for multiple or frequent injections, to prevent tissue damage.

PROCEDURE 28-10   **Administer Parenteral (Excluding IV) Medications: Give a Z-Track Intramuscular Injection into the Dorsogluteal Site**

Goal: *Inject 1 mL of medication into the gluteus medius muscle via Z-track injection using a 23-gauge, 2-inch needle.*

Order: Administer 1 mL of INFeD Z-track into the dorsogluteal site to Carlos Langa, age 63.

EQUIPMENT and SUPPLIES

- Patient's health record
- Written provider's order, including the drug name, strength, dose, and route of administration
- Vial containing the ordered medication
- Alcohol wipes
- Gauze square
- Disposable gloves
- Sharps container
- Sterile needle and syringe unit with safety needle cover
- Additional sterile needle
- PDR, online drug reference, or package insert

PROCEDURAL STEPS

Z-track injections are used for medications that irritate or stain the surface tissues.

1. Read the order and clarify any questions with the provider.
   PURPOSE: The medical assistant should never dispense or administer a drug without making sure the provider's order is legible and the details of the drug are known.
2. If you are unfamiliar with the medication, refer to the PDR, online drug reference, or package insert to determine the purpose of the drug, common side effects, typical dose, and any pertinent precautions or contraindications. Be prepared to answer any questions the caregiver may have about the medication. Use the Seven Rights to prevent errors.
3. Perform calculations needed to match the provider's order. Confirm the answer with the provider if you have any questions.
4. Dispense the medication in a well-lit, quiet area.
   PURPOSE: To prevent distractions and possible errors.
5. Assemble the equipment and sanitize your hands. Choose the correct syringe and needle unit, depending on the site of administration, patient characteristics, and the amount of medication to be injected.
6. Compare the order with the label on the vial of medicine when you remove it from storage. Check the quality of the medication and the expiration

date on the container and dispose of the medication if it appears contaminated, contains sediment, or has expired.
   PURPOSE: To compare the medication label and the provider's order the first of three times.
7. Warm refrigerated medications by gently rolling the vial between your palms.
8. Compare the order with the label on the vial of medicine just before drawing the ordered dose into the syringe unit. Make sure the strength on the label matches the order or that you dispense the correctly calculated dose.
   PURPOSE: To compare the medication label and the provider's order the second of three times.
9. Draw up the ordered amount of medication into the syringe unit following the steps in Procedure 28-3.
10. Replace the needle cover and give a slight turn to loosen the needle. Secure a new needle, still in its sheath, to the tip of the syringe, being careful to not contaminate the needle or hub of the syringe. Discard the contaminated needle in the sharps container with the needle first.
    PURPOSE: The needle that was used to withdraw the medication is covered with the drug, which might be irritating to the skin and subcutaneous tissues.
11. Compare the order with the label on the vial before disposing of the vial or replacing a multidose vial to storage to complete the third label check.
12. Take the medication to the patient.
13. Greet the patient, and identify him by name and date of birth (DOB); compare his name and DOB to those on the order.
    PURPOSE: To make sure you have the right patient.
14. Position the patient comfortably in Sims position.
15. Put on gloves and loosen the needle cover while keeping the needle within the cover and maintaining the sterility of the unit. Open alcohol wipes so that they can be grasped with one hand.
    PURPOSE: To be able to remove the needle cover with one hand and prevent contamination of the needle; you will need to grasp alcohol wipes

PROCEDURE 28-10 —*continued*

with one hand while the other hand holds tissue up and away from the injection site.

16. Expose the dorsogluteal site. This site is found by placing the palm of the nondominant hand on the greater trochanter of the femur, while pointing your fingers toward the posterior superior iliac spine and index finger toward the anterior iliac spine. The injection site is in the upper outer area of the gluteus medius. Visualize the area for the Z-track injection.

17. Apply pressure to the tissue at the dorsogluteal site and push it up and to one side; hold it firmly in place. If the skin is slippery, use a dry gauze sponge to hold the skin in place.
    PURPOSE: Displacing the skin prevents medication from leaking back to the surface.

18. Clean the patient's skin with the alcohol wipe, using a circular motion and moving outward from the center. Make sure to clean the actual area of injection.

19. Remove the cap from the needle by gently shaking the loosened cover free while maintaining the sterility of the needle unit. Grasp the syringe as you would a dart and with one swift movement, insert the entire needle up to the hub at a 90-degree angle into the upper outer area of the gluteus medius muscle.
    PURPOSE: The depth of the injection is determined by the choice of needle length, not by how far you insert the needle. Once the needle is at the tissue layer, do not move it while injecting the medication. Inserting the needle as far as the hub helps keep the needle in place.

20. Aspirate; withdraw the plunger slightly to make sure no blood enters the syringe. If blood appears, immediately withdraw the syringe, apply the needle safety device and dispose of the syringe unit in the sharps container, and compress the injection site with a gauze square. Begin again with step 5.
    PURPOSE: Blood in the syringe means that the needle is in a blood vessel and not in the muscle tissue. You may not administer an intramuscular medication by the IV route.

21. If no blood appears in the syringe, push in the plunger slowly and steadily until all medication has been administered.

22. Wait 10 seconds for the medication to be dispersed, then withdraw the needle at the same angle used for insertion. As the needle is withdrawn, release the displaced tissue to prevent the tracking of medication to the surface.

23. Immediately cover the contaminated needle with the syringe unit safety device and dispose of the needle and syringe unit in a sharps container with the needle first.

24. If the manufacturer recommends it, gently massage the site with the gauze square or a cotton ball. Many medications requiring Z-track administration should not be massaged.

25. Make sure your patient is comfortable and safe.

26. Dispose of your gloves and sanitize your hands.

27. Observe the patient for any adverse reaction. You may need to keep the patient under observation for 20 to 30 minutes.

28. Record the drug administration in the patient's health record, including the exact site of injection.

7/13/20–1:25 PM: 1 mL INFeD administered Z-track in ® dorsogluteal site per Dr. Thau order. Injection site not massaged after administration. No evidence of skin discoloration after administration. Dorothy Gaston, CMA (AAMA)

CLOSING COMMENTS

Patient Education

It is extremely important to coach the patient in how to take a prescribed drug and to make sure he or she understands the purpose of the medication. The provider initially educates the patient, but the medical assistant should be prepared to reinforce the provider's information or to explain parts of the information the patient did not understand. When a patient does not understand the need for the medication or the directions for taking it, the risk is greater that the medication will be taken incorrectly. As a result, the provider's orders will not be carried out, and the desired therapeutic effect will not be achieved. The patient should fully understand the type of medication, its route of administration, its desired effect, and the side effects that need to be reported if they occur.

If the patient receives medication in the facility, he or she should understand the expected results or possible side effects. For example, if a patient is given a diuretic in the office, he or she needs to know what the immediate effect is going to be; this prepares the patient for the urinary urgency and **polyuria** that will occur within a relatively brief period. When a pain medication is given, the patient should have full knowledge so that the possibility of personal injury can be prevented. Any medication given in the ambulatory care setting that affects the patient's ability to walk or drive must be used with caution. The patient must be able to get home safely, and if that is not possible, the medication should not be given.

The medical assistant should coach the patient to comply with the treatment plan and take all of the medication as prescribed. Often if a prescription is not completed, the treatment objectives may not be achieved. Patients should also be coached to take their medication in the time sequence prescribed. This keeps the optimum level of the drug circulating in the bloodstream.

When sample medications are dispensed to the patient in the facility, the package contains inserts that can be helpful in education efforts. Suggest the patient review important parts of the insert and highlight this information for quick reference. If the provider has specific written instructions for the patient to follow, read over the material with the patient before discharge so that any areas of confusion can be cleared up before the patient leaves the office. Make sure that all of the adaptations that are relevant to individual patient needs are considered. For example, if the patient is hard of hearing, make sure you get feedback that the patient understands how to take his medication. Including written instructions will help confirm accuracy in medication administration. Always remember that the more the patient knows and understands about how to take the medication and why it has been prescribed, the greater the likelihood that the patient will comply with medication therapy, and the more likely it is that the drug treatment will be successful.

This also would be a good time to suggest that the patient check the status of medications at home. The National Community Pharmacists Association (NCPA) recommends that the medicine cabinet be checked once a month to determine the age and quality of medications. At that time, the patient should discard any medications that fall into the following categories:

- Medicines for past illnesses
- Any expired medicines, unidentified medications, or medications that are more than 2 years old
- Hydrogen peroxide (H_2O_2) that no longer bubbles or has changed color (H_2O_2 typically has a shelf life of at least 1 year if the bottle is unopened but lasts only 30 to 45 days once the seal has been broken); ointments or salves that have separated or are crumbly; vinegary smelling aspirin; antiseptic solutions that are cloudy or have a solid residue on the bottom; and any medicine of uncertain quality

The NCPA also suggests the following:

- Keep medicines stored away from light, heat, air, and moisture.
- Use medicine from the original container until it is completely used or expired.
- Do not combine medicines from several containers.
- Keep medicine locked away from children.
- Make sure childproof medicine caps are used properly.

Legal and Ethical Issues

A medical assistant must be extremely knowledgeable when administering medications in the ambulatory care setting. Follow all the provider's orders exactly as documented. If you have a question about the order, ask for clarification before you proceed. It is advisable to give a medication only after the order has been written in the patient's record. If the provider gives you a verbal order to administer medication, write it down and review it with the provider before completing the order. This helps eliminate errors and possible omissions in medication therapy.

Legal responsibilities in medication practice include preventing errors by carefully following safe practice procedures while dispensing and administering drugs. Always implement the Seven Rights and perform the three drug order and label checks. Anyone administering a drug must know the possible serious complications related to the drug and must be alert for side effects. The medical assistant must demonstrate compliance with individual state laws regulating scope of practice regarding medications and their administration. Precise documentation of the administration

of medications and of the management of prescriptions cannot be overemphasized.

The administration of drugs involves ethical principles. The patient always comes first. With that foremost in mind, never risk giving an incorrect medication. There is no such thing as a small error because any mistake may result in serious harm or possibly death. If an error is made, it must be reported immediately to the provider so that measures can be taken to help the patient. It is difficult to admit that a mistake has been made, but it is absolutely necessary. For this reason, be sure to double-check your calculations with a co-worker or the provider before dispensing the drug. If a mistake is made, most facilities require the person who made the mistake to complete an incident report. The incident must be documented completely, including the details of the error, to whom the error was reported, any action taken, and subsequent observations of the patient (Procedure 28-11).

Professional Behaviors

The importance of accuracy and accountability cannot be overstated when it comes to the responsibility of being involved in drug treatment. A single mistake could be devastating for the patient. A professional medical assistant recognizes the seriousness of accurately completing medication orders. Do not hesitate to ask for assistance or clarification if you have any doubts about how to follow a medication order or if you are concerned about patient safety. As the patient's advocate it is your responsibility to raise questions as needed to ensure healthy outcomes for your patients.

Medication Errors

According to the U.S. Food and Drug Administration (FDA), medication errors result in at least one death every day and injure more than 1 million people annually in the United States. Medication mistakes can occur at any point in the process between the provider's order up to and including administration of the medication. If a medication error occurs, most facilities require completion of a medication error incident form. An incident report is not part of the patient's record, but it is used by the facility to prevent similar incidents and is kept as a record in case of litigation in the future.

Common causes of medication errors include:

- Poor communication
- Unclear or mistaken product names, directions for use, medical abbreviations, or writing
- Poor procedures or techniques when dispensing or administering the drug
- Inadequate patient preparation and education on the use of the medication
- Job stress in healthcare facilities and/or pharmacies
- Lack of product knowledge or training for healthcare workers
- Medication labeling or packaging that is too similar to another drug product

Data from Pullen RL Jr: Administering a transdermal drug, *Nursing* 38(5):14, 2008.

PROCEDURE 28-11   Complete an Incident Report Related to an Error in Patient Care

Goal: *To promptly report a medication error to your supervisor and complete an incident report form according to the facility's policies and procedures.*

Scenario: *Dr. Thau writes the following order: Administer Ventolin HF, 2 puffs, to Simon Alesiam STAT. You administer 2 puffs of Spiriva, thinking it is the same drug. The patient notices you used a different inhaler from the one he uses at home, and he asks the provider about this. Your office manager tells you to complete the required Medication Error Incident Report Form.*

EQUIPMENT and SUPPLIES

- Patient's health record
- Written provider's order, including the drug name, strength, dose, and route of administration
- PDR, online drug reference, or package insert
- Facility Medication Error Incident Report Form

PROCEDURAL STEPS

1. Complete the facility's Medication Error Incident Report Form (Figure 1).

Northeast Family Practice

1099 McKnight Road

Pittsburgh, PA 15210

MEDICATION ERROR INCIDENT REPORT

EMPLOYEE: Return this COMPLETED FORM to the Office Manager as soon as possible.

Name of Patient Involved: _____

Address: _____ City: _____

Phone Number: _____ Email _____

Age: _____ DOB: _____ Sex: M _____ F _____

Patient ID#: _____ Date of Incident: _____ Time: _____ am/pm

Check Type of Error:

- ❏ Medication given to the wrong patient
- ❏ Wrong medication given
- ❏ Wrong dose of medication given
- ❏ Wrong route of administration
- ❏ Proper technique not followed when administering the medication resulting in patient injury
- ❏ Medication not given at the right time
- ❏ Medication not given
- ❏ Medication not documented accurately
- ❏ Patient education not given resulting in patient administration error
- ❏ Administration of medication resulted in an allergic reaction
- ❏ Other _____

EMPLOYEE Involved in the Incident:

Name: _____

Title: _____

Information about the drug **ordered**:

Brand name: _____

Dosage: _____

Route of administration: _____

Contraindications: _____

Adverse reactions: _____

1

PROCEDURE 28-11 *—continued*

Information about the drug **administered**:

Brand name: _____

Dosage: _____

Route of administration: _____

Contraindications: _____

Adverse reactions: _____

Description of Incident (Who, What, Where, How, Why; Include sequence of events, personnel involved, reason incident occurred):

_____

_____

Actions Taken by Staff Members: _____

_____

Details of patient injury or adverse reactions:

_____

Witness Name: _____ Phone Number: _____

Address: _____

Corrective Action Taken/Follow-Up (Things that have been or will be done to prevent recurrence):

_____

_____

Office Manager Comments:

_____

_____

Office Manager Signature: _____ Date: _____

Provider Comments:

_____

_____

Provider Signature: _____ Title: _____ Date: _____

1   *Adapted from the Kentucky Cabinet for Health and Family Services at http://chfs.ky.gov/. Accessed June 2, 2015.*

2. If you are unfamiliar with the drug, refer to the PDR, online drug reference, or the package insert to determine the purpose of the drug, common side effects, typical dose, and any pertinent precautions or contraindications.

3. Which of the Seven Rights did you not use to prevent the error?
4. What did you learn from this experience?

SUMMARY OF SCENARIO

Dorothy understands the importance of careful management of medications. Because of her concern for patient safety, she asks Dr. Thau to check all her calculations and confers with her if she has any questions about medication orders or patient education. Dr. Thau is a primary care physician, so it is important for Dorothy to understand the factors that affect the administration of medication to patients in all age groups. She routinely uses the standard three label checks when dispensing medications and implements the Seven Rights throughout medication administration procedures.

Dorothy recognizes the importance of complete and accurate documentation of medications, whether they are administered in the facility or given to the patient as a prescription order. In addition, she consistently applies the rules of Standard Precautions when preparing and administering parenteral medications. All those administering a drug must know the possible serious complications related to the drug and must be alert for side effects. Precise documentation of the administration of medications and of the management of prescriptions cannot be overemphasized.

SUMMARY OF LEARNING OBJECTIVES

1. **Define, spell, and pronounce the terms listed in the vocabulary.**
   Spelling and pronouncing medical terms correctly reinforce the medical assistant's credibility. Knowing the definitions of these terms promotes confidence in communication with patients and co-workers.

2. **Do the following related to safety in drug administration:**
   - *Follow safety precautions in the management of medication administration in the ambulatory healthcare setting.*
     The three label checks and Seven Rights must always be performed. Medications are prepared in a quiet, well-lit area. A substitute is never used for the ordered drug or drug strength. Medications are stored as ordered on the package. Medical assistants must never administer a medication they have not prepared personally. If preparing a medication for the provider to administer, the medical assistant places the container with the dispensed drug. Only written provider's orders are followed. The medical assistant must check expiration dates and discard expired drugs. Medications with damaged labels are discarded. Dispensed medication that is not given is discarded. Patients must be consistently asked about drug allergies. Patients are observed for at least 20 minutes after administration of a drug. Drug reactions are reported and documented. Patient education about drug therapy is provided and documented.
   - *Analyze safety guidelines for specific patient populations.*
     Safety precautions in the management of medication administration should be applied consistently. Safe drug administration includes understanding the provider's order, looking up the drug if the medical assistant is unfamiliar with it, and using the three label checks and the Seven Rights every time a drug order is completed.
   - *Document the administration of a medication accurately in the health record.*
     Immediately after administering a drug, the medical assistant should document the date and time of administration; the drug's name, strength, dose, and route of administration; any reactions the patient has to the drug; and patient education about the medication. For parenteral medications, the exact site of administration must be recorded.

3. **Summarize patient assessment factors that can affect medication administration.**
   Such factors include continual evaluation of the patient's physical condition, in addition to holistic factors, such as the patient's history, an accurate list of drug allergies, the patient's ability to understand the drug regimen and to afford the treatment, and special factors based on age, weight, and condition.

4. **Identify various drug forms and their administration guidelines, and administer oral medications.**
   Drugs are packaged in a variety of forms with a variety of administration guidelines. Oral medications include both solid and liquid preparations; mucous membrane medications are absorbed rectally, vaginally, orally, nasally, or topically through the skin. Each form of medication has specific guidelines for administration, but all require consistent use of the three label checks and the Seven Rights. (See Procedure 28-1 for the steps in administering oral medications.)

5. **Do the following related to parenteral administration of drugs:**
   - *Specify parenteral administration equipment, including details about needles and syringes.*
     Parenteral medications are manufactured in ampules and in single-dose or multidose vials. The ordered route of administration, the drug's characteristics, and individual patient factors determine the correct gauge and needle length used for administration. The appropriate syringe is determined by the type of medication ordered and the amount of drug to be administered. Specialty syringe units, such as the insulin pen and the EpiPen, are designed for quick administration of certain medications. Table 28-1 provides further details.
   - *Follow OSHA guidelines in the management of parenteral administration.*
     OSHA guidelines include using syringe units with safety needle covers; wearing disposable, nonsterile gloves and other appropriate protective gear when administering any medication that involves coming into contact with blood or body fluids; never recapping a contaminated needle, applying the unit's needle safety device, and immediately discarding it into a sharps container with the needle first; disposing of contaminated nonsharp materials in biohazard containers; disinfecting contaminated work areas; and washing hands before and after procedures.
   - *Describe and demonstrate the types and locations of parenteral administration with proper use of sharps containers.*
     Parenteral routes of administration include intradermal (ID), subcutaneous (SC), and a variety of intramuscular (IM) sites. The type

Continued

of medication, the provider's order, and the unique characteristics of individual patients determine the route and site of administration. Each requires specific administration practices, which are described in Procedures 28-2 through 28-10.

6. **Recognize the medical assistant's role in coaching patients about the administration of drugs.**

Patient education is crucial if patients are to administer medications correctly at home. The patient should understand the purpose of the drug; the time, frequency, and amount of the dose; any special storage requirements; and the typical side effects. The more the patient knows and understands about how to take the medication and why it has been prescribed, the greater the chance that drug treatment will be successful.

7. **Assess legal and ethical issues in drug administration in the ambulatory care setting, and complete an incident report related to an error in medication administration.**

The medical assistant must be extremely knowledgeable when preparing and administering medications in the ambulatory care facility. If

any questions arise about the order, the medical assistant must ask for clarification before proceeding. Legal responsibilities include preventing plural—errors by carefully following safe practice procedures in dispensing and administering drugs. The medical assistant must comply with individual state laws regulating medications and their administration. Precise charting of the administration of medications and the management of prescriptions cannot be overemphasized.

According to the FDA, medication errors result in at least one death every day and injure more than 1 million people annually in the United States. Medication mistakes can occur at any point in the process between the provider's order up to and including administration of the medication. If a medication error occurs, most facilities require completion of a medication error incident form. An incident report is not part of the patient's record, but it is used by the facility to prevent similar incidents and is kept as a record in case of litigation in the future. (Refer to Procedure 28-11.)

CONNECTIONS

Study Guide Connection: Go to the Chapter 28 Study Guide. Read and complete the activities.

evolve Evolve Connection: Go to the Chapter 28 link at *evolve.elsevier.com/kinn* to complete the Chapter Review Quiz. Check out the other resources listed for this chapter to make the most of what you have learned from Administering Medications.

SAFETY AND EMERGENCY PRACTICES

29

SCENARIO

Cheryl Skurka, CMA (AAMA), has been working for Dr. Peter Bendt for approximately 6 months. During that time, a number of patient emergencies have occurred in the office, and even more potentially serious problems have been managed by the telephone screening staff. Cheryl is concerned that she is not prepared to assist with emergencies in an ambulatory care practice. She decides to ask Dr. Bendt for assistance, and he suggests that she work with the experienced screening staff to learn how to manage phone calls from patients calling for assistance.

Dr. Bendt is participating in a community-wide preparedness effort focused on both natural and human-made disasters, and he expects his practice and employees to be ready to respond if needed. This includes creating plans both to maintain the safety of patients and employees in the facility and to provide assistance as needed in a community emergency.

While studying this chapter, think about the following questions:

- What should Cheryl learn about the medical assistant's responsibilities in an emergency situation?
- What are some of the general rules for managing a medical emergency in an ambulatory care practice?
- What types of questions does the telephone screening staff ask if a patient calls with a medical emergency?
- What information from these phone calls should be documented?
- Is it important for Cheryl to be able to recognize life-threatening emergencies and to be prepared to respond to them? Why?
- What are some of the typical patient emergencies that occur in a healthcare facility?

- How should Cheryl instruct a patient to control bleeding from a hemorrhaging wound?
- What safety practices should be followed in the healthcare facility to protect patients and employees from potential harm?
- What is the medical office's responsibility in preparing for community emergencies?
- Are there common health emergency topics for patient education that Cheryl should be prepared to present?
- What legal factors should Cheryl keep in mind when handling ambulatory care emergencies?

LEARNING OBJECTIVES

1. Define, spell, and pronounce the terms listed in the vocabulary.
2. Describe patient safety factors in the medical office environment.
3. Interpret and comply with safety signs, labels, and symbols and evaluate the work environment to identify safe and unsafe working conditions for the employee.
4. Do the following when it comes to environmental safety in the healthcare setting:
   - Identify environmental safety issues in the healthcare setting
   - Discuss fire safety issues in a healthcare environment
   - Demonstrate the proper use of a fire extinguisher
5. Describe the fundamental principles for evacuation of a healthcare facility and role-play a mock environmental exposure event and evacuation of a provider's office.
6. Discuss the requirements for proper disposal of hazardous materials.
7. Identify critical elements of an emergency plan for response to a natural disaster or other emergency.
8. Maintain an up-to-date list of community resources for emergency preparedness.

9. Describe the medical assistant's role in emergency response.
10. Summarize typical emergency supplies and equipment.
11. Demonstrate the use of an automated external defibrillator.
12. Summarize the general rules for managing emergencies.
13. Demonstrate telephone screening techniques and documentation guidelines for ambulatory care emergencies.
14. Recognize and respond to life-threatening emergencies in an ambulatory care practice.
15. Describe how to handle an unresponsive patient and perform provider/professional-level CPR.
16. Discuss cardiac emergencies and administer oxygen through a nasal cannula to a patient in respiratory distress.
17. Identify and assist a patient with an obstructed airway.
18. Discuss cerebrovascular accidents and assist a patient who is in shock.
19. Determine the appropriate action and documentation procedures for common office emergencies, such as fainting, poisoning, animal bites, insect bites and stings, and asthma attacks.

LEARNING OBJECTIVES—*continued*

20. Discuss seizures and perform first aid procedures for a patient having a seizure.
21. Discuss abdominal pain, sprains and strains, and fractures, and perform first aid procedures for a patient with a fracture of the wrist.
22. Discuss burns and tissue injuries, and control of a hemorrhagic wound.

23. Discuss nosebleeds, head injuries, foreign bodies in the eye, heat and cold injuries, dehydration, and diabetic emergencies; also, perform first aid procedures for a patient with a diabetic emergency.
24. Apply patient education concepts to medical emergencies.
25. Discuss the legal and ethical concerns arising from medical emergencies.

VOCABULARY

arrhythmia (uh-rith′-me-uh) An abnormality or irregularity in the heart rhythm.

asystole (ay-sis′-toh-le) The absence of a heartbeat.

cyanosis (si-an-oh′-sis) A blue coloration of the mucous membranes and body extremities caused by lack of oxygen.

diaphoresis (di-uh-fuh-re′-sis) The profuse excretion of sweat.

ecchymosis (eH-kih-moh′-sis) A hemorrhagic skin discoloration commonly called bruising.

emetic (eh-met′-ik) A substance that causes vomiting.

fibrillation Rapid, random, ineffective contractions of the heart.

hematuria (he-muh-tuhr′-e-uh) Blood in the urine.

idiopathic (ih-dee-oh-path-ik) Pertaining to a condition or a disease that has no known cause.

mediastinum (me-de-ast′-in-um) The space in the center of the chest under the sternum.

myocardium (my-oh-kar′-de-um) The muscular lining of the heart.

necrosis (neh-kroh′-sis) The death of cells or tissues.

photophobia An abnormal sensitivity to light.

polydipsia Excessive thirst.

Safety Data Sheets (SDSs) Documents that accompany hazardous chemicals and substances and outline the dangers, composition, safe handling, and disposal of these items. Safety Data Sheets must be formatted to conform to the Globally Harmonized System (GHS), which mandates that SDS have 16 standardized sections arranged in a strict order.

thrombolytics Agents that dissolve blood clots.

transient ischemic attack (TIA) Temporary neurologic symptoms caused by gradual or partial occlusion of a cerebral blood vessel.

The medical assistant typically is responsible for making the healthcare facility as accident proof as possible. This requires attention to a number of factors. For example, cupboard doors and drawers must be kept closed; spills must be wiped up immediately; and dropped objects must be picked up. The medical assistant also should make sure that all medications are kept out of sight and away from busy patient areas. If children are in the office, all sharp objects and potentially toxic substances must be kept out of reach. In addition, the medical assistant should never leave a seriously ill patient or a restless, depressed, or unconscious patient unattended.

SAFETY IN THE HEALTHCARE FACILITY

Patient Safety

Patient safety is a critical component of the quality of care provided in a healthcare facility. The U.S. Department of Health and Human Services (DHHS) has conducted extensive research on the features of safe patient environments in providers' offices. The DHHS has found the following factors to be crucial to patient safety.

- Open lines of communication must be established among all employees about possible safety issues, and employees must work together to solve these problems before a patient is injured.
- If an injury occurs (e.g., a medication is administered to the wrong patient), policies and procedures must be in place so that all employees recognize the potential for an error and protocols are established for preventing a similar problem in the future.
- Procedures must be standardized in the facility's policies and procedures manual so that all employees can refer to specific guidelines on how procedures should be performed. For example,

in the case of a blood spill, the policies and procedures manual must outline a specific, step-by-step procedure for cleaning up the spill that safeguards both patients and staff members.

- The facility must provide ongoing staff training in patient safety factors.
- Staff members must work as a team to maintain a safe environment for patients. For example, all staff members must follow Standard Precautions to prevent the spread of disease in the facility.

Throughout this text, you have learned about situations that could result in serious harm to your patients. You must constantly be on guard to protect patients from possible injury. For example, studies have shown that healthcare workers frequently confuse drug names, which results in administration of the wrong medication; they also fail to identify a patient correctly before performing a procedure and neglect to perform hand sanitization consistently, thus promoting the spread of infectious diseases. The medical assistant is an important link in the delivery of quality and *safe* care. Can you think of anything you have learned thus far in your studies that could help keep patients safe in the provider's office?

Employee Safety

The healthcare facility should safeguard patients as well as staff members from the possibility of accidental injury. This includes making sure the facility has appropriate safety signs throughout the building as well as appropriate symbols and labels that identify potentially dangerous items (Figure 29-1). Data compiled by the Occupational Safety and Health Administration (OSHA) reveal that the leading causes of accidents in an office are slips, trips, and falls. You must think and work safely to prevent accidents. The following

FIGURE 29-1 *Safety signs, symbols, and labels.*

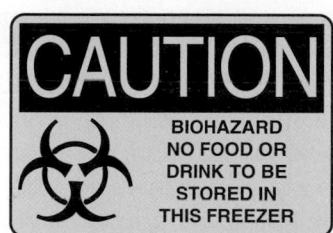
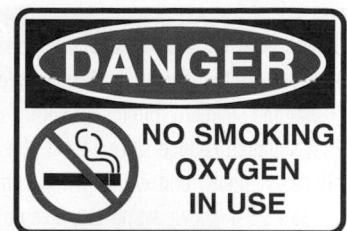

Fire extinguisher

Manual Station
Pull Station/
Fire Alarm Box

Fire hose
or standpoint

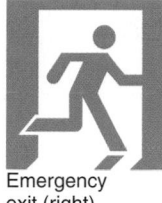
Emergency
exit (right)

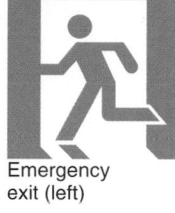
Emergency
exit (left)

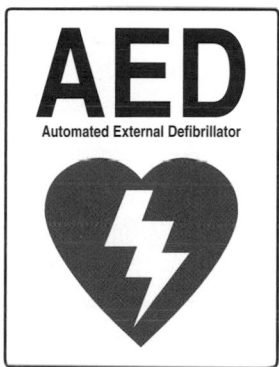
Automated External Defibrillator (AED)

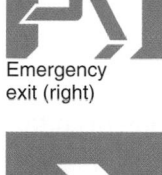

Emergency exit directional arrows
(Can be rotated in increments of 45 degrees)

are some suggestions from OSHA for vigilant accident prevention methods (Procedure 29-1).

1. Use proper body mechanics in all situations. For example, bend your knees and bring a heavy item close to you before lifting rather than bending from your back; push heavy items rather than pulling them; and use a gait belt or ask for assistance when transferring patients.
2. Constantly check the floors and hallways for obstructions and possible tripping hazards, such as telephone and computer cables or boxes.
3. Store supplies inside cabinets rather than on top, where they can fall off and injure someone; store heavier items on lower shelves so they do not have to be lifted any higher than necessary.
4. Clean up spills immediately; slippery floors are a danger to everyone.
5. Use a step stool to reach for things, not a chair or a box that could collapse or move.
6. Have handrails and grab bars available as needed in the facility; use them, and encourage patients to use them.
7. Do not overload electrical outlets.
8. Perform a safety check of the facility routinely; look for unsafe or defective equipment, torn carpeting that could catch heels, adequate lighting both inside and outside the facility, and so on.

A primary concern for personnel and patient safety is infection control. Standard Precautions protocols require employers to provide appropriate and adequate personal protective equipment (PPE). The goal is to protect staff members from occupational exposure to blood-borne pathogens while at the same time safeguarding patients in the facility. OSHA's guidelines include managing sharps and providing current safety-engineered sharps devices; providing hepatitis B immunization free of charge to all employees at risk of exposure to blood and body fluids; using latex-free supplies as much as possible to prevent allergic reactions in both staff members and patients; identifying all chemicals in the facility with **Safety Data Sheets (SDSs)** and adequately storing potentially dangerous substances; and performing proper hand hygiene consistently throughout the workday.

Another serious concern that faces all of us today is the prevention of workplace violence. Unfortunately, rarely does a week go by without reports of violence in a public place. Employees in a healthcare facility are no exception. We started the text with information about and exercises in communication techniques in the workplace: problem solving, therapeutic communication, and assertive behavior. All of these are helpful in dealing with a difficult patient. Employers should provide training on how to identify potentially violent patients and should discuss safe methods for managing difficult patients. Many employers offer training on how to manage assaultive behaviors. Procedure 29-2 presents a scenario that deals with employee safety. Follow the steps of this procedure to learn how to handle such a situation.

OSHA Updates for Signs, Symbols, and Labels

In September, 2013, the Occupational Safety and Health Administration (OSHA) updated standard formats for safety signs, symbols, and labels. This is the first standard change since 1971. The revised standards regulate the color, shape, symbols, and wording that can be used on safety signs and labels. Figure 29-1 shows some examples of the types of signs, symbols, and labels that should be used in an ambulatory care office. The four major types of signs are:

- *Danger signs* (identify the most severe and immediate hazards)
- *Caution signs* (warn of possible hazards that require added precautions)
- *Safety instruction signs* (communicate directions for safety actions)
- *Biologic hazard signs* (identify an actual or potential biohazard)

OSHA specifies the format of each type of sign, the information that must appear, and where each type of sign must be used. Tags or labels must contain a signal word ("Danger," "Caution," "Biologic Hazard," "BIOHAZARD," or the biologic hazard symbol) and a major message, which states a specific hazard or safety instruction. Employers are required to train workers about the information conveyed on safety signs and labels. The signs and labels use graphic symbols and specific colors to explain the sign's warning or message so that the problem of language barriers is minimized (see Procedure 29-1).

PROCEDURE 29-1   **Evaluate the Work Environment to Identify Unsafe Working Conditions and Comply With Safety Signs and Symbols**

Goal: *To assess the healthcare facility for possible safety issues and develop a safety plan.*

Scenario: *Work with a partner to evaluate environmental safety in the laboratory at your school. Record your results and discuss them with the class. After all members of the class have shared their observations, develop a safety plan for your laboratory.*

EQUIPMENT and SUPPLIES

- Pen and paper
- Document or manual on policies and procedures for environmental safety issues in the facility

PROCEDURAL STEPS

1. Check the floors and hallways for obstructions and possible tripping hazards, including torn carpets, possible spills, protruding electrical cords, and so on.
   PURPOSE: To prevent accidental falls.
2. Check storage areas to make sure the tops of cabinets are clear and heavier items have been stored closer to the floor.
   PURPOSE: To prevent injuries from items falling off shelves and to limit the lifting of heavy items.
3. Assess the location and security of handrails and grab bars placed around the facility. They should be placed at all stairs, in restrooms, and in any other areas where staff members or patients may need assistance.
   PURPOSE: Handrails and grab bars help safeguard staff members and patients and provide assistance where needed.
4. Examine all electrical plugs and outlets to prevent electrical overload.
   PURPOSE: Overloading electrical outlets could cause a fire.
5. Check all equipment to make sure it is in safe working condition.

6. Make sure all lights are working (both inside and outside the facility), that lighting is adequate, and that light fixtures are in good condition.
   PURPOSE: Adequate lighting both inside and outside the facility helps prevent accidents, and faulty fixtures can be a fire hazard.
7. Check the working condition of smoke alarms, and examine all fire extinguishers.
   PURPOSE: To monitor the function of smoke detectors and make sure fire extinguishers are charged.
8. Make sure evacuation routes are posted throughout the facility, along with floor plans with clearly marked exit routes.
   PURPOSE: Every room in the facility must have a map with exit routes marked on it to make sure that even those who are unfamiliar with the facility's floor plan can safely reach an exit in case of an emergency.
9. Assess the laboratory's compliance with the safety signs, symbols, and labels required by the Occupational Safety and Health Administration (OSHA). Are all signs, symbols, labels in place and posted properly?
10. Record your observations and share them with the class.
    PURPOSE: To compile a comprehensive list of problem areas.
11. Based on group discussion, develop a plan of action for improving the safety of the laboratory.
    PURPOSE: The student-generated safety plan can be incorporated into the laboratory's policies and procedures manual.

PROCEDURE 29-2 | Manage a Difficult Patient

Goal: *To communicate with an angry patient in a safe, therapeutic manner. The following procedure is part of an overall employee safety plan.*

Scenario: *You are working at the admissions desk when an extremely angry patient comes storming into the office, screaming about a mistake on his bill. Although the facility uses an outside billing center, you recognize that you should attempt to help the patient and try to defuse the situation. Remember: Call 911 immediately and alert any available security if you or one of your co-workers is threatened with violence.*

EQUIPMENT and SUPPLIES

- Patient's record
- Telephone
- Facility's policies and procedures manual

PROCEDURAL STEPS

1. Although it is important to safeguard patients' privacy, do not ask an angry patient into an isolated room; do not close the door.
   <u>PURPOSE</u>: To protect yourself, remain in an open area. If you are in a room with an angry patient, keep the door open and stand close to the door so that you can leave the room quickly if necessary.

2. Alert other staff members to the situation, if possible.
   <u>PURPOSE</u>: To have assistance nearby; call 911 immediately if you feel physically threatened.

3. If you do not feel physically threatened, allow the patient to blow off steam.
   <u>PURPOSE</u>: Attempting to interrupt the patient to give a logical reason for the problem will only make him angrier. Allowing him to continue to yell helps him release the anger so that you can work on a reasonable solution to the problem. Call 911 if at any time you feel threatened.

4. When the patient begins to slow down, offer supportive statements, such as, "I understand it is frustrating to receive a bill you think is unfair." Continue to make supportive statements until the patient is calmer (think of it as the patient screaming his way up a mountain; sooner or later, he is going to run out of steam; when he begins to slow down, you can then start offering supportive statements).

   <u>PURPOSE</u>: Providing verbal support helps defuse the situation and gives the patient the opportunity to become calmer and reach a rational level where you can discuss the problem.

5. Once you can discuss the situation, ask the patient for the details of the problem. Gather as much information as possible so you can work together on a possible solution.

6. After determining the problem, suggest a possible solution to the patient. For example, tell him that you will contact the billing office with the information and will make sure they get back to the patient as soon as possible.
   <u>PURPOSE</u>: Use therapeutic techniques, including restatement, reflection, and clarification, to gather details and work on a possible solution with the patient. Make sure you follow up with the action to prevent future outbursts.

7. Report the incident to your supervisor and document the patient's problem and the agreed-upon action in the patient's health record, taking care not to use judgmental statements.
   <u>PURPOSE</u>: Documenting the patient's problem and the agreed-upon solution allows for continuity of care if follow-up is needed. The patient's medical record is a legal document, and all judgmental statements must be avoided.

8. Discuss your approach to managing the difficult patient at the next staff meeting. With your supervisor's permission, summarize your approach and include it as part of the facility's Employee Safety Plan.
   <u>PURPOSE</u>: The safety plan should be reviewed frequently, and revisions should be made as needed.

Environmental Safety

Environmental safety guidelines include numerous work safety practices, such as office security, management of smoke detectors and fire extinguishers, posting of designated fire exit routes, and securing certain items (e.g., narcotics, dangerous chemicals) in locked storage areas in the facility. In addition to these concerns, staff members should constantly be on the alert for possible safety hazards in and around the building, such as improper lighting, unlimited access to the facility, and inadequate use of security systems.

The medical assistant must be prepared to use a fire extinguisher to prevent injury to patients and to protect the medical facility (Procedure 29-3). An ABC fire extinguisher is effective against the most common causes of fire, including cloth, paper, plastics, rubber, flammable liquids, and electrical fires. Most small extinguishers empty within 15 seconds, so it is important to call 911 immediately if the facility fire is not small and confined. If the fire is small, no heavy smoke is present, and you have easy access to an exit route, use the closest fire extinguisher. However, do not hesitate to evacuate the facility if you believe any danger exists to yourself or others.

Methods of Fire Prevention and Response

- Store potentially flammable chemicals and supplies according to the manufacturers' guidelines.
- Inspect electrical equipment and cords throughout the facility; take care not to overload outlets.
- If a fire is suspected, immediately disconnect oxygen supplies or turn off oxygen tanks to prevent an explosion.
- Smoke alarms should be located throughout the facility, checked periodically, and replaced as needed.
- Fire safety equipment should be available and current. Fire extinguishers must be inspected at least annually. If an extinguisher is discharged, it must be replaced immediately.
- Fire extinguishers should be located in multiple sites throughout the facility and mounted on the wall for easy access.
- If you smell smoke or suspect a fire, immediately notify the fire department (or call 911) and evacuate the facility. Do not use elevators if a fire is suspected.

CRITICAL THINKING APPLICATION   29-1

Cheryl is in the middle of a busy day; patients are in all of the examination rooms, and the waiting room is full. She walks past the patient bathroom and smells smoke. She opens the door and sees smoke and flames coming from the wastebasket. What should she do? Write down your response to this scenario and share it with your classmates.

PROCEDURE 29-3   Demonstrate the Proper Use of a Fire Extinguisher

Goal: *To role-play the safe and proper use of a fire extinguisher.*

EQUIPMENT and SUPPLIES

- Portable, office-size ABC fire extinguisher that has been discharged

PROCEDURAL STEPS

Role-play the following with a discharged ABC fire extinguisher.
1. Pull the pin from the handle of the extinguisher.

2. Aim the discharge from the extinguisher toward the bottom of the flames. <u>PURPOSE:</u> Aiming the fire extinguisher directly onto the fire may spread the flames.
3. Squeeze the handle of the extinguisher so that it begins to discharge.
4. Sweep the extinguisher from side to side toward the base of the fire until it is out or until fire officials arrive.
5. Check on the safety of all patients and other personnel.

Each facility should have a policy and procedure in place for evacuating the building. According to OSHA, the facility's plan first should identify the situations that might require evacuation, such as a natural disaster or a fire. The following provisions should be included in the facility's evacuation plan.

- An emergency action coordinator must be designated, and all employees must know who this individual is. This person (usually the office manager) is in charge if an emergency occurs.
- The coordinator is responsible for managing the emergency at the facility and for notifying and working with community emergency services.
- Evacuation routes with clearly marked exits must be posted in multiple locations throughout the facility. Maps of floor diagrams with arrows pointing to the closest exits are an easy means of

finding the closest door out, even for individuals unfamiliar with the facility.
- Exit doors must be clearly marked, well lit, and wide enough for everyone to evacuate.
- Hazardous areas in the facility that should be avoided during an emergency evacuation must be identified, such as areas where chemicals and oxygen tanks are stored.
- A meeting place outside the facility must be designated for all those evacuating to make sure everyone got out of the facility safely.
- Employees should be trained to assist any co-worker or patient with special needs.
- A designated individual must check the entire facility, including restrooms, before exiting. He or she must make sure to close all doors (especially designated fire doors) when leaving to try to contain the fire or other disaster (Procedure 29-4).

Evacuation Levels

Four levels of evacuation are possible, depending on the severity of the need for evacuation:

Shelter in place: Staff stops all routine activities in preparation for possible evacuation of the facility; close doors/windows for initial protection from fire and smoke.

Horizontal evacuation: Patients and staff move away from immediate danger, but if the facility is located in a multifloor structure, everyone remains on that floor until it is determined that the entire building should be evacuated.

Vertical evacuation: A specific floor in a building is evacuated vertically (i.e., toward the ground level) to prepare for evacuation outside.

Total or full evacuation: The facility is completely evacuated (this is used only as a last resort).

PROCEDURE 29-4 Participate in a Mock Environmental Exposure Event: Evacuate a Provider's Office

Goal: *To role-play an environmental disaster and implement an evacuation plan.*

Scenario: *Role-play the following scenario with your lab group: The building next door to the provider's office where you work is on fire. One member of the group is the designated emergency action coordinator, two individuals are responsible for helping patients with special needs out of the facility, and one person is designated to be the last to leave after the building is clear. In a community emergency situation, certain staff members may be designated to provide immediate assistance to survivors. Two medical assistants are sent to help with fire victims. How could medical assistants help in this situation? After the evacuation is complete, meet in a designated spot to discuss the process and see whether any aspects of the evacuation plan could be improved. Document the steps taken throughout the mock environmental event.*

EQUIPMENT and SUPPLIES

- Pen and paper
- Document or manual on policies and procedures for evacuation of the facility and response to an environmental disaster

PROCEDURAL STEPS

1. In an actual emergency, an emergency action coordinator is in charge.
   PURPOSE: All employees must know who this individual is (usually it is the office manager) and must follow his or her lead in safely responding to the emergency situation.
2. The student who is role-playing the emergency action coordinator is responsible for managing the emergency at the facility and for notifying and working with community emergency services.
   PURPOSE: The coordinator or someone designated by the coordinator must notify community emergency services of the fire; the coordinator works with emergency services to provide care at the scene.
3. Fire victims are being cared for across the street, where a triage and treatment center has been set up by the police, fire, and emergency responder units in the city. Two students role-play staff members who are sent to assist with the victims:
   - Use therapeutic communication techniques to calm and care for victims
   - Implement appropriate Standard Precautions
   - Monitor and record vital signs
   - Gather pertinent health histories
   - Observe victims for possible complications, such as breathing problems, shock, angina, and so on
   - Immediately report to emergency responders any life-threatening changes in a patient's status
   - Use first aid skills as needed

4. The coordinator designates an employee to shut down immediately any combustibles (e.g., oxygen tanks).
   PURPOSE: To prevent an explosion if the fire spreads.
5. Using the posted evacuation routes, role-play staff members following floor plan diagrams to the closest safe exit. Identify any hazardous areas in the facility that should be avoided during the emergency evacuation. Role-play staff members assisting patients, especially those with special needs (e.g., individuals in wheelchairs) during the building evacuation.
   PURPOSE: Evacuation routes must be posted throughout the facility, and exit doors must be clearly marked, well lit, and wide enough for everyone to evacuate. The doors facing the building on fire should not be used because this could be a hazard.
6. Role-play the staff member delegated to check that everyone has left the facility and that fire doors have been closed before he or she leaves the building.
   PURPOSE: To make sure the building is clear and that any fire is contained. This person should leave immediately if there is danger.
7. Role-play evacuated personnel and patients meeting in a designated area to count heads and make sure everyone exited the facility safely.
   PURPOSE: To make sure everyone safely evacuated the facility.
8. After everyone has been accounted for and the patients are secure, role-play staff members reporting to the emergency triage area to provide assistance to rescue workers and victims.
9. Discuss with the class the evacuation exercise and response to a community disaster.
10. Document the specific steps taken during the facility evacuation and your role in the exercise. What were the strengths and weaknesses of the group's response to an environmental emergency?
    PURPOSE: To reflect on the learning activity.

DISPOSAL OF HAZARDOUS WASTE

The chapter on Infection Control explained the management of biohazardous waste; the use of PPE when the potential exists for exposure to blood and body fluids; the importance of flushing the eyes with an eye wash unit if they are exposed to potentially infectious or toxic material; and the consistent use of sharps containers. Regardless of individual responsibilities in the facility, all employees must be aware of potentially dangerous situations and must comply with all safety measures to protect themselves and their patients.

OSHA defines regulated waste as any contaminated item that might release blood or other potentially infectious material; contaminated supplies with dried blood or other potentially infectious material on their surfaces; contaminated sharps; and waste products that contain blood or other potentially infectious material. Healthcare facilities must make special arrangements for the disposal of regulated waste, which often costs as much as 10 times more than regular garbage disposal. It therefore is important to put only supplies contaminated with blood or body fluids into red bag collection systems and sharps containers. The following measures should be used for proper disposal of hazardous materials in the provider's office.

- Place signs on or near the biohazard container to identify its purpose and the materials that should be deposited in it. All biohazardous waste containers should display a biohazard label.
- Make sure all biohazardous waste containers are covered and have a foot pedal for opening and closing the container. This prevents the spread of infectious material and reduces the likelihood that noninfectious material will be tossed inside. Biohazard containers should be kept only in treatment areas where contaminated materials are likely to be produced.
- Place a regular garbage container next to a biohazard container to encourage staff members to use the biohazard bags only as needed.
- Place only sharps in sharps containers; gauze, bandages, and so on belong in a contaminated waste container. Noninfectious items, such as patient gowns that are not contaminated with body fluids, and packaging material, belong in the regular trash.

EMERGENCY PREPAREDNESS

Ambulatory care centers and hospitals may be the first to recognize and initiate a response to a community emergency. If an infectious outbreak is suspected, Standard Precautions should be implemented immediately to control the spread of infection. If the problem has the potential to affect a large number of individuals in the community (e.g., suspected food contamination), a communications network should be established to notify local and state health departments and perhaps federal officials. Your employer may participate in an annual community disaster preparedness drill designed to help facilities improve their response to natural disasters and other emergencies.

Community preparation and response to emergencies are managed by several agencies, including the Office of Civil Defense,

Local Emergency Management Agency (LEMA), Emergency Services, or Homeland Security. Local governments are responsible for creating a system that coordinates police, fire, emergency medical services, public health, and area healthcare response to community-wide emergencies. These agencies develop an all-hazards response plan that would be appropriate for any community emergency. Local officials can turn to state, regional, or federal officials for assistance as needed.

Every healthcare facility should have a policy that includes specific procedures for the management of emergencies on site. When a new employee starts on the job, part of the orientation process is to review the site's policies and procedures manual. As a new employee, be sure to get answers to any questions you have about emergency management in that particular facility.

Staff members should discuss emergencies that may occur and should have an emergency action plan for rapid, systematic intervention. For instance, local industries may present unique problems that call for very specialized care. Plan for these, and ask the provider's advice on the procedures to follow and the supplies to have on hand. If the facility has several employees, each should be assigned specific duties in the event of an emergency. Organization and planning make the difference between systematic care for patients and complete chaos.

Emergency Plan for a Natural Disaster or Other Emergency in an Ambulatory Care Facility

- Evacuate the facility as needed.
- Include procedures for the protection of patients' health records. If the facility uses electronic health records (EHRs), make sure this information is backed up on offsite systems.
- In the case of a community emergency, provide care to the extent possible within the facility.
- Coordinate services between the ambulatory facility and other local healthcare systems, including hospitals and public health departments.
- Provide staff and supplies as needed to help in a community emergency.
- Maintain up-to-date phone trees to notify staff members of an emergency.
- Educate patients in emergency preparedness.

CRITICAL THINKING APPLICATION   29-2

A chemical plant is located about three blocks from Dr. Bendt's office. The office staff is brainstorming ideas about what should be done if an accident occurs at the plant. Based on what you have learned so far about emergency preparedness, what do you think should be included in the office's emergency plan?

Community Resources for Emergency Preparedness

Most communities have an emergency medical services (EMS) system. This system includes an efficient communications network (e.g., the emergency telephone number 911), well-trained rescue personnel, properly equipped ambulances, an emergency facility that is open 24 hours a day to provide advanced life support, and a hospital intensive care unit for victims.

More than 100 poison control centers in the United States are ready to provide emergency information for the treatment of victims of poisoning. Every healthcare facility is required to post a list of local emergency numbers. This list should be kept in plain sight and should be known to all office personnel. A good place to post this vital information is next to all the phones in the facility. Include on the list the numbers for the local EMS system, poison control center, ambulance and rescue squad, fire department, and police department (Procedure 29-5).

Contact Information for Emergency Preparedness

Keep the following telephone numbers readily available in the facility:
- Local hospital numbers, including the emergency department, infection control officer, administration contacts, and public affairs office
- Local and state health department numbers
- Centers for Disease Control and Prevention (CDC) Emergency Response Office
  - Telephone: 800-232-4636
  - Website: www.cdc.gov/phpr/index.htm

The Centers for Disease Control and Prevention (CDC) recommends that all healthcare facilities be aware of possible agents of bioterrorism, including anthrax, botulism, plague, and smallpox. The provider is responsible for diagnosing and reporting any suspected cases, but the medical assistant may be involved in patient care and certainly will participate in preventing the spread of infection in the facility. As with any suspected infectious disease, Standard Precautions should be used to control disease transmission. These precautions should be implemented with all patients, regardless of their diagnosis or possible infection status.

Infection control procedures for bioterrorism threats include the following:
- Sanitize your hands routinely.
- Wear disposable gloves when contamination with blood and body fluids is possible.
- Use masks/eye protection or face shields if you may be splashed by secretions or blood and body fluids.
- Wear impermeable gowns to protect your skin and clothes as needed; remove them promptly and wash your hands to prevent transmission of infectious material.
- Sanitize, disinfect, and sterilize equipment, supplies, and environmental surfaces.
- Dispose of contaminated waste in appropriate biohazard containers.

Another resource that can aid with community emergency preparedness is the Laboratory Response Network (LRN), which coordinates with the DHHS, the CDC, the Federal Bureau of Investigation (FBI), and the Association of Public Health Laboratories (APHL) to ensure an effective laboratory response to bioterrorism threats. The LRN links state and local public health laboratories, and veterinary, agriculture, military, and water- and food-testing laboratories to protect U.S. citizens from bioterrorism, chemical terrorism, and other public health threats.

Community emergency preparedness plans are required by the federal government so that a coordinated response is in place if a natural disaster occurs. The federal government requires all healthcare facilities, including private providers' offices, to be prepared to provide medical services and to contribute medical supplies if a natural disaster or other emergency occurs in the area.

Emergency preparedness plans are designed to coordinate the care provided by all healthcare facilities and agencies in the community, including local emergency management agencies, EMS, fire departments, law enforcement agencies, the American Red Cross, and the National Guard. Each of these groups can provide crucial services during a community emergency.

Medical assistants also can contribute to rescue and emergency efforts. Services that might be performed by trained medical assistants include providing emergency first aid at the site of a disaster; conducting patient interviews in an empathetic manner while using therapeutic communication to help calm victims and gather important health-related information; helping with mass vaccination efforts or antibiotic distribution; performing documentation and electronic health record management; ensuring compliance with the procedures required by Standard Precautions; assisting with patient education efforts; and performing phlebotomy and laboratory procedures according to their skill level.

Psychological Aspects of an Emergency Situation

Everyone involved in an emergency situation experiences a certain amount of anxiety and stress. The Centers for Disease Control and Prevention (CDC) recommends that the following actions be included in a facility's emergency preparedness plan to minimize these negative psychological effects on both healthcare workers and patients:
- Provide fact sheets for employees and patients to help them understand the dangers of certain emergencies, and encourage employee participation in disaster drills.
- Plan in advance for effective communication and action in response to an emergency; the plan should include methods for coordinating a response with local and state agencies and media sources.
- Put into place a method for clearly explaining emergency situations to patients and healthcare workers; offer immediate evaluation and treatment of an infectious outbreak.
- Treat acute anxiety with reassurance and explanation; provide follow-up counseling for employees as needed.

Further information on emergency preparedness can be found at the following CDC websites:
- Emergency preparedness planning: www.bt.cdc.gov/planning
- Coordinating Office for Terrorism Preparedness and Emergency Response (COTPER): www.bt.cdc.gov

---

PROCEDURE 29-5 | Maintain an Up-to-Date List of Community Resources for Emergency Preparedness

Goal: *To develop and maintain a list of community agencies that would respond to a natural disaster or other emergency.*

Scenario: *Your employer asks you to develop a list of groups in your community that are part of the community-wide emergency preparedness plan that has been mandated by the state and federal governments. Using multiple resources, develop a comprehensive list of emergency services for your area.*

EQUIPMENT and SUPPLIES

- Telephone
- Internet access
- Pen and paper
- Electronic record

PROCEDURAL STEPS

1. Start with an online search for the area office of the Local Emergency Management Agency (LEMA), which is sponsored by the Department of Homeland Security. If available, investigate the LEMA website for information about the emergency preparedness plan in your community. You can begin the search at the website *www.ready.gov*, the Federal Emergency Management Agency (FEMA) website is *www.fema.gov*.
   PURPOSE: To develop emergency preparedness plans by starting with the federal and state governments.

2. Gather contact information for local police, fire, and emergency medical services (EMS); post this information next to all telephones in the facility.
   PURPOSE: To ensure that emergency services contact information is immediately available in case of an emergency in the facility.

3. Investigate services provided by your local Public Health office and the American Red Cross.
   PURPOSE: To coordinate services available to potential victims in the community.

4. Organize the information gathered about community resources for emergency preparedness. With your supervisor's approval, post a copy of this information in all appropriate locations in the facility. Prepare a database in the computer that can be updated as the information changes.

ASSISTING WITH MEDICAL EMERGENCIES

First aid is the immediate care given to a person who has been injured or has suddenly taken ill. Knowledge of first aid and related skills often can mean the difference between life and death, temporary and permanent disability, or rapid recovery and long-term hospitalization. The medical assistant may be responsible for initiating first aid in the office and continuing to administer first aid until the provider or the trained medical team arrives. Every medical assistant should successfully complete a course for the professional in cardiopulmonary resuscitation (CPR) and should continue to hold a current CPR card as long as he or she is employed.

Basic knowledge of CPR and life support skills needs to be updated regularly, because procedures change as new techniques are developed. For example, both the American Red Cross and the American Heart Association (AHA) now recommend training on automated external defibrillators (AEDs) for all healthcare workers.

Medical assistants need up-to-date training in current emergency practices. They should encourage their local professional chapters to offer workshops on the management of emergencies in an ambulatory care practice, in addition to community-wide emergency preparedness. Being prepared for both types of emergencies is important. The facility's employees must be ready to respond both to emergencies on site and to natural disasters or other emergencies that affect the community.

Medical assistants are not responsible for diagnosing emergencies, especially over the telephone, but they are expected to make decisions about emergency situations on the basis of their medical knowledge and training. If any doubt exists about how to manage a particular situation or emergency phone call, the medical assistant should not hesitate to consult the provider, the office manager, or some other, more experienced member of the healthcare team.

The Medical Assistant's Role in Performing Emergency Procedures

- Perform only the emergency procedures for which you have been trained.
- If an emergency occurs in the facility, notify the provider.
- If a provider cannot be located, immediately contact the local emergency medical services team (EMS or 911).

Emergency Supplies

Emergency supplies consist of a properly equipped "crash cart" or box of items needed for a variety of emergencies (Figure 29-2). The contents vary to some degree, depending on the types of emergencies the particular office might expect to encounter and whether pediatric patients are seen in the practice. Emergency supplies should be kept in an easily accessible place that is known to all personnel in the office, and the supplies should be inventoried regularly. Expiration dates of medications and sterile supplies must be checked weekly or monthly, along with the status of available oxygen tanks and related

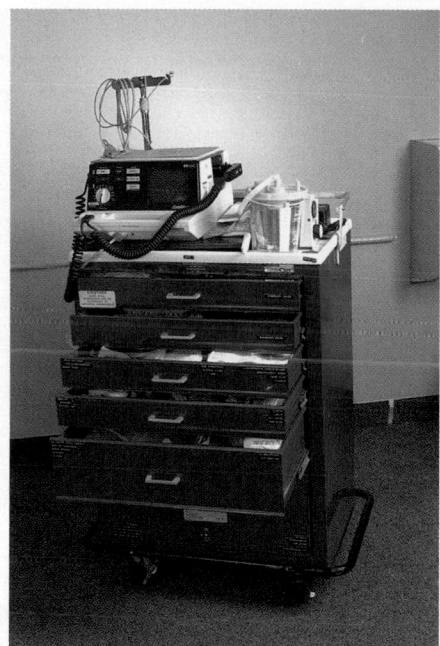

FIGURE 29-2 Office emergency cart with defibrillator. Drawers are marked for easy retrieval of emergency supplies.

materials. The cart should be replenished with fresh supplies after every use. Each time crash cart supplies are checked, a log must be completed and signed for legal purposes.

Emergency pharmaceutical supplies should include certain basic drugs, such as epinephrine, which has multiple uses in emergency situations. As a vasoconstrictor, it controls hemorrhage, relaxes the bronchioles to relieve acute asthma attacks, is administered for an acute anaphylactic reaction, and is an emergency heart stimulant used to treat shock. Epinephrine should be available in a ready-to-use cartridge syringe and needle unit. These units are supplied in 1-mL cartridges.

Other drugs used include atropine, digoxin (Lanoxin), nitroglycerin (Nitrostat), lidocaine (Xylocaine), and sodium bicarbonate. Atropine reduces secretions, increases the respiratory rate and heart rate, and is a smooth muscle relaxant. It is administered in a cardiac emergency for **asystole**, or it can be used to treat bradycardia. Digoxin is a cardiac drug used to treat **arrhythmia** and congestive heart failure (CHF); it is good for emergency use because it has a relatively rapid action. Nitroglycerin is a vasodilator that is given to relieve angina; it acts by dilating the coronary arteries so that an increased volume of oxygenated blood can reach the **myocardium**. Lidocaine is used intravenously to treat a cardiac arrhythmia and locally as an anesthetic, and sodium bicarbonate corrects metabolic acidosis, which typically occurs after cardiac arrest. Many of the medications administered during a medical emergency are given intravenously (IV), which is outside of the medical assistant's scope of practice.

Emergency medical supplies also should include an **emetic**, such as syrup of ipecac, which causes vomiting soon after the syrup is swallowed, and activated charcoal, an antidote that is swallowed to absorb ingested poisons. Narcan, an antidote given intravenously for narcotic drug overdoses, is administered when indicated to raise blood pressure and increase the respiratory rate. Antihistamines for the treatment of allergic reactions and for anaphylaxis need to be available to treat any allergic responses to medications administered in the facility. Such antihistamines include Benadryl for minor reactions and Solu-Medrol, a corticosteroid, for severe anaphylactic reactions.

Other medications also may be found in a crash cart. For example, isoproterenol (e.g., Isuprel, Medihaler-Iso, Norisodrine), an antispasmodic used to treat bronchospasms (e.g., as in an asthma attack), also is effective as a cardiac stimulant. Phenobarbital and diazepam (Valium) are used for convulsions and/or sedative effects. Furosemide (Lasix) is used for CHF. Glucagon is used primarily to counteract severe hypoglycemic reactions (low blood glucose) in patients with diabetes who are taking insulin.

Basic Emergency Supplies

Equipment
- Adhesive tape in 1- and 2-inch widths
- Airways (variety of types and sizes)
- Alcohol wipes
- Ambu bag with assorted sizes of facial masks
- Antimicrobial skin ointment
- Bandage scissors
- Cotton balls and cotton swabs
- Cardiopulmonary resuscitation (CPR) masks (adult and pediatric)
- Defibrillator
- Elastic bandages in 2- and 3-inch widths
- Filter needles
- Flashlight with batteries
- Gauze pads, 2 × 2- and 4 × 4-inch widths, and roller bandage (sterile and nonsterile)
- Gloves (sterile and nonsterile) in multiple sizes
- Hot and cold packs (instant type)
- Intravenous catheters, tubing, solutions (variety of types, including D_5W and Ringer's lactate), and tourniquet
- Laryngoscope with blades
- Lubricant
- Endotracheal tubes (variety of sizes with stylets)
- Personal protective equipment (PPE), including impervious gowns, splash guards or goggles, and booties
- Portable oxygen tank with regulator, mask, and nasal cannula
- Roller gauze (Ace bandages and gauze dressing) in various sizes
- Sharps container
- Sphygmomanometer (pediatric and adult regular and large sizes)
- Splints (various sizes)
- Sterile dressings (miscellaneous sizes, including two abdominal pads)
- Steri-Strips, dermal glue, or suturing material
- Suction machine and catheters
- Syringes and needles (assorted sizes and gauges)
- Tongue blades
- Tubex cartridge system
- Venipuncture supplies and butterfly units

Medications

- Activated charcoal (bottle of 29 to 50 g)
- Antihistamine (injectable and oral)
- Atropine
- Dextrose
- Diazepam (Valium)
- Digoxin (Lanoxin), injectable
- Diphenhydramine (Benadryl)
- Epinephrine (Adrenalin), injectable
- Furosemide (Lasix)
- Glucagon and/or glucose tablets
- Ipecac syrup
- Isoproterenol (Isuprel), injectable
- Lidocaine (Xylocaine), injectable and spray
- Naloxone (Narcan), injectable
- Nitroglycerin tablets
- Phenobarbital, injectable
- Sodium bicarbonate, injectable
- Methylprednisolone (Solu-Medrol), injectable
- Sterile water and saline for injection

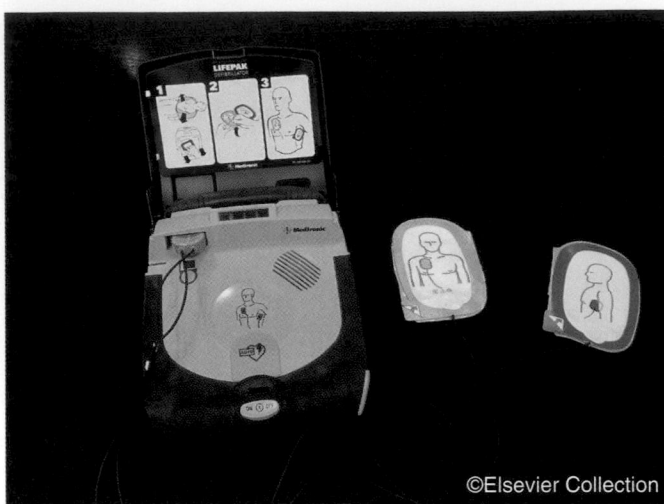

FIGURE 29-3 Fully automated external defibrillator (AED).

Defibrillators

The medical assistant may be required to assist the healthcare team with defibrillation of emergency patients. Defibrillation is indicated when a patient is in ventricular **fibrillation** (VF). VF is a severe cardiac arrhythmia that is caused by uncoordinated, rapid firing of the electrical system of the heart, which makes it impossible for the ventricles to empty. In the absence of ventricular emptying, the patient has no pulse, blood pressure drops to zero, and the patient could die within 4 minutes unless help is given immediately.

Defibrillators are devices that send an electrical current through the myocardium by means of handheld paddles (in a healthcare facility) or self-adhesive pads applied to the chest. This electrical shock causes momentary asystole, giving the heart's natural pacemaker an opportunity to resume the heart rate at a normal rhythm.

An automated external defibrillator has a computerized system that analyzes a cardiac rhythm and delivers voice-prompt instructions on how to operate the device (Figure 29-3 and Procedure 29-6). AEDs use self-adhesive pads that record and monitor the cardiac rhythm, and the device instructs the rescuer when to deliver the electrical charge. The apex-anterior position is the most commonly used pad position, with the anterior (sternum) pad placed to the right of the upper sternum, and the apex pad placed under the individual's left nipple at the left middle axillary line (Figure 29-4). To defibrillate a female individual, the apex pad is placed next to or underneath the left breast. The AED self-adhesive pads are packaged with expiration dates so these should be checked periodically.

Precautions for Automated External Defibrillators

- Neither the individual nor the rescuer should be in contact with any metal during defibrillation. Do not place the AED pad over jewelry, and remove the patient's glasses to prevent injuries.

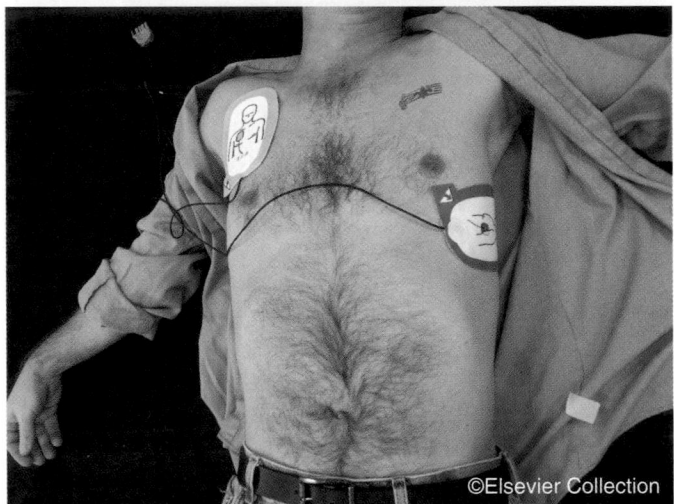

FIGURE 29-4 Connect the adhesive pads to the automated external defibrillator (AED) cables; apply the pads to the patient's chest at the upper right sternal border and at the lower left ribs over the cardiac apex.

- When available, a pediatric-dose AED system should be used for children 1 to 8 years of age (it should not be used on infants younger than 1 year old). These systems deliver a reduced shock dose for victims up to about 8 years old or weighing 55 pounds.
- All clothing (including bras) must be removed; pads must be applied directly to the skin. If the individual has a great deal of hair on the chest, try to push the hair aside before applying the pads; or, apply the pads and quickly remove them to remove hair from the area, then reapply new pads. The machine will prompt you by stating "Check electrode" if the connection is poor.
- To prevent burns, make sure the individual is lying on a dry surface and the chest is dry before applying the pads.
- If the patient has an implanted defibrillator or pacemaker, it will be obvious from the bulged area under the surface of the skin on the chest. Apply the AED pads at least 1 inch away from implants to prevent interference.

| PROCEDURE 29-6 | Maintain Provider/Professional-Level CPR Certification: Use an Automated External Defibrillator (AED) |

Goal: *To defibrillate adult victims with cardiac arrest. Most adult victims in sudden cardiac arrest are in ventricular fibrillation. The survival rate for victims with ventricular fibrillation is as high as 90% when defibrillation occurs within the first minute of collapse; however, the survival rate declines 7% to 10% with every minute defibrillation does not occur.*

EQUIPMENT and SUPPLIES

- Automated external defibrillator (AED) for practice
- Approved mannequin

PROCEDURAL STEPS

These steps are to be performed only on an approved mannequin.

If the healthcare worker witnesses a cardiac arrest, an automated external defibrillator (AED) should be used as soon as possible. If cardiopulmonary resuscitation (CPR) has already been started, continue performing CPR until the AED machine is turned on, pads are applied, and the machine is ready.

1. Place the AED near the victim's left ear. Turn on the AED.
2. Attach electrode pads to the victim's bare dry chest as pictured on the AED. Place the electrodes at the sternum and apex of the heart. Make sure the pads are in complete contact with the victim's chest and that they do not overlap (see Figure 29-4).
3. All rescuers must clear away from the victim. Press the ANALYZE button. The AED analyzes the victim's coronary status, announces whether the victim is going to be shocked, and automatically charges the electrodes (Figure 1).

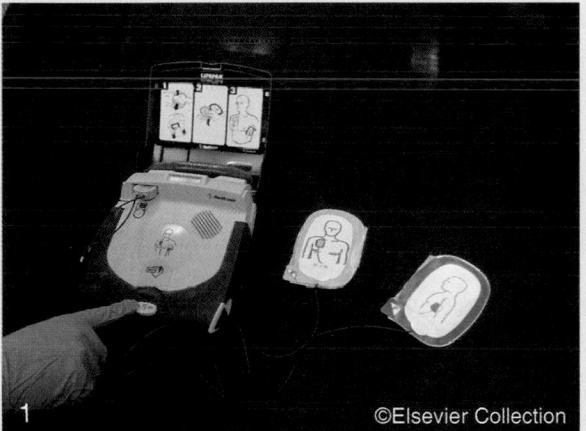
©Elsevier Collection

4. All rescuers must clear away from the victim. Press the SHOCK button if the machine is not automated. You may repeat 3 analyze-shock cycles.
5. Deliver 1 shock, leaving the AED attached, and immediately perform cardiopulmonary resuscitation (CPR), starting with chest compressions.
6. After 5 cycles (about 2 minutes) of CPR, repeat the AED analysis and deliver another shock, if indicated. If a nonshockable rhythm is detected, the AED should instruct the rescuer to resume CPR immediately, beginning with chest compressions.
7. If the machine gives the No Shock Indicated signal, assess the victim. Check the carotid pulse and breathing status and keep the AED attached until emergency medical services (EMS) arrives.
   <u>PURPOSE</u>: Continue to monitor breathing and circulation because these can stop at any time. Keep the AED pads in place to diagnose ventricular fibrillation quickly if it occurs.

GENERAL RULES FOR EMERGENCIES

A medical assistant will face two types of emergencies in an ambulatory care practice: office emergencies and home emergencies. Common office emergencies and their management are discussed later in this chapter. Besides dealing with actual emergency situations on site, a medical assistant frequently is the first person to interact with patients facing potential emergencies at home. It is estimated that one third of the telephone calls received in a provider's office involve some type of problem that requires attention. An immediate decision must be made on how

to manage that problem: by giving home care advice, scheduling an appointment, or, in life-threatening cases, notifying EMS. Many facilities, under the direction and approval of the provider, create a reference list of appropriate questions for specific patient complaints.

Regardless of how emergency phone calls are managed in the facility where you work, consider the following general rules when faced with an emergency:

- It is most important to stay calm. Reassure the patient and make him or her as comfortable as possible.

- Assess the situation to determine the nature of the emergency. Decide whether the need is immediate. This decision requires calm judgment and medical knowledge.
- Obtain as much information as possible to determine the appropriate action.
- Immediately refer any concerns to the office supervisor or provider.

Telephone Screening

Each time the phone rings in a healthcare facility, a person with a possible life-or-death situation may be on the other end of the line. One of the most important tasks performed by medical assistants every day is answering the phones and managing patients' needs efficiently and appropriately. The following emergency action principles serve as a guide for managing emergency phone calls in an ambulatory care practice.

- If the patient's situation is life-threatening, activate EMS/911.
- *Never put a caller with a life-threatening emergency on hold, and always be the last to hang up.*
- Remain on the line until help arrives and you have talked to EMS personnel.
- Immediately record the names of the caller and the patient, the location, and the phone number in case the connection is lost.
- If you are unsure how to manage the emergency situation, contact the provider.
- If the patient is referred to an emergency department (ED), call the ED to notify the staff of the patient's arrival, and make a follow-up call to determine the patient's condition.
- Gather as much information as possible about what is wrong with the patient and when the problem started. Obtain details about the patient's condition, including the following:

- What is the patient's level of consciousness? Alert, responsive, lethargic, or confused? Did the patient lose consciousness at any time? If so, for how long?
- What is the character of the patient's respirations (and pulse, if the caller is able to determine this): normal, rapid, shallow, or difficult?
- Is there bleeding? If so, how much and from where?
- Is there a suspected head or neck injury? If so, has the patient been moved? Is there a suspected fracture? Where?
- Does the patient have a history of this problem?
- Any there other symptoms, such as fever, vomiting, diarrhea, or pain?
- Obtain details about what has been done for the patient. For example:
  - Medication—What, when? Dose, effectiveness? Current allergies?
- Thoroughly document the information gathered and any actions taken, including notification of EMS, whether the patient was sent to the ED or an appointment was scheduled, all home care recommendations, and whether the provider was notified and when.

Based on the outcome of the telephone interaction, a decision is made on when the provider will see the patient (Procedure 29-7). Emergency calls require activation of EMS or immediate attention as soon as the patient arrives. Urgent calls require a same-day appointment if the patient has an acute condition or is in severe discomfort. Such cases would include a young child with a high fever or a patient who complains of moderate to severe abdominal pain. A new patient will have to be worked into the day's schedule, which may cause a delay in currently scheduled appointments. Patients with other, less urgent problems can be scheduled for appointments within the next 3 to 4 days.

PROCEDURE 29-7 | **Perform Patient Screening Using Established Protocols: Telephone Screening and Appropriate Documentation**

Goal: *To assess the direction of emergency care and to document information appropriately in the patient's record.*

Scenario: *Cheryl is working with the telephone screening staff members when they receive a call from the mother of a 5-year-old patient. The mother reports that her son fell and cut his arm. What type of information should Cheryl gather about the injury? What action should be taken? How should the incident be documented?*

EQUIPMENT and SUPPLIES

- Patient record
- Notepad and pen or pencil
- Facility's emergency procedures manual
- Computer scheduling program
- Area emergency numbers

PROCEDURAL STEPS

1. Stay calm and reassure the caller.
   PURPOSE: To enable you to gather accurate details about the patient's condition.

2. Verify the identity of the caller and the injured patient.
3. Immediately record the name of the caller and the patient, their location, and the phone number.
   PURPOSE: To be able to contact the caller if the connection is lost.
4. Determine whether the patient's condition is life-threatening. Quantify the amount of blood loss, whether the patient is alert and responsive, and whether breathing is normal. Notify emergency medical services (EMS) if necessary.
   PURPOSE: Notify emergency services immediately if the patient is in danger.

PROCEDURE 29-7 —continued

5. If EMS is notified, stay on the line with the caller until EMS personnel arrive at the scene.
   <u>PURPOSE</u>: Never break a phone connection in the case of a life-threatening emergency.
6. If EMS is not needed, gather details about the injury to determine whether the patient can be seen in the office or should be referred to an emergency department (ED). Consider the following questions:
   - Is there a suspected head or neck injury? Has the patient been moved?
   - Is there a possible fracture? If so, where?
   - Is bleeding present? Can it be easily controlled?
   - Are there any other symptoms?
   - Is there anything pertinent in the patient's health history that would complicate the situation?
   - Has the caller administered any first aid? If so, what was done?
7. Based on the information gathered, determine when the patient should be seen in the office if he or she has not been referred to an ED.

<u>PURPOSE</u>: Most emergencies are scheduled for an immediate office visit. This may require altering the current appointment schedule.
8. At any point in this process, do not hesitate to consult the provider or experienced staff or refer to the facility's emergency procedures manual to determine how to manage the patient's problem.
9. Always allow the caller to hang up first, just in case more information or assistance is needed.
10. Document the information gathered, the actions taken or recommended, any home care recommendations, and whether the provider was notified.
    <u>PURPOSE</u>: To have a legal record of the management of the emergency and a comprehensive description of the patient's condition and the recommended management.

7/13/20– 1:25 PM: Pt's mother reports child fell against a window and lacerated his arm. Bleeding is moderate but controlled. No reported signs of dyspnea or altered consciousness. Mother will bring child to office immediately for provider assessment. Cheryl Skurka, CMA (AAMA)

Management of On-Site Emergencies

An emergency can occur at any time to anyone. Always follow Standard Precautions when you are at risk for coming into contact with blood or body fluids. When an emergency occurs, it is impossible to determine the level of infection. All body fluids must be considered infectious, and appropriate precautions must be taken to prevent cross-contamination. If the situation is life-threatening, notify EMS and stay with the patient until you are relieved by the EMS provider or the provider in your office. It is important to document all details of the incident in the patient's health record.

Documentation of an On-Site Emergency

1. Patient's name, address, age, and health insurance information
2. Allergies, current medications, and pertinent health history
3. Name and relationship of any person with the patient
4. Vital signs and chief complaint
5. Sequence of events, beginning with how the problem occurred, any changes in the patient's overall condition, and any observations made about the patient's condition
6. Details about procedures or treatments performed on the patient

CRITICAL THINKING APPLICATION   29-3
Cheryl is working the front desk when a patient comes into the office limping. She tells Cheryl that she fell in the parking lot and hurt her ankle. Cheryl helps the patient into an exam room and begins to interview her. Role-play the situation with a classmate and make a list of at least 10 questions Cheryl should ask the patient.

Life-Threatening Emergencies

If a patient in the facility shows any signs of unresponsiveness, the provider must be brought to the patient immediately. If no provider is available in the facility, EMS must be activated. Even when a provider is present, the provider may order you to call 911 for immediate emergency care. Put on gloves before you begin to assess the patient, because any emergency situation may involve exposure to blood or body fluids.

Unresponsive Patient

If a patient is able to talk to you, he or she has an open airway. If the patient does not respond to a simple question (e.g., "Are you OK?"), gently shake the person's shoulder to check responsiveness. If the patient does not respond, you must assume that the patient is unconscious. Immediately call for help and activate EMS if that is office policy.

To care for an unresponsive patient, first assess the patient's respirations to determine whether the person is breathing. When the patient collapsed, the tongue may have gone limp and occluded the trachea. Just by changing the individual's position and opening the airway, you may provide all the assistance the patient needs to breathe independently.

If the patient is face down, roll the victim onto his or her back while supporting the head, neck, and back. Apply the head tilt–chin lift movement to open the airway. The tongue is attached to the lower jaw, so moving the jaw forward automatically opens the patient's airway. If a head or neck injury is suspected, the neck should be manipulated as little as possible; therefore, the airway should be open with the jaw-thrust maneuver. Both of these actions relieve possible obstruction of the trachea by the tongue.

Check for breathing or only gasping for breath while checking the carotid pulse at the same time for 10 seconds. Look for a rise in the chest while listening or feeling for air exchange (Figure 29-5). Breathing may stop suddenly for a variety of reasons, including shock, disease, and trauma. If no breaths are detected but there is a pulse, artificial ventilation must be started immediately because death can occur within 4 to 6 minutes. Barrier devices should be kept on hand for artificial respiration (Figure 29-6), and these should be used if rescue breaths are required (Procedure 29-8).

Administer one breath every 5 to 6 seconds (about 10 to 12 breaths per minute). Check the carotid pulse about every 2 minutes. If there is no pulse, begin chest compressions immediately at a ratio of 30 compressions to 2 breaths with about 100 to 120 compressions per minute.

The AHA uses the acronym CAB (*c*ompressions, *a*irway, *b*reathing) to help people remember the order for performing the steps of CPR (see Procedure 29-8).

When both breathing and pulse stop, the victim has suffered sudden death. Sudden death has many causes, including heart disease, choking, drowning, poisoning, suffocation, electrocution, and smoke inhalation. CPR must be started immediately to attempt to revive the patient and to prevent permanent damage to body organs, especially the brain. Continue CPR until the victim begins to move, an AED is available and ready to use, professional help arrives, or you are too exhausted to continue. If the patient has a pulse but is not breathing, continue rescue breathing and occasionally monitor the pulse until help arrives.

For specific procedures and precautions in the management of respiratory and cardiac emergencies, refer to the *Standard First Aid Manual* of the American Red Cross or the *American Heart Association CPR Manual*, or those organizations' websites. As stated earlier, all healthcare workers should have a current Certification for the Professional in CPR.

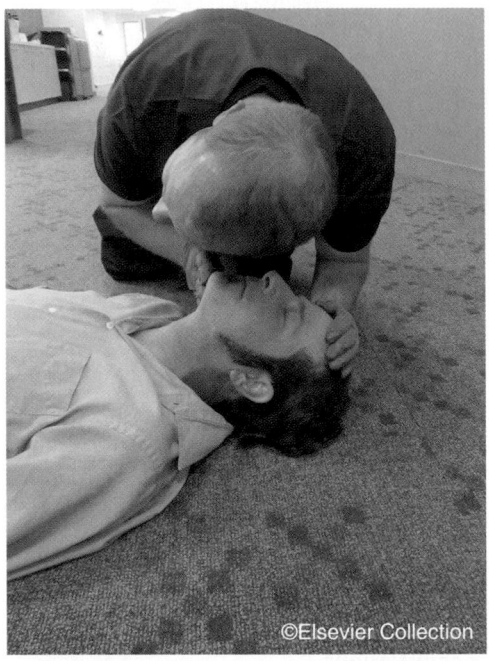

FIGURE 29-5 Checking for breathing in an unconscious patient.

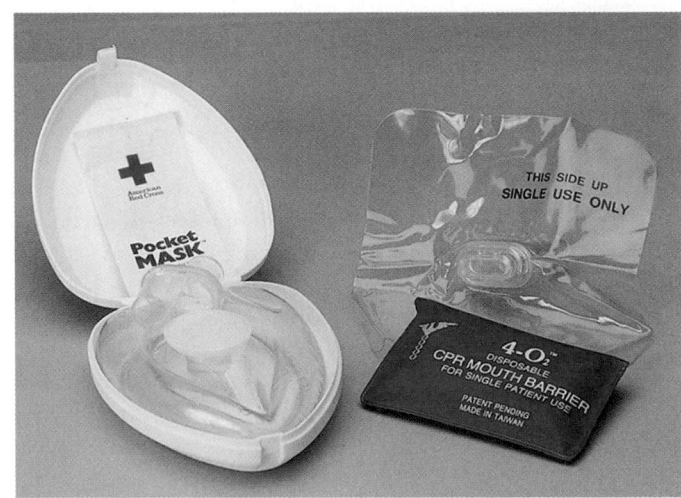

FIGURE 29-6 Cardiopulmonary resuscitation (CPR) mouth barriers.

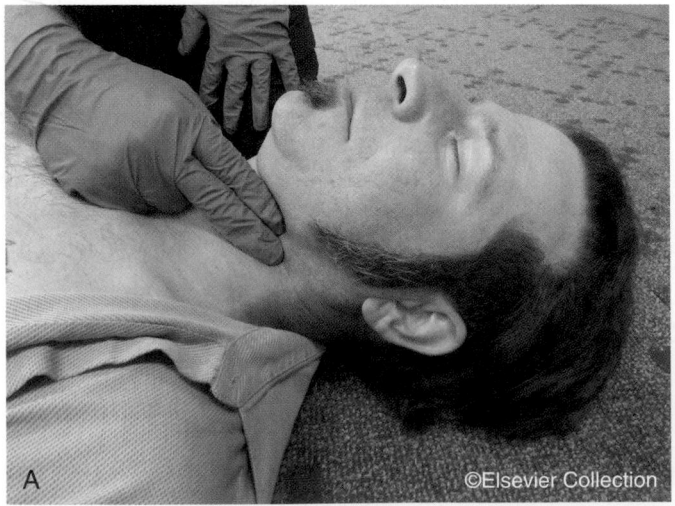
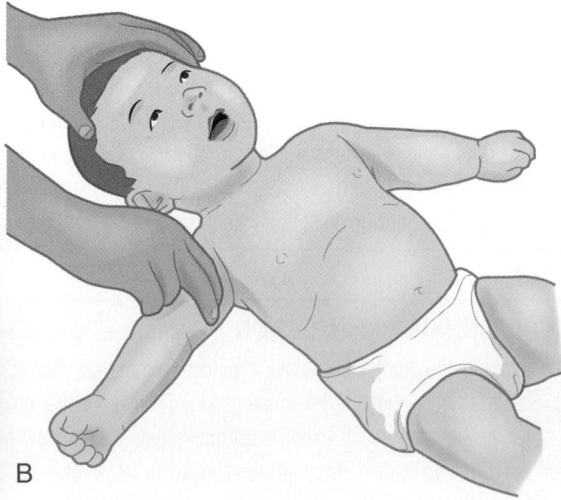

FIGURE 29-7 A, In an adult, check for a carotid pulse. **B,** In an infant, check for a brachial pulse.

PROCEDURE 29-8	Maintain Provider/Professional-Level CPR Certification: Perform Adult Rescue Breathing and One-Rescuer CPR; Perform Pediatric and Infant CPR

Goal: *To restore breathing and blood circulation when respiration or the pulse (or both) has stopped.*

EQUIPMENT and SUPPLIES

- Disposable gloves
- Cardiopulmonary resuscitation (CPR) ventilator masks for adults, children, and infants
- Approved mannequins

PROCEDURAL STEPS

These steps are to be performed only on approved mannequins.

CPR on an Adult

1. Establish unresponsiveness. Tap the victim and ask, "Are you OK?"
   PURPOSE: To determine whether the victim is conscious.
2. If unresponsive, shout for help. Activate the emergency response system. Put on gloves and get a ventilator mask.
   PURPOSE: As soon as it is determined that an adult victim requires emergency care, activate emergency medical services (EMS). Most adults with sudden, nontraumatic cardiac arrest are in ventricular fibrillation. The time from collapse to defibrillation is the single most important predictor of survival.
3. Put the person on his or her back on a firm surface.
4. If an AED is immediately available, deliver 1 shock if instructed by the device, then begin CPR.
5. If an AED is not available, check for breathing or only gasping to breathe while at the same time checking the carotid pulse for 10 seconds.
6. If there is no pulse, start chest compressions. Kneel at the victim's neck and shoulders a couple of inches away from the chest. Place the heel of the hand over the lower part of the sternum, between the nipples but above the xiphoid process.
7. Place your other hand on top of the first and interlace or lift your fingers upward off the chest (Figure 1).
   PURPOSE: This position gives you the most control, allowing you to avoid injuring the victim's ribs as you compress the chest.

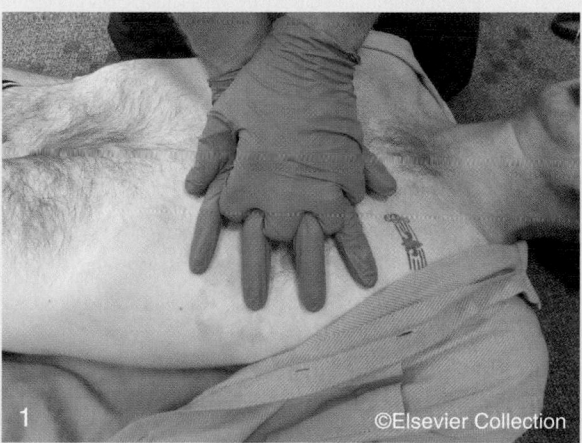

©Elsevier Collection

8. Bring your shoulders directly over the victim's sternum as you compress downward, keeping your elbows locked (Figure 2).

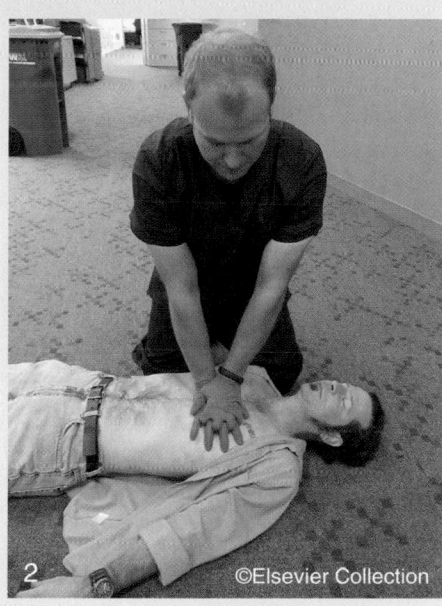

©Elsevier Collection

9. Use your upper body weight (not just your arms) as you push straight down on the sternum at least 2 inches but no more than 2.4 inches in an adult victim. Relax the pressure on the sternum after each compression, but do not remove your hands from the sternum.
   PURPOSE: The depth of compression is needed to circulate blood through the heart. Movement of the hands may injure the victim. Relieving the pressure on the chest between contractions allows the heart to completely fill with blood before the next compression.
10. After performing 30 compressions (at a rate of about 100-120 compressions per minute), perform the head tilt–chin lift maneuver to open the airway. Tilt the victim's head by placing one hand on the forehead and applying enough pressure to push the head back; with the fingers of the other hand under the chin, lift up and pull the jaw forward. Look, listen, and feel for signs of breathing. Place your ear over the mouth and listen for breathing. Watch the rising and falling of the chest for evidence of breathing. If breathing is absent or inadequate, open the airway and place the ventilator mask over the victim's mouth and nose (Figure 3)
    PURPOSE: To open the airway and determine whether the victim is breathing. Give 2 breaths, each breath delivered over 1 second, holding the ventilator mask tightly against the face while tilting the victim's chin up to keep the airway open. Remove your mouth from the mouthpiece between breaths to allow time for the patient to exhale between breaths.

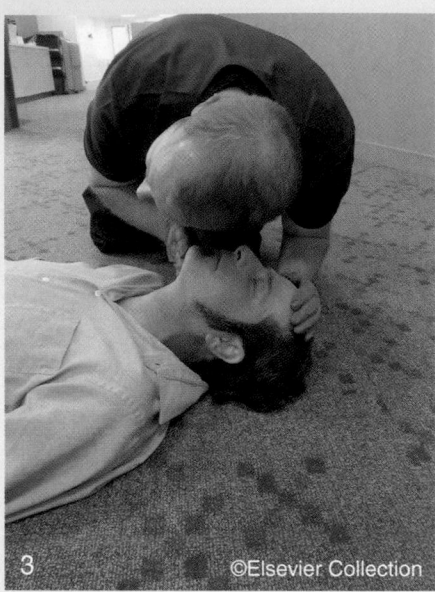

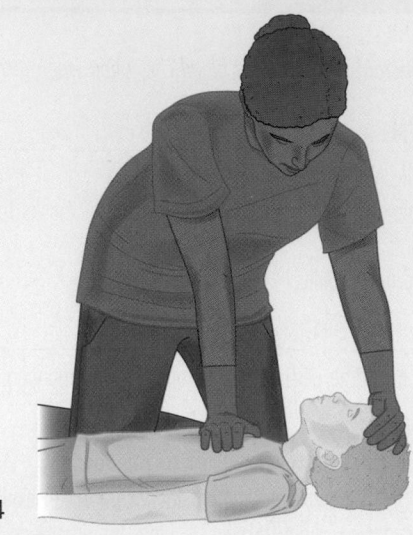

11. Check the patient's pulse (at the carotid artery for an adult or older child; at the brachial artery for an infant). If a pulse is present, continue rescue breathing (1 breath every 6 seconds—about 10 breaths per minute). If no signs of circulation are present, begin cycles of 30 chest compressions (at a rate of about 100-120 compressions) followed by 2 breaths.

12. If the person is still not responding after 5 cycles (about 2 minutes) and an AED is now available, apply it and follow the prompts. Administer 1 shock, then resume CPR, starting with chest compressions, for 2 more minutes before administering a second shock. Continue 30:2 cycles of compressions and ventilations. If an AED is not available, continue CPR until the person shows signs of movement or EMS personnel take over.

CPR on a Child

The procedure for giving CPR to a child ages 1 through 8 is essentially the same as that for an adult. The differences are as follows:

- Perform 5 cycles of compressions and breaths on the child (30:2 ratio, about 2 minutes) before calling 911 or the local emergency number or using an AED. If another person is available, have that person activate EMS while you care for the child.
  PURPOSE: It is important to provide immediate circulation of oxygenated blood to a child to prevent brain damage. Most pediatric cardiac arrests occur because of a secondary problem, such as airway occlusion, rather than a cardiac problem. If you know there is an airway obstruction, clear the obstruction and then proceed with CPR (Figure 4).

- Use only one hand to perform chest compressions.
  PURPOSE: The pediatric sternum requires less force to achieve the needed depression.
- Breathe more gently.
- Use the same compression-to-breath ratio as used for adults (30 compressions followed by 2 breaths per cycle); after 2 breaths, immediately begin the next cycle of compressions and breaths.
- After 5 cycles (about 2 minutes) of CPR without response, apply an AED if available. Use pediatric pads for children ages 1 through 8; if pediatric pads are not available, use adult pads. Do not use an AED on children younger than age 1. Administer 1 shock, if instructed to do so, then resume CPR, starting with chest compressions, for 2 more minutes before administering a second shock.
- Continue until the child responds or help arrives.

Infant Cardiac Arrest

Infant cardiac arrest typically is caused by lack of oxygen from drowning or choking. If you know the infant has an airway obstruction, clear the obstruction; if you do not know why the infant is unresponsive, perform CPR for 2 minutes (about 5 cycles) before calling 911 or the local emergency number. If another person is available, have that person call for help immediately while you attend to the baby.

CPR on an Infant

- Draw an imaginary line between the infant's nipples. Place two fingers on the sternum just below this intermammary line.
- Gently compress the chest at a rate of 100 to 120 per minute.
- Administer 2 breaths after every 30 compressions.
- After about 5 cycles of a 30:2 ratio, activate EMS.
- Continue CPR until the infant responds or help arrives.

PROCEDURE 29-8 —*continued*

Rescue Breathing for an Infant

Use an infant ventilator mask or cover the baby's mouth and nose with your mouth.

13. Give 2 rescue breaths by gently puffing out the cheeks and slowly breathing into the infant's mouth, taking about 1 second for each breath (Figure 5).

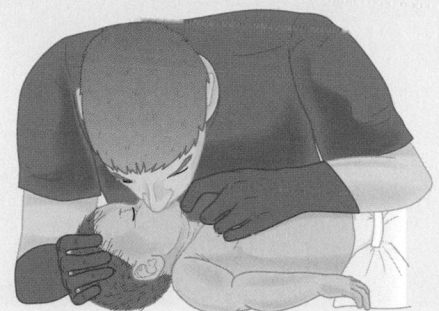

5

14. Remove your gloves and the ventilator mask valve, and discard them in the biohazard container. Disinfect the ventilator mask per the manufacturer's recommendations. Sanitize your hands.

15. Document the procedure and the patient's condition.

Cardiac Emergencies

Chest pain or angina can be associated with heart and lung disease, in addition to a few other conditions. It can be quite serious; a patient with chest pain is treated as a cardiac emergency until a provider has ruled this out. A heart attack, or *myocardial infarction,* usually is caused by blockage of the coronary arteries, which reduces the amount of blood delivered to the myocardium. The most common signal of a heart attack is an uncomfortable pressure, squeezing, fullness, or pain in the center of the chest (symptoms in women, which may be different, are presented in the following box). This may spread to the shoulder, neck, jaw, or arms. The pain may not be severe. The lips and fingernails may turn blue, which is a sign of **cyanosis** (Figure 29-8), or the patient may have a gray, ashen appearance. Frequently the patient clutches the chest in pain. This pain may radiate from the **mediastinum** down the left arm and up the left side of the neck. The pulse may be rapid and weak, and the patient often complains of nausea. Other symptoms include sweating (**diaphoresis**); indigestion; shortness of breath (SOB); cold, clammy skin; and a feeling of weakness (*general malaise*). Unfortunately, most people deny that the problem is serious until they require immediate medical attention.

Signs and Symptoms of Myocardial Infarction in Women

Women may experience symptoms that are different from those traditionally associated with a heart attack. Women's symptoms include a combination of the following:

- Back pain or aching and throbbing in the biceps or forearms
- Shortness of breath (SOB)
- Clammy perspiration
- Dizziness (vertigo): Unexplained lightheadedness or syncopal episodes
- Edema, especially of the ankles and/or lower legs
- Fluttering heartbeat or tachycardia
- Gastric upset
- Feeling of heaviness or fullness in the mediastinum

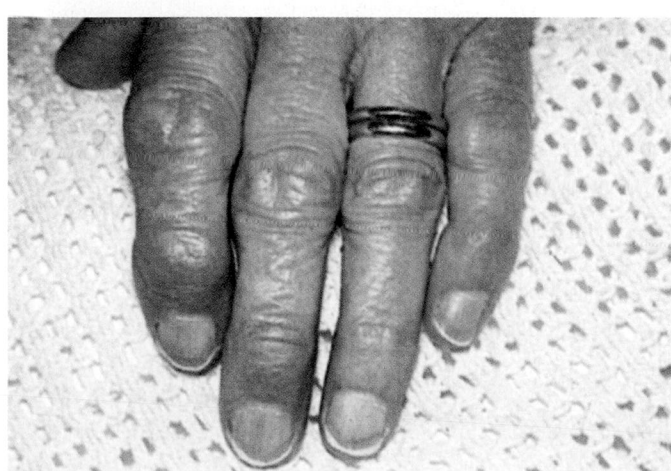

FIGURE 29-8 Cyanosis of the nail beds. (Kamal A, Brockelhurst JC: *Color atlas of geriatric medicine,* ed 2, St Louis, 1991, Mosby.)

Immediately report any of these signs or symptoms to the provider. If the provider is not available, activate EMS. Use a wheelchair to move the patient to an examination room. Breathing will be easier if the patient's head is slightly elevated or if the patient is in a Fowler's or semi-Fowler's position. Keep the patient quiet and warm. Loosen all tight clothing. Take vital signs, including both apical and radial pulses. The provider may order oxygen started on the patient to relieve dyspnea (Procedure 29-9). Bring the emergency cart into the room and open the medication drawer so that the provider can quickly prepare the medications needed. These may include epinephrine (adrenaline), atropine, digitalis, calcium chloride, or morphine.

If the patient is conscious, ask about any medication that he or she has recently taken or is carrying. If the patient has an established heart disorder, the person may be carrying nitroglycerin tablets; these tablets are administered sublingually and may be given with the patient's consent (Figure 29-9). If the provider is in the office or is on the way, connect the patient to the electrocardiograph machine and record a few tracings. If the patient becomes unresponsive before the provider or EMS arrives, it may be necessary to start rescue breathing if no evidence of respirations is noted. If chest pain progresses to cardiac arrest and loss of circulation, CPR must be performed until help arrives.

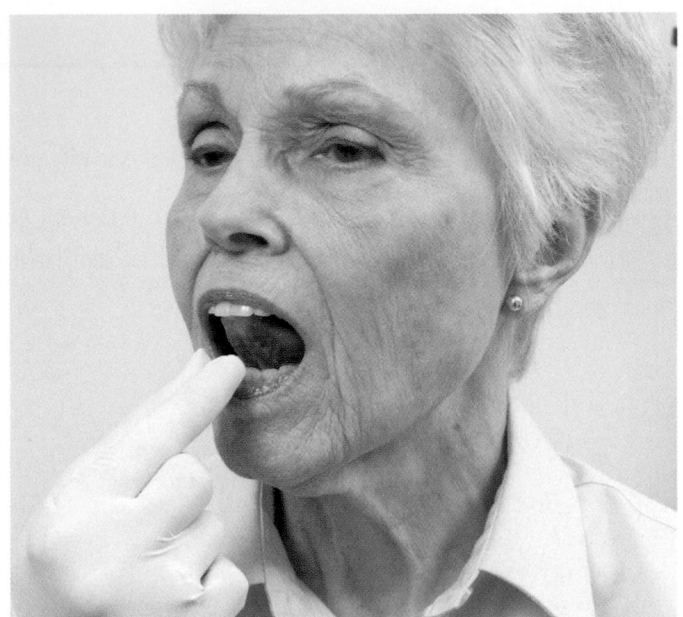

FIGURE 29-9 Nitroglycerin is administered beneath the patient's tongue.

PROCEDURE 29-9   Perform First Aid Procedures: Administer Oxygen

Goal: *To provide oxygen for a patient in respiratory distress.*

EQUIPMENT and SUPPLIES

- Provider's order
- Patient's health record
- Portable oxygen tank
- Pressure regulator
- Flow meter
- Nasal cannula with connecting tubing

PROCEDURAL STEPS

1. Gather equipment and sanitize your hands.
2. Greet and identify the patient, introduce yourself, and explain the procedure.
   PURPOSE: A nasal cannula is applied with a nasal prong in each nostril and the tab resting above the upper lip. Patients who will be using oxygen at home need to be taught how to open an oxygen tank or to use an oxygen compressor. It is vital that patients and their families understand the dangers of oxygen use in the home. They must avoid open flames and must not smoke when oxygen is in use because it is combustible. The provider typically writes an order for the number of liters of oxygen to be delivered and for home healthcare services to set up the equipment in the patient's home.
3. Check the pressure gauge on the tank to determine the amount of oxygen in the tank.
4. If necessary, open the cylinder on the tank one full counterclockwise turn, then attach the cannula tubing to the flow meter.
5. Adjust the administration of the oxygen according to the provider's order. Usually the flow meter is set at 1 to 4 liters per minute (LPM). Check to make sure oxygen is flowing through the cannula.

6. Insert the tips of the cannula into the nostrils and adjust the tubing around the back of the patient's ears (Figure 1).

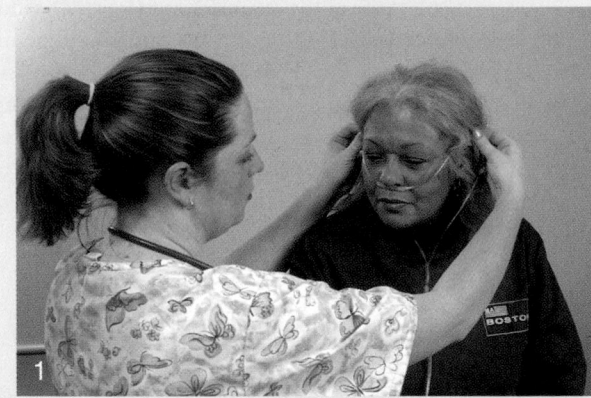

7. Encourage the patient to breathe through the nose with the mouth closed.
8. Make sure the patient is comfortable, and answer any questions he or she may have.
9. Sanitize your hands.
10. Document the procedure, including the number of liters of oxygen being administered and the patient's condition. Continue to monitor the patient throughout the procedure and document any changes in condition.

7/24/20– 3:05 PM: R 28 and labored. Oxygen initiated at 4 LPM via nasal cannula per provider order. Pt observed for signs of dyspnea and tachypnea. Cheryl Skurka, CMA (AAMA)

Choking

Choking is usually caused by a foreign object, often a bolus of food, lodged in the upper airway. The victim may clutch the neck between the thumb and the index finger (Figure 29-10); this universal distress signal should be viewed as a sign the victim needs help. If the victim has good air exchange or only partial airway obstruction and can speak, cough, or breathe, do not interfere, but encourage the patient to continue coughing until the object is expelled. Monitor the patient for signs of respiratory distress, such as pallor and cyanosis. If the patient has a pronounced wheeze or a very weak cough, he or she has a partial airway obstruction with poor air exchange and may need help. If the patient is unable to speak, breathe, or cough, a complete airway obstruction exists, and quick action must be taken to clear the airway. With complete obstruction, the patient eventually loses consciousness from lack of oxygen to the brain. This condition may lead to respiratory and cardiac arrest. If the object is not removed, the victim may die within 4 to 6 minutes. Procedure 29-10 presents the steps involved in clearing an obstructed airway in an adult. The procedure for removal of a foreign airway obstruction is exactly the same for a child older than 1 year of age.

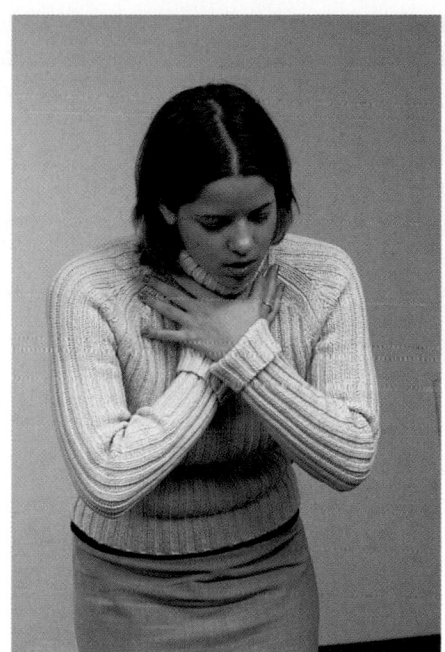

FIGURE 29-10 Universal sign of choking.

PROCEDURE 29-10   Perform First Aid Procedures: Respond to an Airway Obstruction in an Adult

Goal: *To remove an airway obstruction and restore ventilation.*

EQUIPMENT and SUPPLIES

- Disposable gloves
- Ventilation mask (for unconscious victim)
- Approved mannequin for practicing removal of a foreign body airway obstruction (FBAO) in an unconscious person

PROCEDURAL STEPS

Responsive Adult

1. Ask, "Are you choking?" If the victim indicates yes, ask, "Can you speak?" If the victim is unable to speak, tell the victim you are going to help.
   <u>PURPOSE</u>: If the victim is unable to speak, is coughing weakly, and/or is wheezing, he or she has an obstructed airway with poor air exchange, and the obstruction must be removed before respiratory arrest occurs.
2. Stand behind the victim with your feet slightly apart.
   <u>PURPOSE</u>: With an obstructed airway, the victim may lose consciousness at any time. The rescuer must be prepared to lower the unconscious victim to the floor safely.
3. Reach around the victim's abdomen and place an index finger into the victim's navel or at the level of the belt buckle (Figure 1). Make a fist of the opposite hand (do not tuck the thumb into the fist) and place the thumb side of the fist against the victim's abdomen above the navel. If the victim is pregnant, place the fist above the enlarged uterus. If the victim is obese, it may be necessary to place the fist higher in the abdomen. It may be necessary to perform chest thrusts on a victim who is pregnant or obese.
   <u>PURPOSE</u>: The fist should be placed in the soft tissue of the abdomen to avoid injury to the sternum or rib cage.

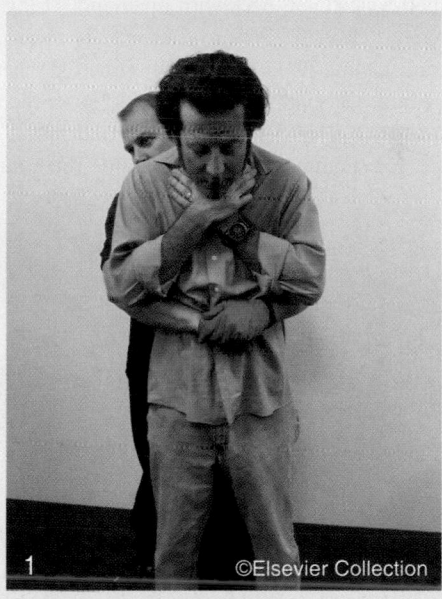

1   ©Elsevier Collection

4. Place the opposite hand over the fist and give abdominal thrusts in a quick inward and upward movement.
   <u>PURPOSE</u>: Abdominal contents pushing against the diaphragm force trapped air out of the lungs, and with it the obstruction.
5. Repeat the abdominal thrusts until the object is expelled or the victim becomes unresponsive.

PROCEDURE 29-10   *—continued*

Unresponsive Adult Victim

The technique for an unresponsive victim is to be practiced only on an approved mannequin.

1. Carefully lower the patient to the ground, activate the emergency response system, and put on disposable gloves.

2. Immediately begin cardiopulmonary resuscitation (CPR) at cycles of 30:2 (compressions to breaths) using the ventilator mask.
   PURPOSE: Higher airway pressures are maintained with chest compressions than with abdominal thrusts.

3. Each time the airway is opened to deliver a rescue breath during CPR, look for an object in the victim's mouth and remove it if visible. If no object is found, immediately return to the cycle of 30 chest compressions.

4. A finger sweep should be used only if the rescuer can see the obstruction.

5. Continue cycles of 30 compressions to 2 rescue breaths until the obstruction is removed or emergency medical services (EMS) arrives.

6. If the obstruction is removed, assess the victim for breathing and circulation. If a pulse is present but the patient is not breathing, begin rescue breathing.

7. Once the patient has been stabilized or EMS has taken over care, remove your gloves and the ventilator mask valve and discard them in the biohazard container. Disinfect the ventilator mask per the manufacturer's recommendations. Sanitize your hands.

8. Document the procedure and the patient's condition.

7/22/20— 8:35 AM: Pt in waiting room, clutching throat and coughing weakly. After confirming pt choking, abdominal thrusts performed until foreign body expelled. Pt breathing without difficulty; R 18 and regular. Incident reported to provider. Cheryl Skurka, CMA (AAMA)

To dislodge a foreign object from the airway of an infant up to 1 year of age, place the baby face down over your forearm and across your thigh. The head should be lower than the trunk, and you should support the baby's head and neck with one hand. Using the heel of your other hand, deliver 5 blows to the back, between the infant's shoulder blades (Figure 29-11, *A*). Holding the baby between your arms, turn the infant face up, keeping the head lower than the trunk. Using two fingers, deliver 5 thrusts to the midsternal area at the infant's nipple line (Figure 29-11, *B*). Examine the infant's mouth, and if the object is visible, pluck it out with your fingertips. *Never perform a finger sweep on an infant.* A baby's oral cavity is too small for a finger sweep, and such an action may only push the obstruction farther into the airway. If the obstruction is not visible, administer 2 rescue breaths by covering the baby's nose and mouth with your mouth, or use a pediatric ventilator mask if available. Repeat the sequence until the foreign body is expelled or help arrives.

If a choking victim is in the late stages of pregnancy, chest compressions should be delivered by placing your cupped hands above

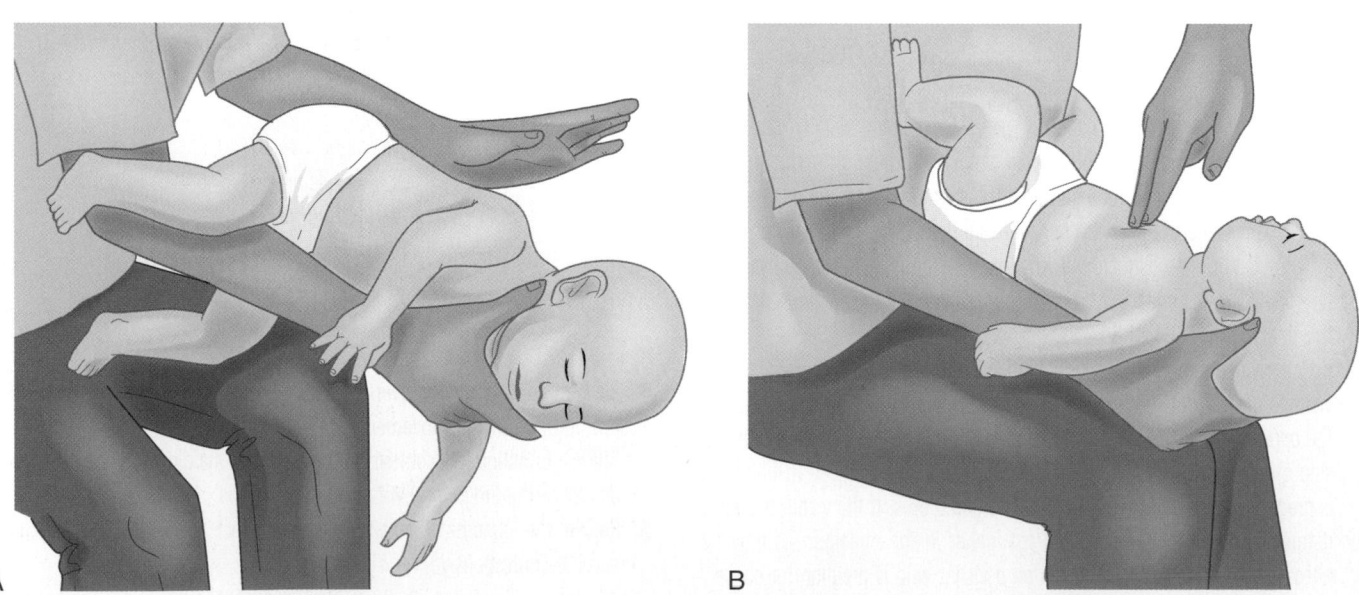

A   B

FIGURE 29-11 A, Back blows are administered to an infant supported on the arm and thigh. **B,** Chest thrusts are administered in the same position as for cardiac compressions.

the uterus to prevent possible trauma to the infant. If the patient is obese and you are unable to wrap your arms around the abdomen, perform chest compressions as you would for a pregnant woman.

The abdominal thrust maneuver also can be performed on yourself if you are choking and no one is nearby to help you. Press your fist into your upper abdomen with quick, upward thrusts, or lean forward and press the abdomen quickly against a firm object, such as the back of a chair.

Cerebrovascular Accident (Stroke)

A cerebrovascular accident (CVA), or stroke, is a disorder of the cerebral blood vessels that results in impairment of the blood supply to part of the brain. This interruption in normal circulation of blood through the brain leads to some degree of neurologic damage, temporary or permanent, depending on the severity of oxygen deprivation to the brain cells.

A minor stroke, or **transient ischemic attack (TIA)**, usually does not cause unconsciousness, and symptoms depend on the location of the circulatory problem in the brain and the amount of brain damage. TIA symptoms are temporary and may include headache, confusion, vertigo, ringing in the ears *(tinnitus)*, temporary paralysis or weakness of one side of the body, transient limb weakness, slurred speech, and vision problems. TIA episodes indicate that the patient is at risk for a major stroke.

Symptoms of a major stroke include unconsciousness, paralysis on one side of the body, difficulty breathing and swallowing, loss of bladder and bowel control, unequal pupil size, and slurring of speech.

Home recommendations for a patient who has suffered a major stroke should begin with notifying the provider and/or activating EMS. Keep the patient lying down and lightly covered. Maintain an open airway. To prevent choking, position the head so that any secretions drain from the side of the mouth. If the patient is lying on the floor, did not fall, and shows no indications of a head or neck injury, he or she can be placed in the recovery position as follows (Figure 29-12):

1. Place the patient's arm that is farthest from you alongside and above the head; place the other arm across the chest.
2. Bend the leg that is closest to you, and after placing one arm under the patient's head and shoulder and the other hand on

the flexed knee, roll the patient away from you while you stabilize the head and neck. The patient's head should be resting on the extended arm.

The recovery position uses gravity to drain fluids from the mouth and keep the trachea clear. Keep the patient in this position until the person is alert or help arrives. Do not give the patient anything to eat or drink. Vital signs should be measured at regular intervals and recorded for the provider.

Advances in early treatment of strokes show great promise in preventing long-term neurologic deficits. However, to prevent permanent brain damage, **thrombolytics** must be administered intravenously within 3 hours of the onset of symptoms. If a patient does not know when the symptoms began (e.g., the person woke up with the symptoms) or cannot accurately tell the provider when the symptoms started, the time allotted for administration begins from the point at which the patient last was known to be asymptomatic. Intracranial hemorrhage must be ruled out before treatment begins. The earlier the treatment starts, the better the neurologic outcomes. The best possible outcomes are seen in patients who receive thrombolytic therapy within 90 minutes of the onset of symptoms.

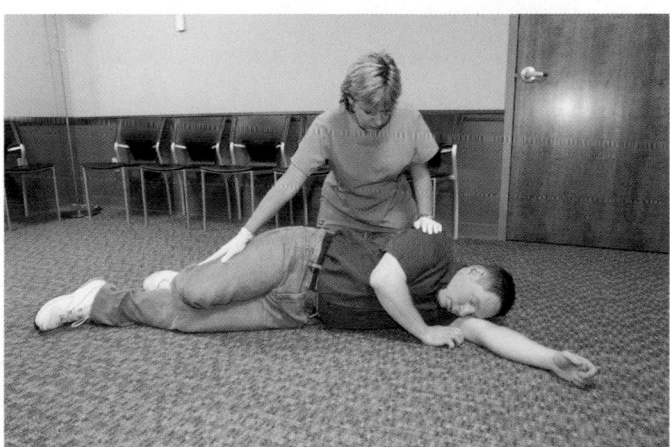

FIGURE 29-12 Recovery position.

Warning Signs of Stroke: *FAST*

The American Stroke Association developed the mnemonic FAST to help people spot the signs of a sudden stroke. If any of these are present, 911 should be called immediately.

Face drooping	• Does one side of the face droop or is it numb? • Ask the person to smile. Is the person's smile uneven?
Arm weakness	• Is one arm weak or numb? • Ask the person to raise both arms. Does one arm drift downward?
Speech difficulty	• Is speech slurred? Is the person unable to speak or hard to understand? • Ask the person to repeat a simple sentence, such as, "The sky is blue." Is the sentence repeated correctly?
Time to call 911	• If someone shows any of these symptoms, even if the symptoms go away, call 911 and get the person to the hospital immediately. Note the time the first symptoms appeared.

Source: American Heart Association and The American Stroke Association.

CRITICAL THINKING APPLICATION   29-4

Thomas Antonio, a 67-year-old patient, calls to report that when he woke up this morning, the left side of his face was drooping and he had difficulty seeing out of his left eye. The symptoms went away in about 2 hours, and he is feeling fine now. The schedule does not show any openings for 2 days. When should Cheryl make an appointment for Mr. Antonio? What questions should Cheryl ask him?

Shock

Shock is a state of collapse caused by failure of the circulatory system to deliver enough oxygenated blood to the body's vital organs. Injury, hemorrhage, infection, anesthesia, drug overdose, burns, pain, fear, or emotional stress can cause this physiologic reaction. Shock can be immediate or delayed, and it is potentially fatal. Many different types of shock can occur, but the signs and symptoms are universal. The most common indicators are a pale, gray, or cyanotic appearance; moist but cool skin; dilated pupils; a weak, rapid pulse; marked hypotension; shallow, rapid respirations; lethargy or restlessness; nausea and vomiting; and extreme thirst.

If a patient shows signs of shock, maintain an open airway and check for breathing and circulation. Place the patient supine with the legs elevated approximately 1 foot to return the blood from the legs to vital organs. Loosen all tight clothing and cover the patient with a blanket for warmth (Procedure 29-11). Do not move the patient unnecessarily. Fluids may be given by mouth if the patient is alert. Because shock can evolve into a life-threatening situation, only basic first aid should be administered, and the patient should be transported to the hospital as soon as possible.

Types and Causes of Shock

Anaphylactic: A severe allergic reaction

Insulin: Severe hypoglycemia caused by an overdose of insulin

Psychogenic or *mental:* Excessive fear, joy, anger, or emotional stress

Hypovolemic or *hemorrhagic:* Excessive loss of blood

Cardiogenic: Myocardial infarction, pulmonary embolism, or severe congestive heart failure

Neurogenic: Dilation of blood vessels as a result of brain or spinal cord injury

Septic: Systemic infection

PROCEDURE 29-11   Perform First Aid Procedures: Care for a Patient Who Has Fainted or Is in Shock

Goal: *To assess and provide emergency care for a patient who has fainted.*

EQUIPMENT and SUPPLIES

- Patient's record
- Sphygmomanometer
- Stethoscope
- Watch with second hand
- Blanket
- Footstool or box
- Pillows
- Oxygen equipment, if ordered by provider:
  - Portable oxygen tank
  - Pressure regulator
  - Flow meter
  - Nasal cannula with connecting tubing

PROCEDURAL STEPS

1. If warning is given that the patient feels faint, have the patient lower the head to the knees to increase the blood supply to the brain (Figure 1). If this does not stop the episode, have the patient lie down on the examination table or lower the patient to the floor. If the patient collapses to the floor when fainting, treat with caution because of possible head or neck injuries.

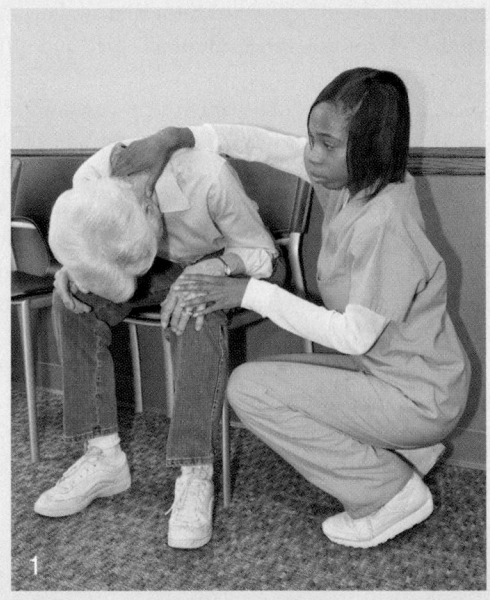

2. Immediately notify the provider of the patient's condition and assess the patient for life-threatening emergencies, such as respiratory or cardiac arrest. If the patient is breathing and has a pulse, monitor the patient's vital signs.
3. If the patient has fainted and vital signs are unstable or the patient does not respond quickly, activate emergency medical services (EMS).
   <u>PURPOSE</u>: Fainting may be a sign of a life-threatening problem.
4. Activate EMS if the patient shows signs of shock—pale, gray, or cyanotic appearance; moist but cool skin; dilated pupils; a weak, rapid pulse; marked hypotension; shallow, rapid respirations; or lethargy or restlessness.

PROCEDURE 29-11 *—continued*

5. Look, listen, and feel for breathing and check the pulse. Maintain an open airway and continue to monitor vital signs.

6. Loosen any tight clothing and keep the patient warm, applying a blanket if needed.

7. If a head or neck injury is not a factor, elevate the patient's legs above the level of the heart using a footstool with pillow support if available (Figure 2).
   PURPOSE: Elevating the legs assists with venous blood return to the heart. This may relieve symptoms of fainting or shock by elevating the blood pressure and increasing blood flow to vital organs.

8. Continue to monitor vital signs, and apply oxygen by nasal cannula if ordered by the provider until the patient recovers or EMS arrives.

9. If the patient vomits, roll the patient onto his or her side to prevent aspiration of vomitus into the lungs.

10. If the patient completely recovers, assist the patient into a sitting position. Do not leave the patient unattended on the examination table.

11. Document the incident, including a description of the episode, the patient's symptoms and vital signs, the duration of the episode, and any complaints. If oxygen was administered, document the number of liters and how long oxygen was administered.

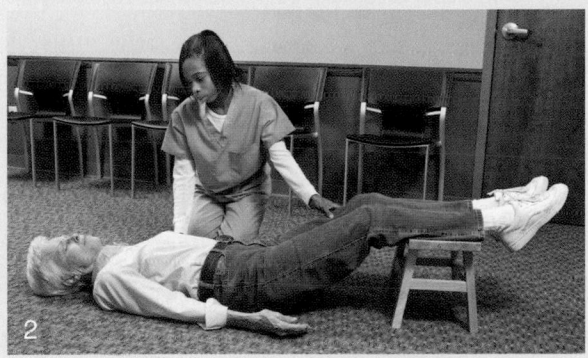

7/29/20– 4:18 PM: Pt in waiting room states she feels faint. Pt lowered to floor, clothing loosened, legs elevated. Provider notified. P 88 and regular, R 22, BP 112/60. Syncopal episode persisted for 90 sec, feeling of vertigo lasted 10 min post syncope. Pt transferred to exam room via wheelchair after recovery. Cheryl Skurka, CMA (AAMA)

COMMON OFFICE EMERGENCIES

The remainder of this chapter highlights typical emergencies seen in an ambulatory care practice or in telephone triage situations. Table 29-1 summarizes common emergencies, the questions that should be asked, and possible actions for home care.

Fainting (Syncope)

Fainting, or *syncope*, is a common emergency. It usually is caused by a transient loss of blood flow to the brain (e.g., a sudden drop in blood pressure), which results in a temporary loss of consciousness. It can occur without warning, or the patient may appear pale; may feel cold, weak, dizzy, or nauseated; and may have numbness of the extremities before the incident. The greatest danger to the patient is an injury from falling during the attack. Therefore, if a patient has syncopal symptoms, immediately place the individual in a supine position. Loosen all tight clothing and maintain an open airway. Apply a cold washcloth to the forehead. Measure and record the patient's pulse, respiratory rate, and blood pressure, and report the findings to the provider. Keep the patient in a supine position for at least 10 minutes after the person regains consciousness. A complete patient history can help determine the possible causes of the attack (e.g., a history of heart disease or diabetes). Document the details of the episode and how long it took the patient to recover completely (see Procedure 29-11).

If the patient does not recover quickly, the provider may activate EMS for transport to the hospital. Syncope might be a brief episode in the development of a serious underlying illness, such as an abnormal heart rhythm or shock, that could lead to sudden cardiac death.

Poisoning

Poisonings are considered medical emergencies and are the sixth leading cause of accidental pediatric death in the United States. Poisoning can occur by oral intake, absorption, inhalation, or injection. Over-the-counter (OTC) medications (e.g., acetaminophen); detergents and bleach; plants; cough and cold medicines; and vitamins cause most cases of poisoning seen in young children. Other typical household poisons include drain cleaner, turpentine, kerosene, furniture polish, and paint (Figure 29-13). Signs and

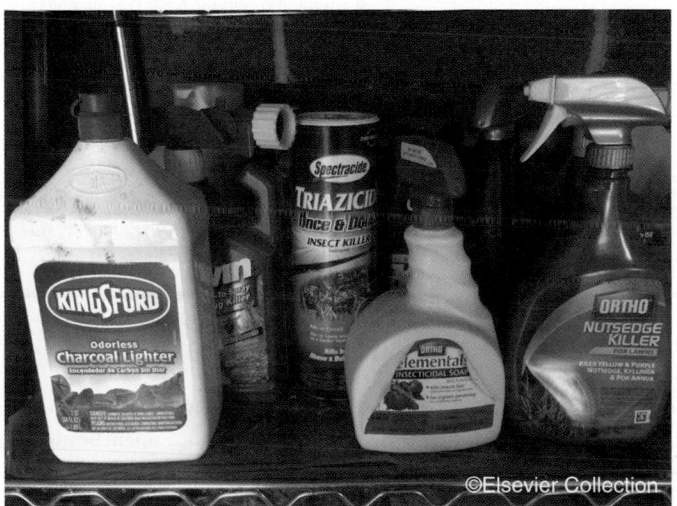

FIGURE 29-13 Hazardous household materials.

TABLE 29-1   Telephone Screening of Possible Emergency Situations

EMERGENCY SITUATION	SCREENING QUESTIONS	HOME CARE ADVICE
Syncope	• Was the patient injured? • Does the patient have a history of heart disease, seizures, or diabetes?	• Syncope does not necessarily indicate a serious disease. If injured by a fall, the patient may need to be evaluated and treated. • The patient should get up very slowly to prevent a recurrence; he or she should then take it easy and drink plenty of fluids. • If the patient is to be seen, someone should accompany him or her to the provider's office.
Animal bites	• What kind of animal (pet or wild)? • How severe is the injury? • Where are the bites? • When did the bites occur?	• The health department or police should be notified. Every effort must be made to locate the animal and monitor its health. • If the skin is not broken, wash the area well and observe for signs of infection.
Insect bites and stings	• Does the patient have a history of an anaphylactic reaction to insect stings? • Does the patient have any of these: difficulty breathing, a widespread rash, or trouble swallowing?	• If the patient has a history of anaphylaxis and has an EpiPen, the EpiPen should be used immediately and emergency medical services (EMS) notified. • Activate EMS if the patient is having systemic symptoms. • An antihistamine (Benadryl) relieves local pruritus.
Asthma	• Does the patient show signs of cyanosis? • Has the patient used prescribed inhalers?	• If a patient with asthma is unable to speak in sentences, has poor color, and is struggling to breathe even after using an inhaler, he or she should be seen immediately or EMS should be activated.

Burns	• Where are the burns located, and what caused them?
	• Are signs of shock present—moist, clammy skin; altered consciousness; and rapid breathing and pulse?
	• If the burn is more than 2 days old, are signs of infection present—foul odor, cloudy drainage?
		• Activate EMS for the following:
		  • Burns on the face, hands, feet, or perineum
		  • Burns caused by electricity or a chemical
		  • Burns associated with inhalation
		  • Signs of shock are present
		• The patient must receive a tetanus shot if he or she has not had one in more than 10 years.
		• Schedule an urgent appointment if signs of infection are reported.

Wounds	• Is the bleeding steady or pulsating? • How and when did the injury occur? • Does the patient have any bleeding disorders, or is the patient taking anticoagulant drugs? • Is the wound open and deep?	• Pulsating bleeding usually indicates arterial damage; activate EMS. • If the injury was caused by a powerful force, other injuries also may have resulted. • Patients taking anticoagulants or who have diabetes or anemia require an urgent appointment. • A gaping, deep wound requires sutures.
Head injury	• Did the patient pass out or have a seizure? Is the patient confused or vomiting? Is a clear fluid draining from the nose or ears?	• If the answer is yes to any of these questions; activate EMS.

symptoms of poisoning, which vary greatly, include burns on the hands and mouth, stains on the victim's clothing, open bottles of medicines or chemicals, changes in skin color, nausea or stomach cramps, shallow breathing, convulsions, heavy perspiration, dizziness or drowsiness, and unconsciousness.

If you receive a phone call about a suspected poisoning, tell the caller not to hang up and not to leave the victim unattended. Call the local poison control center and forward all directions to the caller. Syrup of ipecac has been recommended in the past for home use when a child ingests a poisonous substance, but the

American Academy of Pediatrics now recommends that syrup of ipecac not be kept in the home. There are several reasons for this decision:

- Ipecac should not be given if the child swallowed chemicals that cause burns on contact because the substance can burn the gastrointestinal tract again when it is vomited.
- People with eating disorders often use ipecac to make themselves throw up.
- Ipecac may make it difficult to keep down other drugs that are needed to treat the poison.

If parents believe a child has ingested a poisonous substance, they should call the national poison control center at 1-800-222-1222, or call 911. (Always remember, though, that the best treatment is prevention; parents should be reminded to keep poisonous substances out of sight and out of reach of children). If the patient is to be seen by the provider or sent to the hospital, tell the caller to bring the container of poison or a sample of the vomitus so that the chemical contents of the substance can be verified.

What to Ask When a Poisoning Is Reported

- Victim's name, weight, and age
- Name of the poison taken and any information on the label
- How much was taken
- How long ago the poison was ingested
- Whether vomiting has occurred
- Whether the person has any pertinent symptoms, such as difficulty breathing or an altered state of consciousness
- Whether any first aid has been given, and if so, what

CRITICAL THINKING APPLICATION 29-5

A young mother calls in a panic to report that her 18-month-old daughter swallowed at least half a bottle of cough syrup. The child is fussy and very sleepy, and the mother wants to give her ipecac immediately. What should Cheryl do?

Animal Bites

Possible complications from animal bites include rabies, tetanus, and local skin infection. Any animal bite that is extensive or deep should be seen by a provider. Human infection with rabies is rare; however, if the bite is made by a domestic animal, the animal should be kept quarantined and under observation for 10 days to be monitored for signs of the disease. The animal should not be killed, because a positive finding of rabies is almost impossible to make if the animal has been dead for an extended time. If the bite is made by a bat, raccoon, or any other wild animal, the animal is assumed to be rabid, and the patient must undergo a series of rabies vaccine injections. Local skin infection can be prevented by immediately cleansing the area with antimicrobial soap and water. If the bite breaks the skin (including human bites), the patient's tetanus immunization status must be checked and, if needed, a booster or the entire four-dose tetanus series must be administered as indicated.

Insect Bites and Stings

The bite or sting of an insect can be irritating and painful because of the chemical toxin injected by the insect, but it usually is not serious. Typical symptoms—inflammation, itching *(pruritus)*, and edema—are local and are confined to the area of the bite. In rare cases, a severe allergic reaction may occur; this is a potentially dangerous situation that can lead to anaphylaxis. Signs and symptoms of a systemic allergic reaction include a dry cough, a feeling of tightening in the throat or chest, swelling or itching around the eyes, widespread hives *(urticaria)*, wheezing, dyspnea, and hypotension. Difficulty talking is a sign of urticaria or edema in the throat and may indicate the onset of complete airway obstruction. This is a sign of a true emergency. Epinephrine and oxygen should be ready for immediate administration on the provider's orders. Antihistamines and corticosteroids may be used, but these agents act considerably slower than epinephrine. If acute anaphylactic shock develops, death may occur within 1 hour without medical intervention.

If the stinger is still lodged in the skin, scrape it off with a dull knife, a credit card, or a fingernail. Be careful not to squeeze the stinger, because this injects more venom into the skin. Apply an ice bag to the site to relieve pain and slow absorption of venom. Calamine lotion or hydrocortisone cream may be applied to relieve itching. If the patient has a history of allergies, especially to insect venom, he or she should have access to an EpiPen injection system; this should be used immediately after the sting. In this case, the patient should be transported to the nearest hospital for immediate care.

Removal of a Tick

Ticks can cause a number of diseases, including Rocky Mountain spotted fever and Lyme disease. The tick embeds its head into the skin to obtain blood, and it should be removed intact by the following method:

1. Do not handle ticks with uncovered fingers; use tweezers to prevent personal contamination.
2. Place the tips of the tweezers as close as possible to the area where the tick has entered the skin.
3. With a slow, steady motion, pull the tick away from the skin. Try not to squeeze or crush the tick. If the tick's entire body is not removed, make an appointment with a provider to have the site evaluated.
4. After removal, place the tick directly into a sealable container. Disinfect the area around the bite site using standard procedures.
5. If the tick is removed at home, the provider may suggest that it be brought to the office to be tested for disease.

Asthma Attacks

Asthma is characterized by expiratory wheezing, coughing, a feeling of tightness in the chest, and shortness of breath. During an asthma attack, two different physiologic responses occur. The lining of the respiratory tract becomes inflamed and edematous and produces mucus, which results in narrowing of the air passages. At the same time, bronchospasms occur, which also constrict the airways. The quality and severity of attacks vary greatly among patients, and treatment must be individualized to minimize or eliminate chronic symptoms. If the patient is prescribed a bronchodilator inhaler, it should be used at the first indication of symptoms. Depending on the severity of the attack, give the patient an appointment for the same day as the call, or consult the provider. The provider may recommend that the patient go directly to the ED for emergency respiratory care.

Seizures

Seizures may be **idiopathic**, or they may result from trauma, injury, or metabolic alterations, such as hypoglycemia or hypocalcemia. A *febrile* seizure is transient and occurs with a rapid rise in body temperature over 101.8°F (38.8°C). Febrile seizures typically occur in children between 6 months and 5 years of age. Many different types of seizures occur, but all are caused by a disruption in the electrical activity of the brain.

If a patient suffers a grand mal seizure, which involves uncontrolled muscular contractions, the most important point is to protect the patient from possible injury. Clear everything away from the patient that could cause accidental injury, and observe him or her until the seizure ends. Do not place anything into the person's mouth, because it may damage the teeth or tongue and force the tongue back over the trachea. Do not hold the patient down, because this may result in muscle injuries or fractures. If unconsciousness persists after the seizure has subsided, place the patient in the recovery position to maintain an open airway and allow drainage of excess saliva. After the seizure is over, let the patient rest or sleep, but never leave the person alone. If the provider is not in the office, check the office policies and procedures manual to determine how to manage the situation (Procedure 29-12).

Call 911 for emergency assistance in any of the following situations:

- The patient does not regain consciousness within 10 to 15 minutes.
- The seizure does not stop within a few minutes.
- The patient begins a second seizure immediately after the first one.
- The patient is pregnant.
- Signs of head trauma are present.
- The patient is known to have diabetes.
- The seizure was triggered by a high fever in a child.

PROCEDURE 29-12 Perform First Aid Procedures: Care for a Patient With Seizure Activity

Goal: *To assess and provide emergency care for a patient who has a grand mal seizure.*

EQUIPMENT and SUPPLIES

- Patient's record
- Sphygmomanometer
- Stethoscope
- Watch with second hand
- Blanket
- Pillows

PROCEDURAL STEPS

1. If warning is given that the patient might have a seizure, help lower the patient to the floor. If the patient collapses with a seizure, clear everything away from the patient that could cause accidental injury. If you cannot remove all hard items (e.g., the examination table), pad the hard edges with a blanket or pillow.
   PURPOSE: The patient could be injured when uncontrollable muscular contractions occur with the seizure.
2. Immediately check the time on your watch and call for help.
   PURPOSE: To time the length of the seizure and alert the provider of the patient's seizure activity.
3. Observe the patient throughout the seizure but do not restrain or confine the patient's movements.
   PURPOSE: Stay with the patient for the entire seizure, but do not restrain movement. Restraining the patient may cause musculoskeletal injury.
4. Do not place anything in the patient's mouth during the seizure.
   PURPOSE: The patient's jaw is typically clamped tight during the seizure and trying to force something between the teeth can cause injury.

5. After the muscular contractions have ended, roll the patient into the recovery position on his or her side, with the top knee bent and the head resting on the extended arm closest to the floor.
   PURPOSE: This position helps maintain an open airway.
6. Loosen any tight clothing and keep the patient warm, using a blanket if needed. Let the patient rest, but never leave the patient alone.
   PURPOSE: To maintain patient safety and comfort.
7. If the provider is not in the facility, check the policies and procedures manual to determine how to follow up with the patient.
8. Activate emergency medical services (EMS) if any of the following conditions are present:
   - The patient does not regain consciousness within 10 to 15 minutes.
   - The seizure does not stop within a few minutes.
   - The patient begins a second seizure immediately after the first one.
   - The patient is pregnant.
   - Signs of head trauma are present.
   - The patient is known to have diabetes.
   - The seizure was triggered by a high fever in a child.
9. If the patient completely recovers, assist him or her into a sitting position, check vital signs, and make sure there is someone to accompany the person home.
10. Document the incident, including a description of the episode, the patient's symptoms and vital signs, the duration of the seizure activity, and any complaints.

Abdominal Pain

Abdominal pain is a symptom caused by many different problems, which can range from acute discomfort to life-threatening complications. The clinician should see every patient who reports abdominal pain; the question is how soon the patient should be seen. A patient with acute onset of severe, persistent abdominal pain, especially when this is accompanied by fever, should receive medical attention as soon as possible. Abdominal pain has a variety of causes, including intestinal infection, appendicitis, ectopic pregnancy, inflammation, hemorrhage, obstruction, and tumor.

Treatment in the ambulatory care office depends on the cause of the pain; however, the medical assistant should follow these general guidelines:

- Keep the patient warm and quiet.
- Have an emesis basin available.
- Administer nothing by mouth (NPO).
- Do not apply heat to the abdomen unless so instructed by the provider.
- Administer analgesics as ordered.
- Check and record the patient's vital signs and follow the provider's orders.

Screening Guidelines for Assessing Abdominal Pain

- Assess for shock-related signs and symptoms: diaphoresis; cold, clammy skin; cyanosis or gray pallor; rapid respirations; altered state of consciousness.
- Is the pain severe and constant, or does it come in waves?
- Has the patient had any bloody or tarry stools?
- Is the patient's temperature higher than 101°F (38.3°C)?
- Could the patient be pregnant or has she missed a menstrual period?
- Has the patient experienced continuous vomiting or severe constipation?
- Are any urinary symptoms present, such as frequency, **hematuria**, or flank pain?

- Does the patient have chest pain, shortness of breath, or a continuous cough?
- Does the patient have a history of serious illness, such as diabetes, heart disease, or cancer?

Sprains and Strains

Sprains are tears of the ligaments that support a joint; *strains* are injuries to a muscle and its tendons. Both types of injury may damage surrounding soft tissues and blood vessels and nearby nerves. With a sprain, the victim develops edema and **ecchymosis** around the injury, and any movement of the joint, especially a twisting one, produces pain. Usually no swelling or discoloration is seen with a strain, and only mild tenderness is noted unless the injured muscle or tendon is used.

Tendon strains and ligament sprains take several weeks to heal, whereas muscle tears usually heal in 1 to 2 weeks because muscle has such a rich blood supply. These injuries are treated by elevating the affected area and applying mild compression and ice. Swelling is reduced if ice is applied within 20 to 29 minutes of the injury. After 24 to 36 hours, alternating applications of mild heat and ice usually are indicated. The patient may be advised to immobilize the part.

Fractures

A fracture is a break or crack in a bone, which can result from trauma or disease. Fractures are very painful and affect the patient's ability to freely move the injured part. When a patient with a fracture is brought into the office, the medical assistant should make the patient as comfortable as possible. Place the patient in a position that supports the affected area at the joints above and below the suspected fracture and does not place strain on the injury. Notify the provider immediately and proceed according to the orders given. Emergency treatment for fractures includes preventing movement of the injured part through splinting, elevation of the affected extremity, application of ice, and control of any bleeding (Procedure 29-13). If a patient with an open fracture (i.e., the bone is protruding through the skin) is seen in an ambulatory care office, he or she should be transported to the ED.

PROCEDURE 29-13 | Perform First Aid Procedures: Care for a Patient With a Suspected Fracture of the Wrist by Applying a Splint

Goal: *To provide emergency care for and assessment of a patient with a suspected fracture of the wrist.*

EQUIPMENT and SUPPLIES

- Patient record
- Sphygmomanometer
- Stethoscope
- Watch with second hand
- Splint with padding
- Ace or roller bandage material
- Gloves and sterile dressing (if any open areas on the skin)

PROCEDURAL STEPS

1. Gather equipment and sanitize your hands.
2. Greet and identify the patient, introduce yourself, and explain the procedure.
   PURPOSE: To relieve the patient's anxiety and earn his or her cooperation with the procedure.
3. Obtain vital signs.

PROCEDURE 29-13 —*continued*

4. Assess the area of the suspected fracture for swelling, bleeding, bruising, or protruding bones.
5. If the skin is broken, put on gloves and cover the area with a sterile dressing.
   PURPOSE: Infection control and compliance with Standard Precautions procedures.
6. Moving the limb as little as possible, place the padded splint under the lower arm and wrist.
   PURPOSE: Avoid moving the limb any more than necessary to prevent movement of the fracture and further pain.
7. The area must be immobilized by the splint above and below the suspected fracture.
   PURPOSE: Immobilizing the joint above and below the injury keeps the joint in place, preventing further injury and pain.
8. Secure the splint in place by rolling an Ace bandage or roller bandage around the splint and arm, starting at the arm and rolling down to the wrist and hand.

9. Check the pulse in the affected arm. Note the color and temperature of the skin and the color of the nails.
   PURPOSE: To make sure the splint and bandage have not been applied too tightly.
10. Make sure the patient is comfortable, and answer any questions he or she may have.
11. Sanitize your hands.
12. Document the procedure, including the condition of the patient, the reported pain level, and application of the splint.

7/24/20– 1:05 PM: Temporary splint applied to Ⓛ wrist per provider order. Pt reports some relief of discomfort, with pain at 6 on a 1-10 scale. Hand warm and normal color, nail beds pink, and radial pulse easily palpated. BP 132/80, P 88 and regular, R 22. Cheryl Skurka, CMA (AAMA)

Burns

Burns are among the most common causes of injury in the United States. Burn injuries can result from flame, heat, scalds, electricity, chemicals, or radiation. The skin surface may be reddened, blistered, or charred. The depth and extent of a burn are the major determinants in classifying its severity. The extent of the pain is directly proportional to the extent of the surface area burned and the depth and nature of the burn.

To screen a burn injury, the medical assistant must know what caused the burn, its location and approximate size, the depth of the burn, and whether any additional injuries occurred. If the patient reports a chemical burn, it is important to have the person immediately remove all clothing that may have come into contact with the chemical and flood the affected area with running water to flush the irritant off the skin. If the chemical is not quickly flushed away or remains in the patient's clothing, the agent will continue to burn the skin and may do very serious damage.

The percentage of the body surface area burned can be estimated using the Rule of Nines (Figure 29-14). With this assessment tool, the amount of burned tissue can be quickly calculated. The Rule of Nines divides the body into areas approximately equal to 9% of the total body surface area. When a burn victim is assessed, the affected regions are combined to yield an estimate of the total percentage of burned tissue. Partial-thickness burns over 15% of the total body surface and full-thickness burns of less than 2% can be treated in the ambulatory care office if the patient can be seen immediately. Patients with larger body surface area involvement or other complications should be transported immediately to a hospital, preferably one with a burn unit.

Tissue Injuries

Patients may report any of several different types of wounds. A *contusion* is a closed wound with no evidence of injury to the skin; it typically is caused by blunt trauma, appears swollen and discolored,

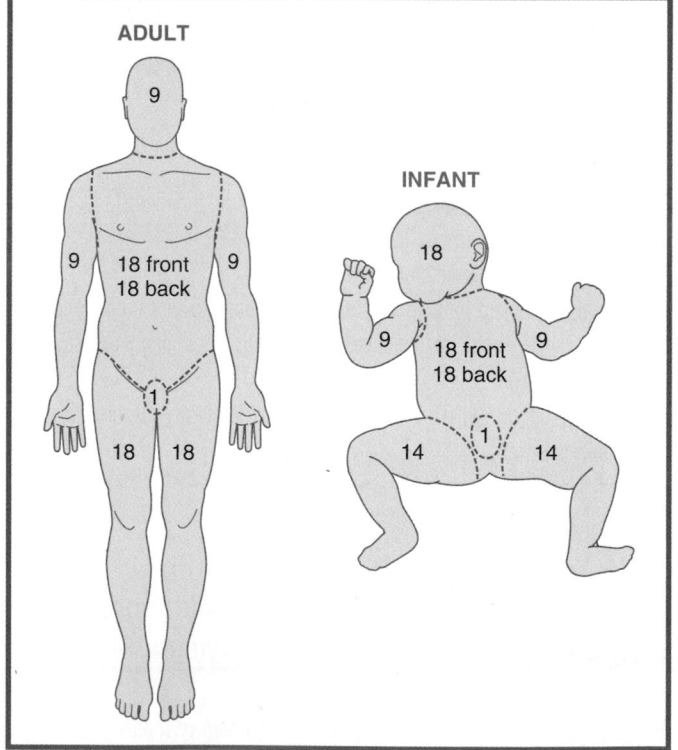

FIGURE 29-14 Rule of Nines classification of burns.

and is painful. A contusion results in a painful bruise, but the skin remains intact. A scrape on the surface of the skin (e.g., a skinned knee, rug burn) is called an *abrasion*. A deeper, jagged wound is called a *laceration*. Additional tissue damage may occur around a laceration; depending on its depth, the wound may need to be repaired surgically. A *puncture* wound occurs when an object is forced into the body (e.g., stepping on a nail). If an object is lodged in body tissues, the best course is to leave it there, stabilize it as much as possible with rolled-up material, and transport the individual to a clinic or ED. The puncture may have severed blood vessels, and if the object is removed, considerable bleeding may occur. An injury in which tissue is torn away (e.g., complete or partial removal of a finger) is known as an *avulsion*.

Lacerations are common presentations in a primary care provider's office. A lacerated wound shows jagged or irregular tearing of the tissues. The severity depends on the cause of the laceration, the site and extent of the injury, and whether the area is contaminated. The injury that caused the laceration also may have damaged blood vessels, nerves, bones, joints, and organs in the body cavities.

When the patient arrives at the facility, put on gloves and notify the provider immediately. Have the patient lie down, and cover the injured area with a sterile dressing (use a dressing that is thick enough to absorb the bleeding) (Procedure 29-14). Reassure the patient and explain your actions as much as possible. Ask the patient when he or she last received a tetanus inoculation, and record the date in the patient's record. If it has been longer than 10 years, the provider probably will want a booster injection given.

Wounds that are not bleeding severely and that do not involve deep tissue damage should be cleaned with antimicrobial soap and water to remove bacteria and other foreign matter. If the laceration is extremely dirty, the provider may want the area irrigated with sterile normal saline solution.

A butterfly closure strip may be used over small lacerations to hold the edges together. If the wound is superficial and has straight edges, it may be closed with a microporous tape (e.g., Steri-Strips)

(Figure 29-15), which eliminates the discomfort of suturing and suture removal. Another wound closure option is a tissue adhesive product (e.g., Dermabond fluid or LiquiBand), which forms a strong, flexible closure similar in strength to nylon suture material. Tissue adhesive products are very useful for closing simple lacerations in children; they provide an antimicrobial and waterproof coating to the wound site that lasts several days, even with repeated washing.

After the clinician closes the wound, the medical assistant typically applies a sterile dressing to the site. The size and thickness of the dressing depend on the type of wound.

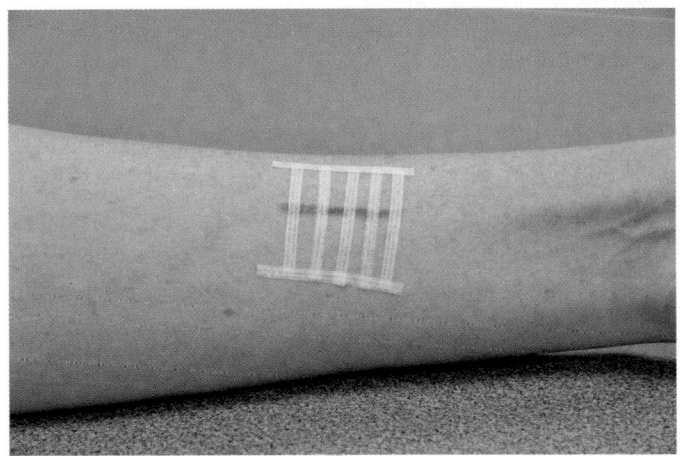

FIGURE 29-15 Steri-Strips.

PROCEDURE 29-14 Perform First Aid Procedures: Control Bleeding

Goal: *To stop hemorrhaging from an open wound.*

EQUIPMENT and SUPPLIES

- Patient's record
- Gloves (sterile if available)
- Appropriate personal protective equipment (PPE) as specified by Occupational Safety and Health Administration (OSHA) guidelines, including:
  - Impermeable gown
  - Goggles or face shield
  - Impermeable mask
  - Impermeable foot covers, if indicated
- Sterile dressings
- Bandaging material
- Biohazard waste container

PROCEDURAL STEPS

1. Sanitize your hands and put on appropriate PPE.
   PURPOSE: To follow Standard Precautions.
2. Assemble equipment and supplies.
3. Apply several layers of sterile dressing material directly to the wound and exert pressure.
   PURPOSE: Direct pressure to a wound slows or stops the bleeding. Sterile supplies are needed to prevent wound infection.

4. Wrap the wound with bandage material. Add more dressing and bandaging material if the bleeding continues.
5. If bleeding persists and the wound is on an extremity, elevate the extremity above the level of the heart. Notify the provider immediately if the bleeding cannot be controlled.
6. If the bleeding still continues, maintain direct pressure and elevation; also apply pressure to the appropriate artery. If the bleeding is in the arm, apply pressure to the brachial artery by squeezing the inner aspect of the middle upper arm. If the bleeding is in the leg, apply pressure to the femoral artery on the affected side by pushing with the heel of the hand into the femoral crease at the groin. If the bleeding cannot be controlled, activate emergency medical services.
7. Once the bleeding has been brought under control and the patient has been stabilized, discard contaminated materials in an appropriate biohazard waste container.
8. Disinfect the area, then remove your gloves and discard them in a biohazard waste container.
9. Sanitize your hands.
10. Document the incident, including details of the wound, when and how it occurred, the patient's symptoms and vital signs, treatment provided by the provider, and the patient's current condition.

Nosebleeds (Epistaxis)

A nosebleed, or *epistaxis*, is a hemorrhage that usually results from the rupture of small vessels in the nose. Nosebleeds can be caused by injury, disease, hypertension, strenuous activity, high altitudes, exposure to cold, overuse of anticoagulant medications (e.g., aspirin), and nasal recreational drug use. Bleeding from the anterior nostril area usually is venous, whereas bleeding from the posterior region usually is arterial and is more difficult to stop. Treatment of epistaxis varies according to the amount of bleeding and the presence of other conditions, and whether the patient is taking anticoagulant medications.

If the bleeding is mild to moderate and from one side of the nose, the patient should sit up, lean slightly forward, and apply direct pressure to the affected nostril by pinching the nose. Constant pressure should be continued for 10 to 15 minutes to allow clotting to take place. If the bleeding cannot be controlled, insert a clean gauze pad into the nostril, and notify the provider. If the provider is not available, proceed with standard EMS protocols. Bleeding should be considered a medical emergency if it is bilateral and continuous or if it occurs in a patient who has a bleeding disorder or has been prescribed anticoagulants.

Head Injuries

The severity of head injuries can vary greatly. The history of the injury (i.e., details about what it is and how it happened) is crucial for determining appropriate management. With a head injury, the patient may appear normal; may experience dizziness, severe headache, mental confusion, or memory loss; or may even be unconscious. Loss of consciousness may be brief or prolonged; it may appear immediately or may be delayed. The victim may experience vomiting; loss of bladder and bowel control; and bleeding from the nose, mouth, or ears. The pupils of the eyes may be unequal and nonreactive to light.

All head injuries must be considered serious. Notify the provider or contact EMS immediately. If evidence of a neck injury is seen, stabilize the neck and do not attempt to move the victim. Do not administer anything by mouth. Keep the patient warm and quiet. Watch the pupils of the eyes and record any changes. Measure vital signs and record the extent and duration of any unconsciousness. If the patient is at home or is sent home after the provider's assessment, he or she should be watched closely for 24 hours after the injury for any change in mental status.

Foreign Bodies in the Eye

The eye is a delicate organ with a unique structure that demands special handling. This kind of emergency is uncomfortable, and it often is extremely difficult to keep the patient from rubbing the eye. Tell the patient not to touch the eye in any way. The provider may order ophthalmic topical anesthetic drops to relieve pain. The patient should be placed in a darkened room to wait for the provider because **photophobia** is common with eye irritations. If a contusion and swelling are present, cold, wet compresses can help. Ask the patient to close both eyes and cover them with eye pads until the provider arrives. The provider may order an eye irrigation to remove the object. The medical assistant should not attempt to search for or remove an object in the eyes.

Heat and Cold Injuries

Exposure to extremes in temperature can cause minor to severe injuries. Heat injuries occur most often on hot, humid days and result in cramps, heat exhaustion, or heatstroke. Heat-related muscle cramps may be the first sign of *heat exhaustion,* which is a serious heat-related condition. Patients with heat exhaustion appear flushed and report headaches, nausea, vertigo, and weakness. *Heatstroke,* the most dangerous form of heat-related injury, results in a shutdown of body systems. Patients with heatstroke have red, hot, dry skin; altered levels of consciousness; tachycardia; and rapid, shallow breathing. This is a true medical emergency. If heat-related problems are recognized in the early stages and are adequately treated, the patient does not usually develop heatstroke. Management of heat-related conditions includes getting the person out of the heat; loosening clothing or removing perspiration-soaked clothing; and giving the person cool electrolyte drinks if he or she is alert. An effective way to lower the victim's temperature is to apply cool, wet cloths and then fan the moist skin so that heat is released from the body by evaporation.

The two types of cold-related injuries are frostbite and hypothermia. *Frostbite,* which is the actual freezing of tissue, occurs when the skin temperature falls to a range of 14° to 25°F (−10° to −3.9°C). Prolonged exposure of the skin to cold causes damage similar to a burn. The tissue may appear gray or white, may be swollen, and may have clear blisters; in full-thickness frostbite, the skin may show signs of tissue **necrosis**, including blackened areas and severe deformity. The more advanced the frostbite, the more serious the tissue damage and the more likely the body part will be lost. Frozen tissue has no feeling, but as thawing occurs, the patient reports itching, tingling, and burning pain. Mild frostbite can be managed by applying constant warmth to the affected areas; this can be done by immersing the area in warm water (no warmer than 105°F [40.6°C]) or by wrapping it in warm, dry clothing. Friction should never be used because this could increase tissue damage. If blisters have formed or if evidence of full-thickness frostbite is seen, the patient should be transported to the nearest ED.

Hypothermia is a medical emergency that may result in death unless the patient receives immediate assistance. Systemic hypothermia occurs when the core body temperature drops below 95°F (35°C). Signs and symptoms of hypothermia include shivering, numbness, apathy, and loss of consciousness. If hypothermia is suspected, activate EMS and provide care for any life-threatening conditions until help arrives. Remove the victim's wet clothing and wrap the victim in blankets while moving him or her to a warm place. If the victim is alert, give warm liquids and apply heating pads (using a barrier to prevent burns) or chemical hot packs to help slowly raise the core body temperature.

Dehydration

A person dehydrates when more water is excreted than is taken in. Dehydration can be a very serious health emergency, leading to convulsions, coma, and even death. Infants, young children, and older adult patients are at greatest risk of developing serious complications from dehydration. Severe dehydration may be caused by excessive heat loss, vomiting, diarrhea, or lack of fluid intake. Symptoms include vertigo; dark yellow urine or no urine output for 8 to

10 hours; extreme thirst; lethargy or confusion; and abdominal or muscle cramps. If the patient shows any of these symptoms and is unable to retain fluids, schedule an urgent appointment or recommend that the patient be taken to the ED. Replacement of lost fluids is vital, so the patient should be encouraged to drink water, tea, sports drinks, fruit juice, or Pedialyte.

Diabetic Emergencies

Diabetes mellitus is caused by a malfunction in the production of insulin in the pancreas or by an inability of the cells to use insulin. Insulin is required on the cellular level so that glucose can be used for energy. Two different diabetic emergencies can occur, one caused by *hyperglycemia* (high blood glucose levels) and the other by *hypoglycemia* (low blood glucose levels).

Insulin shock is caused by severe hypoglycemia, which results when a patient with diabetes takes too much insulin, does not eat enough food, or exercises an unusual amount. Signs and symptoms, which have a rapid onset, include tachycardia, profuse sweating (diaphoresis), headache, irritability, vertigo, fatigue, hunger, seizures, and coma. It is important to provide glucose immediately, preferably in the form of glucose tablets, which have a known, concentrated quantity of glucose.

Diabetic coma results from severe hyperglycemia, which develops because the body is not producing enough insulin; the patient eats too much food or is very stressed; or the patient has an infection. The symptoms of impending diabetic coma, which develop more slowly than those of insulin shock, include general malaise, dry mouth, polyuria, **polydipsia**, nausea, vomiting, SOB, and breath with an acetone (or "fruity") smell. If the patient or caregiver calling for an appointment reports these symptoms, notify the provider immediately because the patient typically would be admitted to the hospital.

In an emergency situation, if a patient diagnosed with diabetes mellitus shows signs and symptoms of a diabetic emergency, the patient should be given glucose. If the problem is caused by insulin shock (hypoglycemia), the patient will improve quickly after receiving glucose; if it is caused by diabetic coma (hyperglycemia), a small amount of added glucose will not affect the patient's condition, and he or she must be transported to the hospital regardless (Procedure 29-15).

PROCEDURE 29-15 **Perform First Aid Procedures: Care for a Patient With a Diabetic Emergency**

Goal: *To provide emergency care for and assessment of a patient with insulin shock or a pending diabetic coma.*

EQUIPMENT and SUPPLIES

- Patient record
- Sphygmomanometer
- Stethoscope
- Watch with second hand
- Disposable gloves
- Glucometer
- Disposable lancet
- Glucose tablets
- Insulin
- Insulin syringe unit
- Alcohol swabs
- Sharps container

PROCEDURAL STEPS

1. Gather equipment and sanitize your hands.
2. Greet and identify the patient and introduce yourself.
   PURPOSE: To relieve patient anxiety and earn patient cooperation.
3. Obtain vital signs.
4. If the patient is known to have diabetes, observe for signs and symptoms that indicate a diabetic emergency.
   - Signs and symptoms of insulin shock or hypoglycemia: Rapid onset of vertigo, fatigue, hunger, tachycardia, profuse sweating, headache, irritability, seizures, and coma.
   - Signs and symptoms of impending diabetic coma or hyperglycemia: Symptoms develop more slowly than those of insulin shock; these include general malaise, dry mouth, polyuria, polydipsia, nausea, vomiting, shortness of breath (SOB), and breath with an acetone (or "fruity") smell.
5. Immediately report patient's condition to the provider and follow his or her orders.
   PURPOSE: A diabetic emergency can be life-threatening.
6. In an emergency situation, if a patient diagnosed with diabetes mellitus shows signs and symptoms of a diabetic emergency, the patient should be given glucose.
   PURPOSE: If the problem is caused by insulin shock (hypoglycemia), the patient will improve quickly after receiving glucose; if it is caused by diabetic coma (hyperglycemia), a small amount of added glucose will not affect the patient's condition, and he or she must be transported to the hospital regardless.
7. Follow the provider's orders and administer 15 g of carbohydrate immediately, preferably in the form of glucose tablets because they have a known concentrated quantity of glucose. If glucose tablets are not available give the patient ½ cup of fruit juice or 5 or 6 pieces of hard candy.
   PURPOSE: To quickly stabilize the patient's blood glucose level
8. Check the patient's blood glucose levels with a glucometer and monitor vital signs.
   PURPOSE: To monitor the patient's current blood glucose level and the patient's condition so the provider can determine appropriate treatment.
   - If the blood glucose level is below 80 mg/dL (insulin shock), administer another 15 g of carbohydrate. Wait 15 minutes and check the glucometer reading again. If the level is still low, repeat steps 7 and 8.

PROCEDURE 29-15   *—continued*

- If the patient's blood glucose levels are elevated (diabetic coma) administer insulin as ordered by the provider

  <u>PURPOSE</u>: To lower blood glucose levels to within a normal range.

9. Continue to monitor the patient and follow the provider's orders for continued care.
   - A patient with insulin shock can be stabilized by continued monitoring of the blood glucose level and administration of glucose every 15 minutes until levels reach normal.
   - A patient with pending diabetic coma may need to be transported to the hospital.

10. Dispose of used supplies and gloves in the appropriate biohazard containers (sharps containers for used lancets and injection unit).
11. Sanitize your hands.
12. Document the actions taken and the patient's condition, including vital signs, glucometer readings, administration of glucose and/or insulin, and whether the patient was stabilized and discharged or emergency medical services (EMS) were activated and the patient was transported to the hospital.

CLOSING COMMENTS

Patient Education

Emergencies can occur anywhere. Patients need to learn how to handle emergency situations both by the example of healthcare workers and through instruction. The medical assistant must remain calm, screen the situation, call for help, and be prepared to administer appropriate first aid. Brochures on home safety can be used to help teach patients methods for preventing accidents in the home.

All patients, even children, should understand how to contact EMS. This is especially important for families with members who have chronic diseases that can be life-threatening, such as heart conditions, severe allergic reactions, diabetes, and asthma. Patients should be encouraged to post important numbers next to the telephone; these include emergency numbers (local EMS and poison control center) and the primary care provider's number. Families with young children must childproof their homes, taking special care to keep potentially poisonous substances stored where children cannot get into them. Placing "Mr. Yuk" stickers on containers of poisonous substances can be an excellent educational tool for young children.

Medical assistants must remember to keep their American Red Cross or AHA certifications current, and they should take advantage of community workshops to maintain and extend their skills. Also, a list of community safety workshops should be posted in an area where patients can see it, and they should be encouraged to attend. Your participation in emergency care workshops, in addition to encouraging others to participate, may help to save lives.

Legal and Ethical Issues

The medical assistant works in the healthcare environment as the provider's agent. Although you are responsible for your own actions, the provider is legally responsible for the care you administer to patients while working in the healthcare facility. You are responsible for knowing the limitations placed on medical assistants in your state and for adhering strictly to your employer's emergency care policies and procedures. Medical assistants are not qualified to diagnose a patient's problem, but they are responsible for acting appropriately in a medical emergency.

Most states have enacted Good Samaritan laws to encourage healthcare professionals to provide medical assistance at the scene of an accident without fear of being sued for negligence. These statutes vary greatly, but all have the intent of protecting the caregiver. A provider or other healthcare professional is not legally obligated to provide emergency care at the site of an accident, regardless of the ethical and moral considerations. Legal liability is limited to gross neglect of the victim or willfully causing further injury to the victim. As a caregiver, you are required to act as a reasonable person and cannot be held liable for personal injury resulting from an act of omission. Good Samaritan statutes provide for evaluation of the caregiver's judgment but are in effect only at the site of an emergency, not at your place of employment.

If you have not been trained in CPR, you cannot be expected to perform the procedure at the emergency site. However, in many states, a healthcare provider with CPR training and skills who is present at the scene can be declared negligent if cardiac arrest occurs and he or she does not administer CPR to the victim.

If the victim is conscious or if a member of his or her immediate family is present, obtain verbal consent to perform emergency care. Consent is implied if the patient is unconscious and no family member is present.

Medical assistants also can play a key role in the community response to natural or human-caused disasters. The medical assistant is cross-trained to perform multiple administrative and clinical duties that would prove very useful in an emergency. These include management of medical records, interacting professionally with patients, performing diagnostic tests, performing phlebotomy and administering medications, assisting with procedures, and administering first aid and CPR as needed. Because of their wide range of skills, medical assistants serve as useful volunteers on local emergency response teams. Investigate agencies and organizations that are committed to emergency preparedness in your community and see how a medical assistant could help these organizations if an emergency arises.

Professional Behaviors

In addition to legal responsibilities, you have an ethical responsibility to your patients to provide the highest standard of care. Always act in the best interest of the patient, and never hesitate to ask the provider and/or the office manager for immediate assistance when faced with a medical emergency. Many types of emergencies can be handled in the provider's office. In an emergency situation, decisions that must be made quickly can determine whether the patient lives. A medical assistant must be prepared to act calmly and efficiently in all emergency situations.

Critical thinking is a crucial part of managing medical emergencies. The ability to ask pertinent questions, consider all available information, and distinguish between relevant and irrelevant patient feedback can make the difference in the immediate management of an emergency situation. Both the provider and the patient rely on the professional medical assistant when he or she is managing potentially serious phone calls and/or caring for a patient with a medical emergency in the healthcare setting.

SUMMARY OF SCENARIO

Cheryl has learned through her work with the telephone screening team and involvement with emergencies in the office how important it is to gather complete information about emergency situations and to act calmly and knowledgeably when managing patient problems. She knows she needs to maintain her certification in CPR for the Professional and to continue to participate in workshops on emergency care so she is prepared for the wide variety of patient problems seen in the ambulatory care practice. Working with the screening staff has reinforced the importance of documenting all interactions on the telephone and all information gathered during patient visits.

Cheryl recognizes that medical assistants in the office must follow the facility's policies and procedures manual for handling emergencies. They must plan ahead and complete their designated duties if an emergency occurs; use community emergency services as needed; and keep emergency supplies and equipment well stocked and ready for any possible emergency. She recognizes that understanding first aid practices for common patient emergencies allows her to assist patients by providing instruction on the phone or by performing specific skills when emergencies occur in the facility.

Cheryl has investigated her legal standing as a medical assistant in her home state and recognizes her responsibilities when a patient calls or shows up at the office with a medical emergency. She will continue to refer to the more experienced screening staff members or to Dr. Bendt when she has questions, but she now feels more confident in managing emergency situations at work. She also recognizes her role as part of the healthcare team if an emergency situation arises in her community.

SUMMARY OF LEARNING OBJECTIVES

1. **Define, spell, and pronounce the terms listed in the vocabulary.**
   Spelling and pronouncing medical terms correctly reinforces the medical assistant's credibility. Knowing the definitions of these terms promotes confidence in communication with patients and co-workers.

2. **Describe patient safety factors in the medical office environment.**
   The medical assistant must be constantly on guard to protect patients from possible injury. Methods for achieving this goal include communicating openly about patient safety issues, following standard procedures when delivering patient care, and working as part of a team to ensure patients' safety.

3. **Interpret and comply with safety signs, labels, and symbols and evaluate the work environment to identify safe and unsafe working conditions for the employee.**
   The four major types of signs are danger signs (identify the most severe and immediate hazards); caution signs (possible hazards that require added precautions); safety instruction signs (designed to communicate directions for safety actions); and biologic hazard signs (identify an actual or potential biohazard). OSHA specifies the format of each type of sign, the information that must appear, and where each type of sign must be used (see Figure 29-1 and Procedures 29-1 and 29-2).

4. **Do the following when it comes to environmental safety in the healthcare setting:**
   - Identify environmental safety issues in the healthcare setting
   - Discuss fire safety issues in a healthcare environment
   - Demonstrate the proper use of a fire extinguisher

   Medical assistants must be constantly on the alert for potentially unsafe conditions; must consistently follow the guidelines established by OSHA for infection control; and must follow safety procedures to prevent workplace violence. Combustibles should be stored properly; electrical equipment must be monitored for safety; smoke detectors and fire extinguishers should be checked routinely; and the facility should be evacuated if a fire breaks out. Procedure 29-3 details the proper use of a fire extinguisher.

5. **Describe the fundamental principles for evacuation of a healthcare facility and role-play a mock environmental exposure event and evacuation of a provider's office.**
   An emergency action coordinator should be designated. This person is in charge of delegating duties to staff members. Exit maps should be posted in multiple areas around the facility. Patients and staff members should be evacuated safely and should meet in a designated

Continued

spot to make sure all staff members and patients have escaped (see Procedure 29-4).

6. **Discuss the requirements for proper disposal of hazardous materials.**

   OSHA has established specific rules about biohazard waste disposal, including the use of sharps containers and red bag collection systems, which must be used properly to avoid disease transmission.

7. **Identify critical elements of an emergency plan for response to a natural disaster or other emergency.**

   Ambulatory care centers may be the first to recognize and initiate a response to a community emergency. Standard Precautions should be implemented immediately to control the spread of an infection. A communication network should be established to notify local and state health departments and perhaps federal officials. Every healthcare facility should have a standard policy with specific procedures for the management of emergencies on site. The CDC recommends that a facility's safety plan include multiple steps to minimize the negative psychological effects of an emergency situation.

8. **Maintain an up-to-date list of community resources for emergency preparedness.**

   See Procedure 29-5.

9. **Describe the medical assistant's role in emergency response.**

   Medical assistants can provide considerable help in a community emergency. They can use therapeutic communication to gather patient data; monitor injured victims; perform first aid and monitor vital signs; and help with any medically related service.

10. **Summarize typical emergency supplies and equipment.**

    A provider's office must have a centrally located crash cart or emergency bag stocked with all emergency supplies, equipment, and medication. This material must be inventoried consistently and maintained. This chapter provides a detailed list of materials that should be readily available for an on-site emergency, including a defibrillator if indicated by the provider's practice.

11. **Demonstrate the use of an automated external defibrillator.**

    See Procedure 29-6.   .

12. **Summarize the general rules for managing emergencies.**

    Management of emergencies requires a calm, efficient approach. The medical assistant should assess the nature of the emergency and determine whether EMS should be activated, or whether the patient requires an immediate or urgent appointment. As many details about the situation as possible should be gathered, and the provider should be consulted when the medical assistant is in doubt.

13. **Demonstrate telephone screening techniques and documentation guidelines for ambulatory care emergencies.**

    Telephone screening is one of the medical assistant's most important tasks. Emergency action principles should be used to determine the level of a patient's emergency. These include determining whether the situation is life-threatening and obtaining the patient's contact information, in addition to all pertinent information about the injury and the patient's signs and symptoms. This information must be shared with the provider, and all details must be documented in the patient's record (see Procedure 29-7).

14. **Recognize and respond to life-threatening emergencies in the ambulatory care practice.**

    Life-threatening emergencies require immediate assessment, referral to the provider or, if the provider is not present, activation of EMS. While waiting for assistance, the medical assistant should check for breathing and circulation. Rescue breaths or CPR is administered if indicated. Depending on the patient's signs and symptoms, the person should be monitored for signs of a heart attack; the Heimlich maneuver is performed for an airway obstruction; the patient is evaluated for signs of a CVA and is assessed for shock. The medical assistant should ask for help when indicated and should perform appropriate procedures based on the patient's presenting condition.

15. **Describe how to handle an unresponsive patient and perform provider/professional-level CPR.**

    See Procedure 29-8 for instructions on performing adult, pediatric, and infant rescue breathing and CPR.

16. **Discuss cardiac emergencies and administer oxygen through a nasal cannula to a patient in respiratory distress.**

    See Procedure 29-9.

17. **Identify and assist a patient with an obstructed airway.**

    Procedure 29-10 presents instructions for assisting an adult with an obstructed airway. Infants with an obstructed airway should receive alternating back blows and chest thrusts with attempted rescue breaths until the item is dislodged or help arrives.

18. **Discuss cerebrovascular accidents and assist a patient who is in shock.**

    A stroke is a disorder of the cerebral blood vessels that results in impairment of the blood supply to part of the brain. Symptoms of a major stroke include paralysis on one side of the body, difficulty swallowing, loss of bladder and bowel control, and slurring of speech. Procedure 29-11 explains how to assist a patient in shock.

19. **Determine the appropriate action and documentation procedures for common office emergencies, such as fainting, poisoning, animal bites, insect bites and stings, and asthma attacks.**

    The medical assistant should always follow Standard Precautions when caring for a patient with a medical emergency. Documentation of emergency treatment should include information about the patient; vital signs; allergies, current medications, and pertinent health history; the patient's chief complaint; the sequence of events, including any changes in the patient's condition since the incident; and any provider's orders and procedures performed (see Table 29-1).

20. **Discuss seizures and perform first aid procedures for a patient having a seizure.**

    See Procedure 29-12.

21. **Discuss abdominal pain, sprains and strains, and fractures, and perform first aid procedures for a patient with a fracture of the wrist.**

    See Procedure 29-13.

SUMMARY OF LEARNING OBJECTIVES—*continued*

22. **Discuss burns and tissue injuries, and control of a hemorrhagic wound.**
    See Procedure 29-14.

23. **Discuss nosebleeds, head injuries, foreign bodies in the eye, heat and cold injuries, dehydration, and diabetic emergencies; also, perform first aid procedures for a patient with a diabetic emergency.**
    See Procedure 29-15.

24. **Apply patient education concepts to medical emergencies.**
    Patients should know how to contact emergency personnel, and families with young children should have telephone numbers for poison control posted. Educating patients in how to care for minor emergencies at home is an important part of telephone triage in the ambula-

tory care practice. Encouraging patients to participate in community safety workshops and to become certified in CPR may help prevent emergencies and save lives.

25. **Discuss the legal and ethical concerns arising from medical emergencies.**
    Good Samaritan laws, which vary from state to state, are designed to protect any individual from liability, whether a healthcare professional or a layperson, if he or she provides assistance at the site of an emergency. The law does not require a medically trained person to act, but if emergency care is given in a reasonable and responsible manner, the healthcare worker is protected from being sued for negligence. This protection, however, does not extend to the workplace.

CONNECTIONS

Study Guide Connection: Go to the Chapter 29 Study Guide. Read and complete the activities.

evolve Evolve Connection: Go to the Chapter 29 link at *evolve.elsevier.com/kinn* to complete the Chapter Review Quiz. Check out the other resources listed for this chapter to make the most of what you have learned from Safety and Emergency Practices.

30

ASSISTING IN OPHTHALMOLOGY AND OTOLARYNGOLOGY

SCENARIO

Kim Tau, CMA (AAMA), works in an outpatient clinic that specializes in the diagnosis and treatment of eye and ear disorders. Kim has been asked by her supervisor to help orient Amy Ling to the practice. Amy recently graduated from a medical assistant program and is familiar with basic eye and ear procedures, but she has many questions about her responsibilities at the clinic. Amy will be responsible for performing initial Snellen and Ishihara screening examinations on new patients and for assisting the ophthalmologist and the optician in the practice. She also must become proficient in conducting audiometry screening tests on pediatric patients, performing ear irrigations, and administering otic medications. Kim recognizes that it is important for Amy to be able to perform these skills with accuracy and confidence; however, she also must develop a sensitivity to the communication and patient education needs of patients with eye and ear disorders.

While studying this chapter, think about the following questions:

- What is the basic anatomy and physiology of the eye and of the ear?
- What are the major types of refractive errors?
- With what disorders of the eye and ear does Amy need to be familiar?
- How is a Snellen test performed?
- What are the important steps Amy should follow in performing eye and ear irrigations and medication applications?
- How is an examination with an audiometer conducted?
- How should Amy perform a throat culture?
- How should Kim prepare Amy to care for patients with sensory loss?

LEARNING OBJECTIVES

1. Define, spell, and pronounce the terms listed in the vocabulary.
2. Explain the differences among an ophthalmologist, an optometrist, and an optician.
3. Identify the anatomic structures of the eye.
4. Describe the process of vision.
5. Differentiate among the major types of refractive errors.
6. Summarize typical disorders of the eye and eyeball other than refractive errors.
7. Do the following related to diagnostic procedures for the eye:
   - Define the various diagnostic procedures for the eye.
   - Perform a visual acuity test using the Snellen chart.
   - Assess color acuity using the Ishihara test.
8. Explain the purpose of and the proper procedure for eye irrigation and the instillation of eye medications.
9. Identify the structures and explain the functions of the external ear, middle ear, and inner ear.
10. Describe the conditions that can lead to hearing loss, including conductive and sensorineural impairments.
11. Define other major disorders of the ear, including otitis, impacted cerumen, and Ménière's disease.
12. Do the following related to diagnostic procedures for the ear:
    - Explain diagnostic procedures for the ear.
    - Use an audiometer to measure a patient's hearing acuity accurately.
    - Identify the purpose of ear irrigations and instillation of ear medications.
    - Demonstrate the procedure for performing ear irrigations.
    - Accurately instill medicated ear drops.
13. Summarize the nose and throat examination and perform a throat culture.
14. Describe the effect of sensory loss on patient education.
15. Discuss legal and ethical issues that might arise when caring for a patient with a vision or hearing deficit, in addition to requirements established by HIPAA and the Americans with Disabilities Act Amendments (ADAA).

VOCABULARY

accommodation Adjustment of the eye that allows a person to see various sizes of objects at different distances.

amblyopia (am-ble-o'-pe-uh) Reduction or dimness of vision with no apparent organic cause; often referred to as *lazy eye syndrome.*

audiologist (aw-de-ah'-lah-jist) Allied healthcare professional who specializes in evaluation of hearing function, detection of hearing impairment, and determination of the anatomic site of impairment.

cones Structures in the retina that make the perception of color possible.

evert To turn the eyelid inside out; this typically is done by the provider to inspect the area for foreign bodies.

fovea centralis (fo'-ve-uh/sen-trah'-lis) A small pit in the center of the retina that is considered the center of clearest vision.

gonioscopy (goh-ne-os'-kuh-pe) A procedure in which a mirrored optical instrument is used to visualize the filtration angle of the anterior chamber of the eye; the procedure is used to diagnose glaucoma.

hertz The unit of measurement used in hearing examinations; a wave frequency equal to 1 cycle per second.

miotic (mi-ah'-tik) Any substance or medication that causes constriction of the pupil.

mydriatic (mid-re-at'-ik) A topical ophthalmic medication that dilates the pupil; it is used in diagnostic procedures of the eye and as treatment for glaucoma.

optic disc The region at the back of the eye where the optic nerve meets the retina; it is considered the blind spot of the eye because it contains only nerve fibers and no rods or cones and thus is insensitive to light.

optic nerve Cranial nerve II, which carries impulses for the sense of sight.

otosclerosis (o-tuh-skluh-ro'-sis) The formation of spongy bone in the labyrinth of the ear, which often causes the auditory ossicles to become fixed and unable to vibrate when sound enters the ears.

ototoxic (o-tuh-tahk'-sik) A medicine or substance capable of damaging cranial nerve VIII or the organs of hearing and balance.

photophobia Abnormal sensitivity to light.

psoriasis (suh-ri'-uh-sis) A usually chronic, recurrent skin disease marked by bright red patches covered with silvery scales.

rods Structures in the retina of the eye that form the light-sensitive elements.

seborrhea (seh-buh-re'-uh) An excessive discharge of sebum from the sebaceous glands, forming greasy scales or crusty areas on the body.

tonometer (toh-nom'-ih-ter) An instrument used to measure intraocular pressure.

A medical assistant is responsible for performing a wide variety of procedures in an ophthalmologic or otorhinolaryngologic practice. First, the medical assistant must be familiar with the normal anatomy and physiology of the eyes, ears, nose, and throat. With an understanding of how these specialty sensory organs function, the medical assistant can master the skills needed to become a valuable asset to providers who specialize in the treatment of eye and ear disorders.

This chapter covers the conditions most frequently seen in the ambulatory care setting. Many subspecialty areas are available to medical assistants in the fields of ophthalmology (eye) and otolaryngology (ear, nose, and throat [ENT]). Learning the fundamental procedures now provides you with a base on which to build the advanced techniques you will need if you choose to concentrate your expertise in these areas.

EXAMINATION OF THE EYE

Ophthalmology is the science of the eye and its disorders and diseases. A physician who specializes in the diagnosis and treatment of disorders and diseases of the eye is an *ophthalmologist.* An ophthalmologist is a licensed medical physician who can diagnose eye disorders, prescribe medication, conduct eye screenings, prescribe glasses or contact lenses, and perform optic surgery. An *optometrist* is not a medical doctor, but he or she is licensed and has earned a degree as a Doctor of Optometry (OD). An optometrist can perform eye examinations, diagnose vision problems and eye diseases, prescribe ophthalmic medications, and treat visual defects through corrective

lenses and eye exercises. *Opticians* are trained to fill prescriptions written by ophthalmologists and optometrists for corrective lenses by grinding the lenses and dispensing eyewear.

Anatomy and Physiology of the Eye

The eyes are the smallest, yet the most detailed and complex, organs of the body. Each is located within a bony cavity (or *orbit*) in the skull. The bony orbit protects and supports the eye. Only approximately one sixth of the eye lies outside the orbit. The eyelid helps protect the eye from trauma. The eyebrows help keep irritants out of the eyes. The eyelashes line the margins of the eyelids and help trap foreign particles.

The conjunctiva is a thin mucous membrane that lines the eyelid and covers the outside of the eyeball except for the most central portion, which is covered by the cornea. The mucus secreted from the conjunctiva helps keep the eye moist. The eye blinks every 2 to 3 seconds, causing the lacrimal gland, located in the superior outer portion of the upper eyelid, to secrete tears. Tears move across the eyes, cleansing and moistening the surface, and drain into the lacrimal canals in the medial corner of the eye. The tears then drain into the nasal cavity through the nasolacrimal duct. Consequently, when a person cries, the excess tears ultimately empty into the nose, producing a watery nasal discharge.

The Eyeball

The eyeball consists of three layers. The outermost layer is made up of the white, opaque sclera and the transparent cornea. The sclera is a tough, fibrous lining that protects the entire eyeball lying within the orbit, whereas the transparent cornea covers the exposed one sixth of the eyeball. The cornea acts as a clear window that allows light to enter the eye. The cornea also *refracts,* or changes, the direction of light rays after they enter the eye. The cornea was one of the first tissues to be transplanted, and corneal transplants now are common. Long-term success after corneal implant surgery is excellent.

The choroid is the posterior portion of the middle layer of the eye. It is the eye's vascular layer, and it contains many blood vessels that supply nutrients to the outer layers of the retina. The choroid also has a brown pigment that absorbs excess light rays that could interfere with vision. In the anterior part of this layer, the choroid creates the iris and the ciliary body. The iris is the colored portion of the eye. It is doughnut shaped, with the opening of the pupil in the center. The iris contains muscles that regulate the size of the pupil according to the intensity of the light; it becomes smaller in bright light and opens wider in dim light. The ciliary body contains both the ciliary muscle, which regulates the shape of the lens, and the ciliary processes, which secrete aqueous humor.

The inner layer of the eye includes the retina in the posterior portion and the lens in the anterior portion. The **rods** and **cones**, **optic nerve**, **optic disc**, and **fovea centralis** are located in the retina. The delicate tissue of the retina is composed of light-sensitive neurons that convert light into neurologic impulses. These impulses travel by means of the optic nerve to the brain, where they are converted into a visual form. Any damage to the retina has the potential to cause partial or complete blindness because the neurologic center of vision is located in the retina.

The lens is a transparent, biconvex body that helps focus light after it passes through the cornea. The lens and the ciliary body divide the eye into two cavities. The posterior cavity, which is between the lens and the retina, contains the transparent, gel-like vitreous humor. Vitreous humor maintains the shape of the posterior eyeball. The anterior cavity, between the cornea and the lens, is filled with aqueous humor, which is continuously produced by the ciliary processes. Aqueous humor helps maintain normal pressure within the eye and provides nutrients to the lens and the cornea (Figure 30-1).

Vision

Vision requires light and depends on the proper functioning of all parts of the eye (Table 30-1). A visual impulse begins with the passage of light through the cornea, where the light is refracted; it then passes through the aqueous humor and the pupil into the lens. The ciliary muscle adjusts the curvature of the lens to again refract the light rays so that they pass into the retina, triggering the photo-receptor cells of the rods and cones. At this point, the light energy is converted into an electrical impulse, which is sent through the optic nerve to the visual cortex of the occipital lobe of the brain; there, the light impulse is interpreted and a picture is created.

Disorders of the Eye

Refractive Errors

Four major types of refractive errors result when the eye is unable to focus light effectively on the retina. *Refraction* is the ability of the lens of the eye to bend parallel light rays coming into the eye so that the rays are focused simultaneously on the retina. An *error of refraction* means that the light rays are not refracted or bent properly and

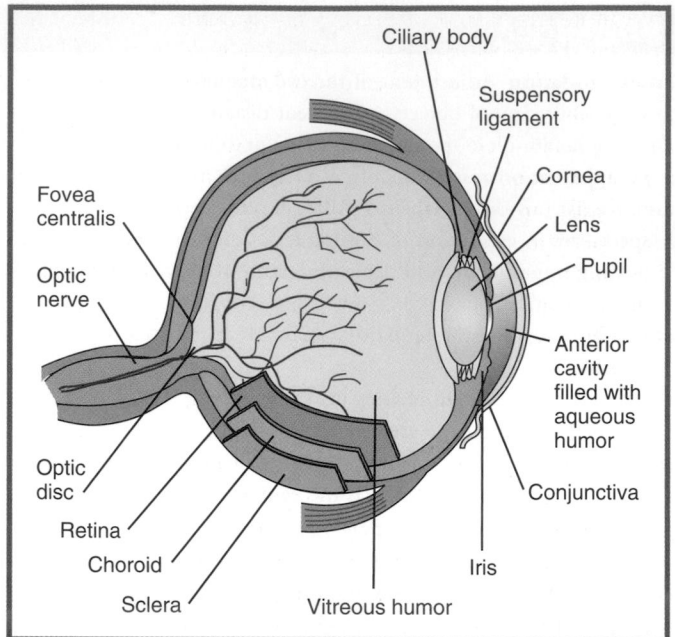

FIGURE 30-1 Anatomy of the eye.

TABLE 30-1 Functions of the Major Parts of the Eye	
STRUCTURE	**FUNCTION**
Sclera	External protection
Cornea	Light refraction
Choroid	Blood supply
Iris	Light absorption and regulation of pupil width
Ciliary body	Secretion of vitreous fluid; changes the shape of the lens
Lens	Light refraction
Retinal layer	Light receptor that transforms optic signals into nerve impulses
Rods	Distinguish light from dark and perceive shape and movement
Cones	Color vision
Central fovea	Area of sharpest vision
Macula lutea	Center of the retina; contains the fovea centralis, the area of most highly acute vision
External ocular muscles	Move the eyeball
Optic nerve	One of a pair of nerves that transmit visual stimuli to (cranial nerve II) the brain
Lacrimal glands	Produce tears
Eyelid	Protects eye

Modified from Damjanov I: *Pathology for the health-related professions,* Philadelphia, 1996, Saunders.

consequently do not focus correctly on the retina. Defects in the shape of the eyeball can cause a refractive error. Most refractive errors can be corrected with corrective lenses, contacts, or surgery (Figure 30-2).

Hyperopia (Farsightedness). When light enters the eye and focuses behind the retina, a person has *hyperopia.* This disorder occurs when the eyeball is too short from the anterior to the posterior wall. An individual with hyperopia has difficulty seeing objects that are close, at reading or working level. A convex corrective lens helps the eye's internal lens place objects directly on the retina and creates a sharp, detailed image, or refractive surgery may be done to correct the shape of the lens.

Myopia (Nearsightedness). *Myopia* occurs when light rays entering the eye focus in front of the retina, causing objects at a distance to appear blurry and dull. Objects viewed at reading or working level are seen clearly. In this disorder, the eyeball is elongated from the anterior to the posterior wall, and the image cannot be sharpened by the internal lens of the eye. A concave corrective lens is used to focus the light rays on the retina, or surgery can be done to change the shape of the cornea. However, the surgery is performed only on adults who have had a stable eye prescription for at least 1 year.

Presbyopia. As people age, the lens of the eye becomes less flexible, and the ciliary muscles weaken; consequently, changing the point of focus from distance to near becomes difficult. This is called *presbyopia.* The condition results in difficulty seeing at reading level. A combination corrective lens, known as a *bifocal lens* or a *progressive lens correction,* is used to focus both distal and proximal objects directly on the retina. Presbyopia actually starts at approximately age 10, but most people do not report an alteration in vision until their early forties. Conductive keratoplasty is a laser surgical procedure used to treat presbyopia.

Astigmatism. *Astigmatism* occurs when light rays entering the eye are focused irregularly. This usually occurs because the cornea or the lens is not a smooth sphere, but rather has an irregular shape. Ophthalmologists describe the lens as being shaped like a football rather than a sphere, such as a basketball. This causes light rays to be unevenly or diffusely focused on the retina, resulting in blurred vision. It is like attempting to focus on objects seen through a wavy piece of window glass. Astigmatism can be corrected with glasses, contacts, or surgery. Surgical correction attempts to reshape the cornea into a more spherical or uniformly curved surface.

Signs and Symptoms of Refractive Errors

Refractive errors in vision can lead to squinting, frequent rubbing of the eyes, and headaches. The individual notices blurred vision or fading of words at reading level, or both. Some refractive errors are familial in nature.

Treatment of Refractive Errors

Eyeglasses and contact lenses are the traditional treatments for visual acuity problems caused by refractive errors. However, problems with the shape of the lens can be corrected surgically. Surgery is performed on an outpatient basis and requires only a short stay in the facility. Medical assistants employed in an outpatient eye surgery facility must be trained to fulfill this specialized role.

CRITICAL THINKING APPLICATION   **30-1**

Amy is assisting Dr. Hanser with visual acuity examinations. He asks her whether she understands the causes of refractive errors. Amy has difficulty explaining why refractive errors occur, so she tells Dr. Hanser she will research the topic and get back to him. What have you learned about the different refractive disorders and why they occur?

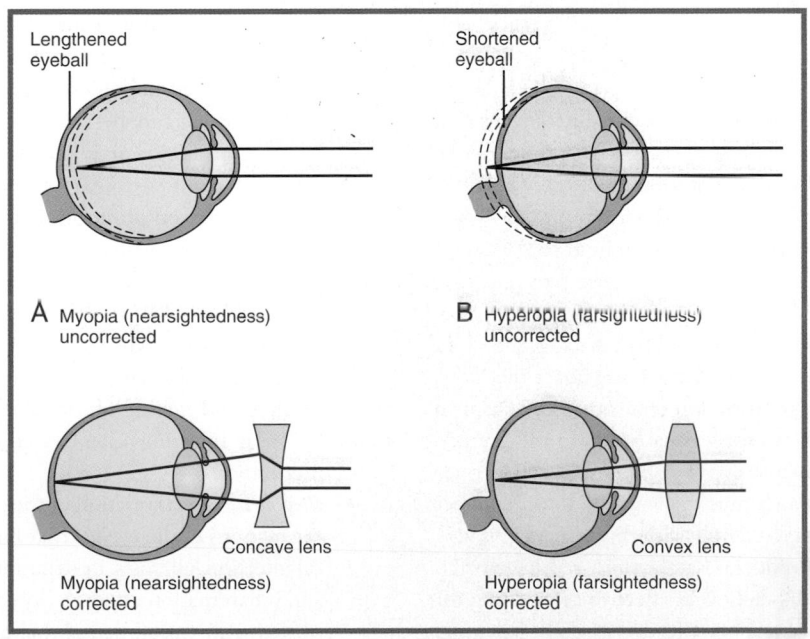

FIGURE 30-2 Errors in refraction. **A,** Myopia. **B,** Hyperopia.

Surgical Correction of Refractive Errors

Most types of health insurance do not cover surgery for refractive corrections. On average, each eye costs $1,500 to $2,200. The following are some of the surgical procedures performed to correct refractive errors.

- *Photorefractive keratectomy (PRK):* The first surgical procedure developed to reshape the cornea with a laser. The same type of laser is used for PRK and LASIK. The major difference between the two types of surgery is the way the middle layer of the cornea is exposed before it is vaporized with the laser. In PRK, the top layer of the cornea (the epithelium) is scraped away to expose the stromal layer underneath. In LASIK, a flap is cut in the stromal layer.

- *Laser-assisted in situ keratomileusis (LASIK):* LASIK uses an excimer laser to reshape the central cornea to treat myopia, hyperopia, and astigmatism. A thin, hinged flap of cornea is created, the flap is lifted, and the exposed surface of the cornea is reshaped. After the corneal curvature has been corrected, the flap is replaced, and the area heals without stitches.

- *Laser-assisted epithelium keratomileusis (LASEK):* In LASEK surgery, the surface epithelial cells of the eye are softened with an alcohol solution, allowing the epithelial layer to be rolled back and the cornea to be exposed. A laser then is used to reshape the cornea and treat myopia, hyperopia, and astigmatism. The epithelial flap is returned to its original position, and a contact lens is placed on the cornea as a bandage for several days to aid healing and reduce pain.

- *Conductive keratoplasty (CK):* CK uses heat created by a laser to reshape the cornea. Heat is applied to the cornea's outer edge to tighten and steepen the cornea. CK is used in patients older than 40 years of age who need correction for hyperopia, presbyopia, and myopia. The procedure causes little or no discomfort and improves vision almost instantly. The corneal changes are not permanent, and retreatment may be required.

Strabismus

Strabismus is failure of the eyes to track together, which means that both eyes do not look in the same direction at the same time. Adults can develop strabismus because of a condition or disease elsewhere in the body, such as diabetes mellitus, muscular dystrophy, or hypertension, or as the result of a head injury. In children, strabismus is caused by weakness in the muscles that control eye movement. If the condition appears in infancy or childhood, it is most commonly associated with **amblyopia**. Treatment involves having the child wear a patch over the unaffected eye so that the muscles of the "lazy" eye are strengthened and/or administration of atropine eye drops to the unaffected eye to medically decrease visual acuity in the "sound" eye, thereby forcing the amblyopic eye to compensate. It was once standard therapy that an eye patch must be worn up to 6 hours per day, but getting young children to comply with this treatment is very challenging. In children with moderate amblyopia, recent research shows that patching for 2 hours daily is as effective as patching for 6 hours daily, and daily atropine is as effective as daily patching.

Children older than 7 years may still benefit from patching or atropine, particularly if they have not previously received treatment for amblyopia. Amblyopia recurs in 25% of children after patching is discontinued; however, slowly reducing the amount of time the patch is worn each day at the end of treatment reduces the risk of recurrence. The main symptom in all age groups is *diplopia* (double vision).

Nystagmus

A constant, involuntary movement of one or both eyes is called *nystagmus*. The eye can move in any direction, and the movement is accompanied by blurred vision. A child may be born with the problem (congenital nystagmus), or the condition may be acquired as a result of a brain tumor, an inner ear lesion, multiple sclerosis, or substance abuse. Nystagmus is caused by an abnormal function in the part of the brain that controls eye movements. Congenital nystagmus is more common than acquired nystagmus, is usually milder, does not worsen over time, and is not associated with any other disorder. A patient with signs and symptoms of nystagmus should initially have a neurologic evaluation to determine the cause of the disorder, with treatment based on those findings. However, congenital nystagmus has no cure. Affected individuals typically are not aware of the eye movements, but they may have a decrease in visual acuity that can be corrected with surgery or corrective lenses.

Infections of the Eye

Many acute disorders of the eye are seen in the ophthalmologist's office. These include the following:

- *Hordeolum* (stye): A localized, purulent infection of a sebaceous gland of the eyelid. The area is inflamed, swollen, and painful. The infection usually is caused by staphylococci, and it is treated with warm compresses and topical or systemic antibiotics.

- *Chalazion:* A small cyst that results from blockage of a meibomian gland (sebaceous gland) that lubricates the posterior margin of each eyelid. The cyst can become infected, inflamed, swollen, and painful. It may disappear spontaneously or may need to be removed surgically.

- *Keratitis:* Inflammation of the cornea that results in superficial ulcerations. It can be caused by the herpes simplex virus, bacteria, or fungi, or it may develop as a result of corneal trauma (e.g., intense light). Symptoms include inflammation, tearing, pain, and **photophobia**. The condition is treated with ophthalmic ointments, eye drops, and use of an eye patch.

- *Conjunctivitis:* Inflammation of the conjunctiva caused by irritation, allergy, or bacterial infection. Bacterial conjunctivitis (pinkeye) is highly contagious and produces a purulent discharge. Symptoms include inflammation, swelling and itching of the sclera, photophobia, and tearing. Bacterial infections are treated with antibiotic ophthalmic preparations.

- *Blepharitis:* Inflammation of the glands and lash follicles along the margins of the eyelids that may be caused by staphylococcal infection, allergies, or irritation. Symptoms include itching and inflammation along the eyelash margins; the condition is treated with antibiotic ophthalmic ointment.

Disorders of the Eyeball

Corneal Abrasion

The cornea, the transparent outer covering of the eye, is prone to abrasion because of its location. Symptoms of corneal abrasion include pain, inflammation, tearing, and photophobia. The abrasion usually is caused by a foreign body in the eye or by direct trauma, such as from poorly fitting or dirty contact lenses. A corneal ulcer may form and become infected.

Diagnosis is based on the patient's signs and symptoms, but it can be confirmed with the instillation of fluorescein stain (Figure 30-3). After instillation of the stain, the provider uses a cobalt blue filtered light to visualize the abrasions, which appear green (Figure 30-4). If the abrasions are caused by a foreign body, it must be removed first; the eye then can be treated with antibiotic ophthalmic ointment to prevent infection. Although patching the affected eye has been recommended in the past, studies now show that patching does not reduce the patient's pain and may actually prolong healing time. Corneal abrasions are quite painful, so the patient may be prescribed topical nonsteroidal antiinflammatory ophthalmic drops, such as diclofenac (Voltaren) and ketorolac (Acular), in addition to oral analgesics. Most corneal abrasions heal in 24 to 72 hours, but the patient should be aware that symptoms can worsen if the affected

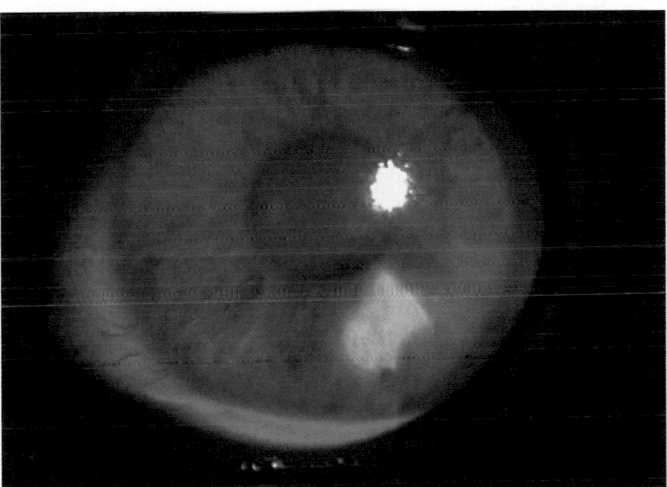

FIGURE 30-3 Corneal abrasion stained with fluorescein.

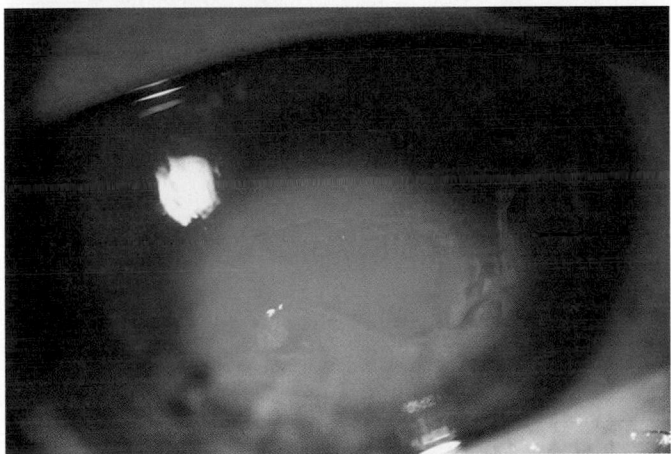

FIGURE 30-4 Corneal abrasion stained with fluorescein and highlighted by cobalt blue light.

eye is exposed to bright light, if excessive blinking occurs, or if the patient rubs the injured surface of the cornea against the inside of the eyelid. Because the patient may develop a secondary infection from the corneal injury, topical antibiotics, including ciprofloxacin 0.3% (Ciloxan) ointment or drops and gentamicin 0.3% ointment or drops, may be prescribed. Patients with contact lenses may be prescribed oral antibiotics and should not wear their contacts until the abrasion has healed and the course of antibiotics has been completed.

Cataract

A cataract is a cloudy or opaque area in the normally clear lens of the eye that blocks the passage of light into the retina, causing impaired vision. This condition may result from injury to the eye, exposure to extreme heat or radiation, or inherited factors. However, most cataracts develop slowly and progressively as a result of the natural aging deterioration of the lens of the eye and typically occur after age 60. With advanced cataracts, the pupil of the eye appears white or gray.

A cataract scatters the light as it passes through the lens, preventing a sharply defined image from reaching the retina resulting in blurred and dimmed vision. The patient may need a brighter reading light or must hold objects closer to the eyes for better viewing. Continued clouding of the lens may cause diplopia. The patient also needs frequent changes of eyeglass prescriptions. Patients with cataracts report difficulty with night vision (nyctalopia), seeing halo images around lights, and increased sensitivity to glare. If left untreated, cataracts ultimately can lead to blindness.

When the patient's vision becomes distorted or appears to be deteriorating, the ophthalmologist performs a *slit lamp* procedure, in which he or she examines the structures at the front of the eye using a combination of a low-power microscope and a high-intensity light that shines into the eye as a slit beam.

The symptoms of early cataract may be improved with new eyeglasses, brighter lighting, and antiglare sunglasses. If these measures do not help, surgical removal of the lens is the only effective treatment. This is performed as an outpatient procedure in a clinic or hospital. After the eye has been anesthetized, the inner portions of the lens (the nucleus and the cortex) are removed. The provider may use an extracapsular extraction, in which the cataract is removed in one piece, or phacoemulsification, in which an ultrasonic probe is used to break up the cataract and the pieces are aspirated, before an artificial intraocular lens (IOL) is implanted. The incision may be closed with fine sutures, or it may be sutureless and self-sealing. The procedure usually takes 15 minutes, and the patient typically can leave the facility after 1 hour. Patients should be aware that they will not be able to drive until cleared by the ophthalmologist, and that they may need help at home until their vision is clear.

The patient is seen in the office the day after surgery and as frequently as needed for the next month. Vision gradually improves until it stabilizes, usually within 2 to 6 weeks; the patient then is fitted with new corrective lenses to match the improved vision.

Glaucoma

One of the most common and serious ocular disorders is a group of diseases known as *glaucoma*. Glaucoma is characterized by increased intraocular pressure (IOP), which damages the optic nerve and causes blindness if left untreated. It rarely occurs in people younger than age 40 and usually is seen in individuals older than age 60. The cause is unknown, but a hereditary tendency toward development of the most common forms has been noted. Glaucoma is responsible for approximately 12% of all cases of blindness. After cataracts (which are typically age related and can be resolved surgically), glaucoma is the leading cause of blindness among African-Americans. It is estimated that more than 3 million Americans have glaucoma, but only half of those know they have it.

The ciliary body constantly produces aqueous humor, which should circulate freely between the anterior and posterior chambers of the eye and eventually empty into the general circulation. A healthy eye is filled with fluid in an amount carefully regulated to maintain the shape of the eyeball. In chronic open-angle glaucoma, the channels that drain the fluid malfunction, and over time aqueous humor builds up, resulting in increased pressure, which affects the blood supply to the retina and the optic nerve. With acute closed-angle glaucoma, the opening of the drainage system narrows or closes completely, causing a sudden increase in IOP (Figure 30-5).

Patients can have chronic open-angle glaucoma for a long time before symptoms occur. Early detection through regular ophthalmic examinations that include IOP measurements is crucial to prevent permanent vision loss. The need to change eyeglass prescriptions frequently, loss of peripheral vision (often called "tunnel vision"), mild headaches, and impaired adaptation to the dark are some of the signs and symptoms that may be seen with chronic glaucoma. Acute closed-angle glaucoma has more obvious symptoms; the patient complains of severe pain, headaches, inflammation, photophobia, and seeing halos around lights. If left untreated, acute glaucoma can cause permanent blindness in a matter of days (Figure 30-6).

Screening for glaucoma is conducted during a complete eye examination. The ophthalmologist first uses a **tonometer** with a slit lamp to measure IOP. The air puff tonometer records the degree of indentation of the cornea from a puff of pressurized air without touching the eye. An applanation tonometer records the pressure needed to indent the cornea when the instrument is applied to the front surface of the eye. Electronic tonometry is the most recently developed technique. The ophthalmologist gently places the rounded tip of a tool that looks like a pen directly on the cornea, with results evident on a small computer panel. **Gonioscopy** also can be used to examine the aqueous fluid drainage system and to determine whether the glaucoma is the open- or closed-angle type. In addition, an ophthalmoscopic examination can identify cupping of the optic disc, which indicates atrophy of the optic nerve.

Diagnosis and immediate treatment for early stage, open-angle glaucoma can delay progression of the disease. Open-angle glaucoma can be relieved with **miotic** and beta blocker eye drops. The combinations of drugs used to treat glaucoma can vary considerably. Miotic medications increase the outflow of aqueous humor, and beta blockers reduce the production of aqueous humor (Table 30-2). It is imperative that the patient use prescribed eye drops and take oral medications daily to prevent further damage to the optic nerve. Laser surgery may be performed to create an opening or to build a new channel for drainage of the aqueous humor. The goal of treatment in any type of glaucoma is to diagnose the disease early and to effectively treat its progression because any loss of sight that has occurred as the result of increased IOP cannot be regained. In closed-angle glaucoma, medications to lower IOP are prescribed so that surgery can be performed to create a channel in which aqueous fluid can circulate. This is a medical emergency because the pressure must be relieved within a few hours or permanent vision damage occurs.

Macular Degeneration

The macula lutea, the part of the retina near the optic nerve, defines the center of the field of vision. Macular degeneration is progressive deterioration of the macula lutea, which causes loss of central vision; the patient can see only the edges of the visual field (Figure 30-7).

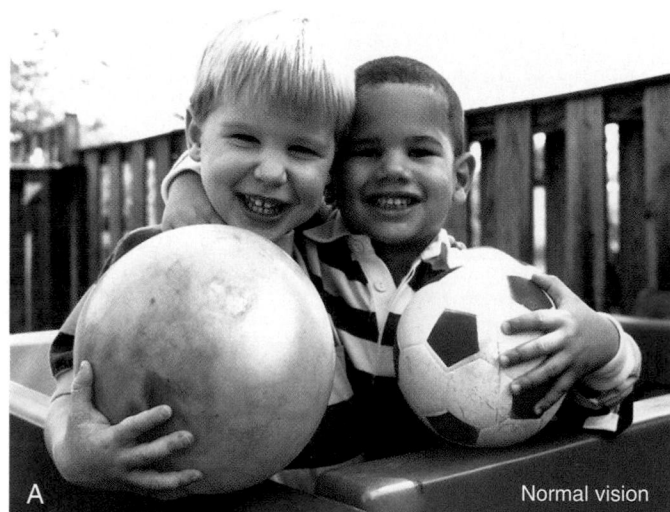

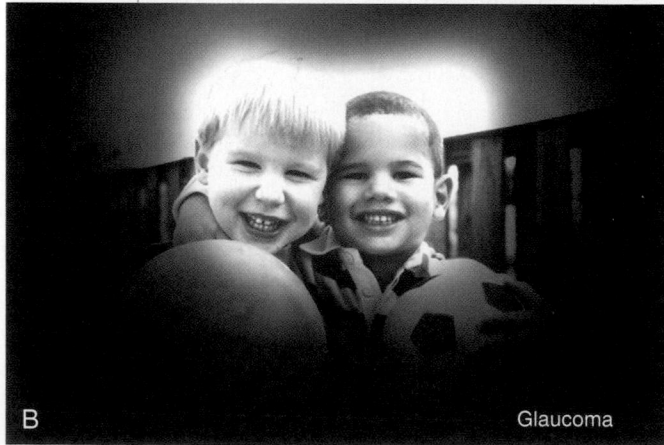

FIGURE 30-6 A, Normal vision. **B,** The same picture as seen by a person with glaucoma, showing loss of peripheral vision (i.e., "tunnel vision"). (From the National Eye Institute: Age-related macular degeneration: what you should know, National Institutes of Health, Bethesda, Md.)

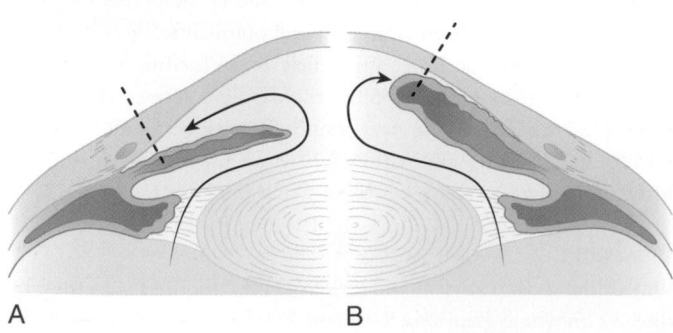

FIGURE 30-5 A, Open-angle glaucoma. **B,** Closed-angle glaucoma.

TABLE 30-2 Ophthalmic Medications

DRUG NAME	CLASS AND USE
Chloroptic, Ciloxan, erythromycin, Neosporin and Garamycin ung	Topical antibiotic ointments
Viroptic	Antiinfective, antiviral
AK-Pred, Durezol	Antiinflammatory agents, corticosteroids
Ocufen, Acular, Voltaren	Topical antiinflammatory agents, nonsteroidal antiinflammatory drugs, analgesics
Isopto Atropine, Cyclogyl	Mydriatic eye drops; eye examinations
Betoptic	Beta blocker eye drops; glaucoma treatment
Alphagan	Alpha-adrenergic agonist eye drops; glaucoma treatment
Rescula, Travatan, Lumigan	Prostaglandin analog eye drops; glaucoma treatment
Isopto Carpine, Pilocar	Miotic eye drops; glaucoma treatment
Alrex, Alocril, Zaditor	Treatment of seasonal allergies

ung, Unguent or ointment.

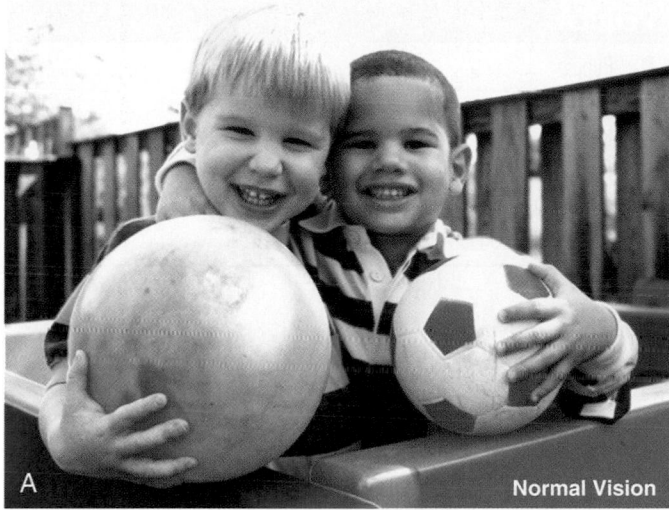

A Normal Vision

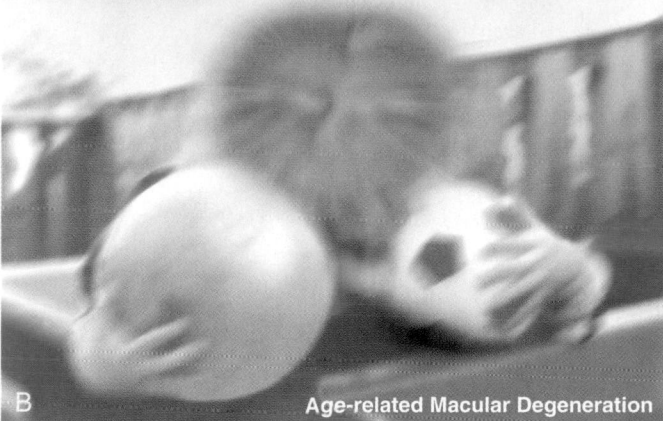

B Age-related Macular Degeneration

FIGURE 30-7 Visual field for a patient with macular degeneration. (From the National Eye Institute: Age-related macular degeneration: what you should know, National Institutes of Health, Bethesda, Md.)

The condition affects more than 10 million Americans and is a leading cause of blindness in those older than 50.

Two types of macular degeneration can occur. The dry form accounts for most cases; it is painless and develops slowly, affecting sharp vision over time, so that reading and other activities that require fine, detailed vision become impossible. Wet macular degeneration causes 90% of all severe vision losses from the disease and has a very acute onset and rapid progression. Dry macular degeneration is caused by the breakdown of light-sensitive cells in the region of the macula; the wet form is seen when new blood vessels behind the retina form and leak blood and fluid into the macula. The condition is age related, but additional risk factors include cigarette smoking, obesity, family history, cardiovascular disease, elevated blood cholesterol levels, light eye color, and excessive sun exposure. The disease has no known cure, but recent research indicates that antioxidants, including beta carotene and vitamins C and E with zinc and copper, may prevent the condition or may help treat the disease in people who have intermediate macular degeneration.

Diagnostic Procedures

A complete examination of the eye is technical and requires expensive equipment and the expertise of an ophthalmologist or optometrist. However, a primary care provider performs some basic examinations and treatments of the eye. The ophthalmoscope is used to examine the interior of the eye. It projects a bright, narrow beam of light through the lens and illuminates the interior parts of the eye and retina. It is helpful for detecting disorders of the eyes and certain systemic disorders, such as capillary changes that occur with diabetes mellitus.

The eyelids are examined for edema, which may be the result of nephrosis, heart failure, allergy, or thyroid deficiency. *Blepharoptosis,* also called *ptosis,* is drooping of the upper eyelid that can be caused by a disorder of the third cranial nerve, muscular weakness as seen in muscular dystrophy, or myasthenia gravis.

The pupils of the eyes are normally round and equal. Normal pupils constrict rapidly in response to light. This is demonstrated by shining a bright, pinpoint light into one eye from the side of the patient's head. The pupil of an illuminated eye constricts, and the pupil of the other eye constricts equally. This test is called *light and* **accommodation** (L&A). An older patient's eyes do not accommodate as well as those of a younger person. Each eye is checked this way. The patient then is asked to look at the provider's finger as it is moved directly toward the patient's nose to check for eye coordination. If the pupils are equal and round, respond normally to light, and adjust and focus on objects at different distances in a reasonable length of time, the provider charts the acronym PERRLA.

PERRLA

P	Pupils
E	Equal
R	Round
R	Reactive to
L	Light [and]
A	Accommodation

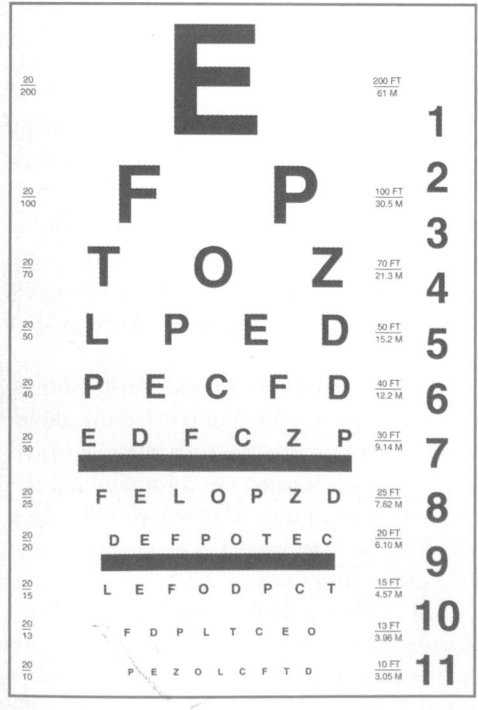

FIGURE 30-8 Slit lamp.

Special techniques used in the ophthalmologist's office include examinations performed with a slit lamp biomicroscope (Figure 30-8). This device is used to view fine details in the anterior segments of the eye. It may be used to view a foreign body because it gives a well-illuminated and highly magnified view of the area. For this examination, the provider first orders administration of a **mydriatic** eye drop to dilate the pupil and enhance visualization of eye structures.

A patient with *exophthalmia* (abnormal protrusion of the eye, possibly resulting from an overactive thyroid or a tumor behind the eyeball) is checked with an exophthalmometer. This instrument measures how far the eye protrudes beyond the edge of the eye socket and helps determine the level of tissue swelling and enlargement behind the eye.

Distance Visual Acuity

Determining distance visual acuity frequently is part of a complete physical examination (Procedure 30-1). It is widely used in schools and industry and is the best single test available for vision screening. Many cases of myopia, astigmatism, and hyperopia have been detected with this routine test. The chart most commonly used is the Snellen alphabetical chart (Figure 30-9, A). This chart displays various letters of the alphabet, which the patient must identify in ever smaller font sizes. Patients with limited knowledge of the English alphabet can be tested with the **E** chart (Figure 30-9, B). In addition, a chart that uses pictures as symbols is available. This chart is used for young children or individuals who do not know the alphabet (Figure 30-9, C). To avoid patient confusion over the **E** chart or the symbol chart, the medical assistant should review the

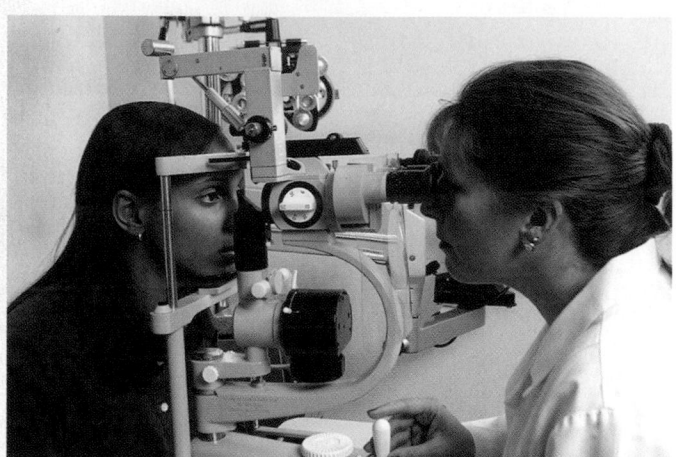

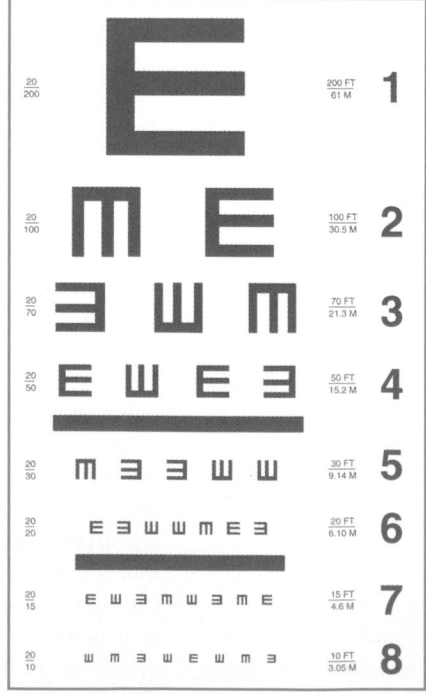

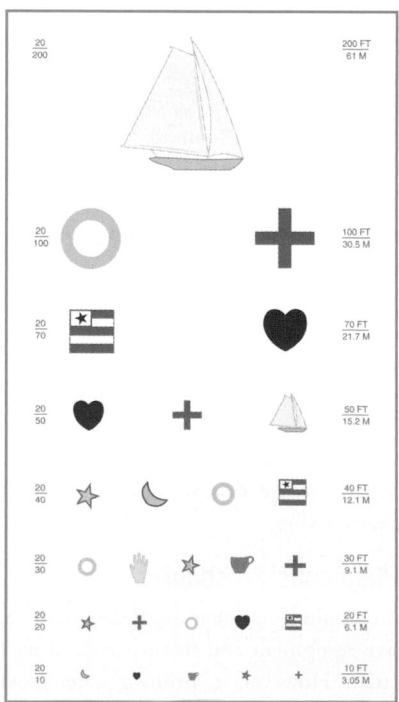

A   B   C

FIGURE 30-9 Different types of Snellen charts.

charts with patients first to make sure they know how to demonstrate the E visualized or the meaning of each picture or symbol. The symbol on the top line of the chart can be read at 200 feet by people with normal vision. In each of the succeeding rows, from the top down, the size of the symbols is reduced so that a person with normal vision can see them at distances of 100, 70, 50, 40, 30, and 20 feet, consecutively.

The patient must not be allowed to study the chart before taking the test. The room or hall should be long enough that the 20-foot distance can be marked off accurately and without interruptions from patient and staff traffic. The chart should be hung at the patient's eye level and illuminated with maximum light, without glare on the chart. Most adults do not need the standard Snellen chart explained, but if the E chart is used, an explanation must be given as to how the E's are to be read. The patient may point up or down or right or left toward the part of the letter that is open. If the E chart is to be used for a child, practice with an index card that has a large E drawn on it before the child is tested. Turn the card in different directions to simulate the position of the "fingers" of the E on the chart, and give the child the opportunity to demonstrate the direction of the E fingers by pointing his or her own fingers in the same direction (Figure 30-10).

Because this is a gross screening of distance visual acuity, the eyes typically are tested with corrective lenses; the patient therefore should not remove glasses or contact lenses unless the provider requests it. Indicate in the patient's health record whether the assessment was done with or without corrective lenses. Record the results of each eye separately and as fractions. The numerator (top number) is the distance of the patient from the chart (always 20 feet), and the denominator (bottom number) is the lowest line read satisfactorily by the patient. For example, if the patient reads the 20 line at 20 feet, the fraction 20/20 is recorded for that eye. *The last line the patient can read without squinting or straining and with no more than two mistakes is the line recorded in the patient's record for that eye.* The medical assistant should document the outcomes of the test, specifying the results for each eye and for both eyes. The Joint Commission no longer recommends the use of medical abbreviations for the eyes and ears because they are frequently confused or misinterpreted; therefore, the medical assistant must now document right eye, left eye, and both eyes.

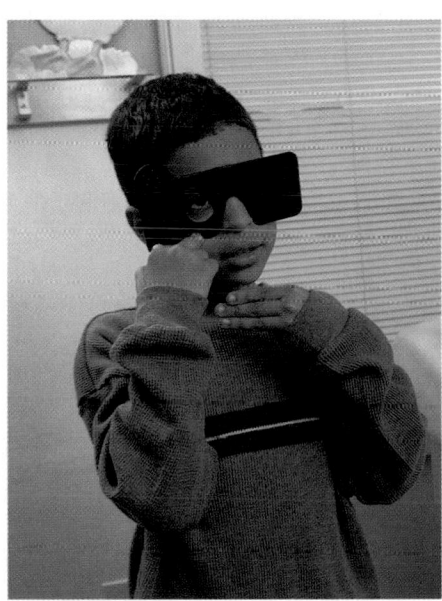

FIGURE 30-10 Visual acuity test with the E chart.

Interpreting Snellen Results

- The patient always stands 20 feet from the chart.
- Each result is a record of how well the patient can see compared with normal vision.
- Example: A patient with a 20/40 reading can see that line correctly standing at 20 feet, but an individual with normal vision can see the same line correctly at 40 feet, so the patient's vision is not as acute as someone with normal vision.
- Example: A patient with a 20/15 reading can see that line accurately standing at 20 feet, but a person with normal vision must stand at 15 feet to have the same vision, meaning the patient's vision is better than someone with normal vision.

CRITICAL THINKING APPLICATION   30-2

Susie Anthony, a 19-year-old patient, is seen today for a general eye examination. The provider orders a routine Snellen test, and Kim administers it. Susie wears contacts. With her right eye, she reads without errors to the 20/25 line; however, she squints and makes three errors at the 20/20 line. With her left eye, Susie makes two mistakes at the 20/30 line; with both eyes she reads the 20/25 without errors. How should Kim document this procedure?

PROCEDURE 30-1 | **Perform Patient Screening Using Established Protocols: Measure Distance Visual Acuity with the Snellen Chart**

Goal: *To determine the patient's degree of visual clarity at a measured distance of 20 feet using the Snellen chart.*

EQUIPMENT and SUPPLIES

- Patient's health record
- Provider's order

- Snellen eye chart
- Disposable eye occluder or an alcohol wipe to clean the occluder before use
- Pen or pencil and paper

PROCEDURE 30-1　—continued

PROCEDURAL STEPS

1. Sanitize your hands.
   PURPOSE: To ensure infection control.
2. Prepare the area. Make sure the room is well lit and that a distance marker is 20 feet from the chart.
3. Identify the patient by name and date of birth and explain the procedure. Instruct the patient not to squint during the test because this temporarily improves vision. The patient should not have an opportunity to study the chart before the test is given. If the patient wears corrective lenses, they should be worn during the test.
   PURPOSE: Explanations help gain the patient's cooperation and alleviate apprehension.
4. Position the patient in a standing or sitting position at the 20-foot marker.
   PURPOSE: Twenty feet is the standard testing distance.
5. Check that the Snellen chart is positioned at the patient's eye level.
6. If the occluder is not disposable, disinfect it before the procedure starts. Then, instruct the patient to cover the left eye with the occluder and to keep both eyes open throughout the test to prevent squinting (Figure 1).
   PURPOSE: Traditionally, the right eye is tested first.

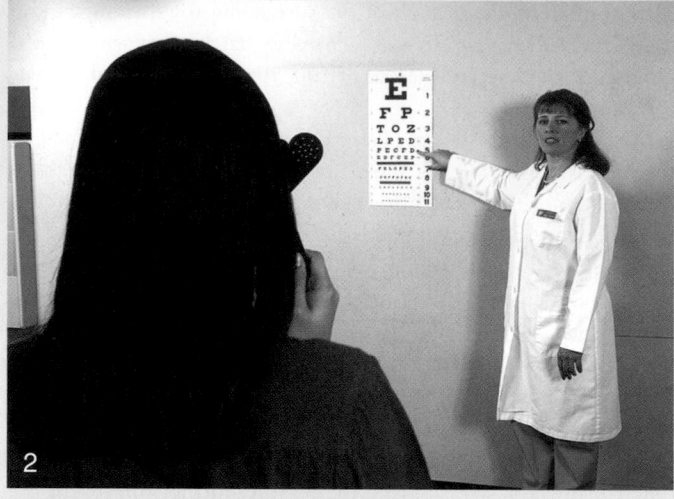

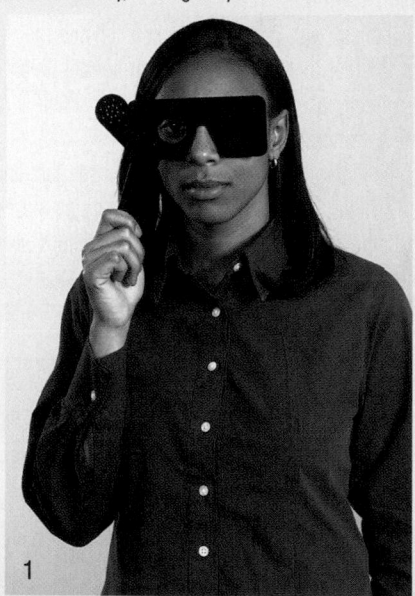

7. Stand beside the chart and point to each row as the patient reads it aloud, starting with the 20/70 row (Figure 2).
   PURPOSE: Starting with larger letters gives the patient confidence and allows for accommodation of vision.

8. Proceed down the rows of the chart until the smallest row the patient can read with a maximum of two errors is reached. If one or two letters are missed, the outcome is recorded with a minus sign and the number of errors (e.g., 20/40−2). If more than two errors are made, the previous line should be documented.
9. Record any of the patient's reactions while reading the chart.
   PURPOSE: Reactions such as squinting, leaning, tearing, or blinking may indicate that the patient is having difficulty with the test.
10. Repeat the procedure with the left eye, covering the right eye.
11. Repeat the procedure with both eyes uncovered.
12. Disinfect the occluder, if it is not disposable, and sanitize your hands.
    PURPOSE: To follow infection control procedures.
13. Document the procedure in the patient's record, including the date and time, visual acuity results, and any reactions by the patient. Also record whether corrective lenses were worn.
    PURPOSE: Procedures that are not recorded are considered not done.

Documentation Exercise: The medical assistant conducted a Snellen exam on Carlene Anderson, who wears contacts. The results were: right eye 20/60; left eye 20/30, but she missed one letter at the 20/30 line; both eyes 20/40. Carlene did not squint or strain during the exam.

Correct Documentation:
8/01/20− 2:20 PM: Visual acuity completed c̄ Snellen chart. Right eye 20/60, left eye 20/30−1, both eyes 20/40 c̄ corrective lenses. No squinting noted. Kim Tau, CMA (AAMA)

Near Visual Acuity

Near visual acuity can be tested with the near vision acuity chart (Figure 30-11). This test is given to screen for presbyopia or hyperopia. If the patient wears corrective lenses, they should be worn during the test. The size of the type on the card varies from newspaper headlines to print similar to that found in telephone books. The test should be given in a well-lit room, with the patient holding the card approximately 14 to 16 inches away. As with the Snellen examination, the near visual acuity test is given for each eye, starting with the right eye. The eye not being tested should be covered with an occluder but left open. The patient should be monitored for indications of difficulty, such as squinting or tearing. The patient reads the card, starting at the top, until reaching the smallest print that can be read. The medical assistant should document the number at

```
                          60

Nothing can take the place of "the only
pair of eyes you will ever have." That is
why you are exercising such good
judgment in taking care of them as you
are now doing.

                          50

For this reason, you will welcome the suggestion
about lenses which are designed and made to
give you "greater comfort and better appearance."
In man's earliest days he had little use for glasses.
He used his eyes chiefly for long distance.

                          40

He worked by daylight and at tasks with little detail. But
now, you use your eyes for much close work—reading,
writing, sewing and many other uses which the eyes of
primitive man did not know. Now your eyes meet all
sorts of lighting conditions, artificial and natural.

                          30

Many of these conditions produce "overbrightness" or glare.
Sometimes it is the direct or reflected glare of sunlight; often it
is direct or reflected from artificial light. And very often this
glare is uncomfortable—impairs your efficiency. But special
lenses, developed by America's leading optical scientists,
combat this glare.

                          25

These lenses give you more            commend them because they will
comfortable vision and blend          give you greater comfort and
harmoniously with your com-           better appearance. Thousands of
plexion. These lenses are less        satisfied wearers testify to their
conspicuous. We are glad to rec-      real benefits.

                          20

You are wise in taking good care of "the     suggestion about lenses which are
only pair of eyes you will ever have."        designed and made to give you "greater
You know how valuable they are, that          comfort and better appearance." In
you can never have another pair. For          man's earliest days he had little use for
this reason, you will welcome the             glasses.

         The above letters subtend the visual angle of 5' at the designated distance in inches.
```

FIGURE 30-11 Near vision acuity chart.

which the patient had no more than two errors for each eye and also the two eyes together; whether corrective lenses were worn; and any signs of eye strain.

Ishihara Color Vision Test

Defects in color vision are classified as congenital or acquired. Congenital defects are caused by an inherited color vision defect and are found most often in males. Acquired defects are caused by eye injury or disease. The Ishihara test is a simple, convenient, and accurate procedure that detects total color-blindness, in addition to the red-green blindness prevalent in congenital blindness (Procedure 30-2). The test assesses the perception of primary colors and shades of colors.

The test booklet contains polychromatic plates made up of colored dots in numeric patterns. The numbers are one color, and the background dots are a different color. Patients with average visual acuity can read the number within the dot matrix without difficulty. Patients with color vision defects are unable to read the number, or they see a totally different number. A section of plates is included that contains colored line trails through a background of dots. These plates are designed to be used with children and adults who are unable to read numbers. In this situation, the patient uses a finger to follow the dotted trail through the picture.

The test should be administered in a quiet room that is well illuminated by sunlight, not by artificial lighting. If this is not possible, create the best situation possible by adjusting lights to resemble the effect of natural daylight. The test uses 14 color plates. The basic test consists of plates 1 through 11. Plates 12 through 14 are used if the patient appears to be having difficulty with red-green differentiations. The medical assistant records the number of plates read correctly. If the score is 10 or higher, the patient is within the average range. If the score is 7 or lower, the patient is suspected of having a color deficiency, and the ophthalmologist performs additional assessment tests using more precise color vision testing equipment.

| PROCEDURE 30-2 | **Instruct and Prepare a Patient for a Procedure: Assess Color Acuity Using the Ishihara Test** |

Goal: *To assess a patient's color acuity correctly and record the results.*

EQUIPMENT and SUPPLIES

- Patient's health record
- Provider's order
- Room with natural light if possible
- Ishihara color plate book
- Pen, pencil, and paper
- Watch with a second hand

PROCEDURAL STEPS

1. Assemble the equipment and prepare the room for testing. The room should be quiet and illuminated with natural light.
   <u>PURPOSE</u>: Natural light is needed to test colors correctly.

2. Check the provider's order. Then introduce yourself and verify the patient's identity by name and date of birth. Explain the procedure. Use a practice card during the explanation and make sure the patient understands that he or she has 3 seconds to identify each plate.
   <u>PURPOSE</u>: To make sure you have the right patient. Also, an informed patient is a cooperative patient. The first plate is a practice plate and is designed to be read correctly.

PROCEDURE 30-2 *—continued*

3. Hold up the first plate at a right angle to the patient's line of vision and 30 inches from the patient. Be sure both of the patient's eyes are kept open during the test (Figure 1).

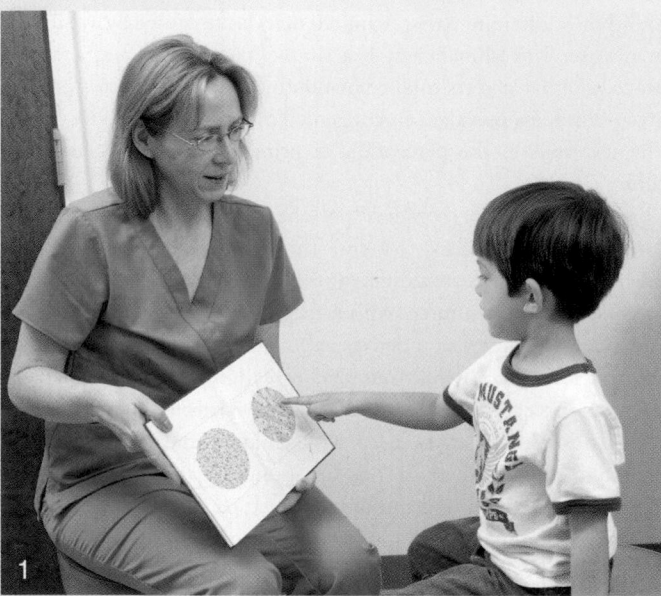

4. Ask the patient to tell you the number on the plate. Record the plate number and the patient's answer (Figure 2).

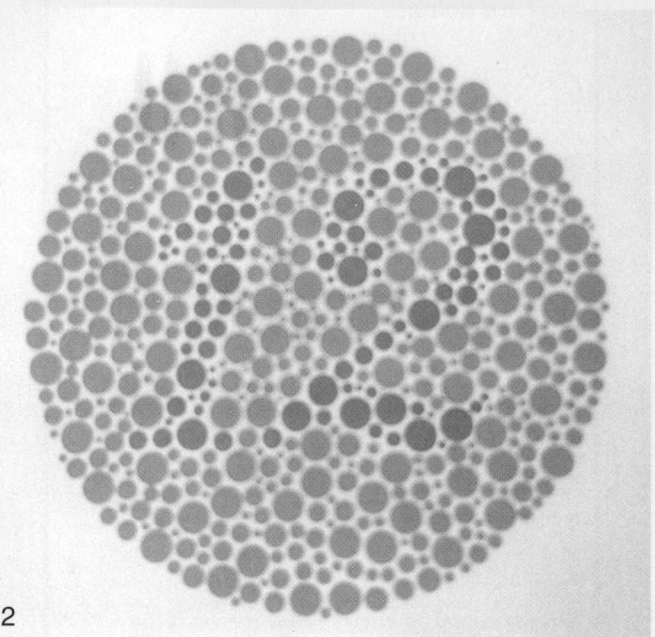

5. Continue this sequence until all 11 plates have been read. If the patient cannot identify the number on the plate, place an X in the record for that plate number. Your record should look like this:
   Plate 1 = pass, Plate 2 = pass, Plate 3 = X, Plate 4 = pass, and so on.
6. Include any unusual symptoms in your record, such as eye rubbing, squinting, or excessive blinking.
7. Place the book back in its cardboard sleeve and return it to its storage space.
   <u>PURPOSE</u>: The Ishihara color plates must be stored in a closed position away from external light to protect the colors.
8. Document the procedure in the patient's health record, including the date and time, the testing results, and any patient symptoms shown during the test.
   <u>PURPOSE</u>: Procedures that are not recorded are considered not done.

Treatment Procedures

Eye Irrigation

The eye is irrigated to relieve inflammation, remove drainage, dilute chemicals, or wash away foreign bodies. Sterile technique and equipment must be used to prevent contamination (Procedure 30-3). Follow the procedure as ordered, making sure the patient is comfortable. Record the treatment in the patient's health record immediately after it has been determined. Remember, if it is not recorded, it has not been done.

Foreign bodies in the eye are very irritating and may cause considerable pain. Most foreign bodies are superficial and can be removed easily. Occasionally, a foreign particle may be deeply embedded, requiring eye surgery. Notify the provider immediately if a patient comes into the office with something in his or her eye.

The first objective of the provider's examination is inspection. The patient is asked to look to either side and up and down so that the anterior surface of the eye can be inspected. For the provider to fully inspect under the upper lid, the patient must cooperate by looking downward while the provider **everts** the upper lid using a cotton-tipped applicator. While the lid is maintained in an everted position, any foreign materials may be rinsed away with sterile water or saline solution. If the provider's order is for you to remove the foreign body, do so with irrigation only. If this technique is unsuccessful, cover both of the patient's eyes with a gauze dressing and notify your supervisor immediately. The eyes track each other, so to prevent movement in the affected eye, both eyes must be covered to prevent possible eye trauma.

Safety Alert

Never attempt to remove a foreign body from the cornea using a cotton-tipped applicator. Scratches to the cornea may result, causing scar formation and impaired vision.

CRITICAL THINKING APPLICATION   30-3

The provider tells Kim to irrigate the left eye of a 22-year-old patient to remove a foreign body. She is to irrigate the eye with sterile normal saline solution until clear. How should Kim document this procedure?

PROCEDURE 30-3   Instruct and Prepare a Patient for a Procedure or Treatment: Irrigate a Patient's Eyes

Goal: *To cleanse one or both eyes as ordered by the provider.*

EQUIPMENT and SUPPLIES

- Patient's health record
- Provider's order
- Prescribed sterile irrigation solution
- Sterile irrigating bulb syringe and sterile basin or prepackaged solution with dispenser
- Basin for drainage
- Sterile gauze squares
- Disposable drape
- Towel
- Nonsterile disposable gloves
- Biohazard waste container

PROCEDURAL STEPS

1. Sanitize your hands.
   PURPOSE: To ensure infection control.
2. Check the provider's orders to determine which eye requires irrigation (or whether both eyes require it) and the type of solution to be used.
3. Assemble the materials needed.
4. Check the expiration date of the solution. Follow medication safety procedures and check the label of the solution three times: (1) when you remove it from the shelf; (2) when you pour it; and (3) when you return it to the shelf.
   PURPOSE: To follow the rules for safely administering medications.
5. Identify the patient by name and date of birth and explain the procedure.
   PURPOSE: To make sure you have the right patient. Also, explanations help gain the patient's cooperation and ease apprehension.
6. Assist the patient into a sitting or supine position, making sure that the head is turned toward the side of the affected eye. Place the disposable drape over the patient's neck and shoulder.
   PURPOSE: This position causes the solution to flow away from the unaffected eye, reducing the chance of cross-contamination of the healthy eye.
7. Put on gloves and rinse your gloved hands under warm water to remove all powder from the gloves, or wear powder-free gloves.
   PURPOSE: Gloves help hold the eye open, but powder may irritate the eyes.

8. Place (or have the patient hold) a drainage basin next to the affected eye to receive the solution from the eye. Place a poly-lined drape under the basin to prevent the solution from getting on the patient.
9. Moisten a gauze square with solution and cleanse the eyelid and lashes. Start at the inner canthus (near the nose) and move to the outer canthus (farthest from the nose). Dispose of the gauze square in the biohazard waste container after each wipe (Figure 1).
   PURPOSE: Debris on the lids or lashes must be cleaned away before the conjunctiva is exposed.

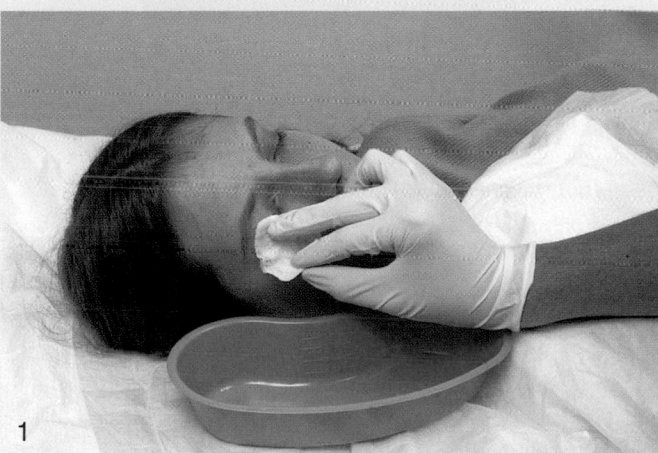

1

10. If you are using a bulb syringe, pour the required volume of room-temperature irrigating solution into the basin and draw the solution into the bulb syringe. If an irrigating solution in a prepackaged dispenser is used, remove the lid.
    PURPOSE: Cold solution causes the patient pain and discomfort
11. Separate and hold the eyelids with the index finger and thumb of one hand. With the other hand, place the syringe or dispenser on the bridge of the nose parallel to the eye.
    PURPOSE: To support and steady the dispenser.

PROCEDURE 30-3   —continued

12. Squeeze the bulb or dispenser, directing the solution toward the lower conjunctiva of the inner canthus; allow the solution to flow steadily and slowly from the inner to the outer canthus. Do not touch the eye or eyelids with the applicator (Figure 2).
PURPOSE: To prevent possible injury to the eye.

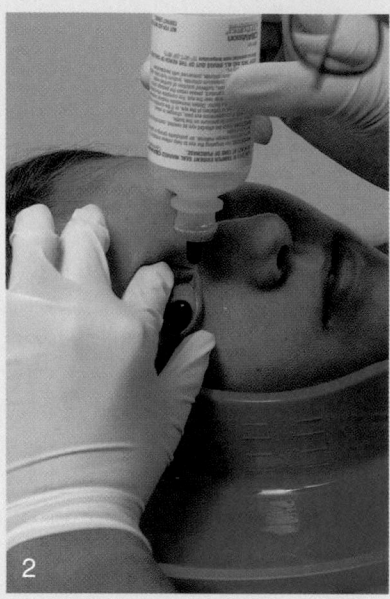

13. Refill the syringe or continue to gently squeeze the prepackaged bottle, and continue the procedure until the amount of solution ordered by the provider has been administered or until drainage from the eye is clear.
14. Dry the eyelid with sterile gauze, moving from the inner canthus to the outer canthus. Do not use cotton balls because fibers might remain in the eye.
15. Dispose of the irrigation results and disinfect the work area.
16. Remove your gloves, dispose of them in the biohazard waste container, and sanitize your hands.
PURPOSE: To ensure infection control.
17. Document the procedure in the patient's health record; include the date and time, the type and amount of solution used, which eye was irrigated, any significant reactions by the patient, and the results.
PURPOSE: Procedures that are not recorded are considered not done.

DOCUMENTATION EXERCISE

Eye irrigations until clear are ordered for Toby Kramer because of sand in both eyes. You use 50 mL of irrigation solution in the right eye and 125 mL in the left eye. After the procedure is complete, the sclera appears red, and Toby complains of irritation in both eyes.

Correct Documentation:
8/06/20– 9:00 AM: Right eye irrigated c̄ 50 mL normal saline sol and left eye c̄ 125 mL. Postprocedure sclera appears inflamed and pt c/o bilateral irritation. Kim Tau, CMA (AAMA)

Instillation of Eye Medication

Medication may be instilled into the eye to treat an infection, soothe an eye irritation, anesthetize the eye, or dilate the pupils before examination or treatment (Procedure 30-4). Ophthalmic medications are available in several forms. Liquid drops usually are supplied in small squeeze bottles with tips that allow one drop at a time to be dispensed, or the bottle may contain a dropper with a small rubber attachment used to dispense the medication by drops. Eye ointments are dispensed in small metal or plastic tubes with an ophthalmic tip that allows them to be dispensed in a small ribbon of ointment directly into the bottom eyelid (see Table 30-2).

Safety Alert

Whatever the medication, the dispenser should never touch the eye while the prescribed amount of medication is administered. This can traumatize the eye and can contaminate the medication applicator. If the tip of the dispenser touches any surface, dispose of it in a biohazard waste container because it is contaminated.

CRITICAL THINKING APPLICATION   30-4

Amy is ordered to administer Xalatan, 1 drop each eye, to a 75-year-old patient recently diagnosed with glaucoma. How should Amy document this procedure?

PROCEDURE 30-4   Instruct and Prepare a Patient for a Procedure or Treatment: Instill an Eye Medication

Goal: *To apply medication to one or both eyes as ordered by the provider.*

EQUIPMENT and SUPPLIES

- Patient's health record
- Provider's order
- Sterile medication with sterile eye dropper or ophthalmic ointment

- Disposable drape
- Sterile gauze squares
- Disposable nonsterile gloves
- Biohazard waste container

PROCEDURE 30-4 —*continued*

PROCEDURAL STEPS

1. Sanitize your hands.
   PURPOSE: To ensure infection control.
2. Check the provider's order to determine which eye requires medication (or whether medication is ordered for both eyes) and the name and strength of the medication to be used.
   PURPOSE: To prevent a medication error.
3. Assemble the equipment and supplies.
4. Check the expiration date of the solution. Follow medication safety procedures and check the label of the medication three times: (1) when you remove it from the shelf; (2) when you pour it; and (3) when you return it to the shelf.
   PURPOSE: To follow the rules for safely administering medications.
5. Introduce yourself, identify the patient by name and date of birth, and explain the procedure.
   PURPOSE: To make sure you have the right patient. Also, explanations help gain the patient's cooperation and ease apprehension.
6. Put on nonsterile gloves and rinse your gloved hands under warm water to remove all powder from the gloves or wear powder-free gloves.
   PURPOSE: Gloves help hold the eye open, but powder may irritate the eyes.
7. Assist the patient into a sitting or supine position. Ask the patient to tilt the head backward and look up.
   PURPOSE: Looking up helps prevent the applicator's tip from touching the cornea. It also helps keep the patient from blinking as the medication is instilled. For eye drops, draw the medication into the dropper. For an eye ointment, remove the cap.
8. Pull the lower conjunctival sac downward (Figure 1).
   PURPOSE: To create a pocket for the medication.

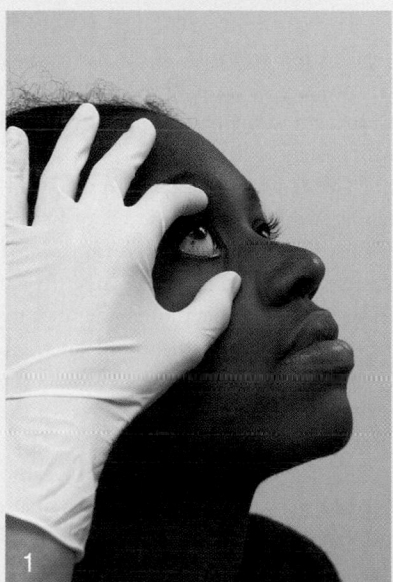

9. Administer the prescribed number of drops or amount of ointment into the eye. For eye drops, place the drops in the center of the lower conjunctival sac, with the tip of the dropper held parallel to the eye and $\frac{1}{2}$ inch above the eye sac. For eye ointment (ung), squeeze a thin ribbon along the lower conjunctival sac from the inner canthus to the outer canthus, making sure not to touch the eye with the applicator.
   PURPOSE: Placing the medication in the conjunctival sac rather than on the eyeball prevents injury to the cornea. Touching the eye with the applicator could injure the eye and contaminates the applicator (Figure 2).

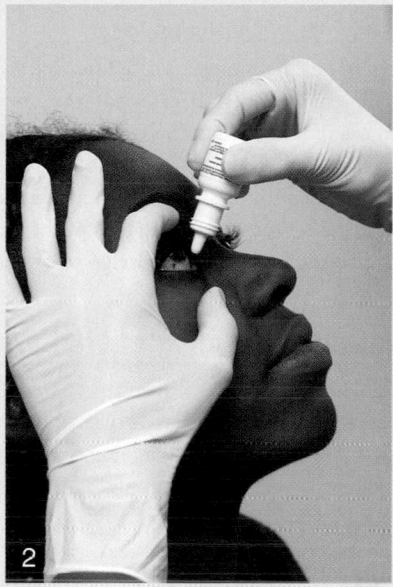

10. Instruct the patient to close the eye gently and rotate the eyeball.
    PURPOSE: Gently closing the eye prevents the medication from being dispelled, and rotating the eyeball distributes the medication evenly (Figure 3).

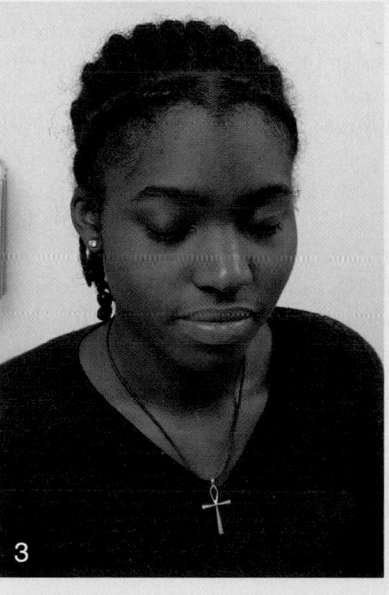

PROCEDURE 30-4   *—continued*

11. Dry any excess drainage from the inner canthus to the outer canthus, and explain that the medication may temporarily blur vision.
12. Discard the unused medication, and disinfect the procedure area.
13. Remove your gloves, dispose of them in the biohazard waste container, and sanitize your hands.
    PURPOSE: To ensure infection control.
14. Record the procedure in the patient's health record, including date and time, name and strength of the medication, dose administered, eye

treated, teaching instructions given (if treatment is to continue at home), and any observations.
PURPOSE: Procedures that are not recorded are considered not done.

8/8/20– 1:45 PM: Thin ribbon of Neosporin ophthalmic ung applied in lower conjunctival sac of right eye. No pt complaints. Pt instructed on home care application of med, including washing hands before and after procedure and taking care not to touch eye c̄ applicator. Kim Tau, CMA (AAMA)

Aseptic Procedures in Ophthalmology

A major concern in ophthalmologic procedures is the contamination of eye medication applicators. Because of the concern of cross-contamination, use of stock ophthalmic medications is discouraged. The sterility of all eye medications is critical for good patient care. Newly opened sterile solutions should be used for each patient and should be discarded after instillation or given to the patient for home use. All instruments used to remove a foreign body should be sterile.

EXAMINATION OF THE EAR

Otorhinolaryngology is the medical specialty that deals with the ear, nose, and throat. It frequently is referred to as *otolaryngology* or even as a single specialty of otology or laryngology. Usually, the specialty otorhinolaryngology is referred to simply as *ear, nose, and throat* (ENT).

Anatomy and Physiology of the Ear

The visible portion of the ears is only a small part of the actual organ of hearing. Most of this structure lies hidden in the temporal bone. Anatomically, the organ of hearing is divided into three sections: the outer ear, the middle ear, and the inner ear (Figure 30-12).

Outer (External) Ear

The outer ear consists of the auricle, or pinna, the fleshy part of the ear that can be seen on the side of the head, and the external auditory canal, the tube that extends from the auricle to the tympanic membrane (eardrum).

The auricle collects sound waves and sends them down the auditory canal. The skin that lines the auditory canal contains numerous hair follicles and many nerve endings, in addition to ceruminous glands that secrete cerumen (commonly called *earwax*), which lubricates the canal. Both the hair and the waxy cerumen help prevent foreign objects from reaching the eardrum. The canal has a slight S shape and is approximately 1 inch (2.5 cm) long.

Middle Ear

The middle ear, sometimes called the *tympanic cavity,* is an air-filled chamber that begins with the tympanic membrane and terminates at the oval window. The middle ear contains the auditory ossicles or bones: malleus, incus, and stapes. These three tiny bones are linked by minute ligaments to form a bridge across the space of the

tympanic cavity. The malleus is next to the tympanic membrane, and the stapes is against the oval window. The eustachian tube opens into the middle ear cavity and connects to the nasopharynx. It is designed to equalize pressure in the middle ear with that in the external auditory canal. This equalized pressure makes hearing possible. Upper respiratory infections may spread to the middle ear through the eustachian tube; this is a very common occurrence in young children.

The tympanic membrane is a thin, disk-shaped tissue that seals off the outer ear from the middle ear. Sound waves conducted through the external auditory canal hit this membrane and cause it to vibrate. These vibrations are picked up by the three ossicles and are changed from air-conducted sound waves to bone-conducted sound waves. The ossicles transmit the bone-conducted sound waves through the middle ear to the oval window, which is the membrane that connects the middle ear and the inner ear. At the oval window, the sound waves move into the fluids of the inner ear. This fluid motion excites the receptors, changing the bone-conducted sound into sensorineural impulses.

Inner Ear

The inner ear, called the *labyrinth,* is divided into the cochlea and the semicircular canals, which are joined by the vestibule. The semicircular canals function to maintain equilibrium, and the cochlea is responsible for the sense of hearing.

The organ of Corti, which contains the receptors for sound, is located within the cochlea. It is made up of hairlike sensory cells surrounded by sensory nerve fibers that form the cochlear branch of the eighth cranial nerve. Sound impulses cause the hairs to bend and rub against the nerve fibers, which initiate stimuli to travel through the cochlear nerve into the brain for sound interpretation.

The eighth cranial nerve transmits auditory impulses to the medulla oblongata. These impulses then travel to the thalamus and on to the auditory cortex of the temporal lobe of the brain, where they are interpreted into audible sound and speech patterns.

The semicircular canals are responsible for evaluating the position of the head in relation to the pull of gravity. The three canals are positioned at right angles to one another, on different planes (Figure 30-13). When the head turns rapidly, these fluid-filled canals must rapidly adjust and send the stimulated change into the central nervous system, which interprets the information and initiates the desired response to maintain balance. With repetitive or excessive

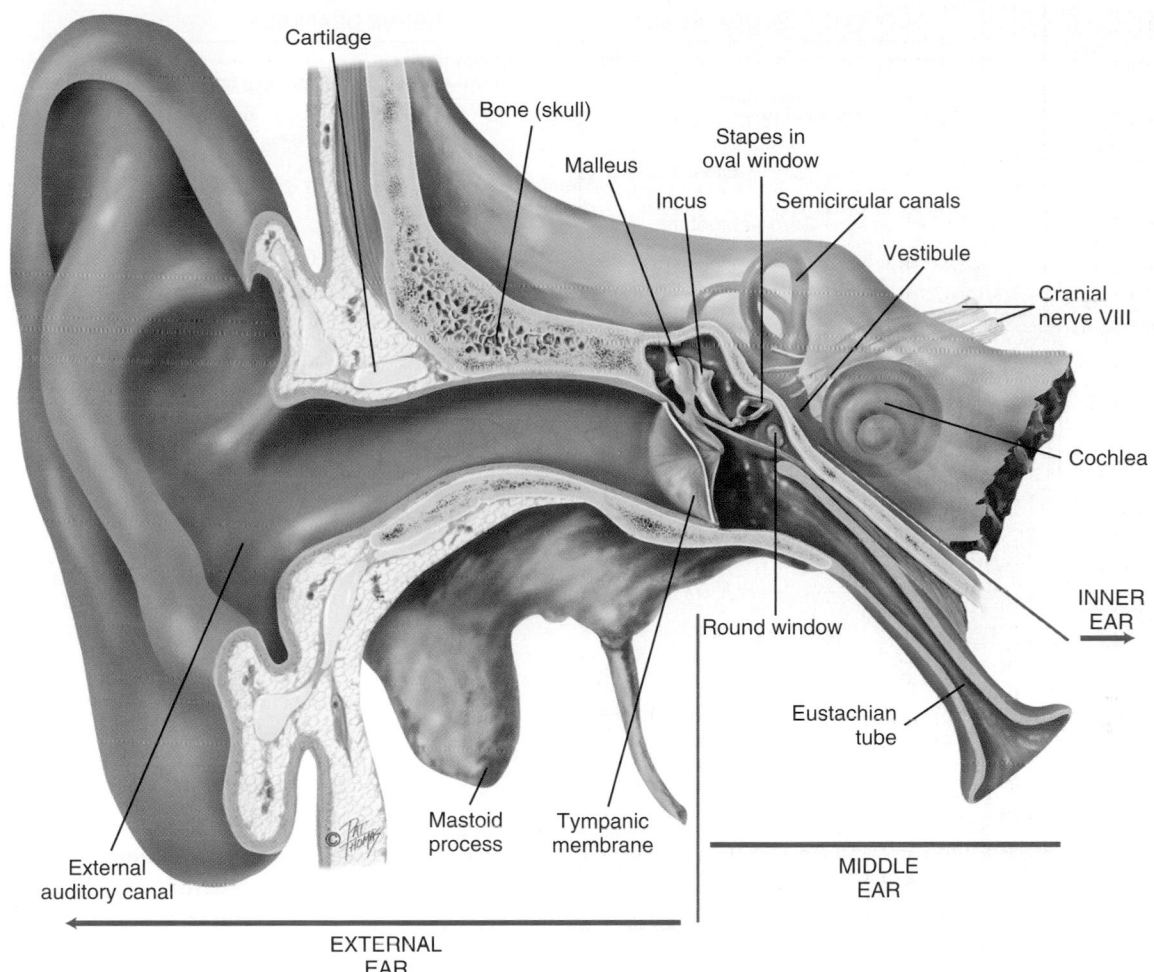

FIGURE 30-12 Anatomy of the ear. (From Jarvis C: *Physical examination and health assessment*, ed 7, Philadelphia, 2016, Saunders.)

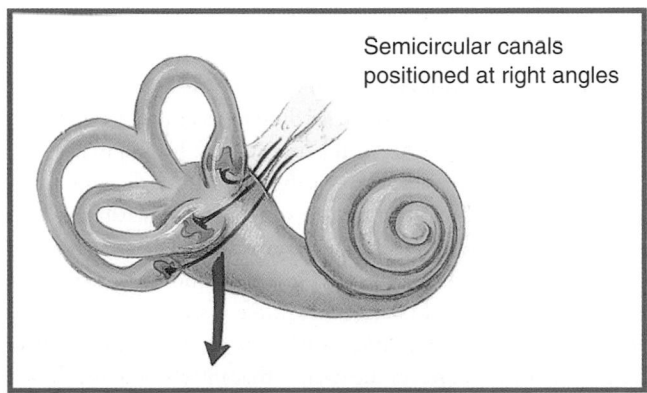

Semicircular canals
positioned at right angles

FIGURE 30-13 Semicircular canals. (From Applegate EJ: *The anatomy and physiology learning system*, ed 4, Philadelphia, 2011, Saunders.)

stimulation to the equilibrium receptors, some people become nauseated and may vomit. This condition is known as *motion sensitivity* or *motion sickness*.

Disorders of the Ear

Hearing Loss

Two problems result in hearing loss: a conduction problem and a sensorineural impairment. Some individuals have both conditions.

Conductive hearing loss is caused by a problem originating in the external or middle ear that prevents sound vibrations from passing through the external auditory canal, limits the vibration of the tympanic membrane, or interferes with the passage of bone-conducted sound in the middle ear. Some common causative factors in conductive hearing loss include impacted cerumen; trauma to the tympanic membrane, especially with scar formation; hemorrhage or fluid in the middle ear; **otosclerosis**; and recurrent chronic ear infections. Patients with conductive hearing loss receive the greatest benefit from a hearing aid. If the hearing loss is caused by a malfunction or congenital abnormality of the ossicles, a surgical procedure can be performed to replace the damaged ossicles with manufactured models.

A sensorineural hearing loss results from an abnormality of the organ of Corti or of the auditory nerve. Viral infection (e.g., rubella, influenza, herpes) can result in hearing loss, as can head trauma or certain **ototoxic** medications. The first sign of ototoxic drug complications usually is *tinnitus*, a ringing in the ears. This sometimes occurs with high doses of aspirin, certain antibiotics (erythromycin and vancomycin), and chemotherapeutic agents. A sensorineural hearing loss also can occur because of prolonged exposure to loud noise, such as repetitive noise in the workplace, or loud music, which damages the delicate cilia lining the organ of Corti.

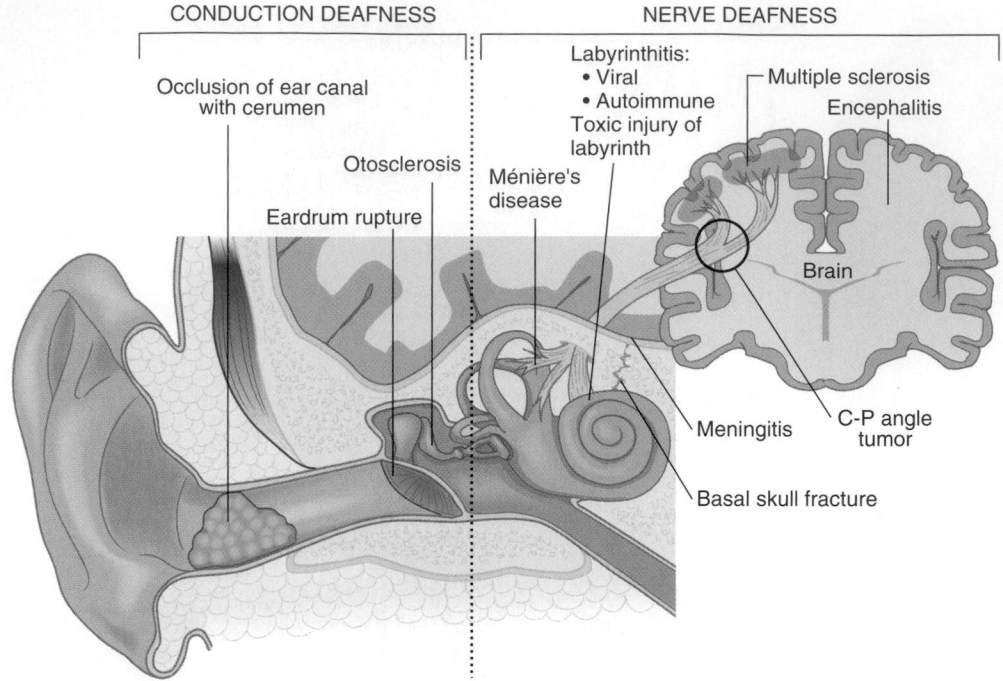

FIGURE 30-14 Causes of deafness.

Presbycusis, the hearing loss that affects aging people, is caused by a reduction in the number of receptor cells in the organ of Corti and also is classified as a sensorineural loss. Children can be born with a congenital hearing deficit or deafness because of an intrauterine infection, such as measles (rubella) (Figure 30-14).

If the sensorineural hearing loss cannot be improved by hearing aids, an option is surgical implantation of an artificial cochlea. Cochlear implants are complex devices that use electrical impulses to stimulate the auditory nerve, which then carries the current to the brain to be interpreted as sound. Cochlear implants bypass damaged portions of the ear and directly stimulate the auditory nerve. These implants do not create normal hearing but provide increased sound for a person with profound or complete hearing loss.

Mixed hearing loss is a combination of conductive and sensory deafness. This type of loss can result from tumors, toxic levels of certain medications, hereditary factors, and stroke.

Otitis

Two common types of otitis are seen in patients in an otology or family practice. The first affects the external ear canal and is called *otitis externa,* or swimmer's ear. Otitis externa may be caused by dermatologic conditions, such as **seborrhea** or **psoriasis**, trauma to the canal, or continuous use of earplugs or earphones. Swimmers frequently have otitis externa because water collects in the ears and mixes with cerumen to form an ideal culture medium for bacteria and fungus. Patients with otitis externa complain of severe pain and have inflammation and swelling of the external auditory canal, hearing loss, and possibly purulent (containing pus) or serous drainage. The inflammation is treated with antibiotic or steroid ear drops, and the canal must be kept clean and dry, or the condition can become chronic.

Otitis media is an inflammation of the normally air-filled middle ear that results in a collection of fluid behind the tympanic membrane. Otitis media can be serous or suppurative. Serous otitis media occurs because of a buildup of clear fluid in the middle ear; patients complain of a full feeling and some hearing loss. In suppurative otitis media, purulent fluid is present in the middle ear, and the patient has fever, pain, and hearing loss. Otitis media often is associated with an upper respiratory tract infection caused by a virus or an allergic reaction that results in swelling and inflammation of the sinuses and eustachian tubes. A child's eustachian tube is shorter, narrower, and more horizontal than that of an adult. The small size and decreased angle for drainage increases the chance that inflammation will block the tube and cause fluid to collect in the middle ear, which not only is uncomfortable but also interferes with the conduction hearing process (Figure 30-15).

Risk Factors for Otitis Media

Factors That Cannot Be Controlled
- Gender (male)
- Age (infants and younger children [6 to 18 months])
- Premature birth

- Family history
- Siblings with infections
- Seasonal factors (most common during cold and flu season), seasonal allergies

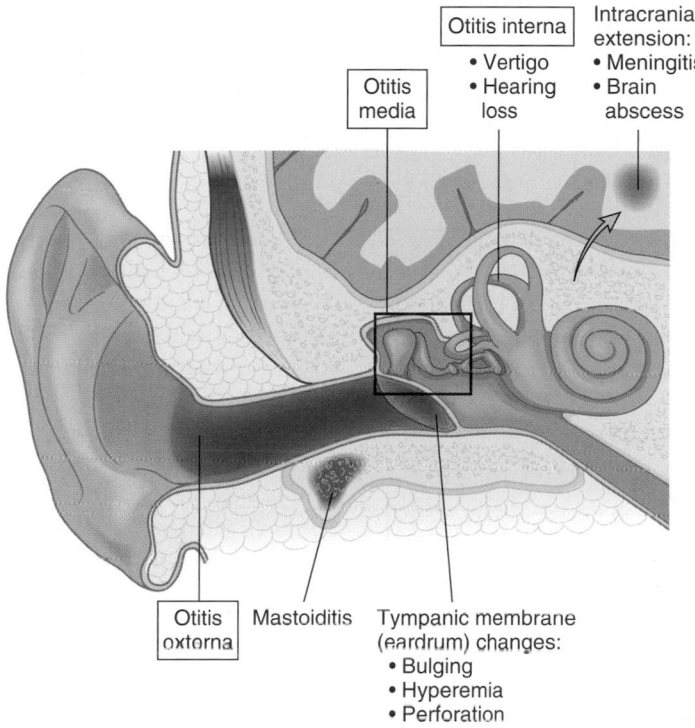

FIGURE 30-15 Inflammation and infection of the ear and surrounding tissues.

An otoscopic examination reveals that the normally pearly gray tympanic membrane is inflamed (bright pink or red) and bulging (Figure 30-16). Areas of fluid or pus may be visible through the membrane. A *tympanogram* may be done to determine the air pressure of the middle ear and the mobility of the tympanic membrane. During a tympanogram test, a small earphone is placed into the ear canal and the air pressure is gently changed. This test is helpful for showing whether an ear infection or fluid is present in the middle ear (Figure 30-17). A tympanic membrane responding normally to an increase in air pressure will move, resulting in a peaked tympanogram. If fluid or pus in the middle ear is putting pressure on the tympanic membrane, the membrane moves only slightly or not at all, resulting in a slight peak or a flat tympanogram recording.

Treatment of otitis media may be a conservative "watch and wait" approach. However, if a fever and pronounced pain are present, the individual may be given antibiotics and told to take over-the-counter analgesics such as acetaminophen or ibuprofen. If this condition becomes chronic, the provider may recommend a *myringotomy*,

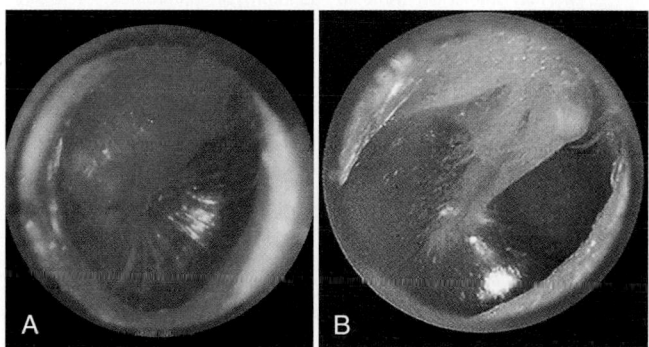

FIGURE 30-16 A, Tympanic membrane with otitis media. **B,** Normal tympanic membrane. (From LaFleur Brooks M: *Exploring medical language,* ed 9, St Louis, 2014, Mosby.)

which is the creation of a surgical incision in the tympanic membrane to drain the fluid, followed by insertion of a tympanostomy tube to continually drain the middle ear of fluid. This may be necessary to prevent permanent hearing loss caused by damage to the ossicles (Figure 30-18).

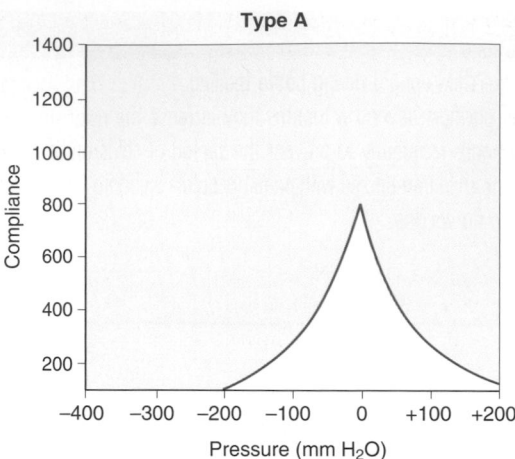

FIGURE 30-17 A normal tympanogram shows a peak at normal pressure (0). An ear with fluid produces a flat tympanogram.

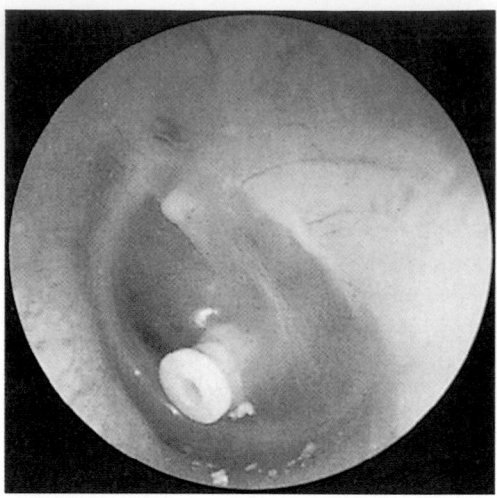

FIGURE 30-18 Tympanic membrane with a tympanostomy tube. (From Frazier MS, Drzymkowski JW: *Essentials of human diseases and conditions,* ed 5, St Louis, 2013, Saunders.)

Recommendations for Treating Otitis Media

The development of drug-resistant strains of bacteria as a result of overprescription of antibiotics is a growing concern. The American Academy of Pediatrics recommends the following for the treatment of otitis media:

- Treatment with antibiotics should be delayed, giving the child's immune system a chance to fight the infection by itself. This delay should last 24 hours in children 6 to 24 months old and 72 hours for older children. Approximately 61% of children improve within 24 hours, regardless of whether they are treated. If the child's condition does not improve, an appropriate antibiotic can be prescribed.
- The child typically improves within 48 to 72 hours, but the parent should understand how important it is to complete the antibiotic medication as ordered to prevent the infection from recurring.
- The provider may decide to treat otitis media with a short course of antibiotics (i.e., 5 days) but at a higher dose. The drugs of choice include amoxicillin (Amoxil), azithromycin (Zithromax), and cefuroxime (Rocephin).
- Antibiotics will not help if otitis is caused by a virus. The child should be observed for possible complications, and analgesics should be administered for pain control. Viral otitis media typically resolves within 7 to 14 days.

The medical assistant plays a key role in helping parents understand why antibiotic therapy may not be recommended. They also must educate parents about the importance of administering a prescribed antibiotic at the time ordered, using the correct dose, and completing the entire prescription.

Impacted Cerumen

Cerumen normally is a soft, yellowish, waxy substance that lubricates the external auditory canal. Excessive secretion of cerumen can gradually cause hearing loss, tinnitus, a feeling of fullness, and *otalgia* (ear pain). Impacted cerumen that has been pushed up tightly against the eardrum is a common cause of conductive hearing loss because sound vibrations cannot pass through the cerumen to initiate movement of the tympanic membrane. Individuals with psoriasis, abnormally narrow ear canals, or an excessive amount of hair growing in the ear canals are more prone to this condition.

An otoscopic examination quickly reveals this problem. If impacted cerumen is found, it must be removed. This can be done by softening the wax with oily drops, such as carbamide peroxide (Debrox), and then irrigating the ear with warm water until the plug is removed. Because this condition can recur, the patient may need to schedule periodic examinations. If the patient is experiencing hearing loss because of the impaction, it is immediately remedied with removal of the cerumen.

Ménière's Disease

The semicircular canals of the inner ear, in coordination with the eighth cranial nerve, control balance and give a sense of how the body is positioned. The canals contain fluid (the endolymph), the filtration and excretion of which are controlled by the part of the canal called the *endolymphatic sac.* Ménière's disease causes swelling and edema in this part of the semicircular canals, along with an overproduction or collection of excess endolymph. When this occurs, the patient shows signs. Although the cause of this problem is unknown, Ménière's disease is a chronic, progressive condition that triggers episodes of recurring attacks of *vertigo* (dizziness), tinnitus, a sensation of pressure in the affected ear, and advancing hearing loss. During an acute attack, patients experience nausea, vomiting, and problems with balance. These attacks can last a few hours to several days, and they increase in severity over time.

During active periods of the disease, the patient is treated symptomatically with medications for nausea and vomiting. A salt-restricted diet, diuretics, and antihistamines may be prescribed to control edema in the labyrinth. Surgical destruction of the affected labyrinth is an option. Although this relieves symptoms, it may also result in permanent deafness if the cochlea is damaged.

Useful Questions for Gathering a History of Ear Problems

- Are you experiencing nausea, vomiting, dizziness, ear pain, fever, headache, upper respiratory infection, ringing of the ears, drainage, loss of balance, or hearing loss?
- What are the onset, duration, and frequency of symptoms?
- Have you taken any medication for the symptoms? If so, what medication? Has it been helpful?
- Do you have the problem in both ears?
- Are you experiencing pain? On a scale of 1 to 10, with 10 being the worst pain, how would you rate the pain? Is it localized or radiating, in one ear or both?
- Has anything you have tried relieved the symptoms?

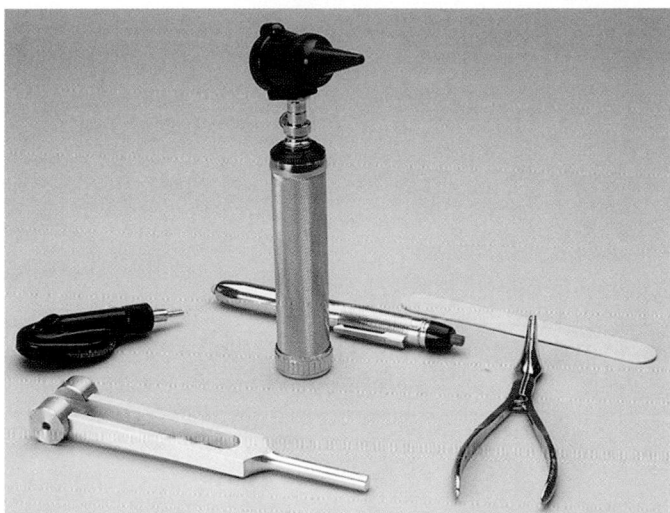

FIGURE 30-19 Instruments used in an otoscopic examination.

Diagnostic Procedures

An ear examination involves viewing the external auditory canal with an otoscope covered by an ear speculum (Figure 30-19). Disposable plastic speculum covers should be used each time to prevent disease transmission. A normal otoscopic examination reveals an external auditory canal with a small amount of cerumen and a pearly gray and concave tympanic membrane. In addition to performing the otoscopic examination, the provider palpates the area around the pinna for abnormalities or sensations. A number of tests are used to assess hearing acuity, ranging from simple tuning fork tests to quantitative and qualitative audiometric testing. If a hearing loss is suspected, the next test usually is performed with a tuning fork.

Tuning Fork Testing

Tuning fork tests measure hearing by air conduction and bone conduction. Remember that in bone conduction, the sound vibrates through the cranial bones to the inner ear. Tuning forks are available in different sizes, each with a different frequency. The most

commonly used tuning fork is the 512 Hz **hertz** (Hz), which means that it vibrates 512 cycles per second, the level of normal speech patterns. To activate the fork, the provider holds it by the stem and strikes the tines softly on the palm of the hand. Striking the tines too forcefully creates a tone that is too loud for diagnostic use. The two tests used to evaluate hearing are the Weber and Rinne tests. Both of these procedures are commonly used to evaluate conductive and sensory losses.

The Weber test is used if the patient reports that hearing is better in one ear than in the other. The vibrating fork is placed in the center of the top of the head, and the patient is asked in which ear the tone is louder, or if the tone is the same in both ears. Because the patient is hearing the tone by bone conduction through the head, a normal result is hearing the sound equally in both ears.

The Rinne test is designed to compare air conduction sound with bone conduction sound. In this test, the stem of the vibrating fork is placed on the patient's mastoid process, and the patient is instructed to raise a hand when the sound disappears. The fork is quickly inverted so that the vibrating tines are approximately 1 inch in front of the external ear canal. If hearing is normal, the patient should still hear a sound. In normal hearing, the sound is heard twice as long by air conduction as by bone conduction.

Audiometric Testing

An audiometric test may be done in an otology or a family practice and is performed by medical assistants who have received additional training. Audiometry measures the lowest intensity of sound an individual can hear (Figure 30-20). The patient, frequently a child, is assisted in placing headphones over the ears.

Newer machines give the operator the choice of performing a traditional manual hearing test or an automated one. In the automatic mode the patient is prompted through the ear phones to press a hand button as soon as he hears a tone. The advantages of automated machines are that voice prompts are available in multiple languages and the test requires less time to complete. The medical assistant can watch the progress of the test on the audiometer's LCD screen. Whether the test is delivered manually or with an automated model, each ear is tested by delivering a single frequency at a specific intensity, starting with low-frequency tones and going up to very high frequencies. The patient is asked to signal when he or she hears the sound. The results are printed on a graph, called an *audiogram*, or the medical assistant charts the results on a graph sheet (Procedure 30-5). An adult with normal hearing can hear tone frequencies below 25 decibels, and children with normal hearing can hear those below 15 decibels.

If initial screening indicates a hearing deficit, the provider may recommend an appointment with an **audiologist** for audiometric evaluation. The evaluation consists of a battery of tests that assesses the level of hearing impairment and provides valuable information as to how the patient may be helped. The first test evaluates speech comprehension and assesses the patient's ability to follow verbal instructions. Once this evaluation is complete, the patient is placed in a soundproof booth with earphones over the ears. From this point on, the audiologist speaks to the patient and conducts all testing through the earphones. The assessment includes testing the frequency, intensity, and audibility of sound. This process takes approximately 1 hour.

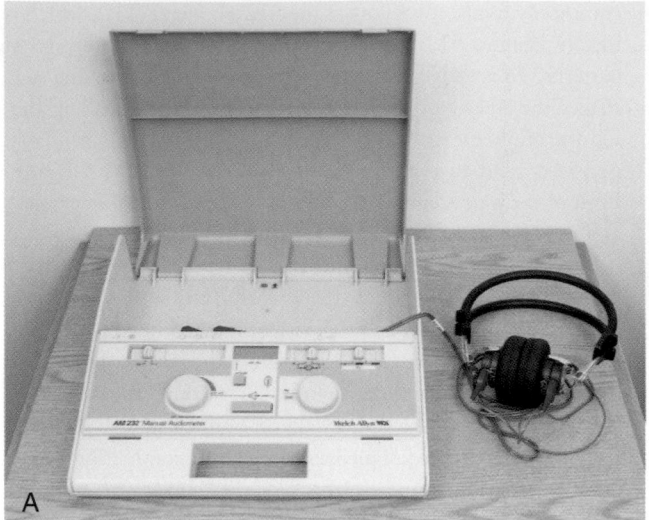
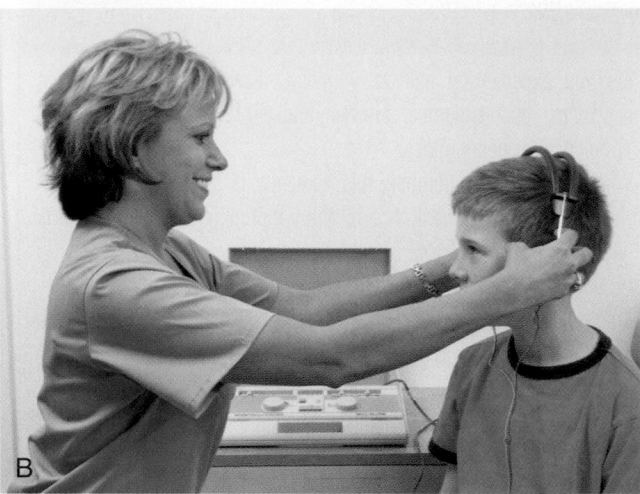

FIGURE 30-20 Audiometer with headset.

PROCEDURE 30-5	Perform Patient Screening Using Established Protocols: Measure Hearing Acuity with an Audiometer

Goal: *To perform audiometric testing of hearing acuity.*

EQUIPMENT and SUPPLIES

- Patient's health record
- Provider's order
- Audiometer with adjustable headphones and graph paper
- Quiet area

PROCEDURAL STEPS

1. Sanitize your hands, assemble the equipment, and bring the patient into a quiet area (see Figure 30-20).
   PURPOSE: The testing room should be free of distractions and noise so the patient can concentrate completely on the hearing evaluation.
2. Introduce yourself, identify the patient by name and date of birth, and explain the procedure.
   PURPOSE: To make sure you have the right patient. Also, explanations help gain the patient's cooperation and ease apprehension.
3. Explain that the audiometer measures whether the patient can hear various sound wave frequencies through the headphones. Each ear is tested separately. When the patient hears a frequency, he or she should raise a hand or push the button to signal the medical assistant.
   PURPOSE: Patient education is needed for compliance with the examination.

4. Place the headphones over the patient's ears, making sure they are adjusted for comfort.
5. The audiometer tests each ear separately, starting at a low frequency. If the results are not automatically recorded by the machine, the medical assistant documents the patient's response to the frequencies on a graph or audiogram. Results for the left ear are marked with an X, and those for the right ear are marked with an O (see the following figure) (Figure 1). More advanced machines automatically record the results. The medical assistant must have specialized training to conduct this test.
6. Frequencies are increased gradually to test the patient's ability to hear. Each response by the patient is documented.
7. After one ear has been tested, the other ear is then tested, and the results are documented.
8. The results are given to the provider for interpretation or downloaded into the patient's electronic health record for the provider to review.
9. The equipment is sanitized and disinfected according to the manufacturer's guidelines.
10. Sanitize your hands.

PROCEDURE 30-5   *—continued*

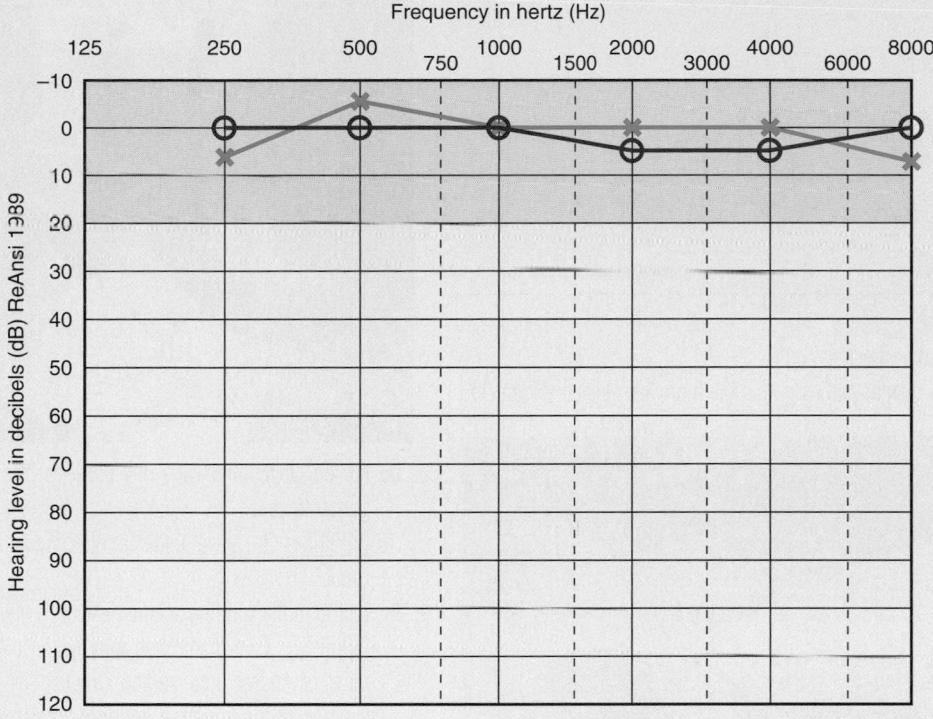

Aseptic Procedures in Otology

Routine examination instruments should be disinfected or sterilized after each use according to office policy and stored in a clean area. Surgical asepsis must be practiced when dressings are changed and minor surgery is performed. Medications, such as ear drops and nose drops, must be handled carefully to prevent contamination.

Treatment Procedures

Ear Irrigation

Irrigation of the ear is done to remove excessive or impacted cerumen, to remove a foreign body, or to treat the inflamed ear with an antiseptic solution (Procedure 30-6). When an ear irrigation is ordered by the provider, the medical assistant may perform the procedure if he or she has had the proper training and is competent in the technique. To prevent discomfort for the patient, it is important to administer the irrigating solution with the applicator tilted up, toward the top of the external canal, so that the solution is not directed at the tympanic membrane. Some discomforts the patient may experience during ear irrigation include vertigo, ear discomfort, coughing, or a tickle in the back of the throat. Perform the procedure as prescribed, making sure the patient is comfortable. Always document the treatment and its results immediately after completion.

CRITICAL THINKING APPLICATION   **30-5**

Kim is instructed to perform a bilateral ear irrigation on a 68-year-old patient with impacted cerumen. Before the procedure, she uses an otoscope to check the auditory canal and sees a large amount of dark brown cerumen in the right ear, completely covering the tympanic membrane. The left ear has a moderate amount of golden brown cerumen covering the bottom half of the tympanic membrane. After the procedure, both membranes are visible, and the patient tolerated the procedure without complaints. How should Kim document the procedure?

PROCEDURE 30-6   **Instruct and Prepare a Patient for a Procedure or Treatment: Irrigate a Patient's Ear**

Goal: *To remove excess or impacted cerumen from one or both of the patient's ears.*

EQUIPMENT and SUPPLIES

- Patient's health record
- Provider's order
- Irrigating solution
- Basin for irrigating solution
- Bulb syringe or an approved otic irrigation device

PROCEDURE 30-6 —*continued*

- Gauze squares
- Otoscope
- Drainage basin
- Disposable drape with poly-lined barrier
- Cotton-tipped applicators
- Disposable gloves
- Biohazard waste container

PROCEDURAL STEPS

1. Sanitize your hands.
   <u>PURPOSE</u>: To ensure infection control.
2. Check the provider's order and assemble the materials needed (Figure 1).

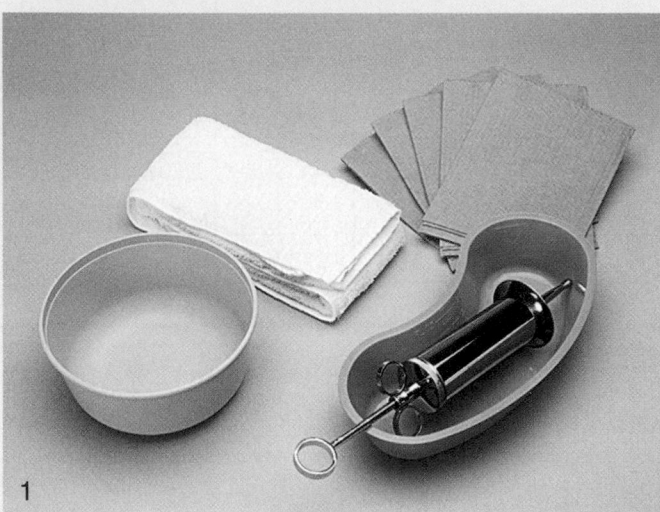

3. Check the label of the solution three times: (1) when you remove it from the shelf; (2) when you pour it; and (3) when you return it to the shelf.
   <u>PURPOSE</u>: To prevent a medication error.
4. Prepare the solution as ordered. The solution should be kept at body temperature to help loosen the cerumen.
5. Introduce yourself, identify the patient by name and date of birth, and explain the procedure.
6. Inspect the affected ear with an otoscope to locate the cerumen impaction.
7. Place the patient in a sitting position with the head tilted toward the affected ear. Place a water-absorbent towel over a poly-lined barrier on the patient's shoulder, and the collecting basin on the towel at the base of the ear. The patient can assist you by holding the collecting basin in place (Figure 2).
   <u>PURPOSE</u>: To minimize the risk of getting the patient's clothing wet and to direct the flow of water into the collecting basin.

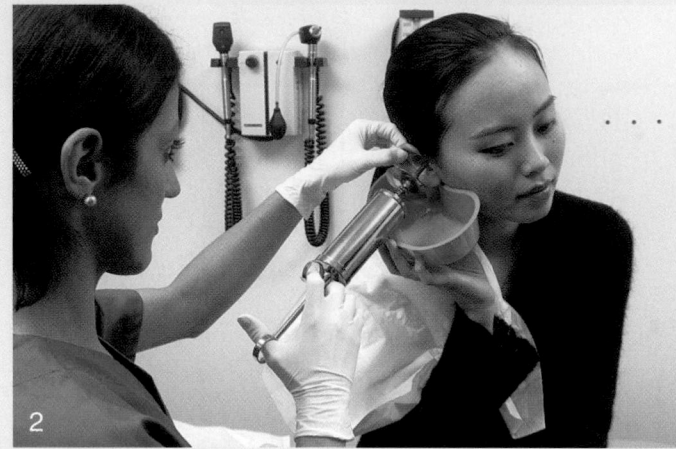

8. Put on gloves and wipe any particles from the outside of the ear with gauze squares.
   <u>PURPOSE</u>: To prevent the introduction of foreign material into the ear canal.
9. Test to make sure the solution is warm; then fill the syringe and expel air.
   <u>PURPOSE</u>: Cold medication may increase the pain level or cause symptoms of nausea and vertigo; trapped air in the syringe increases the pressure of the irrigation, causing discomfort.
10. Straighten the external ear canal. For adults and children older than age 3, gently pull the pinna of the ear up and back; for children younger than age 3, pull the earlobe down and back (Figure 3).
    <u>PURPOSE</u>: Straightening the canal allows the irrigating fluid to circulate through it.

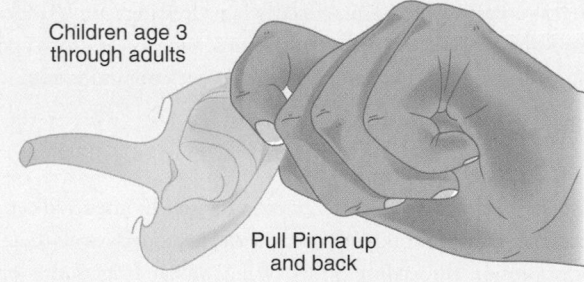
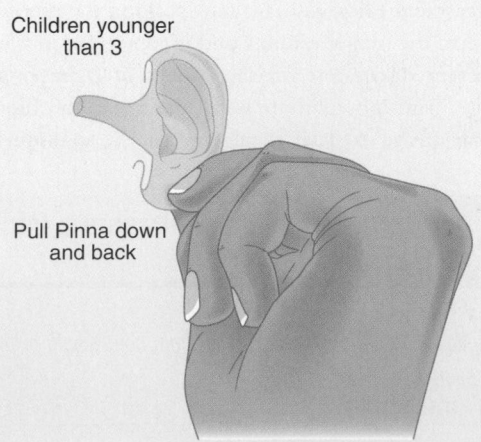

Children age 3 through adults

Pull Pinna up and back

Children younger than 3

Pull Pinna down and back

PROCEDURE 30-6 —continued

11. Place the tip of the syringe into the meatus of the ear.
12. Gently direct the flow of the solution toward the roof of the external auditory canal.
    PURPOSE: This helps prevent injury to the tympanic membrane, aids in the removal of embedded material, and provides the most comfort for the patient.
13. Refill the syringe with warm solution and continue until the material has been removed. Note the particles in the collecting basin to be evaluated when the material has been successfully removed.
14. Dry the patient's external ear with gauze squares and the visible ear canal gently with cotton-tipped applicators.
    PURPOSE: Inserting the applicator into the canal may cause serious trauma.
15. Inspect the ear with an otoscope to determine the results (Figure 4).

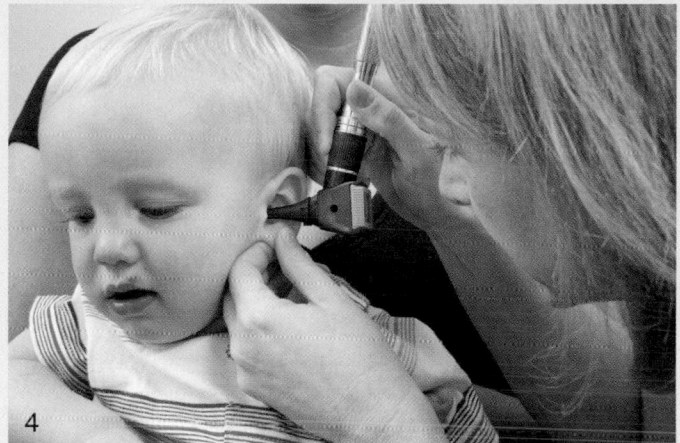
4

16. Place a clean, absorbent towel on the examination table and allow the patient to rest quietly with the head turned to the irrigated side while you wait for the provider to return to check the affected ear.
17. Disinfect the work area and the equipment. Dispose of your gloves in the biohazard container, and sanitize your hands.
    PURPOSE: To ensure infection control.
18. Document the procedure in the patient's health record, including the date and time; the ear irrigated; the type and amount of irrigating solution used; the characteristics of the material returned from the irrigation; the visibility of the tympanic membrane after irrigation; and any reactions by the patient.
    PURPOSE: Procedures that are not recorded are considered not done.

Documentation Exercise: You are ordered to perform an irrigation of both ears on Mrs. Ophelia Black because of impacted cerumen. Otoscopic examination before the irrigation revealed a large amount of dark brown ear wax in both ears. After irrigation, both tympanic membranes were visible, and Mrs. Black had no complaints of discomfort.

Correct documentation:
8/12/ 20– 10:15 AM: Right and left ears irrigated c̄ 500 mL saline sol bilaterally. Lrg amt dark brown cerumen expelled; post irrigation both TMs visible and pearly gray. No c/o discomfort. Kim Tau, CMA (AAMA)

Instilling Otic Medications

Medication ordered for ear instillation is given to soften impacted cerumen, to relieve pain, or as an antibiotic drop for an infectious pathogen (Procedure 30-7). Patients with ear conditions may be in considerable pain and may have difficulty hearing, which makes health teaching a challenge. Wait until after the procedure has been completed and the patient is more comfortable to reinforce health behaviors.

PROCEDURE 30-7 | **Instruct and Prepare a Patient for a Procedure or Treatment: Instill Medicated Ear Drops**

Goal: To instill the correct medication in the accurate dose directly into the external auditory canal.

EQUIPMENT and SUPPLIES

- Patient's health record
- Provider's order
- Prescribed otic drops in dispenser bottle
- Cotton balls
- Disposable gloves
- Biohazard waste container

PROCEDURAL STEPS

1. Sanitize your hands and gather the equipment and supplies.
   PURPOSE: To control infection and to reduce procedure time.
2. Check the medication label three times: (1) when you remove it from the shelf; (2) when you prepare it; and (3) when you return it to the shelf.
   PURPOSE: To prevent a medication error.

PROCEDURE 30-7   —continued

3. Introduce yourself, identify the patient by name and date of birth, and explain the procedure.

4. Have the patient sit up and tilt the head away from the affected ear, or lie down on the side with the affected ear upward.
   PURPOSE: To expose the ear for treatment, allow gravity to help the medication flow into the canal, and ensure the patient's comfort.

5. Check the temperature of the medication bottle. If it feels cold, gently roll the bottle back and forth between your hands to warm the drops.
   PURPOSE: Cold medication may increase the pain level or cause symptoms of nausea and vertigo.

6. Hold the dropper firmly in your dominant hand. With the other hand, gently pull the pinna up and back if the patient is older than age 3 or the earlobe down and back if the patient is younger than age 3.
   PURPOSE: To straighten the ear canal and make it easier for the medication to reach the target tissue.

7. Place the tip of the dropper in the ear canal meatus and instill the number of ordered medication drops along the side of the canal making sure that the tip of the dropper does not touch the ear canal (Figure 1).

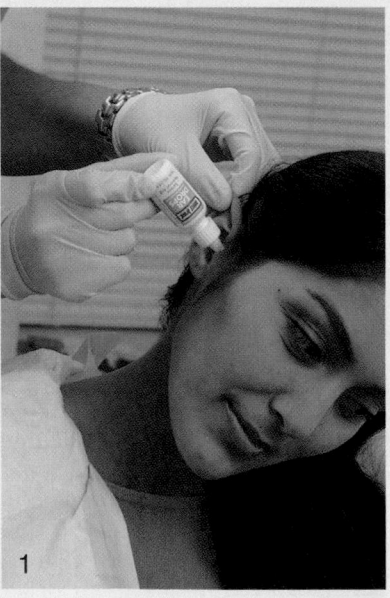

8. Instruct the patient to rest on the side opposite the affected ear and to remain in this position for approximately 3 minutes.
   PURPOSE: To help the medication reach the base of the canal and prevent it from immediately running out of the ear (Figure 2).

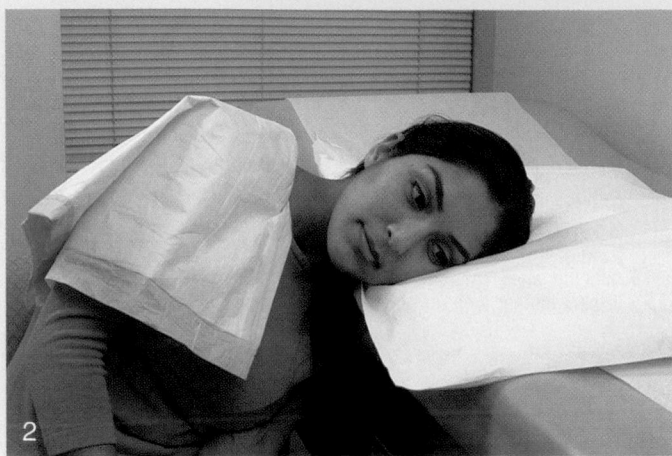

9. If instructed by the provider, place a moistened cotton ball into the ear canal.
   PURPOSE: To protect the ear canal and prevent medication from leaking out of the ear.

10. Disinfect the work area. Dispose of your gloves in the biohazard waste container, and sanitize your hands.
    PURPOSE: To ensure infection control.

11. Document the procedure in the patient's health record, using the appropriate abbreviations; include the date and time; name, dose, and strength of the medication; the ear treated; and any reactions by the patient.
    PURPOSE: Procedures that are not recorded are considered not done.

8/12/20– 3:22 AM: ii gtts Auralgan otic sol administered to right ear. No c/o discomfort. Pt instructed on home use. Kim Tau, CMA (AAMA)

EXAMINATION OF THE NOSE AND THROAT

If you are working in an ENT specialty office, you also will assist in the examination of the nasal cavity and the throat. The nasal cavity is examined to inspect the mucous membrane of the nostrils. The common cold and allergies are the main causes of changes in the mucosa. The provider may use a nasal speculum to visualize the nostrils and examines the nasal sinuses by palpation and transillumination.

The throat is the area that includes the larynx and pharynx; it can be viewed with the aid of a mirror and either a tongue depressor or a gauze square for grasping the tongue. In the nasopharynx, the provider looks for enlarged adenoids (pharyngeal tonsils) and for the orifices of the eustachian tubes. The provider may spray the patient's throat with a topical anesthetic before the examination to prevent the gag reflex.

Throat specimens frequently are collected in the provider's office to assist in the diagnosis of strep throat infections. Strep throat is caused by the group A beta-hemolytic streptococcal bacteria; if left untreated, it can cause serious complications. Throat cultures are collected by gently swabbing the back of the throat and the surfaces of the tonsils with a sterile swab. The mouth and tongue should be avoided to prevent contamination of the swab with the normal flora of the mouth (Procedure 30-8).

PROCEDURE 30-8	Perform Patient Screening Using Established Protocols: Collect a Specimen for a Throat Culture

Goal: *To collect a throat culture, using sterile technique, for immediate testing or for transportation to the laboratory.*

EQUIPMENT and SUPPLIES

- Patient's health record
- Provider's order
- Laboratory requisition
- Nonsterile gloves
- Face protection barrier
- Sterile swab
- Sterile tongue depressor
- Transport medium
- Biohazard waste container

PROCEDURAL STEPS

1. Sanitize your hands.
   PURPOSE: To ensure infection control.
2. Gather the materials needed.
3. Introduce yourself, identify the patient by name and date of birth, and explain the procedure.
4. Put on gloves and face protection.
   PURPOSE: To follow Standard Precautions.
5. Position the patient so that the light shines into the mouth.
   PURPOSE: To illuminate the area to be swabbed.
6. Remove the sterile swab from the sterile wrap with your dominant hand and grasp the sterile tongue depressor with your nondominant hand.
   PURPOSE: To achieve better control of the swabbing process.
7. Instruct the patient to open the mouth and say "Ah." Depress the tongue with the depressor.
   PURPOSE: Saying "Ah" helps elevate the uvula and reduces the tendency to gag. The tongue is depressed so that you can see the back of the throat and prevent contamination of the sterile swab.
8. Swab the back of the throat between the tonsillar pillars, especially any reddened, patchy areas of the throat, white pus pockets, purulent areas, and the tonsils; take care not to touch any other areas in the mouth (Figure 1).
   PURPOSE: Pathogenic organisms are found in the back of the throat and on the tonsils.

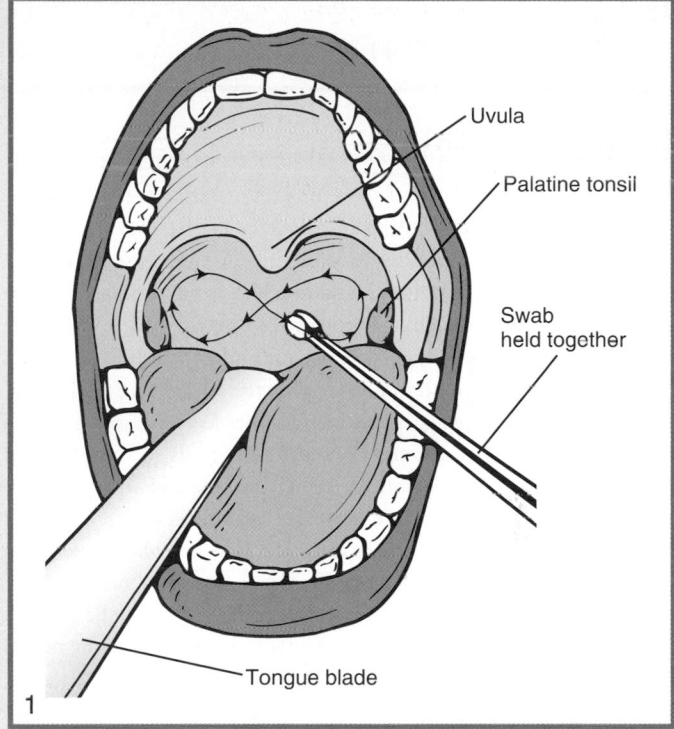

Uvula
Palatine tonsil
Swab held together
Tongue blade
1

9. Place the swab in the transport medium, label it, and send it to the laboratory (Figure 2). If direct slide testing is requested, return the labeled swab to the laboratory.
   PURPOSE: A transport medium prevents the swab from drying. Labeling immediately after collection prevents specimens from becoming mixed up.

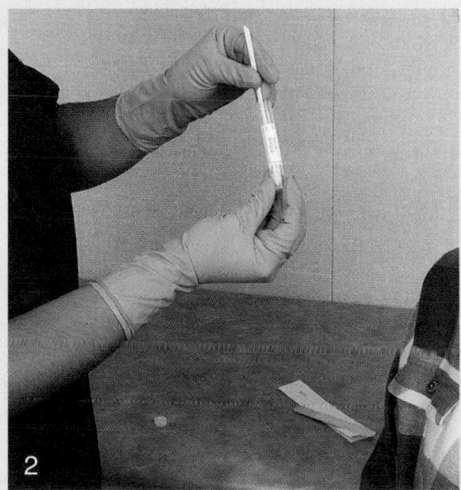

2

10. Dispose of contaminated supplies in the biohazard waste container.
    PURPOSE: To prevent the spread of infection.

PROCEDURE 30-8   *—continued*

11. Disinfect the work area.
12. Remove your gloves and discard them in the biohazard waste container.
13. Sanitize your hands.
    PURPOSE: To ensure infection control.

14. Document the procedure in the patient's health record.
    PURPOSE: Procedures that are not recorded are considered not done.

8/14/20– 8:35 AM: Throat specimen collected via swab from tonsillar area. Sent to University Laboratories for strep testing. Kim Tau, CMA (AAMA)

CLOSING COMMENTS

Patient Education

Patients with vision or hearing impairment face serious challenges. For these patients, the medical assistant must use good listening skills, appropriate nonverbal methods, and touch to communicate empathy and understanding. Teaching may have to be adapted to meet the special needs of these patients. A person with a vision loss benefits from large-print forms and handouts, increased lighting, and verbal rather than written instructions to reinforce learning. For an individual with a hearing deficit, printed instructions, demonstrations of how to manage treatments, or even sign language interpretation should be available to ensure accurate communication. Including family members in the patient's treatment plan and offering referrals to appropriate community or professional resources may be very beneficial to a patient with sensory loss. Each patient must be assessed individually to determine the type of adaptation that he or she needs.

An important part of patient education for those administering eye medications at home is stressing the need to maintain the sterility of the medication. Patients and/or family members must be taught how to apply the medication while preventing trauma to the eye and contamination of the applicator. Patients administering ear treatments also must understand how to instill the medication.

CRITICAL THINKING APPLICATION   **30-6**

Mr. Samuel Langton is a 77-year-old patient with profound hearing loss and severe glaucoma. How would you suggest that Amy communicate therapeutically with this patient? Role-play this interaction with one of your classmates.

Legal and Ethical Issues

Diminished sight or hearing may render a patient seriously impaired. To prevent accidents and office injuries, always ask a sight- or hearing-impaired patient whether he or she requires assistance. When you escort the patient to an examination room, offer your arm and tell the patient the approximate distance you will be walking. If the patient is to have an examination that involves local anesthesia or eye drops that dilate the pupil, be sure the patient has recovered and someone is available to take the patient home before allowing him or her to leave the facility. Never assume that the patient is capable of leaving alone. If the patient insists on leaving before the designated recovery time, inform the provider and record the time and circumstances surrounding the event in the patient's health record. This information should be signed and witnessed. The provider may want a refusal of care form signed by the patient and placed in the health record.

HIPAA Requirements

Regardless of the patient's disability, the ambulatory care center must follow the guidelines for Notice of Privacy Practices (NPP) established by the Health Insurance Portability and Accountability Act (HIPAA). The NPP is a form developed by the facility that outlines the patient's rights and the facility's legal responsibilities to safeguard the patient's protected health information. The facility must give the NPP to each new patient at the first office visit. To comply with HIPAA guidelines, the document must be in a language the patient easily understands. The staff is responsible for obtaining the patient's signature on the form, which indicates the patient's agreement with the stipulations of the facility's privacy practice. An individual with a vision deficit may require a large-print form, or a staff member may need to read the document to the person and answer any questions. The staff must make sure that patients with hearing deficits have had time to read the document before signing.

Americans with Disabilities Act Requirements

The Americans with Disabilities Act (ADA) was passed in 1990, and amendments were added in 2008. The Americans with Disabilities Act Amendments (ADAA) prohibits discrimination based on disability. An individual with a disability is defined by the ADAA as a person who has a physical or mental impairment that substantially limits one or more major life activities; a person who has a history or record of such an impairment; or a person who is perceived by others as having such an impairment. Public facilities, including ambulatory care facilities and other healthcare buildings, must comply with ADAA requirements for physical accommodations. Public medical facilities must provide individuals with disabilities access to communication devices if they have a problem with vision, hearing, reading, or comprehension. Additional details can be found at *http://www.ada.gov/nprm_adaaa/adaaa-nprm-qa.htm*.

Professional Behaviors

Patients with vision and hearing problems require an extra level of professional courtesy and respectfulness. Imagine what it would be like if you could not see clearly or if you had difficulty understanding what your provider is saying to you. How would you like a family member who has sensory difficulties treated when he or she visits the provider? Focus on how you can adapt the facility's environment to accommodate the needs of these patients. Is there adequate lighting? Are patient education materials available that have been adapted for individuals with vision impairment? How can you most effectively and respectfully communicate with a patient who has a hearing loss? Many times, just the act of empathy—imagining yourself in the place of the patient—can help guide you to treat patients with the respect and courtesy they deserve.

SUMMARY OF SCENARIO

After observing Kim and asking many questions, Amy is beginning to understand her special responsibilities in the ophthalmology and otorhinolaryngology clinic. She recognizes the need to be familiar with the anatomy and physiology of both the eye and the ear, in addition to the importance of being able to perform specialty-related skills, such as irrigations, medication instillations, and diagnostic procedures. Amy has become quite proficient at performing Snellen and Ishihara screening examinations and accurately documenting the results of each. Kim has taught her to use the audiometer and assisted her with the first few screenings, so she is now ready to do hearing tests on her own.

Although she learned about eye and ear medications in her medical assistant program, Amy found that instilling these medications in an actual patient is different from working on mannequins and classmates. Kim has reinforced the skills she learned in her program, continually emphasizing infection control procedures and reinforcing patient education information. Amy realizes that she needs to understand the pathologic conditions that can occur in the sensory organs so that she can assist the provider as needed and answer patients' questions.

After working with patients who have vision and hearing deficits, Amy understands the importance of adapting communication techniques to meet the needs of each patient. She has decided to take advantage of educational opportunities at the hospital and through her professional organization to continue to learn about this special area of practice.

SUMMARY OF LEARNING OBJECTIVES

1. **Define, spell, and pronounce the terms listed in the vocabulary.**
   Spelling and pronouncing medical terms correctly reinforce the medical assistant's credibility. Knowing the definitions of these terms promotes confidence in communication with patients and co-workers.

2. **Explain the differences among an ophthalmologist, an optometrist, and an optician.**
   An *ophthalmologist* is a medical doctor who specializes in the diagnosis and treatment of the eye; an *optometrist* can examine and treat visual defects; an *optician* fills prescriptions for corrective lenses.

3. **Identify the anatomic structures of the eye.**
   The anatomy of the eye begins with the outer covering, the conjunctiva, and three layers of tissue: sclera, choroid, and retina. The retina is where light rays are converted into nervous energy for interpretation by the brain.

4. **Describe the process of vision.**
   Vision begins with the passage of light through the cornea, where it is refracted. The light rays then pass through the aqueous humor and pupil into the lens. The ciliary muscle adjusts the curvature of the lens to again refract the light rays so that they pass into the retina, triggering the photoreceptor cells of the rods and cones. Light energy is converted into an electrical impulse that is sent through the optic nerve to the brain, where interpretation occurs. Table 30-1 shows how vision requires light and depends on the proper functioning of all parts of the eye.

5. **Differentiate among the major types of refractive errors.**
   Refractive errors include hyperopia, myopia, presbyopia, and astigmatism. All are caused by a problem with bending light so that it can be accurately focused on the retina. These conditions usually are caused by defects in the shape of the eyeball and can be corrected with glasses, contacts, or surgery.

6. **Summarize typical disorders of the eye and eyeball other than refractive errors.**
   Eye disorders can range from problems with eye movement, as in strabismus and nystagmus, to infections of the eye, including hordeolum, chalazions, keratitis, conjunctivitis, and blepharitis. Disorders of the eyeball include corneal abrasions, cataracts, glaucoma, and macular degeneration.

7. **Do the following related to diagnostic procedures for the eye:**
   - *Define the various diagnostic procedures for the eye.*
     Diagnostic procedures for the eye begin with a visual examination of the eye with an ophthalmoscope. Next, the eyelids are examined for abnormalities, and the pupils are tested for PERRLA. More advanced techniques include the use of a slit lamp to view the fine details of the eye and an exophthalmometer to measure the distance of the eyeball from the orbit. Distance visual acuity typically is assessed with a Snellen chart; near visual acuity is tested with a near vision acuity chart. A patient can be tested for a color vision defect with the Ishihara test.
   - *Perform a visual acuity test using the Snellen chart.*
     Procedure 30-1 explains the Snellen evaluation.
   - *Assess color acuity using the Ishihara test.*
     Procedure 30-2 outlines the color acuity examination.

8. **Explain the purpose of and the proper procedure for eye irrigation and the instillation of eye medication.**
   Eye irrigation relieves inflammation, removes drainage, dilutes chemicals, or washes away foreign bodies. Sterile technique and equipment must be used to prevent contamination. Medication may be instilled into the eye to treat an infection, soothe an eye irritation, anesthetize the eye, or dilate the pupils before examination or treatment. Procedure 30-3 describes the method for eye irrigation, and Procedure 30-4 explains how to administer eye medications.

9. **Identify the structures and explain the functions of the external ear, middle ear, and inner ear.**
   The external ear consists of the auricle, or pinna, and the external auditory canal, which transmits sound waves to the tympanic membrane. The middle ear is an air-filled cavity that contains the ossicles. The sound vibration passes through the tympanic membrane, causing the ossicles to vibrate. This bone-conducted vibration passes through the oval window into the inner ear. The organ of Corti, in the cochlea of the inner ear,

Continued

SUMMARY OF LEARNING OBJECTIVES—*continued*

converts sound waves into nervous energy, which is sent to the brain for interpretation. The semicircular canals in the inner ear maintain equilibrium.

10. **Describe the conditions that can lead to hearing loss, including conductive and sensorineural impairments.**
Conductive hearing loss is caused by a problem that originates in the external or middle ear and prevents sound vibrations from passing through the external auditory canal, limiting tympanic membrane vibrations or interfering with the passage of bone-conducted sound in the middle ear. A sensorineural hearing loss results from damage to the organ of Corti or the auditory nerve and prevents vibrations from being converted into nervous stimuli.

11. **Define other major disorders of the ear, including otitis externa and media, impacted cerumen, and Ménière's disease.**
Otitis externa is an inflammation of the auditory canal, and otitis media is an inflammation of the normally air-filled middle ear, resulting in the collection of serous or suppurative fluid behind the tympanic membrane. Impacted cerumen is a common cause of conductive hearing loss. Ménière's disease is a chronic, progressive condition that affects the labyrinth and causes recurring attacks of vertigo, in addition to tinnitus, a sensation of pressure in the affected ear, and advancing hearing loss.

12. **Do the following related to diagnostic procedures for the ear:**
    * *Explain diagnostic procedures for the ear.*
      The ear examination begins with an otoscopic examination. It can include various tuning fork tests to detect conductive or sensorineural hearing deficits and more advanced audiometric testing.
    * *Use an audiometer to measure a patient's hearing acuity accurately.*
      Procedure 30-5 explains the audiometry examination.
    * *Identify the purpose of ear irrigation and instillation of ear medications.*
      Irrigation of the ear is performed to remove excess or impacted cerumen, to remove a foreign body, or to treat the inflamed ear with an antiseptic solution. Medication is instilled into the ear to soften impacted cerumen, relieve pain, or treat an infectious pathogen.

* *Demonstrate the procedure for performing ear irrigations.*
  Procedure 30-6 describes how to perform an ear irrigation.
* *Accurately instill medicated ear drops.*
  Procedure 30-7 explains how to administer otic drugs.

13. **Summarize the nose and throat examination and perform a throat culture.**
Examination of the nose and throat begins with inspection of the nasal cavity; this is followed by visual examination of the throat and the nasopharynx. Throat cultures may be done to determine whether a streptococcal infection is present. The anterior and posterior neck regions are palpated for abnormalities. Procedure 30-8 explains how to perform a throat culture.

14. **Describe the effect of sensory loss on patient education.**
Patients with vision and hearing impairments face serious challenges and require individualized attention to meet their health education needs. Patients with vision loss may need large-print forms and handouts, increased levels of lighting, or verbal instructions rather than written ones. Individuals with hearing deficits may benefit from printed instructions, demonstrations on how to manage treatments, or even sign language interpretation. Family members should be included in the patient's treatment plan, and referrals to appropriate community or professional resources may be very beneficial.

15. **Discuss legal and ethical issues that might arise when caring for a patient with a vision or hearing deficit, in addition to requirements established by HIPAA and the ADAA.**
Diminished sight or hearing may render a patient seriously impaired. To prevent accidents and office injuries, the medical assistant should always ask a sight- or hearing-impaired patient whether he or she requires assistance. Regardless of the patient's disability, the ambulatory care center must follow the guidelines for Notice of Privacy Practices (NPP) established by HIPAA. Public facilities also must comply with ADAA requirements for physical accommodations. If appropriate, assistive devices must be provided for individuals with vision or hearing impairments.

CONNECTIONS

Study Guide Connection: Go to the Chapter 30 Study Guide. Read and complete the activities.

evolve Evolve Connection: Go to the Chapter 30 link at *evolve.elsevier.com/kinn* to complete the Chapter Review Quiz. Check out the other resources listed for this chapter to make the most of what you have learned from Assisting in Ophthalmology and Otolaryngology.

ASSISTING IN DERMATOLOGY

31

SCENARIO

Dr. Sam Lee is a dermatologist who employs several medical assistants in his busy private practice. Melissa Bauman, CMA (AAMA), has worked for Dr. Lee since graduating from a medical assisting program last year. Melissa works as a clinical specialist, whose primary responsibilities are to perform telephone screening, prepare patients for procedures, and assist Dr. Lee as needed. To fulfill her responsibilities in the dermatology practice, Melissa must be familiar with common diseases and disorders that affect the skin, assist with dermatologic procedures, and be prepared to reinforce patient education about the treatment and prevention of dermatologic conditions.

While studying this chapter, think about the following questions:

- What are the basic anatomy and physiology of the integumentary system?
- What are common diseases and disorders that affect the integumentary system?
- How can Melissa determine the difference between the levels of burn injuries?

- Why is it important that Melissa understand the concepts of staging and grading of malignant tumors?
- What are the primary malignancies of the skin?
- What dermatologic procedures should Melissa be prepared to be prepared to assist with in a dermatology practice?

LEARNING OBJECTIVES

1. Define, spell, and pronounce the terms listed in the vocabulary.
2. Explain the major functions of the skin.
3. Describe the anatomic structures of the skin.
4. Compare various skin lesions and give examples of each.
5. Describe typical integumentary system infections and infestations.
6. Differentiate among various inflammatory and autoimmune integumentary disorders.
7. Recognize thermal and cold injuries to the skin.
8. Compare the characteristics of benign and malignant neoplasms.
9. Do the following relating to benign and malignant neoplasms:
   - Explain the grading and staging of malignant tumors.
   - Conduct patient education on the warning signs of cancer.

- Describe skin malignancies and their treatment.
- Define the ABCDE rule for identifying a malignant melanoma.
10. Do the following relating to dermatologic procedures:
    - Discuss how to assist with a dermatologic examination.
    - Summarize allergy testing procedures.
    - Describe the diagnosis and treatment of allergies.
11. Explain dermatologic procedures performed in the ambulatory care setting.
12. Discuss the medical assistant's role in patient education, in addition to legal and ethical issues that would apply to a dermatology practice.

VOCABULARY

alopecia (al-o-pe'-se-uh) Partial or complete lack of hair.

anaplastic Relating to an alteration in cells to a more primitive form; a term that describes cancer-producing cells.

basement membrane A deep layer of the skin that secures the epithelium to underlying tissue; separates the epidermis from the dermis.

benign A tumor or tissue growth that is not cancerous; it may require treatment or removal, depending on its location and/or for cosmetic reasons.

bilirubin (bih-luh-roo'-bin) An orange pigment in bile; its accumulation leads to jaundice.

cryosurgery The technique of exposing tissue to extreme cold to produce a well-defined area of cell destruction.

débridement The removal of foreign material and dead, damaged tissue from a wound.

ecchymosis Discoloration of the skin caused by the escape of blood into the tissues from ruptured blood vessels; typically caused by bruising.

electrodesiccation The destruction of cells and tissue by means of short high-frequency electrical sparks.

eschar Devitalized skin that forms a scab or a dry crust over a burn area.

exacerbation An increase in the seriousness of a disease, marked by greater intensity of the signs and symptoms.

excoriated Skin that has been injured by scratching; abraded.

glomerulonephritis (glo-mer′-yoo-loh-nih-fri′-tis) Inflammation of the glomerulus of the kidney.

hyperplasia An increase in the number of normal cells.

jaundice A yellow discoloration of the skin and mucous membranes caused by deposits of bile pigments; these deposits occur because of excess bilirubin in the blood.

keloid A raised, firm scar formation caused by overgrowth of collagen at the site of a skin injury.

keratin A very hard, tough protein found in the hair, nails, and epidermal tissue.

keratinocytes The skin cells that synthesize keratin.

leukoderma Lack of skin pigmentation, especially in patches.

malignant A term describing tumor or tissue growth that is cancerous, anaplastic, invasive, and can metastasize.

opaque Not translucent or transparent; murky.

petechiae (peh-te′-ke-uh) Small, purplish hemorrhagic spots on the skin.

postherpetic neuralgia Pain that lasts longer than a month after a shingles infection and is caused by damage to the nerve; the pain may last for months or years.

recessive A gene that only produces a particular condition if both the mother and the father carry that particular gene; neither of the parents have the condition.

teratogen (te-rah′-tuh-jen) Any substance that interferes with normal prenatal development, resulting in a developmental abnormality.

The skin is the largest organ of the human body. In an average-size adult, it covers a total area of about 20 square feet. Forming the outer boundary of the body, the skin performs several essential functions: it acts as a barrier to protect vital internal organs from infection and injury; it helps dissipate heat and regulate body temperature; and it synthesizes vitamin D when exposed to ultraviolet (UV) light. In addition, various sensory receptors present throughout the skin enable it to respond to such sensations as heat, cold, pain, and pressure.

The specialty of dermatology deals with the skin and its accessory structures: hair, nails, and sweat glands, and the subcutaneous tissue that lies beneath the skin. A physician who specializes in dermatology is called a *dermatologist*.

ANATOMY AND PHYSIOLOGY

The integumentary system is composed of the skin and its accessory organs. Each square inch of the skin contains millions of cells,

numerous specialized nerve endings, hair follicles, muscles, sweat glands to cool the body, and sebaceous glands, which release *sebum*, an oily substance that lubricates the skin. These diverse structures and glands are nourished by a permeating, elaborate network of blood vessels. The thickness of human skin varies markedly at different parts of the body, ranging from fairly thin over protected areas (e.g., the eyelids) to very thick over areas subject to abrasion (e.g., the palms and soles).

Skin is composed of three layers: the epidermis (the thin, uppermost layer); the dermis (the thicker layer beneath that makes up about 90% of the skin mass and often is referred to as the *true skin*); and the subcutaneous layer (the layer composed primarily of fatty, or adipose, tissue) (Figure 31-1).

Epidermis

New skin cells, called **keratinocytes**, are found in the basal cell layer of the epidermis and migrate upward over about 4 weeks. As the cells move toward the surface, they grow flatter and scalier,

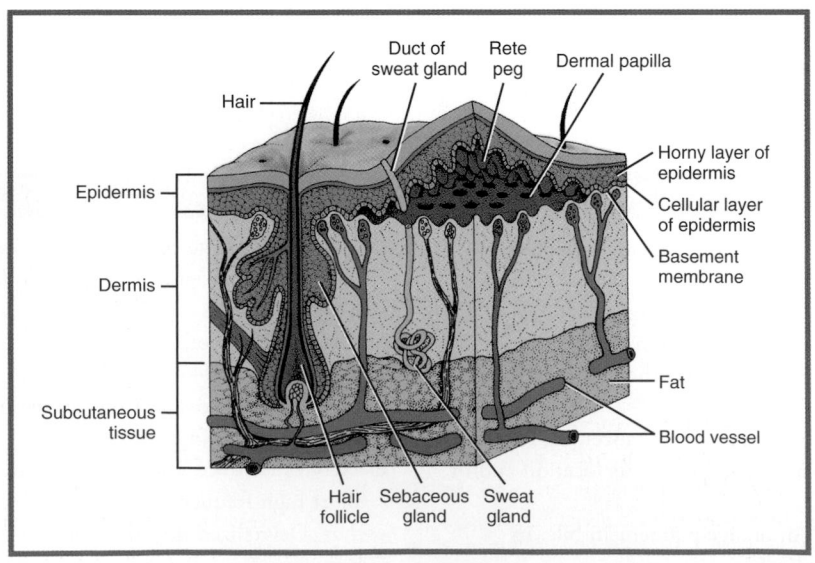

FIGURE 31-1 The three layers of the skin.

eventually losing their nuclei and changing into dead skin cells that contain an inert protein called **keratin**. Keratin makes up the outermost layer of the epidermis and forms a protective barrier across the surface of the skin that helps control water loss from the body. Ultimately, the outermost keratin layer sloughs off as a result of washing and friction. Hair and nails, which are also composed of keratin, are products of the epidermis.

About 95% of the cells in the epidermis are keratinocytes. The other 5% of epidermal cells are pigmented cells, or melanocytes. Melanin is a protein manufactured in the body that gives coloring to the skin and protects the body from UV radiation. Skin coloring is determined not by the total number of melanocytes, which is relatively constant for all races, but rather by the rate at which these cells produce melanin. The amount of melanin produced depends on genetics and exposure to UV light. Individuals with albinism, an inherited **recessive** trait, are unable to produce melanin, so they have white hair and skin and lack pigment in the iris. Because they have no protection from UV light, they must either stay out of the sun or routinely protect themselves with sunglasses and high level USB sunscreen.

Dermis

The underlying dermis is a thick layer of connective tissue that contains collagen and elastin fibers, in addition to water and jelly-like materials that make the skin compressible. Collagen fibers help prevent tearing of the skin; elastin is a flexible fiber that makes the skin resilient. Distributed throughout the dermis are blood vessels, lymph vessels, muscle cells, hair follicles, and sebaceous and sweat glands. Sweat glands are exocrine glands. The two types of sweat glands are *eccrine glands* and *apocrine glands.* Eccrine glands, the most numerous, are present over most of the body; they regulate body temperature by excreting water (sweat) through the skin pores to release heat. *Apocrine glands,* which open into hair follicles and are located in specific areas, including the axilla, scalp, face, and genitalia. Apocrine glands secrete a fatty sweat in response to stress. This sweat is odorless when excreted; bacterial action results in odor.

A variety of microorganisms, called *normal* or *resident flora,* are found on the skin and may increase the risk of integumentary system infection. Healthcare workers are encouraged to sanitize their hands before and after each procedure to prevent transient microbes picked up throughout the day from becoming resident flora. If transient microorganisms are not destroyed and/or removed by good hand sanitization techniques, they eventually become part of the individual's resident flora. Sensory receptors for the nervous system that detect pain, temperature, pressure, or texture also are located in the dermis.

Subcutaneous Layer

The subcutaneous layer contains fat cells, which provide insulation and serve as a depository for reserve calories. It also contains blood vessels, nerves, and the base of the appendages of the skin (e.g., hair follicles). Subcutaneous tissue is distributed unevenly, and as the human body ages, it thins considerably, which can make administering injections or drawing blood more difficult in aging patients. This loss of subcutaneous tissue is one reason elderly people are unable to compensate for changes in temperature, so they are colder when temperatures drop and hotter when temperatures rise. Aging skin is very fragile; it is easily traumatized and damaged by items such as the tourniquets used for drawing blood and bandage adhesives. The medical assistant must be very careful to avoid injuring the skin of an elderly person.

DISEASES AND DISORDERS

Skin is continuously exposed to the environment and may be affected by a wide range of disorders, including infections, inflammatory processes, allergic reactions, and tumors. Many skin problems resolve spontaneously; others can be managed with drug therapy; and still others, such as tumors, large cysts, or moles, may require surgical intervention.

Skin Lesions

Skin lesions can be caused by a systemic problem, such as an allergic reaction to medication, or they may develop from a localized infection. When communicating with the provider and documenting in the patient's health record, always use correct medical terminology to describe skin lesions, such as, "The patient reports a widespread maculopapular rash across the anterior trunk" rather than "The patient has a red, raised rash on his stomach."

When you gather details from the patient about the characteristics of lesions, some elements you should consider include the following:

- Describe the color, elevation, and texture of the lesion.
- Does the patient have any pain or *pruritus* (itching)? If pruritus is present, is the area **excoriated** or inflamed?
- Is any drainage present? If so, what are its characteristics?
- What is the exact anatomic location of the lesion? Have changes occurred over time?

Primary lesions are those that appear immediately. Macules, papules, plaques, nodules, cysts, wheals, and pustules all are primary lesions. *Secondary lesions* are the result of alterations in a primary lesion. Examples of secondary lesions include scales, crusts, fissures, erosions, ulcerations, and scars (Figure 31-2). For instance, vesicles (blisters) from a partial-thickness burn are primary lesions, but if the blisters break and ulcerations form, healing ends in a scar. Ulcerations and scars are secondary lesions.

CRITICAL THINKING APPLICATION   **31-1**

Using the pictures and definitions in Figure 31-2, identify the correct medical term for the following skin lesions:

- Crack in the skin that can occur with athlete's foot
- Small blister
- Vesicle filled with pus
- Large blister that can occur with burns
- Flat lesion that has changed color (e.g., freckles)
- Raised lesion (e.g., eczema)

Infections

Bacterial Infections

Impetigo. Impetigo is a common, superficial infection caused by streptococci or *Staphylococcus aureus* that usually affects children. Initially impetigo looks like small vesicles on the face (especially

PRIMARY LESIONS

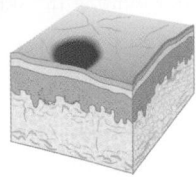

MACULE
Flat area of color change (no elevation or depression)

Example: Freckles

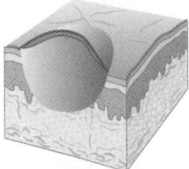

PAPULE
Solid elevation less than 0.5 cm in diameter

Example: Allergic eczema

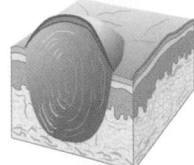

NODULE
Solid elevation 0.5 to 1 cm in diameter. Extends deeper into dermis than papule

Example: Mole

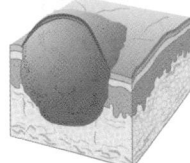

TUMOR
Solid mass—larger than 1 cm

Example: Squamous cell carcinoma

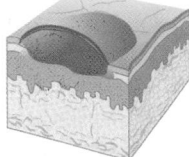

PLAQUE
Flat elevated surface found on skin or mucous membrane

Example: Thrush

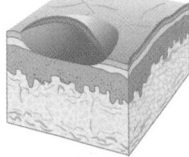

WHEAL
Type of plaque. Result is transient edema in dermis

Example: Intradermal skin test

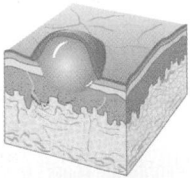

VESICLE
Small blister—fluid within or under epidermis

Example: Herpesvirus infection

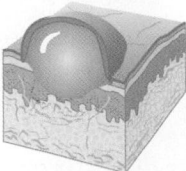

BULLA
Large blister (greater than 0.5 cm)

Example: Burn

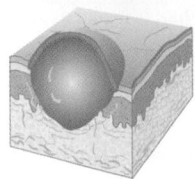

PUSTULE
Vesicle filled with pus

Example: Acne

SECONDARY LESIONS

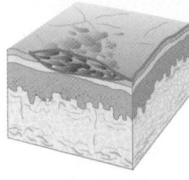

SCALES
Flakes of cornified skin layer

Example: Psoriasis

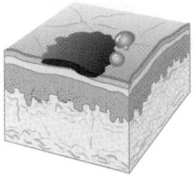

CRUST
Dried exudate on skin

Example: Impetigo

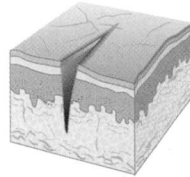

FISSURE
Cracks in skin

Example: Athlete's foot

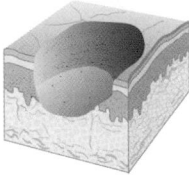

ULCER
Area of destruction of entire epidermis

Example: Decubitus (pressure sore)

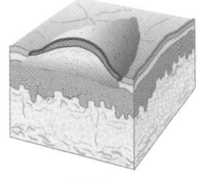

SCAR
Excess collagen production after injury

Example: Surgical healing

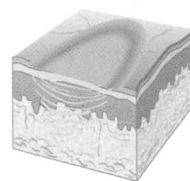

ATROPHY
Loss of some portion of the skin

Example: Paralysis

FIGURE 31-2 Different types of skin lesions.

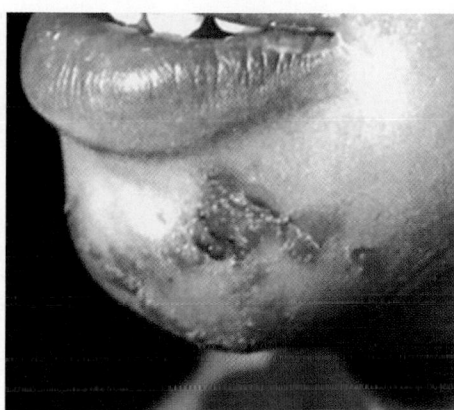

FIGURE 31-3 Impetigo. (From Marks J, Miller J: *Lookingbill and Marks' principles of dermatology,* ed 5, Philadelphia, 2014, Saunders.)

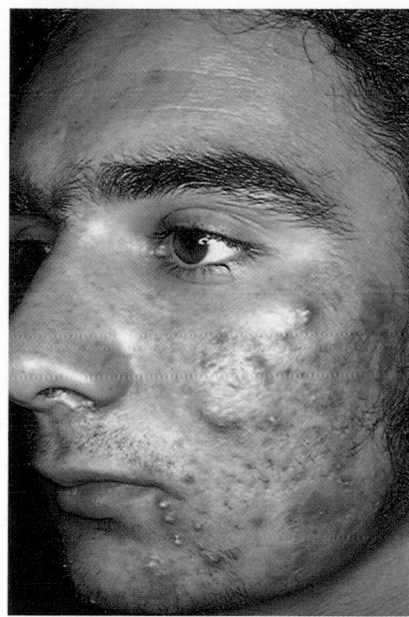

FIGURE 31-4 Acne. (From Paller A, Mancini A: *Hurwitz clinical pediatric dermatology: a textbook of skin disorders in childhood and adolescence,* ed 4, Philadelphia, 2011, Saunders.)

around the nose and mouth) that quickly enlarge and rupture, excreting a honey-colored exudate. The exudate forms crusty lesions, and beneath the crust, the area is inflamed and moist (Figure 31-3). Pruritus accompanies the infection, and scratching helps spread the lesions at the site. Impetigo is contagious, and bacteria are transmitted by direct contact with the drainage, whether at other sites or with other children through the sharing of toys and touching. Consistent hand washing is required to help break the chain of infection. It also is important to keep personal items that may be contaminated, such as washcloths, linens, and drinking glasses, away from other members of the family. If the areas of infection are limited, topical treatment with an antibiotic ointment may be effective. However, impetigo caused by streptococci may result in **glomerulonephritis**; more involved infections may require treatment with oral antibiotics.

CRITICAL THINKING APPLICATION   31-2

Mrs. Allio calls the office because she is concerned that her children have been exposed to a child in the neighborhood who was diagnosed with impetigo. She tells Melissa that her 3-year-old woke up this morning with blisters around his mouth. Dr. Lee prescribes polymixin-bacitracin-neomycin (Neosporin) ointment to be applied three times daily to the affected areas. What should Melissa tell Mrs. Allio about preventing the spread of infection to her other children?

Acne. *Acne vulgaris* typically begins at puberty and is caused by a number of factors, including inherited predisposition, hormonal fluctuations, exposure to heat and humidity, and the use of oily creams (Figure 31-4). Acne is a disorder of the hair follicle and sebaceous gland unit. It develops when sebum, which reaches the skin surface through the hair follicles, stimulates the follicle walls, causing more rapid shedding of skin cells. Cells and sebum stick together and form a plug that promotes the growth of staphylococcal organisms in the follicles. The result is the formation of comedones (blackheads and whiteheads), pimples, pustules, or larger abscesses at the site.

Acne treatment begins with twice-daily face washes with benzoyl peroxide or salicylic acid. Medications include topical antibiotic cream (e.g., erythromycin) or application of a retinoid, such as Retin-A (tretinoin) or adapalene (Differin). Minocycline (Solodyn) is an extended-release drug that offers a continuous but very low dose of the antibiotic minocycline. It is used to treat moderate to severe acne in patients 12 years of age or older. Severe cystic acne can be treated with isotretinoin (Claravis), but this drug is a strong **teratogen** and should never be prescribed for pregnant women or women who are not using contraceptives. The use of oral contraceptives (e.g., Ortho Tri-Cyclen and Estrostep) also may reduce acne outbreaks. Laser resurfacing can be performed to smooth out shallow acne scars that form as the result of extreme cases of acne vulgaris.

Acne conglobata is a severe form of acne that typically occurs later in life and results in lesions across the back, buttocks, thighs, face, and chest. Abscesses or cysts may form between affected sites, and healing frequently results in **keloid** formation. This type of acne requires more aggressive treatment with systemic corticosteroids (e.g., prednisone), oral antibiotics, oral retinols, and laser resurfacing or **débridement** to treat excessive scarring.

Rosacea. Rosacea is a chronic disease seen most frequently in women between the ages of 30 and 60. It causes inflammation and pustule formation and begins as frequent flushing across the nose, forehead, cheeks, and chin. As the condition progresses, capillaries of the face dilate and are visible across affected areas as small, red, edematous lines; these are accompanied by eye inflammation and photosensitivity. Over time, the face appears red, eye inflammation is more apparent, and painful nodules and pustules form. Men with rosacea may develop rhinophyma, a large, inflamed, bulbous nose caused by **hyperplasia** of sebaceous nasal tissue (Figure 31-5). Individuals with rosacea eventually may develop an obvious thickening of the skin across the forehead, nose, cheeks, and chin. The condition is treated with topical antibiotics and, as symptoms progress, with oral antibiotics, such as doxycycline (Oracea), which helps reduce

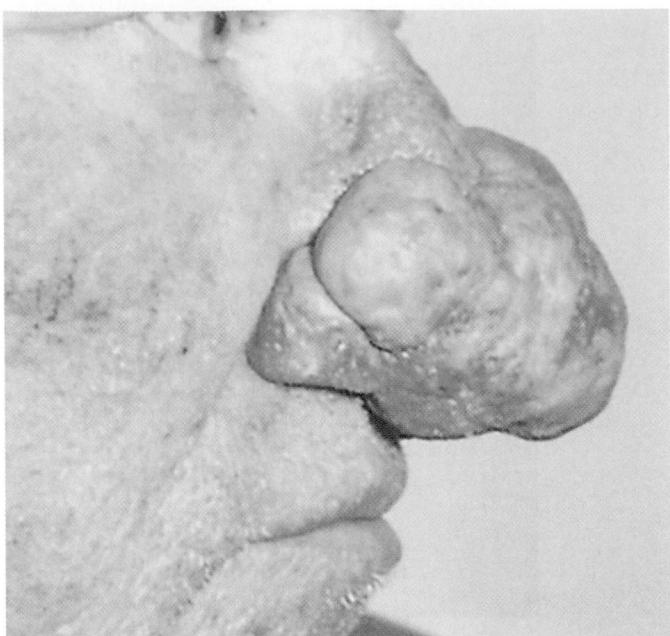

FIGURE 31-5 Rhinophyma. (Courtesy Michael O. Murphy, MD.)

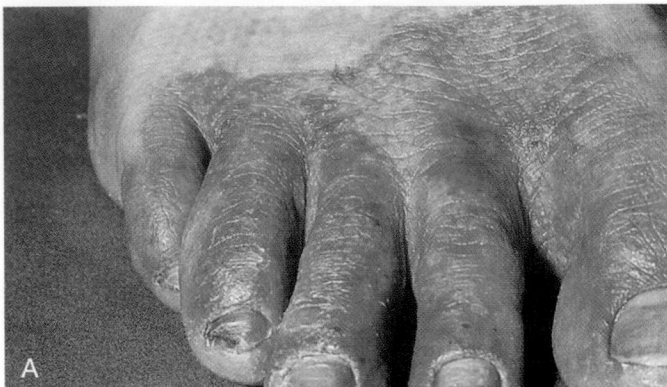

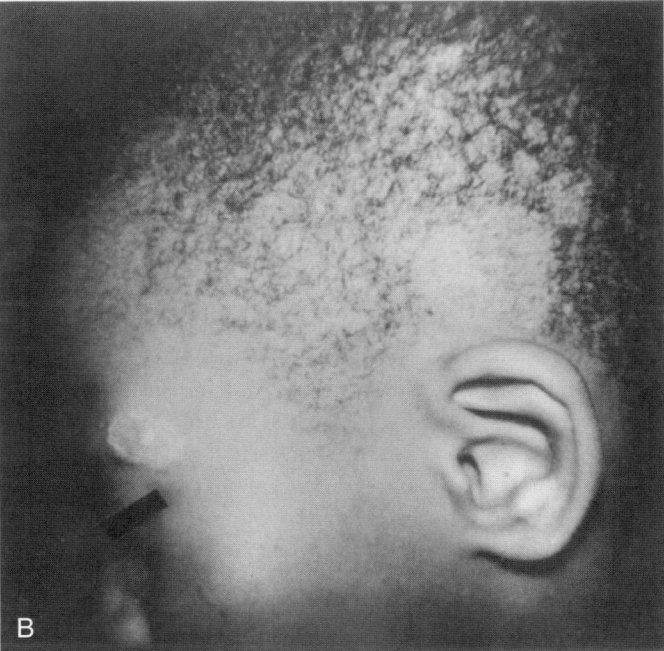

FIGURE 31-6 Fungal infections. **A,** Tinea pedis. **B,** Tinea corporis. (**A** from Gawkrodger D: *Dermatology*, ed 5, New York, 2012, Churchill Livingstone; **B** from Mahon CR et al: *Textbook of diagnostic microbiology*, ed 5, Philadelphia, 2015, Saunders.)

the number of pimples and bumps on the face; however, it may not reduce the redness and flushing.

Furuncles and Carbuncles. A *furuncle,* or boil, is a localized staphylococcal infection that begins as inflammation of a hair follicle *(folliculitis)* or skin gland. The affected area is raised, inflamed, and painful and eventually may produce purulent drainage. A *carbuncle* is a collection of furuncles that have joined to form a large infected area that may drain through multiple sites or form an abscess. Both infections are treated with oral antibiotics, frequent cleansing of the area, application of an antibiotic ointment and, in some cases, surgical incision and drainage of the purulent material.

Cellulitis. Cellulitis is an acute infection of the skin and subcutaneous tissue caused by staphylococci or streptococci. It begins from a small cut or as a result of a skin injury, or it develops at the site of a furuncle or ulcer. The area surrounding the site becomes inflamed, edematous, and painful with red streaks along the lymph vessels that lead from the infection. The condition is treated with oral antibiotics. Warm compresses applied locally aid healing, and analgesics may be needed to relieve discomfort. It is important that patients with cellulitis are treated appropriately because a systemic infection can develop if the lymph glands become involved.

Fungal Infections (Dermatophytoses)

Fungal, or mycotic, infections, such as *tinea pedis* (athlete's foot) (Figure 31-6, *A), tinea cruris* (jock itch), and *tinea corporis* (ringworm) (Figure 31-6, *B)* are extremely common. These pathogens, which tend to live off dead tissue in the keratin layer of the epidermis, the hair, or the nails, cause almost no inflammation in the underlying skin. The fungus invades the skin where it has been damaged or is consistently moist. All of these lesions are pruritic and are characterized by a distinct border with scaling areas that have a clear center. Secondary bacterial infections may occur with excoriation.

The provider typically diagnoses a fungal infection by noting the way the skin looks and the patient's complaints of pruritus. The skin may be scraped to obtain cells for examination under a microscope, and sometimes the provider may order a skin culture, for which a suspicious area is swabbed or scraped using sterile technique. The sample is sent to the laboratory for analysis. Treatment consists of topical antifungal agents, such as clotrimazole (Lotrimin), ketoconazole (Nizoral), econazole, or nystatin (Mycostatin). Antibiotics may be necessary if a secondary infection occurs. Because mycotic infections thrive in dark, moist areas, the patient should be advised to keep the site clean and dry and to wear loose clothing if possible. All types of dermatophytoses can become chronic infections if not managed carefully.

Tinea unguium, or *onychomycosis* (Figure 31-7), is a fungal infection of the toenails and fingernails. Unlike athlete's foot, which occurs on the skin's surface, nail fungus lives in the nail bed and the nail plate. The nail provides the fungus with an extremely well-protected place to live, which is why nail fungus may be especially difficult to treat. The primary sign of nail fungus is the appearance of the nail,

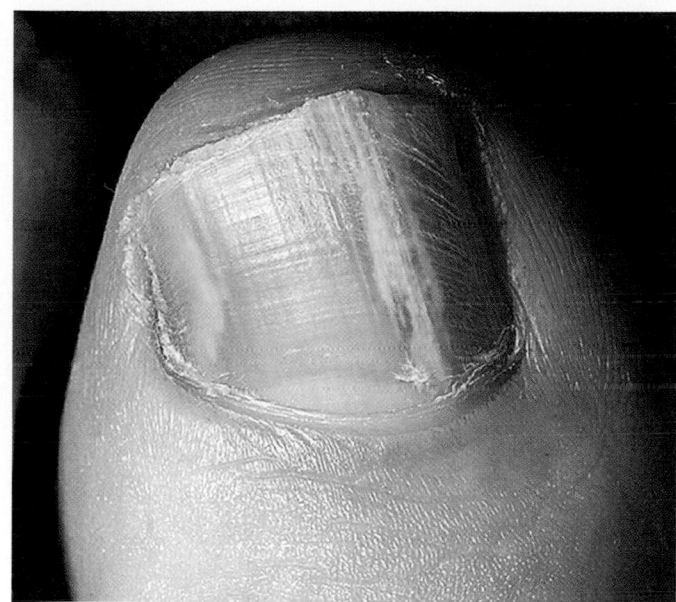

FIGURE 31-7 Tinea unguium. (From Habif TP: *Clinical dermatology*, ed 5, St Louis, 2010, Mosby.)

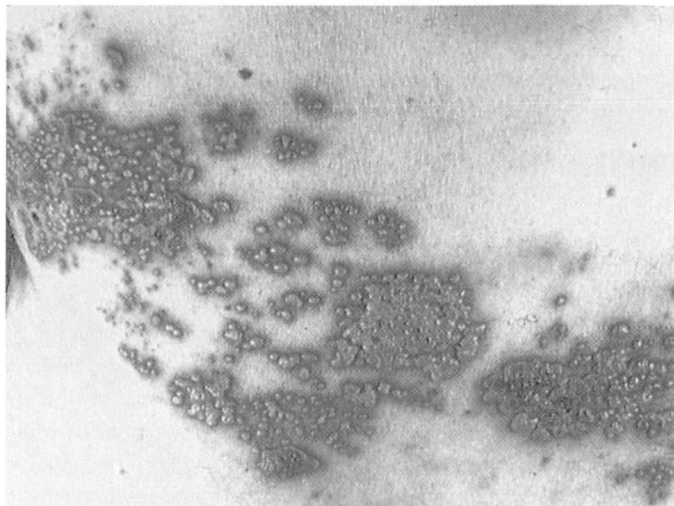

FIGURE 31-8 Herpes zoster (shingles). (From Swartz MH: *Textbook of physical diagnosis*, ed 7, Philadelphia, 2014, Saunders.)

which turns yellow, white, or **opaque**. The texture also changes, and the nail becomes thick and brittle. If the fungus has been present for a long time, the nail can become twisted or distorted. The most effective treatment for nail fungus is oral terbinafine hydrochloride (Lamisil) or itraconazole (Sporanox), which inhibit the production of fungal cells. However, the drug must be taken for 6 weeks to treat fungal infection of a fingernail and for 12 weeks for infection of a toenail; treatment carries the risk of liver complications.

Viral Infections

Warts. Warts, or verrucae, are caused by the human papillomavirus (HPV). Infection with HPV results in hyperplasia of the epidermis and a raised, cauliflower-like appearance. Verrucae can develop anywhere, but the most common sites are the fingers and the soles (plantar warts). Most warts resolve over time, but they can be treated with topical chemicals, excised surgically, vaporized with lasers, or removed with **cryosurgery**.

Herpes Simplex (Cold Sores). Cold sores, or fever blisters, are caused by herpes simplex virus type 1 (HSV-1). The initial infection may be asymptomatic or may cause painful ulcers along the gum lines of the mouth or on the lips. After the primary infection, the virus remains dormant in the trigeminal nerve and can be reactivated by exposure to the sun or to cold; by the presence of another infection, such as an upper respiratory infection; or when the patient is under stress. The patient reports a feeling of burning, tingling, or numbness before the eruption of vesicles. The blisters heal in 2 to 3 weeks, but the process may be speeded up by the use of topical antiviral drugs, such as acyclovir (Zovirax), docosanol (Abreva), or penciclovir cream (Denavir), or with oral antivirals, including famciclovir (Famvir), acyclovir, or valacyclovir (Valtrex). If started at the first indications of a cold sore, antiviral medications can limit the duration and severity of the outbreak.

Herpes Zoster (Shingles). Herpes zoster is an acute inflammatory disorder characterized by highly painful vesicular eruptions on the trunk of the body and occasionally on the face (Figure 31-8). The lesions develop on one side of the body and follow the course of the peripheral nerve, or dermatome, that has been infected by the varicella virus, the same virus that causes chickenpox. The virus lies dormant in a dorsal root ganglia and is reactivated in later years. The cause of this reactivation is unclear, although it appears to be related to stress, immune system problems, and aging.

The onset of the disorder usually is marked by pain along the nerve pathway, and lesions appear in approximately 3 days. Inflammation lasts 10 days to 5 weeks. The patient is diagnosed by the characteristic pattern of painful lesions. Patients complain of burning or tingling pain or in some cases numbness or itching on one side of the body. The most common location for shingles is a band that spans one side of the trunk around the waistline. It may also occur on the forehead, cheek, nose, and around one eye, which may threaten vision. Besides the characteristic rash and associated pain, shingles is diagnosed by isolating the virus in cell cultures and by the presence of varicella zoster antibodies in the blood.

Treatment focuses on promoting the patient's comfort with analgesic and antipruritic medications. Corticosteroid medications (prednisone) and antiviral drugs (e.g., topical or oral Zovirax, and oral Famvir or Valtrex) also can be prescribed. Antiviral medications help shorten the length and severity of the shingles outbreak, but they must be started as soon as possible after the rash appears to be most effective. Therefore, individuals who think they might have shingles should call their provider as soon as possible. One of the most serious complications of herpes zoster is **postherpetic neuralgia**, which causes chronic pain after resolution of the initial outbreak. The condition may require treatment with a combination of medications, including lidocaine skin patches (Lidoderm), narcotics, antidepressants (duloxetine [Cymbalta]) or venlafaxine [Effexor XR]), and the anticonvulsant gabapentin (Horizant).

Two vaccines are available that may help prevent shingles. The chickenpox (varicella virus) vaccine (Varivax) is given to babies 12 to 18 months old and to older children and adults who have not had chickenpox; this vaccine reduces the risk and severity of both chickenpox and shingles. The herpes zoster vaccine (Zostavax) is recommended for all adults 60 years or older, regardless of whether they have had shingles. This vaccine does not guarantee protection against shingles, but it can reduce the duration and severity of the outbreak, and it helps prevent postherpetic neuralgia.

Parasites

The itch mite (which causes scabies) and lice (which cause pediculosis) are the two most common parasites that infest human beings. Both scabies and pediculosis are highly contagious. Scabies mites are tiny organisms, barely visible to the eye, that burrow into the epidermis (Figure 31-9). Diagnosis of scabies may require scraping of the skin at an inflamed area and examination of the mites under a low-power microscope. Patients describe symptoms of intense itching, possibly a body rash, and a sensation of something crawling on the skin. Treatment consists of ridding the body of the parasite, controlling the pruritus, and disinfecting the home environment to prevent reinfestation. There are usually no symptoms during the first 2 to 6 weeks of a scabies infestation, but affected individuals can spread the scabies mite during this time. Scabies treatment is recommended for all household members and sexual contacts in the past month; all of these individuals should be treated at the same time to prevent reinfestation. No over-the-counter products have been approved for scabies treatment, so the patient must get a prescription.

Scabies is treated with a single application of 5% permethrin (Elimite) or crotamiton (Eurax) creams all over the body, from the neck down. Because the medication should be left on for a minimum of 8 hours, it typically is applied before bedtime. Treatment must be repeated in 7 to 10 days to destroy the nits (eggs). If a secondary infection occurs, antibiotics may also be prescribed. Lindane lotion (Kwell) is no longer recommended because of widespread resistance and the potential of severe neurologic side effects.

Pediculosis (infestation with lice) can be caused by three different types of lice: head lice (*Pediculus humanus capitis* [Figure 31-10, *A*]); body lice *(Pediculus humanus corporis);* and pubic lice (*Pthirus pubis* [Figure 31-10, *B*]). Lice are large enough to be seen on the hair shafts.

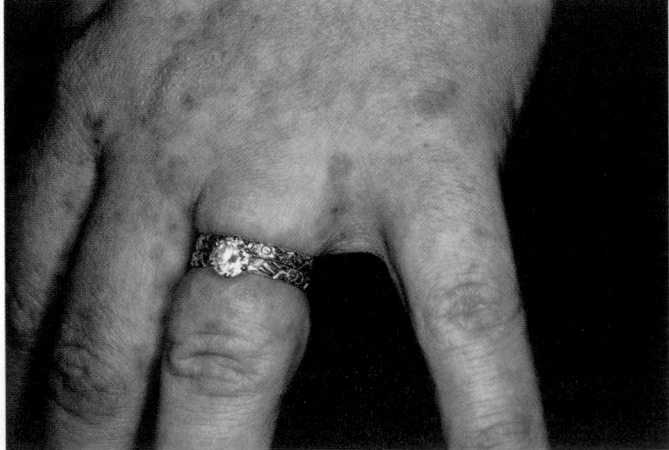

FIGURE 31-9 Scabies rash of the hand. (From James WD et al: *Andrews' diseases of the skin,* ed 11, Philadelphia, 2011, Saunders.)

CDC Recommendations for Treating Lice

The Centers for Disease Control and Prevention (CDC) has established the following recommendations for treating lice:
1. All infested persons (household members and close contacts) and their bedmates should be treated at the same time.
2. Apply a lice medicated shampoo (Nix or Ovide). Do not use cream rinse or a conditioner before applying the medication. Do not rewash the hair for 1 to 2 days after treatment.
3. The American Academy of Pediatrics no longer recommends the use of Lindane shampoo since it can be toxic to the brain and other parts of the nervous system.
4. After treatment, check the hair and use a nit comb to remove nits and lice every 2 to 3 days. Continue to check for 2 to 3 weeks to make sure all lice and nits are gone. Head lice survive less than 1 to 2 days, and nits die within 1 week if they are not on a person.
5. Retreatment is recommended after 9 to 10 days to kill any surviving hatched lice before eggs are produced.
6. The following measures should be taken to prevent reinfestation:
    - Machine wash in hot water and dry on high heat: all clothing, bed linens, and other items worn or used for 2 days before treatment; and dry-clean items that cannot be washed; or seal all exposed items in a plastic bag for 2 weeks.
    - Soak combs and brushes in hot water for 5 to 10 minutes.
    - Vacuum floors and furniture.

Centers for Disease Control and Prevention. *www.cdc.gov/parasites/lice/head/ treatment.html.* Accessed April 26, 2015.

CRITICAL THINKING APPLICATION   **31-3**

Melissa's daughter brought home a note today warning of a scabies outbreak in her school. Melissa has a few red marks on her forearms, and the areas are quite itchy. Dr. Lee does a skin scraping of one of the areas and views itch mites under the microscope. How should Melissa and her family be treated? Should Melissa remain at work?

Inflammatory Skin Disorders

Seborrheic Dermatitis

Seborrheic dermatitis is one of the most common chronic inflammatory conditions of the sebaceous glands. It alters the amount and quality of the sebum, resulting in dry or moist, greasy-appearing scales and yellowish crusts on the scalp, eyebrows, eyelids, and sides of the nose, behind the ears, and in the middle of the chest. The condition has many different forms, including cradle cap in infants and dandruff in adults. Seborrheic dermatitis of the scalp can be treated with tar- or sulfur-based shampoos; inflammations of the skin usually are treated with topical corticosteroids, such as generic triamcinolone diacetate or betamethasone valerate, or fluocinolone acetonide (Synalar). Seborrheic keratosis (age spots) is characterized by benign, slightly raised, tan to black lesions that occur with aging.

Contact Dermatitis

Contact dermatitis is an acute inflammatory response to a skin irritant or from exposure to a substance that causes an allergic

FIGURE 31-10 Types of lice. **A,** *Pediculus humanus capitis* (head louse) and lice in the hair. **B,** *Phthirus pubis* (pubic or crab louse) and pubic lice rash. (**A** from Lissauer T et al: *Illustrated textbook of paediatrics,* ed 4, London, 2012, Mosby; **B** from Long SS et al: *Principles and practice of pediatric infectious diseases,* ed 4, Philadelphia, 2012, Saunders.)

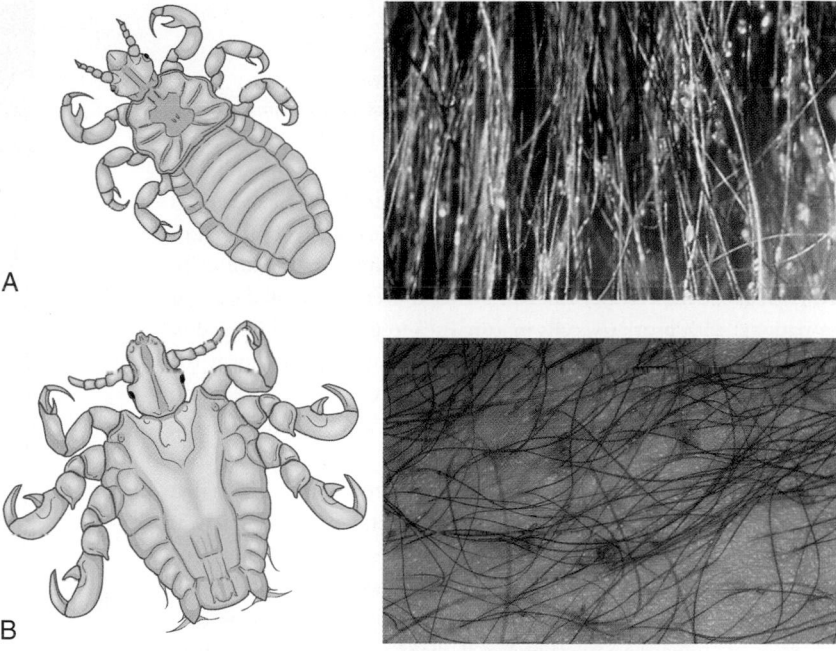

reaction. An individual who is allergic to latex gloves or who has been exposed to poison ivy shows the signs and symptoms of contact dermatitis. The individual complains of redness (erythema), edema, pruritus, and vesicles. The patient should be encouraged to wash the affected area immediately after exposure to remove the irritant. Medical treatment includes application of a corticosteroid cream or the use of oral corticosteroid medications (e.g., prednisone, methylprednisolone [Medrol]) if the symptoms are severe.

Eczema (Atopic Dermatitis)

Eczema is an idiopathic inflammatory skin disease that tends to occur in patients with a family history of allergies. In young children, it may be caused by food allergies, and in older children, stress or temperature extremes can trigger flare-ups. The condition usually improves and may disappear as the child ages. Eczema is characterized by a vesicular rash on the face, neck, and elbows and behind the knees and ears. It causes pronounced pruritus that if left untreated results in excoriation of the affected area from constant scratching. Eczema is not contagious.

Eczema is diagnosed with a comprehensive family history and examination of the skin. The patient may be asked to investigate possible allergens by making a list of all items that might be responsible for the outbreak, or the provider may recommend allergy testing. The goal of treatment is to reduce the frequency and number of eruptions and to relieve the pruritus so that affected areas do not become excoriated. The primary inflammation usually is treated with topical corticosteroids and oral antihistamines (e.g., diphenhydramine [Benadryl], cetirizine [Zyrtec], fexofenadine [Allegra]) to control itching. The provider may recommend controlled exposure to sunlight or UV rays to prevent and treat outbreaks. Psoralens are a group of light-sensitive drugs that absorb ultraviolet (UVA) light and are combined with UVA to treat skin conditions such as eczema and psoriasis. An example of a drug in this classification is methoxsalen (Uvadex). Inflammation of eczema plaques typically indicates a secondary staphylococcal infection, which should be treated with an oral antibiotic.

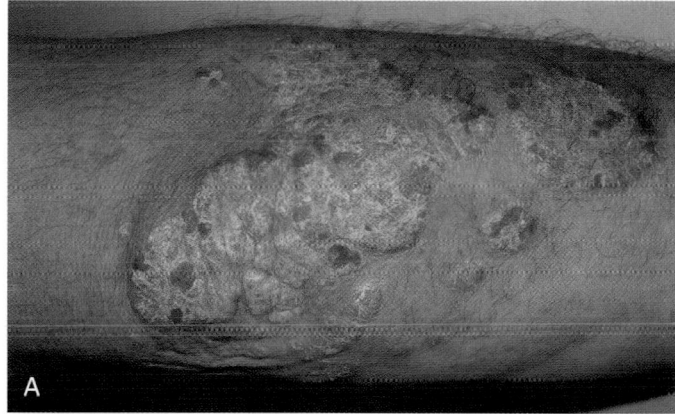

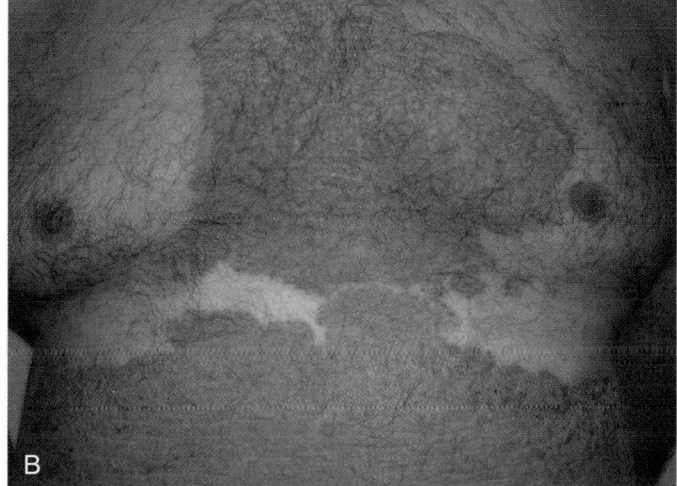

FIGURE 31-11 Psoriasis. (From Marks J, Miller J: *Lookingbill and Marks' principles of dermatology,* ed 5, Philadelphia, 2014, Saunders.)

Autoimmune Skin Disorders

Psoriasis

Psoriasis is a chronic skin disease that produces discrete pink or red lesions covered with silvery scales (Figure 31-11). The disease may begin at any age, although most patients develop the problem before age 40. The lesions are not infectious, and the disease is characterized by periodic flare-ups throughout life. Psoriasis is caused by an autoimmune reaction that speeds up the maturation rate of skin cells. Normal skin cells mature, die, and are shed every 28 to 30 days, but in patients with psoriasis, cells mature in 3 to 6 days, and instead of sloughing off the surface of the skin, they build up and form the classic psoriatic silvery patch. The affected skin is dry, cracked, and encrusted. Lesions may appear on the scalp, chest, buttocks, and extremities.

Outbreaks of psoriatic plaques are associated with triggers that the patient may be able to identify and therefore avoid, such as infection (e.g., strep throat); an injury to the skin or a bug bite; stress; cold weather; smoking and heavy alcohol consumption; and certain medications, such as lithium for mood disorders or beta blockers for hypertension. Psoriasis is diagnosed by observation of the skin, a careful patient history (a familial link has been established), and/or a skin biopsy. Treatment is palliative because the disease has no cure. Exposure to UV light may slow cell production, and coal tar preparations help relieve irritation when applied to affected areas. The provider also may order a combination of therapies, including methotrexate (Rheumatrex); a retinoid, such as acitretin (Soriatane); the immunosuppressant cyclosporine (Neoral); low-dose antihistamines; and oatmeal baths to promote the patient's comfort. Biologic medications, which target the body's immune system, are very effective treatments for moderate to severe psoriasis. Research shows infliximab (Remicade) is the most effective biologic agent for psoriasis. Excimer laser treatments that localize high-intensity wavelengths of UV light to targeted plaques, reducing both cell production and inflammation, may also be effective.

Systemic Lupus Erythematosus

Systemic lupus erythematosus (SLE) is a chronic autoimmune inflammatory disease of the connective tissue. The cause is unknown, although women are 10 times more likely to develop the disease than men. It can affect any connective tissue in the body but typically causes inflammatory changes in the skin, joints, muscles, and kidneys. SLE usually involves more than one organ, and the patient experiences periods of **exacerbation** and remission. A diagnostic characteristic of the disease is a butterfly-shaped rash that stretches from one cheek across the nose to the other cheek (Figure 31-12). Other integumentary system symptoms include erythematous patches and plaques, **alopecia**, and photosensitivity.

The prognosis for SLE depends on organ involvement; patients who develop renal, cardiovascular, or neurologic complications have a poor prognosis. Treatment includes the use of nonsteroidal antiinflammatory drugs (NSAIDs), including ibuprofen (Advil) and diclofenac (Voltaren), or controlled low doses of corticosteroids (prednisone) when needed. Serious cases are treated with cytotoxic drugs (cyclophosphamide [Cytoxan]) and antimalarial drugs, such as hydroxychloroquine (Plaquenil) as needed to control inflammatory reactions.

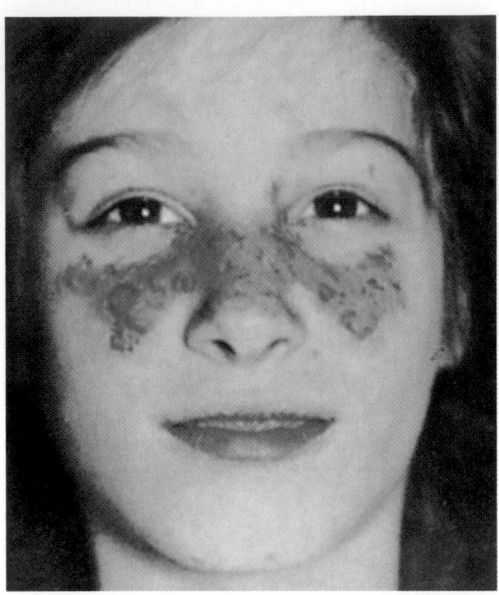

FIGURE 31-12 Butterfly rash of systemic lupus erythematosus (SLE). (Modified from Kliegman RM et al: *Nelson textbook of pediatrics,* ed 18, Philadelphia, 2007, Saunders.)

Diagnosis of Systemic Lupus Erythematosus

The American Rheumatism Association has developed 11 criteria for the diagnosis of systemic lupus erythematosus (SLE):
- Malar or "butterfly" rash
- Discoid skin rash—patchy redness with hyperpigmentation and hypopigmentation
- Photosensitivity—skin rash in reaction to sunlight
- Mucous membrane ulcers of the lining of the mouth, nose, or throat
- Arthritis
- Pleuritis or pericarditis—inflammation of the tissue that lines the heart or lungs
- Kidney abnormalities
- Brain irritation—seizures and/or psychosis
- Low blood cell counts
- Abnormal immune studies
- Positive antinuclear antibodies (ANAs) in the blood

Thermal Injuries

Skin can be damaged and injured by exposure to moderately high or low temperatures over an extended period. It also can be injured in a relatively short time when exposed to very high or low temperatures. The most common thermal injuries are burns, which are classified as superficial thickness (first degree), partial thickness (second degree), or full thickness (third degree), depending on the depth of the wound (Figure 31-13). With severe burns, all three types commonly are seen in the same location: superficial burns along the edges, partial-thickness burns with vesicles closer to the center, and full-thickness burns at the center of the area.

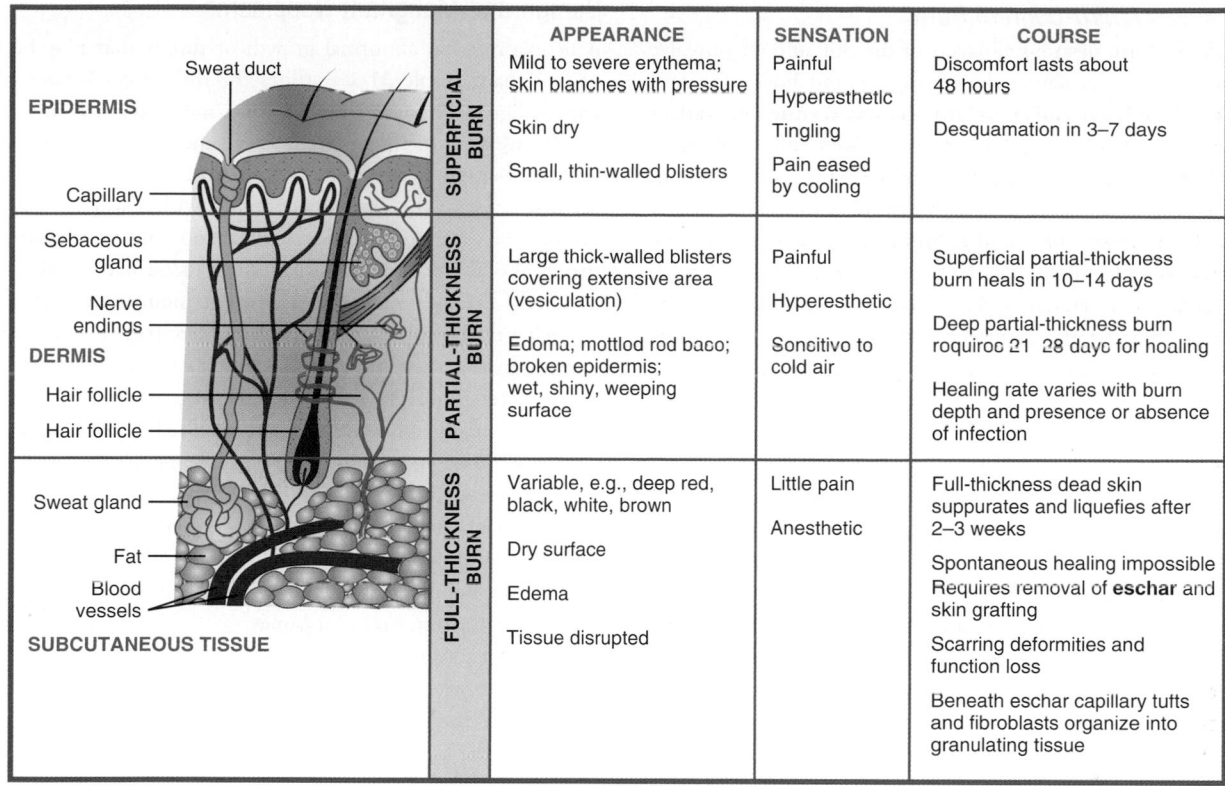

		APPEARANCE	SENSATION	COURSE
EPIDERMIS — Sweat duct, Capillary	SUPERFICIAL BURN	Mild to severe erythema; skin blanches with pressure Skin dry Small, thin-walled blisters	Painful Hyperesthetic Tingling Pain eased by cooling	Discomfort lasts about 48 hours Desquamation in 3–7 days
Sebaceous gland — Nerve endings — DERMIS — Hair follicle — Hair follicle	PARTIAL-THICKNESS BURN	Large thick-walled blisters covering extensive area (vesiculation) Edema; mottled red base; broken epidermis; wet, shiny, weeping surface	Painful Hyperesthetic Sensitive to cold air	Superficial partial-thickness burn heals in 10–14 days Deep partial-thickness burn requires 21–28 days for healing Healing rate varies with burn depth and presence or absence of infection
Sweat gland — Fat — Blood vessels — SUBCUTANEOUS TISSUE	FULL-THICKNESS BURN	Variable, e.g., deep red, black, white, brown Dry surface Edema Tissue disrupted	Little pain Anesthetic	Full-thickness dead skin suppurates and liquefies after 2–3 weeks Spontaneous healing impossible Requires removal of **eschar** and skin grafting Scarring deformities and function loss Beneath eschar capillary tufts and fibroblasts organize into granulating tissue

FIGURE 31-13 Classification of burns.

Superficial (First-Degree) Burn

A superficial burn affects only the epidermis, is erythemic (red), blanches with pressure, and is painful but does not have blisters at the site. Mild sunburn and a steam burn without vesicle formation are examples of superficial burns.

Partial-Thickness (Second-Degree) Burn

A partial-thickness burn destroys the entire epidermal layer and varying depths of the dermis and causes blister formation and subcutaneous edema and pain. The danger of infection in the blistered area also is a concern. If a burn is deep enough, some destruction of the hair follicles and the sebaceous glands may occur.

Treatment of Minor Burns

Because burns damage the natural protection of the skin, preventing infection at the site is a primary concern. Superficial-thickness burns typically heal on their own within a week, as long as they are kept clean and infection does not occur. Medical treatment of partial-thickness burns includes gentle cleansing of the site with a bactericidal solution and débridement of broken blisters or dead skin. Intact blisters should be left alone. Partial-thickness burns may be treated with a thin layer of silver sulfadiazine cream and application of a nonadherent, multilayered dressing for several days to 1 week. The patient's tetanus immunization status should be reviewed, and a tetanus injection should be given if needed. The provider also may order analgesics to relieve pain. Patients with partial-thickness burns (those reporting blisters at the site of the burn) should be seen by the provider for treatment.

Patient Education for Burn Care

- Warning signs of infection include fever, malaise, inflammation, swelling, increased pain, odor, and drainage from the burn area. Any of these should be reported to the provider immediately.
- Review wound care with the patient, including gentle cleansing with bactericidal solution (e.g., povidone-iodine solution [Betadine]) and covering the wound with an antibiotic ointment (silver sulfadiazine) so that the dressing does not stick to the burn.
- The patient should eat a high-calorie, high-protein diet to maintain weight and promote healing.
- For partial-thickness burns, the development of new skin takes 6 weeks, and complete healing occurs in 6 to 12 months, depending on the extent of the burn.

CRITICAL THINKING APPLICATION 31-4

Thomas Rangoso, a 66-year-old patient, calls the office to report a burn on his right hand and forearm. He fell while passing the stove and burned himself on the hot surface. Mr. Rangoso tells Melissa that the area is very red and painful and has blisters in the center. He wants to break the blisters and put butter on the burn. Should Mr. Rangoso be seen by Dr. Lee? What should Melissa tell him about how to care for the burn until he is seen by the physician?

Full-Thickness (Third-Degree) Burn

A full-thickness burn destroys all layers of the skin and may involve underlying fat, muscle, nerves, blood supply, and bone. The area appears charred or white and has a firm, leathery texture. The patient feels no pain because nerve endings have been destroyed. Full-thickness burns have the potential to cause major complications, including dehydration, circulatory collapse, respiratory distress, and septic shock. Treatment of major burns includes maintaining the patient's airway, replacing fluids, preventing infection, and administering oxygen. Débridement of affected tissue, including areas of **eschar**, and skin grafts are required for wound healing. Depending on the extent of the burns, the patient may be hospitalized in an intensive care unit or a specialty burn unit.

Burns are classified according to the percentage of body surface involved, based on the Rule of Nines. The Rule of Nines is an assessment tool that helps caregivers quickly calculate the amount of burned tissue. The body is divided into sections equal to about 9% of the total body surface area (TBSA). When a burn victim is assessed, the affected regions are combined to yield an estimate of the total percentage of burned tissue. Partial-thickness burns over 15% of the total body surface and full-thickness burns of less than 2% can be treated in the ambulatory care setting if the patient can be seen immediately. Patients with larger body surface area involvement or other complications should be transported immediately to a hospital.

Cold Injuries

Cold injuries usually are less severe than burns, but prolonged exposure to cold temperatures can result in infection, gangrene, amputation and, in severe cases, death. Frostbite is caused by exposure to subfreezing temperatures. Damage occurs at the level of the capillaries, which become permanently dilated and unable to regulate local blood flow. Signs and symptoms of superficial frostbite include burning, tingling, numbness, and a white or grayish color of the skin. With deep frostbite, blisters form and the area is hard, mottled, edematous, and blue or gray after thawing.

The extent of injury is determined by visual examination and the history of the exposure. Treatment consists of warming the area with immersion in warm water (100° to 106°F [38° to 41°C]). The affected site should never be rubbed because this increases cellular destruction. The person's vital signs should be monitored, and the provider's orders should be followed explicitly.

Benign and Malignant Neoplasms

A neoplasm is an abnormal growth or tumor that may be benign or malignant. Table 31-1 outlines the differences between benign and malignant tumors. Invasion and metastasis are the principal criteria used to distinguish between cancerous and noncancerous tumors. **Benign** masses are encapsulated, and although they may increase in size, they remain confined within a shell; **malignant** tumors, on the other hand, invade and take over surrounding tissues. Local invasion of surrounding tissue occurs when malignant cells break through the **basement membrane** that separates epithelial cells from connective tissue. Here the cancerous cells can invade blood and lymph vessels, which carry the malignant cells to organs throughout the body. Patients diagnosed with *carcinoma in situ* have a malignant tumor that is confined to the original site of growth without invasion of the basement membrane. Patients with *regional spread* have evidence of malignant cells in surrounding tissues but no evidence of lymph node involvement. Patients with distant spread, or *metastasis,* show lymph node involvement locally and the development of secondary tumors in other organs, including the lungs, liver, brain, or bones.

Malignant tumors are classified according to their grade and stage. A biopsy sample of the tumor is obtained and sent to a pathologist. The pathologist examines the cells under a microscope and *grades* the sample according to its histologic, or cellular, classification of differentiation. *Differentiation* is the process that normal cells go through to mature. Immature, or primitive, cells never mature and are classified as **anaplastic**, or cancerous. Therefore, the more poorly differentiated the cells (i.e., the less they look like normal cells), the more likely it is that the tissue is cancerous.

If the provider receives a grading report that indicates anaplastic cancerous cells, the next step is to determine whether the cancerous cells have spread from the original site; this is called *staging* the tumor. With staging, a physical examination and diagnostic tests (e.g., bone, liver, or positron emission tomography [PET] scans) are done to determine the degree of tumor spread to a secondary location. The size and depth of the primary tumor, the degree of lymph node involvement, and the presence of metastatic spread determine whether the patient has carcinoma in situ (i.e., a tumor localized to the organ of origin), direct spread beyond the primary organ, lymph node metastasis, or confirmed secondary tumor growth in a distant metastatic site. Grading and staging determine the extent of malignant involvement, which allows the provider to plan appropriate treatment.

TABLE 31-1	Differences Between Benign and Malignant Tumors	
CHARACTERISTIC	**BENIGN TUMOR**	**MALIGNANT TUMOR**
Cellular structure	Same as surrounding tissue	Anaplastic changes and poor cellular differentiation
Type of growth	Encapsulated mass that expands over time	Infiltrates and metastasizes; distant spread through the bloodstream or lymph system to other body tissues and organs can occur
Rate of growth	Usually slow; rarely fatal	May be slow, rapid, or very rapid; almost always fatal if left untreated
Destruction of localized tissue	None	Common; ulceration and necrosis of surrounding tissue

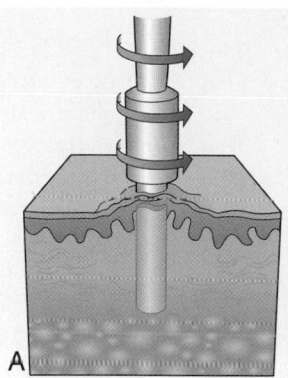 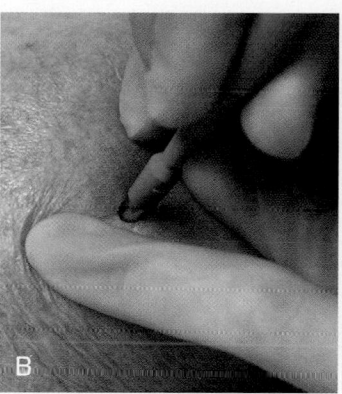 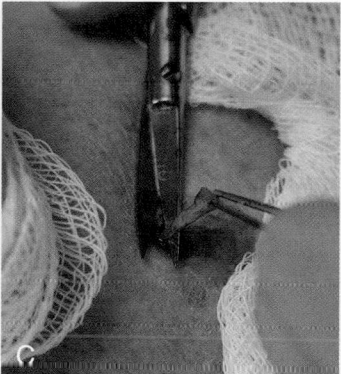 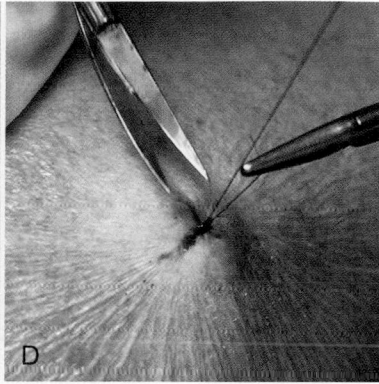

FIGURE 31-14 A, Punch biopsy. **B,** Punch biopsy instrument rotated into the skin. **C,** Cutting the base of the specimen. **D,** Closure of the biopsy wound with a simple epidermal stitch. (Modified from Bolognia J: *Dermatology*, ed 2, Edinburgh, 2008, Mosby.)

Three methods are used to obtain a small piece of tissue for examination under a microscope. In an *excision biopsy*, such as removal of a mole, the entire lesion may be removed for analysis. A *punch biopsy* involves removal of a small section from a designated location in the lesion; the center usually is the optimum site. If the lesion is on the surface of the skin (e.g., a mole), this is done with a scalpel-like circular punch instrument (Figure 31-14); in other cases, a large-gauge needle and syringe unit is used to aspirate cells and fluid from a suspicious area (e.g., a breast biopsy). A *shave biopsy* is performed with a scalpel or razor by cutting or shaving off the growth or lesion for a thin specimen of combined epidermis and upper dermis cells. This method is used to biopsy a possible squamous cell carcinoma lesion. The medical assistant may help the provider perform these biopsy procedures.

The protocol for the treatment of cancer depends on the stage, grade, and type of carcinoma. Possible treatments include surgical removal of the tumor, radiation therapy, chemotherapy, hormone therapy, and immune system boosters. These approaches may be used singly or in combination and usually are determined by an *oncologist,* a physician specialist in the study and treatment of cancer.

Assisting with a Tissue Biopsy

1. Assemble the necessary supplies for the procedure.
2. Prepare the patient with proper gowning, draping, and positioning and make sure the patient understands the procedure.
3. Confirm that the provider has obtained the patient's informed consent.
4. Prepare the site of the biopsy according to office protocol.
5. Assist the provider as needed, using appropriate personal protective equipment according to Standard Precautions.
6. Label the sample container and prepare it for transport to the testing laboratory. Remember to include laboratory request forms.
7. Clean the procedure area, properly dispose of all waste materials, and disinfect and sterilize equipment used in the procedure.
8. Sanitize your hands and document the procedure, including the patient education provided on biopsy site care.

Patient Education: *Cancer's Seven Warning Signs*

The initial letters of the warning signs spell out the word CAUTION. Any of these warning signs should be reported to the provider immediately. Early detection and self-examination are crucial to cancer survival.

- Change in bowel or bladder habits
- A sore that does not heal
- Unusual bleeding or discharge
- Thickening or a lump in the breast or elsewhere
- Indigestion or difficulty in swallowing
- Obvious change in a wart or mole
- Nagging cough or hoarseness

Neoplasms of the Skin

Neoplasms of the skin may be benign or malignant. Examples of benign tumors include birthmarks and moles (nevi). However, a tumor may be benign but have a predisposition to be cancerous, which means that it can change from a benign state to a malignant one. Whenever a neoplasm is discovered, the provider usually performs a biopsy of the lesion to establish the type of cells involved.

Three cancerous lesions of the skin can occur: basal cell carcinoma, squamous cell carcinoma, and malignant melanoma. Basal cells line the deepest layer of the epidermis. Basal cell carcinoma is very slow growing and is the most frequently seen form of skin cancer. The most common sites are areas of the body exposed to the sun, such as the face and forearms. The typical basal cell carcinoma appears as a small, pearly, dome-shaped nodule with small, visible blood vessels called *telangiectasias*. However, it also can appear as a persistent sore, with a reddish, irritated appearance (Figure 31-15), that does not heal.

Squamous cell carcinoma grows rapidly and is more serious because it has a tendency to metastasize. It appears as a firm, red nodule with visible scales, and it may ulcerate and form a crust (Figure 31-16). Patients typically report both basal and squamous cell skin cancers as sores that persist and never heal.

Malignant melanoma develops from a change in a mole. Sunburns increase the risk of melanoma, and individuals with more moles than average (more than 100) are at greater risk. Individuals with congenital nevi (moles present at birth) are more likely to

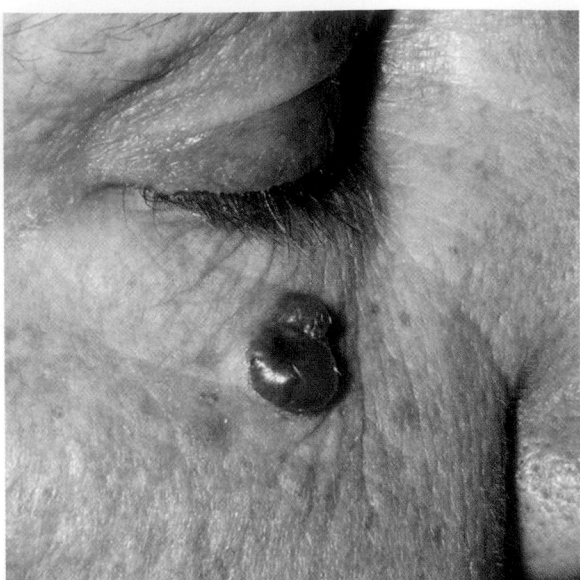

FIGURE 31-15 Basal cell carcinoma. (From James WD et al: *Andrews' diseases of the skin,* ed 11, Philadelphia, 2011, Saunders.)

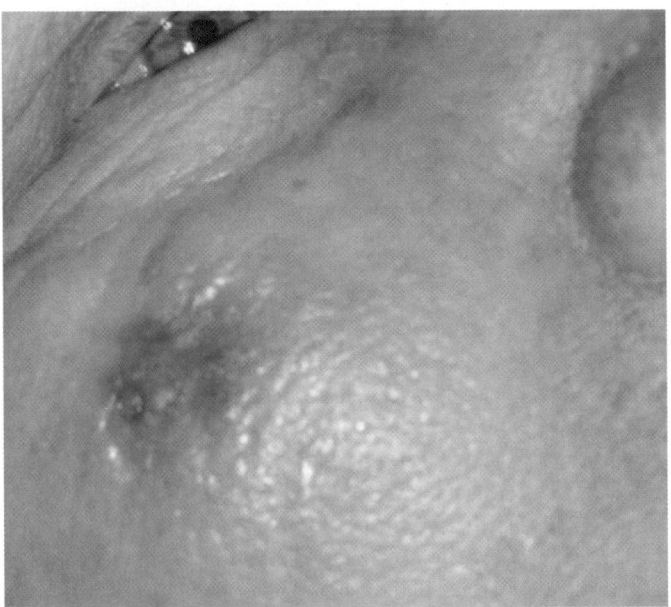

FIGURE 31-16 Squamous cell carcinoma. (From Pfenninger JL, Fowler GC: *Pfenninger and Fowler's procedures for primary care,* ed 3, Philadelphia, 2011, Saunders.)

develop a melanoma. Additional risk factors include an inability to tan, light or red hair, fair skin, family history, and a large number of childhood sunburns. Many forms of melanoma occur, but all are pigmented lesions (usually brown, tan, blue, red, black, or white) that are asymmetric (i.e., have irregular borders) and usually are larger than 6 mm (Figure 31-17). Staging of the disease depends on the depth of the mass, not on the surface size of the mole. If cancerous cells have invaded the basement membrane, the risk of metastasis via the blood and lymph vessels in the dermis is greater. The incidence of malignant melanoma has doubled in the past 10 years, and the disease causes more deaths than all other skin diseases. Melanomas often recur or metastasize within 5 years of diagnosis. The patient should be examined routinely for at least 10 years after removal of a melanoma.

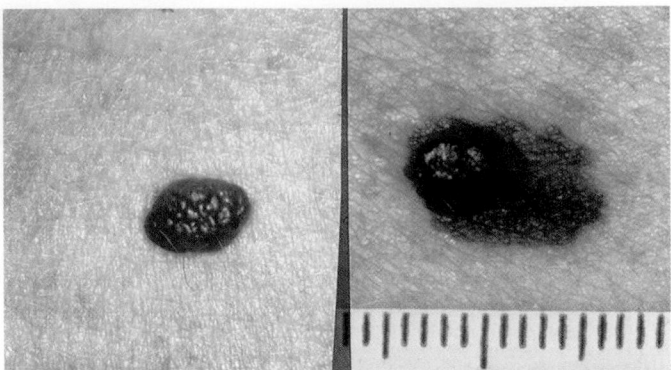

FIGURE 31-17 Pigmented skin lesions. *Left,* Benign pigmented nevus (mole). *Right,* Malignant melanoma. (Courtesy National Cancer Institute, Bethesda, Md.)

All skin cancers are diagnosed by the appearance of the lesions, and the diagnosis is confirmed by biopsy. Treatment depends on the type, the level of invasion, and the location of the mass. The provider may choose to remove the tumor surgically or eradicate it with cryosurgery, **electrodesiccation**, or application of topical chemotherapeutic agents. Ipilimumab (Yervoy) is used to treat melanoma that cannot be removed by surgery or that has metastasized. Yervoy helps the immune system recognize and kill cancer cells. A microscopic surgical procedure (Mohs surgery) is an effective, precise method for treating and removing basal and squamous cell carcinomas. The Mohs technique is performed by specially trained dermatologists, who use a microscope to systematically trace the cancerous lesion down to its roots and remove the tumor layer by layer; this minimizes the chance of regrowth and reduces scar formation.

The National Cancer Institute has stated that the best way to prevent skin cancer is to protect the skin from the sun, starting at an early age. People of all ages should do the following:

- Stay out of the midday sun (10 AM to 4 PM).
- Use protection against UV rays reflected off water and snow.
- Use protection against UV rays even on cloudy days, on which exposure can still occur.
- Wear protective clothing and a wide-brimmed hat when in the sun and protect the eyes with sunglasses.
- Use a sunscreen that filters both UVB and UVA rays with a sun protection factor (SPF) of at least 15.
- Avoid using artificial sun lamps and tanning beds.

Early Warning Signs of Malignant Melanoma: *ABCDE Rule*

If a mole displays any of the following characteristics, a dermatologist should examine it immediately.

A	Asymmetry	One half of the mole does not match the other half.
B	Border	The edges of the mole are blurred or irregular.
C	Color	The mole is not the same color throughout and has shades of tan, brown, black, red, white, or blue.
D	Diameter	The mole is larger than 6 mm, about the size of a pencil eraser.
E	Elevation	A mole that once was flat against the skin now is raised and elevated.

DERMATOLOGIC PROCEDURES

The integumentary system can reflect both internal and external reactions and disease processes. The skin holds information about the body's circulation and nutritional status, and signs of systemic diseases. It also acts as a mirror, reflecting aging changes that occur in all organs of the body. For many people, self-esteem is linked to a youthful appearance, and dermatologic conditions may be very threatening to feelings of self-worth. As you prepare patients for a dermatologic examination, allow them to express their anxieties. The impairments that most frequently bring a patient to the dermatologist's office are cosmetic disfigurements caused by a skin disease, pain and pruritus, and interference with sensations or movements.

Assisting with a Dermatologic Examination

During a dermatologic examination, the provider inspects the entire body, beginning with the scalp and continuing to the soles, including the genital area. Inspection of the skin is followed by detailed examination of suspicious areas through palpation, diascopy, and special tests. A diascope is a glass plate held firmly against the skin to permit observation of changes produced in underlying areas when pressure is applied. Inspection may include the use of a magnifying lens and a bright light to closely examine a suspicious lesion or growth. The dermatologist frequently asks the medical assistant to take photographs of moles and/or to document specific measurements and locations of suspicious lesions. These are placed in the health record for comparison when the patient returns for follow-up visits.

In the physical examination, concerns about the integumentary system include abnormal coloring, such as cyanosis, pallor, erythema, **leukoderma**, or excessive brown patches. **Jaundice** may indicate an increase in the level of **bilirubin** in the blood. Decreased pigmentation is found in *vitiligo*, an acquired loss of melanin characterized by blotchy white patches on the skin. Lesions, ulcers, and bruises may be the result of pathologic conditions. Localized red or purple changes may be caused by vascular neoplasms, birthmarks, or subcutaneous hemorrhages (**petechiae** and **ecchymosis**). Palpation helps confirm findings of the inspection. Therefore, inspection and palpation are interrelated in confirming the diagnosis of an integumentary system disorder. Palpated findings may include the skin's texture or elasticity or the presence of edema or a neoplasm.

Gowning and draping a patient for a skin examination depend on the area to be examined. Remember to expose the area adequately but also to protect the patient's privacy. Try to make the patient as comfortable as possible and offer support when it is needed.

Skin Testing for Allergies

Skin testing to detect allergies requires percutaneous application or intradermal injection of a small amount of antigen (or groups of antigens) and later examination of the test sites for a visible reaction. The larger the localized skin reaction, the more profound the patient's allergic response to the tested allergen.

Percutaneous Test. A percutaneous, or scratch, test may be performed on the forearm, upper arm, or back. The back is favored in young children because of the large area of skin available. It also is easier to immobilize the child in this position. The skin surface is labeled or numbered in rows 1½ to 2 inches apart, and a small amount of allergen is placed on the skin, which is then scratched

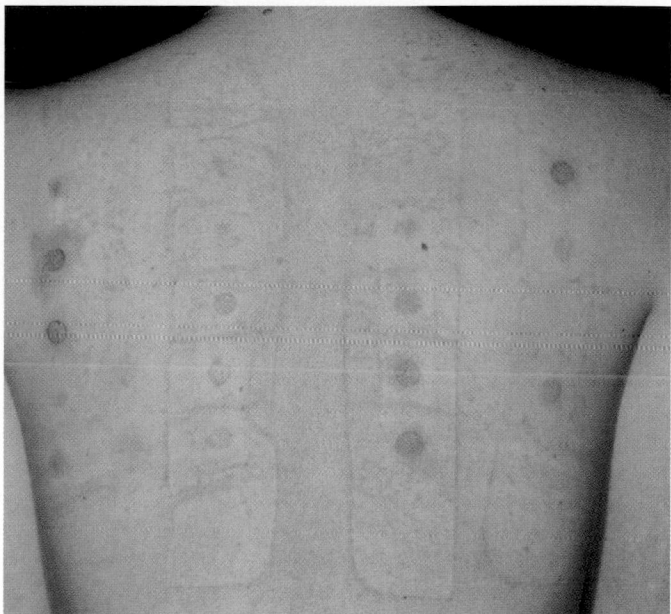

FIGURE 31-18 Results of allergy testing. (From Habif TP: *Clinical dermatology*, ed 5, St Louis, 2010, Mosby.)

or pricked to place the allergen just under the skin surface. Many allergists use a plastic device that is dipped into the designated allergens and lightly pressed into the skin so that the prick and allergen deposition occur at the same time. Seventy or more tests may be done at one time. It is essential to follow a pattern so that the site of each allergen can be easily identified. This type of allergy testing is used for allergic rhinitis, asthma, and detection of food allergies.

A reaction usually occurs within 10 to 30 minutes of exposure to the allergen. If the reaction is positive, a wheal (hive) forms at the site of the scratch (Figure 31-18). Interpretation of the test result should always be based on a comparison of this reaction with that of the control, which is a scratch with a plain fluid free of any allergy-producing extract.

The interpretation, or reading, of the skin tests is performed by the provider or a trained technician. Reactions commonly are graded from 2 to 4. No precise definition of a reaction can be given, and the intensity of the response may vary among individuals. However, as a general rule, a 2 reaction implies a wheal that is definitely larger than that of the control. A larger wheal is interpreted as a 3, whereas the presence of pseudopods (fingerlike extensions around the periphery of the wheal) may be read as a 4. If a strong reaction occurs, the allergen extract should be carefully wiped off to prevent any further exposure. Frequently, large or significant reactions are accompanied by local itching. Patients should remain in the office for at least 30 minutes after completion of the test in case a delayed systemic allergic response occurs.

Patch Test. This test uses an allergen that is applied to a patch that is placed on the skin. Patch testing helps detect delayed allergic reactions associated with contact dermatitis. The patches are placed on the arms or back and must remain in place for 48 hours. The patient needs to avoid bathing and activities that cause heavy sweating. The patches are removed at a subsequent office visit. Skin irritation at the patch site indicates an allergy to that particular substance.

Guidelines for Allergen Skin Testing

- The patient should stop taking all antihistamines or allergy medications 3 to 10 days before testing to prevent false-negative results.
- Recommended sites for injection or application of the allergen are the anterior forearm, the upper arm, and the back.
- Allergen sites must be specifically labeled and spaced approximately $1\frac{1}{2}$ to 2 inches apart.
- If the patient shows signs of anaphylaxis, notify the provider immediately and prepare emergency supplies. Allergy testing should be performed only when the provider is on site.
- Skin testing may cause a mild systemic allergic response, resulting in rhinitis, wheezing, and sneezing. The patient should contact the provider if a more severe reaction occurs.

Intradermal (Intracutaneous) Test. The intradermal test is more sensitive than the percutaneous test and usually is used to diagnose allergies to penicillin and insect venom, such as from bee stings. Extracts are injected into the intradermal layer of the skin in doses of 0.1 to 0.2 mL. This method also is used for the tuberculin (purified protein derivative [PPD]) test and the Valley Fever coccidioidomycosis test. When intradermal injections are used for allergy testing, 10 to 15 allergens may be tested at one time on each arm. The reaction time is identical to that of the scratch test; however, the antigen is more dilute.

Radioallergosorbent Test. The radioallergosorbent test (RAST) measures the level of antibodies created when a sample of the patient's blood is mixed with allergens in the laboratory. The RAST is easier to perform than skin testing because it requires a single venipuncture. Although skin testing remains the preferred method of diagnosing hypersensitivity, the RAST may be indicated when the patient cannot stop antihistamine medications, when a skin disorder makes accurate interpretation of skin test results difficult, or when skin test results are negative but the patient's signs and symptoms support further investigation. RAST blood tests are primarily used to identify food allergies.

CRITICAL THINKING APPLICATION   31-5

A new employee in the practice asks Melissa's help in understanding the different methods of testing for allergies. What should Melissa tell her about the various skin tests performed in the office and the venipuncture RAST test?

Treatment of Allergies

The classic treatment of allergies is to encourage the patient to avoid known or suspected allergens. Unfortunately, this is not always possible, so the provider may prescribe antihistamine medications, such as levocetirizine (Xyzal), for relief of allergy symptoms. Over-the-counter antihistamines include Allegra, Zyrtec, and Claritin. Another option is the use of immunotherapy, a series of injections in which minute doses of known allergens are administered subcutaneously over time to desensitize the patient's immune system and ultimately develop a resistance to the immune response. This usually requires weekly or bimonthly injections over several years. Some patients are cured, whereas others have only a minor reduction in allergic symptoms. Immunotherapy is controversial because it is an expensive, invasive, and potentially dangerous treatment with unpredictable results. It is recommended only for patients with severe allergic symptoms that are not relieved by antihistamine medications.

If you are responsible for administering allergen injections, you must take great care to dispense the correct dose of each allergen; administer each subcutaneous injection in a separate site; accurately document the procedure and the exact location of each injection; record any local or systemic reactions; and observe the patient for at least 20 to 30 minutes after the injections to detect possible systemic allergic responses, including urticaria (hives), wheezing, or hypotension. If the patient shows any localized or systemic reactions, the provider should be notified.

Appearance Modification Procedures

Chemical Peel (Chemexfoliation). Topical agents are used in chemical peels to minimize or remove minor skin features, such as acne scars, hyperpigmentation, and fine wrinkles. Agents used for chemical peels include tretinoin cream 0.05% to 0.1% concentration (Retin-A) and a number of different acidic preparations. During application, care must be taken to prevent the solution from entering the eyes. The use of chemical exfoliating agents may cause the skin to appear inflamed and dry with crusting and edema. The patient may complain of stinging and burning at the beginning of the treatment regimen. The patient should avoid sun exposure for the length of treatment and should use a sunscreen with a minimum SPF of 15 because photophobia (light sensitivity) is a typical side effect of treatment.

Dermabrasion. A dermabrader is a handheld device that mechanically evens the layers of dermal tissue. It is effective in the treatment of scars from acne vulgaris. Topical anesthetics (e.g., ethyl chloride) or locally injected anesthetics are used for the procedure. Besides the dermabrader, the dermatologist may use a variety of wire brushes, abrasive disks, or other devices to smooth scar tissue. Standard Precautions must be followed, including the use of face and eye guards, to prevent aerosol or splatter contamination from the site. The patient should be educated about wound care, signs of infection, and the presence of photophobia for 6 to 12 months after the procedure.

Laser Resurfacing (Photothermolysis). Laser therapy may be used for fine lines and wrinkles, pigmented areas, shallow scars, and tattoo removal. Typically, the patient is instructed to prepare the site 3 to 6 weeks before the procedure with tretinoin (Retin-A), alpha hydroxy solutions, or bleaches. Laser procedures are performed with the patient under local, regional, or general anesthesia. During the procedure, it is extremely important that the patient and all personnel wear the type of eye protection recommended by the laser manufacturer. After the procedure, cool packs are applied to help reduce swelling, and topical antibiotic ointment is used to prevent infection. The treated area appears inflamed and edematous and can take up to 2 weeks to heal; it can take as long as 6 months for the inflammation to fade.

Botox Injections. Botox is a strong neurotoxin (a substance toxic to nerves) produced by *Clostridium botulinum,* a bacterium that causes food poisoning. Two strains of the botulism bacterium are used in dermatologic procedures for appearance modification. Botox treatments involve injection of the substance around the eyes, mouth, and forehead. The toxin interferes with nervous stimulation, which temporarily paralyzes the muscles of the face that cause wrinkles to form. It also smoothes out the skin and makes it look younger and fresher. The effects are short term, so treatments must be repeated every 3 to 4 months, and some patients complain of an inability to show facial expression because of muscle paralysis.

CLOSING COMMENTS

Patient Education

The field of dermatology offers medical assistants many opportunities and topics for patient education. Skin care products are advertised in the newspaper, online, in magazines, and on television. Consult the dermatologist for whom you work and get approval of skin care products the provider recommends to patients.

Another area of patient education involves the potentially dangerous effects of sunlight and tanning beds. Obtain literature showing how UV rays cause premature aging and may cause cancerous lesions later in life. Tanning beds should be avoided, especially by individuals with a skin disorder and by those taking medications that cause photophobia. Providing patients with information about the warning signs of cancer also is a vital part of patient education in a dermatology practice.

Legal and Ethical Issues

While working in a dermatology practice, you will hear many patients express concern about skin disorders. Allow patients to express their concerns. Use therapeutic listening techniques, but be careful when offering encouragement about the course and outcome of treatment. The improvement made with treatment of a skin disorder may be slow and gradual. Keep encouragement on a positive level. Help the patient recognize small improvements, but remember that it is the provider's role to explain potential treatment outcomes. Promising outcomes could lead to a lawsuit.

Professional Behaviors

The medical assistant must develop the ability to interact therapeutically with patients, families, co-workers, and other members of the healthcare team. When interacting with patients in a dermatology practice, the medical assistant needs to be especially sensitive to the patient's nonverbal behaviors and emotions. Many of the conditions seen in a dermatology practice affect how patients look and how they view themselves. Sensitivity to the importance of appearance, especially when skin conditions and/or treatments might alter a patient's appearance, is a crucial trait for healthcare professionals working in a dermatology practice.

SUMMARY OF SCENARIO

Melissa enjoys her work with Dr. Lee, and she recognizes that she needs to keep up with new developments in the field of dermatology. She has learned the importance of giving patients accurate information while conducting telephone screening and always refers questions or concerns to Dr. Lee. Melissa especially enjoys the patient education aspects of working for a dermatologist,

including teaching patients the importance of using sunscreen, controlling sun exposure, and checking for the warning signs of cancer. Melissa also has learned how to assist Dr. Lee with dermatologic procedures, including allergy skin testing and assisting with biopsies, chemical peels, dermabrasions, and laser resurfacing.

SUMMARY OF LEARNING OBJECTIVES

1. **Define, spell, and pronounce the terms listed in the vocabulary.**
   Spelling and pronouncing medical terms correctly reinforce the medical assistant's credibility. Knowing the definitions of these terms promotes confidence in communication with patients and co-workers.

2. **Explain the major functions of the skin.**
   The skin acts as a barrier to protect vital internal organs from infection and injury. It also helps dissipate heat and regulate body temperature, and it synthesizes vitamin D when exposed to UV light. In addition, various sensory receptors all over the skin enable the body to respond to heat, cold, pain, and pressure.

3. **Describe the anatomic structures of the skin.**
   The skin is made up of three layers: the epidermis, which is the thin, uppermost layer; the dermis, the thicker layer beneath, which makes up approximately 90% of the skin mass; and the subcutaneous layer, which consists primarily of fatty or adipose tissue.

4. **Compare various skin lesions and give examples of each.**
   Figure 31-2 shows different types of skin lesions. The diagnosis of skin lesions is based on the color, elevation, and texture of the lesion; whether

pruritus, excoriation, pain, or drainage is present; and whether the lesion is a primary or secondary growth.

5. **Describe typical integumentary system infections and infestations.**
   Integumentary system infections include bacterial infections, such as impetigo, acne vulgaris, furuncles, carbuncles, and cellulitis; fungal infections, including a variety of tinea growths; viral infections, which cause warts, herpes simplex, and herpes zoster outbreaks; and scabies or lice infestations.

6. **Differentiate among various inflammatory and autoimmune integumentary disorders.**
   Inflammatory and autoimmune integumentary system disorders include a variety of seborrheic dermatitis inflammations, contact dermatitis, eczema, and the autoimmune disorders psoriasis, SLE, and scleroderma.

7. **Recognize thermal and cold injuries to the skin.**
   The most common thermal injuries are burns, which are classified as superficial, partial-thickness, or full-thickness, depending on the depth of the wound. The most important concern in the treatment of burns is the

Continued

SUMMARY OF LEARNING OBJECTIVES—*continued*

prevention of infection. Cold injuries usually are less severe than burns, but prolonged exposure can result in infection, gangrene, amputation, and death.

8. **Compare the characteristics of benign and malignant neoplasms.**
Benign masses are encapsulated, whereas malignant tumors invade and take over surrounding tissues. Local invasion of surrounding tissue occurs when malignant cells break through the basement membrane that separates epithelial cells from connective tissue. This allows the cancerous cells to invade blood and lymph vessels, and blood and lymph then can carry the malignant cells to organs throughout the body.

9. **Do the following relating to benign and malignant neoplasms:**
   - *Explain the grading and staging of malignant tumors.*
     Grading is the histologic, cellular classification of a tumor. The more poorly differentiated the cells, the closer the biopsy sample is to an anaplastic cancerous mass. Staging involves using physical examination and diagnostic tests (e.g., bone or liver scans) to determine the presence of tumor spread.
   - *Conduct patient education on the warning signs of cancer.*
     The warning signs of cancer include any change in bowel or bladder habits; a sore that does not heal; unusual bleeding or discharge; a thickening or a lump in the breast or elsewhere; indigestion or difficulty swallowing; an obvious change in a wart or mole; or a nagging cough or hoarseness. Any of these warning signs should be reported to the provider immediately. Early detection and self-examination are crucial to cancer survival.
   - *Describe skin malignancies and their treatment.*
     Three cancerous lesions of the skin can occur: basal cell carcinoma, which is very slow growing and the most frequently seen form of skin cancer; squamous cell carcinoma, which grows rapidly and is more serious because it has a tendency to metastasize; and melanomas, which are pigmented lesions that are asymmetric, have irregular borders, and usually are larger than 6 mm. Treatment depends on the type of lesion, the level of invasion, and the location. The provider may surgically remove the tumor or may destroy it with cryosurgery, electrodesiccation, laser treatment, the application of chemotherapeutic agents, or Mohs surgery.
   - *Define the ABCDE rule for identifying a malignant melanoma.*
     The ABCDE rule includes examination of the site for any of the following: *a*symmetry, irregular *b*order, *c*hange in color, increase in *d*iameter, and *e*levation. If a mole displays any of these characteristics, a dermatologist should check it immediately.

10. **Do the following relating to dermatologic procedures:**
    - *Discuss how to assist with a dermatologic examination.*
      During a dermatologic examination, the dermatologist frequently asks the medical assistant to take photographs of moles and/or to document specific measurements and locations of suspicious lesions.
    - *Summarize allergy testing procedures.*
      Allergy testing is done by exposing the patient to suspected allergens through a scratch on the skin or an intradermal injection and then observing the exposure site to see whether a localized allergic reaction develops. The patient must be off antihistamine drugs for several days before testing. Sites for allergen exposure include the upper arms, anterior forearms, and back. A provider must be present in the facility while allergy testing is done because of the potential for local or systemic allergic reactions in sensitized individuals. Patch testing can be done for contact dermatitis. The radioallergosorbent test (RAST) measures the level of antibodies created when a sample of the patient's blood is mixed with allergens in the laboratory.
    - *Describe the diagnosis and treatment of allergies.*
      Skin testing to detect allergies requires percutaneous application or intradermal injection of a small amount of antigen and later examination of the test sites for a visible reaction. The larger the localized skin reaction, the more profound is the patient's allergic response to the tested allergen. The classic treatment of allergies consists of avoiding known or suspected allergens and prescribing antihistamine medications or immunotherapy.

11. **Explain dermatologic procedures performed in the ambulatory care setting.**
    Dermatologic procedures that can be performed in ambulatory care practices include allergy skin testing, which can be done with scratch, patch, or intradermal tests; drawing blood for a RAST test; treating allergies with immunotherapy; performing a biopsy or procedure to remove a cancerous area; and appearance modification procedures, including chemical peels, dermabrasion, laser resurfacing, and Botox injections.

12. **Discuss the medical assistant's role in patient education, in addition to legal and ethical issues that would apply to a dermatology practice.**
    Areas for possible patient education include dermatologist recommendations for skin care products, the dangers of UV exposure, and information about the warning signs of skin cancer.

CONNECTIONS

Study Guide Connection: Go to the Chapter 31 Study Guide. Read and complete the activities.

evolve Evolve Connection: Go to the Chapter 31 link at *evolve.elsevier.com/kinn* to complete the Chapter Review Quiz. Check out the other resources listed for this chapter to make the most of what you have learned from Assisting in Dermatology.

ASSISTING IN GASTROENTEROLOGY 32

Joan Rothman, CMA (AAMA), was recently hired by United Community Hospital to work for a group of internists. Joan works primarily with Dr. Raj Sahani, a provider who specializes in gastroenterology. Although Joan did very well in school, she has had to learn more advanced information about disorders of the gastrointestinal (GI) tract so that she can answer patients' questions and understand the diagnostic procedures ordered by Dr. Sahani.

Dr. Sahani has asked Joan to research and develop educational packets for common gastrointestinal diagnostic studies and to work with other staff members on understanding procedures related to the GI system. Part of the role of the medical assistant working in a gastroenterology practice is to make sure that patients are properly prepared for diagnostic procedures. Joan also is expected to help in the orientation of new staff members.

While studying this chapter, think about the following questions:
- What does Joan need to include in the educational packets so that patients are prepared for GI examinations?
- What are some of the GI disorders Joan can expect to see in this specialty practice?
- What information should be included in a pamphlet on infectious viral hepatitis?
- What should a new medical assistant know about the GI examination, including instructions for patients on how to collect fecal specimens?

LEARNING OBJECTIVES

1. Define, spell, and pronounce the terms listed in the vocabulary.
2. Describe the primary functions of the GI system.
3. Identify the anatomic structures that make up the GI system and describe the physiology of each.
4. Differentiate among the abdominal quadrants and regions.
5. Summarize the typical symptoms and characteristics of GI complaints and perform telephone screening for patients with GI complaints.
6. Distinguish among cancers of the GI tract.
7. List common esophageal and gastric disorders; also, describe the signs and symptoms, diagnostic tests, and treatments of each.
8. List intestinal disorders; also, describe the signs and symptoms, diagnostic tests, and treatments of each.
9. Do the following related to diseases of the liver and gallbladder:
   - Classify disorders of the liver and gallbladder, and list the signs and symptoms, diagnostic tests, and treatments for each.
- Describe the similarities and differences among the various forms of infectious viral hepatitis.
10. Summarize the medical assistant's role in the GI examination.
11. Do the following when it comes to assisting with gastroenterology diagnostic procedures:
    - Explain the common diagnostic procedures for the GI system.
    - Demonstrate the procedure for assisting with an endoscopic colon examination.
    - Perform the procedural steps for assisting with the collection of a fecal specimen.
12. Describe the medical assistant's role in the proctologic examination.
13. Describe patient education, in addition to legal and ethical issues, related to assisting in gastroenterology.

VOCABULARY

adhesions (ad-he′zhuns) Bands of scar tissue that bind together two anatomic surfaces that normally are separate.

anastomosis (uh-nas-tuh-mo′-sis) Creating a surgical connection between two body structures, such as blood vessels or loops of intestine.

anorexia (a-nuh-rek′-se-uh) A lack or loss of appetite for food.

ascites (ah-si′-tez) An abnormal collection of fluid in the peritoneal cavity containing high levels of protein and electrolytes.

carcinogens (kar-sih′-nuh-jehns) Substances or agents that cause the development of cancer or increase its incidence.

dysphagia Difficulty swallowing

endemic (en-deh′-mik) A term describing a disease or microorganism that is specific to a particular geographic area.

esophageal varices (uh-sah-fuh-je′-uhl var′-uh-sez) Varicose veins of the esophagus that occur as a result of portal hypertension; these vessels can easily hemorrhage.

fecalith (fe′-kuh-lith) A hard, impacted mass of feces in the colon.

fissures Narrow slits or clefts in tissue such as the mouth or the anal area.

fistula (fis′-chuh-luh) An abnormal, tubelike passage between internal organs or from an internal organ to the body's surface.

flatus Gas expelled through the anus.

gangrene The death of body tissue as a result of loss of nutritive supply, followed by bacterial invasion and decay.

hematemesis (he-muh-tem′-uh-sis) Vomiting of blood; may be obviously red (from esophageal varices or a peptic ulcer) or contains partially digested blood and looks like coffee grounds.

hematocrit The percentage by volume of packed red blood cells in a given sample of blood after centrifugation.

hemoglobin (he′-muh-glo-buhn) A protein found in erythrocytes that transports molecular oxygen in the blood.

hepatomegaly (heh-pah-to-meh′-guh-le) Abnormal enlargement of the liver.

ileostomy The surgical formation of an opening of the ileum onto the surface of the abdomen, through which fecal material is emptied.

jaundice Yellowing of the skin and mucous membranes caused by the deposition of bile pigment. Jaundice is not a disease, but rather a sign of a number of diseases, especially liver disorders.

lymphadenopathy (lim-fa-duh-nah′-puh-the) Any disorder of the lymph nodes or lymph vessels.

peristalsis The rhythmic, involuntary serial contraction of the smooth muscles lining the GI tract.

polyps (pah′-lips) Outgrowths of tissue found in the mucosal lining of the colon. Polyps are considered precancerous.

portal circulation The pathway of blood flow through the portal vein from the GI system to the liver.

portal hypertension Increased venous pressure in the portal circulation caused by cirrhosis or compression of the hepatic vascular system.

pyloric sphincter A muscular ring at the distal end of the stomach that separates the stomach from the duodenum of the small intestine.

sclerotherapy (skleh-rah-ther′-ah-pe) The treatment of hemorrhoids or varicose veins by means of injection of sclerosing solutions.

Valsalva maneuver The act of attempting to exhale forcibly while keeping the nose and mouth closed, such as occurs when a person strains to defecate or urinate; uses the arms and upper trunk muscles to move up in bed; or strains during laughing, coughing, or vomiting. This causes trapping of blood in the great veins, preventing the blood from entering the chest and right atrium.

Internal medicine is a nonsurgical specialty consisting of several subspecialties. Gastroenterology, one of these subspecialties, covers an extremely wide area known as the *gastrointestinal (GI) system*, or the *alimentary canal.* Gastroenterologists are concerned with diseases and disorders of the stomach, small intestine, large intestine (colon), appendix, and accessory organs of the liver, gallbladder, and pancreas. Proctology, a subspecialty of gastroenterology, is concerned with disorders of the rectum and anus. The major purpose of the GI system is to prepare, digest, and absorb the necessary nutrients to maintain homeostasis and excrete waste products through the feces.

ANATOMY AND PHYSIOLOGY

The GI system is basically a long, hollow tube with the same structural organization from its beginning to its termination (Figure 32-1). The muscles lining the GI tract are closely regulated by the autonomic nervous system, which gives the entire system its unique ability to move slowly in some locations and to have increased movement in other sections.

The GI system is divided into two parts: the upper digestive system, which includes the mouth, esophagus, and stomach, and the lower digestive system, which consists of the small and large intestines. The GI tract is rich in lymphatic tissue, which is very important for the absorption of nutrients from ingested food. Unfortunately, the lymphatic vessels also are the main route for the spread of cancer.

As mentioned, the GI organs have three primary functions: digestion, absorption, and elimination. When food is taken in through the mouth, it is chewed, or *masticated,* and moistened with saliva. Salivary amylase, an enzyme released by the salivary glands, mixes with the food and begins carbohydrate digestion. This mass, now called a *bolus,* is swallowed, and the food enters the esophagus. Contractions of the smooth muscles are activated, and the bolus is moved by **peristalsis** down the esophagus and into the stomach.

At the distal end of the esophagus is the gastroesophageal, or cardiac, sphincter, which relaxes as the bolus is swallowed so that it can pass into the stomach. The muscular walls of the stomach overlap in folds, or *rugae,* which permit the stomach to expand and to hold as much as 1 to 1.5 L of food and liquid. The gastric glands in the stomach mucosa secrete hydrochloric acid, pepsinogen (which begins the digestion of protein), and intrinsic factor, which is needed for the absorption of vitamin B_{12}. The gastric contents, called *chyme,* are slowly emptied through the **pyloric sphincter** into the small intestine. The small intestine is made up of the duodenum at the proximal end, the jejunum, and the ileum at the distal end.

The common bile duct delivers bile, which is produced in the liver and stored in the gallbladder, to the duodenum. Bile acids *emulsify* fat; that is, they break down large fat molecules into smaller molecules that can be chemically digested by fat enzymes. The pancreatic duct delivers digestive enzymes to the duodenum, including amylase for carbohydrate digestion, trypsin for protein breakdown, and lipase for fats. This mixture of bile and pancreatic enzymes in the duodenum completes the digestion of nutrients, converting carbohydrates into glucose, protein into amino acids, and fats into fatty acids and glycerol.

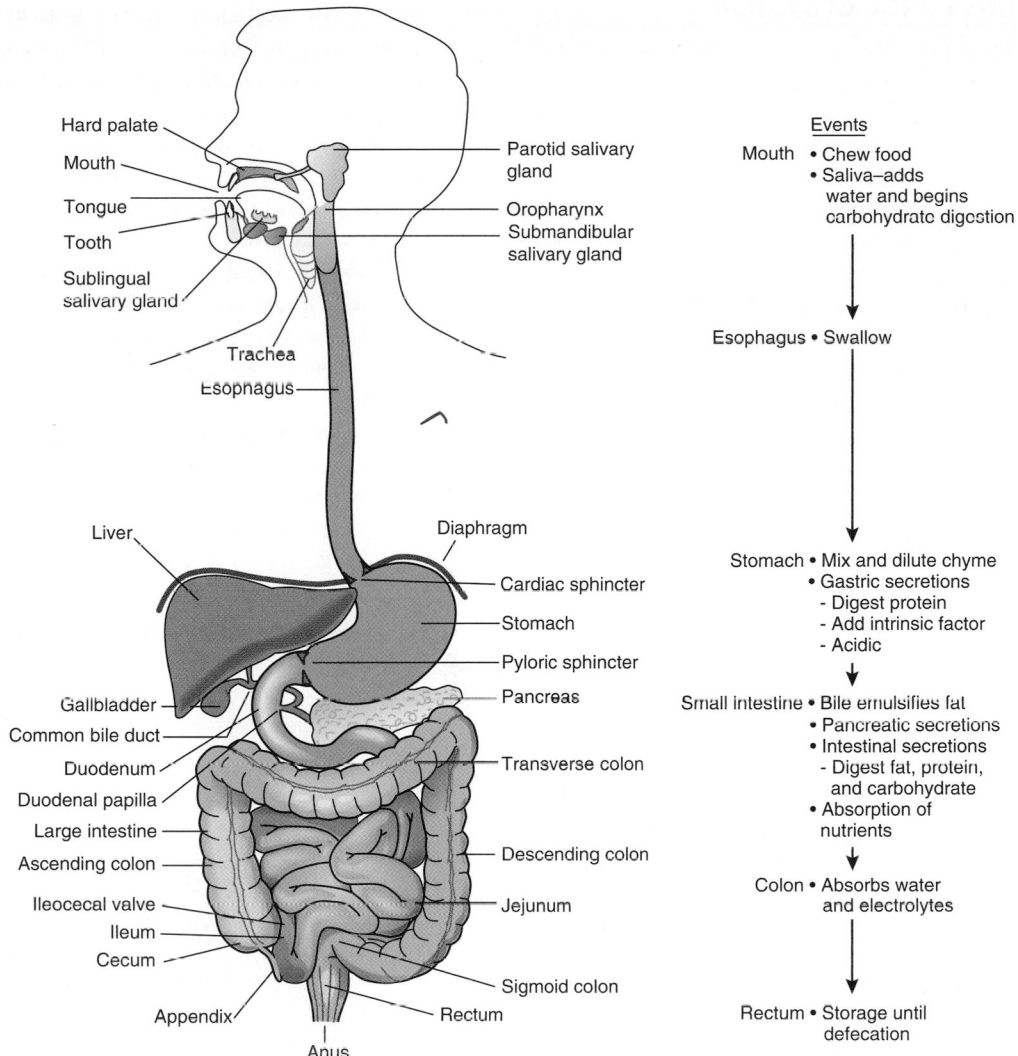

Events

Mouth
• Chew food
• Saliva–adds water and begins carbohydrate digestion

Esophagus • Swallow

Stomach
• Mix and dilute chyme
• Gastric secretions
  - Digest protein
  - Add intrinsic factor
  - Acidic

Small intestine
• Bile emulsifies fat
• Pancreatic secretions
• Intestinal secretions
  - Digest fat, protein, and carbohydrate
• Absorption of nutrients

Colon
• Absorbs water and electrolytes

Rectum
• Storage until defecation

FIGURE 32-1 Anatomy of the digestive system, with associated events. (From VanMeter KC, Hubert RJ: *Gould's pathophysiology for the health professions*, ed 5, Philadelphia, 2015, Saunders.)

Once digestion has been completed in the duodenum, the second function of the GI tract, absorption of nutrients, begins. The small intestine is lined with transverse folds of tissue called *villi.* Approximately 25,000 of these overlapping projections greatly increase the surface area available in the small intestine for nutrient absorption. Each villus is rich with blood vessels that absorb digested nutrients into the **portal circulation** system and carry them directly to the liver for processing. Lymph vessels along the villi absorb fat and deposit it into the systemic circulation. By the time the chyme reaches the terminal end of the small intestine, every nutrient the body needs should have been absorbed. This mass enters the colon, or large intestine, which is made up of the cecum (extending from it is the vermiform appendix), ascending colon, transverse colon, descending colon, sigmoid colon, rectum, and anus. The colon absorbs large amounts of fluids and electrolytes to prevent dehydration of body tissues. Once fluid has been reabsorbed, the remaining solid waste materials, called *feces,* are moved into the sigmoid colon and rectum, and elimination occurs through the anus. This final function is called *defecation.*

CRITICAL THINKING APPLICATION   **32-1**

Summarize what you have learned about the anatomy and physiology of the GI system. Why are the villi of the small intestine so important? If a patient is diagnosed with celiac disease (a condition that causes destruction of intestinal villi because of an immune reaction to gluten), why can this cause malnutrition in an otherwise well-nourished individual?

DISEASES OF THE GASTROINTESTINAL SYSTEM

GI disorders probably are the most common problems seen in a medical office. Most conditions of the GI system are managed by a primary care provider. About 5% to 10% of patients with GI problems are referred to a gastroenterologist for diagnosis and treatment. It is assumed that problems that stem from dental disorders are treated by dental professionals. This chapter concentrates on the GI problems most frequently seen, diagnosed, and treated in an ambulatory care center.

CHARACTERISTICS OF THE GI SYSTEM

The following are the primary structures and functions of the GI system.

The abdominal cavity can be divided into four quadrants or nine regions.

- The quadrant system is more general than the nine-region system. However, patients understand quadrants more easily, and using these terms can help you locate a symptomatic area, such as the site of abdominal pain.
- The four quadrants are identified with abbreviations: The right upper quadrant (RUQ), left upper quadrant (LUQ), right lower quadrant (RLQ), and left lower quadrant (LLQ).
- Figure 32-2 shows the organs located in each quadrant and region. When documenting in the health record, you should use correct medical terminology to detail the location of the patient's complaints. For example, if the patient complains of

pain in the stomach, document it as RUQ pain using an appropriate pain scale (e.g., 1 to 10); a complaint of heartburn would be documented as epigastric distress using the regions identifier.

- The *peritoneum* is a membrane that lines the abdominal wall and covers the organs of the abdominal cavity.
- The *mesentery* is a dorsal peritoneal fold that attaches the jejunum and ileum to the posterior abdominal wall.
- The *omentum* is a fold of fatty peritoneal tissue with multiple lymph nodes. It hangs from the stomach like an apron, covering the anterior transverse colon and the small intestine. Inflammation of the omentum results in the formation of scar tissue and adhesions.
- The GI system digests and absorbs nutrients for the entire body and excretes waste materials in the feces; if it becomes diseased, all other systems are affected.

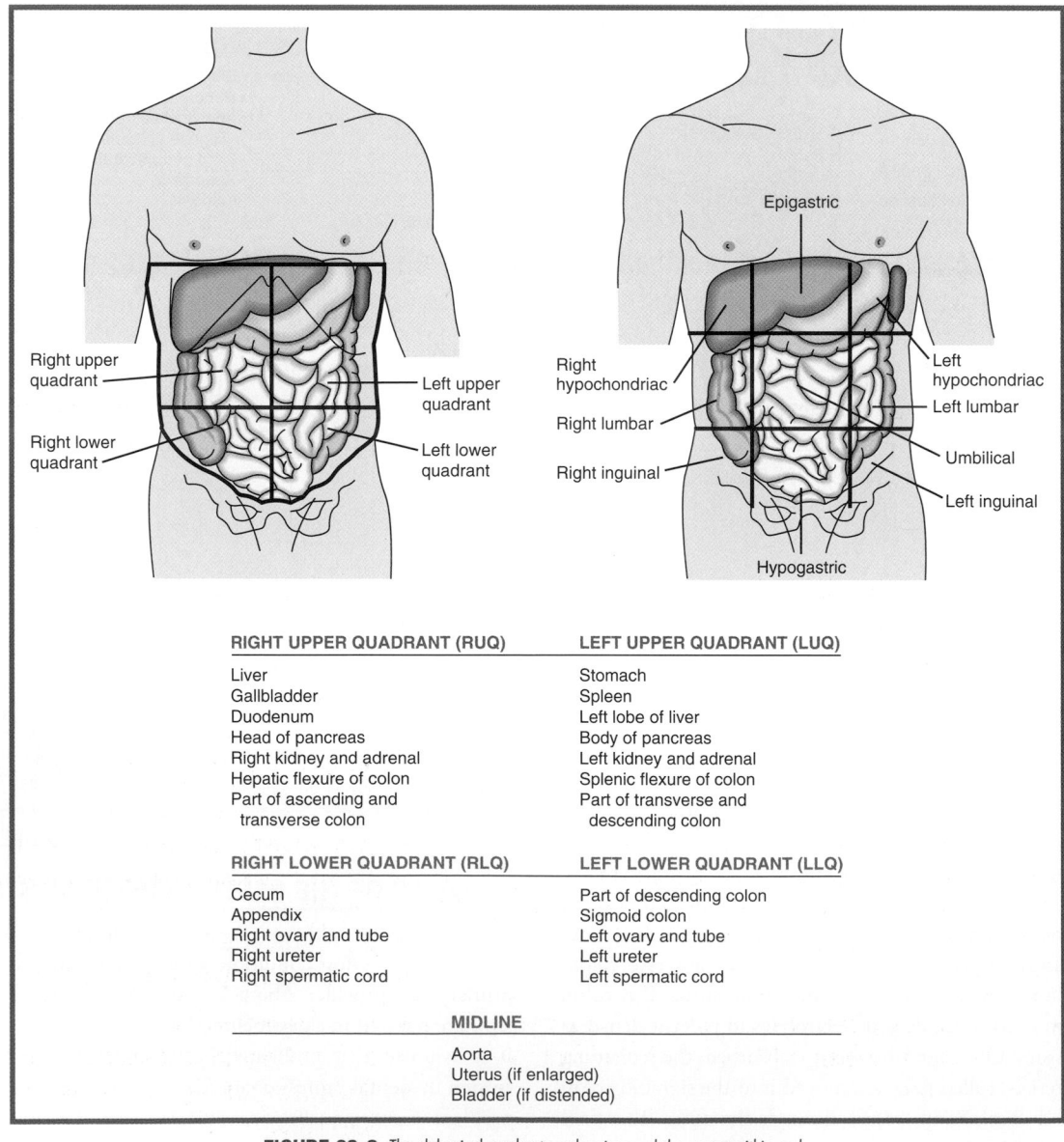

FIGURE 32-2 The abdominal quadrants and regions and the organs within each.

Common Signs and Symptoms of a Gastrointestinal Disorder

A patient with a gastrointestinal (GI) problem may complain of multiple discomforts, including nausea, vomiting, **anorexia**, diarrhea, constipation, and abdominal pain. The medical assistant may find it difficult to identify the exact location and quality of the patient's discomfort. When you discuss abdominal pain with the patient, ask him or her to point to or touch the area where the pain is located. This is one way of making sure the correct quadrant or region is identified, and the patient is properly prepared for the provider's examination. If possible, document the location of the patient's complaint using the abdominal regions (see Figure 32-2) because this is most accurate. For example, if the patient complains of heartburn after eating, this can be charted as: Pt c/o epigastric discomfort after meals; 6 on a pain scale of 10.

Table 32-1 outlines the typical signs, symptoms, and characteristics seen in patients with GI complaints. Telephone screening for GI complaints involves following the facility's policies and procedures manual for management of disorders; gathering detailed information about the onset, duration, and frequency of the problem and the pertinent patient history; and recording the interaction in the patient's health record (this should include the use of medications for relief; a pain scale, if appropriate; and the course of action based on the provider's recommendations). Using Procedure 32-1, outline how you would respond to the scenarios in the following Critical Thinking Application box.

CRITICAL THINKING APPLICATION 32-2

Two days a week, Joan works in the telephone screening area of the practice, where she is responsible for the initial management of calls from Dr. Sahani's patients. The following problems are typical of a call day. What are some questions Joan should ask and subsequently document in each patient's health record?

- The mother of a 7-year-old patient is concerned because her son has been vomiting since yesterday.
- The father of an 18-month-old infant reports that the child has had diarrhea for 2 days.
- A 72-year-old patient is concerned about constipation that has not been relieved by laxatives.

TABLE 32-1 Characteristics of Common Gastrointestinal Complaints

COMPLAINT	CAUSE	CHARACTERISTICS TO REPORT AND RECORD
Vomiting (emesis)	GI irritation, pain or stress, inner ear disturbance, increased intracranial pressure (ICP), food-borne illness	• Onset, frequency, and duration of the problem • Yellow or greenish color (indicates bile from the duodenum) • Pyloric stenosis (causes vomiting of undigested food) • Projectile vomiting (may indicate pyloric stenosis or increased ICP) • **Hematemesis**
Diarrhea	Infection or inflammation, food allergies, food-borne illness, malabsorption syndromes	• Onset, frequency, and duration of the problem • Dehydration (may occur if diarrhea is persistent; occurs more often in infants and older adults) • Presence of blood, mucus, or pus in the stool • Steatorrhea (large, foul-smelling, greasy stools) • Melena (tarry stools from bleeding higher in the digestive tract)
Constipation	Lack of dietary fiber; inadequate intake of fluids, lack of exercise; neurologic disorders, including spinal cord injury and multiple sclerosis; side effect of medications (e.g., codeine, iron, antacids); bowel obstruction or tumor	• Onset, frequency, and duration of the problem • Treatment and effectiveness of over-the-counter (OTC) medications • Diet and fluid intake • Presence of watery diarrhea (may indicate fecal impaction)
Abdominal pain	Ulcerative disease, tumor, appendicitis, bowel obstruction, food-borne illness, infection or inflammatory process	• Onset, frequency, and duration • Exact location (using quadrants or abdominal regions) • Quality of the pain (e.g., burning, cramping, sharp, dull) • Degree of pain (scale of 1 to 10)

PROCEDURE 32-1	Perform Patient Screening Using Established Protocols: Telephone Screening of a Patient with a Gastrointestinal Complaint

Goal: *To answer the telephone professionally and to manage patients' phone calls according to the provider's guidelines.*

Scenario: *With a fellow student, role-play a telephone call from a 22-year-old woman who reports acute abdominal pain.*

EQUIPMENT and SUPPLIES

- Access to the patient's health record
- Access to the appointments schedule
- Telephone
- Message pad
- Pen
- Facility's policies and procedures manual for managing patients' phone calls

PROCEDURAL STEPS

1. Answer the telephone by the third ring, speaking directly into the mouthpiece.
   PURPOSE: Answering promptly conveys interest in the caller. Proper positioning of the mouthpiece allows for an audible tone.

2. Speak distinctly, using a pleasant tone and expression, at a moderate rate, and with sufficient volume.

3. Greet the caller, identify the office and/or the provider and yourself, and offer to help the caller.
   PURPOSE: So the patient knows she has reached the correct number, in addition to the name of the staff member to whom she is speaking.

4. Verify the identity of the caller and his or her date of birth; access the patient's record.
   PURPOSE: To have the patient's health record ready for reference about the health history and recent care.

5. Determine the caller's needs using therapeutic communication skills.
   PURPOSE: To gather comprehensive information about the caller's complaint and to communicate empathetically about the caller's needs.

6. Upon learning the patient's complaint, formulate questions designed to gather the information required to make a decision about when the patient should be seen and the provider notified. On the basis of the patient's gender, age, and complaint of acute abdominal pain, consider the following questions:
   - What are the onset, frequency, and duration of the abdominal pain?
   - What is the exact anatomic location of the discomfort?
   - What is the quality of the pain (e.g., sharp, dull, stabbing)?
   - On a scale of 1 to 10, with 10 being the worst pain, how does she rate the pain?
   - Does the patient have a history of this occurrence? Does she have a history of gynecologic or pelvic disorders?
   - Has she taken any medication for the discomfort and has it been effective?

7. Refer to the facility's policies for patients' phone calls as needed.
   PURPOSE: The medical assistant is not qualified to diagnose the patient. The policies and procedures manual developed by the facility should be used to guide appropriate management of individual patient problems.

8. Depending on the patient's answers to your questions and the facility's policies for the management of abdominal discomfort, refer to the appointment schedule and make an appointment or take a message for the provider to return the patient's call.

9. Document the details of the interaction and the results in the patient's health record.
   PURPOSE: All communications with a patient, including phone calls, are part of the record of care.

In the space below, document the interaction based on the role-play answers given to the questions in step 6.

DOCUMENTATION PRACTICE

_____
_____
_____
_____
_____
_____
_____
_____
_____

Cancers of the Gastrointestinal Tract

Any organ of the digestive tract can develop cancer. Malignant tumors can invade surrounding tissues and metastasize through the blood or lymph system, regardless of their location. Table 32-2 describes some of the common malignant tumors found in the GI system. The exact cause of a malignancy may not be known, but exposure to **carcinogens** increases the risk of developing a cancerous tumor. Examples of carcinogens include tobacco and alcohol, in addition to exposure to chemicals and radiation. A family history and lifestyle factors, such as consuming a diet high in fat and low in fiber, also can increase a person's risk of developing certain types of cancer.

Disorders of the Esophagus and Stomach

Hiatal Hernia

A *hernia* is the abnormal protrusion of part of an organ or tissue through the structures that normally contain it. These protrusions can develop in various parts of the body but most frequently are seen

TABLE 32-2	Cancers of the Gastrointestinal Tract	
TUMOR	**CHARACTERISTICS**	**CAUSE OR CONTRIBUTING FACTORS**
Oral tumor	White mass in or on the mouth that bleeds easily (the mass usually is not painful); ulcer or fissure that does not heal	Cancer of the lip (pipe smoking), cancer of the tongue or gums (chewing tobacco)
Esophageal cancer	Typically found in the distal esophagus; initial sign is dysphagia (difficulty swallowing)	Associated with chronic irritation resulting from chronic esophagitis, alcohol abuse, or smoking
Gastric cancer	Asymptomatic in early stages; usually not diagnosed until well advanced; poor prognosis; marked by anorexia, indigestion, weight loss, fatigue; positive test result for occult blood in the stool	Food preservatives, long-term use of nitrates, smoked foods; genetic association; chronic gastritis
Liver cancer	Primary malignant tumors rare, usually a metastasized secondary tumor; initial symptoms mild; anorexia, vomiting, weight loss, fatigue, **hepatomegaly**, splenomegaly, portal hypertension; usually advanced when diagnosed	Primary tumor caused by cirrhosis from hepatitis or chemical exposure
Pancreatic cancer	Weight loss, jaundice; usually advanced when diagnosed; metastasis occurs early; no effective treatment	Cigarette smoking; increased risk for African-Americans and individuals who are overweight, obese, diabetic, or have chronic pancreatitis
Colorectal cancer	Usually develops from polyps in the colon; metastasis to the liver common; initial signs depend on location of tumor, may include changes in the character of stool, iron-deficiency anemia, fatigue, weight loss, or melena (black, tarry, bloody stool)	Genetic or familial link; diet high in fat, sugar, and red meat and low in fiber; usually occurs in patients over age 55

in the abdominal region. Causes of herniation include congenital weakness of the structures, trauma, relaxation of ligaments and skeletal muscles, and increased upward pressure from the abdomen. Herniation most often is found in middle-aged or older individuals.

The location of the hernia determines the term by which the protrusion is identified. In patients with a *hiatal hernia*, the upper part of the stomach protrudes through the esophageal opening, the hiatal sphincter of the diaphragm (Figure 32-3). With a *sliding hiatal hernia*, part of the stomach moves above the diaphragm when the individual is supine and slides back down into the abdominal cavity when the person stands. Part of the fundus of the stomach moves through the weakened hiatus in a *paraesophageal hiatal hernia*. Food may lodge in the herniated part of the stomach, causing reflux of highly acidic stomach contents into the esophagus, **dysphagia**, and chronic esophagitis, which may cause fibrosis and stricture. Patients complain of heartburn, frequent belching, and increased discomfort when they cough, bend over, or lie down after eating.

Patients with hiatal hernias can be treated with over-the-counter (OTC) medications such as Tagamet, Pepcid, Prilosec, or Prevacid. Treatment may involve dietary modifications, such as avoiding caffeine, cigarettes, and alcohol; eating six small meals a day; losing weight; avoiding lying down after meals; and raising the head of the bed 6 to 8 inches.

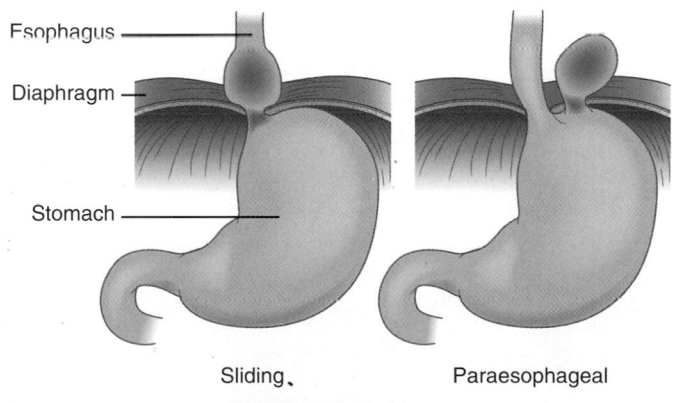

FIGURE 32-3 Hiatal hernias.

Gastroesophageal Reflux Disease

Gastroesophageal reflux disease (GERD) occurs when the gastroesophageal sphincter (cardiac sphincter) at the distal end of the esophagus does not close properly, allowing acidic stomach contents to leak back, or reflux, into the esophagus. The regurgitated acidic contents of the stomach irritate the esophageal lining, causing heartburn symptoms. Occasional heartburn is not a problem, but a patient who experiences heartburn more than twice a week is diagnosed with GERD. All age groups can be diagnosed with GERD; however, it is seen most frequently in adults and is associated with alcohol use, pregnancy, and smoking; it is very common in overweight patients. Besides persistent heartburn, patients may report chest pain, hoarseness in the morning, difficulty swallowing, a feeling of tightness in the throat or a choking sensation, dry cough, and bad breath from the reflux of partly digested food. GERD frequently is seen in patients with hiatal hernias, and treatment protocols are similar in the two conditions.

Laparoscopic repair of the gastroesophageal sphincter may be recommended if lifestyle changes and medication are not effective in curing the problem. The U.S. Food and Drug Administration (FDA) has approved two different implant systems, LINX and Enteryx, which are designed to improve the function of the sphincter muscle. The most important concern with chronic GERD is the potential for developing Barrett's esophagus, a precancerous condition caused by long-term exposure of esophageal cells to gastric contents. Patients diagnosed with GERD are followed regularly by a gastroenterologist so that abnormal cells can be detected early and removed before cancerous changes occur.

Gastric and Duodenal Ulcers

Peptic ulcers occur most frequently in the proximal duodenum (duodenal ulcer) but may also be found in the stomach (gastric ulcer). Both types are characterized by an area of breakdown of the mucosal membrane, which leads to ulceration of the epithelial lining of the duodenum or stomach (Figure 32-4).

The first sign of a peptic ulcer may be iron-deficiency anemia or a positive stool test for occult blood, which results from erosion of blood vessels in the organ wall. Patients typically complain of gnawing or burning pain in the epigastric area between meals. Gastric ulcers may cause weight loss, whereas duodenal lesions often cause nausea and vomiting. If the ulcerative area is bleeding internally, the patient may have hematemesis or melena (dark, sticky feces containing partly digested blood).

The description of the patient's pain gives the provider a suspicion of the disorder. Examination often shows that the patient is guarding the painful area; this is characterized by clutching the upper abdominal area and drawing the knees up toward the chest. A definitive diagnosis is based on an upper GI series (x-ray evaluation) or endoscopy (visualization) of the upper GI tract (Figure 32-5). A biopsy sample of the affected area may be taken during the endoscopy to rule out cancer. A stool test may be ordered to check for occult blood. Blood tests also are ordered to establish the **hemoglobin** and **hematocrit** levels.

Peptic ulcers can appear under a variety of predisposing circumstances, including use of alcohol, smoking, use of nonsteroidal antiinflammatory drugs (NSAIDs) or corticosteroids (e.g., prednisone), and genetic predisposition. However, research indicates that 80% of gastric ulcers and 90% of duodenal ulcers are caused by the *Helicobacter pylori* bacterium. *H. pylori* can be diagnosed either by a blood test that measures the presence of antibodies to the bacteria or by a breath test that is done after the patient swallows a drink containing urea and carbon. Expired air is examined to detect the bacteria. The diagnosis is confirmed with biopsy samples of the gastric and duodenal mucosa obtained during an endoscopic examination.

Peptic ulcers caused by *H. pylori* are treated with a combination of medications, including antibiotics to kill the bacteria and drugs to reduce the production of hydrochloric acid and protect the stomach lining. The most effective treatment is a triple therapy method that lasts 2 weeks and includes two antibiotics (a combination of amoxicillin, Flagyl, or Biaxin) and either a histamine blocker (e.g., Tagamet, Zantac) or a proton pump inhibitor (e.g., Prilosec, Prevacid). Surgery may be indicated in severe cases, such as with perforation of the gastric wall. Any ulcer that does not heal is reevaluated periodically through gastroscopy to rule out cancer.

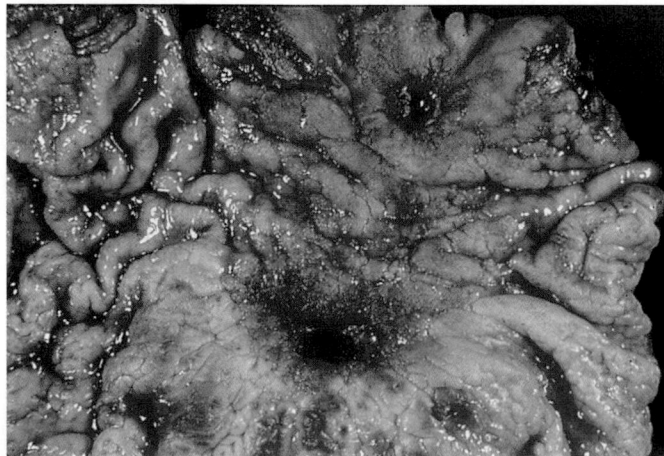

FIGURE 32-4 Peptic ulcer. (From Frazier MS: *Essentials of human diseases and conditions,* ed 4, Philadelphia, 2009, Saunders.)

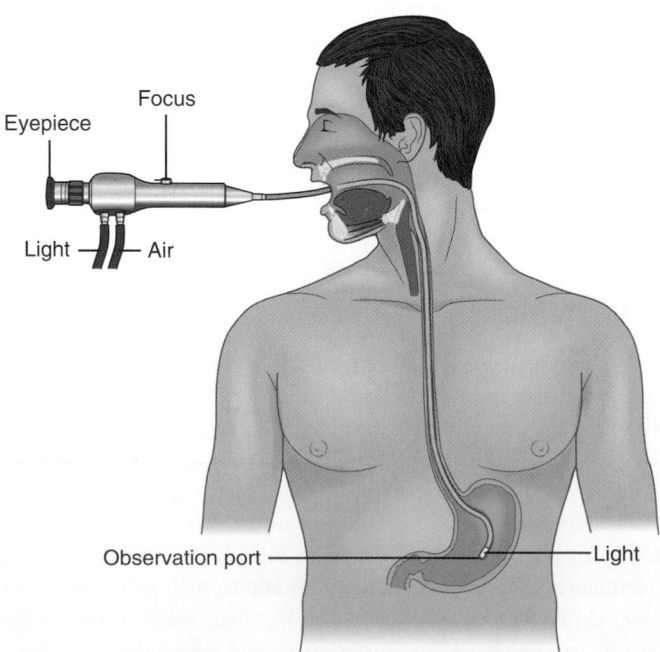

FIGURE 32-5 Fiberoptic endoscopy of the stomach.

Medications for Disorders of the Esophagus and Stomach

- Histamine stimulates acid-secreting cells to release hydrochloric acid; histamine (H$_2$)-blockers reduce the amount of hydrochloric acid released into the stomach. Over-the-counter (OTC) H$_2$-blockers include ranitidine (Zantac), famotidine (Pepcid), and cimetidine (Tagamet).
- OTC antacids (Maalox, Mylanta, Tums) neutralize existing stomach acid and provide rapid pain relief.
- Proton pump inhibitors (PPIs) reduce acid by blocking the action of "pumps" within acid secreting cells; these drugs include omeprazole (Prilosec), lansoprazole (Prevacid), rabeprazole (Aciphex), esomeprazole (Nexium), and pantoprazole (Protonix).
- Cytoprotective agents help protect tissues lining the stomach and small intestine; they include Pepto-Bismol and the prescription medications sucralfate (Carafate) and misoprostol (Cytotec).

Pyloric Stenosis

Pyloric stenosis, which is narrowing and hardening of the pyloric sphincter at the distal end of the stomach, can be caused by scar tissue produced by chronic conditions but typically is seen as a congenital defect in infants. The difficulty becomes apparent in newborns within 2 to 6 weeks of birth because the infant has projectile vomiting immediately after feeding, as a result of the stomach's inability to empty effectively. Consequently, the baby displays symptoms of failure to thrive, becomes dehydrated, has small and infrequent stools, and is very irritable. Congenital pyloric stenosis typically occurs in first-born males and can be corrected by surgery.

Intestinal Disorders

Food-Borne Illness

Eating or drinking contaminated food can result in a food-borne disease (Table 32-3). Each year, 1 in 6 Americans gets sick from consuming contaminated foods or beverages. Many different types of bacteria, viruses, and parasites can contaminate food, but the most common are *Escherichia coli* and *Salmonella* and *Campylobacter* organisms. Patients may experience a variety of symptoms, but the first typically are gastrointestinal: nausea, vomiting, stomach pain, and/or diarrhea. Usually a delay of several hours to days occurs after ingestion of the contaminated substance before symptoms begin. This is the *incubation period*, when the microbes are attaching to the intestinal wall and beginning to multiply. The condition usually is self-limiting and subsides within 48 hours. Occasionally, it can be much more severe and even life-threatening. The more severe cases usually are seen in young children and in individuals in a weakened state of health.

A complete patient history is crucial in determining the diagnosis. Stool and blood cultures may be performed to verify the causative pathogen. If the patient has a remaining portion of the suspected ingested food, it should be sent to the laboratory for analysis. In severe cases, the provider may order an endoscopic examination of

TABLE 32-3   Food-Borne Illnesses

MICROORGANISM	CAUSE	INCUBATION PERIOD	SIGNS AND SYMPTOMS
Staphylococcus aureus	Improper hand washing by food handlers; insufficient refrigeration of salads or improper cooking of meats	4-6 hours	• Low body temperature • Hypotension • Acute, severe nausea • Vomiting • Cramps
Escherichia coli	Fecal contamination of food or water; improper cooking of meat or washing of fruits and vegetables	24-72 hours	• Vomiting • Abdominal cramps • Diarrhea, may contain blood or mucus
Salmonella sp.	Fecal contamination of food; contaminated work areas; undercooked or raw poultry, eggs, or shellfish	8-48 hours	• Acute diarrhea • Sometimes vomiting • Abdominal cramping and pain • Fever
Campylobacter jejuni	Consumption of contaminated food or water; often raw poultry, fresh produce, or unpasteurized milk	2-4 days	• Cramping abdominal pain • Watery diarrhea • Fever
Clostridium botulinum	Bacterial spores in improperly canned or prepared food	12-36 hours	• Vomiting or diarrhea possible • Neurologic complications (e.g., vision problems, paralysis, respiratory failure)

the GI system to determine the extent of the damage or the condition of the mucosal lining of the system.

Treatment of a food-borne disease depends on the microorganism causing the illness and the patient's symptoms. The patient's condition is stabilized and symptoms are treated so that dehydration is minimized and electrolyte balance is maintained. Antiemetics, such as Granisetron or Ondansetron (Zofran), may be prescribed to control nausea and vomiting. Other medications, such as loperamide (Imodium) or diphenoxylate with atropine (Lomotil), may be used to control diarrhea. Antibiotics may shorten the length of the disease but are only prescribed if the organism causing the infection can be identified and will respond to antibiotic therapy. If vomiting and diarrhea cannot be corrected within a reasonable time (as determined by the patient's age, body size, and health condition), the patient may be hospitalized so that intravenous (IV) fluid replacement can be administered.

Irritable Bowel Syndrome

Irritable bowel syndrome (IBS) is a recurrent functional bowel disorder; this means that the bowel does not work as it should, but diagnostic studies fail to show an organic cause for the symptoms. The diagnosis of IBS is made if the patient complains of recurrent abdominal discomfort of at least 3 months; abdominal pain that is relieved by defecation; feeling bloated; a change in bowel habits with constipation, diarrhea, and mucous discharge; and increased flatulence. The most common site of abdominal pain is the left lower quadrant. Diagnostic studies, such as a complete blood count, stool testing for occult blood, urinalysis, barium enema, and colonoscopy, are performed to rule out other GI diseases that have an organic cause.

IBS is more common in women. Symptoms usually appear in late adolescence or early adulthood. The condition seems to have a familial pattern. IBS may account for up to 50% of referrals to gastroenterologists because of concern about possible organic disease. IBS is quite common; an estimated 9% to 20% of the adult population is affected. The syndrome is associated with food intolerances, menstruation, and stress levels.

Treatment is primarily pharmaceutical, with bulk-forming agents (e.g., Metamucil) given for constipation; Imodium or Lomotil for diarrhea episodes; Lactaid if the patient is lactose intolerant; antispasmodic agents (dicyclomine [Bentyl]) for cramping; and anticholinergic agents (hyoscyamine) and simethicone (Mylicon) for bloating and flatulence. Lubiprostone (Amitiza) may be indicated for IBS with constipation. It increases fluid secretion in the small intestine to help relieve constipation.

Alternative therapies for IBS include acupuncture to relieve cramping and improve bowel function; the herb peppermint to relax intestinal smooth muscles; and probiotic foods, such as yogurt, to provide bacteria that make up the natural flora of the intestinal tract to help relieve symptoms. The patient should be encouraged to keep a food diary in an effort to identify foods that exacerbate the symptoms; to increase fluid and fiber intake; and to avoid spicy and fatty foods and caffeine. Routine exercise also can be very helpful in relieving symptoms.

Patients with IBS can become very frustrated and need confirmation that this is a real problem, even though no organic or anatomic changes are apparent. Patients should be encouraged to follow

lifestyle recommendations, including actively working to reduce stress. The medical assistant plays an important role in providing understanding and support to the patient with IBS.

CRITICAL THINKING APPLICATION   **32-3**

Dr. Sahani frequently sees patients with IBS. He asks Joan to prepare a handout for patients describing the disorder, making sure to include possible treatments. What should Joan include?

Weight Loss Surgery

Several different types of bariatric surgery can be performed to help individuals lose weight. One of the most common types is the Roux-en-Y gastric bypass procedure in which surgical staples or a plastic band is used to create a small pouch at the top of the stomach (about the size of an egg); this technique bypasses the duodenum, where most of digestion is completed. The smaller stomach empties directly into the jejunum so that food has limited exposure to digestive enzymes and therefore cannot be easily absorbed. After the surgery, patients can eat only small amounts of food at one time, which reduces the number of calories consumed. This surgery can be done either as an open procedure or with a laparoscope, although the laparoscopic procedure is preferred because it is associated with fewer surgical risks and complications.

Bariatric surgery is an option for patients with a body mass index (BMI) of 40 or higher or those with a BMI of 35 or higher who have a serious medical condition, such as diabetes, hypertension, or sleep apnea. Patients interested in the procedure must undergo a battery of examinations, including a psychological evaluation, and must show that they have been unable to lose weight with other methods. The average cost of a bariatric procedure is $20,000 to $25,000. Medical insurance coverage varies by insurance provider and from state to state. The medical assistant may work as a patient navigator to help surgical candidates investigate insurance coverage.

Recent studies indicate that weight loss after stomach-reduction surgery can drastically improve diabetes mellitus; the greater the weight lost, the more likely the patient is to improve.

Patients begin to lose weight shortly after the procedure and continue to lose for approximately 12 to 24 months. Most individuals lose 60% to 80% of their excess body weight, and most experience resolution of weight-related health issues as the weight comes off, including relief of heartburn, reduced musculoskeletal discomfort, improved breathing, reduced sleep apnea, and lower blood pressure. Because of malabsorption problems, patients may be prone to vitamin B_{12} deficiency (which may necessitate either large oral doses or vitamin B_{12} intramuscular injections on a regular basis); iron-deficiency anemia; lack of calcium absorption, which may contribute to osteoporosis; and other vitamin and mineral deficiencies. Patients should take daily vitamin and mineral supplements to reduce the effects of these malabsorption problems.

The U.S. Food and Drug Administration (FDA) has also approved a weight loss procedure, the adjustable gastric band (AGB), for patients with a BMI of 30 or greater who also have at least one condition linked to obesity, such as heart disease or diabetes. With the AGB, the amount of food that can be consumed at one time is reduced by placing a small bracelet-like band around the top of the stomach. A circular balloon inside the band can be inflated or deflated with saline solution, allowing the surgeon to control the size of the opening into the stomach.

A postsurgical complication of weight loss surgery is rapid gastric emptying, or *dumping syndrome*. This occurs when the contents of the stomach empty too quickly into the small intestine, resulting in distention and increased intestinal motility. Signs and symptoms include nausea, abdominal cramps, diarrhea, vertigo, tachycardia, and diaphoresis (sweating). The condition typically occurs after the individual eats sweets or high-fat foods. Patients undergoing weight loss surgery should be instructed to eat frequent, small meals that are high in protein and low in simple sugars and to drink fluids between meals rather than with meals. These dietary modifications usually can prevent dumping syndrome.

Acute Appendicitis

The vermiform appendix is a narrow pouch, approximately 3½ inches long, that extends off the cecum of the large intestine. It has no known function but can become inflamed and ultimately infected because of obstruction by a **fecalith** or foreign material. As bacteria multiply, the appendix becomes inflamed and swollen, causing ischemia and necrosis of the appendix wall. If the infectious material leaks out or bursts from the appendix, a localized infection forms that may become regional if the abdominal peritoneum becomes involved, resulting in peritonitis. Peritonitis is a serious infection that may become life-threatening.

Classic signs of appendicitis include right lower quadrant pain; nausea and vomiting; tenderness at McBurney's point, which is located between the umbilicus and the right anterior superior iliac spine; low-grade fever; and leukocytosis (an increase in the white blood cell count). Other conditions that might cause similar symptoms include ectopic pregnancy or ovarian cyst, a kidney stone lodged in a ureter, and Crohn's disease. Appendicitis is confirmed with computed tomography (CT) or ultrasound. The infected appendix is removed surgically (appendectomy), typically in a laparoscopic procedure, in which a pencil-thin tube with its own lighting system and a miniature video camera is inserted through a small incision in the abdomen to visualize the area. The surgeon removes the appendix with tiny instruments that are inserted through one or two other small abdominal incisions. However, if the appendix has ruptured, a larger incision is needed to clean the abdominal cavity. After surgery, the patient is treated with broad-spectrum antibiotics to prevent or treat infection at the site.

Crohn's Disease

Crohn's disease, also called *regional ileitis* or *regional enteritis*, is an inflammation that may be located anywhere in the alimentary tract but most commonly is found in the ileum. The inflammation begins with a localized area of ulcer development, with healthy tissue interspersed with areas of affected tissue. Inflammation results in the formation of ulcers that eventually invade deeper into the walls of the intestine, creating scar tissue and partial or complete obstruction at the affected site. If this occurs in the small intestine, the damaged wall reduces the intestine's ability to digest and absorb nutrients; if it occurs in the colon, increased motility prevents reabsorption of fluids. Scar tissue from the localized ulceration ultimately can lead to a bowel obstruction, or the ulcer may completely invade the intestinal wall, resulting in perforation and leakage of intestinal contents into the abdominal cavity. **Adhesions** may develop from chronic inflammation, or **fistulas** may form between two loops of the intestine or between the intestine and adjacent organs.

Signs and symptoms of Crohn's disease include loose, semiformed stool; melena if the ulcers break through blood vessels; pain or tenderness in the right lower quadrant; anorexia; weight loss; anemia; and fatigue. Most patients cycle through periods of remission and relapse. The cause of the disease is unknown, although some theories associate the disease with an autoimmune response, genetic predisposition, or a combination of environmental factors, including certain medications and a high-fat diet. Risk factors include age (most cases are diagnosed between 15 and 35 years of age), smoking, Jewish or European descent, a family history of the disorder, and residence in a developed country or urban area. The diagnosis is made from a barium enema, a small bowel series, abdominal CT scan, and colonoscopy and is confirmed with a biopsy.

The goals of treatment are to reduce inflammation, manage symptoms, and provide nutritional support. Antiinflammatory drug therapy includes sulfasalazine (Azulfidine), mesalamine (Asacol), and corticosteroids (e.g., prednisone, budesonide [Entocort]), which are used during the acute phases. Immune system suppressors, such as infliximab (Remicade), also are recommended to control the immune system's reaction to the inflammatory process. Flagyl and Cipro are antibiotics prescribed for fistulas, and antidiarrheal agents (e.g., Imodium, Lomotil) may provide symptomatic relief. Certolizumab (Cimzia) is used to treat the symptoms of Crohn's disease if other drugs have failed to control the inflammatory process.

Surgical intervention involving resection of the diseased bowel and **anastomosis** may be necessary if an intestinal obstruction occurs; a fistula is present; or abscess formation is seen. Unfortunately, the disease usually recurs at the site of the anastomosis. The patient may require dietary supplements with a high-protein, high-caloric diet to maintain a normal weight, and vitamin B_{12} shots if ulcerations occur in the distal ileum, where the vitamin is absorbed.

Ulcerative Colitis

Ulcerative colitis causes inflammation that usually starts in the rectum and moves proximally through the colon, affecting the lining of the colon in a continuous pattern. The disease causes the formation of ulcers that invade the mucosal and submucosal layers but do not advance through the entire wall of the colon (Figure 32-6). Ulcerative colitis can affect people of any age; although a familial tendency exists, the cause is unknown. The patient complains of abdominal pain, mucoid stools, and intermittent episodes of bloody diarrhea. As the disease progresses, the patient may experience as many as 10 to 20 stools a day, along with weight loss, fever, and general malaise.

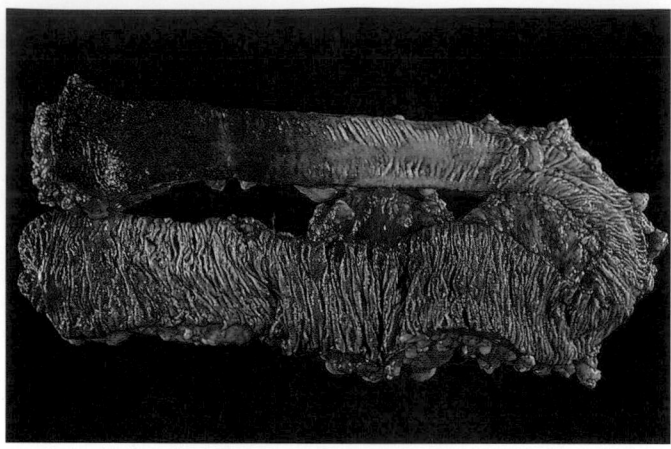

FIGURE 32-6 Ulcerative colitis. (From Hagen-Ansert SL: *Textbook of diagnostic sonography,* ed 7, St Louis, 2012, Mosby.)

is present in the diet, or it may develop after some form of traumatic event, such as infection, injury, pregnancy, severe stress, or surgery. Gluten is found in all grains, including any products made from wheat, barley, rye, and possibly oats. If the affected individual eats a product that contains gluten, even a small amount, an antigen-antibody reaction occurs that causes destruction of the villi in the small intestine. The intestine is unable to absorb nutrients, and the result is malnutrition. The patient has steatorrhea, abdominal pain, and weight loss. Celiac disease can be treated with strict adherence to a gluten-free diet; rice, soy, corn, and potato flours can be substituted for gluten products. Although oats may not be harmful, oat products frequently are contaminated with wheat, so these also should be avoided. Gluten-free products, identified by food label claims, are becoming more widely available.

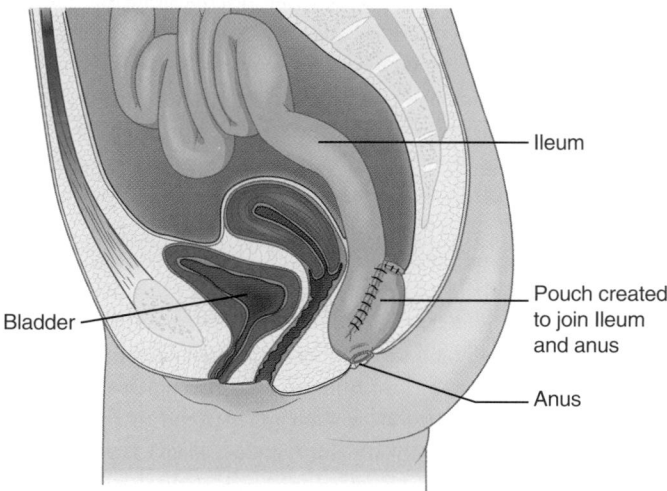

FIGURE 32-7 Ileoanal Anastomosis. Surgical procedure for advanced ulcerative colitis.

Gluten Sensitivity

Until recently, gluten intolerance was believed to be similar to celiac disease or a wheat allergy. However, recent research indicates that gluten intolerance can affect people who do not have either celiac or an allergic response to wheat. The new syndrome, now identified as non-celiac gluten sensitivity (NCGS) or gluten sensitivity (GS), is included in a revised list of gluten-related disorders. Unlike celiac disease, gluten sensitivity does not cause damage to the villi, and the patient's symptoms are similar but less severe. No accepted medical test yet exists for gluten sensitivity. GS is diagnosed by first ruling out a wheat allergy and celiac disease and then using an elimination diet, meaning removing all food containing gluten from the diet, and slowly reintroducing it to see if symptoms recur. If the patient reports relief of symptoms after gluten is removed from the diet, that is how the syndrome is managed.

Drug therapy for ulcerative colitis is similar to that for Crohn's disease, but surgical removal of the colon with an **ileostomy** is considered curative for ulcerative colitis. The problem with this approach is that the patient must wear a bag on the abdomen to collect drainage from the ileum. The procedure of choice for patients who must have the colon removed for treatment of severe Crohn's disease is an ileoanal pouch anastomosis (Figure 32-7). In this procedure, a pouch is formed out of the ileum and then is connected directly to the anus. This results in multiple watery bowel movements a day because the colon is not there to absorb fluid; however, the patient has a continuous GI tract and does not need to wear a collection bag on the abdomen. Patients with ulcerative colitis must be screened annually with a colonoscopy because they have an increased risk of colon cancer.

Celiac Disease

Celiac disease, also known as *celiac sprue,* is a malabsorption syndrome caused by a genetic defect in the intestinal enzyme that metabolizes gluten. Celiac disease can occur at any age once gluten

Diverticular Disease

Diverticula are outpouchings or herniations of the muscular lining of the colon, usually the sigmoid colon. Diverticula develop because of chronic constipation and muscular hypertrophy in the colon and become more common as people age. *Diverticulosis* is an asymptomatic diverticular disease in which multiple diverticula are present in the colon, but the patient has no complaints other than mild discomfort, diarrhea, constipation, or flatulence. However, if the herniations become blocked with feces and inflammation develops, *diverticulitis* occurs. Signs and symptoms include lower left quadrant cramping, tenderness, or pain; nausea and vomiting; low-grade fever; and leukocytosis. A barium enema or colonoscopy may be done to confirm the presence of diverticula.

Patients with diverticulosis are encouraged to eat a high-fiber diet, take a fiber product such as methylcellulose (Citrucel) or psyllium (Metamucil) one to three times a day, and drink plenty of fluids. The goals of dietary management are to prevent the collection of waste in the herniations and to encourage regular, soft bowel movements. If diverticula become inflamed, antibiotics are prescribed to treat the infection. An acute attack with severe pain and

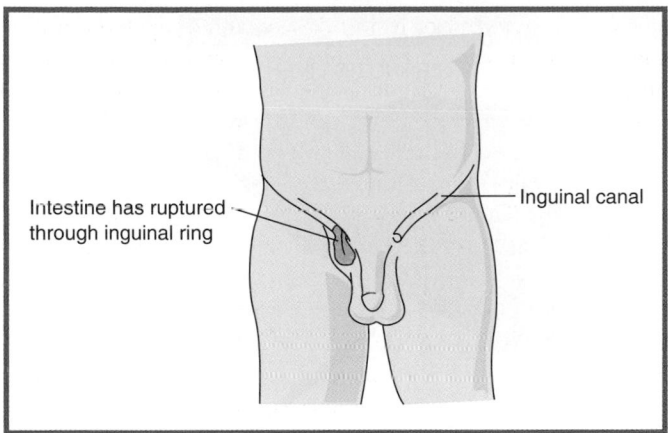

FIGURE 32-8 Herniated inguinal canal.

infection may require hospitalization, IV antibiotic therapy, and pain management. Surgery may be necessary if the colon perforates.

Hernias of the Abdomen

Hernias can develop in various parts of the body but most frequently are seen in the abdomen when an organ or part of an organ protrudes through a weakened area in the abdominal muscle wall. The causes of herniation include congenital weakness of the structures, trauma, relaxation of ligaments and skeletal muscles, and increased upward pressure from the abdomen. They most often are found in middle-aged or older individuals. The location of the hernia establishes the term by which the protrusion is identified. Types of hernias include umbilical hernias; incisional hernias at the site of a previous surgery; and inguinal hernias, in which a loop of the bowel protrudes into the inguinal canal (Figure 32-8).

The usual sign of an abdominal hernia is an abnormal lump or bulge that the patient finds while bathing. This bulge is tender, but the pain is mild. The patient also may discover that the bulge can be pushed back into the abdomen, where it remains until movement or lifting causes it to push through again. If severe pain is present, the bulging tissue (usually a piece of the intestine) may be trapped or strangulated if blood flow has been compromised. If immediate surgical intervention is not performed, the tissue may die, and **gangrene** will set in.

The provider uses palpation to assess an abdominal or inguinal hernia for size and inspects the area with the patient standing and lying down. An inguinal hernia can be detected in a male by having him perform the **Valsalva maneuver**. The most common treatment is surgical repair in the form of a herniorrhaphy or a hernioplasty.

Hemorrhoids

Hemorrhoids are varicose veins of the anus and rectum. They affect approximately 5% of all adults. The disorder has a familial, hereditary predisposition, and it is common in people with varicose veins of the lower extremities and inguinal hernias. Hemorrhoid formation is related to increased pressure in the rectum, often caused by

constipation. If the swollen veins are within the rectal wall, they are considered internal hemorrhoids, which usually do not cause uncomfortable symptoms; if they are firm and protruding and can be felt and/or seen, they are external hemorrhoids, which usually prompt complaints of pain and itching.

Some patients experience no pain, and other patients experience rectal irritation and discomfort. Frequently, the patient reports that anal itching and burning occur immediately after a bowel movement. If the patient must strain to defecate, bleeding and protrusion of the swollen mass can occur. Patients often state that the anal area must be bathed or even soaked in warm water after every bowel movement to relieve the itching and pain.

A proctologic examination and inspection of the anal area reveals external hemorrhoids. Proctoscopy is performed to detect internal hemorrhoids of the rectum. A hemoglobin level and red blood cell count may be ordered to determine whether any significant blood loss has occurred. Hemorrhoids are treated with stool softeners (e.g., docusate sodium [Colace]); fiber supplements (e.g., Metamucil, Citrucel); a high-fiber diet; increased fluid intake; and an analgesic ointment applied locally or by suppository to relieve swelling. If these measures do not correct the problem, the next step may be **sclerotherapy** with a chemical injection, cryosurgery, infrared coagulation to burn hemorrhoidal tissue, ligation, or hemorrhoidectomy.

DISEASES OF THE LIVER AND GALLBLADDER
Cirrhosis

The liver is located in the right upper quadrant of the abdomen. Its primary functions are to metabolize nutrients and detoxify drugs or other harmful substances. The liver also excretes proteins that aid in blood clotting and produces bile for fat metabolism. Cirrhosis is a chronic liver disease in which the lobes of the liver become fibrous and hard, and liver cells degenerate, causing deterioration of liver function. Cirrhosis and chronic liver disease are the twelfth leading cause of death by disease and the fourth most common cause of death in men 40 to 60 years of age. The primary causes of the disease in the United States are chronic alcoholism and hepatitis C. Cirrhosis also can be caused by chronic hepatitis B; nonalcoholic steatohepatitis (NASH) (sometimes called *fatty liver disease,* which is characterized by a buildup of fat in the liver that eventually causes scar formation and loss of liver function); blocked bile ducts; and severe reactions to prescription drugs or exposure to environmental toxins.

The patient is asymptomatic in the early stages of cirrhosis, but as scar tissue replaces normal hepatocytes, the liver begins to fail and the patient experiences fatigue, anorexia, weight loss, and abdominal pain. Complications associated with advanced cases of liver failure include dependent edema (fluid retention in the legs); **ascites** (Figure 32-9); bleeding abnormalities; **jaundice**; pruritus from deposits of bile salts on the skin; sensitivity to medication because the liver is unable to metabolize drugs; **portal hypertension**; **esophageal varices**; insulin resistance, with the development of diabetes mellitus type 2; and cancer of the liver. Treatment is based on the cause of the problem, but avoiding alcohol and eating a nutritious diet are key factors. With advanced cases, the only cure is liver transplantation.

Nonalcoholic Fatty Liver Disease

- The medical term for nonalcoholic fatty liver disease is *nonalcoholic steatohepatitis (NASH);* the condition is similar to alcoholic liver disease but occurs in people who drink little or no alcohol.
- Fat accumulates in the liver and causes inflammation, which may lead to scar formation and cirrhosis.
- The condition is very common and affects all age groups, including children, but is seen most often in middle-aged people who are overweight or obese and have high blood cholesterol and diabetes.
- Symptoms are rare in the early stages. The disease often is detected because of abnormal liver blood test results, and it is diagnosed by a liver biopsy.
- Treatment includes weight loss, exercise, improved diabetes control, and anticholesterol medications.
- The disease can be life-threatening. Not every person with NASH develops cirrhosis, but once serious scarring is present, little can be done to stop the progression of liver failure. The only treatment for advanced cirrhosis with liver failure is liver transplantation.

Hepatitis

Inflammation of the liver, called *hepatitis,* may be caused by a localized infection (viral hepatitis), a systemic infection, chemical exposure, or a complication of drug metabolism. Mild inflammation temporarily impairs function, but severe inflammation may lead to necrosis and serious complications.

Viral Hepatitis

Acute viral hepatitis is an infection of the liver that causes a sudden onset of hepatocyte inflammation. Several forms of the hepatitis virus are categorized as hepatitides A (HAV), B (HBV), C (HCV), D (HDV), and E (HEV) (Table 32-4). Hepatic cells can regenerate; therefore, depending on the degree of liver involvement, the patient may recover completely from the viral infection or could develop widespread necrosis, cirrhosis, and liver failure.

Chronic inflammation, defined as the presence of the disease for longer than 6 months, can occur with HBV, HCV, or HDV. This usually results in permanent liver damage and an associated increased risk of liver cancer. Individuals infected with these three types of hepatitis may become lifelong carriers of the disease. Hepatitis carriers are asymptomatic but can transmit the virus to others.

HAV is transmitted through contaminated water or shellfish. Some parts of the world are **endemic** for the disease. HAV immunization is part of the pediatric and adult immunization schedules. HBV has a relatively long incubation period, which makes tracking the source of the infection difficult. Because the virus is found in all blood and body fluids, it can be transmitted in many ways, including needlesticks, human bites from individuals infected with the virus, sexual contact, and from mothers to babies. Immunization of individuals at increased risk is highly recommended. All healthcare personnel are included in this group because they are at increased risk for infection through exposure to blood or blood products and body fluids. HBV immunization is part of the pediatric and adult immunization sequence.

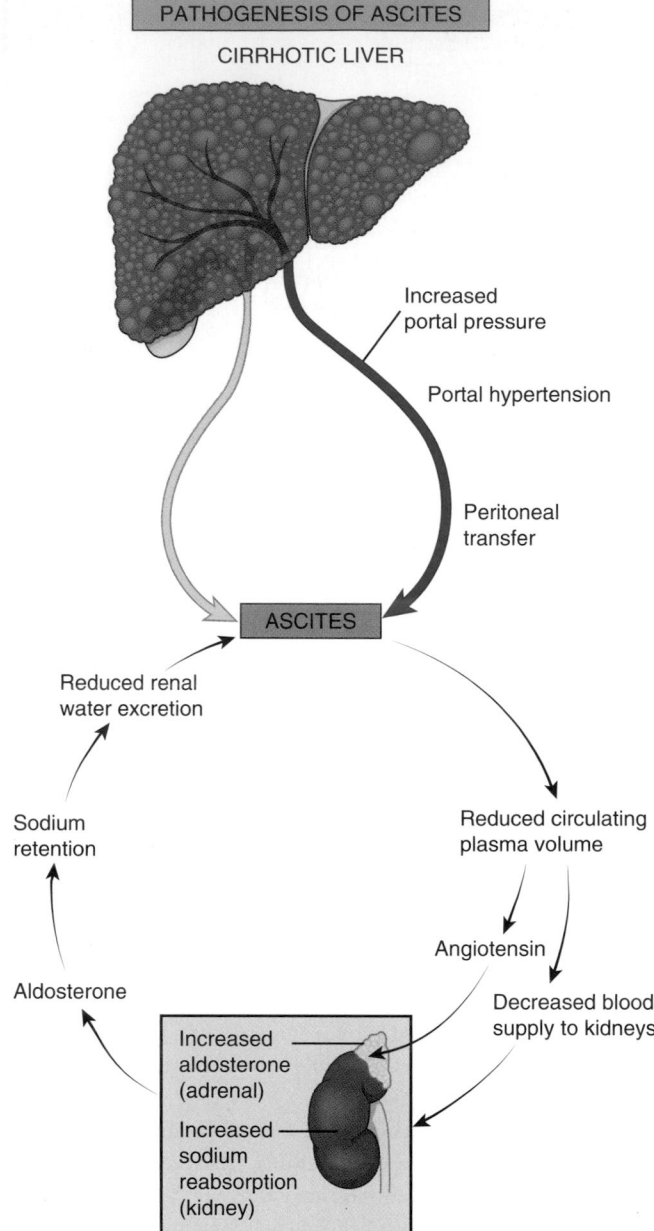

FIGURE 32-9 Pathology of ascites.

As a healthcare professional, the medical assistant cares for sick people on a daily basis who may be carriers of the hepatitis virus. Changing dressings, collecting specimens, holding a patient's hand that was just used to cover the mouth, and discarding a wet baby diaper all are possible ways that exposure can occur. The first line of defense, regardless of whether the medical assistant has been immunized, is frequent sanitization of the hands and wearing gloves when exposure to blood or body fluids is possible.

Diagnosis and Treatment

HAV, HBV, and HCV are diagnosed through identification of the virus or antibodies to the virus in the blood. Another useful diagnostic test is a liver biopsy. Once the infection has been diagnosed, liver function tests are done periodically throughout the course of the disease to determine the degree of liver damage. Patients with

TABLE 32-4 Characteristics of the Viral Hepatitides

TYPE	TRANSMISSION	INCUBATION	SYMPTOMS
A (HAV)	Fecal-oral (food or water contaminated by feces from infected person); contaminated raw shellfish; infected household members or sexual partners	2-7 weeks	• Fatigue • Weakness • Anorexia • Sometimes joint pain hepatomegaly, lymphadenopathy, jaundice
B (HBV; serum hepatitis)	Blood and body fluids; placental transfer	1-6 months	• General malaise • Joint swelling • Pruritic rash • Hepatomegaly • Anorexia • Nausea, vomiting • Dark yellowish-brown urine • Jaundice • May become chronic
C (HCV; non-A non-B)	Blood and body fluids; frequently seen in intravenous drug users and is the most common type of posttransfusion hepatitis	2 weeks–6 months	• Acute onset of fever, chills, malaise, nausea, vomiting • Frequently becomes chronic
D (HDV; delta virus)	Blood and body fluids	Seen only in patients with HBV	• Similar to those of HBV • Increases the severity of HBV
E (HEV)	Fecal-oral	2-9 weeks	• Similar to those with HAV • Seen in India, Asia, Africa, and Central America • Mild form but can cause death in pregnant women

HBV, HCV, or HDV must be monitored for possible chronic hepatitis and the development of a carrier state. Prescription medications include interferon (peginterferon), which stimulates the immune response, and antiviral drugs (Ribavirin) to prevent viral cell replication. Otherwise, the treatment for all forms of hepatitis generally consists of bed rest and a high-protein diet.

The HBV vaccine is given intramuscularly in three doses to prevent the development of hepatitis B. The first two doses are given 30 days apart, and the third is given 6 months after the first. The Occupational Safety and Health Administration (OSHA) requires healthcare employers to offer the vaccine to employees free of charge. Medical assistant programs encourage students to be vaccinated because they also are at risk for acquiring the disease.

Groups at Risk for Hepatitis A, B, and C

- **Hepatitis A (HAV):** Day care workers and clients, institutionalized residents, individuals traveling to infected areas
- **Hepatitis B (HBV):** Intravenous (IV) drug users, homosexual men, hemodialysis patients, hemophiliac individuals, healthcare workers, individuals with a history of frequent sexual partners
- **Hepatitis C (HCV):** Patients receiving frequent blood transfusions, homosexual men, IV drug users, healthcare workers

CRITICAL THINKING APPLICATION   **32-4**

As a healthcare worker who may be exposed to blood and body fluids, Joan is quite concerned about contracting viral hepatitis. For what types of hepatitis is she at risk in Dr. Sahani's office? What can she do to reduce her risk and protect herself from contracting these diseases?

Cholelithiasis (Gallstones)

The gallbladder is an accessory organ of the GI system that stores the bile excreted by the liver. Cholelithiasis, or gallstones, form in the gallbladder from insoluble cholesterol and bile salt. These stones vary in size and number. The reasons for formation are not always clear, although gallstones are more common with a diet that is high in calories and saturated fat; they also are associated with obesity (Figure 32-10). About 20% of people older than age 65 develop cholelithiasis, and the risk is three times higher for women than for men.

Signs and Symptoms

Most gallstones are asymptomatic and are discovered during a routine x-ray. Pain usually occurs when the stones move and obstruct the cystic or common bile ducts. The pain is felt in the epigastric region and the right upper quadrant, often radiating into the right upper back area, and is worse after a high-fat meal. Nausea and vomiting may accompany the pain. The pain hits in a wavelike pattern and is called *colicky pain* or *biliary colic*. If the obstruction is not removed, jaundice may develop.

Diagnosis and Treatment

The provider bases the preliminary diagnosis on the patient's symptoms and on the signs noted on palpation of the upper right quadrant. To confirm the diagnosis, blood tests may be done to detect signs of infection, obstruction, pancreatitis, or jaundice, and an abdominal sonogram is performed to visualize the stones. CT scan may show gallstones, and magnetic resonance (MR) cholangiography may be ordered to diagnose blocked bile ducts. In addition, a hepatobiliary iminodiacetic acid (HIDA) scan can be ordered to diagnose problems in the liver, gallbladder, and bile ducts. The patient is given an IV injection of HIDA, which is taken up by the liver and excreted into the biliary tract. A nuclear scanner then takes pictures of the biliary tract over 2 to 4 hours.

Treatment involves surgical removal of the gallbladder (cholecystectomy), which usually is done laparoscopically.

THE MEDICAL ASSISTANT'S ROLE IN THE GASTROINTESTINAL EXAMINATION

Emotional factors play an important part in many GI problems, often making the separation of functional and organic disorders difficult. Some forms of GI disease may demand immediate attention, such as acute appendicitis or acute gastritis with possible hemorrhage. Both may require surgical therapy. Careful questioning is needed to guide the patient to a precise description of the symptoms. In the role of liaison between the patient and the provider, the medical assistant can help the provider make the diagnosis so that the patient receives the treatment needed.

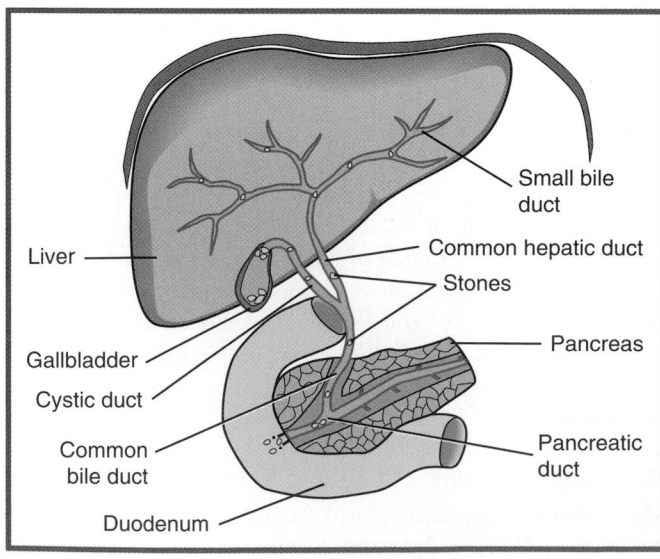

FIGURE 32-10 Gallstones.

Assisting with the Examination

When a patient describes and points to the location of the pain, the medical assistant must know the underlying organs that may be involved. Record the quadrant or region in which the pain is located so that the provider can immediately assess this area when the examination begins. The provider's inspection of the abdomen begins with noting any change in skin color, such as jaundice. Striae (silver stretch marks), petechiae (small, purple hemorrhagic spots), scars, and visible masses may be seen. The contour of the abdomen may be flat, rounded, or bulging in localized areas.

The provider uses palpation and percussion to evaluate the entire abdominal area. As this is done, the medical assistant should remove the drape from the area to be examined and should redrape the patient once this segment of the examination is completed. In addition, the provider may want the medical assistant to document findings as the examination progresses. If the provider wants to examine the anal area, have the patient turn onto his or her left side, and then assist the patient into the Sims position. As this is done, make sure the patient remains draped. After the patient is in the Sims position, adjust the drape on an angle so that it can be easily lifted for the final part of the examination.

CRITICAL THINKING APPLICATION   32-5

Joan is responsible for initially questioning patients about complaints and clearly documenting this information in the patient's record. What information should Joan include that details each patient's GI problem and would be helpful for the provider in determining the patient's diagnosis?

Diagnostic Procedures

Typical diagnostic procedures for the GI system are summarized in Table 32-5. Although most of these procedures are not performed in the ambulatory care setting, the medical assistant must understand the procedure and the recommended patient preparation so that adequate patient education can be provided. If the patient does not prepare adequately for these procedures, the results will be inconclusive, and an expensive, time-consuming, uncomfortable test may have to be rescheduled. It is very important that patients completely understand what is required; the patient should be given a handout to review at home that repeats the verbal instructions given in the office. Providers may vary in their preferences for patient preparation for GI diagnostic tests. It is important that the medical assistant refer to the office policies and procedures manual or ask the provider his or her preference before providing patient education.

The most conclusive diagnostic procedure of the GI system is an endoscopic analysis. In this procedure, the upper GI system is examined by passing a soft, flexible tube down the esophagus into the stomach. The colon is examined through an ascending technique, with entrance through the anus. Fiberoptic technology allows the examiner to view the tissues, take images, and collect laboratory samples during the procedure (e.g., biopsied tissue, gastric fluid, pathogens, bile crystals, cytology samples) with only minor discomfort to the patient.

TABLE 32-5	**Common Diagnostic Procedures for the Gastrointestinal System**	
TEST	**DESCRIPTION AND PURPOSE**	**PATIENT PREPARATION**
Barium swallow	X-ray or fluoroscopic examination of the pharynx and esophagus after the patient swallows barium sulfate; to diagnose hiatal hernia, esophageal varices, strictures, and tumors; takes 15-20 min.	• NPO after midnight • Remove all metal objects • Do not take medication for GERD Laxatives are given after examination to help with excretion of barium.
Upper gastrointestinal (UGI) and small bowel series; air-contrast UGI	X-ray and fluoroscopic examination of the esophagus, stomach, and small intestine after patient swallows barium sulfate; to diagnose ulcers, tumors, regional enteritis, and malabsorption syndrome; takes approximately 30 min.	• Low-fiber diet 2-3 days before • NPO after midnight • No smoking before test • No medications after midnight unless approved by provider • Remove all metal objects • Explain to patient that he or she will swallow a carbonated powder that creates carbon dioxide in the stomach, which helps in visualizing the stomach mucosa Stool will be chalky and light colored for 24-72 hr after test. Laxatives are given after examination to help with excretion of barium.
Barium enema; air-contrast barium enema (ACBE)	X-ray evaluation of large intestine after rectal instillation of barium sulfate; to diagnose colorectal cancer, inflammatory disease of the colon; to detect polyps, diverticula, or obstructions; takes approximately 45 min.	• No dairy products and only liquid diet 24 hr before test • Take bowel preparation as supplied by radiology department; enemas until clear in the morning • No breakfast • Explain to patient that air is insufflated into the colon after instillation of the barium to aid visualization of the colonic mucosa Mild laxative or enema is given after procedure to remove barium. Stools will be light colored for 24-72 hr after test.
Hepatobiliary (HIDA) scan	Nuclear scan after IV injection of radioactive material. Pictures of biliary tract are taken over time to determine whether an obstruction caused by cholelithiasis exists. Best tool for diagnosing acute cholecystitis in patients with acute RUQ pain. Gallbladder visualized 60 min after injection of radionuclide; takes 4 hr to get all images. IV morphine during nuclear scanning speeds up bile movement to reduce scanning time to 1 hr.	• NPO 2 hr before test (ensures that patient's exposure to radioactivity during procedure is minimal) Patient may be given a fatty meal during scanning to determine gallbladder ejection fraction (measures percentage of isotope ejected when gallbladder empties).
Ultrasonography of the liver, gallbladder, biliary system, pancreas	High-frequency sound waves from a transducer penetrate the organ, bounce back to the transducer, and are electronically converted into an image that is recorded on film. Used to diagnose neoplasm of the liver; cholelithiasis in the gallbladder or ducts; pancreatic tumor, abscess, or inflammation.	• Fast before gallbladder and biliary ultrasound • Must be performed before barium contrast studies (barium and gas distort sound waves and alter test results) Does not use contrast or radiation; useful for patients who are allergic to contrast media or are pregnant.

Continued

TABLE 32-5   Common Diagnostic Procedures for the Gastrointestinal System—*continued*

TEST	DESCRIPTION AND PURPOSE	PATIENT PREPARATION
Sigmoidoscopy	Endoscopic examination of distal sigmoid colon, rectum, and anal canal. Used to diagnose inflammatory, infectious, and ulcerative bowel disease and tumors; and to detect hemorrhoids, polyps, fissures, fistulas, and abscesses in the rectum and anal canal. Air insufflated to distend and visualize the lower intestinal tract. Biopsy specimens may be collected and polyps removed; takes 15-20 min.	• Clear liquids day before • NPO night before • Laxatives and 2 Fleet enemas night before Usually done without sedation in the provider's office or outpatient clinic. Patient may experience gas pains after procedure from air instillation and may have slight rectal bleeding if specimen is collected.
Colonoscopy	Endoscopic examination of the large intestine to detect or monitor inflammatory or ulcerative disease; to locate the site of GI bleeding; and to diagnose tumors or strictures. Air insufflated for better visualization. Biopsy samples collected and polyps removed. Recommended for patients with positive fecal occult blood test result and for those at high risk for colon cancer; takes 30-60 min.	• Clear liquid diet for 48 hr before test • Laxatives, enemas until clear, or 1 gallon of Colyte day before • NPO night before • Must drink large amount of fluid after procedure to prevent dehydration from test preparation Large intestine must be completely cleansed. Monitor vital signs before and during procedure. Done with IV sedation in a hospital or outpatient clinic. Patient may experience gas pains after procedure from air instillation and may have slight rectal bleeding if specimen is collected.
Endoscopy	Fiberoptic view of the esophagus and upper GI tract to diagnose or monitor cancer, Barrett's esophagus, peptic ulcers, polyps. Biopsy samples collected and polyps removed; takes 45-60 min.	• No food or fluids for 8 hr before test Back of throat is sprayed with a local anesthetic to reduce gag reflex as tube is passed.

GERD, Gastroesophageal reflux disease; *GI*, gastrointestinal; *HIDA*, hepatobiliary iminodiacetic acid; *IV*, intravenous; *NPO*, nothing by mouth; *RUQ*, right upper quadrant.

Endoscopic procedures are performed to allow the clinician to observe the function of the gallbladder, biliary ducts, and pancreatic ducts. A dye is injected directly into the ducts of the gallbladder and the pancreas, and examination confirms ductal patency and functioning of the organs.

Sigmoidoscopy and Colonoscopy Examinations

Sigmoidoscopy is used to diagnose hemorrhoids, **polyps**, and diverticular disorders. Examination with a flexible sigmoidoscope can be performed in the provider's office because the patient does not undergo anesthesia for the procedure. The patient is positioned in a left-lying Sims position and is draped appropriately. The provider inserts a short, flexible, lighted tube into the rectum and slowly guides it into the sigmoid colon. The scope transmits an image of the inside of the rectum and colon, allowing the provider to examine the lining of these organs carefully. The scope also blows air into the colon to inflate the organ and improve visualization. The provider may remove polyps or biopsy tissue samples during the procedure. The procedure takes 10 to 20 minutes, during which time the patient may complain of pressure and slight cramping in the lower abdomen (Procedure 32-2).

A colonoscope is used to examine the entire length of the large intestine and can be used to remove polyps and collect tissue samples throughout the exam (Figure 32-11). Colonoscopy procedures are performed in a hospital outpatient area or specialty clinic because

they require IV sedation. The American Cancer Society recommends that everyone at average risk for developing colorectal cancer should have a colonoscopy beginning at age 50. Colorectal cancer screening should begin before age 50 if the individual has a personal history of polyps, ulcerative colitis, Crohn's disease, or a strong family history of colorectal cancer or polyps.

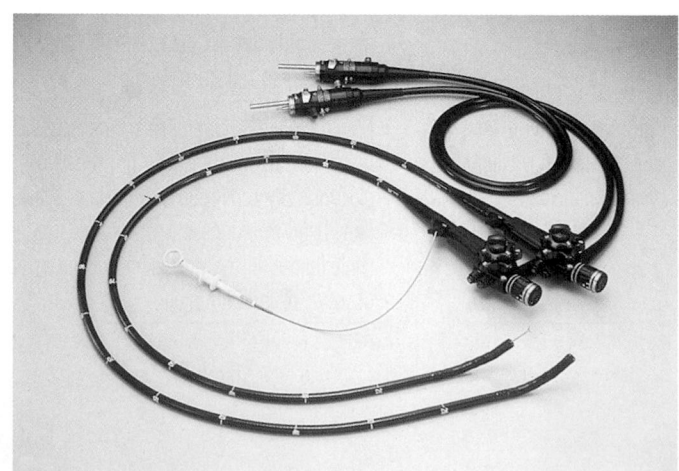

FIGURE 32-11 Flexible colon fiberscopes. (Monohan FD et al: *Phipps' medical-surgical nursing: health and illness perspectives*, ed 8, Philadelphia, 2007, Saunders.)

<table>
</table>

PROCEDURE 32-2	Assist the Provider with a Patient Examination: Assist with an Endoscopic Examination of the Colon

Goal: *To assist the provider with the examination, to prepare collected specimens as requested, and to ensure the patient's comfort and safety.*

EQUIPMENT and SUPPLIES

- Patient's health record
- Laboratory requisition forms
- Nonsterile gloves (for the medical assistant and the provider)
- Appropriate instrument (sigmoidoscope or proctoscope)
- Water-soluble lubricant
- Drape and patient gown
- Long cotton-tipped swabs
- Suction source
- Sterile biopsy forceps
- Rectal speculum
- Specimen containers (with appropriate preservative added)
- Tissue wipes
- Biohazard waste container

PROCEDURAL STEPS

1. Sanitize your hands and assemble all required equipment and supplies.
   PURPOSE: To ensure infection control.
2. Identify the patient by obtaining his or her full name and date of birth; introduce yourself; and explain the procedure. Make sure the patient has completed the proper preparation measure.
3. Ask the patient to empty the bladder.
   PURPOSE: To aid patient comfort during the examination.
4. Give the patient an examination gown. Instruct him or her to remove all clothing below the waist and to put on the gown with the opening to the back. Provide a drape for additional privacy.
5. Obtain and record the patient's vital signs.
   PURPOSE: Baseline vital signs allow detection of variations that might occur during the examination.
6. Assist the patient onto the table. When the provider is ready, place the patient in Sims position.
7. Drape the patient so that only the anus is exposed. A fenestrated drape (a drape with a circular opening over the anus) may be used in place of the rectangular drape.

8. Put on gloves and assist the provider as requested during the examination, including:
   - Lubricating the provider's gloved index finger for the digital examination
   - Lubricating the obturator tip of the instrument before insertion
   - Plugging in the scope's light source when the provider is ready
   - Handing supplies to the provider
   - Collecting specimens by holding the container to accept the sample
   - Labeling specimens immediately because several specimens may be taken from different areas
   - Disposing of contaminated supplies in the biohazard waste container as you are given them by the provider
9. Throughout the examination, observe the patient for any undue reactions. Encourage the patient to breathe slowly through pursed lips to facilitate relaxation.
10. On completion of the examination, provide the patient with tissues to cleanse the anal area. Remove your gloves and dispose of them in the biohazard waste container, then sanitize your hands. Assist the patient into a resting position. Allow the patient time to recover from the procedure. Monitor the patient's blood pressure if indicated.
    PURPOSE: A drop in blood pressure, which often occurs after an invasive procedure, may cause fainting.
11. Once the patient's condition has stabilized, assist the patient off the table and instruct him or her to get dressed. Show the patient where the sink, towels, and tissues are and provide assistance if needed.
12. Complete all laboratory request forms and specimen container labels, and place specimens in the appropriate location for laboratory pickup.
13. Put on gloves and sanitize and disinfect the work area and all equipment used. Carefully follow the manufacturer's recommendations for sanitization and chemical sterilization of the endoscope. Dispose of your gloves in the biohazard waste container and sanitize your hands.
    PURPOSE: To ensure infection control.
14. Record the procedure and any pertinent information in the patient's health record.
    PURPOSE: Procedures that are not recorded are considered not done.

Laboratory Tests

Many of the diagnostic tests for GI disorders are noninvasive. Urine is tested for bilirubin and urinary amylase levels. The stool is tested for occult blood, intestinal ova and parasites, fat excretion, and color.

Occult Blood Screening

Fecal examination is one means of evaluating patients with GI bleeding, obstruction, parasites, dysentery, colitis, or increased fat

excretion. The American Cancer Society recommends that all patients age 50 or older be screened for occult blood in the stool. This test may be performed on younger patients if a family history indicates a need. Blood is not found in the stool of healthy individuals. If the person is experiencing bleeding of the intestinal wall, the blood is likely to be *occult,* or hidden, which means that it cannot be seen with the naked eye. A fecal occult test is done to screen for microscopic bleeding that might occur because of precancerous or cancerous changes in the bowel.

The provider may collect a random stool sample during a routine examination. However, if GI bleeding is suspected, the recommendation is to test three different samples for occult blood. Seven days before the test, the patient should stop taking aspirin and NSAIDs, such as ibuprofen and naproxen (Naprosyn). Starting 72 hours before the stool collections, the patient should not take any more than 250 mg of vitamin C a day; should not eat red meat, including processed meats and cold cuts; and should not eat raw fruits and vegetables, especially melons, radishes, turnips, and horseradish. These restrictions should continue throughout the time the patient is collecting the ordered fecal samples (Procedure 32-3). Failure to follow dietary guidelines or instructions on the use of identified medications can cause false-positive test results.

CRITICAL THINKING APPLICATION   **32-6**

Dr. Sahani wants to update the patient handouts on the preparations necessary for common GI diagnostic procedures. He asks Joan to do the initial research and gather pertinent information that should be included. What should Joan include about patient preparation for these examinations?

PROCEDURE 32-3	Instruct and Prepare a Patient for a Procedure: Instruct Patients in the Collection of a Fecal Specimen

Goal: To assist the provider with the collection of a fecal sample, to process the sample for fecal occult blood screening, and to instruct the patient in fecal occult blood screening at home.

EQUIPMENT and SUPPLIES

- Patient's health record
- Fecal occult blood cards
- Fecal occult blood developer
- Applicator sticks
- Disposable examination gloves
- Biohazard waste container

PROCEDURAL STEPS

1. Sanitize your hands and assemble all required equipment and supplies.
   PURPOSE: To ensure infection control.
2. Identify the patient by obtaining his or her full name and date of birth; introduce yourself; and explain the procedure.
3. Give the patient an examination gown. Instruct him or her to remove all clothing below the waist and to put on the gown with the opening to the back. Provide a drape for additional privacy.
4. Assist the patient onto the table. When the provider is ready, place the patient in the appropriate position for the type of examination ordered.
5. Drape the patient so that only the anus is exposed. A fenestrated drape (drape with a circular opening over the anus) may be used in place of the rectangular drape.
6. Put on gloves and assist the provider as requested during the examination, including:
   - Handing the provider supplies
   - Collecting specimens by holding the fecal occult blood card to accept the sample
   - The provider placing a thin smear of fecal material inside Box A
   - The provider applying a second sample from a different part of the stool inside Box B
   - Closing the cover and disposing of contaminated supplies in the biohazard waste container as you are given them by the provider
7. On completion of the examination, remove your gloves and dispose of them in the biohazard waste container. Sanitize your hands, and assist the patient into a sitting position.

8. Wait 3 to 5 minutes before developing the sample.
9. Put on gloves and open the flap in the back of the card. Apply 2 drops of fecal occult blood test developer directly over the smear.
10. Interpret the results in 60 seconds.
    PURPOSE: The fecal occult blood test is negative if no trace of color is detectable on or at the edge of the smear; it is positive if any trace of blue is seen on or at the edge of the smear (see the following figure).

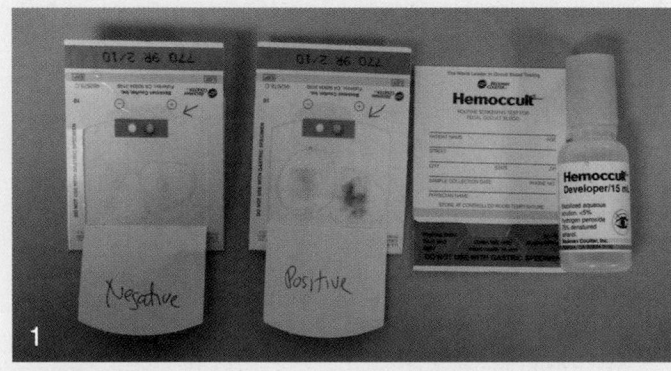

(From Roberts J, Hedges J: *Clinical procedures in emergency medicine*, ed 5, Philadelphia, 2010, Saunders.)

11. Sanitize and disinfect the work area and all equipment used. Dispose of the gloves in the biohazard waste container and sanitize your hands.
    PURPOSE: To ensure infection control.
12. Record the procedure and any pertinent information in the patient's health record.
    PURPOSE: Procedures that are not recorded are considered not done.

PATIENT INSTRUCTIONS FOR HOME COLLECTION OF FECAL OCCULT BLOOD SAMPLES

1. Give the patient a kit for collecting stool samples as ordered by the provider. Typically, the provider orders a sample from three different bowel movements. The patient must follow the recommended medication

restrictions and dietary guidelines throughout the testing period because false-positive results can occur if the recommended medication and dietary restrictions are not followed. These include:
- No aspirin or nonsteroidal antiinflammatory drugs (NSAIDs) for 7 days before the test
- No more than 250 mg of vitamin C per day
- Avoid eating red meat, including processed meats or cold cuts, and raw fruits and vegetables, especially melons, radishes, turnips, and horseradish, for 72 hours before the stool collections

The patient then is instructed as follows:

2. Store the kit in the bathroom at home or carry it with you while you are away from home until the three different stool samples have been collected.
3. Write your name and other required information on the front of the collection cards.
4. Cover the toilet with plastic wrap or use a toilet cap to collect the stool specimen.
   PURPOSE: Stool samples from toilet bowl water can cause errors in the test result.

5. Use one of the applicator sticks to collect a small fecal sample and apply a thin smear inside Box A.
6. Reuse the applicator to obtain another sample from a different part of the stool and apply it to Box B.
7. Close the cover and label the card with the date and time collected.
8. Store cards away from heat, light, and strong chemicals (e.g., bleach). Do not place in a plastic bag.
   PURPOSE. Strong chemicals can affect the slide. The stool sample must air dry to be processed properly.
9. Repeat this procedure for the next two bowel movements, as ordered by the provider, using a different card for each sample.
   PURPOSE: To test multiple stool samples for minute amounts of bleeding.
10. After collecting all samples as ordered, seal the test envelope and return the kit to the provider's office. Do not send stool samples in the mail unless you have a special envelope from the provider.
    PURPOSE: To prevent contamination of the mail.

Proctologic Examination

Proctology is the branch of internal medicine that is concerned with diseases and disorders of the colon, rectum, and anus. The anal area is examined with a proctoscope, which allows detection of hemorrhoids, polyps, **fissures**, fistulas, and abscesses. The rectum and the sigmoid colon are examined with a flexible sigmoidoscope, and the descending, transverse, and ascending colon sections (or the entire colon) are examined with a colonoscope.

Many people are apprehensive about colorectal examinations. To alleviate this anxiety, instruct the patient in exactly what to do before the examination, and provide support during the procedure. Let the patient know that some discomfort, such as cramping, may be experienced. Furthermore, the sensation of expelling **flatus** or of an impending bowel movement may be felt. These sensations are caused by the instrument and the procedure.

The patient must be given specific instructions on how to prepare the colon for any endoscopic examination (see Table 32-5). Refer to your employer's policies and procedures manual to determine the preferred method of patient preparation for each test because providers' orders may vary.

CLOSING COMMENTS

Patient Education

The GI system is responsible for the nourishment of the entire body. When disease interferes with this process, the individual may become ill and develop serious pathologic disorders. Listen for patients' concerns that may indicate a problem within the system and its accessory organs. Report these concerns to the provider or note them in the patient's health record for the provider to read. If the office

has information that may assist the patient in dealing with a particular problem, lay out the information for the provider to give to the patient; or, with the provider's authorization, talk to the patient and offer suggestions that might help the person deal with a particular concern. Learning to perform and assist with diagnostic procedures allows the medical assistant to aid in the diagnostic sequence and to assist the patient in maintaining a healthy GI system.

Legal and Ethical Issues

Legally and ethically, the medical assistant's responsibility is to assist the provider and act as the patient's advocate. All information discussed between the patient and the provider, and all testing procedures ordered and done, must remain confidential. Confidentiality and trust are very closely linked, and these two issues form the basis of a sound patient-provider relationship. The medical assistant is an important part of that relationship and can strengthen it through ethical, professional conduct.

Professional Behaviors

Diagnostic procedures and treatment protocols, especially medications, are constantly changing. The professional medical assistant must be committed to lifelong learning to keep up with the rapid changes in the medical field. Maintaining a current understanding of the human body, the disease process, and how specific GI system diseases are diagnosed and treated requires a willingness to learn and adapt over time. This commitment to lifelong learning is a crucial part of becoming a professional medical assistant.

SUMMARY OF SCENARIO

Joan enjoys working with Dr. Sahani and his patients with GI disorders, but she is constantly challenged to learn and update information about diseases and disorders of the GI system, in addition to their diagnosis and medical management. Joan must consistently work at applying correct medical terminology when documenting patients' complaints and must use her knowledge of GI disorders to ask pertinent, detailed questions when gathering patient information.

Joan has also had to update her knowledge of patient preparation for diagnostic procedures so that patients are adequately educated and prepared

for scheduled examinations. She participates in workshops offered by her local professional organization to stay up-to-date on medications and treatments for GI diseases, especially current research on infectious hepatitis. Joan is looking forward to active involvement in patient care as she continues to prepare patient education materials and to assist Dr. Sahani as needed in providing high-quality patient care.

SUMMARY OF LEARNING OBJECTIVES

1. **Define, spell, and pronounce the terms listed in the vocabulary.**
   Spelling and pronouncing medical terms correctly reinforce the medical assistant's credibility. Knowing the definitions of these terms promotes confidence in communication with patients and co-workers.

2. **Describe the primary functions of the GI system.**
   The GI system is responsible for the digestion of food, the absorption of nutrients, and the excretion of waste materials.

3. **Identify the anatomic structures that make up the GI system and describe the physiology of each.**
   The GI system begins at the mouth and ends at the anal canal. The digestive process starts in the mouth with mastication and enzyme action; the bolus of food is swallowed and passes from the esophagus into the stomach, where digestion continues with the addition of hydrochloric acid and further enzyme action. Digestion ends in the duodenum, with pancreatic juices and emulsification of fat by bile, which is excreted by the liver and stored in the gallbladder. Absorption of nutrients takes place in the ileum and jejunum, and fluids are absorbed in the large intestine. Ultimately, waste materials are excreted through the anus. (See Figure 32-1.)

4. **Differentiate among the abdominal quadrants and regions.**
   The abdominal cavity can be divided into four sections, or quadrants: the right and left upper quadrants and the right and left lower quadrants. More specifically, the abdominal cavity can be divided into nine regions: the right hypochondriac, epigastric, and left hypochondriac regions; the right lumbar, umbilical, and left lumbar regions; and the right inguinal, hypogastric, and left inguinal regions. These anatomic markers are important for clearly identifying the location of a GI problem. (See Figure 32-2.)

5. **Summarize the typical symptoms and characteristics of GI complaints and perform telephone screening for patients with GI complaints.**
   Patients with GI disorders may complain of vomiting because of pain, stress, GI upset, or an inner ear or intracranial pressure disturbance; diarrhea caused by an infection, an allergy, or a malabsorption problem; constipation that occurs because of a low-fiber diet or inadequate fluids,

   as a side effect of medication, or because of a bowel obstruction or tumor; and abdominal pain that varies in intensity and quality. It is important for the medical assistant to identify the location of the patient's discomfort, using either the abdominal quadrants or the abdominal regions, and to note the onset, duration, and frequency of all symptoms. (See Table 32-1.)

   Telephone screening for GI complaints involves following the facility's policies and procedures manual for management of disorders; gathering detailed information about the onset, duration, and frequency of the problem and the pertinent patient history; and recording the interaction in the patient's record, including use of medications for relief; a pain scale, if appropriate; and the course of action based on the provider's recommendations. (See Procedure 32-1.)

6. **Distinguish among cancers of the GI tract.**
   Cancers of the GI tract can occur in any of the primary or accessory organs of the system. These can include oral tumors, which manifest as a white mass or as an ulcer; esophageal tumors, which cause dysphagia; gastric tumors, which cause anorexia and weight loss but are difficult to diagnose in the early stages; liver tumors, which usually occur secondary to metastasis from another cancerous site, accompanied by hepatomegaly and portal hypertension; pancreatic cancer, which usually is advanced when diagnosed; and colorectal cancer, which causes changes in bowel function and anemia. (See Table 32-2.)

7. **List common esophageal and gastric disorders; also, describe the signs and symptoms, diagnostic tests, and treatments of each.**
   Esophageal and gastric disorders include hiatal hernias, in which part of the stomach pushes through the hiatal sphincter of the diaphragm, causing GERD; peptic ulcers, associated with *H. pylori* infections, which are treated with a combination of antibiotics and proton pump inhibitors; and pyloric stenosis, seen most frequently in firstborn male infants, which causes projectile vomiting and must be corrected by surgery. These disorders usually are diagnosed symptomatically and with the use of a barium swallow or an upper GI series of x-ray films. Medical treatment includes the use of Prilosec, Nexium, or Pepcid. Surgery may be indicated for repair of a hiatal hernia or gastric ulcers if perforation occurs.

SUMMARY OF LEARNING OBJECTIVES—*continued*

8. **List intestinal disorders; also, describe the signs and symptoms, diagnostic tests, and treatments of each.**

Intestinal disorders include a variety of conditions. Food-borne illnesses cause mild to severe gastroenteritis, and the symptoms are controlled with antiemetics and antidiarrheal medications. (See Table 32-3.) Dumping syndrome, which may occur as a postsurgical complication of weight loss surgery, results in widespread GI complaints. IBS is a recurrent functional bowel disorder that causes alternating bouts of diarrhea, flatulence, and constipation; it is treated pharmaceutically with bulk-forming agents, antidiarrheals, antispasmodics, and anticholinergics. Acute appendicitis is diagnosed through a positive McBurney's sign and ultrasonography or CT scan and is treated surgically. Regional enteritis, or Crohn's disease, causes localized areas of ulceration in the intestinal tract and is treated medically to reduce inflammation, manage symptoms, and maintain nutritional status. Ulcerative colitis causes inflammatory ulcers that typically start in the anus and move proximally through the colon; treatment is similar to Crohn's disease, but surgical removal of the colon is curative. Celiac disease is a malabsorption disorder caused by a genetic defect in the ability to metabolize gluten. Gluten sensitivity does not cause damage to the villi, and the patient's symptoms are similar but less severe. Diverticular disease consists of small herniations of the muscular lining of the colon and is managed with dietary changes and surgery if diverticulitis is advanced. The abdominal musculature can become weakened and hernias that require surgical repair can develop. Hemorrhoids, which are varicose veins of the anus, are treated with stool softeners, a high-fiber diet, or surgical repair.

9. **Do the following related to diseases of the liver and gallbladder:**
   - *Classify disorders of the liver and gallbladder, and list the signs and symptoms, diagnostic tests, and treatments for each.*

   Disorders of the liver include hepatitis from either viral infection or a chemical reaction, such as alcohol abuse, or as a complication of drug metabolism. Mild inflammation temporarily impairs liver function, but severe inflammation may lead to necrosis and serious complications, including jaundice, cirrhosis, and portal hypertension. The gallbladder stores bile that is excreted by the liver to aid in fat metabolism. If cholelithiasis or cholecystitis develops, the gallbladder may have to be removed surgically to relieve symptoms.
   - *Describe the similarities and differences among the various forms of infectious viral hepatitis.*

   Viral hepatitis is an infection of the liver that causes acute inflammation of hepatocytes. Five forms of this virus exist: A, B, C, D, and E. Hepatic cells can regenerate; therefore, depending on the degree of liver involvement, the patient may either recover or may develop widespread necrosis, cirrhosis, and liver failure. Chronic inflammation can occur with hepatitis HBV, HCV, or HDV. This usually results in permanent liver damage and an associated increased risk of liver cancer. Vaccinations are available for HAV and HBV. (See Table 32-4.)

10. **Summarize the medical assistant's role in the GI examination.**

The medical assistant provides patient support and education, gathers and records specific details about the patient's complaints, and assists the provider with the examination and diagnostic procedures performed in the ambulatory care setting.

11. **Do the following when it comes to assisting with gastroenterology diagnostic procedures:**
   - *Explain the common diagnostic procedures for the GI system.*

   Diagnostic procedures for the GI system include laboratory studies, such as liver panels and urinary tests for bilirubin and amylase, and stool tests for occult blood, intestinal parasites, and fat excretion. Radiologic and endoscopic tests include barium swallow, upper GI series, barium enema, HIDA scan, sigmoidoscopy, and colonoscopy. (See Table 32-5.)
   - *Demonstrate the procedure for assisting with an endoscopic colon examination.*

   The endoscopic colon examination is described in Procedure 32-2. The medical assistant prepares the room, equipment, and patient for the procedure; assists the provider throughout the procedure by positioning the patient, monitoring vital signs as indicated, helping with equipment, and labeling specimens for transport to the laboratory; assists the patient after the examination; sanitizes and disinfects the equipment and the room; and documents the procedure in the patient's health record.
   - *Perform the procedural steps for assisting with the collection of a fecal specimen.*

   Procedure 32-3 presents the steps for collecting a fecal specimen. Patient education includes information on proper dietary and drug restrictions and collecting three different stool specimens for analysis for hidden blood in the stool.

12. **Describe the medical assistant's role in the proctologic examination.**

The medical assistant supports and prepares the patient; positions and drapes the patient for the procedure; monitors vital signs before and during the procedure; and assists the provider with the procedure.

13. **Describe patient education, in addition to legal and ethical issues, related to assisting in gastroenterology.**

The GI system is responsible for the nourishment of the entire body. Listen for concerns the patient expresses that may indicate a problem in the system or its accessory organs. All information discussed between the patient and the provider must remain confidential.

CONNECTIONS

Study Guide Connection: Go to the Chapter 32 Study Guide. Read and complete the activities.

evolve Evolve Connection: Go to the Chapter 32 link at *evolve.elsevier.com/kinn* to complete the Chapter Review Quiz. Check out the other resources listed for this chapter to make the most of what you have learned from Assisting in Gastroenterology.

33

ASSISTING IN UROLOGY AND MALE REPRODUCTION

SCENARIO

Sara Ricci, CMA (AAMA), who has 10 years of experience, works for Dr. Samuel Fineman, a urologist who also manages male reproductive disorders. Dr. Fineman relies on Sara to handle telephone calls from patients, to have a clear understanding of the anatomy and physiology of the renal system, and to assist him in the clinical area of the practice. Although Sara has worked for Dr. Fineman for almost 2 years, occasionally problems still arise that she is not sure how to manage. Sara attends workshops and conferences to earn continuing education units to maintain her CMA credential and tries to choose topics that focus on urologic issues. In addition, she keeps up to date on new diagnostic procedures and treatments for sexually transmitted infections (STIs), including human immunodeficiency virus (HIV) infection and acquired immunodeficiency syndrome (AIDS). Sara helps train other medical assistants in the practice and makes sure adequate patient education supplies are available for self-testicular examination.

While studying this chapter, think about the following questions:

- What is the basic anatomy and physiology of the renal and male reproductive systems?
- What should Sara know about common adult and pediatric urologic disorders so that she can both assist the provider in the practice and answer patients' questions?
- What are some of the pathologic genital conditions seen in men?
- What are the typical signs, symptoms, and treatments for sexually transmitted infections in men?
- How can Sara provide patient education and support for individuals with renal and male reproductive system disorders?

LEARNING OBJECTIVES

1. Define, spell, and pronounce the terms listed in the vocabulary.
2. Describe the anatomy and physiology of the urinary system.
3. Do the following related to disorders of the urinary system:
    - Explain the susceptibility of the urinary system to diseases and disorders.
    - Identify the primary signs and symptoms of urinary problems.
    - Detail common diagnostic procedures of the urinary system.
4. Discuss the causative factors of urinary incontinence, in addition to the various treatments and medications used to treat it.
5. Compare and contrast infections and inflammations of the urinary tract.
6. Describe urinary tract disorders and cancers.
7. Summarize the causes of renal failure and how it is treated.
8. Summarize the typical pediatric urologic disorders.
9. Describe the anatomy and physiology of the male reproductive system.
10. Determine the causes and effects of prostate disorders.
11. Outline common types of genital pathologic conditions in men, and perform patient education for the testicular self-examination.
12. Analyze the effects of sexually transmitted infections in men and summarize the characteristics of HIV infection, including diagnostic criteria and treatment protocols.
13. Describe the medical assistant's role in urologic and male reproductive examinations.
14. Discuss patient education, legal and ethical issues, and HIPAA applications in the urology practice.

VOCABULARY

albuminuria (al-byu-mih-nur'-e-uh) The abnormal presence of albumin protein in the urine.

azotemia (a-zo-te'-me-uh) The retention of excessive quantities of nitrogenous wastes in the blood.

casts In kidney disease, fibrous or protein material molded to the shape of the part in which it has accumulated that is thrown off into the urine.

copulation Sexual intercourse.

creatinine (kre-ah'-tuhn-in) Nitrogenous waste from muscle metabolism that is excreted in urine.

dyspepsia An uncomfortable feeling of fullness, heartburn, bloating, and nausea.

dysuria Painful or difficult urination.

erythropoietin (eh-rith-ruh-poi'-eh-tin) A substance released by the kidneys and liver that promotes red blood cell formation.

VOCABULARY—*continued*

Kaposi's sarcoma A malignant tumor of endothelial cells that begins as red, brown, or purple lesions on the ankles or soles.

leukocytosis An abnormal increase in the number of circulating white blood cells; it often occurs with bacterial infections but not viral infections.

renin An enzyme produced and stored in the glomerulus; it is released by a homeostatic response to raise the blood pressure when needed.

urgency A sudden, compelling desire to urinate and the inability to control the release of urine.

wasting syndrome Physical deterioration resulting in profound weight loss, fatigue, anorexia, and mental confusion.

Urology is the study of the urinary tract in both male and female patients. A physician who specializes in the diseases and disorders of the urinary system is a *urologist*. Urologists also specialize in conditions associated with the male reproductive system.

ANATOMY AND PHYSIOLOGY OF THE URINARY SYSTEM

The urinary tract consists of bilateral kidneys and ureters, the urinary bladder, and the urethra (Figure 33-1). The main function of the urinary system is to remove waste products from the body. Waste materials are byproducts of the body's metabolic processes, and if left to accumulate in the bloodstream, they can become toxic. The urinary system removes salts and nitrogenous wastes (nitrogen is the product of protein metabolism) from the blood, forming urea, which is excreted. Besides excreting waste material, the urinary system performs other functions, such as:

- Helping to maintain homeostasis by regulating water, electrolyte, and acid-base levels
- Activating vitamin D, which is needed for calcium absorption
- Producing **erythropoietin**, which helps control the rate of red blood cell formation

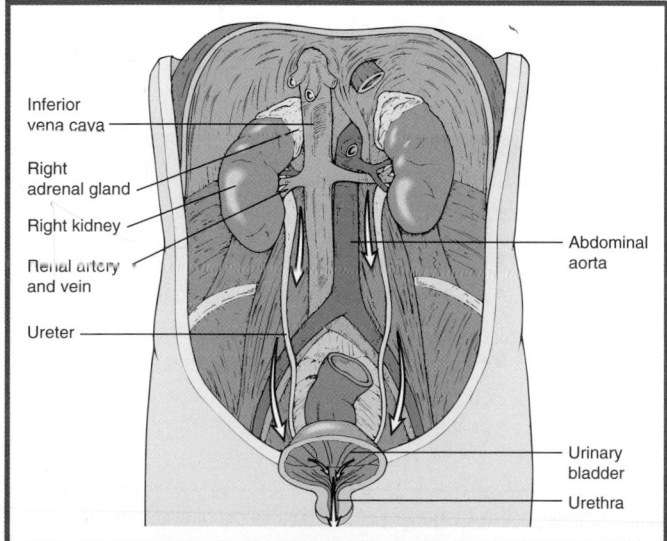

FIGURE 33-1 The urinary system. (From Frazier MS, Drzymkowski JA: *Essentials of human diseases and conditions*, ed 5, St Louis, 2013, Saunders.)

- Helping to maintain blood pressure by secreting the enzyme **renin**

The kidneys are red-brown, bean-shaped glandular organs. They are located posterior to the peritoneum (retroperitoneal) and against the muscles of the back, roughly between the T12 and L3 vertebrae. The left kidney is situated about 1 inch (2 cm) higher than the right because of the location of the liver.

The kidneys remove unwanted substances from the blood and form urine for excretion. For this crucial function, a great deal of blood circulates through the kidneys—approximately 15% to 30% of the total cardiac output. The blood is delivered to the two kidneys by the renal artery and is distributed through the kidneys by a highway of smaller arteries. The blood then is returned through a pathway of veins, including the renal vein, which flows into the inferior vena cava in the abdominal cavity.

The outer layer of the kidney, the cortex, contains the functional unit of the kidney, the *nephron,* where urine is formed as fluid and dissolved substances move between its vascular and tubular structures. Three processes are involved in urine formation: *filtration, reabsorption,* and *excretion.* The nephron consists of the *glomerulus,* a cluster of capillaries extending from the distal renal artery that is partly surrounded by *Bowman's capsule.* Fluid and dissolved substances are filtered from the glomerulus to Bowman's capsule and then into the proximal convoluted *tubules,* where most of the fluid is reabsorbed by venules and arterioles surrounding the tubules and sent back into the general circulation. Based on the homeostatic needs of the body, the kidneys determine the type and quantity of substances reabsorbed. Finally, the remaining substances are excreted through the distal convoluted tubules to the collecting tubules and then on to the *medulla* of the kidney. The medulla contains the *renal pelvis,* where the urine is deposited before passing down the *ureters.* The distal collection area of the renal pelvis is made up of fingerlike projections, called the *calyces,* where urine is first deposited when it leaves the nephron units of the renal cortex (Figure 33-2).

The bilateral ureters are tubular organs approximately 10 inches (25 cm) long; with the aid of peristaltic waves generated by the ureter's muscle layer, the bilateral ureters move the urine from the kidneys to the *urinary bladder.* The urinary bladder is a hollow organ lined with smooth muscle that overlaps in rugae formation, which enables the bladder to expand as it fills. When the bladder is full, the sphincter opens and urine flows into the *urethra.* The urethra is lined with a mucous membrane, and in males it functions both as

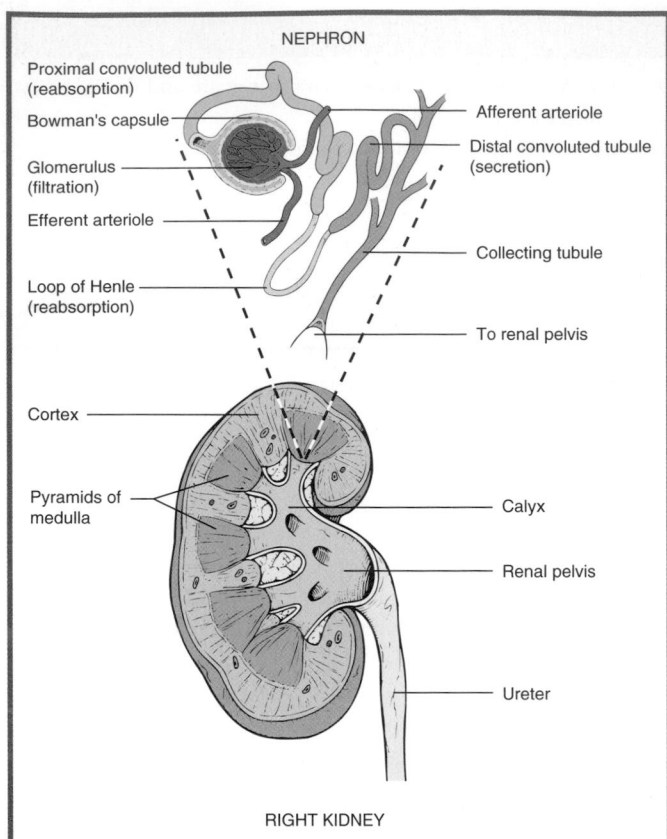

NEPHRON

Proximal convoluted tubule (reabsorption)

Bowman's capsule

Glomerulus (filtration)

Efferent arteriole

Loop of Henle (reabsorption)

Afferent arteriole

Distal convoluted tubule (secretion)

Collecting tubule

To renal pelvis

Cortex

Pyramids of medulla

Calyx

Renal pelvis

Ureter

RIGHT KIDNEY

FIGURE 33-2 The kidney. (From Frazier MS, Drzymkowski JA: *Essentials of human diseases and conditions,* ed 5, St Louis, 2013, Saunders.)

the urinary canal and as a passageway for cells and secretions from various reproductive organs. The male urethra is about 8 inches (20 cm) long and is divided into three sections: the prostatic urethra (which passes through the prostate gland at the base of the bladder), the membranous urethra, and the penile urethra. In a female, the urethra is about 1 to 1½ inches (3 to 4 cm) long. Its proximity to

the vagina and anus exposes the renal system to microorganisms that can cause infection. The urethra passes the urine from the bladder to the urinary meatus and outside the body. The process of urination is known as *voiding* or *micturition.*

CRITICAL THINKING APPLICATION   **33-1**

Dr. Fineman wants Sara to review a number of pamphlets on the anatomy and physiology of the urinary system to be used for patient education. Sara has researched the available pamphlets and must decide which is best suited to the practice. What material should be included in a comprehensive pamphlet? Are diagrams important for patient understanding?

DISORDERS OF THE URINARY SYSTEM

The urinary tract is made up of a continuous mucosal lining that gives organisms entering the urethra a direct pathway through the system. Of the wide range of symptoms that occur in patients with disorders of the renal system, the most common involve changes in the frequency of urination. **Dysuria**, **urgency**, retention, and incontinence all are common symptoms. Abnormal functions of any part of the urinary tract often can be determined through urinalysis, blood urea nitrogen (BUN) levels, and analysis of **creatinine** clearance. Radiologic and endoscopic studies also are important in detecting urinary tract diseases. Table 33-1 summarizes common diagnostic tests of the urinary system.

CRITICAL THINKING APPLICATION   **33-2**

Sara is responsible for scheduling and providing patient preparation instructions for diagnostic radiologic and endoscopic procedures. With Dr. Fineman's approval, she has prepared patient handouts that summarize the correct procedures to follow when a patient is scheduled for specific urologic tests. Today she has a patient who needs to be scheduled for both a cystogram and an intravenous pyelogram (IVP). How should the patient prepare for both of these examinations?

TABLE 33-1	Common Diagnostic Tests of the Urinary System	
TEST	**DESCRIPTION**	**PATIENT PREPARATION**
Uroflowmetry	Patient urinates into a funnel connected to a measuring instrument, which calculates the amount of urine, rate of flow in seconds, and length of time until completion of the void. Evaluates function of the lower urinary tract or helps determine whether an obstruction of normal urine outflow is present.	• Bladder should be full • Drink about four glasses of water several hours before test • Do not push or strain with urination and remain as still as possible during test
Kidney-ureter-bladder (KUB) x-ray	Flat plate films of the abdomen show size, shape, location, and any malformations of the kidneys and bladder. Used to visualize calculi.	No specific patient preparation; contraindicated in pregnancy.

TABLE 33-1   Common Diagnostic Tests of the Urinary System—*continued*

TEST	DESCRIPTION	PATIENT PREPARATION
Renal scanning	Nuclear scans to determine the size, shape, and function of the kidney or to diagnose obstruction or hypertension; radioisotope is administered intravenously (IV), and images are taken to show distribution.	• Void before procedure • Drink 2 or 3 glasses of water before scan • Contraindicated in pregnancy • No sedation or fasting required
Cystography and voiding (cystourethrogram)	X-ray evaluation with contrast dye to study bladder structure or function.	• Foley catheter inserted for a cystourethrogram • Contraindicated in pregnancy • X-ray films may be taken while patient is voiding (voiding cystourethrogram) • After procedure, patient forces fluids to eliminate dye and prevent infection
Intravenous pyelography; may be called *intravenous urography* (IUG)	Dye injected IV, then x-ray films taken at intervals to show passage through kidneys and ureters into bladder. Used to diagnose tumors, calculi, obstructions, and congenital renal problems.	• Contraindicated in pregnancy and with iodine allergies • Liquid diet 8 hr before • Laxative taken evening before • May have enema morning of study • Adequate fluids afterward
Arteriography (angiography)	Dye injected into the renal artery, computed fluoroscopy allows visualization of the blood flow of the kidneys, and serial x-ray films are taken. Used to diagnose stenosis of the renal artery and highly vascular renal cancers.	*Check for allergies to iodine and shellfish.* • Nothing by mouth (NPO) 2-8 hr before • Preprocedural medications administered as ordered • Void before study • Warm flush may occur when dye is injected • Contraindicated in pregnancy
Renal computed tomography (CT)	Can be done with or without contrast dye; transverse views of kidney are taken to detect tumors, abscesses, cysts, and hydronephrosis.	*Check for allergies to iodine and shellfish.* • Remove all metal objects • If contrast medium will be used, fast 4 hr before procedure • Scanner may make loud clicking sounds • Dye may cause flushing, metallic taste, and headache • Contraindicated in pregnancy
Renal ultrasonography	High-frequency sound waves transmitted through kidneys to detect abnormalities. Used to determine kidney size and to diagnose hydronephrosis, polycystic kidneys, and obstructions of ureters and bladder.	No food or fluid restrictions; noninvasive and painless
Cystoscopy	Endoscopic view of urethra and bladder for biopsy. Used to measure bladder capacity, to find or remove calculi, for dilation of urethra and ureters, and for placement of ureteral stents.	• Enemas to clear bowel • Local anesthetic: Force fluids before procedure • General anesthesia: NPO after midnight • Preprocedural sedative to reduce bladder spasms Aftercare: Monitor urinary output for 24 hours.
Retrograde pyelography	Dye injected through cystoscope into bladder, ureters, and kidneys to detect stones and other obstructions; procedure can replace intravenous pyelogram (IVP) for patients with renal failure, obstructions, or allergies to IV dye.	Same as cystoscopy; *check for iodine and shellfish allergies.*

Urinary Incontinence

Urinary incontinence, which is a temporary or chronic loss of urinary control, can be the result of many conditions, including urinary tract infections, brain disorders, and tissue damage. Incontinence also can be caused by straining or coughing in post-surgical patients and in female patients with weak pelvic musculature; in such situations, the condition is called *stress incontinence*.

The treatment of incontinence depends on the causative factor. Behavioral approaches include bladder or habit training that teaches the patient to urinate according to an established schedule rather than when he or she has the urge to void. This is helpful for patients who are incontinent as a result of strokes, Parkinson's disease, Alzheimer's disease, central nervous system (CNS) lesions, or cystitis. Pelvic muscle exercises (Kegel exercises) that strengthen the muscles of the pelvic floor are helpful for women with stress incontinence. Patients are trained to simulate stopping the flow of urine and holding that contraction for 10 seconds. To strengthen the pelvic floor, this exercise should be done in sets of 20 three times a day. A method for managing male incontinence is with an external catheter. External catheters are a type of urine collection device that resembles a pouch or condom, which is securely placed around the penis. They are often called condom catheters. The tip of the device is connected to a drainage tube that empties into a storage bag. Condom catheters are typically used in long-term care facilities but are associated with an increased incidence of urinary tract infections (UTIs).

Patients with neurogenic bladder, who have lost control of urination because of CNS trauma or disease, may have to be catheterized to remove urine from the bladder. Intermittent catheterization to empty the bladder is preferable to indwelling catheters, which often lead to infection. Clean intermittent catheterization can be done using medical aseptic techniques on a schedule at home, usually every 4 to 6 hours. If possible, the patient should be taught to perform routine catheterization throughout the day, or a family member may be involved in care.

Chronic incontinence can be treated pharmacologically with anticholinergics that act to relax the smooth muscle of the urinary bladder and prevent uncontrolled bladder contractions that cause urine to leak out of the bladder (Table 33-2). These medications are used to treat stress incontinence and urgency.

When all other treatments have failed, surgical intervention for urinary incontinence may be the answer. Several different suburethral sling procedures have proved successful in treating female incontinence. An artificial urinary sphincter is helpful for men with incontinence. A device shaped like a doughnut is implanted around the neck of the bladder; it keeps the urinary sphincter closed until the patient presses a valve implanted under the skin. This deflates the ring and releases urine from the bladder.

Urinary Tract Infections and Inflammations

UTIs occur frequently, especially in women, because the urinary system has a direct opening to the outside, and urine is an excellent medium for bacterial growth. Most UTIs are ascending; that is, they start in the perineal area with exposure to pathogens, which infect the continuous mucosa of the urinary system, which in turn allows the pathogen to travel up through the urethra, bladder, and ureters to the kidneys. Infection and inflammation of the urethra is called

TABLE 33-2   Anticholinergic Medications for Treatment of Incontinence, Urinary Bladder Spasms, and Urgency

GENERIC NAME	BRAND NAME	ADVERSE EFFECTS
darifenacin	Enablex	Dry mouth, constipation, **dyspepsia**
dicyclomine	Bentyl	Dizziness, blurred vision, drowsiness
fesoterodine	Toviaz	Dry mouth, constipation
oxybutynin	Ditropan, Gelnique, Oxytrol	Dry mouth, constipation, drowsiness, nausea
solifenacin	Vesicare	Dry mouth, constipation, abdominal pain
tolterodine	Detrol	Dry mouth, blurred vision, constipation

urethritis and that of the bladder is *cystitis.* The resident flora of the colon, *Escherichia coli,* is the usual causative agent.

Women are more susceptible than men to UTIs because of the female anatomy (i.e., a short urethra and the proximity of the anus) and as a result of irritation caused by tampon use and sexual activity. Older men with prostatic hyperplasia and resultant urinary retention also are at risk for frequent urinary tract infections.

General Signs and Symptoms of Urinary Tract Infection

- Overwhelming urge to urinate *(urgency)*
- Burning on urination *(dysuria)*
- Urgency with frequent, small amounts of urine
- Blood in the urine *(hematuria)* or a cloudy, dark, foul-smelling urine
- Frequent urination at night *(nocturia)*

Urethritis

Urethritis, or inflammation of the urethra, is more common in men. It typically is caused by chlamydia or gonorrhea bacteria. Symptoms include the discharge of pus, an itching sensation at the opening of the urethra, and burning on urination. Infectious urethritis can cause cystitis in women, so sexual partners also should be treated. Urinalysis may show hematuria and pyuria (pus in the urine).

Cystitis

Cystitis, an infection of the urinary bladder, causes inflammation of the bladder wall and urinary urgency. Symptoms include very mild to acute discomfort in the lower abdomen, urinary frequency, and painful urination (dysuria). The patient may have signs of a systemic infection, including fever, general malaise, and **leukocytosis**. A positive diagnostic urinalysis shows a bacteria level in the urine of more than 100,000/mL, pyuria, and hematuria. An infection of the urinary bladder is especially difficult to eliminate because of the bladder's overlapping rugae walls. It is very important that patients understand that, to prevent a recurrence of the infection, they must complete the entire antibiotic prescription to destroy all the bacteria in the folds of tissue.

Pyelonephritis

Pyelonephritis, an inflammation of the renal pelvis and kidney, is the most common type of renal disease. It is caused by bacteria that ascend from the lower urinary tract and is associated with conditions such as urinary retention or obstruction that promotes urinary stasis and the growth of bacteria. It frequently is preceded by urethritis and cystitis. With pyelonephritis, pus collects in the renal pelvis, and abscesses form. Symptoms include fever, chills, nausea, vomiting, and flank (lateral lumbar) pain. The patient reports foul-smelling, dark urine with frequency and urgency.

Diagnostic studies include urinalysis of a clean-catch urine sample. It reveals hematuria, pyuria, increased white and red blood cells, **albuminuria**, **casts**, and bacteria. Urine cultures usually are done to determine the causative agent.

Treatment of Urinary Tract Infections

UTIs are treated with antibiotics, such as ciprofloxacin (Cipro), nitrofurantoin (Macrodantin, Furadantin), sulfamethoxazole (Bactrim, Septra), and levofloxacin (Levaquin). Patients may also be prescribed a urinary tract analgesic, such as phenazopyridine hydrochloride (Pyridium), which is rapidly excreted in the urine and has a topical analgesic effect that helps relieve pain, burning, urgency, and frequency. However, Pyridium gives the urine an orange to red color, which initially may be misinterpreted as hematuria. Patients diagnosed with UTIs are encouraged to force fluids to dilute the urine and flush the urinary tract. A follow-up urinalysis should be run to confirm the effectiveness of antibiotic therapy in curing the infection. UTIs tend to recur unless the cause of the infection is removed.

The medical assistant should instruct the patient to finish the entire antibiotic prescription as ordered, to maintain proper hygiene, to empty the bladder completely when the urge to void arises and, for female patients, to wipe the perineal area from front to back to discourage the spread of *E. coli* from the anal area toward the urethral region. Cranberry juice has been recommended for years to help prevent repeat UTIs. However, the American College of Obstetrics and Gynecology (ACOG) states that drinking cranberry juice can decrease the symptoms of UTIs, but there is insufficient evidence to recommend its use to prevent them.

CRITICAL THINKING APPLICATION   33-3

Tabitha Allison, a 22-year-old patient of Dr. Fineman, was diagnosed today with her third UTI in as many months. Patient education on prevention and treatment of UTIs is needed. What information should Sara go over with Ms. Allison?

Glomerulonephritis

Many conditions can cause glomerulonephritis, the inflammation of the glomerulus of the nephron units. Acute glomerulonephritis, or sudden inflammation of the glomeruli, usually develops in children and adolescents about 2 weeks after a streptococcal infection, such as strep throat or scarlet fever. In adults it may also be associated with infections, including hepatitis B and C, or other conditions, such as lupus. Symptoms include low-grade fever, anorexia, general malaise, and flank pain. Hypertension and edema may occur because of reduced renal function. Urinalysis shows hematuria and proteinuria. Diuretics, such as triamterene and hydrochlorothiazide (Dyazide) or furosemide (Lasix), may be given to control hypertension and reduce edema. The prognosis usually is good; most patients recover spontaneously, but in some patients, the condition progresses to a chronic state.

Chronic glomerulonephritis may also be called *nephritis* or *nephrotic syndrome*. It typically develops over many years and may be associated with chronic diseases that affect the blood vessels, such as systemic lupus erythematosus (SLE) and diabetes mellitus. Chronic glomerulonephritis causes progressive, irreversible nephron damage that frequently results in renal failure. At first the patient is asymptomatic, but as the disease progresses and more glomerular damage occurs, the patient develops anorexia, fatigue, hypertension, hematuria, proteinuria, oliguria (scanty urination), and edema. The cause of chronic glomerulonephritis is unknown, but it may be associated with an antigen-antibody reaction in the glomerular capsule that ultimately destroys the nephron unit. Treatment is supportive and involves an attempt to control symptoms by administering antihypertensives and diuretics, in addition to prescription of a diet low in protein with limited sodium and potassium to slow the progression of the disease. Glomerulonephritis is a leading cause of kidney failure; ultimately, many patients require kidney dialysis. The only cure for the disease is kidney transplantation.

Urinary Tract Disorders and Cancers
Renal Calculi

Renal calculi, or kidney stones, are created when crystals in the urine (e.g., calcium, oxalate, uric acid) collect in the kidney or when fluid intake is low, creating a highly concentrated filtrate. The tendency to develop kidney stones runs in families, and patients with a history of renal calculi are at increased risk for developing more stones in the future. Small stones usually do not cause any difficulty until they grow large enough to lodge in the ureters or renal pelvis. If a stone blocks the flow of urine, infection can develop from the resultant stasis. This blockage also can result in hydronephrosis, a backup of urine that causes dilation of the ureters and calyces and increases pressure on the nephron units. Other signs and symptoms include hematuria; cloudy, foul-smelling urine; nausea and vomiting; a persistent urge to urinate; and fever and chills if an infection is present.

If stones are located in the kidney or bladder, the patient often is asymptomatic, and frequent infections are the only presenting problem. If the calculi begin to move or are lodged in the ureters, the patient experiences renal colic, which is severe pain in the flank region that fluctuates in intensity over periods of 5 to 15 minutes. As the calculi progress down the ureter, the pain radiates to the lower abdomen, groin, and genital areas on the affected side. If the stone stops moving, the pain stops until it starts to move again. This pattern, referred to as *renal colic*, continues until the stone is passed or it is treated medically. The patient may be able to pass small stones by drinking large amounts of fluid (2 to 3 quarts of water a day). However, larger stones or calculi that cause bleeding, kidney damage, or persistent infection require medical intervention.

The provider may perform a cystoscopic examination to visualize the urethra and bladder and to remove any stones found (Figure 33-3). The most common procedure for treating calculi is extracorporeal shock wave lithotripsy (ESWL), in which vibrations of powerful sound waves are used to break the stones into fragmented pieces that can be passed through the renal system. Diagnostic studies are performed to identify the exact location of the calculi, and x-rays or ultrasound is used during the procedure to keep track of the calculi and to monitor treatment progress. The patient lies on a water-filled cushion as high-energy sound waves are passed through the body toward the exact location of the calculi (Figure 33-4). The procedure causes moderate pain, so the patient usually is presedated or given a light anesthetic. The patient wears earphones during the treatment because of the loud noise created each time a shock wave is generated. Side effects of the treatment include flank tenderness, hematoma formation across the treatment site, and hematuria. Measures for preventing recurrence include drinking 3 to 4 quarts of fluid a day, preferably water, and following a diet that is low in sodium and animal protein.

Hydronephrosis

Hydronephrosis, or swelling of the kidney caused by inability of urine to drain from the renal pelvis, usually results from blockage caused by renal calculi, but it may also be caused by an enlarged prostate or a tumor. Hydronephrosis can occur bilaterally or unilaterally. The condition frequently is asymptomatic, or patients may complain of mild flank pain as the renal capsule is distended. Urine testing detects hematuria, and, if infection develops from stagnant urine, pyuria. It is important to treat hydronephrosis aggressively because continued pressure from blocked urine flow can cause tissue necrosis and ultimately can lead to irreversible kidney damage. Removing the blockage corrects the condition (Figure 33-5).

Polycystic Kidneys

Polycystic kidney disease is an autosomal dominant genetic disorder, which means that one parent has the disease and each child has a 50% chance of inheriting it. No indications of the disease occur in

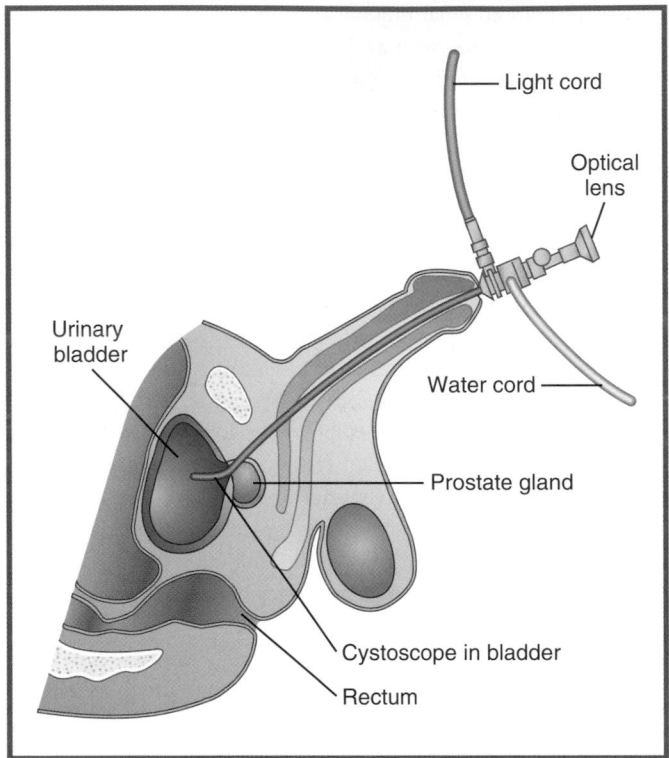

FIGURE 33-3 Cystoscopy.

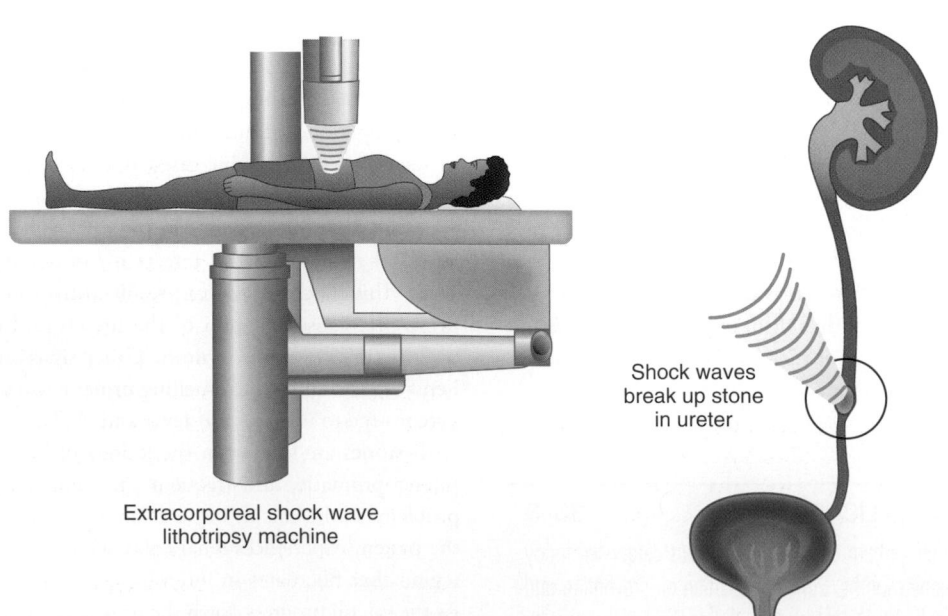

FIGURE 33-4 Extracorporeal shock wave lithotripsy. (From Linton AD: *Introduction to medical-surgical nursing*, ed 6, Philadelphia, 2016, Saunders.)

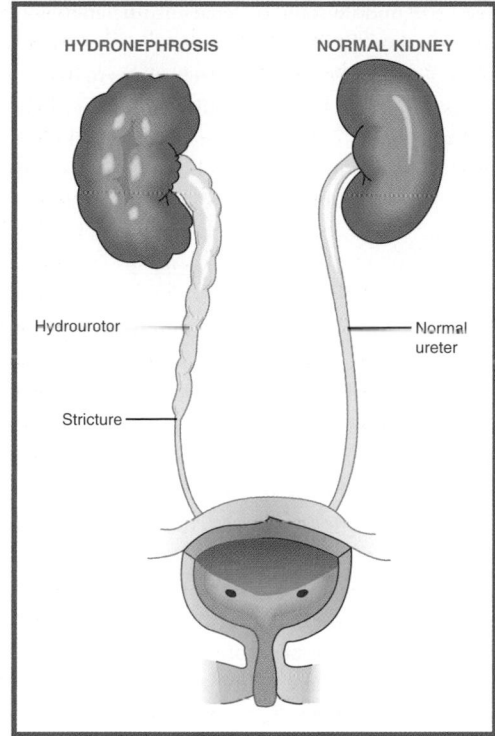

FIGURE 33-5 Hydronephrosis.

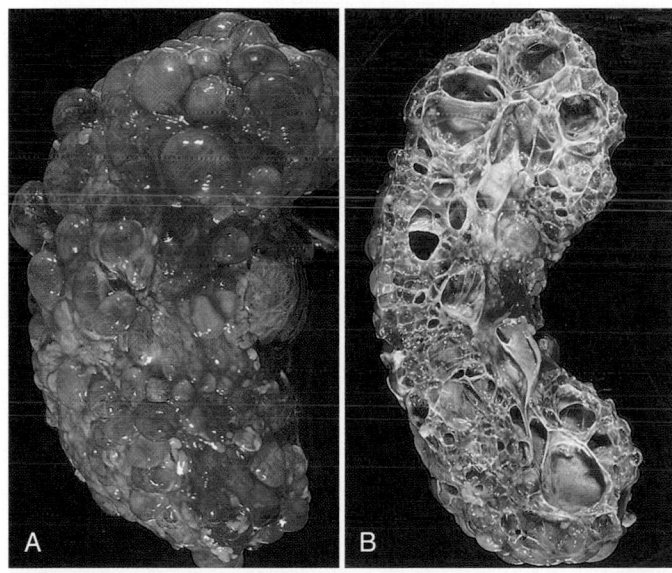

FIGURE 33-6 Polycystic kidney (adult autosomal dominant). **A,** Cysts on the external surface of the enlarged kidney. **B,** Bisected kidney showing large interior cysts. (From Cotran RS, Kumar V, Collins T: *Robbin's pathologic basis of disease,* ed 6, Philadelphia, 1999, Saunders.)

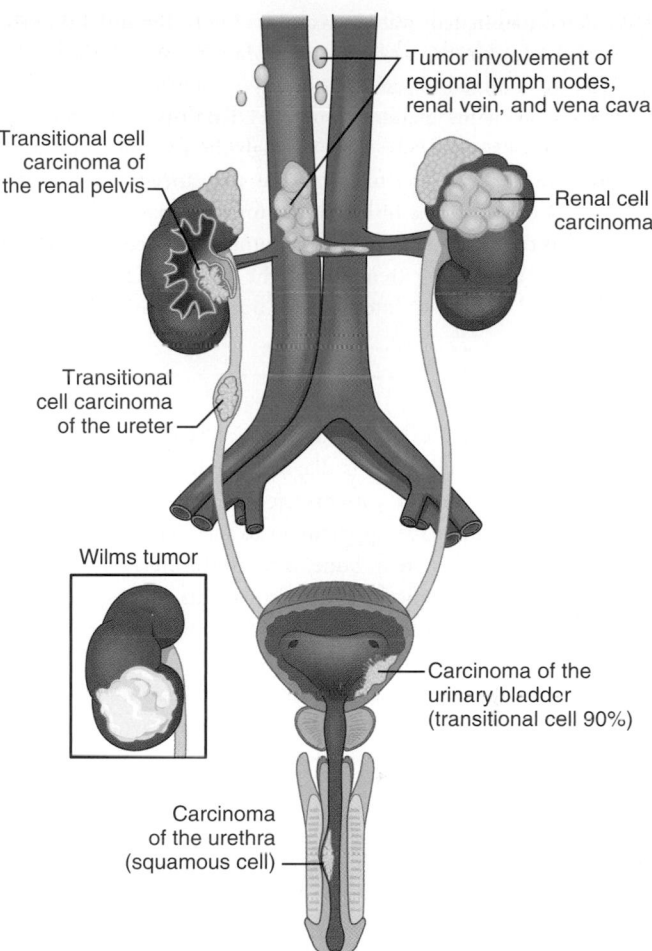

FIGURE 33-7 Neoplasms of the urinary tract.

children, but as time goes on, normal renal tissue in both kidneys is replaced by multiple, benign, fluid-filled cysts (Figure 33-6). The nephrons and collecting tubules become dilated, fused, and infected. As the cysts enlarge, they compress the surrounding tissue, causing necrosis, uremia, and renal failure. Symptoms do not usually become apparent until the individual reaches adolescence or adulthood. Patients with polycystic disease have a family history of kidney disease or renal failure, flank pain, hematuria, and hypertension. They also are more likely to develop UTIs and renal calculi. Because

cyst formation is progressive, most of these patients eventually require renal dialysis or kidney transplantation.

Bladder Cancer

The most common cancer of the urinary tract affects the bladder (Figure 33-7). It is two to three times more common in men than in women. Bladder cancer is characterized by one or more tumors that can metastasize through the blood or surrounding pelvic lymph nodes. Because 50% to 90% of patients experience a recurrence of bladder tumors, follow-up testing that can identify recurrence is extremely important. NMP22 is a urine test that screens for recurrence of the disease. It identifies a protein in bladder cells that are either precancerous or cancerous. Ninety percent of bladder cancers are attributed to these particular cells, which are called *transitional cells* because they are cubelike when the bladder is empty and flat when it is full. The test can be performed in the provider's office, and the results are available in 1 hour. If the NMP22 test result is positive, cystoscopy is performed to confirm the presence of abnormal cells.

Smoking is the greatest single risk factor for the development of bladder cancer. The carcinogens from tobacco become concentrated in the bladder and eventually cause cellular changes in the walls of the organ. Other risk factors include occupational exposure to chemical carcinogens (e.g., oil, rubber, dyes), drinking pesticide-contaminated water, treatment with certain anticancer drugs, and recurrent parasitic infections of the bladder. If the cancerous cells are confined to the inner lining of the bladder, a transurethral resection of the bladder tumor (TURBT) is performed. The provider passes a small wire loop through the urethra and uses an electrical current or a laser to burn away the cancer cells. The procedure may cause dysuria or hematuria for a few days. If the tumor has invaded the walls of the bladder, treatment may require a partial or complete cystectomy (removal of the bladder), chemotherapy, radiation, and the use of interferon to boost the patient's immune system.

Renal Carcinoma

Adenocarcinoma of the kidney, or renal cell cancer, is a primary tumor that can be cured if it is diagnosed and treated in the early stages. However, affected patients frequently are asymptomatic, which gives the tumor the opportunity to metastasize to the lungs, liver, male urogenital system, bone, or brain before it is diagnosed. Renal cell carcinoma typically occurs in patients over age 50 and is seen more often in men and in smokers. Signs and symptoms of the disease include flank pain, anorexia, anemia, hematuria, and an increased white blood cell count. Surgical nephrectomy is the treatment of choice. Although the prognosis for patients with the tumor has improved, the 5-year survival rate is still only approximately 40%.

Wilms Tumor

Wilms tumor, or nephroblastoma, is cancer of the kidney in children. Although the condition appears to be caused by a genetic defect, very few of the children diagnosed with Wilms tumor have a family history of the disease. It usually occurs unilaterally, is diagnosed most frequently at age 3, and rarely occurs after age 8. The tumor may be noticed by parents as a mass in the child's abdomen or by a provider during a routine physical examination. The preferred treatment is a partial or complete nephrectomy combined with chemotherapy. The survival rate for children diagnosed and treated for Wilms tumor is greater than 90%.

Renal Failure

Acute renal failure has a sudden, severe onset caused by exposure to toxic chemicals; circulatory collapse from serious burns or heart disease; acute bilateral kidney infection or inflammation; occlusion of the renal arteries; or complications from surgery. Blood tests show high BUN and creatinine levels, and the patient experiences acute onset of oliguria. The primary problem must be resolved as quickly as possible to prevent necrosis and permanent kidney failure.

Chronic renal failure is a slowly progressive process caused by gradual destruction of the kidneys' ability to filter waste materials. Diabetes mellitus is the leading cause of chronic renal failure in the United States, but it also may be caused by hypertension, glomerulonephritis, polycystic kidneys, long-term hydronephrosis resulting from urinary obstruction, lead poisoning, or renal artery stenosis. Symptoms of the condition may not be evident until as much as 75% of the kidney is no longer functioning.

Patients with chronic renal failure pass through several stages, starting with an early stage of decreased reserve in which no clinical signs are apparent but serum creatinine levels are consistently higher

than average. The middle stage of renal insufficiency is marked by hypertension, elevated BUN and creatinine levels, and a low urine specific gravity. End-stage renal failure (uremia) is marked by oliguria that progresses to anuria (no urine output), edema, hypertension, acidosis, and **azotemia**. The end result is that the kidneys can no longer remove waste products from the blood, and toxicity develops. To survive, the patient must be placed on dialysis or receive a kidney transplant.

Treatment

Dialysis, or cleansing of the blood, is used to treat acute renal failure until the problem is reversed or, for patients in end-stage renal disease, until they receive a transplant. The two forms of dialysis are hemodialysis and peritoneal dialysis. Hemodialysis is typically done in an outpatient clinic or dialysis center, but it can be done at home with the proper equipment and training. The process uses a machine known as an *artificial kidney,* or *dialyzer,* to filter waste products from the blood and return the cleansed blood to the body (Figure 33-8). A surgically placed cannula or shunt creates an internal fistula between an artery and a vein. During the procedure, approximately 1 cup of blood at a time passes from the shunt through a tube to the semipermeable membrane of the dialysis machine. The membrane filters the waste out of the blood, which then is returned to the patient's vein. Patients on hemodialysis require anticoagulant therapy to prevent clots from forming during the blood transfer process. Hemodialysis in a clinic setting usually is needed three times a week; the procedure takes approximately 3 to 4 hours each time.

Peritoneal dialysis uses the capillaries in the peritoneal cavity to filter the blood by infusing the patient's abdomen with a dialyzing fluid through a surgically implanted catheter. The dialysate solution contains a mixture of minerals and sugar dissolved in water that flows through the implanted catheter into the abdomen. The concentrated sugar draws wastes, chemicals, and extra water from the tiny blood vessels in the peritoneal membrane into the dialysis solution. After several hours, the used solution is drained from the abdomen through the tube, taking the waste material with it. Then the abdomen is refilled with fresh dialysis solution, and the cycle is repeated (Figure 33-9).

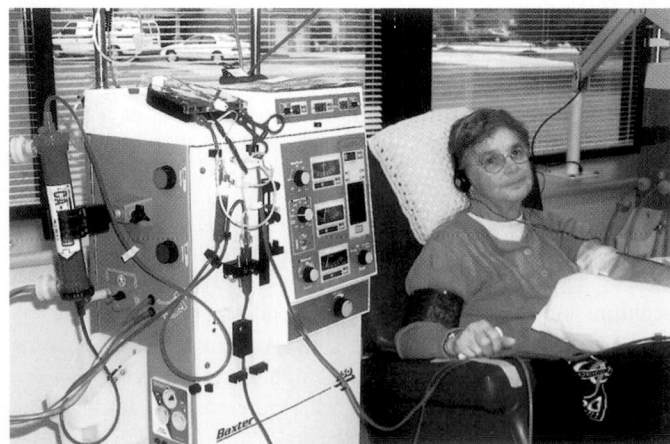

FIGURE 33-8 Hemodialysis. (From Ignatavicius D: *Medical-surgical nursing: patient-centered collaborative care,* ed 6, St Louis, Saunders.)

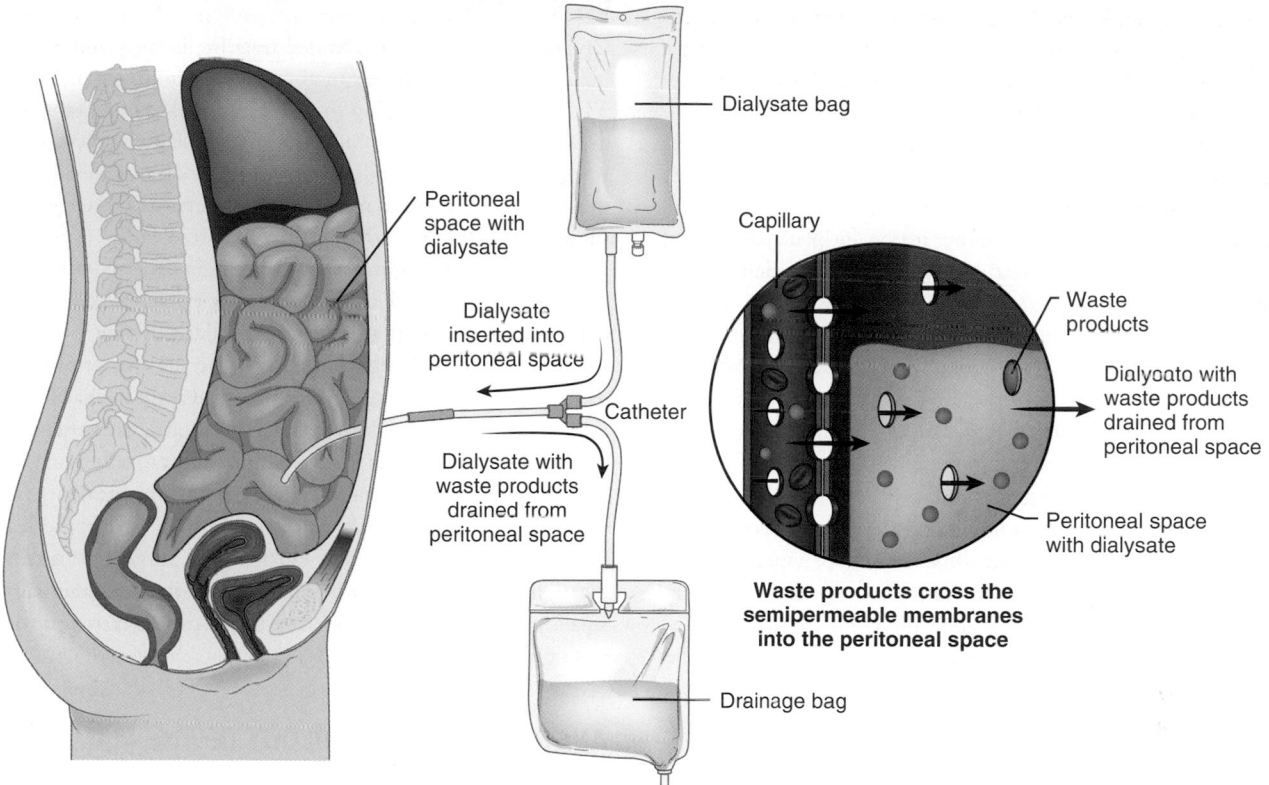

FIGURE 33-9 Peritoneal dialysis.

Peritoneal dialysis can be done at home in two different ways. With continuous ambulatory peritoneal dialysis (CAPD), the patient exchanges the dialysis solution in the abdomen four times a day, 7 days a week. Continuous cycling peritoneal dialysis (CCPD) uses a cycler machine at night to automatically infuse the dialysis solution into and out of the peritoneal cavity. This process takes 10 to 12 hours but can be done while the patient is sleeping.

Although successful kidney transplantation is curative for end-stage renal failure, finding the right donor can be a problem. Donors are matched by blood type, cell surface proteins, and antibodies. Siblings are the best donors, but other blood relatives may also match. If no blood relative donors are available, an adult donor who matches the patient's criteria is the next best fit.

CRITICAL THINKING APPLICATION   **33-4**

Aloysius Gonzales, a 59-year-old patient, is in chronic renal failure. His family is trying to decide whether their father should be brought to the dialysis clinic for hemodialysis, or whether they should try to keep him at home and assist with peritoneal dialysis. Sara will be explaining the mechanism of each procedure to the family. What should she include in her description?

PEDIATRIC UROLOGIC DISORDERS

Early detection and treatment of urologic disorders in children can drastically reduce permanent physical damage to the urinary system.

Nocturnal Enuresis

One of the most common reasons parents bring a child to a pediatric urologist is enuresis, or bed-wetting. Enuresis is the lack of voluntary control of urination at night or during the day by a child considered to be beyond the age when control should have been acquired (usually after age 6). This problem has a familial tendency and is more common in boys than in girls. The urologist first determines whether the problem is physical or psychological. With primary enuresis, bladder control was never established in the child. It may be caused by a physiologic problem with bladder control, such as an immature bladder with small capacity, a neurologic deficit, diabetes mellitus or insipidus, a UTI, or sleep apnea, or it may be a result of stressful events. Secondary enuresis, in which loss of bladder control occurs in a child who has been consistently dry for at least 6 months, can develop because of stressful events, UTIs, diabetes, or sexual abuse.

A physical and neurologic examination and urinalysis with a urine culture help determine whether any physical abnormality or disease process is causing the problem. If a psychological problem is suspected, help from a pediatric mental health professional may be needed. If no known causative factors are present, medications that relax the bladder muscles or that reduce urine production at night may be useful. Unfortunately, these may have side effects, so parents may refuse drug therapy. Parents should positively reinforce dryness and should not punish or embarrass the child. A moisture alarm can be used to help train the child to get up at night to go to the bathroom. This is a small, battery-operated device that connects to a moisture-sensitive pad placed in the pajamas or on the bed that beeps when the pad becomes wet. The goal is to wake the child just as he or she starts to urinate so that the child can stop urinating and get to a toilet. The success rate is high (80%), but the device must be used for at least 2 weeks before any change occurs and for up to 12 weeks to stop accidents.

Urinary Reflux Disorder

Urinary reflux disorder may be another reason for pediatric urology referrals. Reflux nephropathy occurs if the kidneys are damaged by a backward flow of urine. Each ureter has a one-way valve where it enters the bladder that is designed to prevent urine from flowing backward. Reflux may be caused by faulty formation of or damage to the valves, or it may be associated with cystitis, neurogenic bladder, or bladder overfilling because of an obstruction. It may be detected with ultrasonography, a computed tomography (CT) scan of the kidneys, or a voiding cystourethrogram (VCUG) (Figure 33-10). A VCUG is performed by placing a urinary catheter in the bladder and injecting a contrast medium that helps visualization of the bladder and the flow of urine. X-ray films are taken in several positions, the catheter is removed, and the child is asked to void. X-ray films are taken while the bladder empties to determine whether urinary reflux is present. Although a VCUG can be an uncomfortable procedure, the benefit of early detection and reduced damage to the kidneys makes the screening worthwhile. Untreated reflux nephropathy can lead to renal failure.

The treatment for urinary reflux usually is determined by grading its severity on a scale of 1 to 5, with 5 being the most severe. Prophylactic antibiotics may be given daily in low doses to prevent damaging kidney infections, which can cause low-grade reflux. However, with higher grade reflux that persists after 4 or 5 years of age, or for patients who have breakthrough infections despite the antibiotics, surgical repair of the valves of the ureters is necessary. Parents and providers also may opt for surgery because the procedure has a 95% success rate and poses little risk.

Cryptorchidism

Cryptorchidism, or undescended testicles, is fairly common in premature infants and occurs in about 4% of full-term infants (Figure 33-11). The testes develop in the abdominal cavity of the fetus and descend into the scrotum near the end of the pregnancy. If an infant is born with an undescended testicle, the testicle usually drops without treatment by 9 months of age. However, persistent cryptorchidism should be treated because infertility may result from exposure of the sperm to the slightly warmer temperature in the abdominal cavity. In addition, it increases the risk of testicular cancer in adolescence. The current recommendation is that surgical attachment of the testicle should be done by 1 year of age to reduce the chance of permanent testicular damage. Parents need to recognize that this child is considered at increased risk for testicular carcinoma even after treatment and should be taught testicular examination procedures.

The outpatient surgical procedure known as *orchiopexy* involves suturing the undescended testicle in the scrotum. If the testicle is impalpable (cannot be felt), laparoscopic surgery is necessary to locate it. The laparoscope is inserted into the abdomen through a small incision near the navel, and the testicle is moved into proper position or is removed.

ANATOMY AND PHYSIOLOGY OF THE MALE REPRODUCTIVE SYSTEM

The male reproductive system plays an important role in the continuation of the human species (Figure 33-12). Although not necessary for individual survival, the production, sustenance, and transport of male sex cells are vital to the creation of life.

The primary reproductive organs in the male are a pair of testes. The testis is an oval structure about 1⅗ to 2 inches (4 to 5 cm) long and 1 to 1⅕ inches (2.5 to 3 cm) in diameter. Each testis is surrounded by a white, fibrous capsule, and the two testes are contained together in the retractable, saclike scrotum. Lobules in the testes hold

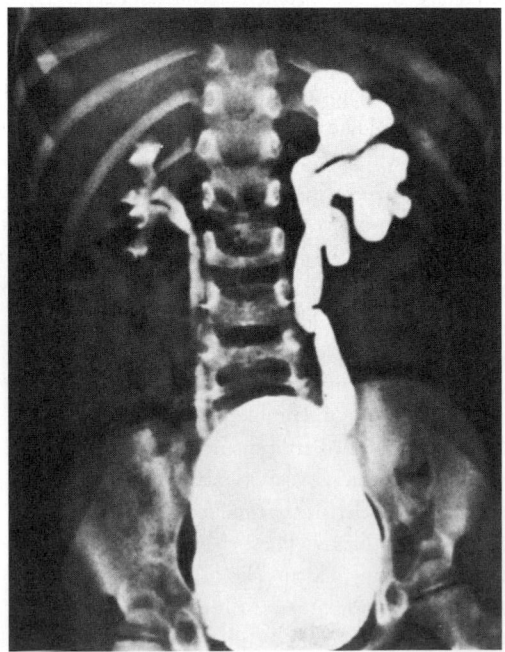

FIGURE 33-10 Voiding cystourethrogram. (From James AE Jr, Squire LF: *Nuclear radiology,* Philadelphia, 1973, Saunders.)

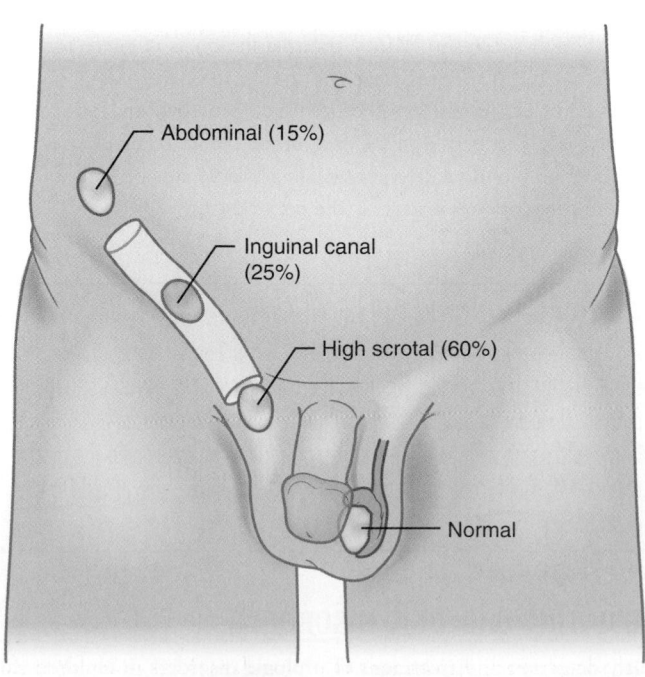

FIGURE 33-11 Cryptorchidism.

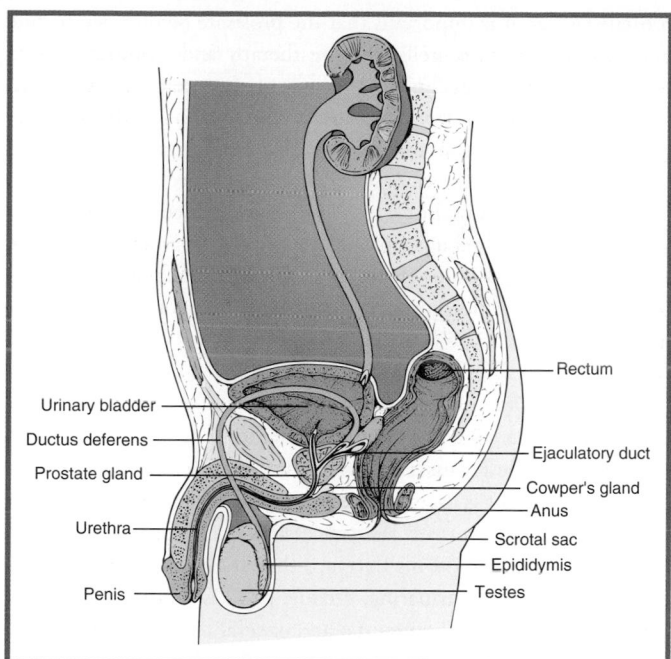

FIGURE 33-12 Male reproductive anatomy. (From Frazier MS, Drzymkowski JA: *Essentials of human diseases and conditions*, ed 5, St Louis, 2013, Saunders.)

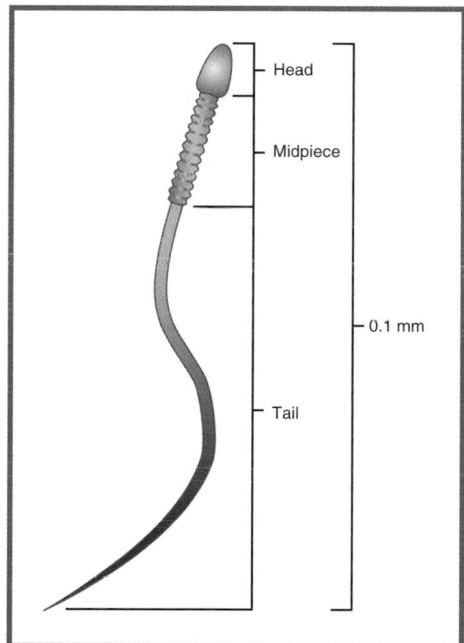

FIGURE 33-13 Sperm.

the seminiferous tubule, where spermatozoa, the male sex cells, are produced. These cells have 23 chromosomes, or half of the deoxyribonucleic acid (DNA) chain needed to form a complete cell. Sperm cells are tadpole-like structures less than 0.1 mm long that are carried to the epididymis for maturation (Figure 33-13).

The epididymis is a coiled tube almost 20 feet (6 m) long that rests on the top and lateral side of each testis. Peristaltic waves in the epididymis help the sperm move into the vas deferens, where the spermatozoa, which are now capable of movement, are stored until ejaculation. Each vas deferens is a muscular tunnel about 18 inches (45 cm) long that connects to the epididymis at the base of that

structure and passes along the side of the testes. The vas deferens becomes the spermatic cord that passes through the pelvic cavity and ends behind the urinary bladder. Uniting there with the seminal vesicle just outside the prostate gland, it passes through the prostate and into an ejaculatory duct that empties its contents into the urethra. The male urethra is an organ of two body systems: the urinary and reproductive systems.

The adult prostate gland is roughly 1⅗ inches (4 cm) wide and 1⅕ inches (3 cm) thick. It surrounds the urethra at the base of the bladder. The prostate gland is about the size of a pea at birth, but it grows rapidly at puberty to its full size (about the size of a walnut) by age 20. The central part of the gland may start to grow again after age 45. The primary function of the prostate gland is to secrete a thin fluid with an alkaline pH that neutralizes vaginal secretions to provide the optimum pH for fertilization. Secretions from the prostate gland, vas deferens, seminal vesicles, and bulbourethral glands combine with sperm cells to form semen. The volume of semen in one ejaculate ranges from 2 to 6 mL and averages roughly 100 million to 200 million sperm cells.

The Penis

The organ of male **copulation** is the penis. It is a cylindrical organ consisting of an elongated body with a slightly enlarged end, called the *glans penis*. Around the glans penis is a fold of skin that begins just behind the glans and extends forward to cover it like a sheath. This is called the *prepuce*, or foreskin, which sometimes is removed in a surgical procedure known as *circumcision*. The penis carries both urine and semen through the urethra and outside the body. When transmitting semen to the female tract, the penis must enlarge and stiffen for insertion. This occurs when three columns of erectile tissue in the penis become stimulated. The arteries in the penis dilate, and the veins compress; this compression reduces blood flow away from the penis, causing it to swell. Motor impulses are stimulated by swelling of the urethra as a result of semen collection, and contraction of the urethra causes ejaculation of the semen through the penis.

Hormone Production

Hormone production is also an important aspect of the male reproductive system. As a group, the male sex hormones are called *androgens*. Testosterone is the primary male hormone. During pubescence, when the male becomes reproductively functional, the anterior pituitary gland produces gonadotropic hormones that stimulate the testes to produce testosterone. Testosterone stimulates enlargement of the testes, growth of body hair, thickening of the skin and bones, increased muscle growth, and maturation of sperm cells.

DISORDERS OF THE MALE REPRODUCTIVE TRACT

Many diseases and disorders of the male reproductive tract are known. The most common of these involve enlargement or inflammation of certain organs and malignant tumors. The prostate is the most widely affected organ.

Diseases of the Prostate

Prostatitis

The cause of inflammation of the prostate is not always known, but it usually develops in the presence of infection. Bacterial causes may be *E. coli* or, in patients with gonorrhea, gonococci. Infection or inflammation of the prostate gland puts pressure on the urethra, causing dysuria, tenderness, and secretion of pus from the tip of the penis. The condition usually is treated with an antibiotic such as penicillin. Chronic prostatitis may develop as a result of repeated UTIs, urethral obstruction, or urinary retention.

Benign Prostatic Hyperplasia

As men age, the cells of the prostate gland that surround the urethra can start to reproduce more rapidly, causing the organ to enlarge (hyperplasia). This nonmalignant process, also known as *benign prostatic hyperplasia* (BPH), is seen in about half of men over age 50 and in more than 90% of men in their 70s and 80s. Enlargement of the prostate gland partly blocks the flow of urine, creating a medium for bacterial infection that can lead to cystitis. Signs and symptoms include urinary urgency and frequency; difficulty starting urination; hematuria; and repeated UTIs. The diagnosis is made from the patient's complaints and a digital rectal examination (DRE), during which the provider can palpate the enlarged gland (Figure 33-14).

Treatment includes the use of alpha-adrenergic blockers, such as doxazosin mesylate (Cardura), tamsulosin (Flomax), or alfuzosin (Uroxatral), which relax the smooth muscles of the bladder, making it easier to urinate. Finasteride (Proscar) or dutasteride (Avodart) may also be prescribed to reduce the size of the prostate, increasing urine flow and providing symptomatic relief. Nonsurgical therapies include laser treatment or placement of a prostatic stent to keep the urethra open. Because enlargement of the gland can be a sign of prostate cancer, it is important that the prostrate be biopsied to rule out possible cancerous cells. If drug therapy and alternative treatments are not successful in relieving the prostate enlargement, surgery is recommended. Transurethral resection of the prostate (TURP), the most common surgical treatment, involves threading a small instrument (a resectoscope) through the urethra to the prostate and scraping away the excess tissue. Laser procedures and microwave therapy can also be performed in the provider's office to remove or destroy obstructing prostate tissue. These outpatient procedures typically have less bleeding and a quicker recovery than TURP but may not be as effective over the long term.

Prostate Cancer

Cancer of the prostate is common in men over age 50 and ranks as the second highest cause of cancer deaths in men, behind lung cancer. The patient is asymptomatic in the early stages and may not become symptomatic until the cancer has spread outside the prostate gland. Once symptoms develop, they include urinary obstruction, with difficulty urinating, frequent UTIs, and nocturia (the need to void at night); hematuria; and generalized pain in the pelvic region. Prostate cancer spreads locally to the bladder, rectum, and lymph nodes of the pelvis, causing metastasis to the bones, lungs, and brain. The prognosis is poor unless the tumor is discovered in the early stages of development, when it is still confined to the prostate gland.

The first indication of a problem may come with a routine DRE, when the provider notices a firm or irregular area in the prostate.

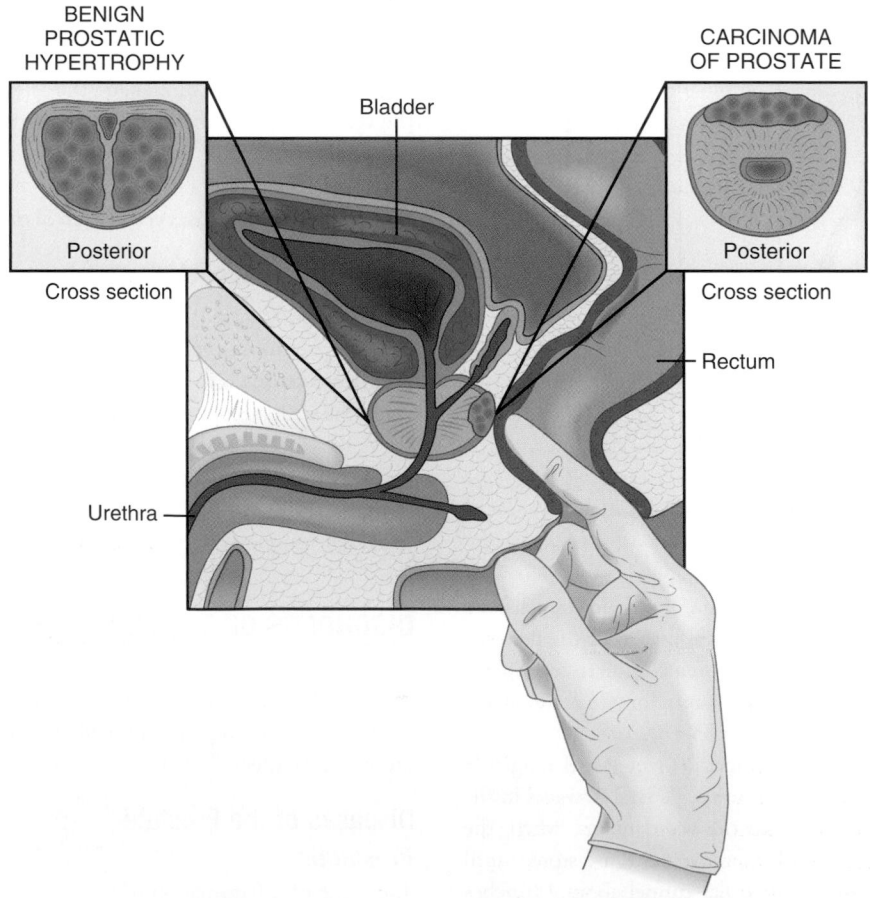

FIGURE 33-14 Digital rectal examination to diagnose benign prostatic hyperplasia and carcinoma of the prostate.

The primary screening tool for cancer of the prostate is the prostate-specific antigen (PSA) blood test. Blood levels of PSA, a protein produced by the prostate, are elevated with prostatitis, BPH, and cancer of the prostate. The higher the PSA level, the more likely it is that the patient has prostate cancer. However, because the PSA level can be elevated with other disorders, one abnormal screening value is not enough to diagnose cancer. The test should be repeated over time, and if levels continue to rise, further diagnostic studies should be done. If tests indicate cancer, the provider may order a transrectal ultrasound, which involves inserting a small transducer into the rectum to bounce sound waves off the prostate, creating a picture. The ultrasound pictures are used to help pinpoint areas of concern during a tissue biopsy. If the transrectal ultrasound does not indicate any suspicious areas, the provider takes multiple biopsies (usually eight) from different sections of the prostate gland. Tissue samples are sent to the pathologist for analysis and diagnosis.

A diagnosis of cancer of the prostate results in a complex decision about treatment because there is no way of knowing how dangerous the cancer is. Some types of prostate cancer grow slowly and never metastasize, whereas others are quite aggressive. The patient's decision to pursue treatment is complicated by the concern over possible side effects, including impotence and incontinence. Because of these difficult issues, the American Cancer Society (ACS) recommends that providers educate patients about prostate cancer screening so they can make informed decisions about testing. The ACS recommends that men with no symptoms of prostate cancer receive education and make informed decisions about screening starting at age 50. Because research indicates that the risks of screening outweigh the benefits in men without symptoms who are not expected to live longer than 10 years (because of age or poor health), these patients should not be offered prostate cancer screening. The ACS continues to recommend that men at high risk—African-American men and men who have a father, brother, or son who was diagnosed with prostate cancer before age 65—begin conversations with their providers earlier, at age 45. Men at higher risk—those with multiple family members affected by the disease before age 65—should start even earlier, at age 40.

The treatment for prostate cancer depends on its stage of spread. Radiation may be delivered directly to the cancer cells through external beam radiation therapy (EBRT), which uses high-powered x-rays to kill the cancer cells. An alternative procedure is implantation of radioactive seeds, a variant of radiation therapy. In this procedure, 40 to 100 rice-sized radioactive seeds are implanted directly into the prostate gland through a precisely placed hollow needle. The radiation is quite strong but has a very short range; this allows it to destroy the tumor but minimizes damage to surrounding tissue. Testosterone can stimulate growth of the tumor, so hormone therapy frequently is prescribed to block the action of testosterone or to stop its production.

Surgical treatment options include removal of the prostate gland by transurethral resection; orchiectomy, in which the testosterone-producing testicles are removed; and radical prostatectomy, in which the prostate and local lymph nodes are removed. These are debilitating surgical procedures that have serious side effects, including urinary incontinence and erectile dysfunction; therefore, they typically are used as a last measure. As with all cancers, chemotherapy may be prescribed for advanced cases or for recurrence.

Pathologic Conditions of the Genital Organs

Epididymitis

Epididymitis is an inflammation of the tubular epididymis. It most often is attributed to a UTI in men over age 40; in younger men, the most common cause is a sexually transmitted infection (STI). Patients experience severe low abdominal and testicular pain, in addition to swelling and tenderness of the scrotum. If abscesses form and produce scar tissue, sterility can occur. Antibiotics, including cefuroxime (Ceftin), ciprofloxacin (Cipro), doxycycline (Vibramycin), and azithromycin (Zithromax), are prescribed for treatment.

Balanitis

Inflammation of the glans penis and the mucous membrane beneath it is known as *balanitis*. It occurs most often in uncircumcised patients with narrow foreskins that do not retract easily and in men with diabetes. It has many causes, including an allergic reaction to certain chemicals (e.g., contraceptive foam), poor personal hygiene that results in a buildup of skin secretions (smegma) around the glans penis, and urinary tract and yeast infections. Treatment depends on the cause of the problem: antibiotics are used for infections, and cleansing is used for smegma buildup; avoiding chemicals that cause reactions can help prevent the problem.

Hydrocele

During the descent of the testes, a small canal develops for them to pass through. If the canal does not close after birth, fluid from the peritoneal cavity may pass through and collect in the scrotum. This is called a congenital *hydrocele*, which must be corrected surgically (Figure 33-15). Acquired hydroceles usually occur after middle age because of a scrotal injury or tumor and can form in men who sit for extended periods (e.g., aging men in long-term care facilities), causing painful scrotal swelling.

Testicular Cancer

Testicular carcinoma is the most common cancer in Caucasian men 15 to 33 years of age. The cause is unknown, but the primary

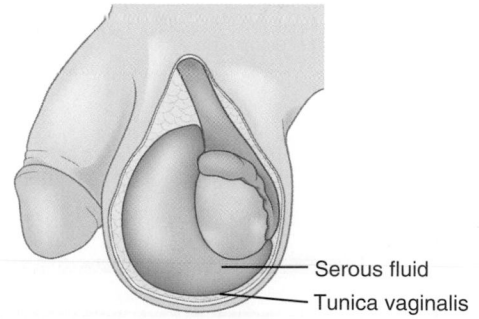

Serous fluid
Tunica vaginalis

FIGURE 33-15 Hydrocele.

predisposing factor is cryptorchidism. The patient complains of a mass in either testicle; a heavy sensation in the scrotum accompanied by a sudden collection of fluid; pain in a testicle or in the scrotum, abdomen, or groin; and unexplained fatigue. Testicular cancer can be treated successfully if diagnosed early; the survival rate for stage I testicular cancer is approximately 95%. Unfortunately, because young men may hesitate to go to the provider to report a mass in the testicle, the cancer may have reached an advanced stage before it is diagnosed. In advanced stages, treatment usually involves a combination of orchiectomy, radiation therapy, and chemotherapy.

The American Cancer Society recommends a testicular exam by a physician as part of a routine cancer-related checkup; however, routine self-exams have not been found to lower the risk of dying from this cancer. Nevertheless, the practitioner may still recommend routine self-screening, beginning in puberty or by age 15 (Procedure 33-1). The practitioner may provide pamphlets or a shower card showing the steps of testicular self-examination (Figure 33-16). The medical assistant can approach this teaching intervention in two ways. One way is to take the information to the patient and tell him to follow the pictures, and if he has any questions, he should call for clarification. Will he call? Would you? The second way is to go over the instructions with the patient. Demonstrate the procedure on a model, if one is available, or a male medical assistant could observe the patient doing the examination for the first time and provide feedback to answer any questions.

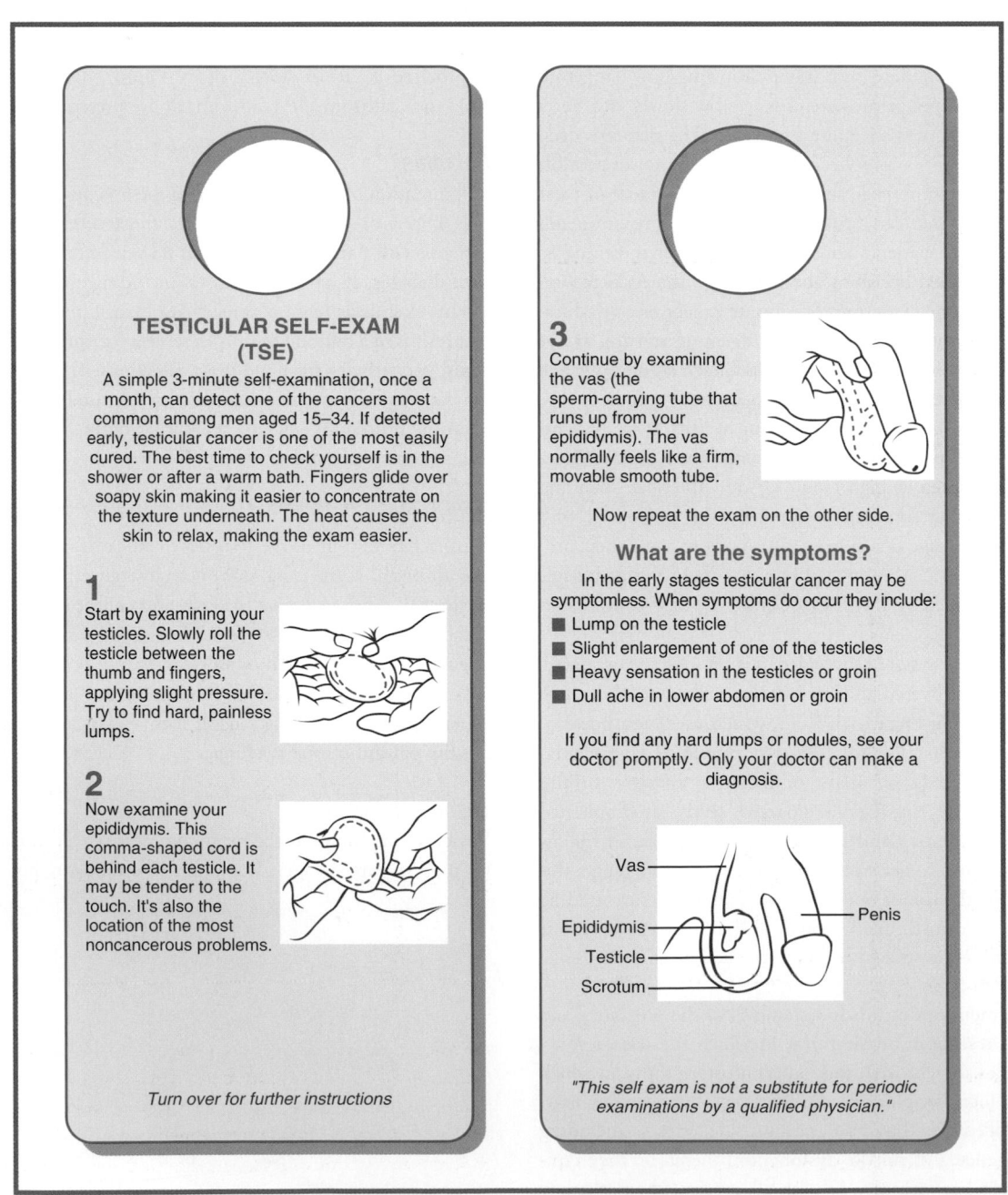

FIGURE 33-16 Testicular self-examination shower card.

PROCEDURE 33-1   Coach Patients in Health Maintenance: Teach Testicular Self-Examination

Goal: *To instruct the patient in the steps of testicular self-examination.*

EQUIPMENT and SUPPLIES

- Patient's health record
- Testicular self-examination pamphlet and shower card
- Demonstration model

PROCEDURAL STEPS

1. Sanitize your hands and collect the required supplies.
   PURPOSE: To ensure infection control.
2. Verify the patient's identity by name and date of birth and explain what you are going to do.
   PURPOSE: Understanding helps promote patient cooperation.
3. Begin by explaining to the patient that testicular cancer may cause no symptoms in the early stages, so it is important to examine the testes once a month for abnormal changes and early detection of the disease. This should begin at puberty, or approximately 15 years of age. It is best to do the examination in the shower or in a warm bath. The total examination takes about 3 minutes.
   PURPOSE: Heat causes the scrotal skin to relax, making the examination easier.
4. *Examination of the testis:* Using the demonstration model, start by holding the scrotum in the palms of the hands. Then feel one testicle. Apply a small amount of pressure. Slowly roll it between the thumb and fingers and feel for any hard, painless lumps (Figure 1).

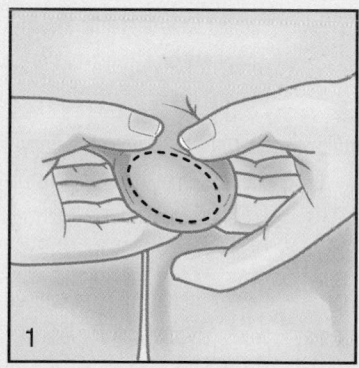

5. *Examination of the epididymis:* This comma-shaped cord is found on top of and behind the testis. Its job is to store and transport sperm. Tender when touched, it is the location of most noncancerous problems. Check for hard spots and lumps (Figure 2).

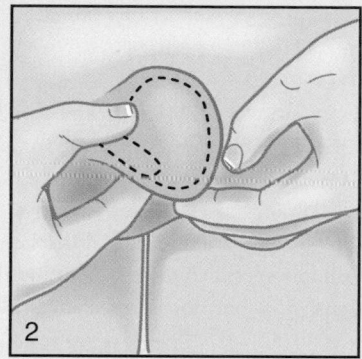

6. *Examination of the vas deferens:* Continue by examining the sperm-carrying tube that runs up the epididymis. Normally the vas feels like a firm, movable, smooth tube (Figure 3).

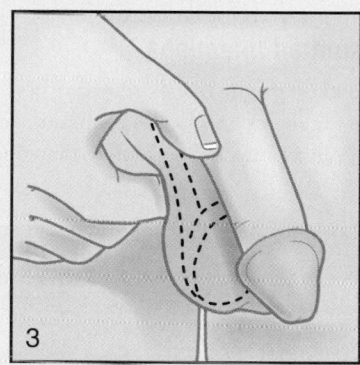

7. Now repeat the entire examination on the other testis.
8. After completing the examination on the model, ask the patient to do a return examination using the model. A male assistant can have the patient do a self-testicular examination.
9. Give the pamphlet to the patient, along with the shower card, with instructions to hang it in the shower as a monthly reminder and guide.
10. Document the instructional interaction in the patient's health record.
    PURPOSE: If it is not documented, it was not done.

8/19/20– 11:12 AM: Pt shown and successfully demonstrated testicular self-exam on model; no questions. Pt given pamphlet and shower card for home use. Dorothy Gaston, CMA (AAMA)

Erectile Dysfunction

The inability to achieve and maintain an erection sufficient for sexual intercourse is a condition known as erectile dysfunction (ED). It has many causes, both psychological and physiologic. Stress, anxiety, fear of unsatisfactory performance, and physical diseases that affect the vascular system, including arteriosclerosis, alcoholism, and diabetes mellitus, all can lead to ED. Changes in erectile function are normal as men age. Also, impotence is a side effect of certain medications, such as some hypertensive drugs. ED can be treated pharmaceutically with sildenafil (Viagra), tadalafil (Cialis), or vardenafil (Levitra). However, these medications are contraindicated in patients with a history of uncontrolled hypertension, myocardial infarction (heart attack), a cerebrovascular accident (stroke), or a life-threatening arrhythmia. In addition, they cannot be taken if the patient is prescribed nitrate drugs, such as nitroglycerin, because the combination of these medications can cause heart complications. If the patient is taking an alpha blocker (e.g., Flomax, Cardura) for treatment of an enlarged prostate, ED drugs must be used with caution because the combination of these medications can cause dangerous hypotension.

Infertility

Fertility peaks in men at age 25. Infertility can be caused by a problem in the man, a problem in the woman, or a combination of the two. About 10% to 20% of male infertility cases have no known cause. For the remaining cases, many causative factors may be involved. Cryptorchidism, stricture, and varicoceles (dilated spermatic cord veins); a low sperm count and poor motility; obstruction of the vas deferens; and hormonal imbalances all are factors in infertility.

Examination of semen specimens is helpful in making a diagnosis of infertility. These tests determine the presence of sperm, the number of sperm in an ejaculation, and the health and motility of the sperm. Ultrasonography also is helpful for detecting blockage of the vas deferens.

Sexually Transmitted Infections

Diseases of the male reproductive system can be acquired during sexual intercourse (Table 33-3). No one is immune to these diseases, and an individual can be infected with more than one at a time. No cure is available for viral STIs, such as human immunodeficiency virus (HIV) infection, herpes, and venereal warts. Bacterial infections are increasingly becoming resistant to antibiotic therapy. STIs frequently are asymptomatic in men, although they can cause serious health problems and are infectious regardless of whether symptoms are present.

Bacterial Sexually Transmitted Infections

STIs caused by bacterial infections include chlamydia, gonorrhea, and syphilis. Gonococci and chlamydiae tend to coexist, so a patient who has tested positive for one of the organisms typically is treated for both. Symptoms are similar to those for urethritis and epididymitis, such as painful and frequent urination, discharge from the penis, and lower abdominal pain. Chlamydia is resistant to penicillin; therefore, a regimen of antibiotics other than penicillin (e.g., Zithromax, doxycycline, erythromycin) is prescribed if the patient has both conditions. Sexual partners must also be treated, or the infection will continue to be transmitted back and forth.

A syphilitic lesion, called a *chancre,* develops on the male genitalia, usually the penis, a few days to a few weeks after exposure (Figure 33-17). Syphilis initially is diagnosed through the Venereal Disease Research Laboratory (VDRL) or the rapid plasma reagin (RPR) antibody blood test. If the results of these are positive, the diagnosis is confirmed with a fluorescent *Treponema* absorption (FTA) test, which is specific for antibodies to the *Treponema* microorganism.

TABLE 33-3   Sexually Transmitted Infections in Men

DISEASE	CAUSATIVE ORGANISM	SIGNS AND SYMPTOMS	TREATMENT
Chlamydia	*Chlamydia trachomatis* (bacterium)	May be asymptomatic; dysuria; itching and white discharge from penis; testicular pain.	Curable with antibiotic therapy: single dose of Zithromax or 1 week of doxycycline (Vibramycin).
Genital herpes simplex virus	Herpes simplex virus type 2 (HSV-2)	Painful genital vesicles and ulcers; erythema and pruritus; tingling or shooting pain 1-2 days before episodes. Viral shedding may occur during asymptomatic periods.	No cure, but antiviral therapy during episodes shortens duration of lesions: acyclovir (Zovirax), famciclovir (Famvir), or valacyclovir (Valtrex).
Genital warts	Human papillomavirus (HPV)	Most prevalent sexually transmitted disease; period of communicability is unknown; pinhead lesions may or may not be visible; warts tend to recur.	Goal of treatment is to remove symptomatic warts; cryotherapy for lesions; podofilox (Condylox) solution or imiquimod (Aldara) cream for lesions.
Gonorrhea	*Neisseria gonorrhoeae* (bacterium)	Dysuria and urinary frequency; thick, cloudy, or bloody discharge from penis.	Curable with antibiotic therapy: azithromycin, doxycycline.
Syphilis	*Treponema pallidum* (spirochete bacteria)	Six stages that can affect multiple body systems; 10- to 90-day incubation; initial sign is a painless lesion, or chancre, at the exposure site (penis); serous discharge from chancre; lymphadenopathy; if left untreated, advances to later stages.	Penicillin G (Wycillin); if patient is allergic to penicillin, doxycycline or tetracycline.
Trichomoniasis	*Trichomonas vaginalis* (protozoon)	Asymptomatic in most men; may feel itching or irritation inside penis, burning after urination or ejaculation, or some discharge from penis.	Single oral dose of metronidazole (Flagyl).

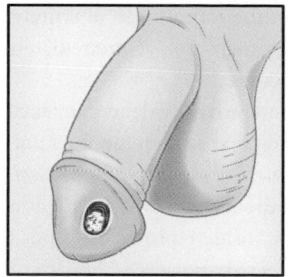

FIGURE 33-17 Syphilitic chancre.

Syphilis can be treated successfully with penicillin but may go unnoticed or unreported. Without treatment, it advances to a secondary phase, which is marked by low-grade fever, headache, and sore throat, in addition to a rash that does not itch but can affect any part of the body. In the secondary phase, the disease is highly contagious but still can be treated with penicillin. The more advanced stages of the disease can remain undetected or dormant for years. Symptoms that appear years after the primary infection show multisystem involvement, including neurologic and cardiovascular complications. Syphilis is not curable in advanced stages.

Viral Sexually Transmitted Infections

Viral STIs include hepatitis B, C, and D; genital herpes; genital warts (caused by the human papillomavirus [HPV]); and HIV infection. With genital herpes, the herpes simplex virus (HSV) enters the body through small breaks in the skin or mucous membranes. Most individuals with HSV infections are asymptomatic, or signs and symptoms are so mild that they go unnoticed. If symptoms are experienced, the first episode typically is the worst, with the formation of a blistered, inflamed, painful rash on the penis, scrotum, or urethra. After several days, the vesicles rupture, resulting in painful, ulcerated areas. The lesions heal in 3 to 4 weeks, but the herpes virus then migrates to a nerve dermatome. Many factors can reactivate the disease at any time (e.g., stress, upper respiratory infection), making the individual infectious again. However, HSV can be spread even when sores are not present.

Genital warts often are asymptomatic in men and require preliminary treatment with acetic acid to be seen. The incubation period for HPV infection may be as long as 6 months. In women, these infections greatly increase the risk of cervical cancer. The Centers for Disease Control and Prevention (CDC) recommends that routine HPV vaccination be initiated at age 11 or 12 years for both male and female children.

Human Immunodeficiency Virus

HIV infection is the most deadly STI. If not treated, HIV infection can develop into AIDS. The virus invades the CD4 T lymphocytes, destroying their ability to fight infection on the cellular level. Within 2 to 4 weeks after HIV infection, many individuals (but not all) experience flulike symptoms, including fever, arthralgia (joint pain), myalgia (muscle pain), lymphadenopathy (enlarged lymph nodes), rash, night sweats, and malaise. In 2013 a new blood test was approved that can detect the virus during this early stage of infection. However, with or without symptoms, an individual newly infected with HIV has a high risk of transmitting the disease to sexual or needle-sharing partners because viral levels are very high at this time.

The U.S. Food and Drug Administration (FDA) now recommends pre-exposure prophylaxis (PrEP) with Truvada for individuals who are HIV negative and in an ongoing sexual relationship with an HIV-positive partner. Truvada (emtricitabine and tenofovir) is a combination of two HIV medications that block important pathways the virus uses to start an infection. If taken as prescribed, the drug lowers the risk of contracting an HIV infection by up to 92%.

Postexposure prophylaxis (PEP) should start as soon as possible after occupational exposure to HIV (at least within 72 hours of exposure) and continue for 4 weeks. PEP medication regimens should include three (or more) antiretroviral drugs to reduce the chance of the person becoming HIV positive. Any healthcare worker who has an accidental exposure (e.g., a needlestick) from an individual who may be HIV positive should receive PEP.

HIV is transmitted when infected blood or blood products, semen, or vaginal secretions come in contact with the mucous membranes or the broken skin of an uninfected person. It also can be passed in utero from an infected mother to her fetus, during delivery, or by breast-feeding. Intravenous drug users who share needles and anyone who has unprotected sex of any kind are at increased risk for contracting HIV. Healthcare workers are also at risk for accidental exposure in the workplace and should consistently follow Standard Precautions to protect themselves and their patients from this deadly disease. HIV is a fragile virus; it cannot survive outside the body, and it is easily destroyed by chemical disinfectants, such as household bleach.

All HIV tests screen for antibodies to the virus. The most widely used screening test for HIV infection is the enzyme immunoassay (EIA; also called the *enzyme-linked immunosorbent assay* [ELISA]), which typically is performed on a venous blood sample. EIA also can be done on other body fluids, including oral fluid and urine, although urine screening is not as accurate or as sensitive to antibody levels. The provider may also order a viral load test, which reflects the amount of HIV in the blood. Generally, the higher the viral load, the more aggressive the HIV infection.

Newer developments in rapid HIV screening use either blood or oral fluid (not the same as saliva; the gums are swabbed) and can produce results within 20 to 60 minutes with accuracy rates similar to those of traditional EIA screening. The FDA has approved the OraQuick Advance HIV1/2 Antibody Test for use on both oral fluid and plasma specimens. For the oral test, a single gentle swab is taken around both the upper and lower outer gums. The swabbing device is inserted into a vial containing a developer solution, and the result is positive if two reddish purple lines appear in a small window after 20 minutes. This test is not designed for home screening because it is restricted to use by trained individuals, such as medical assistants. However, an FDA-approved home test, the Home Access HIV-1 Test System, is available at most drugstores or online. The kit provides the materials for collection of a specimen at home rather than in a healthcare facility. To perform the test, the individual pricks a finger, places a blood drop on a specially treated card, and then mails the card to a licensed laboratory for testing. The individual uses an identification number provided with the kit to call the laboratory for results. According to the CDC, it can take up to 6 months to develop antibodies to HIV, although most people (97%) develop detectable antibodies within the first 3 months after infection.

The goal of treatment of HIV infection is to reduce the amount of virus in the body with antiretroviral drugs, thereby slowing the destruction of the immune system and the onset of AIDS. Currently, 31 antiretroviral drugs (ARVs) have been approved by the FDA to treat HIV infection. These treatments do not cure HIV or AIDS, but they suppress the virus so that people infected with HIV can lead longer and healthier lives. It is important to note, though, that even when treated with ARVs, a person who is HIV positive remains infectious and can transmit the virus for the remainder of his or her life. To prevent the development of resistant HIV strains, a combination of antiretroviral drugs from at least two different classes are prescribed in an approach called *highly active antiretroviral therapy* (HAART). Recent research indicates that individuals who are HIV positive and taking antiretroviral medications are less contagious than those who are not being treated.

Once patients begin antiretroviral treatment, they should continue to take these drugs for the rest of their lives. The medications must be taken at the time and frequency prescribed to be effective in controlling the spread of the virus and to prevent drug-resistant strains from developing. Unfortunately, HIV medications can cause multiple side effects, including fever, nausea, fatigue, liver abnormalities, diabetes mellitus, hypercholesterolemia, decreased bone density, skin rash, pancreatitis, and neurologic disorders. Patients must be educated on the importance of strictly following their prescribed treatment regimen and of immediately reporting any side effects to the provider.

AIDS is diagnosed when evidence appears of a wide range of opportunistic infections that develop because of depressed T-cell counts. These include *Pneumocystis jiroveci* (PJP), candidiasis (yeast infection), **Kaposi's sarcoma**, dementia, and **wasting syndrome**. A patient is considered to be HIV positive when antibodies to the virus are detected; however, the diagnosis of AIDS is not made until the CD4 T-cell count drops below 200 mm^3 (the normal count is 500 to 1,000 mm^3) and/or opportunistic infections have been diagnosed. Current HIV management includes monitoring of CD4 T-cell counts at diagnosis and every 3 to 6 months thereafter.

The psychosocial needs of a patient diagnosed with HIV infection are far-reaching. Treatment is designed to control duplication of the virus in the body, but the patient will always be infectious. Transmission of the disease is prevented by sexual abstinence or consistent use of condoms and precautions with blood spills; these options must be discussed and consistently reinforced with the patient. Community organizations can serve as a source of counseling and support for patients who test HIV positive and for their families. As mandated by federal law, the medical assistant must remember that all information about a patient's HIV status must be kept in strict confidence, and no documentation in the health record can indicate the patient's HIV or AIDS status.

Trends in Reportable Sexually Transmitted Infections

- The Centers for Disease Control and Prevention (CDC) estimates that nearly 20 million new STIs occur every year, costing the healthcare system an estimated $16 billion annually.
- Many cases of chlamydia, gonorrhea, and syphilis are undiagnosed and unreported, and data on several STIs, including human papillomavirus, herpes simplex virus, and trichomoniasis, are not routinely reported.
  - An estimated 24,000 women become infertile each year because of undiagnosed STIs.
  - Chlamydia is the most frequently reported infectious disease in the United States, with more than 1.4 million cases reported in 2014; it is estimated that twice that number are infected but are not diagnosed or treated; improved testing and treatment among men could help reduce transmission to women. The infection can be diagnosed with a urine test, and complications among men are rare.
- Gonorrhea is the second most commonly reported infectious disease in the United States; more than 350,000 cases were reported in 2014. The CDC estimates that twice as many new infections occur each year. The number of reported cases is 19 times higher in African-Americans than in Caucasians. Antibiotic resistance (especially to such drugs as ciprofloxacin [Cipro] and Levaquin) is a serious concern; if the disease goes untreated, epididymitis and possibly infertility can result. Studies indicate that the presence of gonorrhea increases the likelihood of HIV transmission.
- Syphilis is highly infectious in the early stages but is easily curable; left untreated, it can lead to serious long-term complications, including nerve, cardiovascular, and organ damage and even death. Seventy-five percent of syphilis cases occur in men who have sex with men. Syphilis infection can also place a person at increased risk for acquiring or transmitting HIV infection.
- Males typically are asymptomatic or have minimal signs or symptoms of herpes infection. With symptoms, the initial outbreak consists of one or more blisters on or around the genitals that break, leaving tender ulcers that last 2 to 4 weeks. The outbreaks may lessen in severity over time. The virus is present in the body indefinitely, but the frequency of outbreaks declines over time. The virus can be transmitted by an infected partner who does not have a visible sore and who may not know that he or she is infected.
- Herpes simplex virus type 1 (HSV-1) can cause genital herpes, but it more commonly causes oral herpes or cold sores. HSV-1 infection of the genitals can be caused by oral-to-genital contact with a person who has an HSV-1 infection. Condoms do not completely prevent the transmission of genital herpes.
- Most human papillomavirus (HPV) infections are asymptomatic in males; the man may be unaware of the infection but can transmit it to a sex partner. Genital warts may disappear without treatment. Because no diagnostic test for HPV is available for men, the diagnosis is based on

Trends in Reportable Sexually Transmitted Infections—*continued*

evidence of wart development. Condoms do not completely prevent transmission of HPV. New research indicates that the rising rate of oral and throat cancers can be linked to the oral transmission of one of the cancer-causing types of HPV.

- HIV cannot reproduce outside a living host, and no record exists of infection from environmental contact. Also, no evidence indicates that the virus can be transmitted by insects. Latex or polyurethane condoms used consistently and correctly provide a highly effective mechanical barrier to

HIV. Although the number of new HIV infections per year, about 50,000 cases, has stabilized over recent years, the number of cases in men who have sex with men (MSM) continues to increase. The MSM population represents about 4% of the males in the United States, but this group accounts for 78% of new HIV infections and 63% of all HIV cases. The estimated number of new HIV infections is greatest among MSM in the youngest age group (13 to 24). The greatest number of new HIV infections is seen in young African-American MSM.

From STD Trends in the US. *www.cdc.gov.* Accessed February 9, 2016.

CRITICAL THINKING APPLICATION   33-6

The number of patients seen weekly in Dr. Fineman's practice who have STIs continues to rise. Sara is responsible for telephone screening and for clinical medical assisting practices. She is constantly being asked questions about the signs and symptoms of STIs and their treatment. What should Sara know about bacterial and viral STIs and their treatment?

THE MEDICAL ASSISTANT'S ROLE IN UROLOGIC AND MALE REPRODUCTIVE EXAMINATIONS

Much of the diagnosis of urinary dysfunction depends on the patient's history, which may include frequency or urgency of urination, dysuria, or incontinence. A major part of the urologic examination is urinalysis, and the medical assistant must be able to instruct the patient in how to obtain a clean-catch urine specimen. It is best to have the patient collect the specimen during an office visit so that it can be examined immediately. The urologist may need to examine a catheterized specimen, which is collected using sterile technique. This procedure requires advanced training.

Assisting with a Urologic Examination

No special instrument setup is required for a routine urologic examination unless a special procedure is ordered, such as obtaining a catheterized urine specimen or a specimen for culture. Most offices use prepackaged, disposable packs for catheterization and bladder irrigation.

Both male and female patients disrobe and are given a gown. A woman is placed in the dorsal recumbent position, and a man is seated on the examining table. The provider explains what is required to the patient. The primary responsibility during the examination process is to assist the provider with any supplies and equipment needed and to maintain proper draping of the patient.

Assisting with a Male Reproductive Examination

The medical assistant needs to understand the male reproductive system and to provide patient support throughout the examination. The patient should empty his bladder and disrobe before the provider begins the examination. A drape sheet is placed around the patient's waist, covering the lower extremities. A female medical assistant is present only if requested by the provider. The provider inspects the foreskin (if the patient has not been circumcised) and

the glans penis. The penis and scrotum are palpated for possible masses and tenderness. The patient also is examined for possible inguinal hernias. A DRE completes the physical assessment.

A male medical assistant may assist the provider with the examination and help with patient draping and positioning. The medical assistant should watch the patient for signs of discomfort or anxiety, answer the patient's questions, and reinforce the provider's orders as needed.

Vasectomy

A vasectomy is a surgical procedure for sterilizing a male patient (Figure 33-18). It is performed by surgically removing a section of each vas deferens to stop sperm from reaching the prostate and mixing with semen. Sexual function is not affected by the procedure.

The procedure can be performed in a provider's office using a local anesthetic agent, such as lidocaine (Xylocaine). In the standard procedure, which takes approximately 30 minutes, the provider makes a small incision on both sides of the scrotum with a scalpel, clips both vasa deferens, and closes the site by cauterization or with sutures.

The no-scalpel vasectomy is another technique that takes approximately 10 minutes. The provider palpates and clamps the vas deferens under the scrotal sac, makes a tiny puncture through the skin, pulls the vas deferens out and cuts it, replaces the tube, and seals the site. The procedure is repeated on the other side. Patients must be

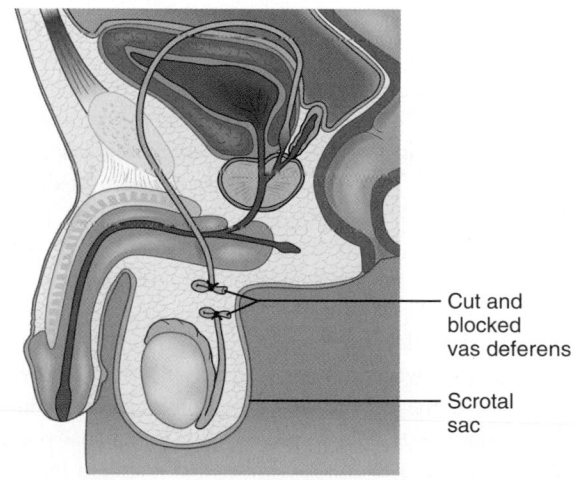

Cut and blocked vas deferens

Scrotal sac

FIGURE 33-18 Vasectomy.

informed that sterility is not achieved immediately because sperm may be present in the ducts; it may take as long as 1 month for the semen to be sperm free. Patients should use a backup method of birth control until two sperm counts 4 to 6 weeks apart show no evidence of sperm.

CRITICAL THINKING APPLICATION   **33-7**

Sara routinely assists Dr. Fineman with urologic and male reproductive examinations. She is also responsible for orienting new employees and helping them learn the procedures that typically are performed in the office. Summarize the role of a medical assistant in helping with these examinations.

CLOSING COMMENTS

Patient Education

Most men younger than 50 years of age have not seen a provider in years. Medical studies reveal that attitude, not biology, has a lot to do with the difference between men's and women's life spans. Men just do not go to the doctor as often as women and tend to ignore symptoms of disease. The solution to maintaining good health is preventive care, and the first step is establishing a good rapport with a provider of choice. As a general rule, a man in good health should have three checkups in his twenties, three to four checkups in his thirties, and a checkup every other year in his forties. After the age of 50, a yearly checkup is recommended. In addition to testing for conditions such as cancer, heart disease, and diabetes, patient education can help male patients make responsible healthcare decisions.

The urinary system is a very private, personal part of the patient's body. Patients often feel embarrassed to ask questions about how to obtain the requested urine or semen sample. The medical assistant can provide this information in a sincere, confidential manner to relieve the patient's anxiety and worry. Diagrams, models, and handouts help the patient understand disease processes and treatments and also encourage patient compliance.

Legal and Ethical Issues

When working in a urology office, the medical assistant must be very careful to ensure that patients have provided informed consent for ordered procedures. If the patient refuses a procedure, the assistant must have the patient sign the appropriate informed refusal forms, which are then included in the medical record. All patient education should be done after the provider has completed the explanation and has given the assistant instructions to do so. Never diagnose, prescribe, or offer comment about a patient's condition. Medical assistants who overstep their professional boundaries may place the provider and themselves in legal jeopardy. Remember that the patient who is legally informed and satisfied with the care received is less likely to take legal action.

Each state has developed special legal guidelines regarding patients diagnosed with HIV that must be strictly followed to prevent litigation. The medical assistant caring for patients with HIV naturally is concerned about possible exposure. Discuss your concerns with your employer and remember that Standard Precautions have been developed to prevent the accidental spread of communicable diseases. If you strictly follow the standards established by the CDC, you need not fear contamination.

Local, state, and national public health agencies require that certain diseases be reported when they are diagnosed by providers or laboratories. All states have a "reportable diseases" list. Many diseases on the lists must also be reported to the CDC, including chlamydia; gonorrhea; the hepatitides A, B and C; syphilis, and HIV/AIDS cases.

HIPAA Applications

Staying up-to-date on confidentiality restrictions covering a patient's HIV status is a major challenge. The Health Insurance Portability and Accountability Act (HIPAA) provides minimum requirements for protecting personal health information, but state laws can override HIPAA regulations if the state law is considered more stringent. In addition, individual healthcare institutions (hospitals, universities, providers' practices) may have their own policies and procedures for managing confidential information about HIV and AIDS. For example, if a provider believes that a person who tests positive for HIV will not disclose his or her HIV status to significant others, most states permit the provider to act. First, the provider must attempt to notify the patient that the information is going to be disclosed. Then the provider can inform the patient's spouse, sexual partner or partners, child, or needle-sharing partner or partners at risk of being infected with HIV about their risk of exposure. However, the state may limit this disclosure by not permitting the provider to identify the name of the individual who is HIV positive.

- Confidential HIV information includes any records that could reasonably identify the individual as a person who has had an HIV test, is HIV positive, has opportunistic diseases related to HIV, or has AIDS.
- The medical practice must report the names of persons who have a positive HIV test to public health authorities for infectious disease surveillance. Some states require that the names of HIV-positive sexual partners also be reported.
- The patient's medical information can be shared with the patient's other medical providers to coordinate care and to manage HIV/AIDS as a chronic condition.
- Depending on state law, written consent may not be needed to release HIV information if a court order for the information is issued or if the information will be provided to certain employees of correctional institutions or residential treatment facilities, funeral directors, or emergency personnel.

Professional Behaviors

A urology practice manages many sensitive patient issues that require strict adherence to confidentiality guidelines. This is especially true for a patient who has a functional disorder with the reproductive system or who has been diagnosed with an STI. HIPAA protects the patient's confidential information, not just the paper or electronic records of that information. This means that verbal disclosure of an individual's HIV and AIDS status is limited to only the personnel who have the right to that information according to individual state laws. For example, if you learn about your neighbor's HIV status at work and you go home and discuss it with your family, your employer is responsible for your disclosure of this information, and both you and your employer may be fined by the state or sued by the patient.

SUMMARY OF SCENARIO

Sara enjoys working with Dr. Fineman and the patients seen in his urology practice. She recognizes the need to stay current with information about disorders of the urologic system and their treatment. Sara continues to learn on the job and through workshops about the urinary system and current therapies. Her expertise is constantly growing, and she uses this knowledge to help with patient education, manage telephone screening, and assist Dr. Fineman with procedures in the office. She also is working on building a database with local resources, support groups, and Internet sites that could be helpful for patients confronted with urologic or male reproductive system problems.

SUMMARY OF LEARNING OBJECTIVES

1. **Define, spell, and pronounce the terms listed in the vocabulary.**
   Spelling and pronouncing medical terms correctly reinforce the medical assistant's credibility. Knowing the definitions of these terms promotes confidence in communication with patients and co-workers.

2. **Describe the anatomy and physiology of the urinary system.**
   The urinary system is made up of two kidneys, the ureters, the urinary bladder, and the urethra. The functions of the urinary system include removing waste products; regulating water, electrolyte, and acid-base levels; activating vitamin D; and secreting erythropoietin and renin. The three processes involved in urine formation are filtration, reabsorption, and excretion. The cortex contains the nephron unit, where urine is formed; the medulla is the collection site for urine.

3. **Do the following related to disorders of the urinary system:**
   - *Explain the susceptibility of the urinary system to diseases and disorders.*
     The urinary tract is made up of a continuous mucosal lining, which gives organisms that enter the urethra a direct pathway through the system.
   - *Identify the primary signs and symptoms of urinary problems.*
     The most common signs and symptoms of urinary problems include changes in the frequency of urination, dysuria, urgency, retention, and incontinence. Abnormal function of any part of the urinary tract can be determined with urinalysis, BUN levels, and creatinine clearance.
   - *Detail common diagnostic procedures of the urinary system.*
     Diagnostic procedures are summarized in Table 33-1.

4. **Discuss the causative factors of urinary incontinence, in addition to the various treatments and medications used to treat it.**
   Urinary incontinence is the temporary or chronic loss of urinary control, and the treatment depends on the causative factor. Options include behavioral techniques, pelvic muscle exercises, external catheters, and condom catheters. Table 33-2 lists various medications used to treat stress incontinence and urgency.

5. **Compare and contrast infections and inflammations of the urinary tract.**
   Most UTIs are ascending; they start with pathogens in the perineal area and infect the continuous mucosa, up through the urethra, bladder, and ureters to the kidneys. Infections and inflammations include urethritis, cystitis, pyelonephritis, and acute or chronic glomerulonephritis.

6. **Describe urinary tract disorders and cancers.**
   Renal calculi are created when salts in the urine collect in the kidney or when fluid intake is low. They can block the flow of urine, causing hydronephrosis. Polycystic kidney disease, a slowly progressive and irreversible genetic disorder, causes the formation of multiple, grapelike cysts in the kidney. Bladder cancer is invasive and can metastasize through the blood or surrounding pelvic lymph nodes. Adenocarcinoma of the kidney initially is asymptomatic and therefore frequently has metastasized before it is diagnosed. Wilms tumor is cancer of the kidney in children.

7. **Summarize the causes of renal failure and how it is treated.**
   Acute renal failure has a sudden, severe onset caused by exposure to toxic chemicals, severe or prolonged circulatory or cardiogenic shock, or acute bilateral kidney infection. Chronic renal failure is a slowly progressive process caused by gradual destruction of the kidneys' ability to filter waste materials. Dialysis is used to treat acute renal failure until the problem is reversed or, for patients in end-stage renal disease, until transplantation can be performed. The two forms of dialysis are hemodialysis and peritoneal dialysis.

8. **Summarize the typical pediatric urologic disorders.**
   Pediatric urologic disorders include enuresis, urine reflux disorder, and cryptorchidism.

9. **Describe the anatomy and physiology of the male reproductive system.**
   The male reproductive system is made up of a pair of testes that contain the seminiferous tubule, where spermatozoa are produced and carried to the epididymis for maturation and into the vas deferens for storage. The prostate gland secretes seminal fluid, which is ejaculated with sperm by the penis. Testosterone stimulates the development of secondary male characteristics and matures sperm.

10. **Determine the causes and effects of prostate disorders.**
    Inflammation of the prostate usually develops because of an infection, such as an STI. Common symptoms are dysuria, tenderness, and secretion of pus from the tip of the penis. Benign prostatic hyperplasia partially blocks the flow of urine and is diagnosed from patient complaints and with a DRE. Treatment includes the use of medication or surgery. Cancer of the prostate is common in men older than age 50 and is the second highest cause of male cancer deaths; complaints include urinary obstruction, UTIs, and nocturia. Prostate cancer is diagnosed by a DRE, elevated PSA level, and biopsy; treatment includes radioactive seed implantation, hormone therapy, or prostatectomy.

11. **Outline common types of genital pathologic conditions in men, and perform patient education for the testicular self-examination.**
    Male genital pathologic conditions include epididymitis, balanitis, prostatitis, and STIs. Testicular tumors usually occur in young men and

Continued

SUMMARY OF LEARNING OBJECTIVES—*continued*

generally are malignant. Erectile dysfunction (ED) typically is treated with medication. Male infertility may be caused by cryptorchidism, stricture, varicoceles, low sperm count and motility, and hormonal imbalances. Patient education for performing a testicular self-examination is summarized in Procedure 33-1.

12. **Analyze the effects of sexually transmitted infections in men, and summarize the characteristics of HIV infection, including diagnostic criteria and treatment protocols.**

Table 33-3 summarizes the signs, symptoms, and treatment of STIs in men. There is no cure for viral STIs, and bacterial causes of infection are becoming increasingly resistant to antibiotic therapy. STIs in male patients frequently are asymptomatic. Bacterial STIs include gonorrhea, chlamydia, and syphilis. Viral infections include genital herpes, genital warts, and HIV. Trichomoniasis is a protozoal infection that is asymptomatic.

HIV invades the CD4 T lymphocytes, destroying their ability to fight infection on the cellular level. Initial exposure may cause flulike symptoms, but after this it could be many years before clinical symptoms of AIDS occur. A patient is considered to be HIV positive when antibodies are detected, and to have full-blown AIDS when T-cell counts are below 200 mm^3 and/or opportunistic infections are diagnosed. HIV is transmitted when infected blood or blood products, semen, or vaginal secretions come in contact with the mucous membranes or broken skin of an uninfected person. It also is transmitted from an infected mother to her fetus in utero, during delivery, or by breast-feeding. Many methods of HIV testing are available. A combination of antiviral drugs is used to control the virus, but the disease has no cure.

13. **Describe the medical assistant's role in urologic and male reproductive examinations.**

In a urology practice, the medical assistant is responsible for taking a complete patient history that details urinary symptoms, providing patient instruction for diagnostic tests, assisting with a urologic or male reproductive examination, and answering patients' questions.

14. **Discuss patient education, legal and ethical issues, and HIPAA applications in the urology practice.**

Confidentiality restrictions that apply to a patient's HIV status vary from state to state. It is the medical assistant's responsibility to manage HIV/AIDS patient confidentiality according to the laws in the state of practice. State and national laws must be followed regarding reporting of certain diseases.

CONNECTIONS

Study Guide Connection: Go to the Chapter 33 Study Guide. Read and complete the activities.

evolve Evolve Connection: Go to the Chapter 33 link at *evolve.elsevier.com/kinn* to complete the Chapter Review Quiz. Check out the other resources listed for this chapter to make the most of what you have learned from Assisting in Urology and Male Reproduction.

SCENARIO

Betsy Davis, CMA (AAMA), recently was hired by the University Women's Hospital to work for Dr. Erin Bock, an obstetrician/gynecologist for a busy family-centered healthcare facility in her community. Betsy has worked for a family practice provider for 3 years, but this is her first position in a specialty practice. Betsy is excited about the opportunity to focus on women's health issues and is especially interested in helping in the obstetric area of the practice. Betsy's responsibilities will include understanding current methods of contracep-

tion and the patient education factors that are important for each. She also must develop expertise in gynecologic diseases and conditions, including diagnostic and treatment protocols for cancers of the female system. Medical assistants in the practice are expected to be able to teach breast self-examination and to answer the questions of pregnant patients concerning a healthy pregnancy, labor, and delivery.

While studying this chapter, think about the following questions:

- What is the basic anatomy and physiology of the female system?
- What does Betsy need to learn about contraceptives to be able to answer patients' questions?
- Betsy needs to become familiar with which gynecologic disorders?
- What are the primary malignancies of the female system?
- How should Betsy assist Dr. Beck with a Pap test?
- How can Betsy teach patients to perform breast self-examination?
- What are the stages of pregnancy and birth?
- How can Betsy help patients understand issues that can arise with menopause?
- What are the typical diagnostic procedures used in obstetrics and gynecology?

LEARNING OBJECTIVES

1. Define, spell, and pronounce the terms listed in the vocabulary.
2. Explain the anatomy and physiology of the female reproductive system.
3. Trace the ovum through the three phases of menstruation.
4. Compare and contrast current contraceptive methods.
5. Summarize menstrual disorders and conditions.
6. Distinguish among different types of gynecologic infections.
7. Do the following related to benign and malignant tumors of the female reproductive system:
   - Differentiate between benign and malignant neoplasms of the female reproductive system.
   - Prepare for and assist with the female examination, including obtaining a Papanicolaou (Pap) test.
   - Demonstrate patient preparation for a loop electrosurgical excision procedure (LEEP).
   - Teach the patient the technique for breast self-examination.
8. Compare the positional disorders of the pelvic region.
9. Summarize the process of pregnancy and parturition.
10. Describe the common complications of pregnancy.
11. Specify the signs, symptoms, and treatments of conditions related to menopause.
12. Outline the medical assistant's role in gynecologic and reproductive examinations and demonstrate how to assist with a prenatal examination.
13. Distinguish among diagnostic tests that may be done to evaluate the female reproductive system.
14. Summarize patient education guidelines for obstetric patients, in addition to legal and ethical implications in a gynecology practice.

VOCABULARY

adnexal (ad-neks-uhl) Pertaining to adjacent or accessory parts.

Bartholin's cyst A fluid-filled cyst in one of the vestibular glands located on either side of the vaginal orifice.

clitoris (klih'-tuh-ris) A small, elongated erectile body above the urinary meatus at the superior point of the labia minora.

coitus Sexual union between male and female; also called *intercourse*.

colostrum (koh-lahs'-trum) A thin, yellow, milky fluid secreted by the mammary glands a few days before and after delivery.

dilation The opening of the cervix through the process of labor, measured as 0 to 10 cm dilated.

dilation and curettage (D&C) The widening of the cervix and scraping of the endometrial wall of the uterus.

VOCABULARY—continued

dysplasia (diss-play-zha) An alteration in cell growth, causing differences in size, shape, and appearance.

effacement The thinning of the cervix during labor, measured in percentages from 0% to 100% effaced.

endocervical curettage The scraping of cells from the wall of the uterus.

fundus The curved, top portion of the uterus; the fundal height can be used as a measurement of fetal growth and estimated gestation.

human chorionic gonadotropin (HCG) A hormone, secreted by the placenta, found in the urine of pregnant females.

lymphedema (limf-uh-de′-muh) Swelling caused by the accumulation of lymph fluid in soft tissues.

mons pubis The fat pad that covers the symphysis pubis.

multiparous Pertaining to women who have had two or more pregnancies.

neural tube defects Congenital malformations of the skull and spinal column caused by failure of the neural tube to close during embryonic development; the neural tube is the origin of the brain, spinal cord, and other central nervous system tissue.

nonstress tests (NSTs) Fetal monitoring used in combination with maternal reports of fetal movement to evaluate the fetal heart rate response.

parturition (par-too-rih′-shun) The act or process of giving birth to a child.

stereotactic (stare--ee-oh-tak-tik) Pertaining to an x-ray procedure used to guide the insertion of a needle into a specific area of the breast.

teratogen Substance that causes the development of fetal abnormalities.

transvaginal ultrasound A procedure used to examine the vagina, uterus, fallopian tubes, and bladder. An ultrasound transducer (probe) is inserted into the vagina and used to bounce high-energy sound waves (ultrasound) off internal tissues or organs and make echoes that form a picture; the provider can identify tumors by looking at the sonogram.

vulva The external female genitalia, which begins at the mons pubis and terminates at the anus.

The branch of medicine that deals with pregnancy, labor, and the postnatal period is known as *obstetrics,* and the branch of medicine that deals with diseases of the genital tract in women is called *gynecology.* Frequently, a provider practices both specialties and is known as an *OB/GYN provider.* Assessment of the female reproductive system is an important part of healthcare. Patients often are hesitant and uncomfortable about talking about sexual matters, so they wait until symptoms are intolerable or disease is advanced before seeking medical care. In addition to the signs and symptoms of disease, the medical assistant must be aware of the patient's emotional state and must give support when needed.

ANATOMY AND PHYSIOLOGY

Female Reproductive System

The female reproductive system includes both internal and external organs. The internal organs are located in the pelvis and cannot be seen without special instruments, such as a vaginal speculum or a laparoscope. The external organs can be seen during the physical examination.

The primary parts of the female reproductive system are the **vulva**, vagina, uterus, fallopian tubes, and ovaries (Figure 34-1). The vulva includes the **clitoris**, the urethral meatus, and the vaginal orifice. These structures are covered by two sets of lips of tissue. The inner set, the *labia minora,* is a thin layer of skin that extends from the top of the clitoris to the base of the vaginal opening. The external set, the *labia majora,* and the **mons pubis** are covered with hair in the adult.

The vagina connects the internal and external organs. This tube-like structure is constructed to receive the penis during **coitus**. It is lubricated by a mucous membrane lining, and its walls are made up of overlapping tissue in the form of rugae; this allows the vagina to expand during the birth of an infant. At the distal end of the vagina is the cervix, often called the neck of the uterus, which is approximately 1 to 1½ inches long. The uterus is an upside-down, pear-shaped muscular organ, and its sole purpose is to house and nourish the fetus from implantation shortly after conception until **parturition**. The uterine walls have three layers. The inner layer, the endometrium, is rich in blood and changes in consistency during the menstrual cycle. The middle layer, the myometrium, is the powerful muscular layer that contracts to make the birth of a baby possible. The outer layer, the perimetrium, protects the structure and attaches to ligaments that support and hold the uterus in place (Figure 34-2).

On both sides of the **fundus** of the uterus are the fallopian tubes, also called the *oviducts.* These tubes extend from the uterus to the ovaries but do not attach to the ovaries. The distal end of the tube opens freely into the abdominopelvic cavity and acts as a passageway for the ovum to the uterus and for the sperm as they search for the ovum. At the distal end of the fallopian tubes are fingerlike projections, called *fimbriae,* which move in a wavelike pattern to draw the released ovum into the fallopian tube.

The ovaries are almond-shaped organs that produce and release the egg (ovum) and excrete the hormones necessary for the development of secondary sexual characteristics and the maintenance of a pregnancy. The ovaries secrete the hormones progesterone and estrogen, which regulate reproductive function. For pregnancy to occur, the vagina must receive the sperm from the male; the sperm move up through the opening in the cervix (the cervical os), through the uterus, and into the fallopian tubes. As many as 200 million to 600 million sperm can be deposited, and about 100,000

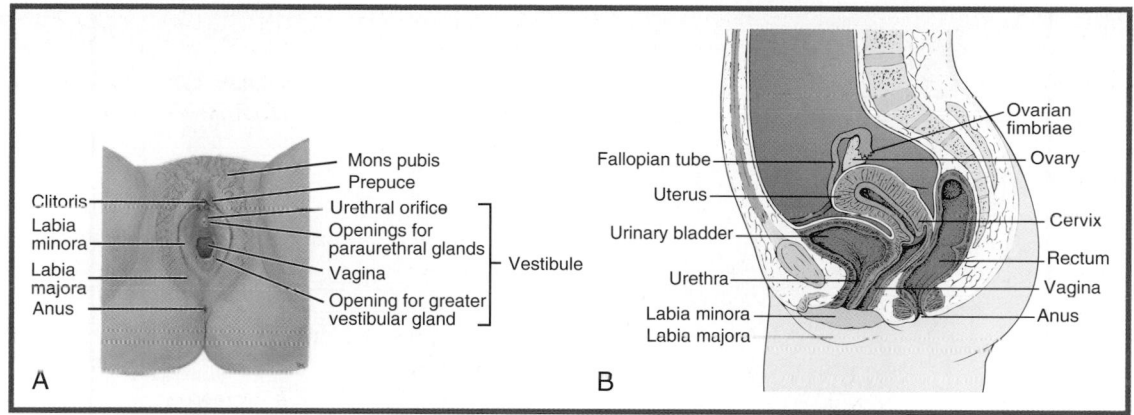

FIGURE 34-1 A, Female external genitalia. **B,** Normal female reproductive system. (**A** from Applegate EJ: *The anatomy and physiology learning system,* ed 4, Philadelphia, 2011, Saunders; **B** from Frazier MS, Drzymkowski JA: *Essentials of human diseases and conditions,* ed 5, St Louis, 2013, Saunders.)

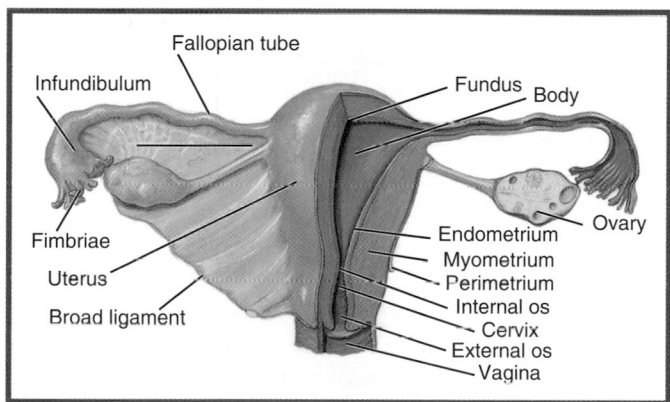

FIGURE 34-2 Uterus and fallopian tubes. (Modified from Applegate EJ: *The anatomy and physiology learning system,* ed 4, Philadelphia, 2011, Saunders.)

survive the acidic environment of the vagina to swim toward the egg.

Fertilization occurs when one sperm cell penetrates and fertilizes an egg. Fertilization usually takes place in the distal third of the fallopian tube. The tiny fertilized ovum, now called a *zygote,* moves by peristalsis and the massaging motion of the cilia that line the fallopian tube into the uterus and implants itself into the uterine wall. After implantation, the placenta forms; this structure supplies the new life with all the nourishment needed for development. Once pregnancy begins, the serum levels of **human chorionic gonadotropin (HCG)** rise, and the hormone spills into the woman's urine, where it can be detected with a pregnancy test.

Breast Tissue

Mammary tissue develops from the increased estrogen secretion that occurs during puberty. In the center of each breast is a nipple surrounded by a pigmented region called the *areola.* Inside the breast are 15 to 20 lobes and their subunits, the lobules of glandular tissue that are separated by connective support tissue and surrounded by adipose tissue. The amount and distribution of adipose tissue determine the size and shape of the breast (Figure 34-3). Breast tissue also contains mammary glands, modified sweat glands that become the

organs of milk production, and a system of ducts for delivery of milk to the nipple. Mammary ducts respond to elevated levels of estrogen and progesterone produced during the menstrual cycle by increasing in size, resulting in premenstrual fullness and tenderness of the breasts.

Four hormones control the mammary glands: *estrogen* is responsible for the increase in size; *progesterone* stimulates the development of the duct system; *prolactin* stimulates the production of milk; and *oxytocin* causes the ejection of milk from the glands.

Menstruation

When a girl enters puberty, one of the many changes that occur is *menarche,* or the beginning of the menstrual cycle. Menstruation is a normal body process that occurs in every female. It is the physiologic means by which the body rids itself of the thickened endometrial wall that develops during the average 28-day cycle. The menstrual cycle involves a series of events controlled by hormones from the pituitary gland and the ovaries. The cycle is divided into three phases: the follicular phase, the luteal phase, and the menstrual phase.

Follicular Phase (Proliferative Phase)

The hypothalamus begins the follicular phase by secreting gonadotropin-releasing hormone (GnRH), stimulating the anterior pituitary to release follicle-stimulating hormone (FSH) and luteinizing hormone (LH). These hormones mature a graafian follicle in an ovary that contains an ovum. The mature ovarian follicle secretes estrogen, which stimulates the growth of the endometrium. It takes approximately 9 days (to day 14 of the menstrual cycle) for the graafian follicle to ripen and bulge out from the ovarian wall. The ovarian wall becomes thinner as the follicle enlarges until it bursts, expelling the ovum into the abdominal cavity. Expulsion of the egg ends the follicular phase. The fallopian fimbriae begin their wavelike motion to fan the ovum into the fallopian tube. The rupture spot on the ovary, now called the *corpus luteum,* begins to secrete progesterone. Ovulation causes a rise in body temperature, and some women experience cramping and tenderness in the lower abdominal area at this time as a result of the rupture of the graafian follicle.

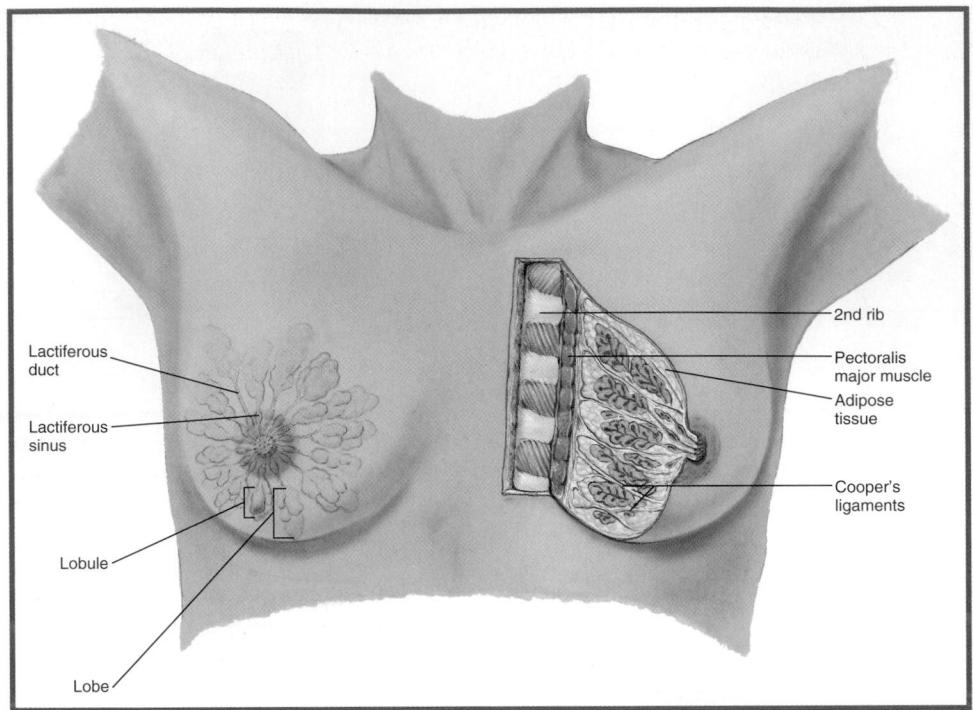

FIGURE 34-3 Normal female breast. (From Jarvis C: *Physical examination and health assessment,* ed 4, Philadelphia, 2004, Saunders.)

Luteal Phase (Secretory Phase)

Once ovulation is complete, the luteal phase begins (day 15). During this phase, progesterone secreted by the corpus luteum causes extensive growth of the endometrium as it prepares for a possible pregnancy. If conception occurs, the corpus luteum continues to secrete progesterone until the placenta is well established and can secrete progesterone and HCG to maintain the pregnancy. If conception does not occur, HCG is not secreted, and the corpus luteum atrophies. Without increased levels of progesterone and HCG, the endometrium breaks down, and menstruation begins.

Menstrual Phase

Menstrual discharge is made up of necrotic endometrial tissue, mucus, and the blood from endometrial engorgement. As the uterus contracts to shed the excess tissue, a woman may experience cramping pain and irritability. This phase usually lasts approximately 5 days, and then the follicular phase begins again.

CONTRACEPTION

A woman's choice of a contraceptive method is based on many factors. To make an informed choice, a patient should know the risks, benefits, side effects, costs, failure rates, and convenience of each available method. In addition, although condoms are only moderately successful at preventing pregnancy, they should be used consistently to prevent transmission of sexually transmitted infections (STIs). The medical assistant may help provide patient education on contraceptive methods. Table 34-1 summarizes the characteristics of various contraceptive methods.

Barrier Methods

Barrier methods of contraception either kill sperm through the use of a chemical spermicide or prevent them from entering the cervical os. These methods, which are relatively inexpensive, include the condom, diaphragm, and cervical cap or sponge. Each method must be used every time the person has intercourse, which means the patient must be motivated to follow through on using it. Patient education on the use of a diaphragm includes the following instructions:

- Examine the diaphragm before each use by holding it up to a bright light to check for holes or cracks.
- Place 1 to 2 tablespoons of spermicidal jelly or cream into the diaphragm dome before insertion.
- Leave the diaphragm in place for 6 hours after intercourse; do not douche until after you have removed it.
- Before repeated intercourse, add spermicide to the outside of the diaphragm with an applicator. Do not remove the diaphragm until 6 hours after the last intercourse.
- After removal, wash the diaphragm with soap and water, allow it to air dry, and inspect it for breaks or holes before storing.
- Have the diaphragm refitted if (1) you gain or lose more than 10 to 15 pounds; (2) you have a miscarriage, give birth, or undergo any type of pelvic surgery; or (3) you have difficulty voiding or moving your bowels with the diaphragm in place.

The cervical cap is a thimble-sized, domed barrier device that fits over the end of the cervix. It also is used with spermicidal jelly (Figure 34-4).

The cervical cap is 92% to 96% effective if used properly. An advantage of this barrier method is that the cap can be inserted up to 12 hours before intercourse and can stay in place up to 72 hours

TABLE 34-1 Commonly Used Contraceptive Methods

TYPE	FAILURE RATE	CHARACTERISTICS	CONTRAINDICATIONS	SIDE EFFECTS
Male or female condom (barrier method)	2%-10%	No prescription or examination needed; easily available; inexpensive	Latex allergy in either partner	Possible allergic response to latex or spermicide
Diaphragm, cervical cap, cervical sponge (barrier method)	2%-19%	Must be fitted by clinician; requires instruction on how to insert and remove; spermicide must be used each time; diaphragm and sponge must be left in place for 6 hours after intercourse	Latex, rubber, or spermicide allergy; uterine prolapse; severe cystocele or rectocele	Increased risk for UTI (diaphragm); increased risk of abnormal Pap test result (cap)
Intrauterine device (IUD)	2%-6%	ParaGard releases copper, which slows sperm in the cervix; Mirena and Skyla release progestin, which reduces sperm mobility and prevents thickening of the endometrial wall	Cervicitis, vaginitis, endometriosis, pelvic infection, history of STI or ectopic pregnancy	ParaGard may temporarily increase vaginal bleeding and menstrual pain; hormonal IUDs (Mirena and Skyla) decrease menstrual flow and cramping
Implanon or Nexplanon	1%	Flexible plastic implant inserted under skin of upper arm; releases progestin to prevent ovulation, thickens cervical secretions to block semen, thins endometrial wall; effective for up to 3 years	Certain antibiotics, HIV drugs, seizure medications may make it less effective; history of blood clots, liver disease, or breast cancer	Irregular bleeding in first 6-12 months; nausea, headache, sore breasts, scarring at implantation site
Depo-Provera (DMPA)	0.5%	Requires 150-mg IM injection every 3 months	Intention of becoming pregnant within 1 year; breast cancer; liver disease	Return of fertility may be delayed 10-18 months; should not be used more than 2 years in a row because it can cause a temporary loss of bone density; headache, weight gain, possibly depression
Oral contraceptives (OCPs) Hormonal patch Vaginal ring	1%	Suppress ovulation; atrophy of the endometrium	Thrombolytic, liver, or coronary artery disease; breast, liver, reproductive tract cancer; smoker over age 35; diabetes; sickle cell disease	Nausea, breakthrough bleeding, breast tenderness, fluid retention; hypertension, elevated lipid levels, blood clots, strokes

HIV, Human immunodeficiency virus; *IM,* intramuscular; *PID,* pelvic inflammatory disease; *STI,* sexually transmitted infection; *UTI,* urinary tract infection.

without decreasing effectiveness or safety. The cervical sponge contains spermicide and also can be inserted hours before intercourse and is effective for 24 hours. The sponge is 80% to 91% effective if always used as directed.

Hormonal Contraceptives

Hormonal contraceptives are a highly effective and reversible form of contraception. They work by inhibiting ovulation, changing the cervical mucosa, affecting sperm mobility, and preventing thickening of the endometrial wall. Hormonal contraceptives include the birth control pill or patch, the vaginal ring, Depo-Provera injections, and hormonal implants.

Besides being a highly effective method of birth control, oral contraceptives can be used to treat a wide range of gynecologic conditions, including menstrual irregularities, premenstrual syndrome (PMS) symptoms, and anovulation; they also can be used to prevent ovarian cysts and may be prescribed to increase bone density. However, to be effective, the pills must be taken daily. Failure rates are associated with noncompliance and can range from less than 1% in highly compliant women to greater than 15% in those who do not take the pills as prescribed. Oral contraceptive pills (OCPs) can have serious side effects, so patients should be informed of conditions that require immediate medical attention. These can be remembered with the mnemonic ACHES: *a*bdominal pain (new and severe), *c*hest pain (new and severe), *h*eadaches (new or more frequent), *e*ye problems (blurred vision or vision loss), and *s*evere leg pain. These symptoms may indicate the formation of a blood clot in the abdomen, chest, or leg, or they may be signs of a stroke;

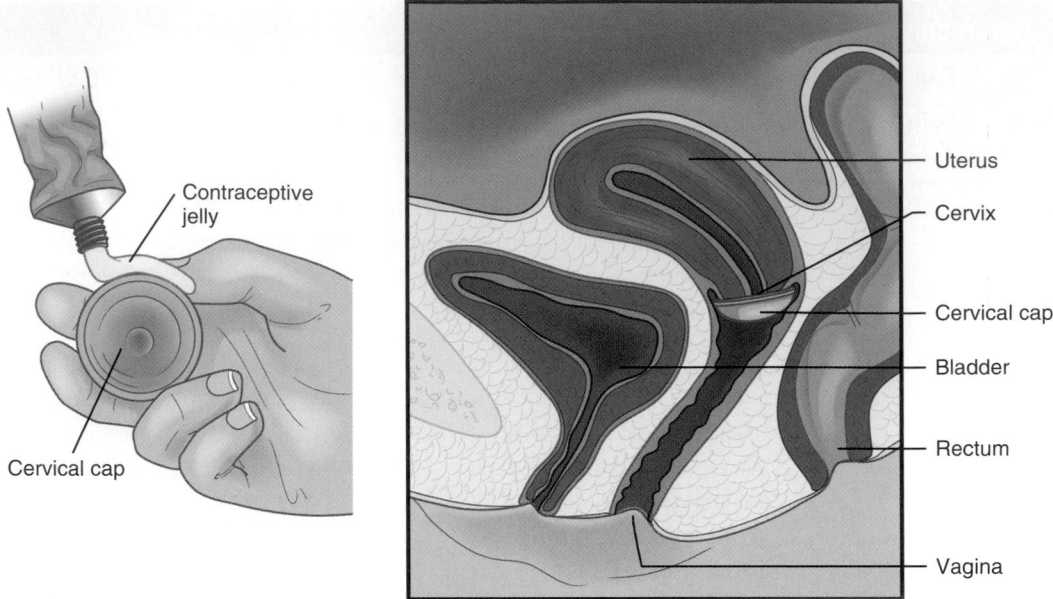

FIGURE 34-4 Cervical cap with spermicide.

blood clot formation and stroke are the most serious complications of OCPs.

A type of oral contraception, Seasonale, limits the number of menstrual periods to four a year, although patients are more likely to have spotting and breakthrough bleeding with this hormone therapy than with the traditional 28-day birth control pill. Seasonale is designed to be taken once a day for 84 days, and then an inactive dose is taken for a week, during which the woman would menstruate. Yaz or Beyaz may be prescribed for women suffering from a severe form of PMS called *premenstrual dysphoric disorder* (PMDD); it also is useful for treating acne in female patients at least 14 years of age who have started menstruating.

As mentioned, hormonal contraception also can be delivered via a transdermal patch, the Ortho Evra patch. The patch is a 1¾-inch square that slowly releases estrogen and progestin through the skin and into the bloodstream. It is considered as effective as oral contraceptives in women who weigh less than 198 pounds; however, the patch is still a very effective method for women who weigh more than this. Current research shows that the risk of blood clots with the contraceptive patch is similar to that observed with oral contraceptives. However, cigarette smoking increases the risk of serious cardiovascular side effects, especially if the patient is over age 35. Patients should be told not to apply any creams or oils at the application site, to change the patch weekly for 3 consecutive weeks, and to go patch free the fourth week, allowing menstruation to occur. The patch can be applied to the buttocks, lower abdomen, and upper body but not to the breasts. The woman can bathe, shower, and swim while wearing the patch, but if it comes off, it should be replaced immediately.

The vaginal ring (NuvaRing) contraceptive device is made of flexible plastic and is inserted into the vagina. The ring slowly releases estrogen and progestin to prevent pregnancy and provide effective contraceptive action for 1 month after insertion. The device is 2 inches in diameter and can be inserted anywhere in the vagina; however, the deeper it is placed, the less likely it is to be felt after insertion. Side effects of the NuvaRing are similar to those of other hormonal contraceptives, and it may increase the risk of heart attack, stroke, and blood clots. When the patient first starts using the ring, an additional method of birth control must be used for the first week. If the ring falls out, it should be rinsed with warm water and reinserted within 3 hours. If it is out for longer than 3 hours, contraception is not certain and the patient should use another birth control method for 1 week.

Depo-Provera is an injectable contraceptive that contains high doses of progestin. Each dose prevents pregnancy for up to 3 months, but women must be compliant in returning to the healthcare facility for follow-up and repeat doses every 9 to 13 weeks. The first injection should be administered within the first 5 days of the menstrual period for birth control coverage. This is a highly effective method of contraception and is ideal for women who either do not comply with a birth control regimen or do not want to take a pill every day. However, using Depo-Provera for 2 years or longer may increase the risk of bone loss and the eventual development of osteoporosis. Almost all patients using the injections experience some menstrual irregularities, but these usually subside after two doses. Women using this form of hormonal contraception are not at risk for the side effects of estrogen exposure, such as increased risk of blood clots and cardiovascular disease.

The Implanon and Nexplanon implants are a single, flexible rod, about the size of a match, that is inserted under the skin of the upper arm. The birth control implant releases a low, steady dose of progestin, which suppresses ovulation, thickens cervical mucus to block the passage of sperm, and thins the endometrial wall to prevent implantation. It prevents pregnancy for up to 3 years after insertion. Hormonal implants have similar risks and contraindications as other hormonal types of contraception.

Intrauterine Devices

The intrauterine device (IUD) (Figure 34-5) is a T-shaped plastic frame with threads attached that is inserted by the provider into the

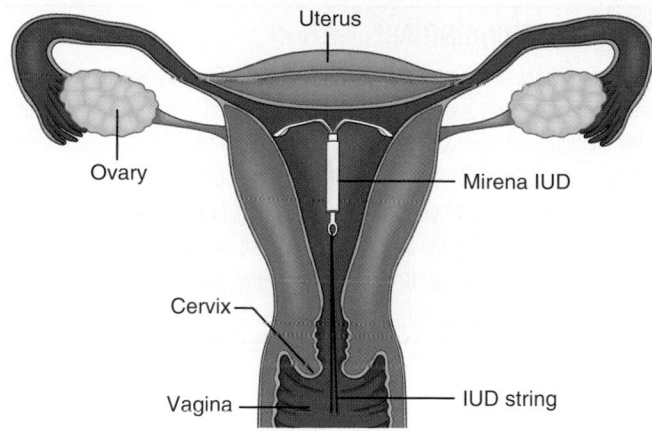

FIGURE 34-5 Mirena IUD.

uterus to prevent pregnancy. Two general types of IUDs are available: the copper type (ParaGard) and the hormonal type (Mirena or Skyla). Both products inhibit fertilization by blocking the sperm's journey to the fallopian tubes, and if fertilization does occur, they prevent the embryo from implanting in the uterine wall. In addition, ParaGard releases copper, which acts to slow sperm in the cervix, whereas Mirena and Skyla release progestin, which reduces sperm mobility and prevents thickening of the endometrial wall during the menstrual cycle. Both types of IUDs are extremely effective at preventing pregnancy (over 99%); the copper type can remain in place as long as 12 years, whereas Mirena IUDs must be replaced every 5 years and Skyla every 3 years. The copper IUD may temporarily increase vaginal bleeding and menstrual pain, but the hormonal IUD results in both decreased menstrual flow and cramping. To remove an IUD, the provider gently withdraws it by pulling on the IUD string. In rare instances, it must be removed surgically.

Permanent Methods

Both male and female patients can undergo surgical procedures that are considered permanent contraceptive methods. Vasectomies in the male were addressed in the urology chapter. For the female, a bilateral tubal ligation can be performed in which a portion of both fallopian tubes is excised or ligated. The cost and rate of complications are higher for tubal ligations than for vasectomies. In addition, tubal ligations must be done on an outpatient basis with general anesthesia, so the woman has that additional risk. Both procedures can be reversed, but not always successfully.

CRITICAL THINKING APPLICATION   **34-1**

Dr. Beck's patients often ask questions about birth control methods, including the pros and cons of each. Although Betsy's former employer also prescribed contraceptives, Betsy was not involved in patient education. Dr. Beck expects Betsy to be aware of all birth control options, their characteristics and side effects, and any patient education details that might be requested or appropriate. Betsy has decided to create a reference sheet for herself that includes all these details. What should she include?

GYNECOLOGIC DISEASES AND DISORDERS

Menstrual Disorders and Conditions

Amenorrhea is the absence of menstruation for a minimum of 6 months; in *oligomenorrhea*, the woman has not experienced a period for 35 days to 6 months. The absence of menstruation outside pregnancy could be the result of a number of factors, including hormonal imbalance, thyroid disease, ovarian failure, or structural defects in the female sex organs. If a patient has established menstruation that stops, this usually is the result of a problem with the hypothalamus or the pituitary. Suppression of the hypothalamus can occur as the result of an eating disorder, stress, or extreme exercise that results in low body fat content.

Women who do not ovulate and therefore do not go through a monthly shedding of the endometrial wall of the uterus are at greater risk for cancer of the endometrium and the breast. Patients usually are started on oral contraceptives that artificially provide the hormones needed to create a monthly menstrual cycle. These women may experience fertility problems and require further testing and medical intervention to become pregnant.

Abnormal menstrual bleeding is a common cause of OB/GYN visits. *Menorrhagia* is excessive menstrual blood loss, such as a menses lasting longer than 7 days. The provider may ask the patient to count the number of tampons or pads used for several cycles to establish a method of determining an estimate of blood loss. Iron-deficiency anemia is a sign that a woman is losing excessive amounts of blood. *Metrorrhagia* is spotting or bleeding between menstrual cycles. The practitioner may prescribe oral contraceptives to atrophy the endometrium and lessen the bleeding. Surgical options for excessive menstrual flow include **dilation and curettage (D&C)** or, in extreme cases, hysterectomy.

Endometriosis

Endometriosis is characterized by the presence of functional endometrial tissue outside the uterus. It commonly is found attached to the ovaries, urinary bladder, fallopian tubes, uterosacral ligaments, intestines, and peritoneum. Many hypotheses have been offered to explain this migration of endometrial tissue, but the most widely accepted is a retrograde flow during menstruation that causes menstrual fluid and stray endometrial cells to migrate out of the fallopian tubes and implant in the pelvic region. The use of tampons has been suggested as a possible cause. A familial tendency also has been noted; a woman with a first-degree relative (a mother or sister) who has the condition has a 10 times greater risk of developing the disorder.

The ectopic endometrial tissue responds to routine hormonal changes; it proliferates, degenerates, and bleeds just as does the endometrium of the uterus throughout the menstrual cycle. This causes inflammation at the site of the implantation that recurs with each cycle, ultimately leading to adhesions and obstruction of the affected tissue. Pain from endometriosis can be severe, interfering with day-to-day activities. The primary symptom of endometriosis is *dysmenorrhea* (painful menstruation). More than one-third of affected patients also report *dyspareunia* (painful intercourse), and others complain of contact pain in the lower abdomen, pelvis, and back beginning 7 days before menses and lasting 3 days after onset. Other symptoms can include profuse menses, hematuria, rectal bleeding, nausea, vomiting, and abdominal cramps. Infertility is a serious problem for approximately 70% of women afflicted with endometriosis because of the buildup of scar tissue and adhesions in and around the fallopian tubes.

Conservative treatment through the use of hormones is recommended when the woman wants to have children. Treatment may consist of a laparoscopy to remove the ectopic endometrial tissue. Pharmaceutical treatment includes continuous use of oral contraceptives to prevent menstruation or Depo-Provera injections. Leuprolide acetate (Lupron) injections may be prescribed intramuscularly every month for 6 months; however, Lupron puts the patient into a state of artificial menopause and can cause menopausal symptoms, including hot flashes, vaginal dryness, and bone density loss. Another medication that causes induced menopause is oral danazol. Danazol lowers estrogen levels and increases androgen levels, which stops ovulation and shrinks endometrial growths; however, it can cause the development of male physical traits, an elevated cholesterol level, and liver disease. In severe cases, a total hysterectomy may be indicated. No cure for endometriosis is known, but pregnancy, breast-feeding, or natural menopause frequently causes remission (Figure 34-6).

CRITICAL THINKING APPLICATION   **34-2**

Melissa Steiner, a 19-year-old patient of Dr. Beck, was diagnosed with endometriosis when she was 17. She has had two laparotomy procedures and continues to complain of moderate to severe pain before and during menstruation. What can Betsy tell her about the disease to help her understand why she has the pain? Melissa also wants to know about long-term complications, including the impact of the disease on fertility. She asks Betsy to help her understand Dr. Beck's explanation of the disease. How should Betsy handle her request?

Infections

Candidiasis

Candida albicans is the yeastlike fungus responsible for candidiasis. *Candida* organisms are commonly part of the normal flora of the mouth, skin, intestinal tract, and vagina. Overgrowth of the organism can be caused by antibiotic use, high estrogen levels, oral contraceptive use, diabetes mellitus, and immunosuppressive disorders, including acquired immunodeficiency syndrome (AIDS).

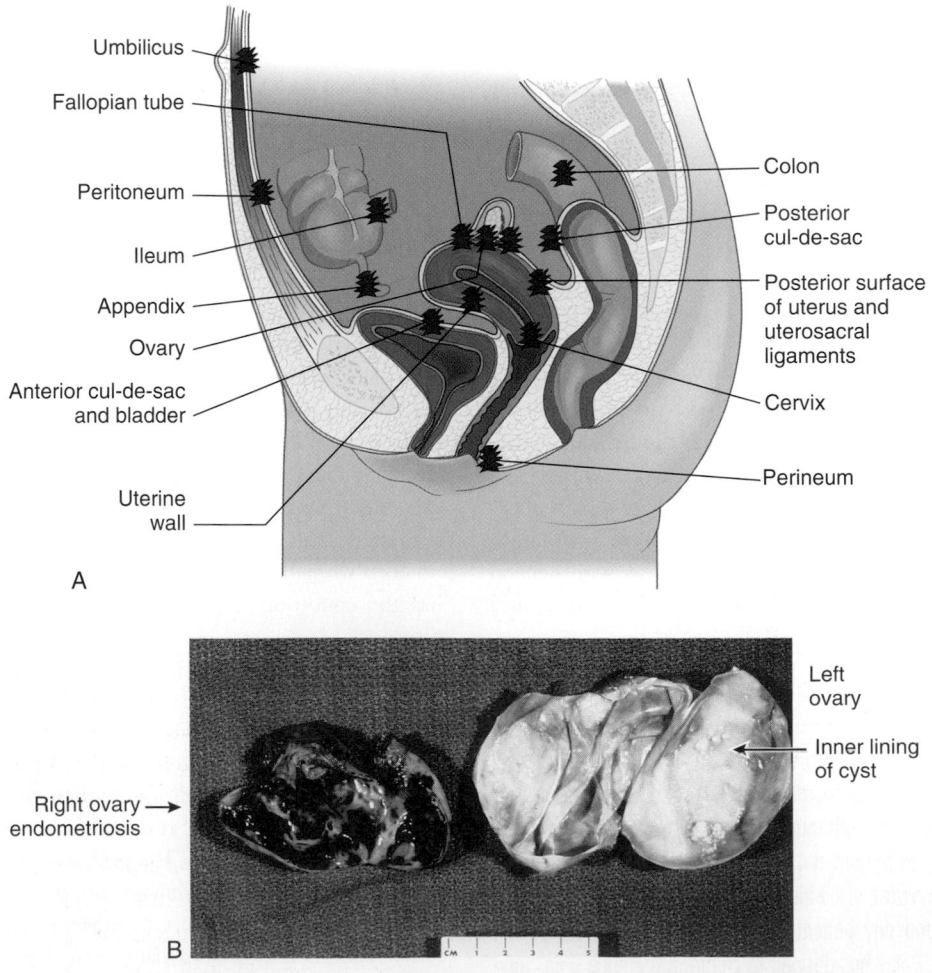

FIGURE 34-6 Endometriosis. **A,** Possible ectopic sites. **B,** Endometriosis involving the right ovary (chocolate cyst) and the left ovary, showing the inner lining of a large cyst with excrescences. (**B** courtesy RW Shaw, MD, North York General Hospital, Toronto, Ontario, Canada.)

Candidiasis also can be spread through sexual contact. Symptoms include vulvovaginal itching; dry, bright red vaginal tissue; and an odorless, white, "cottage cheese" vaginal discharge. This infection can be treated with prescription antifungal medications, such as a single dose of oral fluconazole (Diflucan) or terconazole vaginal suppositories. It also can be treated with over-the-counter (OTC) creams or suppositories, such as Gyne-Lotrimin or Monistat. Women prescribed an antibiotic for an infection may develop vaginal candidiasis as a side effect. Dietary probiotics that are found in yogurt and soy products can help prevent the development of a vaginal fungal infection during antibiotic therapy.

Bacterial Vaginosis

Bacterial vaginosis (BV) occurs when the normal level of bacteria in the vagina is disrupted and secondary bacteria begin to grow and infect the tissue lining. Signs and symptoms include vaginal discharge, odor, pain, pruritus, or burning. Although BV is the most common vaginal infection in women of childbearing age in the United States, it does not usually cause complications. However, an infection of the vagina appears to make women more susceptible to STIs, including infection with the human immunodeficiency virus (HIV); it may lead to pelvic inflammatory disease (PID) if the infection spreads; and in pregnant women, it is associated with a premature or low-birth-weight infant. For these reasons, antibiotic therapy is especially important for pregnant women. The antibiotic of choice is either metronidazole (Flagyl) or clindamycin (Cleocin).

Cervicitis

Cervicitis is an inflammation of the cervix caused by an invading organism. The main sign is a thick, purulent, whitish discharge with an acrid odor. Dysuria may also be noted. Cervicitis can occur after vaginal delivery as a result of an infected cervical laceration, but most cases are caused by an STI. Treatment consists primarily of antibiotics, although cauterization may be indicated if cervical ulcers are present.

Pelvic Inflammatory Disease

PID is any acute or chronic infection of the reproductive system that ascends from the vagina (vaginitis), cervix (cervicitis), uterus (endometritis), fallopian tubes (salpingitis), and ovaries (oophoritis). These infections may cause the fallopian tubes to fill with pus, and chronic episodes can result in scarring of the fallopian tubes and the formation of adhesions. PID is caused by advanced, untreated vaginosis, gonorrhea, or chlamydial infection; or it can develop from infection after pelvic surgery, tubal examination, or abortion. PID is responsible for a large percentage of cases of infertility in women as a result of adhesions that form in the fallopian tubes, preventing the ovum from migrating through the tube. Therefore, it is critical that a woman receive care immediately if she has pelvic pain or other symptoms of PID. The patient may be asymptomatic or may complain of purulent vaginal discharge, fever, malaise, dysuria, lower abdominal pain, bleeding, nausea, and vomiting. Cultures of cervical discharge typically are done to determine the pathogenic organism. Several types of antibiotics can cure PID; however, antibiotic therapy cannot reverse any scarring that has occurred in the fallopian tubes because of an infection. The longer a woman delays treatment for PID, the more likely she is to become infertile or to have a future ectopic pregnancy. Treatment should include broad-spectrum antibiotic therapy, such as Flagyl or ceftriaxone (Rocephin) with doxycycline (Vibramycin). If cultures are positive for an STI, treatment of the patient's sexual partner is necessary to prevent reinfection.

Trends in Sexually Transmitted Infections

- Syphilis, gonorrhea, chlamydia and herpes infections increase the risk of getting the human immunodeficiency virus (HIV).
- Patients infected with gonorrhea frequently are co-infected with chlamydia. Researchers recommend that patients who test positive for either sexually transmitted infection (STI) be treated with a combination of antibiotics such as Rocephin with azithromycin.
- Chlamydia is the most commonly reported notifiable disease in the United States; more than 1.4 million cases were reported in 2014. It is known as the "silent" STI because 75% of infected women and 50% of infected men are asymptomatic. An estimated 40% of women with untreated chlamydia infections develop pelvic inflammatory disease (PID), and infertility results in 20% of those. The condition is diagnosed in African-American women almost seven times more frequently than in Caucasian women. The highest rates are seen in 15- to 24-year-olds. The Centers for Disease Control and Prevention (CDC) recommends yearly chlamydia screening for sexually active women younger than 26 years of age and for those older with risk factors, including new or multiple sex partners. Women infected with chlamydia are up to five times more likely to become infected with HIV if exposed. If chlamydia is diagnosed, the patient and partner should abstain from sexual intercourse until treatment has been completed to prevent reinfection.
- Gonorrhea is a major cause of PID. Most affected women are asymptomatic. Transmission can occur during vaginal birth, causing fetal blindness, joint infection, or a life-threatening blood infection. Pregnant women should be treated as soon as gonorrhea is diagnosed, to reduce these risks.
- Congenital syphilis can cause stillbirth, neonatal death, physical deformities, and neurologic complications.
- Approximately 1 in 5 women 14 to 49 years of age have a genital herpes simplex virus (HSV) infection, which can cause potentially fatal infections in babies. Herpes can be spread by having vaginal, anal, or oral sex with someone who has the disease, and condoms do not completely protect from transmission. Herpes can be contracted from an infected sex partner who does not have a visible sore or who may not know he or she is infected. There is no cure for genital herpes. Treatment with prescription antiviral medications may reduce the frequency, severity, and duration of symptoms in recurrent outbreaks. Antiviral medications include acyclovir (Zovirax), famciclovir (Famvir), and valacyclovir (Valtrex). Studies show

Continued

Trends in Sexually Transmitted Infections—*continued*

that individuals with HSV are more susceptible to HIV infection and that an HIV-positive person with HSV is more infectious.

- At least 50% of sexually active men and women acquire genital human papillomavirus (HPV) infection at some point. By age 50, at least 80% of women will have acquired a genital HPV infection. Each year, about 21,000 women are diagnosed with HPV-associated cervical cancer.
- Trichomoniasis is the most common curable STI in young, sexually active women. Symptoms usually appear in women within 5 to 28 days of

exposure. Pregnant women with trichomoniasis may have premature or low-birth-weight (less than 5 pounds) infants. It is treated with a single dose of either metronidazole (Flagyl) or tinidazole (Tindamax).

- HIV can cross the placenta during pregnancy and infect the baby during birth; it is also found in breast milk. An elective cesarean birth at 38 weeks is recommended to reduce the risk of transmission during the birth process.
- Women who test negative for hepatitis B may receive the hepatitis B vaccine during pregnancy.

Modified from the CDC Sexually Transmitted Diseases (STD) Fact Sheets. *www.cdc.gov/std/healthcomm/fact_sheets.htm.* Accessed May 14, 2015.

Sexually Transmitted Infections

The list of infectious diseases spread by sexual contact continues to grow. These diseases are considered the most common contagious diseases in the United States. All STIs are transmitted from one person to another through body fluids, such as blood, semen, or vaginal secretions during vaginal, anal, or oral sex (Figure 34-7). A summary of STIs and their effect on men was presented in the Urology and Male Reproduction chapter. This chapter focuses on the impact of STIs on women.

The human papillomavirus (HPV), which causes genital warts, is a matter of special concern in women. The infection may be asymptomatic up to 2 years after exposure; however, regardless of whether the virus causes symptomatic wart development, the

infection can lead to serious complications in women. There are more than 40 identified types of HPV, and HPV infection typically is first diagnosed by abnormal Pap test results because the virus can cause such abnormalities. A positive Pap test result is followed up with an HPV DNA test to diagnose the specific strain of HPV that caused the infection. Although most women have a healthy immune system that can successfully clear the virus without the development of future health problems, approximately 13 high-risk HPV types are linked to the development of cervical carcinoma. Women diagnosed with one of these carcinogenic strains must have regular Pap testing, usually every 3 to 6 months, for early detection and treatment of precancerous and cancerous cells of the cervix.

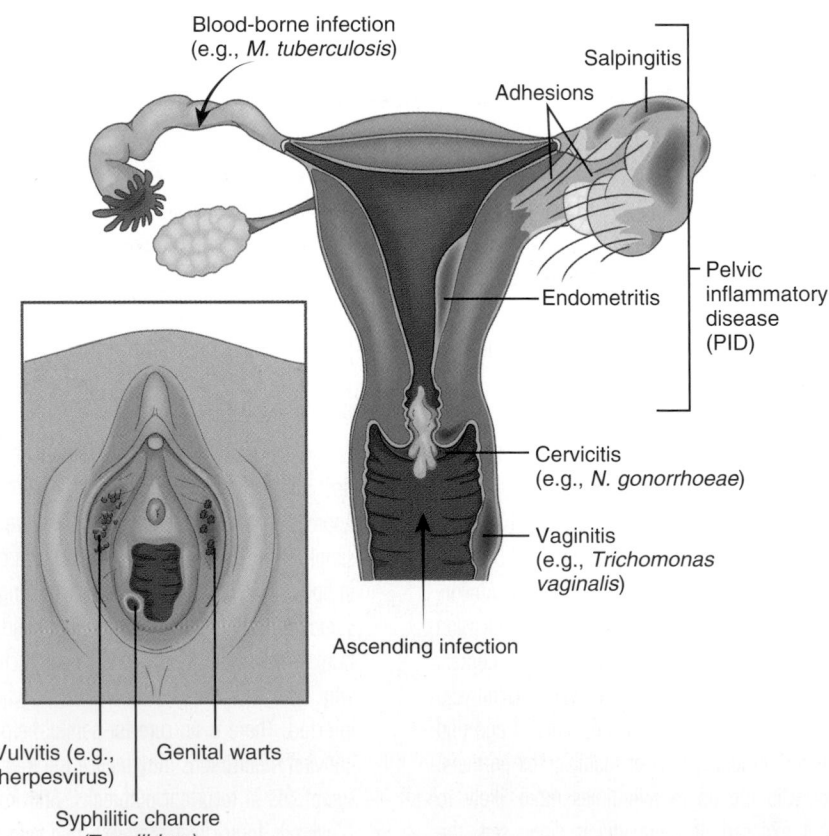

FIGURE 34-7 Ascending infections of the female genital organs are usually caused by sexual contact, pregnancy, or instrumentation. Descending infections usually begin in the blood or lymph nodes.

Three HPV vaccines are available: Cervarix, Gardasil, and Gardasil 9. The vaccines are given in a three-shot series over 6 months to protect girls and young women from HPV infection and the possibility of cervical cancer. Gardasil and Gardasil 9 also protect against genital warts and anal cancer in both females and males. Routine vaccination is recommended for females aged 11 or 12 years, and through age 26 years for those not previously vaccinated. In addition, the vaccines are recommended for routine use in males aged 11 or 12 years and through age 21 years. The goal is to immunize the individual before sexual activity is initiated. The vaccine is also recommended for any man who has sex with men through age 26.

Table 34-2 summarizes the effects of STIs on women. The percentage of women and girls infected with HIV is declining, largely because of educational emphasis on the use of condoms; however, women account for approximately 1 in 4 people living with HIV infection in the United States. Because HIV can be transmitted through the placenta to the developing fetus, it is crucial that women be diagnosed either before pregnancy or as early in the pregnancy as possible. Treatment of pregnant women who are HIV positive with a three-part regimen of zidovudine (ZDV, Retrovir; formerly AZT) can cut the risk of transmission to below 2%. Even where resources are limited, a single dose of medicine given to mother and baby can reduce the risk of HIV infection in the infant by 50%. According to this treatment protocol, the pregnant woman should start taking ZDV at 14 to 34 weeks; it should be administered intravenously during labor and delivery; and it should be given to the infant every 6 hours for 6 weeks after birth. Because some AIDS drugs are very dangerous for developing infants, the medication regimen of a woman currently receiving treatment may be changed during pregnancy. Women who are HIV positive should never breast-feed because the virus is present in breast milk.

CRITICAL THINKING APPLICATION   **34-3**

A 28-year-old patient recently was diagnosed with an acute gonorrheal and chlamydial infection. She first tested positive for HPV when she was 22. Dr. Beck asks Betsy to give the patient educational materials, including information on the potential long-term complications of HPV, and to confirm that she understands the signs and symptoms of STIs in herself and her partner. What should Betsy include in the information?

TABLE 34-2   Sexually Transmitted Infections in Women

INFECTION	CAUSATIVE ORGANISM	SIGNS AND SYMPTOMS	TREATMENT
Chlamydia	*Chlamydia trachomatis* (bacterium)	Often asymptomatic; dysuria; urinary frequency; abdominal pain; increased or decreased vaginal discharge. May cause endometritis, PID, and urethritis. Transmission to newborn can occur during vaginal delivery; causes neonatal eye infections and pneumonia.	Curable with antibiotic therapy; single dose of Zithromax or 1 week of doxycycline (Vibramycin).
Genital herpes	Herpes simplex virus type 2 (HSV-2)	Painful genital vesicles and ulcers; erythema and pruritus; tingling or shooting pain 1-2 days before outbreak; cycle through episodes. Viral shedding may occur during asymptomatic periods. Newborns can be infected by active lesions in vagina at birth. Brain damage, blindness, or death of the newborn may occur. Cesarean section if active lesions at time of birth. Increases risk for cervical cancer.	No cure, but antiviral therapy during episodes shortens duration of lesions; Zovirax, Famvir, or Valtrex
Genital warts	Human papillomavirus (HPV)	Most prevalent STI; period of communicability is unknown; lesions seen more frequently in women; tend to recur; 25% of women with HPV develop invasive cervical cancer; should be followed with routine Pap test (every 3-6 months if diagnosed with one of the carcinogenic strains).	Goal of treatment is to remove symptomatic warts; cryotherapy to lesions; podofilox solution or imiquimod (Aldara) cream to lesions
Gonorrhea	*Neisseria gonorrhoeae* (bacterium)	Dysuria; urinary frequency; abdominal pain; increased or decreased vaginal discharge. May cause endometritis, PID, and urethritis.	Curable with antibiotic therapy; azithromycin or doxycycline
Syphilis	*Treponema pallidum* (spirochete bacterium)	Six stages that can affect multiple body systems; 10- to 90-day incubation; initial sign is a painless lesion, or chancre, at the exposure site (vulva or vagina); serous discharge from chancre; lymphadenopathy. If not treated, advances to later stages. Can infect fetus via the placenta, resulting in congenital syphilis.	Penicillin G; if patient is allergic to penicillin, doxycycline or tetracycline
Trichomoniasis	*Trichomonas vaginalis* (protozoan)	May be asymptomatic; urinary frequency, urgency, and dysuria; frothy yellow-green vaginal discharge; pruritus.	Single dose of metronidazole (Flagyl) or tinidazole (Tindamax); partner must be treated

HPV, Human papilloma virus; *PID*, pelvic inflammatory disease; *STI*, sexually transmitted infection.

Benign Tumors

Fibroid Tumors

Uterine fibroid tumors, also called *fibromyomas, leiomyomas,* or *myomas,* are idiopathic benign tumors composed mainly of smooth muscle and some fibrous connective tissue. These tumors appear to have a genetic link because they tend to run in families. Fibroids vary in number, size, and location in the uterus and are quite common. Menorrhagia is the primary symptom, although the patient may experience bladder or rectal pressure, pelvic pressure, pain, abdominal distortion, and infertility. Fibroid tumors affect premenopausal women because they consist of estrogen-sensitive cells. Fibroid tumors do not recur and do not undergo malignant transformation; therefore, patients with fibroid tumors have an excellent prognosis. Treatment depends on the severity of the symptoms and the patient's age because fibroid tumors tend to become smaller and to calcify after menopause. The masses can be removed surgically, or a hysterectomy may be indicated if bleeding is a serious problem (Figure 34-8).

Ovarian Cysts

Ovarian cysts are sacs of fluid or semisolid material that form on or near the ovaries. They can occur in the follicle or the corpus luteum at any time between puberty and menopause. Most cysts are benign, and small, asymptomatic cysts do not require treatment. Large or multiple cysts may cause discomfort, low back pain, nausea, vomiting, and abnormal uterine bleeding. These can be treated with birth control pills over a period of several months to reduce the size of the cysts or to prevent the development of new cysts. If pharmaceutical therapy is not sufficient, laparoscopic procedures can be done to drain or remove large cysts. Surgery may be indicated if a cyst ruptures, or in cases of torsion of the ovary, in which twisting cuts off the blood supply to the ovary.

Polycystic ovary syndrome is a hormonal problem that may cause cysts to develop over enlarged ovaries. The diagnosis depends on the presence of two or more indicators, including irregular or no menstruation, high testosterone levels, *hirsutism* (excessive body hair in a masculine pattern), acne, and male pattern baldness (androgenic *alopecia*). Women affected by this disorder have unusually high levels of testosterone, estrogen, and LH and decreased amounts of FSH. They initially may be diagnosed because of fertility problems. The combination of hormone irregularities causes the symptoms associated with the disorder; however, some women are diagnosed by menstrual irregularity alone. These women are at greater risk of uterine cancer, because the endometrium does not slough off monthly. Also, there appears to be a link with insulin and cholesterol metabolism, so women with this disorder are at greater risk of developing diabetes mellitus type 2, obesity, and heart disease. The condition is treated with OCPs to stimulate menses artificially, to lower androgen levels, and to reduce masculine-type symptoms if present.

Fibrocystic Breast Disease

Fibrocystic breast disease is characterized by the presence of multiple, palpable nodules in the breasts; these nodules usually are associated with pain and tenderness and fluctuate with the menstrual cycle (Figure 34-9). Over time, the cysts enlarge, and the connective tissue of the breast is replaced with dense, firm fibrous tissue. The masses may be fibrous tumors that have degenerated or sacs filled with fluid. The cysts feel firm and movable, and the degree of tenderness and the size depend on the point in the menstrual cycle, with tenderness peaking just before and during the secretory phase. Several different cellular types of cysts can form, but fibrocystic changes in the breast are not considered precancerous.

Although the risk of breast cancer is not increased with fibrocystic breast disease, the diagnosis of cancerous breast masses becomes more complicated. Because the breasts consistently feel lumpy, breast examinations may not isolate a suspicious mass. In addition, accurate mammography screening is complicated by the dense

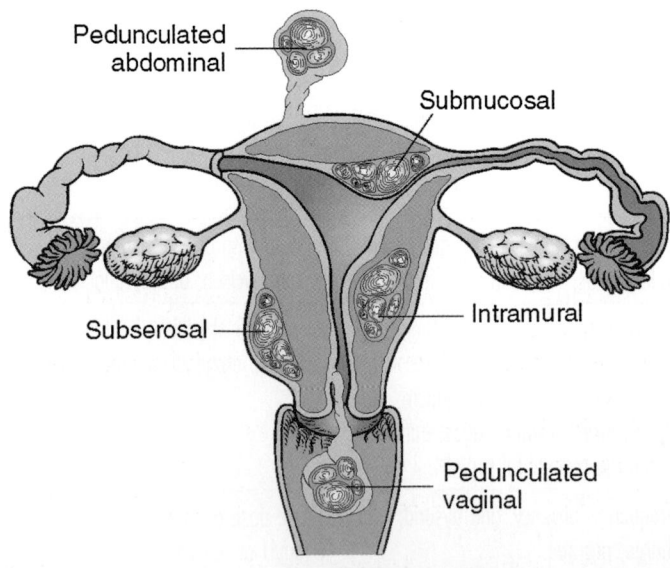

FIGURE 34-8 Uterine fibroid tumors are composed of hormone-sensitive cells and are designated subserosal, intramural, submucosal, or pedunculated, depending on their location. (From Salvo SG: *Mosby's pathology for massage therapists,* ed 2, St Louis, 2009, Mosby.)

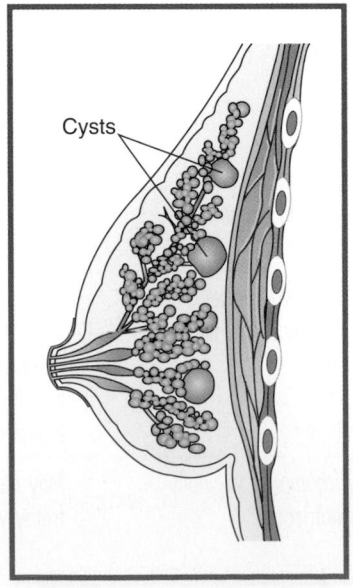

FIGURE 34-9 Fibrocystic breast disease.

nature of the cysts, making visualization of a cancerous area more difficult. Patients should be encouraged to perform monthly breast self-examination (BSE) and to report any changes in the breast immediately.

Malignant Tumors

Most problems with the female reproductive organs are related to abnormal cell growth. Early screening and preventive intervention are essential. Most malignant tumors require surgical removal. Radiation, chemotherapy, and hormone therapy are alternative treatment choices.

Cervical Cancer

Almost all cervical carcinomas are caused by HPV. The first stage of cervical cancer is asymptomatic, but early diagnosis of cervical cellular changes is possible with a Papanicolaou (Pap) test (Procedure 34-1). During the invasive stage, the patient reports abnormal vaginal bleeding and persistent discharge, in addition to bleeding and pain during intercourse. The average age of diagnosis for carcinoma in situ (cancerous cells restricted to the original site) currently is 35; however, it continues to drop because the number of cases in young women is increasing. Women with HPV infection may be tested every 3 to 6 months, depending on previous Pap results.

Pap Test and Other Guidelines for Women

- The first screening Pap test should be performed at age 21 unless the patient has a history of an abnormal Pap test.
- Women ages 21 to 29 should have a Pap test once every 3 years.
- Women ages 30 to 65 who have a history of negative Pap test results should have co-testing (Pap test combined with human papillomavirus [HPV] testing) once every 5 years.
- Women who have had a hysterectomy for noncancerous reasons do not need a Pap test unless they have a cervix.
- Cervical cancer screening with Pap tests should not be done in women older than age 65 if they have no history of cervical cancer and if they

have also had either three consecutive negative Pap test results or two consecutive negative co-test results within the past 10 years.
- These guidelines should be followed regardless of whether the patient has had the HPV vaccine.
- Women should have a yearly physical examination, including breast exam, pelvic exam (with or without a Pap test), and sexually transmitted infection (STI) screening if indicated.
- Patients must have an annual exam to receive birth control.
- Patients with a history of an abnormal Pap test result should consult their provider about how often to schedule Pap tests.

The American Congress of Obstetricians and Gynecologists (ACOG). www.acog.org/About-ACOG/News-Room/News-Releases/2012/Ob-Gyns-Recommend-Women-Wait-3-to-5-Years-Between-Pap-Tests. Accessed May 14, 2015.

PROCEDURE 34-1   Instruct and Prepare a Patient for Procedures and/or Treatments: Assist with the Examination of a Female Patient and Obtain a Smear for a Pap Test

Goal: To assist the provider in the examination of a female patient and in obtaining a diagnostic Pap smear.

EQUIPMENT and SUPPLIES

- Patient's health record
- Laboratory requisition slips
- Patient gown
- Lubricant
- 4 × 4-inch gauze squares
- Drape sheet
- Examination light
- Cervical spatula and Cytobrush
- ThinPrep container
- Vaginal speculum
- Uterine sponge forceps
- Disposable examination gloves
- Urine specimen container, if needed
- Stool for occult blood test cards with developer if needed
- Biohazard waste container
- Appropriate patient education materials

PROCEDURAL STEPS

1. Assemble the materials needed and prepare the room. Prepare the equipment and supplies needed for the Pap test.
2. Sanitize your hands and follow Standard Precautions.
   PURPOSE: To ensure infection control.
3. Introduce yourself, greet the patient and verify her identity by name and date of birth, then, briefly explain the procedure.
   PURPOSE: Explanations gain the patient's cooperation and alleviate apprehension.
4. Instruct the patient to empty the bladder, and collect a urine specimen if needed.
   PURPOSE: The provider's bimanual examination (see Figure 34-18) is performed on an empty bladder.
5. Instruct the patient to disrobe completely and to put on a gown with the opening in the front.
6. Assist the provider with the breast examination. To start, have the patient sit at the end of the examination table. Drape the patient and reassure her as needed.

PROCEDURE 34-1 —continued

7. When the provider is ready to examine the breasts and the abdomen with the patient in the supine position, assist the patient into the supine position and drape as needed.
   PURPOSE: To prevent unnecessary exposure of the patient.

8. When the provider is ready to begin the vaginal examination, assist the patient into the lithotomy position. Have the patient slide down to the end of the table; then adjust the stirrups as needed so that the knees are relaxed and rotated outward. Remember always to position the patient while she is underneath the drape.

9. Direct the light source onto the perineum.
   PURPOSE: To facilitate better viewing of the cervix.

10. Put on gloves. Warm the stainless steel vaginal speculum in warm water (the provider may prefer a disposable plastic speculum). Pass the proper instruments to the provider in the proper sequence. The provider will need the Cytobrush for cervical cells and the spatula for the cervical sample.
    PURPOSE: Teamwork enhances efficiency.

11. Assist the provider with ThinPrep preparation by swirling the cervical specimen in the preservative solution at least 10 times to ensure that the specimen has been mixed with the preservative solution.

12. Label the specimen container and place it in a biohazard bag.

13. Apply water-soluble lubricant to the provider's fingers.
    PURPOSE: To facilitate the bimanual examination.

14. The provider may prepare a stool sample for occult blood testing after the rectal examination. Have the materials ready.

15. Instruct the patient to breathe deeply through the mouth with the hands crossed over the chest.
    PURPOSE: To help relax the muscles.

16. Place the soiled instruments in a basin.
    PURPOSE: To help create better aesthetic surroundings.

17. Assist the patient off the table and with dressing if needed.

18. While the patient is in the dressing room, sanitize and disinfect the examination room, removing used equipment.

19. Sanitize, disinfect, and sterilize stainless steel equipment. Remove your gloves, dispose of them in a biohazard waste container, and sanitize your hands.
    PURPOSE: To ensure infection control.

20. Prepare the Pap test and other samples for transportation to the laboratory. Complete the requisitions, including the date of the patient's last menstrual period (LMP) and whether she is on hormone therapy.

21. Record all procedures in the patient's health record.
    PURPOSE: A procedure is not done until it is entered into the patient's record.

8/23/20—2:00 PM: Pap test and pelvic examination completed by provider. ThinPrep specimen placed for pickup by University Laboratory for cytology. Pt tolerated procedure well. Betsy Davis, CMA (AAMA)

The patient should be informed of factors that can interfere with Pap test results, including menstruation and the use of vaginal creams, spermicidal foams, and douching 2 to 3 days before the examination. Also, the patient should refrain from vaginal intercourse for 24 hours before the examination because it may cause inflammation. The medical assistant should include in the patient history the use of certain medications (e.g., tetracycline), which may interfere with results; whether the patient has a latex allergy; the date of the last menstrual period (LMP); whether the patient has a history of a bleeding disorder or is taking anticoagulant medications; and whether the patient is pregnant or may be pregnant.

The provider obtains the cervical smear with a Cytobrush or a small wooden spatula that is inserted and rotated in the cervical canal to obtain endocervical cells for cytology. A liquid-based cytology exam, such as the ThinPrep Pap test, has replaced the traditional slide preparation method for analyzing these cells because it is more accurate in diagnosing precancerous and cancerous lesions and rarely has to be repeated because of an inadequate cellular sample. The provider uses the same technique to collect the cellular sample, but instead of fixing it onto a glass slide, the collection device is rinsed into a vial containing a preservative solution. In the laboratory, a processor filters the sample and creates a slide with a thin layer of cervical cells that is more uniform and better preserved than is possible with the traditional method.

The pathologist examines the slide to determine whether cellular abnormalities are present. The results are classified into one of five categories: negative or normal, atypical squamous cells, abnormal with low-grade squamous lesions, abnormal with high-grade lesions (precancerous), or carcinoma cells. Inflammation or an STI infection can cause abnormal changes in cervical cells, so the provider decides how to manage abnormal results on the basis of other diagnostic studies.

If the Pap test indicates abnormal cells, the pathologist can grade cervical changes using a cervical intraepithelial neoplasia (CIN) system of I to III, depending on the degree of cellular **dysplasia** (Figure 34-10). CIN I indicates mild to moderate dysplasia; CIN II, moderate and moderate to severe dysplasia; and CIN III, carcinoma in situ. Patients whose Pap tests indicate dysplasia of any severity should have a colposcopy with biopsy if indicated and possibly an **endocervical curettage**. If adequately diagnosed and treated, carcinoma in situ of the cervix has a 100% survival rate at 5 years.

Carcinoma of the cervix is classified into the following stages:
- Stage 0: Carcinoma in situ
- Stage I: Carcinoma of the cervix with no **adnexal** involvement
- Stage II: Carcinoma of the cervix that has not spread into the pelvic wall or vagina

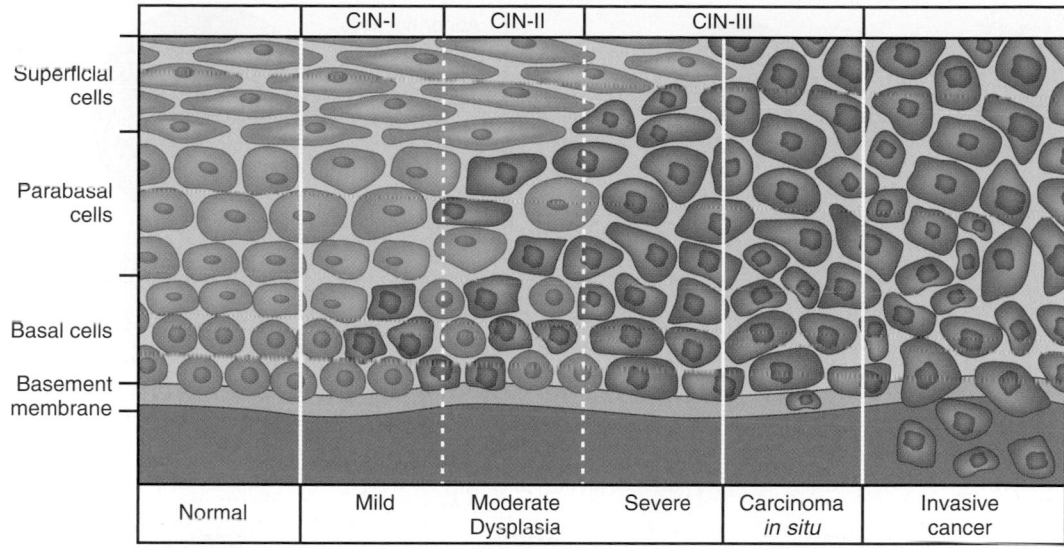

FIGURE 34-10 Cervical dysplasia and carcinoma.

- Stage III: Carcinoma of the cervix that has spread into the lower part of the vagina; may be blocking the ureters
- Stage IV: Carcinoma of the cervix that has spread to nearby organs, such as the bladder or rectum, with involvement of structures outside the pelvic area

Colposcopy is the visual examination of the vagina and cervical surfaces with a colposcope (Figure 34-11). The colposcope is a microscope with a light source and a magnifying lens that can be used during a vaginal examination to locate and evaluate abnormal cells and to detect cancer of the cervix in the early stages, to examine tissue from which an abnormal Pap test has been obtained, and to monitor areas of the cervix where malignant lesions have been removed. A cervical biopsy may be performed in conjunction with a colposcopy. A major advantage of obtaining a biopsy during colposcopy is that the instrument permits visualization of the suspicious area so that the biopsy can be taken from the most atypical site.

Colposcopy is a relatively safe, painless procedure performed in the provider's office. Discomfort may occur when the speculum is inserted into the vagina to improve visualization of the tissue. Discomfort and bleeding can occur when tissue is taken for biopsy. Depending on the results of a previous biopsy, the patient may need a more extensive procedure or conization, in which a cone-shaped wedge of cervical tissue is removed for treatment or further analysis. More often, a less invasive loop electrosurgical excision procedure (LEEP) is performed with injection of a local anesthetic to the cervix and insertion of a wire loop into the vagina. A high-frequency electrical current running through the wire is used to remove abnormal tissue from both the cervix and the endocervical canal. Like conization, LEEP can be used as a diagnostic tool to collect biopsy samples and as a treatment to remove abnormal tissue (Figure 34-12).

Depending on the condition of the cervix, cryosurgery, or the application of freezing temperatures, may be used to treat chronic cervicitis and cervical erosion. Freezing causes cellular necrosis, and

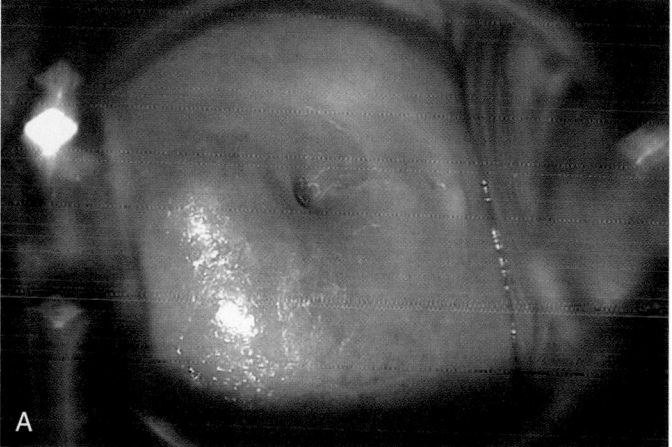

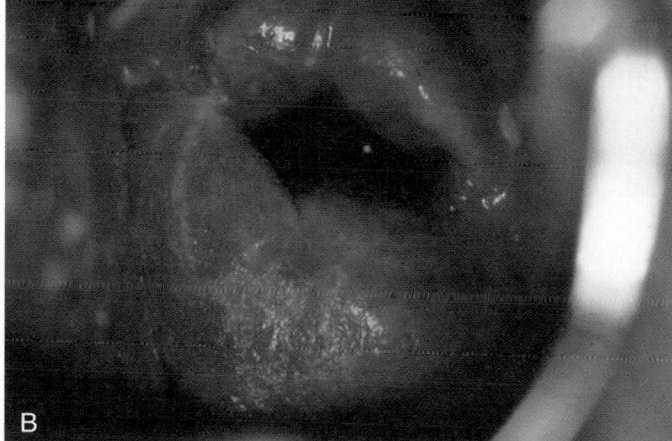

FIGURE 34-11 Colposcopic appearance of normal cervix **(A)** and abnormal cervix **(B)**. (**A** from Swartz MH: *Textbook of physical diagnosis*, ed 7, Philadelphia, 2014, Saunders; **B** from Pfenninger JL, Fowler GC: *Pfenninger and Fowler's procedures for primary care*, ed 3, Philadelphia, 2011, Saunders.)

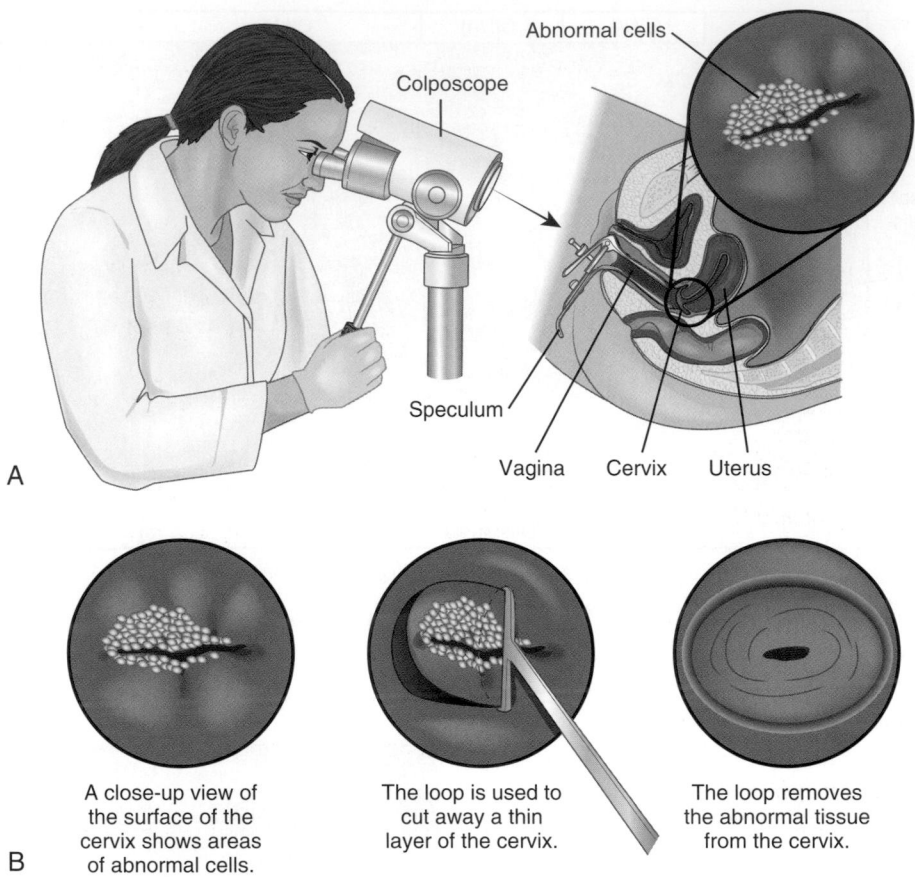

A close-up view of the surface of the cervix shows areas of abnormal cells.

The loop is used to cut away a thin layer of the cervix.

The loop removes the abnormal tissue from the cervix.

FIGURE 34-12 A, Colposcopic view of cervix and LEEP procedure. **B,** LEEP biopsy of abnormal cells.

in approximately 1 month, the dead cells are replaced with healthy cells. The procedure involves placing a probe against the problem area on the cervix and applying liquid nitrogen to the area for approximately 3 to 4 minutes or until the site is frozen (Procedure 34-2). The patient may experience some pain for 30 minutes or so

after the procedure and a slight watery discharge for up to a week. If any signs of infection, foul discharge, or pain develop, the patient should call the provider's office. Advise the patient not to engage in sexual intercourse for 1 month and to expect a heavier than usual menstrual flow for the first cycle after the procedure.

PROCEDURE 34-2	Instruct and Prepare a Patient for Procedures and/or Treatments: Prepare the Patient for a LEEP

Goal: *To prepare the patient and assist the provider in a LEEP.*

EQUIPMENT and SUPPLIES

- Patient's health record
- Cytology request forms
- Colposcope
- LEEP instrument
- Vaginal speculum
- Local anesthetic with syringe unit
- Monsel's solution or similar solution to prevent cervical bleeding
- Disposable examination gloves
- Specimen containers
- Biohazard waste container

PROCEDURAL STEPS

1. Assemble the necessary equipment.
   PURPOSE: To expedite the procedure.
2. Sanitize your hands.
   PURPOSE: To ensure infection control.
3. Greet the patient, introduce yourself, and verify the patient's identity by name and date of birth. Record the patient's vital signs. Check to make sure a signed informed consent form is in the patient's record.
   PURPOSE: To establish a baseline for vital signs and to follow legal protocols.
4. Drape the patient and assist her into the lithotomy position. Put on gloves.

5. Assist the provider with the procedure by handing equipment and supplies as needed.
   - The colposcope is used to visualize abnormal cells.
   - The provider administers a local anesthetic to the cervical area.
   - The LEEP instrument is used to remove abnormal cells.
   - The cervix may be coated with Monsel's solution or a similar solution to prevent cervical bleeding

6. Encourage the patient to take deep breaths to promote relaxation of the pelvic muscles during the procedure. Observe the patient for any signs of distress.
   PURPOSE: To ensure the patient's safety.

7. If a biopsy sample is taken, place the tissue in a specimen cup and label it for the lab.

8. When the procedure is complete, place the patient in a supine position and allow her to rest while you tidy the room and remove the used supplies. Retake her vital signs.
   PURPOSE: To ensure that the vital signs return to baseline levels.

9. Remove your gloves, discard them in a biohazard waste container, and sanitize your hands.
   PURPOSE: To ensure infection control.

10. Help the patient sit up and assist her in dressing if needed.
    PURPOSE: To ensure the patient's safety.

11. Apply gloves and prepare the specimen for lab delivery.

12. Sanitize, disinfect, and sterilize the equipment per the manufacturer's directions and return it to the proper storage area.

13. Remove gloves, dispose in a biohazard waste container, and sanitize your hands. Provide the patient with instructions on follow-up care as ordered by the provider.

14. Record the procedure and the final vital signs measurements in the patient's record.
    PURPOSE: A procedure is not done until it is recorded.

7/22/20–10:25 AM: Cervical LEEP completed by provider without incident. Pt stable, T 98.6°, P 82, R 20, BP 118/72. No c/o discomfort. Pt to call office if any problems noted. Betsy Davis, CMA (AAMA)

Endometrial Cancer

The inner lining of the uterus, the endometrium, is at increased risk for dysplasia in postmenopausal women who have never had children and in those who experienced early menarche and late menopause. Certain conditions, such as obesity, hypertension, and diabetes mellitus, may increase the risk of endometrial cancer. Taking tamoxifen for breast cancer can increase the risk of developing endometrial cancer. This slow-growing cancer begins with hyperplasia of the endometrial wall, followed by dysplasia. Early signs are irregular vaginal bleeding and leukorrhea (white or yellow) vaginal discharge; difficult or painful urination; pain during sexual intercourse; and pelvic pain. The diagnosis usually is made with an endometrial biopsy, **transvaginal ultrasound**, or a CT scan. Treatment involves a complete hysterectomy with radiation therapy and chemotherapy. Because most of these tumors develop after menopause, vaginal bleeding is unusual, and the woman is more likely to seek medical attention. Because of this, early diagnosis and treatment lead to a survival rate of almost 90%.

Ovarian Cancer

Ovarian neoplasms are the most important pathologic disorder of the ovaries. Ovarian cancer causes more deaths than any other cancer of the female reproductive system, but it accounts for only about 3% of all cancers in women. Most of the time the cancer has already metastasized before the tumor is diagnosed. Symptoms do not appear until the tumor has enlarged enough to exert pressure on nearby structures; patients complain of vague abdominal discomfort, bloating, urinary urgency, weight loss, and general malaise.

Researchers are working to perfect a blood test that can be used to screen for ovarian cancer so that the disease can be diagnosed in earlier, more treatable stages. Currently, ovarian cancer is diagnosed by a combination of a pelvic examination that indicates a mass in an ovary; a cancer antigen CA125 blood test, which identifies a protein found in abnormally high levels in women with ovarian cancer (although the test can produce false-positive and false-negative results); and a pelvic or transvaginal ultrasound to evaluate the size and shape of the ovaries. The ultimate diagnosis is based on a biopsy to confirm the presence of cancerous cells.

Little is known about how or why ovarian cancer occurs, but pregnancy, breast-feeding, and oral contraceptive use may reduce the risk. Risk factors include aging (most ovarian cancers are diagnosed in women age 55 or older), family history, genetic mutations, a personal history of breast cancer, and obesity. Treatment consists of a complete hysterectomy (removal of the uterus, fallopian tubes, and ovaries), radiation therapy, and chemotherapy. About 20% of all ovarian tumors are cancerous, and the recovery rate is linked to the location, the stage of tumor development, and the patient's age.

Breast Cancer

Breast cancer is the second leading cause of cancer deaths in women. According to the American Cancer Society, 1 in 8 women have a lifetime risk of developing breast cancer and a 1 in 28 risk of dying from the disease. Predisposing factors include a family history of breast cancer (especially in the mother, sister, or daughter, although fewer than 15% of women with breast cancer have a family history), early menarche and late menopause, first pregnancy after age 30 or no pregnancy, prolonged use of estrogen replacement therapy, excess alcohol intake, smoking, and obesity.

Because research does not link reduced death rates from breast cancer with monthly BSE, the American Cancer Society recommends that women have their practitioner perform a clinical breast examination (CBE) rather than rely on monthly BSEs for early detection. However, although a monthly BSE is now considered optional, women still should be aware of the normal appearance and texture of the breasts and should immediately report to the provider any changes or new breast symptoms. The medical assistant should be prepared to teach the BSE technique (Procedure 34-3). CBEs should be done every 3 years from age 20 to 39 and annually at 40 years of age and older. A mammogram (discussed later in the chapter) should be done annually starting at age 40. If a woman has an increased risk of breast cancer (e.g., family history), the provider may recommend annual mammography screening before age 40 or other diagnostic procedures, such as ultrasound or magnetic resonance imaging (MRI). An MRI scan can reveal tumors too small to detect with a breast examination and that may not show up clearly on a mammogram. The American Cancer Society recommends that those with a high risk for breast cancer have an MRI scan and a mammogram every year.

Women who are genetically predisposed to breast cancer and are at very high risk may opt for a bilateral prophylactic mastectomy, in which both breasts are removed to eliminate the possibility of breast cancer developing in the future. This surgery reduces the risk of breast cancer by at least 95% in women with genetic mutations.

Indications of breast cancer include a palpable breast mass that is firm and immovable, breast pain, tissue thickening, nipple retraction or dimpling, nipple discharge, and axillary lymphadenopathy. If a breast mass is palpated, a mammogram or ultrasound of the area is ordered and, if indicated, a biopsy is performed. The provider may perform a needle biopsy to remove cells and/or tissue from a palpated mass for evaluation by the pathologist. If a nonpalpable mass is found on a mammogram, a **stereotactically** guided needle aspiration is done, and surgical biopsy is a possible follow-up. During this procedure, the provider uses a mammogram to guide the needle toward the suspicious mass, from which a biopsy sample can be taken. If a tissue sample cannot be obtained through a needle, wire localization may be done to pinpoint the areas of concern from the mammogram. During this diagnostic procedure, a thin wire is passed through the breast to the point of concern (based on mammogram visualization). This wire marking is used during a surgical biopsy procedure, to pinpoint tissue that was suspicious on the mammogram.

If a biopsy shows malignant cells, the provider orders an estrogen and progesterone receptor test to determine whether hormones affect the way the cancer grows. If the cancer cells' growth patterns increase when exposed to hormone levels, the provider may recommend treatment with a drug such as tamoxifen, which prevents estrogen from binding to these sites. Tamoxifen may also be prescribed to reduce the risk of breast cancer in high-risk women.

The treatment of breast cancer depends on the type of carcinoma and its staging. Treatment almost always begins with surgery, but the type of surgery and the extent of the tissue removed depend on several factors. One type of breast-saving surgery is *lumpectomy,* in which only the suspicious mass plus a surrounding area of normal tissue is removed; radiation therapy is used as a follow-up to destroy any remaining cancerous cells. A

partial mastectomy may be done for more advanced cases; this procedure involves removal of the tumor and tissue surrounding it, part of the chest muscle beneath the mass, and some of the lymph nodes in the axillary region. A *complete mastectomy,* which involves removal of the entire breast, chest muscle, and axillary lymph nodes, may still be indicated if the mass has spread. However, removal of multiple axillary lymph nodes greatly increases the risk that subsequent **lymphedema** and recurrent infections in the arm on the affected side.

New techniques recommend the removal of the *sentinel lymph node;* this is the first lymph node to receive lymphatic drainage from a tumor and therefore the one most likely to spread cancer cells to other areas of the body. The sentinel node is found by injecting a blue dye near the tumor; the lymph vessels absorb the dye and carry it toward the lymph nodes, and the first node to receive the dye and turn blue is the one that is removed for pathologic testing. If the sentinel node is cancer free, there is very little chance that the breast tumor has metastasized, and no other nodes need to be removed. If cancer cells are evident, further diagnostic procedures are indicated to determine the possible locations of metastatic tumors.

Targeted therapy is a newer type of cancer treatment in which drugs are used to identify and attack cancer cells; as a result, very little damage is done to healthy cells. Targeted therapy is a growing part of many cancer treatment regimens.

Many patients now opt for breast reconstruction after a partial or complete mastectomy. This procedure typically is performed by a plastic surgeon, and a variety of methods can be used to reconstruct breast tissue, including implantation of a silicone or gel material or the use of fat and other tissue from another part of the body, such as the abdomen. Either the surgeon saves a tissue flap that includes the nipple or, after the breast is reformed, tattoo techniques are used to create an areola and nipple. The patient must discuss these options with her surgeon before the mastectomy is performed, and the medical assistant may be involved in the referral process.

Inflammatory Breast Cancer

- Inflammatory breast cancer is a rare, aggressive cancer that causes the sudden onset of discoloration and warmth in the affected breast, along with edema, dimpling of the skin, enlarged axillary lymph nodes, and pain.
- The condition is easily confused with a breast infection, so patients should contact their provider as soon as symptoms appear.
- Cancer cells spread rapidly and block lymph vessels in the skin, which results in the classic symptoms.
- The condition is diagnosed by an excisional biopsy to confirm the presence of clumped cancer cells in the area lymph vessels.
- Inflammatory breast cancer typically is diagnosed as stage III, which means that the cancer has spread to local lymph nodes. However, one third of patients are diagnosed with stage IV carcinoma, in which metastasis already has occurred.

PROCEDURE 34-3	Coach Patients in Health Maintenance and Disease Prevention: Teach the Patient Breast Self-Examination

Goal: *To teach the patient how to palpate her breasts to check for possible abnormalities.*

EQUIPMENT and SUPPLIES

- Patient's health record
- Instruction pamphlet/shower card
- Teaching model (to demonstrate the technique before a return demonstration by the patient)

PROCEDURAL STEPS

1. Assemble the necessary equipment.
2. Sanitize your hands and follow Standard Precautions.
   <u>PURPOSE</u>: To ensure infection control.
3. Greet the patient, introduce yourself, and verify the patient's identity by name and date of birth, then briefly explain the procedure.
   <u>PURPOSE</u>: Explanations gain the patient's cooperation and alleviate apprehension.
4. Instruct the patient to examine her breasts while bathing or showering in warm water because the fingers glide more easily over wet tissue. The best time to perform this examination is immediately after the end of the menstrual period, when breast engorgement is minimal. Nonmenstruating women should examine their breasts the first of each month.
5. Instruct the patient to raise one arm, using the right hand to examine the left breast and the left hand for the right breast. Using the finger pads of the three middle fingers, move in a small circular pattern up and down the breast. Starting at the axillary region, work down the area and back up again from the axillary to the ribs below the breast, back up to the clavicle, and repeatedly across to the sternum bilaterally (Figure 1).

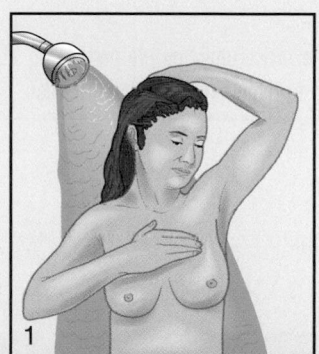

6. After finishing her bath or shower, the patient should continue the examination in front of a mirror with the arms at the sides. Then, with her arms raised above her head, she should look carefully for changes in the size, shape, and contour of each breast. She should look for puckering, dimpling, or changes in skin texture (Figure 2).

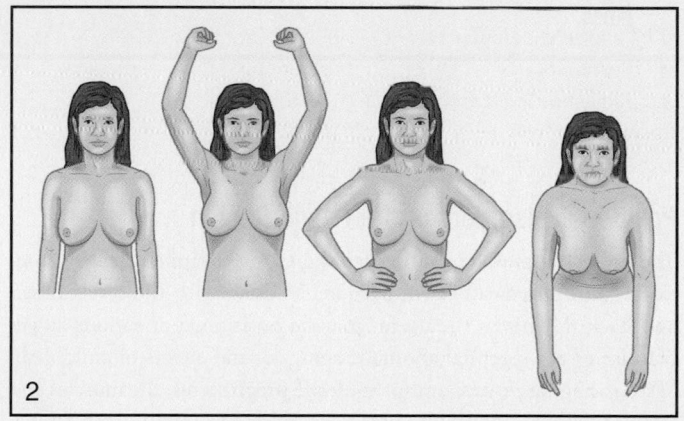

7. Instruct the patient to squeeze both nipples gently and to look for discharge (Figure 3).

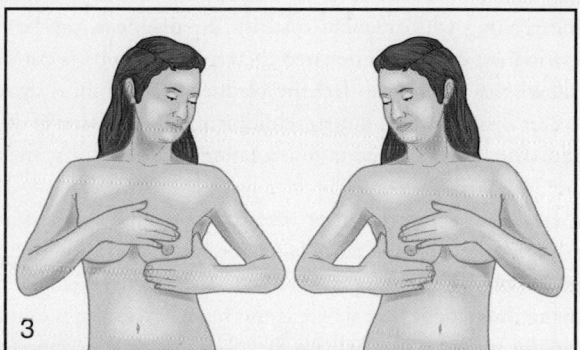

8. Before dressing, the patient should lie on a bed. A towel or pillow is placed under the right shoulder, and the right hand is placed behind the head. The right breast is examined with the left hand. Instruct the patient to press gently in small circles, starting at the top outermost edge, including the axillary region, and spiraling in toward the nipple. This is repeated with the left breast (Figure 4).

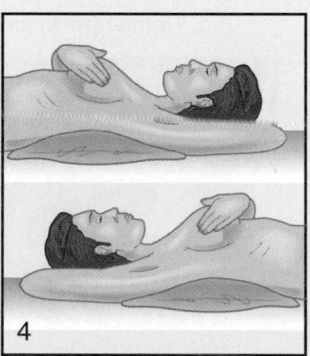

PROCEDURE 34-3   —*continued*

9. The patient should provide a return demonstration using the teaching model to confirm her understanding.
10. Give the patient an instruction pamphlet and/or shower card to use at home.

11. Record the patient education intervention in the patient's health record. <u>PURPOSE</u>: Patient education interventions should always be documented; a procedure is not done until it is entered into the patient's record.

Positional Disorders of the Pelvic Region

The correct anatomic position for the uterus is tipped slightly anteriorly (anteverted) and bent over the bladder, with the cervix down and back. However, the uterus may be positioned at various angles because of a congenital anomaly, aging, or the effects of childbirth. With the aging process and/or multiple pregnancies, the muscles and ligaments that support the uterus, bladder, and rectum can stretch or weaken. This weakening of the supportive structures of the pelvic floor can result in multiple structural disorders.

A *cystocele* is a protrusion of the bladder into the anterior wall of the vagina. The bladder becomes angled, and urinary retention is common, along with frequent cystitis. The diagnosis can be made by having the patient bear down as the vaginal opening is examined; this allows the provider to feel the bladder protrusion. A cystocele can result from injury during childbirth, obesity, heavy lifting, chronic coughing, and poor musculature that occurs with aging (Figure 34-13).

A *rectocele* is a protrusion of the rectum into the posterior wall of the vagina. The patient complains of difficulty with bowel movements and pressure in the pelvic region. The diagnosis can be made by having the patient bear down as the vaginal opening is examined so that the provider can palpate the posterior wall. Rectoceles are most often seen in postmenopausal women. A rectocele may result from pregnancy, difficult delivery, prolonged labor, obesity, chronic coughing, and repeated lifting of heavy objects.

The uterus also may lose supportive structure and drop into the vagina. This structural disorder is called *uterine prolapse*. The prolapse may involve only descent of the cervix into the vaginal area, or it may progress to protrusion of both the uterus and the cervix from the vaginal opening.

The first step in the treatment of pelvic positional disorders is to teach the patient how to perform pelvic floor muscle exercises, or Kegel exercises. The patient may be referred to a physical therapist that specializes in female disorders and uses biofeedback to help train the patient to perform the exercises accurately. If severe, all three of these structural abnormalities can be corrected with surgery.

Kegel Exercises

Kegel exercises help strengthen the pelvic floor muscles. They are done to prevent or treat pelvic organ prolapse and incontinence. The steps are as follows:

1. Contract the muscles that make up the pelvic floor by visualizing that you are stopping the flow of urine midstream.
2. Hold the contraction to the count of 3 and then slowly relax for a count of 3.
3. Repeat the exercise until you are performing 20 contractions in a set, with up to three sets throughout the day.

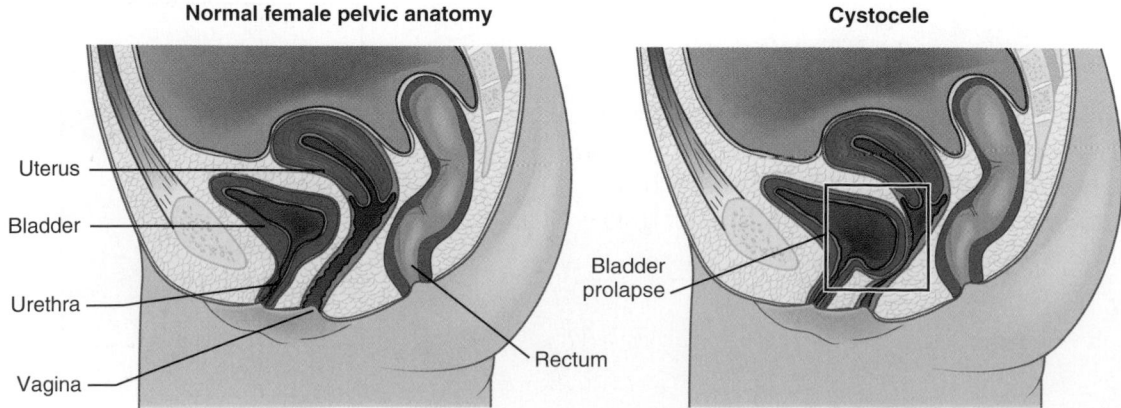

Normal female pelvic anatomy — Uterus, Bladder, Urethra, Vagina, Rectum

Cystocele — Bladder prolapse

FIGURE 34-13 A cystocele is a protrusion of the bladder into the anterior wall of the vagina.

PREGNANCY

Anatomy and Physiology

Fertilization usually takes place in the distal third of the fallopian tube when one sperm cell penetrates and fertilizes an egg, which is then called a *zygote*. The zygote, which is made up of 23 chromosomes from the ovum and 23 chromosomes from the sperm, forms the first complete cell. This cell begins to grow and multiply immediately. The zygote travels down the fallopian tube and reaches the uterus in 5 to 6 days, implanting in the uterine endometrium. Enzymes are secreted by the zygote to aid the implantation process.

After implantation, the placenta forms within the uterine wall. It is derived from maternal endometrial tissue and from the chorion, the outermost membrane that surrounds the developing zygote. The amnion, the innermost layer of the membranes, holds the fetus suspended in an amniotic cavity surrounded by a fluid called *amniotic fluid*. The amnion and the fluid sometimes are called the "bag of water." In about 25% of pregnancies, breaking of the amniotic sac signals the onset of labor.

Within 2 weeks of fertilization, the zygote has undergone mitosis and is well established in the uterus. The next stage of development is the embryonic period, which includes week 3 to week 12 of pregnancy (the first trimester). The embryonic period is a crucial time because this is when all tissues and organs develop. During the second and third trimesters, the embryo becomes a fetus; this is when cells develop and begin their primary functions, organs mature, and the fetus gains weight and grows in length.

Throughout the pregnancy, maternal and fetal blood never mixes. Nutrients and oxygen diffuse from the mother's blood across the placental membrane into the blood vessels of the fetus's umbilical cord. Carbon dioxide and waste materials pass from the umbilical cord, through the placenta, and into the mother's circulatory system for excretion (Figure 34-14).

The placenta also acts as a gland by producing HCG and progesterone to maintain the pregnancy. Low levels of progesterone can lead to spontaneous abortion in pregnant women and menstrual irregularities in nonpregnant women. The average gestation is calculated at 9 calendar months, 10 lunar months, or 266 to 280 days. As previously mentioned, it is divided into three trimesters.

First Trimester

The first trimester is the period from the beginning of the LMP through week 14. It is a time of multiple physical and psychological changes for the woman and a crucial time for fetal organ development. It is essential that the pregnant woman understand the importance of a nutritious diet and of avoiding potential **teratogens**. The woman may complain of breast tenderness, constipation, headaches, urinary frequency, and nausea and vomiting. Rest, relaxation exercises, plenty of fluids, regular exercise, and small, frequent meals help relieve these discomforts. During this time, the obstetrician obtains a complete health history of the patient, including family, medical, menstrual, and obstetric histories. The obstetric history includes the number of times the patient has been pregnant (gravida) and the number of pregnancies carried to more than 20 weeks' gestation (para).

CRITICAL THINKING APPLICATION   **34-4**

You are interviewing a new OB patient. She tells you that this is her fourth pregnancy, and she has two children. She had two early miscarriages. How would you document this obstetric history?

Second Trimester

The second trimester extends from week 15 through week 28 after the LMP. The uterus has enlarged to above the umbilicus, and the patient feels the first fetal movements, called *quickening*. In addition to the basic health history and physical examination, assessment is performed by abdominal palpation and fetal heart monitoring. The height of the fundus may be measured in centimeters from the symphysis pubis to the fundus. At each office visit, a urine sample is screened with a dipstick to detect protein and/or glucose, and the woman's blood pressure is monitored for signs of hypertension. The mother may complain of backache, dizziness, leukorrhea, and leg cramps from the increasing size of the uterus.

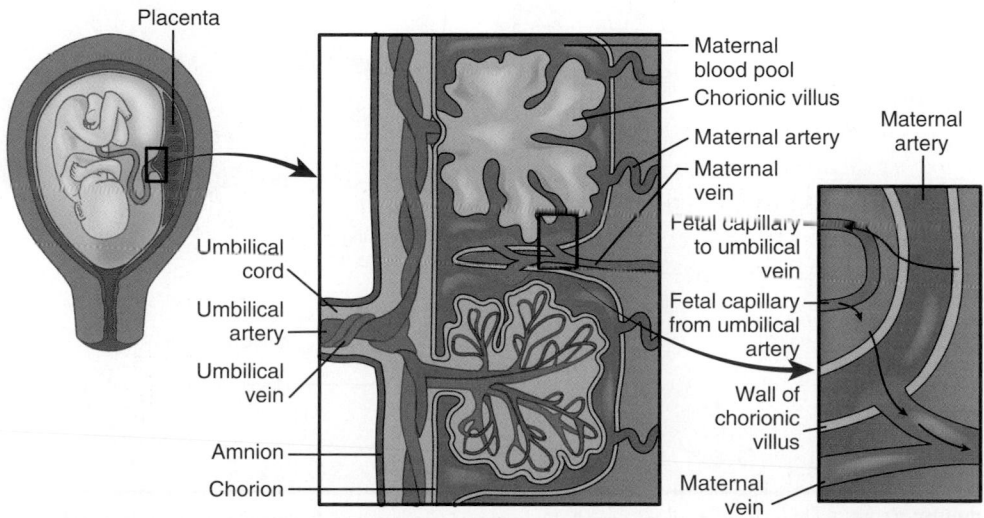

FIGURE 34-14 Structural features of the placenta and exchange of nutrients and wastes between maternal and fetal blood.

Third Trimester

The third trimester begins at week 28 and lasts until delivery. This period is marked by rapid fetal growth, with the baby gaining close to 1 pound per week. The patient continues to be closely monitored. Childbirth preparation classes usually begin during this time. The patient experiences noticeable breast enlargement and may have an occasional discharge from the nipples of the clear, sticky fluid **colostrum**. The pregnant woman may complain of uterine cramping *(Braxton-Hicks contractions)*, heartburn, edema, and frequent urination. *Lightening*, the dropping of the fetus into the pelvis, may occur a few weeks before birth, especially in *primigravidas* (women in their first pregnancy). Tdap (immunization for diphtheria, tetanus, and pertussis [whooping cough]) should be administered between 27 and 36 weeks' gestation to maximize maternal antibody response and passive antibody transfer levels to the baby. Anyone caring for the newborn, including husbands, grandparents, older siblings, and babysitters, should also be vaccinated. This vaccination has become more important because of an increase in whooping cough outbreaks in recent years. Pertussis is a very serious respiratory infection in newborns and young children.

Parturition

Labor is the physiologic process by which the uterus expels the fetus and the placenta (Figure 34-15). To be born vaginally, the baby must

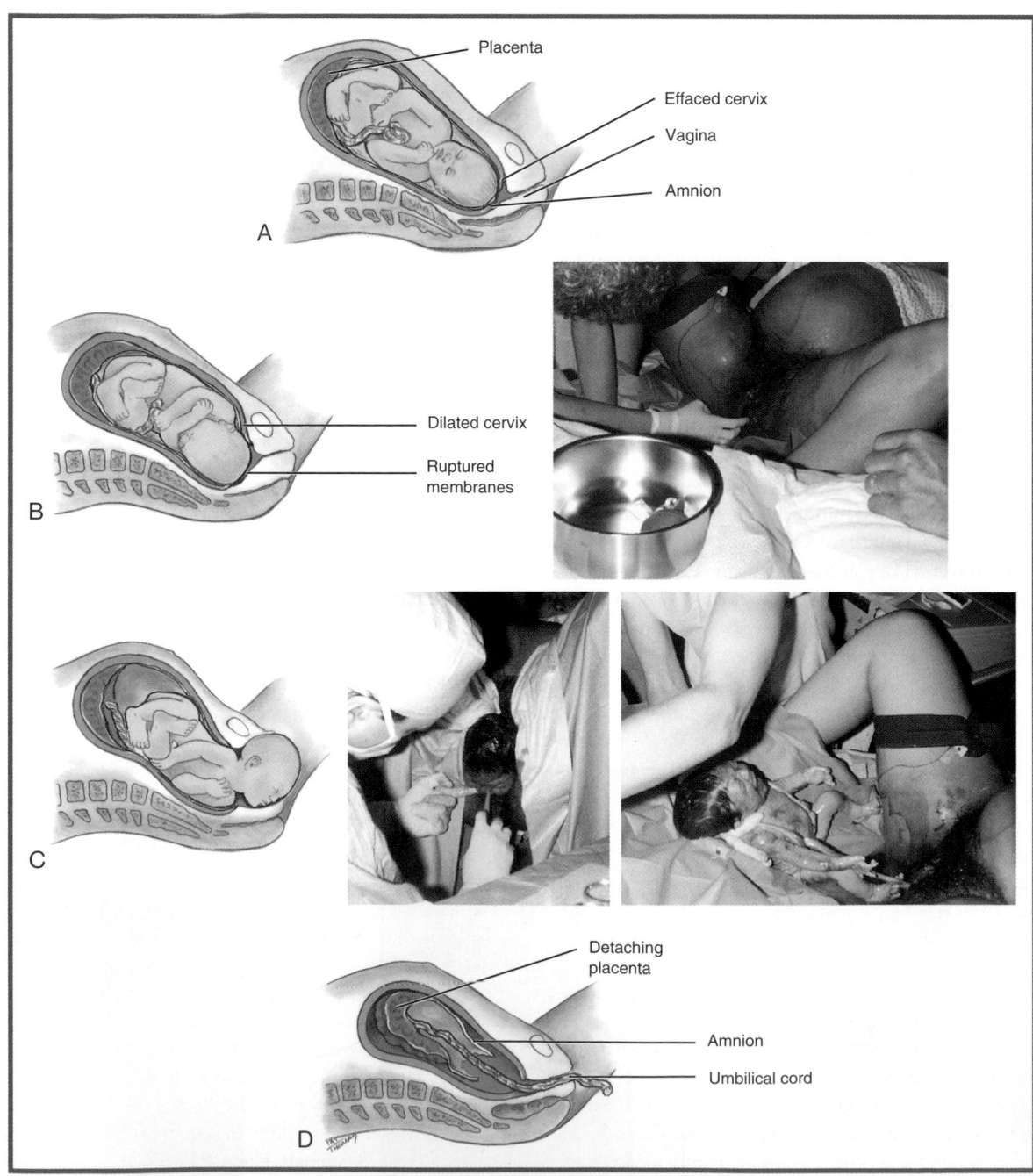

FIGURE 34-15 The labor process. **A,** Effaced cervix. **B,** Dilation stage. **C,** Expulsion stage. **D,** Placental stage. (From Applegate EJ: *The anatomy and physiology learning system,* ed 4, Philadelphia, 2011, Saunders.)

drop down into the pelvic floor, and the cervix must efface (thin out) and dilate (open up). **Effacement** is the thinning of the cervix from its prelabor length of 1 to 1½ inches to a completely thin tissue (Figure 34-15, *A*). This occurs when uterine contractions pull cervical tissue upward as labor progresses so that the bottom uterine segment (the cervix) becomes thinner and the top uterine segment (the fundus) becomes thicker. Effacement is measured as a percentage; the cervix is said to be 0% to 100% effaced. **Dilation** (sometimes called *dilatation*) is the opening of the cervix, which allows the infant to pass out of the uterus and into the vaginal birth canal. Dilation is measured in centimeters, which are estimated during vaginal examinations by manual palpation. Labor is divided into three stages:

- Stage I: Lasts from the onset of labor through complete dilation and effacement of the cervix (Figure 34-15, *B*). During this time, uterine contractions become longer, stronger, and closer together until complete dilation and effacement occur and pushing begins. Stage I is divided into early active (up to 3 cm dilation and 80% to 100% effaced), active (4 to 7 cm dilation and completion of effacement), and transition (8 to 10 cm dilation). The average length of time for primigravidas in stage I is 9 to 11 hours.
- Stage II: Lasts from complete dilation and effacement of the cervix through the birth of the fetus (Figure 34-15, *C*). This is the pushing stage, which lasts approximately 1 hour for primigravidas.
- Stage III: Lasts from the birth of the fetus through expulsion of the placenta (Figure 34-15, *D*). This occurs approximately 20 minutes after the birth of the baby.

Pregnancy Complications

Infertility and Abortions

Fertility problems in women can occur for many different reasons, including a history of STIs that have caused scarring or adhesions of the fallopian tubes, failure to ovulate or irregular ovulation, congenital anomalies of the reproductive organs, endometriosis, medications that reduce fertility, and advancing age.

Problems in becoming pregnant can occur at several points in time, the first being abnormal fertilization. Some couples are unable to have a child because of the inability of the sperm and the ovum to unite. Ovarian factors are not totally understood; however, it is known that as women age, the ova become less viable. If the couple is able to fertilize an egg, another problem that can occur is improper implantation.

An *ectopic* pregnancy is one that occurs outside the uterus. Although an ectopic pregnancy can develop on or near the ovary or in the abdominal cavity, most occur in the fallopian tube. As the zygote develops, the cells that form the placenta begin to erode the muscle layer of the tube, bleeding and destruction of the muscular layer occur, and the tube ruptures. Rupture of the fallopian tube containing an ectopic pregnancy is a serious event that requires immediate surgical intervention to prevent serious hemorrhage.

Once a woman becomes pregnant, problems can occur with carrying the infant to term. Interruption of a pregnancy before the term of fetal viability is called an *abortion,* which is identified in lay terms as a miscarriage. There are several different categories of naturally occurring abortions, including the following:

- Spontaneous: No identifiable cause.
- Complete: Complete expulsion of both fetus and placenta with no medical intervention.
- Incomplete: Expulsion of only parts of the fetus and placenta; a D&C must be done to remove the remaining pieces or the mother will continue to bleed.
- Missed: The fetus dies in utero and must be removed surgically.
- Threatened: Cervical bleeding occurs, but dilation does not, and the pregnancy continues uninterrupted.

It is estimated that 1 in 3 pregnancies terminates by a naturally occurring abortion, and in most cases, the causes are not clear. Chromosomal anomalies frequently are detected in an aborted fetus or placenta and may be the primary reason for the abortion. Spontaneous abortion is the loss of a pregnancy before week 20 of fetal development. Common causes are defective development of the embryo, abnormalities of the placenta, endocrine disorders, malnutrition, infection, drug reaction, blood group incompatibilities, severe trauma, and shock. Symptoms include vaginal bleeding of varying degrees of severity and lower abdominal cramping that progresses to cervical dilation with rupture of membranes and complete expulsion of the products of conception. Induced abortions involve evacuation of the uterus at the request of the mother.

Listeria Infection

Listeria monocytogenes (Listeria) is a bacterium that can be found in soft cheeses, hot dogs, and luncheon meats. Most healthy people exposed to *Listeria* organisms don't become ill. However, pregnant women, newborns, older adults, and people with weakened immune systems are more susceptible. In some cases a *Listeria* infection can lead to life-threatening complications, including the following:

- A generalized blood infection (*septicemia*)
- Inflammation of the membranes and fluid surrounding the brain (*meningitis*)

Complications of a *Listeria* infection may be most severe for an unborn baby; a *Listeria* infection early in the pregnancy may lead to miscarriage. *Listeria* organisms can cross the placental barrier, and infections in late pregnancy may cause stillbirth, or an infant may die shortly after birth. This is why pregnant women must avoid potentially contaminated foods.

Placental Abnormalities

Pregnancy complications can occur because of the site of placental implantation. In *placenta previa,* the placenta implants in the lower uterine segment. If routine sonograms diagnose placenta previa early in a pregnancy, the placenta may migrate upward with uterine wall enlargement. However, if the previa persists throughout the pregnancy and the placenta is implanted on or near the cervix when the mother goes into labor, dilation and effacement of the cervix can cause the placenta to tear loose (Figure 34-16). Complete dilation and effacement cannot progress without serious oxygen deprivation to the fetus and hemorrhaging in the mother. The signs of placenta previa include painless, bright red vaginal bleeding during or near the last trimester. The diagnosis is confirmed with a sonogram. A

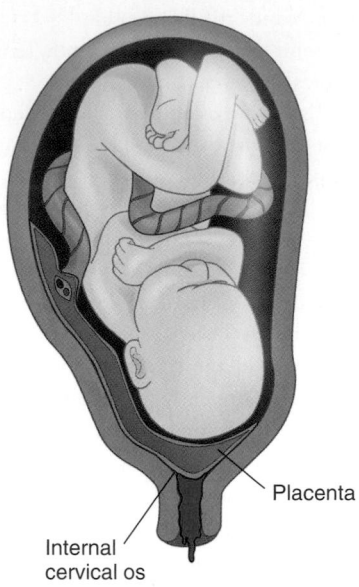

Placenta

Internal
cervical os

FIGURE 34-16 Placenta previa.

cesarean section is done as close to term as possible to prevent complications in both mother and fetus.

Another placental problem, *abruptio placentae,* occurs when the placenta detaches from the uterine wall. The pregnant woman reports an acute onset of severe abdominal pain; firmness on palpation and hemorrhaging from the vagina also are factors. She also shows signs of shock, including tachycardia, a thready pulse, hypotension, and clammy, cool skin. The fetus shows signs of distress from lack of oxygen, including a decreased fetal heart rate and lack of movement. This is a true obstetric emergency and requires immediate cesarean delivery to save the infant and the mother.

Maternal Disorders
Gestational Diabetes. Any degree of impaired glucose tolerance during pregnancy is diagnosed as gestational diabetes mellitus (GDM). Gestational diabetes occurs in 5% to 9% of pregnancies, and the number is growing, primarily because of the increased incidence of obesity. Women at greatest risk are over age 30; have a family history of diabetes mellitus; had a body mass index (BMI) greater than 25 before pregnancy; and are members of certain racial groups, including African-Americans, Hispanics, and Native Americans.

The American Congress of Obstetricians and Gynecologists (ACOG) recommends that all pregnant patients be screened for GDM at 24 to 28 weeks' gestation using a 50-g, 1-hour glucose challenge test. The patient is given a concentrated drink equivalent to 50 g of glucose, and blood is drawn 1 hour afterward to measure blood glucose levels. A level higher than 140 mg/dL indicates GDM, but these patients are retested with a 3-hour glucose challenge. Blood is checked every hour for 3 hours after the patient drinks a concentrated glucose solution, and elevation in two of these blood draws is considered a positive result for GDM.

It is very important that women diagnosed with GDM carefully monitor their blood glucose levels regularly using a glucometer. This requires the patient to place a drop of blood on a machine that

analyzes it and reports the current blood glucose level. Patients may be able to achieve normal glucose levels with diet therapy and exercise. However, studies indicate that the best medical treatment for GDM is insulin therapy. The mother's problem with glucose metabolism typically goes away after the birth of the infant, but these women are at greater risk of developing diabetes mellitus type 2 later in life. Patient education on healthy lifestyles, including the importance of a nutritious diet, weight management, and exercise, is needed to help prevent adult-onset diabetes mellitus type 2.

The medical assistant's responsibilities include performing blood tests as ordered, completing routine urinary dipstick tests at each visit, and providing referral to a dietitian for help with diet therapy management.

Hypertension. Most women who develop hypertension during pregnancy have normal blood pressure before becoming pregnant and also during early pregnancy but develop hypertension in the second half of the pregnancy. Gestational hypertension (pregnancy-induced hypertension) can be mild to severe and occurs in approximately 10% to 15% of pregnancies.

If hypertension is accompanied by proteinuria after 20 weeks of pregnancy, the patient is diagnosed with *pre-eclampsia,* or toxemia, which occurs in approximately 2% to 3% of pregnancies. Pre-eclampsia usually shows up unexpectedly during a routine prenatal visit. The patient has an elevated blood pressure with protein or albumin in the urine and may also have uremia, altered liver function, and a reduced platelet count. The birth of the baby cures pre-eclampsia, with blood pressure returning to normal within a few days of delivery. However, if indicators of pre-eclampsia occur early in the pregnancy, the provider attempts to balance the need to prevent premature birth of the infant with what is best for the mother. The baby is monitored with routine **nonstress tests (NSTs)**, sonograms, and maternal reports of fetal movement. If pre-eclampsia persists, the patient is at risk of severe headaches, vision disturbances, oliguria, and convulsions either before or during labor, and an emergency cesarean section may be required to prevent serious maternal complications.

The medical assistant is responsible for monitoring the pregnant woman's vital signs at each visit, including any report of a sudden weight gain that may indicate edema, and for performing routine urine dipstick tests. Complete and accurate documentation of findings helps alert the provider to possible problems with hypertension.

MENOPAUSE

Menopause is the permanent ending of menstruation as a result of cessation of ovarian function. It usually occurs between 45 and 55 years of age but can occur as early as the 30s and as late as the 60s. Menses may stop suddenly, flow may decrease over time, or the time between menses may lengthen until complete cessation occurs. Menopause can be diagnosed only retrospectively. Only after 12 months of amenorrhea is a woman said to be in menopause, and the years after this are called *postmenopause.*

Perimenopause begins when hormone-related changes start to appear, and it lasts until the final menses; this can be as long as 10 years before menopause. During this time, women are still ovulating, but the uneven rise and fall of estrogen and progesterone may cause symptoms. Some women experience few or no symptoms, whereas others have hot flashes, concentration problems, mood swings, irritability, migraines, vaginal dryness, urinary incontinence, dry skin, and sleep disorders. Treatment focuses on relieving these signs and symptoms. The provider may prescribe very low-dose oral contraceptives (Loestrin 1/20, Alesse) to balance estrogen and progesterone levels or short-term hormone replacement therapy (HRT) (e.g., Premarin, Prempro) to treat symptoms. The provider also may recommend that the patient consume soy products or take soy supplements for a plant source of estrogen. Vitamin E may help alleviate hot flashes, and vitamin B_6 helps create natural serotonin, a neurotransmitter that affects mood. Other methods that help alleviate symptoms include avoiding caffeine and spicy foods to reduce hot flashes, using relaxation techniques to aid with sleep disorders, consuming a low-fat diet high in calcium and vitamin D, and performing regular weight-bearing exercise to help prevent osteoporosis and heart disease.

Medical treatment of menopause focuses on managing uncomfortable symptoms and preventing conditions associated with a drop in blood levels of estrogen, such as osteoporosis and coronary artery disease. Providers traditionally treated perimenopause and menopause with long-term HRT for most women; however, studies indicate that although HRT does protect the menopausal woman from osteoporosis, hip fracture, and colon cancer, at the same time it increases the risk of heart attack, stroke, breast cancer, and blood clotting. It is now recommended that providers prescribe HRT to meet individual patient needs over a short term (i.e., no longer than 5 years) rather than as routine treatment for all menopausal women. Studies show that the risk for heart disease and other complications increases after 5 years of HRT. The medical assistant must be aware of the provider's recommendations regarding HRT.

Other medications that may be prescribed include antidepressants, such as venlafaxine or fluoxetine (Prozac, Sarafem), to prevent hot flashes. Gabapentin (Neurontin) and clonidine (Catapres) also may be prescribed to reduce the frequency of hot flashes. Because the development of osteoporosis is a concern in perimenopausal and postmenopausal women, the provider may prescribe alendronate (Fosamax), risedronate (Actonel), or ibandronate (Boniva) to reduce bone loss and the risk of fracture. Another drug that may be used to improve postmenopausal bone density is raloxifene (Evista); however, hot flashes are a common side effect of this medication. Vaginal dryness can be treated with estrogen administered locally by vaginal tablet, ring, or cream, or the patient can use K-Y Jelly or some other vaginal moisturizer as a lubricant.

CRITICAL THINKING APPLICATION   **34-5**

Rose Conrad, a 53-year-old patient of Dr. Beck, calls because she read recently that the hormone replacement therapy she has been taking for 3 years may be dangerous. Dr. Beck has reviewed her case and agrees that if she is concerned, she can stop taking the medication; however, she recommends that Mrs. Conrad try some alternative therapies. What suggestions might Dr. Beck make for nonpharmaceutical treatment of perimenopausal symptoms?

THE MEDICAL ASSISTANT'S ROLE IN GYNECOLOGIC AND OBSTETRIC PROCEDURES

As the female progresses from menarche through the childbearing years and then into menopause, her medical concerns change, and the focal point of the physical examination may change as well. The overall goal of the medical office is to keep her physically and mentally healthy. Being able to assist the provider in identifying possible problems before the problem becomes a threat to the patient's health is a major priority of care. This is best accomplished by listening to the patient. Remember, to the patient, there is no such thing as a routine examination.

Examination Preparation

An annual or semiannual examination of the female reproductive system is done to ensure normality of the reproductive organs or to diagnose and treat abnormalities of these organs. Before the provider begins the examination, the medical assistant should obtain a complete gynecologic history. After documenting the patient's history and chief complaint, the medical assistant should prepare the room and the patient for the examination (see Procedure 34-1).

The following should be included in the gynecologic history:

- Age at menarche
- Details about the regularity of the menstrual cycle; the amount and duration of menstrual flow; and a history of menstrual disturbances and their treatment
- Any current indicators of infection, including vaginal discharge, pelvic pain, urinary difficulties, and so on
- Feedback on any breast abnormalities and the date of the patient's last mammogram
- Date of the last Pap test
- Sexual history; STI history
- Number of pregnancies and live births
- Date of LMP
- Lifestyle factors, including diet, exercise, smoking, alcohol use, and so on

The physical examination during a first prenatal visit includes an overall assessment of the woman's health status, including vital signs, weight, and urinalysis. The medical assistant must prepare the patient and also the supplies and equipment necessary to obtain pelvic measurements, perform serologic tests, and prepare for laboratory tests (Procedure 34-4). The provider assesses heart, lung, and thyroid function and performs a physical examination to rule out any other abnormality. Next, the provider performs an obstetric examination that includes palpation of the mother's abdomen, measurement of the height of the uterus, and an internal or pelvic examination.

A series of blood tests also is performed during the initial prenatal visit. In follow-up prenatal visits, the medical assistant should collect a urine specimen for urinalysis, weigh the patient, measure her blood pressure, and answer questions about diet and health habits. The mother should gain approximately 10 to 12 pounds in the first half of pregnancy and another 15 to 17 pounds during the second half. Experts believe that a healthy weight gain is somewhere between 25 and 35 pounds. The baby's heart tones can be picked up through a specialized method, called *Doppler ultrasound,* somewhere between 9 and 12 weeks' gestation. Once recorded, the fetal heart rate is assessed at each subsequent visit. Ultrasound exams are typically done once during the first trimester and then again between weeks 18 and 20 to assess fetal development, confirm the age of the fetus and proper growth, and to determine the gender of the baby. Prenatal blood and laboratory tests include the following:

- Hematocrit and hemoglobin levels to check for anemia.
- Blood type and Rh with antibody screening for possible Rh incompatibility.
- Rubella titer to determine whether the mother is immune to German measles; rubella infection during pregnancy can cause multiple birth defects, including deafness, vision disorders, and mental retardation.
- Syphilis screening; if the result is positive, antibiotic treatment is initiated to protect the fetus from congenital syphilis.
- Hepatitis B screening because this virus can be passed to the fetus in utero.
- HIV screening is suggested; if the result is positive, treatment of the mother greatly reduces the risk of transmission to the fetus.
- Pap test to check for abnormal cervical cells.
- Gonorrhea and chlamydia cultures to prevent infection of the baby at birth.
- Urinalysis to detect protein, white blood cells, or glucose.
- Maternal blood screen (at 15 to 20 weeks) to detect any risk of fetal chromosomal disorders.
- Cystic fibrosis carrier screening.
- Group B streptococcus culture of the lower vagina for strep B infection, performed between weeks 32 and 36; if the result is positive, the mother is treated with antibiotics to prevent fetal exposure during vaginal birth.
- If indicated, an NST to evaluate the fetal heart rate; the mother is attached to a fetal monitor, with the goal of seeing accelerations in the fetal heart rate with movement; performed in a hospital.
- Stress test or oxytocin challenge test (OCT) if the NST is abnormal; a small amount of oxytocin (which causes the uterus to contract) is administered intravenously while the mother is attached to a fetal monitor to see how the fetus responds to the normal stresses of labor; this test is performed in a hospital.

Any concerns the patient has should be noted and reported to the provider. The medical assistant should be prepared to suggest community resources that can provide assistance to new parents, such as childbirth and parenting classes; infant cardiopulmonary resuscitation (CPR) courses; nutritional counseling if needed; and contact information for the Special Supplemental Nutrition Program for Women, Infants, and Children (WIC), which helps lower-income expectant mothers get nutritious food.

The examination room must be adequately equipped and the surroundings pleasant. A dressing area with an adjacent toilet should be provided. The dressing area should ensure privacy and should be equipped with tissues and sanitary protection items, in addition to disposable examination gowns and drapes. The medical assistant should restock supplies as needed throughout the day.

PROCEDURE 34-4 Instruct and Prepare a Patient for Procedures and/or Treatments: Assist with a Prenatal Examination

Goal: To promote a healthy pregnancy for the mother and fetus and to screen for potential problems.

EQUIPMENT and SUPPLIES

- Patient's health record
- Scale with height measure
- Sphygmomanometer
- Stethoscope
- Tape measure
- Doppler fetoscope
- Ultrasound gel
- Urine specimen container
- Disposable examination gloves, vaginal speculum, and lubricant if vaginal examination is to be performed
- Sexually transmitted infection (STI) test setups
- Laboratory requisition slips
- Biohazard waste container
- Biohazard bags for specimen transport
- Patient education materials

PROCEDURAL STEPS

1. Sanitize your hands and assemble the necessary equipment.
2. Greet the patient, introduce yourself, and verify the patient's identity by name and date of birth.
3. Weigh the patient and record the weight.
   PURPOSE: An expectant mother's weight reflects both maternal nutritional status and fetal growth; an unusual weight gain may indicate fluid retention.
4. Apply gloves and collect a urine specimen and perform a urinalysis to detect protein, glucose, or ketones in the urine; remove gloves, dispose in a biohazard waste container, and sanitize hands. Record the urinalysis results.
   PURPOSE: Protein, glucose, or ketones in the urine may indicate problems with the pregnancy.
5. Measure and record the patient's blood pressure.
6. Instruct the patient to disrobe from the waist down and to put on a gown open to the front so that the uterine fundal height can be measured.
   PURPOSE: The provider will palpate the abdomen and may use a tape measure to assess the fundal height as a determinant of fetal growth.
7. Assist the patient onto the examination table, if needed, and provide a drape for privacy.
8. Assist the provider as needed throughout the examination. If a Doppler fetoscope is to be used to listen to the fetal heart tones, apply a liberal amount of ultrasound gel to the patient's abdomen and hand the fetoscope to the provider. After the procedure, clean the Doppler head with a paper towel and offer the patient tissues to wipe the gel off her abdomen.

9. After the examination is complete, assist the patient off the examination table; make sure to observe for signs of dizziness or problems with balance.
   PURPOSE: Lying supine or in the lithotomy position puts pressure on the aorta, which may result in momentary vertigo when the patient sits or stands.

10. Answer the patient's questions and provide patient education materials as needed.
    PURPOSE: To take advantage of "teaching moments" to provide information on diet, health habits, and community resources.

11. Apply gloves, collect and package all specimens for transport. Complete labels as needed.

12. Discard supplies and disinfect the equipment according to the manufacturer's guidelines.

13. Remove gloves and dispose in a biohazard waste container. Sanitize your hands.

14. Document the pertinent information in the patient's health record.
    PURPOSE: A procedure is not done until it is recorded.

Assisting with the Examination

The female reproductive system examination is probably the most emotionally charged medical experience the average woman undergoes. Even women with relatively sophisticated attitudes toward their bodies and sexuality may be embarrassed by the casual, impersonal approach of the medical team during this procedure. Many women fear the provider's findings. Anxieties and fears are best handled through explanations and by showing a genuine interest in the patient's concerns. The medical assistant is responsible for supporting the patient and assisting the provider during the procedure. The procedure should be fully explained to the patient to prevent unnecessary embarrassment and discomfort. During the explanation, the assistant has the opportunity to conduct patient teaching.

In preparation for the examination, the patient should empty her bladder, completely disrobe, and put on an examination gown that opens in the front. The patient should have been advised at the time the appointment was made not to douche or have sexual intercourse for 24 hours before the examination so that vaginal discharges can be evaluated properly and to ensure accurate results of cytologic studies.

Breast Examination

Begin the examination by assisting the patient into a sitting position and by adjusting the gown so that the breast tissue can be easily exposed. The provider will instruct the patient to place her arms above her head, and the assistant should be present to assist the patient if she has difficulty following these instructions. When the patient is instructed to assume a supine position, help the patient, adjust the gown, and drape as needed to assist the provider and to protect the patient's privacy. The foot rest should also be extended. A small pillow may be placed under the patient's head for comfort. When the examination is complete, the gown is readjusted to cover the breasts. The provider may choose to discuss breast self-examination with the patient at this time or may inform the patient that the medical assistant will be explaining the technique at the end of the examination (see Procedure 34-3).

Abdominal Examination

After the breasts have been examined, cover them and position the drape to allow the provider to palpate the abdomen; this is done to confirm normal symmetry and to detect any masses. In the case of pregnancy, the level of the fundus is measured to determine fetal growth. For this examination, the patient's arms should be placed at her sides to achieve better relaxation of the abdominal muscles.

Pelvic Examination

The medical assistant should remain in the examination room to provide reassurance to the patient and as legal protection for the provider while the patient's vaginal and perineal areas are examined. Furthermore, the lithotomy position is awkward to assume without assistance and may be embarrassing to the patient. Never place the patient in the lithotomy position until the provider is ready to begin the examination. When you assist the patient into the lithotomy position, always keep her totally covered.

You should stand at the patient's side so that you can observe the patient, yet still be able to move quickly if needed by the provider. First, the provider inspects the external genitalia and palpates the perineal body. The patient may be asked to bear down to show any muscular weaknesses that may be the result of lacerations of the perineal body during childbirth. A third-degree laceration may have involved the rectal sphincter and may cause rectal incontinence.

Next, the vaginal speculum, without lubrication, is inserted for examination of the cervix and the vaginal canal and for obtaining the Pap specimen. The speculum should be prewarmed with warm water. Have the patient take some deep breaths to help relax the abdominal muscles. The normal cervix points posteriorly and has smooth, pink, squamous epithelium. Abnormalities most frequently seen are ulcerations (erosions), **Bartholin's cysts**, and cervical polyps. Because erosions cannot be palpated, inspection is the only method of detecting them. Healed lacerations from childbirth are common in a **multiparous** patient. Pregnancy increases the size of the cervix, and hormone deficiency causes it to atrophy. The vaginal wall is reddish pink and has a corrugated appearance from the overlapping tissue (rugae) lining. Vaginal infections change the appearance of the vaginal mucosa. After the Pap specimen has been obtained, you may be responsible for labeling the specimen and preparing it for transport to the cytology laboratory. Be sure to follow laboratory instructions during the preparation to avoid having to repeat the examination.

After removal of the vaginal speculum, the provider does a bimanual examination; that is, two gloved fingers are lubricated with a water-soluble jelly (lubricant) and inserted into the vaginal canal,

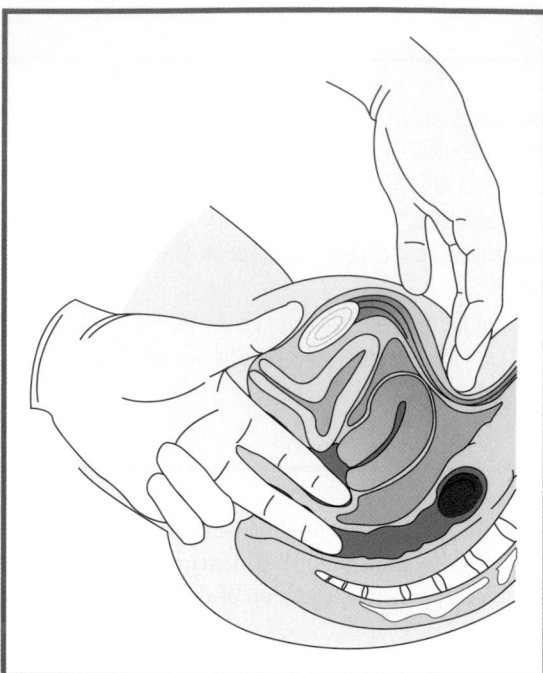

FIGURE 34-17 Bimanual examination.

and the other hand palpates the abdomen over the pelvic organs and the mons pubis (Figure 34-17). The uterus is examined for shape, size, and consistency, and its position is noted. A normal uterus is freely movable with limited discomfort. A laterally displaced uterus usually is the result of pelvic adhesions or displacement caused by a pelvic tumor. The fallopian tubes and ovaries are evaluated. Normal tubes and ovaries are difficult to palpate, which is why the provider may have to press firmly in the pelvic area, causing minor discomfort for the patient. A stool test for occult blood may also be done.

Postexamination Duties

When the examination is finished, help the patient into a sitting position and into the dressing room if needed. Following the Standard Precautions established by the Occupational Safety and Health Administration (OSHA), remove the examination equipment and supplies while the patient is dressing so that when the provider returns to talk to the patient, the room is neat and clean. Once the patient has left, the room should be sanitized, disinfected, and restocked as necessary so it is ready for the next patient.

Safety Alert

Instruments that come in contact with a patient, including vaginal speculums, should be sanitized, disinfected, and sterilized before they are used for another patient. If the instrument does not penetrate tissue, it can be stored under clean or medically aseptic conditions. Some providers prefer to use disposable speculums for routine pelvic examinations. Instruments that penetrate tissue (e.g., uterine biopsy punch, uterine tenaculum, cervical dilators and sounds) must be sterilized, stored, and handled under sterile conditions.

DIAGNOSTIC TESTING

Sonography

Sonography is a technique in which high-frequency sound waves are used to produce images of the body's soft tissues. It can distinguish between cysts and tumors, and it is used during pregnancy to determine the number of fetuses and their age and gender; fetal abnormalities; and the position of the placenta. The skin over the area to be studied is coated with conductive gel or lotion, and the transducer is pressed lightly against the area. Sound waves emitted by the transducer bounce off the structure being studied and are converted into electrical impulses that create a picture for analysis. The mother may be asked to drink several glasses of water 1 hour before the procedure so the full bladder can be used as a reference point.

Sonograph technology is divided into two methods. The grayscale image converts sound wave echoes into graphs or dots that form pictures of organs and blood vessels (Figure 34-18). The Doppler method converts the ultrasound into audible sounds that are heard as pulsations and is used in the obstetrician's office to monitor the heartbeat of the fetus. Color-coded Doppler signals, three-dimensional imaging, and contrast medium enhancement of ultrasound images provide more accurate images and data on organ structure and function.

Fetal Diagnostic Tests

- *Chorionic villus sampling:* Chorionic villi are tiny placental projections, the cells of which have the same genetic material found in fetal cells. Cellular screening at 8 to 12 weeks' gestation provides early detection of genetic or chromosomal disorders. Potential complications include accidental abortion, infection, bleeding, and fetal limb deformities. Results are available within several days.
- *Amniocentesis:* This procedure involves needle aspiration of approximately 2 tablespoons of amniotic fluid after week 14 of pregnancy to detect genetic and chromosomal abnormalities or inherited metabolic disorders (Figure 34-19). Potential complications include miscarriage, fetal injury, infection, premature labor, and maternal hemorrhage. Results take up to 2 weeks.

Mammography

Mammography is a specialized x-ray technique that provides images of breast tissue and is performed to identify abnormal masses that would go undetected in a breast palpation examination (Figure 34-20).

Special x-ray equipment is used that compresses the breast firmly during each exposure. Compression is essential to provide the high degree of detail needed to visualize the significant but often subtle signs of a tumor. This process is not usually painful, but some patients, especially those with fibrocystic breast disease, may find it uncomfortable. If pain persists after the examination, ibuprofen is recommended for relief.

Patients with breast implants should follow routine guidelines for mammography; however, implants may make diagnosing breast cancer more difficult because they tend to obscure the breast image. It is recommended that women with implants have mammograms done at a facility where the radiologist is experienced at interpreting

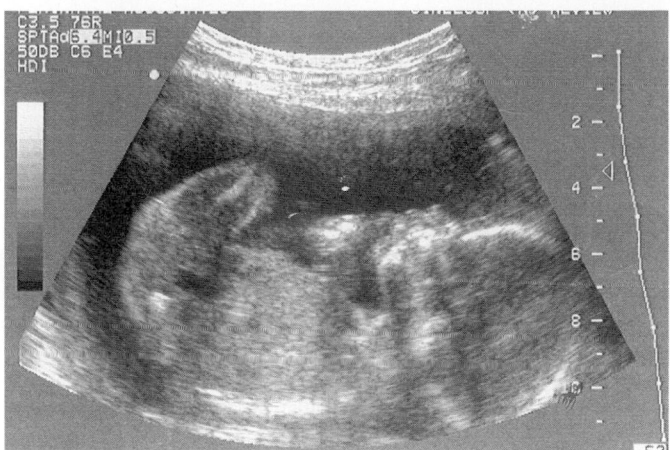

FIGURE 34-18 Sonogram of a fetus.

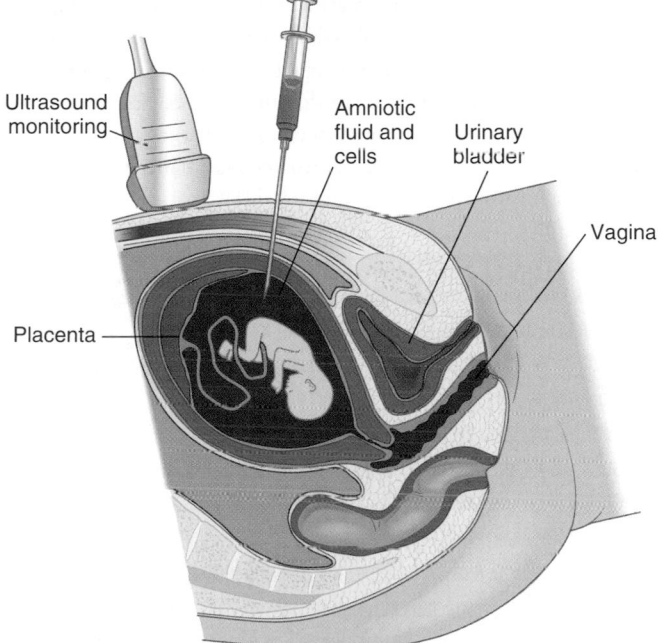

FIGURE 34-19 Amniocentesis.

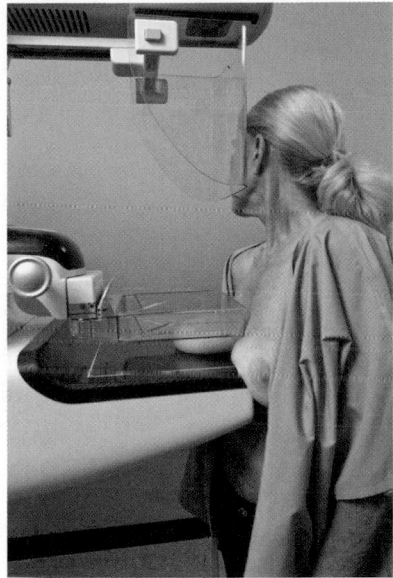

FIGURE 34-20 Proper position of the breast for a mammogram. (From Bontrager KL, Lampignano J: *Textbook of radiographic positioning and related anatomy,* ed 8, St Louis, 2014, Mosby.)

these particular studies. In addition, women with silicone implants should have an MRI examination to check for recurrence or rupture of the implants.

In preparation for mammography, patients are instructed not to use underarm deodorant and not to apply powder or lotion on the breasts or axillary areas. These products may contain ingredients that produce artifacts on mammographic images. This is especially true of antiperspirants that contain aluminum salts. When previous mammograms are available, every effort must be made to obtain them because comparative evaluation often is significant in the radiologic diagnosis.

Pregnancy Testing

Pregnancy tests are designed to detect HCG, which is secreted after the ovum has been fertilized. It appears in the blood and urine of pregnant women as early as 10 days after conception. Once pregnancy has been confirmed, the patient undergoes a complete medical and obstetric examination, which includes a number of laboratory

tests. The estimated date of delivery (EDD) is calculated at the first office visit (the EDD frequently is called the *expected due date*). The EDD typically is determined with a gestational wheel (Figure 34-21), or it may be calculated by the electronic health record (EHR) software. However, most obstetricians rely on fetal sonograms to determine the expected due date.

CLOSING COMMENTS

Patient Education

Depending on the provider's policies, the medical assistant can distribute patient education materials that promote sexual health and prevent gynecologic and obstetric disorders throughout the patient's life.

A woman who is planning a pregnancy or who has just found out that she is pregnant may benefit from some simple guidelines for healthy living.

- *Nutrition:* Before pregnancy, emphasize the need for folic acid to prevent **neural tube defects**. The woman can take a supplement or can eat dark green, leafy vegetables. Many women have iron-deficiency anemia, and eating foods high in iron (red meat, spinach, or enriched cereal) is helpful. A pregnant woman must meet the calcium needs of both herself and her fetus; therefore, she needs about 1,000 mg of calcium a day. Most pregnant women should consume about 2,500 calories a day. Women of average weight should gain 25 to 35 pounds, but underweight women should gain 28 to 40 pounds for a healthy infant.
- *Alcohol:* Alcohol passes through the placenta to the fetus and can cause serious problems. No one knows how much is safe, so it is a good idea for pregnant women to avoid alcohol completely.
- *Smoking:* Smoking can cause premature birth and low-birth-weight full-term infants. Smoking is linked to an increased risk of otitis media, heart problems, and upper respiratory infection in infants, and also to sudden infant death syndrome

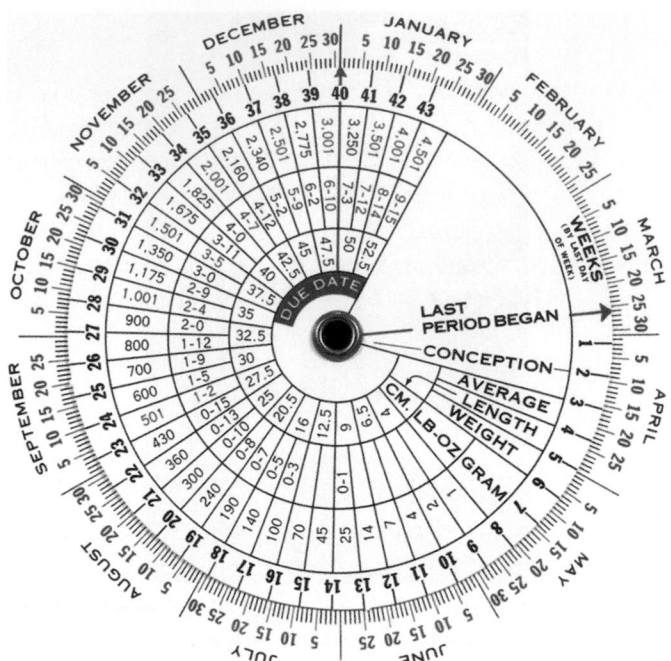

FIGURE 34-21 Gestational wheel. (From Jarvis C: *Physical examination and health assessment,* ed 6, St Louis, 2012, Saunders.)

(SIDS). Pregnant women should not smoke and should not be exposed to secondhand smoke.

- *Medicine:* All chemicals pass through the placenta; therefore, a pregnant woman should never take any medicine (even over-the-counter drugs) without the knowledge and approval of her obstetrician. If the medical assistant is managing telephone screening, having a list of provider-approved medications next to the phone helps in answering patients' questions.
- *STI screening:* STI screening should be done before a woman becomes pregnant. Many STIs are asymptomatic in women but treatable. Infants are at risk for serious health problems if exposed to certain STIs in utero or during the birth process.

Advantages of Breast-Feeding

For the Infant
- Completely digestible nutrition source for the infant
- Protects against gastrointestinal infection
- Protects against food allergies
- Provides newborn with mother's antibodies to infectious disease
- Associated with higher infant IQ
- Promotes muscular eye and facial development
- Promotes maternal-infant bonding

For the Mother
- Simple, safe, and economical
- Promotes uterine involution, which reduces postpartum bleeding
- Reduces the incidence of breast cancer
- Promotes maternal-infant bonding

Pregnant women usually are searching for information about pregnancy and wellness both during and after the birth. Use the waiting room as an education center and provide videos, books, and

pamphlets on health issues and parenting. Keeping an up-to-date list of community education and support programs also is helpful. The obstetric patient who is interested in breast-feeding may need education and support to be successful. The American College of Pediatricians recommends breast milk as the optimum food for newborns. Referral to a breast-feeding support group or a lactation consultant can help a new mother solve her breast-feeding problems and find answers to her questions.

Legal and Ethical Issues

Many ethical and legal issues arise as a result of missed communication. Listen to what every patient reports, and write down any information that will assist the provider in treating the patient. The issue may appear to be an insignificant problem, but to the patient, it may be a major concern. Let the provider be the judge of whether the problem is relevant. As the patient's advocate and the provider's assistant, the medical assistant plays an important role in establishing good communication as a vital link in patient care.

Confidentiality is crucial in dealing with obstetric and gynecologic disorders. Only healthcare professionals directly involved in the patient's care should know the purpose of the patient's visit, diagnosis, or treatment. Maintaining patient confidentiality is not just an ethical responsibility; in the case of HIV status, it is a legal requirement.

Professional Behaviors

The medical assistant may be in the position to recognize and provide assistance to women who are being mistreated. Battered women seldom come forward and tell healthcare workers they are being abused. If the patient reports such problems to the medical assistant, or if an abusive situation is suspected, the medical assistant should not hesitate to report this information to the provider. The American Medical Association (AMA) has developed guidelines to help caregivers recognize victims of abuse.

- *Know what to look for:* Suspicious findings include multiple injuries at different sites, especially areas that normally are covered by clothing. Also, the patient may be frightened, anxious, and passive and may have a history of "accidents."
- *Know what to ask when obtaining a patient history:* Even patients who show no signs of abuse should be asked whether they have ever been in an abusive relationship; if verbal arguments ever become physical; if their partner acts differently when drinking or using drugs; and if their partner is overprotective and jealous.
- *Know what to say and do:* A battered woman suffers both physical and emotional abuse. She may begin to believe that she deserves to be mistreated, and she needs unconditional and nonjudgmental emotional support from the healthcare worker. She needs to be treated with warmth and respect and encouraged to develop a plan of action to deal with the next violent episode. Suggestions include having immediate access to important documents, keys, money, and transportation; the address of a safe house; and phone numbers for the police and local domestic violence hotline, if available. The National Domestic Violence Hotline can be reached at 1-800-799-SAFE (7233) or at www.thehotline.org/. It provides 24-hour help for victims seeking local shelters. Contact information for local shelters or sources of help could be posted in patient bathrooms to encourage those in need to turn to these services.

SUMMARY OF SCENARIO

Having worked with obstetric and gynecologic patients, Betsy has learned that a wide range of disorders and conditions can affect a woman's health and pregnancy. She also has learned how to assist with a number of different diagnostic procedures performed in the ambulatory care setting. An integral role of the medical assistant in the OB/GYN practice is reinforcing the provider's patient education efforts. Betsy enjoys this part of the practice but realizes that it involves extensive reading and discussion with Dr. Beck to determine her preferred method of teaching. Betsy stays up to date on current contraceptive practices by attending local workshops offered by the American Association of Medical Assistants (AAMA), along with regional conferences. She has networked with other CMAs to develop a comprehensive community resource guide for obstetric and gynecologic patients in the practice and has created an educational center in the patient waiting room. Betsy recognizes that she must continue to learn about new practices and recent research to help provide the best possible care for the women in Dr. Beck's practice.

SUMMARY OF LEARNING OBJECTIVES

1. **Define, spell, and pronounce the terms listed in the vocabulary.**
   Spelling and pronouncing medical terms correctly reinforce the medical assistant's credibility. Knowing the definitions of these terms promotes confidence in communication with patients and co-workers.

2. **Explain the anatomy and physiology of the female reproductive system.**
   The female reproductive system is made up of the external genitalia and the internal organs, including the vagina; the cervix, which must dilate and efface for vaginal birth of a child; the uterus; the fallopian tubes; and the ovaries, which mature and produce ova.

3. **Trace the ovum through the three phases of menstruation.**
   The follicular phase matures a graafian follicle so that an ovum can be released at the same time the endometrial wall is thickening; the luteal phase causes extensive growth of the endometrium; if conception does not occur, the menstrual cycle begins with the breakdown of the endometrium and menstrual flow.

4. **Compare and contrast current contraceptive methods.**
   Barrier contraceptive methods include the use of condoms, a diaphragm, a cervical cap, or a cervical sponge; all of these are relatively inexpensive and reversible, but they must be used with each instance of intercourse. Two general types of IUDs are available to inhibit fertilization and prevent the embryo from implanting in the uterine wall. Hormonal contraceptives include Depo-Provera injections, the Implanon or Nexplanon implants, oral and patch contraceptives, and the vaginal ring, all of which are very effective but have side effects and contraindications. (See Table 34-1.)

5. **Summarize menstrual disorders and conditions.**
   Menstrual disorders include amenorrhea and oligomenorrhea; abnormal menstrual bleeding includes menorrhagia and metrorrhagia; endometriosis is characterized by the presence of functional endometrial tissue outside the uterus.

6. **Distinguish among different types of gynecologic infections.**
   Gynecologic infections include candidiasis; BV; cervicitis; and PID, which is any acute or chronic infection of the reproductive system that ascends from the vagina (vaginitis), cervix (cervicitis), uterus (endometritis), fallopian tubes (salpingitis), or ovaries (oophoritis). (See Table 34-2.)

7. **Do the following related to benign and malignant tumors of the female reproductive system:**
   - *Differentiate between benign and malignant neoplasms of the female reproductive system.*
     Benign tumors of the reproductive system include uterine fibroids, ovarian cysts, the hormonal disease of polycystic ovary syndrome, and fibrocystic breast disease, the presence of multiple palpable nodules in the breasts. Malignant tumors include cervical, endometrial, and ovarian cancers that vary in their diagnostic features and symptoms. Breast cancer can have multiple origins. Treatment of all forms of reproductive cancer depends on the staging and grading of the tumors.
   - *Prepare for and assist with the female examination, including obtaining a Papanicolaou (Pap) test.*
     Procedure 34-1 explains the steps for assisting with examination of a female patient.
   - *Demonstrate patient preparation for a LEEP.*
     Procedure 34-2 describes how to prepare a patient for cryosurgery.
   - *Teach the patient the technique for breast self-examination.*
     Procedure 34-3 explains how to teach breast self-examination.

8. **Compare the positional disorders of the pelvic region.**
   Positional disorders of the pelvic region include cystocele or rectocele, which causes protrusion of the bladder or the rectum into the vaginal wall, and uterine prolapse, in which the cervix or uterus drops into the vaginal area. Kegel exercises can help improve these problems, but if they are severe, all three structural abnormalities can be corrected with surgery.

9. **Summarize the process of pregnancy and parturition.**
   Pregnancy occurs when the ovum and the sperm meet in the fallopian tube and a zygote is formed. The zygote implants in the uterine wall, and the placenta begins to form, which provides hormonal support for the pregnancy. The fetus is surrounded by an amniotic sac and floats in amniotic fluid. Oxygen and nutrients for the fetus pass through the placenta to the umbilical cord. The embryonic period ends at 12 weeks; by then, all tissues and organs have developed. During the remainder of the pregnancy, the organs mature and begin to function, and the fetus grows.

Continued

SUMMARY OF LEARNING OBJECTIVES—*continued*

Pregnancy is divided into three trimesters. The first trimester is a crucial time for fetal organ development; the second trimester brings quickening and many physiologic changes in the mother; during the third trimester, the fetal organ systems mature. The three stages of labor are dilation and effacement of the cervix, birth, and expulsion of the placenta.

10. **Describe the common complications of pregnancy.**

    Complications of pregnancy include potential loss of the pregnancy as a result of different types of abortions (miscarriages). Placental abnormalities include placenta previa, in which the placenta covers the cervical os, and abruptio placentae, in which the placenta breaks away from the uterine wall. Both cause maternal hemorrhage, threaten fetal oxygen supply, and require a cesarean birth to protect the fetus and mother. Maternal disorders include GDM, which requires dietary changes and possible insulin therapy, and hypertension, which may progress to pre-eclampsia, a life-threatening rise in blood pressure accompanied by edema, uremia, and possibly seizure activity.

11. **Specify the signs, symptoms, and treatments of conditions related to menopause.**

    Menopause is the permanent ending of menstruation caused by the cessation of ovarian function. Perimenopause begins when hormone-related changes start to appear and lasts until the final menses. Some women experience few or no symptoms, whereas others have hot flashes, concentration problems, mood swings, irritability, migraines, vaginal dryness, urinary incontinence, dry skin, and sleep disorders. The provider may prescribe low-dose oral contraceptives or HRT, weight-bearing exercise, soy products or vitamin supplements, dietary changes, and medication to manage hot flashes, mood swings, vaginal dryness, and to prevent osteoporosis.

12. **Outline the medical assistant's role in gynecologic and reproductive examinations and demonstrate how to assist with a prenatal examination.**

    The medical assistant prepares the patient for the examination, equips the room, makes sure supplies are available and properly prepared, positions and drapes the patient as needed, assists with the Pap smear or any other procedures, and provides support and understanding for the patient. (See Procedure 34-4.)

13. **Distinguish among diagnostic tests that may be done to evaluate the female reproductive system.**

    Diagnostic tests for the female reproductive system include sonography during pregnancy to determine the number of fetuses, fetal age and gender, fetal abnormalities, and the position of the placenta; chorionic villus sampling or amniocentesis; maternal blood tests to diagnose genetic disorders; mammography, which provides an x-ray image of the breast tissue to identify cancerous tumors; colposcopy procedures that permit visualization of abnormal cervical tissue for evaluation or biopsy; and a variety of tests done during pregnancy.

14. **Summarize patient education guidelines for obstetric patients, in addition to legal and ethical implications in a gynecology practice.**

    A woman who is planning a pregnancy or who has just found out she is pregnant may benefit from some simple guidelines about nutrition, alcohol consumption during pregnancy, medications that might affect the developing fetus, STI screenings, and breast-feeding.

    Confidentiality is crucial in dealing with obstetric and gynecologic disorders. Only healthcare professionals directly involved in the patient's care should know the purpose of the patient's visit, diagnosis, or treatment. The medical assistant may be in the position to recognize and provide assistance to women who are being mistreated. If the patient reports such problems to the medical assistant or if an abusive situation is suspected, the medical assistant should not hesitate to report this information to the provider.

CONNECTIONS

Study Guide Connection: Go to the Chapter 34 Study Guide. Read and complete the activities.

evolve Evolve Connection: Go to the Chapter 34 link at *evolve.elsevier.com/kinn* to complete the Chapter Review Quiz. Check out the other resources listed for this chapter to make the most of what you have learned from Assisting in Obstetrics and Gynecology.

ASSISTING IN PEDIATRICS

35

SCENARIO

Susie Kwong, CMA (AAMA), who has 2 years of experience, has accepted a new position with North Hills Pediatrics, a large practice with several physicians. Susie's primary responsibility will be to assist in the clinical area, but she also will have to rotate through the message screening center in the office. Office policy states that telephone screening employees should manage problems as much as possible. However, if patient callbacks are needed, they are to be referred to the physician on call that day by noon for morning calls and no later than 5 PM for afternoon calls. Although the physicians in the practice have developed specific guidelines for managing patient problems, Susie is anxious about this responsibility, so she asks to work with the screening staff for several days before she starts answering incoming calls.

While studying this chapter, think about the following questions:

- What other clinical responsibilities should Susie be prepared to perform?
- Are patient and caregiver health education an important part of delivering high-quality care in a pediatric setting?
- Does Susie need to be clinically competent to perform immunizations and document their administration?
- How can Susie maintain her skill level and continue to learn about patient-centered pediatric care?

LEARNING OBJECTIVES

1. Define, spell, and pronounce the terms listed in the vocabulary.
2. Describe childhood growth patterns.
3. Summarize the important features of the Denver II Developmental Screening Test.
4. Discuss developmental patterns and therapeutic approaches for pediatric patients.
5. Identify four different growth and development theories.
6. Consider the implications of postpartum depression.
7. Explain common pediatric gastrointestinal disorders, in addition to failure to thrive and obesity.
8. Describe disorders of the respiratory system in children.
9. Distinguish among pediatric infectious diseases.
10. Recognize the etiologic factors and signs and symptoms of the two primary pediatric inherited disorders.
11. Summarize the immunizations recommended for children by the Centers for Disease Control and Prevention (CDC).
12. Demonstrate how to document immunizations and maintain accurate immunization records.
13. Compare a well-child examination with a sick-child examination.
14. Outline the medical assistant's role in pediatric procedures.
15. Measure the circumference of an infant's head.
16. Obtain accurate length and weight measurements, and plot pediatric growth patterns.
17. Accurately measure pediatric vital signs, and perform vision screening.
18. Correctly apply a pediatric urine collection device.
19. Describe the characteristics and needs of the adolescent patient.
20. Specify child safety guidelines for injury prevention, and explain the management of suspected child abuse, neglect, or exploitation.
21. Summarize patient education guidelines for pediatric patients.
22. Discuss the legal and ethical implications in a pediatric practice.

VOCABULARY

anomaly (uh-nom'-uh-le) A congenital malformation that occurs during fetal development.

attenuated (uh-ten'-yuh-wat-ed) Weakened or changed; refers to the virulence of a pathogenic microorganism in reference to vaccine development.

autonomy (aw-ton'-oh-me) The ability to function independently.

congenital (kuhn-jen'-ih-tul) An anomaly or defect that is present at birth.

dermatome (dur'-muh-tohm) An area on the surface of the body that is innervated by nerve fibers from one spinal nerve root.

epiphyseal plate (ih-pe-fis'-e-uhl) A thin layer of cartilage located at the ends of a long bone where new bone forms.

excoriation (ek-skawr-e-ay′-shun) Inflammation and irritation of the skin.

fontanelle (fon-tan-el′) A space covered by thick membranes between the sutures of an infant's skull; called the baby's "soft spots"; there are both anterior and posterior fontanelles.

hydrocephaly (hi-dro-seh′-fuh-le) Enlargement of the cranium caused by abnormal accumulation of cerebrospinal fluid in the cerebral system.

laryngoscopy (lar-in-gahs′-kuh-pe) Visual examination of the voice box area through an endoscope equipped with a light and mirrors for illumination.

lymphadenopathy (lim-fad-en-op′-uh-the) An abnormal enlargement of a lymph gland.

microcephaly (mahy-kroh-seh′-fal-e) Small size of the head in relation to the rest of the body.

nonorganic (nahn-or-gan′-ik) Refers to not having an organic or physiologic cause; a disorder that does not have a cause that can be found in the body.

perinatal (per-uh-neyt′-l) The period between the 28th week of pregnancy and the 28th day after birth.

rhonchi (rong′-ki) Abnormal sounds heard on auscultation of an airway obstructed by thick secretions; a continuous rumbling sound that is more pronounced on expiration.

serous (seer′-uhs) A thin, watery, serumlike drainage.

stridor (stri′-der) A shrill, harsh respiratory sound heard during inhalation when a laryngeal obstruction is present.

suppurative (suhp′-yuh-rey-tiv) Characterized by the formation and/or discharge of pus.

urticaria (ur-tih-kair′-e-uh) Hives.

Pediatrics is the medical specialty that deals with the development and care of children and with the treatment of childhood diseases. Pediatric patients range in age from newborn to puberty. Some practices continue to see the child until he or she graduates from high school. Subspecialties within pediatrics include surgery, cardiology, and psychiatry.

Approximately 50% of the patients in a pediatric office are there for well-baby or well-child visits. The roles of the pediatrician and the medical office staff are to supervise and help maintain the health of these patients. Parents must be involved in the care and development of their young children for treatment to be a success. The medical assistant can help by encouraging therapeutic communication among the patient, parents, and medical staff. The trust a child develops in these relationships and the consideration the family receives in the physician's office form the basis of good medical care.

Pediatric care actually starts before the child is born, with the promotion of good general health for mothers before conception and during pregnancy. The confidence and enthusiasm of parents can have a significant impact on an infant's physical and emotional well-being.

NORMAL GROWTH AND DEVELOPMENT

The terms *growth* and *development* often are used together. They refer to the combination of changes a child goes through as he or she matures. *Growth* refers to measurable changes, such as height and weight. The first determinant of these physical characteristics is the genetics inherited from the parents; however, a child's growth can be influenced by many factors, including nutritional status, environmental factors, and the presence of disease. *Development* encompasses qualitative maturation in motor, mental, social, and language skills. A child's development is determined by a combination of prenatal, environmental, and caregiver factors. Each child has his or her own pattern of growth and development. Pediatric assessments are individualized for each child according to age, developmental level, health condition, family characteristics, and past experiences

with healthcare professionals. The pediatrician checks for indications of irregularities in growth and development by comparing a child's physical, intellectual, and social levels with published national standards. This comparison indicates whether the child is at the appropriate stage of growth and development for his or her chronologic age.

Growth Patterns

Physical growth is one of the most visible changes in childhood. The average birth weight is 7 to $7\frac{1}{2}$ pounds, and in 6 months, the baby's birth weight doubles. Growth then slows slightly; by 1 year of age, the birth weight has tripled and length has increased by 50%. By age 2, the child has reached approximately 50% of his or her adult height. Between ages 1 and 2, the child gains approximately $\frac{1}{2}$ pound per month. Between ages 2 and 3, weight gain averages 3 to 5 pounds and height increases 2 to $2\frac{1}{2}$ inches. Most children slim down during this period, so that by the time the third birthday arrives, the potbellied toddler has become the characteristic preschooler.

During the preschool period (ages 3 to 6 years), weight increases 3 to 5 pounds per year; height increases at a slower but steady rate of $1\frac{1}{2}$ to $2\frac{1}{2}$ inches per year. By age 4, the child usually has doubled the birth length. During this time, the legs are the fastest growing part; fatty connective tissue continues to increase slowly until approximately age 7. This same growth rate continues through the school-aged period (6 to 12 years), and as this period of development ends, the child usually is into a growth spurt that indicates impending puberty.

The growth spurt continues for approximately 2 years, and the child then reaches adolescence (ages 12 to 18 years). During this period, the adolescent gains almost half of his or her adult weight, and the skeleton and organs double in size. Weight increases in girls by 20 to 25 pounds and in boys by 15 to 20 pounds. Girls grow 5 to 6 inches, and boys grow 4 to 5 inches. As the growth spurt is completed, the teenager reaches sexual maturity. In girls, sexual maturity is signaled by the onset of the menstrual cycle; in boys, it is determined by the presence of sperm in the semen. The timing of sexual maturity in both genders varies greatly.

Skeletal growth is complete in girls between 15 and 16 years of age and in boys between ages 17 and 18. Skeletal growth is considered complete when the growth plates (**epiphyseal plates**) of the long bones of the extremities have fused completely.

Growth charts that can be used to compare the child's individual growth pattern with national standards have been used since 1977, but in 2000 the Centers for Disease Control and Prevention (CDC) revised the charts to reflect cultural and racial diversity (samples are available at the website *www.cdc.gov/growthcharts*). The CDC charts take into account whether an infant was formula-fed or breast-fed because breast-fed infants may grow differently during the first year of life.

In addition, the CDC growth charts include information on the average body mass index (BMI) for infants and young adults 2 to 20 years of age, giving pediatricians another weapon in the fight against childhood obesity. The BMI is a means of assessing the relationship between height and weight. BMI conversion charts typically are available or they are calculated automatically in electronic health record (EHR) programs, but the BMI can be calculated by dividing the child's weight in kilograms by the height in meters squared:

$$BMI = \frac{Weight\ (kg)}{Height\ (m)^2}$$

Denver II Developmental Screening Test

Each child develops individually and attains developmental plateaus differently. The Denver II Developmental Screening Test is a standardized tool used to screen for developmental delays, to investigate concerns about an infant's development, or to monitor high-risk children for potential problems (Figures 35-1 and 35-2). The Denver Developmental Materials were originally created in the 1960s to help identify children from birth to six years of age with potential developmental delays who then could be referred for assistance and treatment. The test should be given at ages 3 to 4 months, 10 months, and 3 years. Although it is not difficult to administer, only those trained in the procedure and in interpretation of the results should give it. The assessment focuses on four developmental areas:

- *Gross motor skills:* Evaluates the child's ability to control large muscle groups (e.g., sitting, standing, kicking, running, and balance).
- *Language:* Assesses the child's hearing and understanding and use of language (e.g., word comprehension, ability to follow simple commands, use of subjects, and counting).
- *Fine motor skills:* Tests the child's coordination of fine motor muscles and eye-hand coordination (e.g., reaching, grasping, piling blocks, and drawing).
- *Personal skills:* Examines the child's self-confidence, socialization, and ability to care for personal needs (e.g., playing games, using a fork and spoon, dressing, and brushing the teeth).

The results of the test are analyzed and determined to be normal or suspect, or the child is diagnosed as untestable. With an abnormal finding, the child should be rescreened in 1 to 2 weeks to rule out temporary developmental delays caused by fatigue or anxiety. If those results are abnormal, the child may be retested with other developmental tests, either by the pediatrician or by a professional pediatric testing agency.

Developmental Patterns

General patterns of child development occur rapidly during the first year of life as the infant progresses from reflex activities (e.g., grasping fingers and sucking) to learning to manipulate simple objects (e.g., pulling open drawers or throwing toys out of the crib). In addition to these motor skills, the child learns verbal patterns, progressing from cooing and crying for attention to speaking his or her first words.

Therapeutic Approaches for Infants (Newborn to 12 Months)

- Crying is normal; use distraction, but do not overstimulate.
- It is important to keep the infant close to the caregiver; either have the parent hold the infant, or keep the parent in the child's line of vision.
- Involve the parent as much as possible, depending on the task and the parent's level of comfort.
- Place a familiar object near the infant, and keep frightening ones out of view.
- An infant's negative response to strangers usually develops at approximately 8 months; do not take the rejection personally.
- Do not restrain the infant any more than necessary, but be ready to use restraint at times (e.g., when giving an injection) to keep the infant safe.
- Encourage the caregiver to cuddle and hug the child after the procedure is complete.
- Unpleasant procedures are associated with other objects, so do not use play areas for treatment, and do not use a favorite toy or object during the procedure; offer it afterward for comfort.

CRITICAL THINKING APPLICATION 35-1
Susie receives a call from the mother of a 6-month-old child. The woman is concerned that her child may not be reaching his developmental milestones. What type of information about the child's growth and development should Susie gather? If Susie is unable to answer the mother's questions, what should she do?

By age 3, the child is showing increased **autonomy**. Now the child can walk, is toilet trained, sits at the table and eats with the family, can make simple sentences, understands the word "no," and even imitates the parent by using verbal gestures that he or she has seen used. The child's vocabulary consists of up to 900 words.

During the preschool stage the child becomes increasingly independent and initiates activities. Preschoolers have mastered many gross motor skills and are perfecting their fine motor development. Verbal communication has increased to full simple and even complex sentences but remains quite literal. For example, if you tell a preschool child that you are going to fly to visit Aunt Sue, the child

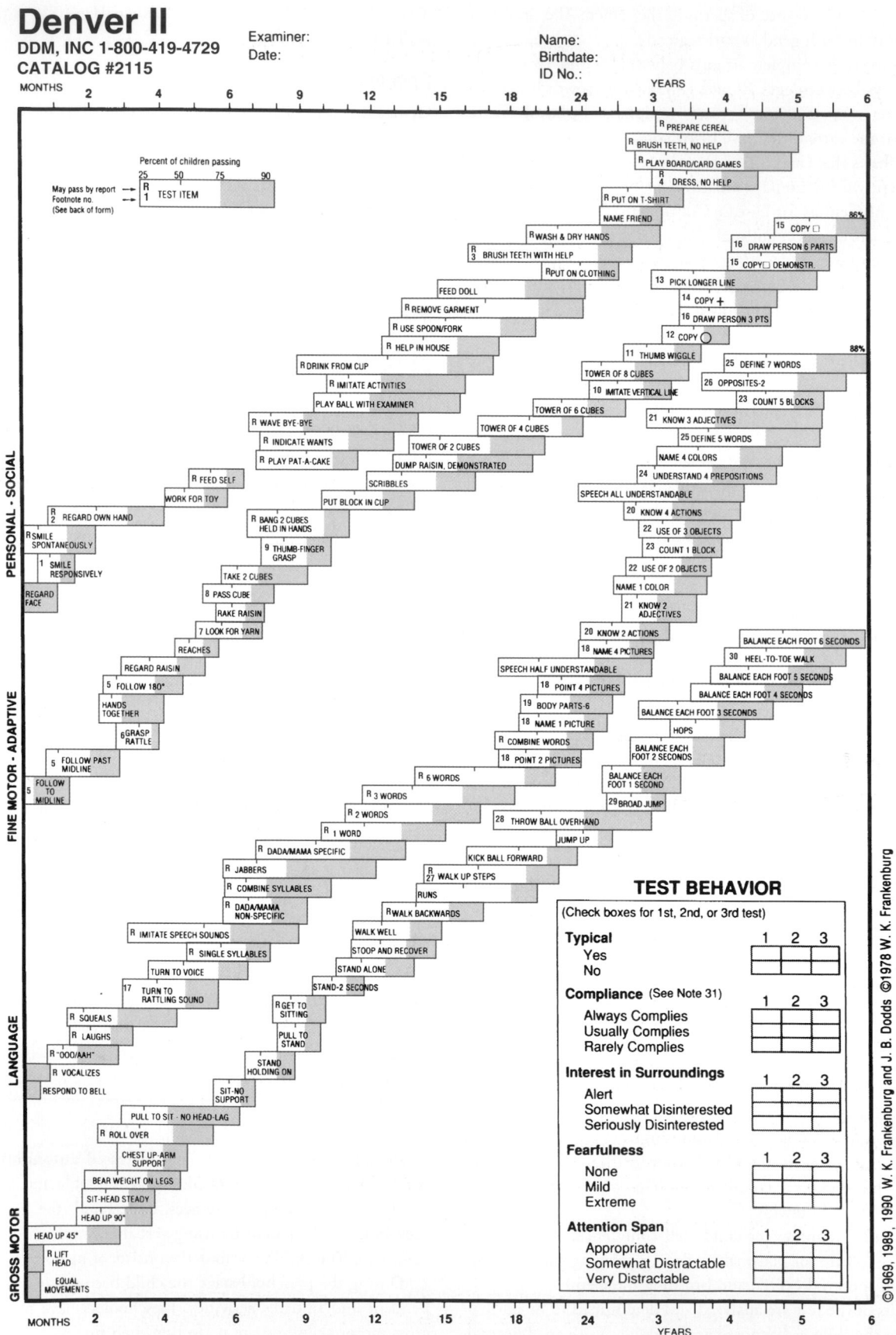

FIGURE 35-1 Denver II Developmental Screening Test (DDST). (From http://www.fpnotebook.com/Peds/Neuro/DnvrPrscrngDvlpmntl Qstnrl.htm.)

DIRECTIONS FOR ADMINISTRATION

1. Try to get child to smile by smiling, talking or waving. Do not touch him/her.
2. Child must stare at hand several seconds.
3. Parent may help guide toothbrush and put toothpaste on brush.
4. Child does not have to be able to tie shoes or button/zip in the back.
5. Move yarn slowly in an arc from one side to the other, about 8" above child's face.
6. Pass if child grasps rattle when it is touched to the backs or tips of fingers.
7. Pass if child tries to see where yarn went. Yarn should be dropped quickly from sight from tester's hand without arm movement.
8. Child must transfer cube from hand to hand without help of body, mouth, or table.
9. Pass if child picks up raisin with any part of thumb and finger.
10. Line can vary only 30 degrees or less from tester's line. /
11. Make a fist with thumb pointing upward and wiggle only the thumb. Pass if child imitates and does not move any fingers other than the thumb.

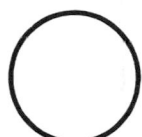
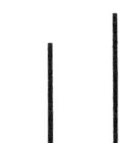
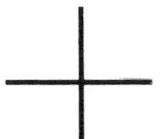

12. Pass any enclosed form. Fail continuous round motions.
13. Which line is longer? (Not bigger.) Turn paper upside down and repeat. (pass 3 of 3 or 5 of 6)
14. Pass any lines crossing near midpoint.
15. Have child copy first. If failed, demonstrate.

When giving items 12, 14, and 15, do not name the forms. Do not demonstrate 12 and 14.

16. When scoring, each pair (2 arms, 2 legs, etc.) counts as one part.
17. Place one cube in cup and shake gently near child's ear, but out of sight. Repeat for other ear.
18. Point to picture and have child name it. (No credit is given for sounds only.)
    If less than 4 pictures are named correctly, have child point to picture as each is named by tester.

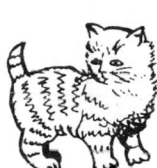
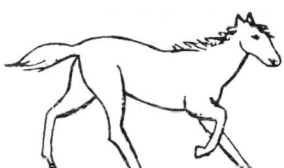
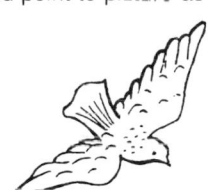
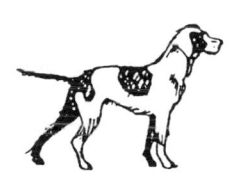
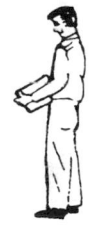

19. Using doll, tell child: Show me the nose, eyes, ears, mouth, hands, feet, tummy, hair. Pass 6 of 8.
20. Using pictures, ask child: Which one flies?... says meow?... talks?... barks?... gallops? Pass 2 of 5, 4 of 5.
21. Ask child: What do you do when you are cold?... tired?.. hungry? Pass 2 of 3, 3 of 3.
22. Ask child: What do you do with a cup? What is a chair used for? What is a pencil used for?
    Action words must be included in answers.
23. Pass if child correctly places <u>and</u> says how many blocks are on paper. (1, 5).
24. Tell child: Put block **on** table; **under** table; **in front of** me, **behind** me. Pass 4 of 4.
    (Do not help child by pointing, moving head or eyes.)
25. Ask child: What is a ball?... lake?... desk?... house?... banana?... curtain?... fence?... ceiling? Pass if defined in terms of use, shape, what it is made of, or general category (such as banana is fruit, not just yellow). Pass 5 of 8, 7 of 8.
26. Ask child: If a horse is big, a mouse is __? If fire is hot, ice is __? If the sun shines during the day, the moon shines during the __? Pass 2 of 3.
27. Child may use wall or rail only, not person. May not crawl.
28. Child must throw ball overhand 3 feet to within arm's reach of tester.
29. Child must perform standing broad jump over width of test sheet (8 1/2 inches).
30. Tell child to walk forward, ⟨⟩⟨⟩⟨⟩⟨⟩→ heel within 1 inch of toe. Tester may demonstrate.
    Child must walk 4 consecutive steps.
31. In the second year, half of normal children are non-compliant.

OBSERVATIONS:

FIGURE 35-2 Instructions for the DDST. (From http://www.fpnotebook.com/Peds/Neuro/DnvrPrscrngDvlpmntlQstnrl.htm.)

thinks you are going to flap your arms and fly. Nonverbal communication skills are also being mastered. The vocabulary now includes more than 2,000 words. During this period, children need to develop social skills, such as sharing and taking part in peer group activities.

Therapeutic Approaches for Toddlers and Preschoolers (2 to 6 Years)

- Toddlers and preschoolers often fear visits to the doctor; ignore temper tantrums and negative behavior.
- Praise the child as much as possible.
- Perform unpleasant procedures as quickly as possible; the fear of the procedure is worse than the actual discomfort.
- Allow the child to keep on as much clothing as possible for security and comfort.
- Use words familiar to the child, and do not use words the child could misinterpret. For example, "The test uses dye" (the child may think you mean "die"); "The doctor will put you to sleep so it doesn't hurt" (the family dog may have been put to sleep).
- Explain a procedure as the child would sense it; that is, what it will look like, how it will smell, how it will feel, and so on.
- Allow the child to handle equipment when possible.
- Do not use the child's favorite doll or stuffed animal to demonstrate; the child may believe the toy feels pain.
- Explain procedures to the parents away from the child when possible; the child may misinterpret the information.

School-aged children have perfected fine motor skills and can paint, draw, and play an instrument. They enjoy team activities and are expanding their reading and writing skills. Their intellectual skills are developing, and social skills are going through refinement as a sense of self-achievement and self-worth is developed. During this time the child learns and tests the rules for socializing outside the immediate family as an independent individual.

Therapeutic Approaches for School-Aged Children (7 to 11 Years)

- Allow choices when possible, such as which arm to use for an injection.
- A parent or caregiver should always be present during examinations.
- Remove only as much clothing as needed for the examination or procedure.
- Explain procedures in concrete terms; use pictures and diagrams when possible.
- Give the child time to ask questions.
- School-aged children often are curious, and they can be cooperative if they know what is expected of them.
- Address the conversation to the child; involve the child in decision making as much as possible.
- Provide privacy.

Adolescence, or the transition stage, is the time when the individual attempts to establish an adult identity. The teenager proceeds by trial and error, experimenting with adult roles and behavior patterns. Traditional values learned in childhood may be questioned, and peer relationships take on new importance. During this time teenagers must develop the emotional maturity and motivation to make reasonable decisions. They look to family members for encouragement and guidance in making decisions that will help them develop self-confidence and to become patient and less impulsive and self-centered.

Therapeutic Approaches for Adolescents (12 to 18 Years)

- Adolescents are self-conscious and strongly influenced by peers.
- Privacy is very important to them.
- Address how a procedure might affect the adolescent's appearance.
- Do not be judgmental; listen without condemning.
- Encourage the adolescent to verbalize his or her concerns and fears.
- The adolescent may regress to more childish behaviors when sick.
- Teenagers want to be treated as adults; they want to know what is being done and why.
- To promote honest discussion about lifestyle issues, encourage the teenager to see the physician without the parent present.

CRITICAL THINKING APPLICATION   **35-2**

Based on what you have learned about therapeutic approaches for the pediatric patient, what would be the best way to deal with the following patient situations?

1. A crying 3-month-old being seen for a well-child visit
2. A 10-month-old with otitis media
3. A 2-year-old who needs the dressing changed on an infected wound
4. A 5-year-old scheduled for vision and hearing screening
5. An 8-year-old who needs a throat culture to rule out a strep infection
6. A 12-year-old who needs a penicillin injection in the dorsogluteal site
7. A 15-year-old girl who complains of abdominal pain and is accompanied by her mother

---

Developmental Theories

Psychologists have been researching and developing theories about human behavior since the beginning of the twentieth century. The first psychologist to gain influence from his theories about human behavior was Sigmund Freud, who believed that the motivating stimulus for human behavior is the libido, which is defined as an individual's pleasure-seeking instincts. Freud's theory describes four major components of the mind: the *unconscious mind,* which cannot be accessed but affects our behavior; the *id,* which focuses on immediate self-gratification; the *ego,* which develops throughout life and balances the immediate desires of the id with the reality of the social world; and the *superego,* the individual's conscience, which helps the child incorporate social expectations and norms. Freud also was the first therapist to identify five developmental stages: the oral, anal, phallic, latency, and genital stages.

The next developmental theory to gain general acceptance was the psychosocial approach of Erik Erikson. Erikson expanded Freud's work to recognize cultural and social influences on individual development. His theory is based on stages of development that the individual must pass through and master. Each stage focuses on a developmental crisis, starting in infancy and ending in old age. According to Erikson, the following are the stages that children must master:

- *Trust versus mistrust:* Infants learn to rely on caregivers; mistrust occurs if needs are not met.
- *Autonomy versus shame and doubt:* Toddlers learn language skills and gain independence; they may feel shame and doubt if they cannot meet parental expectations or are overprotected.
- *Initiative versus guilt:* Preschoolers actively seek out new experiences; children become hesitant if restrictions or reprimands make them feel guilty or afraid to try more challenging skills.
- *Industry versus inferiority:* School-aged children enjoy finishing projects and receiving recognition; they develop feelings of inferiority if not accepted by peers or if they cannot please their parents.
- *Identity versus role confusion:* Adolescents face many physical and hormonal changes in this stage. Teenagers work at figuring out who they are and where they fit; they are looking for a direction for their lives. If they are unable to establish an identity and sense of direction, they become role confused.

Jean Piaget's developmental theory focuses on intellectual growth, with four stages of cognitive development. From birth to 24 months, children progress through the *sensorimotor stage,* which starts with reflexive behavior and advances to learning by doing. The *preoperational stage* (2 to 7 years) is characterized by language development and using play to understand the world. In the *concrete operational stage* (7 to 11 years), children develop logical thinking and become less egocentric. Finally, the *formal operational stage* (11 years or older) brings abstract thinking and deductive reasoning to establish values and determine the meaning of life.

Lawrence Kohlberg's theory, which focuses on moral reasoning, involves levels similar to Piaget's cognitive development theory, yet recognizes the influence of culture and interpersonal relationships on the child's moral development. In *preconventional morality,* the child's behavior is based on the external control of authority figures. The child perceives the goodness or badness of a behavior based on parental reaction. In the *conventional level,* the child wants to follow the rules of the group or society and internalizes the values of others. As the child reaches adolescence, the *postconventional level,* he or she develops individual morality and values, and behavior is regulated internally rather than externally. Table 35-1 summarizes these growth and development theories.

Postpartum Depression

- The incidence of postpartum depression (PPD) is not clear, but an estimated 10% to 20% of women struggle with major depression before, during, and after delivery of a baby. Fewer than half of these are diagnosed in routine office visits.

- Postpartum depression can be diagnosed a month to a year after childbirth. Women with a history of depression during pregnancy should be monitored for signs of postpartum depression for a minimum of 4 months.
- Risk factors include a history of depression, abuse, or mental illness; smoking or alcohol use; anxiety during pregnancy and fears over child care; lack of financial resources and secure relationships; a fussy or colicky infant; and lack of social support.
- Symptoms of postpartum depression include anorexia and insomnia; irritability and anger; overwhelming fatigue; loss of interest in sex and lack of a feeling of joy in life; feelings of shame, guilt, or inadequacy; severe mood swings; difficulty bonding with the baby; withdrawal from family and friends; and thoughts of harming herself or the baby.
- Postpartum depression must be detected as soon as possible so that treatment can begin; untreated postpartum depression may last for a year or longer. Treatment includes both counseling and antidepressant medication.

The 10-question Edinburgh Postnatal Depression Scale (EPDS) is a valuable and efficient way of identifying patients at risk for **perinatal** depression. Healthcare professionals working with the perinatal population should use the EPDS as a routine part of postnatal care because the EPDS is a valid and reliable means of detecting PPD. This screening tool is user friendly, easy to administer, and easy to score. A score of 10 to 12 is considered the cutoff for PPD; the mother should be referred for further evaluation or treatment. Users may reproduce the scale without further permission, providing they respect the copyright by quoting the names of the authors and the title and the source of the paper in all reproduced copies. The EPDS can be accessed at the American Academy of Pediatrics website at: www2.aap.org/sections/scan/practicingsafety/Toolkit_Resources/Module2/EPDS.pdf

From www2.aap.org/sections/scan/practicingsafety/Toolkit_Resources/Module2/EPDS.pdf. Accessed January 12, 2015.

CRITICAL THINKING APPLICATION 35-3
The pediatricians in Susie's office routinely screen new mothers for postpartum depression using the Edinburgh Postnatal Depression Scale (EPDS). Research the EPDS questionnaire online. In Susie's office, the medical assistants perform the assessment. With a classmate, role-play the use of the form.

PEDIATRIC DISEASES AND DISORDERS

The disease process in pediatric patients poses special problems, because children are constantly changing both physically and functionally. As a child grows and develops, the immune system matures, and with the aid of routine prophylactic immunizations, the child acquires long-term protection against certain infectious diseases.

Gastrointestinal Disorders
Colic
Colic usually is seen in the newborn period or in early infancy. The problem is intermittent. The classic situation is an infant

TABLE 35-1   Summary of Growth and Development Theories*

AGE GROUP	FREUD: PSYCHOSEXUAL THEORY	PIAGET: COGNITIVE THEORY	ERIKSON: PSYCHOSOCIAL THEORY	KOHLBERG: MORAL REASONING
Infant	Oral stage; child operates with the pleasure principle, and the id develops.	Sensorimotor level; uses reflexive behavior; has to do things to learn.	Building basic trust versus mistrust; learning drive and hope.	Avoids punishment and obeys for obedience's sake.
Toddler	Passes through oral aggressive stage to anal stage; elimination is used to control and inhibit.	Coordinates more than one thought at a time; uses thought to create new solutions.	Autonomy versus shame and doubt; learning self-control and willpower.	Avoids punishment and the power of authority figures.
Preschool to early school years	From phallic stage, in which the ego (conscious reality) develops, to latent stage, in which the superego (morality) develops.	Intuitive-preoperational; preschoolers are egocentric and have magical thinking. Early school-aged children begin to develop understanding of cause and effect. Child functions symbolically using language; develops understanding of life events and relationships.	Preschoolers process initiative versus guilt and attempt to develop direction and purpose. Children mimic others and are more purposeful in establishing goals.	Develops preconventional morality; follows the standards of others to avoid punishment or to earn a reward; recognizes some things are self-satisfying and some are done to satisfy others.
School age	Latent stage continues; superego develops morality or a conscience; represses the sexual drive.	Concrete operations: uses mental reasoning to solve problems; attempts to reach logical solutions; tests beliefs to establish values.	Industry versus inferiority; establishing methods for solving problems and a feeling of competence; mastering tasks and using hands to create things.	Conventional morality; doing what is expected is important. Children need to be good in their own eyes in addition to doing what they perceive others expect of them; they want to please others.
Adolescence	Genital stage	Formal operations developing; adolescents are determining values that will guide their lives and religious affiliations; they develop abstract ideas that can be based in reality.	Identity versus role confusion; developing self-identity that will determine devotion and fidelity in future relationships.	Postconventional morality; developing respect for the laws of society; learning to consider the greatest good for the greatest number; values are related to one's group. Behavior is controlled internally.

*Freud (1856-1939); Piaget (1896-1980); Erikson (1902-1994); Kohlberg (1927-1987).

between 2 weeks and 4 months of age who has crying episodes that occur at least three times a week for longer than 3 hours a day and lasting 3 weeks. During an attack, the infant draws up the legs, clenches the fists, and cries inconsolably. The abdominal distress of colic usually occurs in the late afternoon and evening. Many theories have been suggested for why infants have colic, but none has been proven correct. If the baby is fed infant formula, pediatricians recommend switching formulas, perhaps to a non–cow's milk type, because this may help relieve the infant's discomfort. Treatment consists of determining the cause; however, the child frequently outgrows the condition before the causative agent can be identified. Drugs are not helpful and in some cases may be dangerous for the infant. Parents need reassurance that they are not responsible for the child's discomfort, and they may find counseling and assistance in developing coping techniques helpful.

Diarrhea

Diarrhea can be caused by a variety of microorganisms, including bacteria, viruses, and parasites. However, children sometimes can have diarrhea without having an infection, such as when diarrhea is caused by food allergies or by certain medications, such as antibiotics. Diarrhea is diagnosed when the child has two or more watery or apparently abnormal stools within 24 hours. The child may not show other signs of illness or may have nausea, vomiting, stomach aches, headache, or fever. If the diarrhea continues for longer than 2 days, medical intervention is needed, because prolonged diarrhea, in which fluid loss becomes excessive, can cause dehydration and electrolyte imbalance. In addition, a resultant diaper rash and **excoriation** can be very painful.

Pediatric diarrhea needs to be followed closely with observation. In the case of bloody stools, laboratory analysis should be ordered to determine the causative factors. Infants and small children should be followed up by telephone in 12 hours and then daily until the diarrhea has stopped. Parents should know the indications of dehydration, including lack of tears when crying, lethargy, fewer wet diapers or decreased urination, dry mouth and lips, and weight loss. The physician may recommend the use of oral rehydration therapy, such as Pedialyte or Infalyte; small amounts (approximately 2 tablespoons) are offered at a time (i.e., every 15 minutes) to prevent vomiting. Soft drinks, juices, sports drinks, and tea should be avoided because they lack electrolytes and may lead to even more diarrhea. Parents should be informed that the child's diarrhea may not stop when the child is given oral rehydration therapy, but the fluids prevent the child from becoming dehydrated. It is important to continue to feed the child because lack of food can damage the villi in the small intestine. If breast-fed, the baby should continue to nurse because breast milk is shown to protect the gastrointestinal lining.

The banana, rice, applesauce, and toast (BRAT) diet has been the traditional approach for children with diarrhea, but it is no longer recommended because there is no evidence that it is useful. In fact, the poor protein content of the BRAT diet may contribute to continued diarrhea and poor nutrition. Pediatricians now recommend that children resume their prediarrhea diet as soon as possible so that they continue to eat something they prefer while the intestine heals. Probiotics found in certain yogurt products can also be helpful in stabilizing the child while the intestinal tract gets back to normal. The child should not be given over-the-counter (OTC) antidiarrheal medications, such as Pepto-Bismol, Kaopectate, Imodium, or Lomotil, because these can cause serious side effects, including decreased motility of the bowel, respiratory depression, and drowsiness. The provider may prescribe antibiotics if stool cultures test positive for pathogens. Children with severe dehydration require hospitalization and intravenous (IV) hydration to replace electrolytes and fluids.

CRITICAL THINKING APPLICATION 35-4
Susie receives a call from the grandmother of a 3-year-old child who has had diarrhea since last night. What are some questions Susie should ask to determine the seriousness of the problem? Should the child be seen today, even though appointments are already overbooked?

Failure to Thrive

Failure to thrive is a symptom more than a disease. Failure to thrive refers to children whose current weight or rate of weight gain is much lower than that of other children of similar age and gender. It is diagnosed in an infant or young child whose weight is consistently below the 3rd percentile on standardized growth charts or one who is 20% below the ideal body weight for length. Physical, mental, and social skills also are delayed in these children. Manifestations include failure to roll over, smile, coo, stand, or walk at age-appropriate developmental levels. Failure to thrive can be caused by a physiologic factor (e.g., malabsorption disease or cleft palate), or it may be

related to a problem with the parent-child relationship. The physician needs an accurately recorded history of the child's birth weight and subsequent length, weight, and head circumference measurements. A comprehensive family history is important to rule out genetic growth abnormalities or a history of malabsorption problems, such as cystic fibrosis or celiac disease.

Children with failure to thrive need more calories than usual—approximately 150% of their normal calorie load—to catch up to their target weight. Both medical and social factors are evaluated in the treatment of children with this problem. Experts believe that infants may suffer from this problem if they are being neglected; however, low weight gains also are possible with extremely attentive and cautious parents. The family must be considered as a whole to treat **nonorganic** causes effectively. Treatment may include the use of support groups and parental counseling.

Obesity

Just as with adult weight patterns, children are assessed according to their BMI. A child's level of body fat varies as the child grows; for example, children normally slim down as they reach school age, and very often their weight increases as they mature from adolescence to adulthood. In addition, body fat levels vary between boys and girls as they reach puberty. Pediatricians use growth charts that plot the child's BMI-for-age to determine whether the child's weight, in comparison with height, is within healthy limits. A child is considered overweight if the BMI-for-age is between the 85th and 94th percentiles; the child is identified as obese if the BMI is at or greater than the 95th percentile. Obesity now affects nearly 18% of all children and adolescents in the United States, and since 1980 the number has almost tripled. Children who are overweight or obese as preschoolers are five times as likely as normal-weight children to be overweight or obese as adults. Studies have shown that a child who is obese between the ages of 10 and 13 has an 80% chance of becoming an obese adult.

The reasons for childhood obesity vary; they include a family history of obesity, inactivity, high-calorie diets, and stress. In rare cases, childhood obesity may be caused by metabolic or endocrine disorders. Overweight and obese children are at greater risk of developing serious health conditions, including asthma, diabetes mellitus type 2, sleep apnea, and hypercholesterolemia, which increases the risk of cardiovascular disease and hypertension. The psychosocial impact of obesity can be overwhelming for many children because isolation, loneliness, and lack of self-esteem are common. The pediatrician can provide assistance by recommending a comprehensive diet and exercise program that emphasizes healthy living. The medical assistant can help by providing educational materials, encouragement for the child and parents, and referral to community education and support programs.

CRITICAL THINKING APPLICATION 35-5
Juanita Johnston is a 12-year-old patient who was recently diagnosed as being obese. You are asked to help Juanita and her mother access online information about healthy nutrition options. What websites would be most appropriate for Juanita and her family? What other community resources can you recommend to support the family in making healthier nutrition decisions?

Respiratory Disorders

Common Cold

The common cold, or infectious rhinitis, has more than 100 causative pathogens and is highly contagious. It is spread through respiratory droplets from rhinitis, sneezing, or coughing, either from direct contact or from touching contaminated items. The signs include nasal congestion, low-grade fever, and general malaise. Most colds are self-limiting and run their course in about a week. In infants and young children, the primary concerns are nasal congestion and loss of appetite. The parent may need to be shown how to use a nasal bulb syringe to suction the nose of an infant (Figure 35-3). Secondary infections in the lower respiratory tract or in the middle ear can occur.

Cautions on the Use of Over-the-Counter Cough and Cold Medicines in Children

The U.S. Food and Drug Administration (FDA) strongly recommends that over-the-counter (OTC) cough and cold products not be given to children under 2 years of age. A number of serious complications may occur, including death, convulsions, rapid heart rate, and diminished levels of consciousness. These medications are given for symptomatic relief and have not been proven to be safe or effective for very young children. Manufacturers have responded to the FDA's recommendation by voluntarily removing the products from shelves.

The FDA also is concerned about the use of these products in children ages 2 to 11 years. Parents need to know that many OTC cough and cold products contain the same active ingredients. Giving a child more than one product that contains the same active ingredient can result in overdose, especially if the wrong dose is given or the product is administered too frequently. Parents of older children are encouraged to read the Drug Facts section on the label of each product to familiarize themselves with the active ingredients in the product and to follow dosing guidelines strictly to reduce the risk of complications.

One of the secondary infections that can occur is strep throat, which is caused by group A *Streptococcus* bacteria. It is easily spread when an infected person coughs or sneezes contaminated droplets into the air and another person inhales them. A person also can become infected by touching such secretions and then touching the mouth or nose. Symptoms of strep throat infections may include severe sore throat, fever, headache, and **lymphadenopathy**; also, the throat appears bright red, and pustules may be present on the tonsils. If they are not treated with antibiotics, strep infections can lead to scarlet or rheumatic fever; infections of the skin, bloodstream, or ears; and pneumonia. Scarlet fever is characterized by a bright red, rough-textured rash that spreads over the child's body. Rheumatic fever is a serious disease that can damage the heart valves.

Otitis Media

Infection or inflammation of the middle ear usually is a side effect of a cold or other upper respiratory tract disorder, but it also can be caused by allergies. Otitis media (OM) usually occurs in children younger than 3 years of age. Signs include inflammation of the middle ear, with fluid building up behind the tympanic membrane. The child may cry persistently, tug at the ear, have a fever, be irritable, and have diminished hearing in the affected ear. These symptoms sometimes may be accompanied by diarrhea, nausea, and vomiting.

Otitis media is classified as either **serous** (Figure 35-4) or **suppurative** (Figure 35-5), depending on the composition of the accumulated fluid in the middle ear. In Figure 35-5, pus is in the middle ear and shows up as white in the image. Because otitis media may be caused by bacteria or a virus, determining the most appropriate treatment can be difficult. Traditionally, children with indications of a middle ear infection were treated with antibiotics; however, if the infection is caused by a virus, antibiotics do not help.

In 2013, the American Academy of Pediatrics (AAP) and the American Academy of Family Physicians (AAFP) released an updated clinical practice guideline for the diagnosis and management of otitis media in children age 6 months to 12 years. Antibiotics should be prescribed for children 6 months or older who have severe signs and symptoms (typically amoxicillin or azithromycin

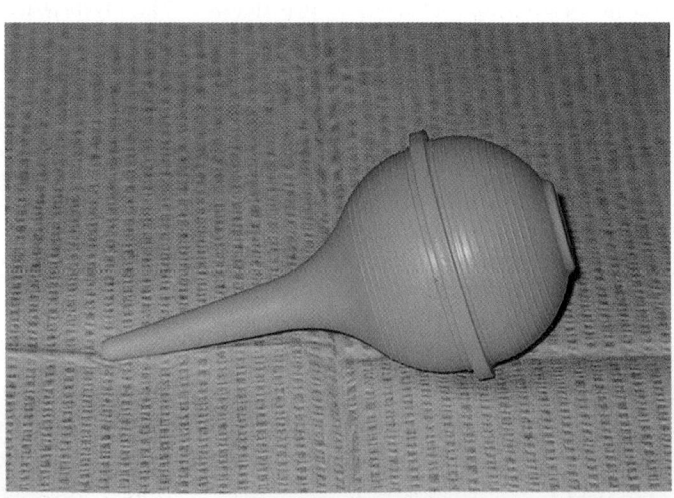

FIGURE 35-3 Nasal bulb syringe.

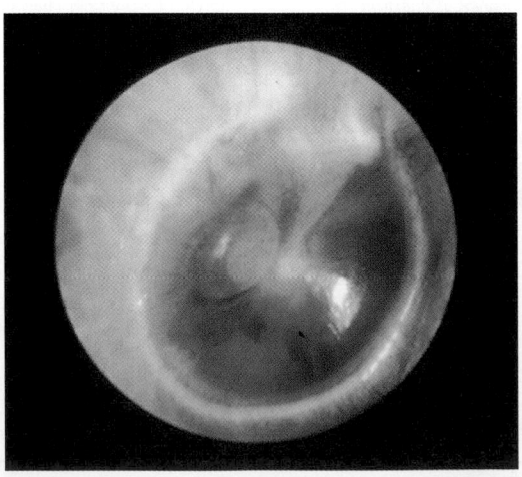

FIGURE 35-4 Serous otitis media. (From Swartz MH: *Textbook of physical diagnosis,* ed 5, Philadelphia, 2006, Saunders.)

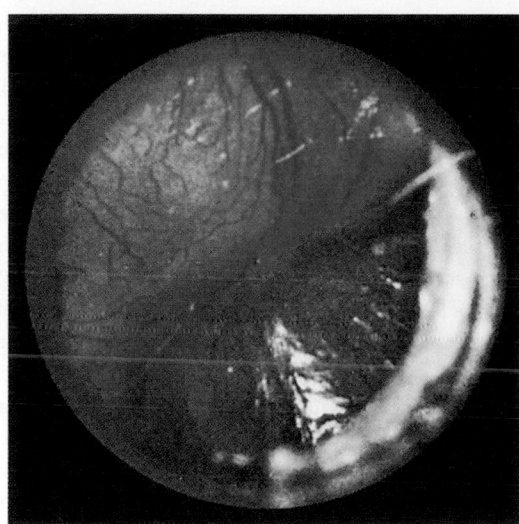

FIGURE 35-5 Suppurative otitis media. (Courtesy Dr. Richard A. Buckingham and Dr. George E. Shambaugh, Jr.)

[Zithromax]). Antibiotics can also be prescribed in patients under 24 months of age who are experiencing nonsevere bilateral infections. However, in children over 6 months with nonsevere symptoms, observation and a follow-up within 48 to 72 hours before initiating antibiotics may be offered to assess patient improvement. If no improvement is noticed or symptoms have worsened, antibiotic therapy should be started. In all cases, if the child has not improved in 48 to 72 hours, the current antibiotic should be switched. Because antibiotics do not provide immediate relief from symptoms, children can be given oral acetaminophen and/or ibuprofen for pain relief.

If fluid in the middle ear persists for longer than 3 months and/or if the child experiences hearing loss, the physician may recommend a *myringotomy*; in this operation, a small incision is made in the tympanic membrane and a tube is inserted to drain the fluid and balance the pressure between the outer and middle ear. The tube typically stays in the eardrum for 6 to 12 months and falls out as the child grows.

CRITICAL THINKING APPLICATION   **35-6**

A young mother calls, extremely upset about her 4-year-old son. His symptoms started 3 days ago with a cold, but now the child complains of a sore throat and an earache. What questions should Susie ask to determine whether the child should be seen today?

Croup

Croup is a viral inflammation of the larynx and the trachea that causes edema and spasm of the vocal cords. This varying degree of obstruction of the cords produces hoarseness; a harsh, barking cough; and **stridor** during inhalation. The episodes usually occur at night, and symptoms ease by morning. The infection usually is self-limiting, and the child typically recovers without treatment. Mild croup can be relieved by using a cool mist humidifier in the child's room, sitting with the child in a steamy bathroom, or even taking the child outside if the air is cool. Children with allergies may require medical treatment. If the problem becomes chronic or continues for a longer period, the child may need to be treated with corticosteroids (e.g., prednisone). The physician may recommend **laryngoscopy** to visualize the vocal cords or may order throat cultures to determine the underlying cause of the inflammation.

Pertussis (Whooping Cough)

Pertussis is a very contagious respiratory illness, commonly known as *whooping cough,* which is caused by bacteria that attach to the cilia (tiny, hairlike extensions) that line part of the upper respiratory system. The bacteria release toxins that damage the cilia and cause inflammation and swelling. Whooping cough is spread by coughing or sneezing while in close contact with others. Infants who get pertussis are typically infected by older siblings, parents, or caregivers who might not even know they have the disease.

Pertussis can cause violent and rapid coughing, over and over, until the air is gone from the lungs and the child is forced to inhale with a loud "whooping" sound. Infants may not exhibit the classic cough associated with pertussis but can develop life-threatening *apnea*, which is a pause in the child's breathing. About half of infants younger than 1 year of age who get the disease are hospitalized. Early treatment with antibiotics, before the coughing fits start, is very important. The best way to prevent pertussis is through vaccination.

The recommended pertussis vaccine for infants and children is DTaP. This is a combination vaccine that protects most children for at least 5 years from three diseases: diphtheria, tetanus and pertussis. However, complete vaccination requires five doses starting at 2 months of age up through 4 to 6 years of age. In addition, vaccine protection for these three diseases fades with time. The CDC recommends that adults get a Tdap booster at least every 10 years. Being up-to-date with the pertussis vaccine is especially important for families with and caregivers of newborns.

Current recommendations are that pregnant women get a dose of Tdap during each pregnancy, preferably at 27 through 36 weeks' gestation. If the expectant woman receives the immunization in her final trimester, maternal pertussis antibodies transfer to the newborn in utero, providing the baby protection against pertussis in early life. In addition, Tdap helps protect the mother, so she does not become infected and transmit the disease to her newborn. All family members and caregivers of the infant also should receive a Tdap booster before coming into contact with the infant.

Bronchiolitis

Bronchiolitis is a viral infection of the small bronchi and bronchioles that usually affects children younger than 3 years of age. The infection varies in severity and is seen in children with a family history of asthma and those exposed to cigarette smoke. The child typically has a previous history of rhinitis and cough, with an acute onset of wheezing and dyspnea. Symptoms occur because of inflammation, edema, increased secretions, and bronchospasm in the respiratory pathway. Treatment includes acetaminophen for discomfort and fever and a bronchodilator inhaler (albuterol sulfate [Proventil]) or nebulizer treatments for relief of wheezing. Most children fully recover in 2 weeks, but as many as 50% have recurrent wheezing and coughing.

Respiratory Syncytial Virus

Respiratory syncytial virus (RSV) infects the lungs and bronchioles. Healthy older children and adults usually experience mild, coldlike symptoms and recover in a week or two. However, RSV can cause a serious respiratory infection in infants and older adults. Premature infants, children younger than 2 years of age with **congenital** heart or chronic lung disease, and children with weakened immune systems are at highest risk for severe RSV infections. RSV is the most common cause of bronchiolitis and pneumonia in children younger than 1 year of age.

Symptoms start out similar to those of the common cold, including runny nose, decreased appetite, coughing, sneezing, and fever. Wheezing associated with bronchiole irritation and inflammation may also occur. In very young infants, irritability, decreased activity, and breathing difficulties may indicate that hospitalization is necessary. Because the infection is caused by a virus, there are no medications that can cure RSV; however, other drugs may be prescribed to help treat symptoms.

Researchers are working to develop a vaccine for RSV. The physician may prescribe the drug palivizumab (Synagis) for infants and children at great risk of developing severe RSV infections. Palivizumab does not cure the infection but can help prevent serious illness by boosting the child's immune system. It is given in monthly intramuscular injections during the fall, winter, and spring, when most RSV infections occur.

Asthma

Asthma is the most common chronic health problem among children. It is the result of two specific reactions, bronchospasm and inflammation. During an asthma attack, the bronchial tubes begin to spasm, which reduces the amount of air that can pass through them. At the same time, the tissue lining the bronchioles becomes edematous and secretes mucus; therefore, in an asthma attack, the smaller airways are filling up with mucus and secretions. Air passing through these secretions causes the classic symptom of asthma, wheezing on expiration. Asthma has a strong hereditary link. Factors that can trigger an attack include:

- Respiratory infections, including infections caused by common cold viruses
- Exposure to cigarette smoke
- Stress
- Strenuous exercise
- Weather conditions, including cold, windy, or rainy days and extreme humidity
- Allergies to animals, dust, pollen, or mold
- Indoor air pollutants, such as paint, cleaning materials, chemicals, or perfumes
- Outdoor air pollutants, such as ozone

Children with asthma have a nonproductive cough accompanied by an expiratory wheeze and shortness of breath. Shallow breathing makes it difficult for the child to speak more than a few words at a time. The child complains of tightness or pressure in the chest, and the provider hears **rhonchi** on auscultation. An asthma attack can last minutes to days and may develop into a medical emergency. Each child and each attack must be evaluated independently.

The therapeutic plan is determined by the severity and frequency of attacks. Children with mild to moderately persistent disease (i.e., symptoms that occur less than twice a week or as often as daily) should be referred to a specialist. A child who experiences symptoms two or more times a week should take daily medication to prevent asthma attacks. Such medications may include inhaled corticosteroids that deliver an antiinflammatory directly to the bronchioles (e.g., fluticasone [Advair Diskus, Flovent]); long-acting bronchodilators, including salmeterol (Serevent); and oral medications, such as montelukast (Singulair) or zafirlukast (Accolate). The child also is prescribed a quick-acting medication, or "rescue inhaler," such as albuterol (Proventil, Ventolin), for acute relief of bronchospasm or exercise-induced asthma; this inhaler should be readily available at all times. (Further management of asthma is covered in the Assisting in Pulmonary Medicine chapter.)

Influenza

Influenza (the "flu") is an acute, highly contagious viral infection of the respiratory tract. The highest incidence is seen in school-aged children, but it is most severe in infants and toddlers. It is transmitted by direct contact with moist secretions. Children tend to have high fevers with influenza and are susceptible to pulmonary complications. Influenza can vary widely in severity, ranging from very mild to life-threatening. The virus can destroy the respiratory epithelium, which is one of the body's defense mechanisms against bacterial invasion. With the loss of this protective mechanism, bacteria can invade any part of the respiratory tract and cause pneumonia.

No medication cures influenza. However, antiviral medications can make the illness milder and make patients feel better faster. They may also prevent serious complications from the flu; however, they work best when started within the first 2 days of initial symptoms. Zanamivir (Relenza), an antiviral, is inhaled every 12 hours, but it cannot be prescribed for children under 5 years of age. In 2012 the U.S. Food and Drug Administration (FDA) approved the use of oseltamivir (Tamiflu) to treat children as young as 2 weeks of age who have shown symptoms of flu for no longer than 2 days.

Antibiotics are prescribed only if a secondary bacterial infection develops, such as sinusitis. The usual treatment for influenza is bed rest, increased fluids, and a nonaspirin analgesic to reduce fever and relieve discomfort.

Flu vaccines are available but are beneficial only if the individual is vaccinated before the onset of the disease. Furthermore, annual vaccines do not provide immunity from all strains of the flu virus. The CDC recommends annual flu vaccinations for all healthy children from age 6 months to 19 years of age and their caregivers. The nasal spray vaccine is approved for use in people 2 years through 49 years of age. The flu shot is recommended for any child over 6 months of age who has a chronic health problem, such as children with chronic heart or lung diseases (including asthma); those undergoing long-term aspirin therapy; children with diabetes mellitus or sickle cell anemia; and those with kidney, blood, or suppressed immune system diseases. The first influenza immunization for children age 6 months to 8 years requires two doses given about 1 month apart. Children 9 years of age or older need only one dose per season. Influenza strains continually change, so the child must receive an updated version of the vaccine each year.

Infectious Diseases

Conjunctivitis

Pinkeye, also called *conjunctivitis,* is discussed in the Ophthalmology chapter. It is a common infection in children and is highly contagious, especially in day care centers and schools. It can be caused by a bacterial or viral infection that produces white or yellowish pus, which may cause the eyelids to stick shut in the morning. Health teaching for caregivers of infected children includes the following:

- Use good hand sanitization practices and hygiene, including proper use and disposal of tissues.
- Do not share towels or any other item that comes in contact with the child's face.
- Disinfect any articles that may have been contaminated.
- Children diagnosed with infectious conjunctivitis should be treated with an antibiotic for at least 24 hours before returning to day care or school.

Tonsillitis

Tonsillitis is caused by many infectious agents, but the most common is *Streptococcus A.* The onset is sudden, and the disorder can cause intense pain within a short time, in addition to fever and general malaise. The tonsils appear enlarged and inflamed and may be covered with pustules. A throat culture usually is performed to determine the causative organism. Treatment consists of bed rest, a liquid to soft diet, an analgesic throat spray, and oral antibiotics if the causative organism is a bacterium. The danger lies in the secondary problems that can occur, which include rheumatic heart disease and kidney disease if the streptococcal infection is not treated with antibiotics.

Fifth Disease

Fifth disease, also called *erythema infectiosum, parvovirus infection,* or *slapped cheek disease,* is an infection caused by parvovirus B19. Outbreaks are most common in the winter and spring. Symptoms begin with a mild fever and general malaise. After a few days, the cheeks take on a flushed appearance, making the face look as if it has been slapped. A lacy rash also may be seen on the trunk, arms, and legs, but not all those infected develop the rash.

Most children who get fifth disease are not very ill and recover without any serious consequences. However, children with sickle cell anemia, chronic anemia, or an impaired immune system may become seriously ill when infected and require medical care. If a pregnant woman becomes infected with parvovirus B19, she has an increased risk of miscarriage, and the fetus may suffer from severe anemia. The woman herself may have no symptoms or may have a mild illness with a rash and/or arthralgia (joint pain).

Fifth disease is spread through direct contact or by breathing in respiratory secretions from an infected person. Patients are most contagious before the onset of the rash; once the rash appears, they are no longer considered contagious. Once individuals recover from fifth disease, they develop immunity that generally protects them from parvovirus B19 infection in the future.

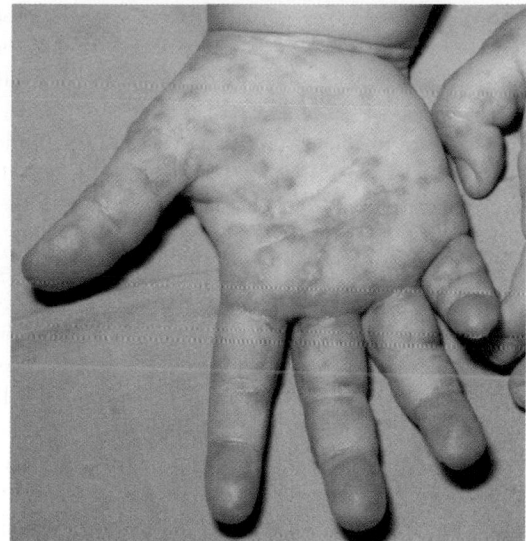

FIGURE 35-6 Vesicular palm lesions in hand-foot-and-mouth disease. (From Schachner LA, Hansen RC: *Pediatric dermatology,* ed 4, St Louis, 2011, Mosby.)

Hand-Foot-and-Mouth Disease

Hand-foot-and-mouth disease is caused by the coxsackievirus, which is transmitted by direct contact with nose and throat drainage, saliva, or the stool of an infected individual. The disease is seen most often in day care settings, where children can easily come in contact with infected bodily secretions. Symptoms include a combination of fever; sore throat; painful red blisters on the tongue, mouth, palms, and soles; headache; anorexia; and irritability (Figure 35-6). Most cases of hand-foot-and-mouth disease are not serious. The most common complication of the infection is dehydration. Young children may stop eating and drinking because sores in the mouth make swallowing painful. Because the infection is caused by a virus, antibiotic therapy is not helpful, and the disease must run its course. Supportive therapy is recommended, consisting of plenty of rest, fluids, and acetaminophen or ibuprofen for fever or discomfort. To prevent the spread of the disease, family members should be instructed to wash their hands thoroughly, especially after diaper changes, and frequently disinfect shared items (e.g., toys). Individuals with the disease are highly contagious during the first week; however, the virus may be spread for weeks after symptoms have cleared. Children with hand-foot-and-mouth disease should be kept out of day care or school until the fever is gone and mouth sores have healed.

Varicella (Chickenpox)

Chickenpox is caused by a member of the herpes virus group and is transmitted by direct or indirect droplets from the respiratory tract of an infected person. The incubation period is 14 to 21 days. Children usually run a slight fever for up to 3 days before the skin eruptions occur, and they are contagious at this time. Skin lesions continue to erupt for 3 to 4 days and cause intense itching. The infection lasts approximately 2 weeks and in most cases leaves the child with lifetime immunity. The disease is so contagious in its early stages that an exposed person who is not immune to the virus has a 70% to 80% chance of contracting the disease.

The varicella virus vaccine, Varivax, is available for protection against chickenpox. Varivax is very effective; 80% to 90% of those vaccinated are completely protected from chickenpox. If a child does get chickenpox after vaccination, it is usually a very mild case, lasting only a few days, and involving limited skin lesions, low-grade or no fever, and few other symptoms.

The CDC recommends that children receive two doses of the vaccine, the first between 12 and 15 months of age and the second between 4 and 6 years. Adolescents and adults who have never had chickenpox also should receive two doses of the vaccine. Varivax has proved to be safe and effective and can be administered at the same time as the measles, mumps, and rubella (MMR) vaccine. An alternative combination vaccine for the measles, mumps, rubella, and varicella (MMRV) is recommended for children between 12 months to 12 years old. It is a single shot that can be used in place of the MMR and MMRV vaccines. Two doses of MMRV are recommended, the first dose at 12 through 15 months of age and the second dose at 4 through 6 years of age. The one MMRV vaccine licensed in the United States is ProQuad.

Chickenpox is not a serious disease for most children. However, newborns and individuals with an impaired immune system (e.g., those undergoing chemotherapy for cancer, those with acquired immunodeficiency syndrome [AIDS], and those who take steroid medications [e.g., prednisone]) may have a severe case or can even die. Chickenpox can be very dangerous for pregnant women, causing stillbirths or birth defects, and can be spread to their babies during childbirth. Occasionally chickenpox can cause serious, life-threatening illnesses, such as encephalitis or pneumonia, especially in adults. After infection, the virus migrates to a **dermatome** and may cause shingles (herpes zoster) later in life.

Meningitis

Meningitis is an inflammation of the membranes that cover the brain and spinal cord. It is caused by a bacterial, fungal, or viral infection. Viral meningitis usually is mild and clears up on its own within 10 to 14 days. Fungal meningitis can be quite serious and typically is seen in immunocompromised individuals, such as those with AIDS. Meningitis caused by a bacterial infection (sometimes called *spinal meningitis*) is one of the most serious types, sometimes leading to permanent brain damage or even death. Bacterial meningitis most often is caused by three different bacteria: *Neisseria meningitidis* (meningococcal meningitis), *Streptococcus pneumoniae,* and *Haemophilus influenzae* serotype b (*H. influenzae* meningitis). These bacteria are carried in the upper back part of the throat (nasopharynx) of an infected person and are spread either through the air (when the person coughs or sneezes) or by direct contact with secretions, such as through kissing or sharing eating or drinking utensils. However, transmission usually occurs only after very close contact with the infected person. Signs and symptoms of bacterial meningitis include a sudden onset of fever, headache, neck pain or stiffness, vomiting (often without abdominal complaints), and irritability. These signs and symptoms may quickly progress to a decreased level of consciousness (the person is difficult to rouse), convulsions, and death. For this reason, if any child displays symptoms of possible meningitis, he or she should receive medical care immediately. Bacterial meningi-

tis is treated with immediate hospitalization and IV antibiotic therapy.

Meningitis caused by *H. influenzae* serotype b (Hib) can be prevented with the Hib vaccine, which is given as part of the routine childhood immunizations in three or four doses starting at 2 months of age. Some cases of meningococcal meningitis also can be prevented by vaccination. However, this vaccine is not used routinely outside of childhood except during outbreaks or for high-risk children who did not receive the original immunization. Many states require reporting of bacterial meningitis cases to the health department, which probably will recommend preventive antibiotics for potentially exposed people.

Hepatitis B

Infection with the hepatitis B virus (HBV) can lead to a serious, chronic infection of the liver. The virus can be transmitted across the placenta or during the birth process if the mother is infected. HBV also can be transmitted sexually, by blood transfusion, or by direct contact. A child can carry the virus for years and only later develop liver failure or liver cancer. Many states now include immunization for HBV in the recommended immunization schedule, which usually is begun in the newborn nursery. The CDC recommends that all infants receive their first intramuscular injection before leaving the hospital, the second dose at 1 to 2 months of age, and the third dose at 6 months. The vaccination schedule most often used for adults and children has been three intramuscular injections, the second and third administered 1 and 6 months after the first.

CRITICAL THINKING APPLICATION   **35-7**

An expectant mother is questioning the administration of her infant's first hepatitis immunization in the newborn nursery. What details can you share with her about the importance of the infant starting the hepatitis B virus (HBV) series? Can you refer her to any online sources of information?

Reye's Syndrome

The cause of Reye's syndrome is unknown, but the disorder has been linked to the use of aspirin during a viral illness. Reye's syndrome is an acute and sometimes fatal illness characterized by fatty invasion of the inner organs, especially the liver, and swelling of the brain. It most often is seen in children from infancy through puberty (age 16).

Prevention is the best treatment, which means children up to age 14 should never be given aspirin unless prescribed by a physician for a chronic condition such as juvenile rheumatoid arthritis. Parents should be advised to use nonsalicylate analgesics and antipyretics (e.g., ibuprofen and acetaminophen) for fevers or discomfort. Parents should also be warned to read the labels of OTC medications carefully because cold and flu remedies may contain aspirin. The syndrome is rare because of well-informed caregivers and a responsive pharmacology industry that no longer puts aspirin into products for children.

Autism Spectrum Disorder

- Children diagnosed with autism spectrum disorder (ASD) show a wide range of neurologic and developmental behaviors. The most severe form is autism, or classical ASD; a milder form may present as Asperger syndrome; and sometimes a child cannot be categorized into a specific diagnosis and so is labeled with a pervasive developmental disorder (PDD).
- ASD occurs in all ethnic and socioeconomic groups and affects every age group.
- The Centers for Disease Control and Prevention (CDC) estimates the prevalence of ASD to be 1 in 68; it is almost five times more common among boys (1 in 42) than among girls (1 in 189).
- Children with autism have impaired social interaction, do not respond to their name, avoid eye contact, and show limited interest in their surroundings. They rarely communicate with others and display repetitive movements or mannerisms, such as rocking or twirling. They may also have self-abusive behaviors, such as biting and head banging. Many children with autism have a very high pain tolerance but are extremely sensitive to noise, touch, or other sensory stimulation.
- The cause of this developmental disorder is unknown, but researchers believe it is due to a combination of genetic errors and environmental factors, perhaps a problem with fetal brain development. Although many parents are concerned about a connection with vaccines, extensive studies have failed to show a link between the two.
- The American Academy of Pediatrics (AAP) recommends a general developmental screening at every well-child visit and a developmental screening using a standardized tool at 9, 18, and 30 months, or whenever a caregiver expresses concern. In addition, autism-specific screening is recommended for all children at the 18- and 24-month visits.
- Treatment involves coordinated educational and behavioral interventions to help the child develop social and language skills. Medications may be prescribed to treat depression, anxiety, and obsessive-compulsive behaviors.

From https://www.aap.org/en-us/about-the-aap/Committees-Councils-Sections/Council-on-Children-with-Disabilities/Pages/Autism.aspx. Accessed February 9, 2016.

Modified Checklist for Autism in Toddlers: *M-CHAT-R*

The M-CHAT-R has been validated to assess risk for autism spectrum disorders (ASDs) in toddlers between 16 and 30 months of age. The M-CHAT-R can be administered and scored as part of a well-child checkup. Caregivers complete the questionnaire based on the child's typical behavior. The medical assistant may be asked questions about the form, so you should be familiar with its purpose and instructions for completion.

The primary goal of the M-CHAT-R is to detect as many cases of ASD as possible. It therefore has a high false-positive rate; this means that not all children who score at risk will be diagnosed with ASD. If the initial tool is positive, the Follow-Up questions (M-CHAT-R/F) should also be administered. If results remain positive, the child should be referred for diagnostic evaluation by a specialist trained to evaluate ASD in very young children. Scoring instructions can be downloaded from the website *www.mchatscreen.com*.

The following are the questions on the M-CHAT-R.

1. If you point at something across the room, does your child look at it?   Yes   No
   (FOR EXAMPLE, if you point at a toy or an animal, does your child look at the toy or animal?)

2. Have you ever wondered if your child might be deaf?   Yes   No

3. Does your child play pretend or make-believe?   Yes   No
   (FOR EXAMPLE, pretend to drink from an empty cup, pretend to talk on a phone, or pretend to feed a doll or stuffed animal?)

4. Does your child like climbing on things?   Yes   No
   (FOR EXAMPLE, furniture, playground equipment, or stairs)

5. Does your child make unusual finger movements near his or her eyes?   Yes   No
   (FOR EXAMPLE, does your child wiggle his or her fingers close to his or her eyes?)

6. Does your child point with one finger to ask for something or to get help?   Yes   No
   (FOR EXAMPLE, pointing to a snack or toy that is out of reach)

7. Does your child point with one finger to show you something interesting?   Yes   No
   (FOR EXAMPLE, pointing to an airplane in the sky or a big truck in the road)

8. Is your child interested in other children?   Yes   No
   (FOR EXAMPLE, does your child watch other children, smile at them, or go to them?)

9. Does your child show you things by bringing them to you or holding them up for you to see—not to get help, but just to share?   Yes   No
   (FOR EXAMPLE, showing you a flower, a stuffed animal, or a toy truck)

10. Does your child respond when you call his or her name?   Yes   No
    (FOR EXAMPLE, does he or she look up, talk or babble, or stop what he or she is doing when you call his or her name?)

11. When you smile at your child, does he or she smile back at you?   Yes   No

Continued

Modified Checklist for Autism in Toddlers: *M-CHAT-R—continued*

12. Does your child get upset by everyday noises?   Yes   No
(FOR EXAMPLE, does your child scream or cry to noise
such as a vacuum cleaner or loud music?)

13. Does your child walk?   Yes   No

14. Does your child look you in the eye when you are   Yes   No
talking to him or her, playing with him or her, or
dressing him or her?

15. Does your child try to copy what you do?   Yes   No
(FOR EXAMPLE, wave bye-bye, clap, or make a funny
noise when you do)

16. If you turn your head to look at something, does your   Yes   No
child look around to see what you are looking at?

17. Does your child try to get you to watch him or her?   Yes   No
(FOR EXAMPLE, does your child look at you for praise,
or say "look" or "watch me"?)

18. Does your child understand when you tell him or her to   Yes   No
do something?
(FOR EXAMPLE, if you don't point, can your child
understand "put the book on the chair" or "bring me
the blanket"?)

19. If something new happens, does your child look at your   Yes   No
face to see how you feel about it?
(FOR EXAMPLE, if he or she hears a strange or funny
noise, or sees a new toy, will he or she look at your
face?)

20. Does your child like movement activities?   Yes   No
(FOR EXAMPLE, being swung or bounced on your knee)

Official M-CHAT Website at http://www2.gsu.edu/~psydlr/Site/Official_M-CHAT_Website.html. Accessed February 9, 2016.

Inherited Disorders

Cystic Fibrosis

Cystic fibrosis (CF) is an *autosomal recessive* genetic disorder (i.e., both parents are carriers, but neither has the disease). CF prevents the normal movement of sodium chloride (salt) into and out of cells. The lungs and pancreas are primarily affected, resulting in a buildup of abnormally thick secretions in the lungs and blockage of the pancreatic ducts, which prevents the excretion of pancreatic digestive enzymes and results in malabsorption problems. The child is prone to developing an emphysema-like lung condition because of the obstruction of the air pathways with mucus. There is also an abnormality in the sweat glands, which produce sweat that is very high in sodium chloride.

Signs and symptoms of cystic fibrosis include a salty taste to the skin, which may be noticed when parents kiss the child, steatorrhea (large, greasy, foul-smelling stools), abdominal distention, failure to thrive, chronic cough, and frequent respiratory infections. All states screen newborns for CF using either a genetic test or a blood test. The genetic test shows whether the newborn has the CF gene, and the blood test evaluates pancreatic function. If either of these tests suggests CF, the diagnosis is confirmed using a sweat test, which shows an elevated chlorine level.

Treatment of the disease is complicated and requires a multispecialty approach because so many systems are involved. The first line of treatment is prevention of bronchial obstruction through routine chest percussion therapy (CPT). Mechanical devices have been developed to assist with CPT. Two examples are an electric chest clapper, known as a *mechanical percussor,* and an inflatable therapy vest that uses high-frequency airwaves to force the mucus that is deep in the lungs toward the upper airways. Medical treatments include bronchodilators and antibiotics for signs of infection. More recent therapies have included medications such as aerosolized dornase alfa (Pulmozyme), which makes mucus thinner and easier to cough up. The child also is given pancreatic enzymes to improve digestion and absorption of nutrients. Ivacaftor (Kalydeco), the first drug to target the genetic cause of CF, was approved by the FDA in 2012 for patients 6 years of age or older who have certain genetic mutations of CF. Ivacaftor, an oral medication taken twice a day, helps improve lung function, lower sweat chloride levels, and help patients gain weight. The drug marks a breakthrough in CF treatment because it is the first to address the underlying cause of the disease.

Cystic fibrosis is a chronic, progressive disease that has no cure; the life expectancy is 35 to 40 years. Genetic testing can identify carriers, and its presence can be detected through prenatal genetic testing with either chorionic villi sampling or amniocentesis. Cystic fibrosis usually occurs without any warning (parents have no idea they are carriers), so families need support and understanding to cope with the demands of caring for a child with the disease.

Duchenne's Muscular Dystrophy

Muscular dystrophy is an X-linked genetic disease (passed from mothers to sons) that causes progressive muscle degeneration. The disease usually develops between 3 and 5 years of age and is marked by progressive muscular breakdown and weakness, frequent falls, a waddling gait, possible swallowing problems, and difficulty climbing stairs. The disorder is diagnosed with a blood test that shows an elevated level of creatine kinase (CK) (an enzyme that leaks out of damaged muscle), electromyography, muscle biopsy, and genetic testing. As the disease progresses and the necrotic skeletal muscles are replaced with fat and fibrous connective tissue, muscle function is gradually lost. Respiratory insufficiency and infections are common because of involvement of the diaphragm and intercostal muscles required for breathing. The disease has no cure and no specific treatment except for supportive care. Family counseling is helpful so that family members can learn to cope with the disease. Because of improved cardiac and respiratory care, life expectancy is increasing. Survival into the early 30s is becoming more common, and some men have lived into their 40s and 50s.

IMMUNIZATIONS

Over the years, immunization has helped dramatically reduce potentially lethal childhood infections. Figure 35-7 summarizes the 2016 immunization recommendations from the CDC for children 0 through 18 years of age. These can be found at the CDC's website: *http://www.cdc.gov/vaccines/schedules/downloads/child/0-18yrs-child-combined-schedule.pdf.*

The schedules are updated periodically as new vaccines become available and/or research indicates a better method for giving the vaccine. The CDC recommends immunization against infectious diseases for all children, except those for whom a particular vaccination would pose a risk. However, each state develops its own immunization program and methods of enforcement.

2016 Immunization Schedule

2016 immunization schedule changes include the following:

- The vaccine order was changed to group them by the recommended age of administration.
- A purple bar was added for *Haemophilus influenzae* type b (Hib) vaccine for children aged 5 to 18 years that recommends vaccination administration to certain high-risk children.
- The inactivated polio vaccine footnote was updated for children who received only the oral poliovirus vaccine and received all doses before age 4.
- The hepatitis B vaccine footnote was revised to clarify when postvaccination serologic testing should be done on infants born to mothers with hepatitis B.
- It includes recommendations for the use of two recently licensed meningococcal B vaccines (Trumenba and Bexsero) and the 9-valent human papillomavirus vaccine (Gardasil 9).

Summary of changes in the 2016 Pediatric Immunization Schedule. http://www.medscape.com/viewarticle/858103?nlid=98844_3901&src=wnl_newsalrt_160201_MSCPEDIT&uac=235043AJ&impID=977298&faf=1. Accessed February 10, 2016.

The vaccines used in immunizations consist of a suspension of **attenuated** organisms or their toxins, which is administered to stimulate an active immune response in the child's body, resulting in the production of antibodies against the specific pathogens. Booster doses usually are equivalent to a single dose of the initial immunization; for some immunizations, such as tetanus, boosters are prescribed at designated intervals to ensure maintenance of immune levels.

Vaccine manufacturers have trade names for each product and have established protocols to ensure potency and stability. All vaccines are tested for safety and effectiveness. In every package of vaccine is an insert that fully describes the vaccine, its use, the route of administration, adverse reactions, and signs and symptoms the parent might observe after immunization that would indicate a potential problem. Untoward responses include high fever, swelling at the site of the injection, **urticaria**, breathing difficulties, severe headache, and convulsions. Any of these should be reported

to the physician immediately. Vaccine storage should follow the manufacturer's guidelines (e.g., some vaccines must be refrigerated; others must not be exposed to sunlight).

Some vaccines are grown in birds' eggs or in a medium made of animal organs or are weakened with chemicals. Therefore, a child who is allergic to eggs cannot receive some of the vaccines, such as the MMR, and the vaccine for varicella. The medical assistant must know the potential allergic problems, common symptoms, and adverse reactions to immunizations and must make sure the parent is informed. Table 35-2 details guidelines for childhood immunizations.

Before a child or adult receives a vaccine, the healthcare provider is required by the National Childhood Vaccine Injury Act (NCVIA) to provide a copy of a Vaccine Information Sheet (VIS) to either the adult patient or the child's parent or legal guardian. A VIS provides information about the risks and benefits of each vaccine. If providing the parent or guardian with the VIS is the medical assistant's responsibility, he or she should do the following (Procedure 35-1):

- Before administering the vaccine, give the parent the most current VIS available for that particular vaccine. Give the parent enough time to review the information and then answer any questions or refer the parent's concerns to the physician before administering the vaccine. VIS forms are available online in a number of different languages to meet the needs of a diverse patient population.
- Document in the child's health record the date the VIS was given and the publication date of the VIS (which appears on the bottom of the form).
- To make sure the office has the most current VIS forms, either call the state health department or refer to the CDC website (*www.cdc.gov/vaccines/hcp/vis/current-vis.html*). Forms can be printed directly from the site.
- An informed consent form must be signed and attached to the child's health record or electronically signed in the child's electronic health record (EHR) before immunizations are given. Documentation of immunization administration must include the date the vaccine was administered, the manufacturer of the vaccine, the manufacturer's lot number, the type of vaccine, the exact site of administration if an injection was given, any reported or observed side effects, the name and title of the person who administered the vaccine, and the address of the medical office where the vaccine was administered.
- An official immunization booklet should be given to the parent and updated as needed to reflect the child's current immunization status. The medical assistant should not only document the required details in the patient's health record, but also complete the parent's immunization booklet each time the child receives another vaccination or booster. These parent records help schools and day care centers determine the child's immunization status. Some states are developing computerized immunization record systems.
- It is very important that vaccine vials be handled and stored properly to maintain the compound's ability to fight disease. The CDC's recommendations for vaccine management practices can be found at http://www.cdc.gov/vaccines/recs/storage/.

Text continued on p. 802

Vaccine	Birth	1 mo	2 mos	4 mos	6 mos	9 mos	12 mos	15 mos	18 mos	19–23 mos	2–3 yrs	4–6 yrs	7–10 yrs	11–12 yrs	13–15 yrs	16–18 yrs
Hepatitis B[1] (HepB)	1st dose	←—— 2nd dose ——→			←————————— 3rd dose —————————→											
Rotavirus[2] (RV) RV1 (2-dose series); RV5 (3-dose series)			1st dose	2nd dose	See footnote 2											
Diphtheria, tetanus, & acellular pertussis[3] (DTaP: <7 yrs)			1st dose	2nd dose	3rd dose		←———— 4th dose ————→					5th dose				
Haemophilus influenzae type b[4] (Hib)			1st dose	2nd dose	See footnote 4		←— 3rd or 4th dose, See footnote 4 —→									
Pneumococcal conjugate[5] (PCV13)			1st dose	2nd dose	3rd dose		←— 4th dose —→									
Inactivated poliovirus[6] (IPV: <18 yrs)			1st dose	2nd dose	←————————— 3rd dose —————————→							4th dose				
Influenza[7] (IIV; LAIV)					Annual vaccination (IIV only) 1 or 2 doses						Annual vaccination (LAIV or IIV) 1 or 2 doses		Annual vaccination (LAIV or IIV) 1 dose only			
Measles, mumps, rubella[8] (MMR)					See footnote 8		←— 1st dose —→					2nd dose				
Varicella[9] (VAR)							←— 1st dose —→					2nd dose				
Hepatitis A[10] (HepA)							←— 2-dose series, See footnote 10 —→									
Meningococcal[11] (Hib-MenCY ≥6 weeks; MenACWY-D ≥9 mos; MenACWY-CRM ≥2 mos)					See footnote 11									1st dose		Booster
Tetanus, diphtheria, & acellular pertussis[12] (Tdap: ≥7 yrs)														(Tdap)		
Human papillomavirus[13] (2vHPV: females only; 4vHPV, 9vHPV: males and females)														(3-dose series)		
Meningococcal B[11]														See footnote 11		
Pneumococcal polysaccharide[5] (PPSV23)												See footnote 5				

Legend:
- Range of recommended ages for all children
- Range of recommended ages for catch-up immunization
- Range of recommended ages for certain high-risk groups
- Range of recommended ages during which catch-up is encouraged and for certain high-risk groups
- Range of recommended ages for non-high-risk groups that may receive vaccine, subject to individual clinical decision making
- No recommendation

This schedule includes recommendations in effect as of January 1, 2016. Any dose not administered at the recommended age should be administered at a subsequent visit, when indicated and feasible. The use of a combination vaccine generally is preferred over separate injections of its equivalent component vaccines. Vaccination providers should consult the relevant Advisory Committee on Immunization Practices (ACIP) statement for detailed recommendations, available online at http://www.cdc.gov/vaccines/hcp/acip-recs/index.html. Clinically significant adverse events that follow vaccination should be reported to the Vaccine Adverse Event Reporting System (VAERS) online (http://www.vaers.hhs.gov) or by telephone (800-822-7967). Suspected cases of vaccine-preventable diseases should be reported to the state or local health department. Additional information, including precautions and contraindications for vaccination, is available from CDC online (http://www.cdc.gov/vaccines/recs/vac-admin/contraindications.htm) or by telephone (800-CDC-INFO [800-232-4636]).

This schedule is approved by the Advisory Committee on Immunization Practices (http://www.cdc.gov/vaccines/acip), the American Academy of Pediatrics (http://www.aap.org), the American Academy of Family Physicians (http://www.aafp.org), and the American College of Obstetricians and Gynecologists (http://www.acog.org).

NOTE: The above recommendations must be read along with the footnotes of this schedule.

FIGURE 35-7 Recommended immunization schedule for children ages birth to 18 years. (From www.cdc.gov/vaccines/schedules/downloads/child-/0-18yrs-child-combined-schedule.pdf. Accessed January 13, 2015.)

5. Pneumococcal vaccines. (Minimum age: 6 weeks for PCV13, 2 years for PPSV23)

Routine vaccination with PCV13:
- Administer a 4-dose series of PCV13 vaccine at ages 2, 4, and 6 months and at age 12 through 15 months.
- For children aged 14 through 59 months who have received an age-appropriate series of 7-valent PCV (PCV7), administer a single supplemental dose of 13-valent PCV (PCV13).

Catch-up vaccination with PCV13:
- Administer 1 dose of PCV13 to all healthy children aged 24 through 59 months who are not completely vaccinated for their age.
- For other catch-up guidance, see Figure 2.

Vaccination of persons with high-risk conditions with PCV13 and PPSV23:
All recommended PCV13 doses should be administered prior to PPSV23 vaccination if possible.
- For children 2 through 5 years of age with any of the following conditions: chronic heart disease (particularly cyanotic congenital heart disease and cardiac failure); chronic lung disease (including asthma if treated with high-dose oral corticosteroid therapy); diabetes mellitus; cerebrospinal fluid leak; cochlear implant; sickle cell disease and other hemoglobinopathies; anatomic or functional asplenia; HIV infection; chronic renal failure; nephrotic syndrome; diseases associated with treatment with immunosuppressive drugs or radiation therapy, including malignant neoplasms, leukemias, lymphomas, and Hodgkin disease; solid organ transplantation; or congenital immunodeficiency:
1. Administer 1 dose of PCV13 if any incomplete schedule of 3 doses of PCV (PCV7 and/or PCV13) were received previously.
2. Administer 2 doses of PCV13 at least 8 weeks apart if unvaccinated or any incomplete schedule of fewer than 3 doses of PCV (PCV7 and/or PCV13) were received previously.
3. Administer 1 supplemental dose of PCV13 if 4 doses of PCV7 or other age-appropriate complete PCV7 series was received previously.
4. The minimum interval between doses of PCV (PCV7 or PCV13) is 8 weeks.
5. For children with no history of PPSV23 vaccination, administer PPSV23 at least 8 weeks after the most recent dose of PCV13.

- For children aged 6 through 18 years who have cerebrospinal fluid leak; cochlear implant; sickle cell disease and other hemoglobinopathies; anatomic or functional asplenia; congenital or acquired immunodeficiencies; HIV infection; chronic renal failure; nephrotic syndrome; diseases associated with treatment with immunosuppressive drugs or radiation therapy, including malignant neoplasms, leukemias, lymphomas, and Hodgkin disease; generalized malignancy; solid organ transplantation; or multiple myeloma:
1. If neither PCV13 nor PPSV23 has been received previously, administer 1 dose of PCV13 now and 1 dose of PPSV23 at least 8 weeks later.
2. If PCV13 has been received previously but PPSV23 has not, administer 1 dose of PPSV23 at least 8 weeks after the most recent dose of PCV13.
3. If PPSV23 has been received but PCV13 has not, administer 1 dose of PCV13 at least 8 weeks after the most recent dose of PPSV23.

8. Measles, mumps, and rubella (MMR) vaccine. (Minimum age: 12 months for routine vaccination)

Routine vaccination:
- Administer a 2-dose series of MMR vaccine at ages 12 through 15 months and 4 through 6 years. The second dose may be administered before age 4 years, provided at least 4 weeks have elapsed since the first dose.
- Administer 1 dose of MMR vaccine to infants aged 6 through 11 months before departure from the United States for international travel. These children should be revaccinated with 2 doses of MMR vaccine, the first at age 12 through 15 months (12 months if the child remains in an area where disease risk is high), and the second dose at least 4 weeks later.
- Administer 2 doses of MMR vaccine to children aged 12 months and older before departure from the United States for international travel. The first dose should be administered on or after age 12 months and the second dose at least 4 weeks later.

Catch-up vaccination:
- Ensure that all school-aged children and adolescents have had 2 doses of MMR vaccine; the minimum interval between the 2 doses is 4 weeks.

11. Meningococcal vaccines. (Minimum age: 6 weeks for Hib-MenCY [MenHibrix], 9 months for MenACWY-D [Menactra], 2 months for MenACWY-CRM [Menveo], 10 years for serogroup B meningococcal [MenB] vaccines: MenB-4C [Bexsero] and MenB-FHbp [Trumenba])

Routine vaccination:
- Administer a single dose of Menactra or Menveo vaccine at age 11 through 12 years, with a booster dose at age 16 years.
- Adolescents aged 11 through 18 years with human immunodeficiency virus (HIV) infection should receive a 2-dose primary series of Menactra or Menveo with at least 8 weeks between doses.
- For children aged 2 months through 18 years with high-risk conditions, see below.

11. Meningococcal vaccines (cont'd)

Catch-up vaccination:
- Administer Menactra or Menveo vaccine at age 13 through 18 years if not previously vaccinated.
- If the first dose is administered at age 13 through 15 years, a booster dose should be administered at age 16 through 18 years with a minimum interval of at least 8 weeks between doses.
- If the first dose is administered at age 16 years or older, a booster dose is not needed.
- For other catch-up guidance, see Figure 2.

Clinical discretion:
- Young adults aged 16 through 23 years (preferred age range is 16 through 18 years) may be vaccinated with either a 2-dose series of Bexsero or 3-dose series of Trumenba vaccine to provide short-term protection against most strains of serogroup B meningococcal disease. The two MenB vaccines are not interchangeable; the same vaccine product must be used for all doses.

Vaccination of persons with high-risk conditions and other persons at increased risk of disease:

Children with anatomic or functional asplenia (including sickle cell disease):

Meningococcal conjugate ACWY vaccines:
1. Menveo
   o Children who initiate vaccination at 8 weeks: Administer doses at 2, 4, 6, and 12 months of age.
   o Unvaccinated children who initiate vaccination at 7 through 23 months: Administer 2 doses, with the second dose at least 12 weeks after the first dose AND after the first birthday.
   o Children 24 months and older who have not received a complete series: Administer 2 primary doses at least 8 weeks apart.
2. MenHibrix
   o Children who initiate vaccination at 6 weeks: Administer doses at 2, 4, 6, and 12 through 15 months of age.
   o If the first dose of MenHibrix is given at or after 12 months of age, a total of 2 doses should be given at least 8 weeks apart to ensure protection against serogroups C and Y meningococcal disease.
3. Menactra
   o Children 24 months and older who have not received a complete series: Administer 2 primary doses at least 8 weeks apart. If Menactra is administered to a child with asplenia (including sickle cell disease), do not administer Menactra until 2 years of age and at least 4 weeks after the completion of all PCV13 doses.

Meningococcal B vaccines:
1. Bexsero or Trumenba
   o Persons 10 years or older who have not received a complete series: Administer a 2-dose series of Bexsero, at least 1 month apart. Or a 3-dose series of Trumenba, with the second dose at least 2 months after the first and the third dose at least 6 months after the first. The two MenB vaccines are not interchangeable; the same vaccine product must be used for all doses.

Children with persistent complement component deficiency (includes persons with inherited or chronic deficiencies in C3, C5-9, properdin, factor D, factor H, or taking eculizumab [Soliris]):

Meningococcal conjugate ACWY vaccines:
1. Menveo
   o Children who initiate vaccination at 8 weeks: Administer doses at 2, 4, 6, and 12 months of age.
   o Unvaccinated children who initiate vaccination at 7 through 23 months: Administer 2 doses, with the second dose at least 12 weeks after the first dose AND after the first birthday.
   o Children 24 months and older who have not received a complete series: Administer 2 primary doses at least 8 weeks apart.
2. MenHibrix
   o Children who initiate vaccination 6 weeks: Administer doses at 2, 4, 6, and 12 through 15 months of age.
   o If the first dose of MenHibrix is given at or after 12 months of age, a total of 2 doses should be given at least 8 weeks apart to ensure protection against serogroups C and Y meningococcal disease.
3. Menactra
   o Children 9 through 23 months: Administer 2 primary doses at least 12 weeks apart.
   o Children 24 months and older who have not received a complete series: Administer 2 primary doses at least 8 weeks apart.

Meningococcal B vaccines:
1. Bexsero or Trumenba
   o Persons 10 years or older who have not received a complete series: Administer a 2-dose series of Bexsero, at least 1 month apart. Or a 3-dose series of Trumenba, with the second dose at least 2 months after the first and the third dose at least 6 months after the first. The two MenB vaccines are not interchangeable; the same vaccine product must be used for all doses.

For children who travel to or reside in countries in which meningococcal disease is hyperendemic or epidemic, including countries in the African meningitis belt or the Hajj:
- administer an age-appropriate formulation and series of Menactra or Menveo for protection against serogroups A and W meningococcal disease. Prior receipt of MenHibrix is not sufficient for children traveling to the meningitis belt or the Hajj because it does not contain serogroups A or W.

For children at risk during a community outbreak attributable to a vaccine serogroup:
- administer or complete an age- and formulation-appropriate series of MenHibrix, Menactra, or Menveo; Bexsero or Trumenba.

For booster doses among persons with high-risk conditions, refer to MMWR 2013 / 62(RR02);1-22, available at http://www.cdc.gov/mmwr/preview/mmwrhtml/rr6202a1.htm.

For other catch-up recommendations for these persons, and complete information on use of meningococcal vaccines, including guidance related to vaccination of persons at increased risk of infection, see MMWR March 22, 2013 / 62(RR02);1-22, and MMWR October 23, 2015 / 64(41); 1171-1176 available at http://www.cdc.gov/mmwr/pdf/wk/mm6441.pdf.

FIGURE 35-7, cont'd

TABLE 35-2   Guidelines for Childhood Immunizations

VACCINE	TRADE NAME	ROUTE OF ADMINISTRATION	CONTRAINDICATIONS*	SIDE EFFECTS
DTaP Diphtheria, tetanus, pertussis (whooping cough)	Daptacel, Infanrix	IM; Td (tetanus and diphtheria) boosters at 11-12 yr if at least 5 yr since last dose; subsequent booster every 10 yr	Moderate or severe acute illness; neurologic problem; complication after previous dose (e.g., fever, convulsions)	Mild fever, anorexia, irritability, drowsiness
HAV Hepatitis A (can use either Havrix or Vaqta)	Havrix, Vaqta	IM; all children 1 yr; 2 doses 6 mo apart	Hypersensitivity to product, acute infection or fever	Localized injection site reaction, fever, headache
HBV Hepatitis B	Engerix-B, Recombivax HB	IM; may give with all other vaccines but at a separate site; requires 3 injections	Moderate or severe acute illness; yeast allergy; severe cardiovascular disease	Fever, pain at site, headache, malaise, vomiting
Hib *Haemophilus influenzae* serotype B meningitis	COMVAX, PedvaxHIB, Pentacel, ActHIB, Men-Hibrix	IM; may give with all other vaccines but at a separate site. Three doses of ActHIB, MenHibrix, or Pentacel at 2, 4, and 6 months or 2 doses PedvaxHib or COMVAX at 2 and 4 months of age; booster dose at 12 through 15 months	Not routinely given to children older than 5; moderate or severe acute illness	Minimal
HPV Human papillomavirus	2vHPV (Cervarix) females only; 4vHPV (Gardasil), 9vHPV (Gardasil 9) males and females	IM; routine vaccination at age 11 or 12 years; second dose 1 to 2 months after first dose; third dose 16 weeks after second dose	Hypersensitivity to ingredients; pregnancy	Relatively few; mild headache and GI upset
Influenza Trivalent inactivated vaccine for 6 months; at 2 years, use live, attenuated vaccine	FluLaval, Fluzone, FluMist (nasal spray)	IM; annually each fall	Allergy to eggs; recent fever	Uncommon; fever, local irritation at injection site, general malaise
IPV Inactive poliovirus for polio	Ipol	SC or IM; 4 doses; may give with all other vaccines but at a separate site	Moderate or severe acute illness; egg allergy	Uncommon
Meningococcal vaccine for meningitis (MCV4)	Menactra, Menveo, Bexsero, or Trumenba	IM; single dose of Menactra or Menveo vaccine at age 11 through 12 years, with a booster dose at age 16 years; aged 16 through 23 years vaccinated with a 2-dose series of Bexsero or a 3-dose series of Trumenba vaccine to provide short-term protection	Moderate or severe acute illness; history of allergic reaction to MCV4	Uncommon
MMR Measles, mumps, rubella	M-M-R II	SC; may give with all other vaccines but at a separate site	Moderate or severe acute illness; immunocompromised patients (may be given if HIV positive); pregnancy or possible pregnancy in 3 mo; egg allergy	Fever

TABLE 35-2 Guidelines for Childhood Immunizations—*continued*

VACCINE	TRADE NAME	ROUTE OF ADMINISTRATION	CONTRAINDICATIONS*	SIDE EFFECTS
Pneumococcal (PCV) Pneumococcal pneumonia	Pneumovax 23, Prevnar 13	IM or SC; all children 2-23 mo; administer every 6 yr for high-risk patients	Moderate or severe acute illness; hypersensitivity	Drowsiness, local irritation at site, mild fever
Rotavirus (Rota) RotaTeq for prevention of rotavirus gastroenteritis	Rotarix	PO; 3 doses at 6-12 wk; subsequent doses at 4-10 wk intervals	Hypersensitivity	GI upset and blood disorders
Varicella (chickenpox)	Varivax	SC; may give with all other vaccines but at a separate site; 2-dose series at ages 12 through 15 months and 4 through 6 years	Confirmed history of chickenpox; pregnancy or possible pregnancy in 1 mo; moderate or severe acute illness; immunocompromised patients; egg allergy	No salicylates for 6 wk afterward to prevent risk of Reye's syndrome
May give combination vaccine: measles, mumps, rubella, varicella (MMRV)	ProQuad	SC; may give with all other vaccines but at a separate site; all susceptible children 12 mo or older	Confirmed history of chickenpox; pregnancy or possible pregnancy in 1 mo; moderate or severe acute illness; immunocompromised patients; egg allergy	No salicylates for 6 wk afterward to prevent risk of Reye's syndrome

GI, Gastrointestinal; *HIV*, human immunodeficiency virus; *IM*, intramuscular; *PO*, oral; *SC*, subcutaneous.
*Mild illness is not a contraindication.

PROCEDURE 35-1   **Verify the Rules of Medication Administration: Document Immunizations**

Goal: *To document accurately the administration of a pediatric immunization.*

Scenario: *Samantha Anderson, a 5-week-old infant, has just received her second dose of the hepatitis B (HBV) vaccine. Document the administration of the vaccine.*

EQUIPMENT and SUPPLIES

- Patient's record
- Vaccine administration record (VAR)
- Parent's immunization booklet (if used in the medical practice)
- Vaccine Information Sheet (VIS) for hepatitis B (a link to the current VIS forms can be accessed at www.cdc.gov/vaccines/hcp/vis/current-vis.html)

PROCEDURAL STEPS

1. Gather the necessary forms.
2. Make sure the provider obtained informed consent from the parent, that the hepatitis B VIS form was given, and that all the parent's questions were answered before the vaccine is dispensed and administered.
   PURPOSE: To follow risk management practices.
3. After dispensing the vaccine dose and before administering it, complete the information required on the VAR, including the name of the vaccine, the date given, the route of administration and site, the vaccine lot number and manufacturer, the date on the VIS form, the date it was given to the parent, and your signature or initials.
   PURPOSE: To meet the legal requirements of the National Childhood Vaccine Injury Act.
4. Administer the vaccine intramuscularly (see the Administering Medications chapter).

5. In the parent's immunization booklet, record the date of administration, the name and address of the physician's practice, and the type of vaccine administered.
   PURPOSE: To maintain an accurate and comprehensive parental record of childhood immunizations for school and/or day care purposes.
6. After administering the HBV vaccine, record the following details in the child's health record:
   - Date the vaccine was administered
   - Vaccine's manufacturer, batch and lot numbers, and expiration date
   - Type of vaccine administered and dose
   - Route of administration and exact site if an injection was given
   - Any reported or observed side effects
   - Publication date of the VIS form given to the parent (on the bottom of the form)
   - Parent education about possible side effects of the vaccine
   - Name and title of the person who administered the vaccine

4/2/20— 3:25 pm: Mother given VIS form for Hep B. Had no questions. Administered second dose of Hep B IM to ⊕ vastus lateralis per Dr. Flint's order. No problems noted after injection. S. Kwong, CMA (AAMA)

PROCEDURE 35-1 ____*—continued*

Vaccine Administration Record for Children and Teens

(Page 1 of 2)

Patient name: _____

Birthdate: _____ Patient ID number: _____

Clinic name and address

Before administering any vaccines, give copies of all pertinent Vaccine Information Statements (VISs) to the child's parent or legal representative and make sure he/she understands the risks and benefits of the vaccine(s). Always provide or update the patient's personal record card.

Vaccine	Type of Vaccine[1]	Date given (mo/day/yr)	Funding Source (F,S,P)[2]	Route & Site[3]	Vaccine		Vaccine Information Statement (VIS)		Vaccinator[5] (signature or initials & title)
					Lot #	Mfr.	Date on VIS[4]	Date given[4]	
Hepatitis B[6] (e.g., HepB, Hib-HepB, DTaP-HepB-IPV) Give IM.[3]									
Diphtheria, Tetanus, Pertussis[6] (e.g., DTaP, DTaP/Hib, DTaP-HepB-IPV, DT, DTaP-IPV/Hib, Tdap, DTaP-IPV, Td) Give IM.[3]									
***Haemophilus influenzae* type b[6]** (e.g., Hib, Hib-HepB, DTaP-IPV/Hib, DTaP/Hib, Hib-MenCY) Give IM.[3]									
Polio[6] (e.g., IPV, DTaP-HepB-DTaP-IPV/Hib, DTaP-IPV) Give IPV SC or IM.[3] Give all others IM.[3]									
Pneumococcal (e.g., PCV7, PCV13, conjugate; PPSV23, polysaccharide) Give PCV IM.[3] Give PPSV SC or IM.[3]									
Rotavirus (RV1, RV5) Give orally (po).[3]									

See page 2 to record measles-mumps-rubella, varicella, hepatitis A, meningococcal, HPV, influenza, and other vaccines (e.g., travel vaccines).

How to Complete This Record

1. Record the generic abbreviation (e.g., Tdap) or the trade name for each vaccine (see table at right).

2. Record the funding source of the vaccine given as either F (federal), S (state), or P (private).

3. Record the route by which the vaccine was given as either intramuscular (IM), subcutaneous (SC), intradermal (ID), intranasal (IN), or oral (PO) and also the site where it was administered as either RA (right arm), LA (left arm), RT (right thigh), or LT (left thigh).

4. Record the publication date of each VIS as well as the date the VIS is given to the patient.

5. To meet the space constraints of this form and federal requirements for documentation, a healthcare setting may want to keep a reference list of vaccinators that includes their initials and titles.

6. For combination vaccines, fill in a row for each antigen in the combination.

Abbreviation	Trade Name and Manufacturer
DTaP	Daptacel (sanofi); Infanrix (GlaxoSmithKline [GSK]); Tripedia (sanofi pasteur)
DT (pediatric)	Generic DT (sanofi pasteur)
DTaP-HepB-IPV	Pediarix (GSK)
DTaP/Hib	TriHIBit (sanofi pasteur)
DTaP-IPV/Hib	Pentacel (sanofi pasteur)
DTaP-IPV	Kinrix (GSK)
HepB	Engerix-B (GSK); Recombivax HB (Merck)
HepA-HepB	Twinrix (GSK), can be given to teens age 18 and older
Hib	ActHIB (sanofi pasteur); Hiberix (GSK); PedvaxHIB (Merck)
Hib-HepB	Comvax (Merck)
Hib-MenCY	MenHibrix (GSK)
IPV	Ipol (sanofi pasteur)
PCV13	Prevnar 13 (Pfizer)
PPSV23	Pneumovax 23 (Merck)
RV1	Rotarix (GSK)
RV5	RotaTeq (Merck)
Tdap	Adacel (sanofi pasteur); Boostrix (GSK)
Td	Decavac (sanofi pasteur); Generic Td (MA Biological Labs)

Technical content reviewed by the Centers for Disease Control and Prevention

For additional copies, visit www.immunize.org/catg.d/p2022.pdf • Item #P2022 (4/14)

This form was created by the Immunization Action Coalition • www.immunize.org • www.vaccineinformation.org

PROCEDURE 35-1 —*continued*

Vaccine Administration Record for Children and Teens

Patient name:_____

Birthdate:_____ Patient ID number:_____

Clinic name and address

Before administering any vaccines, give copies of all pertinent Vaccine Information Statements (VISs) to the child's parent or legal representative and make sure he/she understands the risks and benefits of the vaccine(s). Always provide or update the patient's personal record card.

Vaccine	Type of Vaccine[1]	Date given (mo/day/yr)	Funding Source (F,S,P)[2]	Route & Site[3]	Vaccine		Vaccine Information Statement (VIS)		Vaccinator[5] (signature or initials & title)
					Lot #	Mfr.	Date on VIS[4]	Date given[4]	
Measles, Mumps, Rubella[6] (e.g., MMR, MMRV) Give SC.[3]									
Varicella[6] (e.g., VAR, MMRV) Give SC.[3]									
Hepatitis A[6] (HepA) Give IM.[3]									
Meningococcal (e.g., MenACWY-CRM; Men-ACWY-D; Hib-MenCY; MPSV4) Give MenACWY and Hib-MenCY IM[3] and give MPSV4 SC.[3]									
Human papillomavirus[6] (e.g., HPV2, HPV4) Give IM.[3]									
Influenza (e.g., IIV3, trivalent inactivated; IIV4, quadrivalent inactivated; RIV, recombinant inactivated [for ages 18–49 yrs]; LAIV4, quadrivalent live attenuated) Give IIV and RIV IM.[3] Give LAIV IN.[3]									
Other									

See page 1 to record hepatitis B, diphtheria, tetanus, pertussis, *Haemophilus influenzae* type b, polio, pneumococcal, and rotavirus vaccines.

How to Complete This Record

1. Record the generic abbreviation (e.g., Tdap) or the trade name for each vaccine (see table at right).

2. Record the funding source of the vaccine given as either F (federal), S (state), or P (private).

3. Record the route by which the vaccine was given as either intramuscular (IM), subcutaneous (SC), intradermal (ID), intranasal (IN), or oral (PO) and also the site where it was administered as either RA (right arm), LA (left arm), RT (right thigh), or LT (left thigh).

4. Record the publication date of each VIS as well as the date the VIS is given to the patient.

5. To meet the space constraints of this form and federal requirements for documentation, a healthcare setting may want to keep a reference list of vaccinators that includes their initials and titles.

6. For combination vaccines, fill in a row for each antigen in the combination.

Abbreviation	Trade Name and Manufacturer
MMR	MMRII (Merck)
VAR	Varivax (Merck)
MMRV	ProQuad (Merck)
HepA	Havrix (GlaxoSmithKline [GSK]); Vaqta (Merck)
HepA-HepB	Twinrix (GSK)
HPV2	Cervarix (GSK)
HPV4	Gardasil (Merck)
LAIV (Live attenuated influenza vaccine)	FluMist (ModImmuno)
TIV (Trivalent inactivated influenza vaccine); RIV (Recombinant influenza vaccine)	Afluria (CSL Biotherapies); Agriflu (Novartis); Fluarix (GSK); Flublok (Protein Sciences Corp.); Flucelvax (Novartis); FluLaval (GSK); Fluvirin (Novartis); Fluzone, Fluzone Intradermal [for ages 18–64 yrs] (sanofi)
MCV4 or MenACWY, MenACWY-CRM, MenACWY-D; Hib-MenCY	MenACWY-D = Menactra (sanofi pasteur); MenACWY-CRM = Menveo (Novartis); Hib-MenCY (MenHibrix [GSK])
MPSV4	Menomune (sanofi pasteur)

Technical content reviewed by the Centers for Disease Control and Prevention

For additional copies, visit www.immunize.org/catg.d/p2022.pdf • Item #P2022 (4/14)

This form was created by the Immunization Action Coalition • www.immunize.org • www.vaccineinformation.org

Safe Handling and Storage of Vaccines

The Centers for Disease Control and Prevention (CDC) have devised a list of important rules and steps to ensure safekeeping of a practice's vaccine supply. This list can be used as a checklist in the office.

_____ 1. One person should be in charge of the handling and storage of vaccines at the facility, with a backup person to ensure proper management.

_____ 2. A vaccine inventory log should be maintained that includes the following:

_____ (1) Vaccine name

_____ (2) Number of doses

_____ (3) Date vaccine was received

_____ (4) Condition of vaccine on arrival

_____ (5) Manufacturer

_____ (6) Lot number

_____ (7) Expiration date

_____ 3. Vaccines should be stored in separate, self-contained units that refrigerate or freeze only. A household-style combination unit can be used to store only refrigerated vaccines; frozen vaccines must be kept in a separate, stand-alone freezer.

_____ 4. The vaccine refrigerator and freezer should not be used for food or drinks.

_____ 5. Vaccines should be stored in the middle of the refrigerator or freezer, not in the door.

_____ 6. New supplies should be placed behind the vials with the closest expiration date; the vials with the nearest expiration date should be used first.

_____ 7. A sign should be posted on the refrigerator door identifying which vaccines should be stored in either the refrigerator or the freezer.

_____ 8. One thermometer should be kept in the refrigerator and one in the freezer; the refrigerator temperature should be maintained at 35° to 46° F (2° to 8° C) and the freezer temperature at −58° to 5° F (−50° to 15° C) or colder.

_____ 9. Containers of water should be kept in the refrigerator and ice packs in the freezer to help maintain cold temperatures.

_____ 10. A temperature log should be kept on the refrigerator door; the refrigerator and freezer temperatures should be recorded twice a day: first thing in the morning and at the end of the day.

_____ 11. A "Do Not Unplug" sign should be posted next to the refrigerator's electrical outlet.

_____ 12. If the refrigerator or freezer stops working, the following steps should be taken:

- Immediately place the vaccines in another refrigerator or freezer, and mark them so that they can be separated from vaccines that were not affected.

- Record the temperature of the refrigerator or freezer, and contact the vaccine manufacturer or state health department. Follow their instructions on the use, alteration of expiration dates, or disposal of the vaccines.

_____ 13. The facility should have a copy of the health department's general and emergency vaccine management policies.

CRITICAL THINKING APPLICATION   **35-8**

Susie will be administering pediatric immunizations during the well-baby visits scheduled for today. To prepare for this responsibility, she looked up the primary vaccinations, their routes of administration, contraindications, and possible side effects. The first child arrives for her 4-month checkup. What immunizations should the child receive, and how should they be administered? The baby's father asks whether she will get sick from the vaccines. What should Susie tell him? What does Susie need to do to meet the requirements of the National Childhood Vaccine Injury Act?

THE PEDIATRIC PATIENT

An infant's first physical assessment comes at the time of delivery, when the pediatrician assesses the newborn's ability to thrive outside the uterus. The Apgar score is a system for evaluating the infant's physical condition at 1 and 5 minutes after birth (Table 35-3). Developed by pediatrician Virginia Apgar, the scoring system evaluates the following: *a*ppearance (color); *p*ulse (heart rate); *g*rimace (reflex; response to stimuli); *a*ctivity (muscle tone); and *r*espiration (breathing). These parameters are each rated 0, 1, or 2. The maximum total score is 10. Infants with low scores require immediate medical attention.

Well-Child Visits

The frequency of well-child visits varies with the provider and the community. It may follow this pattern: 2 weeks, 4 weeks, 8 weeks, 4 months, 6 months, 12 months, 18 months, 2 years, 5 years, 10 years, and 15 years. These visits focus on maintaining the child's health through basic system examinations, immunizations, and upgrading of the child's medical history record.

The decision on whether the child is to be seen alone or with the parent depends on the pediatrician and the child's age. Often the child looks to the parent for approval before answering or performing a skill; for this reason, the provider may want to assess the child alone. If this is the case, explain to the parent that the provider wants to evaluate the child's independent abilities and that as soon as testing is complete, the provider will explain the results of the tests.

The medical history is an essential guide to the pediatric examination. With an infant, the provider depends on the caregiver for the history, but as the child gets older, some history may be obtained from the child and clarified or amplified by the parent. Close observation also gives the provider considerable information.

Lead Paint Exposure

Children are especially vulnerable to lead levels in their environment. High blood lead levels can result in serious brain injury, including seizures, coma, and death; lower levels can cause learning problems, stunted growth, and behavior disorders. The most common causes of lead exposure are lead-based paint in homes and on imported toys and chronic exposure to lead-contaminated dust and water. The Centers for Disease Control and Prevention (CDC) recommend a screening blood test for lead levels in all children between 1 and 2 years of age. For children who show elevated levels, follow-up should include home and school environmental testing to determine the cause of lead exposure.

TABLE 35-3   Apgar Scoring System*

	ASSIGNED SCORE		
CLINICAL SIGN	0	1	2
Heart rate	Absent	100	100
Respiratory effort	Absent	Slow and irregular	Good and crying
Muscle tone	Limp	Some flexion of the arms and legs	Active movement
Reflex irritability	No response	Grimace	Coughing and sneezing
Color	Blue and pale	Body pink and extremities blue	Pink all over

*Readings are taken by the pediatrician at 1 minute and 5 minutes after birth. At *1 minute:* If the score is 7 or lower, some nervous system problems are suspected. If the score is below 4, resuscitation usually is necessary. At *5 minutes:* If the score is at least 8, the child probably is reacting normally.

Sick-Child Visits

Sick-child visits occur whenever needed, usually on short notice. For this reason, most pediatric offices keep open appointments in the schedule to accommodate calls for sick-child visits. The length and frequency of this type of visit depends entirely on the child and the illness. The medical assistant frequently is the first point of contact for a sick child and the child's caregiver.

Determining whether the child should be seen immediately or the problem can wait for an opening in the schedule is crucial to pediatric care. The medical assistant should follow established office policies, but when in doubt about the seriousness of the problem, he or she should ask the office manager or physician for advice. Usually the provider prefers to see the child rather than delay seeing a patient with a potentially serious condition. When the medical assistant conducts telephone screening, if the child is young (under 2 years old) and the parent reports frequent cycles of crying, lethargy, vomiting that lasts longer than 24 hours, diarrhea (more than six stools in the past 12 hours), or fever of 101°F (38.3°C) or higher, the best course is to see the child right away. He or she cannot verbalize associated pain or problems.

Table 35-4 summarizes some important questions for telephone screening of an older child who can communicate symptoms. It is important to focus on the *onset* (when symptoms first started), *frequency* (are symptoms constant, or do they cycle through recurrences), and *duration* (how long the episodes last) of the problem, in addition to attempted treatments and their effectiveness. As with any other patient, all telephone communication should be documented to record the reason for the call; the information gathered; the action taken, including whether the provider was consulted; any orders given; and whether and when an appointment was scheduled.

THE MEDICAL ASSISTANT'S ROLE IN PEDIATRIC PROCEDURES

The medical assistant is responsible for assisting the pediatrician with examinations; updating patient histories; performing ordered screening tests (e.g., vision, hearing, urinalysis, and hemoglobin checks); administering immunizations; measuring and weighing children as needed; and providing patient and caregiver support. A medical assistant must develop a relationship with the pediatric patient that encourages cooperation and compliance with tests and treatment plans. If the child becomes upset, everything that needs to be done during that visit will be done under duress, and the chance for future mistrust intensifies.

Interacting with children requires special techniques, depending on the child's age. A calm, unhurried manner is essential to gaining cooperation. The tone of voice should be gentle but confident. Using a firm, direct approach about expected behavior is important in gaining the cooperation of older children. Offer reasonable choices when possible, such as, "Would you like your shot in your left leg or your right leg?" not, "Are you ready for your shot now?" Offering sincere praise for the child during the examination or procedures helps ease anxiety and builds self-esteem. If the child is having an unusually difficult time, try to discover the reason. If he or she has had a bad medical experience in the past, the child may be afraid of what might happen. Each step should be explained in a language the child (and parent) can understand. Children younger than age 2 feel better when the parent holds them or remains very close (Figure 35-8). Preschool children enjoy playing, so making a game out of the situation is helpful (Figure 35-9). Whatever the child's age, the medical assistant should be sensitive to his or her individual needs and should adapt the examination and procedures as much as possible to meet those needs.

TABLE 35-4	Important Questions for Telephone Screening of Pediatric Problems
COMPLAINT	**SCREENING QUESTIONS**
Pain	• What are the onset, frequency, and duration of the pain? • On a scale of 1 to 10, how severe is the pain? • Where is the exact location? • Was any accident involved? (include details). • Has the pain gotten worse over time? • Has the pain interfered with sleep? • Is there associated fever, vomiting, diarrhea, or rash?
Gastrointestinal	• What are the onset, duration, and frequency of the symptoms? Has the child been vomiting longer than 24 hours without improvement? • Is the child drinking and/or eating? • Is the child dehydrated (e.g., dry mouth, no urination in 8-10 hours, listless)? • If the child has diarrhea, have there been more than five or six watery stools in 12 hours? • Does the child have other symptoms (e.g., vomiting, fever of 101° F [38.3° C], rapid breathing)?
Respiratory	• What are the onset, duration, and frequency of the symptoms? • How would you describe the child's breathing? • Has the child been diagnosed with a breathing disorder? • Is a prescribed treatment being used? • Are any other signs or symptoms present (e.g., severe headache, stiff neck, fever, cough)? • If the child is coughing, what does it sound like? • Are there signs of a sore throat or earache?

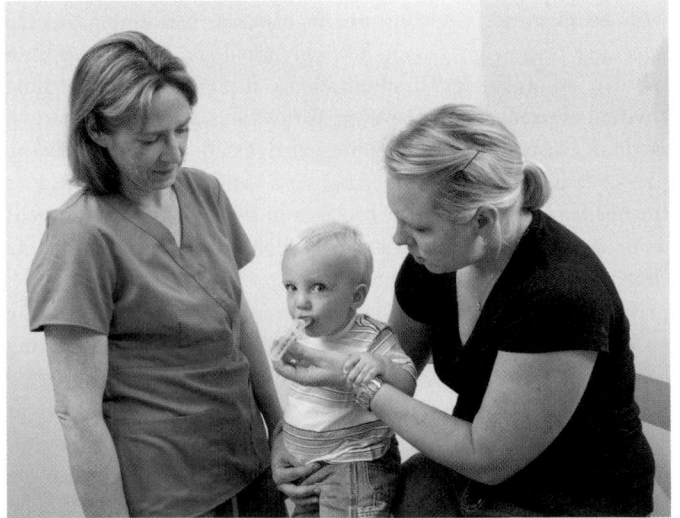

FIGURE 35-8 Sometimes a pediatric patient is more comfortable when held by a parent.

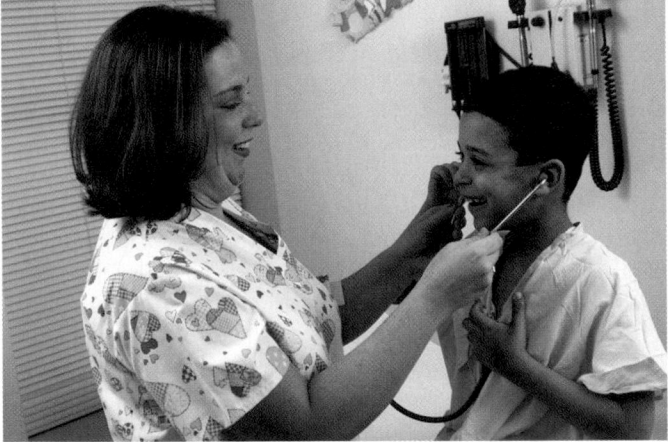

FIGURE 35-9 Making a game out of a procedure.

The sequence of the physician's examination varies and frequently is based on the child's cooperation. The pediatrician probably will leave procedures and tests that are likely to cause the most objections until the end of the appointment. The provider is constantly evaluating the child's growth and development. A child's alertness and responses tell the provider a considerable amount. With infants and young children of preschool age, the parent is closely questioned about the child's eating, sleeping, and elimination habits. A school-aged child usually is a little more cooperative during an examination and can answer most questions without parental assistance. Adolescent patients should be given the option of not having parents present during an examination. This may permit teenagers to respond more honestly about lifestyle factors and also protects their privacy.

Measurement

Examination of the child during routine well-child care includes measurement of the circumference of the infant's head to determine normal growth and development (Procedure 35-2). The size of the child's head reflects the growth of the brain. Brain growth is 50% complete by 1 year of age, 75% by age 3, and 90% by age 6. Routine head measurement is recommended in children until 36 months of age and in older children whose head size is not within norms. If the circumference of the head deviates greatly from normal measurements, **hydrocephaly** or **microcephaly** may be suspected. It is important to discover any congenital problem as early as possible so that appropriate treatment can be started.

Along with the head circumference, the medical assistant should record the child's length (or height) and weight (Procedure 35-3) on growth charts so that the provider can compare the child's measurement statistics with national standards. Growth charts consist of a series of percentile curves that illustrate the distribution of selected body measurements.

The current version of the CDC's growth records consists of 16 charts (eight for boys and eight for girls) (Figures 35-10 and 35-11). These charts, which represent revisions of the 14 previous charts, include the BMI-for-age charts for boys and for girls ages 2 to 20 years. As mentioned previously, the BMI is the recommended method of determining whether children or adults are overweight or obese. The BMI growth charts can be used beginning at 2 years of age, when height can be measured accurately.

The Zika Virus and Microcephaly

The Zika virus is spread to people through mosquito bites. The most common symptoms of Zika are fever, rash, joint pain, and conjunctivitis. Affected individuals typically have mild symptoms that last from several days to a week. The CDC and other world health organizations are investigating a link between pregnant women who have contracted the Zika virus and the risk of having an infant with microcephaly. There is currently no vaccine or specific medicine to prevent Zika infections. The only method for controlling the spread of the disease is through mosquito control. The CDC recommends that pregnant women in any trimester consider postponing travel to areas where there are known Zika virus infections.

Microcephaly is linked with the following problems:
- Seizures
- Developmental delays
- Intellectual disability
- Problems with movement and balance
- Feeding problems, such as difficulty swallowing
- Hearing loss
- Vision problems

Zika Virus. http://www.cdc.gov/zika/index.html. Accessed February 10, 2016.

PROCEDURE 35-2 Maintain Growth Charts: Measure the Circumference of an Infant's Head

Goal: To obtain an accurate measurement of the circumference of an infant's head and plot the result on the patient's growth chart.

EQUIPMENT and SUPPLIES

- Patient's record, with appropriate growth chart
- Flexible disposable tape measure
- Age- and gender-specific growth chart
- Pen

PROCEDURAL STEPS

1. Sanitize your hands.
   PURPOSE: To ensure infection control.
2. Identify the patient by name and date of birth. If he or she is old enough, gain the child's cooperation through conversation.
   PURPOSE: To alleviate anxiety and gain the child's trust.
3. Place an infant in the supine position, or the infant may be held by the parent. An older child may sit on the examination table.
4. Hold the tape measure with the zero mark against the infant's forehead, slightly above the eyebrows and the top of the ears. Ask the parent for assistance if necessary.
5. Bring the tape measure around the head, just above the ears, until it meets (Figure 1).

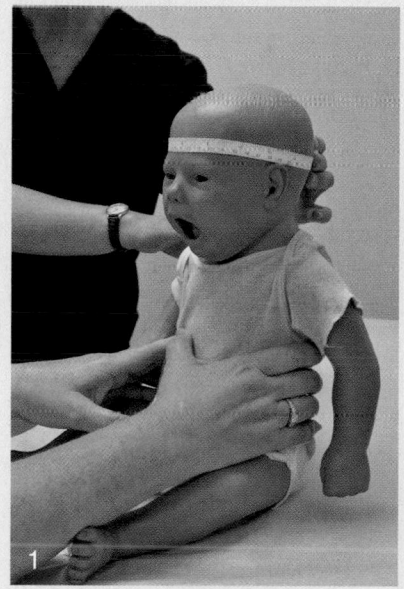

6. Read to the nearest 0.6 cm or ¼ inch.
7. Record the measurement on the growth chart and in the patient's health record.
   PURPOSE: A procedure is not done until it is recorded.
8. Dispose of the tape measure.
9. Sanitize your hands.
   PURPOSE: To ensure infection control.

PROCEDURE 35-3 Maintain Growth Charts: Measure an Infant's Length and Weight

Goal: *To measure an infant's length and weight accurately so that growth patterns can be monitored and recorded.*

EQUIPMENT and SUPPLIES

- Patient's record
- Infant scale with paper cover
- Flexible measuring tape
- Examination table paper
- Pen
- Pediatric length board, if available
- Gender-specific infant growth chart
- Biohazard waste container

PROCEDURAL STEPS

Measuring an Infant's Length

1. Sanitize your hands, identify the child by name and date of birth, assemble the necessary equipment, and explain the procedure to the infant's caregiver.
2. Undress the infant. The diaper may be left on while the length is measured, but it must be removed before the infant is weighed.
3. Cover the examination table with smooth, flat paper. Ask the caregiver to place the infant on his or her back on the examination table. If the table is a pediatric table with a headboard, ask the caregiver to hold the infant's head gently against the headboard while you straighten the infant's leg and note the location of the heel on the measurement area. If there is no headboard, ask the caregiver to gently hold the infant's head still while you draw a line on the paper at the back of the baby's head and at the heel after extending the leg (Figure 1).

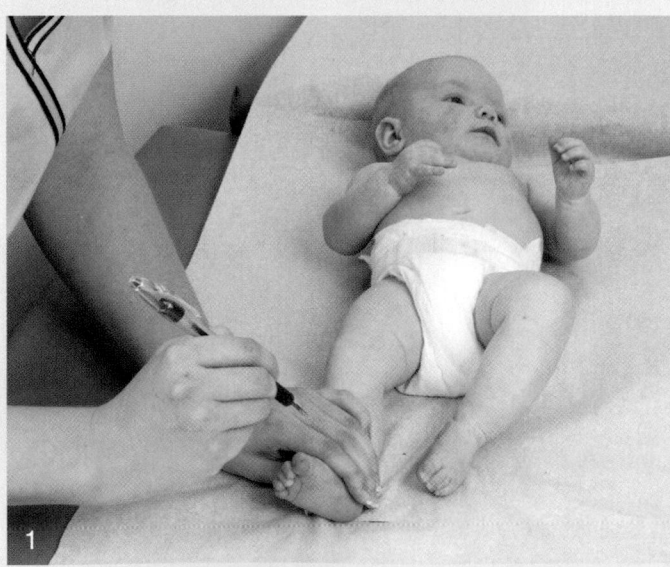

4. Measure the infant's length with the tape measure and record it.
5. Document the results in either inches or centimeters, depending on office policy, on the infant's growth chart, in the progress notes, and in the caregiver's record if requested. Complete the growth chart graph by connecting the dot from the last visit.

Weighing an Infant

1. Sanitize your hands, identify the child by name and date of birth, assemble the necessary equipment, and explain the procedure to the infant's caregiver.
2. If the scale is not a digital model, prepare the scale by sliding weights to the left; line the scale with disposable paper to reduce the risk of pathogen transmission.
3. Completely undress the infant, including removing the diaper.
   PURPOSE: It is important to get the most accurate weight possible and a diaper, especially a wet one, will add to the total weight.
4. Place the infant gently on the center of the scale, keeping your hand directly above the infant's trunk for safety (Figure 2).
   PURPOSE: To protect the infant from possible injury.

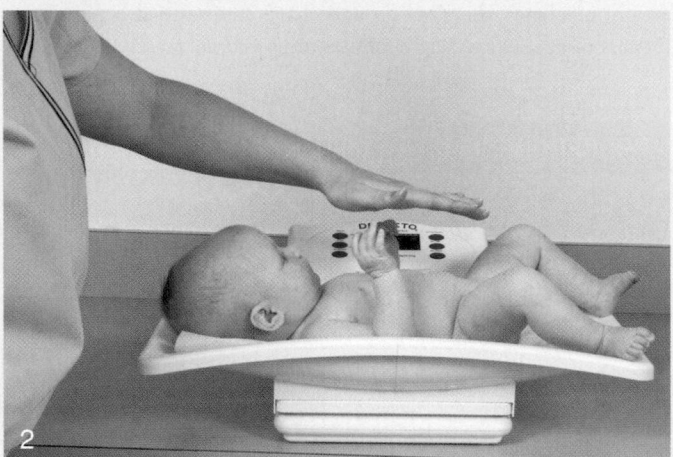

5. If the scale is not a digital model, slide the weights across the scale until balance is achieved. Attempt to read the infant's weight while he or she is still.
6. If the scale is not a digital model, return the weights to the far left of the scale and remove the baby. The caregiver can rediaper the baby while you discard the paper lining the scale. If the scale became contaminated during the procedure, follow Occupational Safety and Health Administration (OSHA) guidelines for use of gloves and disposal of contaminated waste. Disinfect the equipment according to the manufacturer's guidelines.
   PURPOSE: Infection control.
7. Sanitize your hands.
8. Document the results in either pounds or kilograms, depending on office policy, on the infant's growth chart, in the progress notes, and in the caregiver's record if requested. Complete the growth chart graph by connecting the dot from the last visit.

8/24/20–10:20 AM: Wt 17 lb 4 oz. Length 27 in. S. Kwong, CMA (AAMA)

Birth to 36 months: Boys
Length-for-age and Weight-for-age percentiles

NAME _____

RECORD # _____

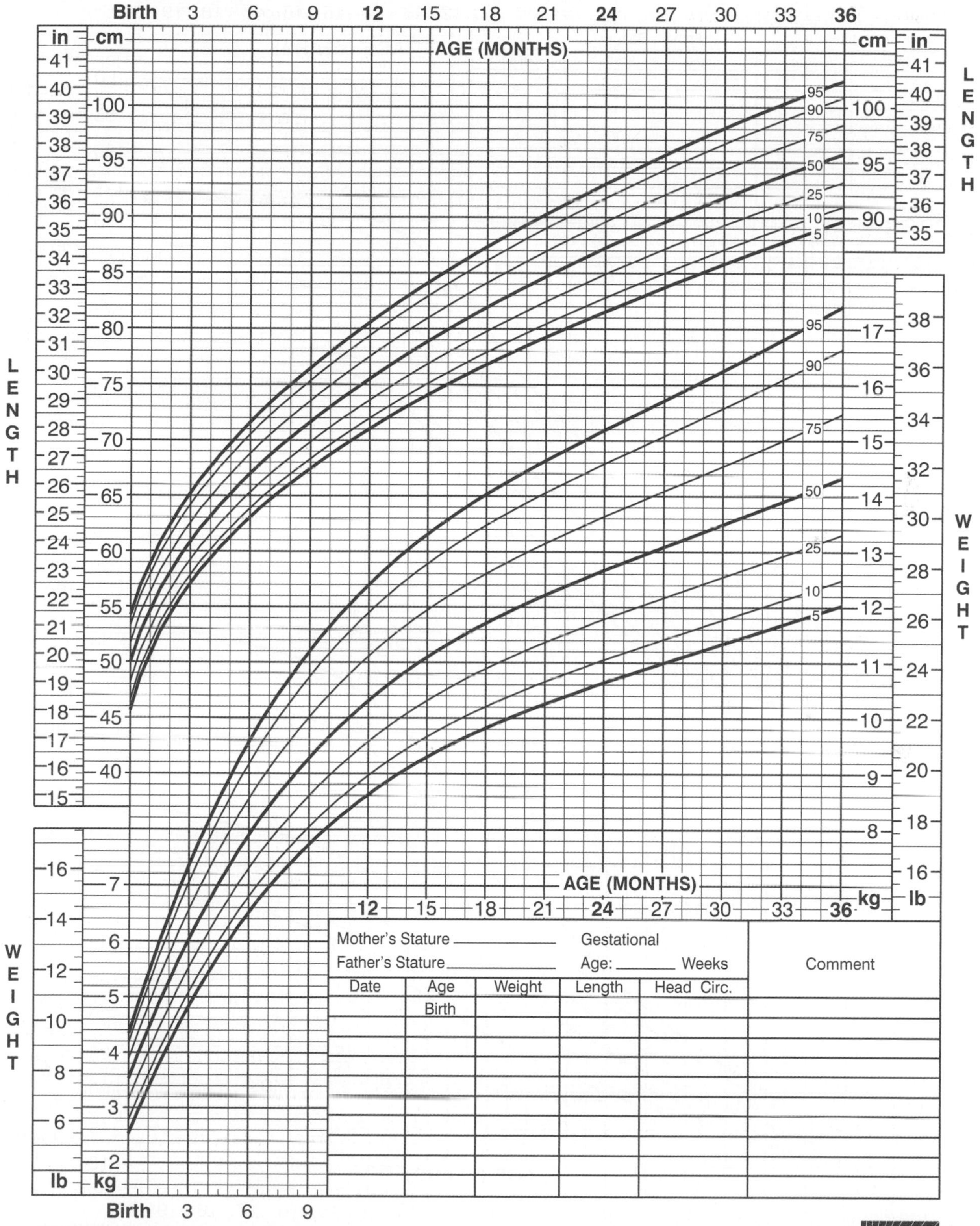

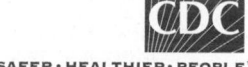

Published May 30, 2000 (modified 4/20/01).
SOURCE: Developed by the National Center for Health Statistics in collaboration with
the National Center for Chronic Disease Prevention and Health Promotion (2000).
http://www.cdc.gov/growthcharts

SAFER · HEALTHIER · PEOPLE™

FIGURE 35-10 Growth chart: males (birth to 36 months).

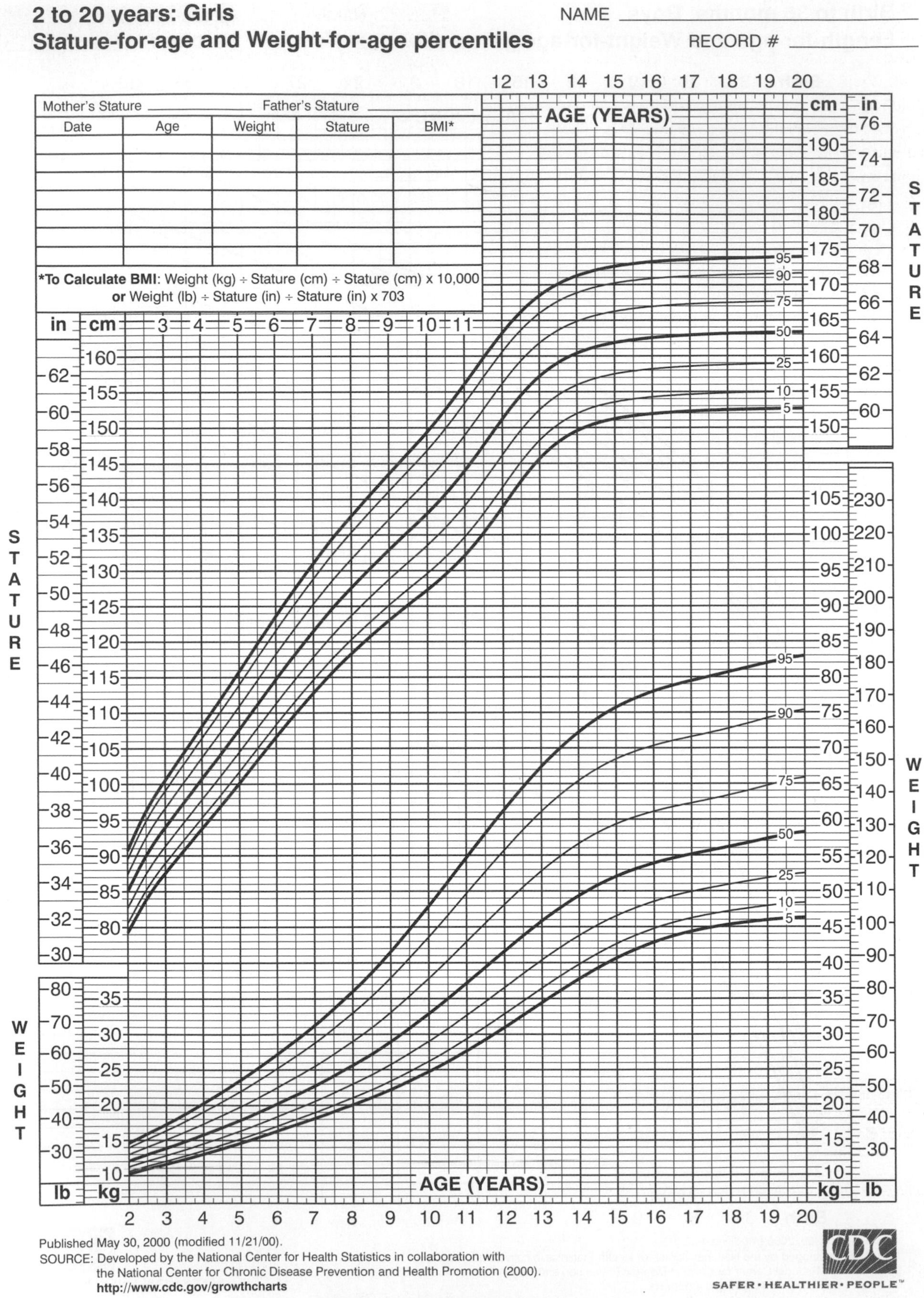

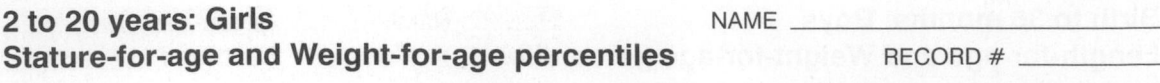

2 to 20 years: Girls
Stature-for-age and Weight-for-age percentiles
NAME
RECORD #
Mother's Stature
Father's Stature
Date
Age
Weight
Stature
BMI*
*To Calculate BMI: Weight (kg) ÷ Stature (cm) ÷ Stature (cm) x 10,000
or Weight (lb) ÷ Stature (in) ÷ Stature (in) x 703
AGE (YEARS)
STATURE
WEIGHT
cm
in
kg
lb
95
90
75
50
25
10
5
Published May 30, 2000 (modified 11/21/00).
SOURCE: Developed by the National Center for Health Statistics in collaboration with
the National Center for Chronic Disease Prevention and Health Promotion (2000).
http://www.cdc.gov/growthcharts
CDC
SAFER • HEALTHIER • PEOPLE™

FIGURE 35-11 Growth chart: females (2 to 20 years).

Assisting with the Examination

The pediatrician will have a designated set of procedures that the medical assistant completes before the physician sees the child (Procedure 35-4). Vital signs are measured first (Table 35-5). Depending on the child's age and level of cooperation, the temperature may be obtained by the axillary, oral, rectal, tympanic, or temporal method. The rectal and temporal methods are considered most accurate in infants; however, the temporal method is easiest, quickest, and less invasive. It is important to remember that the younger the child, the more immature the ability to regulate body heat. Therefore the temperature of an infant may fluctuate easily and rapidly. The child's pulse rate is affected similarly to that of an adult; it can increase as a result of activity, anxiety, illness, and environmental temperature. If the child is younger than age 2, the pulse is measured apically by placing the stethoscope on the left side of the chest medial to the nipple. Always count the beats for 1 full minute for accuracy.

An alternative method of obtaining the pulse of a very young child is to use the brachial artery in the upper arm. After age 2, the child's pulse may be taken at the radial pulse site. Anticipate a pulse rate higher than that of an adult; the younger the child, the faster the pulse. The respiratory rate is easily obtained in a child because the chest can be readily observed. Expect the rate to be increased according to the child's age (the younger the child, the faster the normal respiratory rate) and health. The ratio of four pulse beats to one respiration should remain constant in a healthy child.

Blood pressure measurements are not included in most pediatric examinations. However, if the child has a heart or kidney **anomaly**, a blood pressure reading may be ordered. The cuff must be the appropriate width to obtain an accurate reading, and the bell of the stethoscope must be small enough to seal over the site. It is best to use a pediatric stethoscope with a pediatric bell when obtaining an infant's pressure. Blood pressure readings in a young child are lower than those in an adult.

To prevent a small child or infant from rolling the head from side to side during the provider's examination, stand at the head of the table and support the child's head between your hands, taking care not to press on the ears or on the anterior or posterior **fontanelles**. An infant need not be draped, but privacy is important to an older child. Sincere respect and friendly conversation at the child's level accomplishes a great deal. Always be patient with children. Make sure they understand what is expected. Always involve the parents or caregivers as much as possible.

TABLE 35-5	Reference Ranges for Pediatric Vital Signs
VITAL SIGN	**REFERENCE RANGE**
Temperature	
Oral	98.6°F (37°C)
Aural	100.4°F (38°C)
Axillary	97.6°F (36.4°C)
Pulse	
Newborn	100-180 beats per minute
3 mo-2 yr	80-150 beats per minute
2-10 yr	65-130 beats per minute
Respirations	
Newborn	30-50 breaths per minute
1-3 yr	25-30 breaths per minute
4-6 yr	23-25 breaths per minute
7+ yr	16-20 breaths per minute
Blood Pressure	
Newborn	Systolic 90 mm Hg; diastolic 70 mm Hg
1-5 yr	Systolic 100 mm Hg; diastolic 70 mm Hg
6-12 yr	Systolic 120 mm Hg; diastolic 84 mm Hg
13+ yr	Systolic, 100 mm Hg + age; diastolic, 30-40 mm Hg less

Accurately judging the level of pain a young patient is experiencing can be difficult. If the child is able to communicate, the Wong-Baker Faces Pain Scale could be used, which shows simple drawings of faces that express varying levels of pain on a 0 to 10 scale (Figure 35-12).

PROCEDURE 35-4   Measure and Record Vital Signs: Obtain Pediatric Vital Signs and Perform Vision Screening

Goal: *To accurately obtain vital signs and assess the vision of a pediatric patient.*

EQUIPMENT and SUPPLIES

- Patient's record
- Digital, tympanic, or temporal thermometer
- Pediatric blood pressure cuff
- Wristwatch with sweep second hand
- Weight scale with height bar
- Stethoscope
- Snellen E eye chart and oculator
- Pen

PROCEDURAL STEPS

1. Gather the necessary equipment.
2. Sanitize your hands. Identify the child by name and date of birth.
   <u>PURPOSE</u>: To ensure infection control.
3. Explain the procedure to the parent, and if you want the parent to help by holding the child, explain how you want him or her to do that.
   <u>PURPOSE</u>: Explanations ahead of time save time and improve cooperation.
4. Help the child stand in the center of the scale, then weigh the child. Ask the child to turn around, then measure the child's height. Record your findings.
5. Obtain the tympanic, temporal, or axillary temperature using the procedure explained in the Vital Signs chapter. Vital Signs (Figure 1).

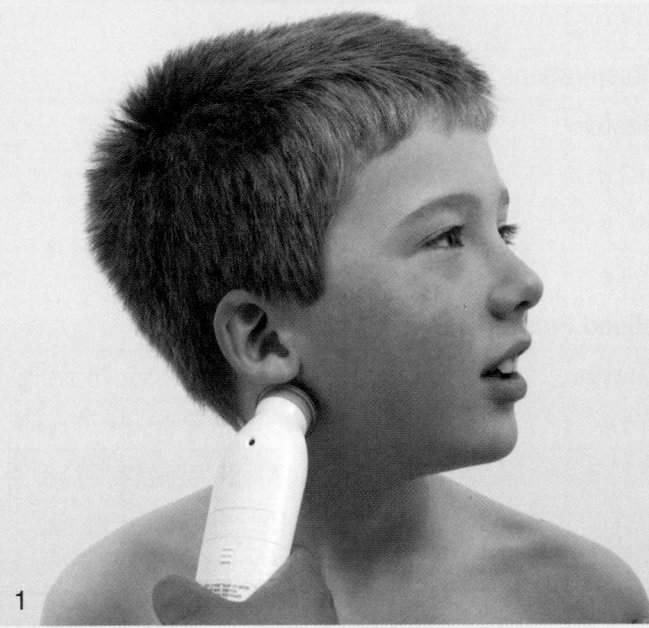

6. Record the temperature and indicate the method used.
   <u>PURPOSE</u>: A procedure is not done until it is recorded in the patient's record.
7. Place the stethoscope on the child's chest at the midpoint between the sternum and the left nipple. Listen for the apical beat (Figure 2).

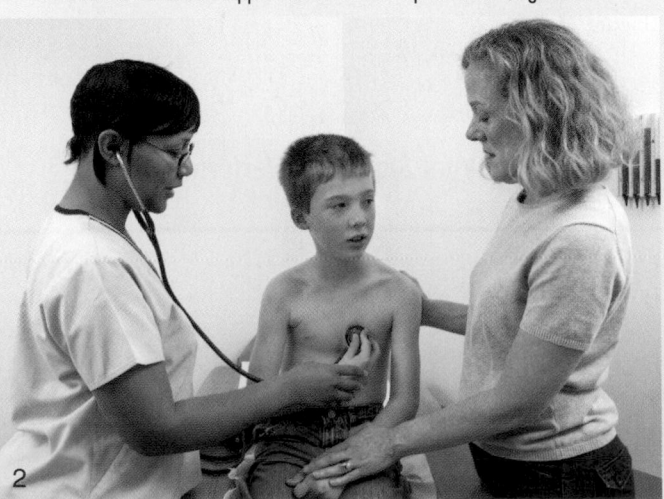

8. Count the apical beat for 1 full minute.
9. Record the apical pulse. Be sure to place "Ap" before the rate to indicate that this is an apical pulse reading.
   <u>PURPOSE</u>: A procedure is not done until it is recorded in the patient's record.
10. Observe the child's chest, or place your palm on the child's chest, and count the respirations for 1 full minute.
11. Record the respiratory rate.
    <u>PURPOSE</u>: A procedure is not done until it is recorded in the patient's record.
12. Check to make sure you have the correct-sized blood pressure cuff and then take the child's blood pressure (see the procedure in the Vital Signs chapter) (Figure 3).

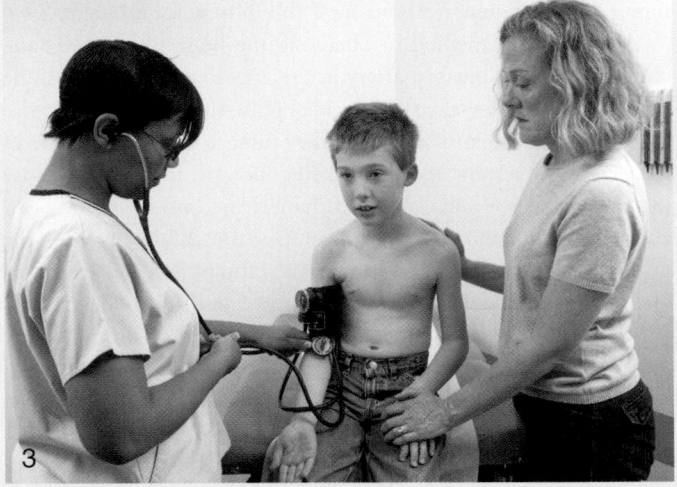

13. Record the blood pressure.
    <u>PURPOSE</u>: A procedure is not done until it is recorded in the patient's record.
14. If vision screening is to be done, familiarize the child with the E chart by asking him or her to make an E that points the same way your E is pointing. Then position the child in front of the pediatric Snellen E chart (Figure 4) and have the child match the E sign (using the fingers) with the E on the chart to which you are pointing.

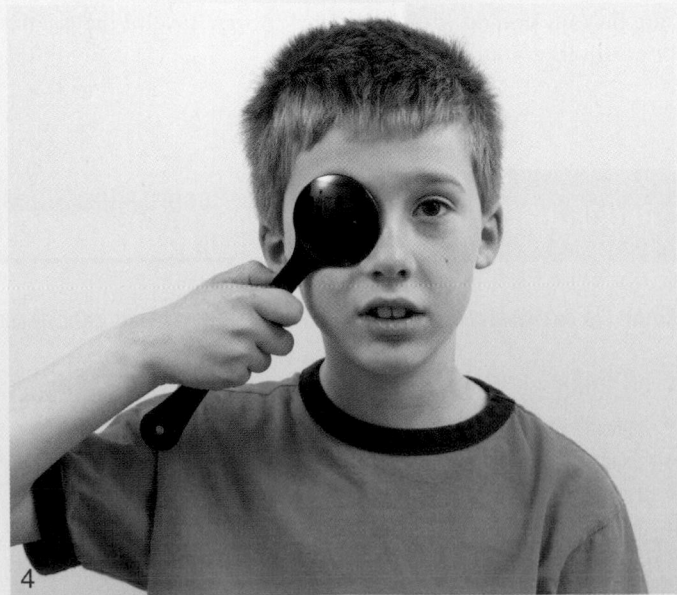

PROCEDURE 35-4 —*continued*

15. Record the vision results.
    PURPOSE: A procedure is not done until it is recorded in the patient's record.
16. Compliment the child on his or her performance, and if the parent is present, share the praise with the parent.
    PURPOSE: To build rapport and encourage self-confidence in the child.

17. Sanitize your hands.
    PURPOSE: To ensure infection control.
18. Perform appropriate disinfection and return all equipment to the proper storage area.

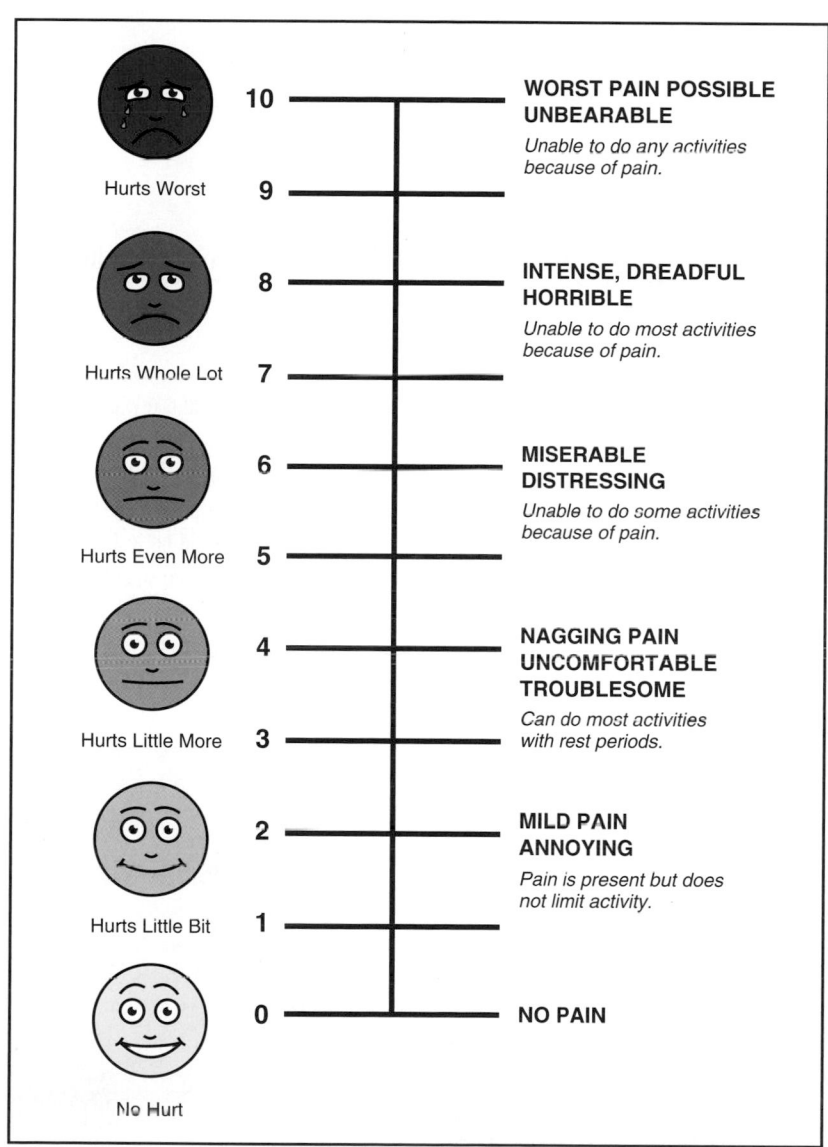

FIGURE 35-12 Wong-Baker Faces Pain Scale for children age 3 to 7 years. (From Hockenberry MJ, Wilson D: *Wong's essentials of pediatric nursing,* ed 8, St Louis, 2009, Mosby.)

Obtaining a Urine Sample

The easiest way to obtain a urine sample from a child who is toilet trained is to give the parent the container and instructions ahead of time. Then, when the child arrives at the office for the examination, the sample is available to be tested. If the sample is needed while the child is at the office, consult with the parent for the best method to use. If the child is not toilet trained, a pediatric urine collection device can be put on him or her to collect the sample (Figure 35-13 and Procedure 35-5). This device is placed as soon as the child is checked in to increase the chance of obtaining the needed sample

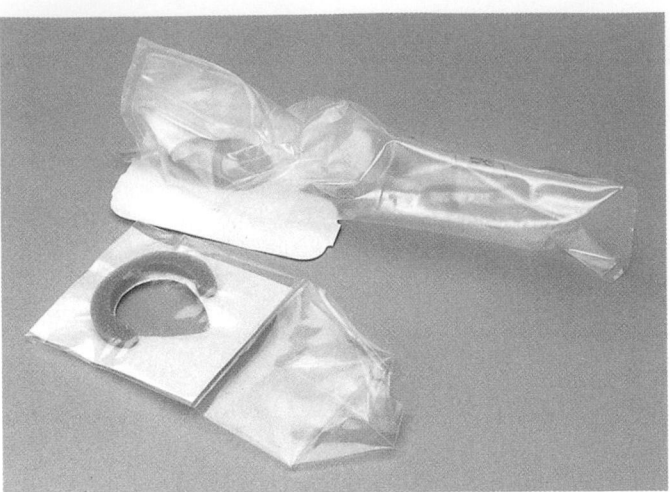

FIGURE 35-13 Urine collection devices.

before the child leaves. Once the device is in place, the child can be diapered to help hold it properly. Make sure the adhesive sticks tightly so that the specimen collects in the device when the child urinates.

In some cases the child may need to be catheterized to obtain the specimen. Pediatric catheterization kits contain all the supplies needed for this procedure. When preparing the kit, always remember that this is a sterile procedure. The pediatrician usually asks the parent to help with the infant while the medical assistant labels and prepares the specimen for the laboratory. In some practices a registered nurse (RN) or a specially trained medical assistant may perform a catheterization procedure to collect a pediatric urine sample.

PROCEDURE 35-5   Assist Provider With a Patient Exam: Applying a Urinary Collection Device

Goal: *To apply a pediatric urinary collection device properly.*

EQUIPMENT and SUPPLIES

- Patient's record
- Pediatric urine collection bag
- Labeled laboratory urinary container
- Laboratory test request form
- Antiseptic wipes
- Biohazard waste container
- Disposable examination gloves

PROCEDURAL STEPS

1. Assemble all needed supplies. Identify the child by name and date of birth.
   PURPOSE: To manage time efficiently.
2. Sanitize your hands and put on gloves.
   PURPOSE: To ensure infection control.
3. Ask the parent to remove the child's diaper, or place the child in a supine position on the examination table and remove the diaper.
4. Cleanse the genitalia with antiseptic wipes.
   Male: Cleanse the urinary meatus in a circular motion, starting directly on the meatus and working in an outward pattern. Repeat with a clean wipe. If the child has not been circumcised, gently retract the foreskin to expose the meatus; using a fresh wipe, cleanse the area around the meatus and return the foreskin to its natural position. Cleanse the scrotum last using a fresh wipe.
   Female: Hold the labia open with your nondominant hand; with your dominant hand, cleanse each side of the inner labia, from the clitoris to the vaginal meatus, in a superior to inferior pattern, using a fresh wipe for each side. With a third wipe, cleanse directly down the middle over the urinary meatus. Discard all wipes in a biohazard container.
   PURPOSE: To prevent contamination of the urine specimen with surface pathogens.

5. Make sure the area is dry. Unfold the collection device, remove the paper from the upper portion, place this portion over the mons pubis, and press it securely into place. Continue by removing the lower portion of the paper and securing this portion against the perineum. In male children the penis and scrotum should be in the opening of the collection bag. Make sure the device is attached smoothly and that you have not taped it to part of the infant's thigh (Figure 1). Rediaper the infant or, if the parent is helping, have the parent rediaper the infant at this time. The diaper will help hold the bag in place.

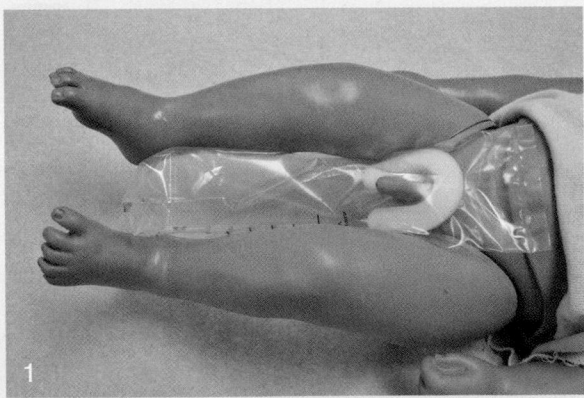

6. If allowed, suggest that the parent give the child liquids (or nurse the infant if breast-feeding); check the bag for urine at 15-minute intervals.
   PURPOSE: Increasing intake helps increase output.
7. When a noticeable amount of urine has collected in the bag, put on gloves, remove the device, cleanse the skin area where the device was attached, and rediaper the child.

PROCEDURE 35-5 ___—continued

8. Pour the urine carefully into the laboratory urine container, and handle the sample in a routine manner.
9. Dispose of all used equipment in a biohazard waste container.
10. Remove your gloves, dispose of them in a biohazard container, and sanitize your hands.

11. Document the procedure in the patient's record.
   PURPOSE: A procedure is not done until it is recorded.

8/24/20–10:45 AM: Urine specimen collected for culture as ordered by Dr. Flint. Placed for pickup by North Hills Laboratory. S. Kwong, CMA (AAMA)

THE ADOLESCENT PATIENT

The adolescent patient may present the greatest challenge to health education and disease management. Adolescence begins with the onset of puberty, a time when the child's reproductive system matures; this is a period marked by rapid changes in the endocrine and musculoskeletal systems. The adolescent undergoes rapid growth spurts and the development of secondary sexual characteristics.

Health examinations for patients in this age group should include screening for height and weight; gathering details about diet and exercise routines; screening for sexually transmitted infections (STIs) (and, for sexually active female adolescents, a Pap test, especially to screen for infection with the human papillomavirus [HPV]); reviewing the vaccination history and administering boosters as indicated; and assessing for high-risk behaviors, such as substance abuse, smoking, and sexual behavior.

Health problems most frequently seen in adolescent patients include eating disorders (anorexia nervosa and bulimia nervosa), obesity, and injury-related problems. Accidents are the leading cause of death and injury in adolescence, and suicide is the third leading cause of death. All healthcare personnel should be on the alert for indicators of suicide, including:

- Signs of depression, such as headaches, abdominal discomfort, anorexia, fatigue, aggressiveness, drug or alcohol abuse, and sexual promiscuity
- Verbal statements that hint at the adolescent's intention to commit suicide; talking about dying
- Actions such as giving away prized objects, withdrawing from social groups, suddenly changing normal behavior patterns, or writing a suicide note

INJURY PREVENTION

Unintentional injuries are the leading cause of death and disability in children in the United States. Injuries cause more childhood deaths than all diseases combined. The primary causes of childhood injuries are motor vehicle accidents, drowning, burns, falls, poisoning, aspiration with airway obstruction, and firearm accidents. Childhood injuries are linked to the child's growth and development level and usually are preventable. Young children are totally dependent on caregivers to keep them safe, so constant supervision and a childproof environment are essential for this age group. Older children need to be aware of health hazards and should be encouraged

to protect themselves from injury (e.g., use bike helmets, protective padding when skateboarding, seat belts, and so on). The highest incidence of accidental injuries is seen in children under age 9, but as children grow older, the percentage of deaths from injuries increases. In the United States, more than 9,000 children die each year—about 25 deaths a day—from injuries. Healthcare workers play a major role in injury prevention. The medical assistant is responsible for making sure the ambulatory care office is safe and parents are educated about potential hazards.

CRITICAL THINKING APPLICATION   35-9

The office manager asks Susie to check the entire office for potential child safety problems. After inspecting the facility, Susie is concerned about some safety issues, so she decides to create a checklist for future use. What precautions or safety features should she include?

CHILD ABUSE

The Child Abuse Prevention and Treatment Act states that all threats to a child's physical and/or mental welfare must be reported. This means that every teacher, healthcare worker, and social worker—in fact, every citizen—who suspects that a child is being neglected, abused, or exploited must report this to the proper authority. The agency must record the report, and after three similar reports, the agency must investigate.

When suspected abuse, neglect, or exploitation are reported, the individual must provide his or her name; however, this is considered confidential information and is not given to the child's parent or guardian, nor is it given to the investigating officer. The individual making the report also is protected under the law from any liability for reporting suspicions of child abuse.

If the medical assistant suspects that a child is a victim of abuse, neglect, or exploitation, he or she should consult with the pediatrician immediately. In most states, the medical assistant and the provider can make separate reports to the authorities. However, state laws vary, so state and local reporting protocols should be outlined in the office procedures manual.

Signs of Child Abuse

Obvious Signs
- Previously filed reports of physical or sexual abuse of the child
- Documented abuse of other family members
- Different stories from the parents and the child on how an accident happened
- Stories of incidents and injuries that are suspicious
- Injuries blamed on other family members
- Repeated visits to the emergency department for injuries

Examination Findings
- Trauma to the nervous system
- Internal abdominal pain
- Discolorations/bruising on the buttocks, back, and abdomen
- Elbow, wrist, and shoulder dislocations

Changes in Child Behavior
- Too eager to please the parent
- Overly passive and too compliant
- Aggressive and demanding
- Parenting the parent (role reversal)
- Delays in the normal growth and development patterns
- Erratic school attendance

Physical Indicators
- Poor hygiene
- Malnutrition
- Obvious dental neglect
- Neglected well-baby procedures (e.g., immunizations)

CLOSING COMMENTS

Patient Education

In a pediatric practice, the child usually is joined by one or both parents during visits to the physician. Parents need reinforcement, praise, and understanding in dealing with the health and welfare of their child. Provide parents with information to help them understand their children's behavior and improve their parenting skills. Understanding the normal behavioral characteristics of a particular developmental stage may increase the parents' confidence and reinforce expectations for the child.

The waiting room is an ideal place for parent education. Use the space and resources available to provide up-to-date information on child health issues and on local resources for support and assistance. If the pediatrician has pamphlets available, discuss them with the parents. Answer questions when possible, or alert the provider so that questions can be answered during the office visit. Every opportunity should be taken to teach parents about sound healthcare. Because so many ambulatory care visits involve infectious disorders, educating children and parents on the following infection control measures may help reduce the spread of disease:

- Children should cover their mouth with a disposable tissue when they cough and/or cough into their bent arm rather than their hands.

- A tissue should be used only once and then immediately thrown away.
- Children should not be allowed to share toys they have put in their mouth.
- After a child has discarded a toy that was in the mouth, it should be placed in a bin for dirty toys that is out of reach of others. Wash and disinfect these toys before allowing children to play with them again.
- Make sure all children and adults follow good hand-washing practices. Have pump hand sanitizers available throughout the office.

Legal and Ethical Issues

In the United States, children are considered persons who are growing and developing physically, emotionally, and mentally. Our laws view children as a distinct group, and laws and customs have been established that deal with the protection of children's rights. Occasionally in the pediatric office, legal and ethical issues arise, and the entire office staff may be faced with an ethical situation. If this type of situation occurs, the first option is to talk it over with the pediatrician. It may be necessary to have an office staff meeting to identify the conflict, note pertinent laws and facts, consider possible options and the consequences of each, and decide on a course of action. Facing ethical issues confidently may reduce the risk of liability. If the pediatrician's feelings are different from yours, this might be a totally separate dilemma with which you will have to deal. Always remember that as your employer, the physician makes the final decision, and as long as you work in that office, you are required to do things according to that decision.

If something happens that you cannot ethically support, seek the help of your local medical assistant organization. You may find that others have been in similar situations and that they can suggest possible methods of solving the problem.

Professional Behaviors

Working as a medical assistant in a busy pediatric practice can be very challenging. In essence, you are faced with two clients: a child who may be frightened and not feeling well, and a caregiver who typically is stressed. When you are dealing with emotionally charged situations, it is very easy to lose patience and act out yourself. Continuing to act professionally can help you manage these difficult situations. Consider the following suggestions:

- Routinely use active listening to get as much information as possible from the parents. Paying attention not only to the parents' words, but also to their feelings, helps the parents feel valued.
- Focus on age-appropriate methods for communicating with the child. Interacting with children on a level that they can understand helps them feel more comfortable and hopefully promotes cooperative behavior.
- Use time management techniques to handle the work challenges you face each day. Staying organized keeps you from feeling overwhelmed.

SUMMARY OF SCENARIO

After working with the telephone screening staff, Susie realizes the importance of becoming familiar with childhood diseases and disorders and the management policy of her physician-employers. Many times Susie has had to refer to the office disease manual to make sure she is asking the right questions and gathering all the information needed for the physician who will make the daily response calls. From working in the clinical area, Susie also has realized that a pediatric practice actually has two groups of patients: the child and the caregivers. She must be sensitive to the needs of both groups and develop communication skills that build trust with the child and his or her parents. Susie is working on developing a comprehensive education site in the office for interested parents and is creating a community resource guide for interested caregivers. She recognizes the need to stay up to date on the CDC's recommendations for childhood immunizations, and routinely refers to the CDC's website to make sure the office has the most recently published VIS forms. Susie regularly attends her local American Association of Medical Assistants (AAMA) chapter meetings to maintain her certification and to continue to learn about the pediatric practice specialty.

SUMMARY OF LEARNING OBJECTIVES

1. **Define, spell, and pronounce the terms listed in the vocabulary.**
Spelling and pronouncing medical terms correctly reinforce the medical assistant's credibility. Knowing the definitions of these terms promotes confidence in communication with patients and co-workers.

2. **Describe childhood growth patterns.**
By 6 months of age, the child's birth weight has doubled; at 1 year it has tripled, and the child's length has increased by 50%. By age 2 the child has reached approximately 50% of adult height. This same growth rate continues through the school-aged period, 6 to 12 years, which leads into a growth spurt that indicates impending puberty. In adolescence, ages 12 to 18 years, the adolescent gains almost half of his or her adult weight and the skeleton and organs double in size.

3. **Summarize the important features of the Denver II Developmental Screening Test.**
The Denver II Developmental Screening Test is a standardized tool used for children between 1 month and 6 years of age to screen healthy infants for developmental delays, to validate concerns about an infant's development, or to monitor high-risk children for potential problems.

4. **Discuss developmental patterns and therapeutic approaches for pediatric patients.**
Using therapeutic approaches for infants, toddlers, school-age, and adolescent patients improves communication with a variety of patient age groups and promotes quality patient care.

5. **Identify four different growth and development theories.**
Table 35-1 summarizes Freud's psychosexual, Piaget's cognitive, Erikson's psychosocial, and Kohlberg's moral reasoning theories.

6. **Consider the implications of postpartum depression.**
The American Academy of Pediatrics recommends that pediatricians perform postpartum screening on all new mothers to promote total child care.

7. **Explain common pediatric gastrointestinal disorders, in addition to failure to thrive and obesity.**
Pediatric gastrointestinal disorders include infant colic; diarrhea, which can be caused by a variety of different microorganisms and is treated medically when it continues for longer than 2 days; failure to thrive caused by a physiologic factor (e.g., malabsorption disease or cleft palate) or a nonorganic cause that is associated with the parent-child relationship; and obesity if the child's BMI is equal to or greater than the 95th percentile.

8. **Describe disorders of the respiratory system in children.**
The common cold may lead to secondary bacterial infections, including strep throat or otitis media; croup is a viral disorder that affects the larynx; pertussis, commonly known as whooping cough, is caused by bacteria that attach to the cilia of the upper respiratory system and can cause violent, rapid coughing and apnea in infants; bronchiolitis is a viral infection of the bronchioles that causes acute onset of wheezing and dyspnea; RSV is a virus that infects the lungs and bronchioles; asthma causes bronchospasms and inflammation of the bronchioles; and influenza is an acute, highly contagious viral infection of the respiratory tract.

9. **Distinguish among pediatric infectious diseases.**
Pediatric infectious diseases include conjunctivitis, caused by a bacterial or viral infection; tonsillitis, typically caused by beta-hemolytic streptococci; fifth disease, also called *erythema infectiosum*, a mild infection caused by parvovirus B19; hand-foot-and-mouth disease, caused by the coxsackievirus, which causes multiple symptoms, including painful blisters on the tongue, mouth, palms of the hands, and soles of the feet; chickenpox, caused by a member of the herpesvirus group; meningitis, an inflammation of the membranes that cover the brain and spinal cord, caused by bacteria or viruses (bacterial meningitis is the more dangerous); HBV, which can lead to serious and chronic infection of the liver and can be transmitted across the placenta; and Reye's syndrome, which is linked with the use of aspirin during a viral illness.

10. **Recognize the etiologic factors and signs and symptoms of the two primary pediatric inherited disorders.**
Pediatric inherited disorders include cystic fibrosis, an autosomal recessive genetic disorder that causes exocrine glands to produce abnormally thick secretions and primarily affects the lungs and pancreas; and Duchenne's muscular dystrophy, an X-linked genetic disease that causes progressive muscle degeneration.

Continued

SUMMARY OF LEARNING OBJECTIVES—*continued*

11. **Summarize the immunizations recommended for children by the Centers for Disease Control and Prevention (CDC).**
    The CDC's recommendations for childhood immunization are summarized in Table 35-2 and Figure 35-7.

12. **Demonstrate how to document immunizations and maintain accurate immunization records.**
    Procedure 35-1 summarizes how to document immunizations in both the official vaccination record and the parent's immunization booklet. Documentation of immunization administration on the VIS form must include the date the vaccine was administered, the vaccine's manufacturer, the manufacturer's lot number, the type of vaccine, the route of administration and exact site if an injection is given, any reported or observed side effects, the name and title of the person administering the vaccine, the address of the medical office where the vaccine was administered, and the date.

13. **Compare a well-child examination with a sick-child examination.**
    Well-child visits are typically scheduled from age 2 weeks through 15 years to focus on maintaining the child's health with physical examinations, immunizations, and upgrading of the child's medical health history record. Sick-child visits occur whenever the child needs to be seen because of illness or injury. Table 35-4 summarizes important questions for telephone screening of pediatric problems.

14. **Outline the medical assistant's role in pediatric procedures.**
    The medical assistant assists the pediatrician with examinations; maintains patient histories; performs ordered screening tests, such as vision, hearing, urinalysis, and hemoglobin checks; administers immunizations; measures and weighs children as needed; documents accurately; and provides support to patients and caregivers.

15. **Measure the circumference of an infant's head.**
    Procedure 35-2 outlines the steps for measuring an infant's head.

16. **Obtain accurate length and weight measurements and plot pediatric growth patterns.**
    Procedure 35-3 outlines the steps for measuring an infant's length and weight and documenting on the child's growth chart.

17. **Accurately measure pediatric vital signs, and perform vision screening.**
    Procedure 35-4 summarizes the steps for obtaining accurate pediatric vital signs and performing vision screening on a child. Tympanic or temporal thermometers are the easiest and quickest method for measuring temperature; the apical pulse should be taken for a full minute, respirations observed and recorded, and blood pressures taken with the appropriate-sized cuff when indicated. After patient education, the Snellen E chart is used to perform vision screening and to record results accurately.

18. **Correctly apply a pediatric urine collection device.**
    Procedure 35-5 summarizes the steps for applying a urinary collection device.

19. **Describe the characteristics and needs of the adolescent patient.**
    Adolescents are going through extreme physical and emotional changes, and an extra measure of patience and understanding is required to establish therapeutic interactions. Ensuring their privacy, giving them the option of being seen without parents, and providing pertinent education materials all are important factors in patient-centered adolescent care.

20. **Specify child safety guidelines for injury prevention, and explain the management of suspected child abuse, neglect, or exploitation.**
    The medical assistant should be involved in parent education on injury prevention for children. Childhood injuries are linked to the child's growth and development level and therefore are often predictable and many times preventable. If the medical assistant suspects that a child is a victim of abuse, neglect, or exploitation he or she should consult with the pediatrician immediately. In most states, the medical assistant and the physician can make separate reports to the authorities.

21. **Summarize patient education guidelines for pediatric patients.**
    Parents need reinforcement, praise, and understanding in dealing with the health and welfare of their child. Provide parents with information to help them understand their children's behavior and improve their parenting skills.

22. **Discuss the legal and ethical implications in a pediatric practice.**
    Occasionally in the pediatric office, legal and ethical issues arise, and the entire office staff may be faced with an ethical situation. If this type of situation occurs, the first option is to talk it over with the pediatrician. It may be necessary to have an office staff meeting to identify the conflict, note pertinent laws and facts, consider possible options and the consequences of each, and decide on a course of action.

CONNECTIONS

Study Guide Connection: Go to the Chapter 35 Study Guide. Read and complete the activities.

evolve Evolve Connection: Go to the Chapter 35 link at *evolve.elsevier.com/kinn* to complete the Chapter Review Quiz. Check out the other resources listed for this chapter to make the most of what you have learned from Assisting in Pediatrics.

ASSISTING IN ORTHOPEDIC MEDICINE

36

SCENARIO

Kaiwan Tillman became interested in orthopedics before he even knew what the word meant. In the sixth grade, he broke his right femur in a bicycle accident. He had to have multiple operations and undergo lengthy rehabilitation to regain complete movement in the leg. On graduation from high school, he attended the local community college and enrolled in a medical assisting program that offered an associate's degree. Since earning his CMA (AAMA),

Kaiwan has worked in a sports medicine clinic. The clinic staff at Sports Medicine Associates includes three orthopedic surgeons, two physical therapists, and two massage therapists. Kaiwan is very excited about working in the clinic, although he initially was somewhat intimidated. Dr. Steve Alexander is the team physician for a local professional baseball team, and Kaiwan's responsibilities include assisting Dr. Alexander with treating the team.

While studying this chapter, think about the following questions:

- What are the primary responsibilities of the medical assistant in an orthopedic practice?
- What clinical skills are required in this specialty practice?
- What are the common musculoskeletal injuries and disorders that the medical assistant should understand?
- What diagnostic and treatment procedures typically are used in an orthopedic practice?

LEARNING OBJECTIVES

1. Define, spell, and pronounce the terms listed in the vocabulary.
2. Describe the principal anatomic structures of the musculoskeletal system and their functions.
3. Differentiate among tendons, bursae, and ligaments.
4. Summarize the major muscular disorders.
5. Identify and describe the common types of fractures.
6. Explain the difference between osteomalacia and osteoporosis.
7. Classify typical spinal column disorders.
8. Differentiate among the various joint disorders.
9. Summarize the medical assistant's role in assisting with orthopedic procedures.
10. Explain the common diagnostic procedures used in orthopedics.
11. Discuss therapeutic modalities used in orthopedic medicine.
12. Apply cold therapy to an injury.
13. Discuss various heat treatments and assist with hot moist heat application to an orthopedic injury.
14. Discuss therapeutic ultrasonography, massage, exercise, and electrical muscle stimulation.
15. Explain the use of common ambulatory devices, properly fit a patient with crutches, and coach a patient in the correct mechanics of crutch walking.
16. Discuss the management of fractures and prepare for and assist with both the application and removal of a cast.
17. Summarize patient education guidelines for orthopedic patients.
18. Discuss the legal and ethical implications in an orthopedic practice.

VOCABULARY

arthritis (ahr-thri'-tis) Inflammation of a joint.

articular (ar-tih'-kyuh-luhr) Pertaining to a joint.

bursae (bur'-suh) Fluid-filled, saclike membranes that provide cushioning and allow frictionless motion between two tissues.

cartilage (kahr'-tl-ij) A rubbery, smooth, somewhat elastic connective tissue that covers the ends of bones.

cervical (ser'-vih-kuhl) Pertaining to the neck region containing seven cervical vertebrae.

corticosteroids (kawr-tuh-koh-ster'-oidz) Antiinflammatory hormones, natural or synthetic.

crepitation (kreh-puh-ta'-shun) A dry, crackling sound or sensation.

diaphysis (di-ah'-fuh-suhs) The midportion of a long bone; it contains the medullary cavity.

endoscope (en'-duh-skohp) An illuminated optic instrument for visualization of the inside of the body; it may be inserted through an incision in minimally invasive surgery.

epiphysis (eh-pih'-fuh-sis) The end of a long bone; it contains the growth (epiphyseal) plates.

goniometer (go-ne-om'-ih-ter) An instrument for measuring the degrees of motion in a joint.

inflammation (in-fluh-ma'-shun) A tissue reaction to trauma or disease that includes redness, heat, swelling, and pain.

VOCABULARY—continued

kyphotic (ki-fot'-ik) Relating to the normal convex curvature of the thoracic spine.

ligaments (lig'-uh-ments) Tough connective tissue bands that hold joints together by attaching to the bones on either side of the joint.

lordotic (lor-do'-tik) Relating to the normal concave curvature of the cervical and lumbar spines.

lumbar (lum'-bahr) Relating to the lower back region that contains the five lumbar vertebrae.

luxation (luhk'-sa-shun) Dislocation of a bone from its normal anatomic location.

malaise (muh-layz') An indefinite feeling of debility or lack of health, often indicating or accompanying the onset of an illness.

medullary cavity (meh-duhl'-a-re) The inner portion of the diaphysis; it contains the bone marrow.

periosteum (per-e-os'-te-uhm) The thin, highly innervated, membranous covering of a bone.

prosthesis (pros-the'-suhs) An artificial replacement for a body part.

range of motion (ROM) The extent of movement possible in a joint; the degree of motion depends on the type of joint and whether a disease process is present; ROM exercises are applied actively (independently) or passively (with assistance) to prevent or treat joint problems.

reduction Return to correct anatomic position, as in reduction of a fracture.

sarcoma A malignant tumor in fibrous, fatty, muscular, synovial, vascular, or neural tissue.

scoliosis An abnormal lateral curvature of the spine.

striated A muscle that contains fibers divided by bands of cross stripes or striations because of overlapping myofilaments.

synovial fluid A clear fluid found in joint cavities that facilitates smooth movements and nourishes joint structures.

tendons Tough bands of connective tissue that connect muscle to bone.

A physician who specializes in orthopedics is responsible for diagnosing and treating diseases and disorders of the musculoskeletal system, especially those affecting the bones. Rheumatologists are specialists in treating inflammatory joint disorders. Chiropractors are doctors of chiropractic (DC) but are not medical physicians; they use manual adjusting procedures to correct subluxations or misalignments of the spine to allow maximum function, thus facilitating the body's ability to maintain homeostasis and prevent disease.

The musculoskeletal system includes all of the skeletal muscles, bones, joints, and supportive connective tissues (**cartilage**, **tendons**, and **ligaments**). The general functions of the musculoskeletal system are to:

* Protect the internal organs
* Support the body in standing erect
* Produce movement
* Perform hemopoietic functions (production of blood cells in the red bone marrow)
* Store the minerals calcium and phosphorus in the bones

ANATOMY AND PHYSIOLOGY OF THE MUSCULOSKELETAL SYSTEM

Muscles

More than 600 muscles attach to the human skeleton (Figure 36-1). These muscles account for approximately half of a person's weight, and they contribute to the body's distinct shape. This chapter discusses the skeletal muscles that attach to bones and allow movement. Skeletal muscle fibers are voluntary and **striated** (Figure 36-2, A). The body has two other types of muscle: smooth muscle (Figure 36-2, B), which lines organs and blood vessel walls and is nonstriated, and cardiac muscle (Figure 36-2, C), a striated muscle in the heart. Both of these types are *involuntary* muscles; that is, the individual cannot control their function. Skeletal muscles are *voluntary*; when they contract or relax can be controlled. Special fibers in

skeletal muscles allow them to shorten (contract) and lengthen (relax), which creates movement (Table 36-1). These muscles are connected to bone with bands of tough, fibrous connective tissues called *tendons*.

Bones

The human skeleton is composed of more than 200 bones (Figure 36-3). Bones provide a framework to protect vital organs. In general, the size and shape of a bone is related either to how much it moves and how much body weight it must carry, or to its protective function for the underlying organs.

Bones generally are categorized by shape: long, short, flat, rounded, or irregular. A long bone is made up of a **diaphysis** (the shaft), which has an expansion at each end (the **epiphysis**) (Figure 36-4). The epiphysis is covered with **articular** cartilage and is attached by ligaments to the epiphysis of another bone, forming a joint. Articular cartilage reduces the stress of weight bearing and the friction of movement. The thickness of the cartilage depends largely on the amount of stress placed on a particular joint. The **medullary cavity**, inside the diaphysis, contains yellow bone marrow.

Bone is living tissue that is constantly being remodeled in response to stress or injury. It also is a storage location for minerals, including calcium and phosphorus. Red bone marrow produces blood cells and is found in the spongy (cancellous) bone of the proximal epiphyses of the humerus and femur, sternum, ribs, and vertebrae of adults. Bones are covered with a thin, membranous tissue, the **periosteum**, which contains many sensory nerves.

CRITICAL THINKING APPLICATION   36-1

In what way does Kaiwan benefit by being familiar with the names and locations of the major bones of the extremities? How might this knowledge make his job at Sports Medicine Associates more interesting? What is the difference between tendons and ligaments?

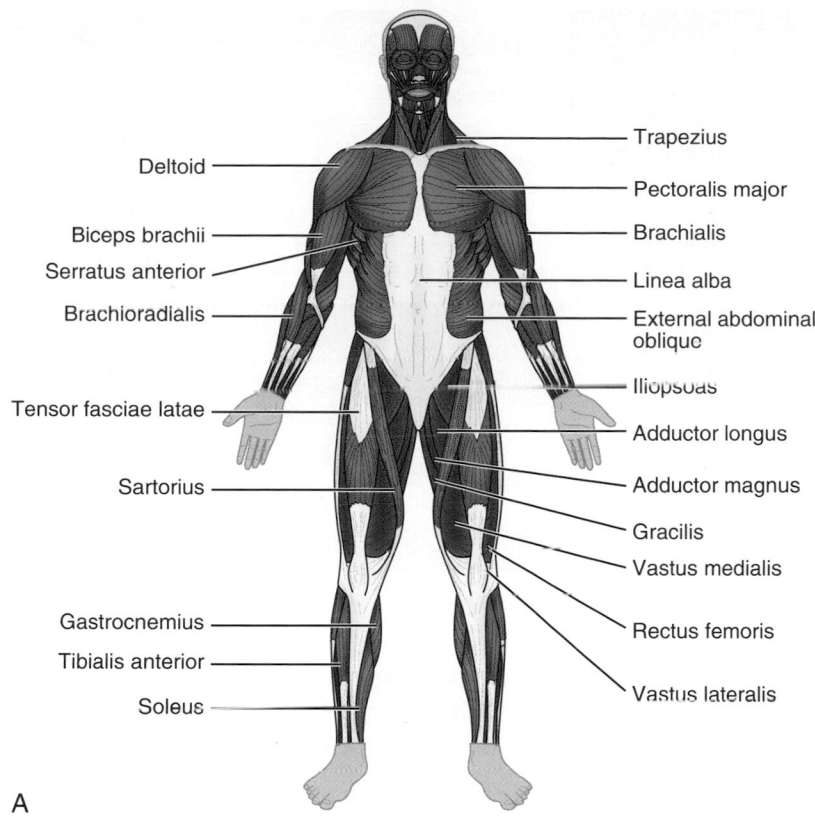

Deltoid

Biceps brachii

Serratus anterior

Brachioradialis

Tensor fasciae latae

Sartorius

Gastrocnemius

Tibialis anterior

Soleus

Trapezius

Pectoralis major

Brachialis

Linea alba

External abdominal oblique

Iliopsoas

Adductor longus

Adductor magnus

Gracilis

Vastus medialis

Rectus femoris

Vastus lateralis

A

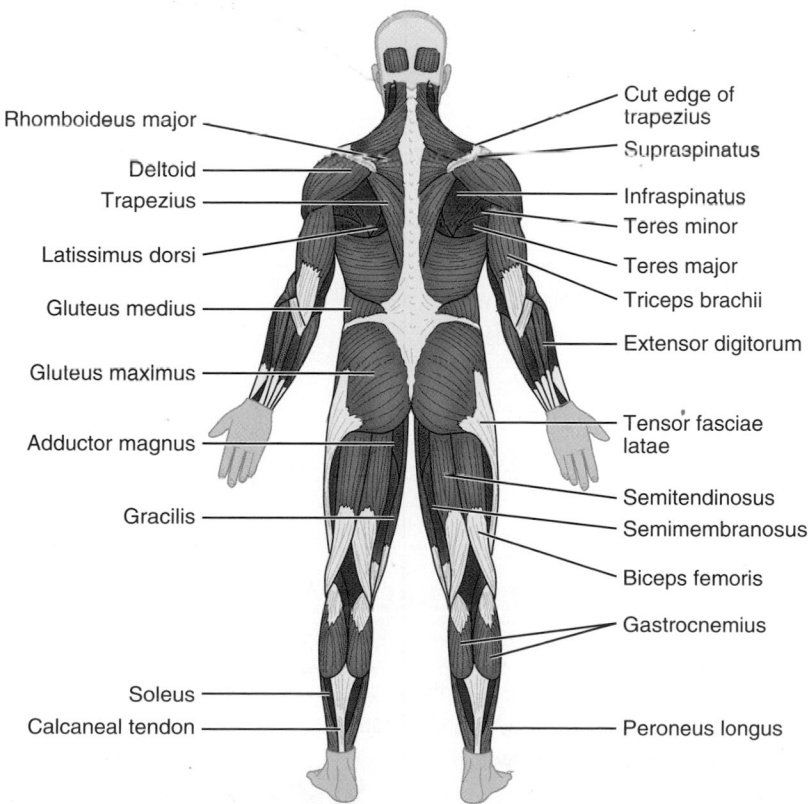

Rhomboideus major

Deltoid

Trapezius

Latissimus dorsi

Gluteus medius

Gluteus maximus

Adductor magnus

Gracilis

Soleus

Calcaneal tendon

Cut edge of trapezius

Supraspinatus

Infraspinatus

Teres minor

Teres major

Triceps brachii

Extensor digitorum

Tensor fasciae latae

Semitendinosus

Semimembranosus

Biceps femoris

Gastrocnemius

Peroneus longus

B

FIGURE 36-1 Muscles of the body. **A,** Anterior view. **B,** Posterior view.

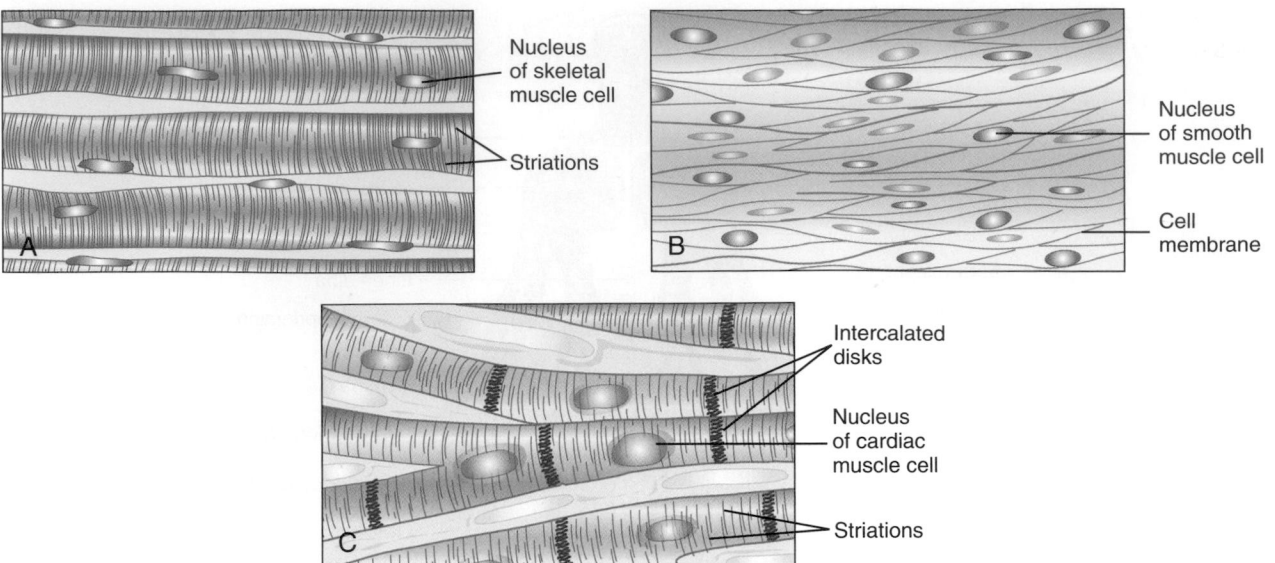

FIGURE 36-2 A, Skeletal muscle. **B,** Smooth muscle. **C,** Cardiac muscle. (From Applegate E: *The anatomy and physiology learning system,* ed 4, St Louis, 2011, Saunders.)

TABLE 36-1	Types of Body Movement		
MOVEMENT	**DEFINITION OR EXAMPLE**	**MOVEMENT**	**DEFINITION OR EXAMPLE**
Flexion 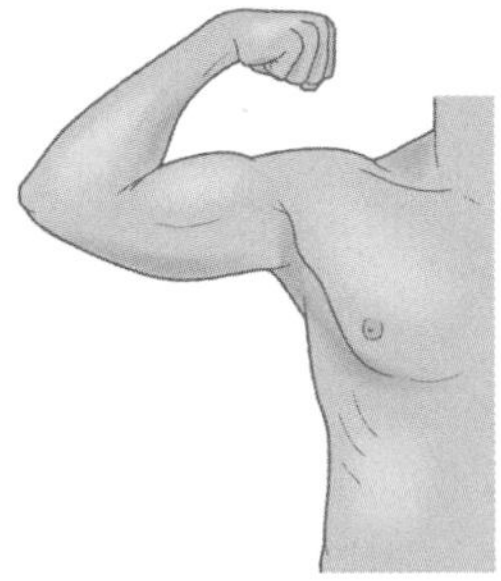	Reduces the angle of the joint and brings the two bones closer together.	Abduction 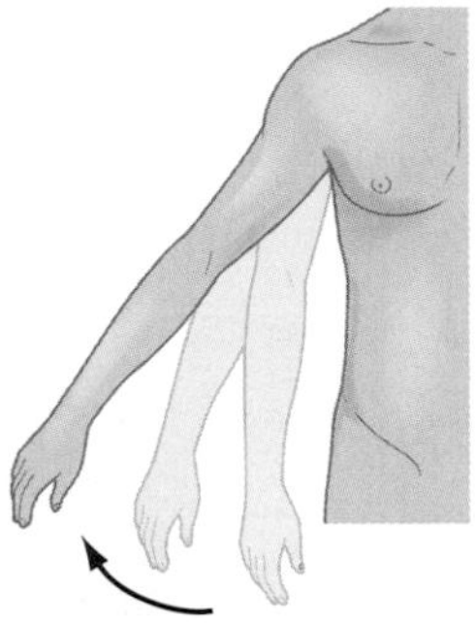	Moving the body part away from the midline or median plane of the body.
Extension 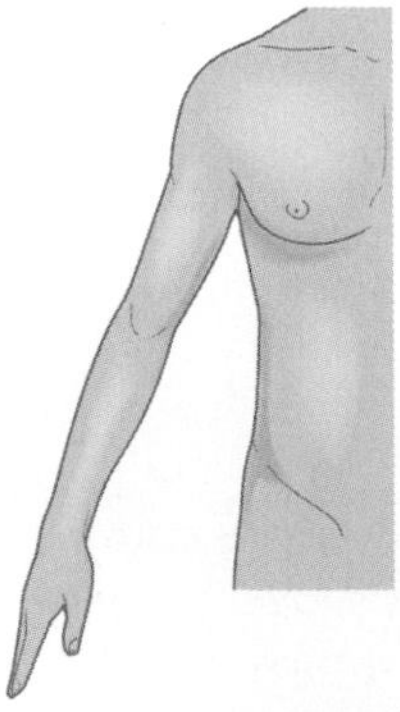	The opposite of flexion; increases the angle or distance between two bones or parts of the body.	Adduction 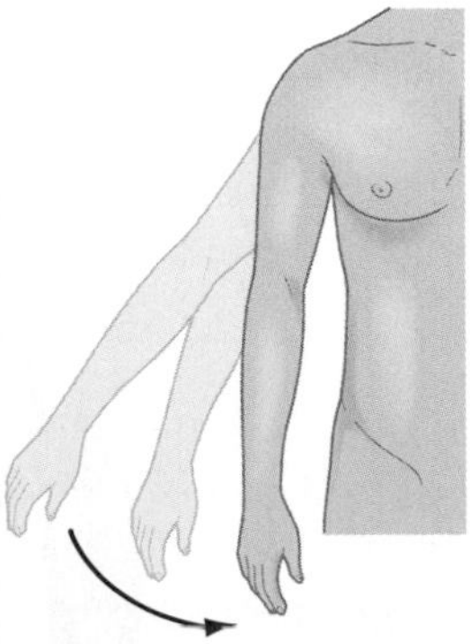	The opposite of abduction; moving the body part toward the midline of the body.
Hyperextension 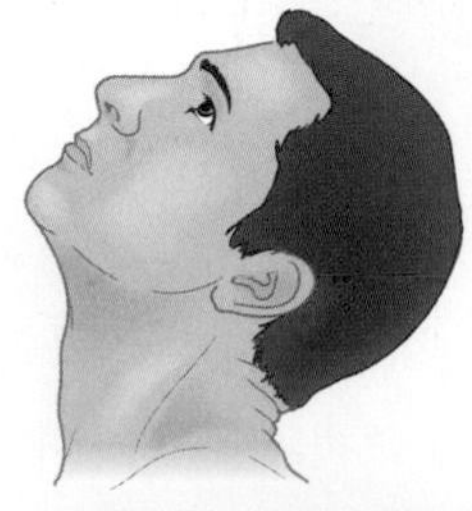	Extension 180 degrees (e.g., the neck is extended backward or the toes are pointed downward).	Rotation 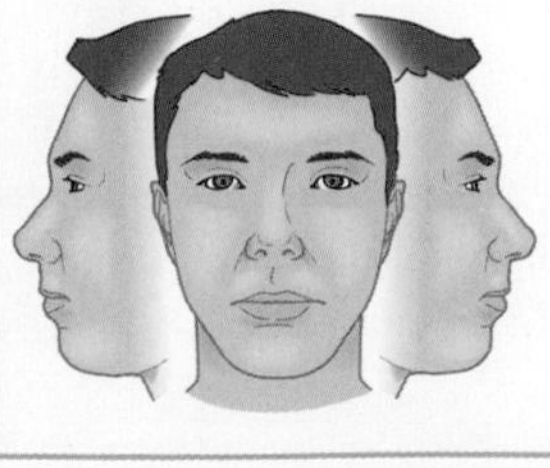	Moving a bone around its central axis; common in ball-and-socket joints.

TABLE 36-1   Types of Body Movement—*continued*

MOVEMENT	DEFINITION OR EXAMPLE	MOVEMENT	DEFINITION OR EXAMPLE
Circumduction	Circular movement of a limb; a combination of abduction, adduction, extension, and flexion.	Eversion	Turning the sole of the foot laterally, or outward.
Dorsiflexion	Moving the instep of the foot up and dorsally, reducing the angle between the foot and the leg.	Inversion	The opposite of eversion; turning the sole of the foot medially, or inward.
Plantar flexion	A toe-down movement of the foot at the ankle; increases the angle of the joint.	Pronation	Rotation of the forearm that turns the palm of the hand downward, or posteriorly.
		Supination	The opposite of pronation; rotation of the forearm that turns the palm of the hand upward, or anteriorly.

Joints

Bones are connected to each other at junctions known as *joints*. The two main kinds of joints are nonsynovial joints and synovial joints. In nonsynovial joints, the bones are joined with fibrous cartilage and are immovable (e.g., the sutures of the skull) or only slightly moveable (e.g., the vertebrae). Synovial joints are freely moveable because the adjacent ends of two bones are covered with cartilage and are enclosed in a joint cavity that contains a viscous, slippery fluid called **synovial fluid**, which is an excellent lubricant. Synovial joints such as the elbow and the knee are hinge joints, which allow movement in only one plane (Figure 36-5). Other synovial joints, such as the hip and shoulder, allow movement in many planes, which permits a wider **range of motion (ROM)** than a hinge joint has.

Types of Joints

As mentioned, joints are classified by the way they are shaped or by their ability to move. The joints of the skull are known as *sutures*. Sutures permit the skull to grow with the child but have very limited flexibility. The hinge joints of the elbow and knee allow for movement in one plane, such as bending back and forth. A gliding joint, as in the wrist and foot, is made up of two flat-surfaced bones that slide over each other, allowing limited movement. Ball-and-socket joints, as in the shoulder and hip, allow for the greatest ROM by permitting the joint to rotate in a complete circle. Artificial joints have been successfully implanted to replace joints that have been damaged by disease or trauma, including the joints of the hip, knee, ankle, shoulder, elbow, wrist, and finger.

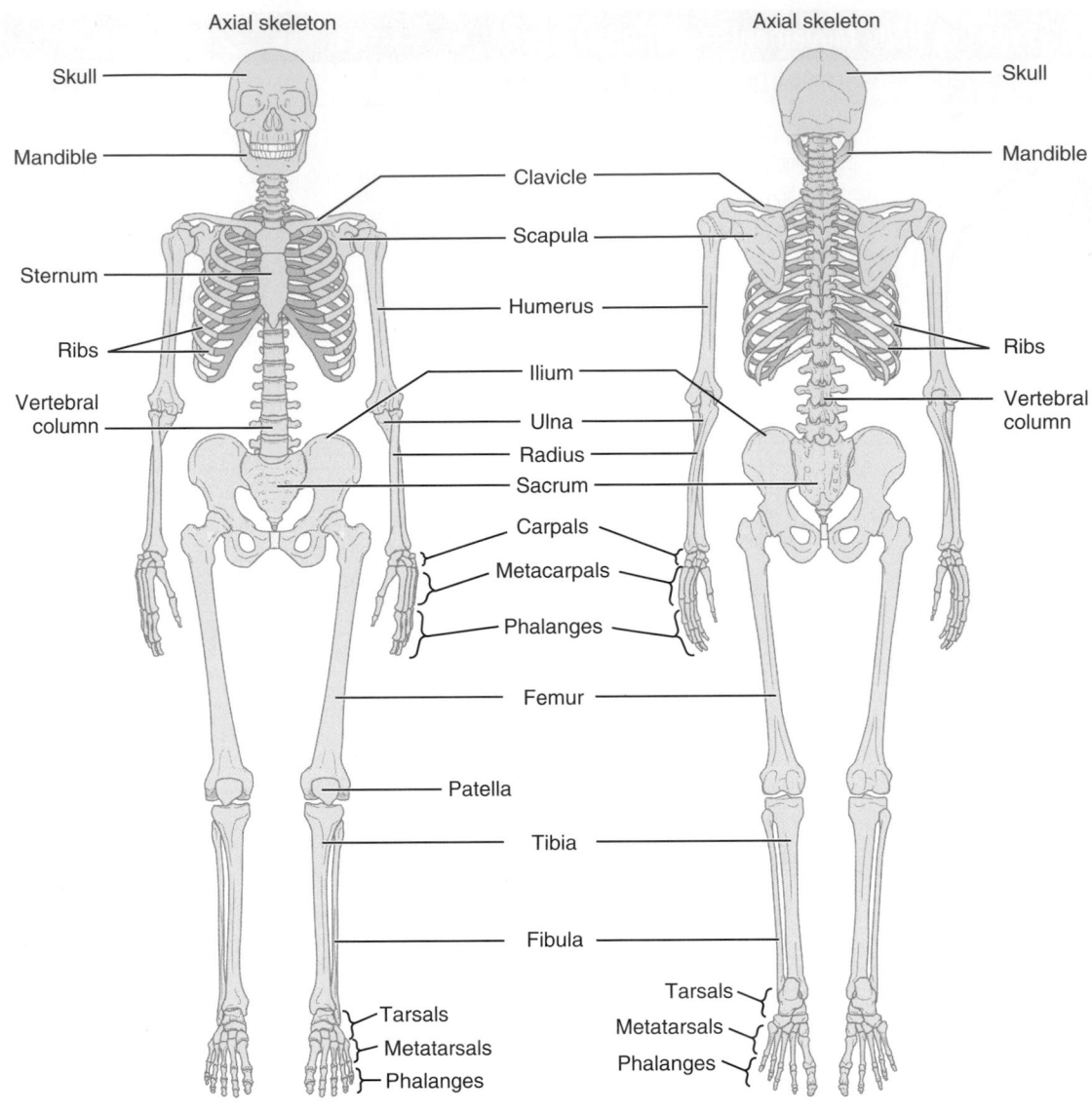

FIGURE 36-3 Axial skeletal bones *(outside columns)* and appendicular skeletal bones *(middle column)*.

Ligaments, Tendons, and Bursae

Ligaments are powerful, strong, fibrous bands of connective tissue that connect bone to bone at the joint and encase the joint capsule. Ligaments allow purposeful joint movement and prevent excessive movement in any particular joint. Ligaments may be oblique or parallel to the joint, as in the knee, or may surround the joint, as in the hip.

Plantar Fasciitis

Plantar fasciitis (pronounced PLAN-ter fash-ee-EYE-tus) is the most common cause of heel pain. The plantar fascia is a flat ligament that connects the heel bones of the foot to the toes. It supports the arch of the foot. If the plantar fascia is strained, it becomes weak, swollen, and inflamed. The primary symptom is pain that radiates from the heel or the bottom of the foot when standing or walking. Risk factors for plantar fasciitis include:

- Excessive pronation (the feet roll inward when walking)
- High arches or flat feet
- Walking, standing, or running for long periods
- Overweight
- Tight Achilles tendons or calf muscles

Most people with plantar fasciitis have pain when they take their first steps after they get out of bed or sit for a long time. Stretching and strengthening exercises or use of specialized devices, such as splints or orthotics (customized arch supports), may provide symptomatic relief.

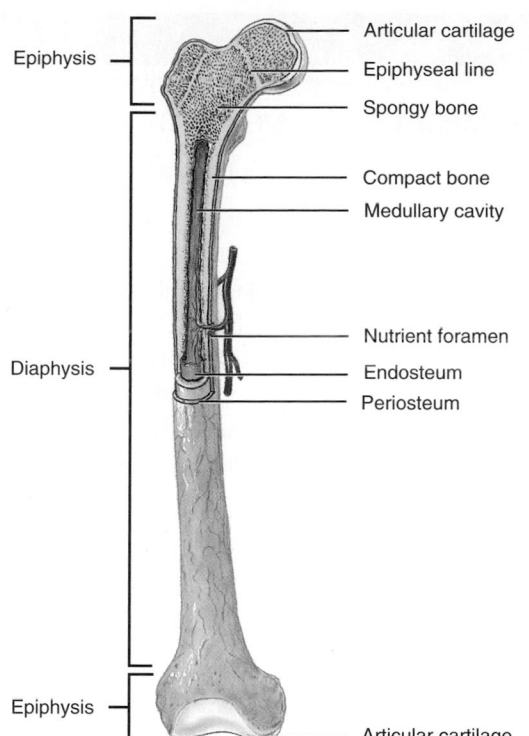

FIGURE 36-4 Long bone features. (From Applegate E: *The anatomy and physiology learning system,* ed 4, St Louis, 2011, Saunders.)

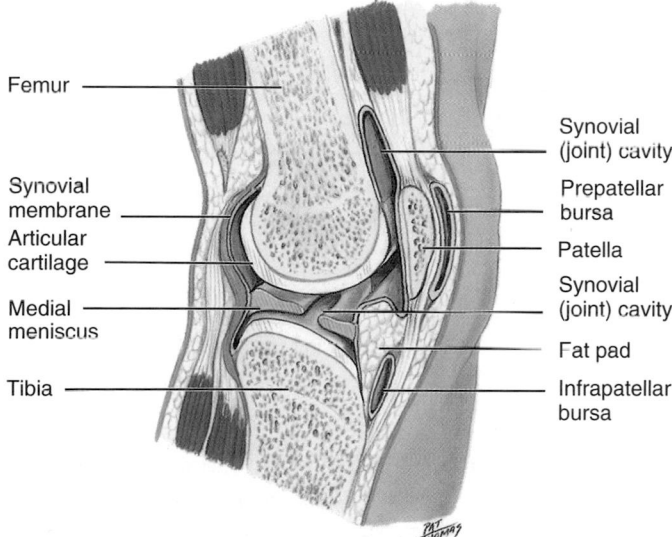

FIGURE 36-5 Sagittal section of the knee joint. (From Applegate E: *The anatomy and physiology learning system,* ed 4, St Louis, 2011, Saunders.)

A tendon is a strong bundle of connective tissue that attaches muscle to bone. Tendons can be flat or round and can pass between muscles, between bones, or through specialized openings between bones; for example, the carpal tunnel is a narrow opening in the bones at the base of the hand.

Bursae are fibrous sacs that lie between tendons and bones; they are lined with synovial membranes that secrete synovial fluid and act as cushions between a bone and a tendon or between a tendon and

a ligament. Bursae reduce friction and help muscles and tendons glide smoothly over bone.

MUSCULOSKELETAL DISEASES AND DISORDERS

Musculoskeletal diseases and conditions can affect any of the muscles, bones, or joints. These problems are common and have a tremendous impact on a person's quality of life. Brittle or deformed bones that are prone to fracture often mark bone disorders such as osteoporosis and osteomalacia. Joint disorders, such as osteoarthritis (OA), rheumatoid **arthritis** (RA), and gout, can lead to painful, swollen, or inflamed joints. Muscle problems, such as sprains and spasms, can bring on sudden pain or cause stiffness (Table 36-2).

Trauma to the musculoskeletal system can quickly lead to **inflammation** in the area of injury. This type of injury is one of the leading causes of time lost from work and for visits to primary care physicians and emergency departments. As soon as possible after injury, even before a patient is seen by a provider, treatment involving rest, ice, compression, and elevation (RICE therapy) should be started. The combination of these measures can help reduce swelling and inflammation and enhance healing.

Using Frozen Peas for an Ice Bag

A bag of frozen peas (or corn) easily conforms to the shape of a body part and serves as an excellent means of immediately applying ice to a musculoskeletal injury. The vegetable ice bag should be wrapped in a towel to protect tissue from overexposure to the cold. It should be applied for 20 minutes, put back into the freezer for 30 to 60 minutes, and applied again.

To maintain musculoskeletal health, a person must have a significant dietary intake of foods rich in calcium and vitamin D; must avoid smoking; and must include weight-bearing exercises (e.g., walking) in the daily routine. In addition to these lifestyle measures, medications sometimes are required for conditions that impair normal functioning of the musculoskeletal system. The conditions discussed in the following sections are typically seen in an orthopedic practice.

CRITICAL THINKING APPLICATION   **36-2**

Why is it important to obtain an accurate history from an injured patient who comes to the office for the first time? What is Kaiwan's responsibility in finding out the reason a new patient is being seen?

Muscular Disorders

Fibromyalgia

Fibromyalgia is a condition of widespread connective tissue and muscular pain and often includes severe fatigue of unknown origin. A patient with fibromyalgia usually complains of diffuse aches and pains all over the body. The disorder can affect people of all ages and is seen more frequently in women than in men. Chronic pain and fatigue are the cardinal signs in the absence of any other known cause. Associated conditions can include sleep disorders, irritable

TABLE 36-2　Common Musculoskeletal Conditions

DISEASE	SYMPTOMS, SIGNS, AND ETIOLOGY	DIAGNOSTIC PROCEDURES	LABORATORY TESTS	TREATMENT AND MEDICATIONS
Bursitis and tendonitis	Painful joint with reduced ROM; caused by overuse of the joint, injury, or disease	History, physical examination, x-ray studies to rule out fracture	CBC to rule out infectious arthritis	RICE, temporary immobilization, NSAIDs
Carpal tunnel syndrome	Hand and finger pain, numbness, tingling, difficulty grasping or holding objects, especially in the morning; caused by compression of the median nerve at the carpal tunnel area	Physical examination; Tinel and Phalen compression tests; NCS and EMG; ultrasonography of the wrist	Routine lab tests to rule out other conditions	Rest and splint wrist; OTC NSAIDs, diuretics, oral prednisone or corticosteroid injections; forearm extensor stretching and strengthening exercises; endoscopic surgical decompression in severe cases
Dislocation	Painful joint that is out of place and has severely reduced ROM; caused by traumatic injury to the joint	History of trauma, physical examination, x-ray studies	None	Reduce and temporarily immobilize joint; analgesics
Fibromyalgia	Chronic, severe musculoskeletal pain, generalized weakness; cause unknown but has contributing factors	History, physical examination to rule out other causes	As appropriate to rule out other conditions	NSAIDs, analgesics, rest, control of stress. Pregabalin (Lyrica); milnacipran (Savella) for pain, fatigue, and depression; zolpidem (Ambien) for sleep; tramadol (Ultram) for relief of pain; and antidepressants duloxetine (Cymbalta) and fluoxetine (Prozac)
Fractures	Severe pain, swelling, reduced ROM	History, physical examination, x-ray studies	None	Reduction, immobilization, analgesics, NSAIDs
Gout	Painful joint inflammation, often affects great toe, very sensitive to touch and movement; metabolic disease caused by buildup of uric acid	History, physical examination, microscopic synovial fluid examination for uric acid crystals	Serum uric acid test	Low purine diet, limit alcohol, NSAIDs, analgesics, prednisone, colchicine (Colcrys); allopurinol (Lopurin, Zyloprim); and probenecid (Probalan)
Herniated disk	Depend on location and severity of herniation; back pain, extremity pain or weakness; caused by trauma or stress	History, physical examination; MRI; EMG or NCS	None	Rest, antiinflammatories, analgesics, physical therapy, epidural corticosteroid injections, surgical laminectomy in severe cases
Infectious arthritis	Severely infected and inflamed joint; usually result of surgery or trauma	History, physical examination, microscopic synovial fluid examination for cell count and presence of bacteria	CBC, culture of joint fluid	NSAIDs, corticosteroids, appropriate antibiotic or antiviral agents
Lupus	Painful or swollen joints and muscle pain; unexplained fever or rash; chest pain with deep breathing; hair loss; Raynaud's phenomenon; sun sensitivity; leg and eye edema; mouth ulcers; swollen glands; extreme fatigue; autoimmune disease	Very careful history and physical examination to rule out possible causes of presenting symptoms; frequently a diagnosis of exclusion	Diagnostic tests as needed to rule out possible causes of symptoms, renal lab tests, blood tests for hemolytic anemia or low platelet and WBCs; antinuclear antibody test	No known cure; type of pharmaceutical treatment depends on organs involved; medications include NSAIDs; antimalarial hydroxychloroquine (Plaquenil); prednisone; immunosuppressives azathioprine (Imuran), cyclophosphamide (Cytoxan); IV belimumab (Benlysta)

TABLE 36-2   Common Musculoskeletal Conditions—*continued*

DISEASE	SYMPTOMS, SIGNS, AND ETIOLOGY	DIAGNOSTIC PROCEDURES	LABORATORY TESTS	TREATMENT AND MEDICATIONS
Lyme disease	Bull's-eye lesion, flulike symptoms, arthritic pain, meningitis, Bell's palsy, memory loss, mood disorders; bacterial infection carried by ticks	Careful history; physical examination to check for tick bite	Two-step blood test; enzyme immunoassay and Western blot test	Initially antibiotics; later stages IV ceftriaxone (Rocephin)
Myasthenia gravis	Profound muscular weakness, frequently starting with facial muscles; can involve any; voluntary muscles; autoimmune neuromuscular disease; unknown cause	History, neurologic examination, EMG	Anti-AChR antibody test	Acetylcholinesterase, steroids; immune inhibitor cyclosporine (Sandimmune), thymectomy
Osteoarthritis	Gradually increasing joint pain; gradually decreasing ROM in affected joint; caused by degeneration of articular cartilage	History, physical examination, x-ray studies, MRI	RA test to rule out rheumatoid arthritis; CBC to rule out infectious arthritis	Exercise and weight control, NSAIDs, physical therapy, analgesics, ambulatory support, intra-articular steroid injections
Osteomalacia	Fractures, muscle weakness, bone pain; metabolic disease caused by vitamin D deficiency or problems with its metabolism	History, physical examination, x-ray studies, bone scan	Serum vitamin D, serum calcium, serum alkaline phosphatase, PTH level, occasionally bone biopsy	Vitamin D and calcium supplements
Osteoporosis	Frequent fractures, exaggerated thoracic kyphosis, reduced height, back pain; multiple risk factors; low calcium/vitamin D diet; lack of exercise; genetic factors	History, physical examination; DXA scan; ultrasound of the heel	None	Weight-bearing exercise; calcium supplementation; pharmaceutical treatment with alendronate (Fosamax), risedronate (Actonel), zoledronic acid (Reclast), and ibandronate sodium (Boniva); raloxifene (Evista)
Rheumatoid arthritis	Severe joint pain and joint deformity; autoimmune response to synovial membrane; unknown cause	History, physical examination, x-ray studies	RF and blood antibody tests	NSAIDs; corticosteroids; methotrexate (Rheumatrex), leflunomide (Arava), hydroxychloroquine (Plaquenil) and sulfasalazine (Azulfidine), etanercept (Enbrel), infliximab (Remicade), and adalimumab (Humira); analgesics; low-impact exercise; joint replacement in severe cases
Scoliosis	Lateral spinal deformity accompanied by back pain; congenital defect	Physical examination, radiographic studies	None	Braces, casts, surgery
Sprain, strain, spasm	Cardinal signs: inflammation, redness, heat, swelling, pain, reduced ROM; caused by trauma	History, physical examination, including active and passive ROM, x-ray studies to rule out fracture	None	RICE and NSAIDs

AChR, Acetylcholine receptor; *CBC,* complete blood count; *DXA,* dual energy x-ray absorptiometry; *EMG,* electromyography; *IV, intravenous; MRI,* magnetic resonance imaging; *NCS,* nerve conduction studies; *NSAIDs,* nonsteroidal anti-inflammatory drugs; *OTC,* over-the-counter; *PTH,* parathyroid; *RA,* Rheumatoid arthritis; *RF,* rheumatoid factor; *RICE,* rest, ice, compression, elevation; *ROM,* range of motion; *WBCs,* white blood cells.

bowel syndrome, chronic headaches, temporomandibular joint (TMJ) problems, painful menstrual periods, increased chemical sensitivity, and other musculoskeletal complaints.

Although the cause remains unknown, fibromyalgia can be triggered by an automobile accident or a bacterial or viral infection, or it can follow the diagnosis of other medical conditions, such as RA, lupus, or hypothyroidism. It is aggravated by changes in the weather or temperature, monthly hormonal variations, stress, anxiety, and depression. In the past, a physical examination for possible fibromyalgia would include a check for 18 specific tender points on a person's body to see how many of them were painful when pressed firmly. However, current diagnostic guidelines no longer suggest checking for tender points. A fibromyalgia diagnosis is made if a person reports widespread pain for longer than 3 months without any other medical condition. There are no blood tests specifically to diagnose fibromyalgia, but the provider may order certain laboratory studies to rule out other possible causes of the widespread pain.

Treatment goals include reducing pain, enhancing sleep, and reducing anxiety and stress. Pregabalin (Lyrica), an antiseizure medication, is the first drug approved by the U.S. Food and Drug Administration (FDA) to treat fibromyalgia. Milnacipran (Savella) may be prescribed to reduce pain and fatigue and help with the depression associated with fibromyalgia. Prescription sleeping pills, such as zolpidem (Ambien), are prescribed only for the short term because the body eventually becomes tolerant to the medication, rendering it ineffective. Other medical treatments include over-the-counter (OTC) analgesics (e.g., Tylenol or ibuprofen) and antiinflammatory agents, including tramadol (Ultram) for relief of pain; and antidepressants, such as duloxetine (Cymbalta) to ease the pain and fatigue associated with fibromyalgia and fluoxetine (Prozac) to help promote sleep. Stress reduction, physical therapy, and relaxation exercises help control symptoms. Fibromyalgia has no known cure.

Myasthenia Gravis

Myasthenia gravis is a chronic autoimmune neuromuscular disease of unknown origin that affects voluntary muscle contraction. It can occur at any age but most frequently affects young adult women (under age 40) and older men (over age 60). Often the patient experiences a sudden onset of weakness in the muscles that control eye and eyelid movement, facial expression, and swallowing. Symptoms vary in type and severity and may include drooping of one or both eyelids (ptosis); blurred or double vision (diplopia) as a result of weakness of the muscles that control eye movements; an unstable or waddling gait; weakness in the arms, hands, fingers, legs, and neck; altered facial expressions; difficulty swallowing; shortness of breath; and impaired speech (dysarthria).

Myasthenia gravis is caused by a defect in the transmission of nerve impulses to muscles. It occurs when a nervous stimulus is unable to stimulate a muscle at the neuromuscular junction, the place where nerve cells connect with the muscles they control. Normally, when impulses travel down the nerve, the nerve endings release acetylcholine (ACh), a neurotransmitter that activates muscular contraction. In myasthenia gravis, antibodies block, alter, or destroy the receptors for ACh at the neuromuscular junction, which prevents the muscle contraction. The condition is diagnosed with a complete history and physical exam, including a neurology exam to detect muscular weakness, especially in the movement of the eyes. Blood tests for certain antibodies are also ordered, but they are not always conclusive. The primary treatment is a medication that inhibits acetylcholinesterase, the enzyme that normally breaks down ACh. This allows ACh to remain at the neuromuscular junction longer than usual so that more of the remaining receptor sites can be activated. Immunosuppressive drugs, such as prednisone or cyclosporine (Sandimmune), may be prescribed to improve muscle strength by suppressing the production of abnormal antibodies. Surgical removal of the thymus gland (thymectomy) reduces symptoms and may cure some individuals. Spontaneous improvement and remissions can occur.

Sprains, Strains, and Spasms

A *sprain* is a wrenching or twisting of a joint in an abnormal plane of motion or beyond its normal ROM that results in stretching and/or tearing of a ligament. Concurrent damage to area blood vessels, muscles, tendons, and nerves may occur. Probably the most common sprain is the ankle sprain (Figure 36-6), which can occur when a person steps off a curb or into a small depression and twists the ankle. Severe sprains are so painful the joint cannot be used, and they are

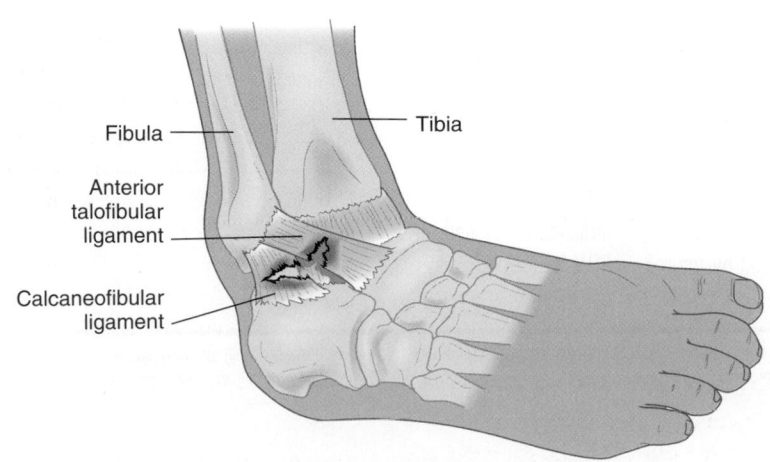

FIGURE 36-6 Ankle sprain.

accompanied by swelling and reddish to bluish discoloration because of ruptured blood vessels in the area.

A *strain* may be a simple overstretching of a muscle or tendon, or it can be caused by partial or complete tearing of the tissue away from the bone.

These soft tissue injuries are diagnosed by a comprehensive history and physical examination. Usually x-ray films are taken to rule out fractures. The treatment includes RICE: *rest* of the injured joint with no weight bearing to prevent further damage; *ice* or cold application for 20 minutes at a time, four to eight times a day, during the first 24 to 48 hours to reduce pain and swelling; *compression* with an elastic wrap or air cast to reduce swelling; and *elevation* of the injured part. The provider also may recommend OTC antiinflammatory drugs (e.g., naproxen or ibuprofen) to help reduce pain and inflammation at the site. A severe soft tissue injury may require the use of crutches to prevent weight bearing, immobilization by casting, or surgical repair.

Treatment of a sprain or strain may also include rehabilitative exercises. The provider typically prescribes an exercise program designed to prevent stiffness, improve the joint's ROM, and restore normal flexibility and strength. Some patients may also be referred to physical therapy for complete return of function after the initial pain and swelling have subsided.

Telephone Screening of Joint Injuries

The following factors can help the medical assistant determine the need for an appointment when a patient calls to report a joint injury:

- Presence of severe pain and inability to put any weight on the injured joint
- Crooked appearance of injured area or unusual lumps and bumps
- Inability to move the injured joint
- Inability to walk more than four steps without significant pain
- Limb buckles or gives way if attempts are made to use the joint
- Numbness in any part of the injured area
- Inflammation that spreads out from the injured area
- History of injury to this particular joint
- Pain, swelling, or inflammation over a bony prominence

CRITICAL THINKING APPLICATION   36-3

A patient comes into the clinic hopping on one foot and holding the other in the air. She says she thinks she broke her ankle when she stepped off the curb wrong and fell. What is the first thing Kaiwan should do for this patient? What tests will Dr. Alexander most likely order? Why?

Muscle spasms occur spontaneously and may persist for hours. They typically are caused by heavy exercise and muscle fatigue, but they also can be caused by dehydration, hypothyroidism, lack of calcium or magnesium, kidney failure, and alcoholism. Muscle spasms can be quite painful. Treatment includes massage, direct pressure, ultrasound therapy, stress reduction, stretching exercises, and muscle relaxants in some cases.

Restless Legs Syndrome

A patient with restless legs syndrome (RLS) reports unpleasant sensations, such as tingling, aching, and twitching of the legs, during periods of inactivity, especially at night. The individual feels an overwhelming urge to move the affected leg (or legs) to relieve these abnormal feelings. Patients with nighttime leg twitching are diagnosed with periodic limb movements of sleep (PLMS), which causes involuntary flexion and extension of the legs during sleep. Most people with this disorder have difficulty getting to sleep or staying asleep.

Initial treatment plans include lifestyle changes, such as relaxation exercises, soaking in a warm bath, cutting back on caffeine, and moderate exercise. If these methods do not relieve the symptoms, patients may be prescribed medications, including ropinirole (Requip), rotigotine (Neupro), or pramipexole (Mirapex) to increase the amount of the neurotransmitter dopamine in the brain; anticonvulsants, such as gabapentin (Neurontin) and pregabalin (Lyrica); or sleep agents, such as zolpidem (Ambien) or eszopiclone (Lunesta).

Skeletal Disorders

Fractures

A fracture is a break or crack in a bone, generally as the result of trauma or disease. Many different types of fractures occur, and each produces its own set of problems (Table 36-3). The common symptom of all fractures is pain. Other symptoms may include swelling, bleeding, inability to move, misalignment of the bone, and discoloration of the immediate area.

When a patient with a suspected fracture comes into the office, you should make the person as comfortable as possible. First aid includes positioning the patient to prevent stress on the injured area; elevating the injured extremity if possible; and controlling any bleeding but never applying pressure over a suspected fracture. Do not attempt to straighten the fracture or move it in any way. If the patient must be moved, either apply a splint or support the joints above and below the suspected fracture before and while moving the patient. The fracture must be confirmed by x-ray examination as soon as possible.

Treatment includes **reduction**, if necessary, and immobilization. Reduction places the fractured bone back into its correct anatomic alignment. Reduction may be closed or open. In a closed reduction, the provider manipulates the bone into its correct position. If this is not possible or if the fractured bones have pierced the skin, an open reduction is required, which is surgical realignment of the bone. During an open reduction, the orthopedic surgeon may have to install metal pins, plates, or screws to facilitate and maintain correct bone alignment. These metal implants may be temporary or permanent, depending on the extent of injury (Figure 36-7). After the fracture has been reduced, it must be immobilized with a brace, splint, or cast to prevent movement of the fracture site and thereby facilitate healing. The duration of immobilization depends on the severity of the fracture.

Osteomalacia

The term *osteomalacia* literally means "softening of the bones." Osteomalacia is a metabolic disease in which inadequate calcium or

TABLE 36-3   Types of Fractures

FRACTURE	DEFINITION	FRACTURE	DEFINITION
Closed, or simple	Broken bone is contained within intact skin.	Comminuted	Break is caused by severe, direct force, which creates a fracture with multiple fragments.
Open, or compound	Skin is broken above the fracture; open to the external environment creating the potential for infection.	Impacted	Break is caused by strong forces that drive bone fragments firmly together.
Longitudinal	Fracture extends along the length of the bone.	Pathologic	Break results from weakening of the bones by disease, as in osteoporosis or **sarcoma**.
Transverse	Break is caused by direct force applied perpendicular to a bone; fracture runs across the bone.	Nondisplaced	Bone ends remain in alignment.
Oblique	Break is caused by a twisting force with an upward thrust; fracture ends are short and run at an oblique angle across the bone.	Displaced	Bone ends are moved out of alignment.
Greenstick	Break is caused by compression or angulation forces in the long bones of children under age 10; because of its softness, the bone is cracked on one side and intact on the other side.	Spiral	Break is caused by a twisting or rotary force, which results in long, sharp, pointed bone ends; suspicious as a child abuse injury.

TABLE 36-3	Types of Fractures—*continued*		
FRACTURE	**DEFINITION**	**FRACTURE**	**DEFINITION**
Compression	Break is caused by forces that drive bones together; typically seen in the vertebrae.	Depression	Bone fragments of the skull are driven inward.
Avulsion	Break is caused by forceful contraction of a muscle against resistance, and a bone fragment tears at the site of muscle insertion.		

From Chester GA: *Modern medical assisting,* Philadelphia, 1999, Saunders.

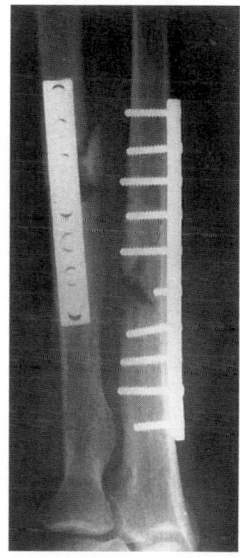

FIGURE 36-7 Orthopedic hardware from open reduction of fractures of the radius and ulna. (From Mettler MA: *Essentials of radiology,* ed 3, Philadelphia, 2004, Saunders.)

phosphorus (or both) is available for building new bone during growth or remodeling. It is caused by either a lack of vitamin D or problems with its metabolism. The skeleton gradually loses calcium, and the bones soften and become more flexible. Weight bearing gradually changes the shape of the softened bones. Symptoms can include reduced endurance, easy fatigability, **malaise,** and generalized bone tenderness and pain. Osteomalacia in children is called *rickets.*

Osteomalacia may be caused by a fat absorption problem in the gastrointestinal tract that prevents adequate absorption of dietary fats, resulting in steatorrhea and vitamin D deficiency. Vitamin D promotes the body's absorption of calcium, which is essential for normal development and maintenance of healthy teeth and bones. Vitamin D can be produced by the body with adequate sun exposure, and nearly all milk sold in the United States is fortified with

vitamin D. Osteomalacia can occur in individuals who use very strong sunscreen, have limited exposure to sunlight, experience short days of sunlight, live in a smoggy environment, or do not drink milk because of lactose intolerance. The condition is treated with vitamin D, calcium, and phosphorus supplements.

Osteoporosis

Osteoporosis is a disease in which calcium deposits in the bone gradually decline, and bones become increasingly weak and brittle so that even small stressors, such as bending over or coughing, can cause fractures. Bone strength depends on the size and density of the bone structure and the amount of calcium, phosphorus, and other materials deposited and maintained in the bone. Bones are constantly changing through a process called *remodeling,* or bone turnover. This process allows bones to grow and heal. As we age, remodeling breaks down bone more quickly than it forms new bone. Peak bone mass is reached by the middle 30s, so a person's risk of developing osteoporosis depends on the bone mass collected by age 25 to 35 and how rapidly bone tissue is lost after that. Lack of vitamin D and calcium in the diet results in a lower peak bone mass and a more rapid onset of bone loss later in life. People over age 50 are particularly at risk, and women are four times more likely to develop osteoporosis than men. Osteoporosis is a major public health threat in the United States; more than 40 million people either already have osteoporosis or are at high risk of developing it because of low bone mass.

Osteoporosis often is called a "silent" disease because the progressive loss of bone density occurs without any symptoms. Osteopenia is mild bone loss that is not severe enough to be called osteoporosis but that increases the risk of osteoporosis. By the time fractures occur, the disease is quite advanced. Patients with osteoporosis complain of back pain because of a fractured or collapsed vertebra; loss of height over time, with stooped posture (kyphosis, or "dowager's hump"); and fractures, typically of the vertebrae, wrists, and hips. Risk factors include being a postmenopausal woman over age 50; a slight build with a family history of osteoporosis; a history of amenorrhea; anorexia nervosa; a low dietary calcium intake; an excessive intake of caffeinated soda; an inactive lifestyle; smoking; alcohol abuse; hyperthyroidism; a reduced lifetime exposure to estrogen; and long-term treatment with certain medications, including antiseizure drugs, corticosteroids, and heparin. Men over age 50 with low testosterone levels also are at risk. Osteoporosis occurs in all races but is slightly more common in Caucasian and Asian individuals.

The diagnosis is made by a specialized form of x-ray evaluation that specifically measures bone density. This study allows the diagnosis of osteoporosis before a fracture occurs and thus intervention to prevent fractures. Readings are repeated annually to determine the rate of bone loss and to monitor the effectiveness of treatment. Intervention and treatment include increasing dietary intake of calcium and vitamin D; increasing weight-bearing exercise; and pharmaceutical treatment with bisphosphonates (alendronate [Fosamax], risedronate [Actonel], zoledronic acid [Reclast], and ibandronate sodium [Boniva]); in addition, hormone therapy, such as estrogen and some hormone-like medications (e.g., raloxifene [Evista]) may be prescribed to slow bone breakdown. The best screening test is a dual energy x-ray absorptiometry (DXA) scan, which measures the bone density of the spine and hip. Ultrasound of the heel can also be used to diagnose osteoporosis.

The National Osteoporosis Foundation recommends that all women have a bone density test if they are not receiving estrogen replacement therapy and are in any of the following categories:

- Undergoing long-term treatment with medications that can cause osteoporosis, such as prednisone
- Have diabetes type 1, liver disease, kidney disease, or a family history of osteoporosis
- Experienced early menopause (in the early 40s)
- Are postmenopausal, over age 50, and have at least one risk factor for osteoporosis
- Are postmenopausal, over age 65, and have never had a bone density test

CRITICAL THINKING APPLICATION   36-4

Mrs. Viola Carson, a 78-year-old patient, is being seen in the office today for follow-up after hip replacement surgery. Mrs. Carson fractured her hip from a simple fall at the grocery store. Why would the physician suspect she has osteoporosis? What treatment might be recommended to prevent further fractures in this patient?

Spinal Column Disorders
Abnormal Spinal Curvatures

When the medical assistant looks at a patient's back, the spine should be vertically straight. Any abnormal deviation or curvature to the right or left is called **scoliosis**. Mild scoliosis generally causes no problems and usually is not even noticeable. When scoliosis is severe, it can cause significant back pain and possibly heart or lung problems because of the diminished space in the thoracic cavity on one side.

When the spine is viewed from a lateral position, four normal curves are seen (Figure 36-8). The **cervical** and **lumbar** regions should have curves toward the front of the body; these are called **lordotic** curves. The normal curves in the thoracic region of the spine and the sacrum are toward the back and are called **kyphotic**

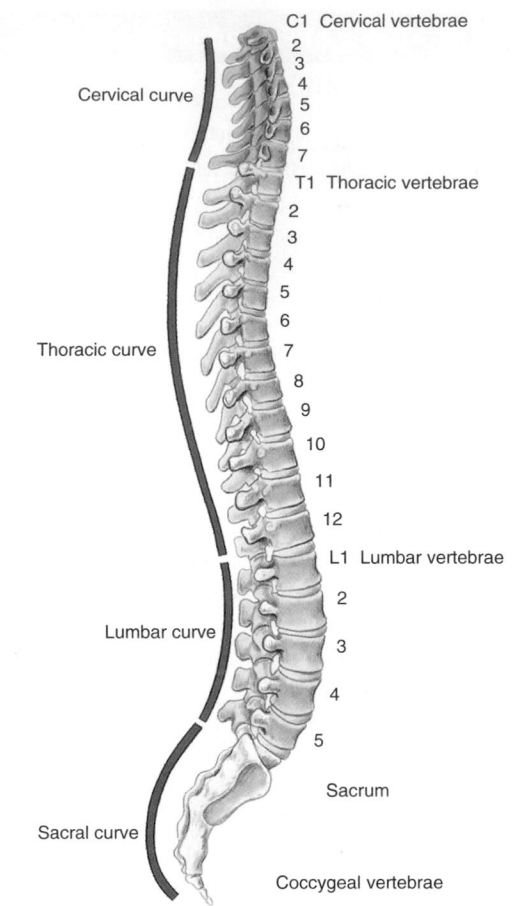

FIGURE 36-8 Normal curves of the spine. (From Applegate E: *The anatomy and physiology learning system*, ed 4, St Louis, 2011, Saunders.)

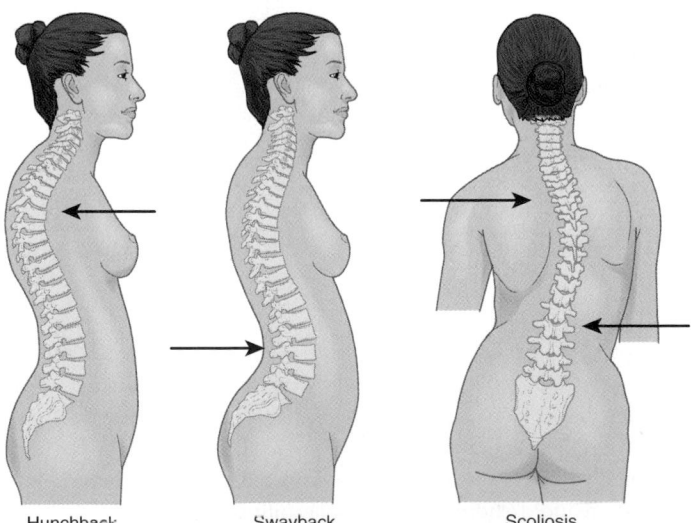

FIGURE 36-9 Spinal curve abnormalities.

curves. Loss of cervical lordosis is called *military neck*. Excessive lumbar lordosis is called *swayback*. Excessive upper thoracic kyphosis is called *hunchback* (Figure 36-9).

These conditions are diagnosed by inspection and palpation and may be confirmed with x-ray studies. Treatment may include chiropractic care, orthopedic devices (e.g., braces), shoe lifts, exercises, and electrical muscle stimulation. In severe cases, rigid casting with or without surgery may be necessary.

Herniated Disk

A herniated disk occurs when the soft nucleus of an intervertebral disk protrudes through a tear or weakened area in its tough outer cartilaginous covering (Figure 36-10). This condition occurs most often in the lumbar region of the spine, frequently in the cervical region, and rarely in the thoracic region. In children and young adults, disks have a high water content. As people age, this water content declines, and the structures begin to shrink and become less flexible. This causes the spaces between the vertebrae to narrow. Factors that can weaken intervertebral disks include improper lifting; smoking; excessive body weight that places added stress on the disks of the lower back; sudden, possibly slight pressure; and repetitive strenuous activities. Herniation may also occur gradually over time as a result of a progressive deterioration of the disks.

Symptoms depend on the location and extent of the protrusion of the nucleus beyond its normal location. If the herniation occurs in the lumbar region, it usually causes severe low back pain that can radiate down the leg and cause difficulty walking. If the herniated disk is in the cervical region, the person usually has a burning pain in the neck that can radiate down the arms to the fingers.

The diagnosis is made from a careful history; physical examination; either magnetic resonance imaging (MRI) or computed tomography (CT) scans to confirm which disk is injured; and electromyography (EMG) or nerve conduction studies (NCS), which measure nervous stimulation of affected muscles. Treatment depends on the severity of the herniation and the symptoms. Conservative treatments include rest and nonsteroidal antiinflammatory drugs (NSAIDs); analgesics for the pain; physical therapy; chiropractic adjustments; and epidural steroid injections into the exact level of the disk herniation to reduce swelling around the disk and relieve symptoms. Spinal injections are usually done in the provider's office under x-ray guidance to the injection site. If these measures are ineffective and the patient has recurring pain, numbness, and progressive weakness, surgery may be necessary.

Joint Disorders

Dislocation

Dislocation of a joint is also called a **luxation**, a condition in which two bones of a joint are no longer in approximation (Figure 36-11). A *subluxation* is an incomplete dislocation of a joint, meaning that the bones are only slightly out of proper alignment and location. It is possible to have a congenital dislocation, especially of the hip. Common dislocations occur in the finger, thumb, and shoulder and usually are caused by trauma, frequently while a person is playing sports. Symptoms include pain, swelling, loss of motion, and sometimes temporary paralysis of the affected part. A dislocation requires immediate reduction and immobilization to prevent permanent injury to nerves and major blood vessels near the joint. Occasionally, surgical reduction and repair may be necessary to stabilize the joint. Chiropractic treatments relieve subluxations.

CRITICAL THINKING APPLICATION   36-5

A patient comes into the office from her weekly softball game. After sliding into home plate, she immediately was unable to move her right arm, and she says that she has a lot of pain in her right shoulder. What steps should Kaiwan take to help this patient?

Gout

Gout, which may also be called *gouty arthritis,* is a metabolic disease involving overproduction or improper elimination of uric acid. Uric acid is a waste product formed from the breakdown of purines, which are found naturally in the body and in certain foods, including organ meats (liver, brains, and kidney), anchovies, herring, asparagus, mushrooms, and dried beans. Drinking too much alcohol is a risk factor because alcohol interferes with the removal of uric acid

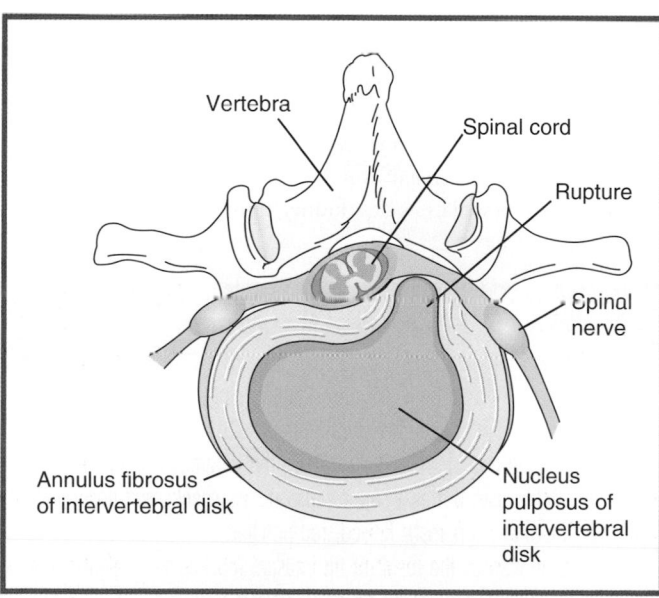

FIGURE 36-10 Herniation of a vertebral disk.

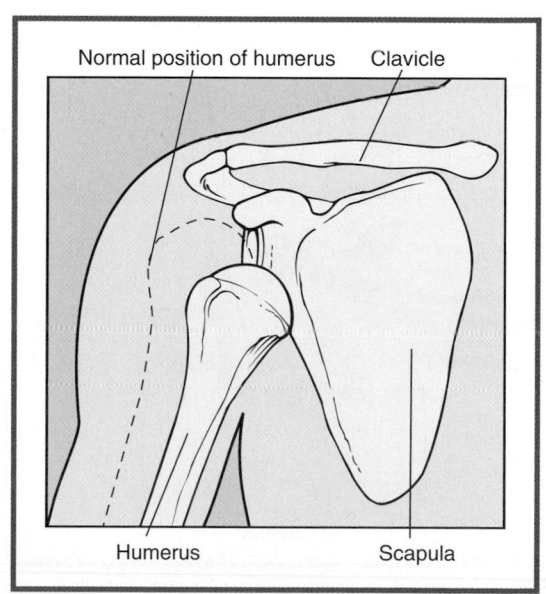

FIGURE 36-11 Luxation (dislocation) of the shoulder. (From Frazier MS, Drzymkowski JW: *Essentials of human diseases and conditions,* ed 3, Philadelphia, 2004, Saunders.)

from the body. Uric acid should dissolve in the blood so that it can be excreted as it passes through the kidneys. However, with gout, uric acid is not effectively excreted, and needle-like crystals of uric acid collect in the synovial fluid of the affected joint, causing extreme sensitivity to touch, pronounced inflammation, and severe pain. The most frequently affected area is the great toe (Figure 36-12). Risk factors include kidney disease, consumption of alcohol, obesity, untreated hypertension, and a family history of the disease. Men are more likely to experience gout than women, but women become increasingly susceptible to gout after menopause.

In general, keeping uric acid levels within a normal range is the key to preventing future episodes of gout. Therefore, long-range treatment includes dietary modifications to eliminate foods containing purine. To treat an acute onset, the patient may take NSAIDs (e.g., ibuprofen and naproxen [Aleve]) for pain and joint inflammation. In severe cases the provider may prescribe prednisone. Pharmaceutical treatment may begin with colchicine (Colcrys), an antiinflammatory medication that is most effective if taken within 12 hours of an attack, to help prevent the buildup of uric acid crystals in the joints. To reduce the risk or lessen the severity of episodes, treatment includes allopurinol (Lopurin, Zyloprim), which slows uric acid production and helps dissolve crystals, and probenecid (Probalan), to increase uric acid excretion through the kidneys.

Lupus

The three main types of lupus are systemic lupus erythematosus (SLE), discoid lupus erythematosus, and drug-induced lupus. Of these, SLE is the most common and serious form of the disease. SLE is an autoimmune disease of unknown cause. It occurs primarily in women 20 to 50 years of age, although it can occur in both younger and older individuals. Other risk factors include recurrent infections caused by the Epstein-Barr virus, a family history of the disease, and African-American race.

SLE is difficult to diagnose and entirely unpredictable. The patient develops autoantibodies (antibodies to self) that can attack any tissue or organ in the body; this may result in severe inflammation with tissue changes and destruction. According to the National Institutes of Health (NIH), the common symptoms of lupus include:

- Painful or swollen joints and muscle pain
- Unexplained fever
- Red rashes, most commonly on the face
- Chest pain upon deep breathing
- Unusual loss of hair
- Pale or purple fingers or toes from cold or stress (Raynaud's phenomenon)
- Sensitivity to the sun
- Edema in the legs or around the eyes
- Mouth ulcers
- Swollen glands
- Extreme fatigue

The progression and severity of the disease vary widely among patients. Furthermore, problems associated with SLE change over time and overlap with those of many other disorders. For these reasons, providers may not initially consider lupus until the signs and symptoms become more obvious. At times the disease may become severe, and at other times it may subside completely.

There is no known cure for lupus; the therapeutic goal is to maintain patient function as much as possible. The type of pharmaceutical treatment prescribed depends on which parts of the body are affected by the disease and the severity of the symptoms. Some medications used to treat SLE include NSAIDs (e.g., naproxen and ibuprofen) to reduce joint pain and inflammation; antimalarials (e.g., hydroxychloroquine [Plaquenil]) to treat skin and joint problems and the ulcers that some people develop in the mouth or nose; **corticosteroids** (prednisone) during acute inflammatory processes; and immunosuppressive medications (e.g., azathioprine [Imuran] and cyclophosphamide [Cytoxan]) to suppress the immune system. Belimumab (Benlysta), which is administered intravenously (IV), may be prescribed for patients receiving other standard lupus medications. The kidneys may fail even with treatment, which may necessitate either kidney dialysis or a kidney transplant.

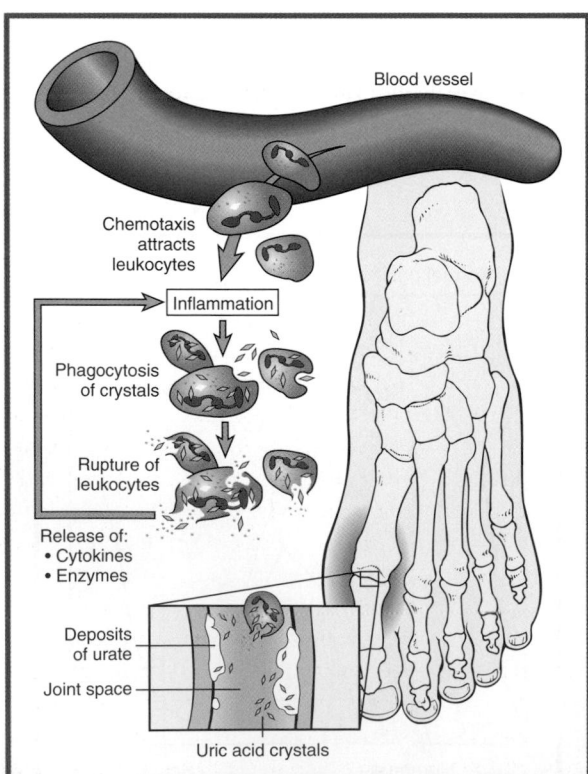

FIGURE 36-12 Gout is characterized by deposits of uric acid crystals in the connective tissue. The inflammation most often affects the joint of the big toe. (From Damjanov I: *Pathology for the health-related professions,* ed 4, St Louis, 2012, Saunders.)

Criteria for Diagnosing Systemic Lupus Erythematosus

Providers use the American College of Rheumatology's 11 criteria of lupus to help diagnose systemic lupus erythematosus (SLE). Four or more of the following criteria must be present to make the diagnosis.

1. Malar rash: Butterfly-shaped rash across cheeks and nose
2. Discoid (skin) rash: Raised, red patches
3. Skin rash as the result of an unusual reaction to sunlight
4. Mouth or nose ulcers: Usually painless

5. Arthritis of two or more joints without bone destruction
6. Inflammation of the lining around the heart (pericarditis) and/or lungs (pleuritis)
7. Neurologic disorder: Seizures and/or psychosis
8. Renal (kidney) disorder: Excessive protein in the urine
9. Hematologic (blood) disorder: Hemolytic anemia or low platelet and white blood cell (WBC) counts
10. Immunologic disorder: Presence of unusual antibodies
11. Elevated antinuclear antibodies: Indicates an autoimmune disease

Lupus Research Institute. http://lupusresearchinstitute.org/lupus-facts/lupus-diagnosis. Accessed January 15, 2015.

Infectious Arthritis

Infectious arthritis usually occurs after some type of systemic or local infection in some other part of the body or after a joint has been exposed to a pathogen by trauma or surgery. The infection can be caused by bacteria, fungi, or viruses. The joint usually shows signs of severe inflammation and significantly reduced ROM. To determine the diagnosis, the provider may order an x-ray evaluation and bone scan and may withdraw synovial fluid for microscopic examination and culture. The goals of treatment are to reduce inflammation, increase ROM, and treat the causative organism with the appropriate medication.

Lyme Disease

Lyme disease is an infection caused by the *Borrelia burgdorferi* and the *Borrelia mayonii* bacteria. It is transmitted to humans by a bite from ticks of the Ixodes family. The disease is named after Lyme, Connecticut, where it was first identified in 1975 in a cluster of children who showed signs of what was thought to be rheumatoid arthritis. Eventually epidemiologists traced the cause of the problem to a bacterial infection. Signs and symptoms may include a "bull's-eye" lesion, called *erythema migrans*, surrounding the area of the tick bite; this lesion can appear within a few days or up to a month after exposure. The rash can last several days to several weeks and occurs in as many as 80% of people infected with Lyme disease. Additional indicators of the disease include flulike symptoms, such as fever, chills, fatigue, body aches, and headache. If the infection remains untreated, the patient can develop arthritic pain in the large joints (e.g., the knees); meningitis; Bell's palsy; numbness or weakness of the limbs; memory loss and difficulty concentrating; and changes in mood or sleep habits.

The diagnosis is made by taking a careful history, including the patient's level of outdoor exposure, locating the tick bite, and ruling out other causes for presenting symptoms. Laboratory blood tests to identify antibodies to the bacterium are used to help confirm the diagnosis. These tests are most reliable a few weeks after an infection because it takes some time for antibodies to develop. The Centers for Disease Control and Prevention (CDC) currently recommends a two-step process using the same blood sample. An enzyme immunoassay (EIA) is done. If the result is negative, Lyme disease is ruled out. If the result is positive, an immunoblot test (e.g., the Western blot test) is done next to confirm the diagnosis. Antibiotics, such as doxycycline (Doryx, Monodox) and amoxicillin (Amoxil), are the standard treatment for Lyme disease in its early stages. If the disease has progressed to a later stage, the patient may be hospitalized for treatment with IV ceftriaxone (Rocephin).

Patient Education for Preventing Lyme Disease

- Wear pants tucked into socks and long-sleeved shirts when walking in wooded or grassy areas.
- Use insect repellents that contain 20% to 30% diethyltoluamide (DEET).
- Tick-proof your yard by clearing brush and leaves, where ticks live.
- Check yourself, your children, and your pets for ticks; deer ticks are no bigger than the head of a pin or a grain of pepper; shower immediately after returning from wooded areas because ticks can remain on the skin for hours before attaching themselves.
- Do not assume you are immune; Lyme disease can occur in the same person more than once.
- Use fine-tipped tweezers to remove a tick. Grasp the tick as close to the skin's surface as possible; pull upward with steady, even pressure; thoroughly clean the bite area and your hands with rubbing alcohol, an iodine scrub, or soap and water; dispose of a live tick by submerging it in alcohol, placing it in a sealed bag/container, wrapping it tightly in tape, or flushing it down the toilet. Never crush a tick with your fingers.
- If you develop a rash or fever within several weeks of removing a tick, see your healthcare provider. Be sure to tell him or her about your recent tick bite and when the bite occurred.

Centers for Disease Control and Prevention (CDC). www.cdc.gov/lyme/. Accessed January 15, 2015.

Osteoarthritis

OA, also called *degenerative joint disease* (DJD), is marked by significant thinning and degeneration of the articular cartilage of synovial joints. The symptoms range from mild to severe, depending on the amount of degeneration. As the articular cartilage disintegrates and wears away, the roughened surface of the bone is exposed, leaving bone rubbing against bone, with resultant pain and stiffness of the involved joint. Commonly involved joints include the fingers, the spine, and the weight-bearing joints of the hips, knees, and feet. Diagnosis frequently includes x-ray films and an MRI, which show degenerative changes in the joint surfaces and uneven joint space narrowing.

Treatment goals include relieving pain, maintaining normal motion in the joint, and attempting to prevent crippling deformities. Exercise and weight control are important components of treatment to keep the joints mobile and prevent additional wear and tear on joint tissues. Medications may include analgesics, NSAIDs, and intra-articular steroid injections. Using a walker or cane may be helpful for maintaining mobility. Severe cases require surgery to remove the affected joint and replace it with a joint **prosthesis.**

Rheumatoid Arthritis

RA is an autoimmune inflammatory condition that involves an immune system response to the synovial membranes, causing synovitis. Proteins are released at the site of the joint inflammation, eventually resulting in thickening of the synovium and damage to the cartilage, bone, tendons, and ligaments of the affected joint. Gradually the joint loses its shape and alignment, causing deformity and pain. Scientists still do not know exactly what causes the immune system to turn against the body's own tissues in RA, but research indicates it is a combination of factors, including genetic predisposition, environmental factors, and hormone interactions, because most individuals with RA are female.

Early symptoms include malaise, fever, weight loss, and morning stiffness of the affected joints. RA typically occurs in a symmetric pattern, meaning that if one knee or hand is involved, the other one also is. The disease often affects the wrist and finger joints. Usually, bouts of arthritis increase in frequency and severity over time. As this occurs, the joints become damaged, and joint swelling and deformity occur. The patient ultimately loses the ability to move the affected joints, and a pronounced loss of strength occurs in the muscles attached to the inflamed joints. Small lumps, called *rheumatoid nodules,* may form at pressure points in the elbows, hands, feet, Achilles tendons, knees, and posterior scalp, and even in the lungs. Patients with RA may appear undernourished and chronically ill because of the formation of degenerative lesions in the collagen (connective tissues) in the lungs, heart, blood vessels, and pleura (Figure 36-13). Periods of increased disease activity, called *flare-ups,* alternate with periods of relative remission, during which the swelling, pain, difficulty sleeping, and weakness fade or disappear. X-ray findings show uniform joint space narrowing, which is different from the degenerative changes seen in OA.

Rest and exercise seem to be the key elements in treating RA. Therapeutic exercises are designed to prevent and correct deformities, control pain, strengthen weakened muscles, and improve joint function. The most frequently prescribed medications are NSAIDs, including aspirin (acetylsalicylic acid), indomethacin (Indocin), diclofenac (Voltaren), naproxen (Naprosyn), and ibuprofen (Motrin). Corticosteroids (prednisone and Medrol) may be prescribed for severe flare-ups. To limit the extent of joint damage early in the disease, the provider prescribes disease-modifying antirheumatic drugs (DMARDs), including methotrexate (Rheumatrex), leflunomide (Arava), hydroxychloroquine (Plaquenil), and sulfasalazine (Azulfidine). Biologics used include etanercept (Enbrel), infliximab (Remicade), and adalimumab (Humira). In severe cases, surgical joint replacement may be necessary.

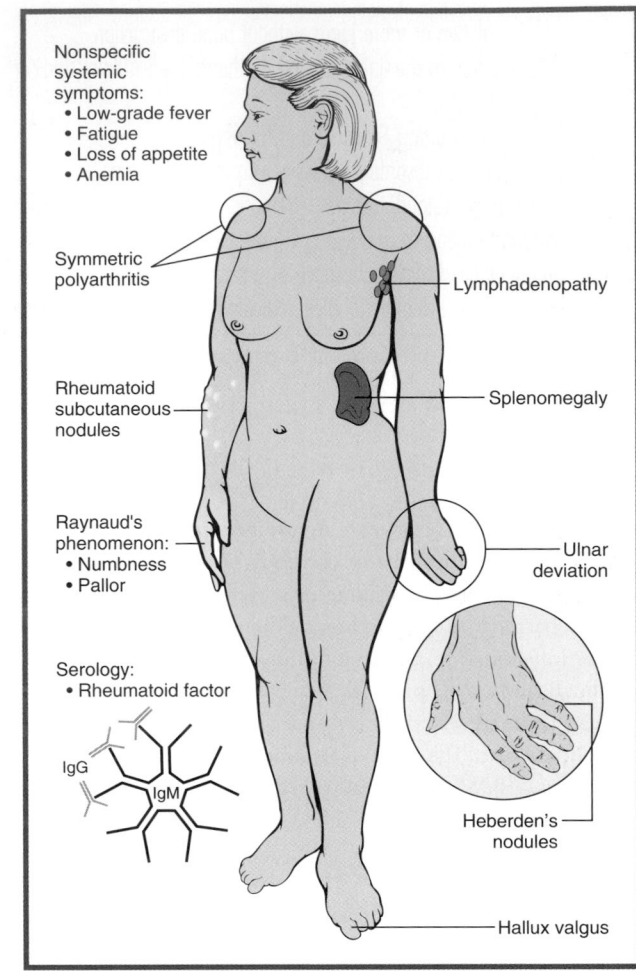

FIGURE 36-13 Signs and symptoms of rheumatoid arthritis. (From Damjanov I: *Pathology for the health-related professions,* ed 4, St Louis, 2012, Saunders.)

CRITICAL THINKING APPLICATION   **36-6**

An 80-year-old male patient with arthritis comes into the office complaining of severe pain in his knees, hips, and lower back. The pain makes it impossible for him to get up onto the examination table. What should Kaiwan do? Is this patient required to get onto the examination table? Why or why not?

Tendonitis and Bursitis

Tendonitis is one of the most common causes of pain in the shoulder and elbow. Inflammation of tendons may be associated with calcium deposits in the bursae around the joint, causing concurrent bursitis. The diagnosis is made if the patient has increased severity of pain when abducting the arm beyond 50 degrees. Treatment includes pain relief and reducing the localized inflammation to make exercise possible and to prevent shoulder immobility, called *frozen shoulder.* Medications might include analgesics, NSAIDs, and injections of long-acting corticosteroids. Cold applications are helpful in relieving pain; heat applications are contraindicated because they tend to aggravate calcium tendonitis.

Bursitis is a painful inflammation of a joint bursa that most commonly follows repetitive movement or prolonged pressure on a joint. The pain is increased with movement of the affected joint. It also can occur from staphylococcal or tubercular infections and with some joint diseases, such as gout and arthritis. Treatment includes preventing the activity that caused the bursitis and protecting the affected site from excessive pressure and movement. NSAIDs may provide pain relief, but corticosteroid antiinflammatories may be needed in severe cases.

Carpal Tunnel Syndrome

As mentioned, the carpal tunnel is a narrow opening in the bones at the base of the hand; this is where the median nerve passes to send nervous stimuli to the hand. Sometimes the passageway becomes narrowed because of inflammation and swelling of the tendons in the area; the result is compression of the nerve, which in turn produces pain, weakness, or numbness in the hand and wrist, radiating up the arm. Symptoms usually start gradually, with frequent burning, tingling, or itching numbness in the palm of the hand and the fingers, especially the thumb and the index and middle fingers. Symptoms are worse in the morning because many people sleep with flexed wrists. As symptoms progress, the individual experiences decreased grip strength, difficulty making a fist and grasping small objects, and problems with fine motor movements.

Carpal tunnel syndrome results from a combination of factors that increase pressure on the median nerve and tendons in the carpal tunnel. Research indicates it may be due to a congenital narrowing of the carpal tunnel area. Contributing factors include trauma or injury to the wrist that cause swelling; hypothyroidism; rheumatoid arthritis; work stress; repeated use of vibrating hand tools; fluid retention during pregnancy or menopause; or the development of a cyst or tumor in the canal. Although carpal tunnel syndrome has long been blamed on repetitive movements of the hand and wrist, there are very limited data to support this belief.

A complete physical examination and routine lab tests to rule out diabetes, arthritis, and fractures are done initially to determine the cause of the discomfort. Diagnostic examinations include the Tinel test, in which pressure on the median nerve in the wrist causes tingling in the fingers or a shocklike sensation in the hand. Another test done during the physical examination is the Phalen, or wrist-flexion, test, in which the patient holds the forearms upright while pointing the fingers down and pressing the backs of the hands together; a positive result is when tingling or increased numbness is felt in the fingers within 1 minute. To confirm the diagnosis the provider typically orders an electrodiagnostic test. In a nerve conduction study, electrodes are placed on the hand and wrist and small electric shocks are applied while a technician measures the speed of the nervous impulses to the area. For electromyography, a fine needle is inserted into a muscle and the patient is asked to contract his or her muscles by moving a small amount. The electrical activity of the muscle is viewed on a screen and can determine the severity of damage to the median nerve. Ultrasounds can also show an impaired median nerve.

Initial treatment recommendations are to rest the hand and wrist for at least 2 weeks, avoiding activities that may worsen symptoms, and immobilize the wrist in a splint to avoid further damage. Patients are told to wear the splint to bed each night to prevent pressure on the median nerve while sleeping. Cool packs to the wrist can help reduce inflammation and swelling in the carpal tunnel area. Treatment includes over-the-counter NSAIDs; diuretics to reduce swelling and fluid accumulation at the site; or corticosteroid injections directly into the wrist or taken orally to provide immediate, temporary relief of symptoms. Once symptoms have been relieved, physical therapy to promote stretching and strengthening can be helpful. Surgery is recommended if symptoms last for 6 months. This is a simple endoscopic procedure in which the carpal ligament is cut and the tunnel area is enlarged. The procedure is generally done with an **endoscope**, using local anesthesia, on an outpatient basis.

THE MEDICAL ASSISTANT'S ROLE IN ASSISTING WITH ORTHOPEDIC PROCEDURES

The role of the medical assistant begins with accurately recording the patient's description of the circumstances surrounding the onset of the problem, what measures were taken to alleviate the problem, and the patient's current concerns. Record the exact anatomic location of the pain and ask the patient to quantify its intensity on a scale of 1 to 10; also ask about both OTC and prescription medications taken, including the names of drugs, the dosage and frequency, the date and time of the last dose, and whether the drug has been helpful in relieving symptoms.

Offer assistance when escorting the patient to the examination room. Use a wheelchair, if necessary. Assist the patient into a comfortable position in the examination room by offering a pillow or folded blanket to support the painful or injured body part. The patient may have limited mobility because of pain, so you may need to provide assistance with disrobing and getting into an examination gown. Make sure the patient is warm enough by offering an additional sheet or blanket. Explain clearly what is happening and what the patient can expect. Notify the provider as soon as the patient is ready for the examination.

Assisting With the Examination

The provider may use inspection, palpation, ROM testing, and muscle testing to examine the major skeletal muscles and joints. Much of the examination involves comparing muscles and joints on the affected side with those on the contralateral side for size, position, and strength. When the patient needs to assume a certain position, demonstrating the position or movement desired may be helpful. Watch the patient during the manipulative and palpatory portion of the examination for a facial grimace or physical jerk or jump, which may indicate pain.

As a general rule, the unaffected side is examined first, then the affected side, and the two are compared. You may be responsible for taking notes during the examination. Keep the patient properly draped and assist the provider by handing equipment as needed. Most examinations require the use of a measuring tape, goniometer, blood pressure cuff, and stethoscope. Be alert and ready to prevent the patient from falling during the examination because some of the requested movements and positions may place the injured patient off balance.

The provider performs a gait analysis by watching the patient walk in a straight line, with or without the patient knowing he or she is being observed. In addition to being associated with disorders of the musculoskeletal system, gait abnormalities may be caused by an associated neurologic condition.

SPECIALIZED DIAGNOSTIC PROCEDURES IN ORTHOPEDICS

Range-of-Motion Evaluation

Often orthopedic injuries severely affect the normal ROM of a joint. Measuring the ROM of specific joints is an objective measure of both the seriousness of an injury and the recovery progress. When the ROM of a particular joint is evaluated, usually both active and passive ROM results are measured and recorded.

The joint movement in a single plane is measured with a **goniometer**. A goniometer has two arms that are fixed together with a hinge joint at one end (Figure 36-14). Each of the arms is lined up with a bone on each side of the joint being tested. The degrees of motion are indicated on a scale on the hinged center of the instrument. To determine the active ROM of a joint, the patient is asked to move the joint as far as possible. For evaluation of passive ROM, the patient is asked to relax, and the provider moves the joint as far as possible. All ROMs are measured in degrees. During these examinations, you may be asked to record the degrees of motion for active and/or passive ROM for specific joints and to note any pain, tenderness, or **crepitation** during the examination.

CRITICAL THINKING APPLICATION   **36-7**

How can Kaiwan best assist Dr. Alexander in testing upper extremity ROM in a new patient? What equipment should Kaiwan have ready? What patient position would best facilitate this examination? Why?

Muscle Strength Evaluation

During the ROM evaluation, the provider also assesses each muscle group for strength. Normal muscle strength allows for complete voluntary ROM despite resistance. This resistance can be gravity, as when rising from sitting to a standing position, or physical, as in pulling, pushing, or lifting an object. Muscle strength is bilaterally equal in normal conditions. The evaluation compares like muscles in each hemisphere of the body, such as using a blood pressure cuff to compare the grip of the right hand with the grip of the left hand (Figure 36-15).

Using a Blood Pressure Cuff to Assess Grip Strength

1. Roll up an aneroid blood pressure cuff and have the patient hold it in one hand.
2. Inflate the cuff to 20 mm Hg of pressure and lock the valve.
3. Ask the patient to squeeze the cuff as tightly as possible.
4. Note the increase in pressure on the dial (a normal grip registers above 150 mm Hg).
5. Record the hand tested and the results of the test.
6. Repeat on the other hand.

RADIOLOGY

Radiology and diagnostic imaging frequently are used to help diagnose orthopedic conditions (Figure 36-16). X-ray evaluation is necessary to diagnose fractures, dislocations, and bone and joint diseases accurately. X-ray films also can be used to track the healing of a fracture.

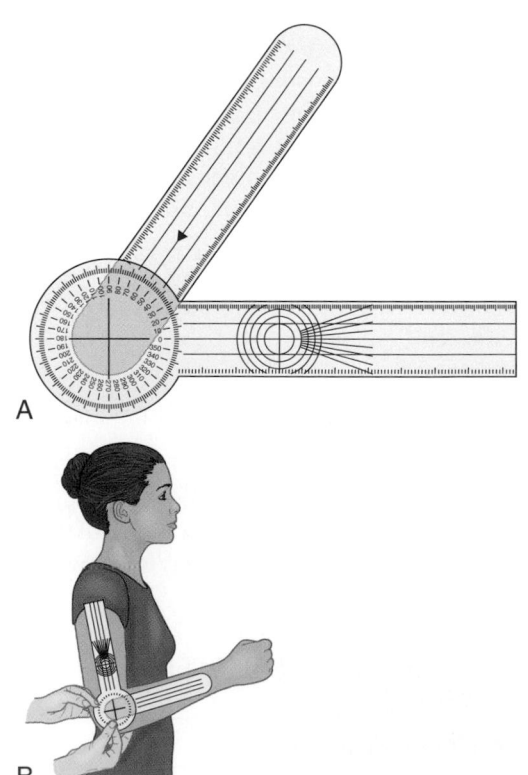

FIGURE 36-14 A, Goniometer. **B,** Correct position of the goniometer on the arm.

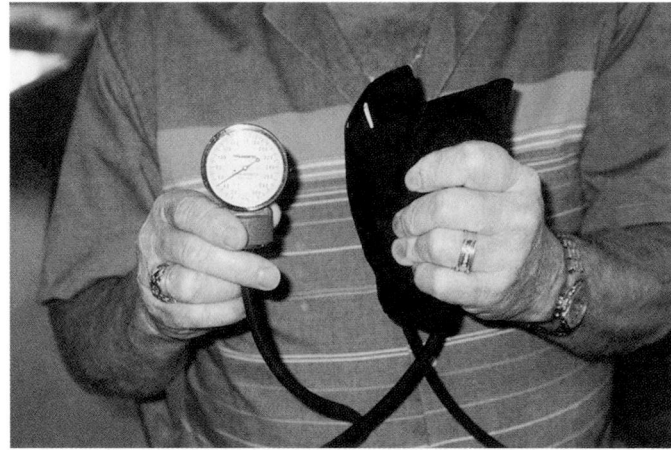

FIGURE 36-15 Assessing grip strength using a blood pressure cuff.

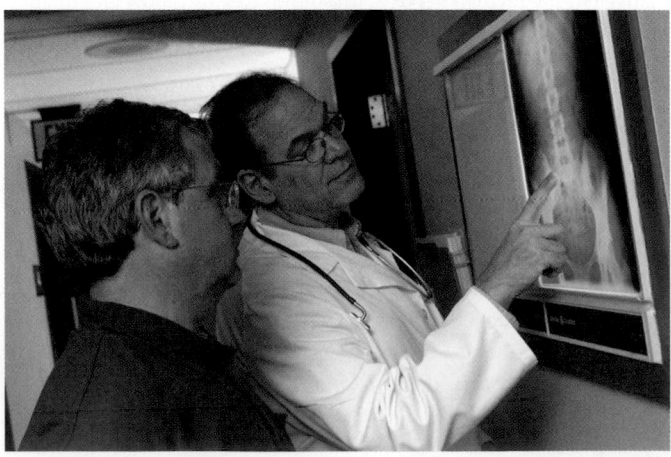

FIGURE 36-16 Reading a lumbar radiograph.

When a diagnostic test is necessary, you should explain the procedure to the patient. Your explanation should include what will be done, how it is done, where it will take place, and approximately how long it will take. Patients always are concerned about whether the procedure will hurt. Tell the truth. If the procedure is painful, let the patient know so that he or she can prepare for it. Discuss the procedure in a professional yet empathetic manner. If the patient wants to talk with the provider about the test, make sure this happens.

Specialized Imaging Techniques Used in Orthopedics

- Arthrogram—Visualizes the joints with an x-ray after the injection of a radiopaque dye.
- Bone scan—Evaluates areas of bone growth, bone tumors, and other bone disease patterns; requires the use of an injected dye or isotope.
- Dual energy x-ray absorptiometry (DEXA or DXA) scan—Specialized x-ray that assesses bone density; used to diagnose and manage osteoporosis.
- Computed tomography (CT) scan—Visualizes multiple planes of soft tissue such as tumors, lesions, or some spinal injuries; usually used with an injected dye.

- Electromyography (EMG) and nerve conduction velocity (NCV) studies—Evaluate muscle and nerve response to stimulus.
- Biopsy of bone and muscle—Tissue is examined by a pathologist to identify cancerous tumors, neoplasms, and pathogens.

THERAPEUTIC MODALITIES

Physical treatment methods called *modalities* often are used in orthopedic, chiropractic, and physical therapy offices to treat orthopedic conditions. These can include the application of cold, heat, baths, electric currents, therapeutic ultrasonography, massage, and therapeutic exercises. Cold applications are recommended for the first 48 hours after an injury to help control pain and swelling. Heat application is used after this to help improve circulation, reduce pain, and maintain muscle and joint function (Table 36-4). *Diathermy* is a technique for creating deep tissue heat through the use of a high-frequency current, ultrasonic waves, or microwave radiation. Deep heat is used to reduce pain, relieve muscle spasms, resolve inflammation, and promote healing. Deep heat may be used to treat chronic arthritis, bursitis, fractures, and other musculoskeletal problems.

General Principles of Cold Application

Cold applications, such as ice packs and cold compresses, act as vasoconstrictors and also cause contraction of the involuntary muscles of the skin ("goose bumps"). These two actions reduce the blood supply to the area and exert a numbing effect on the sensory nerve endings. Cold applications can help control bleeding, prevent further swelling and inflammation, and reduce pain. Disposable, reusable, or homemade ice packs most commonly are used for cold application (Procedure 36-1).

TABLE 36-4	Effects of Heat and Cold Application		
APPLICATION	**CAUSES**	**TISSUE RESPONSE**	**THERAPEUTIC EFFECT**
Heat	Vasodilation, muscle relaxation, increased metabolism, local warmth	Increased blood flow, more white blood cells to area, reduced muscle spasm, decreased pain	• Increased nutrients to site • Faster removal of wastes • Phagocytosis • Faster tissue repair
Cold	Vasoconstriction, numbness of nerve endings, reduced metabolism, increased blood viscosity	Reduced blood flow, local anesthesia, reduced oxygen need, faster blood clotting	• Inhibition of swelling • Reduced inflammation • Reduced pain

PROCEDURE 36-1   Assist the Provider with Patient Care: Assist with Cold Application

Goal: *To apply a cold compress to a body area to reduce pain, prevent further swelling, and/or reduce inflammation.*

EQUIPMENT and SUPPLIES

- Patient's health record
- Small ice cubes or ice chips (at home, patient can use frozen bag of peas or corn)
- Ice bag or closeable disposable plastic kitchen food bag
- 2-3 Towels

PROCEDURAL STEPS

1. Sanitize your hands.
2. Greet the patient, introduce yourself and verify the patient's identity by name and date of birth, and explain the procedure. Answer any questions.
3. Check the ice bag for leaks.
4. Fill the bag with small cubes or chips of ice until it is about two thirds full.
   PURPOSE: Small chips conform more easily to the shape of the body.
5. Push down on the top of the bag to expel excess air and put on the cap or seal the plastic bag.
   PURPOSE: To remove as much air as possible from the bag because air is a poor conductor of cold.

6. Dry the outside of the bag and cover it with one or two towel layers.
7. Help the patient position the ice bag on the injured area.
8. Advise the patient to leave the ice bag in place for about 20 to 30 minutes or until the area feels numb, whichever comes first.
   PURPOSE: Leaving the ice in place for longer than 20 to 30 minutes may cause tissue damage.
9. After removing the ice pack, check the skin for color, feeling, and pain.
   PURPOSE: If the treated area becomes very painful, remains numb, or is pale or cyanotic, the ice bag should be removed and the provider notified.
10. Dispose of ice pack and towels; if supplies are not disposable follow manufacturer recommendations on sanitizing the bag and place towels in facility laundry. Sanitize your hands.
11. Record the procedure in the patient's health record.
    PURPOSE: A procedure is not considered done until it is recorded.

8/27/20—1:45 PM: Ice pack applied to Ⓡ knee for 20 min. No c/o discomfort. Pt instructed to continue ice application at home for 20-30 min q 3 hr while awake for 24 hr as ordered by Dr. Alexander. Call provider if edema persists or pain increases. K. Tillman, CMA (AAMA)

Heat Modalities

Heat produces local vasodilation, which increases circulation. This accelerates the inflammatory process, promotes local drainage, reduces swelling, relaxes muscles, and repairs tissues and cells. The effects of external heat application depend on the type of heat used, the length of time it is applied, the frequency with which it is applied, the patient's general condition, and the size of the area treated. Heat application is an excellent therapeutic modality, but it must be used with caution to prevent overheating and burning of surface tissues. Special care must be taken in patients who have reduced sensation because they may not sense a burn occurring. Therefore, heat application is contraindicated in the following circumstances:

- With acute inflammatory conditions, particularly during the first 48 hours; heat will increase swelling if applied immediately after the injury
- In individuals with severe circulatory problems of any kind
- In those with diminished or abnormal sensation
- Over areas with encapsulated pus
- On blisters from previous burns
- Over scar tissue, which does not have a normal blood supply and easily overheats
- Over the abdomen in a pregnant woman
- Over inflamed skin because the initial erythema caused by a burn cannot be detected
- Over any metal jewelry or any area with metal implants

Body parts may safely be heated to 110°F (44°C) without any tissue damage. Redness appears, because the skin capillaries become congested at the skin's surface. Heat modalities may be either wet or dry and can have either superficial or deep effects. Dry heat therapies include heating pads, infrared radiation lamps, ultraviolet radiation, and hot-water bottles. More penetrating methods of dry heat application include diathermy and ultrasound. Moist heat modalities (Procedure 36-2) include soaks, whirlpool treatments, hot moist compresses (Figure 36-17), and paraffin baths.

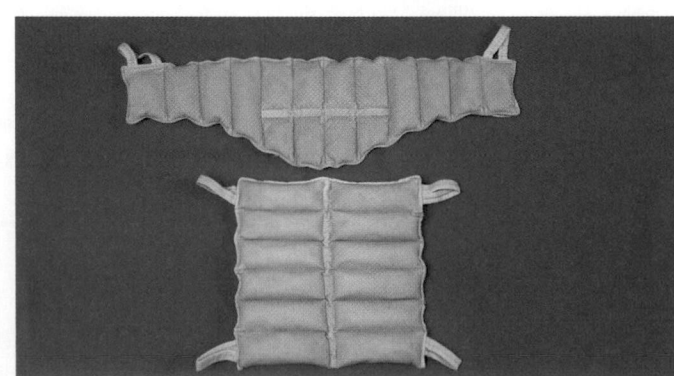

FIGURE 36-17 Commercial hot packs made of canvas containing a silicone gel.

PROCEDURE 36-2 | Assist the Provider with Patient Care: Assist with Moist Heat Application

Goal: *To apply moist heat to a body area to increase circulation, increase metabolism, and relax muscles.*

EQUIPMENT and SUPPLIES

- Patient's health record
- Commercial hot moist heat packs
- 2-3 Towels

PROCEDURAL STEPS

1. Sanitize your hands.
2. Greet the patient, introduce yourself and verify the patient's identity by name and date of birth, and explain the procedure. Answer any questions.
3. Ask the patient to remove all jewelry from the area to be treated.
   PURPOSE: To prevent trauma to the area and the collection of heat at the jewelry site.
4. Place one or two towel layers over the area to be treated.
   PURPOSE: To prevent trauma and a burn in the area.
5. Apply the commercial moist heat packs (Figure 1).
6. Cover with a towel.
7. Advise the patient to leave the heat pack in place no longer than 20 to 30 minutes, off for the same amount of time, and then repeat if needed.
   CAUTION: Monitor the patient for complaints of discomfort or signs of a burn, including erythema and blister formation.

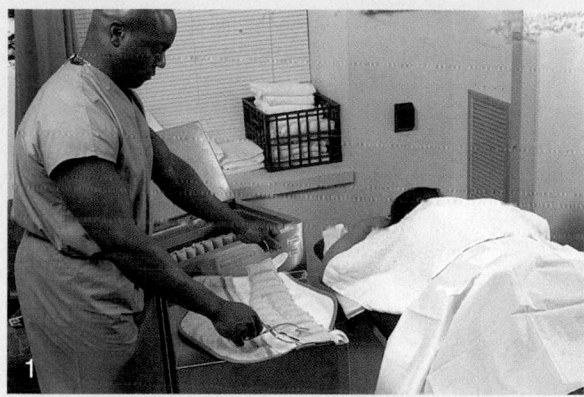

8. Record the procedure in the patient's health record.
   PURPOSE: A procedure is not considered done until it is recorded.

9/2/20–8:35 AM: Commercial moist heat pack applied to cervical/thoracic region as ordered by Dr. Alexander for 20 min. Pt states muscle cramps relieved. Instructed to continue moist heat packs at home q 2 hr for 20 min for relief of muscular pain. Cautioned pt about danger of accidental burn to the area. To return to office 9/6/20 for F/U. K. Tillman, CMA (AAMA)

Paraffin Bath

A paraffin bath is especially useful for treating chronic joint inflammation. A mixture of 7 parts paraffin and 1 part mineral oil is melted and heated to approximately 125° F (52° C). The body part (usually a hand, an elbow, or a foot) is dipped into the warm paraffin mixture and removed immediately, leaving a thin coating on the skin. This dipping is repeated six to 12 times, until a thick coating of paraffin remains on the body part (Figure 36-18). The part then is wrapped with plastic and a towel to allow the heat to penetrate the tissues. The paraffin is kept on for 30 minutes and then is peeled off. The process leaves the skin soft, warm, moisturized, and pliable, with slight erythema. The treatment provides relief from aching joints, especially for patients with rheumatoid arthritis.

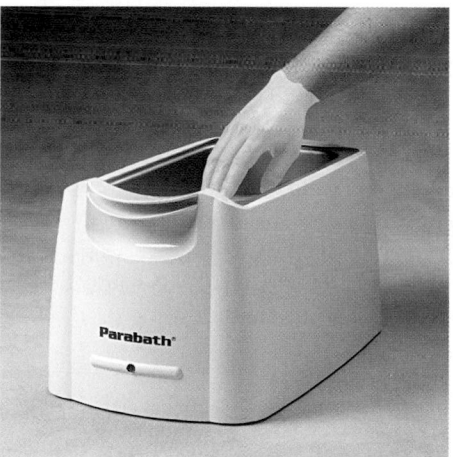

FIGURE 36-18 A paraffin bath is especially helpful for relieving pain in patients with arthritis. The hand is dipped in warm paraffin, which is left on for about 30 minutes and then peeled off.

CRITICAL THINKING APPLICATION   36-9

Kaiwan is helping a 56-year-old patient with RA who is receiving a paraffin bath treatment for both hands. He did not check the temperature before having the patient put her hands in the bath, and when she puts her hands in, she immediately pulls them out and complains that it is too hot. How should Kaiwan handle this situation? What should he say to the patient? What steps should he take to prevent this from occurring with another patient?

Heating Pads

Electric heating pads are often used at home without any concern for correct technique. People consider an electric heating pad a safe household product that is often used to treat sore muscles or joints; however, it can be dangerous for patients with decreased temperature sensation, diabetes, spinal cord injuries, patients who have suffered a stroke, patients taking medication for pain or sleep or those who have consumed alcohol. Prolonged use on one area of the body can cause a severe burn, even when the heating pad is at a low temperature setting. The FDA recommends the following precautions to avoid possible injury when using electric heating pads:

- Inspect the heating pad before each use; throw it away if it looks worn or cracked or if the electrical cord is frayed.
- Keep the removable cover on the pad during use.
- Place the heating pad on top of the body part in need of heat (do not lie or sit on the pad because the temperature increases if heat is trapped).
- Unplug the heating pad when not in use.
- Read and follow all manufacturer's instructions.
- Never use a heating pad on an infant; on a person who is unable to feel the temperature of the pad (e.g., after a stroke); on a sleeping or unconscious person; or near an oxygen tank.
- Electric heating pads should be left in place no longer than 30 minutes.

Therapeutic Ultrasonography

Ultrasound is the energy carried by very-high-frequency sound waves. Audible sounds are the result of sound waves vibrating from 100 to 12,000 hertz (Hz; cycles per second). Ultrasonic waves vibrate at a rate of up to 1 million Hz and cannot be heard by the human ear. The ultrasound transducer contains a quartz crystal that vibrates very rapidly when an electric current is passed through it. It is placed in contact with the body, and the vibrations are passed into the tissues. Because these waves do not travel through air, complete contact with the body must be maintained during treatment by using a coupling agent (a water-soluble gel) between the ultrasound transducer and the skin.

The ultrasound waves cause the tissue to vibrate, generating heat as they penetrate superficial tissues and speeding up circulation to the area. This increases the metabolism in the local area, which has a beneficial effect on the body's healing process. Because ultrasound waves travel best through water, they penetrate deeper into body tissues with high water content, such as muscles. Ultrasonography may reduce pain and increase the rate of collagen synthesis, which promotes healing. It is often used to improve wound healing and relieve the swelling and edema associated with soft tissue injuries. Bone tissue contains almost no water; therefore, ultrasonography must be used very carefully around bony areas because the waves may concentrate and cause damage.

Massage and Exercise

Massage is the systematic, therapeutic stroking or kneading of the body or a body part, which can effectively relieve or significantly reduce both localized and referred pain. Medical assistants are not usually asked to perform therapeutic massage on patients, but you should be familiar with the terminology.

A growing branch of healthcare uses exercise to aid muscle relaxation, promote healing, and provide relief from tension and pain caused by stress or a wide variety of physical disorders. Exercise also can be used to restore mobility, coordination, and strength. If the motion in a joint is restricted even for a short time, the joint tissues become dense, hard, and shortened. These changes can begin to occur in as little as 4 days. This can be prevented or reduced by the use of active or passive exercises.

In active exercise, the patient initiates and controls movements of a particular part of the body. Special equipment may be used,

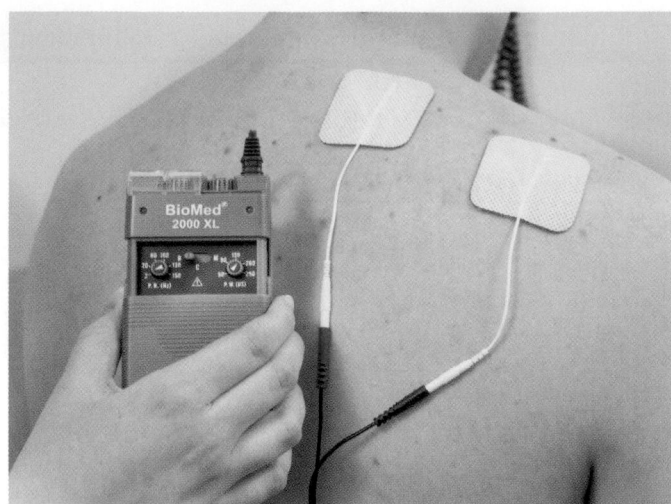

FIGURE 36-19 Application of a transcutaneous electrical nerve stimulation (TENS) unit.

such as stationary bicycles, treadmills, resistance bands, and/or weight machines. In passive exercise, the therapist moves the body part without the voluntary action of the patient. Both active and passive exercises can be performed to maintain normal ROM or to remedy diminished ROM after an injury.

Electrical Muscle Stimulation

A *transcutaneous electrical nerve stimulation* (TENS) unit is a low-voltage machine that creates a controlled electrical current through disposable gel electrodes. The electrodes are typically placed on the area of pain or at a pressure point, creating a circuit of electrical impulses that travels along nerve fibers. This low-voltage current is useful for stimulating the motor and sensory nerves that supply muscles. Stimulation provides a passive means of exercising a muscle when a patient cannot activate the muscle voluntarily because of injury. Electrical muscle stimulation frequently is used to prevent atrophy of a normal muscle. TENS treatments are used most often to treat muscle, joint, or bone problems that occur with illnesses such as osteoarthritis or fibromyalgia, or for conditions such as low back pain, neck pain, tendonitis, or bursitis (Figure 36-19).

AMBULATORY DEVICES

Crutches

Axillary crutches are made of wood or aluminum and must be measured to fit the patient, as described in Figure 36-20 and Procedure 36-3. It is very important to fit the crutches properly and to make sure the patient understands the importance of not bearing weight in the axillary region. If the crutch is too long or the handgrips are too low, or if the patient leans forward bearing weight on the armpit, serious injury can occur to the nerves in the brachial plexus. Patient guidelines for the correct use of crutches include the following:

- Wear flat shoes with nonskid soles to prevent accidents.
- Bear weight on your hands and the handgrips, not on your armpits.
- Report any numbness or tingling of the upper body or arms to the provider; this may indicate nerve damage from axillary weight bearing.
- Keep your elbows close to your body so that the crutches are against your side.

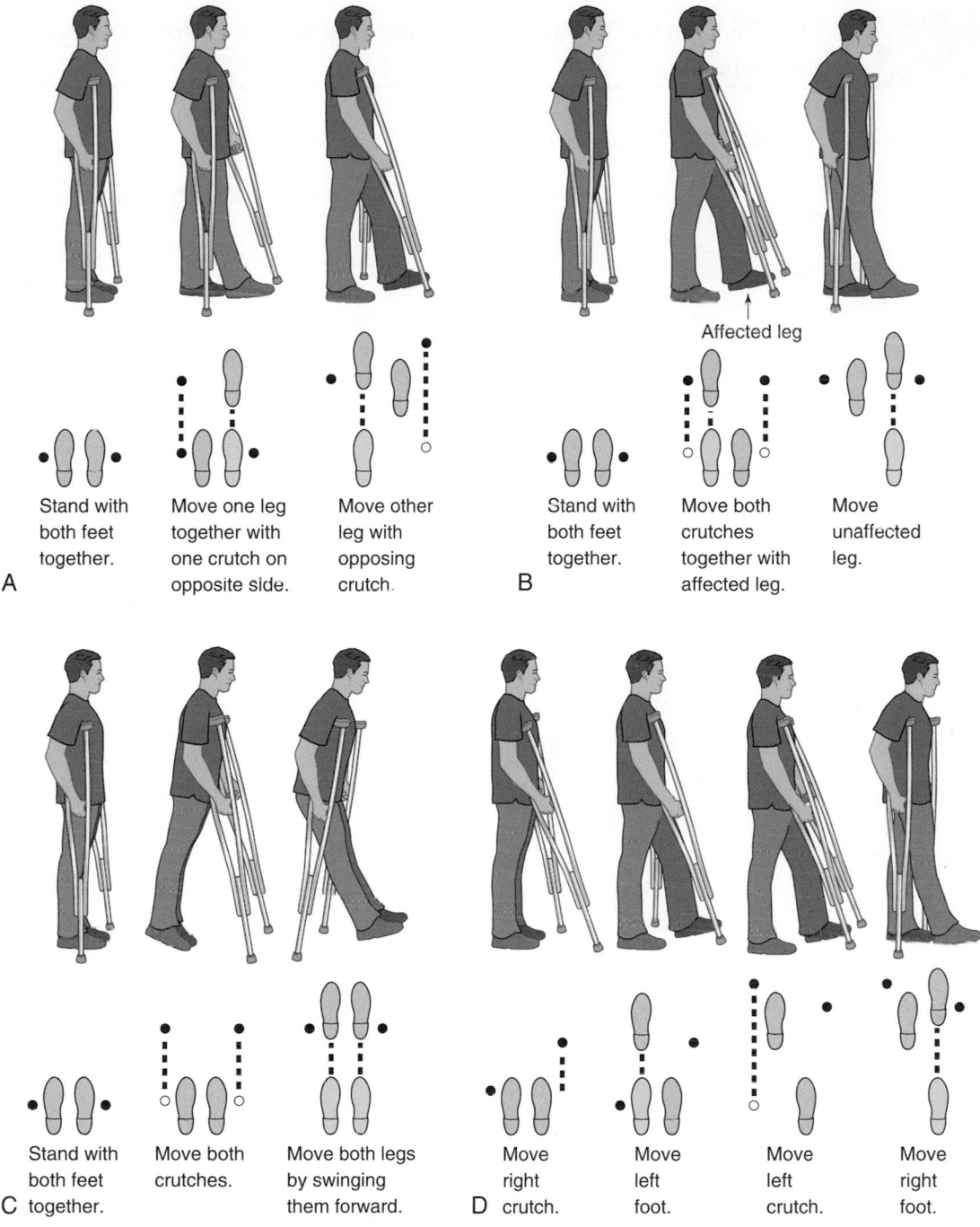

FIGURE 36-20 Crutch gaits. **A,** Two-point crutch gait. **B,** Three-point crutch gait. **C,** Swing-through gait. **D,** Four-point crutch gait.

- Place the crutch tips about 2 inches to the side of each foot so that you do not trip over them.
- Keep your elbows slightly bent when doing crutch walking.
- Keep your head up; do not look at your feet when using your crutches.
- Make sure the crutch tips, handgrip pads, and axillary pads on your crutches are in good condition at all times.
- Remove all throw rugs to keep from tripping or sliding.
- To stand up from a chair: Place both crutches on the injured side, tilt forward and push off with the arm on your uninjured side while bearing weight on the uninjured leg.

- To sit down: Place both crutches on the uninjured side, ease yourself down onto the chair while bearing weight with the uninjured arm and leg.
- To get into and out of a car: Make sure the front seat is moved back as much as possible. Back up toward the seat until you feel its edge; hold both crutches on the side of the body closest to the car door; grab the seat's head rest, tilt your head forward so that you do not bump it, and sit down. Place the heel of your uninjured leg on the car frame and push yourself back into the seat until you can swing the injured leg into the car.

PROCEDURE 36-3	Coach Patients in the Treatment Plan: Teach the Patient Crutch Walking and the Swing-Through Gait

Goal: *To fit crutches accurately and to teach the patient to use the crutches properly in three-point walking.*

EQUIPMENT and SUPPLIES

- Patient's health record
- Crutches with arm pads and foam handgrips

PROCEDURAL STEPS

1. Greet the patient, introduce yourself, and verify the patient's identity by name and date of birth. Explain the procedure, and answer any questions the patient may have. Sanitize your hands.
2. Ask the patient to stand up straight.
3. Fit the crutches to the patient so that they are 1 to 1½ inches (2 finger-widths) below the armpits when they are standing up straight. The handgrips should be even with the top of the hip line (Figure 1).

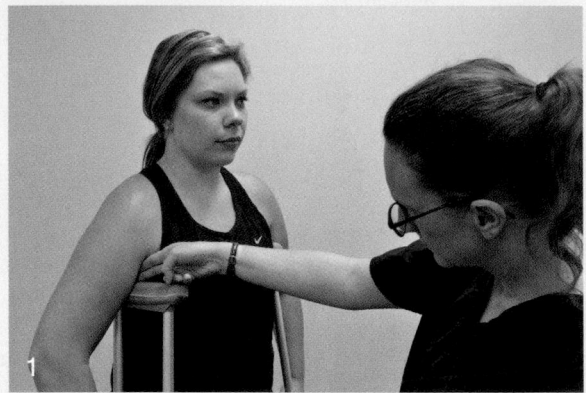

4. Make sure all wing nuts are tight.
5. Make sure the foam pads at the armpits and around the handgrips are comfortable.
6. Instruct the patient to keep the injured leg as relaxed as possible and slightly bent at the knee.
7. Adjust the handgrips on the crutches so that the patient's elbow is bent approximately 30 degrees when he or she is holding the handgrip.
8. Place the crutch tips about 2 inches in front of each foot and approximately 6 inches to the side of each foot before beginning crutch walking.
9. Ask the patient to push down on the crutches and lift the body slightly, nearly straightening the arms. The patient should hold the top of the crutches tightly to the sides and use the hands to absorb the weight. Do not let the tops of the crutches press into the armpits.
   <u>PURPOSE:</u> To prevent injury to the muscles and nerves of the axillary region.

10. Have the patient swing the body forward about 12 inches (see Figure 36-20, *C*).
    <u>PURPOSE:</u> The swing-through gait is one of the fastest crutch gaits that can be used, but it requires a great deal of energy and upper body strength.
11. Instruct the patient to stand on the good leg, then move the crutches just ahead of the good foot, and repeat.
12. Additional crutch gait patterns can be taught as needed.
    - *Two-point crutch gait:* Move the left crutch and the right foot together, then the right crutch and the left foot together. Repeat. This gait is used if both legs are weak; it can be a challenge for the patient to learn the pattern (see Figure 36-20, *A*).
    - *Three-point crutch gait:* Move both crutches and the affected leg forward, then bear weight down through the crutches and move the unaffected leg forward. Repeat. This gait is used if the patient is unable to bear weight on one leg (see Figure 36-20, *B*).
    - *Four-point crutch gait:* Move the right crutch forward, then the left foot, followed by the left crutch and then the right foot. This gait provides the best stability, but it is slow; however, it can be helpful for patients in whom both legs are weak (see Figure 36-20, *D*).
13. *Stairs:* Face the steps, hold the handrail with one hand, and tuck both crutches under the armpit on the other side. To go up the steps, start with the uninjured side, keeping the injured side raised behind. If the stairway does not have handrails, keep one crutch under each arm. With the crutches on the step where you are standing, step up with your stronger leg, push down on the crutches, and then step up with the weaker leg. Once both feet are on the same step, bring the crutches up. To go down steps, hold onto the hand rail with 1 hand with both crutches under the opposite arm. If there is no hand rail, keep 1 crutch under each arm, first place crutches on next step down, step down with weaker leg followed by the strong leg. If necessary, the patient can sit on the stairs and move up or down each step.
14. Document the patient education intervention in the patient's record.
    <u>PURPOSE:</u> A procedure is not considered done until it is recorded.

9/7/20–3:17 PM: Pt instructed in crutch walking using 3-point gait on steps and floor. Pt understands need to avoid weight bearing on ⊕ leg. Pt demonstrated technique s̄ difficulty. K. Tillman, CMA (AAMA)

Walkers

Walkers are used primarily by geriatric patients to help with balance and support. A walker's wide base helps stabilize the gait of weakened patients and can support up to 50% of the patient's body weight. Walkers are made of aluminum and can easily be adjusted to fit an individual. They are lightweight, can fold flat for storage and traveling, and can be equipped with a front pack to carry personal items or supplies. They also can be fitted with a fold-down seat. The disadvantage of a walker is that it cannot be used in small, cramped quarters.

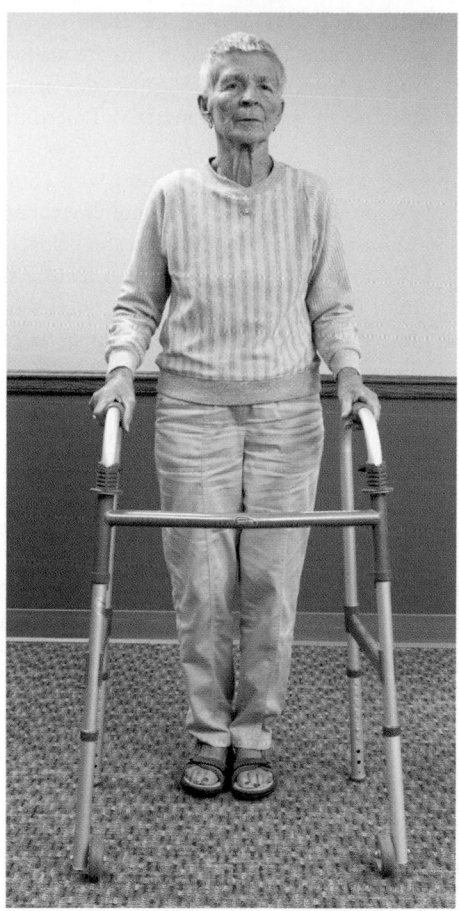

FIGURE 36-21 Properly fitted walker. Note the angle of the arms and the height of the walker.

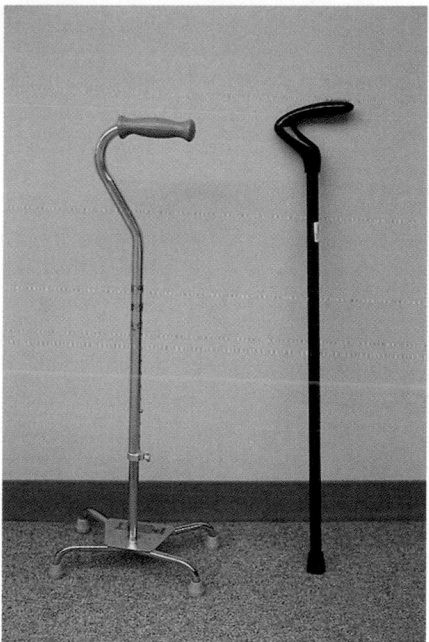

FIGURE 36-22 Types of standard canes. (From DeWit S: *Fundamental concepts and skills for nursing,* ed 4, St Louis, 2014, Saunders.)

To adjust the height of a walker, have the patient stand by the examination table. The top of the walker should be just below the patient's waist at the same height as the top of the hip bone. If the walker has been correctly adjusted to the patient, the patient's elbows will bend about 30 degrees while he or she uses the walker (Figure 36-21). Patient guidelines for walker use include the following:

- Lift the walker (or roll it if it is fitted with wheels) about an arm's length in front of you.
- Take your first step with the weaker leg, using the walker for support. If both legs are weak or you are using the walker for general support, start with either leg.
- Take smaller, slower steps than usual; if you step too close to the front of the walker, you can lose your balance.
- Hold your head up and look straight ahead.
- To sit down, back up with the walker until you feel the back of the chair against your legs; let go of the walker and reach back for the chair; slowly lower yourself into the chair.

Canes

Canes are available in a variety of designs (Figure 36-22). The single-tipped cane with a curved handgrip is indicated for individuals who need only minimal assistance with walking. Another type is the legged cane, which has a tripod or quad base. This base provides greater stability for the patient than does a single-tipped cane.

It is heavier and is recommended for patients who need greater support.

To fit a cane properly, have the patient stand up straight and measure the distance from the wrist crease to the floor. If the patient is age 70 or older or finds that extra length would feel more comfortable, up to 2 inches can be added to the previous measurement. This is the total length of the cane fitted to the patient. The patient's elbow should be bent to approximately 20 to 30 degrees if the cane has been correctly adjusted.

Canes typically are used to help a patient with balance problems, to widen the base of support so that falls are less likely, and to reduce weight bearing on an affected leg. To walk safely with a cane, the patient needs to be taught the following steps:

- Always use the cane on the side opposite the affected leg so that it can provide additional support as you walk through the step.
- The cane and the injured or weak leg should be advanced at the same time so that the cane and the leg are hitting the ground at the same time.
- Start by positioning the cane one small stride ahead on the strong side and step off with the injured leg, finishing the step with the stronger leg.
- Bear weight with the arm holding the cane as needed.
- The unaffected leg should bear the weight through the step.

Wheelchairs

Wheelchairs provide mobility for patients who cannot walk or who are able to walk only short distances. With a manual wheelchair, the patient uses arm muscles for mobility. Wheelchairs also come with motors that can be controlled by the patient. The patient is referred to an orthopedic appliance store, where the appropriate wheelchair is fitted to the individual.

MANAGEMENT OF FRACTURES

When a patient is diagnosed with a fracture or another injury that requires immobilization, the provider must decide whether a traditional cast (typically of fiberglass), a splint, or a brace is most appropriate to promote healing. Splints and braces have a slight opening in the front which allows for possible swelling at the site; these are often used with acute fractures or sprains or for initial stabilization of a fracture before surgery (Figure 36-23). If the patient needs to wear a cast only when using the limb, braces or splints are available in the shape of a boot or sleeve with Velcro fasteners that fit over the fracture to immobilize the area. An air cast is a temporary cast that is inflated around the limb to immobilize it. The type of cast used depends on the location and severity of the injury, the patient's age and occupation, and the provider's preference.

Casts provide superior immobilization because they completely surround the injury, but they are less forgiving if the area swells and could have higher complication rates; for these reasons, they are generally reserved for complex fractures. Casts are made up of fiberglass that has fiber or resin in the roller gauze; this creates a strong, lightweight, and relatively waterproof material (Procedures 36-4 and 36-5).

Before applying a cast, first wrap the area with cotton padding or a stockinette to protect the skin. To immobilize the injured area, the splint or cast must cover the joints above and below the fracture. As a fracture heals, the provider may decide to remove the cast and apply a splint until the fracture has mended completely. A patient may call the office complaining that the splint or cast feels tight. Swelling typically occurs in the first 48 to 72 hours after the injury. The patient should be told to elevate the injured part above the heart to help collected fluid drain from the site; to gently move the fingers or toes at the affected area to improve circulation; and to apply ice around the splint or cast in a plastic bag at the level of the injury to help reduce swelling.

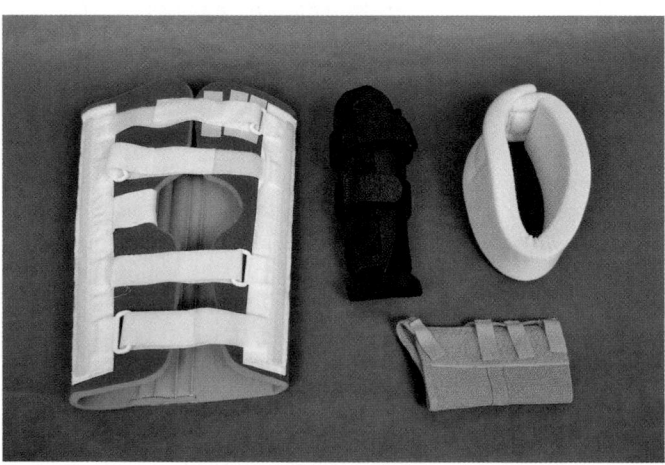

FIGURE 36-23 Examples of braces and splints.

CRITICAL THINKING APPLICATION   **36-10**

Kaiwan has just finished helping Dr. Alexander put a cast on the arm of a 6-year-old girl who fell out of her neighbor's tree house and fractured her radius. Her mother wants to take her home immediately. Should the patient be allowed to leave immediately? Why? What might happen?

PROCEDURE 36-4   Assist the Provider with Patient Care: Assist with Application of a Cast

Goal: *To assist the provider in applying a fiberglass cast.*

EQUIPMENT and SUPPLIES

- Patient's health record
- Rolls of fiberglass
- Basin for casting material
- Bandage
- Stockinette
- Gloves for provider and medical assistant
- Sheet wadding and/or spongy padding
- Stand to support foot (lower extremity)
- Tape
- Scissors
- 2-3 Towels
- Water

PROCEDURAL STEPS

1. Sanitize your hands.
2. Greet the patient, then introduce yourself and verify the patient's identity by name and date of birth.
3. Explain the procedure for applying a cast and answer any questions.
   <u>PURPOSE</u>: Knowing what to expect reassures the patient. Questions about the injury should be directed to the provider.
4. Assemble the necessary equipment.

PROCEDURE 36-4   *—continued*

5. Seat the patient comfortably, as directed by the provider. If the cast is being applied to the lower extremity, the toes must be supported by a stand.
   PURPOSE: The amount of flexion of the ankle can be controlled by supporting the toes so that the patient can more easily maintain the desired position without fatigue.

6. Clean the area that the cast will cover. Note any objective signs and ask about subjective symptoms (chart them at the end of the procedure).
   PURPOSE: The condition of the area under the cast must be noted before the cast is applied so that it can be compared with the site when the cast is removed. Clean the area with a mild soap solution or as directed. Dry thoroughly.

7. Cut the stockinette to fit the area the cast will cover.

8. Apply the stockinette smoothly to the area the cast will cover. Leave 1 or 2 inches of excess stockinette above and below the cast area to finish the cast (Figure 1).

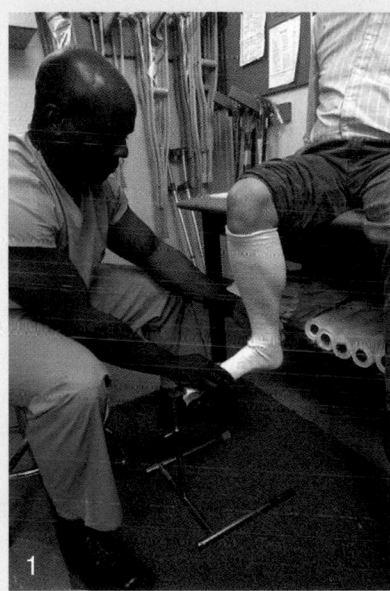

9. Excess stockinette may be cut away where wrinkles form, such as at the front of the ankle (Figure 2).
   PURPOSE: Stockinette must lie smoothly and cannot be too bulky or wrinkled because this may cause a pressure wound.

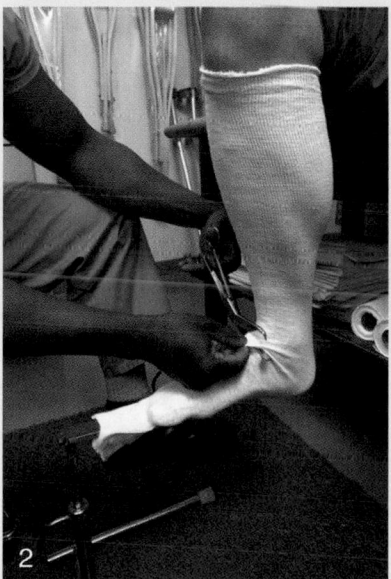

10. Apply sheet wadding along the length of the cast using a spiral bandage turn. Extra padding may be used over bony prominences, such as the bones of the elbow or ankle.
    PURPOSE: Padding the cast helps reduce pressure against bony prominences, which could cause skin breakdown.

11. Put on gloves.

12. With lukewarm water in the basin, wet the fiberglass tape as directed by the provider (Figure 3).
    PURPOSE: Immersing the roll of fiberglass tape in water begins the chemical reaction that will cause the cast to harden. The cast can be shaped while wet and will harden in the shape that is formed.

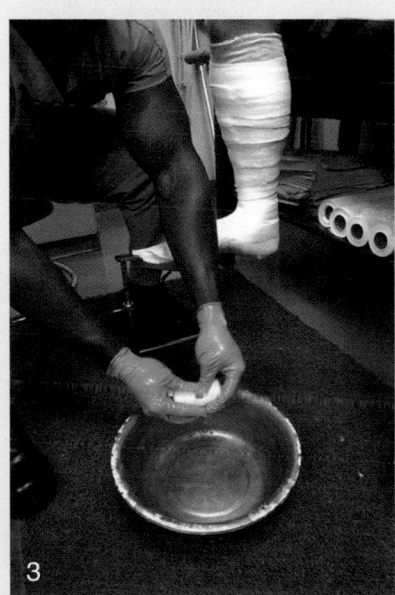

PROCEDURE 36-4   *—continued*

13. Assist as directed as the provider applies the inner layer of fiberglass tape. A length of 1 to 2 inches of stockinette is rolled over the inner layer of the cast to form a smooth edge when the outer layer is applied.

14. As directed by the provider, help to open and apply an outer layer of fiberglass tape (shown in the following figure as blue) (Figure 4).

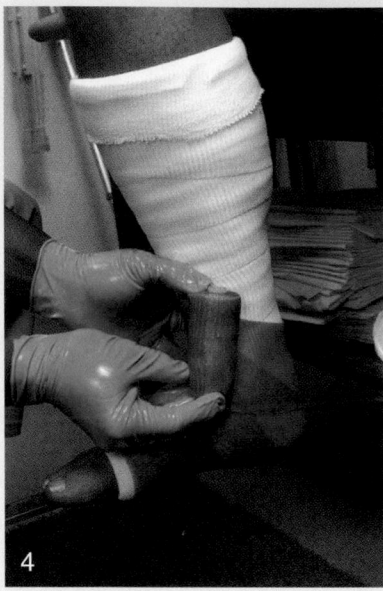

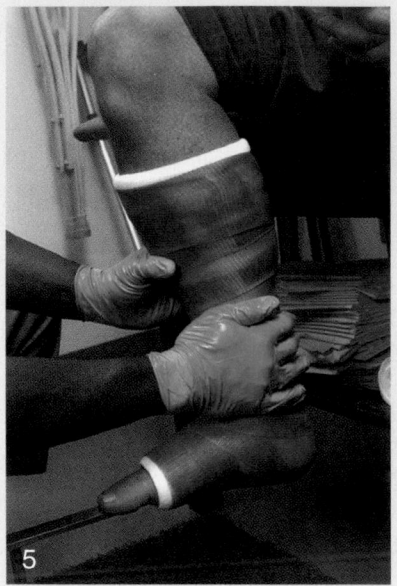

15. Help shape the cast as directed. All contours must be smooth (Figure 5). <u>PURPOSE</u>: If flat or dented areas develop on the cast, they may cause pressure on the skin below.

16. Discard the water and excess materials. Remove your gloves and wash your hands.

17. Reassure the patient, review cast care verbally, and provide written instructions.

18. Document observations and the procedure in the patient's health record. <u>PURPOSE</u>: A procedure is not considered done until it is recorded in the patient's health record.

9/8/20–1 PM: Assisted with application of knee to toe cast to ® leg. Skin under cast dry and intact. Pt given written instructions on cast care. Material reviewed s̄ questions. Instructed to call physician if there is numbness, tingling, swelling of toes, blue discoloration. K. Tillman, CMA (AAMA)

PROCEDURE 36-5   Assist the Provider with Patient Care: Assist with Cast Removal

Goal: *To remove a cast.*

EQUIPMENT and SUPPLIES

- Patient's health record
- Cast cutter
- Cast spreader
- Large bandage scissors
- Basin of warm water
- Mild soap
- Towel
- Skin lotion

PROCEDURAL STEPS

1. Greet the patient, introduce yourself and verify the patient's identity by name and date of birth, and then explain the procedure. Answer any questions the patient may have. <u>PURPOSE</u>: The patient may think cast removal is painful; explain how it is done to allay the patient's anxiety and ensure cooperation.

2. Provide adequate support for the limb throughout the procedure. <u>PURPOSE</u>: To ensure the patient's comfort.

PROCEDURE 36-5 *—continued*

3. Sanitize your hands. Using the cast cutter, make a cut on the medial and lateral sides of the long axis of the cast (Figure 1).

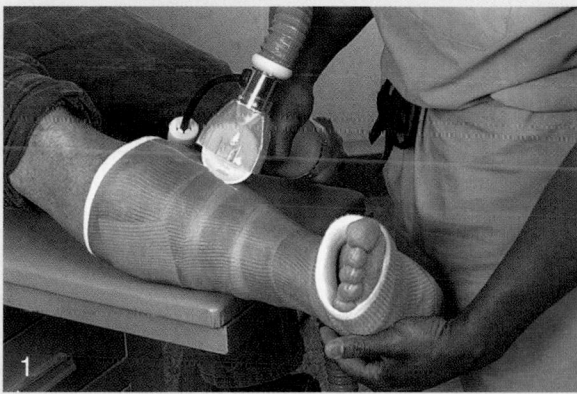

4. Use the cast spreader to pry apart the two halves using the cast spreader (Figure 2).

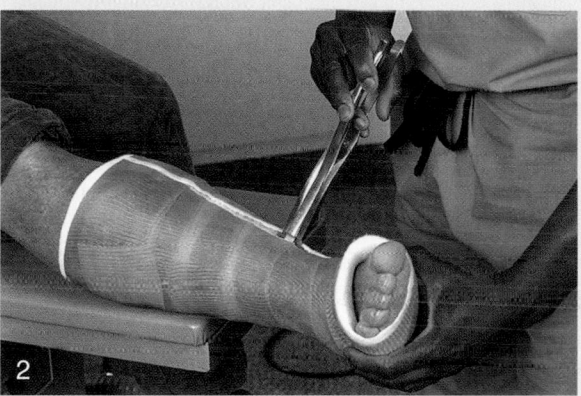

5. Carefully remove the two parts of the cast.
6. Use the large bandage scissors to cut away the stockinette and padding remaining.
7. Gently wash the area that was covered by the cast with mild soap and warm water.
   PURPOSE: To ensure the patient's comfort.
8. Dry the area and apply a gentle skin lotion.
   PURPOSE: To ensure the patient's comfort.
9. Give the patient appropriate instructions about exercising and using the limb, as directed by the provider.
   PURPOSE: To enhance continued healing, restore lost strength, and prevent injury.
10. Record the procedure in the patient's health record.
    PURPOSE: A procedure is not considered done until it is recorded.

CLOSING COMMENTS

Patient Education

An informed patient is better prepared to continue with home care. Musculoskeletal conditions, particularly arthritis, can be so painful and debilitating that these patients may be easy prey for miracle drug promotions. It is important for you to recognize the need for patient education about the condition and to work diligently with the patient and family to encourage participation in effective care programs. When you work with the provider and the physical therapist in helping the patient, you become an important member of the healthcare team. This type of involvement leads to patient satisfaction and to personal satisfaction and a sense of achievement for the medical assistant.

Patient Education for the Care of a Splint or Cast

The American Academy of Orthopedic Surgeons recommends the following measures for caring for a cast or splint:

- Keep the splint or cast dry; moisture weakens the material, and damp padding can irritate the skin. Use two layers of plastic or buy waterproof shields to keep the splint or cast dry while you shower or bathe. In special circumstances, the provider can apply a waterproof cast.
- Do not walk on a "walking cast" until it is completely dry and hard; it takes at least 1 hour for fiberglass to become hard enough to walk on.
- Prevent dirt, sand, and powder from getting inside the splint or cast.

- Do not pull out the padding.
- Do not stick objects (e.g., coat hangers) inside the splint or cast to scratch itching skin; if itching persists, contact your provider.
- Do not break off rough edges of the cast or trim the cast before asking your provider.
- Inspect the skin around the cast; if it is red or raw, contact your provider.
- Inspect the cast regularly; let your provider know if it becomes cracked or develops soft spots.

Legal and Ethical Issues

Working with orthopedic patients may require assisting with assessments and performing procedures that directly involve the patient's recovery plan. Many of the procedures in this chapter are not the basic procedures you will be required to perform when you are first hired as a medical assistant. These techniques all involve additional on-the-job training and practice. Before performing any of the described procedures, you should check with your local and state medical assistant organizations about the laws in your state. Whenever you perform the procedures and techniques described in this chapter, you are responsible for them. The following steps are all required before you perform any procedure on a patient:

- You must have a written order before performing a procedure.
- You must follow the procedure precisely as it is ordered, without variation.

- Never advise the patient without permission.
- Make sure you know what instructions the provider gave the patient and reinforce them.
- If you have any concerns about a procedure, discuss them with the provider privately before proceeding.
- Do not perform a procedure if you are uncomfortable; get someone to help you.

Always remember: You are the assistant, and this is the provider's patient. The physician ultimately is responsible for every aspect of the patient's care. If you feel uncertain or unsure of any order the provider has written for a patient, you must get it clarified before you proceed. Always stay within the legal and ethical guidelines of the medical assisting profession in your state.

Professional Behaviors

Musculoskeletal injuries and disorders are commonplace in the ambulatory care setting. Because of this, patients may ask for your advice on how to manage their health problems. Remember that as the medical assistant you should never diagnose or recommend treatment for a patient. That is the provider's responsibility. Responding professionally to inquiries, offering provider-approved educational materials, and/or referring patients and family members to accepted websites can be very helpful. Respectful and courteous behavior should be standard practice for a medical assistant when he or she interacts with patients and their families.

SUMMARY OF SCENARIO

Kaiwan is becoming more and more comfortable in his position as an orthopedic medical assistant at the sports medicine clinic. His enthusiasm is contagious. Patients consistently comment on his positive, upbeat manner. Kaiwan is motivated to learn new methods of better assisting the providers with routine procedures. He always seeks answers to questions that occur with new patients. He has gained a great deal of confidence and now remembers always to check the temperature of the paraffin bath before starting a treatment. One of the

most enjoyable aspects of his job continues to be assisting Dr. Alexander with treating the team members. Kaiwan has attended two continuing education seminars in sports medicine with Dr. Alexander. He now is thinking about continuing his education part time to become an athletic trainer while still working at the clinic. Kaiwan recognizes the importance of continuing education in maintaining orthopedic skills.

SUMMARY OF LEARNING OBJECTIVES

1. **Define, spell, and pronounce the terms listed in the vocabulary.**
   Spelling and pronouncing medical terms correctly reinforce the medical assistant's credibility. Knowing the definitions of these terms promotes confidence in communication with patients and co-workers.

2. **Describe the principal anatomic structures of the musculoskeletal system and their functions.**
   The main structures of the musculoskeletal system are the skeletal muscles, which provide movement; tendons, which connect muscles to bones; bones, which provide support, protection, mineral storage, and blood cell development; and ligaments, which connect bone to bone.

3. **Differentiate among tendons, bursae, and ligaments.**
   Tendons are the tough bands that connect muscles to bones; ligaments provide support by connecting bone to bone and preventing a joint from

moving beyond its normal ROM. Bursae prevent friction between different tissues in the musculoskeletal system.

4. **Summarize the major muscular disorders.**
   Fibromyalgia is a condition of unknown origin that causes widespread connective tissue and muscular pain, along with sleep disorders and extreme fatigue. Myasthenia gravis is an autoimmune disorder that affects the use of ACh at the neuromuscular junction, resulting in muscular weakness, especially in the face and eyes. A sprain is the tearing of ligaments, and a strain is the overstretching or tearing of a muscle or tendon. (See Table 36-2.)

5. **Identify and describe the common types of fractures.**
   The common types of fractures are explained in Table 36-3.

6. **Explain the difference between osteomalacia and osteoporosis.**

Osteomalacia is softening of the bones, which occurs because of a problem with the metabolism or absorption of vitamin D, calcium, and phosphorus; in children the condition is called *rickets*. Osteoporosis is a reduction in bone density, which can be caused by many factors, including lack of dietary calcium early in life; it leads to brittle bones that fracture easily. (See Table 36-2.)

7. **Classify typical spinal column disorders.**

Spinal column disorders are related to the shape of the spine: scoliosis is a lateral deviation; lordosis (swayback) is a pronounced curve of the lower back; and kyphosis is a pronounced cervical curve, or hunchback. A herniated disk occurs when the soft nucleus of an intervertebral disk protrudes through a tear or weakened area in its tough outer cartilaginous covering.

8. **Differentiate among the various joint disorders.**

Joint disorders include dislocations, in which the two bones of the joint are no longer approximated; gout, which is a form of arthritis caused by the collection of uric acid crystals, most commonly in the synovial membrane of the great toe; SLE, which is a widespread autoimmune disorder that can affect any organ system in the body; Lyme disease, a form of infectious arthritis caused by bacteria transmitted via a tick bite, can cause extensive joint and neurologic problems if left untreated; OA, caused by degeneration of the articular cartilage of synovial joints; RA, an autoimmune disorder that causes crippling pain and deformity of the joints; and tendonitis and bursitis, which are inflammatory reactions of supportive tissue typically caused by overuse of a joint.

9. **Summarize the medical assistant's role in assisting with orthopedic procedures.**

The medical assistant is responsible for gathering and recording a detailed history of the patient's presenting problem; providing the patient with assistance as needed; and assisting with the orthopedic examination.

10. **Explain the common diagnostic procedures used in orthopedics.**

Common diagnostic procedures routinely performed in the orthopedic office include ROM evaluation, inspection, palpation, percussion, muscle strength evaluation, and x-ray studies. Other diagnostic tools include arthrograms, myelograms, bone scans, CT, MRI, electromyography, biopsies, and diagnostic ultrasonography.

11. **Discuss therapeutic modalities used in orthopedic medicine.**

Therapeutic modalities include the application of cold and heat (see Table 36-4); paraffin baths; hot-water bottles and moist heat packs; therapeutic ultrasonography; massage and therapeutic exercise; and electric muscle stimulation.

12. **Apply cold therapy to an injury.**

Cold should be used immediately after an injury to help reduce inflammation, inhibit additional swelling, and help relieve pain. The ice pack should remain in place for 20 minutes at a time, several times a day, and the area should be checked for feeling and color after each application. (See Procedure 36-1.)

13. **Discuss various heat treatments and assist with hot, moist, heat application to an orthopedic injury.**

Heat should be used on injuries after 48 hours to promote circulation and healing, reduce swelling, and promote soft tissue relaxation in the affected area. Care must be taken to prevent burns. (See Procedure 36-2.)

14. **Discuss therapeutic ultrasonography, massage, exercise, and electrical muscle stimulation.**

Therapeutic ultrasound applies deep tissue heat to an injured area. It is important to keep the applicator head constantly moving in a circular fashion over the injured site during the treatment. Massage is systematic stroking of the body or body part. Medical assistants are not usually asked to perform therapeutic massage on patients. A transcutaneous electrical nerve stimulation (TENS) unit is often used to treat muscle, joint, or bone problems that occur with osteoarthritis and fibromyalgia, in addition to neck and back issues.

15. **Explain the use of common ambulatory devices, properly fit a patient with crutches, and coach a patient in the correct mechanics of crutch walking.**

The most common ambulatory assistive devices are crutches, canes, walkers, and wheelchairs. The most important aspects of using these assistive devices in an orthopedic practice are to fit them properly to the patient and to instruct the patient adequately in how to use the device properly and safely. Procedure 36-3 presents the steps for properly fitting a patient with crutches and explaining the correct mechanics of crutch walking. (See Figure 36-20 for various crutch gaits.)

16. **Discuss the management of fractures and prepare for and assist with both the application and removal of a cast.**

The management of fractures includes reduction, immobilization, analgesics, and NSAIDs. The tissue beneath the cast must be safeguarded by applying a stockinette and sheet wadding. The casting material then is immersed in water and carefully rolled around the limb (see Procedure 36-4). The steps for preparing for and assisting with cast removal are shown in Procedure 36-5.

17. **Summarize patient education guidelines for orthopedic patients.**

Musculoskeletal conditions are often painful and debilitating. The medical assistant should recognize the need for patient education and work with the patient, family, and healthcare team to promote recovery.

18. **Discuss the legal and ethical implications in an orthopedic practice.**

Before performing any orthopedic procedures, the medical assistant should check with local and state medical assistant organizations about applicable state laws. Procedures and techniques should be performed only under the direct supervision of the physician.

CONNECTIONS

Study Guide Connection: Go to the Chapter 36 Study Guide. Read and complete the activities.

evolve Evolve Connection: Go to the Chapter 36 link at *evolve.elsevier.com/kinn* to complete the Chapter Review Quiz. Check out the other resources listed for this chapter to make the most of what you have learned from Assisting in Orthopedic Medicine.

37 ASSISTING IN NEUROLOGY AND MENTAL HEALTH

SCENARIO

Mai Lee, CMA (AAMA), has been working in Dr. Kim Song's neurology practice for 2 years. Dr. Song has always been pleased with Mai's professional behavior toward all patients in his practice. She uses therapeutic communication when interacting with the diverse patient population and is conscientious about accurately maintaining electronic health records (EHRs). Dr. Song has just asked Mai to train a new medical assistant in the clinical procedures of the office. He is expanding his clinic hours and wants to have Mai more involved in assisting him with patients, particularly in patient education. She is excited to have additional responsibilities with Dr. Song's patients, and she is quite happy about the raise in salary that goes along with her new position.

While studying this chapter, think about the following questions:
- What is the basic anatomy and physiology of the neurologic system?
- What should Mai know about typical neurologic disorders?
- What are the diagnostic and treatment procedures for common nervous system disorders?
- What is the medical assistant's role in the neurologic examination?
- Is patient education a significant factor when working with patients diagnosed with either nervous system or mental health disorders?

LEARNING OBJECTIVES

1. Define, spell, and pronounce the terms listed in the vocabulary.
2. Summarize the anatomy and physiology of the nervous system.
3. Differentiate between the central and peripheral nervous systems.
4. Distinguish among common nervous system diseases and conditions and identify the typical symptoms associated with neurologic disorders.
5. Describe the pathology of cerebrovascular diseases.
6. Identify the various types of epilepsy.
7. Compare and contrast encephalitis and meningitis.
8. Explain the dynamics of brain and spinal cord injuries.
9. Summarize common central nervous system (CNS) and peripheral nervous system (PNS) diseases.
10. Differentiate among common mental health disorders.
11. Analyze the medical assistant's role in the neurologic examination.
12. Explain the common diagnostic procedures for the nervous system.
13. Outline the steps needed to prepare a patient for an electroencephalogram (EEG).
14. Describe the steps for preparing a patient for and assisting with a lumbar puncture.
15. Discuss the implications of patient education in a neurologic and mental health practice.
16. Explain the legal issues and Health Insurance Portability and Accountability Act (HIPAA) applications associated with neurology and mental health.

VOCABULARY

anomalies (uh-noh'-muh-leez) Deformities or deviations from a normal condition, resulting from faulty development of a fetus.

ataxia (uh-taks'-e-uh) Failure or irregularity of muscle actions and coordination.

aura A peculiar sensation that precedes the appearance of a more definite disturbance; commonly seen with migraines or seizure activity.

benign Not cancerous and not recurring.

blood-brain barrier An anatomic-physiologic structure made up of astrocyte glial cells that prevents or slows the transfer of chemicals into the neurons of the central nervous system (CNS).

bruit (broot) An abnormal sound heard during auscultation of a carotid artery; it is caused by the flow of blood through a narrowed or partially occluded vessel.

coma An unconscious state from which the patient cannot be aroused.

cryptogenic (krip-tuh-jeh'-nik) Pertaining to a disease with an unknown origin.

diplopia (dih-ploh'-pe-uh) Double vision.

embolus A mass of undissolved matter that blocks a blood vessel; frequently a blood clot that has traveled from some other part of the body.

exacerbation (ig-zas'-er-bay-shun) An increase in the seriousness of a disease marked by greater intensity of signs and symptoms.

VOCABULARY—*continued*

ischemic (ih-ske′-mik) Pertaining to a decreased supply of oxygenated blood to a body part.

malaise A generalized feeling of weakness or discomfort; usually marks the onset of a disease.

malignant Cancerous.

myelin sheath A segmented, fatty tissue that wraps around the axon of the nerve cell and acts as an electrical insulator to speed the conduction of nerve impulses.

occlusion Complete obstruction of an opening.

palliative Therapy that relieves or reduces symptoms but does not result in a cure.

papilledema Swelling of the optic disc as a result of increased intracranial pressure.

paresthesia (par-uhs-the′-ze-uh) An abnormal sensation of burning, prickling, or stinging.

paroxysmal (par-ok-siz′-muhl) Pertaining to a sudden recurrence of symptoms; a sudden spasm or convulsion of any kind.

plaque An abnormal accumulation of a fatty substance.

proprioception The sensation of awareness of body movements and posture; nerve impulses that provide the central nervous system with information about the position of body parts.

radiopaque A substance that can easily be visualized on an x-ray film.

thrombus A blood clot.

transection Cross section; a division made by cutting across.

The human brain weighs about 3 pounds, requires about the same amount of energy needed to light a 20-watt bulb, stores more than 100 trillion bits of information, and works better than any computer. The matter that makes up the brain is approximately 85% water and therefore has a soft texture. Early scientists believed that the brain's function was to cool the blood. Today's scientists have shown us that even though the brain receives 20% of the body's blood supply, its function is much more complex than simply cooling blood.

Neurologists specialize in the diagnosis and treatment of medical disorders and conditions of the nervous system. A *neurosurgeon* provides surgical management and treatment for trauma and other conditions requiring surgery. A *psychiatrist* is a physician who treats behavioral disorders and neurologic conditions that affect behavior.

ANATOMY AND PHYSIOLOGY OF THE NERVOUS SYSTEM

The nervous system works with the endocrine system to integrate stimuli, both from within the body and from the outside environment, to regulate body systems; this allows homeostasis to be maintained. The nervous system is divided into two major parts: the *central nervous system* (CNS), which is made up of the brain and spinal cord, and the *peripheral nervous system* (PNS), which includes all the nervous tissue and neurologic responses found outside the CNS.

The brain is the "president" or "chief executive officer" of the body. It constantly receives information from the periphery, including all the organs and systems inside the body and on its surface. This information (i.e., stimuli) is carried to the brain by the peripheral nerves along the *afferent,* or ascending, nerve tract. The brain monitors and interprets the stimuli received from the afferent nerves and sends appropriate responses back along *efferent* pathways to the organs or to the body's surface. These responses from the brain cause a specific reaction in the organ, in the glands, or in skeletal muscles. These reactions keep the body running smoothly and allow it to react instantly to both external and internal stimuli.

The functioning cell of the nervous system is the neuron (Figure 37-1). The brain contains billions of individual neurons. Formation of the nervous system starts very early in embryonic development (i.e., by week 3); it begins as the neural tube, which eventually develops into the brain and spinal cord. Each neuron is made up of a main cell body that contains the nucleus and a relatively long extension of the cell, called the *axon,* which may be covered with a **myelin sheath**. Multiple filaments, called *dendrites,* extend from the neuron body. Dendrites receive the nervous impulse from a preceding neuron and carry it into the cell body. Impulses are carried away from the cell body through the axon to another neuron or to cells in another tissue. This transfer of stimuli begins as an electrical impulse that travels down an axon of one neuron and becomes a chemical impulse while moving across the synapse (the space between two neurons) to the dendrite of another neuron. The transfer of impulses from the end of one neuron to the dendrites of another is enhanced by chemical neurotransmitters, which bind to specific receptor sites on the dendrites of the next neuron. If the nerve impulse is traveling to a muscle or to any other organ or tissue instead of another neuron, the chemical neurotransmitters bind to special receptors in the target tissue. Messages move throughout the entire nervous system in this manner. Impulses in the neuron are electrical; the impulses become chemical as a specific neurotransmitter is released at each synapse, and they become electrical again as they are picked up by the subsequent dendrites of another neuron or by the target tissue.

Supportive cells of the nervous system are called *glial* or *neuroglial* cells. Glial cells do not carry on any of the functions of the nervous system; these specialized cells perform specific functions within the nervous system; for example, Schwann cells form the myelin sheath, and astrocytes help form the blood-brain barrier. The **blood-brain barrier** closely regulates what substances enter the brain tissue. Oxygen, water, and glucose molecules easily pass into the brain, whereas many chemicals and drugs are prevented from moving into brain tissue. Brain inflammation can increase the ability of many drugs to cross the blood-brain barrier because of damage to the specialized glial cells.

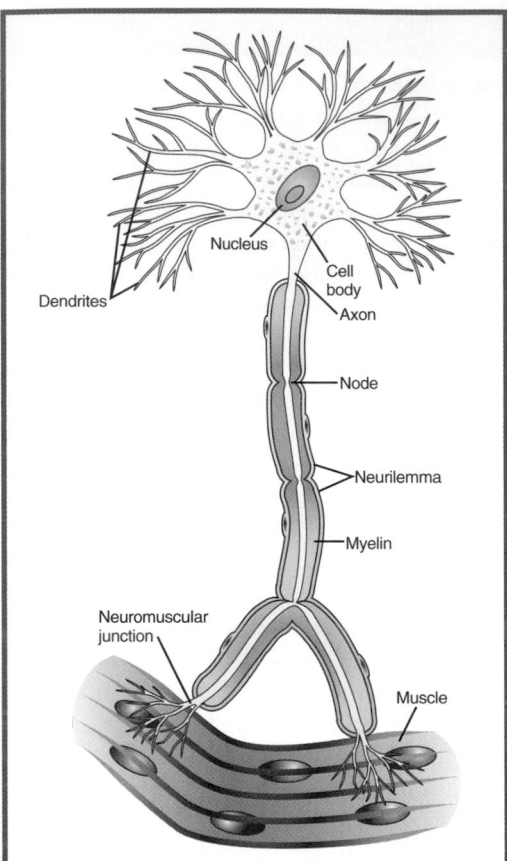

FIGURE 37-1 A neuron.

What Happens When You Accidentally Touch a Hot Pan

1. When your hand comes into contact with a hot pan on the stove, impulses travel from the area of contact to the central nervous system (CNS) along an afferent (sensory neurons) nervous pathway, carrying the information "hot."
2. The CNS performs a hasty analysis and determines that a heat danger is present.
3. The CNS sends a quick, strong message back to skeletal muscles via the efferent (motor neurons) pathway to move the finger immediately.
4. You quickly pull your hand away from the hot pan, preventing a serious burn and maintaining homeostasis.

Central Nervous System

As mentioned, the brain and spinal cord together make up the CNS. The brain is encased within the skull in the cranial cavity. The spinal cord is a bundle of nervous tissue that extends inferiorly from the brainstem at the base of the brain and exits the skull at the foramen magnum. It descends for about 17 inches inside the spinal canal, which courses through the vertebrae of the backbone.

Brain

The brain accounts for only about 2% of a person's weight, but it consumes about 20% of the body's oxygen. The brain is divided into three main areas: the cerebrum, the cerebellum, and the brainstem (Figure 37-2). The cerebrum, the largest and uppermost section of the brain, has multiple convolutions along its surface, called *gyri,* which are formed by the folding in of the cerebral cortex. The gyri are separated by shallow grooves, called *sulci.* The gyri greatly increase the surface area of the cerebrum, which maximizes the potential of the CNS neurons in each area. The cerebrum is divided into lobes, which are named after the region of the skull under which they are located. The cerebrum is separated by a longitudinal fissure into left and right hemispheres. The right hemisphere usually controls artistic functions, such as drawing, rhythm, and picture memory. The left hemisphere controls verbal functions, such as reading, writing, speaking, and mathematic calculations. The two halves of the brain are connected by the corpus callosum. This bundle of nerve tissue facilitates communication between the two sides of the brain. The corpus callosum is the largest collection of white matter within the brain; it has a high myelin content, which allows for quicker transmission of information. Some congenital defects include a complete lack of this neural tissue.

The diencephalon, located deep in the center of the cerebrum near the superior portion of the brainstem, is made up of the thalamus and the hypothalamus. The thalamus acts as a relay station between sensory neurons and the cerebral cortex. The functions of the hypothalamus include controlling the autonomic nervous system; regulating endocrine processes; and managing body temperature, sleep, and appetite to maintain homeostasis. Within the cerebrum are four spaces, called *ventricles,* which contain cerebrospinal fluid (CSF). CSF nourishes, lubricates, and provides some cushioning protection for the brain and the spinal cord.

The cerebellum, which is just inferior to the occipital lobe of the cerebrum, controls balance, equilibrium, posture, and muscle coordination. The brainstem controls reflexes and serves as a sensory relay station for input coming into the brain from the body. The brainstem plays a vital role in vision, hearing, respiration, heart rate, blood pressure, waking, and sleeping.

Spinal Cord

The spinal cord extends from the inferior portion of the brainstem to approximately the second lumbar vertebra. Thirty-one pairs of spinal nerves extend from the spinal cord through openings in the vertebrae. Starting just below the first cervical vertebra in the neck, a nerve extends from the spinal cord on each side; therefore, a pair of spinal nerves originates at each level. Each of these pairs of nerves innervates a specific organ or area of the body. The spinal cord carries messages between the spinal nerves and the brain.

Meninges

Because the brain and the spinal cord are critical to life, they are well protected. They both are encased in some of the thickest bones in the body; they also are surrounded by three membranes, called *meninges;* and they are cushioned by the CSF (Figure 37-3).

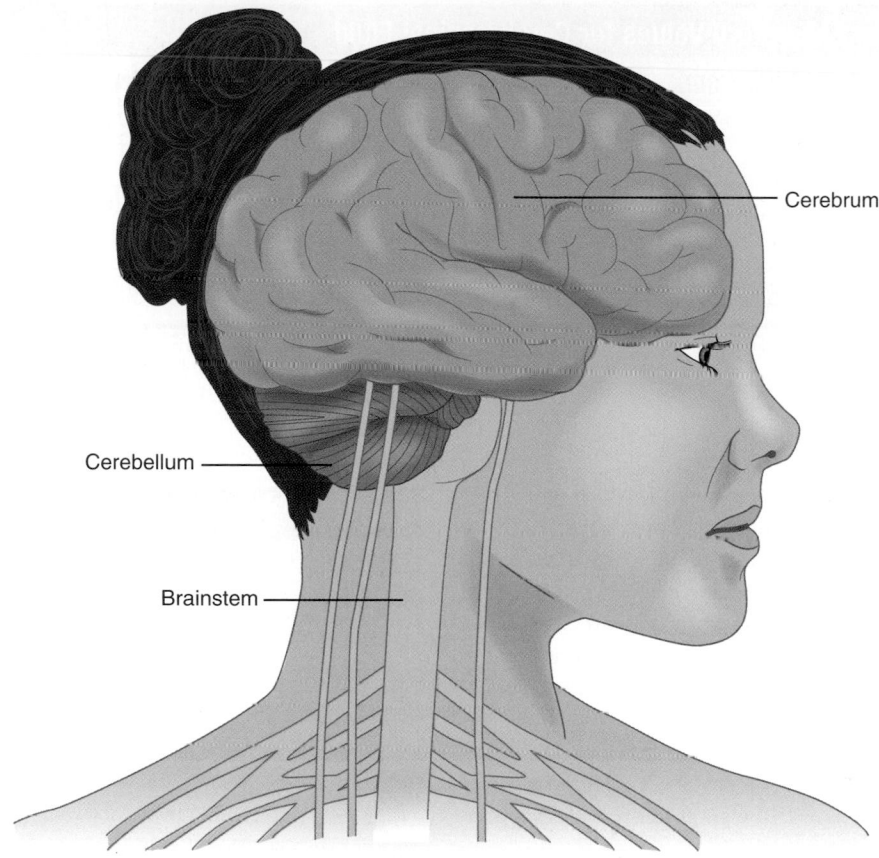

FIGURE 37-2 The brain.

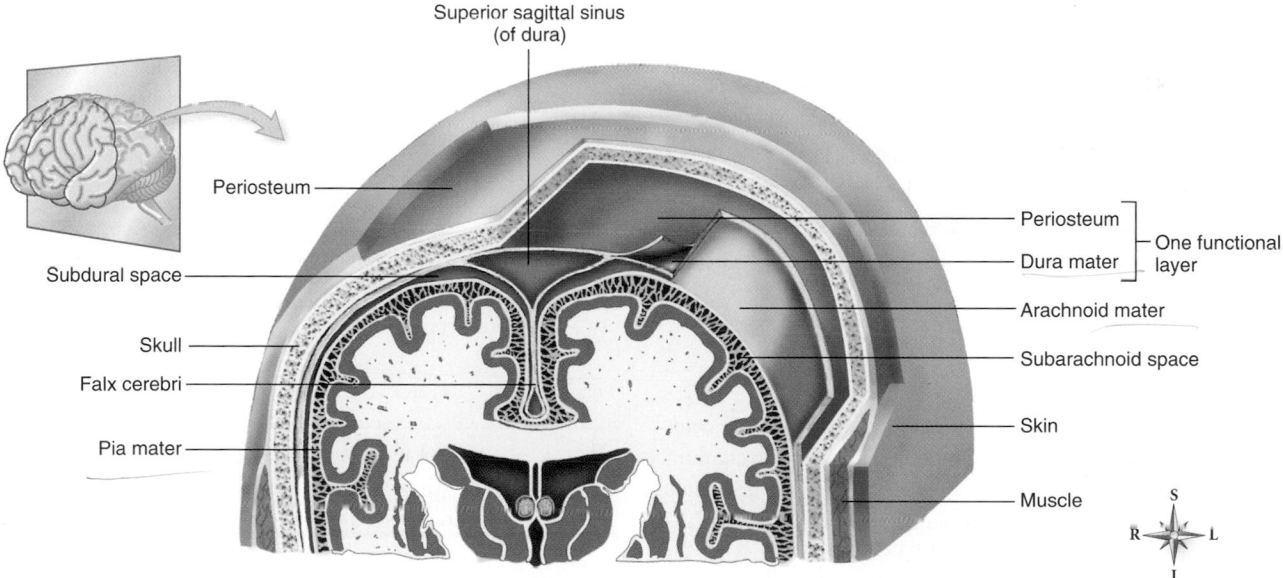

FIGURE 37-3 Protective coverings of the brain. (Modified from Patton K, Thibodeau G: *Anatomy and physiology*, ed 9, St Louis, 2016, Mosby.)

The outer layer of the meninges is called the *dura mater* ("hard mother") because it is a tough membrane, similar to a very strong rubber band. The subdural space lies below the dura mater and contains small veins that have little protection. Trauma to the head can cause bleeding of these tiny vessels, ultimately leading to the development of a *subdural hematoma*. Above the dura mater is the epidural space. The arterial supply to the meninges comes from blood vessels that line the inner aspect of the skull. If the skull is fractured, these arteries can be damaged, resulting in a collection of blood between the skull and the dura mater called an *epidural hematoma*.

TABLE 37-1   Typical Laboratory Values for Cerebrospinal Fluid

CONDITION	PRESSURE (mm)	APPEARANCE	CELLS	PROTEIN (mg/dL)	GLUCOSE (mg/dL)
Normal	50-200	Clear, colorless	0-10 lymphocytes and monocytes	<45	50-80
Acute bacterial meningitis	200-500	Turbid	100-10,000 granulocytic neutrophils	50-500	Absent or low
Subarachnoid hemorrhage	200-500	Bloody	Red blood cells (RBCs)	50-1000	50-80

The middle meningeal layer is the *arachnoid,* which was given that name because of its fine spider-web appearance. Beneath the arachnoid membrane in the subarachnoid space is the cerebrospinal fluid, a clear liquid that contains glucose, protein, and chloride produced by specialized cells in the ventricles (Table 37-1). CSF circulates continuously through the ventricles and around the brain and spinal cord, carrying nutrients and removing wastes.

The innermost meningeal layer, which covers the brain and spinal cord, is the delicate *pia mater* ("tender mother"); it is highly vascular and the thinnest of the three layers. The pia mater provides support for the blood vessels of the brain.

Hydrocephalus

Hydrocephalus is the abnormal accumulation of cerebrospinal fluid (CSF) in the ventricles of the brain. It can be detected in utero with sonography or diagnosed at birth. It is the result either of overproduction of CSF or of failure of the fluid to drain properly. If left untreated, hydrocephalus causes gross enlargement of the skull and severe damage to brain tissue from increased intracranial pressure. The only treatment is surgery to place a shunt (tube) from a ventricle in the brain to the right atrium or to the abdominal cavity. The shunt allows the excess CSF to drain away from the brain.

Peripheral Nervous System

The PNS is made up of the nerves that exit the brain or spinal cord. The peripheral nerves exiting the brain directly through the cranium are called *cranial nerves.* Cranial nerves originate from the underside of the brain and relay information to and from the sensory organs and muscles of the face and neck (Table 37-2). The spinal nerves from the spinal cord enter and exit the spinal canal through spaces between the vertebrae. Spinal nerves carry information to and from the brain through the spinal cord. Sensory fibers in these nerves carry stimuli from the skin and internal organs to the CNS. Motor fibers carry messages from the CNS to skeletal muscles, causing them to contract.

The autonomic nervous system (ANS) is part of the PNS. Autonomic nerves control *homeostasis;* that is, they keep the body running smoothly, much like a thermostat controls the temperature in a

TABLE 37-2   Cranial Nerves and Their Functions

CRANIAL NERVE	NAME	FUNCTION
I	Olfactory	Smell
II	Optic	Vision
III	Oculomotor	Eye movement Pupil constriction and accommodation
IV	Trochlear	Eye movement
V	Trigeminal	Muscles of chewing General sensations from anterior half of head, including entire face and meninges
VI	Abducent	Eye movement
VII	Facial	Muscles of facial expression Tearing, salivation, and taste
VIII	Vestibulocochlear	Hearing and equilibrium
IX	Glossopharyngeal	Swallowing and taste
X	Vagus	Breathing, speech, sweating, regulating heartbeat, stimulating muscles of gastric region
XI	Spinal accessory	Shoulder and head movements
XII	Hypoglossal	Tongue movements

room. The ANS (Figure 37-4) is an automatic system that regulates body functions such as breathing, heart rate, sweating, circulation, and digestion. It also controls the actions of muscles in blood vessel walls, organs, and glands. Just as a thermostat can control both heating and cooling in a room to maintain a comfortable temperature, the autonomic system is made up of two divisions, called the *sympathetic system* and the *parasympathetic system.* The sympathetic system promotes responses geared toward protecting the individual

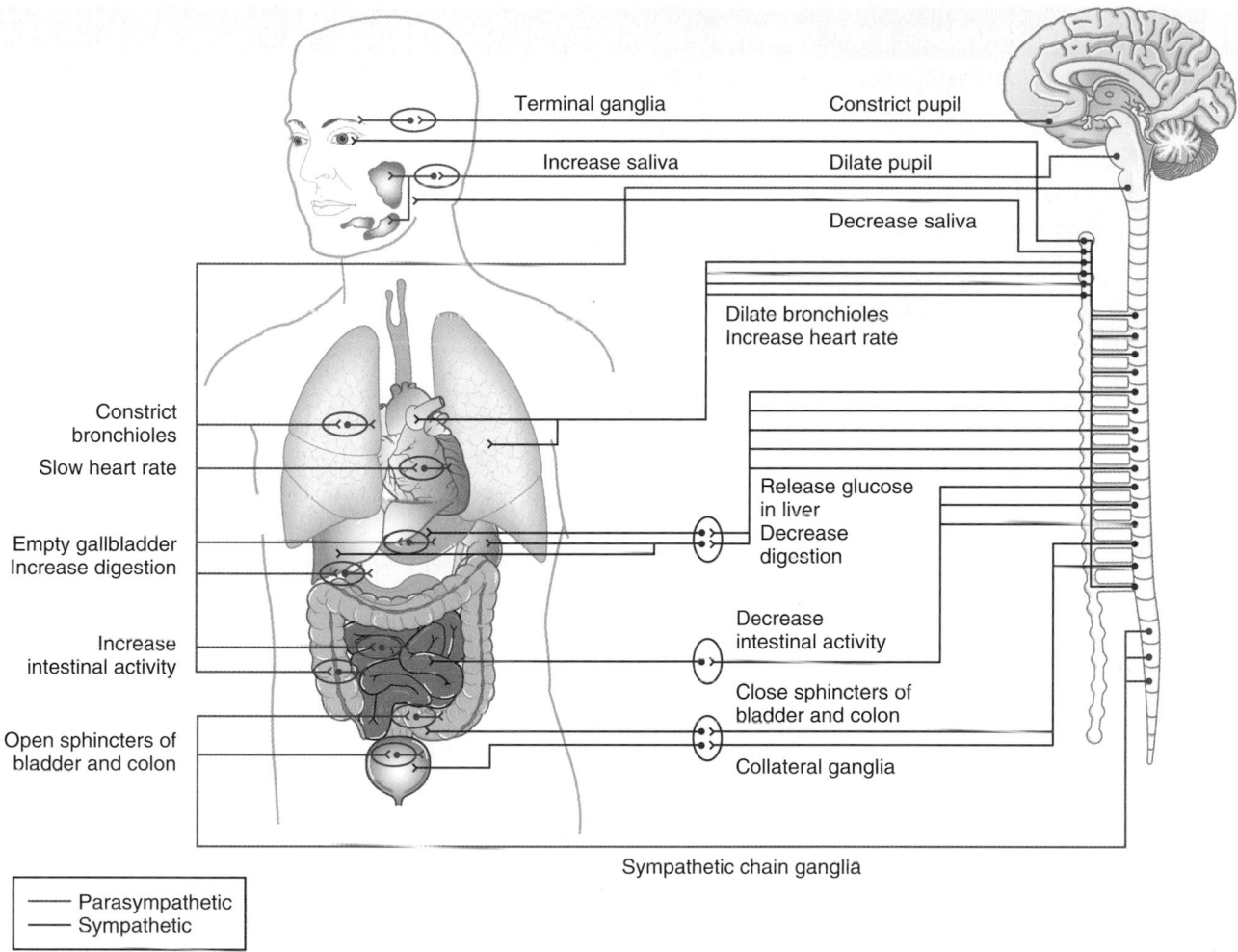

FIGURE 37-4 Structure and function of the autonomic nervous system. (From Applegate E: *The anatomy and physiology learning system,* ed 4, St Louis, 2011, Saunders.)

("fight or flight"), generally causing a stimulating effect: it speeds up the heart, raises blood glucose levels and blood pressure, reduces peristalsis, and widens the bronchioles, allowing more oxygen to enter the body quickly. The parasympathetic system generally promotes rest or a reducing effect: it slows the heart rate, constricts the bronchioles, and increases digestive system function.

CRITICAL THINKING APPLICATION   **37-1**

Dr. Song mentions a patient's nervous system function to Mai. The patient hears this conversation and later asks Mai, "What does my nervous system do?" How should Mai answer this question? What resources could she use to help explain the nervous system to the patient?

DISEASES AND DISORDERS OF THE CENTRAL NERVOUS SYSTEM

Because the CNS and PNS are so complex, diseases and conditions that affect them can produce a wide range of signs and symptoms. Causes include trauma, infection, congenital **anomalies**, degeneration, tumors, and vascular disorders (Table 37-3). The medical

assistant needs to listen carefully when a patient describes his or her neurologic symptoms. Many different types of symptoms can indicate a serious condition of the nervous system.

Cerebrovascular Disease

Cerebrovascular disease (CVD) is the fourth leading cause of death and the most frequent cause of crippling disease in the United States. Generally, CVD is related to arteriosclerosis or atherosclerosis of the cerebral arteries, but it also can be caused by untreated or uncontrolled hypertension, cerebral hemorrhage, thrombi, or emboli. Arteriosclerosis causes progressive loss of elasticity of the arterial wall and is seen in elderly individuals with CVD. Atherosclerosis, the deposit of fatty **plaque** on the inside of the arterial wall, can involve any of the major arteries supplying the brain or any of their branches. Sudden narrowing, or **occlusion**, may occur when an artery becomes blocked by a **thrombus** or an **embolus**.

CVD usually is diagnosed through cerebral arterial angiography, in which a **radiopaque** dye is injected into the suspect vessel and an x-ray film is immediately taken. Other confirming tests include magnetic resonance imaging (MRI), computed tomography (CT), and electroencephalography.

TABLE 37-3   Common Diseases and Conditions of the Nervous System

DISEASE	SIGNS, SYMPTOMS, AND ETIOLOGY	DIAGNOSTIC PROCEDURES	LABORATORY TESTS	TREATMENT AND MEDICATIONS
Alzheimer's disease	Short-term memory loss; progressive, irreversible confusion and disorientation; cause unknown, familial link	History, MRI	None specific; ordered to rule out other causes of dementia	Supportive care, donepezil (Aricept), galantamine (Razadyne), rivastigmine (Exelon), memantine (Namenda)
Brain tumor	Depend on location; generally caused by increased ICP; can be primary tumor but typically metastasis	History, neurologic examination, imaging studies	None	Estrogen, surgery, radiation, chemotherapy
CVA	Depend on severity; speech difficulties, hemiplegia, confusion, loss of muscle coordination; caused by thrombus, embolus, hemorrhage	History, neurologic examination, CT, MRI	MRI, CT, carotid angiogram, echocardiogram, lumbar puncture with CSF pressure and analysis	Thrombolytics within 3 to 4 $\frac{1}{2}$ hours of when the symptoms first started, antiinflammatories, anticoagulants, hyperbaric oxygen, rehabilitation, supportive care
Encephalitis	Increased ICP, cerebral edema; caused by virus	History, lumbar puncture	CSF analysis, blood cultures, routine blood labs	Antivirals, supportive care
Epilepsy	*Grand mal:* Tonic-clonic muscle contractions *Petit mal:* Momentary absence, stare, amnesia; cause unknown	History, neurologic examination, CT, MRI, EEG	Blood work	Anticonvulsants phenytoin (Dilantin), carbamazepine (Tegretol), valproic acid (Depakene), gabapentin (Neurontin), levetiracetam (Keppra), clonazepam (Klonopin), lamotrigine (Lamictal)
Closed head injury caused by trauma	Depend on location and severity of injury; headache, increased ICP; caused by trauma	History, neurologic examination, CT, MRI, cranial x-ray studies, lumbar puncture	CSF analysis	Corticosteroids, diuretics; reduce ICP
Meningitis	Headache, flulike symptoms, nuchal rigidity, seizures	History, neurologic examination, Kernig's and Brudzinski's signs, lumbar puncture	CSF analysis, cultures	Antibiotics, analgesics, drugs to reduce cerebral edema, anticonvulsants, antiinflammatories
Migraine	Unilateral throbbing headache, nausea, vomiting, blurred vision; individual triggers, caused by combination of trigeminal nerve abnormality and imbalance of neurotransmitter serotonin	History, neurologic examination, MRI	Tests to rule out organic causes of headaches	NSAIDs, sumatriptan (Imitrex), rizatriptan (Maxalt), zolmitriptan (Zomig), topiramate (Topamax), gabapentin (Neurontin)
Multiple sclerosis	Problems with vision, sensation, motor function; autoimmune disease, progressive inflammation and deterioration (demyelination) of the myelin sheath	History, neurologic examination, MRI	None	Corticosteroids, interferon (Betaseron, Avonex), glatiramer acetate (Copaxone) fingolimod (Gilenya), and additional medications to treat fatigue, pain, spasticity, and bladder control problems
Parkinson's disease	Resting tremor, shuffling gait, masklike face; combination of genetic and environmental factors, deficiency of neurotransmitter dopamine	History, neurologic examination	None	Carbidopa-levodopa (Sinemet), pramipexole (Mirapex), ropinirole (Requip); surgical destruction of affected area of the brain; deep brain stimulation

CSF. Cerebro spinal fluid; *CT,* computed tomography; *CVA,* cerebrovascular accident; *EEG,* electroencephalogram; *ICP,* intracranial pressure; *MRI,* magnetic resonance imaging; *NSAIDs,* nonsteroidal antiinflammatory drugs.

Signs and Symptoms Suggesting Possible Neurologic Problems

- Recurrent headache
- Periodic memory loss
- Change in sleeping patterns
- Frequently dropping items
- Difficulty with particular speech patterns
- Numbness in a specific body area
- Visual disturbances or abrupt changes in vision
- Loss of consciousness
- Confusion or disorientation as to date, time, and place

Transient Ischemic Attacks

Transient ischemic attacks (TIAs), also called *ministrokes,* occur when the blood supply to a particular part of the brain is inadequate for a limited time, and symptoms typically disappear within an hour. TIAs occur when brain tissue becomes **ischemic** for a short time, causing the same symptoms as a stroke. Because the cause of the ischemia is limited, the symptoms dissipate quickly. Symptoms can include numbness or weakness in the face, arm, or leg or on one side of the body; confusion or difficulty talking or understanding speech; vision abnormalities, including **diplopia**; difficulty walking; and vertigo or loss of balance and coordination.

These episodes may occur in the days, weeks, or months before a stroke. Patients and their families should understand that any strokelike symptom should be taken seriously. Approximately one third of individuals experiencing TIAs have an acute stroke sometime in the future. Therefore, those experiencing TIAs should be seen within 1 hour of the onset of symptoms so that they can be evaluated carefully and treated to prevent a possible stroke. Depending on the person's health history and the results of a medical examination, the provider will recommend medications or surgery to reduce the risk of stroke. Individuals with atrial fibrillation (an irregular, rapid firing of electrical activity in the atria of the heart) may be prescribed anticoagulants (e.g., heparin or warfarin [Coumadin]), or they may be put on daily low-dose aspirin or clopidogrel (Plavix), because these individuals are at increased risk of emboli formation. When TIAs occur, it is time for preventive treatment and patient education, including altering and/or treating such factors as hypertension, smoking, heart disease, diabetes, carotid artery disease (carotid artery occlusion with atherosclerotic plaques), and heavy alcohol abuse.

Cerebrovascular Accident

A cerebrovascular accident (CVA) is the most important clinical manifestation of CVD. A CVA, commonly referred to as a *stroke,* occurs when a vessel in the brain either ruptures or becomes occluded, and brain cells on the other side of the damaged vessel become oxygen deprived. Cerebral artery ruptures are caused by uncontrolled hypertension or hemorrhaging of a weakened section of an artery in the brain. As a result of the rupture, the surrounding brain tissue fills with blood, damaging and possibly destroying the affected tissue. An occlusion occurs when an embolus or thrombus becomes wedged

in an artery and obstructs the flow of blood to an area of the brain (Figure 37-5).

The patient's symptoms depend on the location of the arterial occlusion or rupture. Some of the more common symptoms include slurred speech; unexplained confusion; sudden, severe headache; difficulty swallowing; vertigo; diplopia; loss of consciousness; personality change; loss of bowel or bladder control; and paralysis on one side of the body. The diagnosis of a CVA begins with a physical examination to assess the patient for the signs and symptoms of a stroke. The exam is repeated over time to see whether symptoms are getting worse or improving. The medical assistant should immediately check the patient's blood pressure to determine whether the cause of the CVA is hypertension. The physician will also listen to the carotid arteries with a stethoscope for a bruit. If a **bruit** is present, it indicates atherosclerotic buildup in the carotid arteries. The CVA may have been caused by a piece of the plaque that broke off and became lodged in a cerebral blood vessel.

The type of CVA must be determined as soon as possible so that the best treatment can be provided. The following diagnostic studies are ordered immediately:

- Angiogram of the head to look for a blood vessel that is blocked or bleeding
- Carotid duplex (ultrasound) to see whether the carotid arteries are blocked or narrowed
- Echocardiogram to see whether the stroke was caused by a blood clot from the heart (this frequently occurs with atrial fibrillation)
- Magnetic resonance angiography (MRA) or CT angiography to check for abnormal blood vessels in the brain; this confirms the presence of a vessel bleed

Treatment of a stroke requires immediate emergency transport to the hospital. The initial emphasis is on minimizing the long-term disabilities often seen with strokes by providing immediate treatment to prevent additional brain tissue damage. Thrombolytic drugs to dissolve the clot and anticoagulants may be given if the cause of the stroke was a thrombus or an embolus. However, thrombolytic medication can effectively treat resulting ischemia only if they are given within the first 3 to $4\frac{1}{2}$ hours of when the symptoms first started. The sooner this treatment begins, the better the chance of a good outcome. If cerebral edema is present, the patient is treated with corticosteroids and diuretics to reverse the swelling. Hyperbaric oxygen also can be used to increase oxygenation of the brain. An important part of recovery is extensive treatment in a stroke rehabilitation program that includes physical, occupational, swallowing, and speech therapies.

CRITICAL THINKING APPLICATION 37-2

Mai answers the phone at the clinic. The caller is a patient, an anxious woman who is desperately trying to say something but appears unable to do so. Mai thinks the patient is trying to say something like "Help." Mai checks the number on the caller ID display, looks it up in the office computer, and finds that it belongs to a 50-year-old patient who came in 2 days earlier because of frequent, severe headaches and hypertension. How should Mai handle this situation? Be sure to think about what she should do, why she should do it, and what might happen if she does nothing.

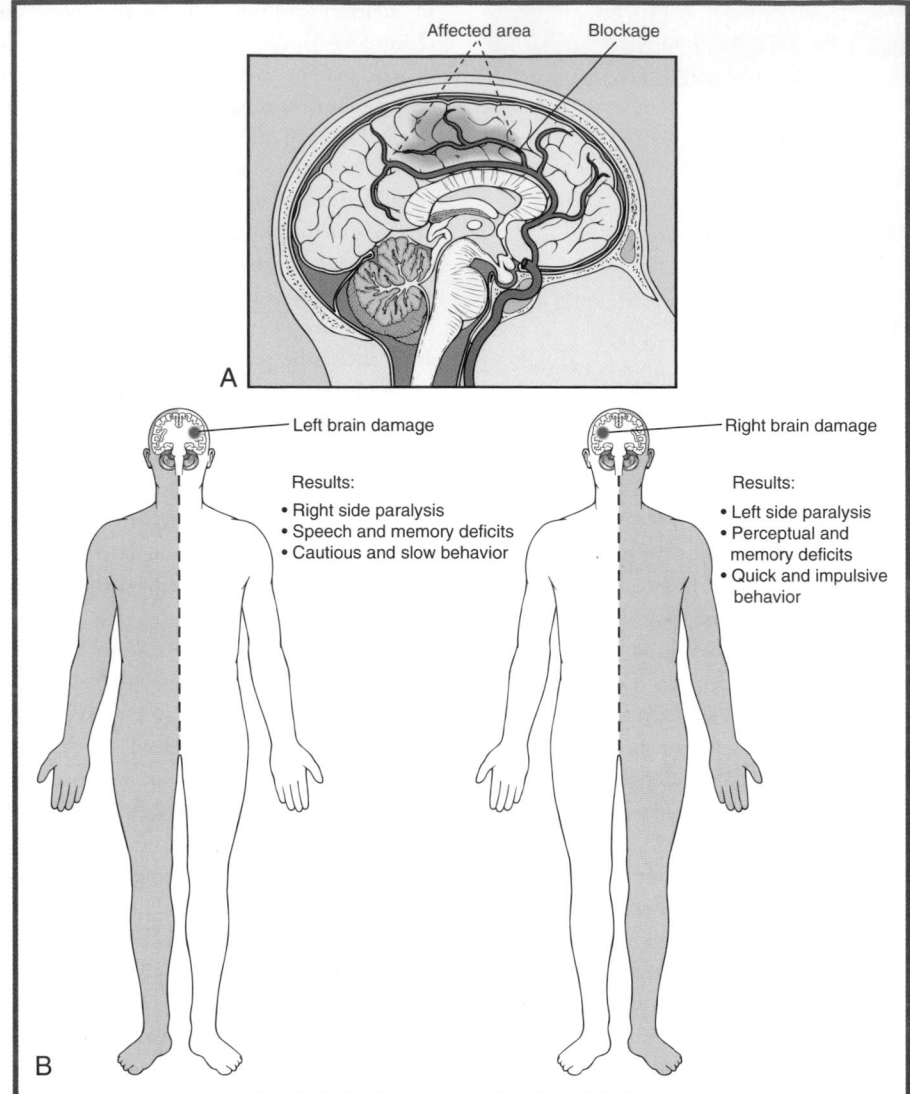

FIGURE 37-5 Cerebral artery occlusion **(A)** and hemiplegia **(B).** (Modified from Frazier MS, Drzymkowski JW: *Essentials of human diseases and conditions,* ed 5, St Louis, 2013, Saunders.)

Types, Causes, and Risks of Cerebrovascular Accidents

Thrombotic stroke: A blood clot (thrombus) forms in a cerebral artery and blocks distal blood flow.

Embolic stroke: A blood clot from elsewhere in the body (e.g., the lower leg) or a piece of plaque (typically from the carotid arteries) breaks away and flows through the bloodstream to the brain; the embolus eventually blocks a cerebral artery, causing distal ischemia.

Cerebral hemorrhage: An artery in the brain ruptures, possibly because of untreated or uncontrolled hypertension or a congenital aneurysm.

Any of the following factors can increase the risk of a stroke:

- Hypertension
- Diabetes (increases the risk by two to three times)
- Hypercholesterolemia
- Cigarette smoking (increases the risk by 50%)
- Obesity
- Family history of stroke; risk of a first stroke is nearly twice as high for African-Americans

- Endocarditis (may promote thrombus formation)
- Arteriosclerosis and atherosclerosis
- Heart disease (e.g., atrial fibrillation, which increases the risk by five times)
- Sleep apnea
- Sickle cell anemia
- Cocaine abuse

Individuals with three or more of the following five health conditions are twice as likely to have a cerebrovascular accident:

- Obesity
- Low level of high-density lipoprotein (HDL) cholesterol
- High triglyceride level
- Blood pressure ≥130/85 mm Hg
- Diabetes and/or prediabetes (fasting blood sugar of 100 to 125 mg/dL)

www.cdc.gov/stroke/facts.htm. Accessed January 19, 2015

Migraine Headache

About 12% of the U.S. population suffers from migraine headaches; three times more women than men are affected. Migraine headaches are **paroxysmal** attacks of headaches that can be completely incapacitating and frequently are associated with other symptoms, such as nausea, vomiting, visual disturbances, and throbbing pain on one side of the head. The manifestations of migraine headaches differ from one individual to another. The patient may experience a sensory warning sign, or **aura**, before the onset of the headache. An aura often consists of some form of visual disturbance, such as dark lines or spots within the visual field or a flash of light.

Medical science has not yet discovered the underlying cause of migraines. However, researchers believe they may be caused by a combination of a problem with the trigeminal nerve and an imbalance of chemicals in the brain, especially the neurotransmitter serotonin. Individuals who suffer from migraine headaches report a number of different triggers, including changes in estrogen levels; certain foods, such as alcohol, chocolate, aspartame, caffeine, and monosodium glutamate (MSG); elevated stress levels; bright lights, sun glare, and certain smells; altered sleep patterns; and changes in the weather, especially with changing altitude levels and barometric pressures. The diagnosis usually is established from a complete medical history. An EEG, a CT scan, or an MRI study may be performed as part of the diagnostic process to rule out other causes of the headaches.

Drugs used to treat migraines include nonsteroidal anti-inflammatory drugs (NSAIDs) and triptans, such as sumatriptan (Imitrex), rizatriptan (Maxalt), and zolmitriptan (Zomig), which mimic the effects of serotonin, causing vascular constriction. These drugs must be taken at the onset of the headache to be effective and can be delivered via different routes: oral medications, nasal sprays, or intravenously (IV). Other medications recommended for the prevention of migraines include beta blockers and antidepressants. Antiseizure medications, such as topiramate (Topamax) and gabapentin (Neurontin), may be effective in reducing the frequency and severity of the headaches. Other treatments include biofeedback techniques and elimination diets to avoid migraine triggers.

Dementia and Alzheimer's Disease

The term *dementia* describes a group of symptoms caused by altered brain function. Dementia symptoms may include short-term memory loss; disorientation about person, time, and place; neglect of personal hygiene, nutrition, and safety; personality changes; and inability to follow simple directions. Dementia can be caused by multiple conditions. Some can be reversed, such as nutrition disorders or disorientation caused by a minor head injury. Others are irreversible, such as multi-infarct (vascular) dementia and Alzheimer's disease.

Multi-infarct dementia is caused by a series of small strokes that interfere with the brain's blood supply, resulting in multiple areas of tissue necrosis. The location of the infarcts determines the degree of disability and the dementia symptoms that might occur. Symptoms of an acute onset of dementia typically are caused by this type of dementia. People with multi-infarct dementia are likely to show signs of improvement or remain stable for long periods and then quickly develop new symptoms if more strokes occur. Untreated or uncontrolled hypertension usually is the cause of this type of dementia.

Alzheimer's disease is the most common form of dementia among older people today. It is a devastating, chronic, progressive, and degenerative disease that begins in the parts of the brain that control thought, memory, and language. The patient exhibits slow, increasing loss of recent memory; loss of recognition of people, places, and events; confusion and disorientation; and physical deterioration that leads to death. The cause remains unknown, and there is no known cure. Treatment is supportive care only. Alzheimer's disease is talked about in more detail in the Geriatrics chapter.

CRITICAL THINKING APPLICATION   **37-3**

Mr. Jackson, a 75-year-old patient with dementia, is coming in for his first visit. He does not respond to verbal commands and is unable to answer direct questions. How can Mai get him into the examination room and into a patient gown while preserving his dignity?

Epilepsy and Seizure Disorders

Epilepsy is a chronic brain disorder associated with abnormal electrical impulses generated by some of the neurons in the brain. These errant impulses cause seizures (Figure 37-6). A seizure is characterized by abnormalities in levels of consciousness, sensory disturbances, and impaired motor function. A diagnosis of a seizure disorder is made if the individual has two or more seizures. Children may have a single seizure associated with a high fever (i.e., febrile seizure), but that alone does not mean that the child has a seizure disorder. However, most individuals with the disorder have an onset of seizures during childhood, although many children grow out of the problem. In many cases the cause is never identified; some known causes include brain tumors, CNS infections, anoxia, CVA, and traumatic head injury.

Seizures are classified as either partial or generalized, based on how much of the brain is involved in the abnormal electrical activity. Partial seizures result from abnormal electrical activity in just one part of the brain, whereas generalized seizures involve most or all of the brain. Seizure classifications are divided into more specific categories. Simple partial seizures originate in a small, localized area of the brain, do not cause loss of consciousness, and are identified by a repetitive action, such as shaking of an arm or a leg or altered speech. Complex partial seizures also begin in a small area of the brain but cause staring and repeated movements, such as hand rubbing, lip smacking, swallowing, and postseizure confusion or amnesia. Generalized seizures include petit mal seizures, which are brief episodes characterized by staring, subtle body movement, and brief lapses of awareness.

Probably the best-known seizure disorder is the generalized tonic clonic form that causes grand mal seizures, with loss of consciousness and tonic (stiffening) muscle contractions, followed by clonic (twitching, jerking) muscle contractions of the limbs, clenched teeth, and/or loss of bowel or bladder control. After the shaking subsides, the individual may fall asleep or appear confused for a few minutes. The patient may experience an aura, usually a sensory warning (e.g., a specific smell or taste) before a grand mal seizure.

Diagnosis depends on an accurate seizure history, EEG, and CT or MRI scans. Seizures cannot be cured but usually can be controlled effectively by pharmaceutical treatment; however, finding the most

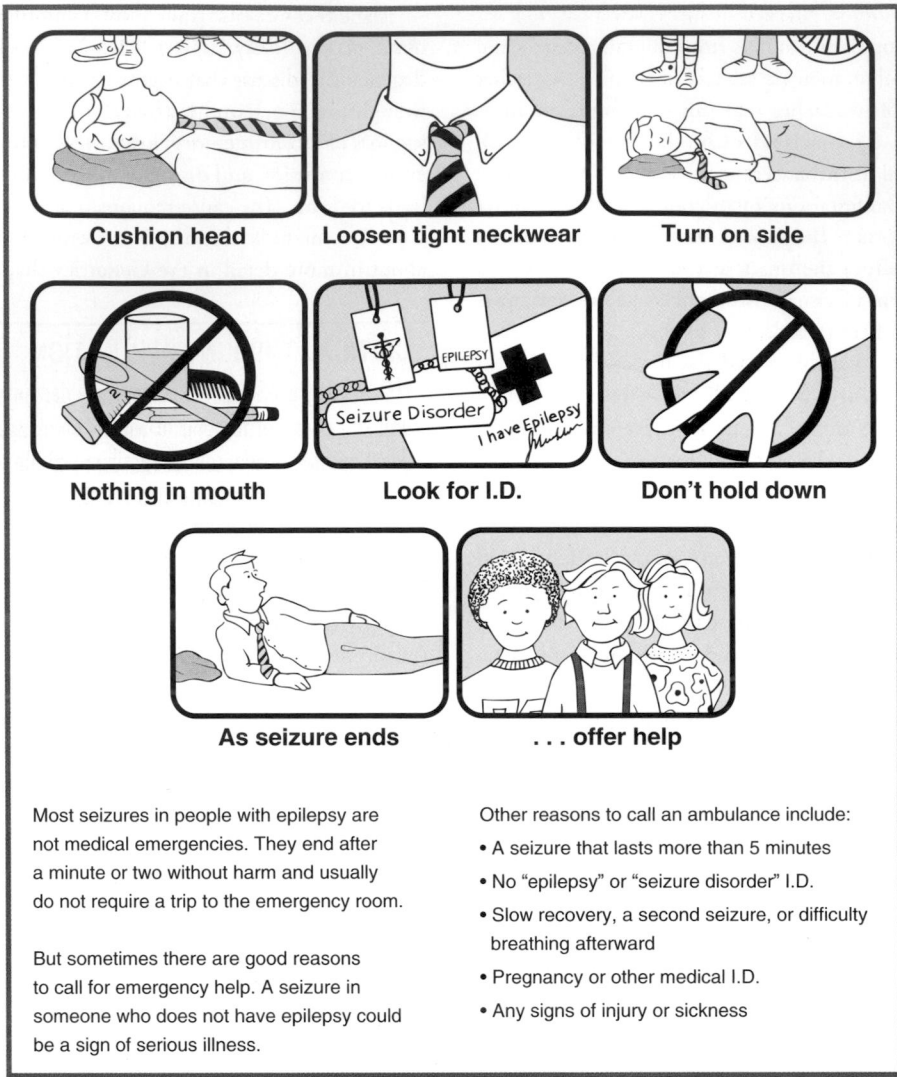

Cushion head   **Loosen tight neckwear**   **Turn on side**

Nothing in mouth   **Look for I.D.**   **Don't hold down**

As seizure ends   **. . . offer help**

Most seizures in people with epilepsy are not medical emergencies. They end after a minute or two without harm and usually do not require a trip to the emergency room.

But sometimes there are good reasons to call for emergency help. A seizure in someone who does not have epilepsy could be a sign of serious illness.

Other reasons to call an ambulance include:

• A seizure that lasts more than 5 minutes
• No "epilepsy" or "seizure disorder" I.D.
• Slow recovery, a second seizure, or difficulty breathing afterward
• Pregnancy or other medical I.D.
• Any signs of injury or sickness

FIGURE 37-6 First aid for seizures. (Modified from *www.epilepsyfoundation.org*.)

effective medication at the right dose can be complex. Depending on the seizure type, different medications are prescribed. Some individuals with epilepsy require more than one drug or have to try multiple medications until the most effective one is found. Antiseizure (anticonvulsant) medications include phenytoin (Dilantin), carbamazepine (Tegretol), valproic acid (Depakene), gabapentin (Neurontin), levetiracetam (Keppra), clonazepam (Klonopin), and lamotrigine (Lamictal). It is very important that patients know never to stop taking their seizure medication without the physician's supervision because this may trigger more frequent and severe seizure episodes.

Central Nervous System Infections

Encephalitis

Most cases of encephalitis are viral in origin and are transmitted to humans from mosquitoes and ticks or are caused by other infections, such as herpes infections. In mild cases symptoms include stiff neck and headache, muscle aches, **malaise**, and general flulike symptoms. In more severe cases, the symptoms can include fever, delirium, seizures, **coma**, and even death.

Encephalitis is diagnosed by an MRI or a CT scan of the brain; lumbar puncture with CSF analysis, including cultures to determine the causative microorganism; EEG; and blood tests to detect viral antibodies. A patient with cerebral inflammation from encephalitis may suffer from confusion, disorientation, and other behavioral changes. These symptoms are part of the disease and usually disappear when the condition improves.

Patient management treats the symptoms and is aimed at controlling fever and seizure activity, in addition to constant monitoring of respiratory and urinary functions. Viral encephalitis is treated with antiviral medications, such as acyclovir (Zovirax) and foscarnet (Foscavir); if the condition is caused by herpes simplex, acyclovir (Zovirax) or ganciclovir (Cytovene) is prescribed; bacterial encephalitis is treated with antibiotics. In patients with severe CNS damage, recovery usually is prolonged, and physical therapy is necessary to overcome the neurologic and musculoskeletal complications.

Meningitis

Meningitis is an infection and inflammation of the meninges and CSF of the brain and spinal cord that can be caused by viruses, bacteria, or fungi. Meningitis is transmitted from an infected individual through coughing, sneezing, kissing, or sharing personal items, such as eating utensils or a toothbrush. Viral meningitis usually is mild and has flulike symptoms that typically resolve in about 2 weeks without treatment. Fungal meningitis is seen in patients with immune deficiencies, such as acquired immunodeficiency syndrome (AIDS), and can be life-threatening. Acute bacterial meningitis can occur as a complication of an earlier infection of the ears, sinuses, or lungs, or it can be transmitted from an infected person.

Distinguishing between the types of meningitis is difficult but extremely important for effective, early treatment. *Haemophilus* meningitis was once the most common form of bacterial meningitis but the *Haemophilus influenzae* b (Hib) pediatric vaccine has greatly reduced the number of cases. Bacterial meningitis can be quite serious; symptoms include a high fever, severe headache, stiff neck, photophobia, confusion, seizures, and positive Brudzinski's and Kernig's signs. The diagnosis is confirmed by analysis of a CSF sample, which is tested for bacteria or blood; glucose levels (low levels occur in bacterial or fungal meningitis); and white blood cells (elevated WBCs indicate infection). The procedure is done in a hospital and takes about 45 minutes. Additional diagnostic tests include a CT scan to identify brain swelling, hemorrhage, or abscess and/or an MRI scan, which produces clearer pictures than a CT scan and can help identify brain and spinal cord inflammation and infection. The individual typically is ordered antibiotics and antiviral medications while waiting for final laboratory results because a delay in treatment can be life-threatening. The patient also is treated with analgesics and medications to reduce cerebral edema. Despite treatment, bacterial meningitis can be fatal or can cause long-term neurologic damage.

Brain and Spinal Cord Injuries

Traumatic brain injuries are caused by a blow or jolt to the head. They may be limited to a particular section of the brain or may result in generalized neurologic damage. Injuries can range from a mild concussion to severe injury, coma, and death. A minor concussion usually has no long-term side effects; however, a moderate to severe brain injury can result in headaches, amnesia, confusion, personality changes, and seizures. Spinal cord injuries usually result from severe, accidental trauma to the back or neck. These injuries are most common in the 16- to 30-year-old age group and are associated with automobile and sports accidents. The higher the damage to the spinal cord, the more serious the injury.

The extent of CNS injury can be limited with the proper use of child car seats, adult safety belts, helmets in childhood sports and activities, and reducing the frequency of drinking and driving. Several types of brain injuries can occur, depending on the type and amount of force with which the head is struck.

Cerebral Concussion and Contusion

Concussion is the mildest and the most common type of brain injury. Trauma from an impact or a sudden change in motion can cause a concussion with loss of consciousness, which may last seconds to several minutes and may be followed by a period of disorientation that lasts up to 24 hours (Figure 37-7). A single concussion may disrupt the normal electrical activity in the brain, but the brain usually is not injured permanently. However, research has shown that the damage from multiple concussions may be

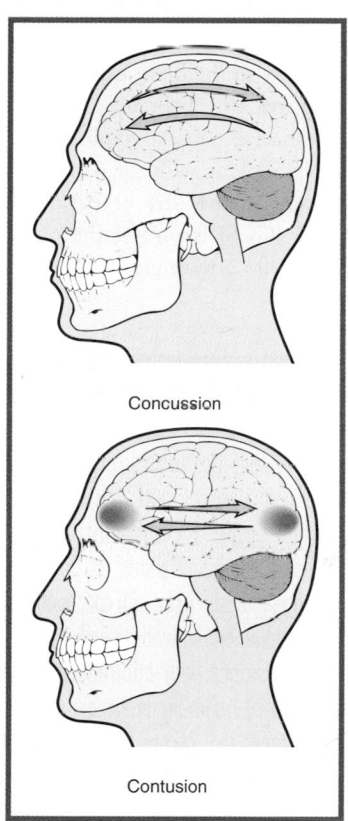

FIGURE 37-7 Brain concussion and contusion. (Modified from Frazier MS, Drzymkowski JW: *Essentials of human diseases and conditions,* ed 5, St Louis, 2013, Saunders.)

Signs of a Concussion

Signs of a concussion that occur seconds to minutes after a head injury include:

- Possible loss of consciousness
- Difficulty focusing, with slowed responses
- Slurred speech
- Nausea and vomiting
- Headache
- Blurred vision
- Confusion and disorientation or amnesia

The patient should be seen immediately if he or she reports any of the following signs and symptoms days or weeks after a head injury:

- Persistent headache
- Vertigo (dizziness)
- Inability to concentrate
- Repeated problems with memory
- Nausea or vomiting (especially if vomiting is projectile)
- Unusual anger, irritability, anxiety, or depression
- Sleep disorders
- Seizures

TABLE 37-4	Glasgow Coma Scale				
SCORE	1	2	3	4	5
Eye opening	No response	To pain	To voice	Spontaneously	
Best motor response (movement of arms and legs)	No response	Extension to pain	Flexion to pain	Localizes to pain	Follows commands
Best verbal response	No response	Incomprehensible sounds	Inappropriate words	Disoriented and converses	Oriented and converses

Scoring: 13 to 15, mild head injury; 9 to 12, moderate head injury; 3 to 8, severe head injury.

cumulative. No one knows how many concussions are too many before permanent damage occurs. The medical assistant should help gather a comprehensive head injury history so that the provider is aware of all previous concussions, including those that occurred outside playing sports, to determine when or if a child should return to sports activities.

A more serious injury to the brain can cause the formation of a contusion, or bruised area, usually because of a skull fracture. Symptoms can include headache, nausea, vomiting, vision disturbances, and sensitivity to light. Talking with the patient may reveal reduced levels of concentration, irritability, or periods of amnesia. The Glasgow Coma Scale (GCS) is one of the most commonly used severity scoring systems for assessing coma and impaired consciousness (Table 37-4).

Brain Injuries

The Centers for Disease Control and Prevention (CDC) has developed a free, downloadable tool kit, "Heads Up: Brain Injury in Your Practice," which is available at the following website: *http://www.cdc.gov/headsup/index .html*. It provides practical, easy-to-use clinical tools for assessing and managing head injuries. Medical assistants should be knowledgeable about the potentially serious damage that can occur with concussions and the importance of early diagnosis. Information on the website includes:

- A booklet for physicians with information on the diagnosis and management of mild traumatic brain injury (MTBI) or concussion
- A patient assessment tool (Acute Concussion Evaluation [ACE])
- A care plan to help guide a patient's recovery
- Fact sheets in English and Spanish on preventing concussion
- A palm card for on-field management of sports-related concussion (ideal for education of coaches)

From *http://www.cdc.gov/headsup/index.html*. Accessed February 11, 2016.

CRITICAL THINKING APPLICATION   37-4

- Mai is putting together information on head injuries for the family of a patient who recently suffered a minor concussion. The family should watch for what symptoms? When should the family seek additional medical care? What resources could Mai use to develop the pamphlet?
- Dr. Song said he would approve the pamphlet after Mai completed it, but he was called away on an emergency before he saw it. A patient sees it behind the desk and asks to take one. Should Mai let him? Why or why not?

Open and Closed Head Injuries

In a closed head injury, a brain injury occurs but the skull is not fractured. A more serious brain injury can occur with an open head injury because the skull is fractured or displaced. A serious head injury can cause life-threatening damage to the intracerebral structures. Subarachnoid hemorrhage may occur when the delicate meningeal blood vessels are ruptured, resulting in the collection of blood in the subarachnoid space. This causes a rapid increase in intracranial pressure, which may give rise to sudden, severe headache; nausea and severe projectile vomiting; motor disturbances; visual disturbances; and seizures. In addition to trauma, other predisposing factors that can cause subarachnoid hemorrhage include hypertension, a family history of the condition, and congenital malformations of cranial blood vessels. Treatment is designed to reduce the intracranial pressure, sometimes surgically.

A subdural hematoma develops when blood collects in the space between the dura mater and the arachnoid layers of the meninges, usually as a result of head trauma that has caused slow bleeding from ruptured blood vessels in the meningeal layers. Symptoms of increased intracranial pressure occur over several days as the hematoma increases in size. Signs and symptoms build over time and include headache, motor disturbances, speech abnormalities, nausea and vomiting, seizures, and a decreased level of consciousness. Treatment requires surgery to stop the bleeding and reduce the pressure inside the skull. People age 75 or older are at greatest risk of developing a subdural hematoma after a minor fall.

Shaken Baby Syndrome

Shaken baby syndrome is the most common reason for serious head injury in infants. It is caused by violently shaking the infant back and forth, forcing the brain against opposite ends of the skull. Shaking is so dangerous for babies because of their small size compared to their relatively large head size, in addition to their undeveloped neck muscles. The typical presentation is a child approximately 6 months old who is brought to the clinic or emergency department because of difficulty breathing or marked lethargy. Usually little or no external bruising or trauma is seen. Physical findings on examination or autopsy include a subdural hematoma and retinal hemorrhages. The history given by the caregiver usually indicates that the baby "fell" from the sofa, coffee table, or bed or was "dropped." Approximately one fourth of these infants die of their injuries.

Spinal Cord Injuries

If a traumatic accident completely transects the spinal cord, all CNS stimulation to nerves distal to the injury stops, resulting in paralysis of the areas below the injury. The most common causes of spinal cord

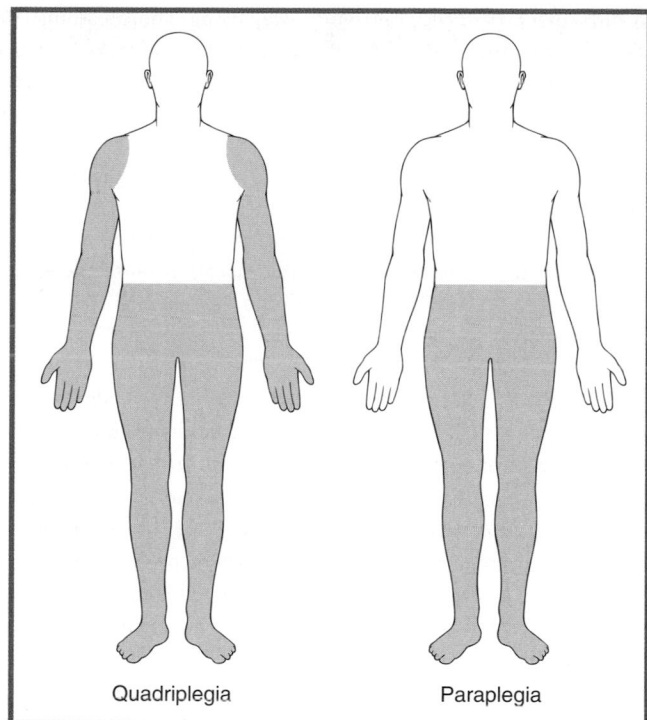

FIGURE 37-8 Types of paralysis: quadriplegia and paraplegia. (Modified from Frazier MS, Drzymkowski JW: *Essentials of human diseases and conditions,* ed 5, St Louis, 2013, Saunders.)

injuries in the United States are car or motorcycle accidents; falls, especially in those over age 65; violence; sports injuries; and diseases that cause inflammation of the spinal cord, including arthritis and cancer. Paralysis from spinal cord **transection** is classified into one of two categories (Figure 37-8). In *paraplegia,* transection occurs below the midpoint of the spinal cord, causing paralysis of both legs; loss of function below the level of injury, including loss of bladder and bowel control; and sexual dysfunction in males. In *quadriplegia,* transection occurs in the upper thoracic or cervical region of the spinal cord, causing paralysis of all four limbs, respiratory difficulty, and loss of function to all muscles below the injury point. *Hemiplegia* is unrelated to spinal cord injury and occurs when a CVA, a vascular injury such as a ruptured aneurysm, or a tumor occurs on one side of the brain, resulting in paralysis on the opposite side of the body.

No surgery or treatment can restore a transected cord, although much research currently is under way, including electrical stimulation of nerves and medications to promote nerve cell regeneration or improve the function of the nerves that remain after a spinal cord injury. Treatment also includes surgical stabilization of the spine, physical and occupational therapy, and the use of assistive devices. If the spinal cord is injured but not completely transected, the degree of paralysis depends on the degree of injury. Such patients usually respond well to physical therapy, and their ability to restore motor function is good, although they may always have some functional limitations.

Additional Central Nervous System Pathologies

Parkinson's Disease

Parkinson's disease (PD) is a chronic, progressive, debilitating disease that affects about 1% of individuals over age 60; more than 50,000 new cases are reported annually in the United States. PD is slightly more common in men than women. The four primary symptoms of

PD are tremors of the hands, arms, legs, jaw, and face; rigidity of the limbs and trunk; bradykinesia, or slowness of movement; and postural instability with impaired balance and coordination. The typical presentation of PD includes a unilateral, pill-rolling tremor; a high-pitched, monotone voice; difficulty swallowing; a masklike facial expression; and bowed head and forward-bent posture. Tremors and rigidity increase in severity over time. Currently there are no laboratory tests specific for PD; therefore, the diagnosis is based on a comprehensive medical history and neurologic examination.

Parkinson's disease is believed to be caused by a combination of genetic and environmental factors that result in a deficiency of the neurotransmitter dopamine in the brain. It is diagnosed with a comprehensive neurologic examination to determine symptoms and their severity. There is no test that clearly identifies the disease. PD has no cure, but the most common medication prescribed for symptomatic relief is carbidopa-levodopa (Sinemet). Levodopa enters the brain and is converted to dopamine; carbidopa increases levodopa's effectiveness and prevents or decreases many of the side effects of levodopa. Dopamine agonists, which mimic the effects of dopamine, are also prescribed; these include pramipexole (Mirapex) and ropinirole (Requip). Although the initial response to medical treatment can reflect dramatic relief of symptoms, over time the body's response to parkinsonian medications declines. Surgical destruction of the most affected area of the brain may produce some relief of symptoms.

Another treatment option is deep brain stimulation (DBS), in which a surgically implanted device similar to a cardiac pacemaker delivers electrical stimulation to specific areas in the brain that control movement; this also blocks the abnormal nerve signals that cause PD symptoms.

Tumors

The symptoms of a brain tumor depend on the type and location of the mass, but generally the initial symptoms are headaches, vomiting, dizziness, diplopia, and alterations in muscle strength and coordination. Changes in personality and mental function, seizures, progressive paralysis, loss of speech, and sensory disorders appear as the tumor enlarges.

CNS tumors can be diagnosed by means of CT, MRI, EEG, or lumbar puncture. Ophthalmoscopic examination may reveal **papilledema**. Accurate diagnosis of a brain tumor includes determining its precise location in the brain and whether it is **benign** or **malignant**. Approximately half of all brain tumors are metastatic growths from other primary cancer sites in the body. Lung cancer, breast cancer, and melanoma frequently spread to the brain by metastasis. Regardless of whether the mass is benign or malignant, as brain tumors grow, they cause serious problems and complications for the patient because of the limited space inside the skull. Treatment of brain tumors can include surgery, chemotherapy, and radiation in any combination.

CRITICAL THINKING APPLICATION   **37-5**

A 34-year-old man has just found out that he has a brain tumor, and Mai is to schedule him for surgery next week. Before he leaves the office, he says he wants to talk to Mai privately. They go into an examination room, and he says, "Tell me the truth; this is cancer, and I'm going to die, right?" How should Mai respond to this frightened patient?

DISEASES OF THE PERIPHERAL NERVOUS SYSTEM

Multiple Sclerosis

The axon of a nerve cell is covered with a myelin sheath to protect and insulate electrical stimulation as it passes to the terminal end of the neuron. Multiple sclerosis (MS) is an autoimmune disease that causes progressive inflammation and deterioration (demyelination) of the myelin sheath; this leaves nerve fibers uncovered, which results in scattering of the nervous message as it passes down the axon. Myelinated axons are commonly called *white matter*. Researchers have learned that MS also damages the nerve cell bodies, which are found in the brain's *gray matter*, in addition to the axons themselves in the brain, spinal cord, and optic nerve. The term *multiple sclerosis* refers to the distinctive areas of scar tissue (sclerosis, or *plaques*) present in the white matter of people who have MS. These areas are visible on MRI brain scans.

There is no single test used to diagnose MS. Diagnosis is difficult because the signs and symptoms of the disease mimic those of other neurologic disorders. Diagnostic studies include a complete history and physical with a detailed neurologic examination and an MRI of the brain and spinal cord to look for distinctive plaques and areas of sclerosis from scar tissue at the inflammation sites. MS frequently is diagnosed by the exacerbation and remission of neurologic symptoms characteristic of the condition. Patients cycle through remission and relapse with an ever-increasing degree of dysfunction after each episode.

Early symptoms may include numbness, **paresthesia**, diplopia, **ataxia**, and bladder control problems. As the disease progresses, patients experience increased spasticity, vertigo, depression, gait problems, joint pain, fatigue, and varying degrees of paralysis. MS most commonly begins in women between the ages of 20 and 40. The cause remains unknown; however, the common belief is that it is due to a combination of genetic and environmental factors, including family history, living in a Northern climate, low vitamin D levels, smoking, and viral infection.

MS has no cure; therefore, treatment focuses on alleviating symptoms and delaying the progression of the disease. Medications used to treat the disease include corticosteroids during periods of **exacerbation**: interferon (Betaseron, Avonex) and glatiramer acetate (Copaxone) to reduce the frequency and severity of relapses; fingolimod (Gilenya) for relapsing forms of MS, and additional medications to treat fatigue, pain, spasticity, and bladder control problems. Some patients live an essentially normal life with only occasional attacks, whereas others experience rapidly progressive incapacitation.

Amyotrophic Lateral Sclerosis

Amyotrophic lateral sclerosis (ALS), or Lou Gehrig's disease, is a rapidly progressive, ultimately fatal neurologic disease that destroys the motor neurons responsible for voluntary muscle control. Without stimulation from motor neurons, muscles cannot function and gradually weaken and atrophy. The cause is unknown. The disease is more common among white males 60 to 69 years of age, but younger and older people also can develop the disease. In about 5% to 10% of individuals with ALS, the disease is inherited, with one parent carrying the faulty gene. The diagnosis is primarily based on symptoms and signs and a series of tests to rule out other diseases.

ALS usually begins with small, local, involuntary muscle contractions in the forearms and hands. As the disease progresses, the patient has difficulty with speech, chewing, swallowing, and breathing. In most cases the disease does not affect a person's personality, intelligence, or memory, nor does it affect the ability to see, smell, taste, hear, or recognize touch. The first drug treatment for the disease is riluzole (Rilutek), which reduces damage to motor neurons and prolongs survival, especially in patients with difficulty swallowing. Other treatments, which are **palliative**, include attempts to keep the individual as comfortable as possible and to help with pain, depression, sleep disturbances, and constipation. Death from failure of the respiratory muscles usually occurs within 3 to 5 years after the onset of symptoms.

Bell's Palsy

Bell's palsy is a temporary facial paralysis. It results from inflammation and edema of cranial nerve VII, which in turn are caused by a viral infection (e.g., herpes simplex or Epstein-Barr virus). The condition occurs suddenly, and symptoms reach their peak within 48 hours. The disorder usually subsides spontaneously over several weeks to months. Symptoms range in severity from mild weakness to complete paralysis on the affected side, depending on the degree of nervous involvement. The patient can experience facial twitching, eyelid drooping, excessive tearing of the affected eye, and drooping of the mouth with drooling of saliva. The patient is unable to close the eye on the affected side completely and may have taste disturbances. The antiviral drug acyclovir may be prescribed, in addition to prednisone to reduce the inflammation and control edema. The physician recommends an eye patch to protect the exposed eye, especially at night, to prevent corneal abrasions.

Peripheral Neuropathy

Peripheral neuropathy is not a disease in itself, but rather a condition of peripheral nerve dysfunction that can have more than 100 different known causes. It can be **cryptogenic**, or idiopathic, which means that the underlying cause cannot be identified. Conditions that can cause peripheral neuropathy include diabetes mellitus, human immunodeficiency virus (HIV) infection, nutritional deficiencies, and neurologic side effects of some medications. Symptoms usually affect the legs and arms and can include muscular weakness and pain or sensory disturbances such as burning, numbness, and tingling.

Symptoms can vary widely from person to person in both number and severity. Patients often feel extremely frustrated when they try to explain to the physician the abnormal sensations they are experiencing. Peripheral neuropathies can result from damage or injury to any portion of the neuron. Treatment of peripheral neuropathy is most effective when the causative condition is diagnosed and then treated successfully. Encouraging a healthy lifestyle, including weight control, exercise, a nutritious diet, and limiting or avoiding alcohol, helps control the physical and emotional effects of peripheral neuropathy.

Mental Health

Each year more than 44 million Americans are affected by a diagnosable mental condition that adversely affects their work, their relationships with family and friends, and their activities of daily living. Mental health disorders can be caused by a number of factors, alone or in combination, including changes in brain chemicals, hereditary makeup, psychological disposition, and life experiences. Emotional and physical symptoms can occur for no apparent reason and can be quite persistent. Emotional symptoms may include panic, apprehension, fear, anxiety, nightmares, withdrawal, flashbacks, and ritualized repetitive behaviors, such as constant hand washing. Possible physical symptoms include tachycardia, shortness of breath, sleep disturbances, gastrointestinal upset, muscular tension, and cold, clammy hands. Patients often do not associate these symptoms with a mental health disorder and therefore do not get the appropriate diagnosis and treatment.

Depressive Disorders

About 10% of adults in America experience depression each year. Almost twice as many women as men are affected by the disorder. Depression interferes with daily activities and causes pain and suffering not only to those who have the disorder, but also to those who care about them. Although multiple medications and psychosocial therapies are available to treat and manage depression, most individuals do not seek treatment. Depressive disorders affect the way a person thinks, feels, eats, and sleeps. People with depression cannot "snap out of it" and without treatment may experience symptoms that persist for weeks, months, or years.

Depressive disorders can be categorized as major depressive disorders, dysthymic disorders, and bipolar disorders. Individuals with major depression show a combination of symptoms that interfere with their ability to work, study, sleep, eat, and enjoy activities they once considered pleasurable. Dysthymic disorders are a less severe type of depression in which patients experience long-term, chronic symptoms that are not incapacitating but that affect their level of performance and daily emotions. Many people with dysthymia also experience major depression at some time in their lives. Individuals with bipolar disorders, also called *mood disorders* or *manic-depression*, cycle through a wide range of moods from extreme highs (mania) to extreme lows (depression). When in the depression cycle, they may show any or all of the symptoms of a depressive disorder. When cycling through mania, they may make decisions or act in a way that can be both embarrassing and dangerous. Manic individuals are extremely energetic and rarely sleep. If left untreated, the disorder can progress to a psychotic state.

Patients must understand that antidepressant medications take a minimum of 3 to 4 weeks for the full therapeutic effects of the drug to occur. Once they start to feel better, many individuals are tempted to stop taking the medication. *It is important to continue treatment for a minimum of 4 to 9 months to prevent a recurrence of the depression.* The patient should never stop taking antidepressant medication suddenly or without the direction of a physician. Individuals with bipolar disorders or chronic major depression may need maintenance therapy indefinitely.

Treatment for depression typically begins with a selective serotonin reuptake inhibitor (SSRI) because these medications have limited side effects. SSRIs include fluoxetine (Prozac), paroxetine (Paxil), sertraline (Zoloft), and citalopram (Celexa). Other medications include duloxetine (Cymbalta), venlafaxine, and bupropion (Wellbutrin). If the patient's symptoms are not relieved, the physician may order an older group of drugs called *tricyclic antidepressants* (TCAs), such as imipramine (Tofranil), which inhibit the reabsorption of serotonin and norepinephrine.

Recently, concern has arisen about the association of suicidal thoughts with antidepressant medications in children and adults in the first few weeks of treatment and also when dosages are altered. The U.S. Food and Drug Administration (FDA) has warned physicians to monitor patients closely when starting antidepressant therapy and to provide patient and family education on the importance of reporting to the physician any changes in symptoms.

Symptoms of Depression

According to the National Institute of Mental Health (NIMH), the severity of depressive symptoms varies among individuals and also with each episode. A discussion of the following symptoms can be found at the NIMH website: *http://www.nimh.nih.gov/index.shtml.*

- Persistent sad, anxious, or "empty" feeling
- Feelings of hopelessness and pessimism
- Feelings of guilt, worthlessness, and helplessness
- Loss of interest or pleasure in hobbies and activities that once were enjoyed, including sex
- Decreased energy and complaints of fatigue
- Difficulty concentrating, remembering, and making decisions
- Insomnia, early morning awakening, or oversleeping
- Either anorexia and weight loss or overeating and weight gain
- Thoughts of death or suicide, with possible suicide attempts
- Restlessness, irritability
- Persistent physical complaints that do not respond to treatment (e.g., headaches, gastrointestinal disturbances, or chronic pain)

Anxiety Disorders

Anxiety disorders affect approximately 19 million American adults. The primary symptoms are an overwhelming, irrational feeling of anxiety and fear. Anxiety disorders include panic disorder, obsessive-compulsive disorder (OCD), post-traumatic stress disorder (PTSD), and phobias. Individuals with panic disorder report feelings of terror that strike unexpectedly and are accompanied by nausea, chest pain, palpitations, diaphoresis, weakness, vertigo, syncope, and a fear of impending doom or loss of control. People with OCD experience anxious thoughts or images (obsessions) that they cannot control, so they resort to performing specific rituals (compulsions) to try to prevent or dispel the obsession. For example, an individual may be obsessed with germs or dirt, so he or she repeatedly washes the hands; or an individual may have to check repeatedly to make sure a door is locked because of fear that it will be left open. Performing the ritual does not bring pleasure, only temporary relief of the anxiety caused by the obsession, which will grow if the compulsion is not performed.

PTSD can occur after a patient is a part of or witnesses some terrifying, horrendous, or violent physical or emotional event, such as assault, battery, rape, war, natural disasters, acts of terrorism, and serious accidents during which many people are killed or injured. The person who survives the ordeal often has flashbacks; feelings of panic, fear, or guilt; constant replaying of the event in his or her mind; or deep feelings of emotional numbness.

As a result, the person is constantly on guard for a possible threat; has an exaggerated reaction when startled; and is frequently irritable, has difficulty concentrating, and experiences sleep problems. Severe depression and inability to function normally in daily activities also may be present.

A phobia is an intense, irrational fear of something that poses little or no actual danger. It may include such things as fear of heights, escalators, tunnels, and water. Although the individual may realize that the fear is unreasonable, just the thought of facing the feared object or situation causes a panic attack or severe anxiety. The two types of treatment for anxiety disorders are antianxiety medication, such as alprazolam (Xanax) or buspirone, and specific types of psychotherapy.

Schizophrenia

Schizophrenia is a chronic, severe, disabling brain disorder with symptoms that include hallucinations and delusions; difficulty speaking and expressing emotions; and cognitive deficits, such as problems with concentration and memory loss. Schizophrenia cannot be cured, but psychotic episodes can be reduced significantly by long-term, consistent pharmaceutical treatment. However, relapses are not unusual, because most individuals with schizophrenia stop taking their antipsychotic medication periodically because they feel better, they do not believe they need the medication, or they do not think that taking it regularly is important. In addition, the earliest antipsychotic medications, such as chlorpromazine (Thorazine) and haloperidol (Haldol), caused disturbing side effects, including rigidity, persistent muscle spasms, tremors, and restlessness. Newer drugs, which have limited side effects, include risperidone (Risperdal), olanzapine (Zyprexa), and aripiprazole (Abilify).

Suicide Facts from the National Institute of Mental Health

- More than 90% of individuals who commit suicide have a diagnosable mental disorder, typically depression, or are substance abusers.
- The highest suicide rate in the United States is seen in Caucasian men ages 45 to 59.
- Suicide is the tenth leading cause of death in the United States, but the third leading cause of death among 15- to 24-year-olds.
- Although women attempt suicide two to three times more often than men, four times as many men are successful.
- Twenty percent of those who commit suicide in the United States are veterans.
- Risk factors vary with age, gender, and ethnic group. They include serious depressive disorders; reduced levels of serotonin (a neurotransmitter); a prior suicide attempt; family violence, including physical or sexual abuse; and exposure to the suicidal behavior of others, including family members and peers.

www.nimh.nih.gov/health/statistics/suicide/index.shtml. Accessed January 20, 2015.

THE MEDICAL ASSISTANT'S ROLE IN THE NEUROLOGIC EXAMINATION

As with other physical examinations, a careful history provides the physician with valuable clues in diagnosing neurologic conditions. Such clues may include a record of seizures, syncope, diplopia, incontinence, or any of the previously mentioned subjective symptoms. The patient's general health often complicates a neurologic diagnosis.

The purposes of a neurologic examination are to determine whether a nervous system problem is present, to discover its location (or locations), and to identify the type and extent of the malfunction. During the examination, the physician may determine the effect of the symptoms on the patient's emotional status, intellectual performance, cognitive ability, and general behavior (Procedure 37-1). The patient's grooming and mannerisms are carefully observed, as is his or her ability to communicate effectively, including the appropriate use of speech, language, and writing skills. The medical assistant should listen carefully for difficulty putting words together, slurred speech, and whether the conversation makes sense. If you notice inappropriate changes in the patient, note them on the patient's record for the physician's attention and evaluation.

The physical examination of the neurologic system includes evaluation of the cranial nerves. You can assist by helping the patient assume the proper position necessary for each test and by having the instruments the physician needs ready for use. For example, cranial nerve I (the olfactory nerve) is tested by determining the patient's ability to identify familiar odors, such as coffee, tobacco, or cloves. Cranial nerve V (the trigeminal nerve) is checked by having the patient differentiate between warm and cold objects held against the right and left cheeks.

Peripheral nerve function is evaluated by examining the motor system, including muscular strength, gait, and movements. The diameters of the upper arms and the calves of the legs may be measured and compared to diagnose muscle atrophy. Motor functioning can be assessed through Romberg's test, in which the patient is asked to stand with the feet together, arms horizontal to the body, and eyes closed. The sensory system is examined by noting the patient's ability to perceive superficial sensations, such as a wisp of cotton brushed on the skin, a light pinprick, or hot and cold touching certain areas. Several deep tendon reflexes (DTRs), such as the patellar and Achilles reflexes, are checked (Figure 37-9). Babinski's reflex is tested by stroking the lateral aspect of the sole of the foot with a dull instrument (e.g., the handle of a reflex hammer or a tongue blade). For a positive Babinski's sign, the great toe dorsiflexes while the other toes fan out. This may indicate a possible stroke or brain lesion. Other diagnostic tests may include a skull radiograph, carotid arteriogram, EEG, and MRI and CT studies.

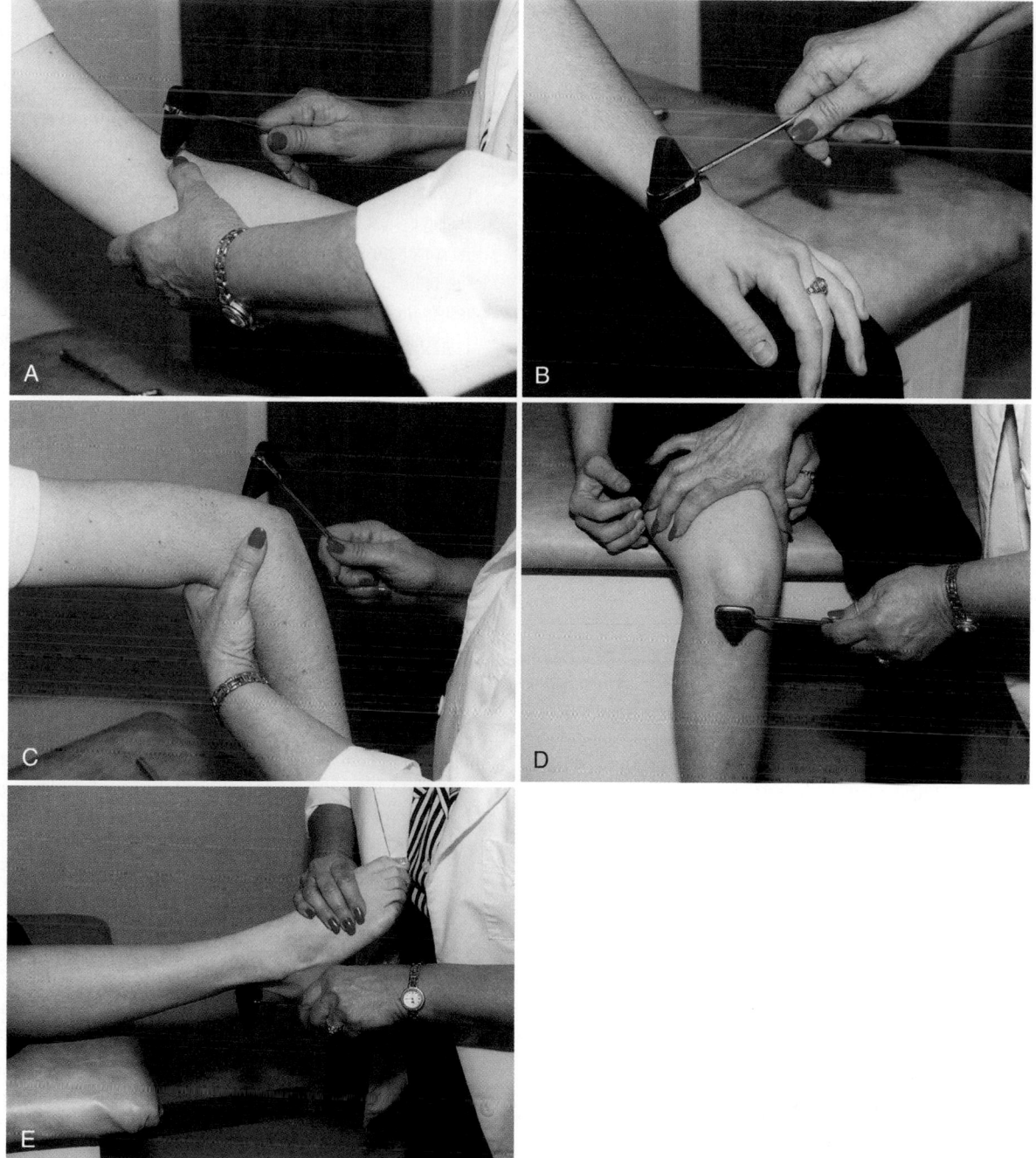

FIGURE 37-9 Testing deep tendon reflexes. **A,** Biceps reflex—results in flexion of the elbow. **B,** Brachioradialis reflex—results in flexion and supination of the forearm. **C,** Triceps reflex—results in extension of the arm. **D,** Patellar reflex—results in extension of the leg. **E,** Achilles reflex—results in plantar flexion of the foot.

PROCEDURE 37-1   Assist the Provider with Patient Care: Assist with the Neurologic Examination

Goal: *To assist the provider in performing a neurologic examination of the patient.*

EQUIPMENT and SUPPLIES

- Patient's record
- Patient gown
- Drape
- Otoscope
- Ophthalmoscope
- Percussion hammer
- Disposable pinwheel
- Penlight
- Tuning fork
- Cotton ball
- Tongue depressor
- Small vials of warm and cold liquids prepared according to the provider's instructions
- Small vials of sweet and salty liquids prepared according to the provider's instructions
- Small vials containing substances with distinct odors (e.g., instant coffee, cinnamon, vanilla) prepared according to the provider's instructions

PROCEDURAL STEPS

1. Assemble and prepare the equipment and supplies needed for the neurologic examination, and prepare the room.

2. Sanitize your hands and follow Standard Precautions.
   <u>PURPOSE</u>: To ensure infection control.
3. Greet and identify the patient by name and date of birth, and introduce yourself. Briefly explain the procedure.
   <u>PURPOSE</u>: Explanations gain the patient's cooperation and ease apprehension.
4. Instruct the patient to disrobe as needed for the examination and to put on an exam gown with the opening in the back.
5. During the examination, be prepared to assist the patient in changing positions as necessary. Have the necessary examination instruments ready for the provider at the appropriate time during the examination. Record all results from the examination as indicated by the provider.
   <u>PURPOSE</u>: To facilitate a thorough, accurate neurologic examination.
6. A neurologic examination proceeds as follows but can be modified according to the provider's preference:
   - Mental status examination
   - **Proprioception** and cerebellar function
   - Cranial nerve assessment
   - Sensory nerve function
   - Reflexes

DIAGNOSTIC TESTING

Several tests are used to help the physician accurately diagnose conditions and diseases of the neurologic system. The most common diagnostic procedures are the lumbar puncture and various radiographic studies (Table 37-5).

Electroencephalography

Electroencephalography is used to record the brain wave activity of a patient suspected of having a seizure disorder or to determine the effectiveness of pharmaceutical treatment to control the brain's abnormal electrical activity. The particular pattern of brainwave activity helps diagnose the seizure disorder type. EEGs also are used to help localize the area of the brain that is causing a partial seizure disorder. To prepare for the test, the patient may be told to stop taking certain medicines (sedatives, muscle relaxants, sleeping aids, or anti-seizure drugs) and to avoid all caffeine for 12 hours before the test. During an EEG, 16 to 25 electrodes are placed on the patient's scalp with either paste or an elastic cap to record the electrical activity of the brain. The patient must remain very still during the examination, even sleep if possible, so that the electrodes can pick up the electrical impulses of the brain without interference. Once the electrodes are in place, an EEG typically takes up to 60 minutes. Sedation may be required for pediatric patients (Figure 37-10).

Every individual has a unique EEG pattern. In a healthy brain, most of the recorded waves are the occipital alpha waves coming

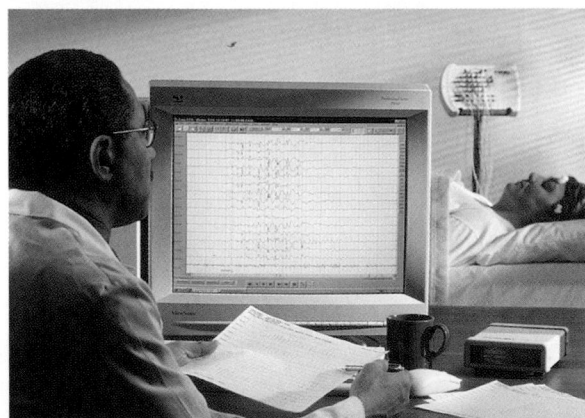

FIGURE 37-10 Patient undergoing electroencephalography. (From Linton A: *Introduction to medical-surgical nursing,* ed 4, St Louis, 2008, Saunders.)

from the back of the head. Irregular slow waves are called *delta waves,* which normally are found in people deeply asleep and in infants and young children. A delta wave pattern is abnormal in an awake adult. Rhythmic slow waves, called *theta waves,* show a decrease in brain activity. Electrical silence (flatline EEG) indicates no evidence of brain activity and is one of the criteria used to determine brain death. EEG is valuable for diagnosing epilepsy, brain tumors, and other brain conditions (Procedure 37-2).

TABLE 37-5 Diagnostic Tests for the Nervous System

TEST	PROCEDURE AND PATIENT PREPARATION	PURPOSE
Arteriography (angiography)	Patient usually is given a sedative. Then, after injection of a local anesthetic, a catheter is threaded into an artery toward the head. A contrast medium is injected, and videofluoroscopic studies are recorded. The patient must remain still during the procedure, which may last up to 1 hour.	To visualize the vertebral and carotid arteries, cerebral arterial circulation, leaking vessels, aneurysms, and occluded vessels
CT scan	Patient's head is strapped into a foam block to prevent movement, and patient lies on a moveable table. The table moves into the CT machine, which converts an x-ray study into a visual image of multiple transverse sections of the test structure. Procedure can last up to 1 hour, and the patient must remain still the entire time.	To visualize multiple, serial, radiographic sections of a structure, differentiating between bone and soft tissues
EEG	Patient relaxes comfortably on a recliner or bed. Electrodes are attached to the head. The examiner may ask the patient questions, give the patient various forms of visual or auditory stimulation, or have the patient sleep.	To record electrical activity of the brain to determine cerebral function or origin of seizure activity, diagnose sleep disorders, or determine lack of brain function
Lumbar puncture	With the patient in a side-lying fetal position, a local anesthetic is injected. A needle then is inserted into the subarachnoid space between the third and fourth lumbar vertebrae; CSF leaks out and is collected for analysis. Patient must remain very still during the procedure, which normally takes 5-20 minutes.	To determine CSF pressure, obtain CSF specimens for testing, reduce intracranial pressure, and inject contrast medium for radiographic studies
MRI	Patient should not have any metal in the body. Patient lies down on a moveable table, and the head is strapped into a foam block to prevent movement. The table moves into the MRI machine, which converts the cells' electromagnetic energy into a visual image. Patient must remain still during the procedure, which lasts up to 1 hour.	As with CT, to visualize multiple, serial, radiographic sections of a structure; shows images of the brain, spinal cord, and surrounding vascular and soft tissue
PET scan	Radioactive isotope is injected into the patient, and the brain is scanned to locate areas of isotope concentration. Patient must remain still during the procedure, which lasts up to 2 hours.	A radionuclide study that can identify areas of increased metabolic activity, vascular abnormalities, and space-occupying lesions
X-ray studies	Patient's head is placed in a specific position in front of the x-ray film; patient must remain still for about 1 minute while x-ray is taken.	Bone studies to identify fractures and other bone pathologies

CSF, Cerebrospinal fluid; *CT,* computed tomography; *EEG,* electroencephalography; *MRI,* magnetic resonance imaging; *PET,* positron emission tomography.

PROCEDURE 37-2   Explain the Rationale for Performance of a Procedure: Prepare the Patient for an Electroencephalogram

Goal: To prepare a patient physically and psychologically so that an accurate, useful electroencephalogram (EEG) can be obtained.

EQUIPMENT and SUPPLIES

- Patient's record

PROCEDURAL STEPS

1. Greet and identify the patient by name and date of birth. Introduce yourself and explain that you will go over what is going to happen step by step to ensure the best results.
2. Explain the purpose of the EEG, how the procedure is performed, and what is expected of the patient during the test.
3. Tell the patient that the electrodes pick up tiny electrical signals from the body and that there is no danger of electrical shock.
4. Explain that the test is painless, because the electrodes are attached to the scalp with paste or an electrode cap is worn.
5. If this is a sleep EEG, suggest that the patient stay up later than usual the night before the test so that it will be easier to fall asleep.
   <u>PURPOSE</u>: Sleep medications usually are not used because they may alter the brain wave pattern.

PROCEDURE 37-2 *—continued*

6. Go over the physical preparation, including the diet to be followed for the 48 hours before the test. This usually includes no stimulants (e.g., coffee, chocolate, or sodas) and no skipping meals.
   PURPOSE: Meal skipping may cause hypoglycemia, which alters brain function.

7. Explain that a baseline EEG will be taken at the beginning of the test and during this time the patient will be asked to avoid all movement, even eye and tongue movement.
   PURPOSE: These activities can be very disruptive to the brain wave tracing.

8. If a stimulation examination is ordered, explain that the patient will be asked to view flickering lights to stimulate the brain. The EEG will measure the brain's response to this stimulation.

9. Ask the patient whether he or she has any questions. If so, answer the questions so that the patient understands the procedure clearly.
   PURPOSE: Patients are more likely to cooperate if they understand the process so that they are not unduly apprehensive before and during the test.

10. Document patient education in the patient's record.

NOTE: Advanced training is required to perform an EEG.

Lumbar Puncture

If the physician suspects that an infection or inflammation of the CNS is present, a lumbar puncture (spinal tap) is ordered to collect a CSF sample for culture and analysis of glucose and protein, or to detect increased intracranial pressure or an area of intracranial bleeding. The patient is placed on the left side in the fetal position; using sterile technique, the physician injects the lumbar puncture site with a local anesthetic, and the puncture is performed by inserting a special needle into the subarachnoid space, usually between the L4 and L5 vertebrae (Figure 37-11). The pressure in the subarachnoid space is recorded, and at least four tubes of CSF are collected for laboratory analysis.

The most common complaint after the procedure is a severe headache. Extended bed rest once was recommended to prevent a spinal headache, but research no longer supports this approach. After the procedure, the patient is encouraged to drink fluids to rehydrate so that the CSF that was withdrawn during the spinal tap is replaced as quickly as possible. Medical practices usually have a specially equipped room where this procedure is performed. If you are working in such an office, you may be responsible both for assisting with the procedure and for monitoring the patient after the procedure until he or she is sent home. Watch for side effects such as severe headaches, visual disturbances, and pain. You also will have particular office protocols to follow regarding the frequency of vital signs, liquid intake, urine output, and visitors. Lumbar punctures usually are performed in hospitals, outpatient clinics, or surgical centers (Procedure 37-3). On discharge, patients should be told to notify the physician immediately if they experience any numbness and tingling of the legs; drainage of blood or liquid from the puncture site; inability to urinate; or a persistent headache.

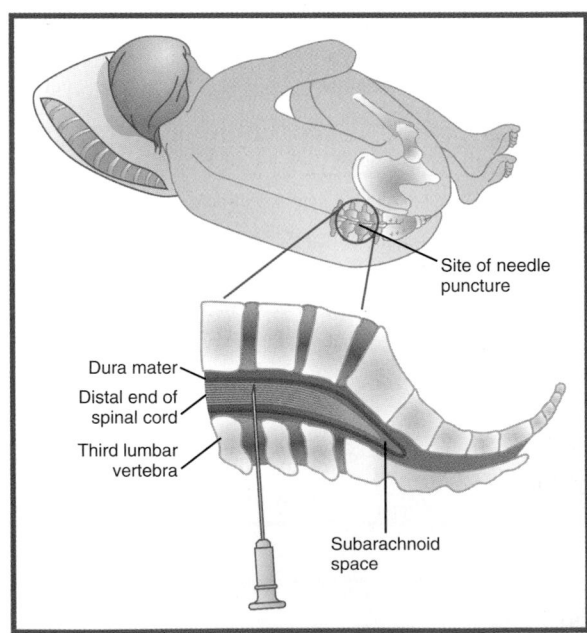

FIGURE 37-11 Lumbar puncture.

CRITICAL THINKING APPLICATION   **37-6**
Dr. Song wants to perform a lumbar puncture on a 10-year-old girl who he suspects has bacterial meningitis. Her mother agreed to the procedure, but while Mai is preparing the girl, the mother changes her mind. She is afraid that inserting a needle into her daughter's spine will paralyze the girl. What should Mai do in this situation?

PROCEDURE 37-3	Assist the Provider with Patient Care: Prepare the Patient for and Assist with a Lumbar Puncture

Goal: *To prepare a patient physically and mentally for a lumbar puncture so that a specimen of cerebrospinal fluid (CSF) can be obtained for testing.*

EQUIPMENT and SUPPLIES

- Patient's record
- Patient gown
- Drape
- Local anesthetic with appropriate syringe unit
- Sterile, disposable lumbar puncture kit with specimen tubes
- Instrument stand
- Sterile gloves
- Permanent marker to label tubes or printed labels
- Laboratory requisitions as needed
- Biohazard laboratory transport bag
- Biohazard waste container

PROCEDURAL STEPS

1. Assemble the materials needed, and prepare the room. Prepare the equipment and supplies needed for the lumbar puncture.
2. Sanitize your hands and follow Standard Precautions.
   PURPOSE: To ensure infection control.
3. Identify the patient by name and date of birth and introduce yourself. Explain that you will go over what will happen step by step to ensure the best results.
4. Make sure the signed consent form is in the patient's record.
5. Have the patient void just before the procedure.
   PURPOSE: To improve the patient's comfort during the procedure.
6. Give the patient a hospital gown and have him or her put it on with the opening in the back.
7. Place the patient in a left side-lying fetal position for the lumbar puncture.
   PURPOSE: To give the provider the easiest access to the lumbar region.
8. Support the patient's head with a pillow as necessary and provide a pillow for between the knees if needed.
   PURPOSE: To make the patient as comfortable as possible for the procedure.

9. Perform a sterile skin preparation of the lumbar region in the usual manner.
   PURPOSE: To prevent bacterial infection at the puncture site.
10. Place the sterile disposable lumbar puncture kit on an instrument stand for the provider's use. Include a syringe with needle for aspiration of the local anesthetic.
11. When the provider is ready to perform the lumbar puncture, cleanse the rubber top of the local anesthetic vial and hold the vial for the provider to aspirate the desired amount of drug.
    PURPOSE: To maintain sterile technique and expedite the procedure.
12. Reassure the patient and help him or her hold still during injection of the local anesthetic and insertion of the spinal needle.
    PURPOSE: To facilitate accurate insertion of the spinal needle.
13. Attach the printed labels to the specimen tubes or, using the permanent marker, label the specimens #1, #2, and #3 in the order in which they are collected. This is a crucial step in the procedure.
    PURPOSE: Different tests are done on different tubes. The accuracy of these tests depends on the tube on which they are performed.
14. Complete the laboratory requisition form and prepare the CSF specimens for transport to the laboratory.
    PURPOSE: To ensure that all the necessary tests are ordered correctly.
15. Apply gloves and clean the area by disposing of sharps, biohazard materials, and regular waste in the normal manner. Sanitize your hands.
16. Monitor the patient and give liquids as directed by the provider.
17. Document the procedure in the patient's health record.
    PURPOSE: A procedure is not complete until it has been documented accurately in the patient's health record.

9/15/20–8:32 AM: Lumbar puncture performed by Dr. Song. 300 cc CSF labeled and placed for pickup by North Hills Laboratory. Pt stable, no c/o discomfort. Pt given instructions for home care before leaving office. M. Lee, CMA (AAMA)

CLOSING COMMENTS

Patient Education

The nervous system is the major communication and control system in the human body. It influences and regulates all mental activity, including thought, learning, and memory. It is responsible for maintaining homeostasis (constant internal environmental conditions that are compatible with life) among the body's systems. Through its many receptors, the nervous system constantly monitors what is going on inside the body and in the environment outside the body.

When the nervous system becomes damaged or diseased, signs and symptoms can appear in every other body system. Motor activity

can become erratic, or the person's activity level can decline to the point where the individual becomes unable to communicate or function normally.

Your main responsibilities as a medical assistant in neurology are to observe, listen, and report any changes in patients. Even signs and symptoms that may seem rather slight can give the physician the one clue needed to put the puzzle together and arrive at a correct diagnosis before proceeding to the appropriate treatment. It is crucial that medical assistants working in a neurology practice recognize the importance and significance of a variety of symptoms. For example, severe headache accompanied by vomiting may indicate a serious intracranial problem that requires immediate attention. The medical assistant in a neurology practice must remain alert to these types of situations at all times, because neurologic emergencies can develop quite rapidly.

Legal and Ethical Issues

In neurology you will be faced with a variety of behaviors and personality changes that frequently are a part of neurologic conditions. Often a patient is not aware of these changes and may appear as though nothing is wrong. You must treat this patient with the same dignity and respect as you would all other patients, despite how the patient may treat you. Some patients are concerned that loved ones have turned against them and are treating them in an abusive manner. A patient's family may be experiencing severe emotional stress in coping with the patient's behavior. You must remember the medical assistant's code of ethics and the need for total confidentiality. Whatever is discussed in the examination room cannot be repeated to other staff members in the office and can never be discussed outside the office. Confidentiality must be strictly maintained.

HIPAA Applications

Under the privacy regulations of the Health Insurance Portability and Accountability Act (HIPAA), patients typically have the right to obtain a copy of their confidential health information. However, access to psychotherapy notes is limited. HIPAA defines psychotherapy notes as the documentation completed by a mental health professional that describes and analyzes the conversations with a patient during counseling sessions. These notes are not supposed to be stored in the patient's general chart and should not be released to third-party payers. Disclosure of psychotherapy notes requires specific permission from the patient before any documentation can be released to an insurance provider. Under federal law, the therapist must decide whether to release the notes to the patient, and if the therapist decides not to release the information, the patient cannot appeal this decision. However, the final authority rests with individual state laws. If a state law is stricter than the federal mandate or gives the patient greater access to psychotherapy notes, state law takes precedence over federal law. Further details about the HIPAA Privacy Rule are available at the following website: *http://www.hhs.gov/hipaa/for-professionals/special-topics/mental-health/index.html.*

Professional Behaviors

The ability to think critically is a crucial component of acting professionally, especially in a neurologic practice, because patients present with a wide variety of signs, symptoms, and mental health states. An important component of critical thinking is the ability to question patients logically and distinguish between relevant and irrelevant information. We must always be on the alert for any personal bias that may prevent us from delivering respectful patient care. This is especially true for interacting with patients who have been diagnosed with mental illness. The medical assistant's ability to conduct a professional and respectful patient history and to use appropriate interpersonal communication skills lays the groundwork for the client's care in the neurology office.

SUMMARY OF SCENARIO

Mai has excelled in her new position as clinical assistant and patient educator. With Dr. Song's approval, she has developed a series of patient information sheets that explain the functions of the nervous system, the symptoms to watch for after a head injury, the kinds and causes of headaches, and infections of the nervous system. Patients often ask for information sheets for other family members and for their friends and neighbors. She also developed a set of information sheets to explain typical neurologic diagnostic tests and how best to prepare for them. Although the patient receives a copy of the information sheet, Mai still talks with each patient to make sure he or she understands exactly what will happen in the test and to answer all questions completely. Mai feels a great deal of personal satisfaction from working with patients and helping them understand their diagnosis and treatment protocols.

SUMMARY OF LEARNING OBJECTIVES

1. **Define, spell, and pronounce the terms listed in the vocabulary.**
   Spelling and pronouncing medical terms correctly reinforce the medical assistant's credibility. Knowing the definitions of these terms promotes confidence in communication with patients and co-workers.

2. **Summarize the anatomy and physiology of the nervous system.**
   The main function of the nervous system is to control body functions so that homeostasis can be maintained. It does this by receiving messages in the CNS from the PNS, then sending a response to the appropriate location in the body, again via the PNS. The neuron is the functional cell of the nervous system, and neuroglial cells support and protect neurons throughout the system. The brain is made up of the cerebrum, cerebellum, and brainstem. The CNS is well protected, first by the skull and then by the dura mater, arachnoid mater, and pia mater meninges.

3. **Differentiate between the central and peripheral nervous systems.**
   The nervous system is made up of two parts: the CNS, which includes the brain and spinal cord, and the PNS, which includes all the nerves outside the CNS.

4. **Distinguish among common nervous system diseases and conditions and identify the typical symptoms associated with neurologic disorders.**

Symptoms of potentially serious neurologic conditions include headache, nausea and vomiting, change in vision, altered level of consciousness, memory loss, sleep disorders, confusion or disorientation, and problems with mobility. Table 37-3 summarizes the most common diseases and conditions of the nervous system.

5. Describe the pathology of cerebrovascular diseases.
CVD may be caused by atherosclerosis, hypertension, thrombi, emboli, or aneurysm. A TIA is a temporary limitation of function as a result of short-term ischemia. A CVA occurs when the blood supply to a particular part of the brain is cut off by an embolus, a thrombus, or an aneurysm that bursts. Migraine headaches are related to a combination of a problem with the trigeminal nerve and an imbalance of chemicals in the brain. Multi-infarct dementia is caused by a series of small strokes that interfere with the brain's blood supply, resulting in multiple areas of tissue necrosis. Alzheimer's disease is the most common form of dementia in older people.

6. Identify the various types of epilepsy.
Seizures are classified as either partial or generalized, based on how much of the brain is involved in the abnormal electrical activity. Partial seizures result from abnormal electrical activity in just one part of the brain, whereas generalized seizures involve most or all of the brain. Generalized seizures include petit mal seizures, which are brief episodes characterized by staring, subtle body movement, and brief lapses of awareness. Probably the best-known seizure disorder is the generalized tonic-clonic disorder, which causes grand mal seizures.

7. Compare and contrast encephalitis and meningitis.
Encephalitis is a viral infection of the brain that can cause serious CNS symptoms. Meningitis may be caused by viruses, bacteria, or fungi. Bacterial meningitis is most serious. Viral meningitis usually resolves without treatment or incident.

8. Explain the dynamics of brain and spinal cord injuries.
Traumatic brain injuries can range from a mild concussion to severe injury, coma, and death. A minor concussion usually causes no long-term side effects; however, a moderate to severe brain injury can result in headaches, amnesia, confusion, personality changes, and seizures. Head injuries can be either open or closed, with possible serious intracerebral damage and potential complications within the meningeal layers. Shaken baby syndrome is caused by violently shaking an infant back and forth, forcing the brain against opposite ends of the skull. The higher the damage to the spinal cord, the more serious the injury.

9. Summarize common central nervous system (CNS) and peripheral nervous system (PNS) diseases.
Parkinson's disease (PD) is a chronic, progressive, debilitating neurologic disease that is caused by a combination of genetic and environmental factors that result in a deficiency of the neurotransmitter dopamine in the brain. Approximately half of all brain tumors are metastatic growths from other primary cancer sites in the body. Multiple

sclerosis (MS) causes progressive inflammation and demyelination of the axon, resulting in a scattering of the nervous message as it passes down the axon. Amyotrophic lateral sclerosis (ALS) is a rapidly progressive, ultimately fatal neurologic disease that destroys the motor neurons responsible for voluntary muscle control. Bell's palsy causes temporary facial paralysis because of damage or trauma to cranial nerve VII. Peripheral neuropathies can result from damage or injury to any part of the neuron and typically are caused by other systemic diseases, such as diabetes.

10. Differentiate among common mental health disorders.
Depressive disorders affect the way a person thinks, feels, eats, and sleeps. People with depression cannot "snap out of it" and without treatment may suffer from symptoms that last weeks, months, or years. Types of depressive disorders include major depression, dysthymia, and bipolar disorders. Anxiety disorders cause an overwhelming, irrational feeling of anxiety and fear; these include panic disorder, obsessive-compulsive disorder (OCD), post-traumatic stress disorder (PTSD), and phobias. Risk factors for suicide include serious depressive disorders; reduced serotonin levels; a previous suicide attempt; family violence; and exposure to the suicidal behavior of others. Schizophrenia is a chronic, severe, and disabling brain disorder with symptoms that include hallucinations and delusions; difficulty speaking and expressing emotions; and cognitive deficits. Suicide is the tenth leading cause of death in the United States. Mental health disorders are treated with psychotherapy and appropriate medications.

11. Analyze the medical assistant's role in the neurologic examination.
When assisting in neurology, the medical assistant must be particularly careful to recognize signs and symptoms, which frequently are quite subtle but yet can be extremely significant in helping to assess and diagnose the neurologic patient accurately (see Procedure 37-1).

12. Explain the common diagnostic procedures for the nervous system.
Diagnostic tests for the neurologic system are summarized in Table 37-5. They include arteriograms; CT, MRI, and PET scans; EEG; lumbar puncture and CSF analysis; and various x-ray studies.

13. Outline the steps needed to prepare a patient for an electroencephalogram (EEG).
Procedure 37-2 outlines the steps for preparing a patient for an EEG.

14. Describe the steps for preparing a patient for and assisting with a lumbar puncture.
Procedure 37-3 describes the procedural steps for preparing a patient for and assisting with a lumbar puncture.

15. Discuss the implications of patient education in a neurologic and mental health practice.
When the nervous system becomes damaged or diseased, signs and symptoms can appear in every other body system. Motor activity can become erratic, or activity level can decline to the point that the person becomes unable to communicate or function normally. Your main

Continued

SUMMARY OF LEARNING OBJECTIVES—*continued*

responsibilities as a medical assistant in neurology are to observe, listen, and report any changes in patients.

16. **Explain the legal issues and HIPAA applications associated with neurology and mental health.**

    Whatever is discussed in the examination room cannot be repeated to other staff members in the office and can never be discussed outside the office. Confidentiality must be strictly maintained. Disclosure of psychotherapy notes requires specific patient permission. Under federal law, the therapist must decide whether to release the notes to the patient, and if the therapist decides not to release the information, the patient cannot appeal this decision. However, the final authority rests with individual state laws.

CONNECTIONS

Study Guide Connection: Go to the Chapter 37 Study Guide. Read and complete the activities.

evolve Evolve Connection: Go to the Chapter 37 link at *evolve.elsevier.com/ kinn* to complete the Chapter Review Quiz. Check out the other resources listed for this chapter to make the most of what you have learned from Assisting in Neurology and Mental Health.

ASSISTING IN ENDOCRINOLOGY

38

SCENARIO

Miguel Vasco has been a certified medical assistant (CMA [AAMA]) for 10 years and has worked for the past 3 years in an endocrinology and internal medicine practice with several physicians. Although he has taken care of patients with many different disorders of the endocrine system, most of the practice's patients arc individuals with diabetes mellitus type 2. One of Miguel's responsibilities is coaching patients newly diagnosed with diabetes in how to monitor their blood glucose levels and maintain a healthy lifestyle.

While studying this chapter, think about the following questions:

- What are the primary responsibilities of a medical assistant in an internal medicine practice?
- What clinical skills are required in this specialty practice?
- What common diseases and disorders of the endocrine system should medical assistants working in this field be able to discuss and explain?
- What diagnostic and treatment procedures typically are used in an endocrinology practice?
- What information should the medical assistant know about the management of diabetes and the possible complications associated with the disease?

LEARNING OBJECTIVES

1. Define, spell, and pronounce the terms listed in the vocabulary.
2. Summarize the anatomy and physiology of the endocrine system.
3. Explain the mechanism of hormone action.
4. Differentiate among the diseases and disorders of the endocrine system.
5. Describe the diagnostic criteria for diabetes mellitus.
6. Do the following with regard to diabetes mellitus:
   - Compare and contrast prediabetes, diabetes type 1, diabetes type 2, and gestational diabetes.
   - Outline the treatment plan and management of the different types of diabetes mellitus.

- Perform blood glucose screening with a glucometer.
- Identify the characteristics of hypoglycemia and hyperglycemia.
- Describe acute and chronic complications associated with diabetes mellitus.
7. Discuss follow-up for patients with diabetes and summarize patient education approaches to diabetes.
8. Discuss legal and ethical issues to consider when caring for patients with endocrine system disorders.

VOCABULARY

adrenocorticotropic hormone (ACTH) (uh-dre-no-cor-tih-ko-tro′-pik) A hormone released by the anterior pituitary gland that stimulates the production and secretion of glucocorticoids.

diabetic retinopathy A condition in which microaneurysms and weakness in the capillary wall within the retina result in ischemia and tissue death.

follicle-stimulating hormone (FSH) A hormone secreted by the anterior pituitary; it stimulates oogenesis and spermatogenesis.

gluconeogenesis (glu-ko-ne-oh-jeh′-nuh-sis) The formation of glucose in the liver from proteins and fats.

glycogen The sugar (starch) formed from glucose; it is stored mainly in the liver.

glycosuria The abnormal presence of glucose in the urine.

growth hormone (GH) Also called *somatotropic hormone;* it stimulates tissue growth and restricts tissue glucose dependence when nutrients are not available.

luteinizing hormone (LH) (lu-te-uh-niz′-ing) A hormone produced by the anterior pituitary gland that promotes ovulation.

nocturia Excessive urination during the night.

polydipsia Excessive thirst.

polyphagia (pah-le-faj′-e-uh) Increased appetite.

prolactin (PRL) A hormone secreted by the anterior pituitary gland that stimulates the development of the mammary gland; it also stimulates the production of breast milk.

satiety The state of being satisfied or of feeling full after eating.
specific gravity The density of urine compared with an equal volume of water.

thyroid-stimulating hormone (TSH) A hormone secreted by the anterior pituitary gland that stimulates the secretion of hormones produced by the thyroid gland.

Individuals with disorders of the endocrine system usually are seen first by the primary care physician (PCP), who may refer them to an internist or an endocrinologist for specialized care. Patients with certain endocrine disorders, such as diabetes mellitus (DM), also may be seen in a specialty clinic for follow-up and treatment. A medical assistant employed in any of these ambulatory care practices assists with diagnostic procedures, specialized examinations, and patient education. It is important that medical assistants recognize the dynamics of endocrine system diseases, so they can help patients understand the importance of lifestyle factors, how to administer their medications, and how to prevent long-term complications from the disease.

ANATOMY AND PHYSIOLOGY OF THE ENDOCRINE SYSTEM

Both the nervous system and the endocrine system control the body's physiologic responses to internal and external stimuli. The nervous system is electrical in nature and sends immediate messages along a nerve pathway to evoke a response; the endocrine system relies on the bloodstream to carry hormonal messages to a target cell for action. Through hormonal action, the endocrine system regulates all body functions. Endocrinology is the study of hormones, their receptor cells, and the results of hormone action.

The word part *endo-* means "in" or "within"; the suffix *-crine* means "secrete." The endocrine system consists of glands located throughout the body that produce and secrete chemicals known as *hormones.* Hormones are excreted directly into the bloodstream, which carries them to the target tissue. They function as the body's chemical messengers, transferring information from one group of cells to another. They control growth, mood, system functions, metabolism, sexual maturity, and reproduction. Hormone levels vary and can be affected by outside factors, such as illness and stress.

Basic Anatomy

Glands are categorized as either exocrine or endocrine. *Exocrine glands,* such as sweat glands and salivary glands, secrete either through a duct or directly onto the surface of the skin or in the mouth. *Endocrine glands* release hormones directly into the bloodstream, which transports the hormones to target cells for action.

The glands of the endocrine system are the hypothalamus, pituitary, pineal gland, thyroid, parathyroids, thymus, and adrenals, and the reproductive glands (i.e., the ovaries and the testes) (Figure 38-1). Some nonendocrine organs, especially the pancreas, also can produce and release hormones. The hypothalamus, located in the inferior midportion of the brain, is the major connection between the nervous and endocrine systems. The hypothalamus controls the action of the pituitary, a pea-sized gland located below the hypothalamus. The pituitary often is called the "master gland" because it secretes hormones that regulate multiple endocrine glands.

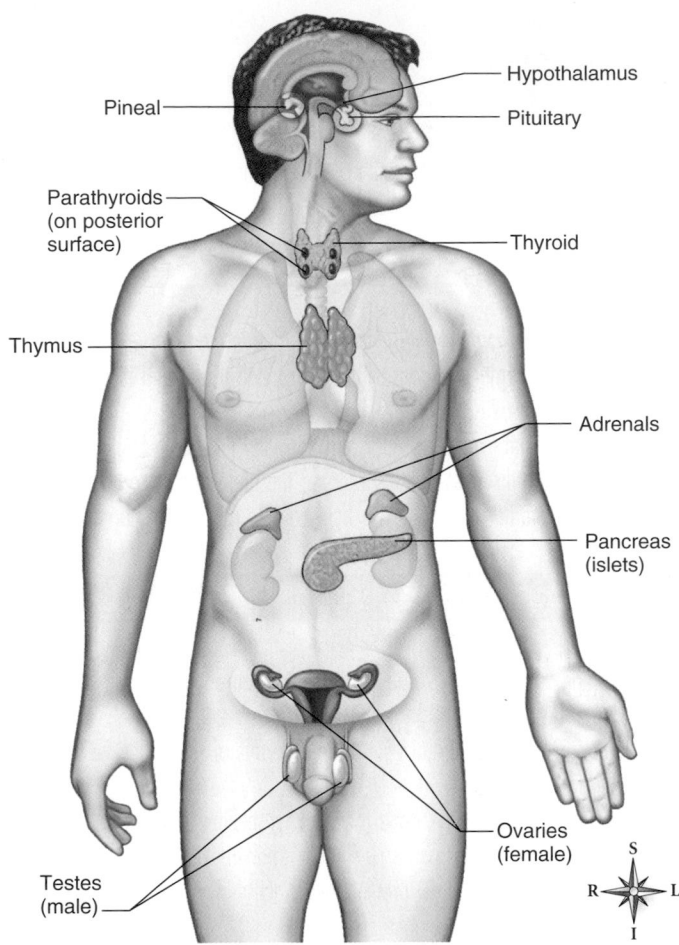

FIGURE 38-1 Location of the endocrine glands. (From Patton KT, Thibodeau GA: *Anatomy and physiology,* ed 9, St Louis, 2016, Mosby.)

The pituitary gland consists of two parts, the anterior and posterior lobes. The anterior pituitary, or adenohypophysis, regulates the functions of the thyroid, adrenals, and reproductive glands. It produces **growth hormone (GH)**, **thyroid-stimulating hormone (TSH)**, **adrenocorticotropic hormone (ACTH)**, **prolactin (PRL)**, **follicle-stimulating hormone (FSH)**, and **luteinizing hormone (LH)**. The posterior lobe of the pituitary, or neurohypophysis, excretes oxytocin, which stimulates the contractions of the smooth muscle of the uterus that occur during labor and the flow of breast milk toward the nipple when an infant breast-feeds. The posterior pituitary also produces antidiuretic hormone (ADH), which helps control fluid balance by acting on the kidneys, causing them to reabsorb fluid as needed to maintain homeostasis (Figure 38-2).

The pineal gland, which is located deep within the brain, excretes the hormone melatonin. Melatonin helps regulate waking and sleeping patterns and also may affect seasonal reactions to alterations in the availability of sunlight.

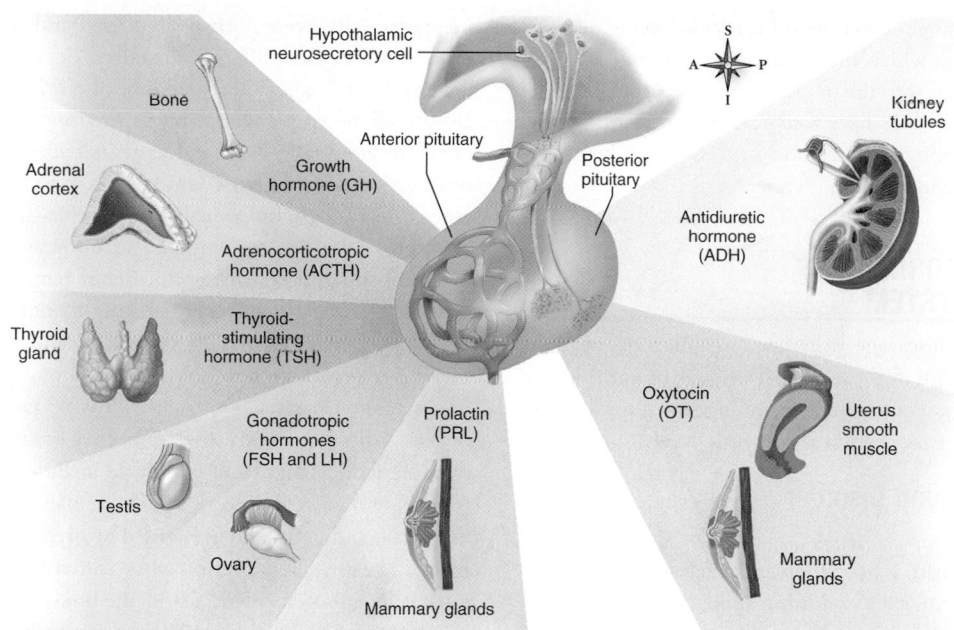

FIGURE 38-2 The principal anterior and posterior pituitary hormones and their target organs. (From Patton KT, Thibodeau GA: *The human body in health and disease,* ed 6, St Louis, 2014, Mosby.)

When stimulated by TSH, the thyroid gland produces the thyroid hormones triiodothyronine (T_3) and thyroxine (T_4), which control the body's metabolic rate and are important factors in bone growth and nervous system development in children. On the dorsal aspect of the thyroid gland are several small parathyroid glands, which release hormones (parathyroid and calcitonin) that regulate the level of calcium in the blood. Parathyroid hormone (PTH) maintains a constant concentration of calcium in the body by regulating the absorption of calcium from the gastrointestinal tract and stimulating the reabsorption of calcium stored in the bone, as needed, to maintain homeostasis. Calcitonin stimulates deposition of calcium into the bone when excess amounts of calcium are available.

The thymus gland, located behind the upper portion of the sternum, produces hormones that stimulate the production of specialized immune system cells called *T cells.* The thymus gland is present at birth and enlarges as the child ages but begins to atrophy as the child reaches puberty. It once was thought that the thymus played no role in the physiology of adults, but we now know that its hormone action is crucial to T-cell maturation.

On top of each kidney are the adrenal glands, which are triangular-shaped glands consisting of an outer layer, called the *adrenal cortex,* and an inner body, called the *adrenal medulla.* The adrenal cortex secretes corticosteroid hormones, including cortisol, aldosterone, and adrenal androgens, all of which influence a wide range of bodily functions. The adrenal medulla produces epinephrine, also called *adrenaline,* which activates the body's reaction to stress.

The gonads produce sex hormones. The male gonads are the testes; they secrete testosterone, which regulates the development of secondary sexual characteristics (e.g., voice changes and the growth of facial and pubic hair) and promotes the production of sperm. The female gonads, the ovaries, produce eggs, or ova (oogenesis), and secrete estrogen and progesterone. The female hormones control the development of breast tissue and other secondary sexual characteristics; they also regulate menstruation and play important roles during pregnancy.

The pancreas performs essential endocrine functions by producing insulin and glucagon, which work together to maintain normal blood glucose levels and store glucose for energy.

CRITICAL THINKING APPLICATION   **38-1**

Miguel is asked to order educational supplies for patients with endocrine system disorders. Because he thinks it is important for patients to understand their health problems, he wants to order a brochure that clearly depicts and describes the anatomy of the endocrine system. What glands and organs should be included in the handout? How can Miguel meet the particular needs of the Hispanic patients in the practice?

Mechanisms of Hormone Action

The goal of hormone regulation is to maintain homeostasis. Hormone secretion is regulated by a number of mechanisms, including nervous stimulation, endocrine control (a hormone from one gland, such as the anterior pituitary, stimulates the release of a hormone from another gland), and feedback systems. An example of nervous system regulation of endocrine function is the release of adrenaline from the adrenal medulla in response to stimulation from the sympathetic nervous system during a stressful episode. In the most common feedback system, negative feedback, an endocrine gland is activated by an imbalance and acts to correct the imbalance by stopping the secretion process. For example, if calcium blood levels fall below normal, the parathyroid glands are stimulated to release PTH. PTH acts to increase blood calcium levels either by stimulating the absorption of calcium from the gut or by demineralizing bone to release stored calcium. This change in the blood calcium level is detected by the parathyroid gland, which then stops production of PTH.

Each hormone released into the bloodstream has particular target cells for action. The target cells have receptors that attract only specific hormones and permit the hormone to pass through the cell membrane and affect cellular action.

DISEASES AND DISORDERS OF THE ENDOCRINE SYSTEM

Faulty secretion of any hormone, whether too much or too little, can cause health problems for patients. The goal of treatment is either to control the hypersecretion of hormones or to replace hormones that are not being secreted at therapeutic levels.

Posterior Pituitary Gland Disorder

Diabetes Insipidus

When ADH, or vasopressin, is not produced or released in sufficient amounts, the patient develops a condition called *diabetes insipidus.* ADH increases the permeability of the renal tubules and the collecting tubules in the kidneys; this permits fluid to be reabsorbed to prevent dehydration and causes the urine to become more concentrated. Without the action of ADH, fluid is not reabsorbed from the renal tubules, resulting in excretion of a large amount of fluid in the urine, with the potential onset of high blood sodium levels and severe dehydration. A lack of ADH can occur because of a tumor (either in the hypothalamus or the posterior pituitary gland) that prevents adequate secretion of the hormone, or it can be induced by trauma, pituitary surgery, or lack of blood supply to that area of the brain. Diabetes insipidus may also develop because of an inadequate response to ADH in the renal tubules, which may be caused by kidney disease or the side effects of certain medications. Diabetes insipidus has no connection to blood glucose levels or diabetes mellitus.

Diabetes insipidus usually has an acute onset, and the patient presents with polyuria, **polydipsia**, **nocturia**, low urine **specific gravity**, and high blood plasma osmolality (concentration). It can result in fatal dehydration if fluid and electrolyte levels cannot be controlled. Diagnostic studies include blood sodium and osmolarity levels, magnetic resonance imaging (MRI) of the head, urinalysis and urine concentration studies, and monitoring of urine output. Replacement therapy with a synthetic vasopressin (desmopressin) nasal spray, oral tablets, or injections is used to treat the disorder.

Diseases of the Anterior Pituitary

Hormones secreted by the anterior pituitary control a number of glandular functions. The effects on the body of changes in anterior pituitary gland secretion depend on whether the hormones are produced at an abnormally low level (hypopituitarism) or at a very high level (hyperpituitarism). A patient diagnosed with panhypopituitarism has a deficiency of all the hormones produced by the anterior pituitary, and the symptoms reflect systemic inactivity of all the glands stimulated by the anterior pituitary hormones.

Growth Hormone Abnormalities

Hypopituitary dwarfism occurs when the pituitary gland fails to produce normal amounts of GH. The child's height is impaired, but he or she will have a normal-sized head and trunk. Hypersecretion of GH causes two different disorders, depending on the patient's developmental age. Oversecretion of GH in childhood, before closure of the epiphyseal plates in the long bones, causes the long bones to grow excessively. Affected individuals may reach a height of 8 feet or taller. Because GH has a secondary effect on the blood glucose level, these individuals may develop diabetes mellitus. Slow-growing, benign anterior pituitary adenomas frequently are the cause of gigantism, and treatment consists of removing the tumor when possible and radiation therapy or drug therapy.

If hypersecretion of GH occurs in adulthood, the disorder is called *acromegaly.* Because the epiphyseal plates are closed, the long bones cannot grow. Consequently, a wide range of manifestations can occur because of excessive connective tissue growth and overproduction of bone. Signs and symptoms include arthralgia, an enlarged tongue, overactive sebaceous and sweat glands, coarse skin, excessive body hair, and nerve damage caused by pressure on peripheral nerves from increasing amounts of bone and soft tissue. A gradual but noticeable enlargement occurs in the bones of the jaw, face, hands, and feet (Figure 38-3). Advanced acromegaly causes complications such as congestive heart failure, DM, cerebrovascular abnormalities, and neurologic symptoms as the tumor grows within the confined space of the hypothalamus. Treatment of acromegaly requires either surgical removal or irradiation of the pituitary tumor.

CRITICAL THINKING APPLICATION   **38-2**

Many different disorders can occur when problems arise with the anterior pituitary gland. Describe two such health problems, using your knowledge of target organ action. What psychosocial issues might patients with growth hormone disorders face?

Disorders of the Thyroid

Hypothyroidism

Deficient secretion of the thyroid hormones may result from a number of factors. One cause of hypothyroidism is endemic iodine deficiency, a lack of iodine in the diet, resulting in the formation of a simple goiter. A *simple goiter* is any thyroid enlargement that has not been caused by an infection or neoplasm. Endemic goiters occur in certain geographic areas. If more than 10% of children 6 to 12 years of age in a particular area have goiters, that geographic location is defined as endemic for goiters.

T_3 and T_4 are produced in the thyroid gland from iodine and are responsible for the regulation of metabolic activities in all body cells. When the thyroid gland is unable to obtain sufficient amounts of iodine from the circulating blood, it enlarges, or hypertrophies, in an attempt to produce the hormones needed by the body. A decreased amount of thyroid hormones results in a lower metabolic rate, heat loss, and poor mental and physical development. The primary sources of dietary iodine are saltwater fish, seaweed, and trace amounts in grains. Iodine deficiency is rare in the United States because of the widespread use of iodized table salt and the distribution of foods from iodine-rich areas. The treatment for a simple goiter is to reduce its size by prescribing dietary supplements of iodine, thyroid hormone replacement, or surgery.

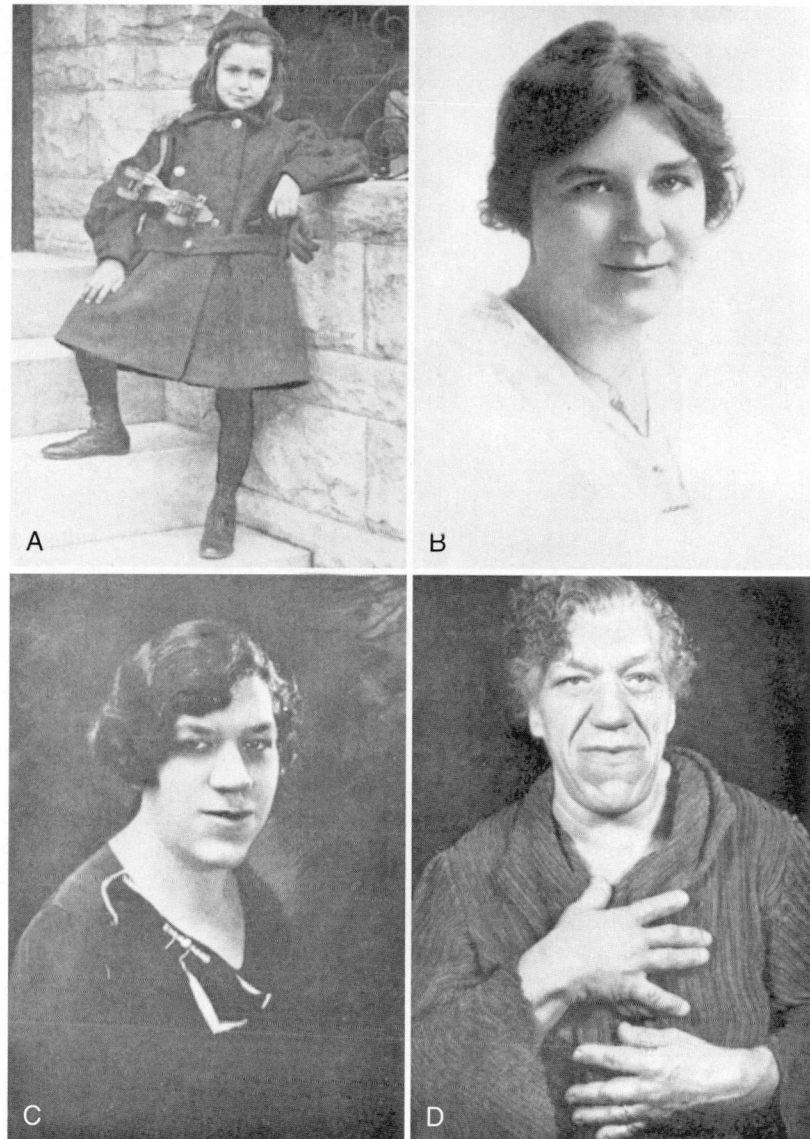

FIGURE 38-3 Progression of acromegaly. **A,** Patient at age 9. **B,** Patient at age 16, with possible early features of acromegaly. **C,** Patient at age 33, with well-established acromegaly. **D,** Patient at age 52, end-stage acromegaly. (From Clinical Pathological Conference, *Am J Med* 20:133, 1956.)

Improper development of the thyroid in an infant or young child usually is congenital. The absence of adequate levels of thyroid hormones results in a condition known as *cretinism*. Newborns have feeding problems, constipation, and a hoarse cry and sleep for extreme lengths of time. Symptoms include lethargy, bradycardia, stunted skeletal growth, and varying degrees of developmental delays, depending on the severity and duration of the hypothyroidism. All newborns in the United States are tested for congenital hypothyroidism. If treatment begins in the first month after birth, infants usually develop normally.

When severe or chronic hypothyroidism occurs in an adult or older child, the condition is called *myxedema*. The patient shows fatigue, weight gain, hair loss, a slower pulse rate, a lowered body temperature, muscle cramps, menorrhagia, and thick, dry, puffy skin. Routine tests to diagnose hypothyroidism include radioimmunoassay (a radiologic blood test) for T_3, T_4, and TSH. Adequate doses of thyroxine (Levothroid, Levoxyl, or Synthroid) restore normal function and appearance. Patients diagnosed with hypothyroidism must take hormone replacement therapy daily for the rest

of their lives, and thyroid function tests are typically rechecked once a year.

Hyperthyroidism

Hyperthyroidism, or thyrotoxicosis, is a condition in which serum levels of thyroid hormones are excessively high. Signs and symptoms include weight loss, tachycardia, palpitations, hypertension, agitation, nervousness, depression, tremor, excessive sweating, goiter, and exophthalmia (protruding eyes) (Figure 38-4). Graves' disease, an autoimmune disorder that stimulates overactive thyroid hormone production, is the most common cause of thyrotoxicosis. The goal of treatment is to control excessive production of thyroid hormone with the antithyroid drugs propylthiouracil (PTU) and methimazole (Tapazole); ingestion of radioactive iodine, which concentrates in the thyroid gland, destroying overactive cells; or surgical thyroidectomy to remove a section of the gland. All of these methods may inadvertently result in hypothyroidism, so the patient's thyroid hormone levels are evaluated after treatment. The patient frequently has to take replacement hormone therapy (Levothroid, Levoxyl, or

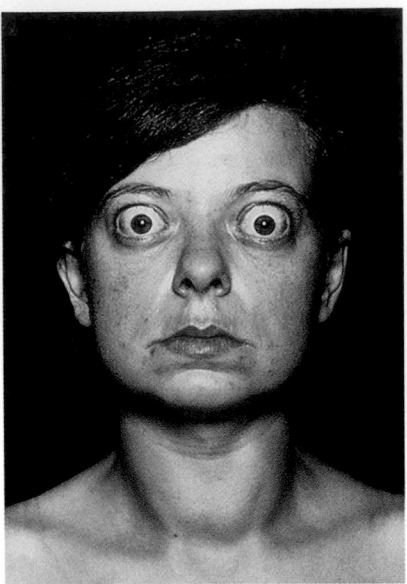

FIGURE 38-4 Exophthalmos in Graves' disease. (From Seidel HM et al: *Mosby's guide to physical examination*, ed 6, St Louis, 2006, Mosby.)

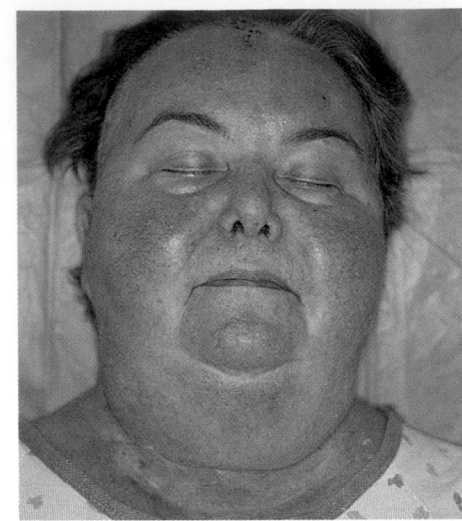

FIGURE 38-5 Cushing's syndrome. (From Seidel HM et al: *Mosby's guide to physical examination*, ed 6, St Louis, 2006, Mosby.)

Synthroid) after treatment to maintain normal thyroid hormone levels. Individuals who develop exophthalmia from hyperthyroidism may require orbital decompression surgery, in which the bone between the eye socket and sinuses is removed, giving the eyes room to return to their normal position.

CRITICAL THINKING APPLICATION   **38-3**

One of the internists, Dr. Misha, asks Miguel if he can describe the signs and symptoms of a patient with hypothyroidism and one with hyperthyroidism. How would you answer this question?

Disorders of the Adrenal Glands

Adrenal insufficiency is called *Addison's disease*. This condition is relatively rare and is caused by an autoimmune reaction that affects the adrenal cortex, which secretes corticosteroid hormones. Symptoms include hypoglycemia, increased pigmentation of the skin, muscle weakness, gastrointestinal disturbances, and fatigue. Cortisol and aldosterone deficiencies lead to retention of potassium and the excretion of water and sodium in the urine. Severe dehydration, low blood volume, low blood pressure, and circulatory shock can occur. Treatment includes replacement of cortisol with the long-term daily administration of glucocorticoids (e.g., prednisone) and replacement of aldosterone with fludrocortisone (Florinef) to control sodium and potassium levels while helping to maintain normal blood pressure levels. Patients should also be encouraged to eat a diet high in complex carbohydrates and protein and to maintain an adequate fluid intake. Patients with Addison's disease are at risk for addisonian crisis, a condition marked by a life-threatening drop in blood pressure, hypoglycemia, and high blood potassium levels. A crisis can be brought on by stressful situations, infections, minor illness, or surgery. Treatment requires immediate administration of an intravenous saline and dextrose solution with corticosteroids.

Hypersecretion of the adrenal cortex, causing increased levels of cortisol, is known as *Cushing's syndrome*. Usually a benign pituitary

tumor causes the release of excessive amounts of ACTH. Symptoms associated with Cushing's syndrome may be seen in individuals taking corticosteroids for medical reasons, such as organ transplantation, severe asthma, or rheumatoid arthritis. Excessive levels of cortisol cause an accumulation of adipose tissue in the trunk; a round, or "moon," face; and fat pads in the cervical spine region, causing the formation of a "buffalo hump" (Figure 38-5). The patient also has glucose intolerance because of insulin resistance at the target cell level.

Additional symptoms include hyperpigmentation, muscle wasting, problems with wound healing, hypertension, kidney stones, and osteoporosis. Female patients have menstrual irregularity, and many patients with Cushing's syndrome experience mental disorders such as irritability, depression, or severe psychiatric disorders. Treatment depends on the cause of the disorder; it includes medication to control cortisol levels, radiation therapy to reduce the size of the tumor, and surgery to remove the tumor.

Endocrine Dysfunction of the Pancreas: Diabetes Mellitus

Diabetes mellitus is a common hormonal imbalance that has reached epidemic proportions in the United States because of the huge increase in the incidence of DM type 2. Approximately 29.1 million Americans, or 9.3% of the population, have DM, and the number is growing. Based on fasting glucose (i.e., A_{1c}) levels, 37% of Americans age 20 or older (86 million people) have prediabetes. In the over-65 age group, this percentage increases to 51%. Diabetes occurs in people of all ages and races but is more common in those over age 60 and in African-Americans, Latinos, Native Americans, and Asian-Americans/Pacific Islanders.

DM is characterized by chronic hyperglycemia and problems with carbohydrate metabolism. This problem with glucose management is caused by a lack of insulin production and/or resistance to insulin at the target cell level. In the pancreas, specialized cells in the islets of Langerhans produce and secrete the hormones insulin and glucagon. When the blood glucose level is too high, beta islet cells secrete insulin, which is sent through the bloodstream to the target

Blood Test Levels for Diagnosis of Diabetes and Prediabetes

	A₁c (percent)	Fasting Plasma Glucose (mg/dL)	Oral Glucose Tolerance Test (mg/dL)
Diabetes	6.5 or above	126 or above	200 or above
Prediabetes	5.7 to 6.4	100 to 125	140 to 199
Normal	About 5	99 or below	139 or below

Definitions: mg = milligram, dL = deciliter
For all three tests, within the prediabetes range, the higher the test result, the greater the risk of diabetes.

FIGURE 38-6 Diagnosis of diabetes and prediabetes. (Data from American Diabetes Association: Standards of medical care in diabetes, 2012, *Diabetes Care* 35 (Suppl 1):S11-63, 2012.)

tissue site to conduct glucose into the cell. When blood glucose levels are low, the alpha islet cells secrete glucagon to stimulate the liver to convert **glycogen** (stored glucose) into circulating glucose.

If there is resistance to insulin at the target cell membrane or if not enough insulin is available to help transport glucose from the blood into the cells, the person experiences a variety of symptoms, including **glycosuria**, polyuria, polydipsia, **polyphagia**, rapid weight loss (DM type 1), drowsiness, fatigue, itching of the skin, visual disturbances, and skin infections. The American Diabetes Association has identified four major types of diabetes: prediabetes, DM type 1, DM type 2, and gestational diabetes. If left untreated or managed poorly, DM can have serious or even life-threatening consequences, such as cardiovascular disease, stroke, hypertension, blindness, kidney disease, nervous system disorders, amputations, pregnancy complications, and diabetic coma. Patient education is crucial for compliance with treatment and prevention of life-threatening complications. Figure 38-6 shows the blood glucose levels for the diagnosis of diabetes in nonpregnant adults and prediabetes.

Diagnostic Criteria for Diabetes Mellitus

- Plasma glucose level ≥ 200 mg/dL (norm is 80 to 120 mg/dL) with the classic symptoms of polyuria, polydipsia, and unexplained weight loss
- Fasting plasma glucose level ≥ 126 mg/dL (norm is 70 to 110 mg/dL) on more than one occasion
- Two-hour oral glucose tolerance test (OGTT) result ≥ 200 mg/dL
- Urinalysis positive for glucose and possibly ketones
- Glycosylated hemoglobin (A₁c or HbA₁c) 6.5% or above (normal is 4% to 6%)

A₁c (HbA₁c), Glycosylated hemoglobin; *PGL*, plasma glucose level; *FPG*, fasting plasma glucose; *OGTT*, oral glucose tolerance test.

Regardless of the type of diabetes, for treatment to be successful, patients must play an active role in the management of their disease. The medical assistant should consistently encourage patients to be active participants in maintaining blood glucose and A₁c levels within the normal range and to constantly be on alert for possible complications of their disease. The ideal is to maintain glucose plasma levels as close to the norm as possible to prevent complications. The American Diabetes Association recommends blood glucose levels between 70 and 130 mg/dL before meals; below 180 mg/dL 2 hours after starting a meal; and an A₁c level below 7%.

Prediabetes

Prediabetes is a condition in which a person's blood glucose level is higher than normal but not high enough for a diagnosis of diabetes type 2. Some of the long-term damage to vascular and cardiac systems may be occurring during prediabetes. Studies indicate that without lifestyle changes to improve health, 15% to 30% of people with prediabetes develop DM type 2 within 5 years. However, if patients lower their blood glucose levels, they can delay or prevent its onset. Experts recommend that patients with prediabetes lose 5% to 7% of their body weight and get at least 150 minutes of physical activity each week, such as brisk walking. A loss of just 10 to 20 pounds can make a huge difference in blood glucose levels.

Blood tests are needed to diagnose prediabetes because no symptoms may be present early in the disease. All diabetes blood tests involve drawing blood at a healthcare provider's office or a commercial facility and sending the sample to a lab for analysis. Lab analysis of blood is needed to ensure that test results are accurate. Glucometers are not accurate enough for diagnosis but may be used as a quick indicator of glucose levels. A₁c results, fasting plasma glucose (FPG) level, and an oral glucose tolerance test (OGTT) are used to diagnose both diabetes and prediabetes (see Figure 38-6 to review diagnostic numbers).

Diabetes Mellitus Type 1

DM type 1 most often develops in children and young adults. This disease previously was known as either juvenile-onset diabetes or insulin-dependent diabetes. In DM type 1 the pancreas is unable to produce insulin because autoimmune, genetic, or environmental factors have destroyed the beta islet cells. The cause is unknown, but experts believe an autoimmune reaction destroys these cells. The most common theory is that a virus stimulates the autoimmune reaction, although genetics may also play a role in triggering the disease. DM type 1 affects about 5% of patients with diabetes. Symptoms usually have an acute onset; the affected child becomes very ill within a short time. Treatment of DM type 1 requires insulin administration. The goal for insulin therapy is to maintain blood glucose levels as close to normal as possible without causing hypoglycemia. Insulin must be injected under the skin with a syringe, an insulin pen (Figure 38-7), or an insulin pump; it cannot be taken by mouth because the acid in the stomach destroys it.

The U.S. Food and Drug Administration (FDA) recently approved the drug Afrezza, a rapid-acting inhaled insulin that is administered at the beginning of each meal. It is not a substitute for long-acting insulin; it is not recommended for patients who smoke; and it should not be used for patients with a chronic lung disease, such as asthma or chronic obstructive pulmonary disease (COPD).

The medical assistant usually is involved in coaching patients on how to administer their insulin accurately (Table 38-1 summarizes the various types of insulin). Manufacturers recommend that insulin be stored in a refrigerator at approximately 36° to 46°F (2.2° to 7.8°C). Unopened and stored in this manner, insulin remains potent until the expiration date on the package.

Although insulin should be stored in the refrigerator, injecting the cold solution may be painful for the patient, and patients who must travel with insulin doses need to understand correct storage procedures. The provider may recommend that the patient store the bottle currently in use at room temperature. Depending on the type of insulin, it can be stored safely at room temperatures for 7 to 28 days. For example, Humalog and Regular insulins can be stored at room temperature for 28 days, whereas NPH and premixed solutions containing NPH can be stored this way only for 7 to 14 days. Extreme temperatures can make the drug less effective, so it should not be frozen (frozen insulin must be discarded), left in the sunlight, or carried in the glove compartment of a car. Temperatures below 59°F (15°C) or above 86°F (30°C) must be avoided. Successful treatment of DM type 1 involves a complicated regimen in which various types of insulin are given in multiple injections (typically three or four) throughout the day. The insulin type and dosage are balanced by the patient's typical exercise regimen and diet. The patient must monitor blood glucose levels with a glucometer periodically throughout the day to determine

whether the levels are within normal range. The provider typically prescribes glucometer testing in the morning before breakfast, before dinner, and possibly before lunch and at bedtime if the patient is having difficulty keeping blood plasma levels stabilized. A range of insulin types and doses are recommended by the provider based on daily glucometer readings. An important responsibility of the medical assistant is to teach the patient how to perform glucometer screening (Procedure 38-1).

Alternative Methods of Insulin Administration

- *Insulin pump:* A computerized device that administers a constant dose of insulin using a small portable pump. The pump is programmed to deliver a measured dose of insulin by continuous subcutaneous infusion through a needle-tipped catheter, which is placed in the abdomen or buttocks area. This method more closely resembles the body's normal surge of insulin and is designed to maintain blood glucose levels consistently within normal limits.
- *Injector pen:* An injection device that is preloaded with insulin cartridges for easy use (see Figure 38-7). Insulin pens are disposable or refillable and easily portable and therefore can be used by patients with diabetes when they are away from home.

Glucometers are palm sized and use very small amounts of capillary blood from a site in the finger (Figure 38-8), forearm, upper arm, or abdomen. Many different types of glucometers are available, but all display test results within seconds, and the results are stored in the memory function of the machine for future reference. Some more advanced features include a blood analysis display that shows a precise evaluation of blood glucose levels. Other glucometers can be directly downloaded to a computer to help the patient and provider monitor test results. Glucometers are frequently used in the healthcare setting to check both fasting blood sugar (FBS) and nonfasting blood sugar (NFBS) levels. The medical assistant should stress that the accuracy of blood glucose results depends on following the instructions for the particular type of glucometer the patient uses. When

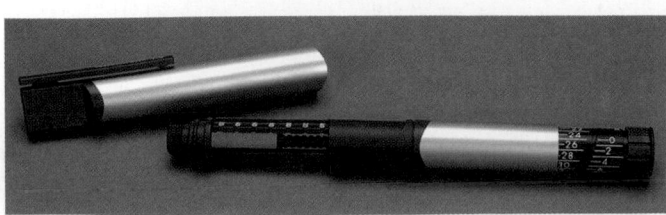

FIGURE 38-7 NovoPen.

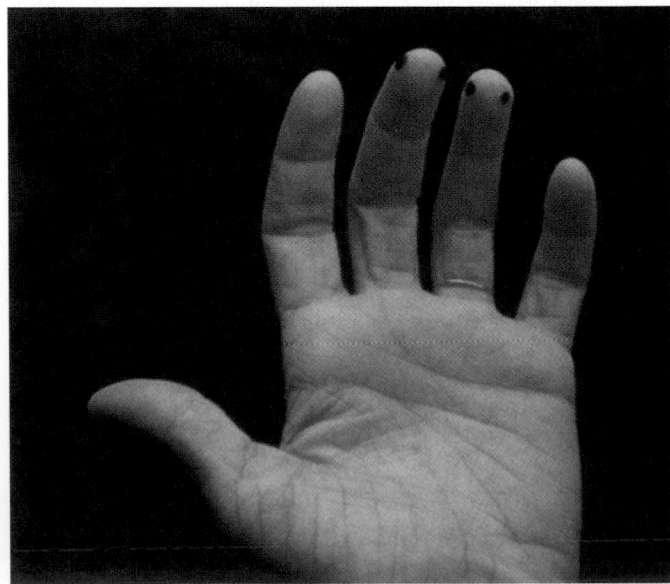

FIGURE 38-8 Capillary puncture sites on the fingers.

TABLE 38-1	Types and Characteristics of Insulin				
TYPE	BRAND NAME(S)	APPEARANCE	ONSET*	PEAK	DURATION
Rapid acting	Humalog, NovoLog, Apidra	Clear	10-30 min	30 min-3 hr	3-5 hr (taken just before or just after meals)
Rapid-acting inhaled	Afrezza	Single-use plastic cartridges used with an Afrezza inhaler	12-15 min	60 min	2.5-3 hr
Short acting	Regular (Novolin R, Humulin R)	Clear	30 min-1 hr	2-5 hr	Up to 12 hr (taken 30 min before meals)
Intermediate acting	NPH (Novolin N, Humulin N)	Cloudy	1.5-4 hr	4-12 hr	Up to 24 hr (taken at bedtime to minimize nighttime hypoglycemia)
Long acting	Lantus,† Levemir	Clear	0.8-4 hr	Minimal peak	Up to 24 hr

*The *onset* is the length of time before the insulin begins to work; the *peak* is the period when the insulin is most effective; and the *duration* is the length of time the insulin exerts an effect in the body.
†Lantus must not be mixed with other insulins.

teaching the patient about glucometer screening, the medical assistant must use the same machine the patient will use at home. Patients should be encouraged to bring their glucometers with them to each office visit so that the provider can review recorded glucose levels.

Patient education for glucometer use should include not only the steps for successfully checking blood glucose levels, but also quality-control mechanisms, as suggested by the manufacturer of the device. Some examples of quality controls include the following:
- Follow the manufacturer's instructions exactly.
- Perform the instrument maintenance specified by the manufacturer, including correct cleaning and storage of the instrument.

- Check the expiration dates on test strips and solutions and store these products correctly.
- Match and correctly enter the test strip code into the instrument before use if required.
- Contact the provider if test results do not match symptoms.

Patients with diabetes also need to find the best method of disposing of their syringes and lancets. Most pharmacies provide a sharps container with a syringe purchase. Local pharmacies or hospitals may offer assistance with disposal of used sharps. If the patient does not have access to a sharps return program, a puncture-resistant container with an opening that can be easily and tightly sealed before disposal is a good choice.

PROCEDURE 38-1   Assist the Provider with Patient Care: Perform a Blood Glucose TRUEresult Test

Goal: *To perform a blood test for diabetes mellitus accurately.*

EQUIPMENT and SUPPLIES
- Patient's record
- TRUEresult glucometer or similar glucose monitoring device
- TRUEtest strip
- Lancet and autoloading finger-puncturing device
- Alcohol preps
- Gauze squares
- Sharps container
- Disposable gloves
- Biohazard waste container

PROCEDURAL STEPS
1. Check the provider's order and collect the necessary equipment and supplies. Perform quality-control measures according to the manufacturer's guidelines and office policy.

2. Sanitize your hands and put on gloves.
   PURPOSE: To ensure infection control.
3. Identify the patient by name and date of birth and ask the person to wash his or her hands in warm, soapy water, then rinse them in warm water, and finally dry them completely.
   PURPOSE: To clean the area that will be punctured; also, warming the fingers may increase peripheral blood flow.
4. Check the patient's index and ring fingers and select the site for puncture (both forearm and fingertip testing can be done).
   PURPOSE: To make sure the site of puncture is free of trauma.
5. Turn on the TRUEresult glucometer by pressing the ON button (Figure 1). No coding is necessary with this monitor; you do not have to match the code on the test strip vial with the code on the glucometer.

PROCEDURE 38-1   *—continued*

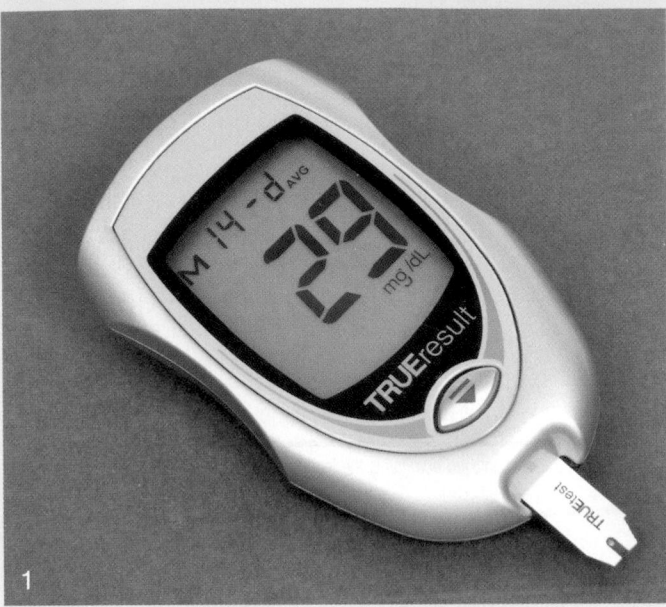

6. The glucometer should be preloaded with test strips. Before doing this, check the expiration date on the container of test strips. Push the test strip release button; a test strip is automatically in place.

7. Cleanse the selected site on the patient's fingertip with the alcohol wipe and allow the finger to air dry (this step is done in the healthcare setting to reduce infections but does not have to be performed by patients at home).

8. Perform the finger puncture and wipe away the first drop of blood.
   PURPOSE: Tissue fluid may be present in the first drop of blood.

9. Apply a small blood sample (0.5 mL) to the end of the test strip (Figure 2).

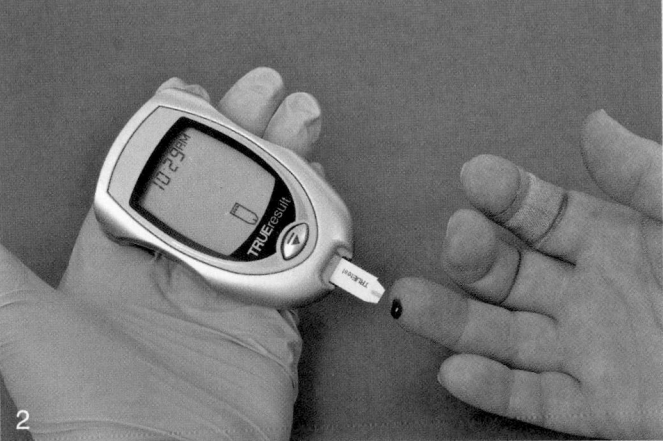

10. Give the patient a gauze square to hold securely over the puncture site; apply an adhesive bandage if needed.

11. The glucometer automatically begins the measurement process, and results are obtained in as soon as 4 seconds.

12. The test result is shown in the display window in milligrams per deciliter (mg/dL).

13. The patient can set up to four testing reminders on his or her personal glucometer; a ketone alarm signals when the blood glucose reading rises above a certain level.

14. The glucometer stores 30 daily average test results, up to 500 individual results, along with the date and time of each recording. Encourage patients to bring their personal glucometer to the clinic so the provider can review daily averages and previous test results.

15. The glucometer automatically turns off.

16. Discard all biohazardous waste in the proper waste containers.
    PURPOSE: To ensure infection control.

17. Clean the glucometer according to the manufacturer's guidelines, disinfect the work area, remove your gloves and dispose of them properly, and sanitize your hands.

18. Record the test results in the patient's health record.
    PURPOSE: A procedure is considered not done until it is recorded.

8/16/20—1:00 PM: Glucometer screening completed as ordered by Dr. Misha. NFBS 144. Pt took routine dose of 10 units Humalog insulin at noon. Pt had no questions. M. Vasco, CMA (AAMA)

Diabetes Mellitus Type 2

DM type 2, once called adult-onset or non-insulin-dependent diabetes, usually develops in adults but may be seen at any age. Factors that increase the risk of DM type 2 include a family history, a history of gestational diabetes, impaired glucose tolerance, physical inactivity, and obesity. In this type of DM, the pancreas produces insulin, but not enough, and/or the target cells are resistant to insulin action. Diabetes type 2 is responsible for 95% of cases of diabetes mellitus.

This form of diabetes frequently goes undetected for many years because of the gradual onset of hyperglycemia and the absence of

Insulin Resistance and Diabetes Type 2 in Children

Factors that affect insulin resistance in childhood include:

- *Puberty:* Growth hormone released during puberty makes it more difficult for the body to use insulin correctly.
- *Female gender:* Girls develop insulin resistance more frequently than boys.
- *Race:* Hispanic, African-American, Native American, Asian-American, or Pacific Island ancestry raises the risk for DM type 2.
- *Diet:* High-carbohydrate and high-fat diets increase the incidence of DM type 2.
- *Obesity:* Insulin resistance increases as the amount of fat around the waist increases.
- *Activity:* Exercise improves how the body's cells use insulin.

Injectable Drugs Used to Manage Diabetes Types 1 and 2

- *Pramlintide* (Symlin): A synthetic form of the hormone amylin that works with insulin and glucagon to maintain normal blood glucose levels. Injections administered before meals help improve A_{1c} levels by reducing the rate at which food moves through the stomach, thereby preventing a sharp increase in blood plasma levels after meals. The drug has been approved for people with DM type 1 who are not achieving the recommended A_{1c} levels and for those with DM type 2 who are using insulin but not achieving A_{1c} goals. The drug improves **satiety**, reduces caloric intake, and may assist with weight loss. Insulin and Symlin dose adjustments, including reducing mealtime insulin doses by 50%, must be managed by the provider to reduce the risk of severe hypoglycemia.
- *Exenatide* (Byetta): Lowers blood glucose levels by increasing insulin secretion. It is injected 60 minutes before breakfast and dinner. The drug helps patients achieve modest weight loss and improves glycemic control. It is not for use by patients with DM type 1. Side effects can include nausea, vomiting, weight loss, heartburn, dizziness, or headache.
- *Dulaglutide* (Trulicity): A drug administered once a week with an injector pen by subcutaneous injection into the abdomen, thigh, or upper arm. It can be given at any time of day, independent of meals. It is used with diet and exercise to improve blood glucose levels in adults with DM type 2. The most common side effects are nausea, diarrhea, vomiting, abdominal pain, decreased appetite, dyspepsia, and fatigue.

classic diabetic symptoms. However, because of the insidious onset over time, patients with diabetes type 2 are at even greater risk of developing vascular complications. Treatment for diabetes type 2 includes weight loss, exercise, dietary restrictions, and oral hypoglycemic medications that act to stimulate insulin production and/or improve tissue response to insulin (Table 38-2). Medications for diabetes type 2 have multiple functions, including stimulating insulin secretion from pancreatic islet cells in patients with some pancreatic function; reducing insulin resistance at the cellular level; improving sensitivity to insulin in muscle and adipose tissue; and inhibiting hepatic **gluconeogenesis**.

As with diabetes type 1, the goal of treatment is to maintain blood glucose levels within the normal range. For some patients, exercise, diet, and weight loss are sufficient to control blood glucose levels. Sometimes just the loss of 10 to 20 pounds is enough to bring blood glucose levels under control. Other patients may need medication to maintain normal blood glucose levels; however, levels must be monitored daily with a glucometer to determine the success of treatment. Over time, the individual with DM type 2 may require insulin to control hyperglycemia.

CRITICAL THINKING APPLICATION   38-4

Carlos Vespa is a 47-year-old patient recently diagnosed with DM type 2. He has a BMI of 32; eats a high-fat, high-carbohydrate diet; and does not exercise. What lifestyle issues should Miguel include in his patient teaching intervention? Mr. Vespa tells Miguel he cannot afford the medication prescribed by the provider or the glucometer needed to monitor his blood glucose levels. Is there anything Miguel can do to help him with these issues?

Gestational Diabetes

A pregnant woman is diagnosed as having gestational diabetes if two or more of the following tests show these results:

- FBS or FPG: Glucose level > 95 mg/dL
- OGTT (using 100 g of glucose):
  - 1-hour glucose level: ≥180 mg/dL
  - 2-hour glucose level: ≥155 mg/dL
  - 3-hour glucose level: ≥138 mg/dL

According to a 2014 analysis by the Centers for Disease Control and Prevention (CDC), gestational diabetes affects approximately 9% of pregnant women in the United States each year and is considered a risk factor for the development of DM type 2 later in life. Factors that increase the risk of gestational diabetes are obesity; maternal age over 38; history of delivering infants who weigh more than 10 pounds at birth; a family history of diabetes; previous, unexplained stillbirth; previous birth with congenital anomalies; smoking; and belonging to certain ethnic groups, including Hispanics, Native Americans, Asian-Americans, and African-Americans. Some women are asymptomatic, whereas others show classic symptoms of diabetes. Because many pregnant women have gestational diabetes without apparent symptoms, all pregnant women are routinely screened between 24 and 28 weeks of pregnancy.

Gestational diabetes is caused by insulin resistance at the cellular level, resulting in hyperglycemia. The elevated glucose in the mother's blood passes through the placenta into the baby, causing hyperglycemia, with increased insulin production in the fetus. The extra carbohydrate energy is stored in the infant as fat and may result in a macrosomic, or "fat" baby, who is at higher risk for breathing problems at birth, obesity, and diabetes type 2.

TABLE 38-2   Oral Hypoglycemics Used in the Treatment of Diabetes Type 2

MEDICATION	CLASSIFICATION	ACTION	SIDE EFFECTS
Tolinase, Diabinese	Sulfonylureas, first generation	Increase insulin production	Hypoglycemia, weight gain
Micronase, Glucotrol, Amaryl	Sulfonylureas, second generation	Increase insulin production	Hypoglycemia, weight gain
Prandin	Meglitinide	Increases insulin release from the pancreas	Hypoglycemia, weight gain
Metformin (Fortamet, Glucophage)	Biguanide	Reduces hepatic glucose production; slightly increases muscle glucose uptake	Nausea, diarrhea, metallic taste
Avandia	Thiazolidinediones	Reduces insulin resistance; increases glucose uptake; redistributes fat; reduces vascular inflammation; preserves beta cells in the pancreas	Minor weight increase; edema
Precose, Glyset	Alpha glucosidase inhibitor	Slow absorption of complex carbohydrates	Gas and bloating, diarrhea
Glucovance (Micronase and Glucophage)	Sulfonylurea and biguanide	Reduces hepatic glucose production and increases insulin secretion	Hypoglycemia, weight gain

The treatment goal for gestational diabetes is to keep plasma glucose levels equal to those of pregnant women without the disorder. The treatment plan always includes diabetic diet counseling and regular physical activity. In obese women, a 30% calorie reduction is effective in reducing hyperglycemia. The American Congress of Obstetricians and Gynecologists (ACOG) now recommends that all pregnant women with fasting glucose levels higher than 95 mg/dL receive daily insulin injections for glucose control. Most women return to normal blood glucose levels after the baby is born; however, two out of three women experience gestational diabetes in future pregnancies. In addition, approximately 50% of women who experience gestational diabetes develop DM type 2 within 5 to 10 years. Because of these risk factors, patient education for women diagnosed with gestational diabetes should stress the following after the baby is born:

- Weight management: If the woman is unable to reach a healthy body mass index (BMI), losing 5% to 7% of her current body weight will lower blood glucose levels.
- Exercise: Minimum of 30 minutes a day.
- Diet: Reduce saturated fat and calorie intake and increase consumption of whole grains, complex carbohydrates, fruits, and vegetables.

Complications of Diabetes Mellitus

Acute Complications. Two acute complications can occur in patients with diabetes, depending on the level of glucose in the bloodstream. If an adult patient's blood glucose level is below 70 mg/dL, the symptoms seen are caused by hypoglycemia (Table 38-3). This reaction, which is related to insulin treatment, may also be called *insulin shock.* The goal is to prevent such episodes with adequate patient education and reinforcement of individualized medical management of diabetes, in addition to frequent blood glucose monitoring. The treatment for hypoglycemia is immediate glucose replacement. The recommended form of sugar supplement is

glucose tablets because each tablet contains a known amount of glucose (5 g). The patient can use other sugar supplements; however, the amount of glucose in these items is unknown, and the patient actually may become hyperglycemic from ingesting too much glucose. After the hypoglycemic crisis has ended, if the next meal is more than 1 hour away, the patient should have a mixed protein and carbohydrate snack (peanut butter crackers, cheese crackers) to maintain blood glucose levels until the next meal.

Treating Hypoglycemia: *the Rule of 15*

Teach patients and their caregivers the following steps for treating hypoglycemia:

1. Treat the hypoglycemia immediately (while the patient remains conscious).
2. If the glucometer reading is below 70 mg/dL, take 15 g of carbohydrate; this is the equivalent of:
   - 3 glucose tablets
   - 1 serving of glucose gel
   - ½ cup of any fruit juice
   - ½ cup of a regular (not diet) soft drink
   - 1 cup of milk
   - 5 or 6 pieces of hard candy
   - 1 tablespoon of sugar or honey
3. Wait 15 minutes, then check the glucometer reading again; if the level is still low, repeat steps 1 and 2.
4. After the symptoms have been relieved, eat a regular meal, as planned, to maintain plasma glucose levels.
5. The provider may order injected glucagon to quickly raise blood plasma levels.

TABLE 38-3	Characteristics of Hypoglycemia and Hyperglycemia		
DISEASE	**CAUSES**	**SIGNS AND SYMPTOMS**	**TREATMENT**
Hypoglycemia (low serum glucose level)	Too much insulin; insufficient calories; excessive exercise; individual with DM type 2 using insulin-boosting medications	Shakiness, vertigo, palpitations, diaphoresis, headache, hunger, pallor, fatigue, confusion, irritability, poor judgment, visual disturbances, seizures, coma	• Ingest sugar (3 glucose tablets recommended); monitor blood glucose level in 15 min • If level still low and symptoms persist, take another glucose tablet • If patient passes out, provider-injected glucagon may be needed; call for emergency services
Hyperglycemia (high serum glucose level)	Too little insulin; body unable to use insulin properly; excessive caloric intake; inadequate exercise; illness; stress	Polyphagia, polyuria, glycosuria, ketonuria, weight loss, pruritus; possibly ketoacidosis, with shortness of breath, "fruity" breath, dry mouth, nausea and vomiting, lethargy	• Exercise if blood glucose level <238 mg/dL • Reduce caloric intake • Provider may alter amount and timing of insulin

A second acute complication of diabetes is diabetic ketoacidosis, or diabetic coma. In this case the person with diabetes is unable to use glucose for energy because insulin is absent or insufficient, or there is resistance to insulin at the target cell site. Hyperglycemia results, with blood glucose levels rising as high as 300 to 750 mg/dL. Because cells cannot use carbohydrates for energy, the body begins to burn fat. Ketones are waste materials from fat metabolism that build up in the bloodstream and cause it to become more acidic. Although the development of ketoacidosis takes longer than insulin shock, it can become a medical emergency if the patient does not recognize the signs, monitor his or her blood glucose levels, and administer insulin as prescribed by the provider.

CRITICAL THINKING APPLICATION   **38-5**

Mr. Vespa returns to the office 1 week later and tells Dr. Misha that he has not been feeling well. Sometimes he feels very shaky, dizzy, and tired; he has been getting headaches and cannot think straight. Dr. Misha orders a glucometer reading, which shows Mr. Vespa's blood glucose level at 65. Dr. Misha's diagnosis is hypoglycemic episodes, and the physician asks Miguel to reinforce patient teaching about hypoglycemic and hyperglycemic signs and symptoms and treatment. What should Miguel include in the teaching intervention? How can he best reinforce the material so that Mr. Vespa will remember how to manage his disease?

Chronic Complications

Microvascular Disease. Arterial changes at the capillary level can occur within 1 to 2 years of the onset of DM. Hyperglycemic episodes combined with the duration of the disease cause degeneration of tissue arterioles, which results in multiple system disorders, including **diabetic retinopathy**. Diabetes is a leading cause of new blindness in people 20 to 74 years of age. Of patients with DM type 1, 90% have retinopathy after 10 to 15 years; of patients with DM type 2 who require insulin therapy, 84% develop retinopathy in 15 to 19 years.

Hyperglycemic episodes damage the blood vessels in the retina; therefore, strict glucose control helps delay the onset of retinopathy and slows its progression. Vision disturbances occur as a result of vascular changes in the capillaries of the retina. These complications can lead to retinal detachment and blindness. In addition, people with diabetes are at much higher risk of developing glaucoma and cataracts; they should have yearly eye screenings and frequent ophthalmologic examinations during routine office visits so that diabetic retinopathy can be diagnosed early.

Microvascular disease also can cause diabetic nephropathy; 20% to 30% of patients with DM type 1 or type 2 have kidney disease. In addition, diabetes is the most common cause of kidney failure in the United States. Diabetic kidney disease is the greatest threat to life in adults with DM type 1. Diabetes damages the small blood vessels in the kidneys and impairs their ability to filter waste from the blood. Degenerative changes cause destruction of the glomerular unit and can lead to renal failure. High blood pressure and smoking often are associated with diabetic nephropathy. Because urinary protein usually is the first sign of kidney damage, frequent testing for albuminuria is suggested. Early treatment slows down the progression of kidney disease. Good glucose control often can reverse early stages of diabetic nephropathy. With disease progression, renal failure may occur, resulting in the need for dialysis and possibly kidney transplantation.

Diabetic Neuropathy. Diabetic neuropathy is the most common complication of diabetes; 60% to 70% of those with diabetes have some form of diabetic nerve damage. This type of nerve damage is caused both by vascular changes and by hyperglycemia. The chief areas that show pathologic changes are the nerves and blood vessels in the eyes, kidneys, legs, and feet. The first signs of diabetic neuropathy usually are numbness, pain, or tingling in the hands, feet, or legs. The loss of sensation in the extremities is important because it affects the patient's ability to be aware of injuries, especially to the feet. Because of peripheral vascular compromise, foot injuries can develop into ulcers, or lesions can become infected and ultimately lead to gangrene and amputation.

Even a minor undetected injury, such as a foot blister, can lead to a serious problem for a patient with diabetes. Individuals with diabetes also may lose temperature sensation and thus are more susceptible to heat or cold injuries, such as burns and frostbite (Figure 38-9). Patients with diabetes should have their feet inspected and a monofilament test done at every clinical visit to ensure early detection and treatment of problems (Procedure 38-2). Healthcare providers should provide patients with verbal and written advice to help prevent or reduce these potentially serious injuries.

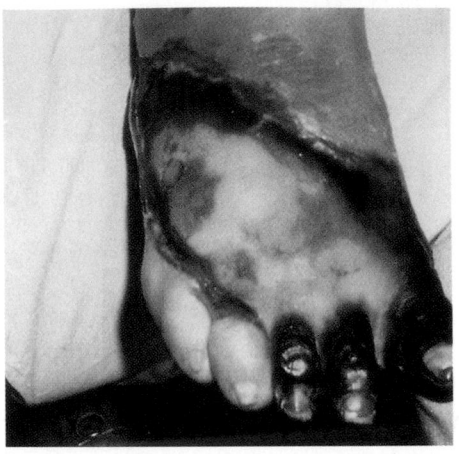

FIGURE 38-9 Patient with diabetes who has peripheral neuropathy and an insensate foot. Cold packs were applied to the patient's foot for treatment of a sprain. Frostbite developed, and the patient required a transmetatarsal amputation. (From Levin ME: Pathogenesis and general management of foot lesions in the diabetic patient. In Bowker JH, Pfeifer MA, editors: *Levin and O'Neal's the diabetic foot,* ed 6, St Louis, 2001, Mosby.)

Questions to Ask When Screening for Diabetic Neuropathy

- Can you feel your feet when walking?
- Have you noticed weakness in the muscles of your feet and legs?
- Do you have problems with balance when standing or walking?
- Do you have trouble feeling heat or cold in your feet or hands?
- Do you have open sores on your feet and legs that heal slowly?
- Have you noticed that your feet have changed shape?
- Do your feet tingle or feel like "pins and needles," or do you have burning or shooting pains in your feet? Do they hurt at night? Are they numb?
- Are your feet very sensitive to touch?
- Do your feet and hands get very cold or very hot?

http://professional.diabetes.org/?loc=rp-slabnav. Accessed January 22, 2015.

PROCEDURE 38-2   Assist the Provider with Patient Care: Perform a Monofilament Foot Exam

Goal: *To assess neuropathy in patients with diabetes.*

EQUIPMENT and SUPPLIES

- Patient's record
- 10-g monofilament tool
- Good lighting
- Disposable gloves
- Paper towels

PROCEDURAL STEPS

1. Check the provider's order and collect the necessary equipment and supplies.
2. Greet and identify the patient by name and date of birth. Introduce yourself and explain the filament testing procedure.
   PURPOSE: To help the patient understand the purpose of the test and to answer any questions.
3. Sanitize your hands and put on gloves.
   PURPOSE: To ensure infection control.
4. Ask the patient to remove socks and shoes and rest the feet comfortably on a stool covered with paper towels or the exam table paper.
5. Using your hand, demonstrate that the monofilament is flexible, not sharp.
   PURPOSE: To alleviate the patient's anxiety.
6. Demonstrate the monofilament on the patient's hand so that there is a point of reference.
   PURPOSE: To help the patient understand what you will be doing when you examine the feet with the filament and what should be felt at each point of assessment.

7. Instruct the patient to close his or her eyes and respond with "yes" when the monofilament is felt on the feet.
   PURPOSE: The patient should have the eyes closed so he or she cannot see where you are touching with the monofilament.
8. Randomly test nine to 12 areas on the anterior and posterior of each foot, according to the instructions on the monofilament tool.
   PURPOSE: To determine areas where the patient has lack of feeling from peripheral neuropathy (Figure 1).

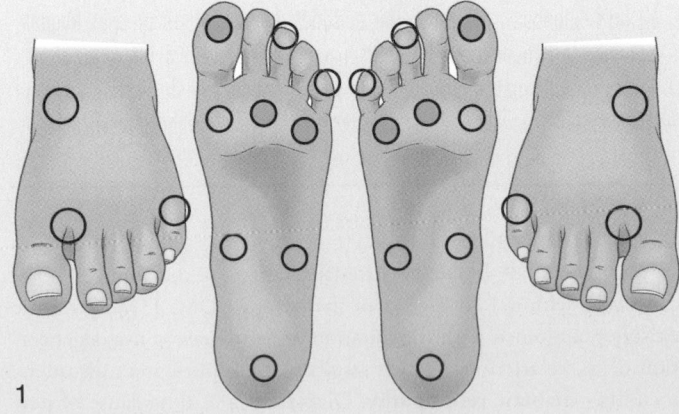

1

9. Starting with the great toe, place the monofilament perpendicular to the skin. Press until the monofilament bends, hold for one second, and then release (Figure 2).

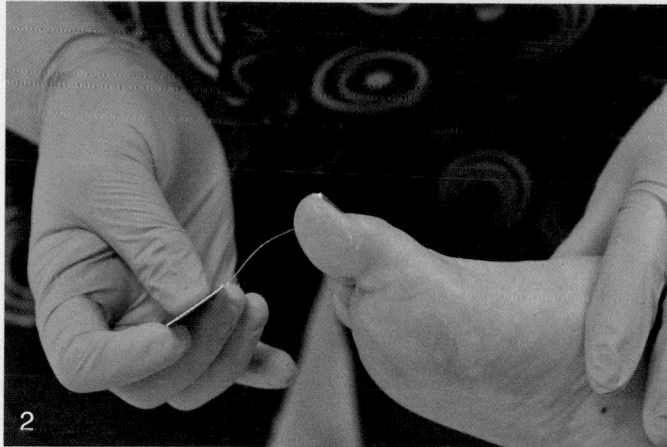

10. The test result is abnormal if the patient cannot feel the monofilament in any one of the areas.

11. Perform the test on both feet and record the number of times the patient felt the monofilament for each foot.

12. Discard all biohazardous waste in the proper waste containers.
<u>PURPOSE</u>: To ensure infection control.

13. Disinfect the work area, remove your gloves and dispose of them properly, and sanitize your hands.

14. Record the number of positive results from the sites tested in the patient's health record. For example, if the filament was used to test 12 locations on each foot, and the patient felt it in 10 of 12 locations on the right foot and in 8 of 12 on the left foot, record those numbers. Also record the locations where an absence of feeling was noted.
<u>PURPOSE</u>: A procedure is considered not done until it is recorded.

8/22/20–10 AM: Bilateral monofilament foot exam completed as ordered by Dr. Misha. Pt did not have feeling in ℝ posterior great toe (11/12) and Ⓛ 4th and 5th posterior metatarsals (10/12). Reinforced pt coaching on adequate blood glucose control and proper foot care. Pt had no questions. M. Vasco, CMA (AAMA)

Macrovascular Disease. Macrovascular disease, in the form of atherosclerosis, is a serious health issue for all patients with diabetes, especially those with DM type 2. People with diabetes are two to four times more likely to have atherosclerotic heart disease or strokes. Coronary artery disease (CAD) is the most common cause of death in people with DM type 2. The longer the patient has had diabetes, the greater the risk of CAD. Strokes occur twice as often in patients with diabetes as in those without the disease. Hypertension is common in patients with diabetes and contributes to the rates of CAD and CVA.

Peripheral vascular disease (PVD), a disease process in blood vessels outside the heart, is associated with atherosclerotic changes in small arteries and arterioles and contributes to the incidence of gangrene and amputations in patients with diabetes. Patients with DM type 2 frequently have signs and symptoms of PVD when first diagnosed. Compromised circulation in the lower extremities causes the formation of ulcers, poor wound healing, and possible progression to gangrene. This progression of PVD may result in amputation of the toes, foot, or leg. An estimated 35% to 75% of men with diabetes experience at least some degree of erectile dysfunction (ED, or impotence) in their lifetime because of vascular and nerve damage.

Infection. All patients with diabetes are at increased risk for infection because of a number of different factors. Those with impaired vision and neuropathies have an increased risk of injury because they may not be able to see or feel potentially dangerous items to prevent injury. Once an injury occurs and the integrity of the skin has been compromised, damaged or atherosclerotic blood vessels are unable to deliver the blood needed for healing, and the thickened blood vessel walls impede the release of white blood cells (WBCs) to the area. The WBCs of patients with diabetes show reduced phagocytosis, so their ability to destroy pathogens is limited. In addition, some pathogens multiply rapidly in the glucose-rich environment of individuals with diabetes. Therefore, the best method of controlling infections in these patients is to control blood glucose levels and prevent skin trauma or damage.

Foot Care for Patients with Diabetes

Patients with diabetes need instruction in foot hygiene and also a foot inspection during each clinical visit, regardless of the reason the patient is being seen. Education guidelines should include the following:

- Wash your feet every day with warm (not hot) water and mild soap.
- Cut your nails straight across to prevent ingrown toenails and possible injuries.
- Apply lotion to your feet, especially the heels. If the skin is cracked or red, speak to your doctor.
- Check your feet every day, using a mirror if necessary. Call your doctor at the first sign of redness, swelling, or numbness.
- Speak with your doctor before seeking treatment of corns, calluses, or bunions.
- Do not go barefoot or allow your feet to get too hot or too cold.
- Check your shoes for foreign objects or rough areas before wearing them.
- Wear comfortable, well-fitting shoes.
- Stop smoking. Smoking causes vasoconstriction, which reduces circulation to the extremities.

CRITICAL THINKING APPLICATION 38-6

Mr. Vespa and his wife are scheduled for a long visit today so that Dr. Misha can review his treatment plan. Dr. Misha asks Miguel to reinforce the possible complications of DM and the elements of foot care. What should Miguel include in his teaching intervention? How can he make sure Mr. and Mrs. Vespa understand the disease, its management, and possible complications? What resources should Miguel use to reinforce the information he is sharing?

FOLLOW-UP FOR PATIENTS WITH DIABETES

Experts agree that the best method of preventing diabetic complications is to maintain blood glucose levels consistently at near-normal ranges. Several laboratory tests can be ordered to monitor a patient's blood glucose levels. The FBS or FPG test measures the glucose levels in a blood specimen after a 12-hour fast. The normal range for an FBS is 70 to 110 mg/dL. Even though the provider may order periodic FBS tests, patients with diabetes still need to check their blood glucose levels as instructed with a home glucometer.

A routine test for monitoring long-term diabetes therapy is the glycosylated hemoglobin (HbA_{1c} or A_{1c}) test. This test has distinct advantages over routine FBS studies because the FBS reflects glucose levels at a given point in time, whereas the glycosylated hemoglobin test reflects serum glucose control over several months. The test measures glucose levels that have been chemically bound to the hemoglobin molecule on the red blood cell (RBC) over a 120-day period (the lifespan of an RBC). The provider can assess average daily glucose levels over the preceding 2 to 3 months and evaluate treatment compliance and results. The patient does not need to restrict food or fluid intake for this test and should continue to take prescribed medication before the blood sample is drawn. The patient's total A_{1c} should be less than 7%. The higher the glycosylated hemoglobin result, the higher the risk the patient will develop diabetic complications.

Developing an Education Plan for Patients Newly Diagnosed With Diabetes

The plan of care for individuals newly diagnosed with diabetes should be developed from a holistic point of view. Holistic care means that the diabetic team (including the medical assistant) considers all

Relationship Between the A_{1c} and Average Plasma Glucose Levels	
A_{1c} (%)	**AVERAGE PLASMA GLUCOSE (mg/dL)**
6	126
7	154
8	183
9	212
10	240

NIH. http://www.niddk.nih.gov/health-information/health-topics/diagnostic-tests/a1c-test-diabetes/Pages/index.aspx#14. Accessed February 11, 2016.

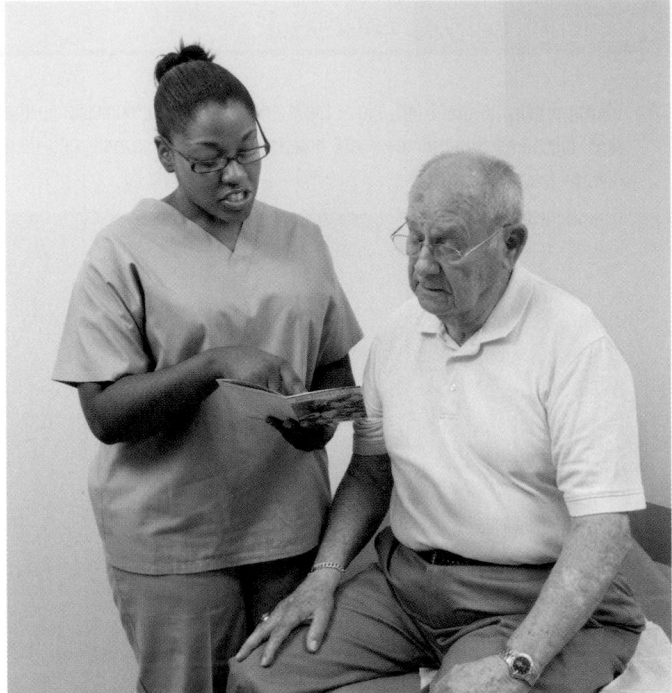

FIGURE 38-10 The medical assistant can use premade educational materials to discuss new lifestyle habits with a patient with diabetes.

aspects of the patient's needs, including lifestyle factors, such as diet and level of exercise; medications and the education needed to comply with their use; education that includes the details of the disease and its possible complications; demonstration and return demonstration as needed until the patient is proficient in glucometer testing and/or insulin administration; family involvement in the treatment process; and the use of community resources (e.g., a diabetic educator, support group, and dietitian) to assist with management of the disease (Figure 38-10). The equipment and supplies needed to treat diabetes effectively can be extremely expensive, so the medical assistant should investigate alternative methods of getting these materials if the patient is unable to afford them. The need for continuous daily glucose control must be emphasized at each patient visit. The medical assistant can also suggest provider-approved online resources that promote information about diabetes.

CLOSING COMMENTS

Patient Education

Because the management of endocrine disorders can be quite complicated, the medical assistant must make sure the patient understands the proper procedures for at-home treatment. By demonstrating a given procedure in the office, the medical assistant can address any inaccurate information or answer any questions the patient may have. Visual materials, such as brochures and procedure cards, also are helpful because they can be taken from the office and used as a reminder. If the patient is taking medication, the medical assistant should review the dosage schedule with the individual, discuss the purpose of the treatment, and clear up any confusion over the provider's instructions. As always, if the medical assistant is uncertain of any procedures or information, he or she should ask the provider for assistance before explaining anything to the patient.

Important Points in Patient Education About Diabetes

- Physical activity (too much or too little), stress, disease, medications, and diet all combine to affect blood glucose levels; following an effective dietary plan is the first step in self-management.
- The medical assistant should weigh the patient and measure his or her height. The medical assistant also should reinforce the body mass index (BMI) recommended by the provider and offer information about the basic nutritional requirements needed to help the individual either maintain his or her ideal body weight or to lose weight.
- The goal of a diet plan is to help maintain a homeostatic blood glucose level. If a healthy blood glucose level is maintained, the patient will avoid complications that can develop with hypoglycemia or hyperglycemia. Basic guidelines, according to the person's ethnic influences, age, gender, and physical activity, are used to establish a therapeutic meal plan. Family members should be involved in dietary health teaching, and appropriate community resources, such as a registered dietitian, should be used to help the patient understand and comply with dietary guidelines.
- The medical management of diabetes can be quite complicated and overwhelming for many patients. People with DM type 2 who are prescribed oral hypoglycemics must understand the drugs' mechanism of action and accurate dosage. Patients with DM type 1 or type 2 who require daily insulin must be able to prepare and administer their medication accurately and must understand the connection between glucometer readings and insulin dosage. All patients with diabetes must be able to use a glucometer accurately and must be aware of the possible complications of the disease. Emergency glucose tablets should be available at all times, and family and friends must be educated about the signs and symptoms of hypoglycemia so it can be treated promptly.

Legal and Ethical Issues

Pathophysiology of the endocrine system can have far-reaching effects on the body's ability to function. Patient education interventions should be documented completely to establish legal proof of the information shared with the patient. Never just assume that the patient understands the disease process and treatment recommendations. The following suggestions can help ensure the patient's welfare and promote risk management:

- Advise patients that a MedicAlert bracelet with their diagnosis and medication information is an important safeguard.
- Patients must take medication as prescribed, following the directions for dosage, route of administration, and storage; they also must be alert for possible side effects.
- Patients newly diagnosed with diabetes should not drive until glycemic control has stabilized. These patients also should be warned about possible visual impairment from the disease.
- Remember that you are always representing your profession and employer, and respond to each situation accordingly.
- Ask for assistance or further information if you feel unprepared to perform a procedure or to give accurate information.

Professional Behaviors

An important part of becoming a professional medical assistant is a commitment to lifelong learning. This chapter focused on the details of diabetes mellitus because it is the most common endocrine system disease and also one of the most serious. Regardless of where you work as a medical assistant, you will end up caring for patients with diabetes and interacting with their families on some level. Diabetes researchers are constantly discovering more information about the disease: how it is diagnosed, the best treatment methods, and the pathophysiology of possible complications. You must commit to continual learning about diabetes so that you are best prepared to care for patients with this life-threatening disorder.

SUMMARY OF SCENARIO

In his interactions with patients, Miguel has learned to pay attention to both verbal and nonverbal messages. He has used this technique consistently when interacting with Mr. Vespa. Miguel recognizes the importance of understanding the anatomy and physiology of the system, the complexity of endocrine system disorders, and the most frequently seen endocrine disorders. As a concerned medical assistant, Miguel continues to read professional journals and attend workshops so that he is prepared to answer questions from patients and assist with current therapies. He is especially interested in DM, because the practice for which he works has so many patients with diabetes. Miguel never hesitates to ask the attending physicians questions about the disease and its management.

SUMMARY OF LEARNING OBJECTIVES

1. **Define, spell, and pronounce the terms listed in the vocabulary.**
Spelling and pronouncing medical terms correctly reinforce the medical assistant's credibility. Knowing the definitions of these terms promotes confidence in communication with patients and co-workers.
2. **Summarize the anatomy and physiology of the endocrine system.**
The endocrine system consists of glands located throughout the body that produce and secrete chemicals known as hormones. The glands of the endocrine system are the hypothalamus, pituitary, pineal, thyroid, parathyroids, thymus, adrenals, and reproductive glands (i.e., the ovaries and the testes). Some nonendocrine organs, such as the pancreas, produce and release hormones. Through hormonal action, the endocrine system regulates all body functions.
3. **Explain the mechanism of hormone action.**
Hormones are chemical transmitters produced by glands and transported to the target tissue by the bloodstream. Hormone secretion is regulated by a combination of nervous stimulation, endocrine control, and feedback systems. Each hormone released into the bloodstream has particular target cells on which it acts.

Continued

SUMMARY OF LEARNING OBJECTIVES—*continued*

4. **Differentiate among the diseases and disorders of the endocrine system.**

   Hypersecretion or hyposecretion of hormones can cause endocrine disorders. When ADH is not produced or is not released in sufficient amounts, the patient develops diabetes insipidus. Gigantism and acromegaly are both diseases of the pituitary gland involving GH. When this condition affects children, gigantism is the result; in adults, acromegaly causes a wide range of manifestations that occur because of excessive connective tissue growth and overproduction of bone. Deficient secretion of thyroid hormone may be caused by an endemic iodine deficiency, resulting in a simple goiter. Improper development of the thyroid in an infant or young child causes cretinism; in an adult or older child, severe hypothyroidism causes myxedema. Hypersecretion of the thyroid gland causes thyrotoxicosis, or Graves' disease. Adrenal cortex insufficiency is called Addison's disease. Hypersecretion of the adrenal cortex, which results in elevated levels of cortisol, is known as Cushing's syndrome.

5. **Describe the diagnostic criteria for diabetes mellitus.**

   Diabetes is diagnosed if the patient has a plasma glucose level of 200 mg/dL or higher with polyuria, polydipsia, and unexplained weight loss; an FPG level of 126 mg/dL or higher on more than one occasion; a 2-hour OGTT of 200 mg/dL or higher; a positive urinalysis result for glucose and possibly ketones; or a glycosylated hemoglobin of 6.5% or higher.

6. **Do the following with regard to diabetes mellitus:**

   * *Compare and contrast prediabetes, diabetes type 1, diabetes type 2, and gestational diabetes.*

     Prediabetes is a condition in which an individual has a higher than normal blood glucose level that is not high enough for a diagnosis of diabetes type 2. Diabetes type 1 is seen in children and young adults and is characterized by a complete absence of insulin production. Patients must receive daily injections of insulin to survive. Diabetes type 2 develops gradually because of an insufficient amount of insulin or resistance to insulin at the target cell site, or both. Weight management, diet therapy, exercise, and medications are used to control glucose levels. Gestational diabetes occurs in approximately 9% of pregnancies but typically resolves after the infant is born. Diet therapy, exercise, and insulin are used for blood glucose control.

   * *Outline the treatment plan and management of the different types of diabetes mellitus.*

     All patients with diabetes must monitor their blood glucose levels regularly to determine the effectiveness of treatment. The goal of treatment is to maintain plasma glucose levels as close to the normal range as possible, as consistently as possible. Management of DM is a complicated interaction involving exercise, therapeutic diet, weight control, and medication. Patients with diabetes type 1 require daily injections of a combination of insulins. Table 38-1 summarizes the types and characteristics of a variety of insulins. Patients with diabetes type 2 may be prescribed oral hypoglycemics or insulin if needed. Table 38-2 explains typical oral hypoglycemics used to treat DM type 2. Diet therapy, exercise, and insulin are used to treat gestational diabetes.

   * *Perform blood glucose screening with a glucometer.*

     Procedure 38-1 describes how to perform plasma glucose screening accurately with a glucometer. Many types of glucometers are available, so it is important that the patient be taught how to perform testing using the type of device that will be used at home.

   * *Identify the characteristics of hypoglycemia and hyperglycemia.*

     With hyperglycemia, the patient experiences a sudden onset of polyphagia, polyuria, glycosuria, ketonuria, weight loss, pruritus, "fruity" breath, dry mouth, nausea and vomiting, and lethargy. This occurs as a result of an inadequate dosage of insulin, target cell resistance, overeating, lack of exercise, illness, or stress. Hypoglycemia causes shakiness, vertigo, headache, hunger, pallor, fatigue, confusion, irritability, visual disturbances, seizures, and possibly coma (see Table 38-3).

   * *Describe acute and chronic complications associated with diabetes mellitus.*

     Complications of DM include hypoglycemia; hyperglycemia and diabetic coma; diabetic neuropathy; microvascular diseases, including diabetic retinopathy and nephropathy; macrovascular diseases, such as atherosclerosis, CAD, CVA, and PVD; and decreased resistance to infection.

7. **Discuss follow-up for patients with diabetes and summarize patient education approaches to diabetes.**

   Patient education for patients with diabetes is an intricate mix of information on the dynamics of the disease; the importance of exercise, diet, and weight control in preventing complications and maintaining health; an understanding of the various types of insulin and when and how they should be administered; and, for patients with diabetes type 2, a knowledge of oral medications, their side effects and dosages; home care management, including proper use of glucometers and insulin administration; prevention of complications through effective control of blood glucose levels; proper foot care; and monitoring for and immediately contacting the provider about infections or other complications. Developing an education plan for patients with diabetes is ideal.

8. **Discuss legal and ethical issues to consider when caring for patients with endocrine system disorders.**

   The pathophysiology of the endocrine system can have far-reaching effects on the body's ability to function. Patient education interventions should be documented completely to establish legal proof of the information shared with the patient. Never assume that the patient understands the disease process and treatment recommendations. Specific risk management procedures may be instituted, depending on the patient's characteristics and diagnosis.

CONNECTIONS

Study Guide Connection: Go to the Chapter 38 Study Guide. Read and complete the activities.

evolve Evolve Connection: Go to the Chapter 38 link at *evolve.elsevier.com/kinn* to complete the Chapter Review Quiz. Check out the other resources listed for this chapter to make the most of what you have learned from Assisting in Endocrinology.

ASSISTING IN PULMONARY MEDICINE

39

SCENARIO

Michael McGuire, CMA (AAMA), works for a primary care physician, Dr. John Samuelson, in the small town in which Michael grew up. Dr. Samuelson's practice is open to all patients, but a large number of individuals with respiratory disease seek his help in managing their pulmonary problems. In the 6 months since he started with the practice, Michael has learned how to assist with pulmonary diagnostic tests and the special needs of patients with respiratory diseases. Michael has become familiar with the diagnosis and treatment of common pulmonary problems and adept at using the practice's new electronic health records (EHR) system. The office manager recently asked Michael to help her orient the staff to the new system so they are able to document respiratory system signs, symptoms, and diagnostic studies accurately. The main employers in the community are coal mining and construction companies, so many patients are at risk for occupation-related respiratory problems.

While studying this chapter, think about the following questions:

- What are the common pathologic conditions of the pulmonary system? What medical terms must Michael know to identify and explain these patient disorders?
- What are the medical assistant's primary responsibilities in working with patients with pulmonary problems?

- What clinical skills are required in this specialty practice?
- What pulmonary complications are associated with smoking and occupational respiratory hazards?
- What diagnostic and treatment procedures typically are ordered for patients with pulmonary disease?

LEARNING OBJECTIVES

1. Define, spell, and pronounce the terms listed in the vocabulary.
2. Describe the organs of the respiratory system and their functions.
3. Explain the process of ventilation.
4. Discuss respiratory system defenses and use correct respiratory system terminology when documenting in the health record.
5. Describe upper respiratory infections (e.g., the common cold, sinusitis, and allergic rhinitis) in addition to lower respiratory infections (e.g., pneumonia).
6. Explain the diagnosis and treatment of tuberculosis.
7. Do the following related to chronic obstructive pulmonary disease:
   - Summarize the disorders associated with chronic obstructive pulmonary disease and their treatments.
   - Teach a patient how to use a peak flow meter.

- Administer a nebulizer treatment.
- Detail patient teaching for the use of a metered-dose inhaler.
8. Discuss obstructive sleep apnea, including causes, risk factors, complications, and treatment.
9. Describe the cancers associated with the pulmonary system.
10. Summarize the medical assistant's role in assisting with pulmonary procedures.
11. Distinguish among common diagnostic procedures for the respiratory system; perform a volume capacity spirometry test and a pulse oximeter procedure; and collect a sputum sample for culture.
12. Discuss patient education, in addition to legal and ethical issues associated with pulmonary medicine.

VOCABULARY

bifurcates Divides from one into two branches.
bronchiectasis (brong'-ke-ek-tuh-sis) Dilation of the bronchi and bronchioles associated with secondary infection or ciliary dysfunction.
cell-mediated immunity An immune response that occurs from the action of T lymphocytes rather than from the production of antibodies.
chronic bronchitis Recurrent inflammation of the membranes lining the bronchial tubes.

cilia (sil'-e-uh) Hairlike projections capable of movement; in the lungs, cilia waves move unwanted substances (e.g., mucus, dust, and pus) upward; cilia are destroyed by smoking.
hypercapnia (hi-per-kap'-ne-uh) Excess levels of carbon dioxide in the blood.
metastatic (meh-tuh-stah'-tik) Pertaining to the process by which cancerous cells spread from the site of origin to a distant site via lymph and blood circulation.

pleurisy Inflammation of the parietal pleura of the lungs; it causes dyspnea and stabbing chest pain, which result in restriction of breathing because of the pain.

pulmonary consolidation In pneumonia, the process by which the lungs become solidified as they fill with exudates.

rhinorrhea (ri-no-re′-uh) The discharge of nasal drainage.

tubercle (too′-buhr-kuhl) A nodule produced by the tuberculosis bacillus.

tracheostomy (tra-ke-os′-tuh-me) A surgical opening made through the neck into the trachea to allow breathing.

virulent (vir′-yoo-lent) Exceedingly pathogenic, noxious, or deadly.

The respiratory system has two primary functions: to exchange oxygen from the atmosphere for carbon dioxide waste and to maintain the acid-base balance in the body.

The two types of respiration are *external respiration,* which brings oxygen into the lungs, where carbon dioxide exchange occurs in the blood vessels surrounding the alveoli, and *internal respiration,* in which oxygen is exchanged for carbon dioxide at the cellular level. Cells soon stop functioning and die if they are deprived of oxygen.

Maintaining the acid-base balance in the body is critical because failure of this function may result in respiratory acidosis or alkalosis. Respiratory acidosis occurs if the patient experiences hypoventilation; carbon dioxide levels increase in the body, causing **hypercapnia**. Respiratory alkalosis occurs with an excess release of carbon dioxide caused by hyperventilation, which may be associated with anxiety or an acute asthma attack. Both conditions can be life-threatening if the underlying causes are not corrected. The respiratory and circulatory systems work together to supply body cells with oxygen and remove metabolic wastes. The ventilation process is controlled by the respiratory center in the central nervous system and assisted by the intercostal muscles and the diaphragm.

THE RESPIRATORY SYSTEM

The thoracic cage, sometimes called the *rib cage,* is a bony structure that is narrower at the top and wider at the base. It is held in place by the thoracic vertebrae of the spine in the center of the back and by the sternum in the center of the anterior aspect of the body. The first seven ribs attach directly to the sternum and are called the *true ribs.* Ribs 8, 9, and 10 fasten one to another, forming the false ribs, and ribs 11 and 12 are the "floating" ribs, or half ribs, because their only attachment is to the thoracic vertebrae. At the base or floor of the rib cage is the diaphragm, a musculotendinous membrane that separates the thoracic cavity and the abdominal cavity (Figure 39-1). The respiratory system is divided into two anatomic regions, the upper respiratory tract and the lower respiratory tract.

Requirements for Normal Respiration

- An open airway leading to the lungs
- Ability of the lungs to expand rhythmically
- Intact alveolar membranes
- Coordination of the intercostal muscles and the diaphragm
- Proper action of the central nervous system's respiratory control center

Upper Respiratory Tract

The upper respiratory tract, which transports air from the atmosphere to the lungs, includes the nose, pharynx (throat), and larynx (Figure 39-2). As air enters the nasal cavity, it is filtered by the **cilia**, warmed by surface capillaries, and moistened by mucous membranes. The paranasal sinuses, hollow cavities that also are lined with mucous cells and cilia, open into the nasal cavity and help warm and moisten inhaled air. The filtered, warmed, and moistened air moves past the tonsils (which have an immunity function and help defend the body from potential pathogens) and through the pharynx. As the air continues toward the lungs, it passes through the larynx. The opening into the larynx is protected by a moveable piece of cartilage, the epiglottis. The larynx, or voice box, is made up of vocal cords, which vibrate when air is exhaled, creating the sound of the voice. Once the air passes through the larynx, it enters the lower respiratory tract.

Lower Respiratory Tract

The lower respiratory tract consists of the trachea, bronchial tubes, and lungs (see Figure 39-2). These structures are also lined with mucous tissue that is covered with cilia. The collection of dust and foreign particles in the cilia initiates the coughing reflex; this helps expectorate mucus and foreign bodies that may contain pathogens. Without these defense mechanisms, pathogens would remain in the lungs and may cause disease. Cigarette smoke and other air pollutants slow or paralyze the cleansing action of the cilia and damage the mucous membrane lining throughout the respiratory tract.

The trachea (windpipe) is a tube that begins at the larynx and extends into the center of the chest, where it divides, or **bifurcates**, into the right and left bronchi. It is about 5 inches long and is surrounded by C-shaped cartilaginous rings. These rings hold the trachea open regardless of changes in air pressure.

It is often said that the bronchial tubes look like a tree hanging in the chest (Figure 39-3). The right bronchus is wider than the left to accommodate the right lung lobes, which also are larger. This means that foreign substances are more frequently seen in the right bronchus. Once the bronchi enter the lungs, they branch into smaller and smaller passageways, much as blood vessels do in the circulatory system. This branching continues until it becomes microscopic. These very tiny bronchi are called *bronchioles.* Every bronchiole terminates in microscopic air sacs called *alveoli.* The alveoli are made of thin tissue, only one cell wall thick, which allows for the exchange of oxygen and carbon dioxide through the cell membrane.

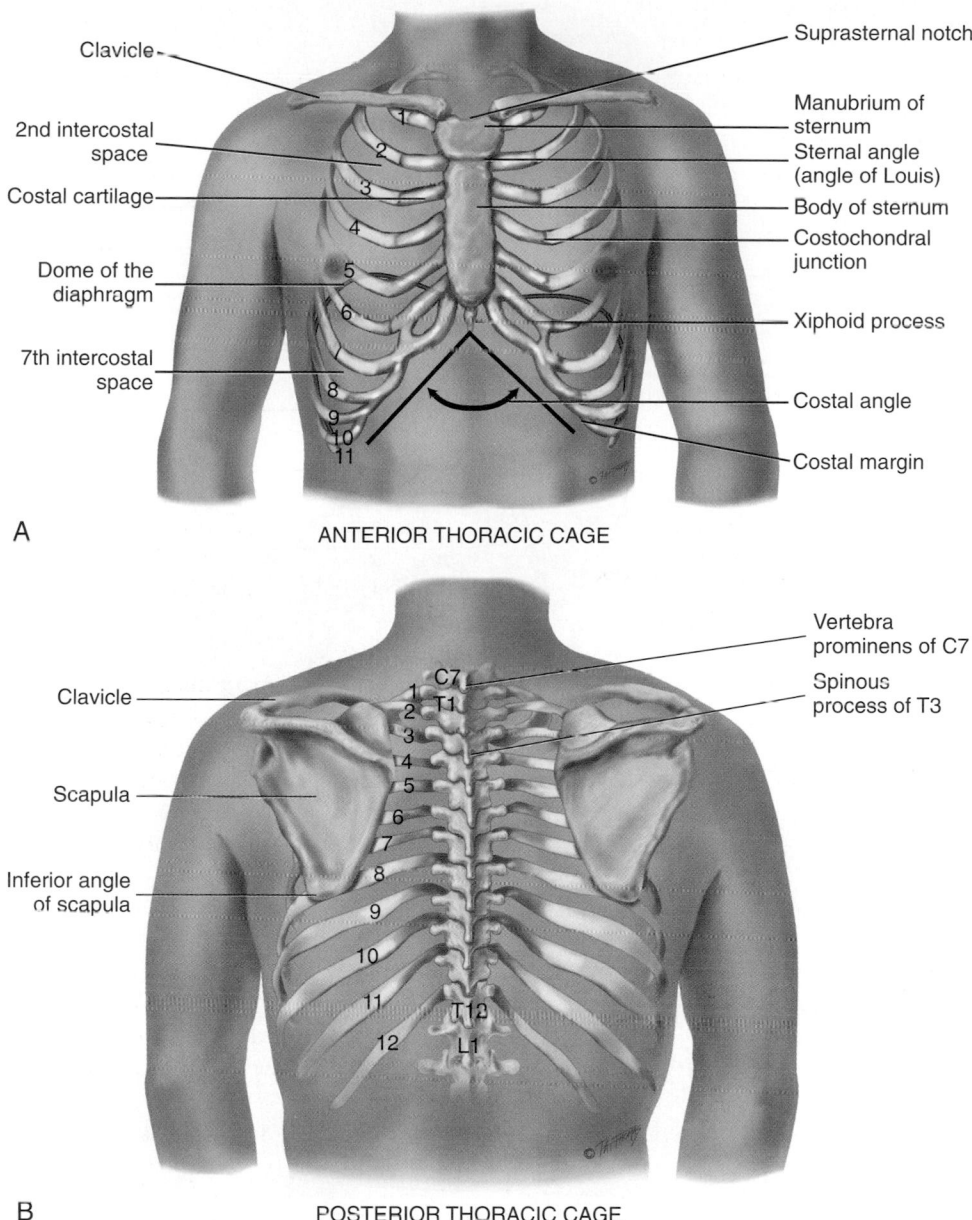

FIGURE 39-1 A, Anterior thoracic cage. **B,** Posterior thoracic cage. (From Jarvis C: *Physical examination and health assessment,* ed 6, St Louis, 2012, Saunders.)

The bronchial tree and alveoli are the major structures in the right and left lungs. The lungs are soft and spongy because of the air sacs that make up most of their mass. They hang in the right and left sides of the chest, separated by the pericardial sac, which contains the heart. The right lung is divided into three lobes and has a greater volume capacity than the left lung. Because each lobe has its own bronchus and blood supply, the removal of one lobe (lobectomy) results in little or no damage to the rest of the lung. The left lung is longer and narrower and has a distinct indentation in its center, known as the *cardiac notch,* where the left ventricle of the heart is located and an apical pulse is heard. The left lung has only two lobes, the upper and lower sections (Figure 39-4).

Each lung is encased in a double-layered sac called the *pleural membrane.* The membrane closest to the lung is called the *visceral pleura,* which doubles back to form the parietal pleural membrane.

Small amounts of pleural fluid fill the space between the two membranes and provide lubrication for the movement of the lungs during inhalation and exhalation.

VENTILATION

In the very delicate lung tissue, the bronchioles deposit oxygenated air into the grapelike structures of the alveoli. Surrounding each alveolus is a network of pulmonary capillaries. The oxygenated air moves through the single-celled walls of the alveoli and into the single-celled walls of the pulmonary capillaries (Figure 39-5). As this is happening, carbon dioxide and other wastes are forced out of the capillaries into the alveoli and then into the bronchioles. This carbon dioxide–oxygen exchange provides oxygen-rich blood that is returned to the heart for distribution throughout the body; carbon dioxide

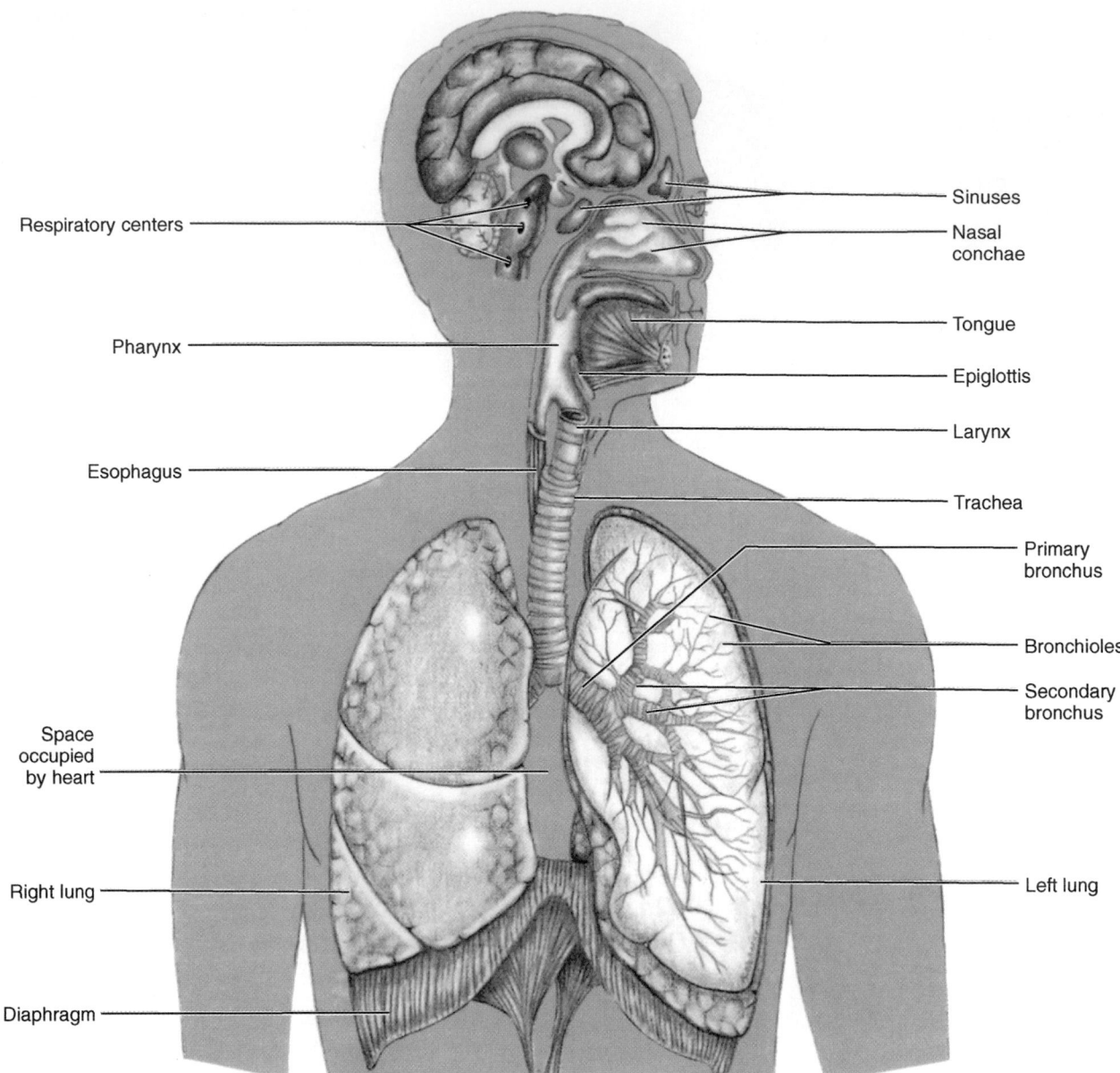

FIGURE 39-2 Anatomic structures of the respiratory system. (From Solomon EP: *Introduction to human anatomy and physiology,* ed 3, St Louis, 2009, Saunders.)

and other waste materials are excreted with exhalation. The process involved in this gaseous exchange is called *ventilation.* The movement of oxygen from the atmosphere into the alveoli is known as *inspiration,* and the movement of waste gases from the alveoli into the atmosphere is called *expiration.*

Inspiration

Inspiration begins with a signal from the medulla oblongata in the brainstem. The signal originates because of an increase in blood carbon dioxide levels, or in the case of patients with chronic obstructive pulmonary disease (COPD), a decrease in blood oxygen levels. The stimulus is carried by the phrenic nerve to the major muscle of inspiration, the diaphragm. When the diaphragm receives the signal, it flattens out and pulls downward. At the same moment, the intercostal muscles between the ribs contract, causing the ribs to move outward and the chest cavity to enlarge. This movement causes the

lungs to expand and increase their volume. The more these muscles are contracted, the deeper the inhalation and the greater the air volume becomes. Respiratory distress occurs when an individual is unable to move an adequate amount of air into the lungs, using the diaphragm and intercostal muscles, to meet the body's needs.

Expiration

The second half of ventilation is expiration. Once inspiration is complete, the diaphragm and intercostal muscles relax, causing the diaphragm to move upward into the thoracic cavity and the ribs to move inward, reducing lung capacity. This movement forces waste air out of the lungs and back into the atmosphere. Expiration requires very little energy and takes place with minimal effort by the body. However, in certain respiratory conditions, such as asthma or emphysema, the person has difficulty getting air out of the lungs, and accessory muscles in the chest and abdomen are needed

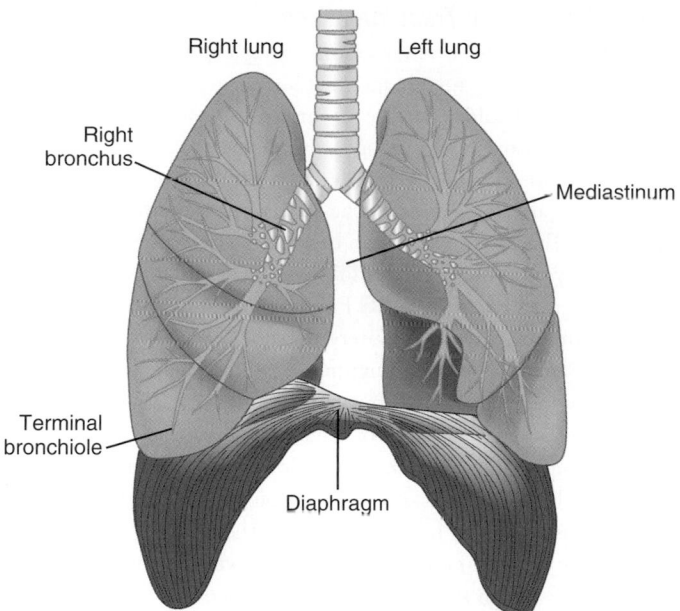

FIGURE 39-3 Bronchial tree.

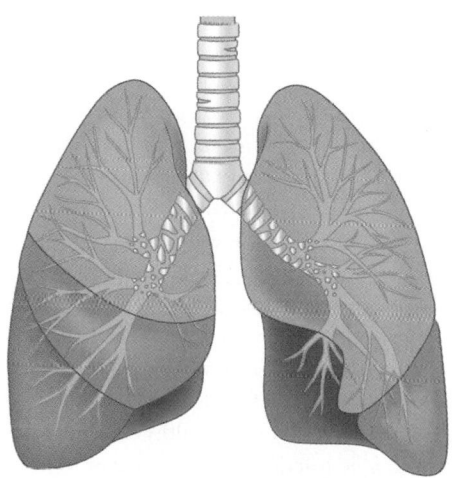

FIGURE 39-4 Lobes of the lungs.

Bronchioles and Alveoli

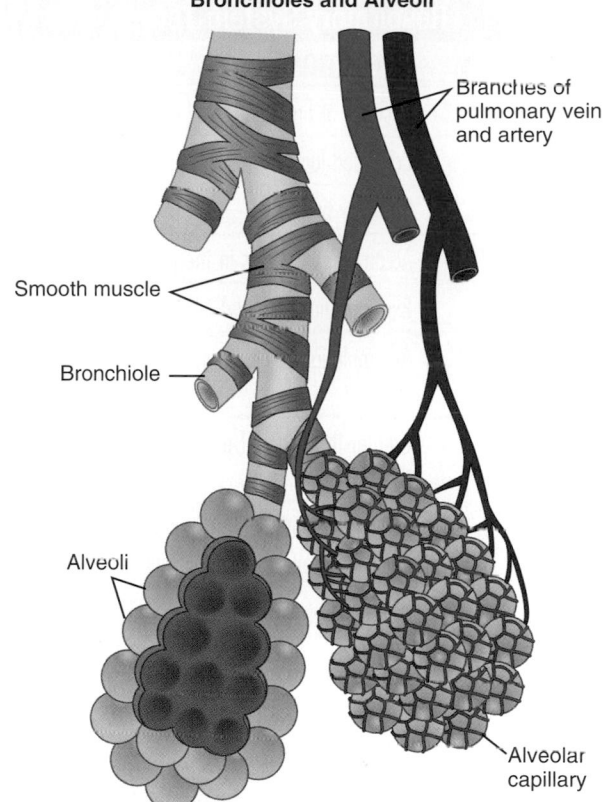

FIGURE 39-5 Alveoli with their capillary network.

to assist the intercostal and diaphragm muscles for complete exhalation.

RESPIRATORY SYSTEM DEFENSES

Every part of the respiratory system has a defense mechanism. In the upper respiratory tract, the mucus-covered ciliated surface of the mucous membranes traps particles and by the continuous flow of the cilia back toward the nasopharynx, the particles are either sneezed outward or swallowed.

The lower respiratory tract is sterile, which is phenomenal considering that each day these airways are exposed to approximately 10,000 L of air containing an endless number of microorganisms and foreign material. The ever-changing airflow, inspiration to expiration, creates a turbulence that makes remaining in the bronchi very difficult for these invading substances. This, combined with coughing, sneezing, and a functioning immune system, protects the

respiratory tract and helps the body maintain homeostasis. Disease occurs when something disrupts the normal homeostatic chain of events.

MAJOR DISEASES OF THE RESPIRATORY SYSTEM

Many diseases affect the respiratory system. The major ones can be divided into infectious diseases, obstructive disorders, and tumors. Chronic lower respiratory diseases (e.g., emphysema) are the third leading cause of death, and influenza and pneumonia are the eighth leading causes of death in the United States. Respiratory diseases cause common symptoms, including sneezing, a productive or nonproductive cough, sore throat or hoarseness, fever, general malaise, altered breath sounds, and changes in breathing patterns. The medical assistant must be familiar with common respiratory terms and use them in documenting a patient's signs and symptoms (Table 39-1).

Infectious Diseases

Respiratory tract infections fall into two categories, depending on their location. Diseases of the nose and upper respiratory tract are more common than diseases of the lower respiratory tract (e.g., pneumonia). Respiratory tract infections account for approximately 75% of all clinically diagnosed infections. Only about 5% of these infections involve the lungs. Most lung infections are seen in hospitalized patients, the elderly, substance abusers, alcoholics, and patients with acquired immunodeficiency syndrome (AIDS).

TABLE 39-1   Respiratory System Terms

MEDICAL TERM	DEFINITION
Apnea	Absence of breathing
Atelectasis	Collapsed lung
Dyspnea	Difficulty breathing
Empyema	Accumulation of pus in the pleural space
Hemoptysis	Expectoration of blood
Hemothorax	Accumulation of blood and fluid in the pleural cavity
Hypercapnia	Greater than normal amounts of carbon dioxide in the blood
Hyperpnea	Deep, rapid, labored respiration that may occur because of exercise or pain and fever
Hypoxemia	Low level of oxygen in the blood
Orthopnea	The need to sit or stand to breathe comfortably
Pleurisy	Inflammation of the parietal pleura, causing dyspnea and stabbing pain; a friction rub may be auscultated
Pneumothorax	Collapse of the lung as a result of the collection of air or gas in the pleural space
Pyothorax	Collection of pus in the pleural cavity, caused by infection
Rales	Bubbling or popping sound heard on auscultation; it is produced by the passage of air through bronchi that are constricted or contain secretions
Rhinoplasty	Plastic surgery to repair or alter the structure of the nose
Rhinorrhea	Excessive drainage from the nose
Rhonchi	Continuous rumbling sound heard on auscultation; it is caused by thick secretions or spasms
Tachypnea	Abnormally rapid rate of breathing
Thoracotomy	Surgical opening into the thoracic cavity

CRITICAL THINKING APPLICATION   39-1

Michael is taking a patient history for a new patient, who reports the following problems: Difficulty breathing; sometimes she has to sit up to breathe comfortably; occasionally she coughs up blood and has excessive nasal drainage. Six months ago, she experienced very rapid breathing and a blue color to her skin, so she was admitted to the hospital. She was diagnosed with blood and fluid around her right lung, which had become infected, causing her lung to collapse. Based on what Michael knows about respiratory system terminology, how should he document this information?

Upper Respiratory Tract Infections

Common Cold. The common cold is an acute inflammatory process affecting the mucous membranes that line the nose, pharynx, larynx, and bronchus. A cold virus spreads through tiny air droplets released when a sick person sneezes, coughs, or blows his or her nose. Usually the term "cold" is used when only the membranes of the nose and pharynx are affected; however, the same virus can affect the larynx and lungs. The viral invasion can be followed by bacterial infections of the pharynx, sinuses, and middle ear. Common signs of an upper respiratory tract infection (URTI or URI) include nasal congestion and **rhinorrhea**, sneezing, watery eyes, pharyngitis (sore throat), laryngitis (hoarseness), and coughing. Nasal discharge usually is clear and watery in the early stage but can become greenish yellow as the virus becomes more **virulent** or when bacteria invade. The patient usually complains of headache, low-grade fever, chills, and anorexia.

Currently there is no cure for the common cold; the infection usually runs its course in 10 to 14 days. The best way to treat it is to get plenty of rest and drink fluids. An over-the-counter (OTC) cold remedy, cough syrup, and acetaminophen may lessen the discomfort of cold-related symptoms; however, OTC cold remedies are not recommended for children under age 4. Antibiotics are prescribed only if there is evidence of a secondary bacterial infection. Echinacea has been promoted as an effective preventive and/or treatment for the common cold, but most studies show little or no evidence that it is effective. However, zinc taken within 24 hours of the onset of cold symptoms may reduce the duration and severity of the common cold in healthy people. In addition, research shows that although vitamin C is not effective at preventing the common cold, taking vitamin C regularly may reduce the duration of cold symptoms in both adults and children, even though it does not diminish the severity of symptoms.

Sinusitis. The paranasal sinuses are air-filled spaces in the skull located in the brow area over the eyes, inside each cheekbone, behind the bridge of the nose, and behind the eyes. Each sinus has an opening into the nose for the free exchange of air and is lined with a continuous mucous membrane. Healthy sinuses are sterile, but an infection or an allergic reaction can cause one or more of the sinuses to become inflamed or infected. Inflammation causes edema and the collection of mucus within the sinus cavity, creating a feeling of pressure, nasal congestion or rhinorrhea, and classic sinus headaches. The location of sinus pain depends on the sinus cavity involved but can be described as pain in the forehead (frontal sinuses), upper jaw and teeth discomfort (maxillary sinuses), pain between the eyes (ethmoid sinuses), and/or an earache and neck pain (sphenoid sinuses). The condition is treated with decongestants, antibiotics for bacterial infections, and analgesics. Sinusitis can be acute, lasting 2 to 8 weeks, or chronic, with symptoms lingering much longer.

Allergic Rhinitis (Hay Fever). Although it is not caused by a pathogenic organism, allergic rhinitis frequently is confused with infectious disease. This disorder affects millions of people every year. It is caused by a reaction of the nasal mucosa to an environmental allergen. The most common allergen is plant pollen; this is where the term "hay fever" originated. Signs and symptoms include sneezing, nasal congestion, nasal itching, and rhinorrhea. Symptoms can be controlled either with OTC antihistamines, such as Sudafed, Zyrtec, and fexofenadine hydrochloride (Allegra), or with prescription antihistamines, such as montelukast (Singulair), and fluticasone (Flonase) and cromolyn sodium nasal sprays. The list of possible allergens is extensive. When this condition is seen in the respiratory practice, the patient usually is referred to an allergist for testing and possible immunotherapy.

Patients may have difficulty determining whether symptoms are caused by a cold or an allergy. The condition usually is an allergy if the eyes, ears, nose, throat, and roof of the mouth (palate) are itchy; the eyes are red and watery; a clear, thin nasal discharge is present; symptoms are seasonal and last for weeks or months; and the individual does not have a fever.

Lower Respiratory Tract Infections

Pneumonia. Pneumonia is both a specific disorder and a general term meaning inflammation of all or part of the lungs (Figure 39-6). Pneumonia can be caused by bacteria, viruses, or other pathogens (Table 39-2). It also can be caused by inhalation of irritants or gas and by aspiration of solids or fluids into the lungs. The most common cause of bacterial pneumonia is streptococci, and influenza is the most common viral cause of pneumonia.

Pneumonia can occur in any age group but most often affects children under the age of 2 and individuals over age 65. It can range from a mild complication to a life-threatening illness. Risk factors include smoking, alcoholism, and immunosuppression caused by diseases or treatment. The patient usually comes to the office with symptoms of high fever, chills, and general malaise. Signs of the illness include dyspnea, tachypnea, chest pain during inspiration, and a relentless cough with possible hemoptysis. Auscultation of the chest reveals rales, rhonchi, and other signs of **pulmonary consolidation**. The infection may spread into the pleural cavity, causing empyema and **pleurisy**.

The diagnosis is confirmed with a chest x-ray evaluation; sputum culture and sensitivity testing to identify the invading organism and determine the appropriate antibiotic therapy; and a white blood cell (WBC) count. A WBC differential is also ordered to determine whether the pneumonia is viral or bacterial. If the pneumonia is viral, the number of WBCs does not increase; if it is bacterial, the greater the invasion, the higher the WBC count. With bacterial pneumonias, the differential count shows elevated neutrophil and monocyte levels. If the invading organism is bacterial, the treatment of choice is antibiotics and lung function therapy until the patient has recovered. If the organism is viral, the patient is given supportive care (e.g., antipyretics, fluids, and oxygen) until the immune system can control the spread of the virus.

Tuberculosis. According to the Centers for Disease Control and Prevention (CDC), approximately one third of the world's population is infected with tuberculosis (TB). TB causes more deaths than any other infectious agent in the world. For more than 50 years, the incidence of TB in the United States steadily declined; however, from the late 1980s through the 1990s, a resurgence in reported cases occurred. This increase was believed to be the result of increased travel and immigration; the number of individuals with AIDS, who have little resistance to disease; an increase in the number of homeless and malnourished people; and the overwhelming proliferation of drug-resistant TB bacilli. An international TB vaccine, bacille Calmette-Guérin (BCG), is available but is rarely used in the United States. The vaccine does not always provide protection from the disease, and those who are vaccinated may show a positive Mantoux test result.

TB is caused by the bacterium *Mycobacterium tuberculosis.* This organism is covered with a waxy substance that enables it to survive outside a living host for a long time. It is transmitted by droplets of sputum expectorated into the environment by an infected host; these droplets are inhaled by another person. In the warm, moist respiratory tract, the organisms again can become active if the individual is susceptible to the disease. TB also can be spread when an infected person coughs or sneezes, releasing airborne infected droplets, which are inhaled and cause an infection if the person is susceptible.

TB develops in two stages. The primary infection occurs when the person is first infected with the bacteria and the lungs become inflamed. **Cell-mediated immunity** ensues, isolating the bacteria and forming a **tubercle**. At this point a healthy individual can stop the spread of infection, causing the TB bacillus in the tubercle to

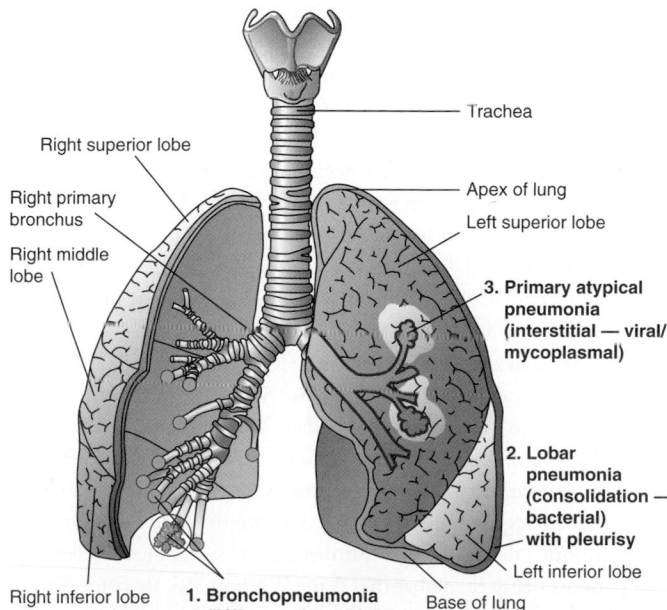

FIGURE 39-6 Types of pneumonia. (From VanMeter KC, Hubert RJ: *Gould's pathophysiology for the health professions,* ed 5, St Louis, 2015, Saunders.)

TABLE 39-2	Pathogens That Cause Pneumonia
PATHOGEN	**TYPE OF INFECTION**
Bacteria	*Streptococcus pneumoniae* *Haemophilus influenzae* *Staphylococcus aureus* *Mycobacteria*
Virus	Influenza virus
Fungi	*Aspergillus fumigatus* *Candida albicans* *Mycoplasma pneumoniae*
Parasite	*Pneumocystis jiroveci* (opportunistic infection, seen in immunosuppressed, debilitated, or terminally ill patients)

become inactive. In this case, the person was exposed to the pathogen but never developed active disease and so is said to have a *latent* TB infection. Individuals with latent TB are asymptomatic and are not infectious. However, because an exposed person develops antibodies to the disease, he or she consistently tests positive on TB skin screening tests. Therefore, rather than the purified protein derivative (PPD), or Mantoux, test, these patients should have chest x-ray studies to diagnose active TB.

At any time the bacilli in the tubercles can be reactivated, and secondary, or active, TB can develop. The patient now is actively infected with the disease, which can spread to the bones, brain, and kidneys (Figure 39-7). Some people develop active TB soon after becoming infected, before the immune system can fight the TB

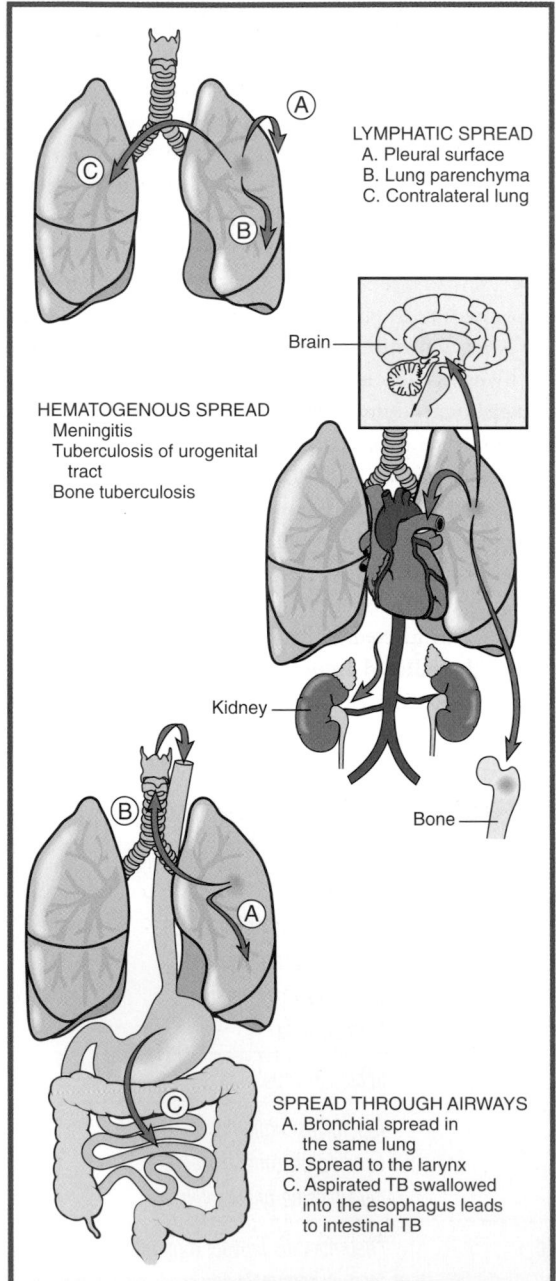

FIGURE 39-7 Spread of tuberculosis. (From Damjanov I: *Pathology for the health-related professions*, ed 4, St Louis, 2010, Saunders.)

bacteria; others develop it later in life, when the immune system is weakened for other reasons.

TB is diagnosed most frequently in people living in crowded conditions with poor hygiene, those who are malnourished, and those who have other chronic conditions. It spreads most rapidly in large cities, in the elderly, alcoholics, and the homeless. Symptoms of an active infection include an intermittent fever that peaks in the afternoon, night sweats, weight loss, and general malaise. As the infection becomes virulent in the host, a productive cough develops, and thick, dark, frequently blood-tinged mucus is expectorated.

The primary diagnosis of TB is established through the patient's signs and symptoms. The infection is suspected with a positive chest x-ray film but is confirmed with a sputum culture. Traditional culture methods originally took 4 to 6 weeks, and this extended period allowed a potentially infectious individual to continue to spread the disease. New culture techniques identify the bacterium in as little as 36 to 48 hours. The practitioner may order the QuantiFERON-TB Gold (QFT) or the T-Spot blood tests to diagnose TB infection. A positive blood test means the person has been infected with TB bacteria, but additional tests must be done to determine whether the person has latent TB infection or TB disease. A negative TB blood test indicates that latent TB infection or TB disease is not likely. Blood tests for TB are preferred if the individual has received the BCG vaccine or if the patient cannot return for a second appointment to look for a reaction to a Mantoux skin test.

A two-step Mantoux test may be ordered for individuals who have lowered immunity (e.g., human immunodeficiency virus [HIV] infection); the elderly who are entering long-term care; and as a baseline for pre-employment testing of healthcare workers and staff members in prisons and long-term care facilities, and those employed in substance abuse centers. Some people infected with *M. tuberculosis* may have a negative reaction to a Mantoux test if many years have passed since they became infected. However, they may have a positive reaction to a second skin test because the initial Mantoux stimulated their immune system's ability to react to the test. If the first test result is negative, the Mantoux should be repeated in 1 to 3 weeks. If the second test result is positive, the person is considered infected and should be treated accordingly. Healthcare providers are required by law to report TB illness to the local health department.

Once a diagnosis of TB has been confirmed, the patient is prescribed long-term treatment with a combination of drugs to eradicate the bacilli. If the patient has tested positive for TB but does not have an active infection, the standard treatment regimen for latent TB is 9 months of daily isoniazid. If the patient is healthy but has recently been exposed to active TB, the provider may opt for a 12-dose regimen of isoniazid and rifapentine (RPT). Rifampin (RIF) may also be prescribed daily for 4 months. All of these treatments are recommended to treat any possible tubercle formations. If the patient has active pulmonary TB, the CDC recommends a four-drug regimen—isoniazid, RIF, pyrazinamide, and ethambutol—daily for 2 months; the regimen then is reduced to two drugs for an additional 4 to 7 months, depending on sputum culture outcomes. It is crucial that patients being treated with TB medications strictly comply with medication orders to prevent the creation of multidrug-resistant TB (MDR-TB). Resistant strains of TB develop because of skipped doses or failure to take the medication as long as prescribed. MDR-TB requires at least 2 years of drug therapy with medications that can cause serious side effects, especially liver damage. All tuberculin-negative healthcare workers should have a PPD test annually; workers who show a positive reaction but are not actively infected with TB should have an annual chest x-ray evaluation to screen for the disease.

Signs and Symptoms of Latent and Active Tuberculosis

Latent Tuberculosis

- Asymptomatic
- Not infectious
- Positive purified protein derivative (PPD) test result
- Positive QuantiFERON-TB Gold blood test result
- Normal chest x-ray studies
- Negative sputum culture

Active Tuberculosis

- Symptoms include cough for 3 weeks or longer, chest pain, hemoptysis, fatigue, weight loss, anorexia, fever with chills, and night sweats
- Infectious (highest risk of infection is with close family members or associates)
- Positive PPD and QuantiFERON-TB Gold blood tests
- Abnormal chest x-ray studies and/or positive sputum culture

Centers for Disease Control and Prevention. Available at *www.cdc.gov/tb/publications/factsheets/general/LTBIandActiveTB.htm*. Accessed January 27, 2015.

CRITICAL THINKING APPLICATION   39-2

Dr. Samuelson is the primary care physician for a nursing home in the area. He is concerned because one of the employees had a positive result on a Mantoux test. What other tests will Dr. Samuelson order to confirm the diagnosis? If those test results come back positive, how will the patient be treated? What about the other employees and residents of the nursing home?

Chronic Obstructive Pulmonary Disease

COPD is a group of diseases with the common characteristic of chronic airway obstruction. COPD is the third leading cause of death in America, and most of those deaths are related to smoking. Among the diseases in this group are **chronic bronchitis**, **bronchiectasis**, asthma, pneumoconiosis, and emphysema. Although the mechanism of the obstruction may vary, a patient with COPD is unable to ventilate the lungs freely, which results in an ineffective exchange of respiratory gases, dyspnea, and productive cough. Over time, eliminating carbon dioxide from the lungs during expiration becomes increasingly difficult. Although COPD can be medically managed, it is not curable.

Asthma

Asthma attacks occur in response to a number of triggers that cause both inflammation and bronchospasm, with resultant airflow obstruction. Asthma can develop into a chronic disease characterized by increased sensitivity of the bronchial tubes to external factors (e.g., environmental irritants, poor air quality, and allergies) or to internal factors (e.g., stress, exercise, infection, and allergen inhalation). Asthma also has a strong hereditary factor.

Asthma attacks can be mild to severe and can last minutes to days. Bronchospasms trap air in the lungs, and the inflammatory response creates edema and causes secretion of mucus into the constricted bronchioles. A patient with asthma complains of a nonproductive cough, dyspnea, expiratory wheezing, and chest tightness. Because the individual has difficulty breathing, tachycardia, pallor, and diaphoresis also may occur. The patient can speak only a few words at a time, stopping intermittently to regulate air intake. When the chest is auscultated, the provider hears diminished breath sounds, with wheezes and rhonchi in the lungs. Peak flow meters and spirometry are used to measure the degree of airflow obstruction. Chest x-ray studies may show changes in the lungs from mucous obstructions. Blood tests include a complete blood cell count with a differential count to determine whether the attack is allergy related (Figure 39-8).

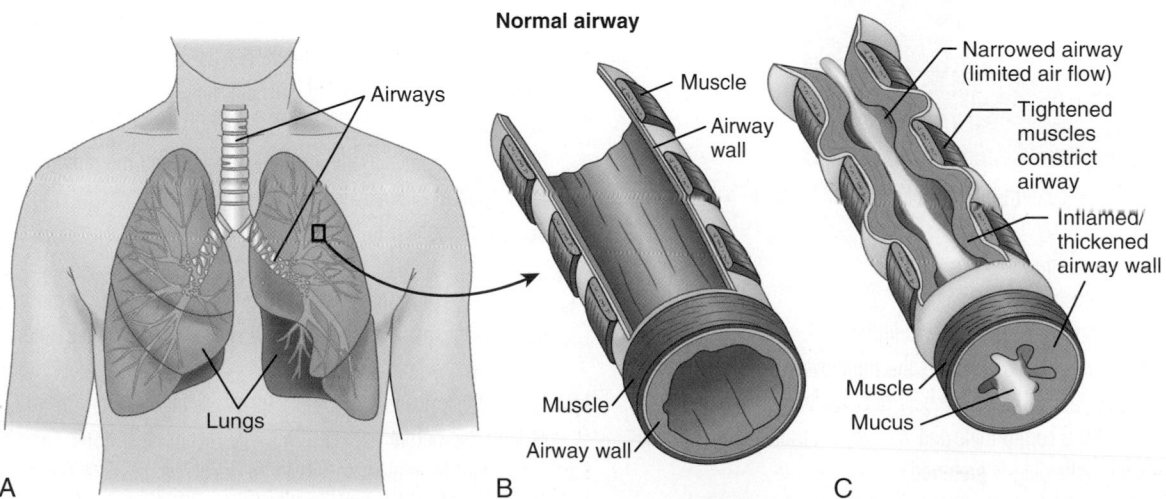

During asthma symptoms

Normal airway

Airways

Muscle

Airway wall

Muscle

Airway wall

Lungs

Narrowed airway (limited air flow)

Tightened muscles constrict airway

Inflamed/thickened airway wall

Muscle

Mucus

A   B   C

FIGURE 39-8 Inflammation and bronchospasm.

Regardless of their age, patients with asthma should be actively involved in the day-to-day management of their disease. The medical assistant may be responsible for teaching the patient how to perform peak flow measurements either daily or at the onset of an attack. Peak flow meters assess the individual's ability to move air into and out of the lungs. The provider may want the patient to keep a log of daily peak flow results or to use the instrument as an at-home monitoring device when chest tightness and wheezing occur. The meter measures the peak expiratory flow rate, which is the fastest speed at which the patient can blow air out of the lungs after taking in as big a breath as possible (Procedure 39-1). Peak flow readings provide an evaluation of bronchiole function that the patient can perform at home with limited assistance. Readings can help predict an asthma attack if levels are falling; measure the degree of bronchospasm; and provide the provider with feedback on the effectiveness of asthma treatment.

PROCEDURE 39-1   Instruct Patients According to Their Needs: Teach a Patient to Use a Peak Flow Meter

Goal: *To instruct the patient in the proper method of performing a peak flow meter test.*

EQUIPMENT and SUPPLIES

- Patient's health record
- Peak flow meter
- Disposable mouthpiece
- Biohazardous waste container

PROCEDURAL STEPS

1. Sanitize your hands.
2. Place the mouthpiece on the peak flow meter and slide the marker to the bottom of the scale.
   PURPOSE: The indicator must be at the bottom of the scale for proper measurement of expiratory effort (Figure 1).

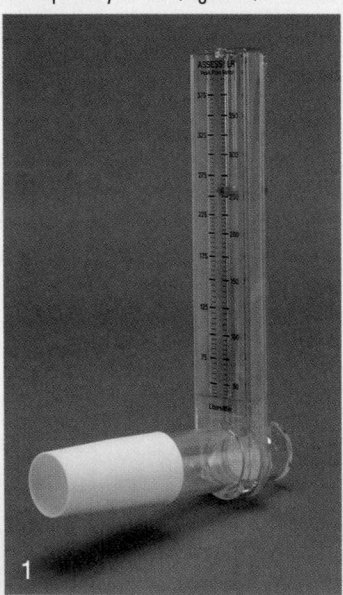

3. Introduce yourself and confirm the patient's identity by name and date of birth.
4. Explain the purpose of the test.
   PURPOSE: To help reassure the patient.
5. Explain the actual maneuver of forced expiration.
   PURPOSE: The patient must understand the maneuver so that he or she can cooperate fully; this produces the best test results.
6. Make sure the patient is comfortable and in a proper position, either sitting upright or standing (standing is preferred).
   PURPOSE: Proper positioning ensures maximum lung expansion and accurate test results.

7. Loosen any tight clothing, such as a necktie, bra, or belt.
   PURPOSE: Tight clothing may restrict breathing capacity.
8. Hold the meter upright, taking care not to block the opening with the fingers (Figure 2).
   PURPOSE: To prevent obstruction of forced exhalation.

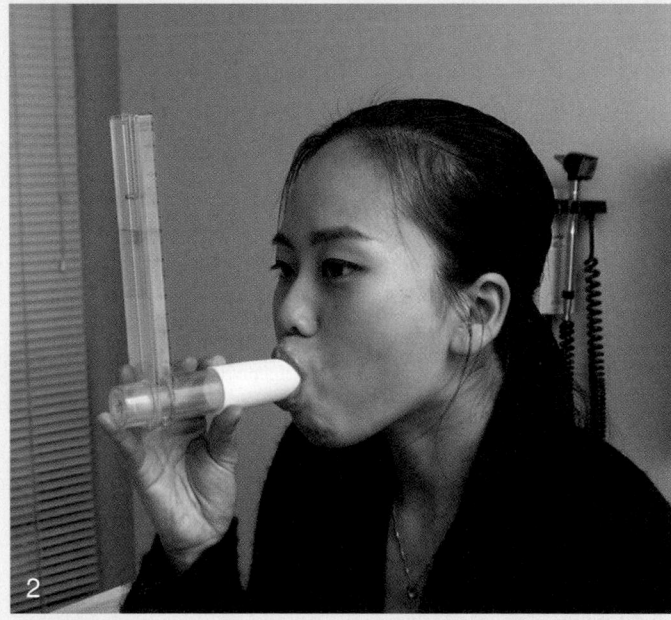

9. Instruct the patient to inhale as deeply as possible, to place the mouthpiece into the mouth beyond the teeth, and to form a tight seal with the lips. Caution the patient not to put the tongue in the mouthpiece when exhaling.
   PURPOSE: To prevent any leakage of air around the mouthpiece and any obstruction of airflow.
10. Instruct the patient to exhale as fast and as forcefully as possible into the peak flow meter.
11. The forced exhalation will move the marker up the scale and stop at the point of the peak expiratory flow. Record this number and return the marker to the bottom of the scale.
12. Repeat the procedure two more times, sliding the indicator to the bottom of the scale before each reading, and record each result.
13. Encourage the patient to inhale as deeply as possible and to exhale as fast and as forcefully as possible with each effort.

PROCEDURE 39-1 *—continued*

14. Place the test results in the patient's record for the provider to review, noting the time and date of the highest reading.
15. Clean and disinfect the equipment, discarding waste in a biohazardous waste container, and give the patient the meter for continued use at home with instructions to follow the manufacturer's cleaning recommendations.
16. Sanitize your hands.
    PURPOSE: To ensure infection control.

17. Record the testing information in the patient's health record.
    PURPOSE: Procedures that are not recorded are considered not done.

CAUTION: Peak flow readings may trigger bronchospasms or severe coughing in patients experiencing an asthma attack. If this occurs, instruct the patient to rest and try again. If the patient is unable to perform three readings because of bronchospasms and/or coughing, follow the provider's guidelines for managing this situation.

Digital peak flow meters are available that automatically record and track peak flow readings (Figure 39-9). However, these models are more expensive, so providers may still use the traditional peak flow meter shown in Procedure 39-1. Three zones of measurement are used to interpret peak flow rates. The green zone is considered normal: the reading is 80% to 100% of normal peak flow rates, indicating the patient's asthma is under control. The yellow zone signals caution: the patient's highest reading is 50% to 80% of normal. The provider makes treatment decisions and recommendations at this point, or the patient may already be instructed on how to manage medications if readings are within this level. The red zone includes readings below 50% of the normal level, and immediate action must be taken to prevent severe bronchospasms.

If the patient is having an asthma attack, the bronchioles are constricting, becoming edematous, and filling up with mucus, so the patient is unable to exhale strongly enough to raise the peak flow indicator to a normal level. If readings are below normal, the provider prescribes a treatment plan that may include contacting the provider when peak flow levels are below a certain point or starting nebulizer treatments. The provider may recommend an increase in antiinflammatory medication if more than a 20% variation from normal is seen in the readings. The medication therapy chosen depends on the severity and frequency of acute attacks, but management is necessary to prevent permanent lung damage and emphysema-like changes in the lungs.

The treatment of asthma consists of a regimen of medications, including "rescue" inhalers (e.g., pirbuterol [Maxair] or albuterol [Ventolin]), which are used to relieve bronchospasms or for exercise-induced asthma (Figure 39-10). Tissue inflammation can be treated with steroid inhalers (e.g., budesonide [Pulmicort Flexhaler], triamcinolone acetonide [Azmacort], or fluticasone [Flovent Diskus]) and/or an oral leukotriene-receptor antagonist taken daily, such as zafirlukast (Accolate) or montelukast sodium (Singulair). Another option is a combination inhaler, such as fluticasone and salmeterol (Advair Diskus), or budesonide and formoterol (Symbicort), to prevent and treat bronchiole inflammation. A severe attack may require injections of epinephrine, oral corticosteroids (prednisone) and/or nebulizer treatments with a bronchodilator (Procedure 39-2). A nebulizer forces compressed air through a medication chamber that converts liquid medication (albuterol or budesonide) into an aerosol or mist that can be inhaled though a mask or mouthpiece.

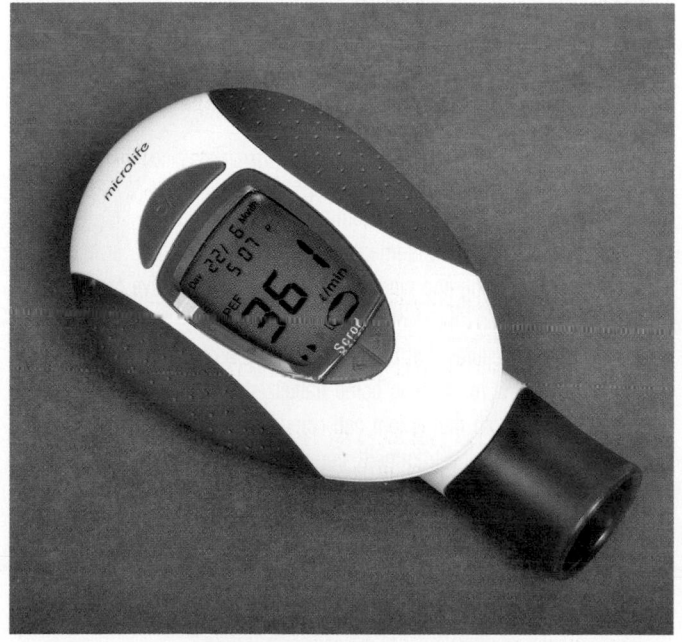

FIGURE 39-9 Digital peak flow meter.

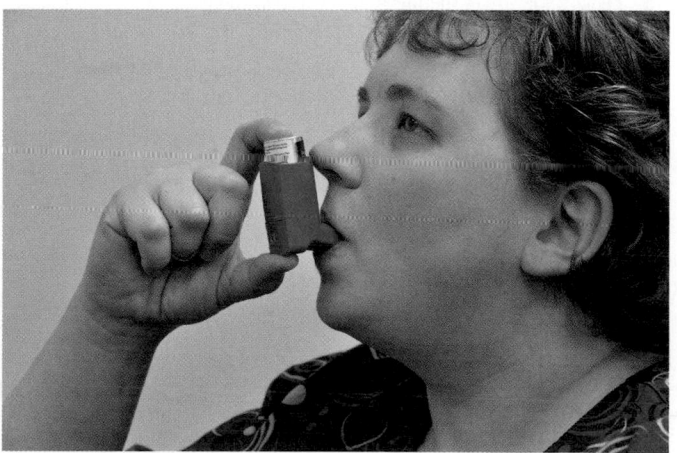

FIGURE 39-10 Use of a metered-dose inhaler.

PROCEDURE 39-2 | **Assist the Provider with Patient Care: Administer a Nebulizer Treatment**

Goal: *To perform a nebulizer treatment.*

EQUIPMENT and SUPPLIES

- Patient's health record
- Nebulizer machine
- Disposable connector tubing with medication dispenser
- Disposable mouthpiece or mask as ordered
- Disposable tissues
- Medication as ordered
- Biohazardous waste container

PROCEDURAL STEPS

1. Plug the nebulizer into a properly grounded electrical outlet.
2. Introduce yourself and confirm the patient's identity by name and date of birth.
3. Explain the purpose of the treatment.
   PURPOSE: To help reassure the patient.
4. Sanitize your hands.
5. Perform the three routine medication checks and measure the prescribed dose of drug into the nebulizer medication cup (Figure 1).

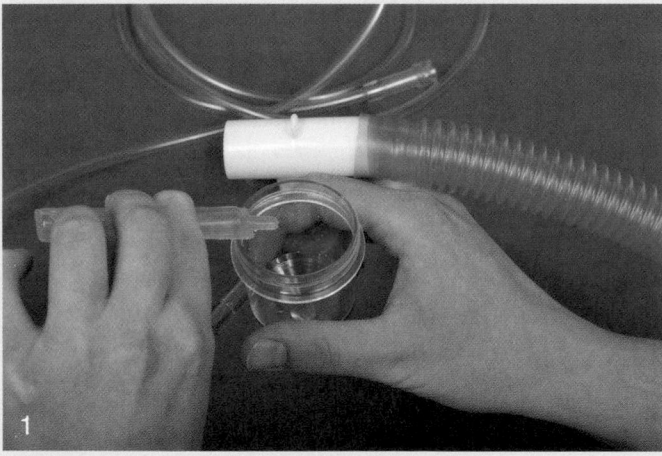

6. Replace the top of the medication cup and connect it to the mouthpiece or face mask.
7. Connect the disposable tubing to the nebulizer and the medication cup.
8. The patient should be sitting upright to allow for total lung expansion.
   PURPOSE: Proper positioning ensures adequate dispersal of the medication.
9. Turn on the nebulizer (a mist should be visible coming from the back of the tube opposite the mouthpiece or into the face mask).
   PURPOSE: The mist is the aerosolized medication.
10. If using a mask, position it comfortably but securely over the patient's mouth and nose.

11. If using a mouthpiece, instruct the patient to hold it between the teeth with the lips pursed around the mouthpiece (Figure 2).

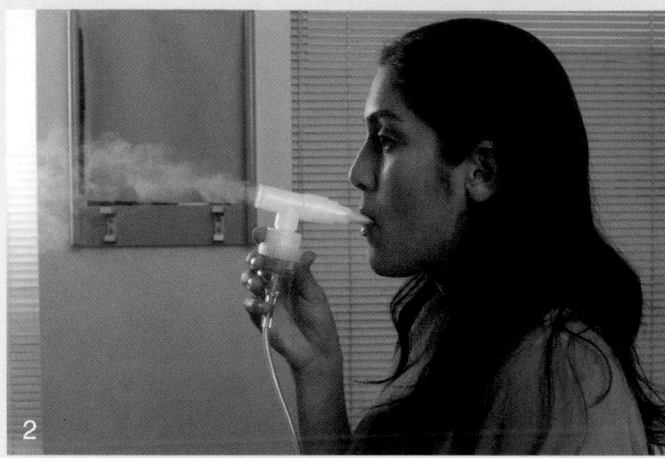

12. Encourage the patient to take slow, deep breaths through the mouth and to hold each breath 2 to 3 seconds to allow the medication to disperse through the lungs.
    PURPOSE: To ensure maximum distribution of the medication in the lung tissue.
13. Continue the treatment until aerosol is no longer produced (approximately 10 minutes).
    CAUTION: If the patient is receiving a bronchodilator (albuterol), he or she may experience dizziness, tremors, or tachycardia. Continue the treatment unless otherwise ordered by the provider.
14. Turn off the nebulizer.
15. Encourage the patient to take several deep breaths and to cough loosened secretions into disposable tissues.
16. Dispose of the mouthpiece or mask and tubing in a biohazard container and instruct the patient also to dispose of the contaminated tissues in the biohazard container.
    PURPOSE: To ensure infection control.
17. Sanitize your hands.
    PURPOSE: To ensure infection control.
18. Record the nebulizer treatment; the patient's response, including the amount of coughing and whether coughing was productive or nonproductive; and any side effects of the medication.
    PURPOSE: Procedures that are not recorded are considered not done.
19. If the patient is to continue home nebulizer treatments, provide patient education for both the patient and caregivers as appropriate. Make sure they demonstrate the treatment steps to confirm understanding.
    PURPOSE: Feedback through demonstration of technique ensures patient follow-through.

The provider prescribes an inhaler dose according to the number of "puffs" of a metered-dose inhaler (MDI) the patient should administer. MDIs consist of a pressurized canister containing medication and a mouthpiece. Most MDIs hold about 200 doses of medication combined with a pressurized gas propellant, which forces the drug out of the canister. When the canister is inverted and depressed, a metered dose (premeasured) is delivered through the mouthpiece in aerosol form. Patient teaching is very important to ensure that the patient operates the device correctly so that the medication can be administered as ordered. If both a steroid and a bronchodilator have been prescribed, the bronchodilator should be taken first, because this opens the airways so that the steroid is better distributed throughout the lungs.

Patient Education for a Metered-Dose HFA Inhaler

The chemical used to deliver medication in most metered-dose inhalers was changed to hydrofluoroalkane (HFA) in 2008. The following are instructions for patients for these devices:

1. The inhaler must be primed (1) before you use it the first time; (2) if it hasn't been used for several days; or (3) if you dropped it. Shake the inhaler and spray into the air (away from your face) up to four times. (See the information that came with your inhaler for exact instructions.)
2. Shake the canister vigorously for 5 seconds.
3. Hold the inhaler upright; put your index finger on the top of the canister, and have your thumb supporting the bottom of the inhaler.
4. Breathe out normally.
5. Place the mouthpiece between your teeth, and close your lips around it; keep your tongue away from the opening of the mouthpiece.
6. Press down the top of the canister with your index finger to release the medication.
7. As you press down on the canister, breathe in deeply and slowly through your mouth until your lungs are completely filled; this should take 4 to 6 seconds (see Figure 39-10).
8. Hold the medication in your lungs for about 5 seconds before breathing out.
9. If you need a second puff, wait about 15 to 30 seconds; shake the canister again before the next puff.
10. Inhalers can be attached to spacers to meet the needs of children or older patients who have difficulty managing the technique. When the canister is depressed, the medication is held in the spacer so the patient has more time to inhale the particles (Figure 39-11).
11. Recap the mouthpiece. HFA inhalers must be cleaned at least once a week to prevent blockage. Remove the medication canister and run warm tap water through the top and bottom of the plastic mouthpiece for 30 to 60 seconds; shake off the excess water and allow the mouthpiece to dry completely (overnight is recommended).
12. After each use of a steroid inhaler, rinse your mouth with water, gargle, and spit out the water to prevent an oral yeast infection (thrush).

NOTE: Follow these steps for a metered-dose inhaler only; to use a dry powder inhaler (e.g., Advair Diskus), close your mouth tightly around the mouthpiece of the inhaler and breathe in quickly.

(Reproduced with permission from Moore RH: Patient information: asthma inhaler techniques in children [Beyond the Basics]. In *UpToDate*: Post TW, editor, UpToDate, Waltham, MA. [Accessed on April 11, 2016.]) Copyright © 2016 UpToDate, Inc. For more information visit www.uptodate.com.

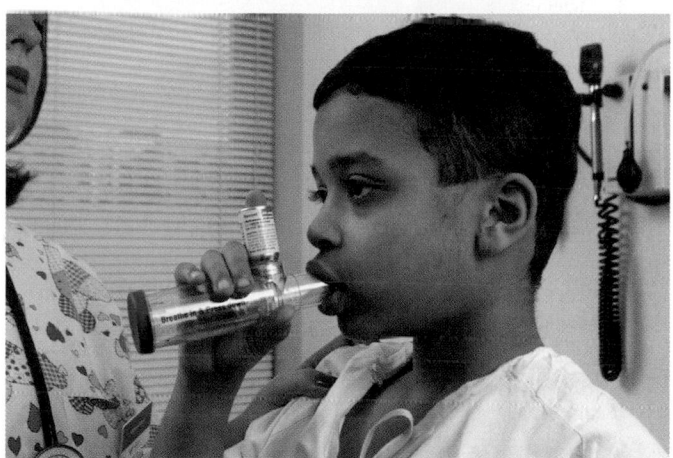

FIGURE 39-11 Use of a metered-dose inhaler with a spacer.

Pneumoconioses

Environmental causes of respiratory diseases include inhaled dusts, fumes, and various kinds of organic or inorganic matter. Most of these respiratory diseases are occupational; a consequence of long-term exposure to unsafe air in the workplace. Although the respiratory system is designed to filter and trap air contaminants, it can become overloaded after intense exposure. Subsequently, irritants enter the lungs, and the damage to pulmonary tissue increases if the particles are very small and can enter the alveoli; if the individual is exposed to a large amount of contaminants over a long period; and if the added irritation of cigarette smoking is a factor.

Some occupations that can cause pneumoconiosis include coal mining (anthracosis); insulation manufacturing and shipbuilding (asbestosis); and stonecutting or sandblasting (silicosis). The tissue changes caused by inhalation of these substances into the lungs are irreversible. Patients develop dyspnea, cough, and emphysema-like changes and have an increased risk of lung cancer.

Emphysema

Emphysema is a progressive obstructive disease of the pulmonary system that is irreversible. Emphysema causes loss of elasticity in the walls of the alveoli. Eventually these one-cell-thick walls stretch and break, creating air spaces that cannot perform oxygen–carbon dioxide exchange. The remaining alveoli become overinflated, and as time progresses, pressure increases in the affected alveoli, and those walls burst. This chain reaction of alveolar destruction causes trapped air to fill the spaces of the no longer functioning alveoli, making complete exhalation very difficult. Cigarette smoking is the primary contributing factor, although patients who develop emphysema at

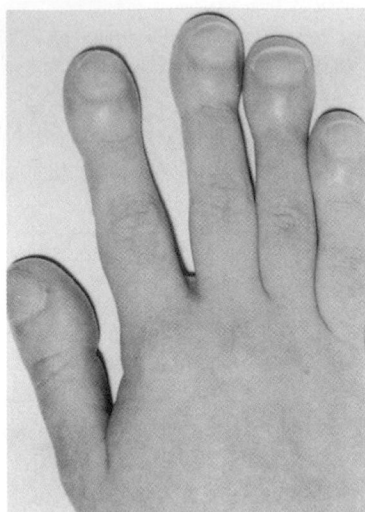

FIGURE 39-12 Clubbing. (From Zitelli B, Davis H: *Atlas of pediatric physical diagnosis*, ed 5, Philadelphia, 2007, Mosby.)

an early age may have a genetic predisposition to the disease. Other contributors include exposure to pollutants (pneumoconioses) or chronic respiratory disorders (chronic bronchitis or uncontrolled asthma).

Symptoms may not be seen until irreversible damage has occurred. When signs and symptoms occur, they include dyspnea, shortness of breath (SOB), wheezing, production of thick mucus, restlessness, fatigue, anorexia, persistent cough (productive or nonproductive), and peripheral cyanosis with clubbing (Figure 39-12). The patient typically is diagnosed from presenting signs and symptoms and a chest x-ray examination, in addition to a pulmonary function test (PFT) that shows increased residual volume and decreased forced expiratory volume (Table 39-3).

Patients with emphysema are encouraged to avoid respiratory irritants and individuals with respiratory infections and to stop smoking. Many of these patients require oxygen therapy and benefit from postural drainage and chest percussion, which help them expectorate trapped mucus. Nebulizer treatments also may be prescribed.

Patients with emphysema expend a great deal of energy just trying to exhale air from the lungs, so they should consume a high-calorie, high-fluid diet and perform certain exercises, such as pursed-lip breathing, to help them conserve energy. Individuals with emphysema require continuous care and support; therefore, encouraging family involvement in the treatment plan is important. Referral to a pulmonary rehabilitation program or support group can benefit both patient and family members.

CRITICAL THINKING APPLICATION   **39-3**

Dr. Samuelson has quite a few patients with either asthma or emphysema. Under Dr. Samuelson's direction, Michael is expected to reinforce patient education and answer patients' and family members' questions. Michael decides to make a file on pertinent health education information and review it with Dr. Samuelson before using it to help coordinate the care of these patients. What information should Michael include in the file? What community resources or groups should be included for patient support?

TABLE 39-3   Pulmonary Function Tests

LUNG FUNCTION	DESCRIPTION	PATIENT INSTRUCTIONS
Tidal volume (TV)	Volume of air inspired and expired during a normal respiration	Patient breathes in and out normally with lips pursed around mouthpiece.
Vital capacity (VC)	Maximum amount of air that can be expired after maximum inspiration	Patient takes deep breath and exhales completely (not forcefully).
Inspiratory capacity (IC)	Maximum amount of air that can be inspired after a normal expiration	Patient breathes in and out normally, then forcibly inhales at the end of the TV.
Expiratory reserve volume (ERV)	Maximum volume of air that can be exhaled after a normal expiration	Patient breathes in and out normally, then exhales forcibly at the end of the TV.
Residual volume (RV)	Volume of air left in lungs after forced expiration	
Functional residual volume (FRV)	Amount of air left in the lungs after a normal expiration	FRV = ERV + RV
Forced vital capacity (FVC)	Amount of air that can be forcefully exhaled from a maximum inhalation	Patient inhales as deeply as possible, then forcibly exhales as much as possible.
Maximum volume ventilation (MVV)	Maximum volume the patient can breathe in and out in 1 minute	Patient breathes in and out as deeply and as frequently as possible for 15 seconds (total volume is multiplied by 4).

Obstructive Sleep Apnea

Obstructive sleep apnea occurs when the muscles in the posterior pharynx that support the soft palate, uvula, tonsils, and tongue relax during sleep. This relaxation causes the trachea to narrow or close with inhalation, momentarily stopping breathing. Blood oxygen levels are lowered, and the brain senses hypoxemia, so it stimulates the patient from sleep to reopen the trachea. The patient is awake so briefly he or she is not aware of the arousal, but this occurs repeatedly throughout the night, preventing the person from achieving a deeper, more restful level of sleep. Because of this interrupted sleep, the individual frequently complains of sleepiness during the day.

Risk factors for developing obstructive sleep apnea include being overweight (a fat or thick neck may narrow the trachea); enlarged adenoids or tonsils; male gender (men develop sleep apnea twice as often as women); a family history of sleep apnea; and alcohol consumption or sedative use, because these chemicals relax throat muscles.

Patients with suspected sleep apnea report chronic fatigue (from the constant startling out of a restful sleep) and pronounced snoring. Sleep apnea is diagnosed after the patient has been monitored during a sleep study, a process called *nocturnal polysomnography*. The patient is connected to equipment that monitors the pulse rate, brain activity, breathing patterns, blood oxygen levels, and limb movements during sleep.

Multiple complications in addition to chronic daytime fatigue can occur because of sleep apnea. Patients are more susceptible to hypertension and resultant heart disease because hypoxic episodes during sleep raise blood pressure and put a strain on the heart. Individuals with sleep apnea also tend to complain of memory problems, morning headaches, depression, and nocturia.

Sleep apnea typically is treated with a continuous positive airway pressure (CPAP) machine (Figure 39-13), which delivers air pressure through a mask placed over the mouth or nose, or through a cannula in the nose. The air pressure created by the machine is greater than that of the surrounding air; this forces the upper airway passages open and prevents tracheal collapse. Although CPAP is the preferred method of treatment, it can be awkward and uncomfortable, making it difficult to sleep. Patients may have to experiment with different types of masks and need to be encouraged to follow through with the recommended treatment. Individuals with mild obstructive sleep apnea can try alternative treatment with a dental device that opens the throat by bringing the jaw forward. Surgery may also be an option to remove the uvula, tonsils, and adenoids, in addition to excess tissue from the nose and back of the throat that vibrates during sleep, resulting in snoring.

Common Signs and Symptoms of Obstructive Sleep Apnea

- Excessive daytime sleepiness (hypersomnia)
- Persistently loud, disruptive snoring
- Snoring, choking, or gasping sounds while asleep
- Episodes of breathing cessation during sleep (apnea)
- Dry mouth or sore throat on awakening
- Morning headache

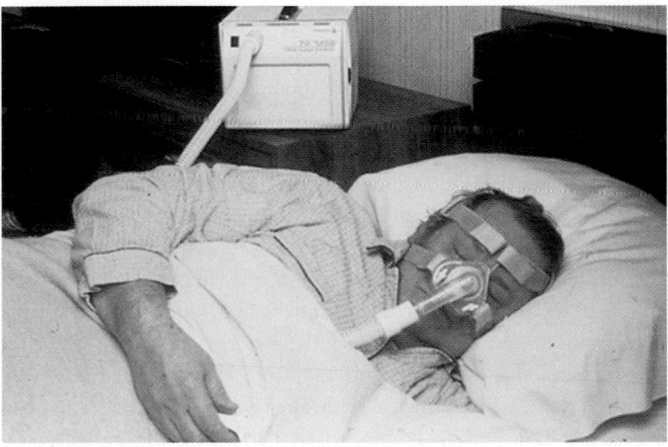

FIGURE 39-13 Patient with a CPAP machine. (Courtesy Respironics, Murrysville, Pa.)

Cancer of the Pulmonary System

The most prevalent neoplasms of the respiratory system are lung cancer and carcinoma of the larynx.

Lung Cancer

Lung cancer is the leading cause of cancer-related deaths for both men and women in the United States. It is estimated that 90% of lung tumors are linked to cigarette smoking; other risk factors include chronic exposure to second-hand smoke, carcinogens (e.g., radon gas and asbestos), and a genetic predisposition. The risk of developing cancer is higher for patients who started to smoke at a young age and who have smoked more than a pack a day for a long period (Figure 39-14). Individuals who quit smoking can significantly lower their risk of lung cancer; after 10 years, the risk of dying from lung cancer is about half that of a person who is still smoking. Female smokers are at greater risk of lung cancer than male smokers.

The lung is a common site of secondary tumors from metastasis in addition to primary carcinomas. Several different cellular types of tumors can develop in the lungs, but the one seen most frequently is bronchogenic carcinoma, which originates in the epithelial lining of the bronchioles (Figure 39-15). The early symptoms of lung cancer (i.e., a chronic, productive cough; SOB; and chest tightness) are masked by symptoms regularly displayed by habitual smokers. A tumor may be discovered accidentally during a routine chest x-ray evaluation or may not be discovered until **metastatic** symptoms (e.g., anemia, weight loss, and fatigue) lead to the diagnosis of a primary lung tumor. Patients who show symptoms usually display local effects of a tumor in the chest, such as bronchial obstruction, atelectasis, hemoptysis, chest pain, and pleural membrane

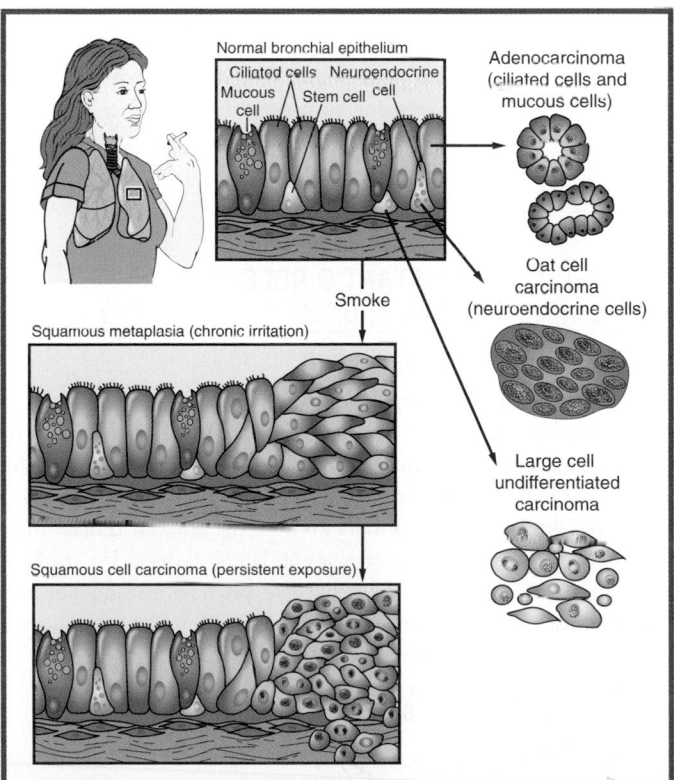

FIGURE 39-14 Classification of lung cancer. (From Damjanov IL: *Pathology for the health-related professions,* ed 4, St Louis, 2010, Saunders.)

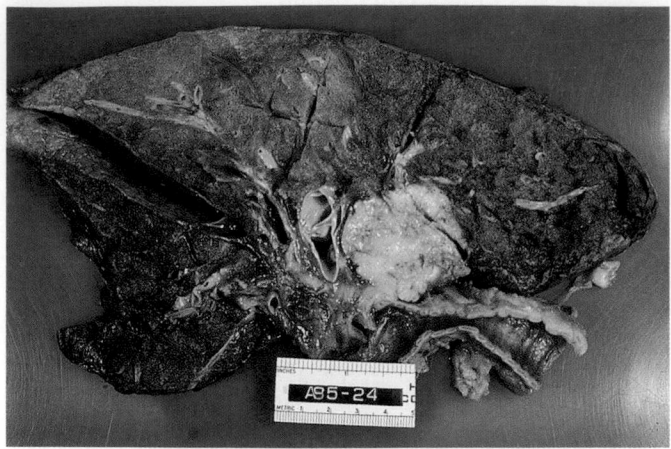

FIGURE 39-15 Lung cancer. (From Damjanov IL: *Pathology for the health-related professions,* ed 4, St Louis, 2010, Saunders.)

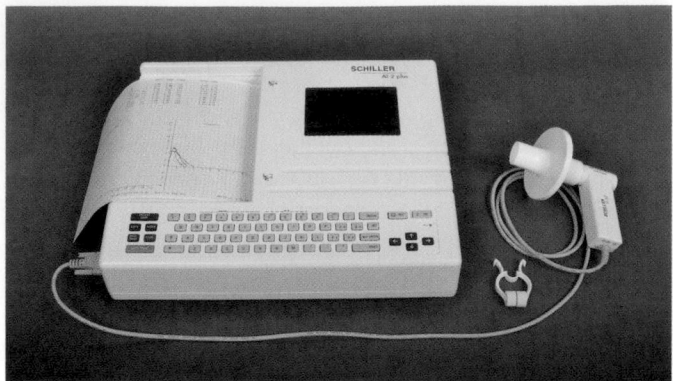

FIGURE 39-16 Spirometer.

involvement. Unless the tumor is diagnosed very early, lung cancer has a poor prognosis. Treatment consists of surgery, radiation therapy, and chemotherapy.

Carcinoma of the Larynx

Carcinoma of the larynx is pathologically linked to tobacco use (including smokeless tobacco) and chronic alcohol consumption. Ninety percent of cases of laryngeal cancer occur in men; most of those affected are 60 to 70 years of age. Patients show early signs of hoarseness, loss of voice, ear pain, and dysphagia (difficulty swallowing); occasionally, respiration becomes impaired. Because of these early symptoms, most laryngeal tumors are discovered in the early stages and can be removed, resulting in a good prognosis. Surgical treatment consists of a partial or total laryngectomy. With a total laryngectomy, the voice is permanently lost, and a **tracheostomy** is performed. Patients undergoing such procedures need comprehensive preparation and benefit from meeting a laryngectomy survivor, in addition to participating in a support group to deal with postsurgical adjustments.

THE MEDICAL ASSISTANT'S ROLE IN PULMONARY PROCEDURES

Assisting with the Examination

Preparing a patient for a respiratory examination includes having the patient disrobe to the waist and put on a gown with the opening in the front or back, depending on the provider's preference. To assess the status of the respiratory system, the provider uses inspection, palpation, percussion, and auscultation on the anterior thorax, then repeats the process on the posterior and lateral thorax. The medical assistant is responsible for assisting the provider throughout the examination, providing privacy and support for the patient, and performing diagnostic tests as ordered.

Diagnostic Procedures

Tuberculosis

If the provider orders TB screening, the medical assistant administers the Mantoux test. An intradermal injection of PPD from a live tuberculin bacillus culture is given to test for the presence of

tuberculin antibodies. A positive Mantoux reaction indicates the possibility of active or latent TB or exposure to the disease. Further testing by chest x-ray examination and sputum culture is required for a definitive diagnosis. Sometimes the provider orders a blood test to diagnose the disease.

Spirometry

PFTs are performed to diagnose a pulmonary abnormality and/or to determine the extent of a pulmonary disease (see Table 39-3). In providers' offices, lung function measurements are taken with a spirometer (Figure 39-16). Successful spirometry requires consistent methods of preparing the patient, explaining and performing the procedure, and determining the results. Patient preparation begins when the procedure is scheduled. The patient should be instructed to wear loose fitting clothing; avoid eating a large meal within 2 hours of taking the test; avoid smoking for at least 1 hour before the test; and avoid taking bronchodilators or nebulizers for 6 hours before the test.

The medical assistant may be responsible for conducting this test in the ambulatory care setting (Procedure 39-3). Before the patient is scheduled for the procedure, the provider considers certain health problems that would contraindicate the test, such as a pneumothorax, a history of angina or recent myocardial infarction, or the presence of vascular aneurysms. When the patient arrives for testing, the medical assistant should explain the purpose of the test, obtain the patient's vital signs (including height and weight), and explain the maneuver. The medical assistant should refer to the patient's health history to make sure that age, gender, and ethnicity have been recorded because these also help determine lung volumes. Spirometry should be described briefly, in simple terms. One explanation that works well is "I am going to have you blow into a machine to see how much air your lungs hold and how fast you can expel it. The test does not hurt, but it does require your cooperation and lots of effort." The patient should be in a comfortable sitting position with the legs uncrossed and both feet on the floor. Dentures that fit poorly may be a nuisance and should be removed if they might interfere. The chin should be slightly elevated and the neck slightly extended. This position should be maintained throughout the forced expiratory procedure. A nose clip is applied to make sure the patient only exhales through the mouth.

PROCEDURE 39-3 | Assist the Provider with Patient Care: Perform Volume Capacity Spirometry Testing

Goal: *To perform volume capacity testing.*

EQUIPMENT and SUPPLIES

- Patient's health record
- Scale with height measuring device
- Sphygmomanometer and stethoscope
- Spirometer with recording paper in place
- External spirometric tubing
- Disposable mouthpiece
- Nasal clip if needed
- Biohazardous waste container

PROCEDURAL STEPS

1. Sanitize your hands and assemble the spirometer.
2. Introduce yourself and confirm the patient's identity by name and date of birth. Determine whether the patient needed any special preparation (e.g., no smoking, not taking bronchodilators) and if so, whether it was done.
   <u>PURPOSE:</u> If special procedures were not followed, the test may have to be rescheduled.
3. Explain the purpose of the test.
   <u>PURPOSE:</u> To help reassure the patient.
4. Measure and record the patient's vital signs, height, and weight.
5. Explain the actual maneuver.
   <u>PURPOSE:</u> The patient must understand the maneuver so that he or she can cooperate fully; this produces the best test results.
6. Make sure the patient is comfortable and either is standing or is sitting (preferred) with the legs uncrossed and the feet on the floor.
   <u>PURPOSE:</u> Proper positioning ensures maximum lung expansion and accurate test results. The test may cause dizziness, so sitting is preferred. If the patient stands, a chair must be next to the person.
7. Loosen any tight clothing, such as a necktie, bra, or belt.
   <u>PURPOSE:</u> Tight clothing may restrict breathing capacity.
8. Show the patient the proper chin and neck position: the chin should be slightly elevated and the neck slightly extended.
9. Practice the maneuver with the patient before beginning the test.
   <u>PURPOSE:</u> To relieve apprehension and enhance understanding.
10. Place a soft nose clip on the patient's nose if this is part of the facility's procedure.
    <u>PURPOSE:</u> To prevent air from escaping through the nose during exhalation.

11. Instruct the patient to place the mouthpiece in the mouth and to seal the lips around it when exhaling (Figure 1).

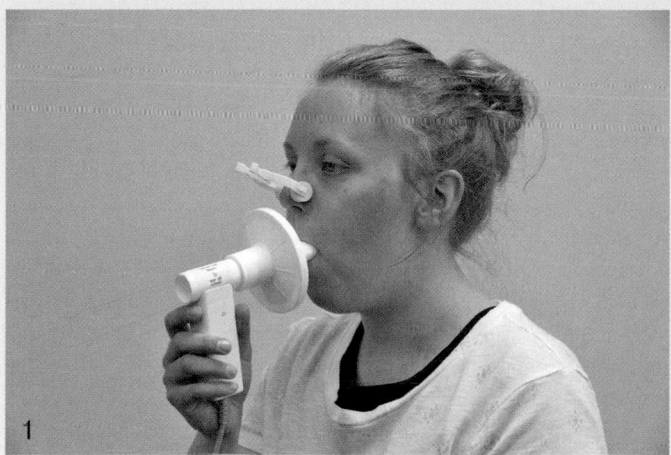

12. Tell the patient to inhale according to instructions; take as deep a breath as possible and blow air out hard and long.
13. Use active, forceful coaching during exhalation. Patient must exhale completely to get accurate test results.
    <u>PURPOSE:</u> Coaching improves performance. The patient should continue to exhale even after he or she thinks the process is complete.
14. Provide the patient with feedback after he or she completes the maneuver.
    <u>PURPOSE:</u> Encouragement and explanations of mistakes in the maneuver can help improve the patient's compliance.
15. Carefully observe the patient for indications of vertigo or dyspnea or any other signs of difficulty. If complications occur, stop the test and inform the provider.
16. Continue testing until three acceptable maneuvers have been performed.
17. Clean and disinfect the equipment. Discard waste, including the disposable mouthpiece and tubing, in a biohazardous waste container.
18. Sanitize your hands.
    <u>PURPOSE:</u> To ensure infection control.
19. Record the procedure in the patient's EHR and/or place the spirometer printout in the records for the provider to review.
    <u>PURPOSE:</u> Procedures that are not recorded are considered not done.

Give specific instructions in simple, direct terms; for example, "I want you to take the deepest breath possible, put the mouthpiece in your mouth and seal your lips tightly around it, and then blow into the tube as hard and as fast as you can in one long, complete breath." An analogy that sometimes is helpful for further explaining the maneuver is "It's like blowing out the candles on a birthday cake when they don't all go out; you need to keep blowing the same breath until they do."

Next, demonstrate the maneuver. Many patients forget some or all of the instructions they have just received, so demonstration reinforces exactly what to do. Show the patient the proper chin and neck position, how to place the mouthpiece at the right time, and how to blow the air out and continue to blow.

When the demonstration is finished, remind the patient of the following points:

- Take as deep a breath as possible.
- Blow air out hard and long.
- Blow until all of the air is out of your lungs.

Use active and forceful coaching while the patient is performing the maneuver. You may need to raise your voice with some urgency to improve the patient's performance, using such phrases as, "Blow, blow, blow!" "Keep blowing, keep blowing!" and "Don't stop blowing!" After the maneuver, give the patient some feedback on the quality of the test and describe what improvements could be made. Continue to repeat efforts until the patient has completed three acceptable maneuvers. The two best efforts are used to calculate pulmonary function. Although most spirometers calculate the normal values for each patient based on the information entered into the machine, the provider can calculate them from the individual's ethnicity, age, height, weight, and gender; the test results are documented as a percentage. If the patient's best efforts are greater than 80% of pretest calculated values, pulmonary function is considered normal. Spirometry tests provide the provider information about the impact of obstruction or pulmonary disease on airflow. If the results are less than 60% of the predicted value, the patient may be given bronchodilators and retested to determine the impact of the inhalant on function.

Test Results. Document the procedure in the patient's EHR and give the provider the printout from the spirometer for review. The results can be uploaded directly into the patient's EHR so a printout may not be necessary. Documentation should include the patient's compliance with preparation, condition during the test, and forcefulness of exhalation when coached during the exam. If any questions arise about the quality of the results, ask the patient to wait while the provider reviews them. If the patient has delayed taking medication, check with the provider as to when the patient should resume taking it.

CRITICAL THINKING APPLICATION   **39-4**

Michael is teaching Cinda, a new employee, how to perform a spirometry test. He has summarized the steps of the procedure on a card, which is kept next to the machine for easy reference. Cinda knows nothing about the procedure. What would be the best way for Michael to teach her about the test? What information should he include? How should she document the procedure in the patient's EHR?

Pulse Oximetry

Pulse oximetry is a noninvasive method of evaluating both the pulse rate and the oxygen saturation of hemoglobin in arterial blood. It identifies the percentage of hemoglobin that is oxygenated compared with the total amount of hemoglobin available. Many ambulatory settings use pulse oximeters to assess a patient's oxygenation status in such disorders as pneumonia, bronchitis, emphysema, or asthma.

To perform the procedure, the medical assistant clips a probe on the patient's earlobe or finger (Figure 39-17). Fingernail polish must be removed before the clip is applied. A beam of infrared light passes through the tissue, and the machine measures the amount of light absorbed by oxygenated hemoglobin, which is displayed on the digital screen as a percentage. At the same time the light measures the patient's pulse rate, which also is shown on the screen. A normal pulse oximetry reading is 95% or higher (meaning 95% of the total available hemoglobin attachments for oxygen are carrying oxygen). Treatment, such as oxygen or bronchodilator therapies, usually is started when readings are 90% to 92% or lower (Procedure 39-4).

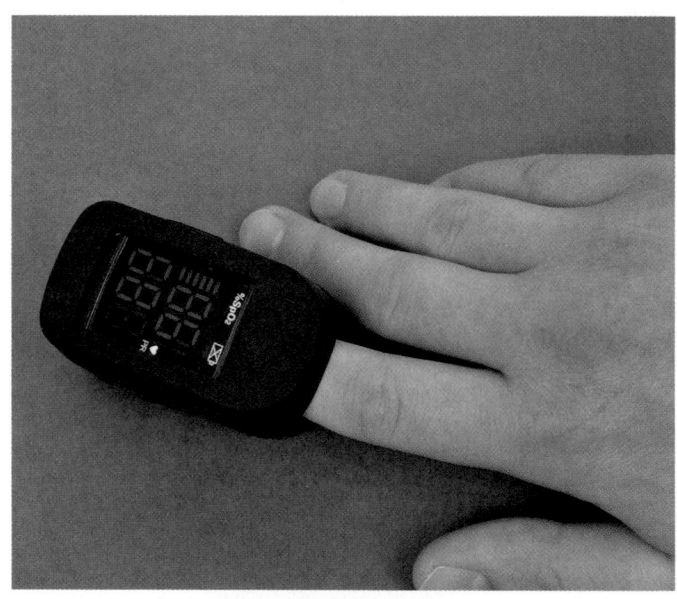

FIGURE 39-17 Pulse oximeter.

PROCEDURE 39-4   Perform Patient Screening Using Established Protocols: Perform Pulse Oximetry

---

Goal: *To assess the adequacy of oxygen levels (or oxygen saturation) in the blood using a pulse oximeter.*

EQUIPMENT and SUPPLIES

- Patient's health record
- Pulse oximeter monitor and appropriate sized probe

PROCEDURAL STEPS

1. Assemble the equipment.

2. Confirm the patient's identity by name and date of birth and explain the procedure.
   PURPOSE: An informed patient is more cooperative.

3. Sanitize your hands.
   PURPOSE: Standard Precautions must be followed to prevent spread of disease.

PROCEDURE 39-4 —continued

4. Turn on the monitor and attach the probe to the finger (preferred) or ear lobe so it is flush with the skin.
5. The light-emitting diode (LED) should be placed on top of the nail. If the patient is wearing nail polish or has artificial nails, these may have to be removed to get a strong pulse signal.
   PURPOSE: To measure the pulse and oxygen saturation level.
6. Record the oxygen saturation percentage and pulse in patient's health record. Include date, time, and if the patient is receiving supplemental oxygen record the amount in liters.
   PURPOSE: Procedures that are not recorded are considered not done.

7. Sanitize the patient probe and the external portion of the monitor with an aseptic cleaner.
   PURPOSE: To follow Standard Precautions.
8. Sanitize your hands.
   PURPOSE: To ensure infection control.

Obtaining Sputum for Culture

A sputum culture is requested when signs and symptoms are accompanied by physical evidence of pneumonia, TB, or other infectious diseases of the lower respiratory tract. The specimen is sent to a laboratory equipped to handle potentially infectious bacteriologic samples. The sample is cultured and incubated, and the pathogenic organism grown in the culture medium is identified. If possible, the provider refrains from starting antibiotic therapy until the sputum has been collected. The sample may also be sent to the laboratory for cytologic analysis, which may indicate a cancerous condition of the lungs or bronchi.

Methods of Collection. In the ambulatory care setting, the primary method of collecting a sputum sample is expectoration (Procedure 39-5). However, sputum also can be collected by tracheal suctioning and bronchoscopy. If the sample is to be collected by expectoration,

most providers have the patient perform the procedure at home with instruction. The medical assistant may be responsible for explaining the procedure to the patient or reinforcing the provider's instructions. The patient should understand that the best time for collecting a sputum specimen is in the morning when the patient first wakes up, before eating or drinking. The patient can rinse out the mouth with water before collecting the sample to reduce contamination from the oropharynx. The sample is collected from sputum coughed up from the lungs, not from saliva, so the patient should be encouraged to cough deeply and forcefully to collect a satisfactory sample. It may help to have the patient take several deep breaths and then cough. At least 1 teaspoon of sputum should be collected in a sterile specimen cup (the patient needs to know how to handle the specimen cup to maintain sterility), which must be returned to the office or laboratory as soon as possible after collection.

PROCEDURE 39-5 Obtain Specimens for Microbiologic Testing: Obtain a Sputum Sample for Culture

Goal: To collect a sputum sample, following Standard Precautions.

EQUIPMENT and SUPPLIES

- Patient's health record
- Sterile laboratory specimen cup, accurately labeled
- Biohazard laboratory specimen bag with laboratory requisition
- Disposable examination gloves
- Face shield with goggles
- Impervious gown
- Biohazardous waste container
- Cup of water
- Ginger ale or juice

PROCEDURAL STEPS

1. Assemble the equipment and label the specimen cup.
2. Identify the patient by name and date of birth and explain the procedure.
   PURPOSE: An informed patient is more cooperative.

3. Sanitize your hands and put on gloves, a face shield with goggles, and an impervious gown.
   PURPOSE: Standard Precautions must be followed when potentially infectious materials are collected.
4. Have the patient rinse his or her mouth with water.
   PURPOSE: Any food particles in the mouth will contaminate the specimen.
5. Carefully remove the specimen cup lid, taking care not to touch the inside of the lid or the inside of the container, and place it upside down on a side table.
   PURPOSE: To maintain the sterile environment of the specimen cup.
6. Instruct the patient to take three deep breaths and then cough deeply to bring up secretions from the lower respiratory tract.
   PURPOSE: The organisms for culture must be from the lung fields in the lower respiratory tract.

PROCEDURE 39-5   —*continued*

7. Tell the patient to spit directly into the specimen container and to avoid getting any sputum on the exterior of the container. Do not touch the inside of the container during the procedure.
   PURPOSE: Sputum on the exterior of the container is considered hazardous. Prevent contamination of the inside of the container.

8. Place the lid securely on the container, taking care not to touch the inside of the lid, and then place the container in the plastic specimen bag.
   PURPOSE: To maintain the sterility of the container and to minimize the chance of spreading the potentially infectious organisms.

9. Offer the patient a glass of juice or ginger ale.
   PURPOSE: The patient may have a bad taste in the mouth after the test, and this may cause nausea.

10. If another sputum test is ordered for the next morning, instruct the patient when to come to the office or explain how to perform the procedure at home. Remind the person to follow the same instructions for preparation. Stress the importance of maintaining the sterility of the container and of collecting the specimen first thing in the morning.

11. Sanitize the work area and properly dispose of all supplies.
    PURPOSE: To follow Standard Precautions.

12. Sanitize your hands.
    PURPOSE: To ensure infection control.

13. Process the specimen immediately to ensure optimum test results or refrigerate the specimen until it is sent to the laboratory for analysis.
    PURPOSE: Microorganisms may propagate or die, which can result in a false-positive or false-negative result.

14. Record the procedure in the patient's health record.
    PURPOSE: Procedures that are not recorded are considered not done.

If the patient is taking antibiotic medications at the time of the specimen collection, this information should be included on the laboratory slip. If the cough does not produce sputum, chest physiotherapy or nebulization may be ordered by the provider to induce it. In some cases the provider may order sputum collection for three consecutive mornings.

CRITICAL THINKING APPLICATION   **39-5**

Tomás Garcia, a 68-year-old patient, has a chronic cough, and Dr. Samuelson orders a sputum culture to rule out an infectious disease. Mr. Garcia is supposed to collect the specimens every morning for the next 3 days, but he is very hard of hearing and does not understand English very well. His daughter, who is bilingual, is with him at today's visit. How should Michael relay the information about how to collect the sputum sample? What important details should be reviewed with Mr. Garcia's daughter?

Bronchoscopy

Bronchoscopy typically is performed in an outpatient clinic or a hospital. However, the medical assistant should be familiar with the procedure because he or she probably will schedule the test, instruct the patient on preparation, and help answer questions from the patient or family.

Bronchoscopy provides an endoscopic view of the larynx, trachea, and bronchi. A pulmonary specialist or surgeon performs the procedure, using a flexible fiberoptic instrument through which the physician can visualize respiratory tissues and collect biopsy specimens or bronchial washings as needed for cytologic evaluation or culture. Laser therapy to treat endotracheal lesions also is possible through the flexible scope.

The patient should remain on nothing by mouth (NPO) status for 6 to 12 hours before the test to reduce the risk of aspiration. Also, the patient should ask the physician whether to continue taking routine medications and when to stop taking aspirin, ibuprofen, or other anticoagulant drugs before the procedure. The patient should perform good mouth care before the procedure to reduce the number of bacteria present, and dentures should be removed. The patient will be given medication before the procedure to aid relaxation and to dry up oral secretions. The medical assistant should reassure the patient the procedure does not interfere with breathing.

Before the instrument is inserted, the physician sprays a topical anesthetic (lidocaine) into the mouth and on the back of the throat to help suppress the gag reflex and reduce any discomfort from passage of the instrument. The tube can be inserted through the nose or mouth, and as it reaches the glottis, more lidocaine is sprayed to control the cough reflex. The physician continues to pass the tube through the bronchi and larger bronchioles, collecting biopsy specimens of any suspicious tissue and obtaining cellular washings if indicated. Because the patient is sedated, it is not an uncomfortable procedure, but the patient may complain of a sore throat and may experience hemoptysis for several hours after the procedure. Biopsy and culture reports usually are available in 2 to 7 days.

CLOSING COMMENTS

Patient Education

It is often said that the greatest fear a person has is the fear of the unknown. Patients frequently worry about tests the physician has ordered. The imagination can create all types of frightening scenarios with even more alarming outcomes. The medical assistant plays a vital role in allaying patients' fears by explaining diagnostic tests, making sure the patient understands how to prepare for the examination and what will be expected of him or her during the procedure. Make sure to give the patient brochures or handouts explaining the procedure that he or she can review at home. Answer all the patient's questions, and consult the provider about questions or concerns you cannot address before the patient leaves the office.

Legal and Ethical Issues

If the pulmonary test ordered is an invasive test, such as bronchoscopy, make sure a written consent form is obtained from the patient and is in the patient's health record. If oxygen therapy is ordered, the physician must write a prescription that specifies the amount of oxygen to be given and the type of device to be used for delivery. The physician also may write an order for a respiratory care practitioner to follow up on the patient at home.

Professional Behaviors

Many of the respiratory conditions you learned about in this chapter have the potential of becoming chronic or lifelong health concerns. A strong link has been established between tobacco use and the development of respiratory disease. It can be quite frustrating for a healthcare professional to work with a patient who continues to smoke despite provider recommendations and the signs of serious respiratory disease. The medical assistant must provide respectful care to all individuals, regardless of their lifestyle choices. Approaching patients with a professional attitude and therapeutic communication techniques can go a long way in strengthening the patient-caregiver relationship.

SUMMARY OF SCENARIO

Michael has become very adept at performing respiratory diagnostic procedures and treatments for ambulatory patients. He enjoys interacting with this special group of patients and works at maintaining an up-to-date file on educational and resource assistance in the community. Michael especially enjoys the patient education aspect of caring for people with respiratory diseases. Many of these patients have chronic diseases that require long-term care by a physician, and Michael attempts to use available "teaching moments" to reinforce healthy lifestyle habits and to confirm patients' understanding of the treatments.

Michael continues to participate in local meetings of the American Association of Medical Assistants (AAMA) to keep up with recent practice trends, and he took a medical terminology refresher course at the local community college to improve his patient interviewing and documentation skills. He is investigating starting a Smoke Stoppers group out of Dr. Samuelson's office to encourage patients to develop a healthier lifestyle, and he emphasizes to his patients who work in the area's coal mines and construction businesses the importance of consistently wearing respirators.

SUMMARY OF LEARNING OBJECTIVES

1. **Define, spell, and pronounce the terms listed in the vocabulary.**
   Spelling and pronouncing medical terms correctly reinforce the medical assistant's credibility. Knowing the definitions of these terms promotes confidence in communication with patients and co-workers.

2. **Describe the organs of the respiratory system and their functions.**
   The respiratory system exchanges oxygen for carbon dioxide waste through external and internal respiration and helps maintain the acid-base balance in the body. It works with the circulatory system to supply body cells with oxygen and remove metabolic wastes. The upper respiratory tract transports air through the nose, pharynx, and larynx. The lower respiratory tract consists of the trachea, bronchial tubes, and lungs.

3. **Explain the process of ventilation.**
   Ventilation is the process by which the bronchioles deposit oxygenated air into the alveoli. A network of pulmonary capillaries surround the alveoli, and oxygenated air moves out of the single-celled walls of the alveoli and into the capillaries. Carbon dioxide is forced out of the capillaries, into the alveoli, and then out through the bronchioles. Inspiration is the movement of oxygen from the atmosphere into the alveoli; expiration is the movement of carbon dioxide from the alveoli into the atmosphere.

4. **Discuss respiratory system defenses and use correct respiratory system terminology when documenting in the medical record.**
   Every part of the respiratory system has a defense mechanism; disease occurs when something disrupts the normal homeostatic chain of events. Table 39-1 defines common terms related to the respiratory system that should be used when charting a patient's signs and symptoms.

5. **Describe upper respiratory infections (e.g., the common cold, sinusitis, and allergic rhinitis), in addition to lower respiratory infections (e.g., pneumonia).**
   URIs include the common cold, which is caused by a virus; sinusitis, which may be a result of an infection or allergic reaction; and allergic rhinitis, which is triggered by multiple factors and causes nasal symptoms. Lower respiratory infections include pneumonia, an infection of the lungs that can be caused by multiple pathogens and that may range from a minor infection to a life-threatening disease.

6. **Explain the diagnosis and treatment of tuberculosis.**
   TB, caused by *M. tuberculosis*, can be either active or latent. Individuals with active TB are infectious and show the symptoms of the disease; those with latent TB have activated tubercles because of a weakened immune system. TB is diagnosed by a combination of PPD testing, chest

Continued

SUMMARY OF LEARNING OBJECTIVES—*continued*

x-ray studies, blood tests, and sputum cultures. It is treated with multiple medications, depending on the type and stage of the disease.

7. Do the following related to chronic obstructive pulmonary disease:

- *Summarize the disorders associated with chronic obstructive pulmonary disease and their treatments.*
  COPD is a group of diseases with the common characteristic of chronic airway obstruction. They include chronic bronchitis, bronchiectasis, asthma, pneumoconiosis, emphysema, and sleep apnea. The mechanism of obstruction may vary, but all these patients are unable to ventilate the lungs freely, which results in ineffective exchange of respiratory gases. Treatments include bronchodilator and corticosteroid inhalers, evaluation of peak flow values, nebulizer treatments, oxygen, chest therapy, and CPAP machines.

- *Teach a patient how to use a peak flow meter.*
  Procedure 39-1 outlines the procedure for teaching a patient how to obtain an accurate peak flow reading.

- *Administer a nebulizer treatment.*
  Procedure 39-2 outlines the procedure for administering a nebulizer treatment.

- *Detail patient teaching for the use of a metered-dose inhaler.*
  Shake the canister, and hold it upright; breathe out normally, place the mouthpiece between the teeth, and close the lips around it; press down on the top of the canister and breathe in deeply and slowly through the mouth until the lungs are completely filled; hold the breath about 5 seconds. Wait about 15 to 30 seconds before the next puff. After using a steroid inhaler, rinse the mouth with water, gargle, and spit out the water to prevent an oral yeast infection.

8. Discuss obstructive sleep apnea, including causes, risk factors, complications, and treatment.
Obstructive sleep apnea occurs when the muscles in the posterior pharynx relax during sleep. Risk factors for developing sleep apnea include being overweight, a family history, and alcohol or sedative consumption. Patients with sleep apnea are more susceptible to hypertension and also could have headaches, depression, and nocturia. Sleep apnea is typically treated with a CPAP machine.

9. Describe the cancers associated with the pulmonary system.
Lung cancer is the leading cause of cancer-related deaths for both men and women; the lung also is a common site of metastatic tumors. The prognosis is very poor for lung cancer because early symptoms mimic chronic conditions present in long-term smokers. Carcinoma of the larynx is linked to smoking and chronic alcohol consumption.

10. Summarize the medical assistant's role in assisting with pulmonary procedures.
Preparing a patient for a respiratory examination includes having the patient disrobe to the waist and put on a gown with the opening in the front or back, depending on the provider's preference. The medical assistant is responsible for assisting the provider throughout the examination, providing privacy and support for the patient, and performing diagnostic tests as ordered.

11. Distinguish among common diagnostic procedures for the respiratory system; perform a volume capacity spirometry test and a pulse oximeter procedure; and collect a sputum sample for culture.
Respiratory diagnostic procedures include the Mantoux intradermal test for TB; PFTs, in which a spirometer is used to diagnose pulmonary abnormalities; pulse oximetry, a noninvasive method of evaluating both the pulse rate and the oxygen saturation of hemoglobin in the arterial blood; culturing of expectorated sputum; and bronchoscopy, in which a flexible fiberoptic instrument is used to view the larynx, trachea, and bronchi endoscopically.

Procedure 39-3 summarizes the steps in spirometry testing. Procedure 39-4 summarizes the steps in performing pulse oximetry. The oximeter probe is placed on the patient's earlobe or finger. An infrared light passes through the tissue, and the machine measures the amount of light absorbed by oxygenated hemoglobin, which is displayed on the digital screen as a percentage. The patient's pulse rate also is displayed. Procedure 39-5 explains how to collect a sputum sample for culture.

12. Discuss patient education, in addition to legal and ethical issues, associated with pulmonary medicine.
If the pulmonary test ordered is an invasive test, written informed consent must be obtained from the patient and filed in the patient's health record. If oxygen therapy is ordered, the provider must write a prescription that specifies the amount of oxygen to be given and the type of device to be used for delivery. The provider also may write an order for a respiratory care practitioner to follow up on the patient at home.

CONNECTIONS

Study Guide Connection: Go to the Chapter 39 Study Guide. Read and complete the activities.

evolve Evolve Connection: Go to the Chapter 39 link at *evolve.elsevier.com/ kinn* to complete the Chapter Review Quiz. Check out the other resources listed for this chapter to make the most of what you have learned from Assisting in Pulmonary Medicine.

40

ASSISTING IN CARDIOLOGY

Adam Stern, CMA (AAMA), has been working for more than 3 years as a medical assistant in a variety of providers' offices. Adam recently was hired to work at City Hospital in the cardiology department. His job description includes working in the clinical area of the practice and assisting the attending physicians with patient education and follow-up. Because Adam has never worked for a cardiologist, he is concerned about his knowledge base and competency in cardiac patient care. Part of Adam's responsibilities will be to help evaluate patient education materials about the warning signs of a heart attack, especially the differences between the symptoms seen in men and those seen in women. The providers expect Adam to be familiar with the electrical conduction system of the heart, typical medications prescribed in a cardiology practice, and common diagnostic procedures that are ordered for patients with cardiovascular diseases.

While studying this chapter, think about the following questions:

- Why is it important that Adam understand the normal anatomy and physiology of the cardiovascular system if he is going to work in a cardiologist's practice?
- What are some common diseases and disorders of the cardiovascular system with which Adam should be familiar?
- What are the common cardiovascular diagnostic procedures that Adam should be prepared to discuss and explain to patients?

LEARNING OBJECTIVES

1. Define, spell, and pronounce the terms listed in the vocabulary.
2. Explain the anatomy and physiology of the heart and its significant structures.
3. Summarize risk factors for the development of heart disease.
4. Do the following related to coronary artery disease and myocardial infarction:
   - Describe the signs, symptoms, and medical procedures used in the diagnosis and treatment of coronary artery disease and myocardial infarction.
   - Summarize metabolic syndrome and associated risk factors.
   - Explain the signs and symptoms of myocardial infarction in women.
5. Compare and contrast the treatment protocols for hypertension.
6. Outline the causes and results of congestive heart failure.
7. Summarize the effects of inflammation and valve disorders on cardiac function.
8. Describe the anatomy and physiology of the vascular system.
9. Differentiate among the various types of shock.
10. Summarize the characteristics of common vascular disorders.
11. Discuss arterial disorders, including causes, risk factors, and common treatments.
12. Outline typical cardiovascular diagnostic procedures.
13. Describe patient education topics, and legal and ethical issues, for cardiovascular patients.

VOCABULARY

ablation (a-blay'-shun) An amputation or removal of any body part.

angioplasty A procedure used to widen vessels narrowed by stenoses or occlusions.

chordae tendineae (kor'-duh/ten'-din-uh) The tendons that anchor the cusps of the heart valves to the papillary muscles of the myocardium, preventing valvular prolapse.

intermittent claudication Recurring cramping in the calves caused by poor circulation of blood to the muscles of the lower leg.

ischemia (is-ke'-mia) A decreased supply of oxygenated blood to an area or body part.

Marfan syndrome An inherited condition characterized by elongation of the bones, joint hypermobility, abnormalities of the eyes, and the development of an aortic aneurysm.

occlude To close off or block (e.g., a blood vessel).

scleroderma (skleh-ruh-der'-muh) An autoimmune disorder that affects the blood vessels and connective tissue, causing fibrous degeneration of the major organs.

statins A class of drugs that lower the level of cholesterol in the blood by reducing the production of cholesterol by the liver; they block the enzyme in the liver that is responsible for making cholesterol.

trans fats Substances that form from hydrogenation of an unsaturated fatty acid; they make a dietary fat more saturated and solid at room temperature.

vegetations Abnormal growth of tissue surrounding a valve consisting of fibrin, platelets, and bacteria.

In the past, cardiac disease was frequently seen in men but seldom in women. That has changed, and today the most common cause of illness and death, regardless of gender, is cardiovascular disease. Medical assistants in all specialties often care for patients with heart disorders. Seldom does the cardiologist discover the heart problem. Most patients who see this specialist already have been diagnosed with a suspected heart disorder and were referred to the cardiologist for verification of the initial diagnosis and specialized treatment.

Because of the overwhelming number of people with cardiovascular problems, all medical assistants must understand the cardiovascular system, be able to recognize early symptoms of potential disorders, perform basic screening tests when ordered by the provider, and assist the provider in the examination of the heart and blood vessels.

ANATOMY AND PHYSIOLOGY OF THE HEART

The heart is a hollow, muscular organ situated in the thoracic cavity in the mediastinal region, between the right and left pleural spaces. It weighs about 9 ounces and is about the size of a fist; approximately two thirds of it is located to the left of the sternum (Figure 40-1). The heart is a pump that provides the force needed to push blood through all the arteries of the body; the blood circulates a continuous supply of oxygen and nutrients to the cells and picks up the metabolic waste products from them. If deprived of these vital functions, the cells die. At the same time, the heart pushes deoxygenated blood through the pulmonary artery to the lungs for oxygen saturation and

receives oxygenated blood back through the pulmonary veins into the left side of the heart. The average adult heart pumps about 5 L of blood every minute. If the heart loses its pumping action for even a few brief minutes, death or permanent damage can result.

Layers of the Heart

The heart is enclosed in a double-membrane sac called the *pericardium*. The outer layer of the pericardial sac, the parietal pericardium, is a tough membrane that connects the heart to the diaphragm and serves as a physical barrier to protect the heart against infection or inflammation from the lungs or pleural space. The inner layer, the visceral pericardium, or *epicardium*, forms the first layer of the heart. Between the two membranes is a small space, the pericardial cavity, which contains about 30 mL of pericardial fluid; this fluid lubricates the internal surfaces of the pericardial membranes, enabling them to slide across each other during heart contractions. The middle layer of the heart, the *myocardium*, is the muscle layer that constitutes the largest percentage of the heart wall. Contractions of this muscle layer force the blood from the heart into the vessels. The inner layer of the heart, the endocardium, includes the heart valves that separate the chambers of the heart and provide a means of blocking the flow of blood from major blood vessels entering and exiting the heart (Figure 40-2).

Heart Chambers and Arteries

The heart is divided into four chambers (Figure 40-3). The atria, the top chambers, receive blood, and the ventricles, the bottom

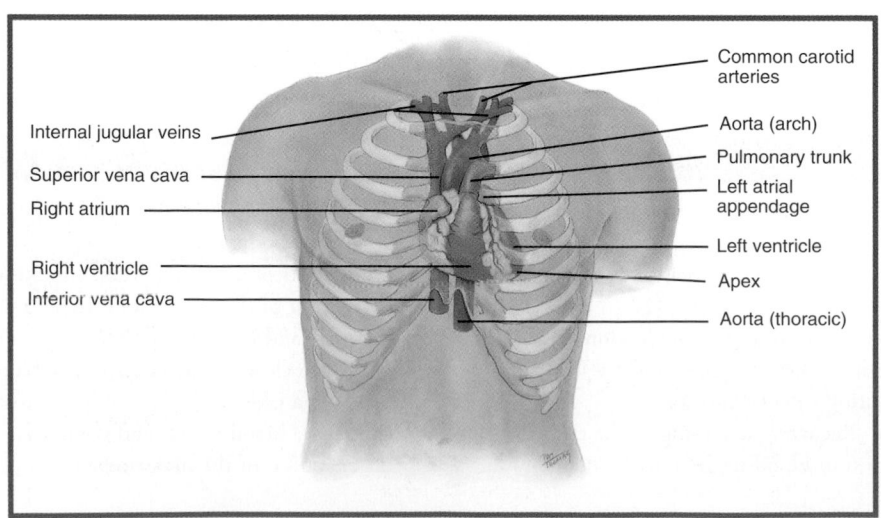

FIGURE 40-1 Location of the heart in the thoracic cavity. (From Applegate EJ: *The anatomy and physiology learning system,* ed 4, St Louis, 2010, Saunders.)

chambers, pump the blood out. The blood flow through the heart begins in the right atrium, which receives deoxygenated blood from the inferior and superior venae cavae. The atria contract, and blood passes through the tricuspid valve into the right ventricle; the ventricles contract, and blood passes from the right ventricle through the pulmonary valve to the lungs via the pulmonary artery (the only artery in the body that contains deoxygenated blood). Oxygenation occurs in the alveoli of the lungs, and the now oxygenated blood returns to the left atria through the pulmonary veins (the only veins

in the body that carry oxygen-rich blood). The atria contract, and blood passes through the mitral (bicuspid) valve into the left ventricle; the ventricles contract, and oxygen-rich blood is sent through the aortic valve out to the body through the aorta (the largest artery in the body).

The myocardium requires a continuous supply of oxygen and nutrients, which are delivered through two coronary arteries that branch off the aorta above the aortic valve (Figure 40-4). The right coronary artery nourishes the anterior and posterior myocardium on the right side of the heart, and the left coronary artery does the same on the left side. The left coronary artery quickly divides and forms the left anterior descending artery and the left circumflex artery. Smaller branches of the coronary arteries feed the myocardium and the endocardium. Any interference in blood flow in any of the coronary vessels can alter the action of the heart.

Heart Conduction

A sophisticated electrical conduction system operated by specialized cells located at various sites in the myocardium stimulates contractions. These muscle contractions move blood through the chambers of the heart and out through the aorta to the rest of the body. Each electrical impulse passes through the heart muscle in a twisting, spiral motion. These rhythmic waves stimulate the cardiac cells to beat, which causes the heart to contract.

The cardiac impulse originates in specialized muscle tissue called the *sinoatrial (SA) node.* The SA node rhythmically initiates impulses 60 to 100 times a minute; because it creates the basic rhythm, it is the pacemaker of the heart. It is located in the posterior, superior

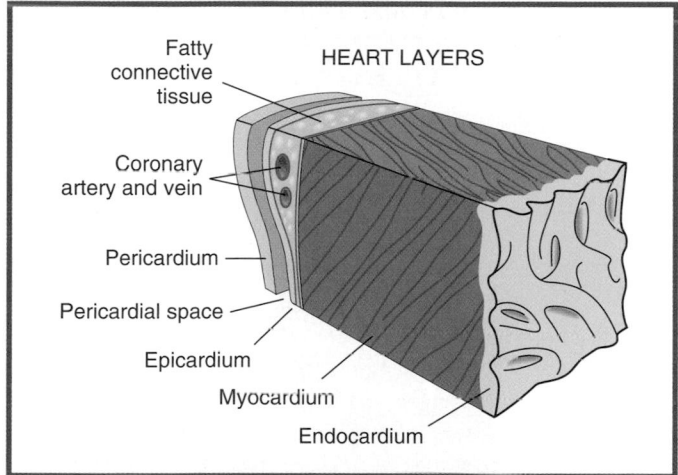

FIGURE 40-2 Layers of the heart. (From Damjanov I: *Pathology for the health-related professions,* ed 4, St Louis, 2012, Saunders.)

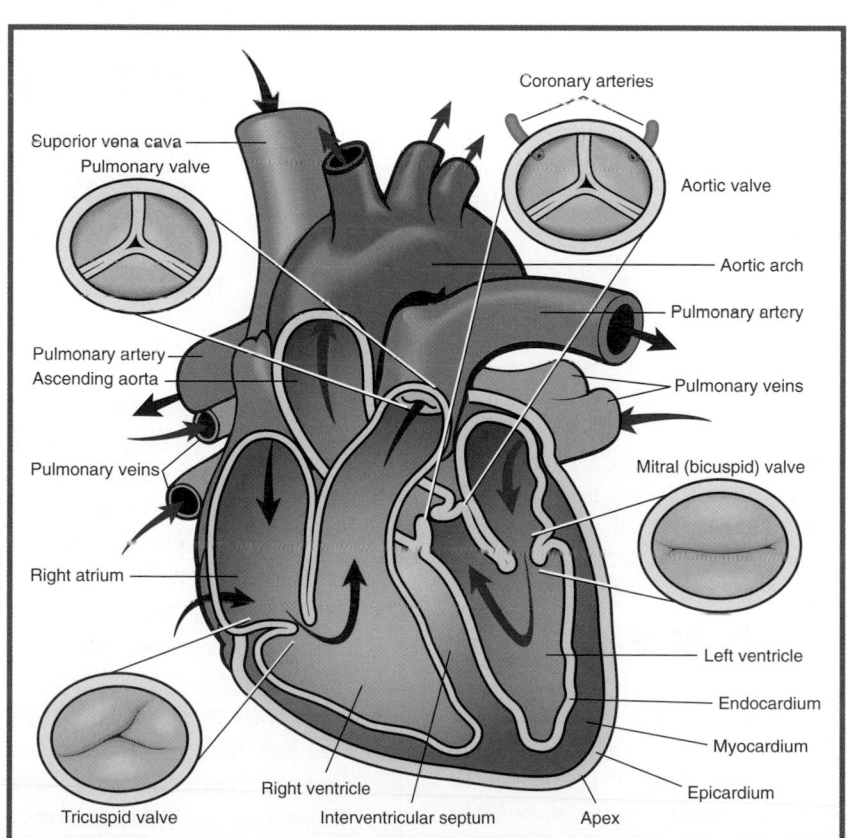

FIGURE 40-3 Chambers of the heart. (From Damjanov I: *Pathology for the health-related professions,* ed 4, St Louis, 2012, Saunders.)

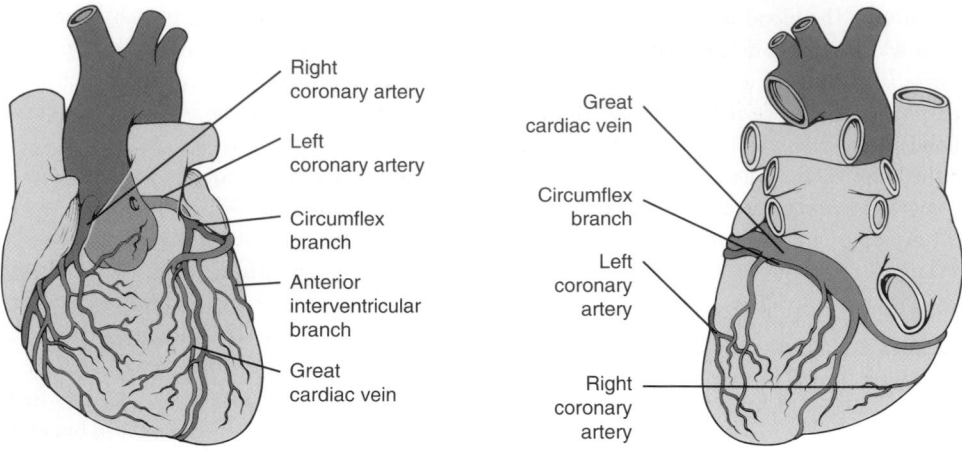

FIGURE 40-4 Coronary arteries. (From Frazier MS, Drzymkowski JW: *Essentials of human diseases and conditions,* ed 5, St Louis, 2013, Saunders.)

wall of the right atrium, at the junction of the superior vena cava and the atrium and just above the tricuspid valve. When the SA node discharges its rhythm pattern into the myocardium, it passes across both atria, resulting in atrial contraction and forcing blood through the valves and into the ventricles. The wave then passes through a second area of specialized muscle tissue on the septal wall between the right atrium and right ventricle, called the *atrioventricular (AV) node.* The AV node holds the impulse for a fraction of a second to prevent inappropriately high atrial rates and to permit the blood to empty from the atria through the tricuspid and mitral valves. At this moment the **chordae tendineae** tightly close the valves between the atria and the ventricles. The AV node then releases the charge, sending it down through the bundle of His, which is located in the septum between the right and left ventricles. This bundle is divided into two main branches: the right bundle, on the right side of the septum, and the left bundle, on the left side. From the bundle branches, transmission of the cardiac wave continues through a mass of cardiac muscle fibers known as the *Purkinje fibers.* The Purkinje fibers completely encase both ventricles, and the cardiac wave causes the ventricles to contract (Figure 40-5).

The electrical impulses that cause the contraction of the atria and the ventricles are called *depolarization.* After depolarization, the cells need a period of electric recovery *(repolarization).* Once recovery is complete, the cells are in a resting phase *(polarization),* and then the entire cycle starts again. The normal cardiac cycle consists of atrial contraction, ventricular contraction, recovery, and heart rest. This cycle maintains the average range of 60 to 100 beats per minute and a normal heart rhythm. It is this electrical force that is traced and evaluated when an electrocardiogram (ECG) is done.

DISEASES AND DISORDERS OF THE HEART

Many diseases and disorders affect the heart and its blood vessels. Disorders that occur when the rhythm of the heart becomes irregular are addressed in the Principles of Electrocardiography chapter. Cardiac disease has multiple risk factors; some of these cannot be changed, and others people can change or seek to have treated. The more risk factors a person has, the greater his or her risk of developing cardiovascular disease.

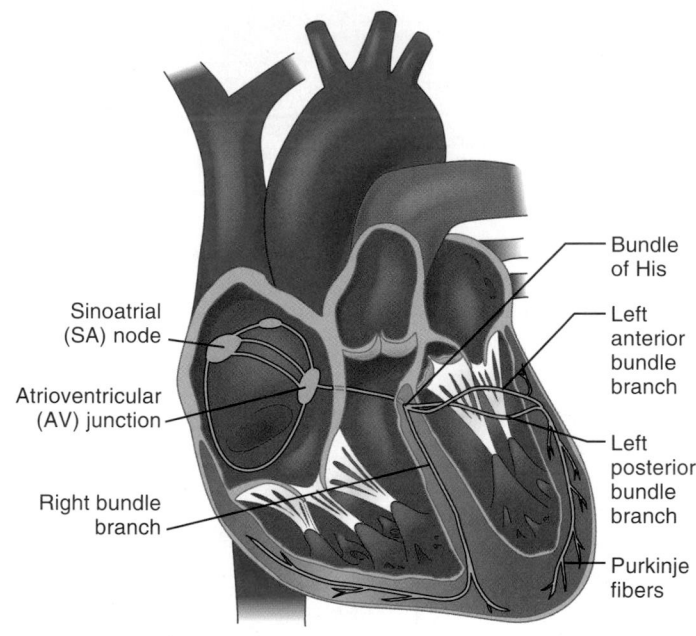

FIGURE 40-5 Cardiac conduction system.

Risk Factors for Heart Disease

Risk Factors That Cannot Be Changed

- *Advancing age:* More than 80% of people who die of coronary heart disease are 65 or older; older women are more likely to die of myocardial infarctions (MIs) than are older men.
- *Gender:* Men are at greater risk of MIs and experience heart attacks earlier in life; women are at greater risk after menopause, but their risk still is not as great as the risk for men.
- *Family history and race:* The children of parents with heart disease are more likely to develop it; African-Americans are at greater risk of developing hypertension and the heart disease associated with it; Mexican-Americans, Native Americans, native Hawaiians, and some Asian-Americans also are at greater risk.

Lifestyle Risk Factors That Can Be Modified or Treated

- *Smoking:* Smokers' risk of developing coronary heart disease is two to four times that of nonsmokers. Male smokers develop heart disease three times more often than women; female smokers develop heart disease six times more often than those who never smoked. Smoking is associated with sudden cardiac death. Exposure to secondhand smoke also increases the risk.
- *High blood cholesterol:* The risk of heart disease rises with rising blood cholesterol levels.
- *Hypertension:* Hypertension increases the amount of work the heart must do to circulate blood throughout the body.
- *Sedentary lifestyle:* Regular exercise helps prevent cardiovascular disease.
- *Obesity and overweight:* Excess weight, especially increased body fat at the waist, is associated with an increased risk of heart disease and stroke; losing as little as 10 pounds can lower the risk.
- *Diabetes mellitus:* The risk of heart disease is even greater if blood glucose levels are not controlled; at least 65% of people with diabetes die of some form of heart or blood vessel disease.

http://www.heart.org/HEARTORG/Conditions/HeartAttack/UnderstandYourRiskofHeartAttack/Understand-Your-Risk-of-Heart-Attack_UCM_002040_Article.jsp#.VsH3EflrKUl. Accessed February 15, 2016.

Coronary Artery Disease and Myocardial Infarction

Coronary artery disease (CAD) causes almost half a million deaths in the United States every year. In CAD the formation of atherosclerotic plaques narrows the arteries supplying the myocardium, which results in a lack of blood supply to the heart muscle and may ultimately lead to a myocardial infarction (MI). Atherosclerotic plaque buildup is primarily related to cholesterol blood levels. Understanding cholesterol levels is crucial for understanding the risk of CAD. To monitor cholesterol levels, the provider will order a complete fasting lipoprotein profile. The profile studies four different levels of fat in the blood:

1. *Total cholesterol:* A score of less than 180 mg/dL is considered optimal.
2. *HDL ("good") cholesterol:* The higher the level the better; a low level of high-density lipoprotein (HDL) cholesterol increases the risk of heart disease. The best levels are 60 mg/dL and above.
3. *LDL ("bad") cholesterol:* A low level of low-density lipoprotein (LDL) cholesterol is considered good for heart health; the recommendations vary based on an individual's heart disease risk. For individuals not at risk, an LDL level of 100 to 129 mg/dL is recommended; for those at very high risk, the LDL level should be below 70 mg/dL. Recent research recommends that individuals with a high risk of heart disease (e.g., LDL level of 190 mg/dL or higher and diabetes type 2) be treated with **statins**. Medications for treatment of hypercholesterolemia are described in Table 40-1.
4. *Triglycerides:* Triglyceride is the most common type of fat in the body; a desirable level is less than 150 mg/dL. High

triglyceride levels combined with low HDL cholesterol or high LDL cholesterol is associated with atherosclerosis and an increased risk for heart attack and stroke.

An atherosclerotic plaque originates at the site of a chronic injury to the endothelial lining of the artery caused by risk factors associated with heart disease (e.g., smoking or hypertension). Platelets attach to the site of the endothelial injury, and lipids begin to accumulate. Eventually an atheroma forms, which is made up of a tough collagen shell covering a fatty center that extends out into the lumen of the vessel, restricting blood flow past the plaque buildup. Inflammation at the site attracts platelets to the surface of the atheroma, resulting in the formation of a clot (thrombus) that can completely block the lumen of the vessel, depriving the myocardium of an adequate nutritious blood supply (Figure 40-6). The cardinal symptom of myocardial **ischemia** is angina pectoris. Angina pectoris is pain behind the sternum that is precipitated by exertion but that can be relieved either by rest or by sublingual nitroglycerin.

Patients may be asymptomatic until the disease becomes fully developed. The first symptom of an MI may be angina, followed by pressure or fullness in the chest, syncope, shortness of breath, edema, unexplained coughing spells, and fatigue. A patient reporting any of these symptoms is considered to have a medical emergency and should be seen by the provider immediately.

Telephone Screening for Chest Pain

The medical assistant should activate emergency medical services if the patient reports any of the following:
- Current chest pain that is crushing, pressing, or radiating to the arms, upper back, or jaw
- Sweating, difficulty breathing, nausea, indigestion, or dizziness
- Any of these symptoms, along with a history of coronary artery disease, myocardial infarction, or angina
- A change in the pattern of the angina
- Chest pain that occurs during rest or with minimum exertion

In recent years the rate of heart disease has declined in men but not in women. Traditional risk factors negatively affect both genders; however, women are at greater risk if they have metabolic syndrome (a combination of hypertension, elevated insulin levels, excess body fat around the waist, and high blood cholesterol levels); if they have increased levels of stress and/or depression; if they smoke (female smokers are at much greater risk than women who do not smoke); and if they have reduced estrogen production before menopause. The difference in female risks and symptoms is associated with the method of plaque buildup in women; the plaque tends to develop as an evenly spread layer along the entire lumen of the blood vessels rather than as a localized plaque buildup, as is seen in men. Women with heart disease typically experience this diffuse atheroma buildup in smaller vessels, which causes more subtle symptoms than the crushing chest pain associated with classic myocardial infarctions.

TABLE 40-1 Prescription Medications to Lower Blood Cholesterol Levels

CLASSIFICATION	ACTION	SIDE EFFECTS AND CAUTIONS
Statins Atorvastatin (Lipitor) Fluvastatin (Lescol) Lovastatin (Altoprev, Mevacor) Pitavastatin (Livalo) Pravastatin (Pravachol) Rosuvastatin (Crestor) Simvastatin (Zocor)	Lower LDL and triglycerides; slightly increase HDL	Headaches, minor itching, constipation, nausea, diarrhea, stomach pain, back pain, pain in the lower legs and arms, liver abnormalities; possible interaction with grapefruit juice
Bile acid–binding resins Cholestyramine (Locholest, Prevalite) Cholestyramine sucrose (Questran) Colesevelam (Welchol) Colestipol (Colestid)	Lower LDL by binding bile acids in the intestine for excretion in the stool; liver converts cholesterol into bile acids, thus lowering the blood cholesterol level	Constipation, bloating, nausea, gas; may increase triglycerides
Cholesterol absorption inhibitor Ezetimibe (Zetia)	Reduces the amount of cholesterol absorbed; lowers total cholesterol and LDL	Fatigue, gas, constipation, abdominal pain, cramps, muscle soreness; possible interaction with grapefruit juice
Fibrates Fenofibrate (Lofibra, Tricor) Gemfibrozil (Lopid)	Lower lipid levels, including cholesterol and triglycerides; reduce production of triglycerides and increase their rate of removal from the bloodstream; modestly increase HDL	Fever or chills, nausea, stomach pain, gallstones, fatigue, vertigo
Statin/niacin combinations Niacin extended release/simvastatin (Simcor) Niacin/lovastatin (Advicor)	Reduce LDL and triglycerides; increase HDL	Muscle, skin and gastrointestinal problems; facial and neck flushing; dizziness, heart palpitations, shortness of breath, sweating, chills; possible interaction with grapefruit juice

HDL, High-density lipoprotein; *LDL,* low-density lipoprotein.

The major concern in heart disease is the lack of blood to the myocardium, which occurs when a vessel becomes totally blocked. Ischemia over a prolonged period leads to necrosis (death) of a portion of the myocardium, resulting in an MI, or heart attack. Symptoms of an MI are similar to those of angina; however, an MI is identified by pain that lasts longer than 30 minutes and is not relieved by rest or nitroglycerin tablets. An MI is a life-threatening event; intervention must begin within the first hour for the best chance for survival.

Metabolic Syndrome

Metabolic syndrome is a group of risk factors that raise the risk of heart disease, diabetes, and stroke. A person with metabolic syndrome is twice as likely to develop heart disease and five times as likely to develop diabetes. To be diagnosed with metabolic syndrome, the patient must have at least three of the following risk factors:
- Abdominal obesity or excess fat in the stomach area (this is a greater risk factor for heart disease than excess fat in other parts of the body, such as on the hips)
- A high triglyceride level
- A low high-density lipoprotein (HDL) cholesterol level (HDL helps remove low-density lipoprotein [LDL] cholesterol from the arteries)
- High blood pressure (hypertension can damage the heart and lead to plaque buildup in the arteries)
- A high fasting blood glucose level (almost 85% of people with diabetes type 2 also have metabolic syndrome)

www.nhlbi.nih.gov/health/health-topics/topics/ms. Accessed February 16, 2016.

Signs and Symptoms of Myocardial Infarction in Women

In addition to angina, the signs and symptoms of a heart attack in women may start weeks before the actual cardiac injury and could include the following:
- Abdominal, neck, shoulder, or upper back pain
- Jaw pain
- Shortness of breath
- Vertigo (dizziness)
- Sweating
- Indigestion or nausea and vomiting
- Extreme fatigue
- Aching in both arms

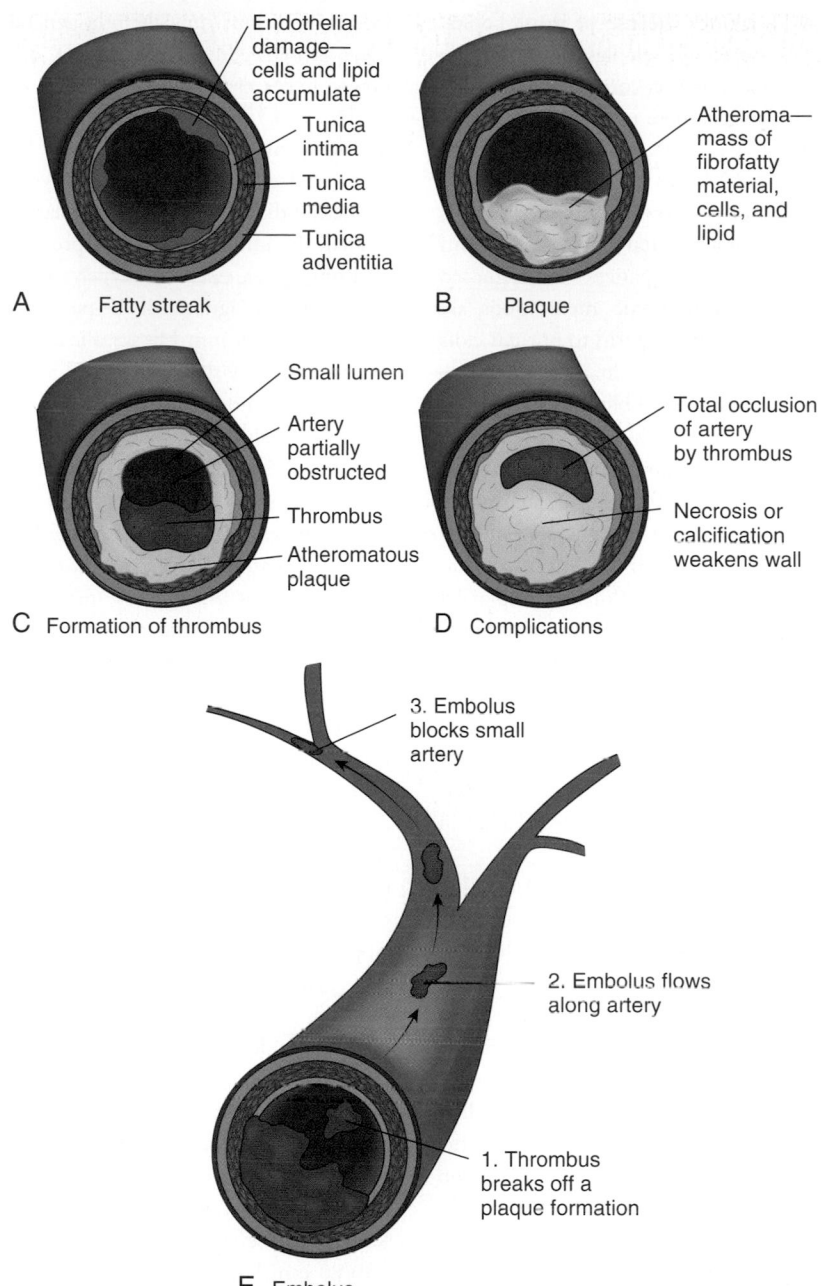

FIGURE 40-6 Development of an atheroma, leading to arterial occlusion.

CRITICAL THINKING APPLICATION   **40-1**

A patient who is scheduled for an appointment in 2 days calls the office and reports that she is not feeling well. She complains that she has a feeling of fullness in the chest, her arms ache, and she is very tired. Although this patient does not have a history of myocardial infarction, what should Adam do?

Diagnostic and Therapeutic Procedures

An MI is diagnosed by ECG changes and elevated cardiac enzymes. The traditional blood test that indicates myocardial damage is the creatine kinase (CK) level. CK levels begin to increase within 3 to 12 hours of the onset of chest pain, reach peak values within 24 hours, and return to baseline after 48 to 72 hours. The more severe the cardiac damage, the longer it takes for CK levels to peak and then return to normal. However, another blood test for possible myocardial damage measures troponin levels. Troponin is a protein that is released into the blood only when myocardial damage occurs. Therefore, even slight elevations may indicate some degree of heart muscle damage. Troponins increase in the bloodstream within 4 to 6 hours after initial myocardial damage and peak in 10 to 24 hours. In the case of minor myocardial damage, troponin levels remain elevated up to 10 to 14 days, allowing for later diagnosis of the event. Patients diagnosed with an MI typically are hospitalized immediately, started on oxygen, and continuously monitored by ECG. (Additional diagnostic procedures, such as an echocardiogram and heart catheterization, are discussed later in this chapter.)

Medical treatment of an MI includes the use of thrombolytic medications, such as alteplase (Activase) and reteplase (Retavase), to dissolve the blood clot that is blocking the coronary artery and prevent permanent myocardial damage. There is a better chance of survival and recovery from certain types of heart attacks if a thrombolytic drug is administered within 12 hours after the heart attack starts. Ideally, the patient should receive thrombolytic medications within the first 30 minutes of arrival at a hospital for treatment. This timetable makes it extremely important that patients be diagnosed and treated as soon as possible. Thrombolytic medications are administered intravenously (IV) along with heparin to prevent clots that are being dissolved from reforming. Aspirin also is used to prevent the formation of blood clots in affected blood vessels. Additional pharmaceutical treatment includes the use of nitroglycerin to dilate the coronary arteries so that more blood can be delivered to the myocardium; beta blockers (atenolol [Tenormin], metoprolol [Lopressor], or propranolol) to slow the heart rate and lower blood pressure; anticoagulants (warfarin [Coumadin]) for 3 to 6 months after the MI to prevent thrombus formation and/or the antiplatelet agent clopidogrel (Plavix); and anticholesterol agents to lower blood cholesterol levels and prevent subsequent formation of atherosclerotic plaques.

When the coronary arteries that supply blood to the myocardium are blocked, or **occluded**, either percutaneous transluminal coronary **angioplasty** (PTCA) or coronary artery bypass grafting (CABG) may be indicated. (These surgical procedures are discussed later in this chapter.)

After discharge from the hospital, patients with CAD that has resulted in an MI face multiple lifestyle changes to prevent another episode. Recommendations include no smoking; regular light exercise, such as walking 30 minutes a day, 5 days a week; a diet low in salt, saturated fat, and cholesterol; maintaining a healthy weight; controlling hypertension; reducing stress; and limiting alcohol intake to one or two drinks a day. The medical assistant should be prepared to provide encouragement and to reinforce the importance of lifestyle changes to prevent future heart problems. If ordered by the provider, professional referrals to a cardiac rehabilitation program and dietitian can also be helpful.

CRITICAL THINKING APPLICATION   **40-2**

Adam receives a telephone call from a patient who complains of nausea and difficulty taking a deep breath; the patient says he feels as if he is going to faint. What questions should Adam ask to determine the seriousness of the problem?

Hypertensive Heart Disease

Chronic elevated blood pressure can result in left ventricular hypertrophy (enlargement), angina, MI, or heart failure. Hypertension also is a major cause of stroke and nephropathy (kidney disease). Some of the risk factors for hypertension include a family history of hypertension or stroke, hypercholesterolemia (high blood cholesterol), smoking, high sodium intake, diabetes, excessive alcohol intake, sedentary lifestyle, obesity, aging, prolonged stress, and race (African-Americans have a higher incidence than Caucasians). Hypertension has an insidious onset, and the patient shows few, if any, signs and symptoms until permanent damage has occurred.

Initial symptoms may include general malaise and headache; epistaxis (nosebleed), vertigo, nausea, or syncope can occur with prolonged hypertension.

The two types of hypertension are primary hypertension and secondary hypertension. Secondary hypertension occurs because of a disease process in another body system, such as renal disease or an endocrine disorder. Before secondary hypertension can be properly treated, the underlying disease process must be resolved.

Primary, or essential, hypertension is idiopathic (of unknown cause) and is diagnosed if the patient's blood pressure is persistently higher than 119 mm Hg systolic and/or 79 mm Hg diastolic at two or more office visits over several weeks or months. If the medical assistant first notes that a patient's blood pressure is elevated, the pressure should be checked in both arms with the patient seated and after the patient has been standing for at least 2 minutes with a cuff that is the proper size for the patient's arm. If the pressure readings are different, the provider uses the higher value for diagnostic purposes. The patient's blood pressures should be checked again after at least 2 minutes. All of these readings must be documented in the patient's record. Some patients have "white coat hypertension," which appears only when they visit the provider. If the patient has a history of this problem, have him or her lie down on the examination table and rest for a few minutes before the blood pressure is taken; this may help in obtaining a more accurate reading.

Hypertension is treated according to the stage of the disease and any accompanying health problems. Table 40-2 summarizes the stages and treatment of hypertension. In all cases the patient needs education and counseling on making lifestyle changes. Components of lifestyle modifications include weight reduction; the Dietary Approaches to Stop Hypertension (DASH) eating plan, which is a diet rich in fruits, vegetables, and low-fat dairy products with reduced saturated and total fat; a reduction in dietary sodium; aerobic physical activity; and moderation of alcohol consumption. It is recommended that patients with diabetes and/or chronic kidney disease start medication therapy if they have a diastolic reading above 130 or a systolic reading above 80 mm Hg. The goal of drug treatment is to stabilize the patient's blood pressure to no more than 140/90 mm Hg; however, in patients with diabetes or chronic kidney disease, the goal blood pressure reading is no more than 130/80 mm Hg.

The medical assistant can play an important role in antihypertensive therapy by teaching the patient how to take his or her own blood pressure at home, providing literature that reinforces the necessity of monitoring the blood pressure, and helping the patient understand that this condition cannot be cured but can be controlled for the rest of his or her life. Continued encouragement and support are needed because compliance with the treatment regimen and making permanent lifestyle changes is difficult for a patient who is not showing any symptoms of disease. Table 40-3 summarizes some of the medications that may be prescribed to manage hypertension.

CRITICAL THINKING APPLICATION   **40-3**

Essential hypertension is a common problem for patients seen in the cardiology department where Adam works. What could Adam do to help patients with primary hypertension? What informational materials or community resources would be helpful in gaining patient compliance with treatment?

TABLE 40-2 Stages and Treatment of Hypertension

BLOOD PRESSURE (mm Hg)	TREATMENT
Prehypertension 120-139 systolic *or* 80-89 diastolic	• Lifestyle modification (reduced sodium, low saturated and trans fat diet; regular aerobic activity; moderate alcohol intake; smoking cessation; weight loss; stress reduction) • Drug therapy for patients with diabetes mellitus or chronic kidney disease
Stage 1 hypertension 140-159 systolic *or* 90-99 diastolic	• Consider coexisting conditions • Thiazide-type diuretics (e.g., furosemide [Lasix] or hydrochlorothiazide plus triamterene [Dyazide]) for most patients
Stage 2 hypertension ≥160 systolic *or* ≥100 diastolic	• Consider coexisting conditions • Two-drug combination for most patients

Seventh Report of the Joint National Committee on Prevention, Detection, Evaluation, and Treatment of High Blood Pressure. Available at *http://www.nhlbi.nih.gov/files/docs/guidelines/jnc7full.pdf.* Accessed February 15, 2016.

Congestive Heart Failure

Congestive heart failure (CHF) occurs when the myocardium is unable to pump an adequate amount of blood to meet the body's needs. Although the onset can be acute, the condition typically develops over time because of weakness in the left ventricle as a result of chronic hypertension, MI of the left ventricular wall, valvular heart disease, or pulmonary complications. Typically, heart failure initially occurs on one side of the heart and then on the other side. Left-sided heart failure usually results from essential hypertension or left ventricular disease, whereas right-sided heart failure can develop as a result of lung disease. Right-sided heart failure that occurs because of pulmonary hypertension associated with chronic obstructive pulmonary disease (COPD) is called *cor pulmonale.*

Consider the blood flow through the heart and what happens if it is blocked or inhibited in some way. In left-sided heart failure, the left ventricle cannot empty completely because of a weakness in the myocardial wall from an MI or because of long-term hypertension. As a result, blood backs up in the left atria, increasing the pressure inside the chamber, and emptying blood from the lungs becomes difficult. Ultimately the lungs begin to fill up with fluid because of the sluggish blood flow, and pulmonary edema results. Signs and symptoms of pulmonary edema include dyspnea, orthopnea, nonproductive cough, rales, and tachycardia. In right-sided heart failure, the right ventricle cannot maintain complete output, and blood backs up in the right atrium; this prevents complete emptying of the vena cava, resulting in systemic edema, especially dependent edema in the legs and feet. Both types of heart failure cause fatigue, weakness, exercise intolerance, dyspnea, and sensitivity to cold temperatures.

TABLE 40-3 Medications Used to Treat Hypertension

CLASSIFICATION	ACTION	TREATMENT PROTOCOL
Thiazide diuretics (Lasix, Aldactone)	Act on kidneys to increase elimination of sodium and water, thereby reducing blood volume	Drugs of choice to treat hypertension; enhance the action of other blood pressure (BP) medications; used in patients with diabetes and those with chronic kidney disease with prehypertension
Beta blockers (Tenormin, Sectral, Lopressor, Ziac)	Reduce the heart rate and cardiac output; reduce the workload of the heart and open blood vessels	May be used with a diuretic for stage 1 and stage 2 hypertension
Angiotensin-converting enzyme (ACE) inhibitors (Lotensin, Capoten, Vasotec)	Cause vasodilation and reduced vascular resistance; reduce the workload of the heart	May be used with a diuretic for stage 1 and stage 2 hypertension; also may be used for hypertension in patients with coronary artery disease, heart failure, or kidney failure
Angiotensin II receptor blockers (Cozaar, Atacand, Avapro, Diovan)	Block the action of chemicals that cause vasoconstriction	May be used with a diuretic for stage 1 and stage 2 hypertension; also may be used for hypertension in patients with coronary artery disease, heart failure, or kidney failure
Calcium channel blockers (Norvasc, Lotrel, Cardizem, Plendil)	Interrupt the movement of calcium into the heart and vessel cells, causing vasodilation	May be used with a diuretic for stage 1 and stage 2 hypertension; also used to treat angina and/or some arrhythmias

Nonpharmaceutical treatment for CHF includes limiting physical activity so that the heart does not have to work so hard, restricting salt, not smoking, reducing stress, and controlling weight. Patient education for an individual with CHF must stress the importance of monitoring weight gain because a sudden increase in weight may indicate fluid retention. Patients should weigh themselves once or twice a week and report any gain of more than 3 pounds to the provider.

Drug therapy for CHF begins with diuretics to treat dyspnea and orthopnea and control edema. Other medications may include an angiotensin-converting enzyme (ACE) inhibitor, a type of vasodilator that widens blood vessels to lower blood pressure and reduce the workload of the heart. Examples of ACE inhibitors include enalapril (Vasotec), lisinopril and captopril (Capoten). Digoxin often is prescribed to increase the strength of myocardial contractions, and beta blockers (carvedilol [Coreg] and metoprolol [Lopressor]) are used to slow the heart rate and improve heart function. Because potassium loss is a common side effect of diuretic and digoxin therapy, patients may also be prescribed a potassium (KCl) supplement. Routine monitoring of serum electrolytes is ordered to determine the need for a potassium supplement so that potential complications can be prevented.

CRITICAL THINKING APPLICATION   **40-4**

Kate Glasgow, a 76-year-old patient with a history of CHF, is in the office today for a checkup. She does not understand why she must stop using salt and start weighing herself regularly at home. What can Adam do to help this patient understand the importance of her treatment regimen?

Orthostatic Hypotension

Orthostatic, or postural, hypotension is diagnosed if the patient experiences a drop in blood pressure when standing, especially when quickly changing from a prone or seated position to an upright one. When we stand, our blood pressure quickly adapts to the pull of gravity by reflexively increasing the heart rate and constricting systemic arterioles. In a patient with orthostatic hypotension, the blood pressure adjusts sluggishly or not at all to rapid changes in position. An acute episode of orthostatic hypotension may be caused by blood pooling in the lower extremities, a reaction to antihypertensive or antidepressant medication, or prolonged immobility. This is a common problem in elderly people and may contribute significantly to falls and related injuries. Patients need to be evaluated for secondary causes and encouraged to adjust from a prone position by sitting on the side of the bed for a bit before standing.

To evaluate orthostatic hypotension, the provider may ask the medical assistant to check the patient's blood pressure while the person is seated, leave the cuff in place, then have the patient stand and immediately check the blood pressure again. Both blood pressure readings should be recorded in the patient's health record for the provider to evaluate. Include in your note any patient complaints after standing, such as dizziness or a feeling of lightheadedness.

Inflammatory and Valvular Disorders

Rheumatic Heart Disease

Rheumatic heart disease develops because of an unusual immune reaction that typically occurs 2 to 4 weeks after an untreated group A beta-hemolytic streptococcal infection. The infection typically starts as "strep" throat or an upper respiratory infection but progresses to the creation of antibodies that react with collagen to cause inflammation in the joints, skin, brain, and heart. About half of those affected develop heart inflammation, but most have a complete recovery. However, in some people the heart is permanently damaged. The disease process in the heart can involve all layers of heart tissue.

Pericarditis, or inflammation of the outer layer of the heart, causes reduced cardiac activity and pericardial effusion (the collection of blood or fluid in the pericardium). Myocarditis, or inflammation of the muscular lining of the heart, usually is self-limiting but may lead to acute heart failure because of weakening of the myocardial wall. Endocarditis, or inflammation of the inner lining of the heart and the heart valves, is the most common heart complication. **Vegetations** form along the outer edges of the valve cusps, causing scarring and stenosis and preventing the damaged heart valve from closing or opening completely. The valvular damage may be asymptomatic at first but eventually can cause serious problems. The mitral valve is affected most frequently, which impairs the ability of the left ventricle to function normally.

Treatment includes the use of antibiotics (penicillin) to eliminate the streptococcal infection completely and antiinflammatory agents for the inflammatory reaction. In 2007 the American Heart Association changed its guidelines on the prophylactic use of antibiotics before a dental or other invasive procedure. No research links dental, gastrointestinal, or genitourinary tract procedures with the development of endocarditis. Therefore, prophylactic use of antibiotics now is recommended only for patients with the highest risk of complications from endocarditis, such as those with artificial heart valves or certain types of congenital heart disease.

Valve Disorders

Disorders of the valves of the heart may be caused by a congenital defect or an infection, such as endocarditis. Two specific problems can occur with valve disease. The valve can be stenosed, or hardened, which restricts the forward flow of blood, or it can be incompetent, which means that it does not close completely, so blood can leak backward, or regurgitate. The most common valve defect is mitral valve prolapse (MVP), an incompetence in the mitral valve caused by a congenital defect or vegetation and scarring from endocarditis.

Valve disorders ultimately can lead to ventricular hypertrophy and cardiomegaly (enlargement of the heart). Severely damaged valves or serious congenital defects may require surgical replacement of the affected valve.

BLOOD VESSELS

Blood vessels are divided into two systems that begin and end with the heart (Figure 40-7). The pulmonary system carries deoxygenated blood from the right ventricle to the lungs and oxygenated blood back to the left atrium. The systemic system carries blood from the left ventricle throughout the entire body and back to the right atrium. The vessels are classified according to their structure and function: *arteries* carry oxygenated blood away from the heart; *capillaries* are the microscopic vessels responsible for the exchange of

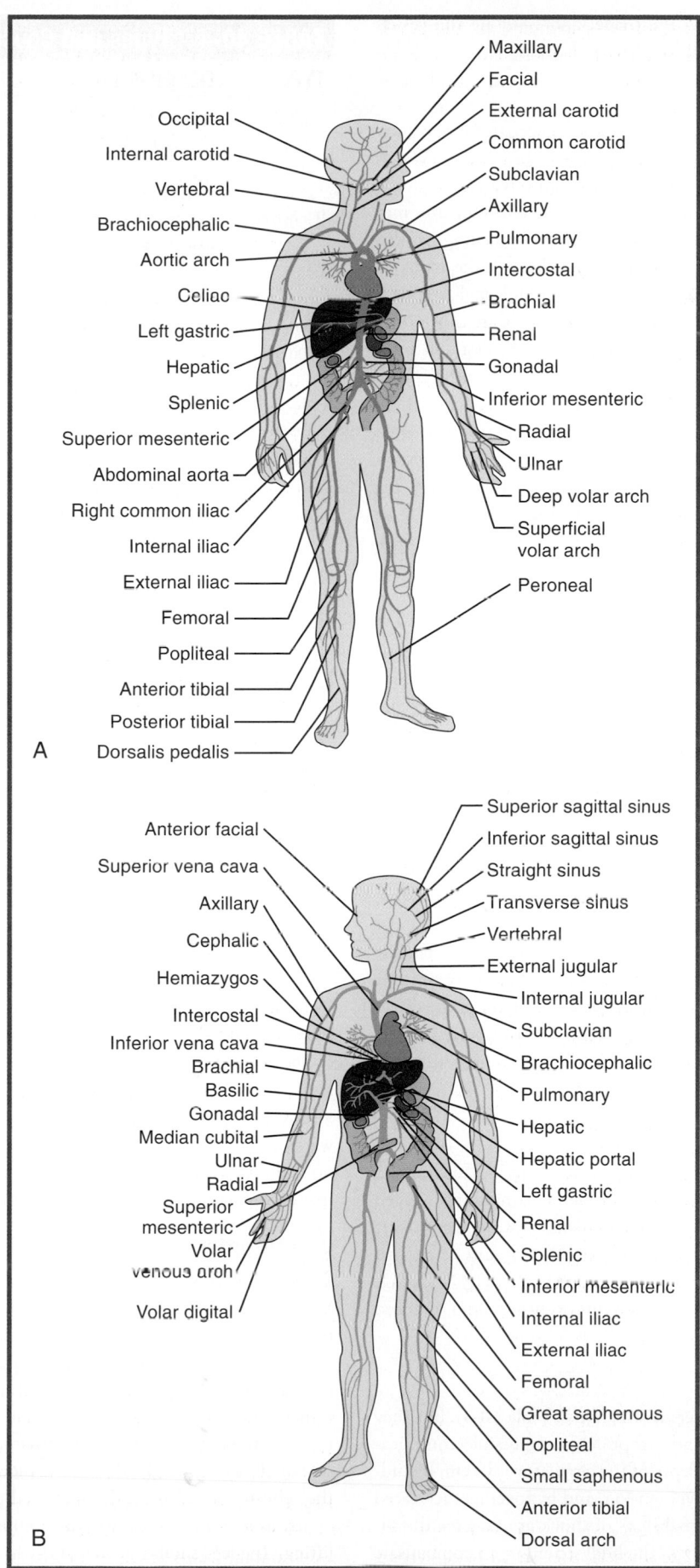

FIGURE 40-7 A, Systemic arteries. **B,** Systemic veins.

oxygen and carbon dioxide in the tissue; and *veins* are the vessels that carry deoxygenated blood back to the heart.

Arteries

All arteries except the pulmonary artery carry oxygenated blood away from the heart to all the cells of the body. The largest of these vessels is the aorta, which starts at the left ventricle and travels through the center of the body into the lower abdomen, where it bifurcates into the right and left femoral arteries, with arteries branching off this system down to the feet. As the aorta passes through the trunk of the body, arteries branch off from it into smaller and smaller vessels, which ultimately become microscopic. These vessels are called *arterioles,* which terminate into tissue capillaries, the smallest and most plentiful of the blood vessels. Capillaries are a single epithelial cell thick, so nutrients and gases can pass through the vessel wall for exchange at the cellular level. Arterioles deliver erythrocytes (red blood cells [RBCs]), which carry oxygen attached to hemoglobin molecules to surrounding tissues. While in the capillary bed, the oxygen that was bound to the RBC hemoglobin is unloaded to the surrounding tissues. When the blood leaves the capillary bed, the oxygen supply has been depleted, and the return portion of the blood cycle now begins.

Veins

As the blood leaves the capillary beds, it enters the smallest veins, called *venules.* From this point on, the blood flows into larger and larger veins until it reaches the largest veins in the body, the inferior and superior venae cavae. The venae cavae deposit deoxygenated blood into the right atrium, where the blood again begins its trip through the heart through the tricuspid valve, into the right ventricle, then through the pulmonary arteries to the lungs, where gas exchange occurs at the alveoli level. Oxygen-rich blood is returned to the left atrium via the pulmonary veins. The walls of veins are thinner than those of arteries because they do not have a muscular lining. Instead, veins have valves that open and close to prevent the backflow of blood. The valves operate by the contraction of muscles around the veins; these contractions massage the blood in the direction of venous flow back to the heart. Venous valves are especially important in the arms and legs because they prevent pooling of blood in the extremities.

VASCULAR DISORDERS

The vascular system constantly supplies blood containing oxygen and nutrients to all the body's tissues and picks up waste from tissue metabolism. For tissues to receive an adequate amount of oxygen and nutrients, the arterial vessels must maintain elasticity, and their linings must remain smooth to prevent occlusion and reduced blood flow.

Shock

Shock can occur in many different situations (Table 40-4), but they all result in the same signs and symptoms and possible complications. Shock is the general collapse of the circulatory system, including reduced cardiac output, hypotension, and hypoxemia (decreased oxygen in the blood). The initial signs of shock are extreme thirstiness, restlessness, and irritability. The body attempts to compensate

TABLE 40-4 Types and Causes of Shock

TYPE	DEFINITION	CAUSES
Cardiogenic	Low cardiac output caused by inability of the heart to pump	Acute MI, arrhythmias, pulmonary embolism, CHF
Hypovolemic	Excessive loss of blood or body fluids	GI bleeding, internal or external hemorrhage, excessive loss of plasma or body fluids, burns
Neurogenic	Peripheral vascular dilation resulting from neurologic injury or disorder	Spinal cord injury, emotional stress, drug reaction
Anaphylactic	Systemic hypersensitivity to an allergen, causing respiratory distress and vascular collapse	Drug, vaccine, food allergies, insect venom, or chemical allergies
Septic (septicemia)	Systemic vasodilation caused by the release of bacterial endotoxins	Systemic infection or bacteremia

CHF, Congestive heart failure; *GI,* gastrointestinal; *MI,* myocardial infarction.

for circulatory collapse with constriction of peripheral blood vessels, allowing blood to pool in the vital organs. This vasoconstriction causes a generalized feeling of cool, clammy skin; pallor; tachycardia; and reduced urinary output. Symptoms progress to a rapid, weak, thready pulse; tachypnea; and altered levels of consciousness. If the process is not reversed, the central nervous system becomes depressed, and acute renal failure may occur.

The cause of the shock must be treated for the patient to survive. If the medical assistant identifies a patient in shock, emergency treatment should be started at once. Do not wait for the first indicators of shock to worsen before calling for help. If the provider is not available, call 911 for emergency medical care. Place the patient in a supine position, assess the vital signs frequently, keep the patient warm, administer oxygen as ordered by the provider, and, if there is no indication of head or neck trauma, elevate the legs about 12 inches to encourage the flow of blood back to the heart.

Vein Disorders
Varicose Veins

Veins have one-way valves that help keep blood flowing toward the heart. Varicose veins are dilated, tortuous, superficial veins in the legs (Figure 40-8). Varicosities can be caused by congenitally defective valves in the saphenous veins and the veins branching off them. Other contributing factors are pregnancy, obesity, prolonged standing or sitting, and heavy lifting. Whatever the cause, the vein valves do not close completely; this allows blood to flow backward, causing the vein to distend from the increased pressure.

Treatment includes consistent aerobic exercise and limiting heavy lifting. The legs should be elevated when possible, and compression

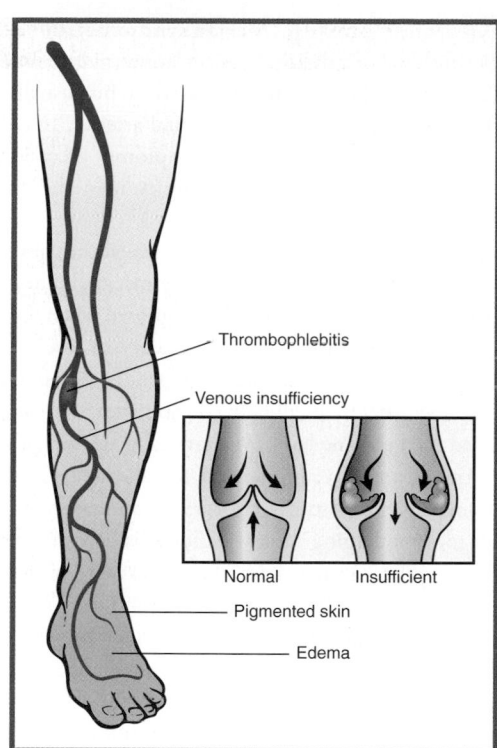

FIGURE 40-8 Varicose veins of the calf. (From Damjanov I: *Pathology for the health-related professions,* ed 4, St Louis, 2012, Saunders.)

stockings should be worn by those who must stand for long periods. Medical intervention includes:

- *Sclerotherapy:* A treatment in which a chemical is injected into the vein to cause irritation and scarring inside the vein, closing it off.
- *Laser surgery:* A procedure in which light energy from a laser is applied to a varicose vein.
- *Endovenous* **ablation** *therapy:* A procedure in which a small incision is made near the varicose vein and a catheter is inserted; a device at the tip of the tube heats up the inside of the vein and closes it off.
- *Endoscopic vein surgery:* An outpatient procedure in which a small incision is made near a varicose vein, and a tiny camera at the end of a thin tube is inserted and moved through the vein; a surgical device at the end of the camera is used to close the vein.
- *Vein stripping and ligation:* This procedure typically is done only in severe cases; the veins are tied shut and removed through small incisions.

Although treatment may be successful, varicosities can recur over time. Patients should be warned to investigate insurance coverage of treatment costs because many insurance companies consider treatment of varicose veins cosmetic surgery. However, if the patient has documented proof of a health risk associated with the varicosities, insurance companies are more likely to pay for treatment.

Deep Vein Thrombosis

Phlebitis is an inflammation of a vein, most commonly seen in the lower legs. When a vein becomes inflamed, a blood clot, or thrombus, may develop at the site. A thrombus is a clot formed by the collection of platelets that attaches to the interior wall of a vessel. Deep vein thrombosis (DVT) is a thrombus with inflammatory changes that has attached to the deep venous system of the lower legs, causing partial or complete obstruction of the vessel. The calf veins are the most common sites of DVT, but it also can develop in the iliac and femoral veins. Risk factors for the formation of a DVT are recent surgery, immobilization, older age (an increased risk is seen after age 50), trauma, obesity, use of oral contraceptives, varicose veins, pancreatic cancer, and pregnancy.

In the early stages, approximately 50% of patients with DVT are asymptomatic. Some patients complain of calf pain or cramping and edema of the affected leg, with warmth and erythema at the site. A thrombus that dislodges and begins to move through the general circulation is called an *embolus.* A pulmonary embolism (PE), which is a thrombus that breaks loose and is carried to the lungs, causing blockage of a pulmonary artery, is the most serious complication and may be the first indication that the thrombus was present. Signs and symptoms of a PE include an acute onset of chest pain that worsens with a deep breath or cough; unexplained shortness of breath; vertigo or syncope (dizziness or fainting); hemoptysis (coughing up blood); and a feeling of anxiety. Patients with any of these indicators should seek immediate medical attention.

DVT typically is diagnosed with venous Doppler studies, which use ultrasound to measure the rate of blood flow through the vessel and can accurately detect venous obstruction. Ultrasound can be used to create an image of the blood flow through the targeted vessel, allowing visualization of the thrombus. Venography also may be ordered; in venography a dye is injected into a large vein of the foot or ankle in the affected leg, and x-ray films of the veins are taken. Once the diagnosis has been confirmed, patients usually are hospitalized for IV anticoagulant therapy (heparin) or subcutaneous (SQ) injections of enoxaparin sodium (Lovenox).

Anticoagulant therapy does not dissolve existing clots; rather, it prevents clots from increasing in size and reduces the potential for additional clots. Oral anticoagulant treatment (warfarin [Coumadin]) is usually continued for 6 months. Patients require regular follow-up, including prothrombin time analysis. The medical assistant may perform venipuncture on these patients, and if so, should follow the office policy for blood draws on patients taking anticoagulants. The medical assistant also should reinforce the provider's recommendations about the prevention of further thrombi and precautions about anticoagulant use.

Patient Education for Prevention of Deep Vein Thrombosis (DVT)

- Take your prescribed medications as directed.
- If you have been prescribed anticoagulants, eat foods high in vitamin K in small amounts (e.g., dark green, leafy vegetables and canola and soy oils).
- Avoid sitting still for long periods; walk around several times during the day or move your legs frequently.
- Alter lifestyle factors such as obesity, smoking, and hypertension, because they increase the risk of DVT.
- Wear compression stockings as ordered by the provider.

Arterial Disorders

Arteriosclerosis and Atherosclerosis

Arteriosclerosis is a general term for the thickening and loss of elasticity of the arterial walls that is associated with aging. Other conditions that can lead to hardening of the arterial wall are hypertension, **scleroderma**, and diabetes mellitus. Arteriosclerosis, which can occur in arteries throughout the body, causes systemic ischemia and necrosis over time.

Atherosclerosis is a form of arteriosclerosis marked by the formation of an atheroma, a buildup of cholesterol, cellular debris, and platelets along the inside vessel wall (Figure 40-9).

Cholesterol is a nonessential nutrient that can be produced in the liver. It forms the base for many of the hormones created in the body. Problems arise from dietary and lifestyle factors that elevate blood cholesterol levels to a dangerous point, causing the formation of atheromas, which ultimately block arteries and cause such disorders as heart attacks and strokes.

Treatment of elevated blood cholesterol levels consists of dietary reductions in saturated and **trans fats**, in addition to aerobic exercise to elevate HDL levels. Patients are encouraged to stop smoking (see Table 42-1 for prescription medications for hypercholesterolemia). The medical assistant can help by educating the patient about risk factors and promoting changes in lifestyle. Referrals to a dietitian may be helpful for patients having a difficult time controlling their saturated fat intake.

Aneurysm

An aneurysm is a ballooning or dilation of a blood vessel wall (Figure 40-10). The patient may have an inherited factor for the development of aneurysms (e.g., **Marfan syndrome**), but a common cause is the buildup of atherosclerotic plaques, which weaken the vessel wall. Aneurysms can occur in any artery but usually develop in either the abdominal aorta or the cerebral arteries. In either case, the patient seldom has any signs or symptoms. Occasionally the patient describes a pounding or pulsating pain in the area of the aneurysm.

Screening is recommended for people between the ages of 65 and 75 if they have a family history of aneurysms, or if they are men who have smoked. An aneurysm can be diagnosed when auscultation of the affected vessel over the area of the aneurysm reveals turbulent blood flow sounds, or a bruit. Radiologic studies, sonography, and computed tomography (CT) all help confirm the diagnosis. Patients are monitored on a routine basis for changes in the size of the aneurysm. Surgical repair is recommended for all aneurysms 6 cm or larger, but smaller ones also can rupture. If an aneurysm is tender and known to be enlarging rapidly, surgery is essential, no matter the size. If a rupture occurs, immediate lifesaving intervention is required.

The medical assistant may aid the provider by observing the patient for signs of pain, mental changes, and changes in pulse and respirations. If any of these signs is observed, the provider must be notified immediately. As with any serious condition, the patient may have a high level of anxiety, and the medical assistant's role is to support the patient and family while encouraging consistent follow-up.

Peripheral Arterial Disease

Peripheral arterial disease develops because of widespread atherosclerotic plaque buildup in the arteries outside the heart, especially in the legs. Plaque deposits reduce the size of the lumen of the blood vessel, thereby reducing the amount of oxygenated blood delivered to the tissues. This lack of oxygen causes symptoms, most notably leg pain when walking, a condition called **intermittent claudication**. Other signs and symptoms of peripheral arterial disease are leg numbness or weakness; persistently cold extremities; sores on the feet or legs that do not heal; and hair loss on the extremities. The most effective methods for controlling intermittent claudication are

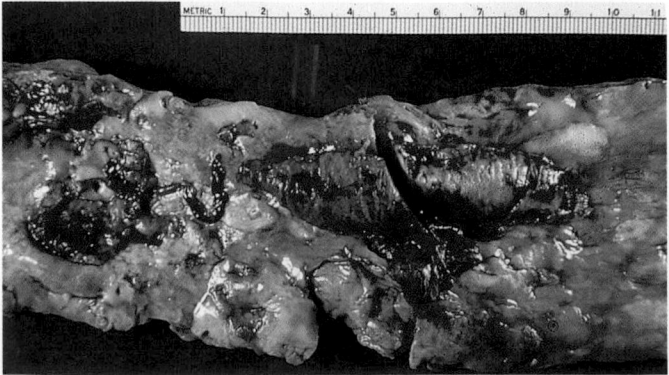

FIGURE 40-9 Atherosclerotic vessel. (From Damjanov I: *Pathology for the health-related professions,* ed 4, St Louis, 2012, Saunders.)

Aneurysm

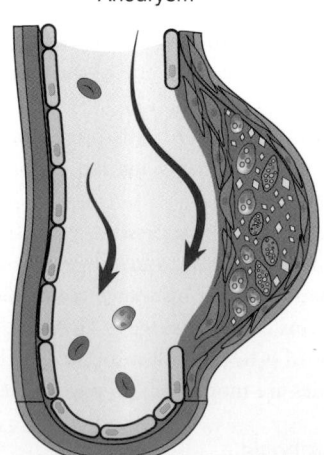

FIGURE 40-10 Aneurysm caused by weakening of the vessel wall. (From Damjanov I: *Pathology for the health-related professions,* ed 4, St Louis, 2012, Saunders.)

regular exercise, smoking cessation, control of hypertension and diabetes, and prescription of statins and antiplatelet drugs. Bypass surgery or angioplasty may be necessary if these methods do not improve blood flow to tissues.

DIAGNOSTIC PROCEDURES AND TREATMENTS

The cardiovascular examination begins with the medical assistant measuring the patient's height and weight, temperature, radial and apical pulses, respirations, and blood pressure in both arms. Most cardiologists also want a complete list of the prescription and over-the-counter (OTC) medications the patient is taking, including the strength and frequency of use for each. A large part of the provider's examination focuses on subjective symptoms. The physical examination covers the chest, heart, and vascular systems. General appearance, color of the skin, symmetry, clubbing of the fingers, jugular vein distention, temperature of the extremities, and breathing patterns are a few of the notations made by the cardiologist.

A very common diagnostic test for the cardiovascular system performed in the ambulatory care setting is the electrocardiogram (ECG), which records the electrical activity of the heart. An ECG is a routine part of many physical examinations, and it also may be ordered if the provider is trying to rule out an MI or to diagnose a cardiac arrhythmia. If the provider wants to evaluate potential cardiac problems in patients over a specific period (usually 24 hours), a Holter monitor may be ordered. The Holter monitor continuously records the patient's cardiac activity, which is compared to symptoms the patient documents during the test period (see the Electrocardiography chapter for further details about diagnostic tools for cardiac conditions). Patient support and education are two very important areas in which medical assistants are deeply involved. When patients understand their condition and are encouraged to take an active role in their treatments, they are inclined to comply with the provider's orders in a more precise and orderly way. Although cardiovascular diagnostic procedures are not typically done in the ambulatory care setting, medical assistants should be familiar with the purpose of the tests so that they can answer patients' questions knowledgeably.

Doppler Studies

Doppler studies can identify occlusions of both veins and arteries from thrombi, emboli, or atherosclerotic plaques. The provider may order arterial Doppler studies for patients with intermittent claudication, lack of a pedal pulse, or leg ulcers that refuse to heal. Venous sonography is ordered to assess patients with pronounced varicosities or those with a swollen, painful leg to rule out the possibility of DVT. For a continuous-wave Doppler study, a conductive gel is applied to the skin over the test site. The Doppler transducer is moved over the site, directing an ultrasound beam at the vessel being checked (Figure 40-11). The sonographic beam picks up the speed of the RBCs as they travel through the vessel; this is heard as a "swishing" sound. The physician listens to the change in the pitch of the sound produced by the transducer to evaluate the blood flow through an area that may be blocked or narrowed. Variations in RBC velocity indicate either partial or complete occlusion of the blood vessel. A two-dimensional image of an artery can be produced with a duplex Doppler scan that directly shows stenosis or occlusion of the artery. These studies usually are conducted in a vascular

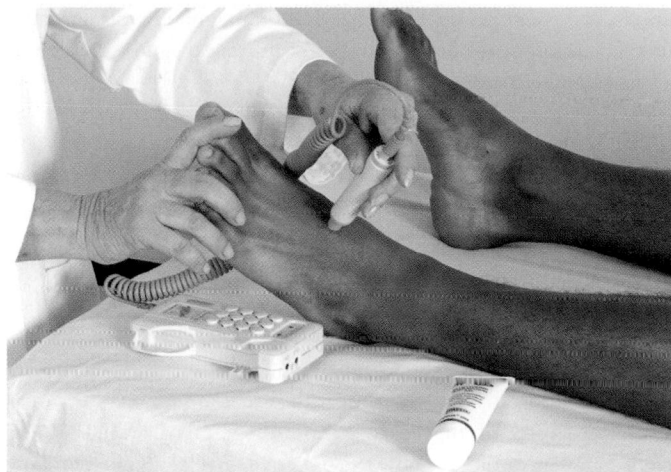

FIGURE 40-11 Doppler study. (From Jarvis C: *Physical examination and health assessment,* ed 7, St Louis, 2016, Saunders.)

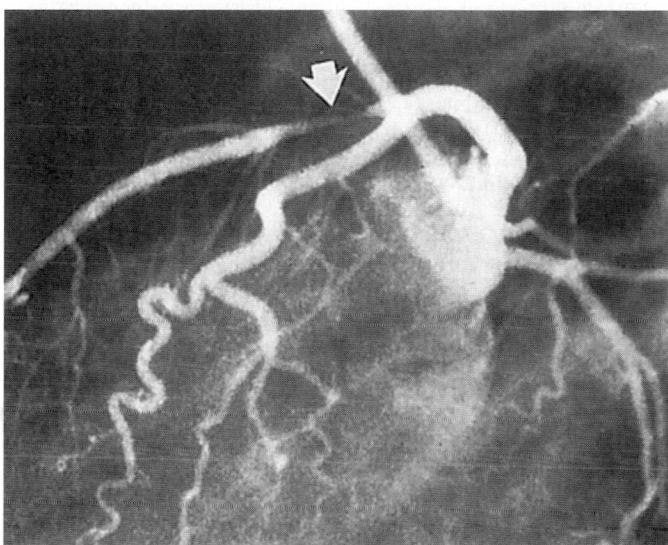

FIGURE 40-12 Coronary angiography showing stenosis *(arrow)* of the left anterior descending coronary artery. (From Braunwald E: *Heart disease: a textbook of cardiovascular medicine,* ed 4, Philadelphia, 1992, Saunders.)

laboratory but may be done in a vascular surgeon's office as an initial assessment of the patient or follow-up after bypass grafting. The medical assistant working in this type of practice requires additional training to perform this procedure.

Angiography

Angiography (arteriography) can be used to evaluate any of the arterial pathways in the body (Figure 40-12). A catheter is inserted into a major artery (usually the femoral artery) and advanced to the artery under study. A radiopaque contrast medium is rapidly injected while x-ray films are taken. The study is used to identify abnormal blood vessels, determine blood flow through the vessel, and diagnose arterial anomalies. Angiography also can be used to identify and locate occlusions of the aorta and arteries of the lower extremities. If the radiopaque substance does not pass through or only partially passes through the vessel, the distal end of the artery will not be visualized or will be only partly visible on the x-ray films. Arteriosclerotic disease can create a total or partial occlusion; emboli typically cause total occlusion of the artery. The study also can diagnose dilation of a vessel caused by an aneurysm.

Echocardiography

Echocardiography is a noninvasive, sonographic procedure that assesses the structure and movement of the various parts of the heart. High-frequency sound waves from a transducer held against the chest wall penetrate the heart. The sound waves bounce off the heart and echo back through the transducer into the machine, where they are converted into a picture that shows the exact size and movement of the parts of the heart being measured. Two-dimensional echocardiography also can be done to provide a spatial picture of the anatomic structures of the heart. Echocardiography usually includes color Doppler studies to show the pattern and velocity of blood flow within the heart and in the great vessels. As with an incompetent valve, backflow of blood can be identified by changes in color (Figure 40-13).

A transesophageal echocardiogram (TEE) uses a long tube with a microphone-like device mounted on one end that the patient swallows into the esophagus. Once in place, the device is very close to the heart, and sound waves emitted by the microphone create high-quality views of the heart and heart valves. Before the patient swallows the device, the mouth and throat are sprayed with medication that numbs the area. The patient may be given a sedative to help him or her relax and remain still during the procedure. Echocardiography is used to diagnose pericardial effusion, valvular heart disease, aneurysms, and myocardial wall abnormalities seen in CHF or MI.

Cardiac Catheterization and Angioplasty

Cardiac catheterization is used to diagnose or evaluate a variety of heart disorders. Patients who have chronic shortness of breath, vertigo or syncope, chest pain, heart palpitations, arrhythmias, or abnormal stress test or echocardiography results or who have recently had an MI all are considered likely candidates for a heart catheterization procedure.

In this procedure, a catheter is passed into the heart through a peripheral vein or artery. If the right side of the heart is to be evaluated, the catheter usually is passed through the subclavian, brachial, or femoral vein; for left-sided views, the right femoral artery usually is used. As the catheter is passed through the vessels into the heart and coronary arteries, pressures are monitored, oxygen levels are measured, and cardiac output is determined. Once the catheter has reached the desired position, a contrast medium is injected and fluoroscopy is used to visualize the heart chambers, valves, and coronary arteries. The cardiologist evaluates the condition of these structures, and any deviation from normal is noted. Cardiac catheterization is performed in a hospital and usually takes 2 to 3 hours. Patients are required to remain immobile and under observation for 4 to 6 hours after the procedure.

During a heart catheterization procedure, if atherosclerotic plaques are discovered to be occluding the coronary arteries, PTCA may be performed. The goals of angioplasty are to restore blood flow to ischemic myocardial tissue, reduce the need for cardiac medication, and eliminate or reduce the number of episodes of angina. When the area of plaque is found, a balloon that surrounds the upper portion of the catheter is inflated and the atherosclerotic material is pressed against the vessel walls, relieving the obstruction. More than one blockage can be treated during a single session, depending on the location of the blockages and the patient's condition. The procedure can take 30 minutes to several hours, depending on the number of blockages treated.

Lasers also may be used to dissolve the obstruction, or a coronary arterial stent (a mesh wire that stretches and molds to the arterial wall) may be inserted and left in place in the vessel to keep it open (Figure 40-14). If multiple coronary artery occlusions are present, the patient may need a CABG procedure. In this surgery, either part of the saphenous vein or an artificial Dacron graft is used to bypass the occluded, diseased section of the coronary artery. The blood flows through the graft to bring nourishment to the ischemic myocardium.

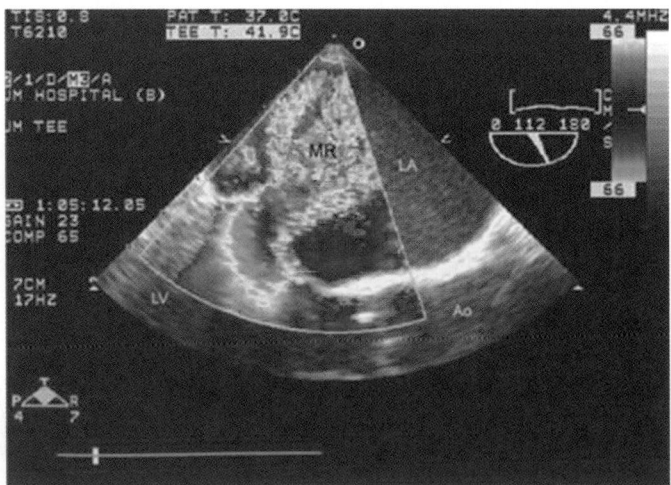

FIGURE 40-13 Transesophageal echocardiogram recorded in a patient with an acute myocardial infarction. Color flow imaging demonstrates the presence of severe mitral regurgitation. *Ao,* Aorta; *LA,* left atrium; *LV,* left ventricle. (From Mann D, Zipes D, Libby P et al: *Braunwald's heart disease,* ed 7, Philadelphia, 2005, Saunders.)

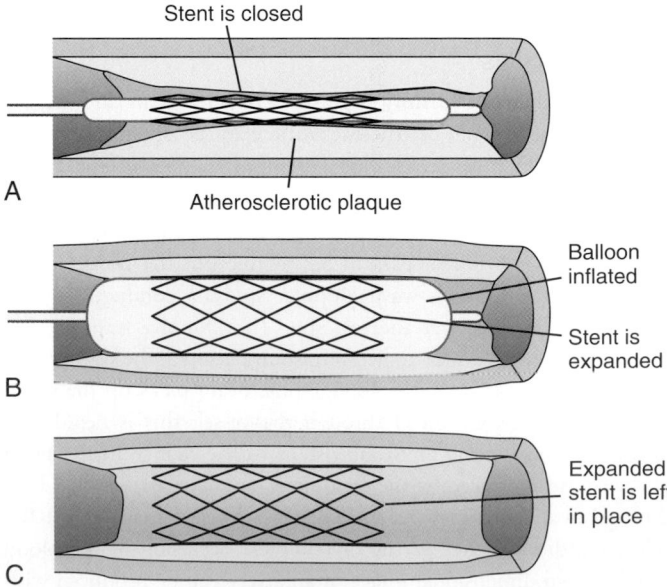

FIGURE 40-14 Angioplasty with stent placement. (From LaFleur Brooks M: *Exploring medical language,* ed 9, St Louis, 2014, Mosby.)

Cardiac Pacemakers

A cardiac pacemaker is a small, battery-powered device that is implanted in the chest wall. It generates an electrical impulse, which is sent to the heart along flexible lead wires (Figure 40-15). Current pacemakers are designed to monitor several different types of data, including blood pressure, temperature, and breathing rate, to determine whether the heart needs to be stimulated to contract more frequently. Patients who require the external electrical stimulation of a pacemaker have an arrhythmia (most often bradycardia) either because of injury to the myocardium or as a consequence of the aging process. Biventricular pacemakers, which deliver electrical impulses to both of the ventricles so that they contract and empty at the same time, are the most recent types. Most biventricular pacemakers can also work as implantable cardioverter-defibrillators, which restore a normal heartbeat.

Pacemakers continually get smaller, from the size of a pack of cigarettes in previous years to models that now are as small as a quarter. The pacemaker must be replaced when the battery pack wears out, and the typical battery life ranges from 5 to 10 years.

Implantable Cardioverter-Defibrillator

An implantable cardioverter-defibrillator (ICD) is a device the size of a pocket watch that is implanted in the chest just below the collarbone and attached to the heart with small wires. It continuously monitors the heart rhythm and is designed to deliver a measured electric shock to the myocardium to correct life-threatening arrhythmias, such as ventricular tachycardia or ventricular fibrillation. ICDs have become the standard treatment for any patient with a serious arrhythmia who is at risk of sudden death from cardiac arrest.

CLOSING COMMENTS

Patient Education

Heart disease and stroke account for more than one third of all deaths in the United States. Genetics, predisposition, and lifestyle factors, such as smoking, lack of exercise, and poor diet, play significant roles in the development of heart disease. Successful management of cardiovascular disease requires major lifestyle changes for most patients. The medical assistant can help by providing encouragement and support and by using community resources to help the patient find assistance with these changes.

Sources for information include the American Heart Association (*www.heart.org/*); workshops and conferences; professional organizations, such as the American Association of Medical Assistants (AAMA); and reputable Internet sites.

Because many patients learn best through visual aids, providing them with pictures, brochures, and pamphlets is an effective means of helping them in this learning process. Always document education interventions so that the provider and/or medical assistant can clarify or expand upon the information on a return visit.

Legal and Ethical Issues

Diagnostic procedures can have a marked effect on the patient's treatment. When entrusted with performing testing procedures, the medical assistant assumes responsibility for the test's accuracy and for performing the test precisely. This is an important role because the results submitted could strongly influence the plan of treatment.

Professional Behaviors

Critical thinking is a crucial part of professional behavior. The ability to question patients logically and comprehensively about possible cardiac signs and symptoms can greatly contribute to high-quality care. The provider relies on the medical assistant for initial information about the patient. Given the seriousness of cardiac conditions, the medical assistant must use his or her knowledge about the topic to gather and analyze the patient's comments so that the provider is better prepared to make an accurate diagnosis and develop an effective treatment plan.

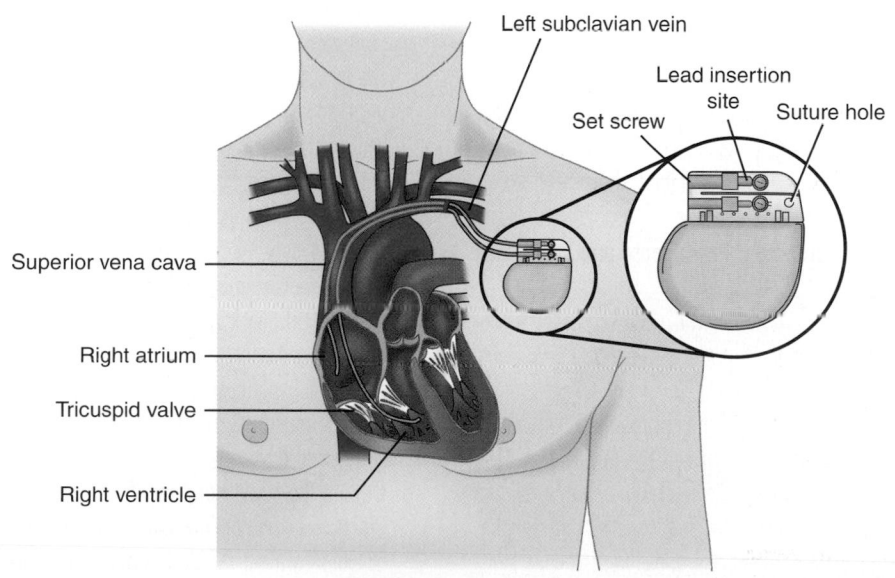

Dual Chamber Pacemaker

FIGURE 40-15 Pacemaker and placement in the chest.

SUMMARY OF SCENARIO

Adam enjoys his new position but recognizes the challenges of interacting with patients who have cardiovascular problems. Most individuals seen at the clinic must make significant changes in their lifestyle to improve their health or prevent further complications. Adam has found it difficult at times to try to help patients who refuse to quit smoking, who do not exercise regularly, and who continue to eat a diet high in saturated and trans fat. He relies on the hospital dietitian for educational support, and he encourages patients who have had an MI to follow the cardiologist's advice and participate actively in the cardiac rehabilitation program offered by the department. He also works hard to stay up to date on cardiovascular medications and treatments because so many of the department's patients have complicated therapeutic plans.

Adam has attended several workshops recently to help him choose education materials that meet the needs of the patients in his practice. He recognizes the need to continue his education in the area of cardiology to stay current with the rapid developments in medication and treatments.

SUMMARY OF LEARNING OBJECTIVES

1. **Define, spell, and pronounce the terms listed in the vocabulary.**
   Spelling and pronouncing medical terms correctly reinforce the medical assistant's credibility. Knowing the definitions of these terms promotes confidence in communication with patients and co-workers.

2. **Explain the anatomy and physiology of the heart and its significant structures.**
   The heart is a muscular organ that pumps blood through all the arteries of the body. It has three layers of tissue surrounded by a double-membrane sac (the pericardium): the epicardium, or first, layer; the myocardium, the middle, muscular layer; and the endocardium, the inner layer, which forms the heart valves. Blood flow through the heart begins in the right atrium, which receives deoxygenated blood from the inferior and superior venae cavae. The atria contract, and blood passes through the tricuspid valve into the right ventricle; the ventricles contract, and the blood passes from the right ventricle to the lungs via the pulmonary artery. Oxygenation occurs in the lungs, and the blood returns to the left atria through the pulmonary veins; the atria contract, and blood passes through the mitral (bicuspid) valve into the left ventricle; the ventricles contract, and oxygen-rich blood is sent out to the body through the aorta.

3. **Summarize risk factors for the development of heart disease.**
   Risk factors for the development of cardiovascular disease that cannot be changed are familial history, aging, and race; factors that can be altered are hypertension, diabetes, elevated blood cholesterol levels, smoking, obesity, lack of exercise, and stress.

4. **Do the following related to coronary artery disease and myocardial infarction:**
   - *Describe the signs, symptoms, and medical procedures used in the diagnosis and treatment of coronary artery disease and myocardial infarction.*
     In CAD, the arteries supplying the myocardium become narrowed by atherosclerotic plaque, resulting in ischemia of the myocardium. The cardinal symptom is angina pectoris, followed by pressure or fullness in the chest, syncope, unexplained coughing spells, and fatigue; however, women may have a different clinical picture. Ischemia leads to necrosis of a portion of the myocardium, resulting in an MI. An MI is characterized by pain that lasts longer than 30 minutes and is unrelieved by rest or nitroglycerin tablets. It is diagnosed by ECG changes and elevated cardiac enzymes. Medical treatment includes thrombolytic medications, aspirin, beta blockers, ACE inhibitors, anticoagulants, and anticholesterol agents. With occlusion, either PTCA or CABG surgery may be indicated. (Table 40-1 reviews medications prescribed to treat hypercholesterolemia.)
   - *Summarize metabolic syndrome and associated risk factors.*
     Metabolic syndrome is a group of risk factors that raise the risk of heart disease, diabetes and stroke. To be diagnosed with metabolic syndrome, the patient must have at least three risk factors, including abdominal obesity, high triglyceride levels, low HDL cholesterol levels, hypertension, and high fasting blood glucose levels.
   - *Explain the signs and symptoms of myocardial infarction in women.*
     The signs and symptoms of a heart attack in women may start weeks before the actual cardiac injury and could include abdominal, neck, shoulder, or upper back pain; jaw pain; shortness of breath; vertigo; sweating; indigestion or nausea and vomiting; extreme fatigue; and/or aching in both arms.

5. **Compare and contrast the treatment protocols for hypertension.**
   The two types of hypertension are primary and secondary hypertension. Secondary hypertension occurs because of a disease process in another body system. Primary hypertension is idiopathic and is diagnosed when the patient's blood pressure is consistently above 119 mm Hg systolic and/or 79 mm Hg diastolic. Table 40-2 summarizes how the varying stages of hypertension are identified and treated, and Table 40-3 lists antihypertensive medications. Chronic elevated blood pressure can result in left ventricular hypertrophy, angina, MI, heart failure, cerebrovascular accident, and nephropathy. Risk factors for hypertension include a family history of hypertension or stroke, hypercholesterolemia, smoking, high sodium intake, diabetes, excessive alcohol intake, aging, prolonged stress, and race.

6. **Outline the causes and results of congestive heart failure.**
   CHF occurs when the myocardium is unable to pump an adequate amount of blood to meet the body's needs. It typically develops over time and initially involves one side of the heart and then the other side. Left-sided

heart failure causes a backup of blood in the left atria and lungs, resulting in pulmonary edema with dyspnea, orthopnea, nonproductive cough, rales, and tachycardia. Right-sided heart failure causes a backup of blood in the right atrium, preventing emptying of the vena cava, resulting in systemic edema, especially in the legs and feet. Both types of heart failure cause fatigue, weakness, exercise intolerance, dyspnea, and sensitivity to cold temperatures.

7. **Summarize the effects of inflammation and valve disorders on cardiac function.**

Rheumatic heart disease develops because of an unusual immune reaction that typically occurs 2 to 4 weeks after an untreated beta-hemolytic streptococcal infection; endocarditis is the most common heart complication, with valve damage. Disorders of the heart valves may be caused by a congenital defect or an infection. Two specific problems can occur with valve disease. The valve can be stenosed, which restricts the forward flow of blood, or it can be incompetent, which allows blood to leak backward. The most common valvular defect is MVP, which results from a congenital defect or vegetation and scarring caused by endocarditis.

8. **Describe the anatomy and physiology of the vascular system.**

Blood vessels are divided into two systems that begin and end with the heart. Vessels are classified according to their structure and function as arteries, which carry oxygenated blood away from the heart; capillaries, the microscopic vessels responsible for the exchange of oxygen and carbon dioxide in the tissue; and veins, the vessels that carry deoxygenated blood back to the heart.

9. **Differentiate among the various types of shock.**

Table 40-4 outlines the various types of shock. All result in the same signs and symptoms and possible complications. Shock is the general collapse of the circulatory system, marked by reduced cardiac output, hypotension, and hypoxemia. Symptoms progress to a rapid, weak, thready pulse; tachypnea; and altered levels of consciousness. If the process is not reversed, the central nervous system becomes depressed and acute renal failure may occur.

10. **Summarize the characteristics of common vascular disorders.**

Varicose veins are dilated, tortuous, superficial veins in the legs that develop because the valves do not completely close, allowing blood to flow backward, thus causing the vein to distend from the increased pressure. Phlebitis is an inflammation of the veins most commonly seen in the lower legs. DVT is a thrombus with inflammatory changes that has attached to the deep venous system of the lower legs and has caused a partial or complete obstruction of the vessel. A thrombus that dislodges and begins to circulate through the general circulation is an embolus. Arteriosclerosis is a general term for the thickening and loss of elasticity of arterial walls; it can occur in arteries throughout the body and cause systemic ischemia and necrosis over time. Atherosclerosis is a form of arteriosclerosis in which an atheroma develops. An aneurysm is a ballooning or dilation of the wall of a vessel caused by weakening of the vessel wall. Peripheral arterial disease affects the vessels outside of the heart, especially the legs and feet, in which circulation is reduced and ischemia can occur.

11. **Discuss arterial disorders, including causes, risk factors, and common treatments.**

Arteriosclerosis can occur in arteries throughout the body and causes systemic ischemia and necrosis over time. An aneurysm is a ballooning or dilation of a blood vessel wall, and peripheral arterial disease develops because of widespread atherosclerotic plaque buildup in the arteries outside the heart.

12. **Outline typical cardiovascular diagnostic procedures.**

Cardiovascular diagnostic procedures include Doppler studies of the patency of blood vessels; angiography to visualize arterial pathways; echocardiography to assess the structure and movement of the parts of the heart, especially the valves; cardiac catheterization to show the heart chambers, valves, and coronary arteries; cardiac pacemaker to monitor blood pressure, temperature, and breathing rate; or placement of implantable cardioverter-defibrillator to monitor the heart rhythm and deliver an electric shock to the myocardium to correct life-threatening arrhythmias.

13. **Describe patient education topics, and legal and ethical issues, for cardiovascular patients.**

Successful management of cardiovascular disease requires major lifestyle changes for most patients. The medical assistant can help by providing encouragement and support and by using community resources to help the patient find assistance with these changes. Sources for information include the American Heart Association, workshops and conferences, professional organizations, and reputable Internet sites.

CONNECTIONS

Study Guide Connection: Go to the Chapter 40 Study Guide. Read and complete the activities.

evolve Evolve Connection: Go to the Chapter 40 link at *evolve.elsevier.com/kinn* to complete the Chapter Review Quiz. Check out the other resources listed for this chapter to make the most of what you have learned from Assisting in Cardiology.

SCENARIO

Bill Novelli, CMA (AAMA), works for Dr. Sara Kennedy, a primary care physician in a small town close to where he grew up. Although patients of all ages are seen in the practice, most patients are age 65 or older. Bill has learned to recognize the unique communication needs of aging individuals and the importance of using family and community resources to maintain optimum health in this special population.

While studying this chapter, think about the following questions:

- Do myths about aging and stereotypes about aging people negatively affect older individuals?
- What are the most common changes that occur in the aging body and what recommendations can be made for health promotion in this age group?
- What suggestions can be made to aging patients and their families to optimize older adults' health and protect them from injury and disease?

- How is Alzheimer's disease diagnosed and what are the stages of its development?
- Why is depression so common in aging individuals and how is it diagnosed and treated?
- How can the medical assistant most effectively communicate with an older person?
- Why is the use of community resources such an important factor in the care of aging people?

LEARNING OBJECTIVES

1. Define, spell, and pronounce the terms listed in the vocabulary.
2. Do the following related to the aging process:
   - Discuss the impact of a growing aging population on society.
   - Identify the stereotypes and myths associated with aging.
   - Role-play the effect of sensorimotor changes of aging.
3. Do the following related to the cardiovascular, endocrine, gastrointestinal, integumentary, and musculoskeletal body systems:
   - Explain the changes in the anatomy and physiology caused by aging.
   - Summarize the major related diseases and disorders faced by older patients.
4. Do the following related to the nervous system, pulmonary system, sensory organs, urinary system, and reproductive systems:
   - Explain the changes in the anatomy and physiology caused by aging.

- Summarize the major related diseases and disorders faced by older patients.
- Describe various screening tools for dementia, depression, and malnutrition in aging adults.
5. Explain the effect of aging on sleep.
6. Differentiate among independent, assisted, and skilled nursing facilities.
7. Summarize the role of the medical assistant in caring for aging patients.
8. Determine the principles of effective communication with older adults.
9. Discuss patient education, as well as legal and ethical issues, associated with aging patients.

VOCABULARY

collagen (kah'-luh-jen) The protein that forms the inelastic fibers of tendons, ligaments, and fascia.

costal Pertaining to the ribs.

decubitus ulcers Sores or ulcers that develop over a bony prominence as the result of ischemia from prolonged pressure; also called *bed sores* or *pressure sores.*

elastin An essential part of elastic connective tissue; when moist, it is flexible and elastic.

lacrimation (lah-krih-ma'-shun) The secretion or discharge of tears.

Ménière's disease (mayn-yayrz') Chronic disease of the inner ear causing recurrent episodes of vertigo, progressive sensorineural hearing loss, and tinnitus.

nocturia Frequent urination at night.

oophorectomy Surgical removal of the ovaries

otosclerosis A condition that causes calcification of the ossicles of the inner ear; the exact cause of otosclerosis is unknown, but it may have a familial or genetic link.

ototoxic Medications that have a harmful effect on the eighth cranial nerve or the organs of hearing and balance.

postherpetic neuralgia Nerve pain that occurs after a shingles outbreak and may become chronic.

According to the Administration on Aging, an agency of the U.S. Department of Health and Human Services, the aging population (those age 65 or older) numbered almost 48 million in 2013. By 2030, almost 1 of every 5 Americans (about 72 million people) will be 65 years or older.

The average life expectancy of an individual who reaches age 65 is an additional 19.3 years (20.5 years for females and 17.9 years for males). A child born in 2013 can expect to live 78.8 years, about 30 years longer than a child born in 1900. Older women outnumber older men; 25.1 million women are over age 65, as are 19.6 million men. About 30% of older people who live outside of institutions live alone; half of women over age 75 live alone. More than half a million grandparents over the age of 65 are the primary caregivers for their grandchildren who live with them. Most older people have at least one chronic medical condition, and many have multiple conditions. Hypertension, arthritis, heart disease, cancer, and diabetes are the health problems most commonly seen in the elderly, and a significant number also suffer from strokes, asthma, emphysema, and chronic bronchitis.

What does all this mean to those who have chosen careers in healthcare? As the aging population expands, it will affect all aspects of society. One area in particular will be these individuals' increased use of health services. To provide quality care to aging patients, medical assistants must understand the aging process, including the physical and sensory changes that occur with aging (Procedure 41-1). This knowledge enables medical assistants to recognize the special needs of the aged and to develop therapeutic management and communication skills that can help them effectively care for the older patient. Ongoing research and education about the aging process have dispelled many of the old stereotypes.

Aging is a complex physiologic, psychological, and social process. Old age is not an illness but a normal life process that people experience in different ways. Lack of exercise, poor nutrition, substance abuse, continual stress, and air pollutants all are factors that cause a person to show the effects of aging decades earlier than someone who has practiced healthy living habits.

As people age, changes occur in their physical appearance and abilities, along with sensory changes in vision, hearing, taste, and smell. These changes do not occur at the same time in everyone; however, sensorimotor changes can have a profound effect on the individual's ability to interact with his or her environment.

Stereotypes and Myths About Aging

- *Most aging people will develop dementia.* Dementia is not part of the normal aging process. However, the older the person, the greater the risk of dementia. About 6% of those over age 65 and almost 50% of those over age 85 are diagnosed with significant memory and disorientation issues.

- *Disease is a normal and an unavoidable part of the aging process.* Recent research verifies that individuals who have established healthy lifestyles as they age remain healthy well into their older years. Aging people are more likely to have health issues, but these are not inevitable for all persons over age 65.

- *Older workers are less productive than younger ones.* Individuals with a strong work ethic continue to perform in this way. It may take aging people longer to learn new material, but they continue to be capable of learning and applying new knowledge.

- *Most older people end up in long-term care facilities.* At any given time, approximately 5% of the aging population lives in long-term care facilities; 80% of aging individuals live independently, with or without a partner.

- *Most aging people have no interest in or capacity for sexual relations.* Sexual interest does not change significantly with age; a decrease in sexual activity is usually related to the loss of a partner.

- *Damage to health because of lifestyle factors is irreversible.* It is never too late to benefit from healthy lifestyle choices.

CRITICAL THINKING APPLICATION   41-1

When Bill first started working with aging patients, he believed many of the stereotypes about people over age 65. Through his work with Dr. Kennedy, he has come to realize that many of these myths have no foundation in actual practice. Based on the myths mentioned in the text, what do you think about these beliefs on aging?

PROCEDURE 41-1 **Demonstrate Empathy: Understand the Sensorimotor Changes of Aging**

Goal: *To role-play an older adult so as to better understand the needs of aging people.*

EQUIPMENT and SUPPLIES

- Yellow-tinted glasses, ski goggles, or laboratory goggles
- Pink, white, yellow "pills" (e.g., various colors of Tic Tacs)
- Petroleum jelly (e.g., Vaseline)
- Cotton balls
- Eye patches
- Tape
- Thick gloves
- Utility glove
- Tongue depressors
- Elastic bandages
- Medical forms in small print
- Pennies
- Button shirts
- Walker

PROCEDURAL STEPS

1. Role-play vision and hearing loss.
   - Put two cotton balls in each ear and an eye patch over one eye. Follow your partner's instructions.
   - *Partner:* Stand out of the line of vision (to prevent lip-reading). Without using gestures or changing your voice volume, tell your partner to cross the room and pick up a book.
2. Role-play yellowing of the lens of the eye.
   - Line up "pills" of different pastel colors.
   - *Partner:* Pick out the different colors while wearing the yellow-tinted glasses.

3. Role-play difficulty with focusing.
   - Put on goggles smeared with petroleum jelly and follow your partner's directions.
   - *Partner:* Stand at least 3 feet in front of your partner and motion for him or her to come to you (your partner is deaf, so talking will not help).
4. Role-play loss of peripheral vision.
   - Put on goggles with black paper taped to the sides.
   - *Partner:* Stand to the side, out of the field of vision, and motion for your patient to follow you.
5. Role-play aphasia and partial paralysis.
   - You are unable to use your right arm or leg. Place tape over your mouth. Let your partner know you need to go to the bathroom.
   - *Partner:* Stand at least 3 feet away with your back to your partner and wait for instructions.
6. Role-play problems with dexterity.
   - Put thick gloves on your hands and try to sign your name, button a shirt, tie your shoes, and pick up pennies.
7. Role-play problems with mobility.
   - Use the walker to cross the room.
   - *Partner:* After your partner starts to use the walker, hand him or her a book to carry.
8. Role-play changes in sensation.
   - Put a rubber utility glove on; turn on hot water; test the difference in temperature between the gloved hand and the ungloved hand.
9. Summarize and share with the group your impressions of the effect of age-related sensorimotor changes.

CHANGES IN ANATOMY AND PHYSIOLOGY

The aging process brings about changes in all of the body's systems. Table 41-1 summarizes these changes and what can be done to promote healthy aging.

Cardiovascular System

Cardiovascular disease is the most frequent cause of illness and disability in the aging population, and congestive heart failure (CHF) is the most common reason for hospitalization. Age-related changes occur in the cardiovascular system, but disease and lifestyle habits such as lack of exercise, poor diet, and stress contribute to these changes. Heart disease is ranked as the leading cause of death among men and women; therefore, proper management of cardiovascular disease can help maintain the health of an aging population and reduce mortality rates.

The aging process causes structural changes in the heart. Myocardial cells enlarge, and deposits of fat and connective tissue increase; these combine to make the myocardial wall stiffer and to lengthen the time needed for the relaxation phase of the cardiac cycle. As a result, cardiac output declines, making aging people more susceptible to CHF. The reduction in cardiac output leads to pooling of blood in the legs, cold extremities, and edema (Table 41-2). In addition, the heart cannot respond as quickly or as forcefully to an increased workload, so exercise, sudden movements, and changes in position can result in dizziness and loss of balance. Aging typically brings with it an increase in blood pressure, requiring the heart to work harder to pump blood into the systemic circulation. Hypertension increases the workload of the left ventricle, and this may result in hypertrophy of the chamber and weakening of the myocardial wall. The valves of the heart tend to thicken and become more rigid, making it more difficult for blood to circulate through the cardiopulmonary vessels. With these cardiovascular problems, arrhythmias become more common.

Aging causes the walls of the veins to weaken and stretch. This damages the valves, especially in the veins of the legs, where the walls are subject to greater pressure as blood struggles to return to the

TABLE 41-1   System Changes with Aging and Measures to Promote Health

SYSTEM	AGE-RELATED CHANGES	HEALTH PROMOTION
Cardiovascular system	Arteriosclerosis and atherosclerotic plaque buildup reduces blood flow to major organs; 50% of the aging population have hypertension; CVD is the number one killer of women and men in their 60s.	Regular exercise; weight control; diet rich in fruits, vegetables, and whole grains; cholesterol, blood glucose monitoring
Central nervous system	Brain shrinks by 10% between ages 30 and 90; takes longer to learn new material; attention span and language remain the same; signs and symptoms may be caused by depression, vascular disease, and drug reactions.	Aerobic exercise to increase blood flow to CNS; maintaining mental activities (e.g., reading, interacting with others)
Endocrine system	After age 50, women have a sharp decline in estrogen; men have a more gradual decline in testosterone.	Possible hormone replacement therapy or natural soy supplements
Gastrointestinal system	Decline in gastric juices and enzymes by age 60; decreased peristalsis with increased constipation; some nutrients are not absorbed as well.	High-fiber diet and adequate fluid intake; regular exercise to prevent constipation
Musculoskeletal system	Muscle mass decreases; tendency to gain weight; gradual loss of bone density; deterioration of joint cartilage.	Strength training to increase muscle mass; stretching to remain limber; exercise; vitamin D and calcium supplements
Pulmonary system	At age 55 the lungs become less elastic and the chest wall gradually stiffens, making oxygenation more difficult.	Quit smoking; regular aerobic exercise
Sensory organs	Hearing is intact through the mid-50s but declines by 25% by age 80; oral problems are common; skin thins and loses elasticity; presbyopia after age 40; cataracts common after age 60.	Avoid exposure to loud noise, use hearing aids; good dental hygiene; prevention of sun damage to the skin; annual eye examinations; diet rich in dark green, leafy vegetables to prevent cataracts and macular degeneration
Urinary system	Kidneys become less efficient; bladder muscles weaken; one third of seniors experience incontinence; prostate enlargement is common.	Pelvic exercises, drugs, or surgery for incontinence; annual PSA with digital rectal exam monitoring for men
Sexuality	*Men:* Impotence is not a symptom of normal aging; men over age 50 may have some altered function. *Women:* Menopause causes vaginal narrowing and dryness, resulting in painful intercourse.	*Men:* Maintenance of cardiovascular health with exercise, weight control, no smoking, diabetes management *Women:* Use of vaginal lubricants or estrogen cream

CNS, Central nervous system; *CVD,* cardiovascular disease; *PSA,* prostate-specific antigen.

TABLE 41-2   Normal Changes in Cardiac Output with Age

AGE	BLOOD PUMPED BY RESTING HEART (quarts/min)	MAXIMUM HEARTBEAT DURING EXERCISE (beats/min)
30	3.6	200
40	3.4	182
50	3.2	171
60	2.9	159
70	2.6	150

American Heart Association. www.americanheart.org. Accessed July 20, 2012.

heart against the force of gravity. As a result, edema and varicose veins of the lower extremities are common in the elderly, increasing the risk of phlebitis and the formation of thrombi in the deep veins, or deep vein thrombosis (DVT).

Arteriosclerosis is considered part of the aging process. The vessel walls thicken and become less elastic as a result of the calcification and buildup of connective tissue. In addition, the artery's ability to dilate and contract diminishes. To maintain an adequate blood supply throughout the body, the heart must work harder to overcome the resistance caused by stiffened vessels. Older adults have a higher incidence of orthostatic hypotension. The clinical criterion for alterations in blood pressure from sitting to standing is a drop of more than 20 mm Hg in the systolic pressure, or more than 10 mm Hg in the diastolic pressure, when the position is changed. When a person with orthostatic hypotension stands, gravity causes blood to pool in the legs resulting in a drop in the amount of blood returning to the heart for circulation. This decrease in circulating blood volume causes a sudden drop in blood pressure. The provider may have the medical assistant take orthostatic blood pressures as part of routine intake protocol for aging patients. To perform this procedure, apply a blood pressure cuff and take the individual's blood pressure while sitting. Leave the cuff in place and have the patient stand. Record the standing blood pressure immediately to document any differences in readings when the position is changed.

Endocrine System

Hormonal changes that occur with aging are related to a general decrease in hormone production combined with changes in tissue receptor binding. The most common endocrine system disorder seen in aging patients is diabetes mellitus (DM) type 2. As a person ages, insulin production by the beta cells in the pancreas decreases and insulin resistance at the tissue level increases. According to the National Institutes of Health, more than half of the 16 million Americans diagnosed with diabetes type 2 are over age 65. Elderly patients with diabetes are at increased risk of developing vascular disease, including renal disorders, retinopathy, neuropathy, myocardial ischemia, angina, myocardial infarction, cerebrovascular accidents, and peripheral vascular disease, such as lower extremity ulcers.

Older patients do not always experience the classic symptoms of diabetes, which are polyuria, polydipsia, and polyphagia. They may show a variety of problems, including unexplained weight loss, slow wound healing, recurrent bacterial or fungal infections, changes in mental state, cataracts, macular disease, muscle weakness and pain, angina, foot ulcers, and uremia. The range of symptoms is due to the insidious onset of diabetes in older people, who may have gradually developing hyperglycemia for years before diagnosis.

The treatment protocol for aging patients with diabetes is the same as for other age groups; however, special consideration must be given to the patient's ability to understand and comply with the therapeutic plan. In addition, because the person may have other health problems that are being treated with medications, an aging patient newly diagnosed with diabetes may face a complicated treatment regimen that requires explicit instruction and continual follow-up in the ambulatory care setting.

The medical assistant must be aware of any sensory abnormalities, such as diminished vision or problems with fine motor skills, which may interfere with the patient's ability to follow treatment guidelines. Teaching and treatment plans must be adapted to meet the individual needs of each patient. For example, if the patient has vision difficulties, an injector pen can be used to deliver a preset amount of insulin.

Factors That Can Affect Diabetes Management in Older People

- Modifying lifestyle risk factors may be more difficult because of poor nutrition, inability to exercise, and long-standing habits, such as smoking and a diet high in saturated fats and calories.
- Previously diagnosed health conditions, such as hypertension and heart disease, in addition to an age-related decline in kidney and liver function, increase the challenge of treating diabetes.

- Older people are more likely to be prescribed multiple medications (polypharmacy), which increases the risk of adverse drug interactions.
- Elderly patients with diabetes are more prone to hypoglycemia and may not recognize and respond quickly to the signs of low blood glucose levels.
- Diabetic complications can develop quickly because of a long history of prediabetes before diagnosis.
- Older people may have decreased physical and/or mental abilities that make it difficult for them to understand and adhere to a complicated treatment regimen.
- Older patients may not be able to afford the medications and supplies needed to maintain health.

CRITICAL THINKING APPLICATION   41-2
Quite a few of the elderly patients in Dr. Kennedy's practice have type 2 diabetes. Based on what you have learned about the difficulty of managing diabetes in aging people, what factors do you need to consider when conducting patient education for an elderly person with diabetes? Are there any community resources that might be useful for patients and their families?

Gastrointestinal System

Age-related changes in the gastrointestinal system begin in the mouth with dental problems, a decrease in the number of taste buds and the production of saliva, and a diminishing sense of smell. Older people generally find eating less pleasurable, have a reduced appetite, and are unable to chew and lubricate their food as well as younger people; this makes dysphagia (difficulty swallowing) a common age-related problem. Aging also brings a decrease in the production of hydrochloric acid, which affects the digestion of calcium and iron. Secretion of intrinsic factor, a protein that is needed for the absorption of vitamin B_{12}, also declines, which affects the function of the nervous system and the formation of red blood cells, resulting in excessive fatigue. It is not unusual for aging patients to be on regular vitamin B_{12} replacement therapy, either through large oral doses or by intramuscular (IM) or subcutaneous (SC) injection.

Food passes more quickly through the small intestine, resulting in poorer absorption of vitamins and minerals. Peristalsis in the colon decreases, making aging patients more susceptible to constipation and diverticular disease. Poor eating habits, a reduced fluid intake, and some medications (e.g., antidepressants, diuretics, antacids containing aluminum or calcium, and medications for Parkinson's disease) also contribute to constipation. The liver decreases in size and weight after age 70. It is still able to perform vital functions, but more time is required to metabolize drugs and alcohol. All of these factors combine to increase the potential for adverse drug reactions in older adults.

Aging individuals have a higher incidence of several gastrointestinal system diseases, such as gastroesophageal reflux disease (GERD), peptic ulcers, diverticulosis (related to lack of dietary fiber and constipation), cholelithiasis, and colorectal cancer. Dietary counseling and annual screenings should be part of the routine care of aging patients.

Integumentary System

The skin is the body's first line of protection against infection, and it also is responsible for preventing the loss of body fluid and regulating body temperature. Changes in the appearance and function of the integumentary system usually are caused by a combination of ordinary age-related changes and environmental factors, especially the amount of sun exposure over time. Exposure to ultraviolet light from the sun frequently is the cause of wrinkles, age spots, blotches, and leathery, dry, loose skin, all of which are associated with aging. Changes caused by the ultraviolet light from the sun or by the normal aging process can affect all three layers of the skin: the epidermis, dermis, and subcutaneous tissue.

The cells in the epidermis reproduce more slowly as people age, and this slower regeneration causes the skin to appear thinner. The skin becomes more prone to tearing and blistering. The risk of infections increases, the healing process takes longer, and older people are more susceptible to bruising. Because the skin can be easily torn, it is important to be very careful when performing phlebotomy or covering a wound on an older patient. Vitamin D synthesis, a major function of the epidermis, significantly declines in aged skin, and a decrease in the number of melanocytes increases photosensitivity.

The dermis loses 20% of its mass during the aging process, resulting in the paper-thin or transparent skin seen in older adults. The number of **collagen** cells in the dermis also declines with age, causing the skin to sag and wrinkle. Because both sweat and sebaceous glands decrease in number, aging people have difficulty tolerating higher temperatures because they perspire less. At the same time, the blood supply to the dermis decreases; this makes it difficult to regulate the body temperature and leads to an increased susceptibility to both hypothermia and heat stroke in aging individuals. Any situation in which an older adult would be exposed to extremes of cold or heat should be avoided. Make sure a blanket is available in the examining room if the air conditioning is on. Ask the person if he or she is too cold or too hot and take the necessary steps to make the patient feel more comfortable.

Atrophy of the subcutaneous layer increases the skin's susceptibility to trauma, so patients bruise much more easily. The skin is denied natural lubrication, and dry skin is one of the most common complaints among older people. In addition, fat deposits increase in the abdomen in men and in the abdomen and thighs in women as they age.

Suggestions that might help older people prevent and treat dry skin include:

- Use a room humidifier to moisten the air
- Bathe less frequently and use warm rather than hot water
- Use a mild soap or cleansing cream (e.g., Aveeno, Basis, or Dove)
- Wear protective clothing in cold weather
- Moisturize dry skin

Pain receptors are distributed throughout the skin. Because of age-related changes in the receptors, older people have a higher pain threshold. They may not notice a cut or burn as quickly as a younger person would, so a more serious burn may occur before it is noticed. In addition, wound healing becomes a problem because of decreased blood flow to dermal tissues.

Other changes occur in the skin's appendages. Hair changes in color, growth, and distribution. Hair grays because of the decreased rate of melanin production and the replacement of pigmented hair with nonpigmented hair. Women lose hair on the trunk and have increased facial hair. Although alopecia (loss of hair) is caused by an inherited trait, aging also causes hair loss. Hair on the eyebrows, nose, and ears becomes coarser and longer in men. The nails of older people take longer to grow and are more brittle. Nails, particularly toenails, thicken as a result of trauma or nutritional deficiencies. It is not unusual for nails to split, making them more susceptible to fungal infections.

Seborrheic keratoses, usually referred to as "age spots," are one of the most common benign skin disorders found in the aging population. They appear as waxy, scaly papules that vary from tan to dark brown (Figure 41-1) and typically are found in areas of sun exposure, such as the trunk, back, face, neck, extremities, and scalp. They are not dangerous but may be removed for cosmetic purposes.

Shingles Risk Reduction

In 2011 the U.S. Food and Drug Administration (FDA) approved a vaccine, Zostavax, developed to reduce the risk of shingles in people age 60 or older. The varicella-zoster virus causes both shingles and chickenpox. After an active chickenpox infection, the virus lies dormant in a nerve dermatome. As people age, their risk increases that the virus will reactivate, causing the formation of blisters and varying degrees of pain along the affected nerve pathway. It is estimated that 2 in 10 people will develop shingles in their lifetime. Zostavax is a live virus vaccine that boosts immunity against the varicella-zoster virus. The vaccine is administered as a single subcutaneous injection. Studies have shown that the vaccine reduces the risk of shingles by about half (51%) and the risk of **postherpetic neuralgia** by 67%; it is most effective in people ages 60 to 69 years. For individuals who develop shingles even though they were immunized, the duration of symptoms is shorter. It is recommended that all individuals over age 60 receive the Zostavax vaccine, even if they have had shingles, to help prevent future occurrences of the disease. Shingles vaccination can be somewhat difficult to get because the vaccine requires storage in a special freezer, and it can be quite expensive ($200 to $250). Therefore, it is important that the patient or the medical assistant first check with the individual's insurance carrier to see whether the injection is covered.

CRITICAL THINKING APPLICATION 41-3

Rose Deluca, a 71-year-old patient of Dr. Kennedy, is unhappy about the changes in her skin that have occurred in the past several years. Based on what Bill knows about the normal changes that occur in the skin as people age, how can he explain these changes to Mrs. Deluca, and what can he suggest to help with dryness and other typical aging changes?

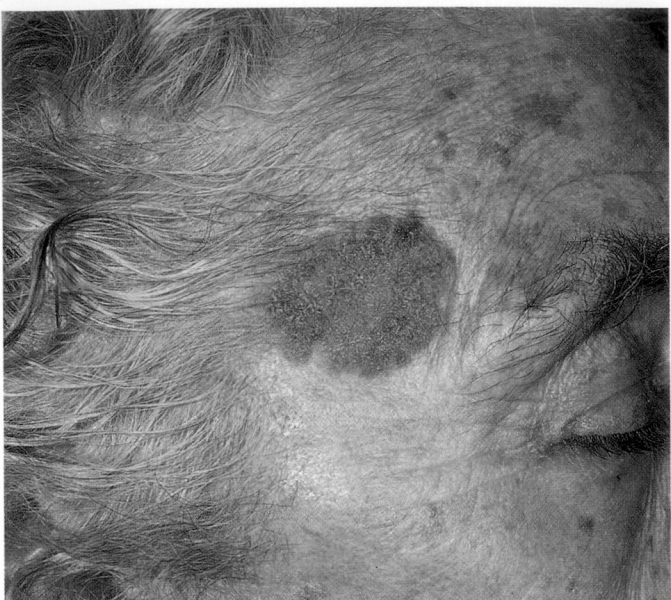

FIGURE 41-1 Seborrheic keratosis. (From Habif TP: *Clinical dermatology: a color guide to diagnosis and therapy,* ed 6, St Louis, 2016, Mosby.)

Musculoskeletal System

As the body ages, changes occur in the muscles, bones, and joints that affect the individual's appearance, strength, and mobility. The extent of change depends on the person's diet, exercise pattern, and heredity. Cartilage loss and degeneration, which produce osteoarthritis, commonly occur in the weight-bearing joints of older people. Joint range of motion is affected, and the intervertebral disc spaces are decreased, causing loss of height as a person ages. A breakdown in joint structures may lead to inflammation, pain, stiffness, and deformity.

Aging brings a decrease in the strength and speed of muscle contractions in the extremities but only a slight decline in overall muscle endurance. Muscular changes in the aging patient are directly related to the individual's activity level. Research shows that musculoskeletal disease is not an inevitable result of the aging process; however, 40% to 50% of women over age 50 have a serious problem with bone demineralization. Men also experience bone loss, but at a later age and a much slower rate than women.

Suggestions for Helping the Older Adult with Mobility, Dexterity, and Balance

- Encourage the person to use assistive devices, such as adaptive silverware, a tub seat or shower chair, electric razor, and reaching devices.
- Assist the person with gripping devices as needed (wait for the patient to place his or her hand around a cup or help him or her with it before letting go).
- Provide older adults with enough time to complete tasks independently.

- Support a post-stroke patient who is ambulatory on the weak side; use a gait belt as needed when transferring a patient from a chair to an examination table.
- The provider may recommend physical therapy for range-of-motion exercises.
- Encourage activity approved by the provider; lack of activity results in a decline in the ability to function.

Osteoporosis

Osteoporosis is the primary cause of hip fractures, which can lead to a loss of independence and also to complications that ultimately can end in death. The spinal vertebrae also can collapse, producing the stooped posture associated with "dowager's hump." Sometimes bones break because of the sheer weight of the body on them. Often people say they fell and broke a bone, when in reality the bone fractured, causing them to fall. Multiple factors contribute to the development of osteoporosis, but it is most common in postmenopausal women. Risk factors for osteoporosis include:

- Female gender (women have a five times greater risk than men)
- Thin; small-boned frame
- Family history of osteoporosis
- Estrogen deficiency before age 45, either from early menopause or **oophorectomy**
- Estrogen deficiency resulting from an abnormal absence of menses (eating disorders, excessive aerobic exercise, fibrocystic ovaries)
- Racial background (Caucasian and Asian women have the highest risk)
- Aging
- Extended use of anticonvulsant drugs, prednisone, and excessive thyroid hormone medications
- Sedentary lifestyle, smoking, excessive alcohol intake, and lack of calcium and vitamin D when growing up

Weight-bearing exercises and calcium and vitamin D supplements are recommended to prevent demineralization of the bones. Medications used to prevent and/or treat osteoporosis include alendronate (Fosamax) and risedronate (Actonel), which reduce the rate of demineralization; raloxifene (Evista), which slows bone thinning and causes some increase in bone thickness; and calcitonin (Calcimar, Miacalcin), which is either injected or inhaled as a nasal spray and results in a decrease in the rate of bone thinning and relieves the pain associated with spinal compression. Another option is an IV medication, zoledronic acid (Reclast), for the once yearly treatment of postmenopausal women with osteoporosis. Reclast helps increase bone density in the spine and hip, thus reducing the risk of fractures.

Falls

The risk of injuries from falls increases with age; falls cause the greatest number of injuries in people over age 70. Aging individuals are at greater risk of falling because of sensorimotor changes in vision and mobility, osteoporosis, and cerebrovascular accidents. Falls in older patients usually result in fractures because a large percentage of these individuals have osteoporosis. Serious fractures, such as those of the hip, require the patient to be immobile for extended periods, and this opens the door to a wide range of debilitating complications, such as **decubitus ulcers**, pneumonia, placement in long-term care facilities, and even death. Falls are largely preventable. The medical assistant can play an active role in helping family members and patients become aware of risk factors and safety measures. Suggestions that can help patients prevent falls are:

- Have regular vision tests.
- Understand the side effects of medications, especially those that cause vertigo.
- If you experience orthostatic hypotension, rise slowly and stand still for a moment with support before moving.
- Limit the use of alcohol.
- If needed, consistently use assistive devices, such as a cane or walker, for support.
- Wear low-heeled, rubber-soled shoes with good support.
- Avoid going outside in icy weather.
- Engage in regular weight-bearing exercise for muscle and bone strength.
- Keep hallways, stairs, and bathrooms well lit.
- Assess the home for possible danger areas; remove throw rugs; use handrails on steps and grab bars in bathrooms; keep emergency numbers handy.

CRITICAL THINKING APPLICATION **41-4**

The family of Rita Schaeffer, a 73-year-old patient, is concerned about the risk of falls. Mrs. Schaeffer recently was diagnosed with osteoporosis, and she lives alone. What information should Bill give the family to help them prevent accidents in their mother's home? Also, Mrs. Schaeffer's 45-year-old daughter is concerned about developing osteoporosis. What steps should the daughter take to prevent the disease?

Nervous System

Cognitive ability (i.e., the ability of a person to think) is influenced by many factors, including a person's general state of health, educational background, and genetic code. The normal process of aging may contribute to a change in the thinking process. The brain begins to get smaller at approximately age 50 and continues to do so as we age because of a loss of fluid within the neurons and shrinkage of dendrites. Thinning of the dendrites makes transmitting messages from one neuron to the next more difficult. As a result of all these factors, the aging brain weighs less, is smaller, and has started to pull away from the sheath or cortical mantle. Older neurons process information more slowly, so retrieving old information and learning new information takes longer. Reaction time also slows, and aging individuals are distracted more easily; however, recent research shows that the loss of brain cells is minimal and that the older brain is still capable of generating new neurons. Researchers believe that continued, moderate physical and mental activity can maintain the cognitive abilities of aging individuals.

Dementia, the severe loss of intellectual ability, is not an inevitable part of aging but rather the result of an organic disorder. Most men and women remain mentally competent until the end of their lives. Sudden loss of memory, disorientation, and trouble performing the daily tasks of life indicate a problem that should be investigated. Many conditions can cause signs and symptoms of dementia, including depression; reactions to prescription and over-the-counter (OTC) drugs; alcoholism; malnutrition; thyroid, liver, heart, and vascular disorders; and Parkinson's disease. Multiple factors can interfere with mental judgment and motor skills, giving the impression of decreased mental status.

The best way to ensure mental functioning in later life is to remain mentally and physically stimulated. Exercise improves memory and thinking because of its positive effect on vascular health, increasing the amount of oxygen delivered to the aging brain. Other ways to maintain mental function are to keep socially active; practice stress-reduction activities; quit smoking; drink alcohol in moderation; use hearing aids and glasses if needed to stay in touch with the world; and receive treatment for depression, diabetes, hypertension, and high cholesterol levels. Risk factors for cognitive decline include:

- Hypertension, diabetes, and heart disease (these reduce blood flow to the brain)
- Environmental exposure to lead
- High stress levels
- Sedentary lifestyle and lack of social interaction
- Low education level
- Smoking and substance abuse

One of the most frequently used screening tools for dementia is the Mini-Mental State Examination, a 5-minute test designed to evaluate basic mental function in a number of different areas. The test assesses the patient's ability to recall facts, write, and calculate numbers. It gives the provider a quick way to determine whether more in-depth testing is needed. Each area of the examination is given a score, and these scores show whether the person is functioning within the expected range for his or her age (Figure 41-2). The medical assistant may be expected to administer this examination.

Alzheimer's Disease

Alzheimer's disease (AD) is a progressive deterioration of the brain caused by the destruction of central nervous system (CNS) neurons, leading to problems with memory, language, thinking, and behavior. Three major changes occur in the brain:

- Amyloid plaques form.
- Neurofibrillary tangles clump together, affecting neuron function (neurons eventually die).
- The connections between neurons that are responsible for memory and learning are lost, resulting in neuron destruction; as neurons die throughout the brain, the affected regions begin to atrophy, or shrink. By the final stage of AD, damage is widespread and brain tissue has shrunk significantly.

Patients who show signs and symptoms of dementia are first evaluated for organic causes, such as systemic disease or depression. AD has no definitive diagnostic test because it can be confirmed only through examination of the brain at autopsy. If the patient shows a gradual onset of progressive difficulty with memory, functional abilities, and behavior and has no evidence of other causes of these disturbances, the physician makes the diagnosis of AD. Imaging studies,

including computed tomography (CT), magnetic resonance imaging (MRI), and positron emission tomography (PET), may help show the structural and functional changes in the brain associated with Alzheimer's disease.

Researchers estimate that about 5 million Americans suffer from AD. The disease typically begins after age 60, and the risk of developing the disorder increases with age, although younger people as early as age 30 have been diagnosed with AD. Research shows that 1 in 9 Americans over age 65 has Alzheimer's disease; almost 50% of people age 85 or older are diagnosed with the disease. Despite these statistics, AD is not considered a normal part of the aging process. Alzheimer's disease is the sixth leading cause of death (across all ages) in the United States and the fifth leading cause of death for those age 65 to 85.

Alzheimer's Disease Warning Signs

1. Memory loss that affects daily life: Forgetting important dates; repeatedly asking the same questions; relying on reminders or family members to remember things.

2. Changes in the ability to follow a plan or solve a problem: Difficulty concentrating on a problem; unable to follow directions; forgetting to pay monthly bills.

3. Changes in the ability to complete familiar tasks: Difficulty completing chores at home, running errands, or performing routine tasks at work.

4. Confusion about time or place: Losing track of time; unable to recall the date or day of the week; forgetting where you are and how you got there.

5. Problems with vision or understanding visual information: Difficulty reading, identifying colors, or judging distances.

6. Problems with words: Forgetting words in the middle of a conversation; repeating parts of a conversation; problems with vocabulary, such as calling things by the wrong names.

7. Misplacing things: Putting things in unusual places or frequently losing things; unable to retrace steps to find a lost object

8. Poor judgment: Paying less attention to appearance or cleanliness and using poor judgment with money.

9. Withdrawal from social activities, work projects, hobbies, or family gatherings.

10. Changes in mood and personality: Confusion, anxiety, depression, or fear, especially when in new or unfamiliar places.

American Academy of Family Physicians. *http://familydoctor.org/familydoctor/en/diseases-conditions/alzheimers-disease/alzheimers-disease-symptoms.html.* Accessed February 15, 2016.

AD is a slowly progressive disease that begins with mild memory problems and ends with severe brain damage. The course the disease takes and how fast changes occur varies among individuals, but on average, patients live for 8 to 10 years after they have been diagnosed. Currently no treatment can stop the progression of the disease. However, a great deal of research on the diagnosis and treatment of AD is under way.

The goal of treatment is to maintain normal activities as long as possible. Currently no medicines can slow the progression of AD,

---

Stages of Alzheimer's Disease

Alzheimer's disease (AD) typically progresses slowly in three general stages. However, each person experiences symptoms and progresses through Alzheimer's stages differently.

- Stage 1 (mild AD): Covers the 2 to 4 years leading up to diagnosis. Memory loss affects the person's job performance, and confusion and disorientation are common. The patient experiences mood or personality changes, has difficulty making decisions and paying bills, gets lost easily, withdraws from others, and loses things.

- Stage 2 (moderate AD): Lasts 2 to 10 years after diagnosis. This stage involves increased memory loss and confusion, a shorter attention span, and restlessness. The patient makes constant, repetitive statements; has problems with reading, writing, and numbers; may be irritable or suspicious; experiences motor problems; and has difficulty recognizing close friends and family members.

- Stage 3 (severe AD): Lasts 1 to 3 years. The patient does not recognize family; experiences weight loss; is unable to care for himself or herself; is incontinent of bladder and bowel; and requires complete care.

---

but the U.S. Food and Drug Administration (FDA) has approved four medications for the treatment of AD symptoms. These drugs help individuals carry out the activities of daily living by maintaining thinking, memory, or speaking skills. They can also help with some of the behavioral and personality changes associated with AD. However, they will not stop or reverse AD and appear to help individuals for only a few months to a few years. Cholinesterase inhibitors improve the production of neurotransmitters in the brain, which helps prevent memory loss from becoming worse for a limited time. These drugs do not help everyone; as many as 50% of patients show no improvement in mental function. Memantine (Namenda) was the first drug to be approved for the treatment of moderate to severe AD, although it also has limited effects (Table 41-3). Individuals with AD frequently experience changes in behavior, so medications may be prescribed to help control sleeplessness, agitation, wandering, anxiety, and depression. Treating these problems helps make the patient more comfortable while easing the burden on caregivers.

Supportive care for family members is absolutely essential because they are faced with caring for a loved one who is suffering progressive memory loss. The medical assistant can be especially helpful in recommending educational workshops, support groups, and stress management skills for caregivers. Multiple resources are available, including online information and support groups, which family members may find helpful.

CRITICAL THINKING APPLICATION   41-5

Maria Angelone, an 86-year-old patient of Dr. Kennedy, is in the second stage of AD. Her husband and children are showing signs of stress from the continuous care Mrs. Angelone requires. Her family still does not understand what is happening to her and what to expect in the future. What information can Bill share with them about the disease, and what resources could be helpful to the family in dealing with the stress of caring for a loved one with dementia?

TABLE 41-3   Medications Approved for the Treatment of Alzheimer's Disease

DRUG	STAGE OF TREATMENT	COMMON ADVERSE EFFECTS
Cholinesterase Inhibitors		
Donepezil (Aricept)	All stages	• Appetite loss
Galantamine (Razadyne)	Mild to moderate	• Dizziness
Rivastigmine (Exelon) tablet, liquid, or topical patch	All stages	• Fatigue • Increased frequency of bowel movements and diarrhea • Insomnia • Muscle cramps • Nausea, vomiting • Weight loss
Receptor Antagonist		
Memantine (Namenda) Prescribed alone or in combination with donepezil	Moderate to severe	• Confusion • Constipation • Diarrhea • Dizziness • Headache

Pharmacy Times: Alzheimer's disease: a disease of deterioration. www.pharmacytimes.com/publications/issue/2014/January2014/Alzheimers-Disease-A-Disease-of-Deterioration. Accessed February 18, 2015.

TABLE 41-4   Age-Related Changes in the Anatomic Structures of the Eye

STRUCTURE	AGE-RELATED CHANGE	EFFECTS
Lens	Thickens, becomes more opaque	Decreased refraction, causing blurred vision; decreased color acuity; cataracts
Anterior chamber	Decrease in size and volume	May develop increased intraocular pressure and glaucoma
Ciliary muscles	Affects pupil constriction and dilation	Limits light accommodation; night blindness
Cornea	Thickens, curve decreases	Problems with refraction
Retina	Decrease in number of rods and nerves	Decreased clarity; requires increase in minimum amount of light needed to see clearly

Pulmonary System

Maximum lung function decreases with age. The rate of airflow through the bronchi slowly declines after age 30, and the maximum force one is able to achieve on inspiration and expiration declines. The lungs lose their elasticity because of changes in **elastin** and collagen. They become smaller and flabbier. The alveoli enlarge, their walls become thinner, and the number of capillaries is reduced. As a result, the effective area for gas exchange in the lungs is reduced. The chest wall may stiffen from osteoporosis of the ribs and vertebrae and calcification of the **costal** cartilage. The respiratory muscles become weaker, making it harder to move air into and out of the lungs. To compensate, older adults rely more on accessory muscles, such as the diaphragm. Weakening of the respiratory muscles and stiffening of the chest wall make it harder to cough deeply enough to clear mucus from the lungs. Pulmonary function tests reveal a decrease in vital capacity and an increase in residual volume. The incidence of sleep apnea and sleep disorders increases, causing a potential problem with nocturnal hypoxemia. All these factors combine to put the older adult at greater risk for pneumonia and aspiration and for reactivation of tuberculosis.

The larynx also changes with aging, causing a change in the pitch and quality of the voice. The voice sounds quieter and slightly hoarse. The individual's voice may sound weaker, but it should not interfere with the ability to communicate effectively.

Sensory Organs

Vision

By the time a person reaches age 50, structural and functional changes in the eye become noticeable (Table 41-4). The eyebrows and eyelashes start to gray. The skin around the eyelids wrinkles, and the loss of orbital fat allows the eye to sink deeper into the orbit. The cornea increases in thickness and has reduced refractive power. A yellow-gray ring (arcus senilis) may develop on the periphery of the cornea. The iris loses pigmentation, and as a result older people appear to have gray eyes.

The lens of the eye continues to grow. As new lens fibers grow, old lens fibers are compressed and pushed to the center, causing the lens to become denser. The lens becomes flatter, thicker, less elastic, and more opaque, progressively yellowing with age. By age 70, the lens has tripled in mass. Clouding of the lens causes light rays to scatter, creating glare.

The pupil is designed to adjust to control the amount of light entering the eye. The ciliary muscle that causes the pupil to dilate weakens during the aging process. As a result, a reduction in the size of the pupil occurs, limiting the amount of light available to reach the retina. Tear production normally decreases. Tear glands do not make enough tears, or the tears are of poor quality and do not keep the eyes wet enough. Eye irritation and excessive tearing are a result of decreased **lacrimation**.

By the early to mid-40s, presbyopia develops, which makes it difficult to focus in detail on objects close at hand. This requires the use of corrective lenses to accommodate age-related farsightedness. The ability to refocus quickly from far to near or near to far decreases. Also, the ability to follow a moving object is decreased. The yellowing of the lens causes it to act like a filter, making it difficult to distinguish certain color intensities. Blues, greens, and violets are hard to differentiate, whereas yellows, reds, and oranges are easier to identify. The loss in the ability to discriminate closely related colors can affect the older person's ability to judge distances or his or her depth perception. This increases an aging person's susceptibility to falls and accidents. Stairs become a potential hazard because the edges of the steps cannot be seen clearly.

Older people need as much as six times more light to read; however, increasing the level of light does not completely compensate for visual decline because the elderly also experience an increased sensitivity to glare. Glare is probably one of the most painful experiences for the aging eye. Exposed light bulbs, such as those used in chandeliers, and light from highly reflective surfaces, such as glass tables and floors, can produce excessive glare. The eye has a decreased ability to respond to abrupt changes from light to dark or dark to light. Going from a well-lit waiting room into a dim hallway or negotiating the way down dimly lit aisles in a movie theater could be treacherous for an older person.

Cataracts, Glaucoma, and Macular Degeneration. Eye diseases and disorders that occur frequently in older individuals are cataracts, glaucoma, and macular degeneration. Cataracts are cloudy or opaque areas in the lens that cause blurring of vision; rings or halos around lights and objects; and a blue or yellow tint to the visual field. Surgical lens extraction and implantation with an artificial lens improves vision in 95% of cases. The procedure, which is performed in an outpatient facility, involves a small incision to remove the lens, laser therapy, or phacoemulsification (ultrasonic vibrations), which breaks up the lens and removes it without the need for an incision. After the procedure, patients must avoid bending or lifting heavy objects for 3 to 4 weeks, and wearing an eye shield at night and glasses during the day helps protect the eye until it heals. Recovery takes about 2 weeks.

Glaucoma is a result of blockage of the outflow of aqueous humor, which causes an increase in intraocular pressure and damage to the optic nerve. If not treated, glaucoma can cause progressive loss of peripheral vision and ultimately lead to blindness; however, it can be treated with medication.

The macula is the part of the eye responsible for sharp vision and color. Damage to or breakdown of the macula is called *macular degeneration,* which causes progressive loss of the central field of vision. Macular degeneration is the leading cause of blindness in aging people, and at this time there is no effective treatment or cure. (All three of these eye disorders are discussed in more detail in the chapter on Assisting in Ophthamology and Otolaryngology).

Suggestions for Helping the Visually Impaired Older Adult

- When escorting an older person, regardless of whether he or she is visually impaired, allow the patient to place his or her hand above your elbow. It is easier for the person to follow your movements. This method also provides a source of support and security.
- Use high levels of evenly distributed, glare-free light.
- Ask the pharmacist to use large lettering when labeling medicine bottles.

- Use paper that has a nonglare finish and large print for forms and educational materials.
- Make distinct differences (e.g., size of containers or color coding with bright primary colors) for pills that are similar in size and color.
- Place all objects within the visual field and prevent clutter.

Hearing

Hearing loss can have a profound psychological effect on aging people, causing depression, social withdrawal, and feelings of isolation. Hearing loss occurs gradually over a long period and may go undetected by the older person and healthcare providers. Lack of attention when addressed, inappropriate responses, asking to have statements repeated, and speaking too loudly or too softly often are signs of hearing loss. Changes in auditory ability begin around age 30; by age 65, one out of three people has a hearing loss, and the number increases to 65% of those over age 80. Age-related hearing loss usually is caused by a dysfunction or loss of cochlear cilia, resulting in an inability to hear high-frequency sounds and difficulty understanding speech. Hearing impairment is compounded by impacted cerumen, otitis media, **otosclerosis**, **Ménière's disease**, long-term exposure to intense noise, and certain **ototoxic** drugs, such as aspirin.

Presbycusis is associated with normal aging and causes a decreased ability to hear high frequencies and to discriminate sounds. Parts of a conversation may be missed because the sound of the word goes above the 2,000-cycle frequency. Often words that sound similar are difficult to differentiate. Consonants such as *g, f, s, sh, t,* and *z* produce high-pitched sounds that are more difficult to hear and differentiate. Low-frequency pitched sounds, such as the vowels *a, e, i, o,* and *u,* may be more easily heard by people with presbycusis. Inability to hear different frequencies combined with low background noise from groups of people talking, noise from appliances, or busy public places compromises an older person's ability to hear clearly. Hearing aids, which can be used to amplify speech, may increase background noises, resulting in sensory overload.

Another hearing disorder common among older people is tinnitus, a ringing or buzzing in the ear. It can be caused by impacted cerumen, an ear infection, use of antibiotics, a reaction to a medication, or a nerve disorder. Tinnitus can cause difficulty understanding conversational speech and can make sleeping difficult because of the continuous sensation of ringing in the ears.

Hearing loss, with its resultant isolation, is directly related to the development of depression in older adults. Treatable depression often is overlooked in elderly people because of coexisting physical illnesses that mask the symptoms of depression. The medical assistant may be able to contribute to information about depression in elderly patients through conversations with the individual and family members. The provider may use or may train the medical assistant to use the Geriatric Depression Scale Short Form, which includes questions for the patient about daily activities, interests, and feelings to help diagnose depression in the ambulatory setting (Figure 41-3).

GERIATRIC DEPRESSION SCALE (SHORT FORM)

Choose the best answer for how you have felt over the past week:

1. Are you basically satisfied with your life? YES / **NO**
2. Have you dropped many of your activities and interests? **YES** / NO
3. Do you feel that your life is empty? **YES** / NO
4. Do you often get bored? **YES** / NO
5. Are you in good spirits most of the time? YES / **NO**
6. Are you afraid that something bad is going to happen to you? **YES** / NO
7. Do you feel happy most of the time? YES / **NO**
8. Do you often feel helpless? **YES** / NO
9. Do you prefer to stay at home, rather than going out and doing new things? **YES** / NO
10. Do you feel you have more problems with memory than most? **YES** / NO
11. Do you think it is wonderful to be alive now? YES / **NO**
12. Do you feel pretty worthless the way you are now? **YES** / NO
13. Do you feel full of energy? YES / **NO**
14. Do you feel that your situation is hopeless? **YES** / NO
15. Do you think that most people are better off than you are? **YES** / NO

Answers in **bold** indicate depression. Although differing sensitivities and specificities have been obtained across studies, for clinical purposes a score >5 points is suggestive of depression and should warrant a follow-up interview. Scores >10 almost always indicate depression.

FIGURE 41-3 Geriatric Depression Scale.

Suggestions for Helping the Hearing-Impaired Older Adult

- Stand in the patient's direct line of vision and gently touch the person to get his or her attention.
- Use gestures, pictures, and large, bold print to communicate.
- Talk in short sentences into the ear with better hearing.
- Do not increase the volume of your speech; this also raises the frequency of the voice, which is the hearing most impaired in aging people. Use expanded speech; lower the tone of your voice and talk in distinct syllables.
- Avoid background noise. Give instructions in a quiet room with the door closed. If the patient has a hearing aid, make sure it is on.

Taste and Smell

During the aging process the abilities to taste and smell decline subtly. Deterioration and atrophy of the taste buds are part of the aging process. The ability to taste salt and sweet flavors is reduced, whereas the ability to detect bitter and sour flavors remains relatively the same. As a result, food frequently tastes bland and unappetizing.

Patients on salt-restricted diets and patients with diabetes must be cautioned about the use of excessive amounts of salt and sugar. A decrease in the sense of smell accompanies the decrease in taste. Not only does this affect the individual's enjoyment of food; it also exposes the person to environmental dangers, such as gas leaks, smoke, and other dangerous odors that may go undetected. Checking for gas leaks around stoves and heaters and using smoke alarms reduce some of the danger. Also, dating food when it is put in the refrigerator is a good idea.

Nutritional Status. Because of the many environmental, social, economic, and physical changes of aging, older people are at greater risk for poor nutrition, which can adversely affect their health and energy level. It is estimated that 25% of the aging population suffers from malnutrition. Nutrition screening should be part of routine primary care to identify nutritional deficiencies and correct them before a disease process develops or to assist in the treatment of chronic disease. Patients with chronic conditions, such as cardiovascular disease, hypertension, and diabetes, can benefit from nutrition assessments and interventions. Malnourished older patients get more infections; their injuries take longer to heal; surgery is riskier for them; and their hospital stays are longer and more expensive.

The most effective method of assessing a patient's nutritional status is through a comprehensive patient interview that considers all potential stumbling blocks to adequate nutrition. The medical assistant can help determine the nutritional status of older patients by considering the following factors when conducting patient interviews:

- *Oral health:* Does the patient wear dentures and if so, do they fit properly? Does the patient have mouth pain? Can he or she swallow without difficulty?
- *Gastrointestinal complaints:* Does the patient have anorexia, nausea, vomiting, diarrhea, or constipation? Is the patient lactose intolerant (the incidence increases with age)?
- *Sensorimotor changes:* Does the patient have loss of vision or hearing or changes in taste and smell? Can the patient feed herself or himself? Does the patient need adaptive utensils?
- *Diet influences:* Can the patient afford, shop for, and prepare food? Are ethnic or religious influences a factor? Does the patient have any disease-related diet restrictions? What is the patient's alcohol consumption?
- *Social and mental influences:* Is the patient depressed, lonely, or isolated? Are support systems available?

CRITICAL THINKING APPLICATION   41-6

Multiple sensory changes occur as people age. Dr. Kennedy asks Bill to develop a handout for patients and family members to help them understand these normal, age-related sensorimotor changes and also adaptations that can improve communication. What information should Bill include?

Urinary System

As the body ages, structural changes in the kidneys cause the urinary system to become less efficient. Between the ages of 40 and 80, the kidney loses about 20% of its mass. The number of functional nephron units decreases. Blood flow to the kidneys is reduced because of a decrease in cardiovascular efficiency. Because of the reduction of blood flow to the kidneys and the decreased number of nephrons, the kidneys become less efficient at filtering waste from the blood. This results in a more diluted, less concentrated urine. The kidneys require more water to excrete the same amount of waste. Medication takes longer to be removed from the body. Older adults are at increased risk for toxic levels of medication in the bloodstream because of this reduced filtration rate.

Fibrous connective tissue replaces the smooth muscle and elastic tissue in the bladder. This thickening of the bladder wall reduces the bladder's ability to expand. The bladder's capacity to store fluid comfortably is reduced from 400 to 250 mL. These structural changes lead to increased frequency of urination and urinary retention. Older adults are at increased risk of urinary tract infections because of residual urine. Sleep is interrupted by the need to void during the night. The sensation of bladder fullness is not recognized as quickly by the older brain. Reduced time between awareness of the need to void and involuntary urination can cause anxiety. Often older adults reduce their fluid intake to prevent possible embarrassment. Unfortunately, this causes dehydration and an increased risk of urinary tract infections. Another change is loss of muscle tone in the urethra. In addition, the pelvic floor muscles in an aging woman relax as a result of decreased estrogen levels or previous pregnancy and childbirth.

Despite these changes, the kidneys have great reserve capacity and are able to continue functioning normally. Urinary incontinence, the involuntary loss of urine, is a significant problem for aging patients but is not a normal part of the aging process. Changes in the urinary system make older people more vulnerable to incontinence, but factors such as infection, confusion, difficulty with mobility, and side effects of medications contribute to the development of the problem. Incontinence is both an emotional and a physical problem. To avoid the risk of an embarrassing accident, people with this problem may avoid social occasions or activities they enjoy. Often people are too embarrassed to admit they have this condition, or they believe it is just part of aging. Once the condition has been diagnosed by a urologist, pelvic floor muscle exercises, medication, or surgery may be recommended.

Reproductive System

Aging brings a decrease in circulating levels of the female hormones estrogen and progesterone, whereas androgen levels increase. The results of this decrease are changes in the genital tract. The vagina diminishes in width and length and becomes less elastic. The cervix, uterus, and ovaries decrease in size. Vaginal secretions decline; therefore, lubrication diminishes, resulting in vaginal dryness. Bacterial or yeast infections may occur because vaginal secretions are less acidic. Estrogen cream applied to vaginal tissue may be prescribed by the provider for help with dryness and thinning of the vaginal tissue. The patient should discuss the benefits and risks of estrogen replacement therapy with the provider to determine whether it should be used.

Even though sperm production may decline in men over age 50, men remain virile well into old age. However, they experience a change in hormonal levels of testosterone, and these changes can affect the prostate gland. The prostate enlarges over time and presses down on the urethra, causing difficulty with urination. Surgery may be required to remove excess portions of the gland. Unfortunately, the operation may cause impotence, which can be treated medically with erectile dysfunction medications.

Men experience some changes in sexual functioning as they age. It takes longer for the penis to become erect, longer for an orgasm to occur, and longer to recover. Direct stimulation may be required before an erection occurs, and when it does, it may be less firm than in younger years.

Some drugs and illnesses can interfere with sexual function. Drugs used to control high blood pressure, antihistamines, antidepressants, and some stomach acid blockers, in addition to the diseases diabetes, arthritis, and arteriosclerosis, can have an adverse effect on sexual function. Often people who have had heart surgery or a heart attack are concerned about sexual activity. Patients need to feel comfortable and should not be embarrassed to discuss their concerns openly with their provider. It is important for healthcare practitioners to dismiss the myth that older patients have lost the desire for and interest in sexual intercourse.

Sleep Disorders

Complaints of sleeping difficulties increase with age. The amount of time spent sleeping may be slightly longer than in a younger person, but the quality of sleep declines. Older people often are light sleepers and have periods of wakefulness in bed. Rapid eye movement (REM) sleep is the stage of sleep when people experience dreaming. Non-REM sleep is the period of deepest sleep. The amount of time spent in the deepest stages of sleep decreases with age. Sleep that is disturbed or that leaves the person feeling tired is not part of the aging process and may indicate some underlying emotional or physical problem. Lack of sleep can result in restlessness, disorientation, "thick" speech, and mispronounced words. Often these symptoms are mistaken as signs of dementia. Other factors that might influence sleep patterns are medications, caffeine, alcohol, depression, and environmental or physical changes.

Common sleep problems in older adults include dyssomnias, such as periodic limb movement disorder (PLMD), in which periodic jerking of the legs occurs during sleep, and sleep apnea, which is common among overweight individuals and can occur frequently during the night, interrupting sleep. Numerous medical conditions can interfere with sleep, including joint and bone pain; Parkinson's disease (because of difficulty changing positions); CHF; chronic obstructive pulmonary disease; diabetes mellitus, which increases **nocturia**; depression; and certain medications (e.g., beta blockers can cause nightmares, antidepressants increase PLMD, and barbiturates may result in nightmares or hallucinations).

It is important to be aware of the effect of sleep problems because often these can be confused with dementia. Patients who are experiencing difficulty with sleeping should be encouraged to document their sleeping patterns, napping patterns, medications, diet, exercise routines, and any events that have resulted in a change of lifestyle. They should discuss this problem with their provider. Simple modification of behavioral patterns may resolve the problem. Taking fewer naps, completing exercise several hours before bedtime, changing eating times, reducing the amount of alcohol and caffeine ingested, drinking a glass of milk before bedtime, or changing medications or the time they are taken all are suggestions that might alter the factors responsible for sleep disturbances.

If behavioral approaches are not effective, medications may be considered for short-term use only, because they have a high incidence of physical and psychological dependence. Elderly people are especially susceptible to side effects from these drugs, such as next-day drowsiness and temporary memory loss. Sedatives or hypnotics that may be prescribed include zolpidem (Ambien), eszopiclone (Lunesta), zaleplon (Sonata), and ramelteon (Rozerem).

Living Arrangements

At any given time, only 5% of the elderly population lives in long-term care facilities. According to information published by the National Institute on Aging, older people live close to their children and are in frequent contact with them. People prefer to age in place; that is, they want to live in their own home environment as long as possible. Individuals are admitted to nursing homes because they are no longer able to perform activities of daily living, such as bathing, dressing, eating, walking, and maintaining bladder and bowel continence. They also have difficulty with grocery shopping, housekeeping, and money management. Chronic health conditions and accidents interfere with the older person's ability to perform these tasks.

Many resources are available to help seniors maintain their independence. Outreach programs, such as Meals on Wheels, deliver nutritious meals to the homes of older adults. Senior centers serve as a focal point for many activities and as a source of information. Transportation services provide rides to doctors' appointments, day care centers, shopping centers, and community events. Home health agencies provide several types of services, including personal care, shopping, transportation, and meal preparation. Some home health agencies provide a range of activities, from patient education to IV therapy; medical-social services; physical, speech, and occupational therapies; and nutrition and dietary counseling. Advanced technology allows people to receive services at home that formerly were provided only at a hospital or a physician's office.

Adult day care centers provide socialization, recreation, meals and, in some centers, physical therapy, occupational therapy, and transportation. These centers offer supervision for older adults who may be taken care of by family members in the evening but need care during the day. They also serve as respite for a caregiver.

Assisted-living facilities can be retirement homes or board and care homes. These facilities are appropriate for older adults who need assistance with some activities of daily living, such as bathing, dressing, and walking. Skilled nursing facilities provide 24-hour medical care and supervision. In addition to medical care, residents receive care that may include physical, occupational, and speech therapies. The objective of treatment is to improve or maintain the person's abilities.

THE MEDICAL ASSISTANT'S ROLE IN CARING FOR THE OLDER PATIENT

Elderly patients in the ambulatory care setting present a specific set of needs that require a certain amount of accommodation by the staff. For example, aging patients typically require more time to perform tasks and have questions answered. The office staff may want to hurry them so that the day's schedule can be maintained. In the best interests of the patient, however, he or she should be treated with respect and given whatever time is needed to prepare for examinations, ask questions and receive answers, and have procedures explained. A system that is sensitive to the needs of older patients schedules longer periods for appointments; has adequate lighting in the waiting room; provides forms in large print; has an examination room equipped with furniture, magazines, and treatment folders especially designed for older adults; and invites a professional in the management of older patients for in-service training.

The primary issue in elder care is effective communication. How you communicate with people is often influenced by what you know or do not know about them. Older people are subject to many changes that affect how they are able to interact with their environment. It is important to recognize these changes and to investigate one's personal perception of older people to break down the barriers that prohibit effective communication.

As people age, they frequently experience a loss of control over their lives because of physical disabilities, economic constraints, and institutional living. Part of the medical assistant's job is to help aging people maintain their dignity and independence while in the ambulatory care setting. Remember, each patient, regardless of his or her education, socioeconomic status, or age, deserves to be treated with compassion and respect. Ask the patient directly what is wrong rather than discussing the patient with family members. It also is important to listen carefully and to be specific and sincere when responding. When a patient is talking, take time to allow him or her to complete the sentence; do not finish it for the person. Give the patient your full attention rather than continuing with other tasks while he or she is speaking. Older people may take a little longer to process information, but they are capable of understanding. Do not hurry through explanations or questions; rather, take time to review a form or give instructions as needed.

Suggestions for Effective Communication With Aging Patients

- Address the patient as Mr., Mrs., or Miss unless the patient has given you permission to use his or her first name.
- Introduce yourself and explain the purpose of a procedure before performing the procedure.
- Face the aging person and softly touch the individual to get his or her attention before beginning to speak.
- Use expanded speech, gestures, demonstrations, or written instructions in block print.
- If the message must be repeated, paraphrase or find other words to say the same thing.
- Observe the patient's nonverbal behavior for cues indicating whether he or she understands.
- Provide adequate lighting without glare.
- Allow patients time to process information and take care of themselves unless they ask for assistance.
- Conduct communication in a quiet room without distractions.
- Involve family members as needed for continuity of care.

- When leaving a telephone message, remember to speak slowly and clearly and repeat the message in the same manner. It is difficult to interpret a message, and even more difficult to write it down, if the message was delivered in a hurried manner.
- Use referrals and community resources for support, such as the following:
  - Alzheimer's Association: *www.alz.org/* (1-800-272-3900).
  - American Council of the Blind: *http://acb.org/* (1-800-424-8666): Provides referrals to state and other organizations that provide services and equipment for the blind.
  - American Speech-Language-Hearing Association: *www.asha.org/* (1-800-638-8255): Offers information on hearing aids, hearing loss, and communication problems in older people and provides a list of certified audiologists and speech pathologists.
  - Arthritis Foundation Information Line: *www.arthritis.org* (404-872-7100): Makes referrals to local chapters and provides information on various types of arthritis.
  - American Diabetes Association: *www.diabetes.org/* (1-800-342-2383): Provides information and support for those with diabetes.
  - Eldercare Locator: *www.eldercare.gov/Eldercare.NET/Public/Index.aspx* (1-800-677-1116): Run by the National Association of Area Agencies on Aging; help line provides information on contacting local chapters that oversee services to older adults.
  - National Institute on Aging Information Center: *www.nia.nih.gov/* (1-800-222-2225): Provides information on aging health issues for patients, families, and healthcare professionals.
  - National Meals-on-Wheels Foundation: *www.mowaa.org/* (1-888-998-6325).
  - National Hospice and Palliative Care Organization: *www.nhpco.org/* (703-837-1500): A nonprofit organization committed to improving end of life care and expanding access to hospice care.

CRITICAL THINKING APPLICATION   **41-7**

New staff members in the practice are complaining of having to repeat information to older patients, who they say do not pay attention when procedures are explained. Dr. Kennedy has decided to invite a gerontologist from the local university to present an in-service workshop on healthy aging. She asks Bill to coordinate the in-service workshop and prepare materials requested by the guest speaker. What information about caring for the ambulatory aging patient should be included in the workshop?

CLOSING COMMENTS

Patient Education

The medical assistant must keep the sensorimotor changes that accompany aging and also respectful patient communication in mind when conducting patient education with older patients. Remember, the aging process does not affect a person's ability to learn; it just may take longer to process the information, and the material may need to be repeated for understanding. Showing

sensitivity to the needs of aging learners ensures successful patient education and improves compliance with prescribed treatment plans. The current aging population generally is respectful toward authority; therefore, if the medical assistant cannot gain the patient's cooperation, the physician may be able to provide authoritative reinforcement of material. General guidelines for effective patient education with older adults include the following:

- The patient may have short-term memory loss, so you may need to repeat the information using different words.
- The patient may be distracted more easily, so learning in a group may be difficult.
- The patient may take longer to process information, so teach at a pace that matches the patient's needs.
- Provide the patient with handouts that have large print and block letters for reviewing information at home.
- Involve family members as needed for continuity of care; provide physician-approved websites for reference.

Legal and Ethical Issues

All patients have the right to know about the medications, treatments, and alternatives available to them. The Patients' Bill of Rights informs the patient of those rights in a healthcare setting. They include the right to privacy about personal and medical information and the right to informed consent, which holds the provider accountable for explaining clearly the advantages and risks of any procedures, tests, or treatments. The patient must give permission for medical care and has the right to refuse treatment. The patient has the right to be informed about his or her condition and treatment and the chances of recovery. The patient also has the right to have advance directives explained to him or her.

Consent must be given by the individual undergoing the procedure, as long as he or she is judged to be competent; that is, as long as the patient is able to understand the consequences of the procedure. In an emergency situation or if a court has ruled that the patient is incompetent, someone else must give consent. This may be a person who already was designated to hold the durable power of attorney, a close family member (spouse, adult child, parent, sibling), or a court-appointed guardian.

Most states have legal documents available that provide written instructions specifying the type of medical care a person wants in the event she or he becomes incapacitated; these are called living wills or *advanced directives*. The document designates a person who has a durable power of attorney; this is an authorization for making medical decisions on an individual's behalf if he or she is unable to make treatment decisions. The document provides a list of specific instructions for the proxy to follow.

Various issues may be covered in these documents. A "do not resuscitate" (DNR) order allows a patient to refuse attempts to restore a heartbeat. The patient also may decide to withdraw life-sustaining treatment, such as respirators or feeding tubes. A copy of the directive should be kept on file as part of the patient's health record. It is important to check the laws of the state in which you practice with regard to advanced directives, because they vary from state to state (Figure 41-4).

Another legal issue in the care of aging patients is the possibility of elder abuse, neglect, and exploitation. Mistreatment of aging people occurs at all social, racial, and economic levels. The abuse

Directive made this _____ th day of _____ in the year _____ .
      (day)   (month)   (year)

I, _____ , being of sound mind, willfully and voluntarily make known my desire that my life shall not be artificially prolonged under the circumstances set forth in this directive.

If at any time I should have
— an incurable or irreversible condition caused by injury,
— disease,
— or illness certified to be a terminal condition by two physicians

and if the application of life-sustaining procedures would serve only to artificially postpone the moment of my death, and if my attending physician determines that my death is imminent or will result within a relatively short time without the application of life-sustaining procedures. I direct that those procedures be withheld or withdrawn, and that I be permitted to die naturally.

In the absence of my ability to give directions regarding the use of those life-sustaining procedures, it is my intention that this directive be honored by my family and physicians as the final expression of my legal right to refuse medical or surgical treatment and accept the consequences from that refusal.

If I have been diagnosed as pregnant and that diagnosis is known to my physician, this directive has no effect during my pregnancy. This directive is in effect until it is revoked.

I understand the full import of this directive and I am emotionally and mentally competent to make this directive. I understand that I may revoke this directive at any time.

I request that only comfort care be provided to me, no antibiotics, no artificial nutrition, no mechanical ventilation, and no hydration. It is my strong preference to be allowed to die outside of a care facility if possible, even if that preference is determined by my physician to shorten my period of dying. The only condition under which I desire these preferences for end of life care to be altered is in the case of possible organ and tissue donation. I request that any and all organs and tissue that may be salvaged be provided for transplant. My remains may then be cremated.

Signed _____ in the City of _____ etc.

I am not a person designated by the declarant to make a treatment decision. I am not related to the declarant by blood or marriage. I would not be entitled to any portion of the declarant's estate on the declarant's death. I am not the attending physician of the declarant or an employee of the attending physician.

I have no claim in against any portion of the declarant's estate on the declarant's death. Furthermore, if I am an employee of the health care facility in which the declarant is a patient, I am not involved in providing direct patient care to the declarant and am not an officer, director, partner, or business office employee of the heath care facility or of any parent organization of the health care facility.

Witness _____

Witness _____

FIGURE 41-4 Sample advanced directive.

may be physical, mental, sexual, material, or financial; it may involve neglect or failure to provide adequate care, or it may involve self-neglect when aging people are unable or refuse to care for themselves. Abuse, neglect, and exploitation of elders by their caregivers may be difficult to identify. The aging victim could feel embarrassed, guilty, or afraid to report the abuse. Indications that a patient may be a victim of elder abuse, neglect, or exploitation are:

• Poor general appearance and poor hygiene
• Pattern of changing doctors and frequent emergency department visits
• Skin lesions, signs of dehydration, bruises (signs of new and old bruising together), abrasions, welts, burns, or pressure sores
• Recurrent injuries caused by accidents
• Signs of malnutrition and weight loss without related illness
• Any injury that does not fit the given history

If abuse, neglect, or exploitation is suspected, interviewing the caregiver and questioning the demands of care and self-reported perceptions of stress levels may help the provider detect the problem. Many states now have laws that require reporting of suspected elder abuse, neglect, or exploitation. Check your state laws to determine the requirements for healthcare workers.

Professional Behaviors

Your future employers will expect you to use problem-solving techniques, including recognizing and defining a problem, analyzing the issue, and developing a plan of action. Elderly patients typically have multiple health problems that are frequently complicated by physical, psychological, and environmental factors. To provide quality care for these individuals, you must look at their health issues in a holistic way, taking into consideration all the factors that affect their eventual ability to follow treatment plans and improve their health status. Part of the process involves identifying resources that might help the aging person be better equipped to take care of himself or herself. Consistently using community and online resources may mean the difference between an aging person being able to stay in her home or having to go to long-term care. The professional medical assistant can play a crucial role in providing assistance to aging clients.

SUMMARY OF SCENARIO

Through his work with Dr. Kennedy, Bill has learned to understand the special needs of aging patients. He used to think that most older people were chronically sick and would ultimately end up in long-term care facilities. Now he understands that most aging people lead healthy, active lives and that the disorders that occur in later life usually are the result of lifestyle factors, such as diet and lack of exercise. Bill also has learned how to communicate effectively with older patients and to conduct patient interviews so as to evaluate the patient's physical, mental, emotional, and nutritional health.

SUMMARY OF LEARNING OBJECTIVES

1. **Define, spell, and pronounce the terms listed in the vocabulary.**
   Spelling and pronouncing medical terms correctly reinforce the medical assistant's credibility. Knowing the definitions of these terms promotes confidence in communication with patients and co-workers.

2. **Do the following related to the aging process:**
   - *Discuss the impact of a growing aging population on society.*
     More than 48 million Americans are 65 years of age or older. By 2030 almost 1 of every 5 Americans (about 72 million people) will be 65 years or older. Most older people have at least one chronic medical condition, and many have multiple conditions. The aging population will affect all aspects of society.
   - *Identify the stereotypes and myths associated with aging.*
     Stereotypes and myths associated with aging include the likelihood of developing dementia, aging and disease development, productivity of older workers, long-term care, sexual activity, and significance of lifestyle factors. To avoid age discrimination and lack of respectful care, the medical assistant should be educated about the realities of aging and the elderly population.
   - *Role-play the effect of the sensorimotor changes of aging.*
     Procedure 41-1 outlines the steps in role-playing the sensorimotor changes that accompany aging.

3. **Do the following related to the cardiovascular, endocrine, gastrointestinal, integumentary, and musculoskeletal body systems:**
   - *Explain the changes in the anatomy and physiology caused by aging.*
     Table 41-1 summarizes changes associated with aging that occur across all body systems. Normal age-related changes are expected, and the individual can compensate for them. However, these changes intensify with poor health habits and chronic disease. Age-related changes can be managed through regular exercise, a healthy diet, prevention of sun damage, and annual physical examinations with health screening.
   - *Summarize the major related diseases and disorders faced by older patients.*
     Major health issues of older people are related to an increase in atherosclerosis and potential cardiovascular disease; hypertension; diabetes mellitus type 2; integumentary system changes; arthritis; osteoporosis; and an increased risk of injury from falls.

4. **Do the following related to the nervous system, pulmonary system, sensory organs, urinary system, and reproductive system:**
   - *Explain the changes in the anatomy and physiology caused by aging.*
     Cognitive ability is influenced by many factors, including the aging process. Maximum lung capacity also decreases with age. By the age of 50, structural and functional changes in the eye become noticeable.

Continued

SUMMARY OF LEARNING OBJECTIVES—*continued*

Hearing loss occurs gradually over a long period and can go undetected. The ability to taste and smell declines subtly as a person ages. As a person ages, structural changes in the kidneys cause the urinary system to become less efficient. Finally, aging brings a decrease in circulating levels of the female hormones estrogen and progesterone and an increase of androgen.

- *Summarize the major related diseases and disorders faced by older patients.*

  Alzheimer's disease is a progressive deterioration of the brain caused by the destruction of CNS neurons; it develops in three stages. Various structures of the eye are affected by aging. Presbycusis, which is associated with normal aging, diminishes the older person's ability to hear high frequencies and to discriminate sounds.

- *Describe various screening tools for dementia, depression, and malnutrition in aging adults.*

  A commonly used screening tool for dementia is the Folstein Mini-Mental State Examination, a 5-minute screening test that is designed to evaluate basic mental function. The provider may use the Geriatric Depression Scale short form, which questions the patient about daily activities, interests, and feelings. Nutritional status can be assessed through a comprehensive patient interview that considers all potential problems preventing adequate nutrition.

5. **Explain the effect of aging on sleep.**

   Complaints of sleeping difficulties increase with age. The amount of time spent in the deepest stages of sleep declines with age. Factors that might influence sleep patterns are medications, caffeine, alcohol, depression, and environmental or physical changes. Common sleep problems in older adults include PLMD and sleep apnea.

6. **Differentiate among independent, assisted, and skilled nursing facilities.**

   Aging people prefer to remain in their home environment for as long as possible. Adult day care centers can provide supervision for older adults who may be taken care of by family members in the evening but need care during the day. Assisted-living facilities are appropriate for older adults who need assistance with some activities of daily living. Skilled nursing facilities provide 24-hour medical care and supervision.

7. **Summarize the role of the medical assistant in caring for aging patients.**

   The medical assistant's role in caring for the older patient is to develop effective communication skills that accommodate age-related sensorimotor changes; to allow time for longer appointments; to provide adequate lighting and forms in large print; and to develop appropriate in-service training as requested by the provider. Examination rooms should have furniture and treatment folders especially designed for the elderly patient. Referrals and community resources should be used for patient and family support.

8. **Determine the principles of effective communication with older adults.**

   Effective communication with aging patients includes addressing the patient with an appropriate title; introducing yourself and explaining the purpose of a procedure before touching the patient; establishing eye contact and getting the patient's attention before beginning to speak; using expanded speech, gestures, demonstrations, or written instructions in block print; repeating the message as needed for understanding; observing the patient's nonverbal behaviors for cues that indicate whether he or she understands; allowing time to process information; preventing distractions; and involving family members as needed.

9. **Discuss patient education, as well as legal and ethical issues, associated with aging patients.**

   Legal and ethical issues associated with aging patients include adequate informed consent, the use of advanced directives, and staying alert for signs of possible elder abuse.

CONNECTIONS

Study Guide Connection: Go to the Chapter 41 Study Guide. Read and complete the activities.

evolve   Evolve Connection: Go to the Chapter 41 link at *evolve.elsevier.com/ kinn* to complete the Chapter Review Quiz. Check out the other resources listed for this chapter to make the most of what you have learned from Assisting in Geriatrics.

PRINCIPLES OF ELECTROCARDIOGRAPHY

42

SCENARIO

Martha Reyes has worked for almost 4 years at a local family practice office, but she has decided to take a new position in the cardiology practice next door, where she will be working for Dr. Julie Lee. Martha is very enthusiastic about the new position, but she realizes that she has a great deal to learn to provide the best patient service possible in Dr. Lee's practice. Although Martha is familiar with general cardiology practices from her previous employment, she must understand and be able to perform procedures specific for cardiac patients, especially electrocardiography.

While studying this chapter, think about the following questions:

- To fulfill her job description with Dr. Lee, what does Martha need to know about the electrical conduction system of the heart?
- How does an electrocardiography machine work?
- How should a patient be prepared for an electrocardiogram?
- How will Martha perform an ECG diagnostic procedure?
- What is the normal appearance of ECG complexes?
- What are the characteristics of common ECG arrhythmias that Martha must be able to recognize?
- What additional cardiac tests should Martha be prepared to assist with and explain to patients?

LEARNING OBJECTIVES

1. Define, spell, and pronounce the terms listed in the vocabulary.
2. Illustrate the electrical conduction system through the heart and discuss the cardiac cycle.
3. Explain the concepts of cardiac polarization, depolarization, and repolarization.
4. Identify the PQRST complex on an electrocardiographic tracing.
5. Summarize the properties of the electrocardiograph and discuss the features of electrocardiograph paper.
6. Describe the electrical views of the heart recorded by the 12-lead electrocardiograph.
7. Discuss the process of recording an electrocardiogram and perform an accurate reading of the electrical activity of the heart.
8. Compare and contrast electrocardiographic artifacts and the probable cause of each.
9. Interpret a typical electrocardiograph tracing.
10. Describe common electrocardiographic arrhythmias.
11. Summarize cardiac diagnostic tests and fit a patient with a Holter monitor.
12. Discuss patient education and the legal and ethical issues involved when performing ECGs.

VOCABULARY

atria The two upper chambers of the heart.

atrioventricular (AV) node The part of the cardiac conduction system between the atria and the ventricles.

bundle of His Specialized muscle fibers that conduct electrical impulses from the AV node to the ventricular myocardium.

cardiac arrest A condition in which cardiac contractions stop completely.

cardioversion The use of electroshock to convert an abnormal cardiac rhythm to a normal one.

defibrillator A machine that delivers an electroshock to the heart through electrodes placed on the chest wall.

diastole The period of relaxation of the chambers of the heart, during which blood enters the heart from the vascular system and the lungs.

ectopic (ek-toh´-pik) Originating outside the normal tissue.

infarction An area of tissue that has died from lack of blood supply.

ischemia (is-ke´-me-ah) Decreased blood flow to a body part or organ, caused by constriction or blockage of the supplying artery.

leads Electrical connections attached to the body to record electrical heart activity; any of the conductors connected to the electrocardiograph, each comprising two or more electrodes that are attached at specific body sites and used to examine and record the electrical activity of the heart.

myocardial (mi-oh-kar´-de-uhl) Pertaining to the heart muscle.

palpitations Pounding or racing of the heart; it may or may not indicate a serious heart disorder.

sinoatrial (SA) node The pacemaker of the heart, located in the right atrium.

systole The period of contraction of the heart.

ventricles The two lower chambers of the heart.

Electrocardiography is the test most frequently used to diagnose heart disease in ambulatory care practices. It is a painless, safe procedure. In electrocardiography, electrodes are attached to the patient's skin and connected to wires that go to the electrocardiograph. Electrocardiography amplifies the electrical impulses from the beating heart, and a pattern of these impulses is recorded on electrocardiographic paper. This record is called the *electrocardiogram* (ECG). The ECG is read and evaluated by the practitioner and becomes a part of the patient's health record (Figure 42-1). Medical practices using electronic health records can record an ECG tracing directly into the patient's electronic record.

To accurately represent the true cardiac activity, the ECG must be performed with a high degree of accuracy and skill. A medical assistant must have an understanding of both the normal cardiac function and the relationship of the ECG recordings to cardiac function. The medical assistant is responsible for ensuring that the patient is prepared mentally and physically for the test and that the equipment is set up properly. When performing electrocardiography, the medical assistant must be able to recognize problems with the recording and make appropriate corrections so that the provider has a clear record of the patient's cardiac activity. The goal is to obtain the most accurate ECG possible.

History of Electrocardiography

Dutch physiologist Willem Einthoven developed techniques to record the electrical activity of the heart in the late 1800s. He called this recording an Electro Kardio Gramm; hence the acronym EKG. Many physicians and other healthcare providers still call the recording an EKG, although the newer, preferred term for an electrocardiogram is ECG.

THE ELECTRICAL CONDUCTION SYSTEM OF THE HEART

The Cardiac Cycle

The cardiac cycle includes all the events that occur in the heart during one single heartbeat. Each chamber of the heart goes through two phases during the cardiac cycle: **systole** and **diastole**. During systole, both the **atria** and the **ventricles** contract and empty of blood. During diastole, the relaxation phase of the heart, the chambers refill with blood. Venous blood from the inferior and superior venae cavae empties into the right atrium during atrial diastole. As the right atrium fills, increased pressure in the chamber causes the tricuspid valve to open, and the right ventricle begins to fill. At the same time, blood returning from the lungs via the pulmonary veins fills the left atrium, causing the mitral valve, or bicuspid valve, to open, emptying blood into the left ventricle. Before systole occurs, the ventricles are already 70% filled. The cardiac cycle for a healthy adult lasts approximately 0.8 second. However, the amount of time it takes for the heart to empty and refill depends on many factors, including the condition of the myocardium and the heart's electrical system.

The electrocardiograph records both the intensity of the electrical impulses and the actual time it takes for each part of the cardiac cycle to occur. It measures the electrical conductive impulses of the heart muscle, allowing the provider to see any disturbances or disruptions in normal heart activity. In addition to being recorded as an ECG, the cardiac cycle can appear as a continuously moving pattern on a monitor screen, accompanied by a sound for each beat.

The specialized electrical conduction system of the heart (Figure 42-2) initiates each heartbeat. The main part of this system is the **sinoatrial (SA) node**, which is located in the upper back wall of the

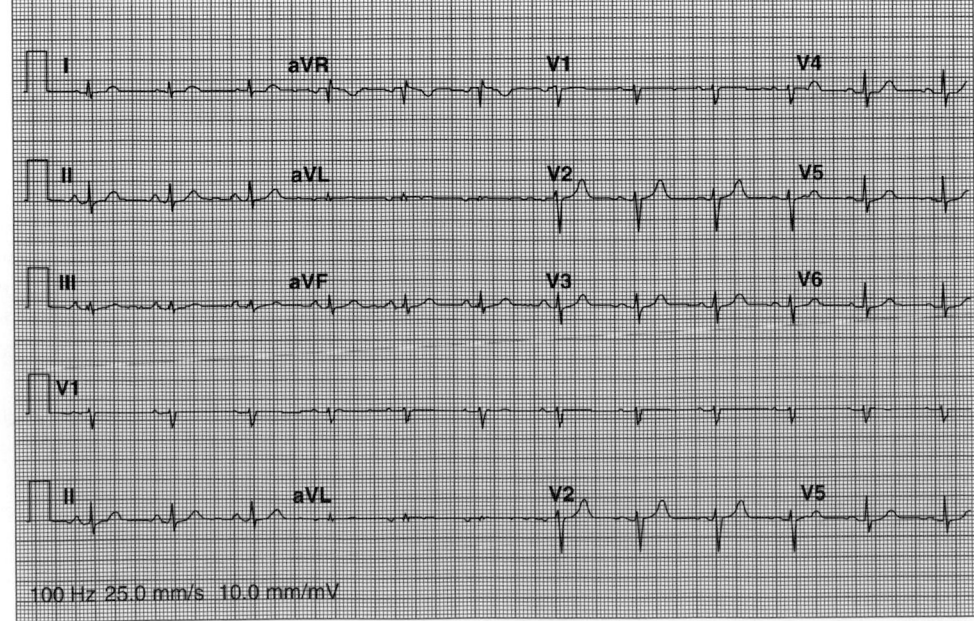

Female	Caucasian	Vent. rate	77 bpm	Normal sinus rhythm
		PR interval	156 ms	Normal ECG
Room:		QRS duration	80 ms	
Loc:		QT/QTc	356/402 ms	
		P-R-T axes	73 56 60	

100 Hz 25.0 mm/s 10.0 mm/mV

FIGURE 42-1 Example of a 12-lead ECG. (Phalen T, Aehlert BJ: *The 12-lead ECG in acute coronary syndromes,* ed 3, St Louis, 2012, Mosby.)

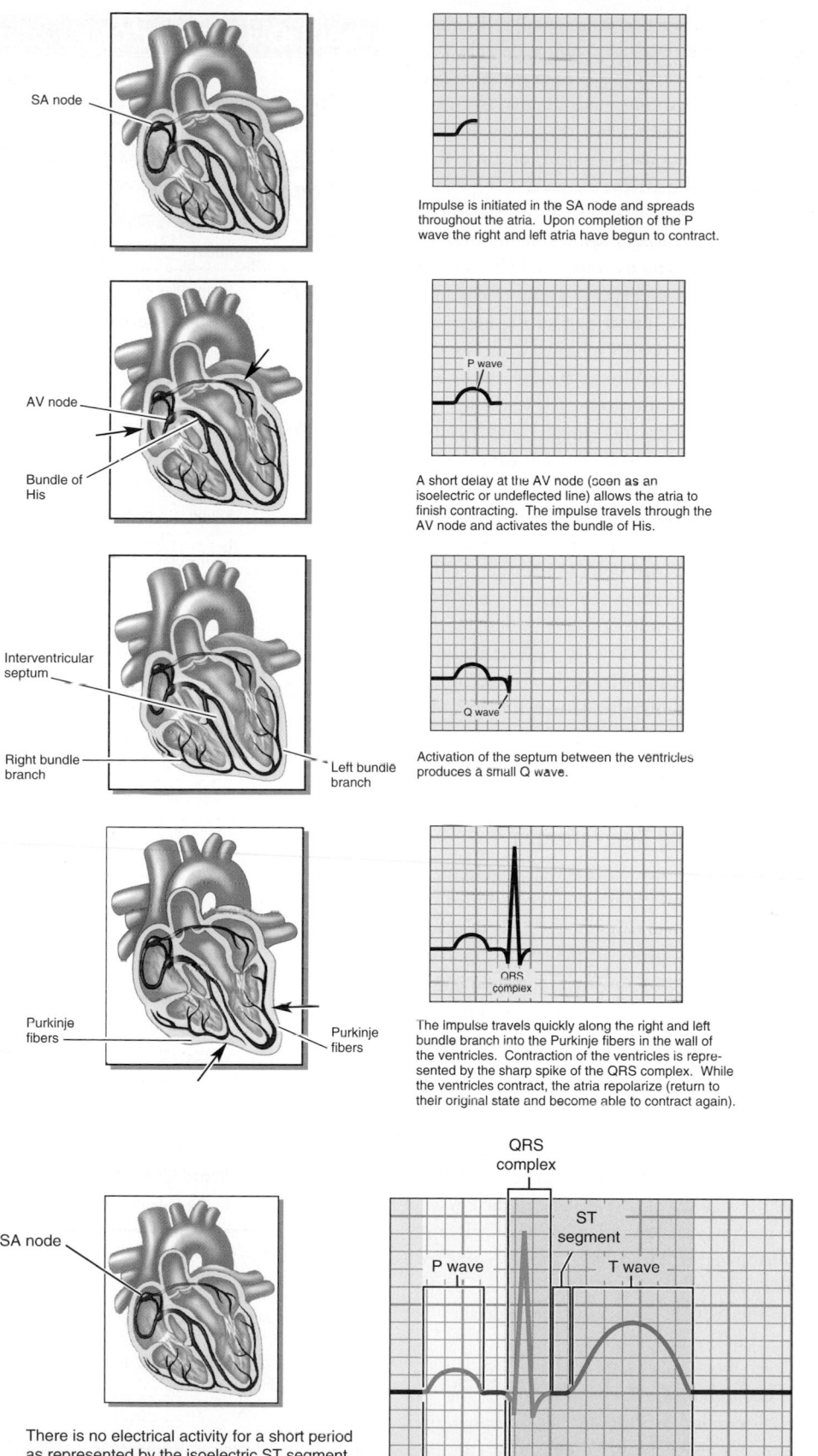

Impulse is initiated in the SA node and spreads throughout the atria. Upon completion of the P wave the right and left atria have begun to contract.

A short delay at the AV node (seen as an isoelectric or undeflected line) allows the atria to finish contracting. The impulse travels through the AV node and activates the bundle of His.

Activation of the septum between the ventricles produces a small Q wave.

The impulse travels quickly along the right and left bundle branch into the Purkinje fibers in the wall of the ventricles. Contraction of the ventricles is represented by the sharp spike of the QRS complex. While the ventricles contract, the atria repolarize (return to their original state and become able to contract again).

There is no electrical activity for a short period as represented by the isoelectric ST segment. Repolarization of the ventricles produces the T wave.

FIGURE 42-2 Electrical conduction system of the heart. (From Hunt SA: *Saunders fundamentals of medical assisting*, revised reprint, Philadelphia, 2007, Saunders.)

right atrium at the junction of the superior vena cava and the right atrium. The SA node controls the rate of heart contractions by initiating electrical impulses 60 to 100 times per minute. Each cardiac cycle, or heartbeat, starts with the SA node generating an electrical impulse that travels in a wavelike pattern across the cardiac muscle of the atria, causing them to contract almost simultaneously. This electrical impulse then stimulates the **atrioventricular (AV) node**, which is located in the posterior, superior portion of the right atrial septal wall, directly behind the tricuspid valve. A slight delay in conduction at this point allows the atria to empty completely. The electrical impulse then is transmitted to a special group of conduction fibers, the **bundle of His**, in the upper part of the interventricular septal wall. The bundle of His divides into two branches; the right bundle branch carries electrical impulses to the right ventricle, and the left bundle branch carries impulses to the left ventricle. The right and left bundle branches divide into smaller and smaller branches, ending in the Purkinje fibers, which spread across the apex of the heart and through the myocardium, stimulating ventricular contraction. The ventricles contract in a twisting sort of action, forcing the blood out of the chambers and into the pulmonary artery on the right side of the heart and the aorta on the left side.

Normal sinus rhythm (NSR) refers to a regular heart rate that falls within the average range of 60 to 100 beats per minute (beats/min). Sinus bradycardia is a heart rate below 60 beats/min; sinus tachycardia is a rate above 100 beats/min. In both of these conditions, the rhythm remains even, but the rate can be a problem. An irregular cardiac rhythm is called an *arrhythmia*. Conditions that interrupt the conduction pathway, SA node to AV node to bundle of His to right and left bundle branches, can cause arrhythmias.

Polarization, Depolarization, and Repolarization

Polarization is the resting state of the **myocardial** wall; no electrical activity occurs in the heart during this phase, which is recorded on the ECG strip as a flatline. In this state the myocardial cells are ready for stimulation. When the electrical system of the heart stimulates myocardial cells, depolarization occurs, resulting in the contraction of the stimulated heart muscle. After depolarization the heart muscle cells must return to a resting state before they can be electrically stimulated again. The process of reaching this resting state is called *repolarization*.

The electrocardiograph records a series of waves, or deflections, above or below a baseline on the ECG paper. Each deflection corresponds to a particular part of the cardiac cycle (Table 42-1). The normal ECG cycle consists of waveforms that are labeled the P wave, the Q wave, the R wave, the S wave, and the T wave. The Q, R, and S waves usually are grouped together; this is called the *QRS complex*. One entire cardiac cycle can be called the *PQRST complex*. In the next section, each part of the ECG is discussed in more detail.

PQRST Complex

The *P wave* signifies the beginning of atrial depolarization. The SA node initiates the electrical impulse, which then moves through the myocardial cells in the atria. Immediately after the electrical stimulation, the cells start to contract, causing the atrial chambers to contract. The P wave is the first deflection from the baseline; it typically is smooth and rounded, and one P wave should occur before each QRS complex. Atrial repolarization is not recorded on the ECG strip

TABLE 42-1	**Cardiac Cycle**	
STAGE	**HEART ACTIVITY**	**ELECTRICAL CURRENT**
P wave*	Atrial contraction	Atrial depolarization
PR interval†	Contraction traversing the atrioventricular (AV) node	Depolarization traversing the AV node
QRS complex‡	Ventricular contraction; electrical stimulation travels from the AV node to the Purkinje fibers	Ventricular depolarization and atrial repolarization
ST segment	Time interval between ventricular contraction and the beginning of ventricular recovery	Time interval between ventricular depolarization and ventricular repolarization
T wave	Ventricular contraction subsides	Ventricular repolarization (electrical recovery); atrial polarization begins
U wave (not always present)	Associated with further ventricular relaxation	Purkinje fibers repolarization
Baseline§	The heart at rest	Ventricular and atrial polarization
PR interval	Time interval between atrial contraction and ventricular contraction; electrical stimulation travels from the SA to the AV nodes	Time interval between atrial depolarization and ventricular depolarization
QT interval	Time interval between the beginning of ventricular contraction and the subsiding of ventricular contraction; electrical stimulation travels from the AV node to the Purkinje fibers	Time interval between the beginning of ventricular depolarization and ventricular repolarization (electrical recovery)

*Wave: A uniformly advancing deflection (upward or downward) from a baseline on a recording.
†Interval: The period of time between two different electrocardiographic events.
‡Complex: The portion of the ECG tracing that represents the sum of three waves (contraction of the ventricles).
§Baseline: A neutral line against which waves are valued as they deflect upward (positive) or downward (negative) from the line.

because its electrical impulse is small and hidden in the QRS complex. When the electrical impulse reaches the AV node, there is a pause in electrical activity. This lack of electrical impulse creates the PR segment, which is a return to baseline. This pause allows the atrial chambers to finish contracting and completely empty.

The electrical impulse then moves from the AV node through the Bundle of His and into the right and left bundle branches. This depolarization of the interventricular septum creates the Q wave, a downward deflection and the start of the QRS complex. As the electrical impulse moves from the bundle branches to the Purkinje fibers, the R wave and the S wave are created. As the ventricular tissue depolarizes, the chambers start to contract, moving the blood out of the heart.

Following the QRS complex, the ST segment is created from the electrical activity generated by the beginning of the repolarization of the ventricular chambers. An upright, slightly rounded asymmetrical wave called the T wave follows the ST segment. This wave is created from the electricity produced from the repolarization of the ventricular chambers. At this time, the atrial chambers are in the polarized state and will remain there until the next heartbeat.

After the T wave, a U wave may be present, though it is not very common. It is thought that the U wave reflects the repolarization of the Purkinje fibers. It can also be seen in patients with potassium imbalances. After the last wave (either T or U), the tracing is an isoelectric line until the next impulse from the SA node. Both chambers are polarized.

The ECG tracing can be divided into two intervals, the PR interval and the QT interval. The term interval reflects a period of time. The PR interval starts at the beginning of the P wave and finishes at the end of the PR segment. During this interval of time, atrial depolarization and contraction occur. The QT interval starts at the beginning of the Q wave and finishes at the end of the T wave. The electrical activities that occur in the heart and conduction system from the Q through the T wave are reflected during this interval.

By measuring the actual configuration and location of each wave in relation to the other waves and to the baseline, in addition to the intervals between waves and segments, the physician can detect rhythmic disturbances of the heart and identify different types of cardiac disorders.

THE ELECTROCARDIOGRAPH

Electrocardiograph machines (Figure 42-3) record 12 **leads** simultaneously and are also referred to as six-channel ECG machines. Four

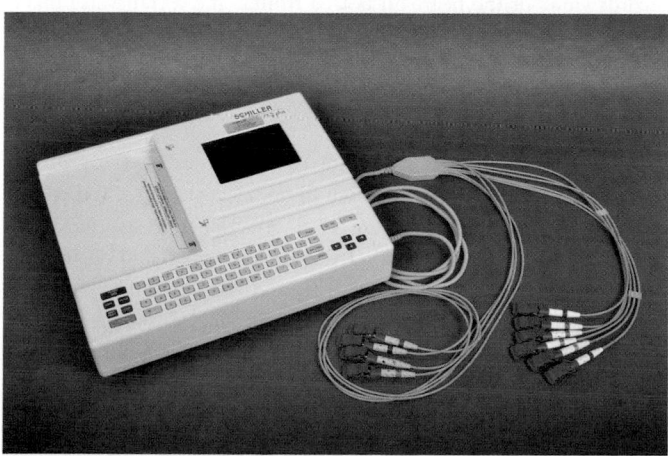

FIGURE 42-3 ECG machine.

limb and six chest electrodes must be placed on the patient at specific anatomic locations before the recording starts. When the ECG is started, the machine records all 12 leads automatically and marks each lead with identifying letters. These multichannel ECG tracings take seconds to perform and can be placed in the patient's health record without mounting, or they can be recorded directly into the patient's electronic health record.

Digital ECGs

Newer versions of ECG machines can be connected into the facility's electronic health record (EHR) system so that ECGs can be recorded directly into a patient's EHR. These machines include advanced technologic functions, such as the following:

- They enable a continuous view of 3-, 6-, and 12-leads of data on the machine's color display.
- They can store up to 300 ECG records.
- They reduce typing mistakes and save time by downloading patient information from the EHR system.
- They eliminate the need for scanning and filing.
- They can recognize and accommodate patients with pacemakers.
- They provide an interpretation of ECGs that considers the patient's gender, age, medication, and so on.
- They include communication tools (e.g., Ethernet), in addition to wireless and Bluetooth technology.
- They can connect with EHR systems to download patient demographics and orders, perform tests, and upload test results to patients' EHRs.

CRITICAL THINKING APPLICATION   42-1

Martha has not yet been taught how to use the ECG machine in Dr. Lee's office. What steps should she take to learn how to use this machine and to feel comfortable and confident using it to obtain ECGs?

Electrocardiograph Paper

Electrocardiograph paper is heat and pressure sensitive, which means that either heat or pressure can cause a mark to appear. The stylus on an ECG machine makes the image on the ECG paper. When the machine is on, the stylus becomes hot and burns a marking on the paper as it moves horizontally past the stylus. Because the paper is pressure sensitive, it must be handled carefully to prevent any additional markings that would blemish the tracing.

ECG paper is graph paper that has horizontal and vertical lines at 1-mm intervals. This is an agreed-on international standard that allows providers anywhere in the world to interpret a patient's ECG in the same manner. A medical assistant needs to know both the size and the meaning of each square on the ECG paper to understand its significance.

The horizontal axis represents time, and the vertical axis represents amplitude. Each small square measures 1 mm on each side. Every fifth line, both vertically and horizontally, is darker than the other lines and creates a larger square measuring 5 mm on each side.

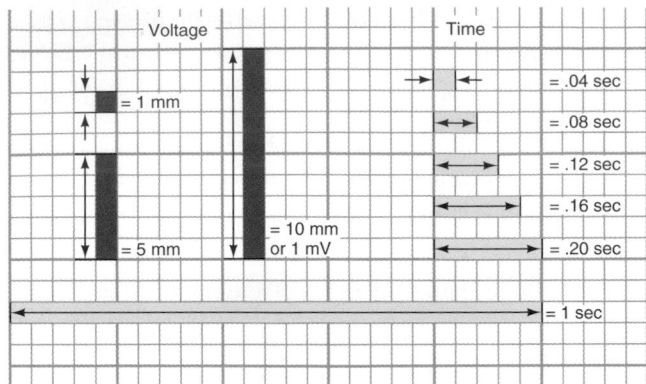

FIGURE 42-4 ECG paper.

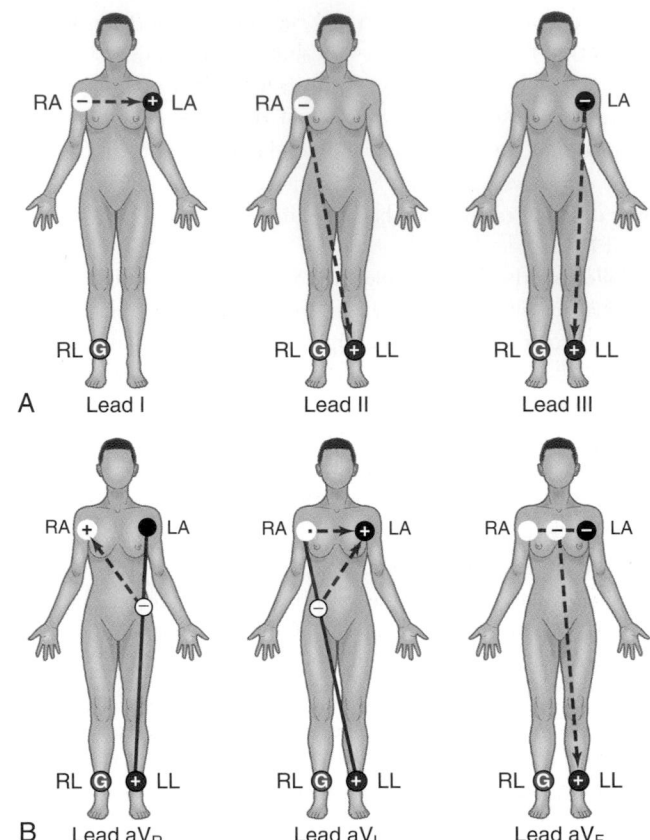

FIGURE 42-5 Standard **(A)** and augmented **(B)** limb leads.

When the electrocardiograph runs at normal speed, one small 1-mm square passes the stylus every 0.04 second, which means that one large 5-mm square passes the stylus every 0.2 second. Continuing this logic, in 1 second, five large squares pass the stylus. Therefore, five sequential large squares show the record of what occurred in the heart during a time span of 1 second (5 large squares × 0.2 second = 1 second). Another way to say this is that at normal speed, the ECG paper travels past the stylus at a rate of 25 mm per second (Figure 42-4).

The voltage, or strength, of the heartbeat also is recorded on the paper. Voltage can be displayed as either a positive or a negative deflection. One millivolt (mV) of electrical activity moves the stylus upward over 10 mm (two large squares). This is the standard normally used for obtaining an ECG, and it can be adjusted to match the strength of the electrical activity of the heart. The machine must be calibrated so that 1 mV of electrical activity produces a deflection that is 10 mm either above or below the baseline. When properly calibrated, the ECG records both the strength of the electrical activity of the heartbeat in millivolts and the speed of the heartbeat over time.

Electrodes and Lead Wires

Ten sensors, called *electrodes,* are placed on the patient's arms (two), legs (two), and chest (six) to pick up the electrical activity of the heart. Electrodes must be applied to specific locations to record the heart's electrical activity from different angles and planes. Ten color-coded and labeled lead wires that end in a small metal clip are attached to the electrodes. The lead wires carry the signal of the heart's electrical activity to the ECG machine. Single-use, self-stick, disposable electrodes, which contain a thin layer of a metallic substance that is a good conductor of electricity, are packaged with conductive jelly in the center. Skin is a poor conductor of electricity, so the conductive jelly serves as an electrolyte that enables the transfer of the electrical activity of the heart into the lead wires of the ECG machine. The electrodes will not work as efficiently if the conductive jelly is dried out, so they should not be used if the package's expiration date has passed.

The *lead wires* to the electrocardiograph carry the cardiac electrical impulses into the machine, where they are magnified by an amplifier. These amplified impulses are converted into mechanical action, which is recorded on the ECG paper by the stylus and/or

shown on a monitor. A single lead records the electrical activity of the heart between two different electrodes, one positive and one negative. The placement of the positive electrode determines the particular view of the heart recorded. If depolarization occurs toward the positive electrode, the deflection is upright; if it moves toward the negative electrode, the waveform is deflected downward. Each lead records the average electrical flow at a specific time in a specific location of the heart.

Lead Recordings

The standard ECG consists of 12 separate leads, or recordings of the electrical activity of the heart, from 12 different angles. The ECG records views of the heart on both a frontal and a transverse plane. The frontal leads include leads I, II, III, aV_R, aV_L, and aV_F. Transverse plane leads include the six precordial, or chest, leads (V_1 to V_6).

Standard Leads

The first three leads recorded are called the *standard* or *bipolar leads* because they each use two limb electrodes to record the heart's electrical activity (Figure 42-5, *A*). The right arm electrode is the negative pole, and the left leg or left arm electrodes are the positive poles. Roman numerals I, II, and III are used to designate these leads.

- Lead I records tracings between the right arm and left arm, recording the electrical activity of the lateral part of the left ventricle.
- Lead II records tracings between the right arm and left leg, recording the electrical activity of the inferior surface of the

left ventricle; this is the lead recorded on a cardiac monitor or on the rhythm strip at the bottom of the 12-lead ECG.

- Lead III records tracings between the left arm and left leg, which reflects the electrical activity of the inferior surface of the left ventricle.

Augmented Leads

The next three leads are the augmented, or combined, leads (Figure 42-5, *B*). These are designated augmented voltage right arm (aV_R), augmented voltage left arm (aV_L), and augmented voltage left leg (aV_F). Because the electrical activity recorded by these leads is relatively small, the ECG machine amplifies (or augments) the electrical potential when recorded. These are all unipolar leads with a single positive electrode that uses the right leg for grounding.

- aV_R records the electrical activity of the atria from the right shoulder; P waves and QRS complexes are deflected below the baseline.
- aV_L records the electrical activity of the lateral wall of the left ventricle from the left shoulder.
- aV_F records the electrical activity of the inferior surface of the left ventricle from the left leg.

Precordial Leads

The precordial, or chest, leads are unipolar and provide a transverse plane view of the heart. They are designated V_1, V_2, V_3, V_4, V_5, and V_6. The V means chest, and each of the numbers represents a specific location on the chest. The QRS complex shows as a negative deflection in V_1 and V_2, and views with each subsequent lead become more positive. Precordial leads measure the electrical activity among six specific points on the chest wall and a point within the heart (Figure 42-6). It is important to avoid placing electrodes directly over a bony prominence.

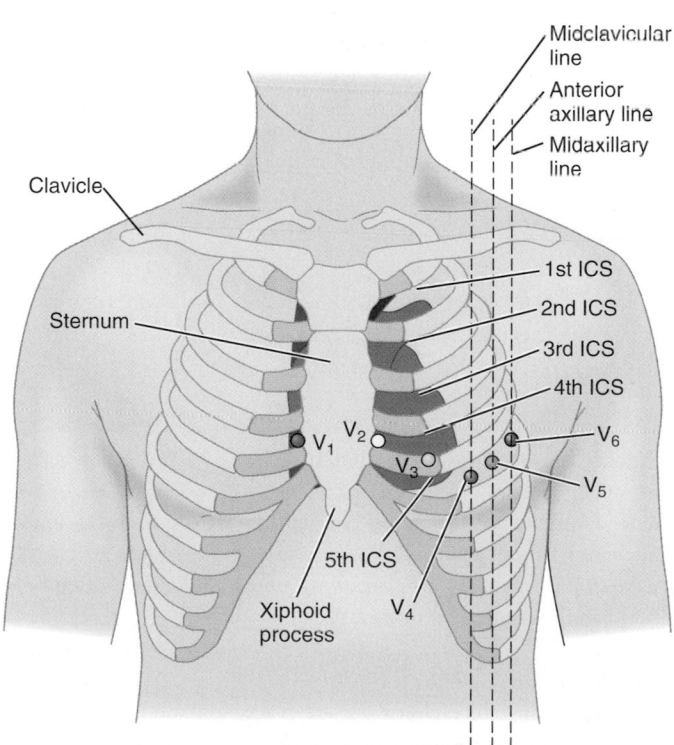

FIGURE 42-6 Chest leads. *ICS,* Intercostal space.

V_1	Placed in the fourth intercostal space, just to the right of the sternum
V_2	Placed in the fourth intercostal space, just to the left of the sternum
V_3	Placed midway between V_2 and V_4
V_4	Placed in the fifth intercostal space, at the left midclavicular line
V_5	Placed horizontal to V_4 in the left anterior axillary line
V_6	Placed horizontal to V_4 in the left midaxillary line

CRITICAL THINKING APPLICATION   **42-2**

Dr. Lee has asked Martha to perform her first ECG on a patient who just came into the office. Martha is not confident that she knows how to place the chest leads properly in the correct locations. How should she handle this situation? Should she perform the ECG procedure as best she can? Why or why not?

PERFORMING ELECTROCARDIOGRAPHY

Preparation of the Room and Patient

The room should be in the quietest location in the office and should be as far as possible from all other electrical equipment, including x-ray machines, diathermy devices, laboratory equipment, centrifuges, fans, refrigerators, and air conditioners. The room should be warm and should have adjustable lighting.

The treatment table should be comfortable and wide enough to provide full support for the patient. The table should be wood or should have an electrically insulated surface. Position the table so that you can work from the side of the patient that is most comfortable for you. Electrocardiographers most often work on the patient's left side, but as long as the electrodes are placed in the proper position, it really makes no difference which side you use.

Small pillows can help the patient relax and provide maximum comfort during the procedure. Offer a pillow for the head and one for under the knees. If a head pillow is used, it should not elevate the patient's shoulders.

The patient should disrobe to the waist and put on the patient gown with the opening in the front; easy access to the patient's extremities must be available. Pantyhose must be removed.

Place the patient in a supine position with the arms comfortably at the sides and the legs not touching one another. If the patient has dyspnea or orthopnea, a semi-Fowler's position should be used, or the patient can be seated on a wooden chair. However, make sure you check with the provider before obtaining an ECG in an alternative position. If a seated position is used, the patient's feet must rest comfortably on the floor or on a footstool. Note any alternative position on the ECG recording.

The patient should empty his or her bladder if needed to help with comfort and relaxation during the procedure. This will help prevent artifacts during the tracing. Check to see whether the patient followed all the instructions provided in Figure 42-7. Record the patient's vital signs and current medications on his or her health record. This information can be programmed into some ECG machines

INSTRUCTIONS FOR PATIENT BEFORE AN ELECTROCARDIOGRAM

Name: _____

Your cardiogram appointment is _____ , _____ at _____ AM / PM
                                   Day   Date   Time

These instructions are simple, but it is important that you follow them. Please call us if you are unable to follow these instructions or keep your appointment so we may make another appointment.

1. There is no discomfort or sensation in having an electrocardiogram. No electricity is put into the patient in any way. Small disposable electrodes are placed on the calf of each leg and on each arm and at different places on the chest. The minute impulse generated by your heart is simply picked up by these electrodes and recorded by the machine.

2. You will be asked to lie down on a comfortable table while the test is being performed by the technician.

3. For your convenience, it is best to wear loose clothing. You will be asked to disrobe to your waist to expose the chest. It will also be necessary to expose your lower legs from the knees down and the upper arms just below the shoulders.

4. The actual test only takes about 5 minutes, but you will be asked to rest for about one-half hour before the test. It is best you do not have a heavy meal for about 2 hours before the test. You should not consume any cold drinks or ice cream or smoke just before the test. It is also advisable to refrain from excessive exercise just before the test. Do not take any medications without the physician's usual instructions and knowledge.

5. During the test, you will be asked to lie absolutely still and relax, because the slightest movement interferes with an accurate tracing. Do not talk.

6. The skin on the legs, arms, and chest must be free from skin ointments, oils, and medications.

7. The technician taking the test is specially trained to perform the test but is unable to tell you the results of the test, because he or she is neither trained nor authorized to make any interpretations of the cardiogram. This is the task of the physician.

FIGURE 42-7 ECG patient instructions.

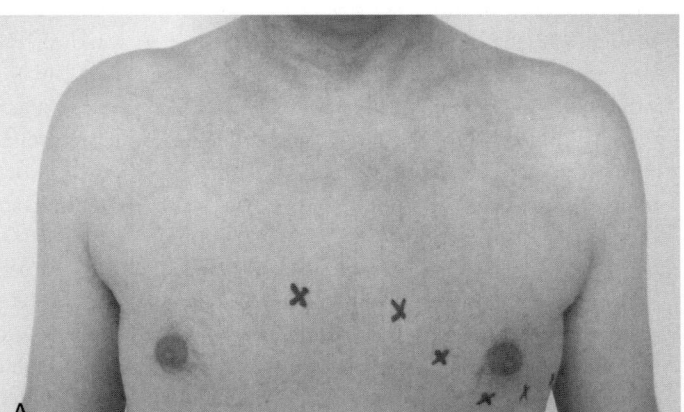
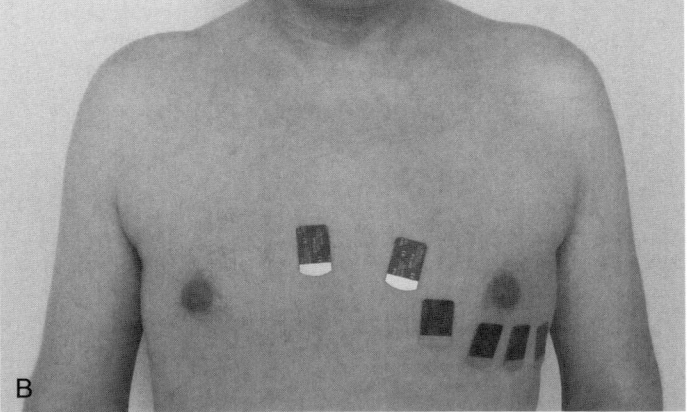

FIGURE 42-8 Chest lead locations. (Thompson P: *Coronary care manual,* ed 2, Australia, 2010, Churchill Livingstone.)

and automatically printed on the ECG recording; if a digital electrocardiograph is used, the information can be recorded directly into the patient's electronic health record (EHR). If the facility where you work does not have a digital machine, then part of your responsibility is to scan the ECG recording into the patient's EHR.

Explain to the patient the nature and purpose of the ECG. Attempt to answer all questions and make the patient as comfortable as possible during the procedure. Stress the importance of not moving during the entire procedure, and assure the patient that there is no danger of shock. Soften the lighting in the room to obtain maximum patient comfort. When you tell the patient to lie still, make sure that he or she is breathing normally. Patients often hold their breath when asked to lie still.

Attaching Leads to the Patient

Disposable, single-use electrodes are placed on the patient's limbs and chest in very specific locations (Figure 42-8). The lead wires from the machine then are connected to the electrodes. Specific lead

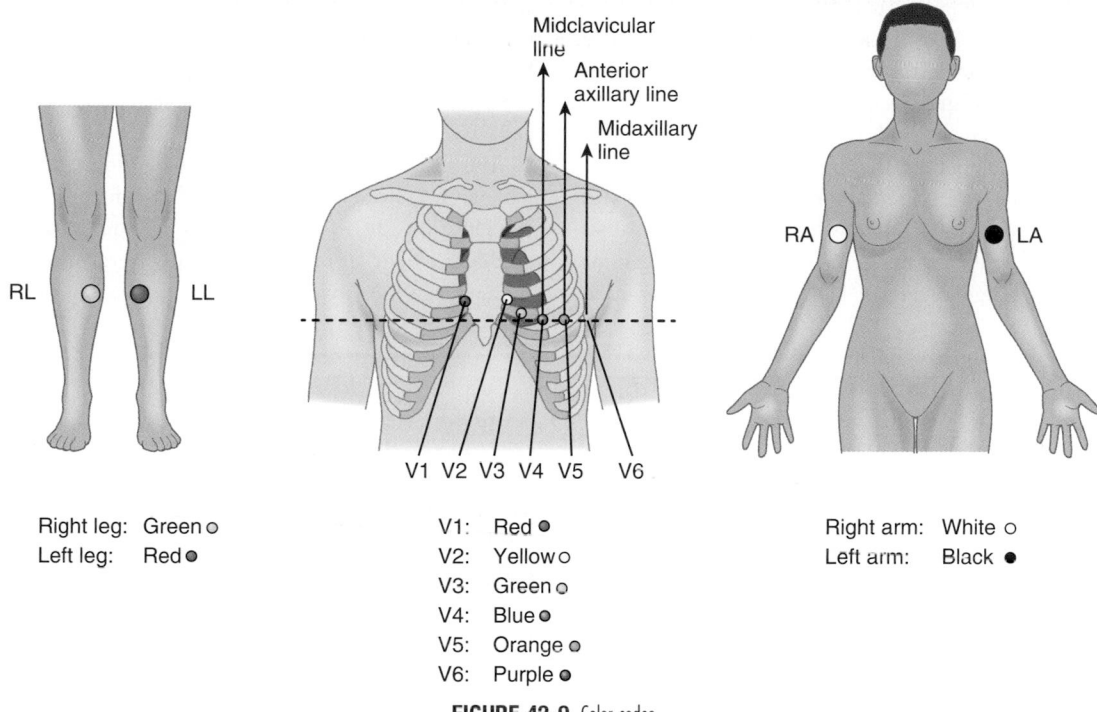

Midclavicular line
Anterior axillary line
Midaxillary line

RA   LA

RL   LL

V1 V2 V3 V4 V5   V6

Right leg: Green ○
Left leg: Red ●

V1: Red ●
V2: Yellow ○
V3: Green ○
V4: Blue ●
V5: Orange ○
V6: Purple ●

Right arm: White ○
Left arm: Black ●

FIGURE 42-9 Color codes.

markings or color coding on the end of each lead wire help ensure that the proper connections are made (Figure 42-9). The leads are attached as follows:

LEAD	ATTACH TO ELECTRODE ON:
RA	Fleshy part of patient's right upper arm
LA	Fleshy part of patient's left upper arm
RL	Fleshy part of patient's right lower leg
LL	Fleshy part of patient's left lower leg

The labeled lead wires then are placed on each precordial electrode.

Special Considerations. If the patient has had a limb amputated, the electrodes are placed above the amputation site. The leg electrodes should be placed on the thighs. With an arm amputation, the electrodes should be placed on the upper arm if it is intact or on the shoulders. The opposite extremity electrode should be in the same location. For people with the heart on the right side, the electrodes are placed in the same locations *except* that those on the left side are placed on the right side, and those on the right are placed on the left. Electrodes should not be placed over a new surgical incision. Place the electrode near the location, but not on the incision. Any changes to electrode placement must be documented on the ECG.

CRITICAL THINKING APPLICATION   **42-3**

Two weeks later, after Martha feels much more confident in her skills for electrode placement and recording an ECG, a new patient, Mr. Sonderford, comes to the office complaining of mild chest pain that he noted when he got out of bed this morning. What concerns might Martha have about Mr. Sonderford? His vital signs are: P 104 weak and irregular; R 24 and quite shallow. Mr. Sonderford is sweating profusely. What should Martha do? Why?

Recording the Electrocardiogram

Procedure 42-1 explains how to record an ECG. It is important that you become familiar with the type of machine used in your practice. Machines vary according to the age and make of the model, but most electrocardiographs currently in use perform standardization functions and labeling automatically. You may have the option of entering specific information about the patient, such as age, gender, prescriptions, and so on. Follow office protocol when performing the procedure. After the machine has been programmed, remind the patient to lie still, and then press the appropriate key to run the ECG strip. Six-channel machines print and label all 12 leads, with a rhythm strip across the bottom of the paper in lead II, in a matter of seconds. Review the printout for clarity, and if it is acceptable, give the recording to the provider for review. If your facility uses a digital electrocardiograph, the ECG is automatically downloaded into the patient's EHR. If a printed ECG is recorded, it may be the medical assistant's responsibility to scan and download the graph into the patient's EHR. Once the provider has approved the ECG and/or the recording is in the patient's EHR, remove the leads and electrodes from the patient, help the person into a sitting position, and provide assistance in getting off the table and dressing if necessary.

Standardization, Sensitivity, and Speed

Standardization has been determined by international agreement so that an ECG can be interpreted in the same way anywhere in the world. This requires the electrocardiograph to be calibrated according to universal measurements. Each time you record an ECG, you must make sure the machine is correctly standardized.

When a machine is in standard mode or set at 1 STD, 1 mV of electricity causes the stylus to move vertically 10 mm, or two large squares. When the machine has been properly set in this way, electrical voltages can be calculated by measuring the vertical movement of the stylus on the paper. The stylus should deflect exactly 10 mm when the standardization button is depressed with a quick pecking motion. The recording of the standardization would be 2 mm wide and rectangular. Each manufacturer's manual explains the exact method of adjustment to obtain a perfect standardization. Most machines have three sensitivity standards that can be selected: ½ STD, which deflects the stylus 5 mm, or one large square; 1 STD, which deflects the stylus 10 mm, or two large squares; and 2 STD, which deflects the stylus 20 mm or four large squares. The appropriate standard is selected as follows: If the QRS complex is too tall and is causing the stylus to move off the paper, the STD should be set to ½ STD. If the QRS complex is too short, the STD should be set to 2 STD. Figure 42-10 shows the three sensitivity standards as they appear when recorded on the ECG paper.

The usual speed for an ECG recording is 25 mm/sec. If the patient's heart rate is very rapid or if certain parts of the complex are too close together, the paper may need to be adjusted to run at double speed, or 50 mm/sec. This extends the recording to twice the normal length. Any change in the speed must be noted on the ECG.

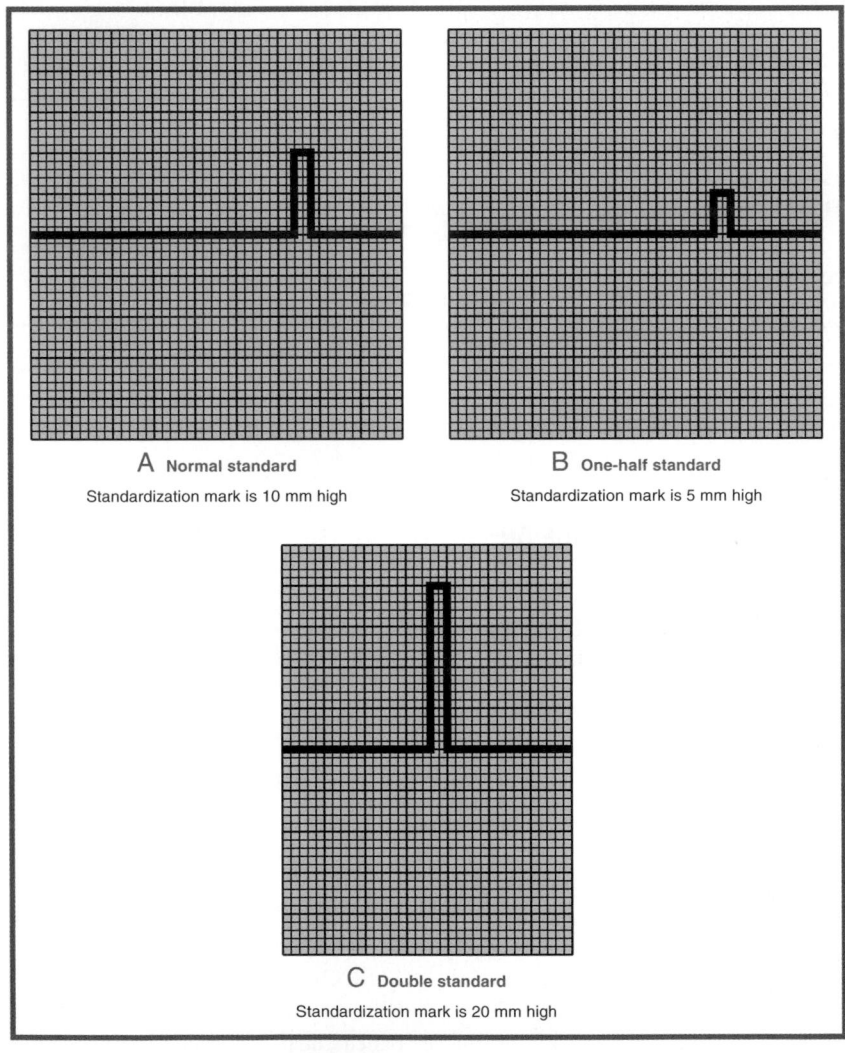

A **Normal standard**
Standardization mark is 10 mm high

B **One-half standard**
Standardization mark is 5 mm high

C **Double standard**
Standardization mark is 20 mm high

FIGURE 42-10 Sensitivity standards.

PROCEDURE 42-1   Perform Electrocardiography: Obtain a 12-Lead ECG

Goal: *To obtain an accurate, artifact-free recording of the electrical activity of the heart.*

EQUIPMENT and SUPPLIES

- Patient's health record
- Three-channel electrocardiograph with patient lead cable and labeled lead wires
- 10 disposable, self-adhesive electrodes
- Patient gown and drape
- Disposable alcohol wipes
- Disposable razor
- Sharps container

PROCEDURE 42-1 *—continued*

PROCEDURAL STEPS

1. Perform the ECG in a quiet examination room away from electrical equipment to avoid artifacts.
2. Sanitize your hands.
   PURPOSE: To ensure infection control.
3. Greet the patient, confirm identity by name and date of birth, and explain the procedure.
   PURPOSE: To alleviate apprehension and gain the patient's cooperation.
4. Ask the patient to disrobe to the waist (including the bra for women) and remove belts, jewelry, socks, stockings, or pantyhose as necessary; have the patient put the exam gown on so that it opens in the front. Provide the patient with privacy while he or she prepares.
   PURPOSE: Electrodes must be applied to bare skin without interference from clothing.
5. Position the patient supine on the examination table and drape appropriately. The table should support the patient's arms and legs.
   PURPOSE: To ensure the patient's modesty and comfort and the accuracy of the recording. Limb support is needed to prevent muscle artifacts.
6. Turn on the machine and enter the patient's demographic information, including name, age, date, time, current medications, and identification number, if this system is used at your facility. If you are using a digital ECG machine, you can download this information onto the ECG recording directly from the patient's EHR.
   PURPOSE: To identify the ECG recording properly.
7. At each location where an electrode will be placed, clean the skin with an alcohol wipe. If the areas are extremely hairy and the electrodes cannot be completely attached to the skin, it may be necessary to shave the areas of electrode attachment.
   PURPOSE: To obtain good electrode adhesion to the skin.
8. After the alcohol has completely dried, apply the self-adhesive electrodes to clean, dry, fleshy areas of the four extremities. The leg electrodes are placed with the tabs facing toward the abdomen on the fleshy part of the calves and the tabs facing down on the inner aspect of the upper arms. The 10 electrodes needed for the procedure are packaged on a card in a multipack, foil-lined envelope. Reseal the envelope after removing the card to prevent the electrolyte gel on the other electrodes from drying out. Apply the self-adhesive electrodes to the clean areas on the chest with the tabs downward. It is important to avoid placing electrodes directly over a bony prominence. Apply the electrodes as follows (Figure 1):
   V_1—fourth intercostal space, just to the right of the sternum.
   V_2—fourth intercostal space, just to the left of the sternum.
   V_3—midway between V_2 and V_4.
   V_4—fifth intercostal space, at the left midclavicular line.
   V_5—horizontal to V_4 in the left anterior axillary line.
   V_6—horizontal to V_4 in the left midaxillary line.

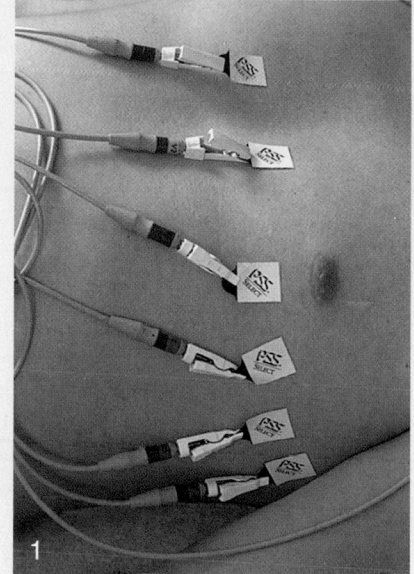

9. Carefully connect the lead wires to the correct electrode with the alligator clips on the end of each lead. The lead wires are color coded and have abbreviations on each clip to match the electrode location. The lead wires should follow the body's contour. Make sure the lead wires are not crossed (Figure 2).
   PURPOSE: To prevent artifacts.

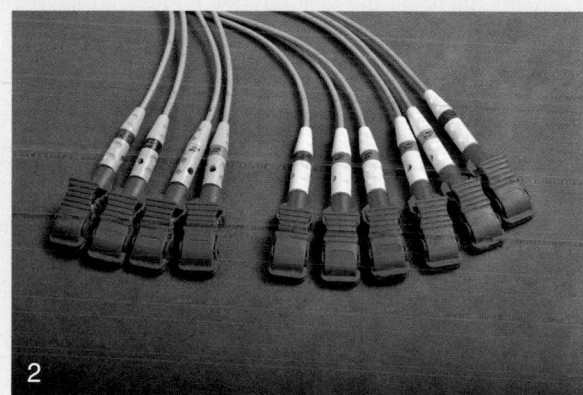

10. Remind the patient to remain still, breathe normally, and not to talk during the recording.
    PURPOSE: To prevent artifacts.
11. Press the AUTO button on the machine and run the ECG tracing. The machine automatically places the standardization at the beginning, and the 12 leads then follow in the three-channel matrix with a lead II rhythm strip across the bottom of the page.
12. Watch for artifacts during the recording. If artifacts are present, make appropriate corrections and repeat the recording to get a clean reading.
13. Remove the lead wires from the electrodes and then remove the electrodes. If the razor was used, dispose of it in the sharps container. Sanitize your hands.
14. Assist the patient with getting dressed as needed. Clean the ECG machine and return it to its storage area.

PROCEDURE 42-1   —continued

15. If a digital machine is used, the ECG recording will be automatically added to the patient's EHR. If not, place the printed recording with the patient's health record for the provider to review. The medical assistant may have to scan the document into the patient's EHR.
16. Document the procedure in the patient's health record.

PURPOSE: Procedures are not considered done until they are documented in the patient's health record.

9/22/20— 3:10 PM: 12-lead ECG recorded per Dr. Lee order without incident. Martha Reyes, CMA (AAMA)

The ECG Tracing and the Health Record

ECG tracings usually are retained in health records for many years to provide a history of the patient's cardiac activity. Paper graphs are typically scanned and downloaded into the patient's EHR. However, if your facility still files paper copies, remember that the ECG paper is both heat, light, and pressure sensitive. Paper clips and staples cannot be used because they scratch and mark a tracing. A single photocopy of the ECG can be made without damaging the original. Many offices routinely put a photocopy in the patient's paper health record because it is less likely to be damaged by handling. If the practice has electronic health records, the tracing is scanned into the patient's electronic record or recorded directly into the patient's EHR.

Regardless of the particular method used, each ECG should be labeled with the following information:
- Patient's full name and identification number if this system is used in the facility
- Gender
- Age
- Date and time of ECG
- List of all medications and/or supplements the patient takes
- Adaptations from normal sensitivity and normal speed

Additional notations should be recorded for any variation from the routine, such as the following:
- Very nervous or anxious patient
- Lack of rest before the test
- Smoking immediately before the test
- Failure to follow any pretest instructions

Interpretive Electrocardiographs

Interpretive electrocardiographs are equipped with a computer that analyzes the recording as it is being run. With this capability, immediate information on the heart's activity is available, which can be valuable for reaching an early diagnosis and initiating immediate treatment. Patient baseline data must be entered into the computer before the ECG is recorded. The computer analysis of the ECG and the reason for each interpretation are then printed on the top of the recording or downloaded directly into the patient's EHR.

Artifacts

An artifact is an unwanted, erratic movement of the stylus on the paper caused by outside interference. The electrocardiograph is extremely sensitive to any kind of nearby electrical activity. Electrical artifacts on the tracing make accurate interpretation of the ECG

difficult. The medical assistant should have a thorough understanding of the causes of and remedies for these artifacts. The main types of artifacts are wandering baseline, somatic tremor, alternating current (AC) interference, and interrupted baseline.

Wandering Baseline

With a wandering baseline, the stylus gradually shifts away from the center of the paper. This usually happens because of slight movement of the patient during the tracing or poor electrode attachment (Figure 42-11). A wandering baseline is resolved by reminding the patient to remain as still as possible; this can be facilitated by keeping the patient comfortable. Make sure electrodes are securely and completely attached to each specific site to eliminate this artifact.

Somatic Tremor

The term *somatic tremor* means muscle movement. Any muscle movement, including movement of skeletal muscle, produces a measurable electrical impulse. This additional input causes unwanted stylus movement during the tracing; this shows up on the recording as jagged peaks of irregular height and spacing with a shifting baseline (Figure 42-12). The most common causes include patient discomfort, apprehension, movement, talking, or a condition that causes uncontrollable body tremors. A patient with uncontrolled tremors must be as calm and comfortable as possible to minimize

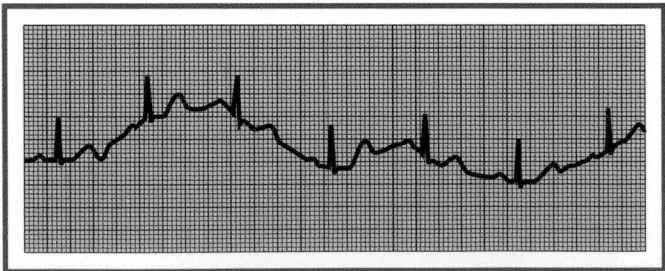

FIGURE 42-11 Wandering baseline.

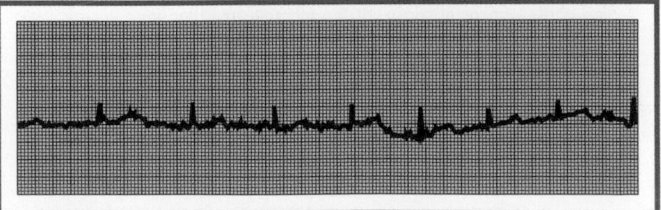

FIGURE 42-12 Somatic tremor.

the somatic tremor artifact. The other causes all can be resolved after they have been identified correctly.

Alternating Current Interference

AC interference appears as a series of uniform small spikes on the paper (Figure 42-13). Electrical currents in nearby equipment or wiring can leak small amounts of electrical energy into the area where the ECG machine is located. The electrocardiograph can pick up this additional electrical energy signal. This can be minimized by making sure the machine is plugged into a three-pronged, grounded outlet; keeping lead wires uncrossed; unplugging other electrical appliances in the room; moving the table away from the wall; and perhaps even turning off overhead fluorescent lights. If all these measures fail, you may need to move to another examination room for the procedure. The last step is to call the manufacturer or your local service representative.

Interrupted Baseline

Baseline interruption occurs when the electrical connection has been interrupted. The stylus moves onto the margin of the paper erratically (Figure 42-14). It moves violently up and down across the paper, or it may record a straight line across the top or bottom of the paper. If the electrodes are dislodged, an interrupted baseline occurs. This cause is virtually eliminated by making sure the electrodes are properly attached to the skin. Other causes include a broken cable wire and cable tips that are attached too loosely or become separated from any electrode.

CRITICAL THINKING APPLICATION   42-4

Dr. Lee asks Martha to explain the causes of artifacts and the methods for correcting ECG recordings that show outside interference. Based on what you have learned about ECG artifacts, what are the typical causes and how would you recommend correcting each?

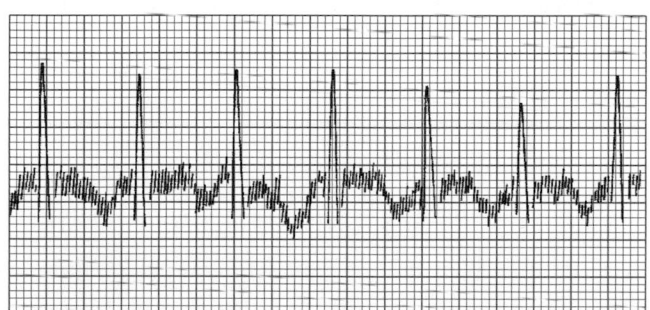

FIGURE 42-13 Sixty-cycle interference. (From Urden L, Stacy K, Lough M: *Thelan's critical care nursing: diagnosis and management*, ed 7, St Louis, 2014, Mosby.)

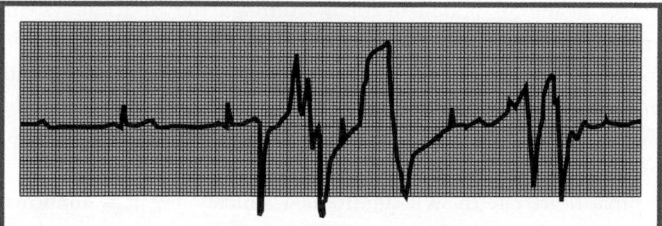

FIGURE 42-14 Interrupted baseline.

THE ECG STRIP

The medical assistant working in a cardiovascular practice must be able to recognize rhythm abnormalities that may appear on the tracing. Alerting the provider to the presence of an arrhythmia while the patient is still connected to the machine may give the provider the opportunity to observe the patient while the machine is running or immediately institute some type of therapeutic or prophylactic intervention. The provider can determine two important heart functions when interpreting the ECG: heart rate and heart rhythm.

Normal Appearance of ECG Complexes

When you examine the ECG recording, first look at the characteristics of each of the waves in the recording (Table 42-2). Are the P waves, QRS complexes, and T waves clearly present? Do they have a consistent appearance, and do they occur at regular intervals? Are any odd beats present that do not fit in with the others? Is the rate normal, fast, or slow? Is the rhythm regular or irregular?

In NSR (see Figure 42-1), each beat of the heart is initiated by an impulse from the SA node that travels without interruption along the normal conduction pathway of the heart. In NSR each beat on the ECG shows a P wave followed by a QRS complex.

Rate

To calculate the heart rate from the ECG recording, count the number of P waves in a 6-second strip (30 large squares) and multiply by 10. In the same manner, you can count the number of P waves in a 3-second strip (15 large squares) and multiply by 20. To get the number of ventricular contractions in 1 minute, you can count the number of complete QRS complexes that occur within 6 seconds and multiply that number by 10.

The heart rate also can be calculated by counting the number of small squares between two R waves and then dividing that number into 1,500 (1 minute on an ECG strip passes 1,500 small boxes). When the number of boxes from one cardiac event to the next same event is divided into 1,500, the result is the patient's heart rate. You can use Figure 42-1 to practice these techniques.

Rhythm

The rhythm of a patient's heartbeat is either regular or irregular. You may pick up an irregular heartbeat when taking the patient's pulse. This same patient will show an irregularity (i.e., a difference in the length of time between cardiac cycles) when an ECG is recorded. If the patient's heart is beating in a regular rhythm, each cardiac cycle occurs within the same time frame, and individual cardiac cycles occur exactly the same length of time apart. To check for ventricular rhythm, you can measure the distance between two consecutive RR intervals. Atrial rhythm is determined by measuring the distance between two consecutive PP intervals. If the heart rhythm is regular, each of these interval measurements is the same.

Calculating a Patient's Heart Rate

To calculate the patient's heart rate from an ECG strip, remember the following:
- 5 large boxes on the graph paper = 1 second
- 15 large boxes = 3 seconds
- 30 large boxes = 6 seconds

Analyzing an ECG Strip

The ECG rhythm strip (lead II view) is evaluated from left to right. Each strip should be assessed for the following:
- Rate
- Rhythm
- P waves (there should be one P wave before each QRS complex; each is a positive deflection, and they are similar in size and shape)

- Intervals (assess for duration and distance)
- Appearance of the segments and waveforms (Are rhythmic PQRST cycles present? Are there any abnormalities, such as more than one P wave, QRS segments without a previous P wave, or an elevated ST segment? Any such abnormalities should be brought to the provider's attention immediately.)

TABLE 42-2 Normal Appearance of ECG Waveforms and Complexes

WAVE OR COMPLEX	DURATION (sec or amplitude)	CHARACTERISTICS TO EXAMINE
P wave	0.06-0.11	• Are P waves present? • Are they normal in shape (not notched or peaked)? • Do all deflect upward (positive)? Is there one for each QRS? Are they evenly spaced from the QRS?
PR interval	0.12-0.20	• Is it constant?
QRS complex	0.08-0.12	• Are the complexes evenly spaced from T waves? • Do all point in the same direction? • Do all appear the same? • Is each preceded by a P wave? • Does the Q wave have a pronounced negative deflection?
ST segment	On baseline (isoelectric line)	• Is it on baseline? • Is it constant? • Is it elevated above the baseline?
T waves	≤5 mm in leads I, II, III ≤10 mm in V_1-V_6	• Are they present? • Are all the same? • Do all show upward deflection (positive)?
QT interval	Should not be more than half the RR interval* if patient has a regular rhythm	• Is it constant?
U wave	Rounded, upright deflection	• Is it present?

*RR interval: Period from onset of one QRS complex to onset of next QRS complex.

TYPICAL ECG RHYTHM ABNORMALITIES

Abnormalities in cardiac rhythm are called *arrhythmias*. These can result from disturbances anywhere along the electrical conduction pathway in the heart from the SA node through the right and left bundle branches. The best way to determine whether an arrhythmia is present is to know what the NSR looks like on an ECG. Study the NSR in the ECG in Figure 42-1. NSR is a heart rate between 60 and 100 beats/min. Any deviations from this should be recognized during the ECG recording, and the medical assistant should notify the physician immediately.

Cardiac arrhythmias commonly fall into one of four broad categories: sinus arrhythmias, atrial arrhythmias, ventricular arrhythmias, and biochemical arrhythmias. The characteristics of

several arrhythmias in each of these categories are compared in Table 42-3.

Sinus Arrhythmias

Sinus rhythm is considered normal; the heart's electrical activity begins in the SA node and follows through the electrical system, ending in atrial and ventricular depolarization. In sinus arrhythmias, the pathway of the electrical charge is normal, but the rate or rhythm of the heartbeat is altered. Sinus arrhythmias may be caused by the SA node firing too slowly or too quickly. In sinus bradycardia, the heart rate is below 60 beats/min. This can be a normal heart rate in well-conditioned athletes, but it is abnormal in other individuals. In sinus tachycardia, the heart rate is above 100 beats/min. This can be a normal heart rate in a person doing

TABLE 42-3 Characteristics of Arrhythmias

TYPE	SIGNS AND SYMPTOMS	ETIOLOGY	ECG CHANGES
Sinus Arrhythmias			
Bradycardia	<60 beats/min	Vagal nerve stimulation; sleep; SA node ischemia; digitalis toxicity; drugs Can be normal in athletes	Essentially "normal" appearing, but slow
Tachycardia	Nonpathologic; heart rate >100 beats/min is pathologic	Increased demand for cardiac output; ectopic pacemaker	P wave can be obscured by ST segment (increasing the ECG speed can reduce this problem)
Atrial Arrhythmias			
PAC	Not pathologic if only several per minute	Increased SA node excitability, causing premature beats of atria Can be caused by nicotine or caffeine	"Extra" P waves
Flutter	200-350 beats/min	Many ectopic atrial pacemakers; normally unstable and progresses to atrial fibrillation if not corrected	Multiple, sawtoothed P waves before essentially normal-appearing QRS complexes
Ventricular Arrhythmias (See Figure 42-16)			
PVC	Generally none	Ectopic pacemakers originating in ventricles from electrolyte imbalance, hypoxia, acute MI	Widened QRS complex
V-tach	Heart rate >100 beats/min, always pathologic	Damaged tissue around one of the "bundles," causing a difference in conduction speed between the two branches or ectopic pacemaker cells	Rapid rate, irregular pattern that includes "extra" or erratic, irregular, or wide QRS complexes
V-fib*	Shock, loss of consciousness, no pulse	Complete loss of synchronization of conduction system	Erratic deflections on the ECG (can be either coarse or fine) No identifiable ECG waves
Asystole	<5 beats/min	Death imminent	Flatline
Biochemical Arrhythmias			
Digitalis toxicity	Abnormal bradycardia, abnormal tachycardia	Digitalis dose that is too high	"Swooping" ST segment depression and/or extended PR intervals
Hypokalemia	Malaise, fatigue, weakness, muscle cramps	Potassium too low, usually from unsupplemented diuresis, from IV fluid administration, or from excessive vomiting	Prominent U waves; T wave and U wave together look like a two-hump camel
Hyperkalemia†	May have none	Potassium too high, usually from IV supplementation	Peaked T wave (can be as tall as R wave) with widening of all waveforms

IV, Intravenous; *MI*, myocardial infarction; *PAC*, premature atrial contraction; *PVC*, premature ventricular contraction; *SA*, sinoatrial.
*Most common life-threatening arrhythmia; frequently precedes asystole if not reversed.
†Life-threatening condition; must be corrected immediately.

aerobic exercise, but it can be abnormal in a resting individual (Figure 42-15).

Atrial Arrhythmias

Problems with electrical discharge of the atria are caused by faulty electrical impulse formation or conduction defects within the atria. Premature atrial contraction (PAC) occurs when the atria contract before they should for the next cardiac cycle. This can appear on the

ECG as an abnormally shaped P wave or an extra P wave. PACs can be seen in smokers and people who consume large amounts of caffeine. Occasional PACs are not abnormal, but they become a medical concern if they regularly occur more than six times a minute. In this situation, the PACs can indicate developing cardiac abnormalities.

Atrial flutter occurs when the atria beat at an extremely rapid rate, up to 300 beats/min. In atrial flutter the impulses come from

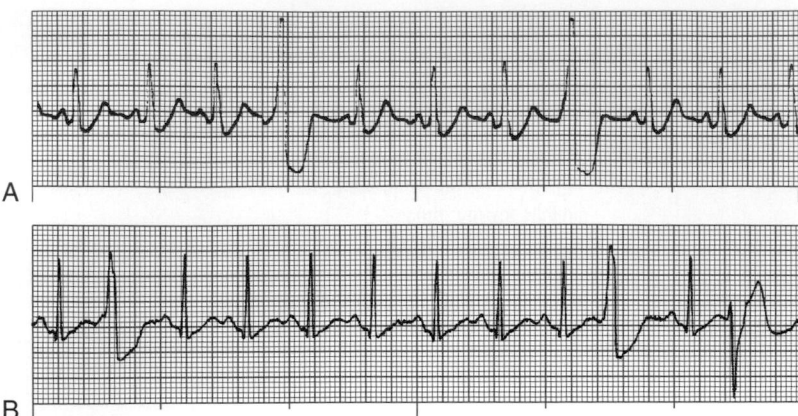

FIGURE 42-15 Sinus tachycardia with frequent, uniform PVCs **(A)** and with multiform PVCs **(B).** (From Aehlert B: *ECGs made easy,* ed 5, St Louis, 2013, Mosby.)

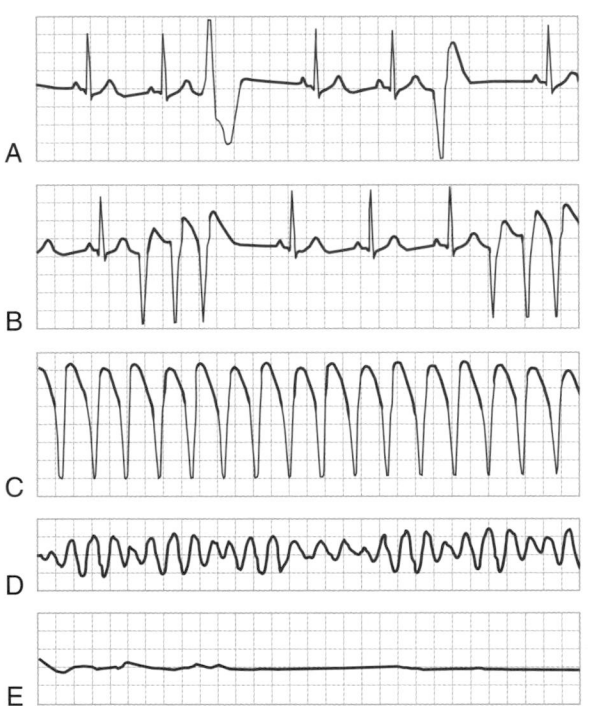

FIGURE 42-16 Ventricular arrhythmias. **A,** PVC. **B,** Three PVCs in a row. **C,** V-tach. **D,** V-fib. **E,** Asystole.

many **ectopic** atrial locations but are blocked at the AV node, which prevents ventricular fibrillation. Atrial flutter is reversed with medication to slow the heart or with **cardioversion** (electrical shock).

Ventricular Arrhythmias

Premature ventricular contractions (PVCs; Figure 42-16, *A* and *B*) occur when the ventricles contract before they should for the next cardiac cycle; that is, a QRS complex appears before a P wave. PVCs occur when an electrical charge originates in either ventricle. This can appear on the ECG as an absent P wave, an abnormally shaped T wave, and a widened QRS complex. This is followed by a pause before the initiation of the next cardiac cycle (see Figure

42-15). PVCs can result from the use of tobacco, alcohol, medications containing epinephrine, and occasionally from anxiety. Infrequent PVCs are not abnormal, but they become a medical concern if they regularly occur more than six times a minute. Pathologic PVCs occur in patients with hypertension, coronary artery disease, and lung disease.

Ventricular tachycardia (commonly referred to as *V-tach*) (Figure 42-16, *C*) is diagnosed when the ventricles beat at extremely rapid rates. It may be seen when multiple PVCs occur in a row or as a short run of fast beats, or it may persist longer than 30 seconds. The patient's heart rate may range from 101 to 250 beats/min. V-tach can precede ventricular fibrillation if not reversed with drugs, cardioversion, or both. V-tach always reflects a pathologic state.

Ventricular fibrillation (commonly referred to as *V-fib*) (Figure 42-16, *D*) is the most critical, life-threatening arrhythmia; it quickly results in death if not treated. V-fib is estimated to precede 85% of cases of **cardiac arrest** in adults. In V-fib, the electrical conduction system of the heart is in total dysfunction. The heart muscle quivers uncontrollably and is essentially ineffective at pumping any blood; therefore, there is no pulse, and the patient is unresponsive and not breathing. Cardioversion with a **defibrillator** is necessary to restore normal function of the electrical conduction system.

Asystole is the result of absence of a heartbeat, or cardiac cessation, which shows as a flatline on the ECG (Figure 42-16, *E*).

Biochemical Arrhythmias

Heart or blood pressure medications may cause an arrhythmia. For example, digitalis, frequently called *dig* (pronounced *dij*), is a common cardiac drug used to slow and strengthen the heartbeat. The heart is quite sensitive to digitalis, and too much can prove toxic and cause changes in the ECG (Figure 42-17). This condition can be reversed by reducing the dosage of digoxin or digitoxin (both are forms of digitalis).

Potassium is a critical mineral for normal cardiac function. Too much potassium in the blood (hyperkalemia) or too little (hypokalemia) can both cause life-threatening arrhythmias that must be corrected quickly.

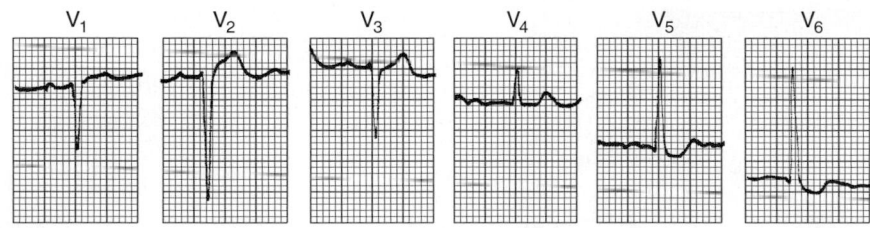

FIGURE 42-17 ECG showing the effects of digitalis. Note the "scooping" of the ST segment, as seen in leads V₅ and V₆. (Goldberger A: *Clinical electrocardiography: a simplified approach,* ed 6, St Louis, 1999, Mosby.)

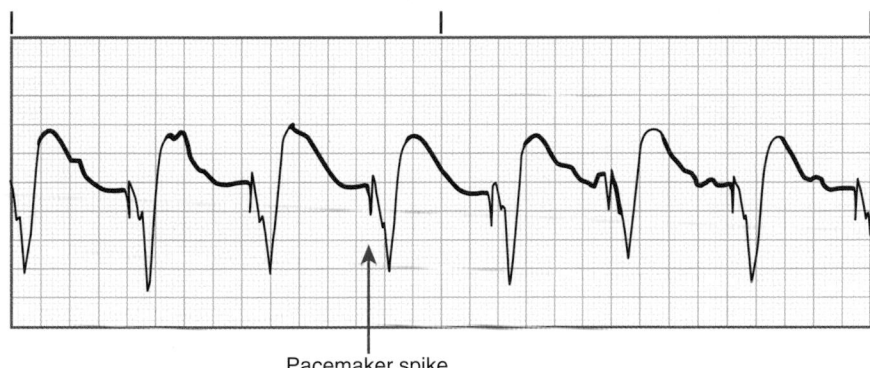

Pacemaker spike

FIGURE 42-18 Pacemaker rhythm strip. (From Lewis S et al: *Medical-surgical nursing,* ed 9, St Louis, 2014, Mosby.)

Pacemaker Rhythms

A pacemaker is a device implanted under the skin that stimulates the electrical activity of the heart. It consists of a small metal pulse generator with a battery and electronic leads that extend from the generator to the myocardium. The entire pulse generator is replaced when the battery wears out, usually every 5 to 10 years.

> ### Pacemakers
>
> A pacemaker is a small device that is placed in the chest or abdomen to help control abnormal heart rhythms. It uses electrical pulses to prompt the heart to beat at a normal rate. Pacemakers can do the following:
> - Speed up a slow heart rhythm.
> - Help control an abnormal or fast heart rhythm.
> - Make sure the ventricles contract normally if the atria are quivering instead of beating with a normal rhythm (atrial fibrillation).
> - Coordinate electrical signaling between the upper and lower chambers of the heart.
> - Cardiac resynchronization therapy (CRT) pacemakers: Coordinate electrical signaling between the ventricles (these are used to treat congestive heart failure).
> - Prevent dangerous arrhythmias.
> - Monitor and record the heart's electrical activity and heart rhythm.
> - Can monitor blood temperature, breathing rate, and other factors (some brands).
> - Adjust the heart rate to changes in activity.
>
> National Heart, Lung, and Blood Institute. *www.nhlbi.nih.gov/health/health-topics/topics/pace.* Accessed February 16, 2016.

Pacemakers are implanted in a hospital, and local anesthesia is used. Before the patient is discharged, the device is programmed to fire according to the needs of the individual patient. The patient is instructed to telephone the physician's office periodically to transmit pacemaker readings across the phone lines; however, this method is being replaced by Internet transmission of data. Internet diagnostic reports can be exported to the patient's EHR. Pacemakers cause wide variations in the appearance of an ECG (Figure 42-18).

Implanted Cardioverter-Defibrillator

An implanted cardioverter-defibrillator, or ICD, monitors the heart rhythm and delivers a shock to the heart if it detects a dangerous ventricular tachycardia or fibrillation (Figure 42-19). It is a small, battery-operated device that is implanted under the skin in the chest or abdomen. An ICD can be used to reverse V-tach and V-fib, especially after the patient has previously had a myocardial **infarction** (MI), or heart attack. The generator is programmed specifically to treat the patient's particular or potential cardiac arrhythmia. An ICD has wires with electrodes on the ends that connect to the heart chambers. If the device detects an irregular rhythm in the ventricles, it uses low-energy electrical pulses to restore a normal rhythm. If the low-energy pulses do not restore normal heart rhythm, the ICD switches to high-energy pulses for defibrillation. The device also switches to high-energy pulses if the ventricles start to quiver rather than contract strongly. The high-energy pulses last only a fraction of a second, but they can be painful.

Just as with pacemakers, the device is programmed to meet the needs of each individual patient. Some ICD functions can be checked over the phone or through a computer connection to the Internet. ICD batteries last 5 to 7 years. The generator and battery are replaced before the battery begins to run down.

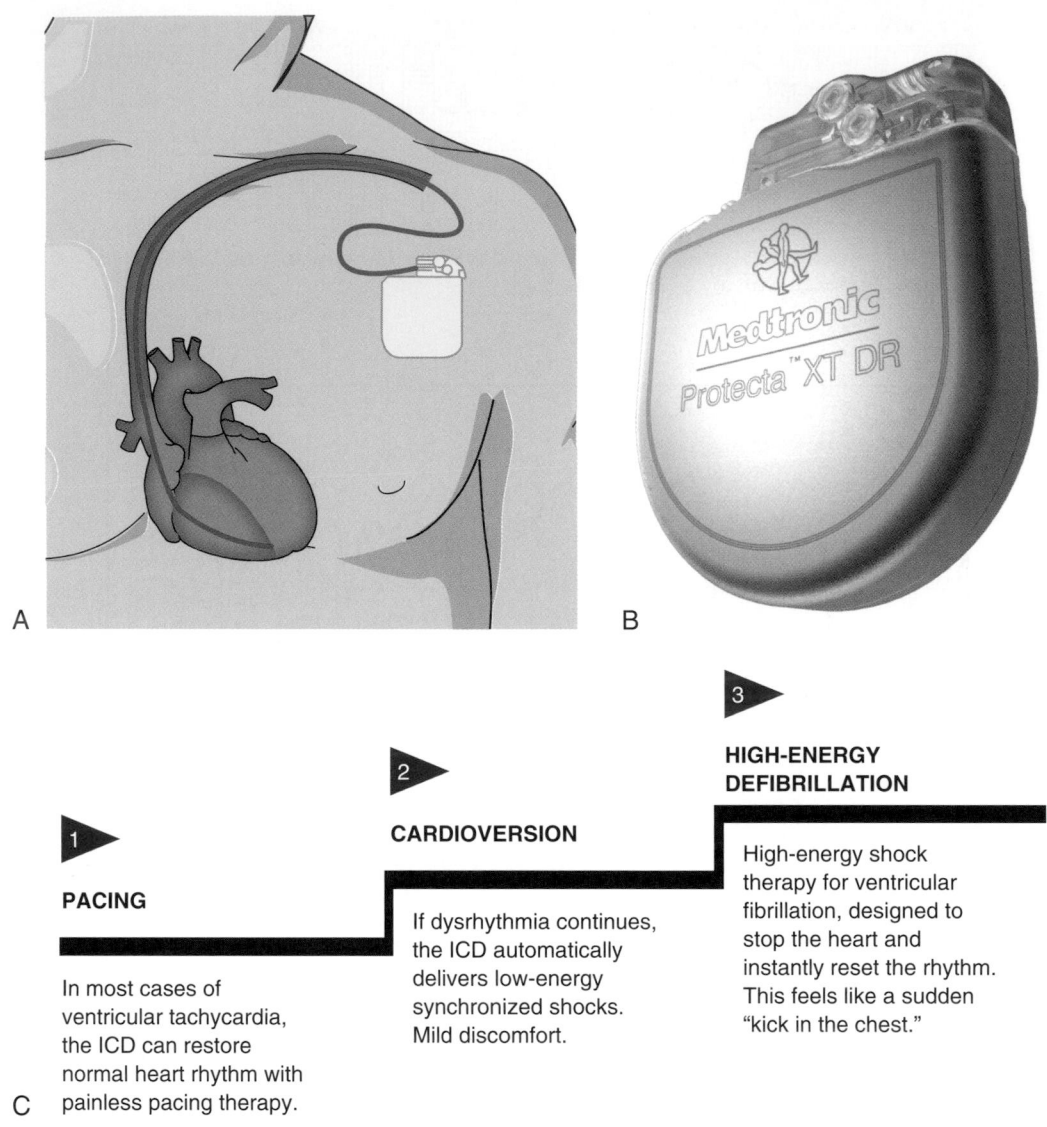

FIGURE 42-19 Implanted cardioverter-defibrillator. (From Urden L, Stacy K, Lough M: *Thelan's critical care nursing: diagnosis and management,* ed 7, St Louis, 2014, Mosby.)

Myocardial Infarction

Sudden heart attack, or MI, occurs in more than 1 million Americans each year, according to the American Heart Association. Approximately 20% of these patients die before reaching the hospital, and approximately 30% die within 30 days of the heart attack. An MI occurs when a portion of the heart muscle becomes ischemic because the blood supply to that area has been interrupted. **Ischemia** eventually leads to tissue necrosis, or infarction.

The heart muscle, the myocardium, receives its oxygen supply from a network of coronary arteries (Figure 42-20) on the surface of the heart. The right coronary artery supplies much of the right side of the heart. The left coronary artery bifurcates into two main branches: the left circumflex artery, which supplies blood principally to the left lateral and posterior walls of the left ventricle, and the left anterior descending coronary artery, which supplies principally the anterior wall of the left ventricle and the interventricular septum. The left anterior descending coronary artery is sometimes called the "sudden death artery" because it feeds such a large portion of the left ventricle.

MI causes specific, recognizable changes on the ECG recording, based on the phase the patient is in when the ECG is recorded (Table 42-4). The three most common changes are elevated ST segments, inverted (upside-down) T waves, and abnormal (pathologic) Q waves (Figure 42-21).

The sooner treatment is initiated after the patient's first awareness of a heart attack, the more effective treatment is and the better the chances for the patient's survival. Immediate treatment for a heart attack includes administration of nasal oxygen, sublingual nitroglycerin (to dilate the coronary arteries), a narcotic analgesic (to eliminate pain), aspirin (to reduce inflammation and decrease clotting time), and possibly a thrombolytic agent to dissolve the clot causing the coronary artery obstruction. Early administration of thrombolytic agents enhances the likelihood of restoring circulation to the myocardium distal to the occluding thrombus (blood clot). After discharge from the hospital, the patient should quit smoking, modify the diet as instructed by a nutritionist, and enter a cardiac rehabilitation program to improve cardiac strength and recovery through exercise.

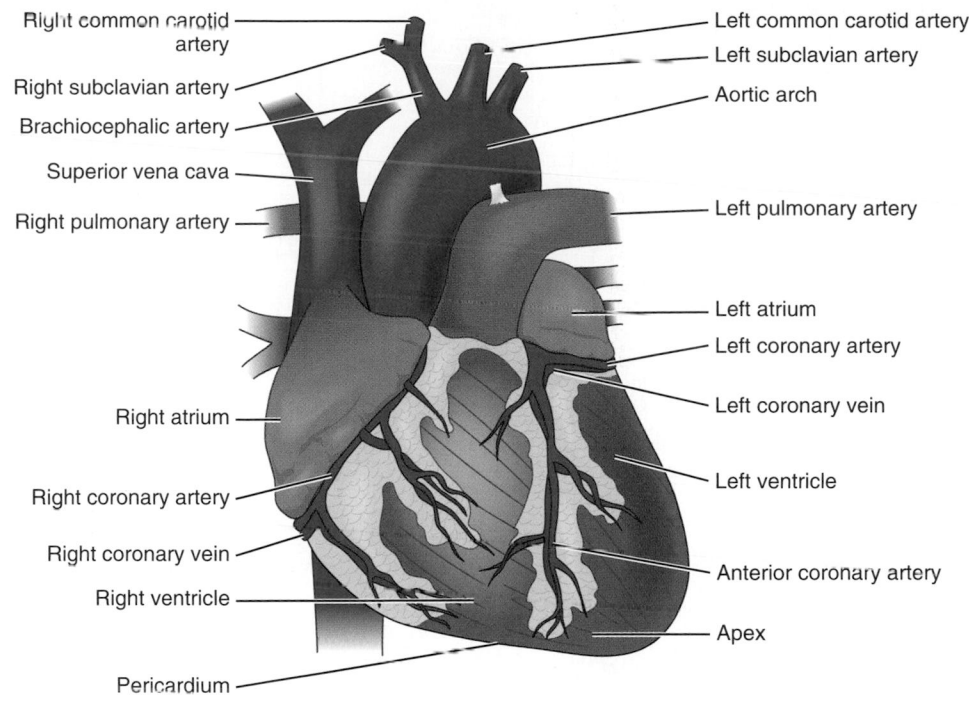

Right common carotid artery
Right subclavian artery
Brachiocephalic artery
Superior vena cava
Right pulmonary artery
Right atrium
Right coronary artery
Right coronary vein
Right ventricle
Pericardium

Left common carotid artery
Left subclavian artery
Aortic arch
Left pulmonary artery
Left atrium
Left coronary artery
Left coronary vein
Left ventricle
Anterior coronary artery
Apex

FIGURE 42-20 Coronary vessels.

TABLE 42-4 Phases of Myocardial Infarction With Electrocardiographic Changes

PHASE	PERIOD OF ECG CHANGES	SPECIFIC ECG CHANGES
I (hyperacute)	First few hours	ST segment elevated from baseline (earliest indication on ECG); peaked "hyperacute" T waves
II (fully evolved)	After hours or days	Deep T waves; pathologic Q waves appear (negative deflection)
III (resolution)	Days to weeks	ST segment returns to normal position; T waves return to normal
IV (stabilized chronic)	Permanent	Negative Q wave deflection remains

Complications of acute MI include a sudden episode of atrial fibrillation, V-fib, or bradycardia that may necessitate implantation of a pacemaker.

RELATED CARDIAC DIAGNOSTIC TESTS

Stress Test

Cardiac stress testing is performed to observe and record the patient's cardiovascular response to measured exercise challenges (Figure 42-22). The goal is to determine if the myocardium is getting enough blood during exercise. A stress test is done to:

- Diagnose cardiac disease that cannot be detected by a standard resting ECG
- Determine abnormal changes in heart rate or blood pressure
- Detect symptoms such as shortness of breath or angina, especially if they occur at low levels of exercise
- Identify and record abnormal changes in the heart's rhythm or electrical activity

A stress test is performed while the patient is exercising on either a bicycle or a treadmill, under careful supervision. The patient must be given the appropriate information explaining the purpose, preparation, and procedure for the test (Figure 42-23).

Myocardial ischemia and even cardiac arrest are serious risks with a cardiac stress test. The medical assistant must be able to recognize symptoms of dyspnea, vertigo, extreme fatigue, severe arrhythmia, and other abnormal ECG readings that may develop during the stress test or immediately after the test during the rest period. All members of a cardiac stress testing team must be prepared to terminate testing immediately if the patient is unable to continue or if abnormalities appear on the monitor. Team members also must be certified in cardiopulmonary resuscitation (CPR) and emergency intervention. The physician must always be present during this procedure. In addition to the routine monitoring equipment, the team must have oxygen, a defibrillator, an endotracheal intubation tray, an artificial breathing bag, and emergency cardiac medications available in case of cardiac crisis. Because of the potential for life-threatening incidents, most physicians have stress tests performed in a hospital or specialized cardiac center, where personnel are trained and ready to assist if a cardiac emergency occurs.

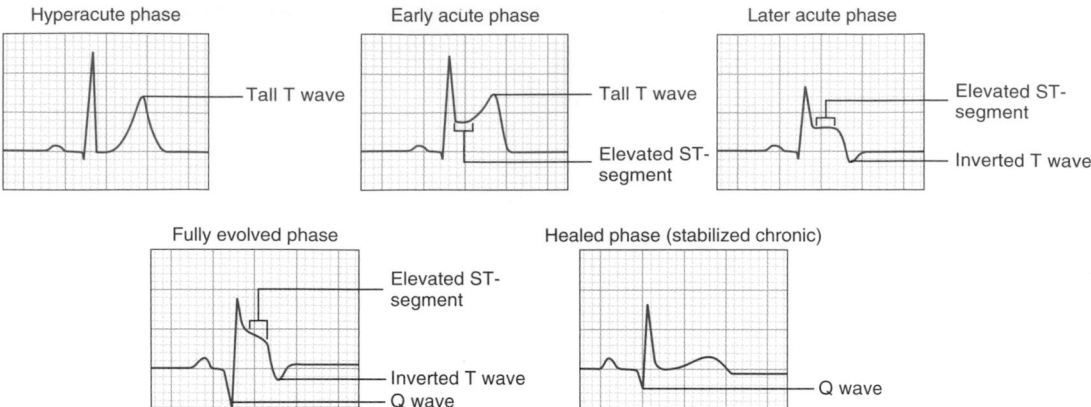

FIGURE 42-21 Changes in the PQRST segment associated with a myocardial infarction. (Butler HA, Caplin M, McCully E et al: *Managing major diseases: cardiac disorders,* vol 2, St Louis, 1999, Mosby.)

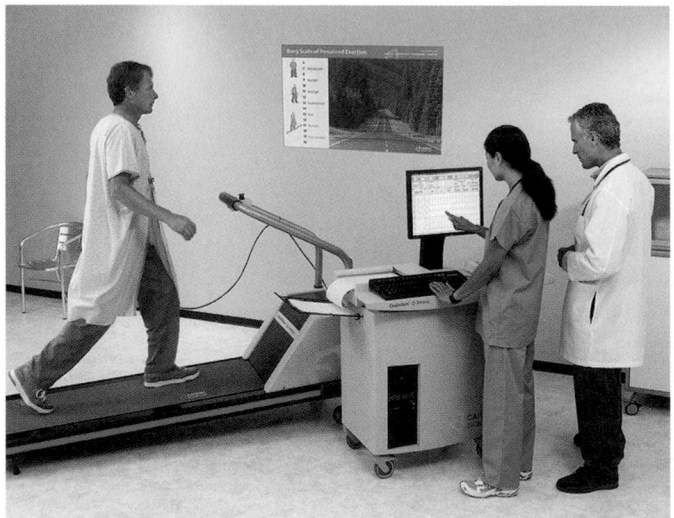

FIGURE 42-22 Cardiac stress test. (Courtesy Cardiac Science, Bothell, Wash.)

CRITICAL THINKING APPLICATION   **42-5**

Mr. Sonderford actually had an MI when he was previously at Dr. Lee's office. He now has completed cardiac rehabilitation and is at the office for a checkup. Dr. Lee wants him to be scheduled for a stress test. Mr. Sonderford has never had one before. He confides to Martha that he is afraid if he does the test, he will die from another heart attack. How should Martha handle this situation?

Holter Monitor

A Holter monitor is a portable system for recording a patient's cardiac activity over a 24-hour period or longer (Procedure 42-2). The monitor is a small, lightweight device that the patient wears while going about usual daily activities. The Holter monitor can be programmed to record cardiac information continuously or periodically, when activated by the patient if symptoms occur, or during periods of stress.

The entire time the monitor is worn, the patient must keep a journal of all stressful events and activities (and also specific details

about activities when any cardiac symptoms occur). Journal entries include the time, duration, and specific activity during the cardiac event, such as rush hour traffic, bowel movements, intercourse, climbing stairs, and periods of anger or emotional distress. Some monitors can even record the patient's voice describing a symptom or event so that it can later be correlated with the ECG recording in the same time frame.

Many cardiologists routinely use Holter monitors in their practices. A medical assistant often is responsible for fitting the monitor on the patient and for removing it after the test period. The patient must have a full understanding of what is required during monitoring, particularly how to use the event marker in case a significant symptom is experienced. The patient also must know how to record the event in a written diary when the event marker is used. The patient may take only sponge baths during the 24 hours of the test. The number of electrodes and leads varies with the number of channels on the particular monitor. Electrode placement is determined by the provider or by the manufacturer's guidelines and should be followed precisely. The skin of male patients may need to be shaved so that the electrodes can be firmly attached. The lead wires are attached to the electrodes and to the Holter monitor, which is worn around the waist or on a belt or in a pouch slung over the shoulder.

At the end of the monitoring period, the patient returns to the clinic, the monitor is disconnected, and electrodes are removed. The recording is placed in a Holter scanner or computer, and the results are analyzed. Any part of the recording can be printed or downloaded into the patient's EHR for further study.

CRITICAL THINKING APPLICATION   **42-6**

Mrs. Jamison was fitted with a Holter monitor at the clinic yesterday at 4 PM. When Martha arrived at 8 o'clock this morning, she found that Mrs. Jamison had left a message with the answering service to call her as soon as possible. When Martha returns the call, Mrs. Jamison tells her that she had taken a shower last night, and she noticed that when she got up to go to the bathroom, "the light was not on" on the monitor. How should Martha handle this situation?

Cardiac Stress Test

Cardiac stress testing (also known as an exercise tolerance test or treadmill test) is a means of observing, evaluating, and recording your heart's response during a measured exercise test. This test determines your capacity to adapt to physical stress.

There are various reasons that your physician may suggest this test for you:

1. To aid in determining the presence of suspected coronary heart disease.
2. To aid in the selection of therapy.
   a. For angina pectoris (tightness or pain in the chest).
   b. Following a myocardial infarction (heart attack).
   c. Following coronary bypass surgery (open heart surgery).
3. To determine your physical work capacity.
4. To authorize participation in a physical exercise program.

Preparation for the Test

1. Avoid eating a heavy meal within 2 hours of your appointment.
2. Take your medications as you usually do, unless your doctor advises you not to take them.
3. Wear a shirt or blouse that buttons down the front with slacks, a skirt, jogging pants, or shorts.
4. Do not wear one-piece undergarments, jumpsuits, or dresses.
5. Tennis shoes are ideal if you have them. Otherwise, wear comfortable flat or low-heeled shoes. Do not wear clogs, sling-backs, crepe soles, boots, or high heels, as they make walking on the treadmill more difficult.

The Procedure

When you arrive in the Cardiology Department, areas of your chest may be shaved (men only) to allow the electrodes to adhere tightly to your chest. A blood pressure cuff will be wrapped around your arm, and an electrocardiogram (ECG) is taken while you are at rest. The technician will then demonstrate how to walk on the treadmill and will answer any questions you may have.

You will then perform a graded exercise test on a motor-driven treadmill. You will begin walking very gradually at a rate you can easily accomplish.

Progressively throughout the test, the speed and grade of the treadmill will be increased, and you will be walking at a faster pace up a slight incline. At no time will you be asked to jog or run, nor will you be asked to exercise beyond your capabilities.

At all times during the test, trained personnel are in the room with you, monitoring your heart rate and blood pressure and observing you for signs of fatigue or discomfort. We do not wish to exercise you to a level that is medically unsafe or physically distressing.

An ECG is taken again when you finish walking. Your cardiologist will immediately interpret the results of the test and explain his or her findings to you. If necessary, medications or treatment will be discussed. A letter with the results of the stress test will be sent to your referring physician.

The entire procedure will take 1 to 1 1/2 hours. If you have any questions regarding the cardiac stress test or any problems with your appointment, please contact us.

FIGURE 42-23 Patient information for a cardiac stress test.

PROCEDURE 42-2	Instruct and Prepare a Patient for a Procedure or Treatment: Fit a Patient With a Holter Monitor

Goal: *To establish a possible correlation between ECG abnormalities and the patient's 24-hour daily activities.*

EQUIPMENT and SUPPLIES

- Patient's health record
- Holter monitor with new batteries
- Disposable electrodes
- Razor
- Sharps container
- Gauze pads or abrasive tool as needed
- Activity diary
- Carrying case with belt or shoulder strap
- Alcohol swabs
- Cloth tape (nonallergenic)

PROCEDURAL STEPS

1. Sanitize your hands.
   <u>PURPOSE</u>: To ensure infection control.
2. Greet the patient and confirm his or her identity by name and date of birth.
3. Assemble the needed equipment, and install batteries in the monitor (Figure 1).

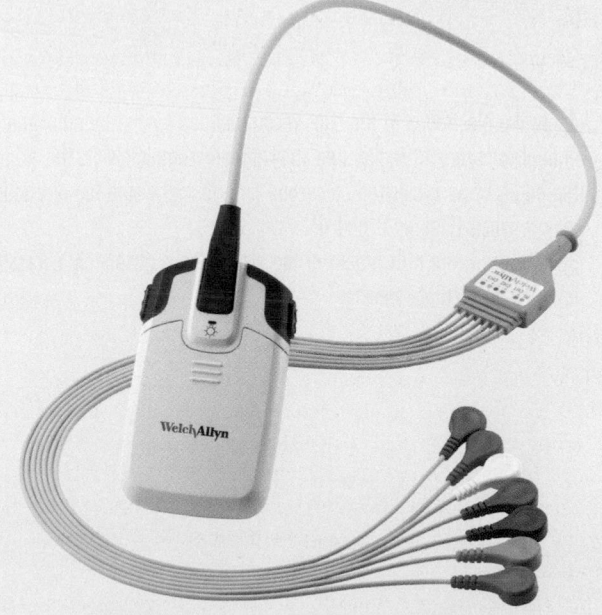

1

(Courtesy Welch Allyn, Skaneateles Falls, NY.)

PROCEDURE 42-2   *—continued*

PURPOSE: New or fully charged batteries ensure accurate monitor function for 24 hours.

4. Explain the procedure. Sanitize your hands.
    PURPOSE: An informed patient helps ensure testing accuracy.

5. Ask the patient to disrobe to the waist and to sit at the end of the examination table or to lie down.
    PURPOSE: This places the patient at the best working level for the medical assistant.

6. Clean each electrode application site with an alcohol swab and allow the sites to air dry.
    PURPOSE: To remove all surface skin oil to ensure maximum electrode adherence. If shaving will be necessary, clean before shaving to prevent irritation and patient discomfort.

7. If the patient has a hairy chest, dry shave the area at each of the electrode sites.
    PURPOSE: The skin must be hairless to provide maximum electrode adherence.

8. Fold a gauze pad over your index finger and briskly rub the sites or use an abrasive tool as indicated (Figure 2).
    PURPOSE: To help electrodes stick more tightly to the skin.

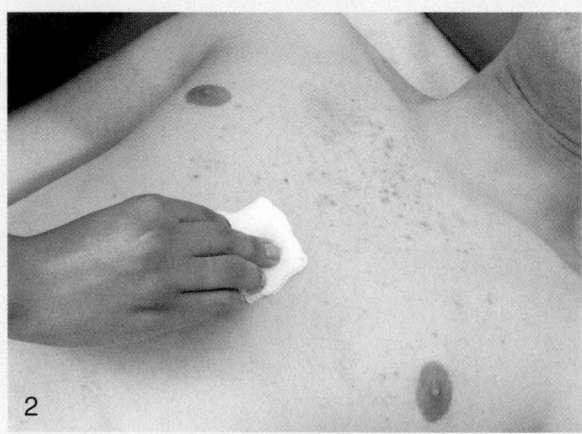

2

9. Apply the electrodes to the sites recommended by the manufacturer; use enough pressure to make sure they adhere completely to the skin. Rub the edges of each electrode a second time to make sure the electrode will stay in place (Figures 3 and 4).
    PURPOSE: Secure attachment of the electrodes is absolutely necessary to produce an accurate tracing.

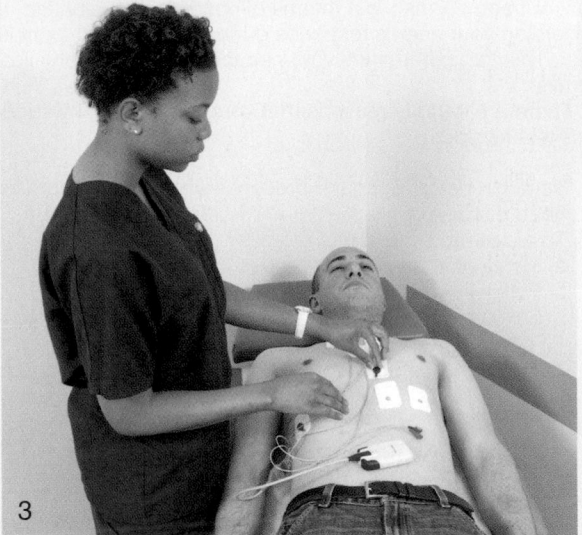

3

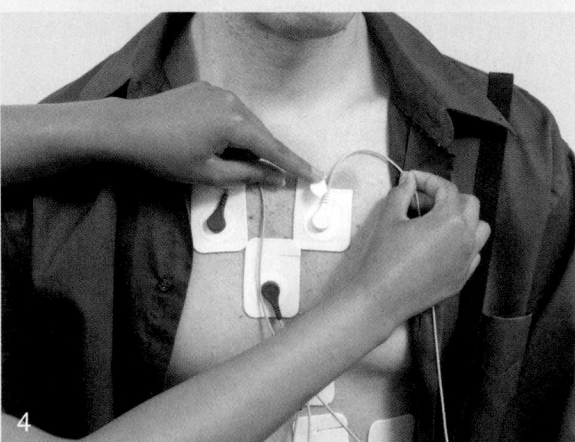

4

10. Attach the lead wires to the electrodes and connect the end terminal to the patient cable.

11. Place a strip of cloth tape over each electrode.
    PURPOSE: To help secure the electrodes in place in case the wires are pulled during the testing period.

12. Attach the test cable to the monitor and plug it into the electrocardiograph. Run a baseline test tracing as directed by the manufacturer's guidelines.
    PURPOSE: To ensure proper connections of the electrodes and running of the monitor.

13. Help the patient get dressed without disturbing the connected electrodes. Make sure the cable extends through the buttoned front or out the bottom of the shirt or blouse.

14. Place the monitor in the carrying case and attach it to the patient's belt or pocket or place it over the shoulder. Be sure the wires are not being pulled or bent.
    PURPOSE: Taut or badly bent wires may loosen or malfunction.

15. Plug the electrode cable into the monitor.

16. Record the patient's name and date of birth and the starting date and time in the patient's activity diary.
    PURPOSE: To establish the starting time of the test and cardiac activity.

17. Give the patient the activity diary and advise him or her to begin by writing in his or her present activity (Figure 5). Include patient education information on the importance of continually recording activities in the diary; using the event marker on the monitor if he or she experiences any symptoms; and correlating the event with a recording in the diary, including the time and details of the related activity before or during the event.
PURPOSE: The diary should correlate the patient's activity with any cardiac symptoms.

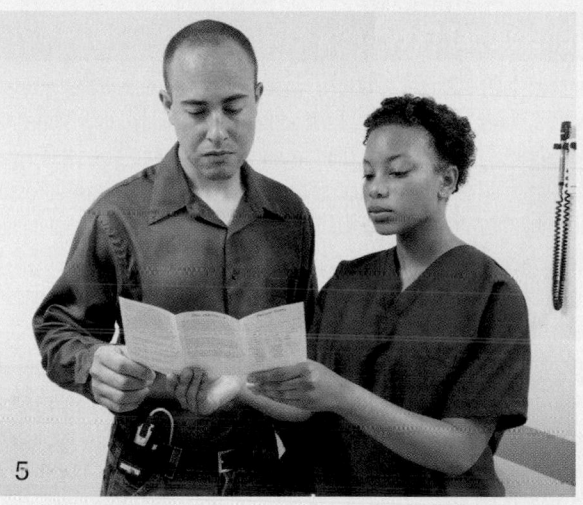

5

18. Schedule the patient for a return appointment in 24 hours.
19. Sanitize your hands.
PURPOSE: To ensure infection control.
20. Record the procedure in the patient's health record.
PURPOSE: A procedure is not considered done until it is documented in the patient's health record.

9/29/20– 3:10 PM: Holter monitor applied per Dr. Lee's order. Pt instructed to leave leads in place until he returns to office tomorrow. Understands to record cardiac symptoms in diary, to use event marker if symptoms occur, and not to shower until monitor is removed. Martha Reyes, CMA (AAMA)

Cardiac Event Monitor

The cardiac event monitor is a small recording device that can be worn up to 30 days to catch events that are difficult to record in a 24-hour period on a Holter monitor, such as chest pain, vertigo, weakness, and **palpitations**. Some monitors have a feature (memory loop recorder) that captures a short period before the moment the recording is triggered and for a short time afterward. This feature can help the provider learn more details about the possible change in the ECG at the time the symptoms started. Other monitors, called "post-event recorders," start recording the ECG from the moment it is triggered. Post-event recorders are quite small and may be worn on the wrist (similar to a wristwatch). Memory-loop recorders are about the size of a pager. Any recordings of cardiac events are sent to either the healthcare facility for the physician to interpret or to a central monitoring center. The transmission is done either over the telephone or wirelessly using cellular technology. Before leaving the office, the patient needs instruction on how to transmit data. The patient is also told to write down all symptoms with whatever activity was occurring at the time (as is done during the Holter monitoring procedure).

Using the information gathered during the recording period, the physician can diagnose heart abnormalities and design the most effective treatment. The monitor must be removed during bathing, so the patient must be taught how to remove and reapply the electrodes throughout the test period. Patient education for using an event monitor includes the following instructions:

- Protect the monitor from damage, and wear it at all times except when bathing.
- Do not alter your lifestyle; regular activities need to be maintained to reflect the cause of cardiac symptoms.
- Trigger the recording by pushing the event monitor when symptoms occur.
- Use the diary to record activities when events occur.
- Change the electrodes daily and the batteries at the same time each day.
- To prevent skin irritation, do not put replacement electrodes in the same spot.
- Put the electrodes on the rib cage under the left breast and in the midaxillary region under the right shoulder.
- If you have any questions, use the contact information provided.

Heart Scan

A noninvasive method of assessing possible cardiac risk is a specialized type of computed tomography called an *electron beam tomography (EBT) heart scan* (also called an *ultrafast CT*). The heart scan takes less than 5 minutes and does not require any needles or injections. It is a screening tool that allows physicians to see the amount of plaque in the coronary arteries by showing the presence of calcium deposits. Calcium makes up approximately 20% of arterial plaque deposits. The EBT heart scan is read, and the physician assigns the patient a calcium score that can be a predictor of future cardiac problems.

CLOSING COMMENTS

Patient Education

Heart disease and stroke account for more than one third of all deaths. Genetic predisposition and detrimental lifestyle habits, such as smoking, lack of exercise, a diet high in saturated fats, and obesity, play significant roles in the development of heart disease. The medical assistant should talk to the patient about factors that can be changed or modified and should encourage any attempt by the patient to make these changes.

Before you can successfully counsel a patient to change a habit, you need to familiarize yourself with possible techniques and approaches to use. Such information can be obtained from the American Heart Association and reputable Internet sites.

Many patients like visual aids when they are learning new information, and brochures with pictures or posters in the office are effective means of promoting learning and eliciting questions from patients. Make a note in the health record of the educational items you give the patient on each visit. On a subsequent visit, ask about the helpfulness of the information, whether the patient tried any modifications, and what the results were. Ask for any suggestions that might help another patient in a similar situation.

Legal and Ethical Issues

An ECG is a valuable diagnostic tool, and it continues to be one of the most common procedures used in the diagnosis of cardiac diseases and conditions. The cardiologist measures the heart's activity and compares the results with known values by analyzing the ECG tracing. Comparing an ECG tracing with previous tracings can identify changes in the condition of the patient's heart.

The provider must be able to interpret the ECG tracing accurately and to establish its value in correctly diagnosing the patient's condition; the medical assistant, therefore, has the ethical obligation to complete the task as accurately and carefully as possible. Diagnostic procedures have a profound effect on a patient's subsequent treatment. When you are entrusted with performing testing procedures, you assume full responsibility for the accuracy and precision of each test you perform. This is a critical role in the medical assisting profession. The results you submit strongly influence each patient's therapeutic treatment plan. No test is ever just routine.

Professional Behaviors

Cardiovascular disease affects a wide variety of individuals across all genders, races, and incomes. Each one of us will likely know someone or have a close personal connection to an individual who has some type of cardiovascular condition. Because of this, it can be very easy to assume you know how to answer patients' questions, and it may be tempting to offer advice about how to manage their conditions. Always remember that medical assistants do not have the knowledge or authority to diagnose or prescribe treatment, regardless of how familiar they are personally with the topic. Refer complex patient questions to the physician, document patients' concerns in the health record, and always follow the practice's policies and procedures when giving the patient information. Professional behavior means being empathetic toward the patient, but always remember that the medical assistant is part of a healthcare team, and restrict your practice to what is ethically and legally permitted.

SUMMARY OF SCENARIO

Martha has worked in Dr. Lee's office for almost 8 months. She has become quite confident in her ability to perform electrocardiography quickly and accurately. She also has learned to communicate effectively with patients about their fears and concerns about various cardiac diagnostic tests. She never forgets to emphasize to a patient the importance of not taking a shower during the

24-hour Holter monitoring period. In 2 months she and Dr. Lee will attend a national meeting of cardiologists in Chicago. Two days of continuing education classes will be offered for medical assistants who work in cardiology. Martha is very excited to be able to continue learning and to sharpen her skills as a medical assistant in cardiology.

SUMMARY OF LEARNING OBJECTIVES

1. **Define, spell, and pronounce the terms listed in the vocabulary.**
   Spelling and pronouncing medical terms correctly reinforce the medical assistant's credibility. Knowing the definitions of these terms promotes confidence in communication with patients and co-workers.

2. **Illustrate the electrical conduction system through the heart and discuss the cardiac cycle.**
   The heart beats in response to an electrical signal that originates in the SA node in the right atrium, spreads over the atria, and causes atrial contraction. This impulse continues to the AV node, through the bundle of His, through the right and left bundle branches, and into the Purkinje fibers, eventually causing ventricular contraction.

3. **Explain the concepts of cardiac polarization, depolarization, and repolarization.**

Polarization is the resting state of the myocardial wall, when there is no electrical activity in the heart. When the electrical system of the heart stimulates a myocardial cell, *depolarization* occurs, resulting in contraction of the stimulated heart muscle. The heart muscle cells must then return to a resting state; the process of reaching this resting state is *repolarization*.

4. **Identify the PQRST complex on an electrocardiograph tracing.**
   The *P wave* shows atrial contraction, the beginning of cardiac depolarization; the *PR segment* is the return to baseline after atrial contraction; the *PR interval* is the time from the beginning of atrial contraction to the beginning of ventricular contraction; the *QRS complex* shows the contraction of both ventricles and the completion of cardiac depolarization; the *ST segment* is the time between the end of ventricular contraction and

the beginning of ventricular recovery; the *T wave* is repolarization of the ventricles; the *QT interval* is the time between the beginning of the QRS complex through the T wave; a *U wave* occasionally can be seen as a small waveform just after the T wave in certain patients.

5. **Summarize the properties of the electrocardiograph and discuss the features of electrocardiograph paper.**

A six-channel ECG machine records all 12 leads simultaneously within seconds. Limb and chest electrodes with leads must be placed on the patient at specific anatomic locations before the recording starts. ECG paper is standardized to represent amplitude and time. The horizontal lines allow determination of the intensity of the electrical activity, and the vertical lines represent time; each of the large squares represents 0.2 second; five of them equals 1 second.

6. **Describe the electrical views of the heart recorded by the 12-lead electrocardiograph.**

Lead I records the electrical activity of the lateral part of the left ventricle; leads II and III record the electrical activity of the inferior surface of the left ventricle. The augmented lead aV$_R$ records the electrical activity of the atria with negative deflection of the P waves and QRS complexes; aV$_L$ records the electrical activity of the lateral wall of the left ventricle; and aV$_F$ records the electrical activity of the inferior surface of the left ventricle. The precordial leads provide a transverse plane view of the heart. They include V$_1$, V$_2$, V$_3$, V$_4$, V$_5$, and V$_6$, with each number representing a specific location on the chest. The QRS complex is a negative deflection in V$_1$ and V$_2$ views, and each subsequent lead becomes more positive.

7. **Discuss the process of recording an electrocardiogram and perform an accurate recording of the electrical activity of the heart.**

Recording an ECG requires knowledge of how to prepare the room and patient; where to place the electrodes and connect the leads to obtain the most accurate recording possible; the ability to recognize and correct the most common types of artifacts on the ECG recording; proper use of the machine available; and knowledge of how best to record ECG tracings in the medical record. Procedure 42-1 outlines the steps for performing a 12-lead ECG recording.

8. **Compare and contrast electrocardiographic artifacts and the probable cause of each.**

An *artifact* is an unwanted, erratic movement of the stylus on the paper caused by outside interference. The main types include *wandering baseline artifacts,* in which the stylus gradually shifts away from the center of the paper because of slight movement or poor electrode attachment; *somatic tremor artifacts,* which are a result of muscle movements in the patient that cause jagged peaks of irregular height and spacing and a shifting baseline; *AC interference,* which causes a series of uniform, small

spikes on the paper because of electrical energy in the area; and *interrupted baseline artifacts,* which occur when the electrical connection between the electrode and the lead is interrupted.

9. **Interpret a typical electrocardiograph tracing.**

Table 42-2 summarizes the normal appearance of ECG waveforms and complexes. The ECG tracing is made up of repeated cardiac cycle (PQRST) recordings. The heart rate is calculated from the ECG recording by counting the number of P waves in a 6-second strip (30 large squares) and multiplying by 10. For the ventricular contraction rate, the number of complete QRS complexes within 6 seconds is counted and multiplied by 10 to get the number of ventricular contractions in 1 minute. The rhythm of the patient's heartbeat indicates whether it is regular. If the patient's heart is beating at a regular rhythm, each cardiac cycle occurs within the same time frame and individual cardiac cycles occur exactly the same length of time apart.

10. **Describe common electrocardiographic arrhythmias.**

In sinus rhythm, the heart's electrical activity begins in the SA node and follows through the electrical system, ending in atrial and ventricular depolarization. In sinus bradycardia, the heart rate is less than 60 beats/min; in sinus tachycardia, the rate is more than 100 beats/min. A PAC occurs when the atria contract before they should for the next cardiac cycle. Atrial flutter occurs when the atria beat at an extremely rapid rate, up to 300 beats/min. PVCs occur when the ventricles contract before they should for the next cardiac cycle. V-tach causes the ventricles to beat at an extremely rapid rate, from 101 to 250 beats/min. V-fib is the most critical, life-threatening arrhythmia and results in death if not effectively treated. Asystole is the result of no heartbeat. Biochemical systemic problems also can cause arrhythmias.

11. **Summarize cardiac diagnostic tests and fit a patient with a Holter monitor.**

Cardiac diagnostic tests include an ECG; a stress test to determine the patient's cardiac response to exercise; a 24-hour Holter monitor to pick up abnormalities during the patient's routine day; a 30-day event monitor to record infrequent cardiac symptoms; and a heart scan to provide noninvasive diagnostic information. Procedure 42-2 explains how to fit a patient with a Holter monitor.

12. **Discuss patient education and the legal and ethical issues involved when performing ECGs.**

Diagnostic procedures have a profound effect on a patient's subsequent treatment. When the medical assistant is entrusted with performing testing procedures, he or she assumes full responsibility for the accuracy and precision of tests performed. This is a critical role in the medical assisting profession. The results you submit strongly influence each patient's therapeutic treatment plan. No test is ever just routine.

CONNECTIONS

Study Guide Connection: Go to the Chapter 42 Study Guide. Read and complete the activities.

evolve Evolve Connection: Go to the Chapter 42 link at *evolve.elsevier.com/kinn* to complete the Chapter Review Quiz. Check out the other resources listed for this chapter to make the most of what you have learned from Principles of Electrocardiography.

Sara Elwood, CMA (AAMA), is employed by Metro Urgicenter, an urgent care clinic in an urban setting. Metro is staffed around the clock and sees patients with urgent problems that are not immediately life-threatening. The facilities at the center include an x-ray department, where images of the spine and the extremities are taken to evaluate for possible fractures. Chest images also are taken to aid the diagnosis of patients with respiratory complaints. The center's staff physicians read the x-ray images as they are taken.

Afterward, the images are sent to a local hospital for formal interpretation by a radiologist. Sara often assists Dr. David Swain, a staff physician, by preparing patients for x-ray examinations and processing images. Sometimes she is responsible for sending the images to the hospital for interpretation. When a patient is sent to another facility for special imaging studies, Sara makes the arrangements and provides the patient with a preliminary explanation of the procedure.

While studying this chapter, think about the following questions:

- To fulfill her job description at Metro Urgicenter, what does Sara need to know about preparing patients for routine x-ray examinations?

- What should Sara know about various diagnostic procedures so that she can effectively provide patient education and answer patients' scheduling questions?
- How are images stored and relayed?

LEARNING OBJECTIVES

1. Define, spell, and pronounce the terms listed in the vocabulary.
2. Discuss basic principles of radiography and the types of x-rays.
3. Identify the principal components of radiographic equipment.
4. Discuss the four prime factors of x-ray exposure.
5. Do the following related to radiographic positioning:
   - Distinguish among the three body planes and use these terms correctly when discussing radiographic positions.
   - Differentiate between anteroposterior (AP) and posteroanterior (PA) projections and describe the lateral and oblique radiographic positions.
6. Discuss fluoroscopy and contrast media.
7. Discuss cardiovascular and interventional radiography, computed tomography, magnetic resonance imaging, sonography, and nuclear medicine.

8. Do the following related to basic radiographic procedures:
   - Explain the patient preparation guidelines for typical diagnostic imaging examinations.
   - Outline the general procedure for scheduling and sequencing diagnostic imagining procedures.
   - Apply patient education principles when providing instructions for preparing for diagnostic procedures.
9. Describe the health risks associated with low doses of x-ray exposure, such as those used in radiography.
10. Describe precautions for ensuring the safety of equipment operators and staff members during x-ray procedures.
11. Summarize the steps for ensuring that patients receive the least possible exposure during x-ray procedures.
12. Explain the legal responsibilities associated with x-ray procedures and the administrative management of diagnostic images.

VOCABULARY

air kerma Kinetic energy released in matter (Gy-$_a$); this is the SI unit term for radiation exposure that represents the amount of radiation in the air to reach the patient. It is measured in Gray, and a subscript "a" is added to indicate that it is a measurement of the radiation in the air.

angiocardiography (an-je-o-kahr-de-og'-ruh-fe) Radiography of both the heart and great vessels using an iodinated contrast medium.

angiography (an-je-og'-ruh-fe) The process of producing an image of blood vessels using an iodine contrast medium.

angioplasty (an'-je-o-plas-te) An interventional technique in which a catheter is used to open or widen a blood vessel to improve circulation.

anterior (an-ter'-e-ohr) The front part of the body or body part while in anatomic position.

anteroposterior (AP) projection (an-tuhr-o-pos-ter'-e-ohr) A frontal projection in which the central ray enters the front of the patient and exits the back to reach the image receptor; the patient is supine or facing the x-ray tube.

aortogram (a-or′-tuh-gram) An image of the aorta, created by using an iodinated contrast medium.

arteriography (ahr-ter-e-og′-ruh-fe) The process of producing an image of arteries using an iodinated contrast medium.

arthrogram (ahr′-thro-gram) Fluoroscopic record of the soft tissue components of joints with direct injection of a contrast medium into the joint capsule.

axial projections Radiographs taken with a longitudinal angulation of the x-ray beam; sometimes referred to as *semiaxial projections.*

Bucky A moving grid device that holds an image receptor and prevents scatter radiation from fogging the image.

cassette A special container that holds either film or a phosphorescent screen inside; it is used to transform an x-ray beam into a visible image; also referred to as an *image receptor* when loaded.

cathartics Laxative preparations.

central ray (CR) An imaginary line in the center of the x-ray beam that leaves the tube and reaches the patient.

computed tomography (CT) A computerized x-ray imaging modality that provides axial and three-dimensional scans.

contrast media Substances used to enhance the visibility of soft tissues in imaging studies.

computed radiography (CR) A modernized x-ray film that uses a reusable cassette-plate image receptor that stores the image much like a flash drive used in household computers.

control booth A separated area or room where the x-ray machine operator can remain safe from radiation while operating radiography equipment. It is protected by a special wall and/or window lined with lead. This area houses the control console, which contains the settings for the machine.

digital radiography (DR) Cassetteless radiography equipment with built-in image receptors that react to radiation and transmit a digital signal directly to the computer.

exposure time The duration of the patient's x-ray exposure, in seconds; the amount of x-rays produced depends on the length of exposure.

dosimeter A badge for monitoring the radiation exposure of personnel.

fluoroscopy (floo-ros′-kuh-pe) Direct observation of an x-ray image in motion.

gantry A doughnut-shaped portion of a scanner that surrounds the patient and functions, at least partly, to gather imaging data.

gray (Gy) The international unit of radiation dose.

image receptor (IR) A device used to transform an x-ray beam into a visible image; it may include a cassette (with either film or a phosphorescent screen inside) or a special detector that is built into the table or Bucky.

intravenous urogram (IVU) Radiographic examination of the urinary tract using intravenous injection of an iodinated contrast medium; also called an *intravenous pyelogram* (IVP).

kilovoltage (kVp) The electrical control setting that determines the penetrating power of the x-ray beam; the higher the voltage, the shorter the x-ray wavelengths and the greater the energy of the x-ray beam.

lateral position A radiographic position labeled according to which of the patient's sides is facing the image receptor.

limited radiography A simplified role in radiography, usually in an outpatient setting; also called *practical radiography.* The limited radiographer may be referred to as a *limited operator* or *basic machine operator.*

lower gastrointestinal (LGI) series Fluoroscopic examination of the colon; barium sulfate usually is used as a contrast medium and is administered rectally; also called a *barium enema.*

magnetic resonance imaging (MRI) An imaging modality that uses a magnetic field and radiofrequency pulses to create computer images of both bones and soft tissues in multiple planes.

milliamperage (mA) The electrical control setting that determines the amount or concentration of the x-rays by controlling how rapidly the radiation is produced; the higher the mA setting, the more x-rays are produced.

myelography (mi-uh-log′-ruh-fe) Fluoroscopic examination of the spinal canal with spinal injection of an iodinated contrast medium.

NPO Nothing by mouth, from the Latin *nil per os.*

nuclear medicine An imaging modality that uses radioactive materials injected or ingested into the body to provide information about the function of organs and tissues.

oblique position Radiographic position in which the body or part is rotated at an angle that is neither frontal nor lateral.

posterior The back portion of the body or body part.

posteroanterior (PA) projection A view in which the central ray enters the back and exits the front of the patient's body; the patient is prone or facing the image receptor.

radiograph An x-ray image taken by a radiographer in the process of radiography.

radiographer One who takes x-rays.

radiography The process of creating an x-ray image to examine internal structures of the body.

radiographic position In radiography, this refers to the placement of a body part, as seen by the image receptor.

radiographic projection In radiography, this refers to the path of the central ray from the radiographic tube, through the patient, and to the image receptor. It is a view, as seen by the x-ray tube.

radiologist A physician who specializes in medical imaging or therapeutic applications of radiation.

sievert (Sv) (se′-vuhrt) The international unit of radiation dose equivalent.

sonography A noninvasive procedure that uses high-frequency sound waves to produce echoes in the body, which are used to create images; common, but not limited to fetal imaging (often referred to as *diagnostic ultrasound*).

source-to-image distance (SID) The distance between the x-ray tube and the film or other image receptor; the greater the distance, the more widely the x-ray beam is spread and the lower the intensity of the beam.

tracers Special radioactive materials that are swallowed or injected intravenously, to track the activity of cells and determine the location of fractures.

upper gastrointestinal (UGI) series Fluoroscopic examination of the esophagus, stomach, and duodenum; barium sulfate is used as a contrast medium and is administered orally.

X-ray images have been used for more than 100 years to examine the internal structures of the body. The fascinating field of medical imaging now includes a wide variety of diagnostic imaging methods. This chapter provides an overview of imaging modalities and introduces you to radiography. Emphasis is placed on x-ray examinations because these are the procedures most commonly performed in the medical assistant's practice setting.

Basic Principles of Radiography

Radiography is the process of creating an x-ray image to examine internal structures of the body. On November 8, 1895, radiography was born when Wilhelm Konrad Roentgen (Figure 43-1) accidentally discovered the first x-ray during an experiment at a German university. Thereafter, scientists and physicians became the first radiographers. Over the years, the process has been further refined, resulting in more advanced discoveries in diagnostic imaging.

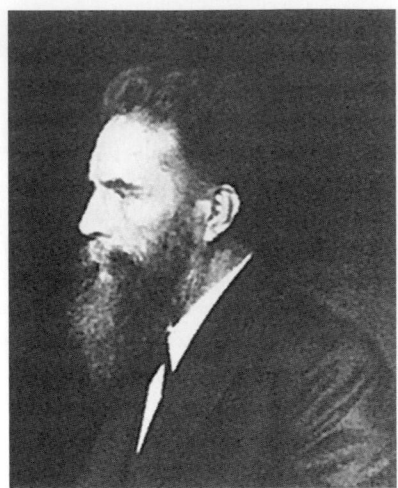

FIGURE 43-1 Wilhelm Konrad Roentgen. (Dibner B: *The new rays of Professor Roentgen,* Norwalk, Conn, 1962, Burndy Library Collection, The Huntington Library, San Marino, Calif.)

How X-Rays Are Created

Ironically, x-rays are created from the tiniest possible particles of matter: atoms. Up close, atoms look a lot like a solar system, with protons and neutrons combining at the core and electrons circling in orbit. When atoms get hot, the orbiting electrons spin faster. The hotter it gets, the faster they spin. Eventually, the force created from the speed causes the electron to break loose and fly out of orbit, producing an energy stream in its wake. When enough electrons are involved and are directed by magnetic pull, a forceful x-ray beam is created.

Because a great deal of heat is needed to create an x-ray beam, a material that can withstand excessive heat must be used. Tungsten metal is the preferred material because it has a very high melting point. As a result, it creates the ability to produce x-rays that are forceful enough to penetrate and exit the body.

It's All in the Name

- Because the process in radiographic imaging is invisible to the naked eye, Wilhelm Konrad Roentgen didn't initially know what kind of ray caused the image he created. Therefore, he called it an "x" ray.
- It is important to note that radio*graphy* is different than radio*logy*, which involves interpretation of images and requires more extensive education in medical school.

A radiographer is much like a photographer who takes a picture with a camera and then processes it (Figure 43-2). In radiography, the camera is larger and more complicated. However, the philosophy is much the same. The radiographer positions a patient in front of the "film" and then directs a beam of radiation onto the targeted area. When the x-ray beam passes through the patient, solid structures (like bones) leave behind a "shadow," or image, known as a **radiograph** (or x-ray).

As with a flashlight beam, when x-rays emerge from the machine, they create a beam in a conelike field that enlarges as it moves farther from the energy source. In radiography, the beam of x-rays is called the *radiation field* (Figure 43-3, *A*). Only items placed within this

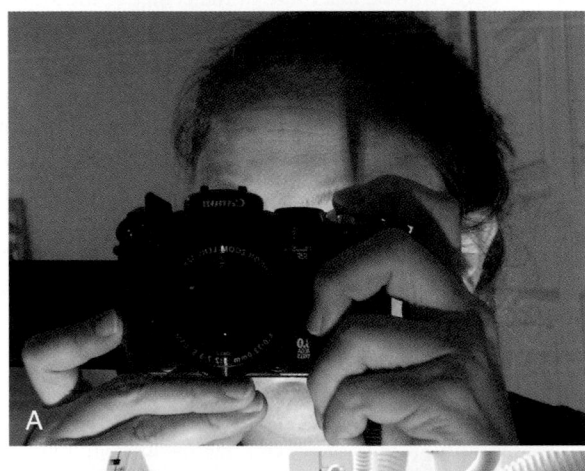

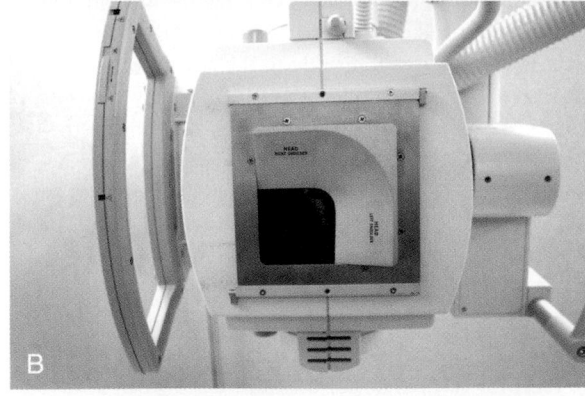

FIGURE 43-2 A, A radiographer is much like a photographer who takes a picture with a camera and then processes it. **B,** The x-ray tube housing and collimator appear somewhat similar to a camera. (**A** courtesy Helen Mills; **B** from Frank ED, Long BW, Smith BJ: *Merrill's atlas of radiographic positioning and procedures,* ed 12, St Louis, 2013, Mosby.)

field can be imaged. The very center of this field is called the **central ray (CR)** (Figure 43-3, *B*). Because it is the most concentrated point of radiation, the targeted part typically is placed in this area. Also similar to a flashlight, the radiation field creates shadows by invisibly "shining" onto the body and penetrating through everything except bone. As a result, the area around the bone is darkened, and the unpenetrated "shadow" remains white (Figure 43-4).

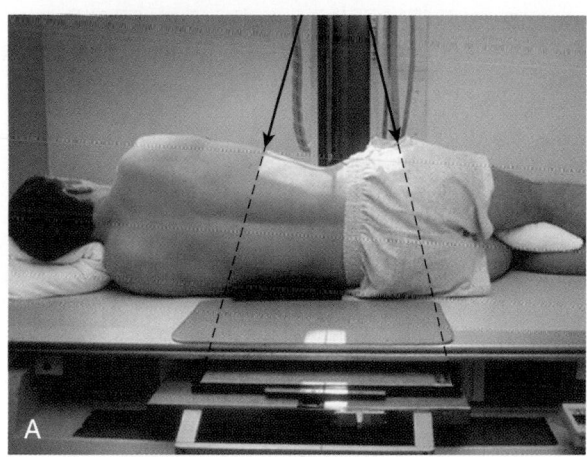
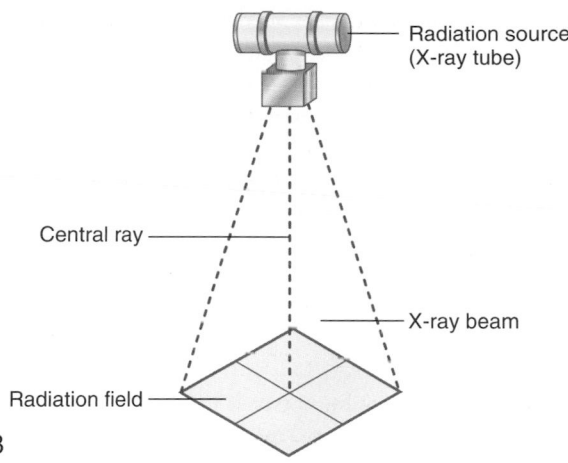

FIGURE 43-3 A, The collimator's light beam demonstrates the radiation field and aids alignment of the image receptor. As does the x-ray beam, the conelike shape of the light becomes larger and less concentrated as it gets farther from the x-ray tube. **B,** The primary x-ray beam leaves the x-ray tube. The useful part of the beam is called the *radiation field.* The center of the beam is called the *central ray.* (**A** from Bontrager KL, Lampignano J: *Textbook of radiographic positioning and related anatomy,* ed 7, St Louis, 2009, Mosby.)

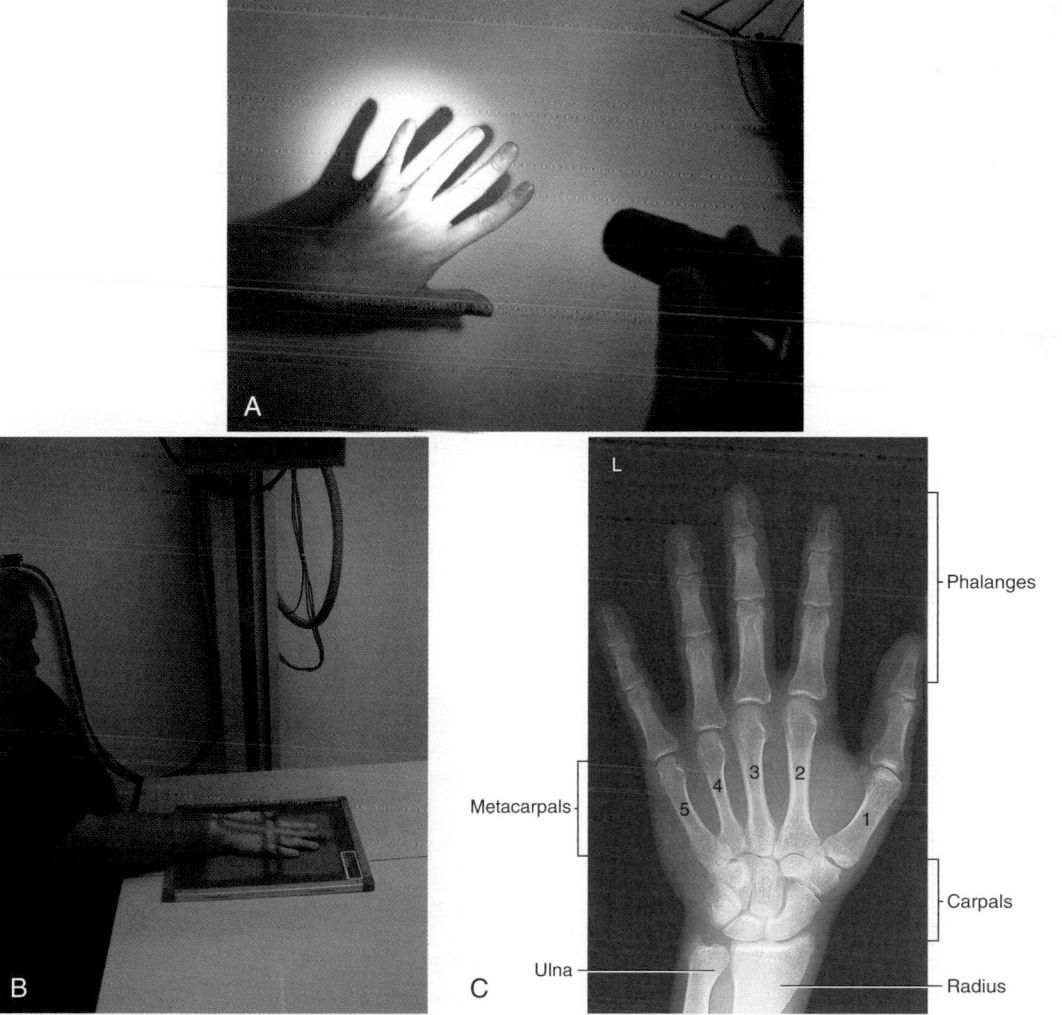

FIGURE 43-4 A, An x-ray creates an image in a manner similar to the way a flashlight beam creates a shadow. **B,** The hand is placed on the film, and invisible radiation shines down from above during exposure, as demonstrated by the light of the collimator. **C,** PA projection of the hand: the bones block x-rays from reaching the film, creating a white shadow. (**A** and **B** courtesy Helen Mills; **C** from Long BW, Frank ED, Ehrlich RA: *Radiography essentials for limited practice,* ed 4, Philadelphia, 2013, Saunders.)

Consider a piece of chicken on your dinner plate. Which is hardest to push a knife through: an area of fat, the thickest area of meat, or bone? Of course, the bone is hardest because it is the most dense. As a result, more force is needed to penetrate bone than muscle or fat. Other factors must be considered, too, such as size. Less power is needed to pierce a thin bone than a thicker bone. X-rays work in much the same way. To determine how to adjust imaging settings, factors such as body size and shape must be taken into account so that the beam properly penetrates the tissues and produces a clear image of the area of concern.

Types of X-rays

Radiation is invisible, and it always travels in straight lines. When an x-ray beam leaves the machine, it is called *primary radiation* (Figure 43-5). After it passes through the patient, it is referred to as *remnant radiation*; this is what creates the image. When an x-ray strikes something and bounces in a different direction, it is referred to as *scatter radiation.*

Not all x-rays that are produced are useful. When a primary x-ray beam reaches a patient, the following may occur:

1. Some of the x-ray beam is absorbed by the body, but enough exits to create an image. This is the main goal in radiography.
2. The x-ray beam is totally absorbed by the body. It does not produce an image and is not useful.
3. The x-ray beam bounces off the patient or table and lands in unintended places (scatter radiation). When it lands around the image, it makes the picture cloudy and more difficult to see. To obtain a clear image, it is important to reduce scatter radiation as much as possible.

Aluminum is the primary filtration material used in radiographic equipment. It is placed between the tube housing port and the patient, to contain and remove useless radiation. This reduces the patient dose and makes the process safer. It also results in a cleaner image, which reduces the likelihood of having to retake a radiograph for better visualization.

Routine plain images are simple radiographs taken of specific body structures, such as the chest or the bones of the extremities or spine. These are the examinations most often performed in ambulatory care centers and most likely to be performed by limited operators, who typically are medical assistants licensed to practice radiography in their state.

Radiographic Equipment

Control Booth

A **control booth** is a separated area or room where the radiographer can remain safe from radiation while operating the equipment. It is protected by a special wall and/or window lined with lead. This area houses the *control console,* which contains the settings for the machine. The control console typically is able to adjust the primary settings: kilovoltage (kVp), milliamperage (mA), and exposure time in seconds (s). It also has a button for turning the power to the console on and off, in addition to two exposure control buttons, which must be pressed in unison to take the x-ray image.

Image Receptor Systems

The **image receptor (IR)** creates the x-ray picture when exposed to radiation. Depending on the type of equipment used, it can take specific forms.

In older x-ray machines, the IR is a special **cassette** that holds traditional film, which must be removed and developed after use (Figure 43-6). This requires special training in handling and processing the film. A separate "light tight" room is used strictly for developing. This room must have enough space to store large chemical tanks, equipment, special lights, unprocessed film, and other materials, in addition to plumbing to provide water for the developing machine. Once processed, the film also must be stored, which requires additional storage space. This is an antiquated method that is being phased out in most offices, but it may still be in use in some cases.

In **computed radiography (CR)**, the image receptor includes a reusable cassette plate, also considered an IR, that stores the image much like a flash drive used in household computers. The x-ray machine operator inserts the CR plate into a reader, which loads the image into the computer (Figure 43-7). A high-intensity laser beam in the processor produces a visible image. This image either is displayed on a monitor or printed with a laser film printer. CR has replaced most film systems to date because it is more convenient and saves time, money, and space. Processing images on the computer

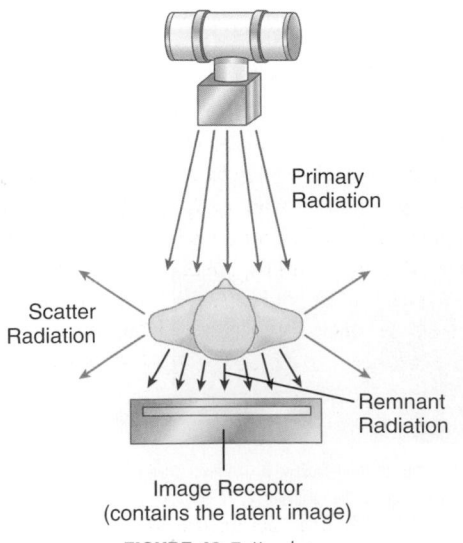

Primary Radiation

Scatter Radiation

Remnant Radiation

Image Receptor
(contains the latent image)

FIGURE 43-5 X-ray beam.

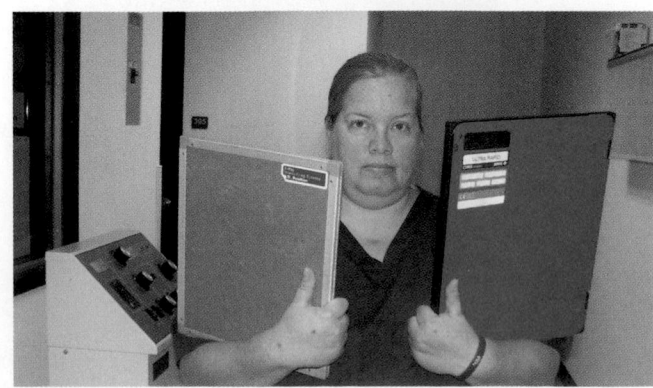

FIGURE 43-6 Image receptors (IRs). Traditional IR *(gray)* and computed radiography IR *(red)*. (Courtesy Helen Mills.)

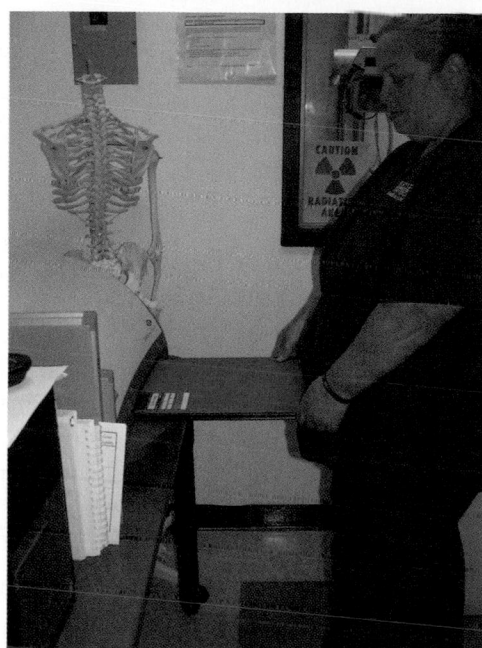

FIGURE 43-7 A computed radiography image receptor (IR) plate is inserted into a reader to load the image into the computer. (Courtesy Helen Mills.)

requires much less room and equipment and allows for electronic storage and transmission.

Digital radiography (DR) is the most modern radiography equipment. With DR, the image receptor is built into the Bucky; thus, this system is considered cassetteless, although cassettes are available for mobile imaging. The digital IR reacts to the radiation shadow and transmits a digital signal directly to the computer. As a result, no cassettes or processing typically are involved. In addition, the computer software may have the capacity to provide further assistance in determining appropriate settings. This is the preferred method of radiography because it provides a multitude of options. As a result of technologic advances, a traditional or computerized Bucky can be converted to DR by inserting a digital detector into the existing equipment. Digital sensor Wi-Fi cassettes can also be used for mobile radiography.

Both CR and DR allow for image adjustments after the x-ray image is taken. This is preferred because it may reduce the number of retakes resulting from operator error and thus reduce the patient's exposure to radiation. Conventional radiographs can be added to the electronic system by scanning them with a laser device called a *film digitizer;* however, both the quality of the images and the ability to adjust them are limited.

Identification. It is essential to label all images with the patient's name and birthdate or medical records ID number, in addition to the date and location of the examination. Serious errors in diagnosis and treatment might occur if images are not correctly identified. When traditional film is used, the identification information is typed on a card that is inserted into the photographic printer in the darkroom. The printer is used to stamp the information on the film after it has been removed from the cassette and before it is processed. With DR and CR, the information is typed into the computer and superimposed on the image.

TABLE 43-1	Essential Elements of Electronic Imaging
DICOM (Digital Imaging and Communications in Medicine)	Standards for exchanging radiographic images
PACS (Picture Archiving and Communication System)	A server that stores radiographic images
Various viewers	Software applications that allow the viewer to study and manipulate images

Technology in Radiography

The computer technology used to store digital images in hospitals and large healthcare systems is the Picture Archiving and Communication System (PACS). Viewer software can be used to connect images with patient database information (e.g., electronic health records [EHRs]), facilitate laser printing of images, and display both images and information at workstations throughout the network as needed. PACS may include transmission equipment for teleradiology, which allows images both to be viewed in remote locations (e.g., a physician's home) and received from remote locations, such as outlying clinics. Through PACS technology, images can be transmitted directly over telephone lines and via the Internet.

The software that accesses the PACS system must conform to specific formats. Digital Imaging and Communications in Medicine (DICOM) is universally accepted (Table 43-1). DICOM is a set of rules or standards set to ensure that the quality of an image stays the same, regardless of the equipment used to take, view, or store it. Because the slightest difference in a radiographic image can have a significant impact on the patient's diagnosis and care, this is essential.

Radiographic Table

During testing, patients remain in the x-ray room. They may be lying on a *radiographic table* (Figure 43-8) capable of sliding around to move them into place. The table either has filmlike elements built into it or a cassette holder that allows an image receptor to be inserted beneath the patient. It also has a *grid,* a device that absorbs unwanted scatter radiation. Together, the grid and image receptor tray are called a **Bucky** (Figure 43-9). Body parts less than 10 cm thick produce relatively less scatter radiation and do not require a Bucky. In this instance, an image receptor would be placed on top of the table, with the body part directly on top of it.

An upright cassette holder or upright IR holder is like a miniature radiographic table that is placed against the wall; with a grid, it is also called a *Bucky.* It is useful for x-ray studies that require a patient to sit or stand.

X-ray Tubes

X-rays are produced in a vacuum-sealed Pyrex glass tube, where all the components can come together without disruption from

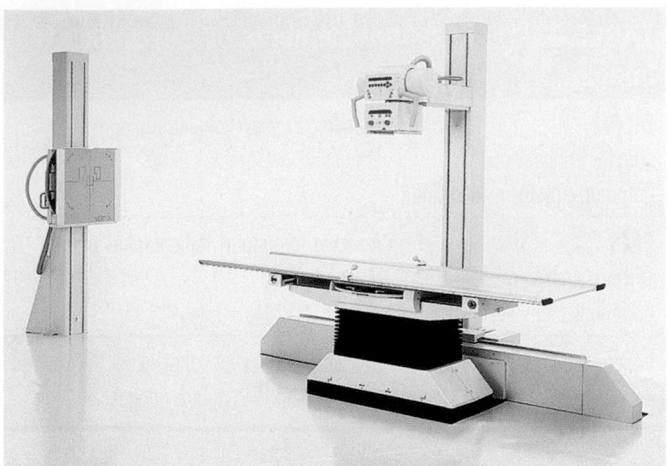

FIGURE 43-8 Radiography table with a tube stand and tube housing; to the side is a standing Bucky. (From Long BW, Frank ED, Ehrlich RA: *Radiography essentials for limited practice*, ed 3, Philadelphia, 2010, Saunders.)

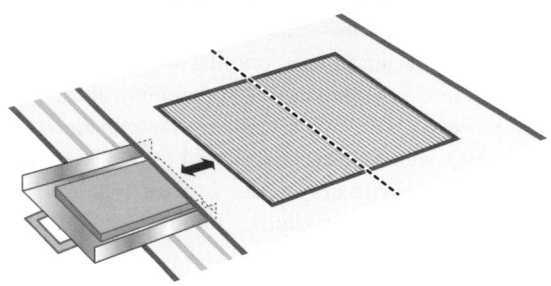

FIGURE 43-9 Bucky grid in place under the surface of the x-ray table.

contaminants in the air. To produce the intense heat needed, high-voltage electrical currents must be created and sent into the tube to heat a tungsten coil. Once the coil is heated, electrons fly out of orbit and are flung into a tungsten target, which directs the flow toward the patient.

The x-ray tube is attached to the wall and/or ceiling to allow it to hover over the radiographic table. It is surrounded by a lead-lined housing, which protects the tube and contains the radiation. Tube supports allow the operator to move the tube in different directions and to adjust its height. The tube automatically locks into place at stopping points, known as *detents*. The lock must be released each time the tube must be moved. The distance from the tube to the image receptor typically is set at 40 or 72 inches, depending on the requirements of the procedure.

Collimator

The collimator is a boxlike device attached beneath the tube housing. It allows the operator to adjust the size of the radiation field. A light at the base of the collimator is used to help the operator see the area that will be affected by radiation, for ease of adjustment. When collimating, it is important to make the field large enough to cover the body part being evaluated, but not so large that it results in unnecessary radiation that can cloud the picture and be absorbed by the patient. Collimation should occur at the center of the image receptor to allow for a clean, complete image.

Power Supply

A *transformer cabinet* typically stands in the corner of the room. It is connected both to the x-ray tube and to the control console by cables. It produces the high voltage required to create x-rays and the low mA needed in the x-ray tube.

X-ray Exposure

Prime Factors

The **radiographer** must take a number of factors into consideration in determining the proper technique and exposure factors for an x-ray examination. The four principal exposure factors are called the *prime factors of exposure*. The interaction of these factors determines the level of x-ray production and ultimately the amount of the patient's x-ray exposure. The prime factors are:

- **Milliamperage (mA):** The electrical control setting that determines the amount or concentration of the x-rays by controlling how rapidly the radiation is produced; the higher the mA setting, the more x-rays are produced.
- **Exposure time** (in seconds [s]): The duration of the patient's x-ray exposure; most exposures are less than 1 second, so the total time a patient is exposed to the x-ray is measured in milliseconds. The amount of x-rays produced depends on the length of exposure.
- **Kilovoltage (kVp):** The electrical control setting that determines the penetrating power of the x-ray beam; voltage controls the speed and power of x-ray beams; the higher the voltage, the shorter the x-ray wavelengths and the greater the energy of the x-ray beam. The following box distinguishes between mA and kVp.
- **Source-to-image distance (SID):** The distance between the x-ray tube and the film or other image receptor; the greater the distance, the more widely the x-ray beam will spread and the lower the intensity of the beam

---

Memory Aids: *kVp versus mA*

kV**p** = **p**ower

m**A** = **A**mount

The total amount of radiation in an exposure is indicated by the milliampere-seconds (mAs), which are determined by multiplying the rate of x-ray current flow (mA) by the exposure time (s). The mAs directly affects the degree of detail or density visible on the image. The operator can adjust the amount of radiation to the patient by adjusting the mA and time settings to administer higher doses of radiation (mA) for shorter periods (s) (especially useful when there is uncontrolled movement, such as with a crying child) or a lower dose for a longer period. The total amount of x-ray exposure used to perform a particular diagnostic study is a combination of kVp, mA, exposure time, and SID.

Technique Charts. A technique chart located near the control console or on the computer screen provides the radiographer with a list of recommended milliampere-seconds, kilovoltage, and source-to-image distance settings for x-ray studies of various body parts in patients of different sizes. The radiographer must refer to technique charts before performing the ordered radiographic procedure. Some control consoles have computerized units that are preprogrammed with the required exposure settings for the selected body part and its size.

Radiographic Positioning

Anatomic Locations

To understand how to read an x-ray order and properly position a patient on the radiographic table, it is essential to understand anatomic terminology. Terms that indicate the surfaces, directions, and planes of various body locations are based on anatomic positioning.

Anatomic position (Figure 43-10) is a view of the body in which the individual is standing, facing the observer, with the palms of the hands forward and the thumbs out. When considering these terms, it is important that you imagine the patient as though standing in this position. It is also important to remember that designations such as "right" or "left" are from the patient's viewpoint (i.e., the patient's right, not the observer's right).

Terms that describe locations on and within the body include the following:

- **Anterior** *(ventral):* Forward or front portion of the body or body part.
- *Cephalic:* Pertaining to the head; toward the head.
- *Caudal:* Toward the tail or end of the body; away from the head; the opposite of cephalic.
- *Distal:* Away from the source or point of origin. For example, the wrist is distal to the elbow, the elbow distal to the shoulder.
- *External:* To the outside, at or near the surface of the body or a body part.
- *Inferior:* Below, farther from the head. For example, the diaphragm is inferior to the lungs.
- *Internal:* Deep, near the center of the body or a part; the opposite of external.
- *Lateral:* Referring to the side or away from the center.

- *Medial:* Toward the center of the body or body part; the opposite of lateral.
- *Palmar:* Referring to the palm (anterior surface) of the hand.
- *Plantar:* Referring to the sole of the foot.
- **Posterior** *(dorsal):* Backward or back portion of the body or body part; the opposite of anterior.
- *Proximal:* Toward the source or point of origin; the opposite of distal. For example, the part of the femur that is attached at the hip is the proximal end of the femur, and the part of the bone that is located at the knee is the distal end of the femur.
- *Superior:* Above, toward the head; the opposite of inferior. For example, the esophagus is superior to the stomach.

Body Planes

Besides anatomic position terms, the planes of the body may be used in radiographic imaging (Figure 43-11). The **sagittal plane** divides the body into right and left parts, and the midsagittal plane divides the body into equal right and left parts. The **coronal plane** (sometimes called the *frontal plane*) divides the body into anterior and posterior parts. The midcoronal or midfrontal plane divides the body into relatively equal parts; it passes through the external auditory meatus (the opening of the ear), the center of the shoulder, the greater trochanter (the bony prominence in the lateral hip area), and the lateral malleolus (the bony prominence on the lateral surface of the ankle). The **transverse plane** divides the body into superior and inferior portions; it may be drawn at any level.

Positions

The medical assistant may assist with radiographic procedures by helping position the patient for a particular x-ray view. Body positions describe the way a patient is placed.

- *Recumbent:* Lying down (in any position); the position may be further described by adding the name of the body surface on which the patient is lying:
  - *Dorsal recumbent:* Lying on the back (supine) with the knees bent and the feet flat on the table

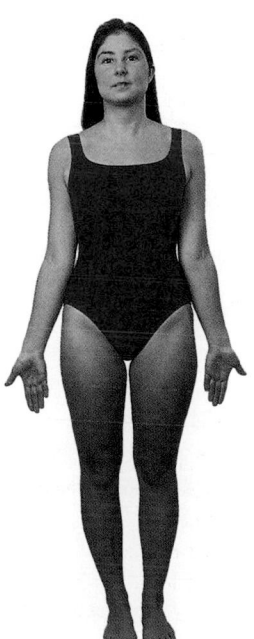

FIGURE 43-10 Anatomical position. (From Frank ED, Long BW, Smith BJ: *Merrill's atlas of radiographic positioning and procedures,* ed 12, St Louis, 2013, Mosby.)

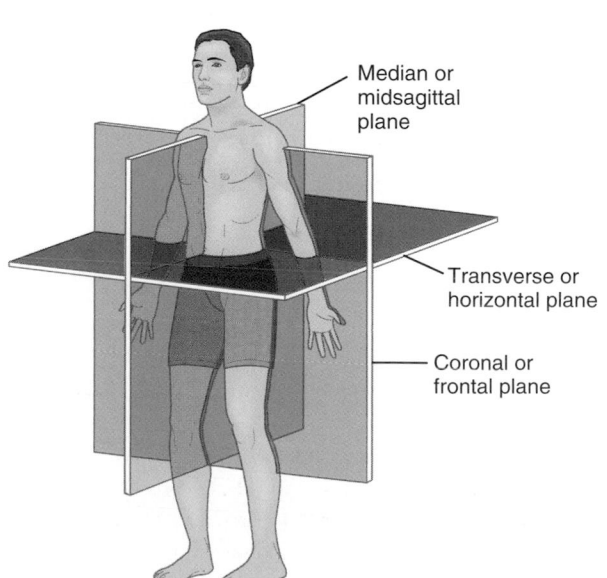

Median or midsagittal plane

Transverse or horizontal plane

Coronal or frontal plane

FIGURE 43-11 Body planes.

- *Lateral recumbent:* Lying on the side
- *Ventral recumbent:* Lying face down, prone
- *Supine:* Lying on the back, face up
- *Prone:* Lying face down
- *Upright:* Standing or seated

Radiographic positions describe how a patient is placed as if seen by the image receptor. These positions can be used as follows in x-ray positioning:

- **Oblique position:** At an angle or a slant (Figure 43-12); always named for the side of the patient nearest the image receptor; further described by combining with projection terms discussed later in this chapter.
  - *Left anterior oblique:* Patient's left side is on the image receptor, with his or her anterior (front) leaning toward the IR.
  - *Right anterior oblique:* Patient's right side is on the image receptor, with his or her anterior (front) leaning toward the IR.
  - *Left posterior oblique:* Patient's left side is on the image receptor, with his or her posterior (back) leaning toward the IR.
  - *Right posterior oblique:* Patient's right side is on the image receptor, with his or her posterior (back) leaning toward the IR.
- **Lateral position:** On the side; always named for the side of the patient nearest the image receptor (Figure 43-13).
  - *Left lateral:* Patient's left side is on the image receptor.
  - *Right lateral:* Patient's right side is on the image receptor.

Radiographic Projections

Sometimes it is helpful to take x-ray images from different views, to get a complete understanding from different angles. A **radio-**

graphic projection (or view) describes the position of the patient as though seen by the x-ray tube. *This is the most accurate term to describe how the patient is placed for the procedure.* It can be used as follows:

- **Anteroposterior (AP) projection:** The x-ray beam leaves the tube, passes through the front of the patient, and exits through the patient's back to reach the image receptor (Figure 43-14). In other words, the patient is supine or facing the x-ray tube.
- **Posteroanterior (PA) projection:** The x-ray beam leaves the tube, passes through the back of the patient, and exits through the patient's front to reach the image receptor (Figure 43-15). In other words, the patient is prone or facing the image receptor.

With both AP and PA projections, the x-ray beam typically reaches the patient at a direct 90-degree (perpendicular) angle. When the beam is tilted slightly, an image can be seen around structures that otherwise would block the view. **Axial projections** (or *semiaxial projections*) are radiographs taken with a longitudinal angulation of the x-ray beam. The beam is projected at an angle, which is further described by the beam's direction (Figure 43-16). If the central ray is described as being cephalad or as having a cephalic angulation, it enters the patient at an angle, directed toward the patient's head.

Memory Aids: *Position versus Projection*
Position: What the image <u>receptor</u> sees
Projection: What the x-ray <u>tube</u> sees

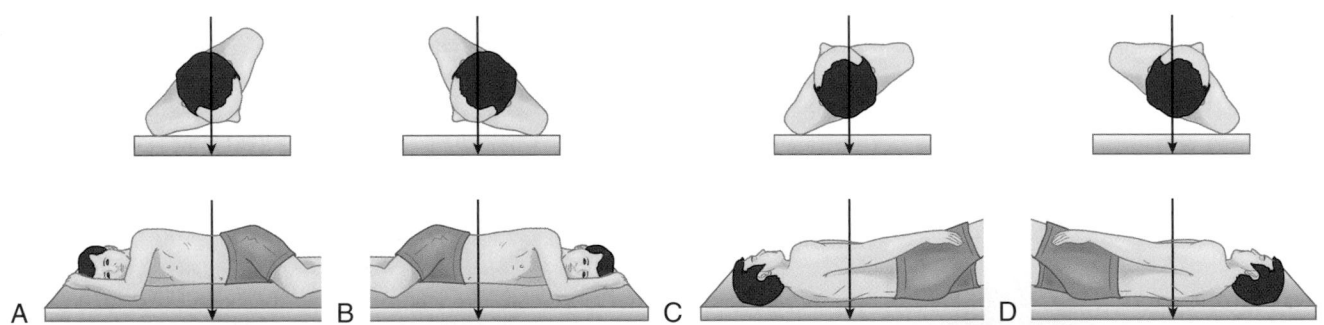

FIGURE 43-12 Oblique positions. **A,** Right anterior oblique (RAO). **B,** Left anterior oblique (LAO). **C,** Left posterior oblique (LPO). **D,** Right posterior oblique (RPO).

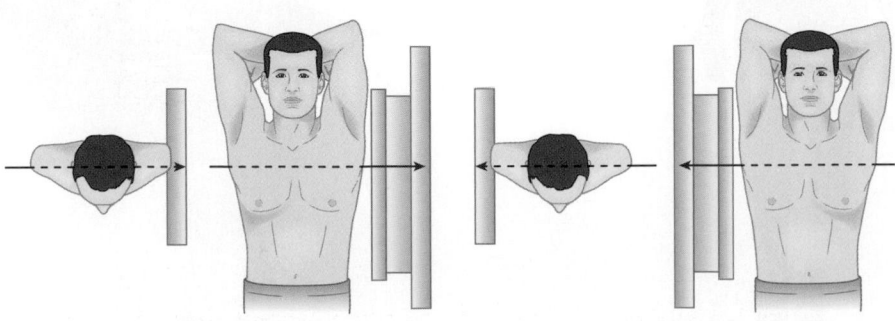

Left lateral   Right lateral

FIGURE 43-13 Lateral positions are named for the side of the body nearer the image receptor.

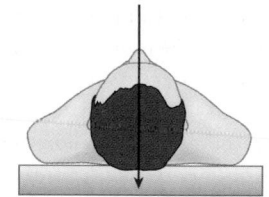

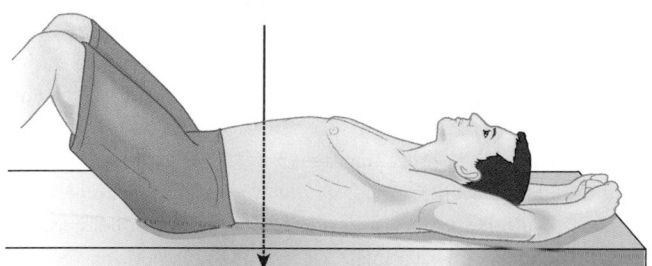

FIGURE 43-14 Anteroposterior (AP) projection.

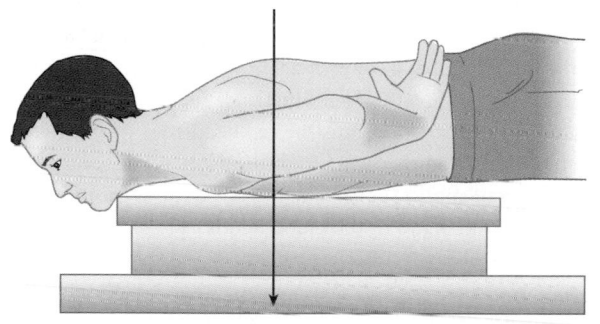

FIGURE 43-15 Posteroanterior (PA) projection.

Axial Projections

If the central ray (CR) is described as being caudad or having a caudal angulation, it enters the patient at an angle that is directed away from the patient's head. This is a method of further detailing both posteroanterior (PA) and anteroposterior (AP) projections.

For example:

- *AP: CR 15-30 degrees cephalad:* The x-ray beam is tilted at a 15- to 30-degree angle, rotated toward the patient's head while the patient is supine or facing the x-ray tube.
- *PA: CR 10-20 degrees caudad:* The x-ray beam is tilted at a 10- to 20-degree angle, rotated away from the patient's head while the patient is prone or facing the image receptor.

Markers

When a patient is positioned for an x-ray image, it is important to align the image receptor, grid, and x-ray beam, with the central ray at the center of the body part to be evaluated. Markers are then used to indicate which side of the body is being imaged. Markers are small squares of plastic with a metal letter in the center that is captured on the image when placed in the radiation field. Right (R) and left (L) are used to indicate the side of the body according to anatomic position (i.e., from the patient's viewpoint). An R or L marker is placed within the radiation field and appears on the image; this helps the viewer identify which part is being viewed.

A technique handbook should be kept on hand to ensure that the correct position is used for the ordered x-ray image.

OTHER DIAGNOSTIC RADIOLOGIC TESTING

Patients typically are sent to another department or facility for more advanced radiologic testing. Although medical assistants do not generally perform the procedures for these tests, it is important that they understand them so that they can educate and prepare the patient. Some tests focus on a specific organ or body part, whereas others create images of a general area. Some tests require the administration of a contrast medium, which enables specific structures to light up and be seen more easily. Some tests involve fluoroscopy, which uses special screens that allow movement to be seen as it occurs.

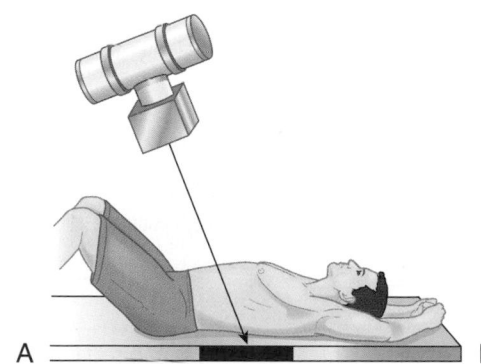
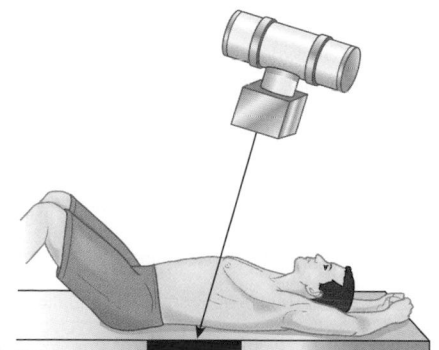

FIGURE 43-16 In axial projections, the x-ray tube is angled to direct the central ray along the long axis of the body or part. **A,** AP projection with a cephalic angulation. **B,** AP projection with a caudal angulation.

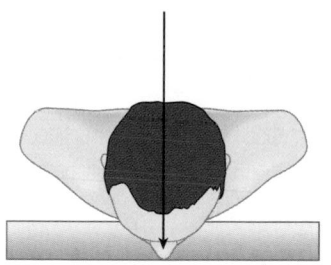

Regardless of the specifics, all tests require patient education to prepare patients and ease their concerns.

Fluoroscopy and X-ray Studies That Use Contrast Media

Fluoroscopy

Fluoroscopy is a technique in which special equipment is used to allow the **radiologist** to view x-ray images in motion. Fluoroscopy also allows the physician to survey an area quickly, without the delay involved in taking and processing images. Most fluoroscopic units are properly called *radiographic/fluoroscopic* (R/F) units because they are designed to take both x-ray images and fluoroscopic views. The x-ray images taken during a fluoroscopic procedure, which are called *spot films,* record the image as seen on the fluoroscope; sometimes the entire fluoroscopic examination is recorded digitally. After the fluoroscopic portion of the study is complete, larger radiographs usually are taken for comprehensive visualization of the entire anatomic region.

An example of a fluoroscopic diagnostic procedure is a barium swallow. If the provider suspects that the patient has difficulty swallowing, a fluoroscope is used to visualize the actual movement of the substance down the esophagus and into the stomach while the patient is in the act of swallowing. Fluoroscopic procedures typically require the use of a contrast medium, such as barium.

X-ray Studies That Use Contrast Media

Although the lungs and bony structures of the body produce clear x-ray images on radiographs, internal organs, such as the stomach and the kidneys, are difficult to see because they absorb radiation to the same degree as the tissues that surround them. To enhance the visibility of these structures, special agents, called **contrast media**, can be used to fill hollow organs and demonstrate their inner contours. Although gases such as air and carbon dioxide sometimes are used as contrast media, radiopaque substances (materials that stop the passage of x-rays, to highlight a particular area), such as barium sulfate or iodine compounds, are used far more often. The agent and the technique vary with the structures to be viewed (Table 43-2).

Among the most common fluoroscopic examinations are studies of the upper and lower gastrointestinal (GI) tract using barium sulfate as a contrast medium. Both require careful patient instruction and advance preparation for a successful study. For an **upper gastrointestinal (UGI) series** (Figure 43-17), the patient swallows a barium sulfate suspension; this study is performed to aid in the diagnosis of ulcers, tumors, and other abnormalities of the esophagus, stomach, and duodenum.

A **lower gastrointestinal (LGI) series** (Figure 43-18) involves a barium enema, which fills the colon and aids visualization of its inner surfaces. This procedure is especially useful in the diagnosis of polyps, tumors, and diverticulosis. For this examination, the inner lining of the large intestine must be clean and free of all fecal matter. The provider prescribes a commercial bowel preparation kit to ensure complete emptying of the large intestine. If the preparation is not adequate, the examination must be rescheduled.

Water-soluble iodine compounds are used as contrast media for a wide variety of applications. When injected intravenously (IV), the contrast agent circulates in the blood and is excreted by the kidneys,

TABLE 43-2 Radiographic Procedures That Use Contrast Media

EXAMINATION	CONTRAST MEDIUM	ROUTE OF ADMINISTRATION	STRUCTURES SHOWN
Angiocardiography	Iodine compounds	Intra-arterial injection via femoral or brachial catheter	Heart and large vessels
Angiography	Iodine compounds	Intra-arterial or intravenous injection	Blood vessels (further defined by region, i.e. renal, cerebral, pulmonary, gastrointestinal [GI], chol/gallbladder)
Arteriography	Iodine compounds	Intra-arterial injection via catheter	Arteries
Arthrography	Iodine compounds	Direct injection into joint capsule	Joints, especially knee, shoulder, and ankle
Hysterosalpingography	Iodine compounds	Direct injection via cannula	Uterus and fallopian tubes
Intravenous urography; intravenous pyelography (IVP)	Iodine compounds, sometimes air	Intravenous injection	Kidneys, ureters, and urinary bladder
Lower gastrointestinal (GI) series (barium enema)	Barium sulfate suspension, sometimes also with air	Rectal catheter	Colon
Lymphangiography	Iodine compounds	Direct injection into lymphatic vessels in the feet	Lymphatic vessels and lymph nodes
Myelography	Iodine compounds	Intrathecal injection (spinal tap)	Spinal canal
Upper GI series (barium swallow)	Barium sulfate suspension	Oral	Esophagus, stomach, and duodenum

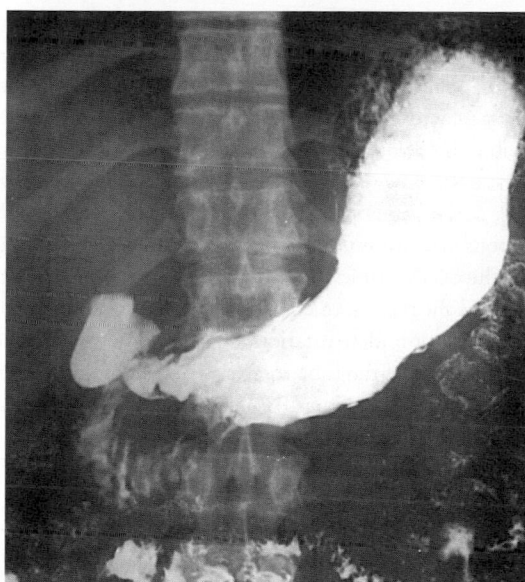

FIGURE 43-17 Radiographic image of the stomach, part of an upper gastrointestinal (UGI) series using oral administration of barium sulfate to provide contrast. (From Ballinger PW, Frank ED: *Merrill's atlas of radiographic positions and radiologic procedures,* ed 10, vol 2, St Louis, 2003, Mosby.)

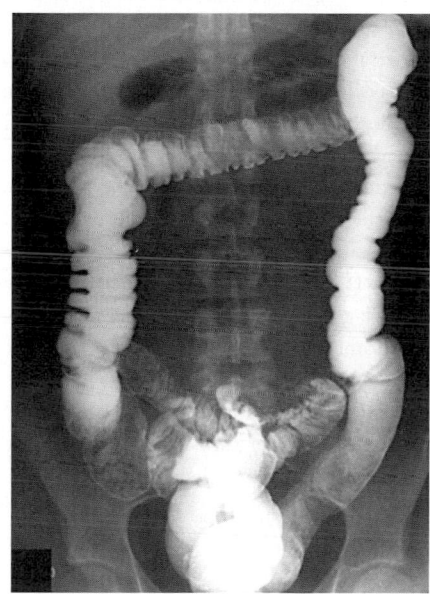

FIGURE 43-18 Lower gastrointestinal (LGI) series. Radiograph of the colon filled with barium sulfate administered by barium enema. (From Ballinger PW, Frank ED: *Merrill's atlas of radiographic positions and radiologic procedures,* ed 10, vol 2, St Louis, 2003, Mosby.)

causing the urine to become radiopaque. Radiography of the kidneys, ureters, and bladder after IV injection of a contrast medium is called an **intravenous urogram (IVU)** (also called an *intravenous pyelogram* [IVP]); this study is useful for identifying kidney stones, tumors, and other abnormalities of the urinary tract. Preparation for an IVU involves fasting and bowel cleansing because material in the colon can obstruct a clear picture of the urinary system.

Iodine contrast agents also can be injected into joint capsules to produce an **arthrogram**, an image of the soft tissue components of joints, especially the knee and the shoulder. **Myelography** involves injection of iodine compounds and sometimes air into the spinal

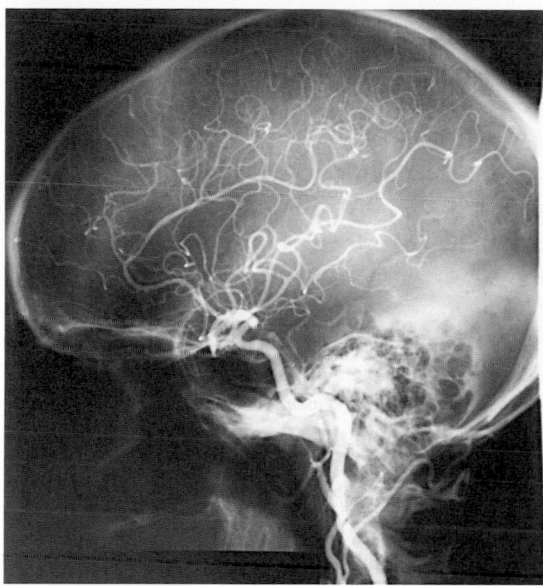

FIGURE 43-19 Cerebral angiogram showing the circulation of the brain enhanced by iodine contrast medium. (From Ballinger PW, Frank ED: *Merrill's atlas of radiographic positions and radiologic procedures,* ed 10, vol 2, St Louis, 2003, Mosby.)

canal to demonstrate pathologic spinal conditions, such as tumors and herniated intervertebral disks. This diagnostic technique is being replaced by magnetic resonance imaging (MRI) and computed tomography (CT) studies, which are less invasive and do not have the potential complications of a myelogram; however, myelography is still useful for patients who cannot undergo MRI or CT for other reasons or if MRI or CT does not provide enough clinical information.

Part of the screening process for diagnostic procedures that use iodine contrast injections is careful questioning of the patient about a history of iodine allergy. All patients who are allergic to shellfish also will be allergic to iodine dye and are at risk for a serious anaphylactic reaction if the contrast agent is injected. The medical assistant is responsible for clarifying allergies with the patient and/or family members and alerting the diagnostic facility if the patient has an iodine allergy. In addition, patients must understand that it is normal to feel flushed or a heat rush when the dye is injected, and some patients initially experience waves of nausea. However, both of these sensations pass quickly.

Cardiovascular and Interventional Radiography

The highly specialized radiographic procedures that display blood vessels are collectively known as **angiography**. A cerebral angiogram, for example, demonstrates the vessels of the brain (Figure 43-19), and renal angiograms show the arteries and veins of the kidneys. An angiocardiogram is a contrast study that shows the interior of the heart chambers and the great vessels that enter and exit the heart, and an **aortogram** demonstrates the aorta. Selective **angiocardiography**, or cardiac catheterization, is used to display the coronary arteries. Arteriograms are pictures of specific arteries, and venograms are studies of veins.

For all these examinations, iodine compounds are injected for radiographic contrast and a rapid series of images are taken or fluoroscopy is used to show the area of concern. Direct injection may be used for some angiographic studies, such as those of the extremities, but the preferred injection method for angiocardiography, aortography, and most **arteriography** procedures is to use a special catheter. A large artery (usually the femoral or brachial artery) is entered with a large-bore needle, and a guidewire is threaded through the needle and into the artery under fluoroscopic control. The needle is removed, the guidewire is left in the vessel, and the catheter is threaded over the wire. The wire then is removed, and the catheter remains in the artery for the duration of the examination. Further manipulation of the catheter may be needed to ensure correct placement in the vessel before injection of the iodine compound. For selective catheterization of smaller vessels, the catheter tip is maneuvered into the root of the vessel of interest, such as the coronary, celiac, renal, or carotid artery.

A timed sequence of images is taken during and after injection of the contrast medium, usually with the aid of an automatic power injector that is electronically coordinated with an automated exposure control. Angiography is used extensively because it provides the best anatomic view of structures within the circulatory system and also offers the opportunity for immediate therapeutic interventions to treat vascular problems as they are identified. Specialized catheter techniques are used for vessel repair, called **angioplasty**, to widen or open arteries that are narrowed or occluded. **Embolization** is a therapeutic intervention technique that reduces or stops blood flow to control hemorrhage, cut off the blood supply to a tumor, or reduce blood loss during surgery.

Computed Tomography

Computed tomography (CT), formerly called *computerized axial tomography* (CAT) scanning, uses a special x-ray scanner to produce detailed pictures of a cross section of tissue. The x-ray studies are taken in the transverse plane and also can be "reconstructed" by the computer to display anatomic structures in other planes. The images are viewed in a variety of formats, called *windows,* which are designed to enhance the views of specific tissues (Figure 43-20). Multiple levels of pictures can be taken in a very short period, with up to 25 continuous images recorded in the time it takes the patient to hold a single breath. Most CT examinations are noninvasive, painless, and do not require any special patient preparation. However, the procedure involves a considerable amount of radiation. Also, patients may feel apprehensive about the equipment because standard machines require the patient enter a tube for the procedure.

Careful explanations are necessary to obtain the patient's cooperation and a satisfactory outcome of the study. The CT scanner consists of a movable table with remote control, a circular **gantry** structure that supports the x-ray tube and detectors, an operator console with a monitor, and a supporting computer system. The CT unit also includes both hardware and software to archive and manage data and to produce hard copies of images. During a scan, the x-ray tube rotates around the patient to collect data. In conventional CT units, the tube makes a complete rotation to gather data for each slice. The table then moves, and the tube rotates again to obtain the next slice. *Spiral* or *helical scanners* scan a spiral path around the patient and can collect data on a larger volume of tissue. These scanners can reconstruct views to create three-dimensional (3D) images. CTs with spectral detectors include the use of color to further enhance visualization for cleaner identification.

The versatility of CT is illustrated by its wide range of applications, including studies of the brain, spine, abdomen, pelvis, chest, neck, and paranasal sinuses. CT is a valuable tool for emergency use, especially in the detection of intracerebral or intra-abdominal hemorrhage. It also is used for orthopedic examinations of the extremities and for contrast-enhanced vascular studies. CT is useful for localizing both lesions and needle position during needle aspiration biopsy, a nonsurgical method of obtaining cells for laboratory examination, and it may be used either in place of or with myelography to expand the range of information available.

More recent advances in CT include the cone beam, which provides high-resolution 3D images of extremities. It uses cone-shaped x-rays to dramatically decrease the radiation dosage, making it faster and safer than standard CT imaging.

Although many CT examinations do not require contrast media, the use of contrast agents vastly increases the scope of CT imaging. Studies of the abdomen usually use oral contrast media to help differentiate the GI tract from the surrounding tissues. The patient ingests a special barium compound or an oral iodine preparation over a specified period before the study. The amount of contrast medium and the time period vary, depending on whether the examination includes only the upper abdomen or the entire abdomen and pelvis. For these studies, the patient is instructed not to eat for 12

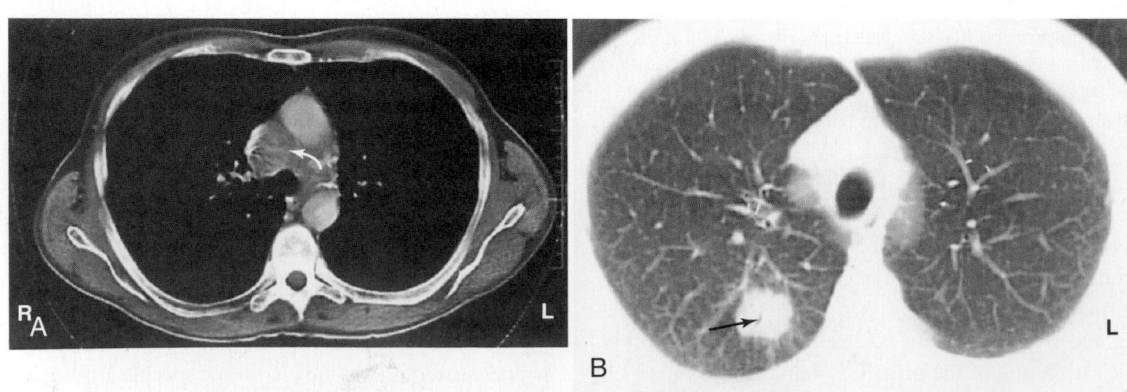

FIGURE 43-20 Two computed tomography (CT) windows demonstrating structures of the chest from the same image. **A,** Mediastinal structures are demonstrated in the center of the field, but the lungs are not well seen. **B,** "Lung window" demonstrates the blood vessels of the lungs and a lung tumor *(arrow).* (From Seeram E: *Computed tomography: physical principles, clinical applications, and quality control,* ed 2, Philadelphia, 2001, Saunders.)

hours and to report to the facility early to drink the contrast preparation before the procedure is scheduled. Some departments have the patient take the contrast medium home, with instructions to drink it before reporting for the appointment.

IV injection of an iodine contrast medium also may be used to increase the contrast level of the patient's tissues. This is advantageous for studies of the chest, abdomen, and soft tissues of the neck because it highlights blood vessels and enhances the visibility of vascular organs such as the liver and spleen. The contrast defines the internal structures of the kidneys, ureters, and bladder as the agent is excreted in the urine. In selected cases, IV contrast agents are used in CT scans of the head to demonstrate brain lesions. Be sure to notify the provider of any iodine or shellfish allergies, and inform the patient not to arrive with a full stomach, which may trigger nausea and vomiting.

Magnetic Resonance Imaging

Magnetic resonance imaging (MRI) is a noninvasive diagnostic modality that allows visualization of anatomic structures without the use of radioactive x-rays. A powerful magnetic field and radiofrequency pulses are combined to produce a radio signal in the body that can be detected and processed electronically to provide images on a computer monitor. The images can be managed in a computer database and can also be stored on magnetic tape and photographed with a special camera to produce film copies that appear similar to x-ray images. The greatest advantage of an MRI is that it can see through bones and focus on specific areas of soft tissue in great detail without the use of radiation (Table 43-3).

The MRI gantry houses the magnet and the main radiofrequency coil. Conventional gantries are tubular, 5 to 8 feet long, and typically require the body part being studied to be placed in the tube during the scanning process. An open gantry design, the open MRI, provides better accommodation for large or claustrophobic patients, but it does not always provide image quality equal to that produced by conventional units. Open gantry units allow for an open view of the four sides surrounding the unit, to feel less confining to patients. Tilting MRI units have an open gantry that can be rotated to allow patients to stand, for weight-bearing images. This is particularly useful for musculoskeletal evaluation.

MRI provides excellent imaging of the soft tissues of the nervous system (Figure 43-21). It is useful in the diagnosis of many types of pathology, including brain and spinal cord tumors and diseases such as multiple sclerosis. MRI also is used for the diagnosis of herniated intervertebral disks and to obtain images of the soft tissue components of joints, particularly the knee, shoulder, and temporomandibular joint. However, it does not generate a clear image of bones.

Magnetic resonance angiography (MRA) is an advanced MRI that focuses specifically on blood vessels and the cardiovascular system. MRA aids in the diagnosis and treatment of heart disorders, stroke, and blood vessel diseases. It is different from traditional angiography because it does not require the insertion of a catheter into the area being imaged. This allows for a faster and more cost-effective diagnosis with less risk to the patient.

The typical scan time for a series of slicelike images ranges from 1 to 10 minutes, and several series, demonstrating different body planes and using a variety of radiofrequency pulse sequences, may be included in an examination. The average time for an MRI study is 30 to 45 minutes. It is critical that the patient remain still, maintaining the desired position, throughout the procedure.

TABLE 43-3   MRI and CT: What's the Difference?

	MRI	CT
Full Name	Magnetic resonance imaging	Computed (axial) tomography
Use	Greatest detail for soft tissues; superior for tumor detection; poor bone imaging	Identifies both bone and soft tissue injuries; used more frequently because of decreased time and cost
Effects	No known biologic hazards	Radiation up to 500× that of x-rays
Cost	Varies by facility from about $400 to $4,000	Varies by facility from about $400 to $3,200
Limits	No metal implants or pacemakers; tattoos may blur images	Not recommended in pregnancy or for children because of high radiation level
Time	Typically less than 30 minutes	Typically less than 5 minutes; speed results in less sensitivity to movement
Contrast	Rare allergic reaction in those with liver or kidney disease	Iodine based; risk of a reaction for those with allergies; may lead to nephropathy

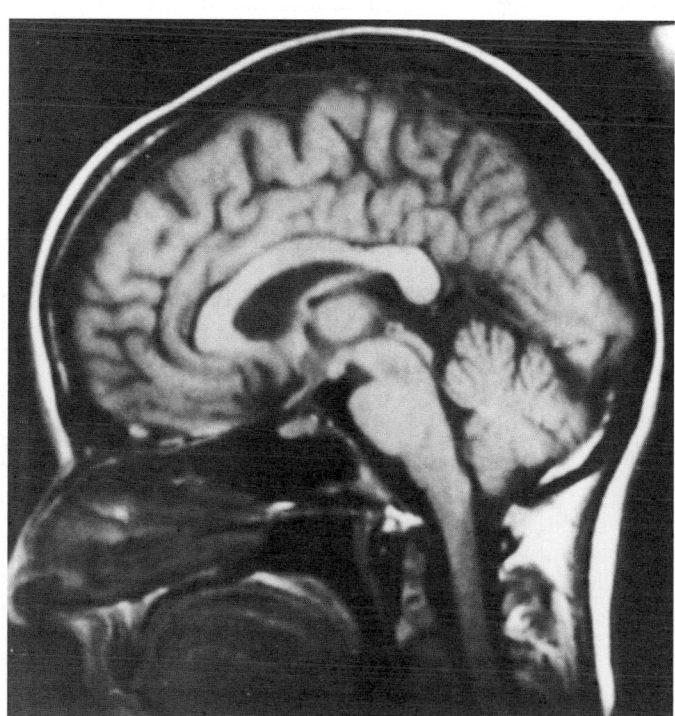

FIGURE 43-21 Midsagittal magnetic resonance image (MRI) of the brain. (From Ehrlich RA: *Patient care in radiography,* ed 8, St Louis, 2013, Mosby.)

Although contrast media are not required for most MRI studies, special paramagnetic agents sometimes are injected intravenously. These agents provide contrast enhancement of certain lesions, particularly brain and spinal cord tumors, and help differentiate disk material from scar tissue in postoperative spinal examinations. Contrast injections also are used in MRA studies. Typically, a series of images is recorded, the contrast agent is injected intravenously, and a second series of images is taken.

The unique MRI environment requires special safety precautions. Conditions that affect patient safety involve both the powerful magnetic field in the gantry and the thermal effects of radiofrequency pulses on certain materials that could overheat and possibly burn the patient. The principal means of ensuring patient safety during an MRI is careful patient screening before the procedure. Although extensive patient interviews are conducted in the magnetic resonance department, preliminary screening of patients should be conducted by the medical assistant before the appointment is made. The magnetic field or the rapid radiofrequency pulses may be hazardous for patients with artificial heart valves, aneurysm clips, neurostimulators, middle ear prostheses, or intrauterine devices. Cardiac pacemakers are a particular hazard, and patients with pacemakers cannot have MRI examinations. Fatalities have resulted from overheating of these implanted devices when patients with pacemakers were scanned.

Other factors that may prohibit the use of MRI technology include patients with orthopedic pins and screws and metal fragments or shrapnel in the soft tissues. Metalworkers who might have steel slivers in their tissues must have a screening x-ray or CT head examination to detect fragments that could damage the eyes or brain, because the pull of the magnetic field is so strong that it could cause the fragments to move. Although the energies involved in MRI have not been demonstrated to cause complications with pregnancy, the current philosophy is to avoid examination of pregnant patients except in urgent cases, especially during the first trimester.

Patients should be assured that everything possible will be done to provide assistance in dealing with both physical and emotional discomfort. Few people are completely comfortable for any length of time in a tightly enclosed space. Even patients with no history of claustrophobia may feel anxious when entering a conventional tubular MRI gantry. Occasionally, this anxiety is so severe that it creates panic, preventing the patient from continuing the examination.

Patients may be reassured if they know what to expect in advance. The procedure requires that the patient lie down on the MRI table, which then automatically moves into the gantry. Plenty of air is available, and there is no physical discomfort except for the need to lie still. The machine makes a very loud "knocking" noise during the scanning process (similar to a jack hammer or heavy machinery). Earplugs or earphones with recorded music may be offered. Patients can communicate with the technologist through an intercom, and the technologist is watching and listening from an adjacent area throughout the procedure. The patient is given a "panic button" to push in case the procedure needs to be stopped because of patient discomfort or anxiety. Because no radiation danger exists, a friend or family member can sit in the room if the patient feels more comfortable with company. Severely claustrophobic patients may be scheduled at a facility with an open gantry MRI or may be given an antianxiety medication before the procedure. Analgesic medications may be administered to patients whose pain makes it impossible to lie still for the duration of the study.

Sonography

Diagnostic medical **sonography** is a noninvasive procedure that is considered very safe for the patient. Sonography is used extensively for fetal imaging. This imaging modality, often referred to as *diagnostic ultrasound,* uses high-frequency sound waves to produce echoes in the body. As the echoes return to the hand-held transducer, their strength and timing are interpreted by a computer to produce a map or graphic image of the echo distribution.

The transducer is covered with a lubricant and moved over the surface of the body so that the image can be viewed in real time on a computer monitor. Special transducer probes can be inserted into body cavities (e.g., the rectum and the vagina) to obtain more detailed examinations of the prostate gland and the uterus. Any interface between substances or tissues of varying density produces an ultrasound echo, which makes sonography an effective technique for showing the shape, size, and condition of organs such as the heart, spleen, gallbladder, breast, and pancreas (Figure 43-22). Sonography, therefore, can be used to diagnose or investigate gallstones or suspicious masses in the breast. For example, if a woman has a suspicious breast mass, the mass can be visualized with a sonogram, and while the radiologist has a clear view of the location of the mass, a needle biopsy sample of the suspicious tissue is collected and sent to the pathologist for examination. This procedure limits the need for invasive surgical biopsies.

Sonography can also be used to detect an abscess, a cyst, or a tumor in adipose tissue. Recent advances in ultrasound technology include computer integration of data to produce 3D images. In addition, Doppler ultrasound is used to detect vascular disease, such as atherosclerosis in the carotid arteries and venous thrombosis of the lower extremities. Echocardiograms involve the use of Doppler ultrasound to evaluate the structure and function of the heart while in motion and can include colorized video to detect the flow of arterial and venous blood.

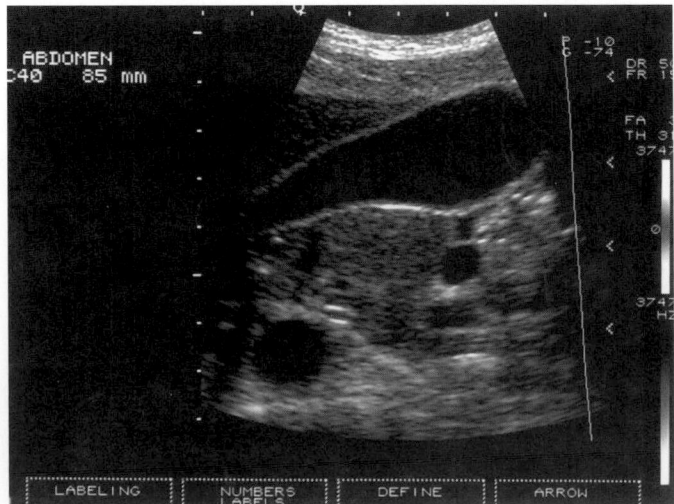

FIGURE 43-22 Abdominal sonogram. (From Ballinger PW, Frank ED: *Merrill's atlas of radiographic positions and radiologic procedures,* ed 10, vol 2, St Louis, 2003, Mosby.)

Ultrasound is also a diagnostic procedure commonly used in obstetrics to evaluate a developing fetus during pregnancy. Recent advances allow for video and still shots of real-time movement in 3D and even 4D, with astounding detail visible. It is used to detect the size and position of the baby and the function of its organs, and placental placement. Ultrasound can also determine the sex of the fetus, in addition to how many fetuses are present in the womb.

Nuclear Medicine

Nuclear medicine images are created by scanning the patient after special radioactive materials, called **tracers**, have been swallowed or injected intravenously (Table 43-4). Tracers are similar to substances that are commonly used by the body, so they enter into the same chemical reactions and are metabolized in a similar way. They are taken up in the target organ or tissue over a period that may vary from half an hour to several days, making cellular activities and even fractures more visible. The tracer then can be detected and its location recorded by a special nuclear medicine scanner, called a *gamma camera*. Two types of tracers used in diagnostic studies are radioactive iodine and radioactive carbon.

Nuclear medicine scans do not provide clear images of anatomic structures. They are used to obtain information about the function of organs and tissues. Abnormal tissues are demonstrated on the image because the tracer is metabolized at a different rate, at a different location, or to a greater or lesser extent than in normal tissue.

Figure 43-23 shows an example of a nuclear medicine bone scan. The tracer is absorbed by the bones and appears in greater or lesser amounts, depending on the level of metabolic activity within the bone. In this scan, the region shows a high level of radioactivity, which indicates an inflammatory process. Tumors of the bone can be diagnosed by "hot spots" in the x-ray image; these show up much more brightly because of rapid cellular division, which results in a higher level of metabolic activity.

Structures visualized with nuclear medicine techniques include the thyroid gland, liver, lungs, brain, skeletal system, kidneys, heart, and blood vessels. Thallium stress studies of the heart are nuclear medicine examinations that permit the physician to view the coronary arteries to diagnose or rule out blockage. Incomplete visualization of the myocardium after administration of a nuclear tracer indicates lack of blood supply to the area and damage to the muscle of the heart.

The radioisotopes used in nuclear medicine decay within a short time (from a few hours to a few days) and are eliminated in the urine or feces. They have a very low level of radioactivity and involve less patient exposure than most x-ray examinations. Positron emission tomography (PET) and single photon emission computed tomography (SPECT) are highly specialized nuclear medicine techniques that use different types of tracers and scanners than conventional nuclear medicine, but the basic principle is the same. Radioactive substances from within the body are detected and mapped by specialized equipment to obtain information about the function of organs, tissues, or systems. Most PET scans today are combined with CT to merge the technology of nuclear medicine procedures with

TABLE 43-4	Common Nuclear Medicine Procedures
PROCEDURE	**PURPOSE**
Bone scan	Helps detect fractures, tumors, and inflammation; used to determine bone growth
Brain scan	Often used with other imaging methods to detect tumors and vascular problems; commonly tested with single photon emission computed tomography (SPECT)
Liver scan	Useful for diagnosing cirrhosis and hepatitis and for detecting tumors and liver abscesses
Lung scan	Often done to detect emboli, blood clots that have traveled through the bloodstream to the lungs
Multiple gated acquisition (MUGA) scan	Evaluates the condition of the heart's myocardium while at rest and/or during stress
Positron emission tomography (PET) scan	Done for cancer investigation; evaluation of myocardial blood supply; investigation of central nervous system disorders by evaluating metabolic activity
Thallium stress test	Used to evaluate cardiac condition and response to stress
Thyroid scan	Rate of contrast uptake is an indicator of thyroid function; scan also is useful for detecting tumors

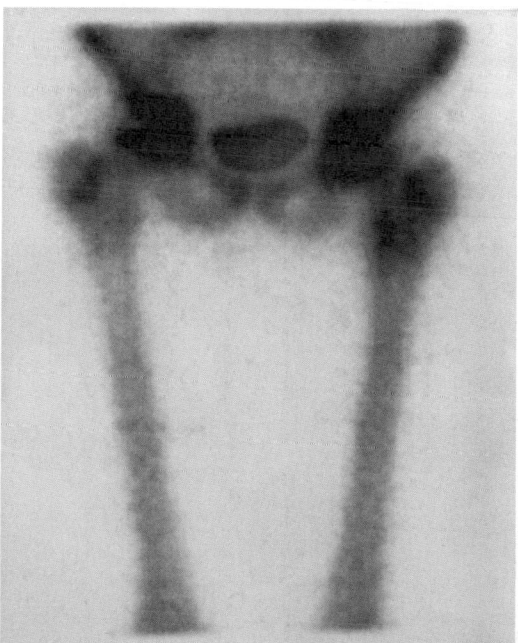

FIGURE 43-23 Bone scan showing increased tracer uptake in the proximal femur. (From Baker A, Macnicol MF: Haematogenous osteomyelitis in children: epidemiology, classification, aetiology and treatment, *Paediatr Child Health* 18(2):75-84, 2008.)

the multiplane view of CT scanners. PET/CT scans are ordered for the following purposes:

- To diagnose a cancerous tumor, evaluate its spread, or determine whether cancer has returned after treatment
- To evaluate the blood flow to the heart
- To determine the extent of damage to the myocardial wall after a heart attack
- To investigate lung lesions visualized with traditional x-ray images
- To diagnose central nervous system disorders, including epilepsy, Alzheimer's disease, Parkinson's disease, and strokes, and to locate brain tumors

Dual Energy X-ray Absorptiometry

Dual energy x-ray absorptiometry (DXA) scans use x-ray technology to evaluate a patient's bone density. A decrease in bone density is diagnostic proof of osteoporosis; evidence of bone density loss (osteopenia) may indicate the individual's risk of developing osteoporosis over time. The test typically evaluates the bone density of the spine and hip. For the examination, the patient lies supine on an x-ray table with the knees flexed and the lower legs elevated (Figure 43-24).

The DXA scanner directs an x-ray from two different sources toward the hip. The greater the mineral density of the bone, the longer the x-ray image is transmitted and the highest test number recorded. The scan is completed within a few seconds and also can be used to evaluate the density of the spine and hips. The patient's density results are compared with standard bone density tables to determine the presence and/or level of demineralization. These numbers are used to predict the patient's risk of an osteoporosis-related fracture. DXA scans are recommended for the following individuals:

- Women with multiple risk factors for osteoporosis
- Women with long-term estrogen deficiencies
- Individuals taking steroids for an extended period
- Individuals taking osteoporosis medications (to evaluate the effectiveness of treatment)
- Patients with unexplained fractures and/or deformities of the vertebra

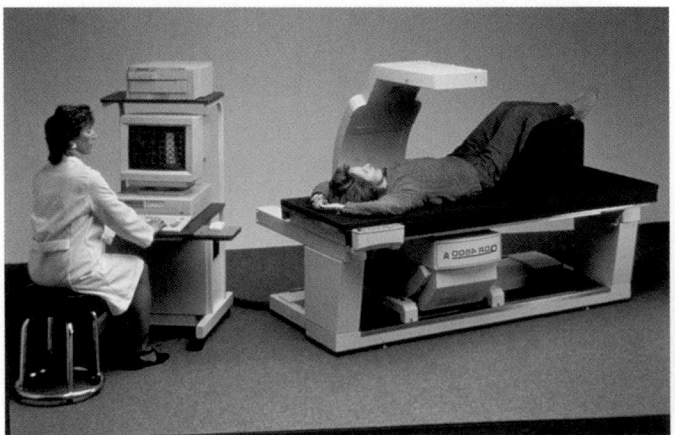

FIGURE 43-24 Patient undergoing a bone density test, or dual energy x-ray absorptiometry (DEXA or DXA).

BASIC RADIOGRAPHIC PROCEDURE

Patient Preparation and Explanation

Before a patient undergoes x-ray studies, a provider examines the individual and orders one or more specific x-ray procedures to help diagnose the patient's problem or to follow up on a previously diagnosed condition. The provider is responsible for getting the patient's informed consent for any procedure, but he or she may ask the medical assistant to make sure the consent form is signed. The patient may not have to sign a consent form for noninvasive diagnostic studies because acceptance of the procedure is adequate evidence of consent. In some facilities, however, patients may be asked to sign a consent form regardless of the type of radiographic procedure. If it is your duty to answer patients' questions about the procedure or to assist with obtaining consent, make sure you are prepared to do so.

Patients often express concern about radiation exposure. You can assure them with confidence that the risks are extremely small and outweigh the health risks of treatment without the information the examination will provide. It may help to point out that the radiographer is well trained in radiation safety and that the equipment is designed to provide good images with the least possible exposure. You can explain that the amount of radiation involved in the procedure is typically less than the exposure to natural background radiation that people in general receive every year.

Patient preparation for routine radiography involves having the patient remove the outer clothing from the area to be radiographed and instructing the person to wear a gown if appropriate. Underwear usually is not a problem. No metal objects should be included in the radiation field because these items appear as artifacts on the images. This includes jewelry (including piercings); zippers, snaps, and other clothing fasteners; underwire bras; and the contents of pockets. Nonmetal objects that are thick or heavy should also be removed. Buttons and the heavy seams in jeans are examples of other clothing items that can cause artifacts on radiographs if they are in the imaging field. Metal items that are not in the radiation field are not a problem, so patients need not remove jewelry or clothing from areas that will not be included in the radiograph.

When the patient is ready, the next step is to assist the patient into the general position required for the x-ray examination. For example, if a hand is to be imaged, the patient can be seated at the end of the x-ray examination table (Figure 43-25 and Figure 43-26, A). For a spinal examination, the patient may need to lie on the table (Figure 43-26, B). If a chest examination has been ordered, the patient stands at an upright image receptor holder (Figure 43-26, C).

The radiographer then selects the correct image receptor, labels it or places a lead marker on it to identify the patient's right or left side, and moves it into position for the exposure (Figure 43-27). Next, the patient is positioned precisely, and the x-ray tube is aligned with the body part and the image receptor at a specific distance (Figure 43-28). The body part must be measured to determine the proper exposure factors according to a technique chart. At this point, lead shields are positioned for radiation protection. The radiographer then goes to the control booth, consults the technique chart, and sets the x-ray control panel to the desired exposure. Final instructions are given to the patient (typically that the patient must remain still

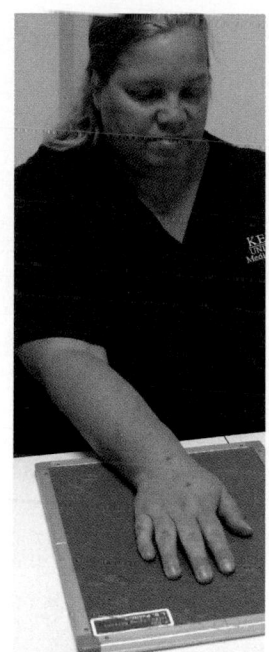

FIGURE 43-25 An x-ray table for an x-ray of the hand. (Courtesy Helen Mills.)

during the x-ray procedure), and the exposure is made. If more than one exposure is needed, the image receptor is changed, the patient is repositioned, and the steps are repeated until the examination is complete.

After the patient's safety and comfort have been ensured, the image is processed. If the image is satisfactory and no further exposures are needed, the patient is returned to an examination room or dressing room. The radiographer or the medical assistant then readies the x-ray room for the next examination.

Although the use of traditional film copies is quickly becoming outdated, some smaller or older offices may still maintain such copies. Traditional films are kept together and given to the provider with the appropriate paperwork. They are kept in large file envelopes that may contain more than one set of films for the same patient. These envelopes must be accurately identified for proper filing. When images are added to the file, notations often are added to the envelope. After the films have been read, they are promptly filed so that they can be retrieved quickly when needed for future reference. Radiology reports also must be filed. Usually the original is filed in the patient's health record; copies may be filed separately or with the films. Digital images are stored in electronic files and can be transmitted electronically or burned onto a CD. However, these images can be viewed only if a viewing software is used.

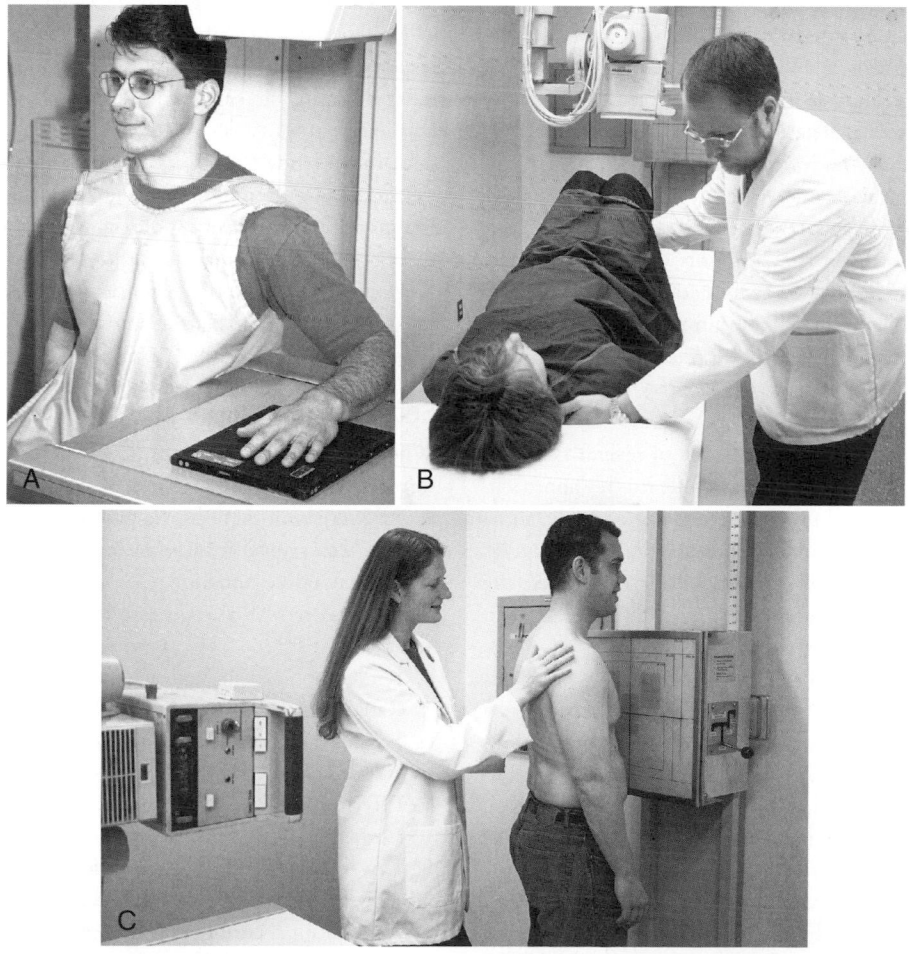

FIGURE 43-26 General positions for radiography. **A,** The patient may be seated at the x-ray table for some upper extremity examinations. **B,** The radiographer helps the patient lie down for spine radiography. **C,** The radiographer assists the patient into position at an upright Bucky for chest radiographs. (From Long BW, Frank ED, Ehrlich RA: *Radiography essentials for limited practice,* ed 4, Philadelphia, 2013, Saunders.)

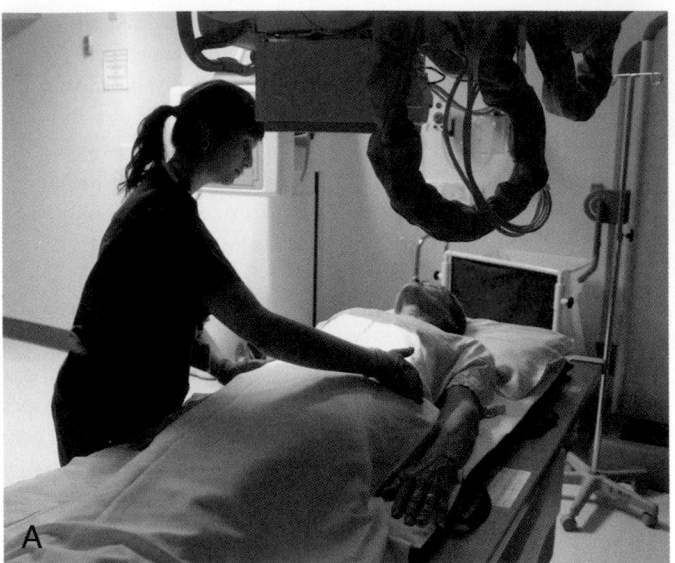

FIGURE 43-27 The cassette or image receptor must be latched securely in the Bucky tray, and the tray must be aligned to the anatomy of interest. (From Ehrlich RA: *Patient care in radiography*, ed 8, St Louis, 2013, Mosby.)

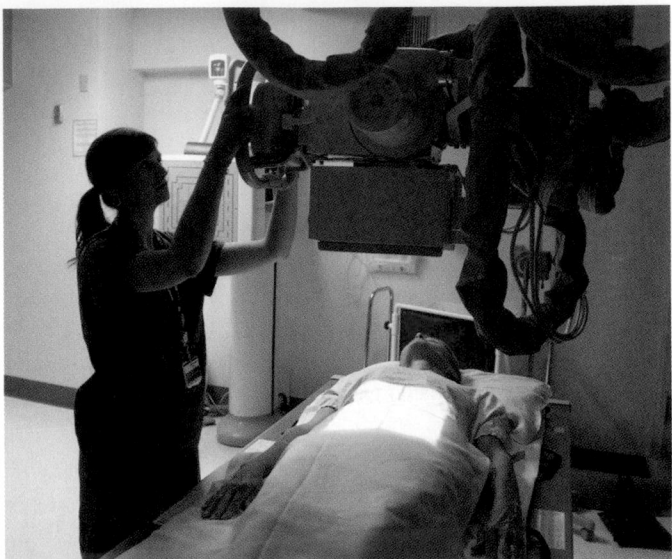

FIGURE 43-28 The x-ray tube must be aligned with the patient and image receptor at the proper distance. (From Ehrlich RA: *Patient care in radiography*, ed 8, St Louis, 2013, Mosby.)

Scheduling and Sequencing Diagnostic Imaging Procedures

One of the most important communications between medical assistants and imaging departments involves the scheduling of multiple diagnostic procedures that may all be ordered at one time by the provider. Consultation often is needed to decide how many procedures can be done in one day and to sequence them in such a way that they will not interfere with one another. For example, a UGI series usually results in barium sulfate scattered throughout the intestinal tract for several days. Even tiny amounts of residual barium cause complications in radiographic examinations of the urinary tract and biliary system, where tiny opacifications are diagnostically significant. Residual barium in the digestive tract also causes unacceptable artifacts on abdominal CT scans. For this reason, barium studies are scheduled last in any series of procedures.

Some imaging departments schedule a series of several examinations in one day for patients who are able to tolerate this approach. Radiologists prefer various scheduling practices. For example, some departments schedule gallbladder and upper and lower GI studies on the same day. Others may insist on 2 or 3 days to complete the same examinations. You should become familiar with the practice in the facility where you usually schedule patients.

Scheduling several examinations on the same day may be less stressful for the patient, resulting in a single bowel preparation, a single period of fasting, and a single trip to the imaging center. However, the number of examinations an individual patient can tolerate varies, especially if the patient is elderly or ill. Make sure you discuss scheduling options with the patient and/or family before planning more than one examination per day.

When fiberoptic studies, such as gastroscopy or colonoscopy, are ordered in conjunction with radiographic examinations requiring barium as a contrast medium, the fiberoptic studies are done first. This avoids the possibility that the barium will interfere with visual assessment during the fiberoptic examination. Patients undergoing gastroscopy usually receive sedation and a muscle relaxant before the physician inserts the gastroscope. When a UGI series is to follow, it should be delayed to allow sufficient time for the patient to become responsive and alert because oral administration of barium to a sedated patient increases the risk that the patient may choke on the barium.

Another study to be considered when sequencing diagnostic procedures is any thyroid assessment test that involves iodine uptake. Because the administration of a contrast medium containing iodine causes inaccurate results in such tests for at least 3 weeks, thyroid assessment blood tests (T_3 or T_4) or nuclear medicine thyroid scans must be performed before any contrast medium with iodine is administered.

Sequencing Order for Diagnostic Studies

When more than one diagnostic study is to be done, they are performed in the following order:
1. All x-ray examinations that do not require contrast media
2. Any laboratory studies or nuclear medicine procedures that involve iodine uptake
3. CT studies with IV contrast any time after iodine uptake blood studies
4. Radiographic examinations of the urinary tract
5. Radiographic examinations of the biliary system
6. Fiberoptic studies (e.g., gastroscopy, endoscopy, sigmoidoscopy, colonoscopy)
7. CT studies of the abdomen or pelvis (done before barium studies)
8. Lower gastrointestinal (GI) series (barium enema)
9. Upper gastrointestinal (UGI) series (barium swallow)

An additional consideration in patient scheduling involves deciding which patients need early morning appointments and which can be scheduled later in the day. Imaging departments always begin the daily routine with patients who must fast in preparation for their examination so that they do not have to go too long without food. When scheduling, request early priority for pediatric and geriatric patients because they have the most difficulty maintaining nothing by mouth (**NPO**) status for long periods, and extended fasting may actually interfere with their recovery.

Patients with diabetes who must postpone their insulin until their morning meal also need priority in scheduling. Outpatients who are diabetic should be reminded to postpone their morning insulin until the examination is complete, even if they have been scheduled for an early appointment. If an emergency should cause a delay, the patient who has had insulin may suffer a reaction. Paperwork done in the office for diagnostic studies needs to include information about patients with diabetes so that the radiology staff is aware of their status.

Although actual scheduling may be done by phone or computer, the patient is typically given a printed copy of the provider's order and any necessary instructions.

CRITICAL THINKING APPLICATION   **43-1**

Mrs. Pellegrini, a 62-year-old patient with diabetes, calls Metro Urgicenter at 8:30 AM to confirm her 10 AM appointment for an outpatient imaging procedure that requires fasting. On speaking with her, Sara learns that Mrs. Pellegrini has already taken her morning insulin. Should Mrs. Pellegrini keep her appointment or be rescheduled? Why or why not?

When you instruct the patient about preparing for an examination, it is important to have printed instructions ready in advance. If more than one alternative is printed on any given paper, be sure to indicate, both orally and in writing, which instructions are to be followed. Review the sheet with the patient slowly, explaining any words or procedures that may not be familiar. Have the patient explain back to you what is to be done (remember the importance of feedback in establishing whether the patient understands). If the patient is too young, too ill, confused, or incapable of understanding and following the instructions, give the instructions (oral and written) to the person who will be responsible for assisting the patient. Be sure to include the telephone numbers of your clinical facility and of the imaging department so that the patient or the patient's family may call if any questions arise after the patient leaves the office.

In preparation for a UGI series, the patient must fast, avoiding water, smoking, and chewing gum. The NPO order usually is for a limited period (commonly 8 to 12 hours) before the procedure. This ensures that the stomach is empty at the time of the examination so that an accurate radiographic image of its inner surfaces can be produced. Chewing gum and smoking are avoided because they tend to increase gastric secretions.

The preparation for a barium enema involves the use of a bowel cleansing kit. These kits usually contain one or more types of **cathartics**, a suppository, a low-volume enema, and illustrated instructions in several languages. Research has demonstrated that increased fluid intake enhances the effectiveness of cathartics and helps minimize the patient's discomfort. For this reason, instructions for cathartics are accompanied by a fluid intake schedule that suggests at least 8 ounces of water or clear liquid every 2 hours between noon and

midnight on the day preceding the examination. The medical assistant should emphasize the importance of fluid intake. The required doses of cathartics have a strong, thorough action that occasionally causes patients to experience painful spasms of the bowel and irritation of the intestinal lining. Persistent diarrhea may last through the night, preventing sleep. Although patients may find this preparation uncomfortable and inconvenient, its effectiveness in cleansing the bowel usually outweighs these considerations.

Caution must be exercised in implementing an aggressive preparation for elderly or frail patients who are likely to be adversely affected. A gentler alternative should be available for these debilitated patients. Those with chronic or acute diarrhea may require a lower dose or less active preparation than is usually given. When the routine strength or amount of cathartics is reduced, several days of a low-residue diet and an increased fluid intake become critical to the success of preparation. Patients should always be advised of the nature of the action expected from the cathartic when it is given. Table 43-5 summarizes common diagnostic procedures and the patient preparation required for each.

CRITICAL THINKING APPLICATION   **43-2**

Dr. Roberts, a physician at Metro Urgicenter, has ordered a barium enema for Mr. Tillman, and Dr. Swain asks Sara to provide Mr. Tillman with the preparation instructions for the procedure. What information should Sara obtain from Mr. Tillman to determine whether the usual bowel preparation is appropriate? If Sara thinks the usual preparation might be too harsh for Mr. Tillman, how should she explain her concern to Dr. Swain and Dr. Roberts? Who should decide whether to implement a variation in protocol: Sara, Dr. Swain, or someone else?

Radiation Safety
Radiation Units

Two systems are used to measure radiation and radiation dose: the conventional (British) system and the international system (Système International [SI]) established in 1981 (Table 43-6). The conventional system includes the roentgen (R), the rad (rad), and the rem (rem), which are all being phased out.

The SI unit for dose measurement is the **gray (Gy)**, which is most commonly used today. **Air kerma** (Gy-$_a$) is the SI unit term for radiation exposure that represents the amount of radiation in the air to reach the patient. The subscript "a" is added to indicate that the radiation in the air is taken into account. The word "exposure" is used to describe air kerma because this is the amount of radiation in the air to which the patient is exposed.

As an x-ray passes through a patient, some of the radiation is absorbed by the patient's tissues; this is referred to as the *absorbed dose* (D). The symbol for absorbed dose (Gy-$_t$) includes a subscript "t" to indicate that it takes into account the radiation remaining in tissue. The absorbed dose is always less than the initial exposure because some of the radiation continues through and exits the patient. References to absorbed dose are often indicated by simply using the word "dose" because this is the dose of radiation that stops in the patient's body.

TABLE 43-5 Diagnostic Procedures and Patient Preparation*

STUDY	PURPOSE	PROCEDURE	PATIENT PREPARATION
Angiography: arteriogram (artery) or venogram (vein)	To aid diagnosis of arterial occlusion, aneurysm, hemorrhage, abnormal vessels, and transient ischemic attacks	Catheter is inserted into femoral, brachial, or carotid artery and advanced under fluoroscopy to site; dye is injected, and x-ray images are taken.	Clear liquids 24 hr before test; nothing by mouth (NPO) 8 hr before test; if abdominal vasculature is to be imaged, patient may need laxative and enemas.
Arthrogram	To detect damage to joint connective tissue and structures	Fluoroscopic and radiographic examination of a joint after injection of air or contrast dye.	NPO 8 hr
Barium enema	To detect bowel obstruction, celiac sprue, colon cancer, polyps, diverticulitis, irritable bowel syndrome	Fluoroscopic and radiographic examination of the colon after barium enema to find internal structural abnormalities; takes approximately 1 hr.	Bowel must be emptied before procedure; clear liquid diet 24 hr before test (no milk); laxatives day before test; enemas morning of test; increase fluids after test—pale stools and constipation are typical.
Barium swallow	To detect esophageal varices, hiatal hernia, pyloric stenosis, obstructions, polyps, tumors, ulcers	Fluoroscopic and radiographic examination as barium is swallowed to detect abnormalities of the pharynx, esophagus, and stomach; takes about 15 min.	NPO and no smoking 8 hr before; if small bowel is included in imaging, instruct on laxative use as prescribed; a barium drink is consumed just before testing; afterward, stools are expected to be white or pale; lower GI tests may require repeat imaging after 24 hr.
Bone scan	To detect bone cancer, bone infection, osteoarthritis, osteomyelitis	Nuclear medicine: Radioactive isotope is injected intravenously (IV), body is scanned, and levels of isotope are imaged. Areas of high metabolism show as "hot spots"; scan is done 1-3 hr after isotope injection.	NPO 4 hr before; must void before scan; radioactive material is excreted in urine within 48 hr and is not harmful to others.
Computed tomography (CT)	Provides detailed, cross-sectional views of all types of body structures; one of the best tools for studying the chest and abdomen	Special x-ray equipment and computers are used to obtain image data from different angles around the body, and multiple cross-sectional views (tomographs) are produced.	NPO 4 hr before if IV contrast medium will be used; no metal objects; must lie very still; advise of confined space and possible claustrophobia.
Intravenous urogram (IVU) or intravenous pyelogram (IVP)	To evaluate structure and function of kidneys, ureters, and bladder	IV contrast medium is injected, and x-ray images are taken of renal structures.	Bowel cleansing and liquid diet 24 hr before with laxatives and possibly enema to prevent obstruction of views; NPO 8 hr.
Magnetic resonance imaging (MRI)	To aid diagnosis of intracranial and spinal lesions, aneurysms, heart defects, multiple sclerosis, and soft tissue abnormalities throughout the body	Magnetic field and radiofrequency energy are transmitted to a computer, which produces cross-sectional images of soft tissue; this may eliminate the need for arthrography and myelography. No radiation exposure is involved. Patient lies on a flat table that moves into a tunnel-shaped scanner; takes 45-90 min.	No caffeine 4 hr before testing; normal diet, unless pelvic testing (6 hr NPO); no eye makeup; must remove all metal; contraindications include tattoos, permanent makeup, and any metallic implants with iron (e.g., pacemakers, artificial heart valves, aneurysm clips, material associated with metal-related occupation); patient will hear loud tapping during test and must remain still; notify provider if patient has iodine allergies or is claustrophobic.

TABLE 43-5   Diagnostic Procedures and Patient Preparation —*continued*

STUDY	PURPOSE	PROCEDURE	PATIENT PREPARATION
Mammography	For early detection of breast cancer and abnormalities through detection of masses	Low-energy x-rays are used to examine the breast; parallel plate compression evens out the thickness of breast tissue for easier viewing.	Scheduled the first week after a menstrual cycle; shower beforehand—no deodorant, talcum powder, or lotion; avoid caffeine 7-10 days before testing. Explain that the position is uncomfortable (breast is sandwiched between two plates) but should take only a short time to complete.
Myelogram	To aid diagnosis of spinal lesions, ruptured disk, spinal stenosis	Fluoroscopic and radiographic examination of the spinal column after injection of contrast medium into the subarachnoid space; takes about 1 hr.	NPO 8 hr
Retrograde pyelography	To evaluate structure and function of kidneys, ureters, and bladder	Contrast medium is injected through a urethral catheter, and x-ray images are taken of renal structures.	Bowel cleansing and liquid diet 24 hr before with laxatives and possibly enema to prevent obstruction of views; NPO 8 hr.
Tomosynthesis	Recent innovation for early detection of breast cancer and breast abnormalities	High-resolution three-dimensional (3D) imaging (similar to a CT scan) used to examine the breast at different angles; parallel plate compression evens out the thickness of breast tissue for easier viewing while the camera makes an arc around the breast, taking multiple images.	Scheduled the first week after a menstrual cycle; shower beforehand—no deodorant, talcum powder, or lotion; avoid caffeine 7-10 days before testing. Explain that the position is uncomfortable (breast is sandwiched between two plates) but should take only a short time to complete.

*With any test that uses contrast dye, ask the patient whether he or she has allergies to iodine, contrast media, or shellfish; if the answer is yes, notify the provider.

TABLE 43-6   Units of Radiation Measurement

	CONVENTIONAL UNITS	NEW SI UNITS
Quantity of radiation exposure in air	roentgen (R)	Air kerma (Gy-$_a$)
Absorbed dose in tissue	rad (rad)	gray (Gy-$_t$)
Type or energy of radiation equivalent dose	rem (rem)	sievert (Sv)

To put it all together: During x-ray imaging, the patient may receive an exposure of 16 mGy-$_a$. From that exposure, he or she may receive an absorbed dose of 1.1 mGy-$_t$. The remaining radiation is the useful remnant radiation that creates the x-ray image.

Memory Aid: *Exposure versus Dose*

Exposure: Radiation in the air.
Dose: The amount of radiation absorbed within the body.

Equivalent Dose

The effect that radiation has on the body depends on the type and characteristics of a particular test. Similarly, occupational radiation can vary based on the type of radiation to which employees are exposed. For example, advanced tests use much higher concentration of radiation and pose a higher risk than a simple x-ray image. Because this difference can have varying levels of biologic effects, it is necessary to clarify the type and energy of exposure to determine an employee's safe level of exposure; this is referred to as *equivalent dose* (EqD). In the SI system, this is called the **sievert (Sv)**. For advanced radiographers, the equivalent dose is evaluated by using a radiation weighing factor to calculate exposure specific to that occupation. However, because limited operators have limited exposure, the absorbed dose and equivalent dose are always the same.

Effects of Low-Dose Radiation Exposure
Cellular Response to Exposure. Most people don't realize that radiation naturally occurs every day in the environment. It seeps out of the ground and settles down from outer space. It is in the food that we eat, the water that we drink, and the homes that we live in. Even our own bodies produce radiation to a certain extent. In fact, according to the U.S. Food and Drug Administration (FDA), in 2½

days of routine activity, we are naturally exposed to the same amount of radiation as we would get with a typical chest x-ray image. This is an important thing to remind patients who are worried about x-ray exposure.

Many cellular effects of radiation exposure are extremely short lived because chemical alterations within the cells are quickly repaired or the cell is replaced. Even if a cell dies, cell death is an insignificant injury unless the number of cells involved is massive. Although most diagnostic x-ray studies are relatively safe, sometimes a cell may be damaged in such a way that its DNA "programming" is changed and the cell no longer behaves normally. This type of injury eventually may result in runaway production of new, abnormal cells, causing a tumor or malignant blood disease.

The relative sensitivity of different types of cells is summarized in the laws of Bergonié and Tribondeau, which state that cell sensitivity to radiation exposure depends on four characteristics of the cell:

- *Age:* Younger cells are more sensitive than older ones.
- *Differentiation:* Simple cells are more sensitive than highly complex ones.
- *Metabolic rate:* Cells that use energy rapidly are more sensitive than those that have a slower metabolism.
- *Mitotic rate:* Cells that divide and multiply rapidly are more sensitive than those that replicate slowly.

According to these laws, blood cells and blood-producing cells are the most sensitive. Cells that are in contact with the environment (e.g., those of the skin and mucosal lining of the mouth, nose, and GI tract) are also fragile. Some glandular tissue also is particularly delicate, especially that of the thyroid gland and the female breast. The tissues of embryos, fetuses, infants, children, and adolescents tend to be more sensitive than those of adults because of their young age and higher metabolic and mitotic rates. Nerve cells, which have a long life and are quite complex, are much less vulnerable to radiation injury.

Somatic Effects.
Radiation effects can be classified as somatic or genetic. *Somatic effects* are those that occur to the body of the person who is irradiated. Whereas the effects of relatively high doses of radiation are immediate and predictable, the effects of the very low doses associated with radiography produce long-term effects. They are not easily identified as a result of radiation exposure because they occur 3 to 30 years after treatment and because the same problems can occur in the absence of radiation exposure. Only extensive research with large populations can demonstrate the role of radiation in causing these effects. In other words, radiation causes increased risk for health problems, but the complications cannot be predicted with respect to any one individual. Although the individual risk is extremely small, increasing exposure to the entire population poses public health risks that require the attention and concern of everyone involved in applying ionizing radiation to human beings.

The documented latent effects of low doses of ionizing radiation include the following:

- *Cataract formation:* This is a risk for radiologists and radiographers who work extensively in fluoroscopy and those who perform other work that involves repeated exposure to the eyes.
- *Carcinogenesis:* Increased risk of malignant disease, particularly cancer of the skin, thyroid, breast, and leukemia.
- *Shortened life span:* A study of the life span of radiologists who died before 1945 showed that they had shorter life spans than

physicians who did not use radiation in their practices. This group included radiologists who had used radiation since the early days of x-ray science. More recent studies show that occupational exposure no longer has a measurable effect on the life span of radiologists. Nevertheless, because radiation exposure has been linked to shortening of the life span, it is a public health concern and another reason to practice a high level of radiation safety.

Genetic Effects.
Genetic effects, in the form of changes or mutations in the hereditary material of reproductive cells, may occur if the ovaries or testes are exposed to radiation. In the female, all the ova cells the individual will ever produce are present at birth. Because no new egg cells are created as the individual ages, the effect of radiation exposure to the ovaries accumulates over time. In addition, the genetic effects of radiation to the testes may include damage to stem cells that produce sperm, resulting in the production of sperm with a genetic mutation. Most genetic mutations threaten the survival of an individual. Even when these changes are recessive (not apparent in the offspring), they may be passed on to future generations.

Radiation and Pregnancy.
Radiation exposure poses risks to the developing embryo or fetus. Research has demonstrated that excessive radiation during pregnancy may result in spontaneous abortion, congenital defects in the child, growth retardation, increased risk of cancer and leukemia in childhood, and an increase in significant genetic abnormalities in the children of parents who were exposed in utero. According to the National Council on Radiation Protection and Measurements (NCRP), studies of women exposed to radiation as a result of diagnostic and therapeutic procedures confirm that radiation to the uterus in excess of 150 mGy$_t$ (5 rad) is cause for concern, with the greatest risk occurring in the first three months of pregnancy. This is more exposure than is received with most x-ray examinations, but these levels may be encountered with direct exposure to the pelvis, especially with CT examinations or fluoroscopic studies. If pregnancy is suspected or likely, always notify the provider and await further orders before proceeding.

Guidelines for Pediatric X-ray Examinations
The following guidelines should be applied for all pediatric x-ray examinations:

- Provide age-appropriate explanations about the procedure and instructions for patient compliance.
- Inform the parents about the procedure and answer questions.
- Give the patient or parents written information when needed about preparation for the examination.
- Explain that allowing parents in the x-ray room will be up to the facility.
- When possible, use commercial immobilization devices to position the child (e.g., restraint board with Velcro closures, papoose board, positioning chair [Figure 43-29]).
- Have a parent help the child maintain a particular position when immobilization devices are not available or are ineffective. The parent must wear the appropriate lead shielding equipment and cannot be pregnant.

Radiation Protection
Clearly, exposure to x-rays creates some risk for both patients and radiographers; therefore, it is essential that those performing

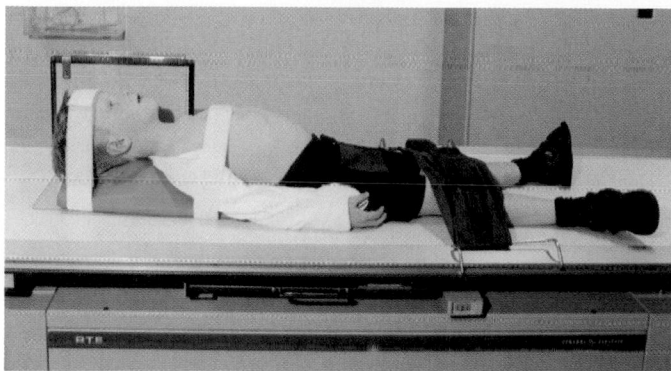

FIGURE 43-29 Immobilization device for a pediatric patient. (From Frank ED, Long BW, Smith BJ: *Merrill's atlas of radiographic positioning and procedures*, ed 12, St Louis, 2013, Mosby.)

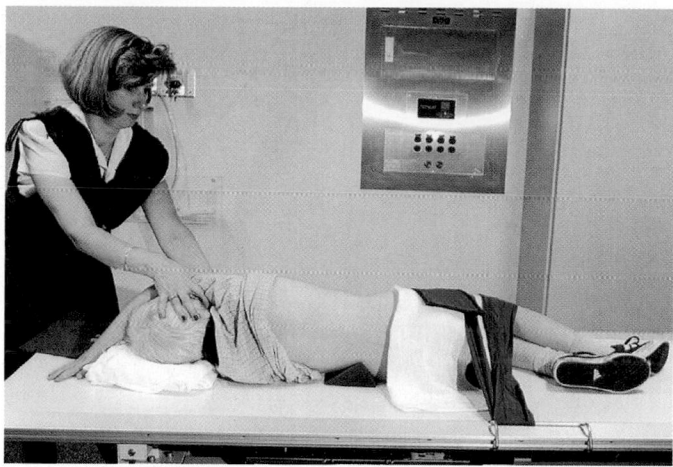

FIGURE 43-30 When holding a child for a radiographic procedure, wear a lead apron and stay as far from the primary x-ray beam as possible. (From Frank ED, Long BW, Smith BJ: *Merrill's atlas of radiographic positioning and procedures*, ed 12, St Louis, 2013, Mosby.)

radiographic studies be knowledgeable about and diligently practice radiation safety. All unnecessary radiation exposure to patients, co-workers, and oneself must be prevented.

Personnel Safety

In diagnostic x-ray departments, radiation hazards exist only in the radiography room and only while the x-ray is being taken. This is due mostly to scatter radiation, which deflects off the patient. X-rays travel at the speed of light. They do not linger in the room after the exposure, and they are not capable of making the objects in the room radioactive. Therefore, the only time a radiation hazard exists is during the x-ray exposure itself.

Because radiographers operate equipment from the protected control booth, their exposure is purposefully limited. However, because radiographers are considered occupationally exposed individuals, they are prohibited from activities that would result in direct exposure to the primary x-ray beam. This means that they are not allowed to hold patients or cassettes during x-ray exposures and must stand clear of the path of the primary x-ray beam during fluoroscopic and mobile radiographic examinations. Whenever possible, patients should be immobilized without someone holding them. When infants or children must be held, a parent (as long as the parent is not pregnant) usually is the appropriate person to perform this duty, with the required lead covering.

Medical assistants may or may not be considered occupationally exposed persons, depending on their work assignments and the frequency with which they are involved with radiation use. Medical assistants who are not routinely exposed occasionally may assist with procedures by holding patients or cassettes. When this is the case, the medical assistant should wear a lead apron and should avoid direct exposure to the primary x-ray beam if possible (Figure 43-30). If the hands will be in the primary beam, lead gloves should also be worn.

Personnel are not exposed to any significant amount of radiation when standing well behind the protective lead barrier of the control booth. X-rays travel in straight lines and do not turn corners. Scatter radiation is not powerful enough to generate additional radiation of concern when it interacts with matter, so the control booth need not be sealed.

Occupational exposure increases when an employee assists with fluoroscopic procedures or uses mobile x-ray equipment. The three principal methods used to protect personnel from unnecessary radiation exposure are time, distance, and shielding.

- Because the amount of exposure received is directly proportional to the time spent in a radiation area, dose is decreased when this time is minimized. For example, you might shorten the time of exposure by stepping into the control booth during fluoroscopic procedures when not required to be near the patient.
- Increasing the distance between yourself and a radiation source reduces your exposure in proportion to the square of the distance; therefore, small increases in distance have a relatively large effect. Mobile x-ray units have long cords on the exposure switches, which allows the radiographer to get as far from the radiation source as possible while making an exposure.
- Shielding is the most common type of personnel protection used in outpatient radiography settings. The lead wall of the control booth provides a radiation safety barrier and is the principal defense for personnel. Other types of shielding include lead aprons, gloves, goggles, and thyroid shields. These types of shielding are worn during fluoroscopic procedures and mobile radiographic examinations.

Pre-exposure Safety Check. Before an x-ray image is taken, double-check to make sure of the following:

- The x-ray room door is closed; a closed door indicates that an exposure is in progress and no one may enter the room.
- No nonessential individuals are in the x-ray room; all essential individuals outside the lead barrier are appropriately shielded.
- All those in the control booth are completely behind the lead barrier.

Personnel Monitoring. A device for monitoring radiation exposure to personnel is called a **dosimeter**. The three basic types of dosimeters are film badges, thermoluminescent dosimeters (TLDs), and optically stimulated luminescence dosimeters (OSLs). OSLs, the most recently developed monitoring dosimeter (Figure 43-31), use aluminum oxide as the radiation detector. OSLs provide greater stability and precision plus the ability to reanalyze and confirm results. For this reason, they are most commonly used.

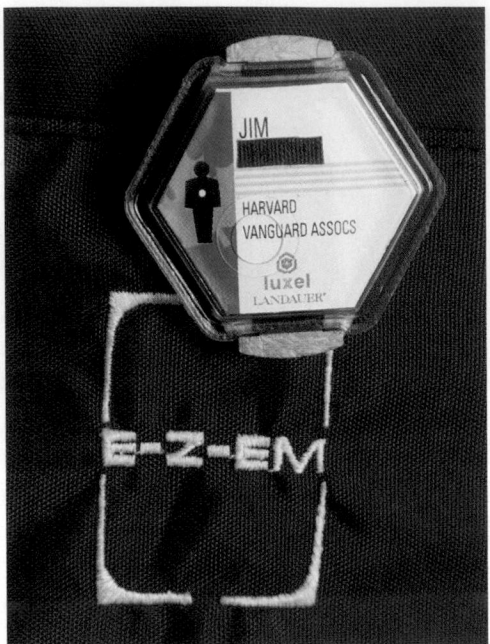

FIGURE 43-31 Optically stimulated luminescence (OSL) dosimeter.

A personnel dosimeter should be worn near the collar, on the front of the body. If a lead apron is worn, the dosimeter should stay on the outside. At the end of the workday, the dosimeter should remain at the medical facility and should not be taken home. Pregnant personnel should also wear a second dosimeter at the waist, which should remain beneath any lead shielding.

Your facility will contract with a radiation monitor badge service laboratory to provide badges, processing services, and reports. The laboratory also is responsible for maintaining permanent records of the radiation exposure of each person monitored. Previously, depending on facility policy, badges were sent for evaluation of radiation exposure on a weekly, monthly, or quarterly basis. Personnel who receive relatively high doses of occupational exposure have historically changed their badges most frequently. Enhanced electronics may allow doses to be automatically read and captured by smart phones and computers, with online report access available for evaluation.

Service companies provide an extra badge in every batch that is marked CONTROL. This badge's purpose is to measure any radiation exposure to the entire batch while in transit. Any amount of exposure measured from the control badge is subtracted from the amounts measured from the other badges in the batch. The control badge should be kept in a safe place, away from anywhere x-ray exposure could occur. *It should never be used to measure occupational dose or for any other purpose.*

Exposure reports are sent to the facility for each batch with an annual summary of personnel exposure. The report sent by the laboratory that processes the personnel dosimeters reports occupational dose in rem. Personnel should be advised of the radiation exposure reported from their badges and should be provided with copies of the annual reports for their own records. Employers are required to provide a complete record of an employee's radiation exposure history to all employees who have radiation exposure records before the individual leaves the employment of that facility.

Effective Dose Equivalent Limits

The effective dose equivalent (EDE) limiting system is used to calculate the upper limit of permitted occupational exposure. For occupationally exposed personnel, the EDE limit is 50 mSv (5 rem) per year. This is assumed to be a whole body dose that affects workers over age 18. These limits apply to occupational exposure only and do not include diagnostic imaging exposure that the worker may receive as a result of tests related to his or her own healthcare.

The established EDE limits ensure that the safety of radiation workers is comparable to that of workers in other, safe occupations. The allowable exposure is considered to be so low as to pose an insignificant risk. The occupational exposure received by radiographers usually is well below the established limit.

Occupational Precautions during Pregnancy

Radiation exposure during pregnancy must be closely monitored because of possible complications for the developing fetus. The National Council on Radiation Protection and Measurements (NCRP) has recommended an equivalent dose (EqD) limit of whole body radiation for the pregnant worker of less than 0.5 mSv per month, with a cumulative total of 5 mSv (0.5 rem) over the 9-month course of the pregnancy. The worker first must submit a written document to her employer declaring the pregnancy. The employer then is responsible for providing fetal radiation monitoring and for ensuring that the occupational dose does not exceed the effective dose equivalent (EDE) limit for pregnant workers. Every effort should be made to minimize exposure, keeping the dose as far below the limit as possible.

For a pregnant radiographer, the safest work assignment is one in which a permanent lead barrier (control booth) always shields the worker during exposures. Pregnant radiographers and those of childbearing age who may be pregnant should pay particular attention to personal safety measures when assisting with fluoroscopy or using mobile x-ray equipment. An additional dosimeter should be worn at waist level, inside of protective shielding.

Patient Protection

The acronym ALARA stands for "as low as reasonably achievable." This is a safety principle in radiography that reminds the radiographer to limit levels of radiation exposure to humans whenever possible. The idea is to use enough radiation to get the job done right the first time, but not more than is needed to obtain a good image. If too low a dose is used and an x-ray must be repeated, the patient is exposed to much more radiation than if a slightly higher dose was used just once. This is the greatest cause of unnecessary radiation that can be controlled by limited radiographers. However, using too high a dose of radiation makes it difficult to see details in a radiograph clearly. This too can lead to repeat exposure and additional radiation. Therefore, it is wise to consult a radiographic chart specifically designed for the radiographic laboratory being used to determine the best setting for the patient's size and position.

The following methods are used to minimize the radiation dose to patients:

- Avoid errors. Double-check requisitions and patient identification so that the right patient gets the right examination.
- Establish good routine procedures and follow them strictly so that errors caused by carelessness do not necessitate repeat exposures.
- Collimate. Use the smallest radiation field needed to fulfill the physician's order. The size of the radiation field should always be less than the size of the image receptor.
- Use the highest kVp consistent with acceptable image quality. This permits use of the least possible mAs to obtain an acceptable exposure.
- Use an SID of at least 40 inches. This limits patient exposure from tube housing leakage and collimator scatter.
- Provide shielding for gonads, eyes, breasts, and thyroid as appropriate.

Gonad Shielding. Lead shields that prevent unnecessary radiation exposure to the reproductive organs are required when the patient is of reproductive age or younger; whenever the gonads are within the primary radiation field; and when the shield will not interfere with the examination. This applies to most patients under age 55.

A shield device consisting of at least 0.5 mm of lead or equivalent is placed between the x ray tube and the patient. Shields attached to the collimator (shadow shields) may be positioned by viewing their shadows within the collimator light field. Shields placed on or near the patient's body are referred to as *contact shields* and are more effective than shadow shields. Both types meet the legal requirements for gonad shielding. The female shield is placed with its lower margin at the level of the pubic symphysis (Figure 43-32). The male shield is positioned with its upper margin about 1 inch below the pubic symphysis (Figure 43-33). It is helpful to note that the pubic symphysis is at about the same level as the greater trochanter of the femur, which prevents the need to palpate the pubic symphysis for proper shield placement.

Pregnant or Possibly Pregnant Patients. The greatest risks for spontaneous abortion, fetal death, and significant birth defects exist when significant levels of exposure occur during the first trimester of pregnancy. The embryo is most vulnerable to radiation insult while tissues are in the process of differentiation. Unfortunately, this creates the greatest hazard at a time when a woman may not yet be aware she is pregnant.

The public is generally aware that x-ray imaging should be avoided during pregnancy, and this may lead to irrational fears on

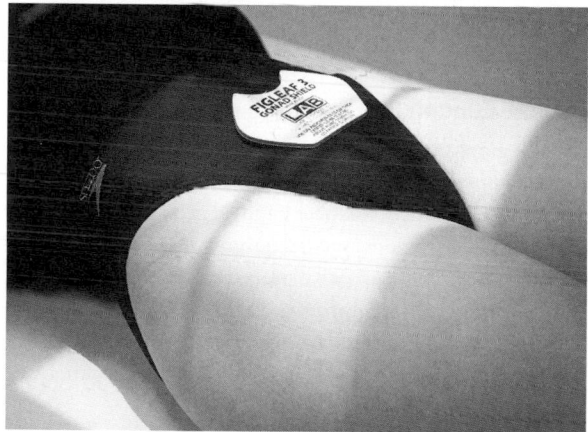
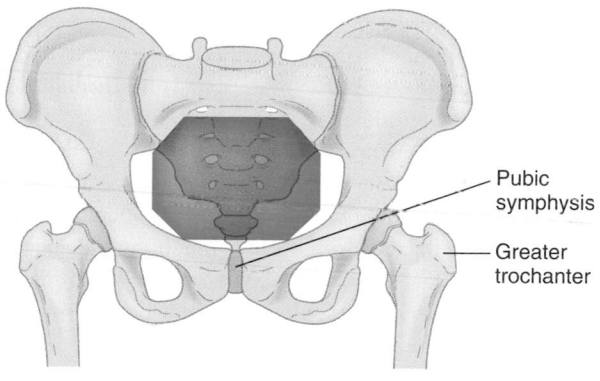

FIGURE 43-32 When precise gonad shielding is required for female patients, place the lower margin of the shield on the upper margin of the pubic symphysis. (Bontrager KL, Lampignano J: *Textbook of radiographic positioning and related anatomy,* ed 8, St Louis, 2014, Mosby.)

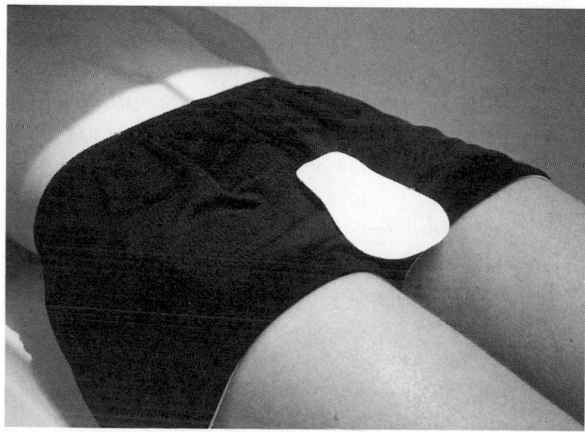
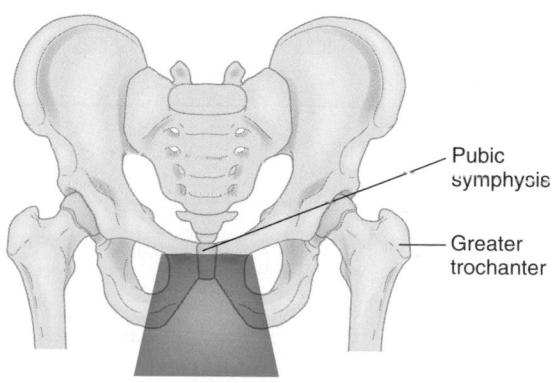

FIGURE 43-33 When precise gonad shielding is required for male patients, place the upper margin of the shield 1 inch below the pubic symphysis. (Bontrager KL, Lampignano J: *Textbook of radiographic positioning and related anatomy,* ed 8, St Louis, 2014, Mosby.)

the part of pregnant women or their families. The chance is extremely remote that a routine x-ray examination of the chest or an extremity would harm the developing child. On the other hand, examinations requiring direct radiation to the pelvis, especially relatively high-dose fluoroscopy studies or CT scans of the abdomen or lumbar spine, may be cause for concern.

Radiation control regulations require that female patients of childbearing age be advised of potential radiation hazards before an x-ray examination. This requirement usually is met by posting signs in the radiology department advising women to tell the radiographer before the examination if they may be pregnant. These signs should be written in all languages commonly used in the community.

The medical assistant should ask specific questions to rule out pregnancy when taking a medical history. If pregnancy is a possibility, an early pregnancy test should be done to rule out the possibility. If the patient is pregnant and the proposed x-ray examination involves direct pelvic radiation, the physician must weigh the potential risks and benefits of the examination and discuss them with the patient before proceeding with the study. In the case of minor or chronic complaints, the examination typically is delayed until after the child is born. In practice, however, the possibility of pregnancy may not even be considered. This is especially true with accident or injury, when the patient is being cared for by unfamiliar physicians in an emergency situation. For this reason, it is essential to consider the possibility of pregnancy in any female of childbearing age and to ask specific questions to determine whether the provider has addressed the issue of pregnancy before proceeding with scheduling or assisting with an x-ray examination.

If an x-ray examination of a pregnant patient must be done, modifications in procedure can help minimize the dose to the embryo or fetus. If the part to be examined is not the abdomen or pelvis, those areas can be shielded with a lead apron. If the abdomen or pelvis is to be evaluated, the number of views or the size of the radiation field may be minimized, resulting in less radiation exposure than that required for a routine procedure.

CRITICAL THINKING APPLICATION   **43-3**

Ingrid White is gowned and ready for a lumbar spine x-ray examination when Sara asks her whether there is any possibility she might be pregnant. Mrs. White confides that she and her husband have been trying to conceive for several months, and she is not sure whether she currently is pregnant. What should Sara do?

CLOSING COMMENTS

Role of the Medical Assistant

Depending on your location, you may or may not be legally permitted to take x-rays. Most states require some sort of license or permit to practice radiography. Some grant licenses only to professional radiologic technologists who have completed at least a 2-year education program and obtained certification in radiography from the American Registry of Radiologic Technologists (ARRT). Other states have a reciprocity policy that allows a medical assistant with a

limited operator's license from another state to work in that capacity.

Limited radiography, sometimes called *practical radiography*, is practiced primarily in clinics and physicians' offices. This field developed as nurses, medical assistants, chiropractic assistants, and other healthcare office personnel were trained to perform basic x-ray procedures in addition to their primary duties. It is called *limited* because the scope of practice is restricted compared with that of registered radiologic technologists. However, the actual title may vary by state. Limited practice does not usually involve the use of contrast media, and additional restrictions may apply, depending on the scope of practice permitted in the states where limited radiography can be legally practiced.

However, even if you are not qualified as a limited operator, it may be helpful to understand the general procedures involved in an x-ray examination and to identify areas where the medical assistant might be of help to the patient or radiographer, or both. The exact nature of your duties will vary with your qualifications, your place of employment, the size of the staff, and the equipment available.

The process of radiography involves validation of orders, patient preparation, image receptor placement, correct positioning of the patient and equipment, measurement of the part to be examined, protective shielding, correct setting of the exposure controls, and identification and processing of the image. These basic procedures vary considerably, depending on the body part to be examined.

Patient Education

In radiography, patient education is the best way to achieve successful participation and to alleviate fears. It is important to tell the patient exactly what to expect in advance. This may require explanation of diet restrictions, medication or contrast usage, the process of imaging itself, and if invasive procedures are included. It is essential to be honest and straightforward with patients, yet to use care and gentleness during the process. Be sure to smile and make good eye contact while discussing details. Always give the patient time to ask any questions or to talk about any concerns.

Legal and Ethical Issues

Only licensed health practitioners are permitted to order x-ray examinations. Interpretation of diagnostic images is part of the professional practice of making a diagnosis and is solely the privilege of specifically trained providers, such as physicians. Although you may learn to recognize certain conditions represented in diagnostic images, you must never discuss your observations with the patient (Figure 43-34).

In most states, x-ray machines must be licensed, and personnel operating this equipment must have a current license or permit. However, according to the American Society of Radiologic Technologists (ASRT), most states allow employees to be trained to operate equipment and position patients, as long as a licensed radiographer supervises and pushes the final exposure button. Always check your specific state standards and institutional policy before engaging in any radiography practice to avoid improperly acting without a license. Practicing without a valid license or permit or practicing outside the scope of one's credentials may result in fines, imprisonment, or both. Employers may also be penalized if their

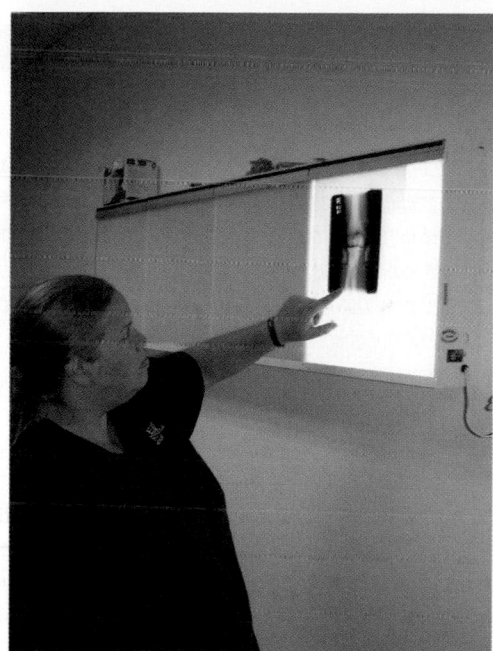

FIGURE 43-34 Although the medical assistant may learn to identify differences in x-ray images, it is important never to discuss them with the patient because this may be considered a diagnosis. (Courtesy Helen Mills.)

employees practice radiography in violation of regulations. Even if you work in a state that currently has no requirements for practicing radiography, you should be aware that the safe practice of radiography requires additional experience, in addition to education beyond that provided in this chapter.

If a patient does not comply with instructions, it is illegal to lay hands on the patient or to hold a patient in position without verbal permission. In legal terms, this is called *battery*, and it is considered a criminal charge. There are only a few exceptions to this law. If a patient is not conscious, consent is not necessary. If a patient is a minor, parental consent is required; however, it is best to have the parent or family member assist. If a patient is mentally confused, a signed order of judgment should be obtained before you assist an unwilling patient.

Patients should never be threatened into compliance. This is considered *assault*, even if the patient is never touched. To avoid this, simply take a few moments to make the patient feel more comfortable by building rapport with him or her. Small talk is a great way to make people relax, particularly if you ask questions that get them to talk about themselves. Then, calmly explain the procedure and offer reassurance. In this instance, a little kindness can go a long way.

X-ray and other diagnostic images are the property of the institution or facility where they are taken. Images are considered part of the health record and are subject to the same kinds of requirements with respect to confidentiality, retention, and availability to the patient. The retention period varies from state to state; usually it is 5 to 7 years. Images may be loaned or transferred to other healthcare providers to assist in the patient's care. The patient should sign a release when images or copies of images are to be sent to another healthcare provider. This process is much less complicated in practices with electronic health records.

CRITICAL THINKING APPLICATION   43-4

One of the new medical assistants at Metro Urgicenter, Carla O'Neal, tells Sara that she is not qualified to practice radiography in the office's jurisdiction. Dr. Swain had instructed her to position a patient and set up the equipment for an x-ray examination. When Carla told him that she was not yet qualified to practice radiography, he replied, "Don't worry. I'll come by in a few minutes and make the exposure." What should Sara and Carla do about this?

Professional Behaviors

Most important in radiographic testing is the rapport that is developed between the medical assistant and the patient. Rushing a patient or being insensitive to his or her fears or needs is likely to cost you more time and effort in gaining cooperation. The best way to get a patient to respond favorably is to look the individual in the eye, smile, and take a little time for small talk.

Patients tend to react to the behavior of the medical assistant in a direct manner. If the radiographer has wrinkled clothing and poor body hygiene, the patient automatically assumes that the provider doesn't care about details, and he or she loses faith immediately. Factors such as gum chewing, untoward body language, and inconsiderate behavior can make a patient distrustful and resistant to cooperation. A professional appearance and a courteous method of communication can go a long way toward helping a frightened patient relax and follow directions.

SUMMARY OF SCENARIO

The providers and radiographer at Metro Urgicenter depend on Sara's assistance to keep the x-ray department running smoothly. Today, for example, she instructed four patients in how to gown and prepare for routine x-ray examinations, and she processed the images after the exams. Greg Nolan had PA and lateral views of the chest because of a persistent cough and fever. Margaret and Jeff Barge both needed spine x-ray studies to rule out possible fractures from a car accident. Dr. Farnsworth, a physician at the practice, ordered AP and lateral views of Ella Jackson's left hip. Sara was proud to see that the images had no handling artifacts after she had processed them. This afternoon, Sara made an appointment for Cecile Marsden to have a bone scan at University Imaging Center. She was able to describe the procedure for Ms. Marsden so that she would know exactly what to expect. Sara recognizes that she must remain up to date on the current radiologic diagnostic procedures to provide assistance when needed and to answer patients' questions. Sara enjoys her work at Metro Urgicenter; she is attending evening classes to become certified as a limited radiographer.

SUMMARY OF LEARNING OBJECTIVES

1. **Define, spell, and pronounce the terms listed in the vocabulary.**
   Spelling and pronouncing medical terms correctly reinforce the medical assistant's credibility. Knowing the definitions of these terms promotes confidence in communication with patients and co-workers.

2. **Discuss basic principles of radiography and the types of x-rays.**
   Radiography is the process of creating an x-ray image to examine internal structures of the body. A radiographer is much like a photographer who takes pictures with a camera and is responsible for processing them. The various types of x-rays are primary radiation, remnant radiation, and scatter radiation.

3. **Identify the principal components of radiographic equipment.**
   The main component of the x-ray machine is the tube in its barrel-shaped tube housing. The collimator is mounted on the tube housing. The tube housing, with its attachments, is mounted on the tube support. The radiographic table and an upright cassette holder provide support for the patient and the image receptor and incorporate a grid device. At the control console, the operator selects the exposure settings and makes the exposure. The collimator is a boxlike device attached beneath the tube housing that allows the operator to adjust the size of the radiation field. The power supply can be controlled in the transformer cabinet.

4. **Discuss the four prime factors of x-ray exposure.**
   The four principal exposure factors are called the *prime factors* of exposure. They include milliamperage, exposure time, kilovoltage, and source-to-image distance. Technique charts provide the radiographer with a listing of recommended millampere-seconds, kilovoltage, and source-to-image distance settings for x-ray studies of various body parts in patients of different sizes.

5. **Do the following related to radiographic positioning:**
   - *Distinguish among the three body planes and use these terms correctly when discussing radiographic positions.*
     The three body planes are the sagittal plane, which divides the body into right and left parts; the coronal plane, which divides the body into anterior and posterior parts; and the transverse plane, which divides the body into superior and inferior parts. For a frontal projection (AP or PA), the coronal plane is parallel to the image receptor and the sagittal plane is perpendicular to it. For a lateral projection, the sagittal plane is parallel to the image receptor and the coronal plane is perpendicular to it. Neither the sagittal plane nor the coronal plane is parallel to the image receptor on an oblique position.
   - *Differentiate between anteroposterior (AP) and posteroanterior (PA) projections and describe the lateral and oblique radiographic positions.*
     - *AP projection:* The patient is supine or facing the x-ray tube. The x-ray beam leaves the tube, passes through the front of the patient, and then exits through the back to strike the image receptor.
     - *PA projection:* The patient is prone or facing the image receptor. The x-ray beam leaves the tube, passes through the back of the patient, and then exits through the front to strike the image receptor.

The oblique and lateral radiographic positions are:
   - *Left anterior oblique:* Patient's left side is on the image receptor with the anterior (front) leaning toward the image receptor.
   - *Right anterior oblique:* Patient's right side is on the image receptor with the anterior (front) leaning toward the image receptor.
   - *Left posterior oblique:* Patient's left side is on the image receptor with the posterior (back) leaning toward the image receptor.
   - *Right posterior oblique:* Patient's right side is on the image receptor with the posterior (back) leaning toward the image receptor.
   - *Left lateral:* Patient's left side is on the image receptor.
   - *Right lateral:* Patient's right side is on the image receptor.

6. **Discuss fluoroscopy and contrast media.**
   Radiography and fluoroscopy are both x-ray imaging procedures with a wide variety of applications. Radiography produces still images; fluoroscopy enables the radiologist to view the x-ray image directly and to observe motion. Contrast media are substances that enhance the visibility of soft tissues. Examples of x-ray studies that use contrast media are an upper gastrointestinal (UGI) series, a lower gastrointestinal series, an intravenous urogram (IVU), an arthrogram, and myelography.

7. **Discuss cardiovascular and interventional radiography, computed tomography, magnetic resonance imaging, sonography, and nuclear medicine.**
   The highly specialized radiographic procedures that display blood vessels are collectively known as *angiography*. Computed tomography uses a special x-ray scanner to produce detailed pictures of a cross section of a tissue. MRI uses a strong magnetic field and radiofrequency pulses to produce images of all parts of the body, including bone, soft tissue, and blood vessels. Nuclear medicine studies demonstrate the function of organs and tissues by mapping the radiation given off within the body when radioactive tracers have been ingested or injected into the patient. Sonography is a very safe imaging method that demonstrates soft tissues using high-frequency sound waves. Nuclear medicine images are created by scanning the patient after special radioactive materials, called *tracers*, have been swallowed or injected intravenously. Dual energy x-ray absorptiometry (DEXA) scans use x-ray technology to evaluate a patient's bone density level.

8. **Do the following related to basic radiographic procedures:**
   - *Explain the patient preparation guidelines for typical diagnostic imaging examinations.*
     Table 43-5 summarizes patient preparation.
   - *Outline the general procedure for scheduling and sequencing diagnostic imaging procedures.*
     When possible, several examinations should be scheduled on the same day if the patient is strong enough. Imaging that requires fasting is easier on the patient if scheduled in the morning. Diagnostic imaging that does not require contrast media or nuclear medicine should be scheduled first. Next are examinations of the urinary tract and biliary system. Fiberoptic studies (e.g., colonoscopy) and CT studies of the abdomen and pelvis should be scheduled before any GI studies that require barium. CT and MRI can be scheduled any time

unless they require IV contrast; if iodine dye is needed, the procedure is scheduled after examinations that do not require visualization. Barium studies are always scheduled last, and a UGI series (barium swallow) is the final procedure.

- *Apply patient education principles when providing instructions for preparation for diagnostic procedures.*
  Table 43-5 summarizes patient preparation guidelines for diagnostic imaging procedures. The patient must be informed of the purpose of the study, how the procedure will be performed, and any important patient preparation steps to make sure the examination can be completed successfully. The healthcare facility should have instruction sheets ready to distribute to patients scheduled for diagnostic studies. The medical assistant must understand diagnostic procedures so that the patient's questions can be answered and informed consent can be obtained. The medical assistant should review instruction sheets with the patient to make sure the preparation is done as recommended. Whenever contrast is to be administered, it is essential to ask the patient about iodine or shellfish allergies and whether he or she has ever had a negative reaction to contrast media; if so, the provider should be informed.

9. **Describe the health risks associated with low doses of x-ray exposure, such as those used in radiography.**
   The health risks associated with radiography are extremely small and consist of a slightly increased likelihood of developing cataracts, cancer, or leukemia. The potential also exists for a minimal decrease in life span and for a negative outcome if the abdominal area is exposed to radiation during pregnancy. Exposure of the reproductive organs may cause genetic changes that can be passed on to future generations.

10. **Describe precautions for ensuring the safety of equipment operators and staff members during x-ray procedures.**
    The principal safety precaution for x-ray equipment operators and staff members is to stay completely behind the lead barrier of the control booth during exposures. Occupationally exposed individuals must not hold patients or image receptors during exposures. Any staff member required to be in the x-ray room during an exposure should be shielded by a lead apron, should stay as far from radiation sources as possible, and should minimize the time spent in the room during exposures.

11. **Summarize the steps for ensuring that patients receive the least possible exposure during x-ray procedures.**
    To ensure that patients receive the least possible exposure during x-ray procedures, radiology personnel should avoid errors that could require repeat exposures; establish good routine procedures and follow them strictly; collimate to the smallest radiation field; use the highest kVp possible; use an SID of at least 40 inches; and shield the reproductive organs and other sensitive organs (e.g., eyes, thyroid, and breasts).

12. **Explain the legal responsibilities associated with x-ray procedures and the administrative management of diagnostic images.**
    Diagnostic images are the property of the facility in which they are made. Only licensed healthcare providers are permitted to order x-ray examinations and/or to interpret x-ray images.

CONNECTIONS

Study Guide Connection: Go to the Chapter 43 Study Guide. Read and complete the activities.

evolve Evolve Connection: Go to the Chapter 43 link at *evolve.elsevier.com/kinn* to complete the Chapter Review Quiz. Check out the other resources listed for this chapter to make the most of what you have learned from Assisting with Diagnostic Imaging.

44

ASSISTING IN THE CLINICAL LABORATORY

SCENARIO

Marsha Rollins, CMA (AAMA), has been employed for 3 years as a Certified Medical Assistant in a medical practice. The providers have a medical laboratory on site, and Marsha has become experienced in collecting specimens, performing laboratory tests, and reporting results. Recently she was offered a position in a smaller practice closer to home; she has accepted the position, knowing that her experience will benefit the practice because the providers would like to expand their on-site medical laboratory testing. One of Marsha's new responsibilities will be equipping the office laboratory.

While studying this chapter, think about the following questions:

- What agencies can assist Marsha as she researches the feasibility of setting up a laboratory in the new office?
- What regulations will guide the testing that can be performed in the laboratory?
- What equipment will Marsha need, and how will she make sure that it stays in good working order?

LEARNING OBJECTIVES

1. Define, spell, and pronounce the terms listed in the vocabulary.
2. Discuss the role of the clinical laboratory personnel in patient care and the medical assistant's role in coordinating laboratory tests and results.
3. Describe the divisions of the clinical laboratory and give an example of a test performed in each division.
4. Explain the three regulatory categories established by the Clinical Laboratory Improvement Amendments (CLIA) and identify CLIA-waived tests associated with common diseases.
5. Identify quality assurance practices in healthcare, document the results on a laboratory flow sheet, and discuss quality control guidelines.
6. Do the following related to laboratory safety:
    - Compare the agencies that govern or influence practice in the clinical laboratory.
    - Discuss the purpose of a Safety Data Sheet.
    - Summarize safety techniques to minimize physical, chemical, and biologic hazards in the clinical laboratory.
7. Describe the essential elements of a laboratory requisition.
8. Discuss specimen collection, including the importance of sensitivity to patients' rights and feelings when collecting specimen. Also, discuss the 8 steps in collecting specimens and informing patients of their results.
9. Explain the chain of custody and why it is important.
10. Describe the differences between Greenwich time and military time.
11. Identify the Fahrenheit temperature and the Celsius temperature of common pieces of laboratory equipment.
12. Name the metric units used for measuring liquid volume, distance, and mass.
13. Do the following related to laboratory equipment:
    - Name the parts of a microscope and describe their functions.
    - Summarize selected microscopy tests that may be performed in the ambulatory care setting.
    - Demonstrate the proper use and maintenance of the microscope.
    - Describe the safe use of a centrifuge.
    - Discuss the use of an incubator.
14. Identify patient education issues, as well as legal and ethical issues, in the clinical laboratory setting.

VOCABULARY

aliquot (ah′-luh-kwaht) A portion of a well-mixed sample removed for testing.
analyte The substance or chemical being analyzed or detected in a specimen.
anticoagulants Chemicals added to a blood sample after collection to prevent clotting.

calibration Determining the accuracy of an instrument by comparing its output with that of a known standard or another instrument known to be accurate.
caustic (kos′-tik) Capable of burning, corroding, or damaging tissue by chemical action.

cytology (si-tah'-luh-je) The study of cells using microscopic methods.

exudates (ek'-syu-dayts) Fluids with high concentrations of protein and cellular debris that have escaped from the blood vessels and have been deposited in tissues or on tissue surfaces.

hemolyzed A blood sample in which the red blood cells have ruptured.

in vitro Latin term meaning "in the laboratory."

preservatives Substances added to a specimen to prevent deterioration of cells or chemicals.

profile testing A series of laboratory tests associated with a particular organ or disease; also referred to as a "panel" of tests.

qualitative A laboratory test result expressed as positive or negative.

quality assurance The process of monitoring all the processes involved before, during, and after a laboratory test is performed in order to produce reliable patient test results.

quality control Manufactured samples with known values used to determine whether a test method is reliable

quantitative A laboratory test result expressed in numeric units of measure.

reagent (re-a'-gent) A testing substance that produces a reaction when interacting with the patient sample

referral laboratory A private or hospital-based laboratory that performs a wide variety of tests, many of them specialized; providers often send specimens collected in the office to referral laboratories for testing.

reference range The numeric range of test values for which the general population consistently shows similar results 95% of the time.

specimen A sample of body fluid, waste product, or tissue collected for analysis.

STAT Immediately.

ROLE OF THE CLINICAL LABORATORY IN PATIENT CARE

Laboratory medicine, or clinical pathology, is the medical discipline that applies clinical laboratory science and technology to the care of patients. The clinical laboratory is the place in which a collected **specimen** is analyzed and evaluated. Tests are performed manually (by hand) or through automation (using specialized instruments).

Personnel in the Clinical Laboratory

Medical laboratories are located in hospitals or in facilities such as providers' offices, clinics, public health departments, health maintenance organizations, and private referral laboratories. The director of a laboratory may be a pathologist, a physician specially trained in the nature and cause of disease, or a clinical laboratory scientist with a doctorate. The laboratory is staffed by various professionally trained individuals, including certified medical technologists (MTs), who have earned a baccalaureate degree, have had additional formal training, and have passed a national certification examination. Other personnel include certified medical laboratory technicians (MLTs) or medical laboratory assistants (MLAs) and credentialed medical assistants (CMAs, RMAs). These employees have completed a 1- to 2-year specialized training program and have passed a national examination. Laboratory assistants and phlebotomists, who have received specialized training in the collection and preparation of laboratory specimens, also work in laboratories. The agencies granting certifications and titles are listed in Table 44-1.

In ambulatory facilities, the lab director may be the physician. These labs are referred to as *physician office laboratories* (POLs). The medical assistant is trained both to perform certain testing procedures in the POL and in methods of collecting specimens that are sent to outside reference laboratories for testing.

Laboratory tests may be used to screen patients for diseases such as diabetes or urinary tract infections. They are also an essential part of a medical diagnosis. In addition, they may be performed to help the provider decide the most appropriate treatment to prescribe and to monitor the effects of medications and/or a disease process. Only healthcare practitioners may request laboratory testing for a patient. The medical assistant may be responsible for a number of these testing procedures. To assume this responsibility, the medical assistant must know proper patient preparation, the procedure for each test, and the normal range of results for the test. The medical assistant must carefully follow all laboratory instructions in obtaining and labeling specimens and sending them to the laboratory. Good communication among the patient, office staff, and laboratory personnel is important. The medical assistant should make the patient feel at ease with these procedures and thus gain the patient's cooperation.

Clinical Laboratory Testing

Clinical laboratory testing is used in conjunction with a thorough health history and physical examination to obtain essential data for screening, diagnosis, and/or management of a patient's condition. The body is considered to be healthy when a state of equilibrium exists in the internal environment. In this healthy state of equilibrium, called *homeostasis,* the physical and chemical characteristics of body substances (e.g., fluids, secretions, and excretions) are within a certain acceptable range, known as the *normal range,* or **reference range**. A change in homeostasis results in abnormal test values that are outside the population's reference range. When a provider uses a laboratory test for diagnosis, the patient's results are compared to the reference range of values. Reference values are also useful for assessing the progress of a patient's course of treatment.

Abnormal values for a particular test may be seen with more than one pathologic condition. For example, a decrease in the hemoglobin level in red blood cells (RBCs) is seen in iron-deficiency anemia, but also in hyperthyroidism and cirrhosis of the liver. Therefore, providers cannot rely solely on one laboratory test to make a diagnosis;

TABLE 44-1   Certifying Agencies for Laboratory Personnel

CERTIFYING AGENCY	TITLE	POSITION
American Society for Clinical Pathologists (ASCP)	MT (ASCP)	Medical technologist
	MLT (ASCP)	Medical laboratory technician—certificate
	MLT-AD (ASCP)	Medical laboratory technician—associate's degree
American Medical Technologists (AMT)	MT (AMT)	Medical technologist
	MLT (AMT)	Medical laboratory technician
	MLA	Medical laboratory assistant
	RMA	Registered medical assistant
Department of Health and Human Services (DHHS)	CLT (HHS)	Clinical laboratory technologist
National Certification Agency for Medical Laboratory Personnel (NCA)	CLS (NCA)	Certified laboratory scientist
	CLT (NCA)	Certified laboratory technician
International Society for Clinical Laboratory Technology (ISCLT)	RMT (ISCLT)	Registered medical technologist
	RLT (ISCLT)	Registered laboratory technician
American Association of Medical Assistants (AAMA)	CMA (AAMA)	Certified medical assistant
National Healthcareer Association (NHA)	CCMA	Certified clinical medical assistant
	CPT	Certified phlebotomy technician
	CMLA	Certified medical laboratory assistant

they must use a combination of data obtained from the health history and physical examination, and a number of diagnostic and laboratory results.

Tests performed in a clinical laboratory range from simple screening of one **analyte** (e.g., measuring glucose to assess for diabetes) to complex **profile testing**, in which more than one analyte is related to a particular organ or disease (e.g., performing a lipid profile to determine the various fats in the blood). A screening test examines a particular specimen for the presence of an analyte that may indicate a disease state. Screening tests are not diagnostic for any particular disease, but rather indicate that the disease state may exist. Screening tests are done routinely on patients on the basis of their age, history, or gender. The results are often **qualitative** in that a numeric value is not attached to the result; they may be simply reported as "positive" or "negative." The fecal occult blood test for blood in the stool (feces) is an example of a screening test. Blood is not normally found in the stool, and its presence may indicate a cancerous lesion in the colon. A positive test result indicates that blood is present, but additional testing is required to determine the source of the blood. For example, in a female patient, further testing or examination may reveal that the patient was having her menstrual period at the time of the first collection of the specimen or that she had bleeding hemorrhoids.

In a **quantitative** test, units of measure are attached to numeric values. These values often are represented as the numeric amount of an analyte per given volume of specimen. It is essential that the quantitative test results be reported with the units of measure. For example, a complete blood cell count for a healthy adult would show these values: RBCs, 5 million per cubic millimeter ($5 \times 10^6/mm^3$);

hemoglobin, 15 grams per deciliter (15 g/dL); and hematocrit, 45%. Generally the units are printed on the laboratory report, but the medical assistant must always make sure that the values are consistent with the test performed.

CRITICAL THINKING APPLICATION   44-1

The **referral laboratory** calls to report the values on several tests performed on the urine of a patient, Cecelia Roberts. Marsha jots down the following: Total protein, 0.12; Occult blood, positive; Albumin, 50; Glucose, 120. What is wrong with the notations she has just made? Are these tests qualitative or quantitative?

DIVISIONS OF THE CLINICAL LABORATORY

Large laboratories are divided into various departments, which may include urinalysis, hematology, chemistry, microbiology, specimen collection and processing, blood bank, coagulation, serology, histology, **cytology**, toxicology, and special chemistry. The small laboratory area in the physician's office provides test procedures in urinalysis, hematology, chemistry, and microbiology.

Urinalysis

Urinalysis includes the physical, chemical, and microscopic examination of urine. In the physical examination, the color, clarity, and specific gravity are noted. The specimen's temperature also may be measured to verify that the sample is a fresh one taken at body temperature, because some individuals may bring a urine sample from elsewhere and try to pass it off as their own. Chemical analysis is performed to measure levels of such analytes as glucose, protein, ketones, blood, bilirubin, urobilinogen, nitrites, and pH. Microscopically, the urine is examined for the visual presence of red, white, and epithelial cells; mucus; casts; crystals; yeasts; parasites; and bacteria. Additional quantitative tests may be performed in the urinalysis department of a reference laboratory to confirm routine screening test results.

Hematology

Hematology is the study of blood cells and coagulation. Laboratory testing in the hematology division may be qualitative or quantitative. Screening tests for hemoglobin and hematocrit are typically performed in the ambulatory setting. Blood cell counts determine the exact number of RBCs, or erythrocytes; white blood cells (WBCs, or leukocytes); and platelets (thrombocytes), either by manual or automated counting. Microscopic tests determine the characteristics of cells, such as size, shape, and maturity. In addition, the hematology department performs tests to determine the coagulating ability of blood components.

Chemistry

The clinical chemistry department analyzes the chemicals found in blood, cerebrospinal fluid (CSF), urine, and joint fluid (synovial fluid). Procedures may include single tests or profiles, which include tests for a number of related analytes. Lipid profiles, for example, include assessments of total cholesterol, triglycerides, and low-density lipoprotein (LDL) and high-density lipoprotein (HDL) cholesterol.

Microbiology

Microbiology involves the study of bacteria, fungi, yeasts, parasites, and viruses. In the microbiology laboratory, microorganisms are grown (cultured) from blood, urine, sputum, CSF, and wound specimens and are identified under the microscope. Sensitivity testing is performed on these organisms to determine the proper antibiotic therapy. Specimens for microbiology must be collected aseptically in sterile containers.

CRITICAL THINKING APPLICATION 44-2

Dr. Watkins has ordered a routine urinalysis (UA), a urine culture and sensitivity (C&S), a blood glucose test, and a complete blood count (CBC) for his patient. Which division of the laboratory is responsible for analyzing the specimens for each test?

GOVERNMENT LEGISLATION AFFECTING CLINICAL LABORATORY TESTING

In 1988 Congress passed the Clinical Laboratory Improvement Amendments (CLIA), establishing quality standards for all clinical laboratory testing to ensure the accuracy, precision, reliability, and timeliness of patient test results, regardless of where the test was performed. A clinical laboratory is defined as any facility that performs laboratory testing on specimens derived from humans for the purpose of providing information about the diagnosis, prevention, and treatment of disease or the impairment of health.

Clinical Laboratory Improvement Amendments

Under CLIA, all entities that perform even one test, including waived tests, must meet certain federal requirements and must register with the Centers for Medicare and Medicaid Services (CMS) as a laboratory. The registration application must be submitted to CMS with information about the laboratory's operations. The type of certificate to be issued and the fees to be assessed are determined from this information. (*Note:* Most POLs are registered as CLIA-waived laboratories.)

CLIA categorization of the commercially marketed tests performed **in vitro** (in a laboratory) is the responsibility of the U.S. Food and Drug Administration (FDA). The FDA has assumed primary responsibility for determining the CLIA complexity categorization of all laboratory tests. Every laboratory test product is assigned to one of three CLIA categories on the basis of the product's potential risk to public health: CLIA-waived tests, moderate-complexity tests, and high-complexity tests.

Common Government Acronyms in the Clinical Laboratory

ACRONYM	TERM	APPLICATION
BBPS	Bloodborne Pathogens Standard	OSHA standard that established precautions for dealing with all blood specimens
CDC	Centers for Disease Control and Prevention	Provides information for CLIA-waived laboratories in *Ready! Set! Test!* booklet
CLIA	Clinical Laboratory Improvement Amendments	Law that regulates all clinical laboratory testing products and sites
CMS	Centers for Medicare and Medicaid Services	Agency with which all labs must register and pay biannual fee based on complexity of tests performed in the lab
CoW	Certificate of waiver	The most common CLIA lab classification for physician office laboratories (POLs)
HHS	Department of Health and Human Services	Federal department that oversees the CMS, FDA, and CDC
FDA	Food and Drug Administration	Approves and categorizes CLIA-waived tests
HCS	Hazard Communication Standard	Standard regulated by OSHA that requires employers to communicate hazards to employees

Continued

Common Government Acronyms in the Clinical Laboratory—*continued*

ACRONYM	TERM	APPLICATION
HIPAA	Health Insurance Portability and Accountability Act	Law that enforces regulations for protected health information
HMIS	Hazardous Materials Information System	Identifies four color-coded chemical hazards (health, flammable, reactive, and other)
OPIM	Other Potentially Infectious Materials	Other materials related to blood-borne pathogens
OSHA	Occupational Safety and Health Administration	Regulates BBPS and HCS to ensure the safety of healthcare workers
PEP	Postexposure prophylaxis	Steps taken if a person is exposed to blood or OPIM
PHI	Protected health information	All test results are considered PHI and must be confidential
POL	Physician office laboratory	Located in ambulatory care facilities
PPE	Personal protective equipment	Gloves, gowns, and face protection worn when dealing with specimens
PPM	Provider-performed microscopy	CLIA moderate to complex microscopy tests available to POLs
QA	Quality assurance	
QC	Quality control	
SDS	Safety Data Sheet (formerly MSDS)	Must be in a uniform format with 16 section numbers, headings, and associated information to inform employees of chemical hazards in the laboratory

CLIA-Waived Tests and Laboratories

CLIA-waived tests are defined as laboratory examinations and procedures that have been approved by the FDA for home use or that are simple laboratory examinations and procedures that have an insignificant risk of an erroneous result, including those that (1) use methodologies so simple and accurate that the likelihood of erroneous user results is negligible, or (2) pose no unreasonable risk of harm to the patient if performed incorrectly. Table 44-2 shows common CLIA-waived tests performed in ambulatory care facilities registered as CLIA-waived laboratories.

The FDA's CLIA-waived database of tests is available to the public on the Internet. This database contains the commercially marketed in vitro test systems categorized by the FDA since January 31, 2000, and tests categorized by the Centers for Disease Control and Prevention (CDC) before that date. The records can be searched by test system name, specialty or subspecialty, the analyte, document number, qualifier, effective date, and complexity.

Moderate- and High-Complexity Tests and Laboratories

The CLIA program oversees the quality of nearly 200,000 different laboratory procedures. An estimated 10,000 different laboratory tests are performed in the United States every day; most of them are categorized by the FDA as moderate-complexity tests. Some of the moderate-complexity tests are performed in POLs, including

TABLE 44-2 CLIA-Waived Tests and Their Purposes

CPT CODES	SPECIMEN AND TEST	PURPOSE
Urine and Feces		
81002	Dipstick or tablet reagent urinalysis (manual or automated)	Urine screening to assess or diagnose diseases such as diabetes mellitus, kidney disease, and urinary tract infection
81025	Urine pregnancy tests: visual color comparison tests	Diagnose pregnancy
82270 82272	Fecal occult blood	Colorectal screening to detect hidden blood in the stool
Blood (Hematology)		
85651	Erythrocyte sedimentation rate, nonautomated	Diagnose inflammatory process; increases in arthritis, infection, leukemia, and most cancers
85013	Spun microhematocrit	Measure RBCs; screening for certain types of anemia
85014QW	STAT-CRIT hematocrit	Screening for certain types of anemia
85018QW	Hemoglobin	Measure hemoglobin level in whole blood

TABLE 44-2   CLIA-Waived Tests and Their Purposes—*continued*

CPT CODES	SPECIMEN AND TEST	PURPOSE
Blood (Chemistry)		
82947QW	Blood glucose by glucose-monitoring devices cleared by the FDA specifically for home use	Monitor blood glucose levels
83036QW	Hemoglobin A_{1c} by single analyte instruments with self-contained or component features to perform specimen-reagent interaction	Measure A_{1c} levels to assess and manage long-term care of patients with diabetes
82465QW, 80061QW	Cholestech LDX	Measure total blood cholesterol, triglycerides, HDL, and glucose levels
80047QW 82330QW 82374QW	Whole-Blood i-STAT Chem8+ Cartridge	Measure ionized calcium, carbon dioxide, chloride, creatinine, glucose, potassium, sodium, urea nitrogen, and hematocrit in whole blood
84443QW	Whole-blood thyroid-stimulating hormone (TSH) assay	Qualitative determination of TSH in whole blood
Blood (Immunology)		
86308QW	Blood mononucleosis antibodies	Rapid whole-blood test to detect heterophile antibodies to help diagnose infectious mononucleosis
86318QW	*Helicobacter pylori* antibodies	Rapid whole-blood test to detect *H. pylori* antibodies to determine the cause of peptic ulcer
86618QW	*Borrelia burgdorferi* antibodies	Rapid whole-blood test to detect *B. burgdorferi* antibodies to diagnose Lyme disease
Microbiology		
86701QW	Trinity Biotech Uni-Gold Recomhigen HIV Test	Detect HIV-1 in a blood specimen
87804QW	Nasal influenza A and B	Quick qualitative diagnosis of influenza antigens in nasal secretions or swab
87889QW	*Streptococcus* A throat swab	Rapid strep test
Toxicology and Gynecology		
G0434QW	Urine and/or blood drug tests	Multiple tests for the presence of a variety of substance abuse agents
83001QW	Urine fertility and menopause	Detect follicle-stimulating hormone in urine
84830	Ovulation tests; visual color comparison tests for luteinizing hormone	Detect ovulation

CLIA, Clinical Laboratory Improvement Amendments; *CPT*, Current Procedural Terminology; *FDA*, U.S. Food and Drug Administration; *HDL*, high-density lipoprotein; *HIV-1*, human immunodeficiency virus type 1.
Centers for Medicare and Medicaid Services. *www.cms.gov/CLIA/downloads/waivetbl.pdf.* Accessed February 6, 2015.

hematology and chemistry testing done on an automated analyzer, Gram staining, and microscopic analysis of urine sediment. High-complexity tests usually are not performed in a POL; these include Papanicolaou (Pap) smear analysis; blood typing and cross-matching; and cytologic testing.

Laboratories that perform moderate- to high-complexity testing must meet rigorous CLIA regulations and are subject to unannounced inspections every 2 years. Each laboratory that performs these tests must establish a system to maintain the integrity and identification of patients' specimens throughout the testing process and to ensure accurate reporting of results. The laboratory also must establish and follow written quality control and quality assurance procedures and must participate in proficiency testing, a form of external quality control. Three times a year, the laboratory must test samples provided by an approved proficiency-testing agency using the same tests the laboratory would use to test a patient's sample. Additionally, CLIA regulations specify qualifications and responsibilities for personnel in the moderate- to high-complexity laboratory, from directors to testing personnel. Personnel requirements are most stringent for high-complexity testing.

Medical assistants may perform all CLIA-waived tests and some moderate-complexity tests with additional training, depending on the certification of the POL in which they are employed. Although medical assistants may not perform high-complexity tests, they are involved in preparing the patient for tests (e.g., explaining the need to fast before blood collection), collecting the specimens required, and recording the results in the patient's health record.

Quality Assurance Guidelines

Quality assurance (QA) is the pledge of healthcare professionals to achieve the highest degree of excellence in the healthcare given to every patient. QA encompasses a comprehensive set of policies developed to ensure excellent documentation and reliability of laboratory testing. These policies benefit the provider by reducing the liability for inaccurate reporting of test results. QA also focuses on establishing a series of operating procedures for the benefit of the patient and the medical assistant who does the laboratory testing. The QA system enables the laboratory to assess, verify, and document the quality of the laboratory process. This documentation is a way of comparing "what is happening" with "what should be happening."

As mandated by law, QA programs monitor all aspects of laboratory activity, from specimen collection through processing, testing, and reporting steps. Programs check supplies, reagents, machinery, and actual test performance. It includes quality control, personnel orientation, laboratory documentation, knowledge of laboratory instrumentation, and enrollment in a proficiency testing program (if the lab performs moderate- or high-complexity tests).

The Three Stages of Quality Assurance in the Laboratory

The overall process required to ensure quality assurance (QA) in the laboratory is divided into three stages, which must be applied to each test or "analytic" procedure. If any of these steps are missed or performed incorrectly, QA has been broken.

Preanalytic Stage
1. The provider orders a test to screen, monitor, or diagnose a patient's condition.
2. A written or an electronic requisition is filled out, showing the test requested, the specimen required, and where the specimen will be tested.
3. The specimen is collected, labeled, and processed (e.g., centrifuged or refrigerated).
4. The specimen is transported to the appropriate laboratory (in the office or pickup for an off-site laboratory).

Analytic Stage
1. Instruments are maintained and calibrated.
2. Controls are run and analyzed for each test method (QC).
3. The specimen is tested, and the results are compared to reference ranges.
4. The test results are logged and documented in the patient's health record.

Postanalytic Stage
1. Specimens are properly discarded.
2. Analyses of control results are compared over time.
3. Patient reports from outside labs are logged.
4. The provider interprets and signs all lab reports.
5. The patient is notified of the results in the office or is contacted by laboratory personnel.
6. The final report and all communication with the patient is documented in the patient's health record.

Accurate record keeping is one of the key responsibilities of a medical assistant. Various forms are available to assist in the recording of laboratory information, although much of this information now can be found online and recorded in an electronic format. If your office uses hard copies (e.g., paper records), the primary record is the laboratory master logbook, in which each procedure performed in the POL is entered, with the dates clearly shown.

POLs are also required to have a procedure manual that describes the processes for testing and reporting patients' results. Personnel are required to perform **calibration** or optic checks on laboratory instruments that utilize light in determining results. In addition, they must run control material each day before patient testing based on the manufacturer's instructions and document the results, and they must perform and document remedial action when errors or problems are identified. Finally, preventive maintenance schedules must be followed and documented. Preventive maintenance prolongs the life of equipment and reduces breakdown; it includes daily cleaning and adjustment and replacement of parts when necessary. Each instrument should have a log or worksheet for recording all changes, including daily maintenance details.

Ready? Set? Test! is an excellent on-line resource provided by the CDC for setting up and maintaining a CLIA-waived laboratory. Figure 44-1 shows the checklist summary of the steps needed to assure proper CLIA-waived testing in a POL.

Quality Control Guidelines

A crucial step in the QA process is the running of **quality controls (QC)** (Procedure 44-1). Specially prepared QC samples are tested daily, along with patient samples. The results of testing performed on QC samples must be within a pre-established range before patient results can be reported. QC samples, called *controls*, usually are supplied with the manufacturer's prepackaged kits, which are intended for use in the small laboratory. These controls should be analyzed at specified intervals. For example, positive and negative controls supplied with pregnancy test kits should be performed with each patient specimen. Urinalysis dipstick controls (used for chemical examination of urine) should be checked daily before patient testing and each time a new **reagent** container is opened. Controls for automated chemistry analyses should be performed at specified intervals during the day. Consistent results of controls ensure constant conditions throughout the testing sequence.

The objective of QC in the laboratory is to ensure the reliability of test results while detecting and eliminating error. *Accuracy* refers

PATIENT TESTING IS IMPORTANT.

Get the right results.

READY?

- Have the latest instructions for ALL of your tests.
- Know how to do tests the right way.
- Know how and when to do quality control.

SET?

- Make sure you do the right test on the right patient.
- Make sure the patient has prepared for the test.
- Collect and label the sample the right way.

TEST!

- Follow instructions for quality control and patient tests.
- Keep records for all patient and quality control tests.
- Follow rules for discarding test materials.
- Report all test results to the doctor.

http://wwwn.cdc.gov/clia/Resources/WaivedTests/

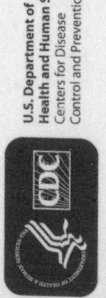

U.S. Department of
Health and Human Services
Centers for Disease
Control and Prevention

FIGURE 44-1 Summary checklist from *Ready? Set? Test?*

to how close the obtained control result is to the manufacturer's control range, and *precision* refers to the consistent reproducibility of the test results. When a series of control results show both accuracy and precision, the test is considered *reliable* and may be used for testing patients. QC monitoring is crucial because patient treatment often is based on or reinforced by the results of laboratory tests. Without QC monitoring, laboratory error is difficult to detect unless the provider notices test results inconsistent with a patient's history. Undetected laboratory errors may result in harm to the patient.

On every day that patient tests are performed, QC tests must also be performed and the results entered on the control flow sheet. When new control vials are opened and used, the results and dates must be entered on a new control flow sheet, along with the expiration dates of the controls. Everyone performing a specific lab test should be "checked out" by performing the test using the manufacturer's control before running patient tests. These records must be retained for several years; the exact number of years is determined by state law and CLIA mandates.

Preventive Maintenance Program for Laboratory Equipment

- Follow the manufacturer's instructions for calibrating instruments (this is also referred to as an *optics check* on instruments dependent on light).
- Read and understand the instructions for routine instrument care.
- Perform all preventive maintenance specified by the manufacturer's instructions.

- Keep spare parts available for immediate use.
- Record the name, address, and phone number of a contact person for maintenance or repair.
- Create a maintenance form or use the one provided.

CRITICAL THINKING APPLICATION   **44-3**

Procedure 44-1 uses the glucose control by which the overall quality control (QC) results for the class will be analyzed. When all the results are logged on the flow sheet, the class will determine whether the glucometer results are accurate, precise, and reliable. Based on the results, may the glucometer be used to test patients? If not, what should be done?

CRITICAL THINKING APPLICATION   **44-4**

Marsha will be performing a hemoglobin test on a blood sample that was collected into a test device. The device will be placed in a HemoCue instrument that produces a digital readout based on the amount of light that passes through the specimen. First, Marsha must perform an optics check, using the control device provided by the manufacturer, to see whether the instrument has been calibrated correctly. If the control does not match the manufacturer's reference value, would Marsha be able to run the patient's test? Why or why not?

PROCEDURE 44-1   Perform a Quality Control Measure on a Glucometer and Record the Results on a Flow Sheet

Goal: *To test and analyze the results of glucometer controls to see whether a glucometer is producing reliable test results, and to record the results on the laboratory flow sheet.*

EQUIPMENT and SUPPLIES

- Disposable gloves
- Glucometer
- Coded test strips designed for the glucometer used
- Control solution provided by the manufacturer
- Package insert showing directions on how to run the glucometer
- Biohazard waste container
- Glucose test control flow sheet

The three color-coded bottles of controls (1, 2, and 3) in the figure will produce high, low, and normal test results. The test strip is to the right of the glucometer, and the container for the test strips is on the far right (Figure 1).

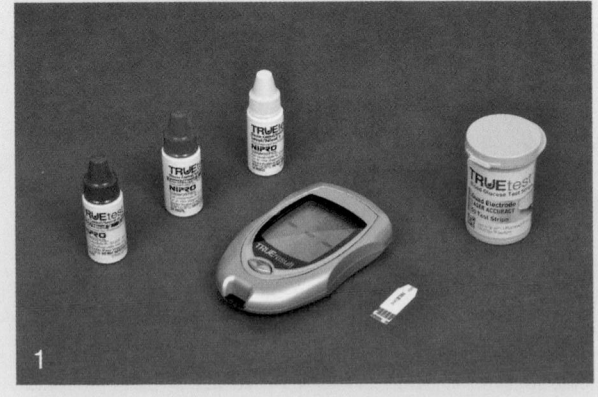

PROCEDURE 44-1 —continued

PROCEDURAL STEPS

The following can be a class exercise in which all the students participate.

1. Sanitize your hands and put on disposable gloves.
   PURPOSE: All controls and specimens are considered biohazardous.

2. Take a coded strip and note the control level and range listed on the control bottle or the strip container.

3. Review the directions on the glucometer package insert and calibrate the meter by inserting the precoded test strip into the monitor or by manually inserting the code number into the monitor (Figure 2).
   PURPOSE: Manufacturers must provide directions on how to calibrate light-sensitive meters every time a new container of test strips is used. *Note:* The newer test strips will code themselves when inserted into the meter.

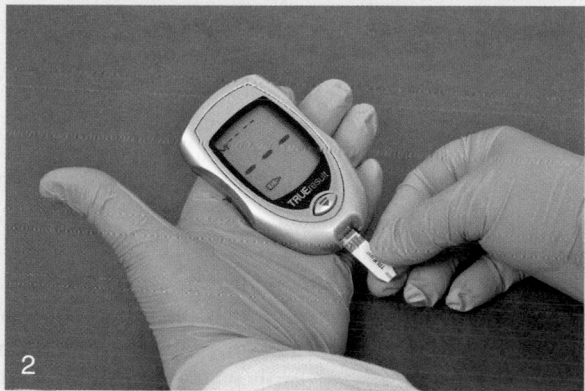
2

4. Check the expiration date on the liquid control bottle and mix well by inverting and rolling the bottle between your hands.
   PURPOSE: If the control bottle date is expired, the control cannot be run. And, it is crucial to have all the reagents in the bottle in suspension to produce reliable results.

5. Complete the top portion of the control log sheet with the test name, control lot number, and expiration date, and also the control's reference range based on whether it is a low-, normal-, or high-level control.
   PURPOSE: All this information is checked each time a control is run to compare the results of the same control.

6. Insert your strip into the glucometer and apply a drop of the liquid control to the strip according to the directions.
   PURPOSE: The manufacturer must supply clear directions that are consistent every time a control or patient specimen is run.

7. Record the result on the glucose test control flow sheet and note whether it falls within the manufacturer's reference range. If not, the test should be repeated with a new strip.
   PURPOSE: An occasional "out of range" result can occur. If the repeated new strip is back in range, proceed with patient testing. If the second strip falls outside the range, the patient may not be tested until the cause of the error is determined.

8. When you have finished running the controls, dispose of the strips, remove your gloves, and sanitize your hands.

9. Observe all the results obtained by the students and compare them to the control ranges provided on the test strip bottle and/or liquid control bottle. Discuss the following:
   - *Accuracy:* Did all the results fall near the middle of the reference range?
   - *Precision:* Were the results consistently close to each other (without extreme highs and lows)?
   - *Reliability:* If both of the previous points are affirmed, the test is reliable and may be used to test patients.

GLUCOSE TEST CONTROL FLOW SHEET

Control Lot #: _____   Expiration Date: _____
Control Range: _____   Level: Low/Normal/High

DATE	STUDENT/MA INITIALS	RESULT	ACCEPT	REJECT	CORRECTIVE ACTION

LABORATORY SAFETY

The importance of safety in the laboratory cannot be overemphasized. Most laboratory accidents can be prevented through the use of proper techniques and common sense. Following safe practices in the laboratory requires a personal commitment and concern for others; an unsafe act may also harm an innocent bystander without harming the person who performs the act.

Safety Standards and Governing Agencies

The U.S. government created a system of safeguards and regulations under the Occupational Safety and Health Act of 1970. This system affects nearly every worker in the United States because the regulations apply to all businesses with one or more employees (the regulations are discussed in detail in the "Safety and Emergency Practices" chapter.). Two programs have been mandated by the Occupational

Safety and Health Administration (OSHA) to ensure the safety of personnel working in clinical laboratories. One covers occupational exposure to chemical hazards; the other covers exposure to blood-borne pathogens.

The CDC also has established recommendations and resources in Standard Precautions and Transmission Precautions as they relate to specimen collection. (These recommendations were discussed in the Infection Control chapter.)

Chemical Hazards

The clinical laboratory is home to chemicals that are flammable, **caustic**, and potentially poisonous. Exposure to these dangerous chemicals can occur through inhalation, direct absorption through the skin, ingestion, entry through a mucous membrane, or entry through a break in the skin. OSHA is involved in regulating the standards directed at minimizing occupational exposure to hazardous chemicals in laboratories. OSHA's Hazard Communication Standard (HCS) (known as the employee "right to know" rule) became law in 1991. It ensures that laboratory workers are made fully aware of the hazards associated with their workplace. The law requires the development of a comprehensive plan to implement safe practice throughout the laboratory with regard to chemicals. All workers must be provided with information and training, and a Safety Data Sheet (SDS; formerly MSDS) must be on file for all chemicals used in the laboratory. OSHA requires the manufacturer of the chemical to make these sheets available, usually as a package insert and/or online.

Since June, 2015, OSHA has required all SDSs to use a uniform format that includes the following section numbers, headings, and associated information:

Section 1. Identification
Section 2. Hazard(s) identification
Section 3. Composition/information on ingredients
Section 4. First-aid measures
Section 5. Fire-fighting measures
Section 6. Accidental release measures
Section 7. Handling and storage
Section 8. Exposure controls/personal protection
Section 9. Physical and chemical properties
Section 10. Stability and reactivity
Section 11. Toxicologic information
Section 12. Ecologic information*
Section 13. Disposal considerations*
Section 14. Transport information*
Section 15. Regulatory information*
Section 16. Other information

Employers must ensure that SDSs are readily accessible to employees.

In the POL, the most common hazardous chemicals are:
- Sodium hypochlorite (bleach) for disinfecting laboratory work areas

---

*Sections 12-15 are regulated by agencies other than OSHA and are required of the manufacturers, not the employees.

- Caviwipes and glutaraldehyde (solutions for disinfection)
- Acetone and dyes used in staining slides

It should be noted that all the above disinfectants and dyes are available in premixed sprays and/or wipes to reduce chemical exposure during dilution. For example, in the past, bleach needed to be diluted daily with water in a 1:10 dilution using 1 part bleach to 9 parts of water. Now, bleach/water sprays are available that make the dilution as they are dispensed.

Following principles of proper handling reduces the risk of harmful effects. If a chemical produces toxic or flammable vapors, work under a fume hood that exhausts air to the outside. In case of accidental exposure of the skin, rinse the affected area under running water for at least 5 minutes. Remove any contaminated clothing. If chemicals are splashed in the eyes, flush the eyes with water from an eyewash station for a minimum of 15 minutes (Figure 44-2). Prompt medical attention must be given to victims of chemical exposure.

Chemicals should be tightly sealed and properly labeled. A hazard identification system, developed by the National Fire Protection Association (NFPA), provides information at a glance on the potential health, flammability, and chemical reactivity hazards of materials. This identification system consists of four small, diamond-shaped, colored symbols grouped into a larger diamond shape. The top diamond is red and indicates flammability (the potential to catch on fire). The diamond on the left is blue and indicates a health hazard such as a dangerous inhalant or corrosive acid. The bottom diamond is white and provides special hazard information, including recommended personal protective equipment (PPE) if biohazards are present, and other dangerous situations. The diamond on the right is yellow and indicates a reactivity or stability hazard. An example of reactivity is mixing an acid (e.g., bleach) with a base (e.g., ammonia), creating a dangerous gas. The four-color system also indicates the severity of the hazard by using numbers imprinted in the diamonds from 0 to 4, with 0 representing no hazard and 4 representing an extremely hazardous substance (Figure 44-3).

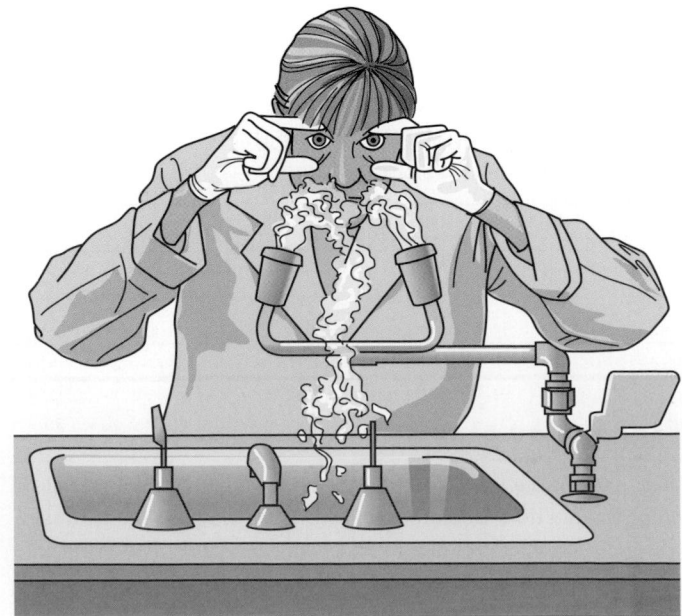

FIGURE 44-2 Eyewash station for chemical exposure.

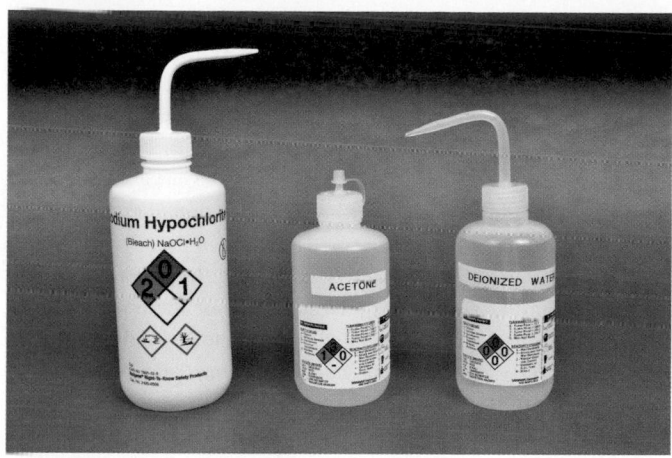

FIGURE 44-3 Three laboratory bottles with chemical labels using the identification system of the National Fire Protection Association. Note the number and color used for bleach, and compare them to the number and color used for water.

Biohazards and Infection Control

Biohazards, or biologic hazards, are materials or situations that present the risk or potential risk of infection. Infection with biohazardous material can occur during specimen collection, handling, transportation, or testing. Specimens with the potential to be infectious include blood, body tissue biopsy specimens, urine, **exudates**, and bacterial cultures and smears. Infection can occur through aspiration of a pathogen, accidental inoculation by a needlestick, aerosols created by uncapping specimen tubes, centrifuge accidents, and entry of pathogens through cuts and scratches.

Standard Precautions

As described in the Infection Control chapter, the CDC continuously monitors infection and disease in the United States and has recommended prevention practices called *Standard Precautions.* These precautions apply to all patient care, regardless of the suspected or confirmed infection status of the patient, in any setting where healthcare is delivered. The precautions are designed both to protect the healthcare provider and to prevent the healthcare provider from spreading infections among patients. Standard Precautions include these five elements: (1) hand hygiene, (2) use of PPE (e.g., gloves, gowns, masks), (3) safe needle practices, (4) safe handling of potentially contaminated equipment or surfaces in the patient environment, and (5) respiratory hygiene/cough etiquette.

Washing or sanitizing your hands is the most effective means of preventing infection. It also is the single most effective way of preventing the spread of all infections. Proper hand sanitation protects you, your patient, and your co-workers because it removes and/or kills organisms. In the laboratory area, it is absolutely essential to sanitize your hands with soap and water or a hand sanitizing product in the following situations:

- When entering and before leaving the area
- Before gloving
- After removing gloves
- After contact with body fluid
- Before and after eating
- Before and after using the restroom

After blood-borne pathogens were identified in the 1970s and 1980s (i.e., hepatitis B virus [HBV], hepatitis C virus [HCV], the human immunodeficiency virus [HIV], and the Ebola virus), the CDC stepped up its infection control recommendations. It acknowledged that all blood in all patients is potentially infectious and therefore required additional monitoring and regulation for the safety of both the healthcare provider and the patient. These guidelines became known as *Universal Precautions.* Regulation of the new law, referred to as the Bloodborne Pathogens Standard (BBPS), was delegated to OSHA.

In 2014 Ebola infection reappeared in Africa and was transmitted to several other continents. The Ebola virus is a blood-borne pathogen that causes bleeding throughout the body. In the United States, a key factor in stopping its spread was the rigorous training in donning and doffing (putting on and taking off) PPE that covered every part of the healthcare worker's body. The CDC provided an Ebola bulletin for ambulatory healthcare practices on the evaluation of patients who may have been infected with the Ebola virus.

Bloodborne Pathogens Standard

OSHA's Bloodborne Pathogens Standard has been law since 1992. It regulates the handling of blood and blood products, but it also includes other potentially infectious materials (OPIM) that may contain blood-borne pathogens. Urine is the only fluid not specifically included in the standard. However, because blood and blood elements frequently are associated with urine, it must be included and considered a possible source of exposure.

The Bloodborne Pathogens Standard covers all employees who could "reasonably anticipate contact with blood and other potentially infectious materials as the result of performing their job duties." HBV, HCV, and HIV are a constant threat to the health and safety of clinical laboratory personnel. Ebola virus infection is a serious concern, although not as common in the United States. These blood-borne pathogens are transmitted through exposure to blood and body fluids, which are the primary substances handled in the laboratory. The Bloodborne Pathogens Standard requires that the laboratory employer have a written exposure control plan that proves the following steps have been taken to protect the lab's employees:

- Written job categories of employees at risk of exposure to blood (laboratory workers are considered "high risk")
- HBV vaccination guidelines and records for each employee at risk
- Record of initial and annual Universal Standard training sessions for blood-borne pathogens and safety training for each employee (including proper use of safety needles)
- Definition and listing of safe work practices: PPE for all lab personnel (fluid-impermeable lab coats that do not leave the laboratory area, disposable gloves, face protection) and labeling of biohazardous sharps and waste containers and their proper disposal
- Sharps injury log of all work-related needlesticks and exposures to blood, with medical intervention after exposure incidents
- Written plan to maintain privacy of the individual exposed to blood
- Documentation of employee input on new safety devices

Safety Guidelines for Other Potentially Infectious Materials (OPIM)

- Handle and process all specimens as if they contained infectious material.
- Wipe the outside of specimen containers with a germicide.
- Dispose of all infectious materials according to state and federal guidelines.
- Clean up spills using a disinfectant (see "Infection Control" chapter).
- Immediately dispose of any chipped or broken glassware into a sharps container using appropriate safety methods to prevent accidental punctures.

Physical Hazards

Physical hazards in the laboratory can be classified as electrical, fire, and mechanical hazards. Electric shock is a threat when any electrical equipment is in use. It is imperative to keep all electrical equipment in proper repair and always to follow manufacturers' instructions.

Use surge protectors, inspect all cords and plugs frequently, never use extension cords, and do not overload circuits. Unplug the electrical device before servicing, and never operate electrical instruments with wet hands. If a sink is nearby, make sure electrical cords do not come in contact with the water supply. Signs and labels should be placed on specific electrical hazards (Figure 44-4).

Open flames are rarely used in a laboratory, but the potential for fire still exists. Fires may be ignited by smoking, heating elements, and sparks. Flammable materials should not be stored near any source of ignition. All laboratory personnel should be familiar with the locations of fire extinguishers and fire safety blankets. Fire extinguishers should be the carbon dioxide (CO_2), dry chemical, or halon type, known as the ABC type of extinguisher. ABC extinguishers can be used on all types of fires. These extinguishers should be inspected regularly by a licensed inspector and replaced or recharged if used. The medical assistant may be responsible for maintaining records on the care and maintenance of fire extinguishers.

Fire safety blankets should be used to smother flames on burning clothing. However, a victim should not be wrapped in a fire blanket, because this may intensify burns. Instead, the flames should be patted out or the victim directed to roll on the blanket.

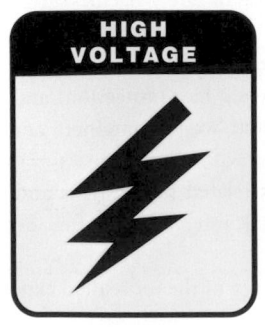 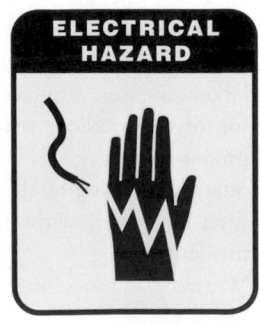

FIGURE 44-4 High-voltage and electrical hazard labels.

Emergency phone numbers should be posted on the wall near the telephone, and all personnel should know the locations of fire alarms, the fire escape routes, and procedures to follow if exits are blocked. Periodic fire drills should be conducted, and hallways and exits should be kept free of clutter.

Mechanical hazards arise from the use of laboratory equipment. Special care should be exercised when using equipment with moving parts, such as centrifuges, and those that rely on pressure, including autoclaves. Centrifuges, devices that separate liquids from solids, present a hazard not only from moving parts but also from glassware that might break during centrifugation and from aerosols that might be created if tubes are not capped tightly. Pressurized types of equipment, such as autoclaves used in sterilization, present a danger if opened prematurely. Although centrifuges and autoclaves often have built-in safeguards, such as locks that prevent entry until the environment is safe, improper care of the equipment can result in failure of the safety measures.

SPECIMEN COLLECTION, PROCESSING, AND STORAGE

Laboratory Requisitions and Reports

When the provider orders laboratory testing that must be done outside the office, an electronic requisition for the work must be sent to the laboratory, or a paper requisition is given to the patient. (It is important to note that the patient's health insurance may only reimburse if specific labs are used.) Paper requisition forms specific to the labs are preprinted, with the most commonly requested tests indicated in a logical sequence (Figure 44-5). Patient information on the requisitions must be complete, accurate, and legible. The patient is then directed to the lab, or the specimen is collected and sent to the lab.

Figure 44-6 shows the electronic lab requisition form used in *SimChart for the Medical Office.* The following information typically is required on the requisition when specimens are sent to a reference laboratory:

- Provider's name, account number, address, and phone number
- Patient's full name, surname first; age, date of birth, and gender; address and insurance information
- Source of specimen
- Date and time of collection
- Specific test (or tests) requested
- Medications the patient is taking
- Whether the patient fasted or followed dietary restrictions if required; time of last intake
- Possible diagnosis
- Indication of whether the test is to be performed **STAT** (i.e., immediately)

When the results of the tests are obtained, a laboratory report is sent to the office. The laboratory reports are typically sent directly from the referral laboratory to the patient's electronic health record (EHR), or they are received electronically as a general electronic record source and then transferred to the correct patient record by practice staff members.

The medical assistant's responsibility is to make sure that all reports are received for the tests performed on the patient outside the provider's office and that the provider has reviewed them, and

Lab Services

IMPORTANT
Patient instructions
and map on back

PHYSICIAN ORDERS

Patient _____ _____ ____
         Last Name   First   M.I.
D.O.B. _____

M ☐ Patient
F ☐ SS# ___ – ___ – ___

Address _____ City _____ Zip _____ Phone # _____

Physician _____

ATTACH COPY OF INSURANCE CARD

Date & Time of Collection: _____

Drawing Facility: _____

Diagnosis/ICD-9 Code _____

(Additional codes on reverse)

☐ 789.00 Abdominal Pain ☐ 414.9 Coronary Artery Disease (CAD) ☐ 244.9 Hypothyroidism
☐ 285.9 Anemia (NOS) ☐ 250.0 DM (diabetes mellitus) ☐ 272.4 Hyperlipidemia
☐ 780.7 Fatigue/Malaise ☐ 401.9 Hypertension
☐ 272.0 Hypercholesterolemia ☐ 485.9 URI (upper respiratory infection)

☐ ROUTINE ☐ PHONE RESULTS TO: # _____
☐ ASAP ☐ FAX RESULTS TO: # _____
☐ STAT ☐ COPY TO: _____

HEMATOLOGY
☐ 1021 CBC, Automated Diff (incl. Platelet Ct.)
☐ 1023 Hemoglobin/Hematocrit
☐ 1020 Hemogram
☐ 1025 Platelet Count
☐ 1150 Pro Time Diagnostic
☐ 1151 Pro Time, Therapeutic
☐ 1155 PTT
☐ 1315 Reticulocyte Count
☐ 1310 Sed Rate/Westergren

URINE
☐ 1059 Urinalysis
☐ 1082 Urinalysis w/Culture if indicated
Urine-24 Hr _____ Spot _____
Ht. _____ Wt. _____
☐ 3033 Creatinine
☐ 3036 Creatinine Clearance (also requires blood)
☐ 3308 Protein
☐ 3096 Sodium/Potassium
☐ Microalbumin 24 Hr _____ Spot _____

SEROLOGY
☐ 8020 ANA (Antinuclear Antibody)
☐ 8040 Mono Spot
☐ 3494 Rheumatoid Factor
☐ 8010 RPR
☐ 5365 Rubella

CHEMISTRY
☐ 5550 Alpha Fetoprotein, Prenatal
☐ 3000 Amylase
☐ 3153 B12/Folate
☐ 3156 Beta HCG, Quantitative
☐ 3321 Bilirubin, Total
☐ 3324 Bilirubin, Total/Direct
☐ 3009 BUN
☐ 3159 CEA
☐ 3348 Cholesterol
☐ 3030 Creatinine, Serum
☐ 3509 Digoxin (recommend 12 hrs., after dose)
☐ 3515 Dilantin
☐ 3168 Ferritin
☐ 3193 FSH
☐ 3066 ▼ Glucose, Fasting
☐ 3061 Glucose, 1° Post 50 g Glucola
☐ 3075 ▼ Glucose, 2° Post Glucola
☐ 3060 Glucose, 2° Post Prandial (meal)
☐ 3049 ▼ Glucose Tolerance Oral GTT
☐ 3047 ▼Glucose Tolerance Gestational GTT
☐ 3650 Hemoglobin, A1C

CHEMISTRY
☐ 5232 HBsAg
☐ 3175 HIV (Consent required)
☐ 3581 Iron & Iron Binding Capacity
☐ 3195 LH
☐ 3590 Magnesium
☐ 3527 Phenobarbital
☐ 3095 Potassium
☐ 3689 Pregnancy Test, Serum (HCG, qual)
☐ 3653 Pregnancy Test, Urine
☐ 3197 Prolactin
☐ 3199 PSA
☐ 3339 SGOT/AST
☐ 3342 SGPT/ALT
☐ 3093 Sodium/Potassium, Serum
☐ 3510 Tegretol
☐ 3551 Theophylline
☐ 3333 Uric Acid

MICROBIOLOGY
Source _____
☐ 7240 Culture, AFB
☐ 7200 Culture, Blood x _____
☐ Draw Interval _____
☐ 7280 Culture, Fungus
☐ Culture, Routine
☐ 7005 Culture, Stool
☐ 7010 Culture, Throat
☐ 7000 Culture, Urine
☐ 7300 Gram Stain
☐ 7355 Occult Blood x _____
☐ 7365 Ova & Parasites x _____
☐ 7400 Smear & Suspension
(includes Gram Stain/Wet Mount)
☐ 7060 Rapid Strep A Screen (Negs confir by cult)
☐ 7065 Rapid Strep A Screen only
☐ 7030 Beta Strep Culture
☐ 5207 GC by DNA Probe
☐ 5130 Chlamydia by DNA Probe
☐ 5555 Chlamydia/GC by DNA Probe
☐ 7375 Wright Stain, Stool

Additional Tests _____

PANELS & PROFILES

☐ X **3309 CHEM 12**
Albumin, Alkaline Phosphatase, BUN, Calcium, Cholesterol, Glucose, LDH, Phosphorus, AST, Total Bilirubin, Total Protein, Uric Acid

☐ ▼ **3315 CHEM 20**
Chem 12, Electrolyte Panel, Creatinine, Iron, Gamma GT, ALT, Triglycerides

☐ ▼ **3357 CARDIAC RISK PANEL**
Cholesterol, HDL, LDL, Risk Factors, VLDL Triglycerides

☐ X **3042 CRITICAL CARE PANEL**
BUN, Chloride, CO2, Glucose, Potassium, Sodium

☐ **3046 ELECTROLYTE PANEL**
Chloride, CO2, Potassium, Sodium

☐ ▼ **3399 EXECUTIVE PANEL**
Chem 20, Iron, Cardiac Risk Panel, CBC, RPR, Thyroid Cascade

☐ **5242 HEPATITIS PANEL, ACUTE**
HAVIgMAb, HBsAg, HBsAb, HBcAb, HCVAb

☐ ▼ **3355 LIPID MONITORING PANEL**
Cholesterol, Triglycerides, HDL, LDL, VLDL, ALT, AST

☐ **3312 LIVER PANEL**
Alkaline Phospatase, AST, Total Bilirubin, Gamma GT, Total Protein, Albumin, ALT

☐ X **3083 METABOLIC STATUS PANEL**
BUN, Osmolality (calculated), Chloride, CO2, Creatinine, Glucose, Potassium, Sodium, BUN/Creatinine, Ratio, Anion Gap

☐ X **3376 PANEL B**
Chem 12, CBC, Electrolyte Panel

☐ ▼ **3382 PANEL D**
Chem 20, CBC, Thyroid Cascade

☐ X **3388 PANEL F**
Chem 12, CBC, Electrolyte Panel, Thyroid Cascade

☐ ▼ **3391 PANEL G**
Chem 20, Cardiac Risk Panel, CBC, Thyroid Cascade

☐ ▼ **3393 PANEL H**
Chem 20, CBC, Cardiac Risk Panel Rheumatoid Factor, Thyroid Cascade

☐ ▼ **3397 PANEL J**
Chem 20, Cardiac Risk Panel

☐ **5351 PRENATAL PANEL**
Antibody Screen ABO/Rh, CBC Rubella, HBsAg, RPR
☐ 1059 with Urinalysis, Routine
☐ 1082 with Urinalysis w/Culture if indicated

☐ X **3102 RENAL PANEL**
Metabolic Status Panel, Calcium, Phosphorus

☐ **3188 THYROID CASCADE**
TSH, Reflex Testing

▼ - patient **required** to fast for 12-14 hours

X - patient recommended to fast 12-14 hours

LAB USE ONLY   INIT _____
☐ SST ☐ PLASMA
☐ PURPLE ☐ SERUM
☐ YELLOW ☐ SWAB
☐ BLUE ☐ SLIDES
☐ GREEN ☐ DNA PROBE
☐ GREY ☐ B. CULT BTLS
☐ URINE
☐ BLACK
☐ OTHER: _____
REC'V. SPECIMEN: ☐ FROZEN
☐ AMBIENT ☐ ON ICE

Special Instructions/Pertinent Clinical Information _____

Physician's Signature _____ Date _____

These orders may be FAXed to: 449-5288

LAB

7060-500 (7/96)

FIGURE 44-5 Laboratory requisition form.

SimChart® for the medical office

| Front Office | Clinical Care | Coding & Billing | | TruCode |

Form Repository   🗓 Calendar   ✉ Correspondence   👥 Patient Demographics   🔍 Find Patient   📋 Form Repository

INFO PANEL
Patient Forms

Advance Directive
Certificate to Return to Work or
School
Disclosure Authorization
Doctor's First Report
General Procedure Consent
Insurance Claim Tracer
Medical Records Release
Neurological Status Exam
Notice of Privacy Practice
Patient Bill of Rights
Patient Information
Patient Records Access Request
Patient Statement
Prior Authorization Request
Referral
⊖ Requisition
    School Physical
    Vaccine Authorization
Office Forms

Requisition
Please perform a patient search to find a specific patient

Requisition Type: [Laboratory ▼]

Patient Name:		Date of Birth:	
Service Date:		Insurance Co:	
Authorization Number (as needed):		Ordering Physician:	

Diagnosis:		Diagnosis Code:	
Diagnosis:		Diagnosis Code:	
Diagnosis:		Diagnosis Code:	
Diagnosis:		Diagnosis Code:	

Laboratory Requisition

☐ **Electrolytes Panel**
  ☐ Sodium
  ☐ Potassium
  ☐ Chloride
  ☐ Carbon Dioxide

☐ **Basic Metabolic Panel**
  ☐ Na, K, CL, CO2
  ☐ BUN
  ☐ Calcium
  ☐ Creatinine
  ☐ Glucose

☐ **Acute Hepatitis Panel**
  ☐ Hepatitis A Antibody IGM
  ☐ Hepatitis B Core Antibody IGM
  ☐ Hepatitis B Surface Antigen
  ☐ Hepatitis C Antibody

☐ **Comprehensive Metabolic Panel**
  ☐ Basic Metabolic Panel
  ☐ Albumin

☐ **Hepatic Function (Liver Panel)**
  ☐ Albumin
  ☐ Bilirubin, Total

☐ **TORCH panel**
  ☐ CMV Ab
  ☐ Herpes Simplex Ab

[Patient Search]   [Print]   [Save to Patient Record]   [Cancel]

FIGURE 44-6 Electronic laboratory requisition form. (From Elsevier: *SimChart for the medical office*, St Louis, 2015, Elsevier.)

the patient has received the results. This can be accomplished by maintaining a master laboratory specimen log sheet that tracks patient specimens, tests ordered, designated lab, results, and provider response.

Specimen Collection

The medical assistant is responsible for the collection of many different types of specimens. It is important to recognize that clinical laboratory results are only as good as the specimen received. The importance of proper specimen collection cannot be overemphasized. If test results are to be accurate indicators of the patient's state of health, it is imperative that the concepts of specimen collection be understood and followed exactly. The most common specimens are blood, urine, and swab samples collected from wounds or mucous membranes. Less often, feces, gastric contents, CSF, tissue samples, semen, and aspirates (e.g., synovial fluid) are submitted for testing. These specimens are analyzed for levels of many chemicals and drugs, types and numbers of cells present, and the presence of microorganisms.

Verifying the patient's identity before the procedure is essential, as is collection of the specimen in an appropriate collection container. For example, blood may be collected using a vacuum tube system. These tubes are available in a variety of sizes, with and without **preservatives** and **anticoagulants**. The tubes are color coded; the color of the stopper denotes which, if any, additive is present (Figure 44-7). Collection in an incorrect tube results in an unacceptable specimen, and recollection is necessary. If the specimen is to be tested for the presence of microorganisms, a sterile container must be used. If the patient is to collect the specimen at home, he or she should be provided with the appropriate container and complete instructions for collection. Bear in mind the principles of patient education, and be sensitive to individual patient factors,

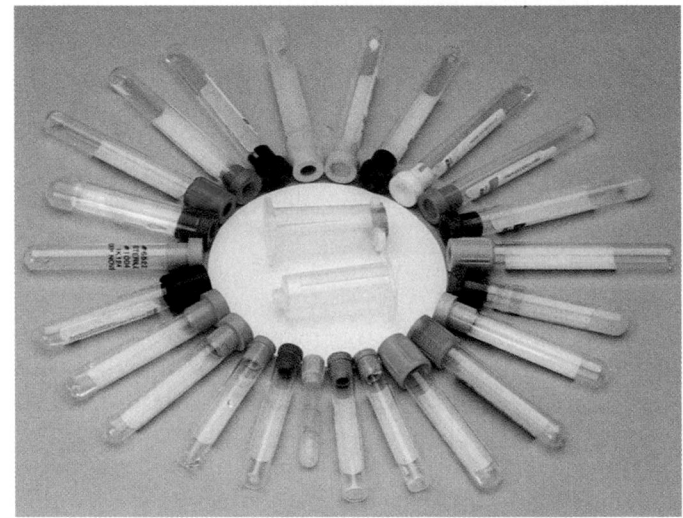

FIGURE 44-7 Vacutainer tubes; note the color-coded tops.

which sometimes can affect the patient's understanding of the instructions and his or her ability to follow through on them.

The medical assistant should always check the laboratory's specimen requirements manual or website for any unfamiliar tests. The manual lists all information on specimen collection. Any unanswered questions should be resolved by calling the laboratory before collecting the specimen. The container must be labeled properly at the time of collection; unlabeled containers are not accepted for laboratory testing. Labels should include the patient's full name, the date and time of collection, and the type of specimen.

Most offices have a laboratory courier service that picks up specimens periodically throughout the day. Specimens should be properly stored (some require refrigeration) until the courier arrives.

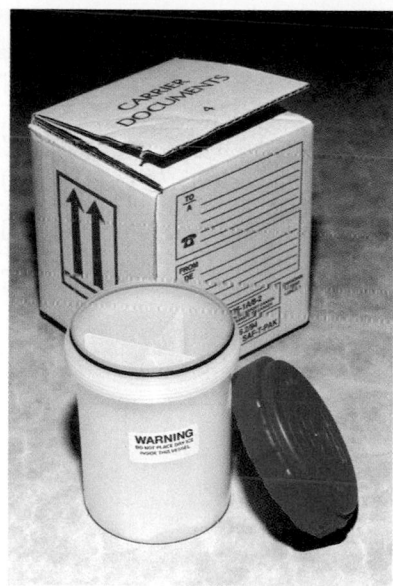

FIGURE 44-8 Specimen mailers.

Instructions for properly obtaining, processing, and preparing a specimen for transport are usually supplied by the testing laboratory. If the instructions are not clear or if you have a question about a particular collection, the laboratory can answer your question over the phone. Criteria for safe shipping of specimens include the length of time acceptable for transport; recommended temperature ranges to maintain the integrity of the specimen; and whether light can affect the specimen.

If the specimen is to be mailed, it must be carefully packaged to prevent breakage, damage, or contamination by all persons handling it. Place specimens in unbreakable tubes with safe-top lids and wrap the containers in absorbent material. Tape the lid of the container shut so that no leakage occurs if the specimen container breaks. Place all specimens in a second container, such as an impervious biohazard bag, for transport. The completed requisition goes inside the outermost wrap. Styrofoam mailers (Figure 44-8) may be used, because they cushion the sample and provide insulation. Styrofoam inserts can be shaped to fit around the specimen container. A warning label specifying the etiologic agent or biologic specimen is placed on the outside of the container.

Preventing Contamination

Medical assistants must take care to prevent contamination of specimens and themselves. Expiration dates on swabs, tubes, transport media, and other collection containers should be checked before these items are used. Any expired materials should not be used and should be discarded properly. An improperly handled specimen may become contaminated or may contaminate the surrounding environment. Standard Precautions should be followed. All blood and other body fluids from all patients should be considered infectious.

Sufficient samples should be collected for the tests requested by the provider. Amounts may vary on the basis of methods used. A report returned from the laboratory marked "QNS" (quantity not sufficient) indicates a request for an additional specimen. Make sure to clarify any questions about the previous specimen by calling the laboratory before collecting a new one.

The specimen collected must be a true representative sample. A swab for a wound culture collected from the surface of the wound generally does not yield the same results as one taken from the depths of the wound. A **hemolyzed** blood specimen or one taken from an atypical area, such as a hematoma or the area above or below an intravenous (IV) drip, shows marked differences in many tests. If a large volume of specimen is collected (e.g., a 24-hour urine specimen), the total volume or weight must be carefully measured and recorded. The specimen must be well mixed before an **aliquot** is removed and submitted for testing.

Handling, Processing, and Storage of Specimens

The specimen must be handled, processed, and stored according to individual guidelines to prevent any alterations that would affect test results. The medical assistant should determine whether the specimen needs to be kept warm or cool. Specimens such as urine require chilling if testing will not be performed immediately. Some cultures or specimens (e.g., gonorrhea cultures and semen analysis) need to be kept at body temperature after collection because cooling kills microorganisms and sperm. When required, serum must be separated from the cells as soon as possible after the specimen has clotted to prevent changes caused by the metabolism of the blood cells. Specimens for bilirubin testing must be protected from light. Some specimens need to be frozen to prevent chemical constituents from changing. Laboratory specimen requirements should be consulted to ensure that each specimen is handled and processed properly.

Chain of Custody

When a specimen may be needed as evidence in a court case, certain procedures must be followed in collecting and handling the specimen. Forensic or medicolegal implications require that any results gathered on testing of a specimen should be obtained in such a fashion that they are recognized by a court of law. Specimen processing must be documented meticulously, ensuring that no tampering with evidence has occurred. *Chain of custody* refers to the stepwise method used to collect, process, and test a specimen. The documentation must be signed by every person who has contact with the specimen, from collection to final reporting of results. Blood alcohol level testing and drug screening often require chain of custody handling. Everything needed for collection of the specimen is provided in a kit—even the gloves, the vacuum tube, and the needle used to collect the blood specimen. Documentation is included and must be signed by all personnel. Medical assistants and phlebotomists have been subpoenaed to testify in court about specimens they have collected; therefore, it is in your best interest to follow chain of custody procedures rigorously.

Steps in Collecting Specimens and Informing the Patient of the Results

1. The healthcare practitioner orders laboratory tests on the basis of physical examination findings and/or to diagnose a disorder.
2. Complete all the fields on the lab requisition or EHR transmission.
3. Collect the specimen after receiving the provider's order, or instruct the patient on how to collect the specimen at home.
4. Label the appropriate specimen container.

5. Process the specimen as you have been trained, or prepare the specimen for transport to a reference laboratory.

6. Properly dispose of specimens collected and tested in the office in biohazard waste containers after tests are completed.

7. Reference laboratory test results are sent to the patient's EHR or provided in an electronic form that the provider reviews and shares with the patient. The results of tests performed in the office are recorded in the patient's EHR and reviewed by the provider, who then shares the results with the patient.

8. Confidentially notify the patient of test results according to office policy, and document in the patient's health record that test results were received and the patient notified of the results.

LABORATORY MATHEMATICS AND MEASUREMENT

All laboratory testing, from specimen collection through reporting of results, relies on the accurate use of values and measurements. For example, values are used for reporting the time the sample was collected, the volume of the specimen, the amount of analyte found in a specimen, and dilutions used in sample preparation and for recording QC results.

Measuring Time

Time of day often is a critical factor in patient care. Medications must be administered, diets must be followed, and specimens must be collected on a particular schedule. Many clinical laboratories use the 24-hour clock when recording time; this method avoids the confusion that comes with the Greenwich clock, which uses AM (morning) and PM (afternoon) designations.

The 24-hour clock system, also known as *military time,* is expressed with four digits in terms of "hundred hours." Noon is referred to as 1200 (twelve hundred) hours; midnight is 0000 (zero hundred), or 2400 hours. The military clock is based on 24 60-minute hours, as is the Greenwich clock; therefore, 5:35 PM is expressed as 1735 (seventeen thirty-five) hours (Table 44-3).

Measuring Temperature

Two scales currently are used for measuring temperature; each is divided into units called *degrees* (Table 44-4). The Fahrenheit scale is considered part of the English system of measurement and is the scale most commonly used in the United States. The Celsius scale, formerly called the *centigrade scale,* is used in countries that apply the metric system. On the Celsius (C) scale, water freezes at 0°C and boils at 100°F. On the Fahrenheit (F) scale, water freezes at 32°F and boils at 212°F.

Units of Measurement

The units of measurement that we commonly use in the United States differ from those used in the clinical laboratory. In everyday life we use the English system of measurement, in which weight is measured in ounces and pounds, length is measured in inches and feet, and volume is measured in cups and quarts. In the laboratory, the metric system and the Système International (SI) are used. It is important that medical assistants memorize and practice these systems so that they can communicate professionally.

TABLE 44-3 Greenwich Time and Military Time	
GREENWICH TIME	**MILITARY TIME**
1:00 AM	0100 hours
3:00 AM	0300 hours
5:00 AM	0500 hours
7:00 AM	0700 hours
9:00 AM	0900 hours
11:00 AM	1100 hours
1:00 PM	1300 hours
3:00 PM	1500 hours
5:00 PM	1700 hours
7:00 PM	1900 hours
9:00 PM	2100 hours
11:00 PM	2300 hours
12:00 AM (midnight)	2400 hours

TABLE 44-4 Common Laboratory Temperatures		
	FAHRENHEIT	**CELSIUS**
Refrigerator	35°-46°	2°-8°
Freezer	32°	0°
Room	59°-86°	15°-30°
Incubator	98.6°	37°
Body temperature	98.6°	37°
Autoclave	254°	121°

The metric system is based on a decimal system, which consists of basic units and prefixes that indicate a system of division in multiples of 10. The basic units of the metric system are the gram (g) for weight, the meter (m) for length, and the liter (L) for volume. Prefixes are added to each symbol to reduce or enlarge them by units of 10. The most common metric units used in the laboratory are millimeters (mm), centimeters (cm), micrograms (mcg), milligrams (mg), grams (g), microliters (mcL), milliliters (mL), liters (L), and cubic centimeters (cc). The cubic centimeter and the milliliter are used interchangeably in the clinical laboratory.

Quantitative test results are reported using the appropriate units of measurement. Some commonly used designations for reporting analytes are mcg, mg, g, dL, and L. Blood glucose, for example, is reported in milligrams per deciliter (mg/dL); hemoglobin levels are reported as grams per deciliter (g/dL).

International organizations, such as the World Health Organization (WHO), officially recognize SI units. Many countries have adopted this system, but the United States has not completely converted to it. The SI is an adaptation of the metric system that uses several of the basic units, although many are different for reporting results. For example, blood glucose is reported in millimoles per liter (mmol/L), and hemoglobin is reported in grams per liter (g/L). Therefore, it is very important that the medical assistant double-check the laboratory's standard and include the appropriate units of measurement when reporting test values.

Measuring Liquid Volume

Test tubes come in many sizes and are typically disposable. Test tubes may be sterile, and some may be calibrated. Micropipettors (Figure 44-9) are used to deliver very small amounts of liquid, from 1 to 1,000 microliters (mcL). It is important to follow the manufacturer's instructions for the device because each may be slightly different. These pipetting devices must be fitted with an appropriate disposable tip. The tips may be sterile, depending on their use. The device is fitted with a piston at the top, which must be depressed before the pipet is filled and when the pipet is drained.

LABORATORY EQUIPMENT

Microscope

Nearly every medical laboratory is equipped with a microscope. This indispensable instrument is used to view objects too small to be seen with the naked eye (Figure 44-10). The microscope is used to evaluate stained blood smears, urine sediment, vaginal secretions, and smears made from body fluids or microbiologic cultures.

Microscopic procedures are not considered CLIA waived because they require judgment and additional training. In addition, an error in reading microscopic findings may have a detrimental effect on the patient's care. Providers petitioned the CMS to create a new laboratory category that would allow them to perform a set of simple microscopic tests that could be performed in the ambulatory setting (Table 44-5). CMS approved the list and created an additional CLIA category called *provider-performed microscopy procedures* (PPMP). Certified CLIA-PPMP laboratories must meet the same quality

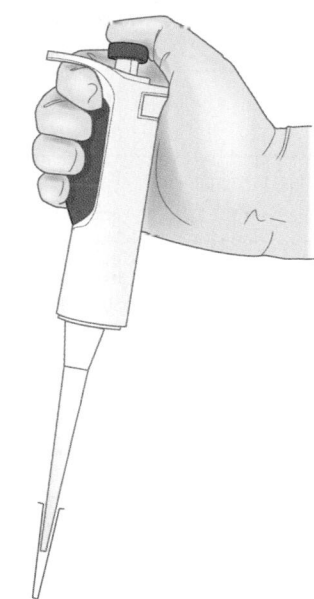

FIGURE 44-9 Piston-type automatic micropipettor.

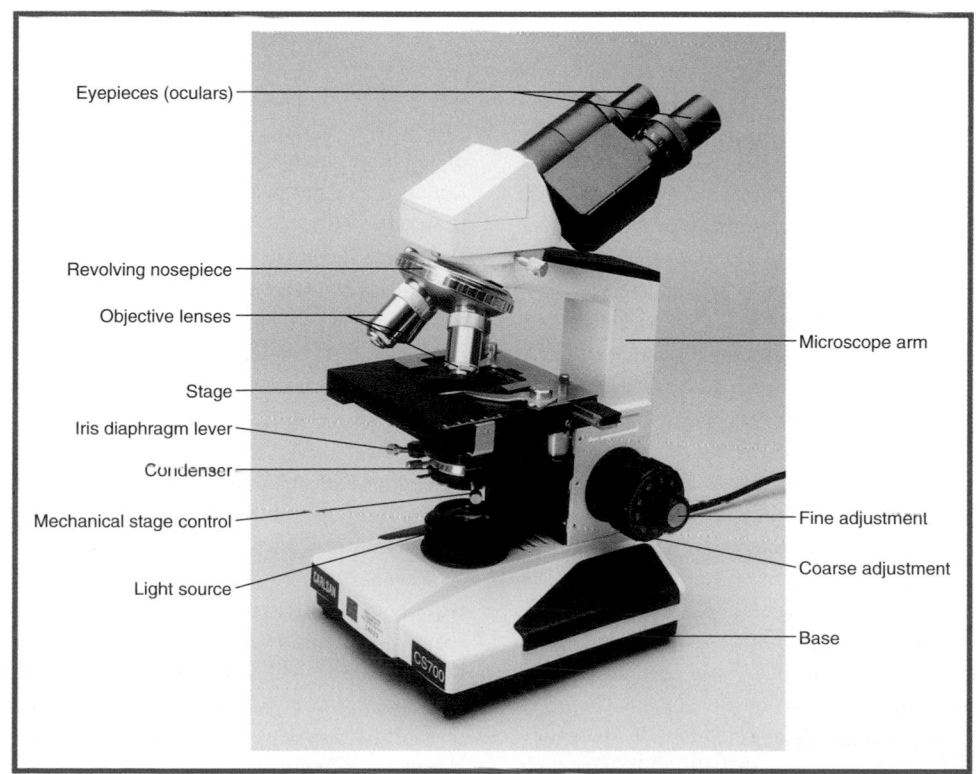

FIGURE 44-10 The parts of a microscope. (Courtesy Cynmar, Carlinville, Ill.)

TABLE 44-5   CLIA-Approved Procedures for PPM (Provider Performed Microscopy)

TEST NAME/CODE*	DESCRIPTION	EXAMPLE
Direct wet mount (Q0111)	Examination of specimens for presence or absence of bacteria, fungi, parasites, and human cellular elements	Observing vaginal secretions for presence of yeast to assist with diagnosis of vulvovaginal candidiasis
KOH preparation (Q0112)	Any preparation using potassium hydroxide	Observing skin scrapings for the presence of fungi
Fecal leukocyte examination (89055)	Simple stain of fecal specimen; assists in diagnosis of diarrheal disease	Leukocytes are found in stool in antibiotic-associated colitis, ulcerative colitis, shigellosis, and salmonellosis
Pinworm examination (Q0113)	Preparations are observed for the presence or absence of *Enterobius vermicularis* eggs	Performing a cellulose tape collection for pinworms
Postcoital direct, qualitative examinations (Q0115)	Vaginal or cervical mucus is examined 4-10 hours after intercourse for presence of live, motile sperm	Assists in the diagnosis of infertility
Qualitative semen analysis (G0027)	Semen is examined for presence or absence of spermatozoa; motility of the sperm is noted	Assists in postvasectomy semen analysis and in the diagnosis of infertility
Urine sediment examination (81015)	Urine sediment is examined for presence or absence of formed elements	Part of a routine urinalysis (see the procedure in the Assisting in the Analysis of Urine chapter for Procedure 45-5, Prepare a Urine Specimen for Microscopic Examination).

*The test's official code for billing purposes is shown in parentheses. Codes that do not begin with a letter are Current Procedural Terminology (CPT) codes; codes that do begin with a letter are Healthcare Common Procedure Coding System (HCPCS) codes, which are used for Medicare patients.
CLIA, Clinical Laboratory Improvement Amendments; *KOH*, potassium hydroxide.

standards as laboratories that perform moderate-complexity tests, including passing three proficiency tests from an outside agency per year. The medical assistant is taught to prepare the microscope slide and bring it into focus, but the final analysis may be made only by a provider, an MA, a dentist, or other highly trained laboratory personnel.

Microscopes have three components: the magnification system, which focuses the image; the illumination system, which brings the image from the slide to the viewer; and the framework, which includes all components responsible for positioning the slide.

The magnification system includes the ocular and the objective lenses plus the fine and coarse knobs to adjust the clarity. Microscopes may be monocular or binocular. A monocular microscope has one eyepiece for viewing, and a binocular microscope has two. The eyepiece, or ocular, is located at the top of the microscope and contains a lens to magnify what is being viewed.

The usual magnification is 10 times (10×). In addition to the ocular, compound microscopes have objective lenses that increase the magnification of the specimen. The objectives are attached to the revolving nosepiece. Most microscopes have four objectives, each with a different magnifying power. The shortest objective has the lowest power (4×) and is called the *scanning lens*. This lens is used to scan the field of interest and then focus on a particular object. Greater detail is observed with the next longest objective, which is low power (10×). The high or high dry objective usually has a magnification of 40× or 45×; the longest objective, oil immersion (100×), allows the finest focusing of the object and requires the use

of a special oil that is placed directly on the slide. This special oil, called *immersion oil*, prevents refraction of the light and improves the resolution (clarity) of the magnified image. Oil immersion is used to view cells and extremely small materials (e.g., bacteria and platelets) and to examine stained specimens.

The total magnification of the specimen is determined by multiplying the magnification of the objective lens by 10 (the magnification of the ocular lens). Therefore, if you have the 10× objective in place when observing blood cells, you are magnifying the image 100 times. Just above the base are the focusing knobs. The coarse adjustment is used only with scanning and low-power lenses, and the fine adjustment is used with high-power and oil immersion lenses.

The arm of the microscope connects the objectives and the oculars to the base, which supports the microscope and contains its light source. The stage of the microscope holds the slide to be viewed. Under the stage is the light source, the condenser, and the iris diaphragm, which make up the illumination system. The condenser directs light up through the slide, and the iris diaphragm regulates the amount of light passing through the specimen.

Microscopes are very precise and expensive instruments that require careful handling. The amount of routine maintenance required depends on the amount of daily use. Dirt is the enemy of the microscope, which must be kept scrupulously clean at all times. Oil, makeup, dust, and eye secretions all can obstruct vision through the lens and may transmit infective organisms. The microscope should always be stored in a plastic dust cover when not in use. Lenses should be cleaned before and after each use with lens paper and lens cleaner. Any other type of tissue scratches the lenses or leaves lint residue behind. Routine use of solvent cleaners, such as xylene, is not recommended, because these cleaners may loosen lenses. The body of the microscope should be dusted with a soft cloth.

The microscope should be placed in a permanent location in the laboratory, on a sturdy table in an area where it cannot be bumped. If a microscope must be moved, it should be carried securely, with one hand supporting the base and the other holding the arm. When the microscope is stored, it should be left covered and with the low-power objective in the highest position. The stage should be centered.

Using a microscope involves focusing and illumination (Procedure 44-2). The image is focused by moving the objectives closer to the specimen using the fine and coarse knobs. Proper focusing begins with the objective at lowest power. The coarse adjustment moves the objective very quickly. This knob is used first to bring the specimen into approximate focus. The fine adjustment focus knob then brings the specimen into precise focus. The fine focus moves the objective more slowly to allow the viewer to zero in on the specimen with greater accuracy. Illumination is accomplished by raising or lowering the condenser and by opening and closing the diaphragm on the condenser.

If the microscope is a binocular model, the eyepieces may need to be adjusted to accommodate the distance between the pupils and the individual's point of greatest visual acuity. A gentle push inward or pull outward adjusts the distance between the eyepieces.

PROCEDURE 44-2 Use the Microscope and Perform Routine Maintenance on Clinical Equipment

Goal: To focus the microscope properly using a prepared slide under low power, high power, and oil immersion, and to perform routine maintenance on the microscope before storing it.

EQUIPMENT and SUPPLIES

- Microscope
- Lens cleaner
- Lens tissue
- Slide containing specimen
- Immersion oil

PROCEDURAL STEPS

1. Sanitize your hands.
2. Gather the needed materials.
3. Clean the lenses with lens tissue and lens cleaner.
   PURPOSE: Dust on lenses can obscure elements in the microscopic field.
4. Adjust the seating to a comfortable height.
5. Plug the microscope into an electrical outlet and turn on the light switch.
6. Place the slide specimen on the stage and secure it.
7. Turn the revolving nosepiece to engage the 4× or 10× lens.
   PURPOSE: Always begin microscopic observations at low power.
8. Carefully raise the stage while observing with the naked eye from the side.
   PURPOSE: Observing from the side prevents breaking of the slide if the coarse adjustment knob is advanced too far.
9. Focus the specimen using the coarse adjustment knob.
   PURPOSE: The coarse adjustment knob quickly brings the specimen into focus.
10. Adjust the amount of light by closing the iris diaphragm, by bringing the condenser up or down, or by adjusting the light from the source.
    PURPOSE: Too much light when the low-power objective is used can be irritating to the eyes.
11. Switch to the 40× lens. Use the fine adjustment knob to focus the specimen in detail.

12. Turn the revolving nosepiece to the area between the high-power objective and oil immersion.
13. Place a small drop of oil on the slide.
    PURPOSE: Immersion oil has nearly the same refractive index as glass and prevents refraction of the light, thus improving resolution.
14. Carefully rotate the oil immersion objective into place. The objective will be immersed in the oil.
15. Adjust the focus with the fine adjustment knob.
    PURPOSE: The fine adjustment knob moves the objective slowly, preventing damage to the microscope and the slide.
16. Increase the light by opening the iris diaphragm and raising the condenser.
    PURPOSE: Lighting is crucial to microscopy; the higher the magnification, the more light that is needed.
17. Identify the specimen.
18. Return to low power but do not drag the 40× lens through the oil.
19. Remove the slide and dispose of it in a biohazard container.
20. Lower the stage.
21. Center the stage.
    PURPOSE: Returning the microscope to this position protects it during storage.
22. Switch off the light and unplug the microscope.
23. Clean the lenses with lens tissue and remove oil with lens cleaner.
    PURPOSE: Dust and oil must be removed from the lenses after a procedure.
24. Wipe the microscope with a cloth.
25. Cover the microscope.
26. Sanitize the work area.
27. Sanitize your hands.

Centrifuge

Centrifugation, which is used when solids must be separated from liquids, involves the application of increased gravitational force achieved by rapid spinning. Centrifugation is used to separate blood cells from serum and also solid materials, such as cells and crystals, from urine.

Centrifuges (Figure 44-11) are designed for specific uses. They may be bench-top or floor models; some may be refrigerated. Some may have rotors or heads that are interchangeable. A typical clinical centrifuge may have a rotor that is set at a fixed angle, in which the specimen cups are held in a rigid position at a fixed angle; another type has a horizontal head with swinging buckets that swing out horizontally during centrifugation; and a third type is used for centrifuging capillary tubes for microhematocrit determination (see the Assisting in the Analysis of Blood chapter). Centrifuges also may be equipped with timers to automatically stop centrifugation at a set time.

Directions for using a centrifuge usually are given in terms of revolutions per minute (rpm). Spinning generates centrifugal force, causing the heaviest particles in a liquid to migrate to the bottom of the tube. Centrifuges can be dangerous if not used correctly. The most important rule is to ensure that the centrifuge is balanced so that tubes of equal size and containing equal volume are directly across from one another in the rotor holders. Therefore, there must always be an even number of tubes in the centrifuge. If a second specimen of the same volume in the same-sized tube is not available for balance, a tube of water may be used to balance the load. Tubes being centrifuged should be capped to prevent emission of aerosols. Rubber cups should be placed in the bottom of the carrier cups to prevent breakage of glass tubes.

Centrifuges should never be opened while they are in operation, nor should you attempt to slow a centrifuge with your hands. Most models are equipped with a brake, which should be used only in an emergency, the most common of which is a broken glass tube. In this case, wait until the centrifuge comes to a complete stop and follow the manufacturer's instructions for disinfecting the unit; also follow Standard Precautions to prevent injury and disease transmission.

Centrifuges should be checked, cleaned, and lubricated regularly to ensure proper operation. A certified technician must use a photoelectric device or a strobe tachometer to ensure the centrifuge's speed to comply with quality assurance guidelines set forth by the College of American Pathologists (CAP).

Incubator

Incubators are cabinets that maintain constant temperatures (Figure 44-12). Generally used in the microbiology laboratory, they maintain a constant temperature of 95° to 98.6° F (35° to 37° C), although other temperatures may also be appropriate. Incubators may have warning alarms that sound if the temperature exceeds or falls below a specified range. The temperature should be checked daily, and the cabinets should be cleaned regularly with a disinfectant approved by the manufacturer.

CLOSING COMMENTS

Patient Education

For many testing procedures, patients must be given a specific set of instructions to follow. For example, patients may be required to fast 8 to 12 hours before blood samples are collected. The consumption of some foods and medication may need to be discontinued prior to laboratory testing. The provider discusses medication alternatives with the patient. In some cases, discontinuing the medication may not be medically advisable, and this must be noted on the laboratory requisition. The laboratory then is alerted to the possibility of drug interference, and an alternative test method may be used.

Often the medical assistant is responsible for explaining to the patient the measures to be taken before laboratory testing. Make sure you have interpreted the provider's orders correctly before explaining

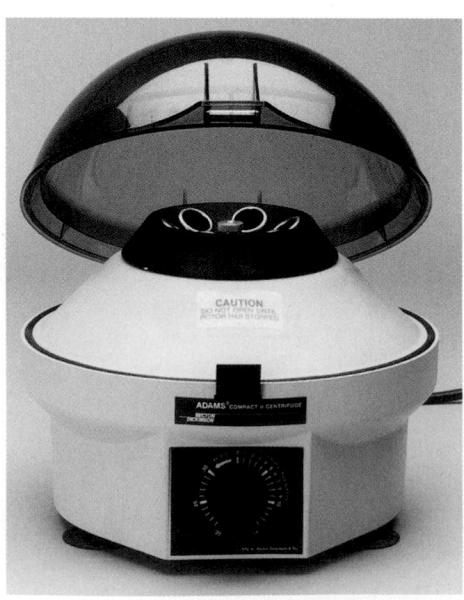

FIGURE 44-11 A centrifuge.

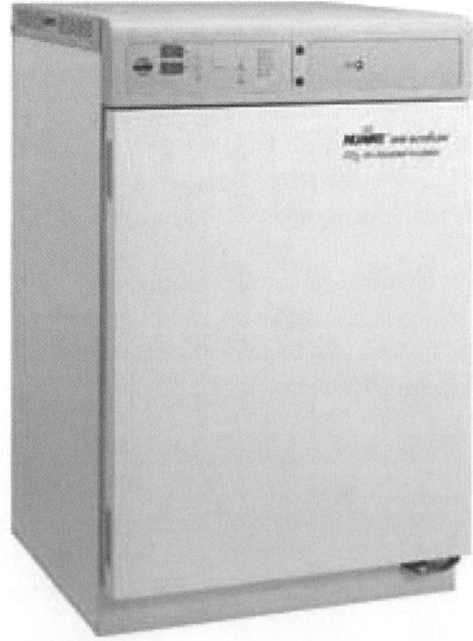

FIGURE 44-12 An incubator. (Courtesy NuAire, Plymouth, Minn.)

the procedure to the patient. The patient should be given written instructions, and a phone number should be included on the instruction sheet so that the patient can call if he or she has questions after returning home.

Legal and Ethical Issues

If disease did not exist, there would be little need for clinical laboratories. The fact that the human body is susceptible to disease necessitates the existence of laboratory testing. All health and safety risks cannot be anticipated or eliminated, but the risks are greatly reduced when everyone who works in the laboratory is conscious of safety guidelines.

Use common sense and document everything. If you are in doubt about the safety of a procedure, ask your supervisor. If you are aware of a potential safety problem, report it to the person in charge. Your welfare, the welfare of the patient, and the welfare of your co-workers may depend on your commitment to safety.

Before the patient receives test results, the medical assistant must make sure the provider has reviewed and signed the results and has given permission for the patient to be told about them. Most providers personally inform patients of laboratory results, but some providers may delegate this duty to office staff. Regardless of who informs the patient of test results, the individual must make sure the specific guidelines for communication are followed as stipulated in the patient's Health Insurance Portability and Accountability Act (HIPAA) release form. Maintaining a patient's privacy and confidentiality are crucial factors that must be considered when dealing with test results.

Professional Behaviors

The next four chapters discuss the most common CLIA-waived tests performed in the POL. They cover patient education, preparation, specimen collection, and testing procedures, which are all aspects of professionalism you must develop as you work with others and document your results appropriately. Look over the Professionalism evaluation form in your study guide to see what actions you should take to become a professional in the laboratory classroom. At the end of the laboratory chapters, your instructor may meet with you one on one to discuss your evaluation results, and/or you may do a self-evaluation of your performance.

SUMMARY OF SCENARIO

Marsha's experience in clinical laboratory testing has made her a valuable asset to her new employer. A thorough understanding of government rules and regulations, including specifics about CLIA, the guidelines published by the CDC, and the regulations established by OSHA have helped Marsha implement laboratory testing in the clinic. Marsha helped the providers design a safe, efficient laboratory space with a refrigerator, a centrifuge, and a biohazard waste station. She developed a rigorous QA program and is now training other medical assistants to perform CLIA-waived testing and daily laboratory maintenance (Table 44-6).

Marsha pays close attention to CLIA regulations and receives regular updates on the tests that can be performed in a POL. She currently is determining the feasibility of performing drug screenings for local businesses. Her employers are pleased with her efforts, and the patients appreciate the convenience of on-site testing.

TABLE 44-6 Laboratory Maintenance Log

	MEDICAL CLINIC							
	DAILY MAINTENANCE CONTROL CHART							
MONTH				YEAR				
	DAILY					MONTHLY		
DAY	REFRIG 2-8° C	FREEZER −0-20° C	ROOM 15-30° C	INCUBATOR 34-36° C	BLEACH COUNTERS	EYE WASH CHECKED	SHOWER CHECKED	BY
1								
2								
3								
4								
5								

SUMMARY OF LEARNING OBJECTIVES

1. **Define, spell, and pronounce the terms listed in the vocabulary.**
   Spelling and pronouncing medical terms correctly reinforce the medical assistant's credibility. Knowing the definitions of these terms promotes confidence in communication with patients and co-workers.

2. **Discuss the role of clinical laboratory personnel in patient care and the medical assistant's role in coordinating laboratory tests and results.**
   Clinical laboratory personnel are responsible for analyzing blood and body fluids and sending the provider the test results, which become part of the essential data for diagnosing and managing a patient's condition. Medical assistants are responsible for collecting specimens, instructing patients, and performing CLIA-waived and some moderately complex testing.

3. **Describe the divisions of the clinical laboratory and give an example of a test performed in each division.**
   Most physician offices that perform laboratory testing do so in the areas of urinalysis, hematology, chemistry, and microbiology. Routine urinalysis, complete blood counts, glucose tests, and throat cultures are some of the tests that might be performed in a POL.

4. **Explain the three regulatory categories established by the Clinical Laboratory Improvement Amendments (CLIA) and identify CLIA-waived tests associated with common diseases.**
   A CLIA-waived test is one that has been approved by the FDA for over-the-counter sales and that may be performed in certified CLIA-waived laboratories (i.e., POLs). The test has been determined to pose no unreasonable risk of harm if performed incorrectly. More complex tests that require additional training or education may be performed only in CLIA-certified moderate- and/or high-complexity laboratories.
   Note: Providers may perform certain microscopic exams if they are certified to perform provider-performed microscopy (PPM).
   CLIA established the standards of quality for laboratory testing. Medical assistants are allowed to perform and monitor all CLIA-waived tests. Table 44-2 summarizes the CLIA-waived tests that may be performed in a registered CLIA-waived laboratory and the common diseases or conditions in which they are used.

5. **Identify quality assurance practices in healthcare, document the results on a laboratory flow sheet, and discuss quality control guidelines.**
   QA involves all the procedures undertaken to ensure that each patient is provided excellent care. QC, which determines whether a laboratory test is accurate, precise, and reliable, is one part of a QA program. Procedure 44-1 outlines the steps for analyzing the reliability of a test based on the results of running its control and documenting the results on a laboratory flow sheet.

6. **Do the following related to laboratory safety:**
   - *Compare and contrast the agencies that govern or influence practice in the clinical laboratory.*
     The federal agencies that regulate clinical laboratories are:
       - Food and Drug Administration (FDA): Regulates the complexity of laboratory tests through the Clinical Laboratory Improvement Amendments (CLIA)

   - Centers for Medicare and Medicaid Services (CMS): Certifies and monitors all clinical laboratories based on the complexity of testing
   - Centers for Disease Control and Prevention (CDC): Oversees the presences of diseases and provides recommendations to prevent the spread of disease
       - Occupational Safety and Health Administration (OSHA): Regulates the Bloodborne Pathogens Standard and the Hazard Communication Standard
       - Environment Protection Agency (EPA) regulates the disposal of biohazard and chemical wastes.
   Although all these agencies provide recommendations for operational procedures in the clinical laboratory, not all have the power to enforce them. For example, the FDA, OSHA and the EPA can impose significant fines for failing to follow regulations, but the Standard Precautions set forth by the CDC are recommended but not enforced.

   - *Discuss the purpose of a Safety Data Sheet.*
     All workers must be provided with information and training, and a Safety Data Sheet (SDS, formerly MSDS) must be on file for all chemicals used in the laboratory. OSHA requires the manufacturer of the chemical to make these sheets available, usually as a package insert and/or online.

   - *Summarize safety techniques to minimize physical, chemical, and biologic hazards in the clinical laboratory.*
     The medical facility must do the following: provide annual formal safety training program to review and update physical, biologic, and chemical hazards that apply to the laboratory; maintain an up-to-date safety procedures manual; provide safety equipment (e.g., fire blankets, fire extinguishers, eyewash stations, and personal protective equipment) to all employees; make sure chemicals are clearly marked with the National Fire Protection Association (NFPA) diamond; make sure SDSs are bound in an accessible manual; and reinforce the principles of Standard Precautions when any biologic material is handled.
     Note: Risks can be minimized in all areas of the laboratory by using common sense.

7. **Describe the essential elements of a laboratory requisition.**
   The laboratory requisition must include all information needed to identify the patient, the ordering provider, the test ordered, insurance information, and the specific details of collection of the specimen (e.g., time and source).

8. **Discuss specimen collection, including the importance of sensitivity to patients' rights and feelings when collecting specimens. Also, discuss the 8 steps in collecting specimens and informing patients of their results.**
   Identification of the patient is the first essential step. If the patient is to collect the specimen at home, he or she should be provided with the appropriate container and complete instructions for collection. Bear in mind the principles of patient education, and be sensitive to factors that can affect the patient's understanding of the instructions for specimen

SUMMARY OF LEARNING OBJECTIVES—*continued*

collection. Review the 8 steps in collecting Specimens and informing Patient of result.

9. **Explain the chain of custody and why it is important.**
   Chain of custody is a method used to ensure that a specimen provided by a patient who may be involved in a legal matter is handled in a fashion that does not compromise the test results. All individuals who handle or test the specimen must be identified in writing and must provide a signature.

10. **Describe the differences between Greenwich time and military time.**
    Greenwich time uses the designations AM and PM, whereas military time uses the 24-hour clock. Therefore, 3:15 PM Greenwich time is 1515 hours in military time. Table 44-3 gives examples of Greenwich time and military time.

11. **Identify the Fahrenheit temperature and the Celsius temperature of common pieces of laboratory equipment.**
    Although the Celsius (centigrade) thermometer is used in the clinical laboratory, in everyday life we commonly use the Fahrenheit system. The incubator is usually set at 37°C (98°F); the autoclave sterilizes at 121°C (254°F); and the refrigerator temperature is 2° to 8°C (35° to 44°F) (see Table 44-4).

12. **Name the metric units used for measuring liquid volume, distance, and mass.**
    Liquid volume is measured in liters; distance is measured in meters; and mass is measured in grams. Prefixes commonly used in the clinical laboratory include *deci-* (0.1), *centi-* (0.01), *milli-* (0.001), *micro-* (0.000001), and *kilo-* (1,000).

13. **Do the following related to laboratory equipment:**
    - *Name the parts of a microscope and describe their functions.*
      The parts of the microscope can be divided into the illumination system (light source, condenser, and iris diaphragm lever), the frame (base, adjustment knobs, arm, stage, and stage control), and the magnification system (objective lenses on the revolving nosepiece and oculars). The illumination system controls the light that passes through the specimen to the eye; the frame provides the structure for the instrument and the components that allow for adjustment of the sample; and the magnification system provides the ground-glass lenses that magnify the specimen.
    - *Summarize selected microscopy tests that can be performed in the ambulatory care setting.*
      Refer to Table 44-5.
    - *Demonstrate the proper use and maintenance of the microscope.*
      Procedure 44-2 outlines the steps for using and maintaining a microscope.
    - *Describe the safe use of a centrifuge.*
      For safe use of a centrifuge, the proper tube must be used and it must be protected from breakage. Centrifuge loads must be carefully balanced, and specimens must be capped to prevent aerosols. Under no circumstances should a centrifuge be opened while it is in operation.
    - *Discuss the use of an incubator.*
      Incubators are cabinets that maintain constant temperatures. They generally are used in a microbiology laboratory. The temperature should be checked daily.

14. **Identify patient education issues, as well as legal and ethical issues, in the clinical laboratory setting.**
    If you are aware of a potential safety problem, report it to the person in charge. Make sure the provider has reviewed and signed test results and has given permission for the patient to be told the results of testing. Follow specific guidelines for communication as stipulated in the patient's HIPAA release form. Maintaining the patient's privacy and confidentiality are crucial factors when communicating with the patient about test results.

CONNECTIONS

Study Guide Connection: Go to the Chapter 44 Study Guide. Read and complete the activities.

evolve Evolve Connection: Go to the Chapter 44 link at *evolve.elsevier.com/kinn* to complete the Chapter Review Quiz. Check out the other resources listed for this chapter to make the most of what you have learned from Assisting in the Clinical Laboratory.

SCENARIO

As part of her duties as a CMA (AAMA), Rosa Gonzales performs tests on patients' urine ordered by her employer, Dr. Ronald Hill. Rosa knows that urinalysis (UA) is a very important part of patient care, and a number of urinary tests are performed in the laboratory in Dr. Hill's busy practice. Dr. Hill most commonly orders routine urinalysis testing, but Rosa also performs some specialized tests. Today Dr. Hill has ordered a UA on a specimen from Mr. Parks; a UA and pregnancy test on a specimen from Mrs. Carpenter; and a UA and culture and sensitivity (C&S) on a specimen from Ms. Hillman.

While studying this chapter, think about the following questions:

- What is involved in a routine urinalysis?
- What quality assurance measures will Rosa follow when performing laboratory tests on urine?
- How are pregnancy and drug tests performed on urine?
- How will Rosa instruct patients in the collection of urine for a routine urinalysis, a urine culture, and other specialized tests such as pregnancy and drug tests?

LEARNING OBJECTIVES

1. Define, spell, and pronounce the terms listed in the vocabulary.
2. Describe the history of the analysis of urine.
3. Describe the anatomy and physiology of the urinary tract, and discuss the formation and elimination of urine by describing the processes of filtration, reabsorption, secretion, and elimination.
4. Do the following related to collecting a urine specimen:
   - Show sensitivity to patients' rights and feelings when collecting specimens.
   - Discuss collection containers.
   - Explain the various means and methods used to collect urine specimens.
   - Instruct a patient in the collection of a 24-hour urine specimen.
   - Instruct a patient in the collection of a clean-catch midstream urine specimen.
5. Examine and report the physical aspects of urine.
6. Perform quality control measures and reassure a patient of the accuracy of the test results based on the steps taken for quality assurance and quality control when performing the chemical urinalysis.
7. Test and record the chemical aspects of urine using CLIA-waived methods.
8. Prepare a urine specimen for microscopic evaluation, and understand the significance of casts, cells, crystals, and miscellaneous findings in the microscopic report.
9. Explain or perform the following CLIA-waived urine tests:
   - Glucose testing using the Clinitest method
   - Urine pregnancy test
   - Fertility and menopause tests
   - Urine toxicology and drug testing
10. List the means by which urine could be adulterated before drug testing.
11. Discuss patient education and legal and ethical issues related to urinalysis.

VOCABULARY

anuria The absence of urine production.

bacteriuria The presence of bacteria in the urine (possible infection).

bilirubinuria (bih-li-roo′-bin-yuhr-e-uh) The presence of bilirubin in the urine (possible liver damage).

cast A protein that has taken on the size and shape of the renal tubules and is washed into the urine. The cast may be identified as hyaline, cellular, granular, or waxy.

Clinitest A test tablet commonly used to screen for and confirm glucose and/or to detect other sugars in urine.

crenate A term describing notched or leaflike, scalloped edges (as seen in shrinking red blood cells).

culture and sensitivity (C&S) A procedure in which a specimen is cultured on artificial media to detect bacterial or fungal growth; this is followed by appropriate screening for antibiotic sensitivity. C&S is performed in the microbiology referral laboratory.

enzymatic reaction A specific chemical reaction controlled by an enzyme.

VOCABULARY—*continued*

filtrate The fluid that remains after a liquid is passed through a filter.

glomerulonephritis A serious kidney condition in which the filtrating capsules are inflamed.

glycosuria An elevated urinary glucose level (possible diabetes mellitus).

hematuria Blood in the urine (possible trauma or infection in the urinary tract).

hemoglobinuria Hemoglobin in the urine (from destruction of red blood cells).

human chorionic gonadotropin (hCG) A substance detected in a positive pregnancy test.

iatrogenic A test result or condition caused by medication or treatment.

ketonuria Ketones in the urine (possible dehydration or diabetic ketoacidosis).

lysed To break open cells (e.g., white or red blood cells).

metabolite The by-product of the metabolism of a substance, such as a drug.

mononuclear white blood cells Leukocytes with an unsegmented nucleus; monocytes and lymphocytes in particular.

myoglobinuria The abnormal presence of a hemoglobin-like chemical of muscle tissue in the urine; it is the result of muscle deterioration.

phenylalanine (fe-il-ahl'-uh-neen) An essential amino acid found in milk, eggs, and other foods. Children unable to metabolize this amino acid eliminate it in the urine.

polymorphonuclear (PMN) white blood cells Leukocytes with a segmented nucleus; also known as *segmented neutrophils,* which appear in the urine during a bacterial infection.

polyuria Excretion of abnormally large amounts of urine in 24 hours.

proteinuria Protein in the urine (possible kidney destruction, especially with casts).

reagent strips Strips used to test the specific gravity, pH, and chemical analytes in urine.

renal thresholds Levels above which substances cannot be reabsorbed into the blood from the renal tubules and therefore are excreted in the urine (e.g., when glucose reaches its renal threshold, the excess glucose appears in the urine).

sediment Insoluble material that settles to the bottom of a urine specimen and to the bottom of centrifuged urine.

supernatant The liquid above the sediment in a centrifuged urine specimen.

urochrome The yellow pigment normally found in urine; it is described as straw, yellow, or amber based on its concentration.

HISTORY OF THE ANALYSIS OF URINE

For centuries abnormalities in the urine have been recognized as possible indicators of a disruption of homeostasis. One of the earliest known tests of urine involved pouring it on the ground to see whether it attracted insects. Such attraction indicated "honey urine," which was known to be excreted by people with skin eruptions. Today, urine is still checked for glucose as a means of detecting diabetes.

During the twentieth century, urinalysis (UA) became a practical laboratory procedure, and today urine is the most commonly analyzed body fluid in the clinical laboratory.

Urine is analyzed for several reasons. First, to detect extrinsic conditions, in which the kidneys are functioning normally but abnormal end products of metabolism are excreted as a result of an imbalance in homeostasis. For example, individuals with diabetes mellitus may excrete glucose in the urine when they are experiencing hyperglycemia. Second, UA is performed to detect intrinsic pathologic conditions that involve the kidneys or the urinary tract, such as the presence of kidney stones or of a urinary tract infection. In addition, because chemicals are excreted through the kidneys, urinalysis can be used to determine the effectiveness of medications and/or the possibility of urinary system side effects from prescribed drugs.

ANATOMY AND PHYSIOLOGY OF THE URINARY TRACT

Medical assistants must have a basic knowledge of kidney structure and urine formation to understand the results of a UA. The urinary tract consists of two kidneys, two ureters, one bladder, and one urethra. The functional unit of the kidney is the nephron (Figure 45-1). Each kidney has more than 1 million nephrons, and each nephron interacts with the blood in the following ways: filtration, reabsorption, and secretion. The kidney selectively excretes or retains substances from the blood according to the body's needs. Approximately 1,200 mL of blood flow through the kidneys each minute.

Formation and Elimination of Urine

Filtration

The blood enters the *glomerulus* of the nephron through the afferent arterioles. The capillary walls of the glomerulus are highly permeable to the water and to the low-molecular-weight components of the plasma (e.g., glucose, urea, electrolytes). These substances filter out of the blood into *Bowman's space* and then into *tubules* of the nephron (see Figure 45-1). Protein and blood cells are too large to be filtrated; therefore, when these substances appear in the urine, it may indicate kidney damage.

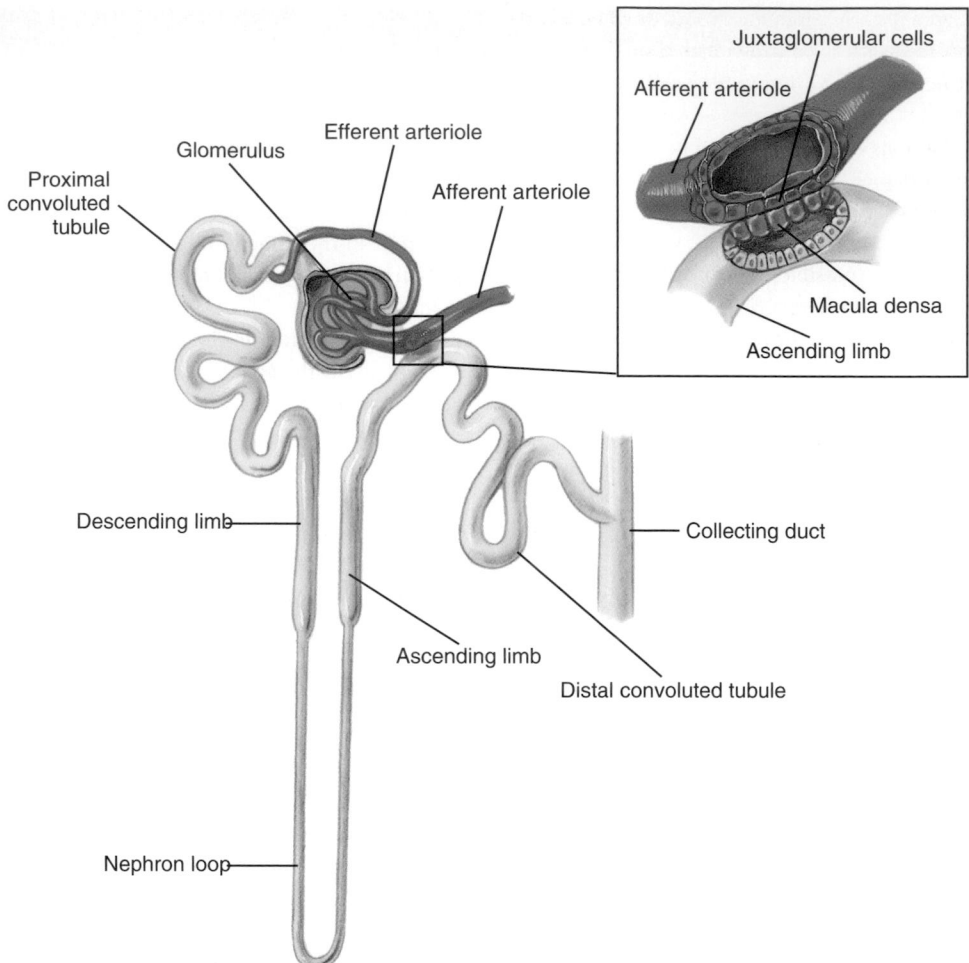

FIGURE 45-1 Nephron. Notice the blood vessels entering and exiting the glomerulus, where the small particles in the blood are **filtered** out of the blood into the surrounding capsule of the nephron. Then, follow the filtrate through the proximal convoluted tubule, the descending limb, the loop of Henle, and the ascending limb of the nephron. This is where water and substances from the filtrate are **reabsorbed** back into the blood vessels. Finally, in the distal convoluted tubule of the nephron, additional waste products are selectively **secreted** into the filtrate by the blood vessels. The collection duct continues to concentrate the filtrate to form urine ready for excretion. (From Applegate EJ: *The anatomy and physiology learning system,* ed 4, Philadelphia, 2011, Saunders.)

Reabsorption

The **filtrate** then travels through the *proximal convoluted tubule* and the *loop of Henle* segments of the nephron, where some of the filtrated products (e.g., glucose) and nearly all of the water are reabsorbed into the blood. The reabsorption of glucose depends on its **renal threshold**; this means that all the glucose will be reabsorbed into the blood if the blood glucose level is below 160 mg/dL. If the blood glucose level is higher than 160 mg/dL, the blood will not reabsorb the glucose. The filtered glucose then remains in the urine, which will test positive for glucose during urinalysis.

Secretion

As the filtrate travels through the last portion of the nephron, known as the *distal convoluted tubule,* the blood vessels selectively secrete additional products into the urine, such as potassium and hydrogen. Some of the secreted substances are the **metabolites** of drugs that may be measured in urine drug testing.

Elimination

The final filtrate formed throughout the nephron drains into a collecting tubule, several of which join to form a collecting duct. The collecting ducts send the filtrate into the renal pelvis, where the filtrate is now called *urine.* Urine passes from the pelvis of the kidneys down the ureters and into the bladder, where it remains until it is voided through the urethra. The kidneys convert nearly 180,000 mL of filtered blood plasma per day into a final urine volume of 750 to 2000 mL, or approximately 1% of the filtered plasma volume.

The largest component of urine is water. The normal waste products found in urine are urea, creatinine, and uric acid, plus the electrolytes chloride, sodium, potassium, phosphate, and sulfate.

COLLECTING A URINE SPECIMEN
Patient Sensitivity

The request for a urine specimen may create an embarrassing moment for the patient. The request should be made in private, such as after the patient is seated in the examination room or while escorting the patient to the restroom. The individual should be given explicit instructions so that he or she understands what is expected. The medical assistant should use therapeutic communication to explain the details of the procedure to the patient and should be observant for indications of confusion. If a language barrier exists, be creative but respectful of the patient's need to follow through correctly on the instructions for collection of the specimen. A picture with directions in a variety of languages could also be posted in the restroom.

Containers

The most important requirement for a collection container is scrupulous cleanliness. The physician office laboratory (POL) should provide the container; patients should not use jars from home. Disposable, nonsterile, plastic, or coated paper containers are the most common and are available in many sizes with tight-fitting lids. Most routine UA testing, pregnancy testing, and tests for abnormal analytes are performed on urine collected in nonsterile containers. Special pliable polyethylene bags with adhesive are used to collect urine from infants and children who are not toilet trained (see the chapter on Pediatrics). For specimens that must be collected over a specified period, large, wide-mouth plastic containers with screw-cap tops are used (Procedure 45-1).

If the sample is being sent to the laboratory for a culture, the specimen must be collected in a sterile container, and the patient must understand how to collect the specimen and how to handle the sterile specimen cup. Such containers are packaged with an intact paper seal over the cap and/or in sterile envelopes (Figure 45-2).

The label on all specimens must include the patient's name, the date and time of collection, and the type of specimen. Always put on gloves before handling filled specimen containers.

Methods of Specimen Collection

Most analyses are performed on freshly voided urine collected in clean containers; this is called a *random specimen*. If the specimen is ordered to be collected when the patient arises in the morning, it is

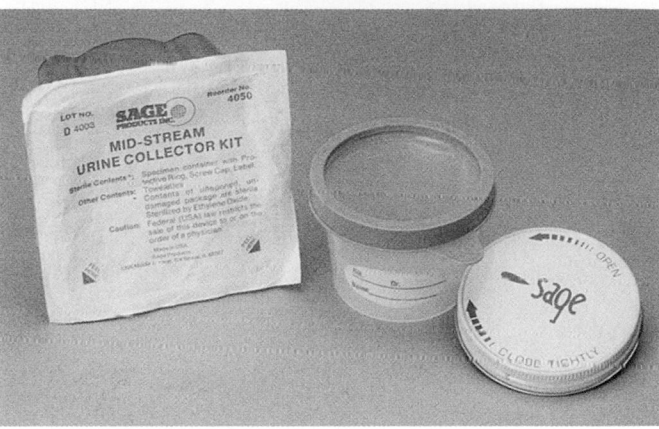

FIGURE 45-2 Sterile container for a midstream specimen.

CRITICAL THINKING APPLICATION   **45-1**

It is 9 AM, and Rosa has received three urine specimens in the laboratory. One of the specimens is in a cup with a paper tab, indicating that the container was sterile, and the other two are in nonsterile containers. What procedures do you think might be performed on the urine collected in the sterile container? What might Rosa do with the other urine specimens? What information should she look for on the label of each specimen?

called a *first morning specimen*. These specimens are most concentrated and are best for nitrite and protein determination, bacterial culture, pregnancy testing, and microscopic examination. *Two-hour postprandial urine specimens*, collected 2 hours after a meal, are used in diabetes screening and for home diabetes testing programs. The *24-hour urine specimen* is collected over 24 hours to provide a quantitative chemical analysis, such as hormone levels and creatinine clearance rates (a procedure for evaluating the glomerular filtration rate of the kidneys). The patient must understand the proper way to collect a 24-hour urine specimen (see Procedure 45-1).

PROCEDURE 45-1   Instruct and Prepare a Patient for a Procedure or Treatment: Instruct a Patient in the Collection of a 24-Hour Urine Specimen

Goal: *To collect a 24-hour urine sample to test for creatinine clearance.*

EQUIPMENT and SUPPLIES

- Patient's health record
- 3-L urine collection container
- Plastic cup or specimen collection pan for collecting urine (which is then poured into the collection container)
- Printed patient instructions
- Laboratory requisition

PROCEDURAL STEPS

1. Greet the patient by name and confirm his or her identity using two identifiers (typically have patients spell their name and give their date of birth).
   <u>PURPOSE</u>: To make sure you have the right patient.
2. Label the container with the patient's name and the current date; identify the specimen as a 24-hour urine specimen; and include your initials.
   <u>PURPOSE</u>: Labeling the container prevents a possible mix-up of specimens.

PROCEDURE 45-1 —*continued*

3. Explain the following instructions to adult patients or to the guardians of pediatric patients.

Patient Instructions: Obtaining a 24-Hour Urine Specimen

(1) Empty your bladder into the toilet in the morning without saving any of the specimen. Record the time you first emptied your bladder on the label.

(2) For the next 24 hours, each time you empty your bladder, all the urine should be collected into the plastic cup or nun's cap that is placed on the toilet. Then pour all the collected urine directly into the large specimen container (Figure 1).
  PURPOSE: Do not urinate directly into the large specimen container because it may have a caustic preservative that you do not want to splash out while urinating.

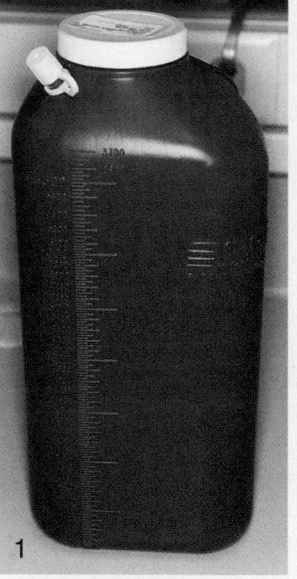

1

(3) Put the lid back on the container after each urination and rinse out the plastic cup or nun's cap and store the container in the refrigerator or at room temperature, as directed, throughout the 24 hours of the study.
  PURPOSE: Refrigeration or the preservative inhibits microbial growth in the specimen.

(4) If at any time you forget to collect your specimen or if some urine is accidentally spilled, the test must be started all over again with a new container and a newly recorded start time.
  PURPOSE: The test will be inaccurate if you fail to collect all urine produced during the designated 24-hour period.

(5) Collect the final urine specimen at the same time the next morning as the first specimen on the previous day was discarded. This last collected specimen is placed in the large container. Collection ends with this voided morning specimen on the second day, which completes the 24-hour period.

(6) As soon as possible after completing collection, return the specimen container to the provider's office or the designated laboratory.

4. Give the patient the specimen container and supplies with written instructions to confirm understanding.

5. Document the details of the patient education intervention in the patient's record.

Processing a 24-Hour Urine Specimen

1. Ask the patient whether he or she collected all voided urine throughout the 24-hour period or whether any problems occurred during the collection process.
  PURPOSE: To confirm the accuracy of the specimen.

2. Complete the laboratory request form and put on disposable gloves before preparing the specimen for transport.

3. Store the specimen in the refrigerator until it is picked up by the laboratory.

4. Document that the specimen was sent to the laboratory, including the type of test ordered, the date and time, the type of specimen, and your initials.

Patient Instructions for Caring for a Urine Specimen Obtained at Home

- Do not put anything but your urine into the container.
- Do not pour out any liquid or powdered preservative from the container.
- If you accidentally spill some of the preservative on yourself, immediately wash with water and call the testing center or designated laboratory.
- Always keep the collection container cool. Refrigerate the container, or keep it in an ice-filled cooler or pail.
- Keep the cap on the container.

A *second-voided specimen* usually is collected to determine glucose levels; the first void of the morning is discarded, and the second void of the day is collected. For a *catheterized specimen*, the provider, nurse, or a specially trained medical assistant inserts a sterile catheter into the bladder to collect the specimen.

The minimum volume needed for a routine UA usually is 12 mL, but 50 mL is preferred. For any type of collection, it is imperative that the patient receive adequate verbal and/or written instructions. The easiest direction to give a patient is "fill the container halfway."

A *clean-catch midstream specimen* (CCMS) is ordered when the provider suspects a urinary tract infection and therefore orders a urine culture for examination of microorganisms. The clean-catch technique is used to remove microorganisms from the urinary *meatus* (opening) by thoroughly cleansing the area around the meatus and then urinating a small amount of urine into the toilet to flush out the distal portion of the urethra. Because the specimen is collected in the medical facility by the patient, the medical assistant needs to give complete, understandable instructions to the patient on the method of collection (Procedure 45-2). Failure to do so may mean that the patient will have to return to the office to provide another specimen. For a *urine culture*, the urine is collected either by catheterization or by the clean-catch method into a sterile container.

PROCEDURE 45-2 | **Instruct and Prepare a Patient for a Procedure or Treatment: Collect a Clean-Catch Midstream Urine Specimen**

Goal: *To collect a contaminant-free urine sample for culture or analysis using the clean-catch midstream specimen (CCMS) technique.*

EQUIPMENT and SUPPLIES

- Patient's record
- Sterile container with lid and label
- Antiseptic towelettes

PROCEDURAL STEPS

1. Greet the patient by name and confirm his or her identity using two identifiers (typically have patients spell their name and give their date of birth).
   PURPOSE: To make sure you have the right patient.
2. Label the sterile, sealed container and give the patient the towelette supplies (Figure 1).
   PURPOSE: Labeling the container prevents a possible mix-up of specimens.

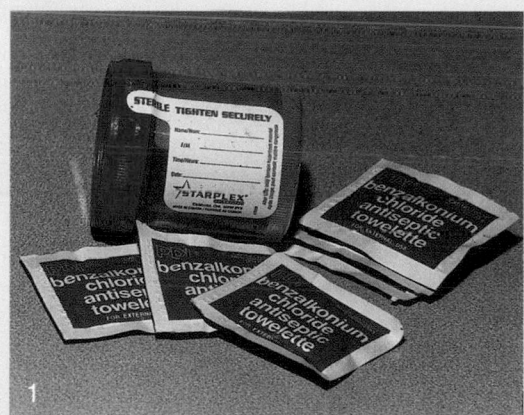

3. Explain the following instructions to adult patients or to the guardians of pediatric patients, making sure you show sensitivity to privacy issues.
   PURPOSE: Instructions must be understood if they are to be followed correctly. By talking to the patient, you can determine whether the patient understands or has any questions.

Patient Instructions: Obtaining a Clean-Catch Midstream Specimen (Female Patient)

(1) Wash your hands and open the towelette packages for easy access.
(2) Remove the lid from the specimen container, being careful not to touch the inside of the lid or the inside of the container. Place the lid, facing up, on a paper towel.

PURPOSE: The lid and the container must be handled carefully to maintain the internal sterility of the container and prevent contamination of the urine sample.
(3) Lower your underclothing and sit on the toilet.
(4) Expose the urinary meatus by spreading apart the labia with one hand (Figure 2, *A*).

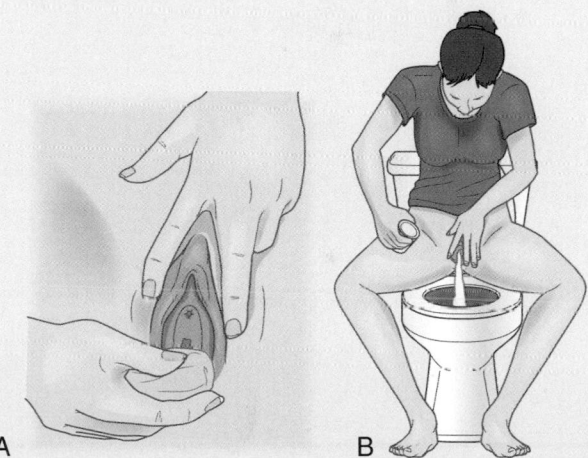

2 A   B

(5) Cleanse each side of the urinary meatus with a front-to-back motion, from the pubis toward the anus. Use a separate antiseptic wipe to cleanse each side of the meatus.
   PURPOSE: Cleansing the area around the urinary meatus prevents contamination of the urine sample. Wiping in one stroke from front to back prevents the passage of microorganisms from the anal region to the area around the urinary meatus.
(6) Cleanse directly across the meatus, front to back, using a third antiseptic wipe (see Figure 2, *A*).
(7) Hold the labia apart throughout this procedure.
(8) Void a small amount of urine into the toilet (Figure 2, *B*).
   PURPOSE: Allowing the initial flow of urine to pass into the toilet flushes the opening of the urethra.
(9) Move the specimen container into position and void the next portion of urine into it. Fill the container halfway. Remember, this is a sterile container. Do not put your fingers on the inside of the container.
(10) Remove the cup and void the last amount of urine into the toilet. (This means that the first part and the last part of the urinary flow

PROCEDURE 45-2   *—continued*

have been excluded from the specimen. Only the middle portion of the flow is included.)

(11) Place the lid on the container, taking care not to touch the interior surface of the lid. Wipe in your usual manner, redress, wash your hands and return the sterile specimen to the place designated by the medical facility.

Patient Instructions: Obtaining a Clean-Catch Midstream Specimen (Male Patient)

(1) Wash your hands and expose the penis.

(2) Retract the foreskin of the penis (if not circumcised).

(3) Cleanse the area around the glans penis (tip of the penis) and the urethral opening (meatus) by washing each side of the glans with a separate antiseptic wipe (Figure 3, *A*).

(4) Cleanse directly across the urethral opening using a third antiseptic wipe.

(5) Void a small amount of urine into the toilet or urinal (Figure 3, *B*).

(6) Collect the next portion of the urine in the sterile container, filling the container halfway without touching the inside of the container with the hands or the penis (Figure 3, *C*).

(7) Void the last amount of urine into the toilet or urinal.

(8) Place the lid on the container, taking care not to touch the interior surface of the lid. Wipe, wash your hands, and redress.

(9) Return the specimen to the designated area.

Processing a Clean-Catch Urine Specimen

1. Document the date, time, and collection type.

2. Process the specimen according to the provider's orders. Perform urinalysis in the office or prepare the specimen for transport to the laboratory. If it is to be sent to an outside laboratory, complete the following steps:

- Make sure the label is properly completed with the patient's information and the date, time, test ordered, and your initials.
- Place the specimen in a biohazard specimen bag.
- Complete a laboratory requisition and place it in the outside pocket of the specimen bag.
- Keep the specimen refrigerated until pickup.
- Document that the specimen was sent.

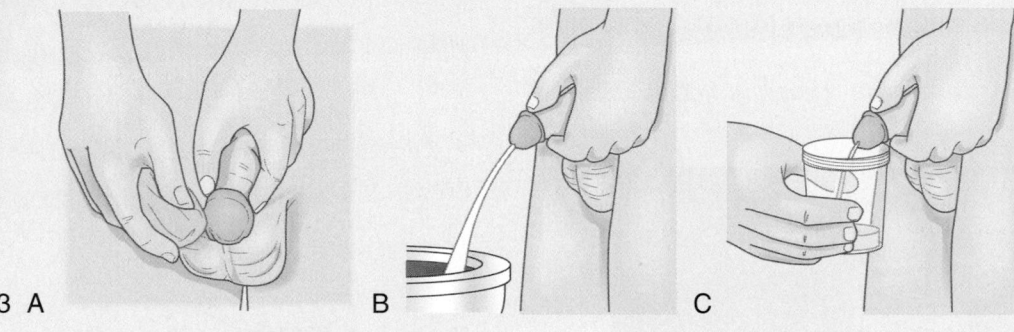

3 A   B   C

Handling and Transportation of a Specimen

Proper handling of specimens is essential. The chemical and cellular components of urine change if the urine is allowed to stand at room temperature (Table 45-1). Urine specimens should therefore be kept refrigerated and should be processed within 1 hour of collection. If the specimen must be transported to a referral laboratory, evacuated transport tubes are available; these contain preservatives and look much like blood collection tubes (Figure 45-3). The vacuum in the tube allows for the delivery of 7 to 8 mL of urine, using a transfer straw or a urine collection cup with an integrated sampling device. Alternatively, the urine can be poured into the tube after the stopper is removed. The preservatives in the BD Vacutainer cherry red/yellow-stoppered tube (i.e., chlorhexidine, ethylparaben, and sodium propionate) prevent the overgrowth of bacteria and inhibit changes in the urine that can affect test results. Chemical reagent strip testing

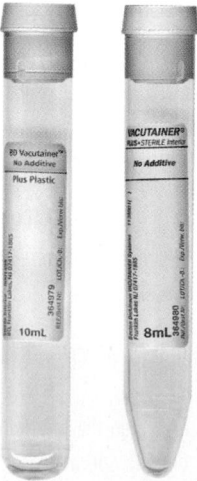

FIGURE 45-3 BD Vacutainer urine preservation tubes. (Courtesy Becton, Dickinson & Co., Franklin Lakes, NJ.)

TABLE 45-1 Changes in Urine after 1 Hour at Room Temperature

CONSTITUENT	CHANGE
Clarity	Urine becomes cloudy as crystals precipitate and bacteria multiply
Color	May change if pH becomes alkaline
pH	Becomes alkaline as bacteria form ammonia from urea
Glucose	Decreases as it is metabolized by bacteria
Ketones	Decreases because of evaporation
Bilirubin and urobilinogen	Undergo degradation in light
Blood	May hemolyze; false-positive results are possible because of bacterial enzymes
Nitrite	Test result may change from negative to positive as bacteria multiply and reduce nitrates to nitrites
Casts	Lyse or dissolve in alkaline urine
Cells	Lyse or dissolve in alkaline urine
Bacteria	Multiply twofold approximately every 20 minutes
Yeasts	Multiply
Crystals	Precipitate as urine cools; may dissolve if pH changes

can be performed on preserved specimens; however, it should be performed within 72 hours. Tubes may be held at room temperature during this time.

A different preservative must be used for urine specimens slated for culture. The BD Vacutainer urine collection kit contains the preservatives sodium formate and boric acid to help preserve the level of bacteria present at the time of collection. This transport system should be used only for urine specimens that will be cultured. Results on the chemical reagent strip may be altered by these preservatives. **Culture and sensitivity (C&S)** testing should be performed within 72 hours. These C&S tubes can be held at room temperature to preserve the bacteria that need to be cultured and then tested for sensitivity.

A laboratory request form must be completed for all specimens that will be transported to another site for analysis. Typical forms include the patient's name and the date; the type of urinalysis ordered; the name of the provider requesting the examination; the appropriate code for the diagnosis that warranted the test according to the *International Classification of Diseases, Tenth Revision, Clinical Modification* (ICD-10-CM); and a line for the provider to

sign after he or she has reviewed the results. Specimens are sent to the laboratory in a plastic biohazard bag that zips closed and has an outside pocket, where the laboratory request is placed. After the test has been performed, the lab sends back the results electronically.

CRITICAL THINKING APPLICATION 45-2

Dr. Hill has ordered a UA on a specimen from Mr. Parks; a UA and pregnancy test on the specimen from Mrs. Carpenter; and a UA and C&S on a specimen from Ms. Hillman. After reviewing the requisitions and entering the patient information into the daily logbook, Rosa notes that Mrs. Carpenter's specimen was collected at 6 AM—3 hours ago. Is this acceptable? Explain your answer. Rosa also notes that the specimen collected in the sterile container from Ms. Hillman is marked "CCMS." Why is this important?

TABLE 45-2 Components of Physical and Chemical Urinalysis

PHYSICAL PROPERTIES	CHEMICAL PROPERTIES
Color	Protein
Clarity	Glucose
Specific gravity	Ketones
Volume*	Bilirubin
Odor*	Blood
Foam*	Nitrite
	pH
	Urobilinogen
	Leukocyte enzyme

*Not always assessed.

ROUTINE URINALYSIS

A complete UA is assessment of the physical properties of the urine and the measurement of selected chemical constituents that are diagnostically important (see Table 45-2).

Physical Examination of the Urine

Appearance

Color. Normal urine is a shade of yellow, ranging from pale straw to yellow to amber. The color depends on the concentration of the pigment **urochrome** and the amount of water in the specimen. A dilute specimen should be pale (straw), and a more concentrated specimen should be a darker yellow (amber). First morning specimens will likely be amber in color due to the concentration of the urochrome during the night. Variations in color may also be caused by diet, medication, and disease. Abnormal colors may be related to pathologic or nonpathologic factors (Table 45-3).

Turbidity. Both normal and abnormal urine specimens may range in appearance from clear to very cloudy. Cloudiness may be caused by cells, bacteria, yeast, vaginal contaminants, or crystals. Often a urine specimen that was clear when voided becomes cloudy as it cools, as crystals form and precipitate.

CRITICAL THINKING APPLICATION   45-3

1. The requisitions accompanying the urine specimens indicate that all three require a UA. Rosa performs the physical analysis and notes that Mrs. Carpenter's urine, which requires the pregnancy test, is amber, whereas the other two specimens are pale yellow. What are possible explanations for Rosa's observations? Should Rosa be concerned about the darker color of Mrs. Carpenter's urine? Should she document this in the patient's electronic health record (EHR) so that Dr. Hill is alerted?
2. Ms. Hillman's urine is turbid, whereas Mr. Parks's urine is clear. What might be causing the cloudiness in Ms. Hillman's urine? Is a cloudy urine cause for concern?

TABLE 45-3   Possible Causes of Urine Colors

COLOR	PATHOLOGIC CAUSE	NONPATHOLOGIC CAUSE
Straw	Diabetes	Diuretics; high fluid intake (coffee, beer)
Amber	Dehydration	Concentrated first morning specimen: Excessive sweating; low fluid intake
Bright yellow	—	Carotene, vitamins
Red	Blood, porphyrins	Menstruation, beets, drugs, dyes
Orange-yellow	Bile, hepatitis	Pyridium (phenazopyridine hydrochloride), dyes, drugs
Greenish yellow	Bile, hepatitis	Senna, cascara, rhubarb
Reddish brown	Old blood, methemoglobin	—
Brownish black	Methemoglobin, melanin	Levodopa (Levodopa, Dopar)
Salmon pink	—	Amorphous urates
White (milky)	Fats, pus	Amorphous phosphates
Blue-green	Biliverdin, infection with *Pseudomonas* organisms	Vitamin B, drugs, dyes

PROCEDURE 45-3   Assess Urine for Color and Turbidity: Physical Test

Goal: *To assess and record the color and clarity of a urine specimen.*

EQUIPMENT and SUPPLIES

- Patient's record
- Urine specimen
- Centrifuge tube
- Fluid-impermeable lab coat and disposable gloves
- Biohazard container

PROCEDURAL STEPS

1. Sanitize your hands. Put on the fluid-impermeable lab coat and disposable gloves.

2. Mix the urine by swirling.
   PURPOSE: Suspended substances settle when urine stands. If urine is not mixed before its appearance is assessed, the finding will be incorrect.
3. Label a centrifuge tube if a complete urinalysis is to be done.
   PURPOSE: If a complete urinalysis is to be done, a portion of the specimen will be centrifuged for microscopic examination. The centrifuged specimen must be labeled to prevent specimen confusion.
4. Pour the specimen into a standard-sized centrifuge tube.
   PURPOSE: Standard-sized containers are better for assessing color and clarity results.

PROCEDURE 45-3 —*continued*

5. Assess and record the color (Figure 1):
- Pale straw
- Yellow
- Amber

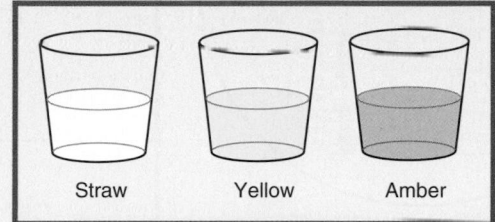

1

Straw   Yellow   Amber

6. Assess the clarity by placing a piece of white paper with fine and dark black print behind the specimen and see if you can see the print:
- Clear—Able to read through the specimen; no cloudiness
- Slightly turbid—Can barely see fine print on white paper through the tube
- Moderately turbid—Cannot see fine print; only dark print can be seen through the tube
- Very turbid—Cannot see any print on white paper through the tube

7. Clean the work area, and dispose of gloves and procedure supplies in the biohazard waste container. Remove lab coat and sanitize your hands.
PURPOSE: To ensure infection control.

8. Record the results in the patient's record.
PURPOSE: A procedure is considered not done until it is recorded.

Volume

The amount of urine is rarely measured in a random specimen. With a timed specimen, volume is measured by pouring the entire collection into a large, graduated cylinder. Generally, it is not accurate enough to use the markings on the side of the collection container. Once the volume has been measured and recorded, a portion of well-mixed specimen, called an *aliquot,* is removed for testing. The remainder is discarded or stored, depending on the preference of the laboratory.

The normal volume of urine produced every 24 hours varies according to the age of the individual. Infants and children produce smaller volumes than adults. The normal adult volume is 750 to 2,000 mL in 24 hours; the average amount is about 1,500 mL. Excessive production of urine is called **polyuria**. This is common in diabetes mellitus, diabetes insipidus, and in certain kidney disorders. Oliguria is insufficient production of urine, which can be caused by dehydration, decreased fluid intake, shock, or renal disease, and urinary tract infections. The absence of urine production, **anuria**, occurs in renal obstruction and renal failure.

Foam

Normally the presence of foam is not recorded, but careful observation of this property can be a significant clue to an abnormality. Foam is seen as small bubbles that persist for a long time after the specimen has been shaken; they must not be confused with any bubbles that rapidly disperse. White foam can indicate the presence of increased protein (Figure 45-4). Greenish yellow foam can mean bilirubinuria. Care should be taken in handling such urine specimens because the greenish yellow color may indicate that the patient has viral hepatitis, which is highly contagious.

Odor

As with foam, odor is not normally recorded but can be an important clue to metabolic disorders. Normal urine is said to be aromatic. Changes in the odor of urine may be caused by disease, the presence

FIGURE 45-4 Dark amber-red urine with foam may indicate an increased protein level and hematuria. *Note:* If the urine were orange-green and the foam greenish yellow, this might indicate bilirubinuria.

of bacteria, or diet. The odor of the urine of a patient with uncontrolled diabetes is described as fruity because of the presence of ketones, which are the products of fat metabolism. An ammonia or putrid smell in the urine can be caused by an infection or may be noted in urine that has been allowed to stand before it is tested. The bacteria break down the urea in the urine to form ammonia. Foods such as asparagus and garlic also can produce an abnormal odor in the urine. Urine from a child with phenylketonuria (PKU) is said to smell "mousy." PKU is a rare hereditary condition in which the amino acid **phenylalanine** is not properly metabolized, which can lead to severe mental retardation. Accumulation of phenylalanine in the blood and urine gives body fluids an odor like wet fur. (Blood sampling for PKU is discussed in the chapter, Assisting in Blood Collection.)

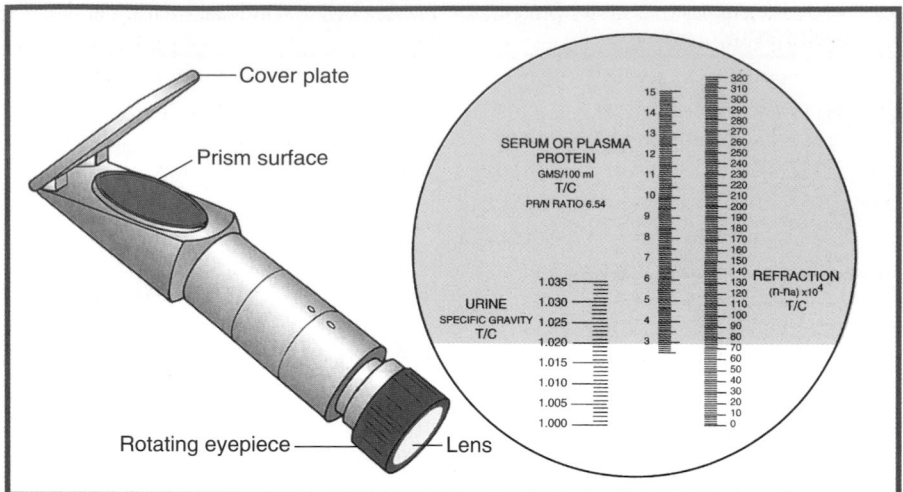

FIGURE 45-5 **Refractometer.** A drop of urine is placed on the prism surface of the refractometer on the left, and the cover plate is closed. When the examiner looks through the lens, the two graphs are seen in the circular field of vision on the right. The urine specific gravity (SG) is read from the left scale, where the blue shadow meets the lighted bottom. The SG is 1.020.

Specific Gravity

The specific gravity is the weight of a substance compared with the weight of an equal volume of distilled water. In UA, it is the rough measurement of the concentration, or amount, of substances dissolved in the urine. The specific gravity of distilled water is 1.000. The normal specific gravity of urine ranges from 1.005 to 1.030, depending on the patient's fluid intake. Most samples fall between 1.010 and 1.025. The urine specific gravity indicates whether the kidneys are able to concentrate the urine. A change in specific gravity is one of the first indications of kidney disease. For example, glomerulonephritis, the presence of glucose, protein, or an x-ray contrast medium used in diagnostic studies may increase the specific gravity of urine, whereas chronic renal insufficiency or diabetes insipidus may lower the specific gravity in urine. To measure the specific gravity, laboratories may use a Clinical Laboratory Improvement Amendments (CLIA)-waived refractometer or a chemical reagent strip.

A *refractometer* measures the refraction of light through solids in a liquid. The result is called the *refractive index,* which for our purposes is the same as specific gravity. The refractometer requires only a drop of urine. One drop of well-mixed urine is placed under the hinged cover of the instrument, and the value is read directly from a scale viewed through an ocular. Figure 45-5 shows the refractometer on the left and the visual results of the urine in the circle on the right. The scale on the left side of the circle shows a urine specific gravity of 1.020. The refractometer must be calibrated daily with distilled water, which should read 1.000 (Figure 45-6). Note that the measurement of specific gravity carries no unit of measure after the number.

The *reagent strip (dipstick) test,* a CLIA-waived test, is the method most commonly used for measuring specific gravity in the POL. The pad on the strip contains a chemical that is sensitive to positively charged ions, such as sodium (Na^+) and potassium (K^+). The pad detects the urine's specific gravity. Various color changes indicate values between 1.000 and 1.030 (see the SPECIFIC GRAVITY row of colors in the second figure in Procedure 45-4).

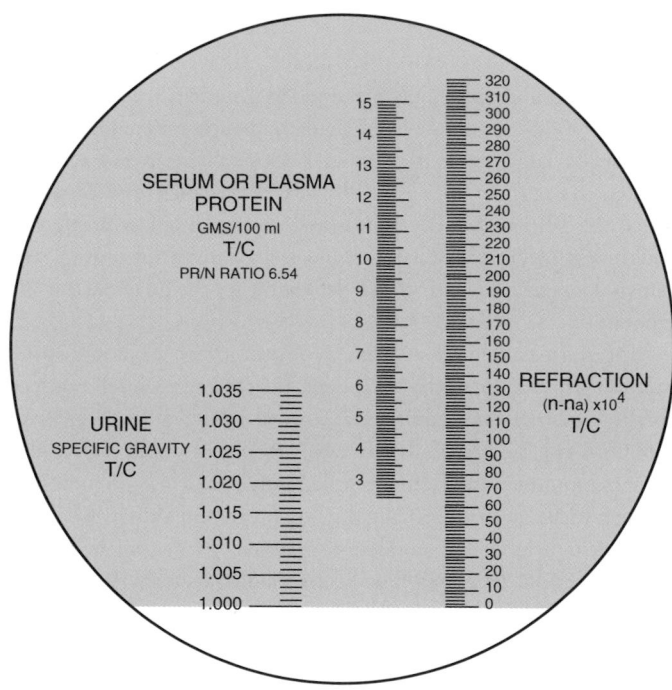

FIGURE 45-6 Refractometer reading using a distilled water control. Note that the urine specific gravity (SG) is 1.000 on both scales.

Chemical Examination of Urine

Tests can be performed on urine to detect the presence of certain chemicals, which can provide valuable information to the provider. In certain situations, these chemical test results can be critical to the diagnosis.

Reagent strip testing is the most widely used technique for detecting chemicals in the urine (Procedure 45-4); these strips are available in a variety of types (Figure 45-7). Generally, they are plastic strips to which one or more pads containing chemical reagents are attached. Test pads are available for measuring pH and specific gravity (physical properties of urine), and for measuring the following chemicals: glucose, ketones, leukocyte esterase, protein, blood, bilirubin, nitrite, urobilinogen, phenylketones, vitamin C, and others. The presence or absence of these chemicals in the urine provides information on the status of carbohydrate metabolism, liver and kidney function, and the patient's acid-base balance.

Reagent strips are designed to be used once and then discarded in a biohazard waste container. The directions for each strip are included inside the package, and these instructions must be followed exactly if accurate results are to be obtained. A color comparison chart is provided on the label of the container. In addition to reagent strips, various tablet tests are available.

All strips and tablets must be kept in tightly closed containers in a cool, dry area and should be removed just before testing. To prevent contamination of the bottle, never touch a strip that has been exposed to urine against the color comparison chart on the bottle. If both a UA and a C&S have been ordered for a specimen, the urine must be cultured or separated into a urine culture tube before the UA is started because introducing a reagent strip into the urine contaminates it.

pH

The pH is a measurement of the degree of acidity or alkalinity of the urine. A urine specimen with a pH of 7 is neutral (Figure 45-8).

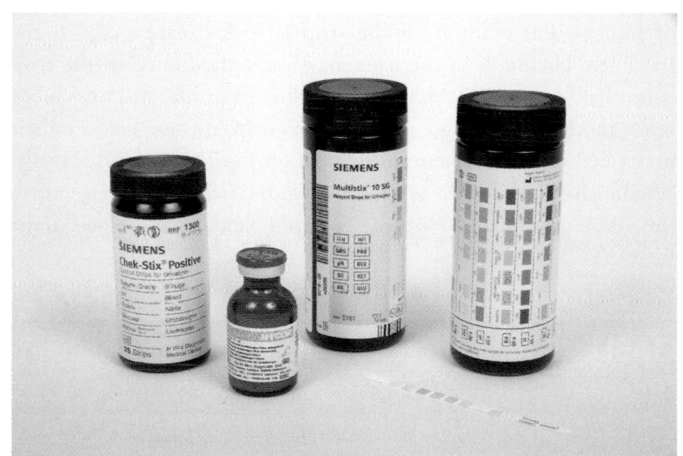

FIGURE 45-7 Examples of two controls *(left)* and two reagent strip bottles for testing various chemicals in urine *(right)*.

A value below 7 indicates acidity, and one above 7 indicates alkalinity. Normal, freshly voided urine may have a pH range of 5.5 to 8. The urinary pH varies with an individual's metabolic status, diet, drug therapy, and disease. In the case of gross **bacteriuria**, the urine pH is alkaline as a result of bacterial conversion of urea to ammonia. Knowing the pH of the urine also assists in identification of crystals if they are found in the urine **sediment**.

Glucose

Glucose is filtered at the glomerulus, but under normal conditions most of it is reabsorbed in the tubules. The minute quantities normally present in the urine are not detected by reagent strips and tablets. Detectable **glycosuria** occurs whenever the filtered glucose in the renal tubules is so high it cannot be reabsorbed into the blood because its renal threshold has been met. The excess glucose is then excreted and detected in the urine specimen. A positive glucose finding is common in urine from patients with diabetes and may be the first indication of the disease. The reagent strip glucose testing method is based on an **enzymatic reaction**. It detects only glucose; in other words, it is specific for glucose.

Ketones

Ketones are the end product of fat metabolism in the body. Acetoacetate, acetone, and beta hydroxybutyric acid are collectively called *ketone bodies*, or *ketones*. **Ketonuria** is common with starvation, low carbohydrate diets, excessive vomiting, and diabetes mellitus. Because ketones evaporate at room temperature, urine should be tested immediately, or the specimen should be tightly covered and refrigerated. The reagent strip detects only acetoacetate. The Acetest, discussed later in this chapter, can be used to detect both acetone and acetoacetate.

Protein

Protein in the urine in detectable amounts is called **proteinuria,** which is one of the first signs of renal disease. We normally excrete a small amount of protein every day; proteinuria may be light to heavy, constant or sporadic. It may be affected by posture. In orthostatic proteinuria, protein is excreted only when the patient is in an upright position. Generally, first morning specimens from these patients are negative, but protein is found in urine passed throughout

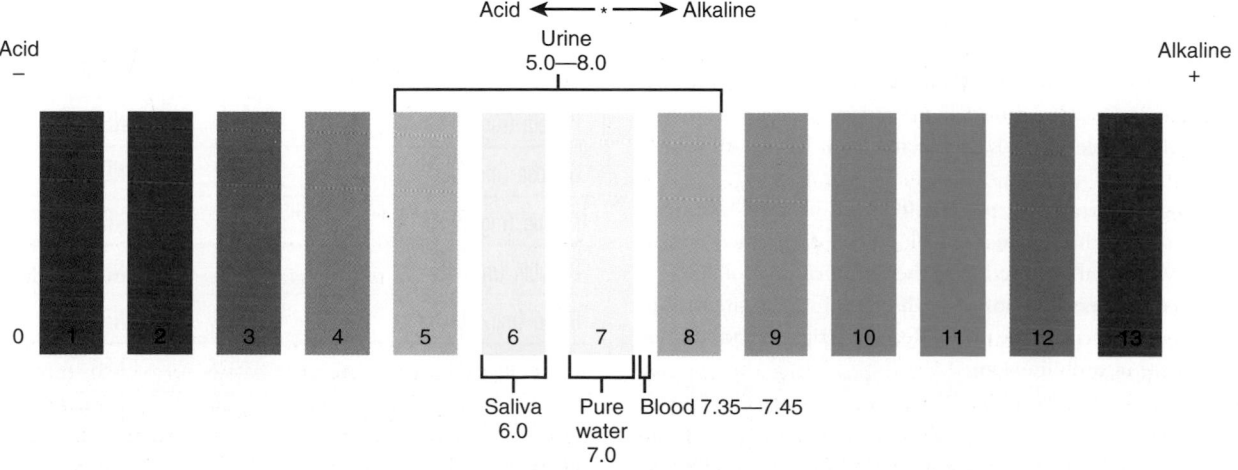

FIGURE 45-8 The pH scale.

the day. Proteinuria is a common finding in pregnancy and must be monitored along with excessive weight gain and increased blood pressure (three possible symptoms of pre-eclampsia). Protein is almost always present in the urine after heavy exercise. The reagent strip is highly sensitive to urinary albumin and is less sensitive to the other proteins: hemoglobin, immunoglobulin, and mucoproteins.

Blood

The presence of blood in the urine may indicate infection or trauma to the urinary tract, resulting in bleeding in the kidneys, bladder, or urethra. The blood test pad on the reagent strip reacts with three different blood constituents: intact red blood cells, hemoglobin from **lysed** red blood cells, and myoglobin, a hemoglobin-like molecule that transports oxygen in muscle tissue.

Hematuria is the presence of intact red blood cells in urine. The color reaction on the reagent strip ranges from yellow through green to dark green when hematuria is present, revealing a speckled appearance. Hematuria can be caused by irritation of the ureters, bladder, or urethra. It also is a common finding in cystitis and in individuals passing kidney stones. A random specimen may contain blood from vaginal contamination if the woman is menstruating.

Hemoglobinuria is the presence of hemolyzed red blood cells. True hemoglobinuria is rare. It occurs as a result of intravascular red blood cell destruction and can be caused by transfusion reactions, malaria, drug reactions, snakebites, and severe burns.

Myoglobinuria occurs when muscle tissue is damaged or injured, as in crushing injuries, myocardial infarctions, and contact sports. Patients with muscular dystrophy often have myoglobinuria. Hemoglobinuria cannot be distinguished from myoglobinuria by reagent strip testing; both cause a uniform change in color from light green to dark green on the strip.

Bilirubin and Urobilinogen

Bilirubin is a product of the breakdown of hemoglobin. Hemoglobin is released from old red blood cells and is gradually converted to bilirubin in the liver. The liver continues to convert bilirubin to urobilinogen, which is sent to the intestines for excretion. Bilirubin is a bile pigment not normally found in urine. Its presence in urine is one of the first signs of liver disease or other diseases in which the liver may be involved.

Bilirubinuria can occur even before jaundice or other symptoms of liver disease are evident. It is the result of liver cell damage or obstruction of the common bile duct by stones or neoplasms (tumors). Excessive bilirubin colors the urine yellow-brown to greenish orange. Because direct light causes decomposition of bilirubin, urine samples must be protected from light until testing is complete.

Urobilinogen normally is present in urine in small amounts. Increases are seen with increased red blood cell destruction and in liver disease. With total obstruction of the bile duct, no urobilinogen is found in the intestines and none is reabsorbed into the circulation; therefore, none is present in the urine. Reagent strip methods cannot detect a decrease in urobilinogen.

Nitrite

Nitrite occurs in urine when bacteria break down nitrate, a common component of urine. A positive nitrite test result may indicate the presence of a urinary tract infection (UTI). However, not all bacteria are able to reduce nitrate to nitrite. Negative nitrite test results also can occur when bacteria are insufficient or when the urine has not incubated in the bladder long enough for the reaction to occur. *Escherichia coli,* the organism that causes most UTIs, reduces nitrate to nitrite. False-positive results can occur if a specimen is allowed to sit at room temperature and contaminating bacteria multiply. False-negative results may occur if the bacteria further metabolize the nitrite and produce ammonia.

Leukocyte Esterase

Leukocytes (white blood cells) are present in urine during infections of the urinary tract. Leukocytes may also be contaminants from the vagina. The leukocyte esterase test pad on the reagent strips takes 2 minutes to **release the esterase in** the lysed **polymorphonuclear white blood cells (PMNs)** before showing a positive reaction. It does not detect **mononuclear white blood cells,** which occasionally are present during infection. The test does not react with small numbers of white blood cells found in normal urine.

Limitations of Reagent Strip Testing

The reagent strip is a reliable method of chemical analysis of urine if used properly. The normal urine reference ranges for a reagent strip are presented in Table 45-4. Errors can arise from a number of sources. For example, if the strip is soaked excessively in the specimen, chemicals in the pads may be overly diluted. If the strip is not held horizontally while read, colors from one pad may bleed onto another. If the test areas on the strip are not read at their prescribed time, the chemical interaction may be misread. Finally, certain chemicals, such as ascorbic acid (vitamin C), may affect the results of nitrite, glucose, bilirubin, and occult blood tests.

TABLE 45-4   Normal Urine Reference Ranges for Reagent Strips

REFERENCE	RANGE
Color	Pale yellow to amber
Clarity	Clear to slightly turbid
Specific gravity	1.001-1.035
pH	4.6-8
Protein (mg/dL)	NEG
Glucose (mg/dL)	NEG
Ketone (mg/dL)	NEG
Bilirubin (mg/dL)	NEG
Blood (mg/dL)	NEG
Nitrite (mg/dL)	NEG
Urobilinogen (Ehrlich units)	0.1-1
White blood cells	NEG

Normal levels of vitamin C do not interfere with analysis, but if a person consumes large amounts of the vitamin, a special strip can be used to detect interfering levels of vitamin C. If an elevated level is found, the patient should be instructed to discontinue vitamin C intake for 24 hours, and then another urine specimen should be collected for testing.

Visual interpretation of color on the reagent strip pads is likely to vary among individuals. Some laboratories use automated instruments to read the strips. Several companies manufacture instruments that use the principle of reflectance photometry in the analysis of reagent strip color. Once the strip has been placed in the instrument, a microprocessor controls the movement of the strip into the reflectometer. Light of a specific wavelength is beamed onto each of the test areas on the strip. Some light is absorbed, and some is scattered or reflected. The amount of reflected light is analyzed by the microprocessor and converted into a digital reading, and the results are printed out (Figure 45-9). The advantage of this method is that timing and color interpretation are consistent. The disadvantage is that the instrument is not able to identify and compensate for highly pigmented urine, leading to false-positive results. The medical assistant should be aware of this and should manually test urine specimens that are darkly pigmented.

Quality Assurance and Quality Control in Urinalysis

The U.S. Food and Drug Administration (FDA) categorizes the chemical analysis of urine performed by an instrument or a reagent strip as a CLIA-waived test. The chemical analysis includes the reagent strip (dipstick) tests for bilirubin, glucose, hemoglobin or blood, ketones, leukocyte esterase, nitrite, pH, protein, specific gravity, and urobilinogen. A commercially available control strip should be used to determine the reliability of the reagent strips used in chemical analysis. One such control strip is the Chek-Stix. The plastic control strip has seven pads, each of which contains synthetic ingredients that mimic human urine when reconstituted in water.

CRITICAL THINKING APPLICATION   45-4

1. Rosa prepares to do the chemical examination of the three urine specimens. (Remember, Dr. Hill has ordered the following:)
   - UA on the specimen from Mr. Parks
   - UA and pregnancy test on the specimen from Mrs. Carpenter
   - UA and C&S on the specimen from Ms. Hillman

   Should Rosa proceed with the chemical analysis of each specimen in exactly the same manner? Explain your answer.

2. After completing the chemical analysis of the three specimens, Rosa notes several differences among the samples:
   - Mr. Parks's test results reveal elevated glucose and ketone levels and an SG of 1.035.
   - Mrs. Carpenter's sample has a high specific gravity (SG).
   - Ms. Hillman's sample reveals an elevated nitrite level, a pH of 8, and an elevated leukocyte esterase reading.

   Based on this information, what are the probable reasons each of these patients visited Dr. Hill today?

After reconstitution, a reagent test strip is immersed in the control solution and the results are compared with a chart that accompanies the Chek-Stix. Both positive and negative Chek-Stix controls are available (Procedure 45-4). The positive reconstituted control shows positive (abnormal) results when a test strip is inserted and read, whereas the negative reconstituted control shows normal urinalysis results along its test strip. It is important to observe and record the abnormal and normal results produced by the positive and negative controls. Also, make sure the test results are consistent with the Chek-Stix charts provided by the manufacturer before testing urine specimens.

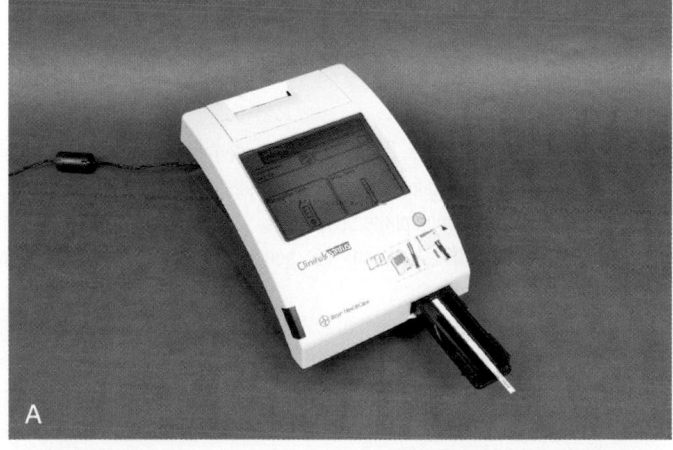

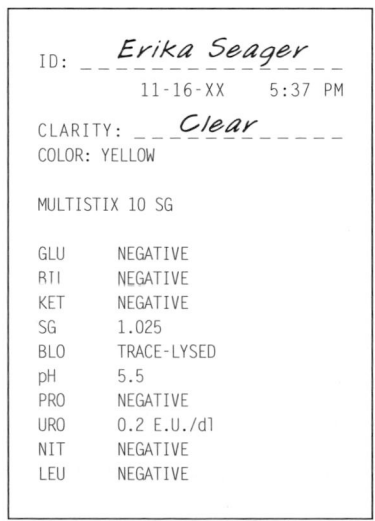

ID: _____Erika Seager_____

11-16-XX   5:37 PM

CLARITY: __Clear_____
COLOR: YELLOW

MULTISTIX 10 SG

GLU	NEGATIVE
BIL	NEGATIVE
KET	NEGATIVE
SG	1.025
BLO	TRACE-LYSED
pH	5.5
PRO	NEGATIVE
URO	0.2 E.U./dl
NIT	NEGATIVE
LEU	NEGATIVE

B

FIGURE 45-9 A, Clinitek 50 Urine Chemistry Analyzer. The reagent strip is placed on the tray before the test is begun. **B,** Sample of the Clinitek results.

PROCEDURE 45-4   Perform Quality Control Measures: Differentiate Between Normal and Abnormal Test Results while Determining the Reliability of Chemical Reagent Strips

Goal: *To reconstitute a control sample and test the reliability of the urinalysis chemical testing strip.*

EQUIPMENT and SUPPLIES

- Chek-Stix Control Strips with reference ranges for urinalysis
- Distilled water
- Capped tube with milliliter markings
- Test tube rack
- Forceps
- Timer
- Urine chemical strips for urine testing
- Color chart for interpreting the chemical strip results
- Fluid-impermeable lab coat and disposable gloves
- Biohazard waste container
- Control reference sheet and control flow sheet

PROCEDURAL STEPS

1. Assemble the equipment and supplies. Record the lot number and the expiration date of the Chek-Stix on the control log sheet.
   PURPOSE: Chek-Stix cannot be used if the expiration date has passed. Recording the lot number and expiration date is an important part of quality assurance.
2. Sanitize your hands. Put on the fluid-impermeable lab coat and disposable gloves.
   PURPOSE: To ensure infection control.
3. Place a conical tube in the rack and remove the cap.
4. Pour 15 mL of distilled water into the tube.
5. Using forceps, remove one strip from the Chek-Stix bottle. Inspect the strips for mottling or discoloration.

PURPOSE: The control strips have chemicals that you should not handle or contaminate with your hands. Any mottling or discoloration may mean that the strips have been exposed to moisture, light, or solvents. Improperly stored control strips should not be used.

6. Place the strip into the water and tightly cap the tube.
7. Invert the tube for 2 minutes.
   PURPOSE: Chemicals embedded in the pads must be thoroughly dissolved in the water.
8. Allow the tube to sit in the rack for 30 minutes.
9. Invert the tube one time and remove the strip with forceps.
10. Discard the strip in the biohazard waste container. Once reconstituted, the control solution is stable for 8 hours at room temperature.
    PURPOSE: To ensure infection control.
11. Perform quality control of the chemical reagent strip by dipping it into the control solution according to Procedure 45-4.
12. Read and record the results.
13. Compare the results with the control reference ranges provided on the Chek-Stix package insert.
    PURPOSE: Results should fall within a given range provided by the manufacturer. If they do not, the chemical reagent strips cannot be used to test patients' urine.
14. Discard the chemical reagent strip and the control solution in the biohazard waste container.
15. Clean up the work area, remove lab coat, and discard gloves in the biohazard waste container, and sanitize your hands.
    PURPOSE: To ensure infection control.

PROCEDURE 45-5   Obtain a Specimen and Perform a CLIA-Waived Urinalysis: Test Urine with Chemical Reagent Strips

Goal: *To perform chemical testing on a urine sample and to reassure the patient of its accuracy.*

EQUIPMENT and SUPPLIES

- Patient's record
- Urine specimen
- Reagent strips
- Timer
- Fluid-impermeable lab coat and disposable gloves
- Biohazard waste container

PROCEDURAL STEPS

1. Sanitize your hands. Put on the fluid-impermeable lab coat and nonsterile gloves.
   PURPOSE: To ensure infection control.
2. Check the time of collection, the container, and the mode of preservation.

PURPOSE: Proper specimen identification and screening of specimens for appropriate collection containers and collection procedures prevent testing of inappropriate specimens.

3. If the specimen has been refrigerated, allow it to warm to room temperature.
   PURPOSE: Certain tests are temperature dependent. Testing of cold specimens may cause false-negative results.
4. Check the reagent strip container for the expiration date.
   PURPOSE: Do not use expired reagents.
5. Remove the reagent strip from the container. Hold it in your hand or place it on a clean paper towel. Recap the container tightly.
   PURPOSE: Test strips are sensitive to moisture and light and must be stored in tightly sealed containers. Contamination from chemical residues on countertops can affect results.

6. Compare nonreactive test pads with the negative color blocks on the color chart on the container.
   PURPOSE: Discolored pads indicate that the product has not been properly stored and must not be used for testing.

7. Thoroughly mix the specimen by swirling.
   PURPOSE: If settling occurs, certain elements may not be detected.

8. Following the manufacturer's directions, note the time, dip the strip into the urine, and then remove it.
   PURPOSE: Tests are time dependent. Some pads darken over time.

9. Quickly remove the excess urine from the strip by pulling the back of the strip across the lip of the specimen container and then blotting the edge of the strip on a paper towel or the side of the specimen container.
   PURPOSE: Excess urine on the strip or prolonged dipping time affects test results.

10. Hold the strip horizontally (Figure 1). At the required time, compare the strip with the appropriate color chart on the reagent container. *Do not touch the strip to the bottle.*

11. Alternately, the strip can be placed on a paper towel.
    PURPOSE: Holding the strip horizontally prevents runover from one test pad to another and prevents interference from mixing of chemicals in the test pads.

12. Read and record the first two results 30 seconds after dipping the strip (the indicated time to read the "Glucose" and "Bilirubin"). Compare the

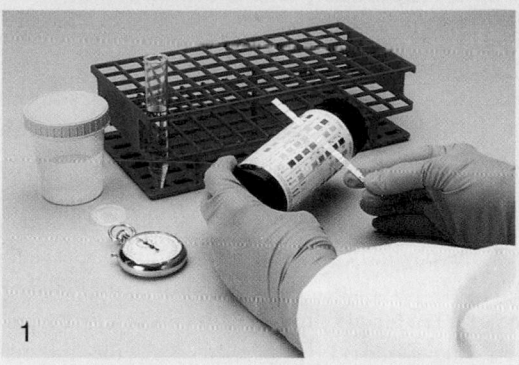

1

two reagent pads closest to your hand with the bottom two rows of the color chart (Figure 2). Continue reading and recording each row of possible results with its appropriate reagent pad at its designated time.
   PURPOSE: Timing is critical. Allowing the strip to come in contact with the bottle contaminates the bottle.

13. Clean the work area and remove gloves. If a paper towel was used, dispose of it, the reagent strip, and the gloves in the biohazard container. Remove lab coat and sanitize your hands.
    PURPOSE: To ensure infection control.

14. Document the results in the patient's record, and reassure the patient of the accuracy of the test results.
    PURPOSE: A procedure is considered not done until it is recorded.

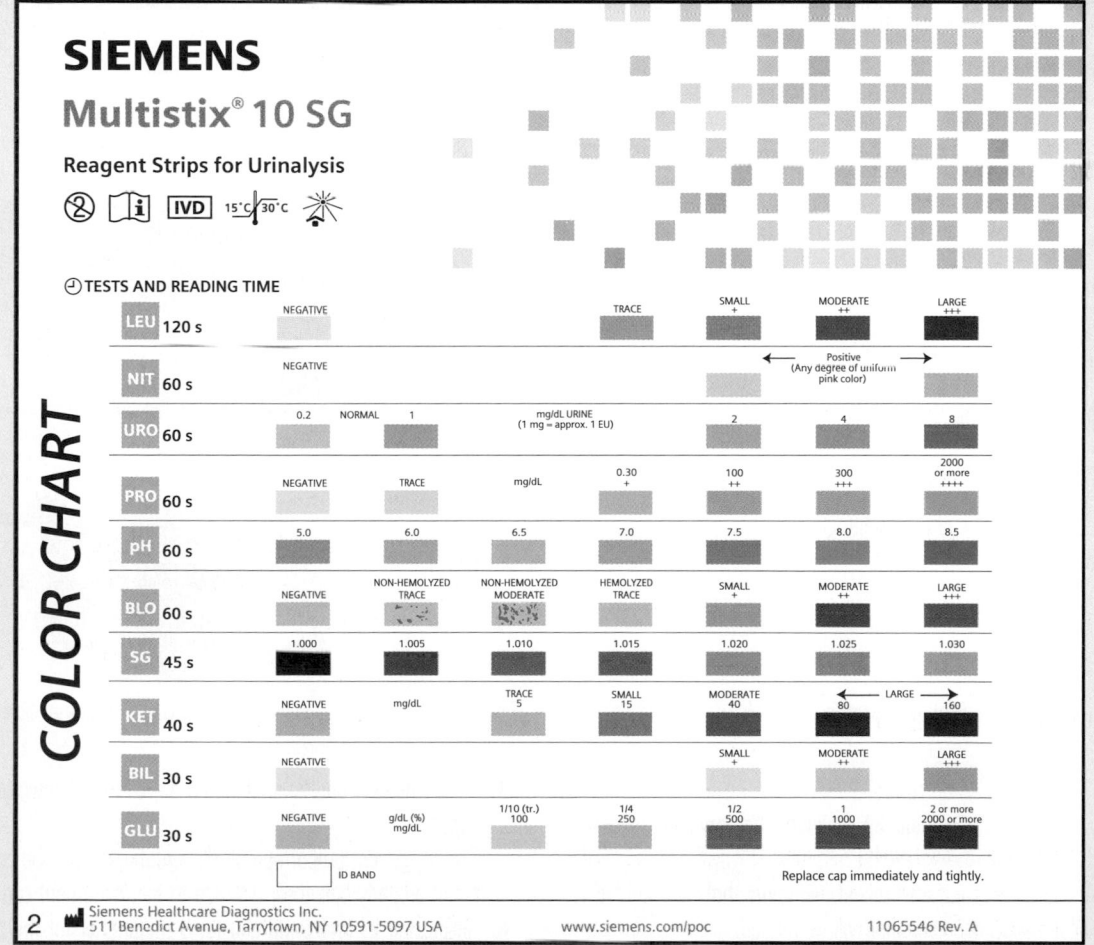

(©Siemens Healthcare 2016. Used with permission.)

Microscopic Preparation and Examination of Urine Sediment

Microscopic examination of urine consists of categorizing and counting cells, casts, crystals, and miscellaneous constituents in the sediment obtained after a measured portion of urine is centrifuged. Many formed elements are found in the urine. Some are significant, and others are not. Most important, the microscopic examination should correlate with the physical and chemical analyses. For example, if the physical examination of the urine appeared pink or red tinged, and the reagent strip tested positive for blood, then one would look for red blood cells during the microscopic examination. Medical assistants should be familiar with the preparation of urine specimens for this test and with the possible test results (Procedure 45-5).

Microscopic Preparation of Urine

To perform the microscopic UA procedure, a laboratory must be certified to perform CLIA Provider Performed Microscopy Procedures (PPMPs), a subcategory of CLIA moderate-complexity laboratories. Quality assurance is as important in the microscopic examination as in the chemical analysis of urine. To ensure consistency and standardization, commercially available systems can be used, such as the KOVA System or the UriSystem. These systems may include specially designed, graduated centrifuge tubes with devices or pipets that allow easy decanting of supernatant and retention of an exact amount of sediment. They also use specially designed plastic slides with wells or coverslips that accept only a given amount of sediment. Control solutions containing preserved cells to be identified are also available from KOVA. Whatever system is used, the Clinical and Laboratory Standards Institute (CLSI) recommends the following:

- The urine volume should be 12 mL.
- The specimen should be centrifuged for 5 minutes at a relative centrifugal force of 400 g (i.e., 400 times normal gravity).
- A standardized slide should be used to view the sediment.
- A consistent reporting format should be used.

When a urine sample is centrifuged, the clear upper portion of the specimen is called the **supernatant**. It is poured off, and a drop of the well-mixed sediment at the bottom of the centrifuged tube is examined under a microscope. The sediment may be stained to give greater contrast to the formed elements. The stain assists in the identification of formed elements by enhancing the detail of internal cellular structure.

PROCEDURE 45-6   Prepare a Urine Specimen for Microscopic Examination

Goal: *To prepare a urine specimen for the provider's microscopic examination to determine the presence of normal and abnormal elements.*

EQUIPMENT and SUPPLIES

- Patient's record
- Urine specimen
- Centrifuge tube
- Centrifuge
- Disposable pipet
- Sedi-Stain
- Microscope slide and coverslip
- Microscope
- Permanent marker
- Fluid-impermeable lab coat and disposable gloves
- Face protection
- Biohazard waste container

PROCEDURAL STEPS

1. Sanitize your hands. Put on the fluid-impermeable lab coat and disposable gloves.
   PURPOSE: To ensure infection control.
2. Gently mix the urine specimen by swirling the covered specimen container.
   PURPOSE: If the urine is not well mixed, elements that have settled to the bottom of the specimen container will be missed.
3. Pour 10 mL of urine into a labeled centrifuge tube and cap the tube.

4. Place the tube in the centrifuge (Figure 1).

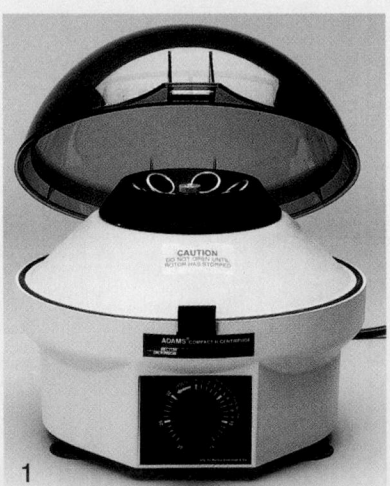

1

(From Stepp CA, Woods MA: *Laboratory procedures for medical office personnel*, Philadelphia, 1998, Saunders.)

5. Place another tube containing 10 mL of urine or water in the opposite cup.
   PURPOSE: For proper operation, centrifuges must be carefully balanced. If not properly balanced, damage to the instrument can occur.
6. Secure the lid and centrifuge for 5 minutes or for the time specified for your instrument.

PROCEDURE 45-6 —continued

PURPOSE: Timing varies according to the speed and the size of the centrifuge head.

7. Remove the tube from the centrifuge after the instrument has come to a full stop.

8. Pour off the clear supernatant from the top of the specimen by inverting the centrifuge tube over the sink drain while allowing the running water from the faucet to flush the urine down. Turn the tube upright when the supernatant has been decanted, allowing a small amount to return to the sediment on the bottom of the tube without losing sediment down the drain (Figures 2 and 3).
PURPOSE: The sediment will be examined under the microscope.

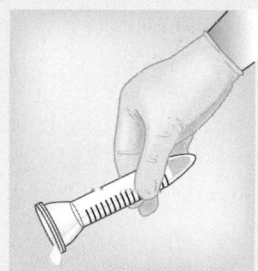

2

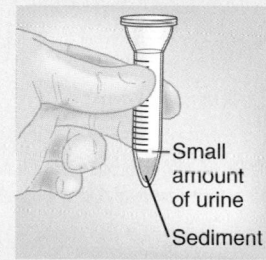

3

Small amount of urine

Sediment

9. Thoroughly mix the sediment with a drop of Sedi-Stain by grasping the tube near the top and rapidly flicking it with the fingers of the other hand until all sediment is thoroughly resuspended.
PURPOSE: Elements centrifuge at different rates. Failure to mix the entire sediment completely results in quantification errors. Sedi-Stain colors the sediment for easier viewing.

10. Transfer 1 drop of sediment to a clean, labeled slide using a clean, disposable transfer pipet.

11. Place a clean coverslip over the drop and place the slide on the microscope stage. Remove face protection.

Note: **The remaining steps typically are performed by the trained healthcare provider.**

1. Focus under low power and reduce the light.
PURPOSE: Mucus and casts are easily missed if reduced light is not used. Constant focusing helps locate them.

2. First, scan the entire coverslip for abnormal findings.
PURPOSE: Casts tend to migrate to the edges of the coverslips.

3. Examine five low-power fields. Count and classify each type of cast seen, if any, and note mucus if present.
PURPOSE: Choose five fields so that one is selected from each corner of the coverslip and the last one is chosen from the middle of the coverslip. If you move to an area and nothing is there, record a zero.

4. Switch to high-power magnification and adjust the light.
PURPOSE: As magnification increases, more light is needed.

5. In five high-power fields, count the following elements: red blood cells, white blood cells, and round, transitional, and squamous epithelial cells.

6. In the same five fields, report the following as few, moderate, or many: crystals (identify and report each type seen separately), bacteria (identify as rods or cocci), sperm, yeast, and parasites.
PURPOSE: "Few," "moderate," and "many" are more easily and universally understood than are exact numbers.

7. Average the five fields and report the results.

8. Disinfect work area and remove gloves. Dispose of them and contaminated materials in the biohazard waste container. Remove lab coat and sanitize your hands.

9. Document the results in the patient's record.
PURPOSE: A procedure is not considered finished until it is recorded.

Microscopic Examination of Urine

The examination of urine is not categorized as CLIA waived; therefore, it cannot be performed by a medical assistant without additional training and rigid compliance with CLIA quality assurance protocols for the laboratory, including periodic proficiency testing.

The three main categories of microscopic findings are casts, cells, and crystals.

Casts

Casts are formed when protein accumulates and precipitates in the kidney tubules and is washed into the urine. The protein takes on the size and shape of the tubules; hence the term *casts*. Casts are cylindric, with flat or rounded ends, and are classified according to the substances observed in them. Certain types of casts are associated with renal pathologic conditions; others are physiologic and are generally caused by strenuous exercise. Because casts dissolve in alkaline urine on standing, examination of a fresh urine specimen is very important.

Hyaline casts are pale, transparent, cylindric structures that have rounded ends and parallel sides (Figure 45-10). Hyaline casts will be missed entirely if the light is not reduced at the condenser. They are formed when urine flow through individual nephrons is diminished.

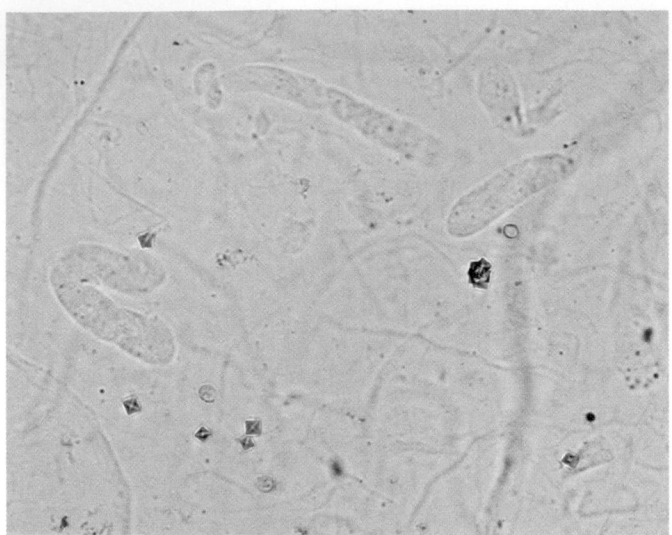

FIGURE 45-10 Hyaline casts. (Brightfield; ×200.) (From Brunzel NA: *Fundamentals of urine and body fluid analysis,* ed 3, Philadelphia, 2013, Saunders.)

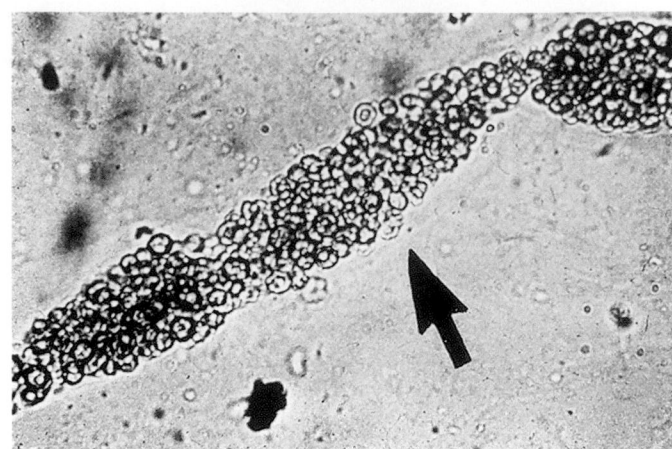

FIGURE 45-12 Red blood cell casts. (From Stepp CA, Woods MA: *Laboratory procedures for medical office personnel,* Philadelphia, 1998, Saunders.)

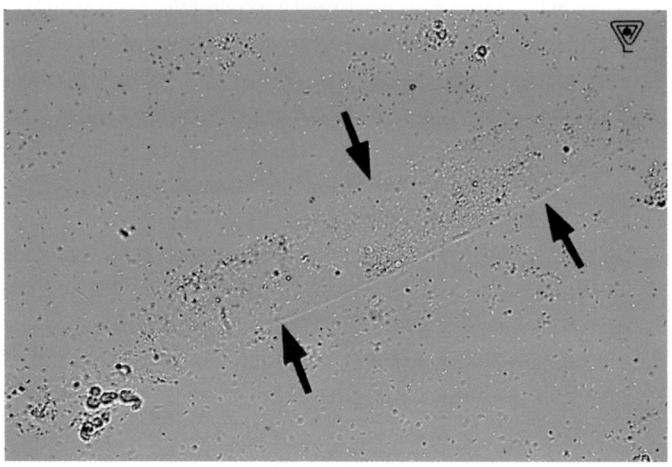

FIGURE 45-11 White blood cell casts. (From Stepp CA, Woods MA: *Laboratory procedures for medical office personnel,* Philadelphia, 1998, Saunders.)

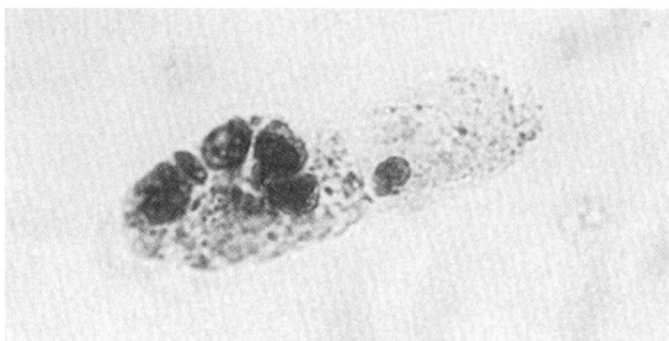

FIGURE 45-13 Renal tubular cell cast, seen with brightfield microscopy. (Sedi-Stain; ×400.) (From Brunzel NA: *Fundamentals of urine and body fluid analysis,* ed 2, St Louis, 2004, Saunders.)

They can be found in the urine of individuals with kidney disease, but also in the urine of people without such disease who have exercised heavily. Occasionally, hyaline casts have granular or cellular inclusions.

White blood cell casts are hyaline casts that contain leukocytes. White blood cells usually have a multilobed nucleus; this differentiates them from renal tubular epithelial cells, which have single, round nuclei. White blood cell casts are seen in pyelonephritis (Figure 45-11).

Red blood cell casts always indicate a pathologic condition and are highly diagnostic. These casts occur in **glomerulonephritis**. They are hyaline casts with embedded red cells, and their presence indicates damage to the glomerular membrane. They may appear brown as a result of the color of the red blood cells present (Figure 45-12).

Renal tubular epithelial cell casts contain embedded renal tubular epithelial cells. These casts are easily confused with white blood cell casts, particularly if the cells have started to degenerate. Renal tubular epithelial cell casts are found when excessive damage has occurred in the kidney. Causes are shock, renal ischemia, heavy-metal poisoning, certain allergic reactions, and nephrotoxic drugs (Figure 45-13).

Finely and coarsely granular casts may indicate renal disease. On close examination, granular casts show a hyaline matrix with coarse or fine granular inclusions. The granules are thought to be caused by protein aggregation or degeneration of cellular inclusions (Figure 45-14).

Waxy casts are rarely seen. They appear as glassy, brittle, smooth, homogeneous structures. They usually are yellowish, have cracks or fissures, and have squared or broken ends. They are considered to be degenerated cellular casts and are found in individuals with severe renal disease (Figure 45-15).

Occasionally more than one type of cell is found in a single cast. Mixed cellular casts have been reported, and absolute identification of the cell types present may be difficult.

Cells

Cells found in the urine include epithelial cells, which are derived from the lining of the genitourinary tract. Red blood cells and white

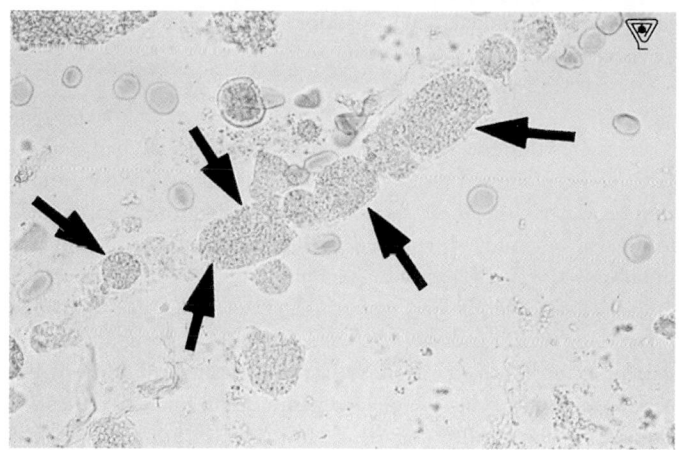

FIGURE 45-14 Granular casts. (From Stepp CA, Woods MA: *Laboratory procedures for medical office personnel,* Philadelphia, 1998, Saunders.)

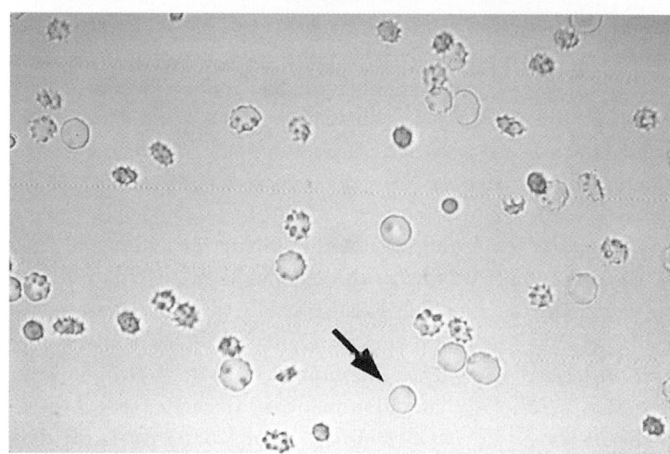

FIGURE 45-16 Red blood cells in the urine. (From Stepp CA, Woods MA: *Laboratory procedures for medical office personnel,* Philadelphia, 1998, Saunders.)

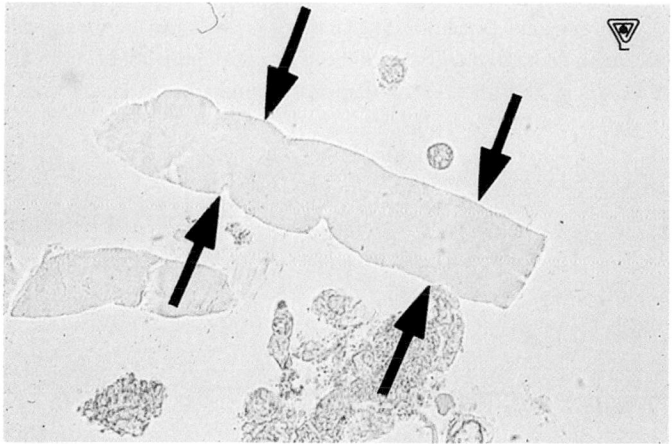

FIGURE 45-15 Waxy casts. (From Stepp CA, Woods MA: *Laboratory procedures for medical office personnel,* Philadelphia, 1998, Saunders.)

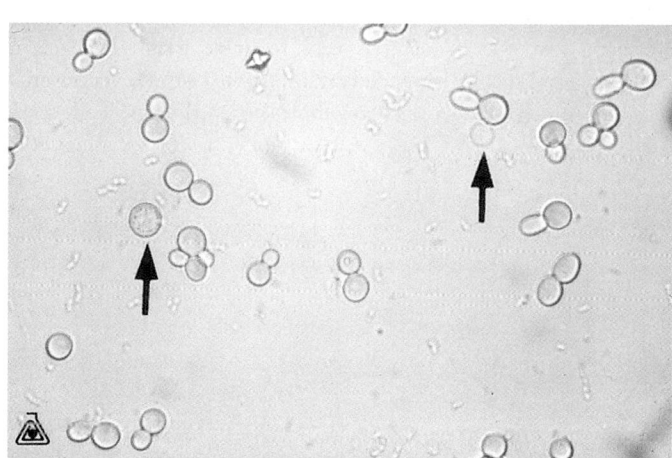

FIGURE 45-17 Yeast in the urine. (From Stepp CA, Woods MA: *Laboratory procedures for medical office personnel,* Philadelphia, 1998, Saunders.)

blood cells are derived from the bloodstream. Cells are classified and counted under high-power magnification.

Red blood cells may enter the urinary tract at any point of inflammation or injury. They may be found in normal urine in small numbers. Persistent hematuria should be investigated. Red blood cells are pale, round, nongranular, and flat or biconcave (Figure 45-16). They are smaller than white blood cells and have no nucleus. In *hypotonic* (dilute) urine, they swell and burst. In *hypertonic* (concentrated) urine, they may **crenate** and wrinkle.

Yeast cells in the urine may indicate vaginal contamination or infection of the urine with yeast (Figure 45-17). Yeast is common in the urine of patients with diabetes. Yeasts are easily confused with red blood cells; they usually are oval and may show budding.

White blood cells, also called *leukocytes,* occasionally may be found in normal urine, but increased numbers are associated with a UTI or with vaginal contamination of the specimen during collection. White blood cells are larger than red blood cells, have a granular appearance, and usually have a multilobed nucleus, although nuclear detail may not be evident. Most white blood cells in the urine are neutrophils (Figure 45-18).

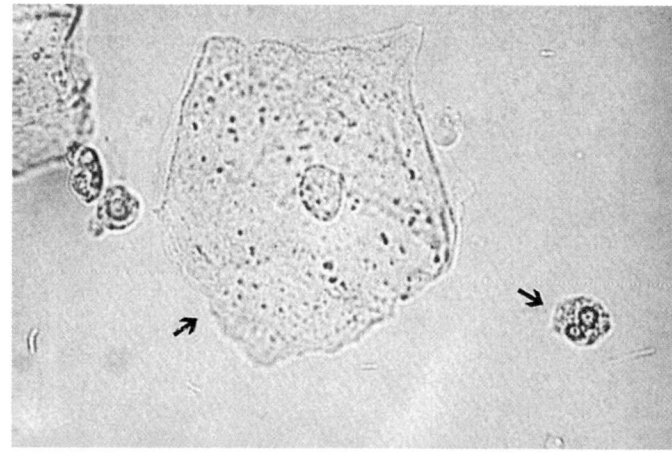

FIGURE 45-18 A large squamous epithelial cell *(left arrow)* and a white blood cell *(right arrow).* (Unstained; ×640.) (From Ringsrud KM, Linne JJ: *Urinalysis and body fluids: a color text and atlas,* St Louis, 1995, Mosby.)

Squamous epithelial cells line the lower portion of the genitourinary tract. When present in large numbers in female patients, they usually indicate vaginal contamination. Squamous epithelial cells are large, flat, irregular cells. They have a single, small, round, centrally located nucleus and often occur in sheets or clumps. Because of their flat nature, the edges of the cells often are rolled or folded (see Figure 45-18).

Transitional epithelial cells line the urinary tract from the renal pelvis to the upper portion of the urethra. They vary from slightly larger than a round epithelial cell to smaller than a squamous epithelial cell. They are round or oval and may have a tail. Occasionally, two nuclei are seen. When transitional cells are present in large numbers, a pathologic condition may exist (Figure 45-19).

Renal tubular or round epithelial cells are somewhat larger than white blood cells, are round or oval, and have a nucleus that is single, large, oval, and sometimes eccentric. A few may be found in normal urine specimens, but their presence in increased numbers indicates tubular damage (Figure 45-20).

To describe epithelial cells, it is helpful to remember the appearance of eggs: Squamous cells resemble fried eggs with a large nuclear "yolk" surrounded by the runny whites; transitional cells are much smaller and resemble poached eggs; and renal tubular round epithelial cells resemble hard-boiled eggs that have been cut in half.

Crystals

Crystals are common in urine specimens, particularly if the specimen has been allowed to cool. Cooling causes solid crystals to precipitate out of the urine, which changes the urine's appearance from clear to cloudy. The presence of most crystals is not clinically significant unless the crystals are found in large numbers. With only very rare exceptions, abnormal crystals are seen in acidic urine. Abnormal crystals may be of metabolic origin and are present because of certain disease states or an inherited metabolic condition, or they may be of **iatrogenic** origin and are present as a result of medication or treatment. Identification of crystals begins with determination of the pH of the urine to ascertain whether the sample is acidic or alkaline. Next, the color, shape, and refractivity are observed. Often a history of medication intake and recent diagnostic testing is helpful.

Crystals are reported as *occasional, few, moderate,* or *many* per high-power field (Table 45-5). At times crystals can be *amorphous* (lacking a defined shape). Amorphous urates (Figure 45-21) are salts of uric acid and are seen as shapeless granulation in acidic urine.

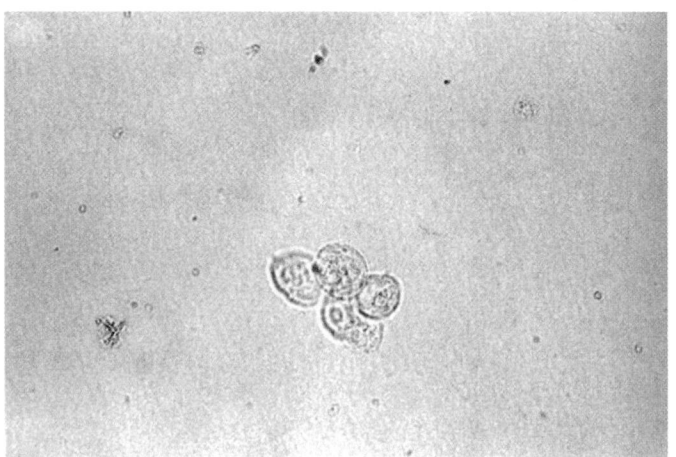

FIGURE 45-19 Cluster of small, unstained transitional epithelial cells. (×400.) (From Ringsrud KM, Linne JJ: *Urinalysis and body fluids: a color text and atlas,* St Louis, 1995, Mosby.)

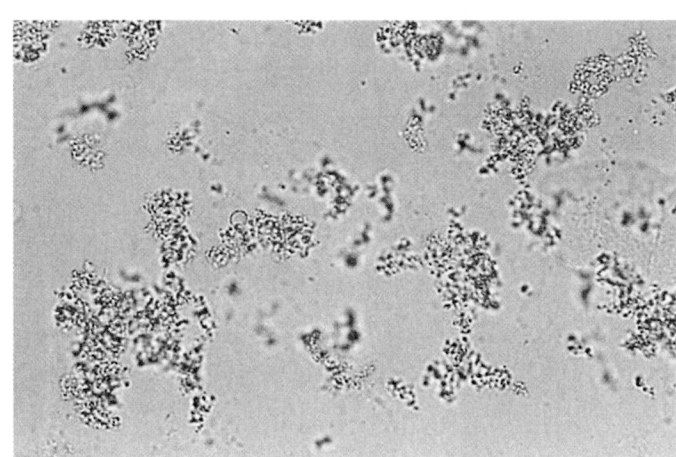

FIGURE 45-21 Amorphous urates. (×400.) (From Ringsrud KM, Linne JJ: *Urinalysis and body fluids: a color text and atlas,* St Louis, 1995, Mosby.)

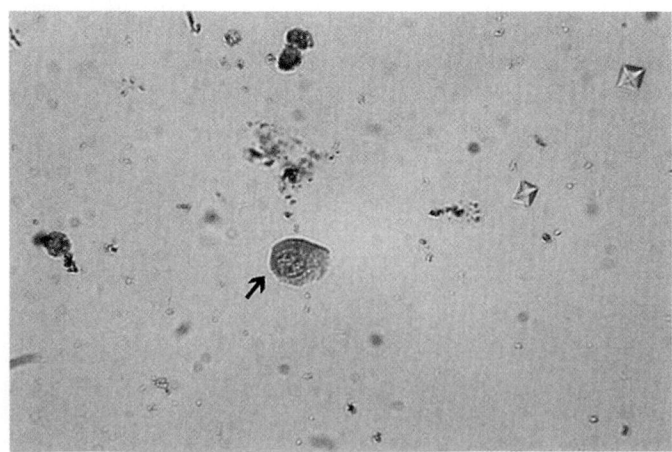

FIGURE 45-20 Renal epithelial cell *(arrow).* (Sedi-Stain; ×400.) (From Ringsrud KM, Linne JJ: *Urinalysis and body fluids: a color text and atlas,* St Louis, 1995, Mosby.)

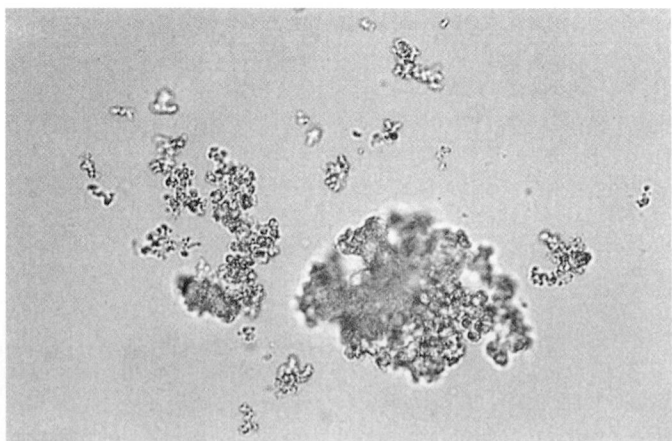

FIGURE 45-22 Amorphous phosphates. (×400.) (From Ringsrud KM, Linne JJ: *Urinalysis and body fluids: a color text and atlas,* St Louis, 1995, Mosby.)

TABLE 45-5 Normal and Abnormal Crystals Found in the Urine

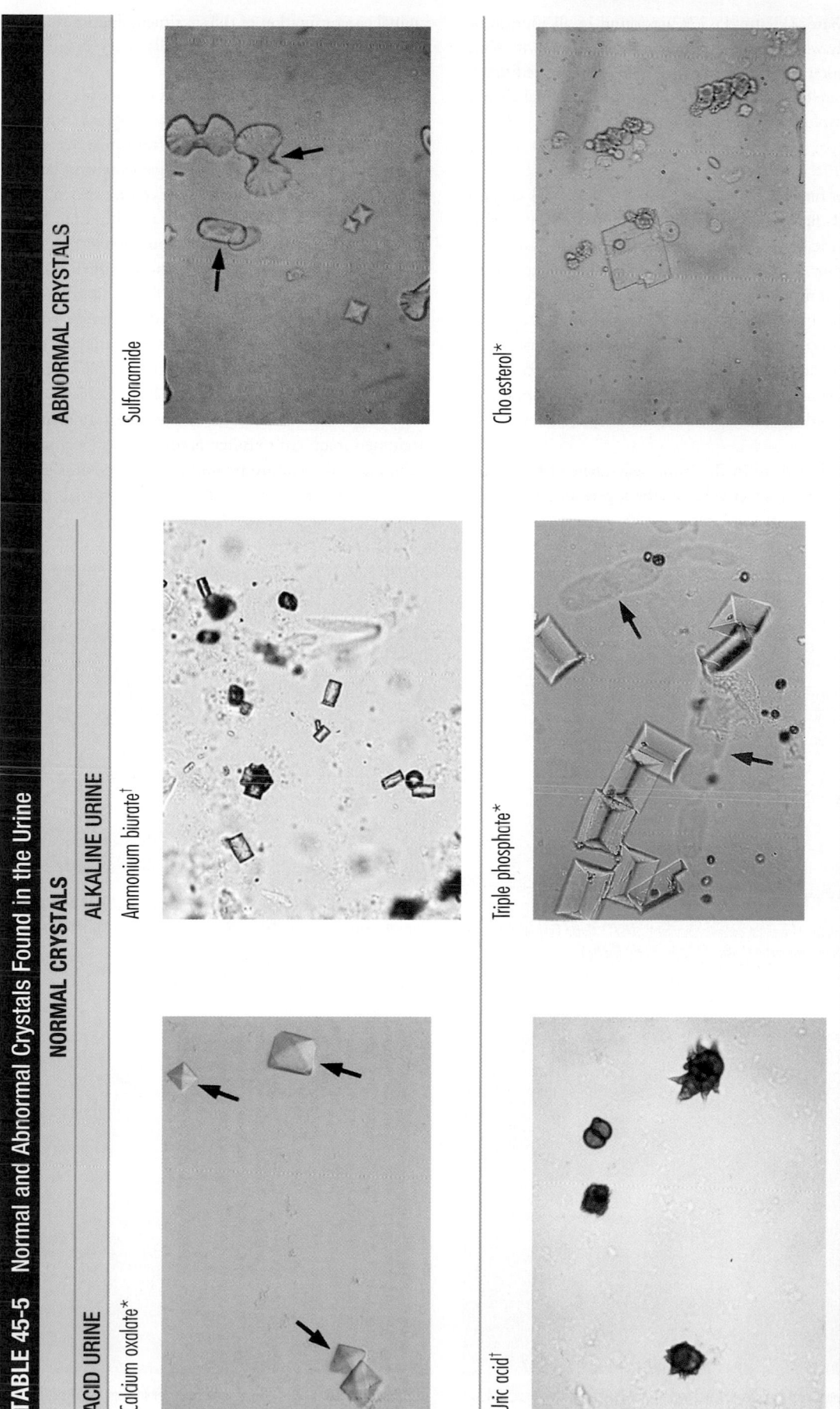

NORMAL CRYSTALS

ABNORMAL CRYSTALS

ACID URINE

ALKALINE URINE

Calcium oxalate*

Ammonium biurate†

Sulfonamide

Uric acid†

Triple phosphate*

Cholesterol*

*From Stepp CA, Woods MA: *Laboratory procedures for medical office personnel,* Philadelphia, 1998, Saunders.
†From Brunzel NA: *Fundamentals of urine and body fluid analysis,* ed 3, Philadelphia, 2013, Saunders.

Amorphous phosphates (Figure 45-22) are found in alkaline urine and are seen as fluffy white precipitate. Amorphous crystals often are so profuse they obscure other formed elements in the sediment. Frequently crystals are difficult to identify without additional chemical testing, such as solubility testing in acid and base.

Miscellaneous Findings

Oval fat bodies are formed when renal tubular epithelial cells or macrophages absorb fats. The fat droplets in the cells vary in size. They are characteristic of kidney distress (Figure 45-23).

A few *bacteria* may be found in normal urine specimens. Heavy bacterial concentrations in the absence of white blood cells may indicate that the specimen was allowed to sit at room temperature and the bacteria multiplied. Urine specimens with a putrid odor, numerous white blood cells, and bacteria (Figure 45-24) are common in UTIs. The bacteria may be bacilli (rod shaped) or cocci (spherical) and are seen under high-power magnification. They are often motile (moving).

Spermatozoa can be found in the urine specimens of both male and female patients. In the latter case, their presence represents vaginal contamination of the specimen. Sperm usually have pointed, oval heads and long, threadlike tails. They may be motile in fresh urine.

Trichomonas vaginalis is the most commonly encountered parasite in urine (Figure 45-25). It is usually a vaginal contaminant but may also be found in urine specimens from male patients. When urine is fresh and warm, *Trichomonas* organisms may be motile and may dart about rapidly when seen under the microscope. *Trichomonas* organisms are pear-shaped protozoa with four flagella. They are larger than round epithelial cells but smaller than squamous cells. *Trichomonas* organisms die when the specimen is cooled.

Mucous threads can be found in most urine specimens. They appear as pale, irregular, threadlike structures with tapered ends. Beginners often confuse hyaline casts with mucous threads. Increased numbers are seen with inflammation and in specimens contaminated with vaginal secretions (Figure 45-26).

Artifacts and contaminants often are found in urine sediment. Training is required to differentiate them. Fibers are common in the sediment and come from clothing, diapers, or digested plant material. Clothing fibers often are long and twisted and sometimes are

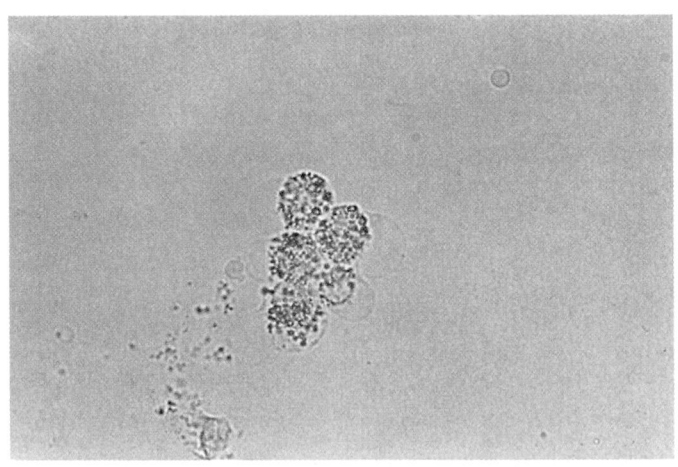

FIGURE 45-23 Small cluster of oval fat bodies. (Unstained; ×400.) (From Ringsrud KM, Linne JJ: *Urinalysis and body fluids: a color text and atlas,* St Louis, 1995, Mosby.)

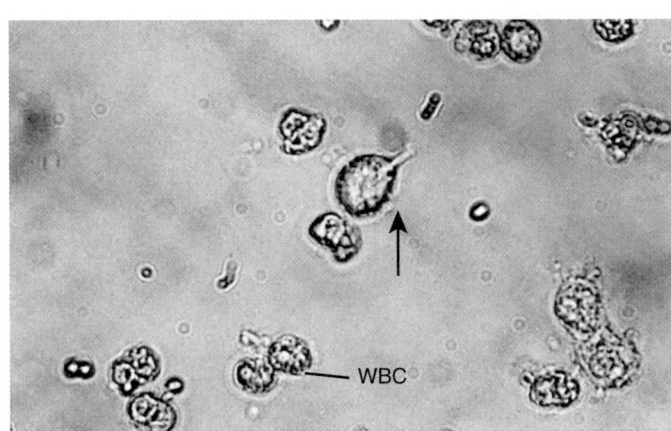

FIGURE 45-25 *Trichomonas* organisms *(arrow)* in the urine. (From Stepp CA, Woods MA: *Laboratory procedures for medical office personnel,* Philadelphia, 1998, Saunders.)

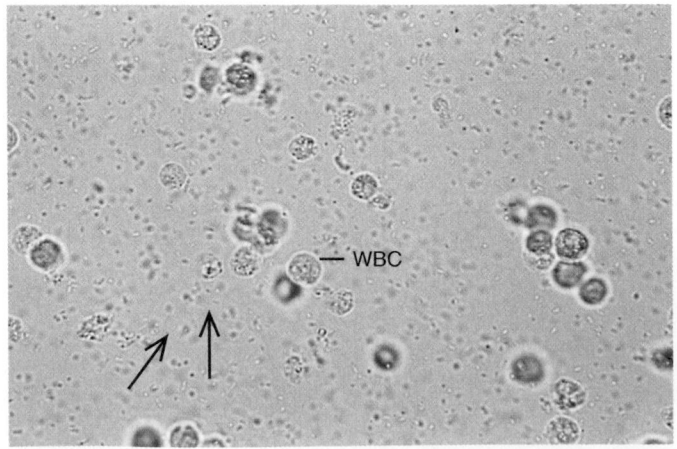

FIGURE 45-24 Numerous small bacteria *(arrows)* and white cells (WBC). (Unstained; ×400.) (From Ringsrud KM, Linne JJ: *Urinalysis and body fluids: a color text and atlas,* St Louis, 1995, Mosby.)

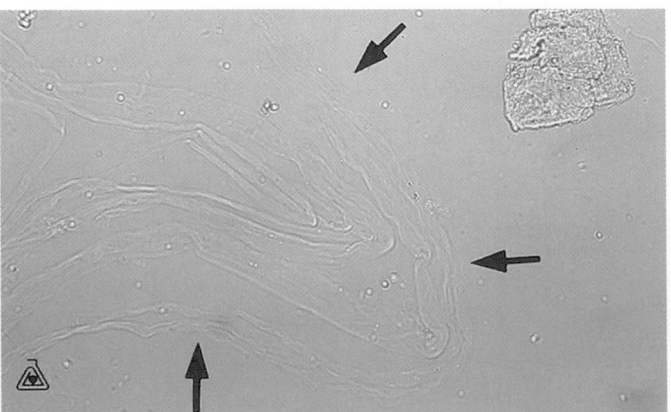

FIGURE 45-26 Mucous threads in the urine. (From Stepp CA, Woods MA: *Laboratory procedures for medical office personnel,* Philadelphia, 1998, Saunders.)

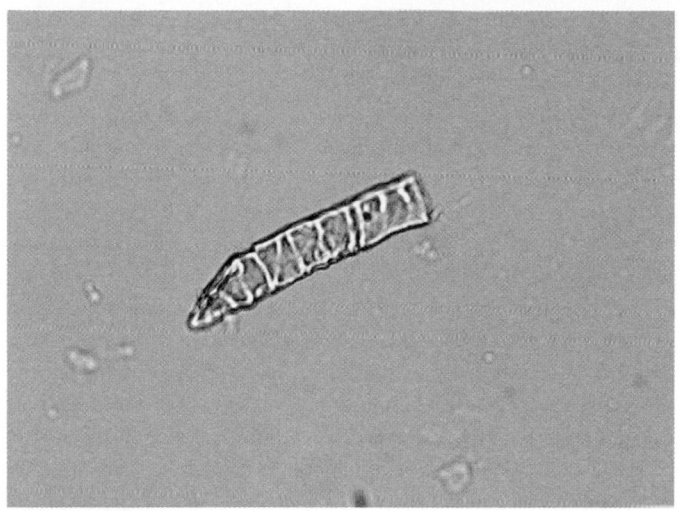

FIGURE 45-27 Diaper fibers. (From Brunzel NA: *Fundamentals of urine and body fluid analysis,* ed 3, Philadelphia, 2013, Saunders.)

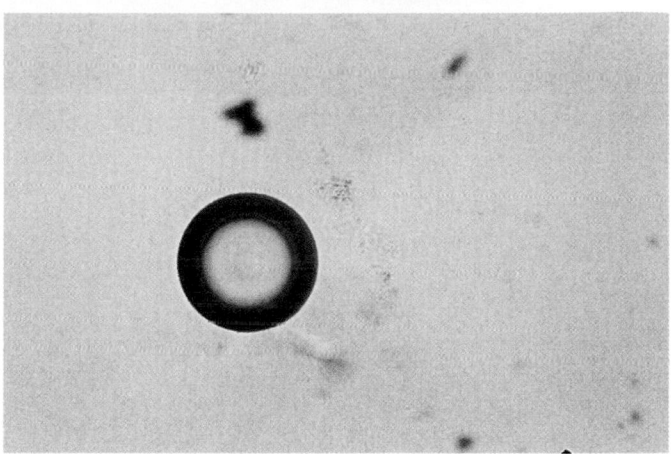

FIGURE 45-30 Large air bubble. (×400.) (From Ringsrud KM, Linne JJ: *Urinalysis and body fluids: a color text and atlas,* St Louis, 1995, Mosby.)

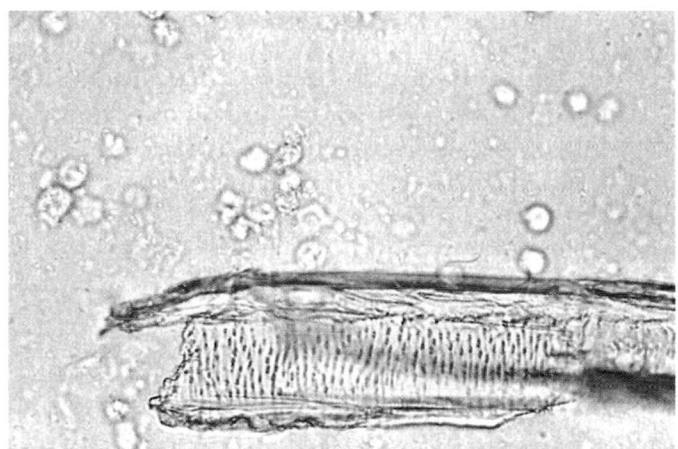

FIGURE 45-28 Plant fiber from fecal contamination; cells and bacteria also are present. (×400.) (From Ringsrud KM, Linne JJ: *Urinalysis and body fluids: a color text and atlas,* St Louis, 1995, Mosby.)

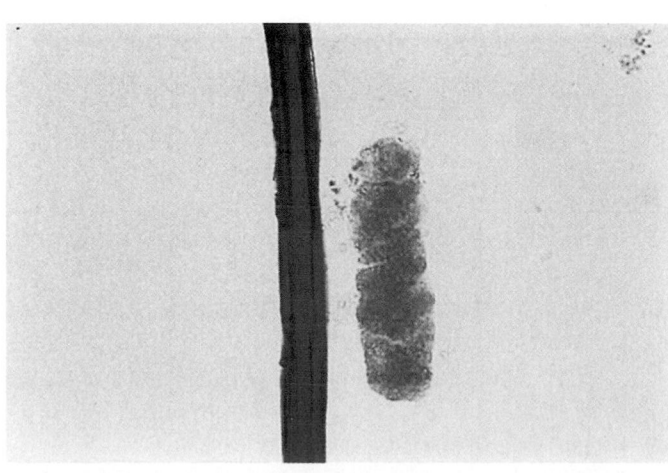

FIGURE 45-29 Fiber, probably hair *(left),* waxy cast *(right).* (Sedi-Stain; ×400.) (From Ringsrud KM, Linne JJ: *Urinalysis and body fluids: a color text and atlas,* St Louis, 1995, Mosby.)

colored. Diaper fibers can be confused with casts (Figure 45-27). Plant fibers appear in the urine as a result of fecal contamination (Figure 45-28). Hair is distinguishable not only because of the visible rough and fragmented cuticle, but also because of the size (Figure 45-29). Air bubbles are common if the coverslip was improperly placed over the sediment. Air bubbles are structureless and refractile (refracting light causing a glow) and have a dark outline (Figure 45-30).

Interpretation of the Microscopic Examination

The medical assistant should understand how the microscopic findings of the sediment are reported. First, the sediment is examined under the low-power objective and low light to locate casts, which generally are found around the edges of the coverslip. Ten to 15 low-power fields are scanned, and the number of casts is counted and reported. The high-power objective and increased light then are used to identify red and white blood cells, epithelial cells, yeasts, bacteria, and crystals. From 10 to 15 high-powered fields should be scanned and the number counted, averaged, and reported. The method of counting varies considerably among laboratories. It is important that all workers in the same laboratory use the same counting and reporting systems. The results of the microscopic examination are reported as follows:

1. The numbers for each element are counted, then averaged. Casts, white blood cells, red blood cells, and the three categories of epithelial cells are counted, totaled, and averaged. Casts, white blood cells, and red blood cells are reported using numeric ranges based on the average:

   0
   0-1
   1-2
   2-5
   5-10
   10-20 and so forth
   TNTC: too numerous to count

Epithelial cells are reported as occasional, few, moderate, or many, as follows:

0	
0-3	Occasional
3-6	Few
6-12	Moderate
≥12	Many

2. The remaining elements are estimated as *occasional, few, moderate,* or *many,* as follows:

Occasional	Not seen in every field
Few	Covers less than a quarter of the field
Moderate	Covers approximately half of the field
Many	Covers the entire field

CRITICAL THINKING APPLICATION   **45-5**

After centrifuging the three urine specimens, Rosa prepares the slides for microscopic examination by a physician. She has learned to correlate the findings from the physician's microscopic findings with the chemical examinations she has already performed on these specimens. She reviews the final results and notes that Mr. Parks's and Mrs. Carpenter's specimens were clear and they had no abnormal microscopic results. Ms. Hillman's specimen was turbid, and Rosa's chemical results showed an alkaline pH, an elevated nitrite level, and an elevated leukocyte esterase reading. What would be the likely microscopic findings for Ms. Hillman's urine?

Additional Tests Performed on Urine
Clinitest

The glucose test on the reagent strip detects only glucose, the most common sugar found in the urine. However, sugars other than glucose also can appear in the urine. Certain metabolic disorders can result in the excretion of sugars such as galactose, fructose, lactose, maltose, or pentose. Galactosemia, a rare pathologic condition, is a congenital deficiency in the body's ability to metabolize galactose to glucose; galactosemia results in excretion of galactose in the urine. Seen in infants, it results in failure to thrive, vomiting, and diarrhea. If detected early, galactose can be eliminated from the diet, and the child develops normally. Lactose may be found in the urine of pregnant women or premature infants. Maltose may be excreted in patients with diabetes. Of the many sugars, only the presence of glucose or galactose signifies possible pathologic conditions.

The **Clinitest**, which is based on the chemical reduction of copper, is commonly used to screen for and confirm glucose and/or to detect other sugars (e.g., galactose in infants) (Procedure 45-7). Copper reduction tests are based on the principle that reducing substances can chemically convert cupric sulfate to cuprous oxide, resulting in a color change. A sugar's reducing ability is determined by the presence of a "chemical reducing group" present in all simple sugars (monosaccharides). The Clinitest tablet is dropped directly into a test tube containing diluted urine. A heat-releasing reaction occurs, and the color of the tube's contents is observed during and after the boiling stops. It is compared with a chart provided by the manufacturer. *Note:* If the color change shows a pass-through that reaches the orange maximum color during the reaction and then ends in a lower color range, the test result is reported as "greater than" the highest positive result.

PROCEDURE 45-7	**Obtain a Specimen and Perform a CLIA-Waived Urinalysis: Test Urine for Glucose Using the Clinitest Method**

Goal: *To perform confirmatory testing for glucose and other simple sugars in the urine using the Clinitest procedure for reducing substances.*

EQUIPMENT and SUPPLIES

- Patient's record
- Urine specimen
- Clinitest tablet, tube, and dropper
- Distilled water
- Test tube rack
- Color chart
- Timer
- Fluid-impermeable lab coat and disposable gloves
- Biohazard waste container

PROCEDURAL STEPS

1. Sanitize your hands. Put on the fluid-impermeable lab coat and disposable gloves.
2. Holding a Clinitest dropper vertically, add 10 drops of distilled water and then 5 drops of urine to a Clinitest tube.
   PURPOSE: Holding the dropper vertically prevents alteration of the size of the drops.
3. Place the prepared tube in the rack (Figure 1).
   PURPOSE: The tube will become too hot to hold after the tablet is placed in the tube.

PROCEDURE 45-7   *—continued*

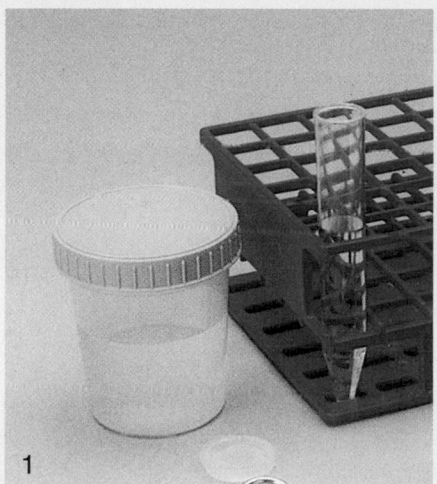

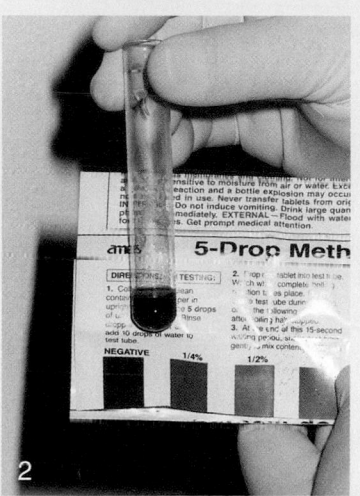

4. Remove a Clinitest tablet from the bottle by shaking a tablet into the bottle cap. (First, make sure your hands are dry and gloved.)
   PURPOSE: Clinitest tablets react with moisture and became caustic. Handling tablets with moist hands could result in hydroxide burns.

5. Tap the tablet into the test tube and recap the container.

6. Observe the entire reaction to detect the rapid pass-through phenomenon, which indicates that the glucose level in the urine is very high (see Note in step 8).
   PURPOSE: If pass-through occurs but is not detected, the reading will be falsely low.

7. When boiling stops, time exactly 15 seconds and then gently shake the tube to mix the entire contents.

8. Immediately compare the color of the specimen with the five-drop color chart and record your findings (Figure 2).

Note: If an orange color briefly develops during the reaction and then converts to a lower, darker color, rapid pass-through has occurred, meaning that the glucose was greater than the highest reading; this is recorded as "greater than 2%."
   PURPOSE: For accurate results, time carefully because all the final color results continue to darken over time.

9. Record the results.

10. Clean up the work area, remove your gloves and fluid-impermeable lab coat, and sanitize your hands.
    PURPOSE: To ensure infection control.

11. Record the results in the patient's record.
    PURPOSE: A procedure is not considered finished until it is recorded.

Urine Pregnancy Testing

All pregnancy tests detect the presence of **human chorionic gonadotropin (hCG)**, a hormone produced by the placenta and present in urine during pregnancy (Procedure 45-8). After the fertilized egg has implanted in the uterus, the hCG levels in serum double every few days. This rapid rise occurs for approximately 7 weeks, and then the level begins to decline. Within 72 hours of delivery, the hormone disappears.

The most common type of test for pregnancy is the lateral flow immunoassay test. Many brands are available for laboratory use and are also available over the counter for home use. These tests can be sensitive enough to detect the presence of hCG as early as 1 week after implantation or 4 to 5 days before a missed menstrual period. The tests can be performed in as little as 5 minutes, and the results are easy to interpret; usually as easy as reading a color change. For optimum results, the test should be performed on the first morning voided specimen because of its higher concentration.

The test is based on reactions that occur between antibodies and antigens. Antibodies are proteins formed in response to antigens; the antibody is specific for the antigen (e.g., as with a lock and key). When antibodies and antigens come in contact, the antibody binds to the antigen, as long as the two are present in sufficient quantity.

The pregnancy test cartridge contains a membrane with an absorbent pad. The urine sample is introduced into the device and wicks through the absorbent pad, reaching the chromatographic (color producing) membrane that will change color in two areas. In a positive sample, the hCG antigen attaches to the antibodies in the test zone (T) forming a pink line. All samples (positive or negative) cause the control zone (C) line to turn blue. The presence of this line indicates that the test has been carried out correctly. If the C control zone does not show a color reaction, the test is considered invalid and must be repeated using another test device. The QuickVue test (see Procedure 45-8) is a lateral flow pregnancy test that can be performed on urine. It is used routinely in many POLs.

PROCEDURE 45-8   Obtain a Specimen and Perform a CLIA-Waived Urinalysis: Perform a Pregnancy Test

Goal: *To perform a pregnancy test on urine using the QuickVue pregnancy test method.*

EQUIPMENT and SUPPLIES

- Patient's record
- Urine specimen
- QuickVue test kit
- Fluid-impermeable lab coat and disposable gloves
- Biohazard waste container

PROCEDURAL STEPS

1. Sanitize your hands. Put on the fluid-impermeable lab coat and disposable gloves.
2. Prepare the testing equipment (Figure 1).

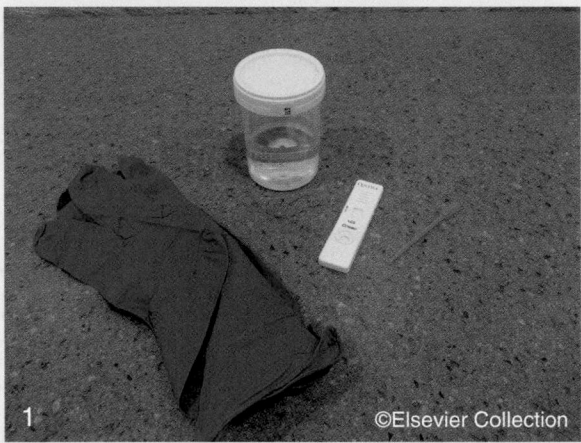

©Elsevier Collection

3. Collect the specimen (preferably a first morning specimen).
4. Remove the test cassette from the foil pouch.
5. Add 3 drops of urine using the pipet (dropper) that accompanies the kit (Figure 2).
   PURPOSE: To ensure accurate test results, the specimen amount must be exact.

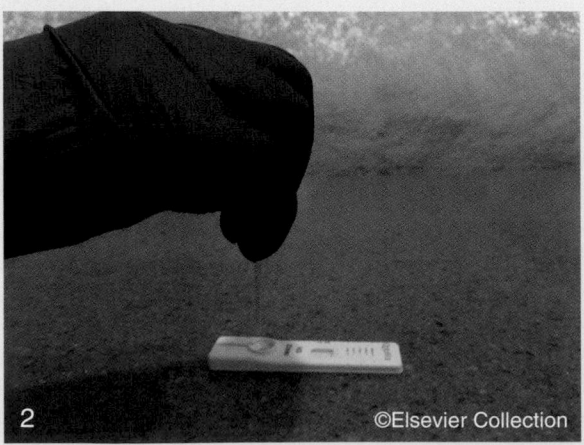

©Elsevier Collection

6. Dispose of the pipet in a biohazard container.
7. Wait 3 minutes and read the test results.
   PURPOSE: To ensure accurate test results, timing must be exact.
8. Interpret the results as:
   - (Figure 3).
   - *Negative:* A blue control line is next to the letter C; no line is seen next to the letter T. (See results below on the left)
   - *Positive:* A blue control line is next to the letter C; a pink line is next to the letter T. (See results below on the right)
   - *Invalid:* If a blue line does not appear in the C area, the test is invalid and the specimen must be retested using another kit. Check the expiration date of the kit before proceeding.

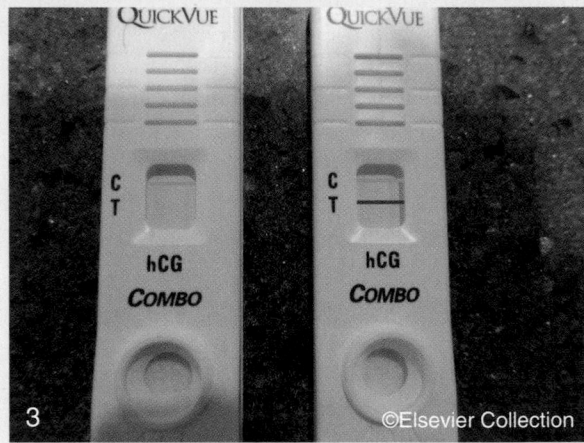

©Elsevier Collection

9. Discard the cassette in the biohazard waste container, remove and discard gloves in the biohazard waste container, then remove lab coat, and sanitize your hands.
   PURPOSE: To ensure infection control.
10. Record the results in the patient's record as either positive or negative for pregnancy.
    PURPOSE: A procedure is not considered finished until it is recorded.

10/2/20 — 3:45 PM: Last menstrual period (LMP) 9/16/20 —. QuickVue pregnancy test: Positive. Rosa Gonzales, CMA (AAMA)

Ovulation Testing

CLIA-waived lateral flow urine tests are available to assist in the prediction of ovulation for women attempting to conceive either naturally or using artificial insemination. During the menstrual cycle, luteinizing hormone (LH) remains at a relatively stable level. Approximately 14 days before menstruation, the body experiences the "LH surge," a brief, rapid increase in LH. This surge triggers the release of the ovum from the ovary. Two to 3 days after the surge, the LH level returns to the base level. Conception is most likely to occur within 36 hours after the LH surge. The principle of this test is similar to that of the pregnancy test: the reservoir pad contains anti-LH antibodies. A positive test result indicates a urine LH level of 20 mIU/mL or higher. Testing usually is performed for 5 consecutive days in the middle of the cycle. Once the surge is detected, ovulation can be expected within 2 to 3 days.

Menopause Testing

A woman is said to have reached menopause when menstruation has not occurred for at least 12 months. The time before menopause, called *perimenopause*, can last for years, bringing with it uncomfortable symptoms such as irregular periods, hot flashes, vaginal dryness, and sleep problems. Some of this may be due to an increase in follicle-stimulating hormone (FSH). Levels of FSH, which is produced by the pituitary gland, increase temporarily each month to stimulate the ovaries. When a woman enters menopause, the ovaries stop producing eggs, and the levels of FSH rise. CLIA-waived lateral flow tests detect FSH in the urine. A positive test result indicates that a woman may be in menopause; a negative test result, along with symptoms of menopause, may indicate that a woman is in perimenopause.

The qualitative lateral flow test should never be used to direct a woman to stop using birth control methods if she does not want to conceive because pregnancy is still possible during perimenopause.

URINE TOXICOLOGY

Toxicology is the study of poisonous substances and drugs, and their effects on the body. The clinical laboratory performs testing on body fluids and tissues to monitor the use of therapeutic drugs such as antibiotics, anticonvulsants, antidepressants, and barbiturates. They may also test for poisoning by herbicides, metals, animal toxins, and poisonous gases (e.g., carbon monoxide).

Laboratory testing for illegal drugs or alcohol is also done, most commonly for employment, insurance, or as a legal requirement (Table 45-6). Although blood serum tests are more accurate for determining current impairment or the time of ingestion, urine is the specimen of choice for most routine screening procedures to determine whether an illegal drug is present. For routine screening, a random specimen is usually collected.

Often, the following safeguards are used to ensure that a specimen is fresh and is truly from the patient: water may be temporarily unavailable in the restroom; bluing agents may be added to the toilets; a sealed container with a temperature-sensitive strip may be provided; and someone may accompany the patient into the restroom during the collection. In some cases a strict chain of custody is required; this means that everyone handling the specimen is documented. The substance for which the test is performed, or its

TABLE 45-6 Commonly Abused Drugs and Body Retention Times	
DRUG	**RETENTION TIME**
Alcohol	2-10 hr
Amphetamine	24-48 hr
Methamphetamine	3-5+ days
Barbiturates	
Phenobarbital	2-6 days
Secobarbital	24 hr
Cocaine, cocaine metabolites	12 hr-3 days
Opiates, heroin, morphine	3-4 days
Phencyclidine (PCP)	3-7+ days
Marijuana (tetrahydrocannabinol metabolites)	2 days-11 wk
Oxycodone	3 days

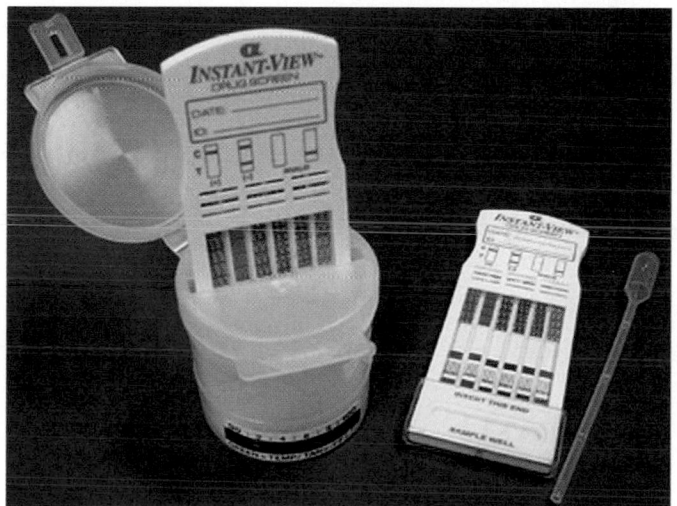

FIGURE 45-31 Instant-View Drug Test. (Courtesy Alfa Scientific, Poway, California.)

metabolite, often remains in urine much longer than the impairment or intoxication lasts. This is one reason urine screening is favored over serum or blood screening.

As a medical assistant, you may be responsible for collecting specimens for toxicology tests and for performing certain tests. Rapid drug screening devices are about the size and shape of a credit card (Figure 45-31). The device is dipped into a urine sample, or urine is directly applied to the device. The results are read according to the manufacturer's instructions in just minutes. Negative results indicate that none of the targeted drugs were detected in the urine sample at specified cutoff levels; inconclusive results indicate that the device reacted with something in the urine and confirmation testing is required.

Urine multidrug screening tests are lateral flow chromatographic immunoassays that test for urine metabolites of a variety of drugs, including amphetamines, barbiturates, benzodiazepines, cocaine, morphine, methadone, phencyclidine (PCP), tricyclic antidepressants, marijuana, Ecstasy, methamphetamines, methadone, oxycodone, and opiates. Available in cartridges that test two to six drugs, the test is a competitive binding immunoassay in which drug and drug metabolites in a urine sample compete with immobilized drug conjugate for antibody binding sites. By using antibodies specific to different drug classes, the test permits independent, simultaneous detection of up to 10 drugs from a single sample in 5 minutes.

In the procedure, urine mixes with a labeled antibody-dye conjugate and migrates along a porous membrane. If the concentration of a given drug is below the detection limit of the test, the antibody-dye conjugate that did not bind to a drug metabolite binds to antigen conjugate immobilized on the membrane, producing a rose-pink band in the appropriate place for that drug. If the level of the drug in the urine is at or above the detection limit, free drug competes with the immobilized antigen conjugate on the membrane by binding to the antibody-dye conjugate, forming an antigen-antibody complex and preventing the development of a rose-pink band (Procedure 45-9).

Note: Unlike with the lateral flow tests for pregnancy, ovulation, and menopause, the appearance of a line in the T band during a drug screening test indicates a negative test result.

PROCEDURE 45-9	Obtain a Specimen and Perform a CLIA-Waived Urinalysis: Perform a Multidrug Screening Test on Urine

Goal: *To screen a urine specimen for drugs or drug metabolites at their specified cutoff levels.*

EQUIPMENT and SUPPLIES

- Patient's record
- Multi-Drug Screen Urine Test in a sealed container
- Freshly voided urine sample
- Timer
- Fluid-impermeable lab coat and disposable gloves
- Biohazard waste container

PROCEDURAL STEPS

1. Sanitize your hands. Put on the fluid-impermeable lab coat and disposable gloves.
2. Assemble the equipment and specimen. Check the expiration date on the test kit.
   <u>PURPOSE:</u> An expired test strip may yield inaccurate results.
3. Determine the temperature of the urine (within 4 minutes of voiding). The temperature should be between 32° and 38° C (90° and 100° F).
   <u>PURPOSE:</u> If the urine temperature is below or above this range, the sample may have been adulterated. Once it has been determined that the sample is at the correct temperature, it may be stored at room temperature for 8 hours or in the refrigerator for up to 3 days before testing.
4. Bring the specimen and the testing device to room temperature.
   <u>PURPOSE:</u> Both the specimen and the device must be at room temperature to ensure accurate results.
5. Remove the device from the foil pouch and label it with the specimen identification.

Dip Method

6. Remove the cap of the specimen and dip the device into the specimen for 10 seconds, making sure the surface of the urine is above the sample well and below the arrowheads in the window (Figure 1).
   <u>PURPOSE:</u> The pads must be saturated with urine.

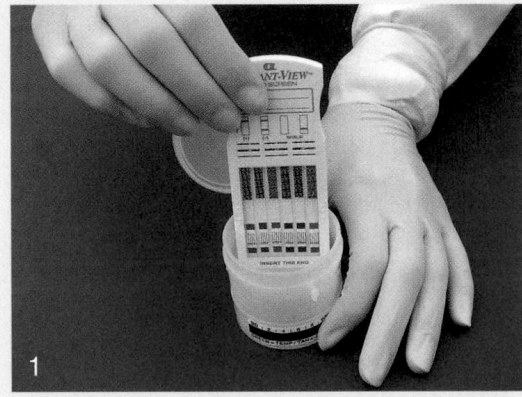

(Courtesy Alfa Scientific, Poway, Calif.)

Alternate Method

7. Remove the pipet from the pouch, and fill it to the line on the barrel with urine. Dispense the entire volume onto the sample well on the testing device (Figure 2).
   <u>PURPOSE:</u> If insufficient urine is available in the cup to use the dip method, this method applies urine to the device.

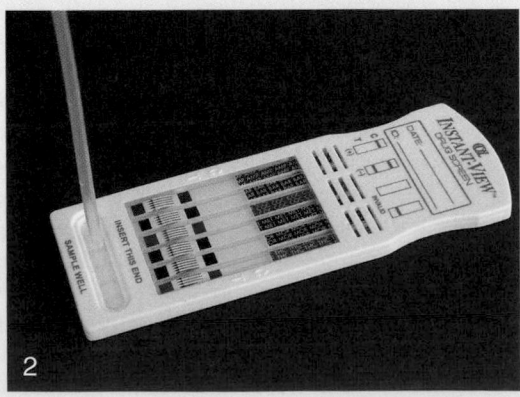

(Courtesy Alfa Scientific, Poway, Calif.)

PROCEDURE 45-9 *—continued*

8. Recap the urine specimen.
9. Set the timer for the designated time: 4 to 7 minutes. Do not read the results until after 7 minutes.
   PURPOSE: Correct timing is essential for reliable, accurate results.
10. Interpret the results (Figure 3):
    - *Positive:* If the C line appears but the T line does not, the result is positive for that drug.
    - *Negative:* If both the C line and the T line appear, the level of the drug or its metabolites is below the cutoff level (i.e., negative for that drug).
    - *Invalid:* If no C line develops within 5 minutes on any test strip, the assay is invalid. Make sure the urine has not been adulterated (see Procedure 45-10) and/or repeat the assay with a new test device.

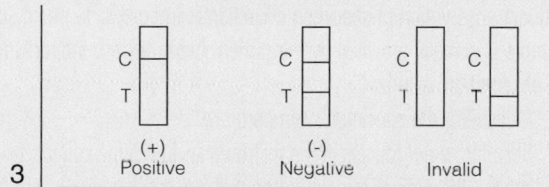

3

(+) Positive   (-) Negative   Invalid

11. Discard the urine and the device in the biohazard container.
12. Disinfect the area. Remove your gloves and dispose in biohazard container. Remove lab coat, and sanitize your hands.
    PURPOSE: To ensure infection control.
13. Record the results in the patient's record.
    PURPOSE: A procedure is not considered complete until it is recorded.

ADULTERATION TESTING AND CHAIN OF CUSTODY

Drug testing has legal ramifications; therefore, additional testing often is necessary to ensure that samples have not been adulterated (Procedure 45-10). Adulteration is the intentional manipulation of a urine sample to allow someone to falsely pass a drug screening test. It may involve using urine from another person or an animal, diluting the sample with water, or adding substances such as bleach, vinegar, eye drops, baking soda, drain openers, soft drinks, or hydrogen peroxide.

Urine collection cups with built-in thermometer panels often are used to ensure that urine has been freshly voided from the bladder. A temperature of 32° to 38° C (90° to 100° F) within 4 minutes of collection is expected. Test strips that detect human immunoglobulins (antibodies) in urine can determine whether the specimen is human in origin and whether it is naturally dilute or has been diluted. Human immunoglobulin G (IgG) is exclusive to humans and is always found at certain levels in urine, even if the urine is naturally dilute. The addition of chemicals to the urine prevents the IgG reaction on the test strip.

Adulteration test strips are also available that detect creatinine, nitrite, pH, specific gravity, glutaraldehyde, and oxidants (see Procedure 45-10).

Creatinine is always present in normal urine because it is excreted from the body at a constant rate. Low or absent levels indicate diluted or substituted nonhuman samples. Urine can be diluted if the person being tested drinks abnormally large amounts of water before the test or if water or another liquid is added to the sample. Creatinine levels usually are checked in conjunction with the specific gravity to screen for dilution or substitution adulteration. Specific gravity readings also determine whether substances such as table salt have been added to the urine.

Nitrites are oxidizing substances that react with the drug or drug metabolite molecules in the urine. Nitrites primarily interfere with antibody binding in lateral flow tests. Nitrates must be added to the urine after voiding. Commercial adulterants (e.g., Whizzies, Klear, and UrineLuck) are tablets or powders that can be added to voided urine. They do not change the color or temperature of the urine. The level of nitrites found in urine with gross bacteriuria or from therapeutic drug metabolites (e.g., nitroglycerin) is below the cutoff for adulteration screening tests.

The *pH* of the sample can affect enzymatic and antibody reactions in lateral flow drug tests. Levels higher than 9.5 or lower than 3 may hamper the enzymatic rate. Alteration of the pH may also affect the stability of the drug or its metabolite. Adulteration of a sample with bleach, drain cleaners, or baking soda changes the pH, but this type of tampering can be detected by an adulteration strip test.

Glutaraldehyde can mask the presence of illegal drugs. Commercially available products such as UrinAid and Clear Choice contain glutaraldehyde intended to adulterate urine. In addition, a 10% solution of glutaraldehyde is sold over the counter for the treatment of warts. This chemical prevents the enzymes in lateral flow tests from reacting properly.

Sensitivity limits for drug screening are set by the U.S. Substance Abuse and Mental Health Services Administration (SAMHSA), the National Institute on Drug Abuse (NIDA), and the U.S. Department of Health and Human Services (DHHS). Positive results on urine samples tested for substances should be confirmed by more specific chemical methods, such as gas chromatography (GC), mass spectrometry (MS), and enzyme-multiplied immunoassay technique (EMIT).

Chain of Custody Rules

1. The individual being tested must provide photo identification.
2. Indirect observation of specimen collection is important to make sure the sample is actually provided by the patient being tested. Indirect methods of observation include:
   - Measuring the specimen's temperature
   - Securing water faucets in the restroom so that urine cannot be diluted
   - Having the patient remove outer clothing and leave personal belongings in the examination room
   - Not allowing water to be run or the toilet to be flushed in the restroom during the collection
   Note: If you suspect the sample has been adulterated, ask the patient to provide another specimen.
3. Within 4 minutes of receiving the specimen, check its temperature (range should be 32° to 38°C [90° to 100°F]) and volume (30 to 45 mL is required), and inspect it for any indications of adulteration (e.g., an unusual color, the presence of foreign materials).
4. Pour the specimen into a specimen bottle and seal the lid with the tamper-evident label/seal provided at the bottom of the chain of custody form with the donor present; include the date and your initials on the label (Figure 45-32).
5. Ship the specimen to the testing laboratory as soon as possible; it must be sent the same day it was collected.
6. Individual results may vary, which can make some results positive at lower substance levels; also, diet, the volume of urine flow, and the amount of substance used can alter results.
7. Because of the legal implications of drug testing, chain of custody must be strictly followed. Each step from collection of the specimen to reporting of test results to the patient must be strictly monitored. Requirements include sealed specimen containers; supervised laboratory analysis throughout the process; and authorized signatures at each step.

PROCEDURE 45-10   Assess a Urine Specimen for Adulteration before Drug Testing

Goal: *To assess a urine specimen for additive adulteration.*

EQUIPMENT and SUPPLIES

- Patient's record
- Adulterant test strips
- Urine sample (freshly voided; urine should be stored at room temperature for no longer than 2 hours or at refrigerator temperature for no longer than 4 hours before testing)
- Paper towels
- Timer
- Fluid-impermeable lab coat and disposable gloves
- Biohazard waste container

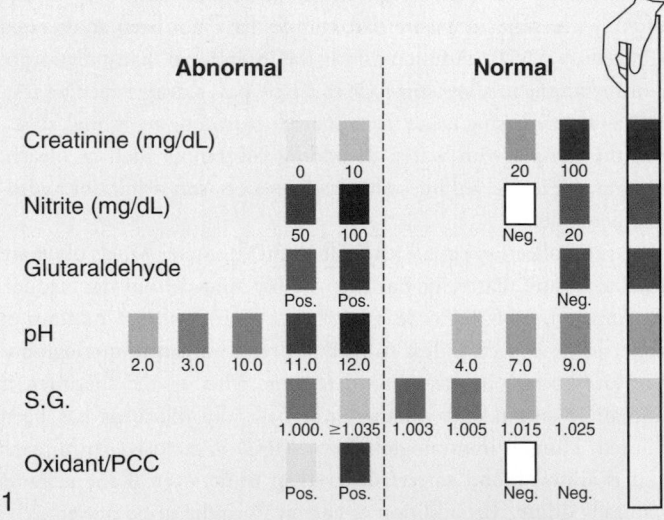

PROCEDURAL STEPS

1. Sanitize your hands. Put on the fluid-impermeable lab coat and disposable gloves.
2. Assemble the equipment and the specimen. Check the expiration date on the test kit.
   PURPOSE: An expired test strip may yield inaccurate results.
3. Remove one strip from the container and recap tightly.
4. Dip the test strip briefly into the urine and then remove it.
5. Blot the strip by touching the side of the strip to a paper towel.
   PURPOSE: Oversaturated strips may not react consistently.
6. Read the results within 1 minute by comparing each pad with the color strips on the canister (Figure 1). These results are for the Quik Test Adulterant Strips. Because the monitor color may vary from manufacturer to manufacturer, always refer to the specific product's package for accurate color reference.
   PURPOSE: Reading the strip results at the incorrect time may result in error.
7. Dispose of the paper towels and the strip in the biohazard container.
8. Disinfect the area, and remove your lab coat. Remove your gloves and dispose of them in the biohazard waste container. Sanitize your hands.
   PURPOSE: To ensure infection control.
9. Record the results in the patient's record.
   PURPOSE: A procedure is not considered complete until it is recorded.

FEDERAL DRUG TESTING CUSTODY AND CONTROL FORM

SPECIMEN ID NO. **1234567** LAB ACCESSION NO.

STEP 1: COMPLETED BY COLLECTOR OR EMPLOYER REPRESENTATIVE

A. Employer Name, Address, I.D. No.   B. MRO Name, Address, Phone and Fax No.

OME No. 0930-0158

C. Donor SSN or Employee I.D. No. _____

D. Reason for Test: ☐ Pre-employment ☐ Random ☐ Reasonable Suspicion/Cause ☐ Post Accident
☐ Return to Duty ☐ Follow-up ☐ Other (specify)_____

E. Drug Tests to be Performed: ☐ THC, COC, PCP, OPI, AMP ☐ THC & COC Only ☐ Other (specify)_____

F. Collection Site Address:

Collector Phone No. _____

Collector Fax No. _____

STEP 2: COMPLETED BY COLLECTOR

Read specimen temperature within 4 minutes. Is temperature between 90° and 100° F? ☐ Yes ☐ No, Enter Remark

Specimen Collection:
☐ Split ☐ Single ☐ None Provided (Enter Remark) ☐ Observed (Enter Remark)

REMARKS

STEP 3: Collector affixes bottle seal(s) to bottle(s). Collector dates seal(s). Donor initials seal(s). Donor completes STEP 5 on Copy 2 (MRO Copy)

STEP 4: CHAIN OF CUSTODY - INITIATED BY COLLECTOR AND COMPLETED BY LABORATORY

I certify that the specimen given to me by the donor identified in the certification section on Copy 2 of this form was collected, labeled, sealed and released to the Delivery Service noted in accordance with applicable Federal requirements.

X_____   AM
PM   **SPECIMEN BOTTLE(S) RELEASED TO:**

Signature of Collector   Time of Collection ▶

_____   / /
(PRINT) Collector's Name (First, MI, Last)   Date (Mo./Day/Yr.) ▶   Name of Delivery Service Transferring Specimen to Lab

RECEIVED AT LAB: **Primary Specimen Bottle Seal Intact**   **SPECIMEN BOTTLE(S) RELEASED TO:**

X_____
Signature of Accessioner ▶   ☐ Yes

_____   / /
(PRINT) Accessioner's Name (First, MI, Last)   Date (Mo./Day/Yr.) ▶   ☐ No, Enter Remark Below

STEP 5a: PRIMARY SPECIMEN TEST RESULTS - COMPLETED BY PRIMARY LABORATORY

☐ NEGATIVE ☐ POSITIVE for: ☐ MARIJUANA METABOLITE ☐ CODEINE ☐ AMPHETAMINE ☐ ADULTERATED
☐ DILUTE ☐ COCAINE METABOLITE ☐ MORPHINE ☐ METHAMPHETAMINE ☐ SUBSTITUTED
☐ REJECTED FOR TESTING ☐ PCP ☐ 6 ACETYLMORPHINE ☐ INVALID RESULT

REMARKS _____

TEST LAB (if different from above) _____

I certify that the specimen identified on this form was examined upon receipt, handled using chain of custody procedures, analyzed, and reported in accordance with applicable Federal requirements.

X_____   _____   / /
Signature of Certifying Scientist   (PRINT) Certifying Scientist's Name (First, MI, Last)   Date (Mo./Day/Yr.)

STEP 5b: SPLIT SPECIMEN TEST RESULTS - (IF TESTED) COMPLETED BY SECONDARY LABORATORY

☐ RECONFIRMED ☐ FAILED TO RECONFIRM - REASON_____

Laboratory Name   *I certify that the split specimen identified on this form was examined upon receipt, handled using chain of custody procedures, analyzed, and reported in accordance with applicable Federal requirements.*

X_____   _____   / /

Laboratory Address   Signature of Certifying Scientist   (PRINT) Certifying Scientist's Name (First, MI, Last)   Date (Mo./Day/Yr.)

PEEL

1234567 A
SPECIMEN ID NO.

PLACE OVER CAP

1234567
SPECIMEN BOTTLE SEAL

/ /
Date (Mo. Day Yr.)

Donor's Initials

PEEL

1234567 B (SPLIT)
SPECIMEN ID NO.

PLACE OVER CAP

1234567
SPECIMEN BOTTLE SEAL

/ /
Date (Mo. Day Yr.)

Donor's Initials

COPY 1 - LABORATORY

PRESS HARD - YOU ARE MAKING MULTIPLE COPIES

0000-0000-0225

Drug Form Part 1
Face Inks: 000 BLK / 000 RED
Date: 05/09/00
Not To Use For Colormatch
Follow PMS Guide For Colors

FIGURE 45-32 First page of the five-page Federal Drug Testing Custody and Control Form.

ALCOHOL TESTING

Alcohol testing is not performed on urine, but CLIA-waived tests are available to detect alcohol using saliva. Saliva-based tests have a high degree of correlation to blood alcohol analysis. The saliva alcohol test uses a Dacron swab saturated with saliva to detect ethanol. The test is used primarily for workplace testing, including the federally mandated testing of transportation workers, but also in private company "drug-free workplace" programs and by emergency departments.

CLOSING COMMENTS

Patient Education

Frequently a medical assistant is called on to explain specimen collection techniques to the patient. Patients want to do the procedure correctly but often lack the knowledge of urinary terminology. They may be embarrassed or may not know how to ask questions about cleaning the genital area. When explaining a urinary collection procedure, you should use pictures and words that the patient will understand. As you explain the procedure in terms the patient knows, he or she will feel comfortable telling you or asking you about pertinent details that may have a definite impact on treatment of the problem. Providing the patient with a clearly written instruction sheet also is helpful. The instruction sheet should be personalized with the patient's name, the time to begin collection or testing (if applicable), what supplies should be used, and a phone number to call if questions arise.

Legal and Ethical Issues

Similar to all other procedures, the test is only as valid as the specimen and the procedure performed on that specimen. You, as the provider's agent, are responsible for that validity when you instruct the patient and when you perform the test.

A medical assistant responsible for office laboratory testing must clearly understand the basic concepts of laboratory medicine. Therefore, you must stay current with the rapid technologic advances in laboratory medicine and help establish a protocol of the tests best suited to your provider-employer.

You are responsible for properly collecting specimens and testing them accurately. In addition, you are responsible for strict adherence to protocol when collecting and testing specimens when legal ramifications are associated with the test results. Patient confidentiality is paramount when drug testing is performed, as is rigid conformation to all established rules and regulations.

Professional Behaviors

Attributes of a laboratory professional performing urinalysis include:
- A discreet, respectful attitude when communicating with patients, co-workers, and supervisors
- Good eyesight and manual dexterity
- Accountability, honesty, and integrity when unsure of the procedure
- Ability to multitask, manage his or her time, pay attention to details, and problem-solve if test results are suspicious

SUMMARY OF SCENARIO

Rosa's skills in the laboratory analysis of urine are highly valued by Dr. Hill. When tests are performed in the office laboratory, Dr. Hill has the results immediately. Dr. Hill's patients also appreciate the convenience of office laboratory testing, in which the physical and chemical analyses are performed by Rosa and other medical assistants. The microscopic analysis is performed by Dr. Hill. Mrs. Carpenter will find out the results of her pregnancy test without having to wait for a call from the laboratory, and UA of Ms. Hillman's CCMS urine sample will help Dr. Hill diagnose a UTI (urinary tract infection) within minutes. Rosa knows that the laboratory services and the quality control measures she takes when performing the complete UA or lateral flow tests are an integral part of the excellent patient care provided by Dr. Hill.

SUMMARY OF LEARNING OBJECTIVES

1. **Define, spell, and pronounce the terms listed in the vocabulary.**
   Spelling and pronouncing medical terms correctly reinforce the medical assistant's credibility. Knowing the definitions of these terms promotes confidence in communication with patients and co-workers.
2. **Describe the history of the analysis of urine.**
   For centuries, abnormalities in the urine have been recognized as possible indicators of disruption of homeostasis. During the twentieth century, urinalysis became a practical laboratory procedure, and today urine is the most commonly analyzed body fluid in the clinical laboratory.
3. **Describe the anatomy and physiology of the urinary tract, and discuss the formation and elimination of urine by describing the processes of filtration, reabsorption, secretion, and elimination.**

The urinary tract consists of two kidneys, two ureters, one bladder, and one urethra. The functional unit of the kidney is the nephron and each nephron interacts with the blood by filtration, reabsorption, and secretion. Urine passes from the pelvis of the kidney down the ureter and into the bladder, where it remains until it is voided through the urethra.

4. **Do the following related to collecting a urine specimen:**
   - *Show sensitivity to patients' rights and feelings when collecting specimens.*
     Requesting a urine specimen from a patient may be an embarrassing moment for the patient. The request should be made in private, and the patient should be given explicit instructions so that he or she understands what is expected.

SUMMARY OF LEARNING OBJECTIVES—*continued*

- *Discuss collection containers.*
  The most important requirement for a collection container is that it be scrupulously clean. The physician's office laboratory should provide the container.

- *Explain the various means and methods used to collect urine specimens.*
  Some urine collections, such as the 2-hour postprandial specimen, must be timed around meals or fasts. Routine UA requires no special preparation, whereas a CCMS requires cleansing of the external genitalia. Only urine that will be cultured must be collected in a sterile container. Urine to be sent to a referral laboratory may require the addition of preservatives.

- *Instruct a patient in the collection of a 24-hour urine specimen.*
  Timed urine specimens are collected to determine the amount of a particular analyte in the urine during a given time frame. Proper patient instruction is necessary to obtain an acceptable specimen (see Procedure 45-1).

- *Instruct a patient in the collection of a clean-catch midstream urine specimen.*
  Proper patient instruction is necessary for an acceptable CCMS. Both men and women are given instructions in cleaning the external genitalia to prevent contamination of the urine. Urine must be collected in a sterile container and refrigerated if it cannot be tested within 1 hour (see Procedure 45-2).

5. **Examine and report the physical aspects of urine.**
   Physical examination of the urine involves determination of the color, turbidity, and specific gravity. Odor and foam color also may be noted (see Procedure 45-3).

6. **Perform quality control measures and reassure a patient of the accuracy of the test results based on the steps taken for quality assurance and quality control when performing the chemical urinalysis.**
   The chemical examination of urine involves determination of the pH level and the levels of glucose, protein, ketones, blood, bilirubin, urobilinogen, and nitrite, in addition to specific gravity and leukocyte esterase, using a reagent strip. The medical assistant should analyze and differentiate the normal and abnormal control results for the reagent strips before running the patient's chemical urinalysis (see Procedure 45-4).

7. **Test and record the chemical aspects of urine using CLIA-waived methods.**
   Perform a chemical urinalysis with a chemical reagent strip. The chemical examination of urine involves determination of the pH level and the levels of glucose, protein, ketones, blood, bilirubin, urobilinogen, and nitrite, in addition to specific gravity and leukocyte esterase, using a reagent strip.

Most chemical urine testing requires reagent strips. It is essential that these supplies be stored in a dark, cool, moisture-free area (see Procedure 45-5).

8. **Prepare a urine specimen for microscopic evaluation, and understand the significance of casts, cells, crystals, and miscellaneous findings in the microscopy report.**
   A complete UA involves physical, chemical, and microscopic assessment. The results of these three assessments must correlate with one another. Refer to Procedure 45-6.

9. **Explain or perform the following CLIA-waived urine tests:**
   - *Glucose testing using the Clinitest method*
     The Clinitest detects reducing sugars in the urine, including glucose and galactose. It is superior to the reagent strip test because it detects sugars other than glucose (see Procedure 45-7).
   - *Urine pregnancy test*
     Pregnancy tests detect hCG, a hormone produced by the placenta. Urine moves through the test (T) and control (C) areas of the test device by lateral absorption. Anti-hCG antibodies embedded in the test cartridge bind to hCG in the urine, causing a color change in the test area (see Procedure 45-8).
   - *Fertility and menopause tests*
     Fertility can be assessed using lateral flow tests that detect LH, which increases in concentration in the urine shortly before ovulation. Menopause can be assessed using lateral flow tests that detect FSH, which increases as menopause approaches.
   - *Urine toxicology and drug testing*
     Drug testing with lateral flow technology is similar to pregnancy testing except that it uses a competitive binding principle. Unlike with the pregnancy test, a line in the T region indicates a negative test (see Procedure 45-9).

10. **List the means by which urine could be adulterated before drug testing.**
    Drinking excessive water before urinating, adding water to a urine specimen, and adding chemicals or products sold specifically to adulterate urine all can render a drug test invalid. Adulteration test strips can detect most methods of adulteration (see Procedure 45-10).

11. **Discuss patient education and legal and ethical issues related to urinalysis.**
    The medical assistant should always carefully explain urinary collection procedures to the patient. Providing a clearly written instruction sheet is also helpful. A medical assistant who is responsible for office laboratory testing must clearly understand the basic concepts of laboratory medicine. He or she is responsible for properly collecting specimens and testing them accurately.

CONNECTIONS

Study Guide Connection: Go to the Chapter 45 Study Guide. Read and complete the activities.

evolve Evolve Connection: Go to the Chapter 45 link at *evolve.elsevier.com/ kinn* to complete the Chapter Review Quiz. Check out the other resources listed for this chapter to make the most of what you have learned from Assisting in the Analysis of Urine.

46 ASSISTING IN BLOOD COLLECTION

SCENARIO

Leah Barney, a recent graduate of a CMA (AAMA) program, is a new employee at the Health Alliance Medical Clinic. The class on medical laboratory procedures was Leah's favorite in her medical assisting program at the community college. In that class, she learned the principles of phlebotomy and performed several phlebotomy procedures both in the school's laboratory and at her externship site. Her employer has arranged for Leah to spend time with an experienced phlebotomist at the clinic so that she is prepared to perform phlebotomy duties in her new position. Nervous but excited, she begins her training.

While studying this chapter, think about the following questions:

- How will Leah know which tubes or which needle size to use?
- How will Leah approach phlebotomy on a child or an elderly person?
- What conditions will require a capillary puncture?

- How can Leah make the clinic patients comfortable and at ease?
- How will Leah handle a difficult "stick"?

LEARNING OBJECTIVES

1. Define, spell, and pronounce the terms listed in the vocabulary.
2. List the equipment needed for venipuncture.
3. Explain the purpose of a tourniquet, how to apply it, and the consequences of improper tourniquet application.
4. Explain why the stopper colors on vacuum tubes differ, and state the correct order of drawing samples for various types of tests.
5. Describe the types of safety needles used in phlebotomy.
6. Explain why a syringe rather than an evacuated tube would be chosen for blood collection.
7. Discuss the use of safety-engineered needles and collection devices required for injury protection.
8. Summarize postexposure management of accidental needlesticks.
9. Do the following related to routine venipuncture:
   - Detail patient preparation for venipuncture that shows sensitivity to the patient's rights and feelings.
   - Describe and name the veins that may be used for blood collection.
   - List in order the steps of a routine venipuncture.
   - Perform a venipuncture using the evacuated tube method.
   - Perform a venipuncture using the syringe method.
10. Do the following related to problems associated with venipuncture and specimen re-collection:
    - Discuss various problems associated with venipuncture.
    - Discuss possible solutions to venipuncture complications.

- Discuss why a specimen may have to be re-collected.
- Describe the major causes of hemolysis during collection.
11. Do the following related to capillary puncture:
    - Explain why a winged infusion set (butterfly needle) would be chosen over a vacuum tube or syringe needle.
    - Perform a venipuncture using a winged infusion set (butterfly needle).
    - List situations in which capillary puncture would be preferred over venipuncture.
    - Discuss proper dermal puncture sites.
    - Describe containers that may be used to collect capillary blood.
    - Explain why the first drop of blood is wiped away when a capillary puncture is performed.
    - Perform a capillary puncture.
12. Discuss pediatric phlebotomy, including typical childhood behavior and parental involvement during phlebotomy and general guidelines for pediatric venipuncture.
13. Describe handling and transport methods for blood after collection.
14. Explain chain of custody procedures when blood samples are drawn.
15. Discuss patient education, in addition to legal and ethical issues, related to assisting in blood collection.

VOCABULARY

anticoagulant An additive that prevents blood from clotting.

antiseptic An agent that inhibits bacterial growth and can be used on human tissue.

hemoconcentration A condition in which the concentration of blood cells is increased in proportion to the plasma.

hemolysis (he-mah′-lih-sis) The destruction or dissolution of red blood cells, with subsequent release of hemoglobin.

phlebotomy The practice of drawing blood from a vein

plasma The liquid portion of a whole blood specimen that has not clotted due to anticoagulant additives. The plasma still contains its natural clotting agents.

serum The liquid portion of a clotted blood specimen that no longer contains its active clotting agents.

syncope Temporary loss of consciousness; also known as *fainting*.

thixotropic gel A material that appears to be a solid until subjected to a disturbance, such as centrifugation, whereupon it becomes a liquid gel that separates blood cells from their serum or plasma.

Phlebotomy is performed primarily to diagnose and to monitor a patient's condition. According to the American Society of Clinical Pathologists (ASCP), nearly 80% of providers' diagnostic decisions are based on the results of laboratory tests, most of which are blood tests. **Phlebotomy** involves highly developed procedures and equipment to ensure the patient's comfort and safety.

Before the 1960s the diseases found in blood were primarily vector transmitted (e.g., malaria from mosquitos). Then several blood-borne viral diseases began to emerge that could be spread by exposure of an infected person's contaminated blood to another person's blood via mucous membranes or a break in the skin. The blood-borne viruses detected were identified as hepatitis B virus (HBV), hepatitis C virus (HCV), human immunodeficiency virus (HIV), and a hemorrhagic virus (Ebola). The diseases caused by these viruses were found in individuals engaged in high-risk sexual behavior; those who had received blood transfusions; and those exposed to blood by contaminated needles or bloody ritual practices.

The high standards necessary for the safe practice of phlebotomy led to the creation of the Bloodborne Pathogens Standard (overseen by the Occupational Safety and Health Administration [OSHA]) and by different organizations that develop additional standards for training. Medical assistants are trained to perform phlebotomy. To be certified as a phlebotomist, however, they must complete course work and training at an accredited institution, perform a specified amount of witnessed "sticks," and then pass a national examination. Some medical assistant programs include this specialized training in their curriculum.

Phlebotomy certifying agencies include the ASCP, the International Academy of Phlebotomy Sciences (IAPS), the National Certification Agency (NCA), and the National Phlebotomy Association (NPA). Continuing education often is required to maintain certification. California and Louisiana were the first states to create state phlebotomy certification requirements. It is important that medical assistants become familiar with the guidelines of the states in which they work because not all states require a certificate to perform phlebotomy.

The most common method of obtaining a blood specimen is venipuncture, in which the blood is taken directly from a surface vein. The vein is punctured with a needle, and the blood is collected directly into a stoppered vacuum tube, or into a syringe and then transferred into the vacuum tube. The procedure is safe when performed by a trained professional, but it must be performed with care. Much practice is required to become skilled and confident in the technique of venipuncture.

VENIPUNCTURE EQUIPMENT

Proper collection of blood requires specialized equipment. A complete list of materials used in routine venipuncture is shown in the following box. Phlebotomists in hospitals generally carry the equipment in a portable tray (Figure 46-1). A physician office laboratory (POL) often has a permanent location where the same supplies are stored and venipuncture is performed. In such cases you likely will seat the patient in a venipuncture chair, which has an adjustable locking armrest to protect the patient if he or she should faint (Figure 46-2). However, if the patient has a history of **syncope**, it is best to perform phlebotomy while the patient is lying on an examination table.

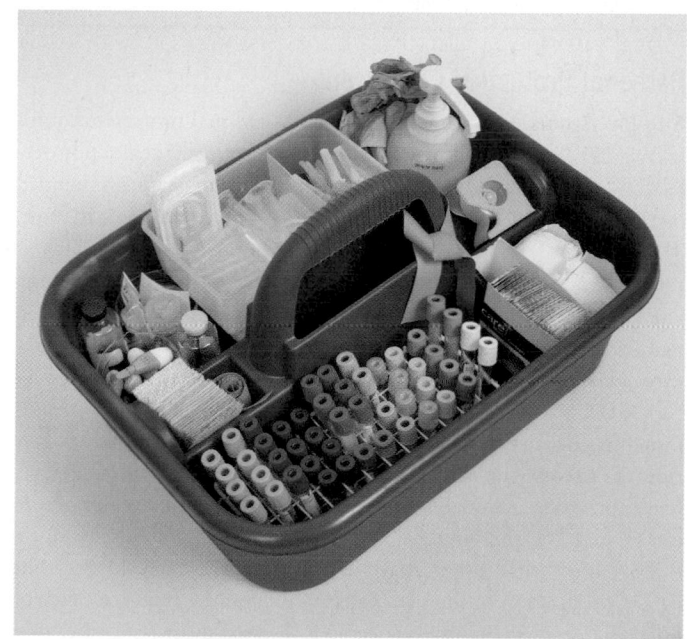

FIGURE 46-1 A fully stocked venipuncture tray.

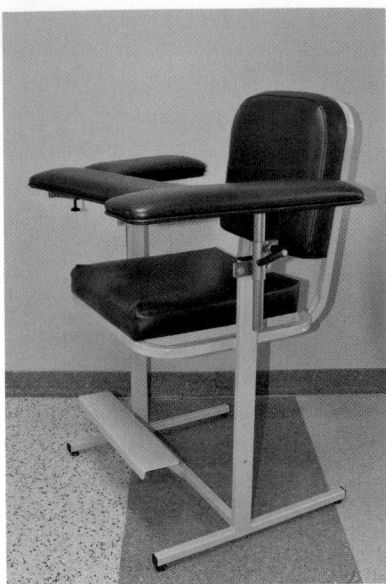

FIGURE 46-2 A phlebotomy chair.

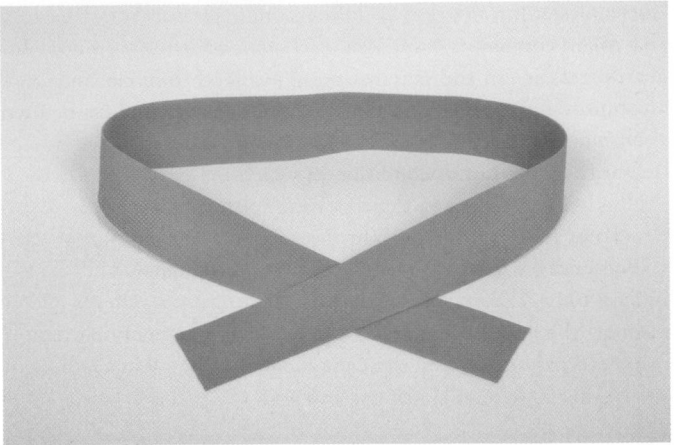

FIGURE 46-3 Example of a latex-free nitrile tourniquet.

Equipment Used in Routine Venipuncture

- Personal protective equipment (PPE): nonlatex gloves, fluid-impermeable lab coat, and face shield (if necessary)
- Marking pen
- Alcohol swabs
- Gauze pads
- Nonlatex bandages
- Nonlatex tourniquets
- Double-pointed safety needles
- Winged infusion sets (butterfly needles)
- Disposable needle holders
- Evacuated, stoppered tubes
- Syringes and removable needles with safety devices
- Biohazard sharps container

Personal Protective Equipment

Employers must provide employees with personal protective equipment (PPE), such as gloves, including the hypoallergenic, powderless, and nitrile or vinyl types. Latex gloves are no longer recommended because the phlebotomist and/or the patient may be allergic to latex. The medical assistant must also use other nonlatex supplies, such as tourniquets and adhesive bandages. All facilities must stock only latex-free supplies because of the potential for allergic responses in workers and patients. Some people with latex allergies can have life-threatening reactions with a latex exposure.

OSHA requires healthcare workers to wear gloves during venipuncture. Because veins can be difficult to locate with gloved fingertips, the site may be palpated before gloves are put on, as long as the hands have been sanitized. The standard procedure for venipuncture established by the Clinical and Laboratory Standards Institute (CLSI) states that gloves may be put on after vein palpation but before preparation of the site. Those who need the final assurance of one last palpation before the needle is inserted must remember that touching the prepared site, even with gloves, contaminates the area.

To help yourself find the vein after the area has been cleansed, make note of certain skin markers, such as creases, freckles, or scars. If the area is touched, it must be cleansed again. Keep in mind that the tourniquet should be tied for no longer than 1 minute at a time.

Tourniquets

Before blood can be drawn, a vein must be located. Application of a tourniquet is the most common way to do this; it prevents venous flow out of the site, causing the veins to bulge. The tourniquet is tied around the upper arm so that it is tight but not uncomfortable and can be released easily with one hand. Single-use, nonlatex tourniquets are available (Figure 46-3) and currently are recommended for reducing cross-contamination between patients and healthcare workers, preventing nosocomial infection, and preventing latex exposure. Other tourniquets with quick-release closures are available and may be more comfortable for the patient, but they must be disinfected after each use.

Tourniquets are applied 3 to 4 inches above the elbow immediately before the venipuncture procedure begins. Because a tourniquet impedes blood flow, leaving it on for longer than 1 minute greatly increases the possibility of **hemoconcentration** and altered test results. The tourniquet should not be tied so tightly as to impede arterial blood flow; this restricts venous blood return, resulting in poor venous distention. Checking the pulse at the wrist ensures that arterial flow is not restricted. Tourniquets also are used when blood is drawn from hand and foot veins and are tied on the wrist or ankle, respectively.

Tourniquets can be uncomfortable for patients, especially those with heavy-set or hairy upper arms, if they are not applied correctly. Make sure the tourniquet is flat against the skin, and if necessary, tie it over the clothing if it is causing the patient discomfort. This may be especially important when blood is drawn in an aging individual because of the fragility of the skin.

Antiseptics

To prevent infection, a venipuncture site must be cleansed with an **antiseptic**. The most commonly used one is 70% isopropyl alcohol, also known as *rubbing alcohol*. Prepackaged alcohol "prep pads" are the product used most often. The square prep pad is rubbed on the skin in a circular motion, and the alcohol is allowed to dry. Alcohol does not sterilize the skin; it inhibits the reproduction of bacteria that might contaminate the sample. To be most effective, the alcohol should remain on the skin 30 to 60 seconds. However, isopropyl alcohol should not be used when a sample for a blood alcohol test is drawn. Sterile soap pads, benzalkonium chloride, or povidone-iodine (Betadine) can be used instead.

If a blood culture is ordered, additional preparation is needed at the venipuncture site to eliminate contaminating bacteria. Povidone-iodine solution commonly is used; chlorhexidine gluconate or benzalkonium chloride can be used for patients who are allergic to iodine. More vigorous cleansing is required for a blood culture sample than for a routine venipuncture. Blood cultures must be drawn into a sterile tube or a bottle specifically designed for the test (Figure 46-4).

Evacuated Collection Tubes

The most common collection system is the evacuated tube system (these tubes are also called *vacuum tubes;* a particular brand is the Vacutainer). It consists of evacuated tubes of various sizes that have color-coded tops, which indicate the tube's contents (Table 46-1). Before the discovery of blood-borne pathogens, tubes were all glass with color-coded rubber stoppers. Now the tubes must be either shatter-resistant glass or plastic, and the rubber tops are being replaced by safer plastic Hemogard colored tops, which do not splatter blood when removed. In Table 46-1, note how the tubes with different-colored stoppers contain different chemical additives, **anticoagulants**, clot activators, and/or **thixotropic gel**. The vacuum in each tube draws a measured amount of blood into the tube. Tube volumes range from 2 to 15 mL.

The size of the tube to be used depends on several factors. Each test performed in the laboratory requires a specific amount of blood. Consult the manual provided by the laboratory to make sure you are drawing the right amount of blood for the test. Tests can often be combined, which reduces the number of tubes that must be drawn. For example, both a complete blood count and an erythrocyte sedimentation rate test (discussed in the next chapter) are performed on a sample from a lavender-topped tube; you need not draw two tubes, because the 7-mL volume is sufficient for both tests. When in doubt, call the laboratory. Keep in mind that blood is approximately half cells and half liquid. If a test requires 3 mL of **serum**, 6 mL of blood must be collected.

Patients often express great concern when several tubes of blood must be drawn. You can allay their fears by explaining that the average adult has a little less than 10 pints of blood (5 L). Most adults can relate to donating a unit of blood, which is around a pint (400 to 500 mL). Because the red-topped tube contains 10 mL, you would have to draw 40 to 50 tubes to remove a pint.

Tube Additives

All plastic vacuum tubes contain an additive. The red-topped plastic tube contains a silicone additive to activate clotting. All the other color-topped plastic tubes contain some form of anticoagulant to prevent blood from clotting. The additive may be a powder, a liquid visible in the tube, or a liquid sprayed inside the tube by the manufacturer and allowed to dry. The choice of anticoagulant depends on the test to be done.

Anticoagulant additives prevent blood from clotting, which allows the contents of the tube to be used in two ways. First, the sample can be used as whole blood; second, the sample can be centrifuged, and the liquid portion, called **plasma**, can be retrieved for testing. Whole blood is used for tests such as a complete blood count (CBC) and blood typing, whereas the plasma is used for STAT (immediate) chemistry testing and coagulation studies.

Ethylenediaminetetraacetic acid (EDTA) is the anticoagulant found in the lavender-topped tube. It prevents platelet clumping and preserves the appearance of blood cells for microscopic examination; however, it is incompatible with the testing reagents used in coagulation studies. Consult the manual provided by the laboratory before obtaining more than one type of specimen from the patient so as to avoid cross-contamination of additives from one tube to another.

Clot activators promote blood clotting in the red plastic tubes. For example, silica particles in the red-topped plastic tubes enhance clotting by providing a surface for platelet activation. Thrombin from the platelets quickly promotes clotting and is used in tubes drawn for chemistry testing or in the event a sample is needed from a patient taking a prescribed anticoagulant, such as heparin.

If blood is allowed to clot and then is centrifuged, the liquid portion is referred to as **serum**. Without a clot activator, blood clots in 30 to 60 minutes, after which it must be centrifuged. The serum must be separated from the cells quickly because cells may continue to metabolize substances such as glucose or may release metabolites that interfere with testing.

Thixotropic gel can be found in some tubes, including the *serum separator tube* (SST). SST tubes are identified by the red-gray (marbled) rubber stopper on glass tubes and the gold Hemogard top on plastic tubes. The *plasma separator tube* (PST) also contains thixotropic gel; the glass tubes have a green-gray (marbled) top, and the plastic tubes have a light green top. Thixotropic gel, a synthetic gel, has a density between that of red cells and plasma or serum; it settles between the two during centrifugation, forming a barrier

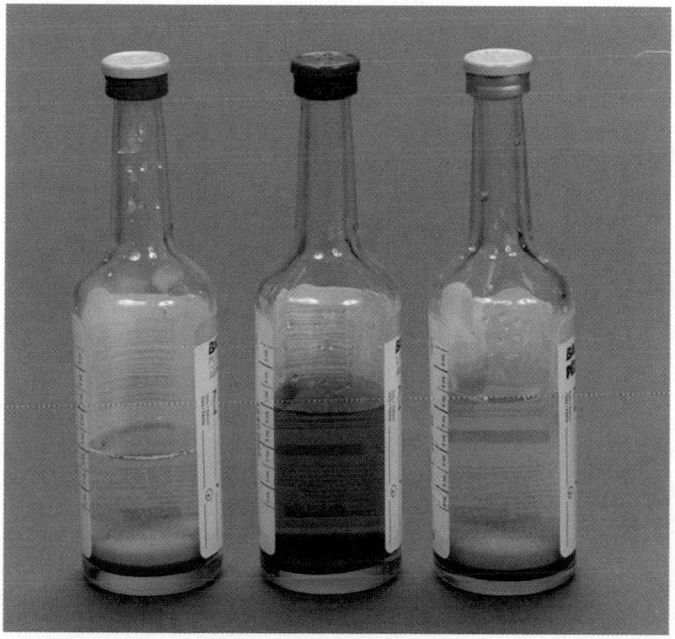

FIGURE 46-4 Bactec blood culture bottles.

that facilitates retrieval of the liquid portion without cellular contamination.

It is important to avoid a "short draw" (i.e., a tube that is not completely filled). Table 46-2 lists the consequences of underfilling tubes. Some tubes are designed to fill only partially, according to their preset vacuum. For example, a 5-mL tube that is set to draw up 3 mL of blood stops drawing up blood when it is a little over half filled. Having the proper ratio of blood to additive is crucial. Always check the tube for an expiration date; outdated tubes may have a diminished vacuum, or the additive may have degraded.

CRITICAL THINKING APPLICATION 46-1

1. Melissa Machen has been assigned to orient Leah to the clinic and her duties as a certified medical assistant. Melissa takes Leah to the laboratory in the clinic, which has a small room with a blood collection chair and a table. What supplies should be on the table for performing venipuncture?

2. What else might Leah find in this room?

TABLE 46-1	Common Stoppers and Additives and Their Laboratory Uses				
VACUUM TUBE COLOR*	COLOR	HEMOGARD COLOR†	ADDITIVE AND ITS FUNCTION‡	LABORATORY USE	OPTIMUM VOLUME/ MINIMUM VOLUME
Adult Tubes					
Pale yellow		Pale yellow	SPS prevents blood from clotting and stabilizes bacterial growth	Blood or body fluid cultures	5 mL/NA
Light blue		Light blue	Sodium citrate; removes calcium to prevent blood from clotting	Coagulation testing	4.5 mL/4.5 mL
Red		Red	None	Serum tests; chemistry studies, blood bank, serology	10 mL/NA
Red-gray (marbled)		Gold	None, but contains silica particles to enhance clot formation	Serum tests	10 mL/NA
Green		Green	Heparin (sodium/lithium/ammonium); inhibits thrombin formation to prevent clotting	Chemistry tests	10 mL/3.5 mL
Green-gray (marbled)		Light green	Lithium heparin and gel for plasma separation	Plasma determinations in chemistry studies	2 mL/2 mL
Lavender		Lavender	EDTA; removes calcium to prevent blood from clotting	Hematology tests	7 mL/2 mL
Gray		Gray	Potassium oxalate and sodium fluoride; removes calcium to prevent blood from clotting; fluoride inhibits glycolysis	Chemistry testing, especially glucose and alcohol levels	10 mL/10 mL
Royal blue		Royal blue	Sodium heparin (also sodium EDTA); inhibits thrombin formation to prevent clotting	Chemistry trace elements	7 mL

TABLE 46-1 Common Stoppers and Additives and Their Laboratory Uses—*continued*

VACUUM TUBE COLOR*	COLOR	HEMOGARD COLOR†	ADDITIVE AND ITS FUNCTION‡	LABORATORY USE	OPTIMUM VOLUME/ MINIMUM VOLUME
Pediatric Tubes					
Red		Red			2 mL/NA 3 mL/NA 4 mL/NA
Lavender		Lavender			2 mL/0.6 mL 3 mL/0.9 mL 4 mL/1 mL
Green		Green			2 mL/2 mL
Light blue		Light blue			2.7 mL/2.7 mL

EDTA, Ethylenediaminetetraacetic acid; *SPS*, sodium polyanethol sulfonate.
*Stopper colors are based on BD Vacutainer tubes.
†Hemogard closures provide a protective plastic cover over the rubber stopper as an additional safety feature.
‡Additives, additive functions, and laboratory uses are the same for both pediatric and adult tubes.

TABLE 46-2 Effects of Underfilling Collection Tubes

STOPPER COLOR	EFFECTS OF UNDERFILLING
Yellow	Reduces possibility of bacterial recovery
Light blue	Coagulation test results falsely prolonged
Red	Insufficient sample
Red-gray, and Gold (SST tubes)	Poor barrier formation; insufficient sample
Green	False results because of excess heparin
Green-gray and light green (PST tubes)	False results because of excess heparin
Lavender	Falsely low blood cell counts and hematocrits; morphologic changes to red blood cells; staining alteration
Gray	False results
Yellow-gray	False results
Royal blue	False results

PST, Plasma separation tube; *SST*, serum separation tube.

Order of Collection

If samples for more than one tube must be drawn during a venipuncture, a specified order must be followed so that material from a previous tube is not transferred to the next tube. Carryover of additives from one tube to the next could cause sample alteration and erroneous results. CLSI has established a set of standards outlining the order of draw for a multitube draw. The same order applies to the filling of tubes when blood is collected in a syringe.

1. *Yellow* top: These blood culture tubes are filled first because they are sterile and should not be contaminated by the other tubes.

2. *Light blue* top: These tubes, which contain sodium citrate, are next because other anticoagulants might contaminate the sample collected for coagulation studies. If no blood culture has been ordered, CLSI recommends that blood for the light blue–topped tube be drawn first if routine coagulation testing has been ordered (i.e., prothrombin time [PT] and activated partial thromboplastin time [APTT]; see next chapter). Some laboratories recommend that a red-topped "waste" tube with no additives be partially filled before the light blue–topped citrate tube to remove any thromboplastin that was released during the venipuncture, because thromboplastin interferes with the coagulation testing. CLSI also recommends that, when a winged infusion set is used, blood be drawn into the red-topped tube even if the order does not call for it. This is done to fill the tubing's dead space with blood before drawing the light blue–topped citrate tube, which must have an exact blood to citrate dilution.. It is not necessary to fill the waste tube to be discarded because it is just removing the air from the tubing.

3. *Red* top: Glass serum tubes without clot activator, or plastic tubes with clot activator, are filled next. These clotted specimens are drawn to test the serum after the specimens have clotted and been centrifuged. SSTs with thixotropic gel are also drawn at this time. Glass SSTs have a red-gray marbled rubber stopper; plastic SSTs have a gold plastic Hemogard top.

4. *Green* top: These tubes are drawn next because the plasma in their anticoagulated specimen is used for testing when STAT results are needed. The dark green tops contain no thixotropic gel. The marbled green-gray rubber tops and the light green plastic Hemogard tops both contain the gel to help separate the plasma from the cells when centrifuged.

5. *Lavender* top: These tubes are now drawn. They contain an EDTA anticoagulant that binds the calcium to prevent clotting and preserves the blood cells. Blood for this tube is drawn near the end because the EDTA additive interferes with the chemistry and coagulation specimens.

6. *Gray* top: This tube is drawn last, and the blood is used to test glucose. Its additives may elevate electrolyte levels and damage cells if passed into the other tubes

To recap, Table 46-1 shows the order of draw of the colored tube tops, in addition to the additives, laboratory uses, and accepted volumes per tube. Table 46-2 lists the effects of underfilling the collection tubes. Table 46-3 shows how many times the various tubes need to be inverted after they have been filled with blood. It is important to mix the contents of the tubes well after collection by inverting them several times (do not shake the tubes).

Types of Needles and Supplies Used in Phlebotomy

A critical part of phlebotomy is knowing which needle and which tube or syringe should be used in each situation. All needles used in phlebotomy are sterile and have a safety device that is activated immediately before or after withdrawal from the vein. The needle is then discarded in a biohazard sharps container. Each needle is housed in a protected cover, which should be inspected before use to ensure that sterility has not been compromised (i.e., the seal should be intact) and that the needle has no manufacturing defects, such as burs or nicks.

Needles have two parts, the hub and the shaft. The hub of the needle is designed to attach the needle to the syringe or the vacuum tube's needle holder. Shafts differ in length, ranging from ¾ to 1½ inches. The length of the shaft has no bearing on the venipuncture procedure. Some phlebotomists prefer a longer needle because it is less likely to slip out of the vein, whereas others prefer a shorter needle because it makes patients less uneasy. One end of the shaft is cut at an angle and forms the bevel, which creates a very sharp point.

The bore, or hollow space, inside the needle is called the *lumen.* Lumen size is important in venipuncture and is referred to as the *gauge.* The gauge is designated by a numeric value. The higher the gauge number, the smaller the lumen. Be sure to match the needle gauge to the size of the tube. A large vacuum tube is more likely to hemolyze the blood if a high-gauge needle (i.e., with a small lumen) is used. For example, a blood bank uses a large, 16-gauge needle to collect pints of blood for transfusions. The lumen is wide, which reduces the chance of **hemolysis.** The small, 23-gauge needle is used to collect blood from small or fragile veins, such as those in elderly and very young patients. Routine adult venipuncture requires a 20- to 21-gauge needle.

Multisample Needles

Multisample needles are commonly used in routine adult venipuncture. They are so called because they are used when several tubes are to be drawn during a single venipuncture. These needles are double pointed (Figure 46-5). One point enters the patient's vein, and the other punctures the rubber stopper of the collection tube. The point that enters the tube is sheathed with a retractable rubber sleeve that allows tubes to be changed without blood leaking into the needle holder or tube holder.

Needle Holders

Double-pointed needles must be firmly placed into a needle adapter or tube holder (Figure 46-6). Usually these are translucent cylinders, and they come in different sizes to accommodate the tube used. The holders often have a ring that indicates how far the tube

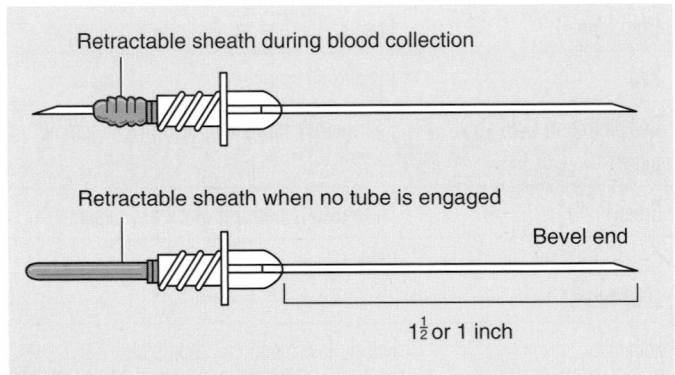

FIGURE 46-5 Multisample needles. The sheathed needle on the left penetrates the vacuum tubes when the needle on the right is in the vein.

TABLE 46-3	Stopper Color and Inversion Mixing
STOPPER COLOR	**MIX BY INVERSION**
Yellow	8-10 times
Light blue	3-4 times
Red or red speckled	5 times
Green	8-10 times
Lavender	8-10 times
Gray	8-10 times

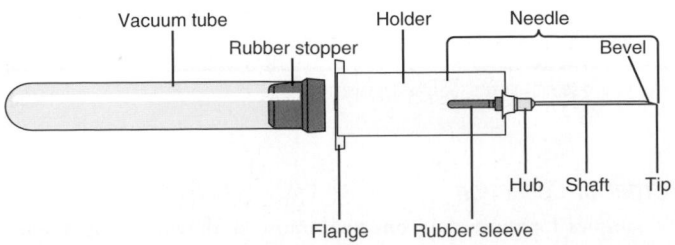

FIGURE 46-6 Vacuum system. *Left,* Vacutainer tube. *Right,* Needle holder with multisample needle attached. (From Hunt SA: *Saunders fundamentals of medical assisting,* Revised reprint, St Louis, 2007, Saunders.)

can be pushed onto the needle without losing the vacuum. OSHA requires that, to prevent accidental needlesticks, the needle holder, with its safety-activated needle still attached, be discarded into the biohazard sharps container immediately after withdrawal from the vein.

Syringes

Syringes are used when there is concern that the strong vacuum in a stoppered tube might collapse the vein. The syringe needle fits on the end of the barrel and also comes in different gauges. The amount of blood drawn into the barrel depends on how much is to be transferred to the stoppered tubes. When blood is drawn into a syringe, it must be transferred immediately to the evacuated tube because the blood will clot in the syringe barrel. In these situations, the syringe's needle safety device must be activated before the needle is discarded in the sharps container. A special transfer tube device is then used to transfer the blood to the vacuum tubes. This device connects to the top of the syringe; it contains an enclosed needle that punctures the vacuum tube's stopper and delivers the blood into the tube (Figure 46-7).

Winged Infusion Sets (Butterfly Needles)

Butterfly needles (Figure 46-8) are designed for use on small veins, such as those in the hand or in pediatric patients. The most common needle size is the small, 23 gauge; the needle is ½- to ¾-inch long and has a plastic, flexible, butterfly-shaped grip attached to a short length of tubing. The hub end is fitted into the syringe or the vacuum tube adapter. Often a syringe is used because pulling in the blood can be controlled more easily. The syringe blood sample must be transferred to the evacuated tubes using the transfer device described previously.

Needle Safety

Healthcare workers who use or may be exposed to needles are at increased risk of needlestick injury. Such injuries can lead to serious or fatal infections with blood-borne pathogens such as HBV, HCV, and HIV. Nursing and phlebotomy staff members are most frequently injured. Needlestick injuries account for most accidental exposures to blood. As is discussed in the Infection Control chapter, used needles should never be recapped except with the appropriate engineered safety devices.

According to OSHA, the best practice for preventing needlestick injuries after phlebotomy is to use safety needles that are activated with one hand immediately after use. The U.S. Food and Drug Administration (FDA), which is responsible for approving medical devices marketed and sold in the United States, recommends devices that provide a barrier between the hands and the needle, after use, in which the phlebotomist's hands remain behind the needle at all times. Safety shields that can be activated before or immediately after removal of the needle from the vein and that remain in effect after disposal also should be an integral part of the device. Finally, these devices should be as simple as possible, requiring little or no training to use. Some examples of needle safety devices are:

- *One-handed vacuum tube needle:* After the needle has been used and removed from the vein, the thumb holding the vacuum tube holder slides under the base of the pink safety device, causing it to snap over the contaminated needle (Figure 46-9, *A*). Or, an orange needle shield on the holder is activated by pressing the device against a surface (Figure 46-9, *B*).
- *Syringe needle safety devices* (Figure 46-10): These devices have a spring-activated shield attached to a disposable syringe needle. After the venipuncture, the phlebotomist activates the device with the thumb holding the syringe, and a spring locks

FIGURE 46-7 BD Vacutainer blood transfer device, showing the blood from the syringe above about to be pulled into the vacuum tube on the bottom when the vacuum tube is pushed into the holder. (Courtesy Becton, Dickinson, Franklin Lakes, NJ.)

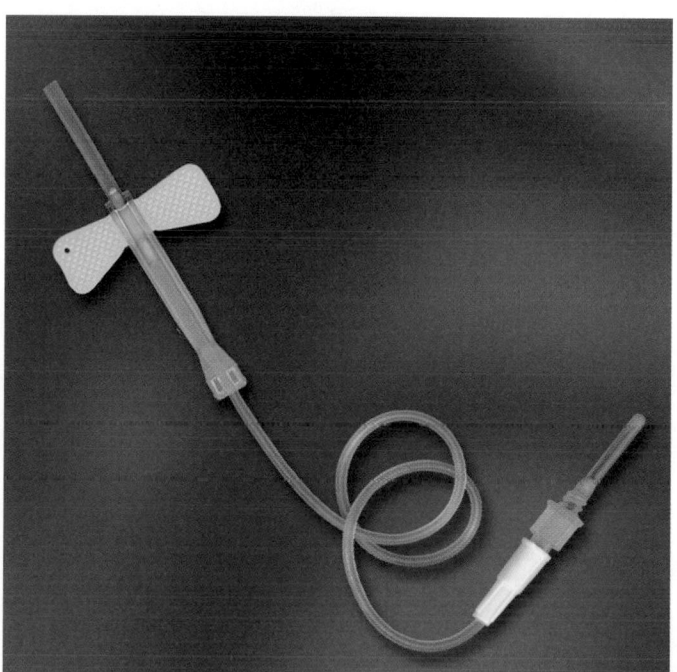

FIGURE 46-8 Winged infusion (butterfly) set with sterile tubing containing a white Luer needle adapter that will attach to a syringe, and a Vacutainer-sheathed needle that will attach to a Vacutainer holder. (Courtesy Becton, Dickinson, Franklin Lakes, NJ.)

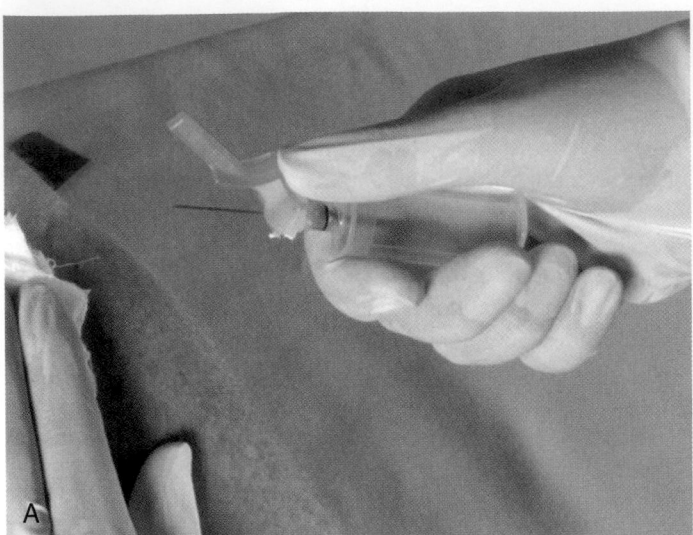
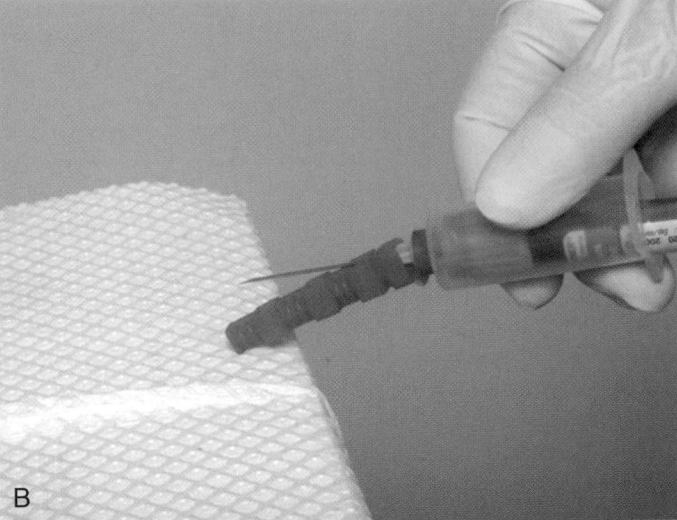

FIGURE 46-9 Hinged or sliding sharps with safety-engineered sharps injury protection (SESIP). **A,** One-handed activation by sliding thumb at the base of device, causing it to cover the needle. **B,** One-handed activation by pressing the orange protective device against an inanimate object. (Modified from Garrels M, Oatis C: *Laboratory testing for ambulatory settings,* ed 2, St Louis, 2011, Saunders.)

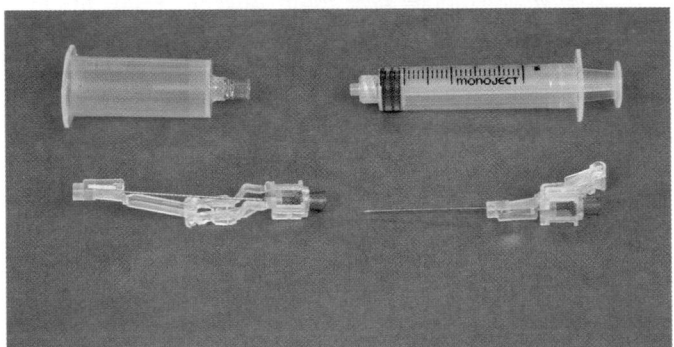

FIGURE 46-10 *Top left,* Blood transfer device for transferring a syringe blood sample to a vacuum tube. Top right is the syringe. *Bottom left,* Syringe safety needle that has been activated. After safety activation, the needle is removed from the syringe, and the blood transfer device is attached to the syringe to transfer blood into vacuum tubes. *Bottom right,* Exposed needle that has not been activated.

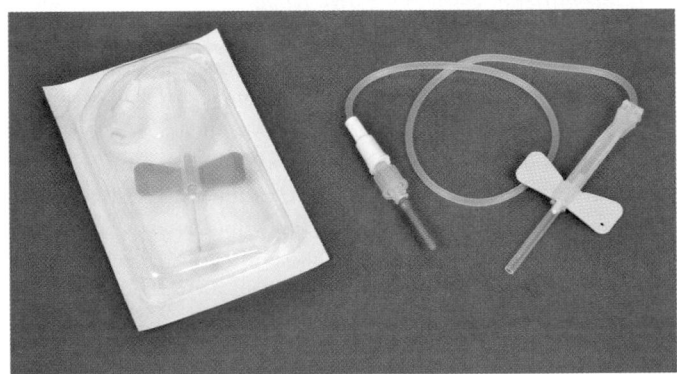

FIGURE 46-11 *The Safety-Lok butterfly needle and the blue "wings" are pulled back into the butterfly body by pulling back on the tubing while holding the "tail" of the butterfly.*

a protective plastic tip into place, protecting the needle. The needle then can be removed and discarded. The syringe is attached to the safety transfer device to deliver the collected blood into the appropriate vacuum tubes (see Figure 46-7).

- *Butterfly needle safety lock* (Figure 46-11): After the venipuncture, the dominant hand holds the butterfly tail while the nondominant hand pulls back on the tubing, causing the needle to slide into the tubing and lock into place.
- *Push-button butterfly safety device* (Figure 46-12): While the needle is still in the arm, the medical assistant grasps the tail of the butterfly with the dominant hand while the nondominant hand presses the button just below the wings, causing the needle to retract into the butterfly body as it leaves the vein.
- *Needle blunting butterfly set* (Figure 46-13): A third "wing" is rotated after collection and before removal of the needle from the vein. As the third wing is rotated, it moves the blunt needle down the shaft before it is removed from the patient.

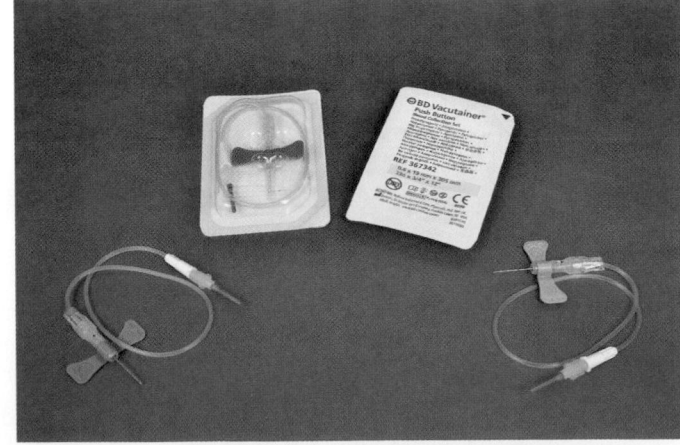

FIGURE 46-12 *The push-button butterfly needle is activated while in the vein. When the black button just below the green wings is pushed, the needle immediately is pulled out of the vein and into the body of the butterfly.*

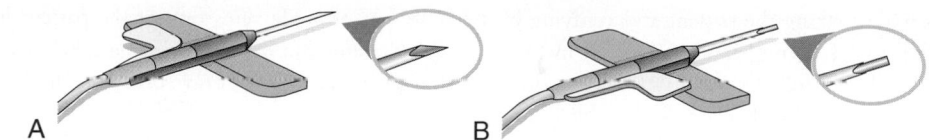

FIGURE 46-13 Needle-blunting sharp with safety-engineered sharps injury protection (SESIP) for winged infusion (butterfly) sets. **A,** Before activation, with needle in vein. **B,** After activation.

It should be noted that OSHA's Bloodborne Pathogens Standard emphasizes that phlebotomists should have direct input on the type of safety needles they will be using. The following steps should be taken to protect against needlestick injuries:

- Help your employer evaluate and select devices with safety features.
- Use devices with safety features provided by your employer.
- Never recap a contaminated needle except with a safety device.
- Plan for safe handling and disposal before beginning any procedure using needles.
- Dispose of used needles and needle holders promptly in appropriate biohazard sharps containers.
- Report all needlestick and other sharps-related injuries promptly to ensure that you receive appropriate follow-up care.
- Tell your employer about hazards from needles that you observe in your work environment.
- Participate in blood-borne pathogen training and follow recommended infection prevention practices, including vaccination against HBV.

OSHA requires employers to establish and maintain a sharps injury log for recording injuries from contaminated sharps. This log should contain information about the device involved in the incident and the department or work area where the incident occurred, in addition to an explanation of the incident. Employee confidentiality must be maintained.

Postexposure Management of Needlesticks

An accidental needlestick is a medical emergency. (OSHA-recommended management procedures are discussed in the Infection Control chapter.) Effective management of an accidental sharps exposure includes the following measures:

- Immediately after injury, the wound is inspected for foreign material, which is removed. The site is washed for 10 minutes with an antimicrobial soap, 10% iodine solution, or chlorine-based antiseptic.
- The injury is reported to the supervisor, and an incident report is completed.
- The employee is referred to a physician for confidential assessment and follow-up. Baseline testing for HBV, HCV, and HIV is recommended for both the employee and the source individual. If the employee has been immunized for HBV and has a positive postimmunization titer, there is no risk of acquiring HBV and no source testing is needed. If the worker has not been immunized or the postimmunization titer is negative, source testing for infection with HBV is recommended if the source is known and can be located. If the source patient tests positive for HBV, the employee should

receive HBV immune globulin (HBIG), and the series of HBV immunizations should be initiated. If the source tests negative, no treatment is indicated. If the source patient cannot be tested, the employee should be treated as if the source patient were positive for HBV. The source should also be tested for HCV. If the source is positive, the employee should be monitored for signs and symptoms of hepatitis for 6 months. No postexposure prophylaxis is recommended for HCV infection. For HIV exposure, most employers recommend a 4-week regimen of antiretroviral drugs. To best protect the victim, antiretroviral therapy should be administered within hours of exposure. Early HIV drug therapy is now recommended for anyone who may be at risk of infection. Because these medications have side effects, the employee is the one who decides whether the medications are started. If the source is found to be negative, antiretroviral therapy can be discontinued.

- Interim testing may be performed if the healthcare worker experiences symptoms of acute HIV exposure or hepatitis. For HIV, antibody testing should be repeated at 6 weeks, 12 weeks, and 6 months if the source was HIV positive or the source's status remains unknown. Confidential follow-up care must include provisions for emotional support and counseling for the healthcare worker.

ROUTINE VENIPUNCTURE

Venipuncture involves several important steps, and the medical assistant must be thoroughly familiar with these steps before attempting the procedure. The first step is to select the proper method for venipuncture (evacuated tube or syringe). Next, the patient must be prepared for the procedure. Patient preparation is followed by the actual venipuncture and specimen collection, and care of the puncture site is provided before the patient is discharged. The final step is proper processing of the specimen.

Patient Preparation

All blood collections begin with a requisition, a form from the patient's provider requesting a test. Requisitions may be computer generated or handwritten and at a minimum must include the following information:

- Patient's name
- Date of birth
- Identification number
- Name of the provider submitting the order
- Type of test requested
- Test status (timed, fasting, STAT, and so forth)

Venipuncture begins with greeting the patient and verifying his or her identity. According to CLSI, proper identification includes asking outpatients to (1) spell their full name and state their address, which are verified on the requisition, and (2) verify their birth date. All the information must be compared with the written information on the requisition. If the patient speaks a different language, has limited language skills (e.g., he or she is a child), or is otherwise unable to communicate, a family member or medical translator must provide the information. The name of this person should be documented.

Introduce yourself and briefly explain the purpose and procedure of the venipuncture. If the patient has questions about the ordered tests, politely request that the patient speak to the provider, and ask whether the individual would like to do so before you collect the sample. Obtain verbal consent to perform the procedure simply by asking whether you have permission to take some blood from the patient's arm. Always ask the patient whether he or she has experienced problems during routine venipuncture in the past, and take steps to prevent such problems. Your self-confidence in the procedure should be evident to the patient and will help allay any fears. Instilling confidence in your patients means acting and speaking professionally. You may want to ask what the patient would prefer to be called, or you can call the person by his or her formal name. Refer to the patient as "Mr. Jones" or "Ms. Smith," not "honey," "sweetie," "Bill," or "Margaret." Being friendly is important, but make sure your patients feel respected and understand that you take your role in their care seriously.

Preparing for the Venipuncture

Seat the patient in a chair; or, if the patient has a history of syncope, have him or her lie down on an examination table. Ask the patient to extend an arm (and place his or her other hand under the elbow to help straighten the venipuncture area). Inspect both arms and ask whether the patient has a preference. Generally, veins in the forearm or the elbow (antecubital area) are used for venipuncture (Figure 46-14). The puncture site should be carefully selected after both arms have been inspected. Alternative sites may be indicated if the area is cyanotic, scarred, bruised, edematous, or burned. You may use veins on the back of the hand or the thumb side of the wrist.

Use foot or ankle veins only if the patient has good circulation in the legs and you have received permission from your supervisor or the physician. Never draw blood from this area if the patient is diabetic.

As mentioned, inspect both arms thoroughly before you choose the venipuncture site. Veins bounce lightly when palpated. The medial veins generally run at a slight right angle to the fold in the antecubital area, whereas the cephalic veins run lateral to the thumb side of the antecubital area. These veins are the veins of choice. The basilic vein, which lies on the inside part of the antecubital area, is very close to the brachial artery and median nerves and should be used only if the medial or cephalic veins are inaccessible. The most common injury patients suffer from phlebotomy is nerve injury. If the patient complains of tingling, numbness, or a shooting pain, discontinue the procedure and choose another site before continuing. Do not probe with the needle under this condition; any attempt at relocating the needle puts the patient at great risk of nerve injury.

To apply a tourniquet, place the tourniquet 3 to 4 inches above the patient's elbow, making sure it is not twisted (Figure 46-15). Grasp the tourniquet ends, one in each hand, at the part of the tourniquet closest to the patient's skin. Pull the ends apart to stretch the tourniquet, then cross one end over the other while maintaining the tension. Tuck the top end of the tourniquet underneath the bottom piece, creating a loop with the upper flap free so that the tourniquet can be released with one hand. The tourniquet should be tight without pinching the patient's skin. Both ends of the tourniquet should be pointing upward so that they do not contaminate the blood draw site.

When the tourniquet is in place, ask the patient to place a fist under the elbow of the arm with the tourniquet and make a fist with the tourniquet arm. Palpate for an acceptable vein using your ungloved, sanitized index finger. If you are able to palpate the vein through gloved fingers, you can continue with the phlebotomy process.

Performing the Venipuncture

When you have located a vein, remove the tourniquet. A tourniquet can remain in place for 1 minute. After its removal, you must wait

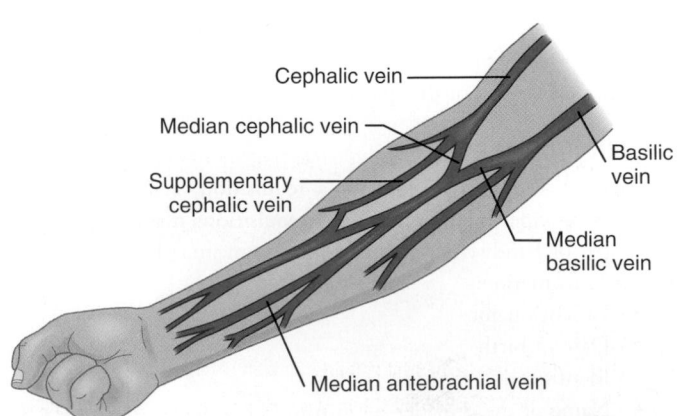

FIGURE 46-14 The veins of the forearm. (From Stepp CA, Woods MA: *Laboratory procedures for medical office personnel*, Philadelphia, 1998, Saunders.)

Cephalic vein
Median cephalic vein
Supplementary cephalic vein
Basilic vein
Median basilic vein
Median antebrachial vein

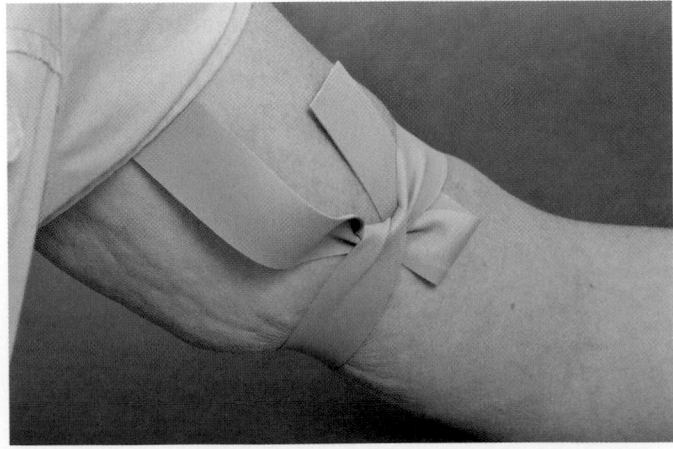

FIGURE 46-15 Placement of a tourniquet.

2 minutes before reapplying it. During this time, sanitize your hands and put on your gloves (if they are not already on) and cleanse the antecubital area with alcohol wipes, starting with a small area and working outward in larger circles. Do not touch this area after cleansing. Assemble the appropriate equipment, making sure everything is within easy reach, that the gauze packets are torn open, and that the contents are easily accessible.

Reapply the tourniquet, ask the patient to reclench the hand into a fist. Do not have the patient pump the fist because this may temporarily increase the level of potassium and ionized calcium in the blood. Relocate the vein (*Note:* If you need to palpate, place your gloved finger on the alcohol wipe first and then palpate with the finger covered by the disinfectant.) Anchor the vein by stretching the skin downward below the collection site with the thumb of the nondominant hand, and swiftly insert the needle into the vein at a 15-degree angle. The bevel should be facing up. If the needle is inserted at an angle greater than 15 degrees, it quickly penetrates the other side of the vein and enters other structures, such as nerves or the brachial artery, and very likely will cause a hematoma or an injury. Push the evacuated tube into the double-pointed needle or pull back on the syringe plunger. When blood enters the tube or barrel, ask the patient to unclench the fist.

Completing the Venipuncture

Continue to draw the specimens, checking periodically on the patient's condition. As you remove each tube from the needle holder, gently invert it several times before you place it in the rack. Tubes with clot activator should be inverted 5 times; light-blue–topped tubes for coagulation studies should be inverted 3 or 4 times; all other anticoagulant tubes should be inverted 8 to 10 times (refer back to Table 46-3). If the tubes are not inverted immediately after collection, small clots can form in the specimen. When you are nearing the end of the draw and the last tube to be collected has been filled, carefully release the tourniquet without jarring the needle, and remove the final vacuum tube. Remove the needle quickly and apply gauze with pressure to the puncture site. Ask the patient to apply direct pressure to the gauze but not to bend the arm.

Immediately activate the safety device to cover the needle and dispose of the entire needle/needle holder unit into a sharps container. While the patient is applying pressure to the site, label the tubes with the labels that accompanied the requisition, or write the following on the vacuum tube's label: patient's last name, then first name; on the next line, write the date and time; on the third line, state whether the patient had been fasting; then sign your initials.

Before putting on the bandage, perform a two-point check to make sure the vein is not leaking. Observe the site for 5 to 10 seconds after releasing pressure and removing the gauze. If visible bleeding occurs or if the tissue around the puncture site rises, continue applying pressure until the bleeding has stopped. Special precautions must be taken for patients taking anticoagulants because the phlebotomy site will bleed longer than is the norm. Put on a pressure bandage by placing a folded gauze pad over the site and then applying the bandage over the gauze. Clean gauze, not a cotton ball, can be held in place by wrapping a stretchy gauze around the arm to hold the gauze in place against the puncture site. Never leave the room or release an outpatient until all the tubes have been labeled. Assess the patient's status one last time, then dismiss the patient or leave the room.

Procedures 46-1 and 46-2 outline the proper procedures for venipuncture using the evacuated tube method and the syringe method. Certain patients, such as those with narrow veins, young children, and aging adults, may require a winged infusion set (butterfly needle) rather than the previously mentioned methods. Butterfly units also can be used to draw blood from the hands of adults. As mentioned, the needle in a winged infusion unit is shorter, and the wings help you grasp and guide the needle more easily. The tubing also minimizes the strength of the vacuum, thus preventing the collapse of fragile veins, which is a common problem with elderly patients (Procedure 46-3).

Text continued on p. 1085

PROCEDURE 46-1 | **Instruct and Prepare a Patient for a Procedure and Perform Venipuncture: Collect a Venous Blood Sample Using the Vacuum Tube Method**

Goal: *To collect a venous blood specimen by the vacuum tube technique.*

EQUIPMENT and SUPPLIES

- Patient's health record
- Provider's order and/or lab requisition
- Vacuum tube needle, needle holder, and proper tubes for requested tests
- 70% isopropyl alcohol pads
- Gauze pads
- Tourniquet
- Hypoallergenic tape or bandage
- Permanent marking pen or printed labels
- Biohazard bag
- Sharps container and biohazard waste container

PROCEDURAL STEPS

1. Check the provider's order and/or requisition form to determine the tests ordered. Gather the appropriate tubes and supplies.
   <u>PURPOSE</u>: Each test requires a specific tube color that is indicated on the requisition.
2. Sanitize your hands and put on the fluid-impermeable lab coat and disposable gloves.
   <u>PURPOSE</u>: To ensure infection control.
3. Verify the patient's identity using two identifiers (e.g., have the person spell his or her last name, state the birth date, and/or show a picture ID). Explain the procedure and obtain permission for the venipuncture.

PROCEDURE 46-1   *—continued*

PURPOSE: To make sure you have the right patient; explanations help gain the patient's cooperation.

4. Assist the patient to sit with his or her arm well supported in a slightly downward position.
   PURPOSE: The veins of the antecubital fossa are more easily located when the elbow is straight.

5. Assemble the equipment. The choice of needle size depends on your inspection of the patient's veins. Attach the needle firmly to the vacuum tube holder. Keep the cover on the needle.
   PURPOSE: If the needle is loose, it may turn during the procedure, causing the bevel of the needle to turn away from its upward position.

6. Apply the tourniquet around the patient's arm 3 to 4 inches above the elbow. The tourniquet should never be tied so tightly that it restricts blood flow in the artery (Figure 1). Tourniquets should remain in place no longer than 60 seconds.
   PURPOSE: The tourniquet is used to make the veins more prominent. A quick check of the radial pulse ensures that the tourniquet has not been applied too tightly.

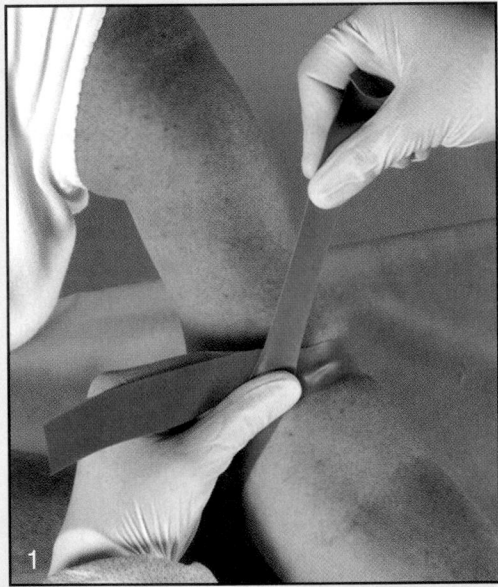

(From Garrels M, Oatis C: *Laboratory and diagnostic testing for ambulatory settings,* ed 3, St Louis, 2015, Saunders.)

7. Ask the patient to make a fist.
   PURPOSE: Clenching the fist produces engorgement of the vein. Do not ask the patient to pump the fist because this may disrupt the blood's electrolyte balance.

8. Select the venipuncture site by palpating the antecubital space. Use your index finger to trace the path of the vein and to judge its depth. The vein most often used is the median cephalic vein, which lies in the middle of the elbow (Figure 2).
   PURPOSE: The index finger is most sensitive for palpating. Do not use the thumb because it has a pulse of its own, which may confuse you.

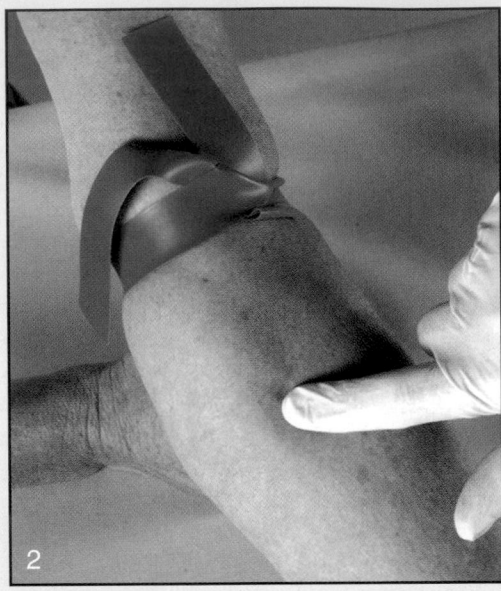

(From Garrels M, Oatis C: *Laboratory and diagnostic testing for ambulatory settings,* ed 3, St Louis, 2015, Saunders.)

9. Cleanse the site, starting in the center of the area and working outward in a circular pattern with the alcohol pad (Figure 3).
   PURPOSE: The circular pattern helps prevent recontamination of the area.

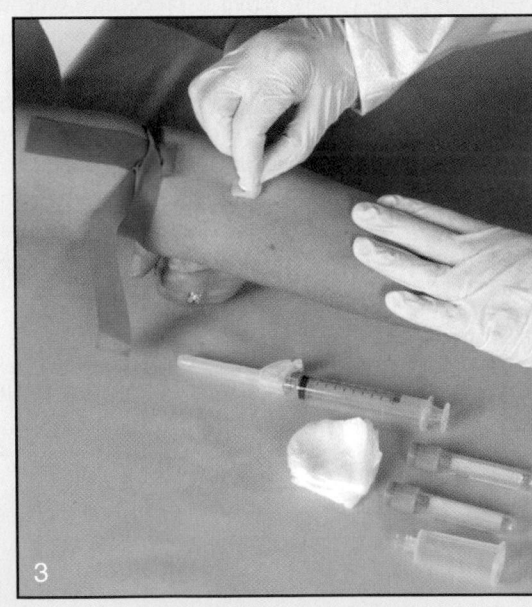

(From Garrels M, Oatis C: *Laboratory and diagnostic testing for ambulatory settings,* ed 3, St Louis, 2015, Saunders.)

10. It is recommended to take the tourniquet off while you assemble your equipment and supplies on the nondominant side of the arm. Then reapply it when the alcohol is dry. Alternatively, dry the site with a sterile gauze pad.
    PURPOSE: Puncturing an area that is still wet with alcohol stings and can cause hemolysis of the sample.

PROCEDURE 46-1 *—continued*

11. Hold the vacuum tube assembly in your dominant hand. Your thumb should be on top and your fingers underneath. You may want to position the first tube to be drawn in the needle holder, but do not push it onto the double-pointed needle past the marking on the holder. Remove the needle sheath.

    PURPOSE: Positioning the hand in this manner provides the best visibility of the needle entering the site and accessibility to insert and withdraw tubes with the nondominant hand. Pushing the tube into the double-pointed needle before it is in the arm causes air to rush into the tube, destroying the vacuum.

12. Grasp the patient's arm with the nondominant hand and anchor the vein by stretching the skin downward below the collection site with the thumb of the nondominant hand.

    PURPOSE: Failure to anchor the vein may cause the vein to move away from the needle as it enters the arm, resulting in a missed vein.

13. With the bevel up and the needle aligned parallel to the vein, insert the needle at a 15-degree angle through the skin and into the vein quickly and smoothly (Figure 4).

    PURPOSE: The sharpest point of the needle is inserted first. Inserting the needle quickly minimizes pain.

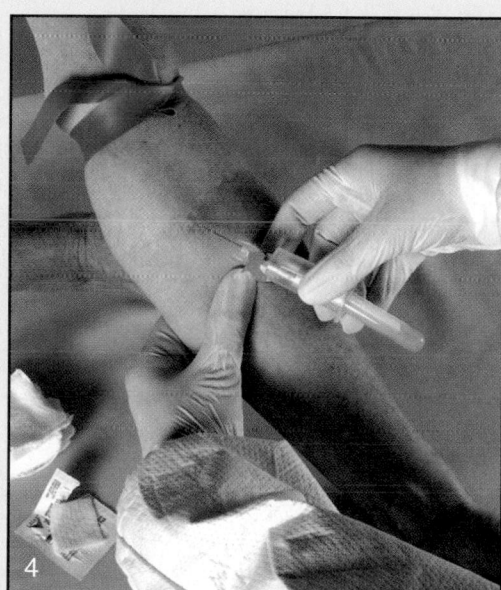

(From Garrels M, Oatis C: *Laboratory and diagnostic testing for ambulatory settings,* ed 3, St Louis, 2015, Saunders.)

14. Place two fingers on the flanges of the needle holder and use the thumb to push the tube onto the double-pointed needle. Make sure you do not change the needle's position in the vein. When blood begins to flow into the tube, ask the patient to release the fist.

    PURPOSE: The thumb has the strength to push the needle swiftly through the stopper. However, if you are not careful, the needle can easily be pushed farther into the site when the tube is pushed.

15. Allow the tube to fill to its maximum capacity. Remove the tube by curling the fingers underneath and pushing on the needle holder with the thumb. Take care not to move the needle when removing the tube. Immediately after removing it from the needle holder, gently invert the tube to mix the additives and the blood.

    PURPOSE: Tubes must be full to ensure the proper anticoagulant-to-blood ratio. Moving the needle may result in inadvertent penetration of the other side of the vein or slipping of the needle out of the vein. Gentle inversion prevents clotting of blood, whereas vigorous mixing may cause hemolysis.

16. Insert the second tube into the needle holder, following the instructions in the previous steps. Continue filling tubes until the order on the requisition has been filled. Gently invert each tube after removing it from the needle holder. As the last tube is filling, release the tourniquet.

    PURPOSE: The tourniquet should remain in place for no longer than 1 minute to prevent hemoconcentration.

17. Remove the last tube from the holder. Place gauze over the puncture site and quickly remove the needle, engaging the safety device (Figure 5). Dispose of the entire unit in the sharps container.

    PURPOSE: The gauze over the puncture site and activation of the safety needle ensure infection control.

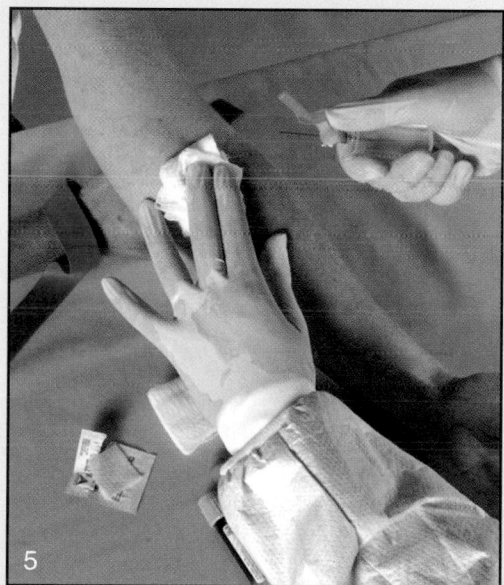

(From Garrels M, Oatis C: *Laboratory and diagnostic testing for ambulatory settings,* ed 3, St Louis, 2015, Saunders.)

18. Apply pressure to the gauze or instruct the patient to do so. The patient may elevate the arm but should not bend it.

    PURPOSE: Applying direct pressure is the best method to stop bleeding. Elevating the arm above the heart also stops bleeding.

PROCEDURE 46-1   *—continued*

19. Label the tubes with the patient's name, the date, and the time, or affix the preprinted tube labels while the patient is applying pressure (Figure 6).

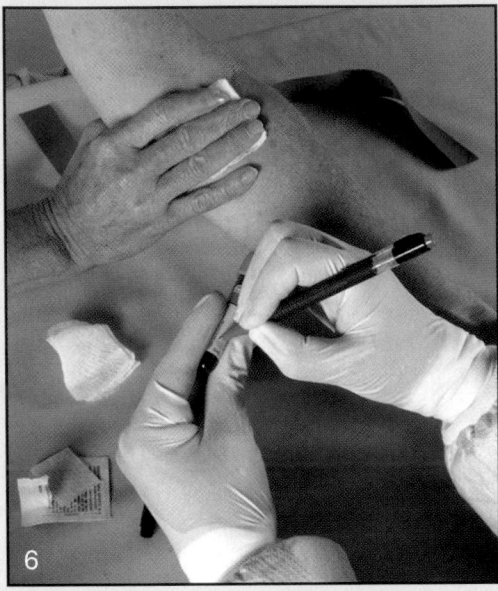

6

(From Garrels M, Oatis C: *Laboratory and diagnostic testing for ambulatory settings,* ed 3, St Louis, 2015, Saunders.)

20. Check the puncture site for bleeding and hematoma formation.
21. Apply a hypoallergenic pressure bandage using a clean, folded gauze pad under the bandage (Figure 7).

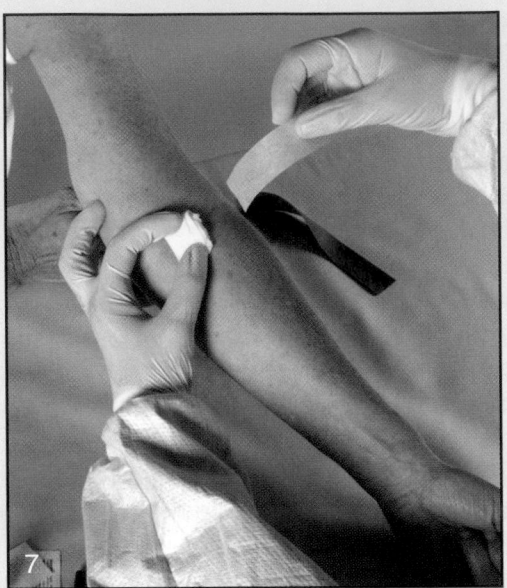

7

(From Garrels M, Oatis C: *Laboratory and diagnostic testing for ambulatory settings,* ed 3, St Louis, 2015, Saunders.)

22. Disinfect the work area. Dispose of blood-contaminated materials (e.g., gauze and gloves) in the biohazard waste container. Remove your lab coat and sanitize your hands.
    PURPOSE: To ensure infection control.
23. Complete the laboratory requisition form and route the specimen to the proper place. Record the procedure in the patient's record.
    PURPOSE: A procedure is considered not done until it is recorded.

10/5/20– 1:45 PM: Venous blood drawn from antecubital space of ℝ arm. Lavender tube for CBC with differential, and gold tube for SMA 12. Placed for pickup by Health Alliance Labs. Leah Barney, CMA (AAMA)

PROCEDURE 46-2   Perform Venipuncture: Collect a Venous Blood Sample Using the Syringe Method

Goal: *To collect a venous blood specimen using the syringe technique.*

EQUIPMENT and SUPPLIES

- Patient's health record
- Provider's order and/or lab requisition
- Syringe with 21- or 22-gauge safety needle
- Vacuum tubes appropriate for tests ordered
- 70% isopropyl alcohol pads
- Gauze pads
- Tourniquet
- Safety transfer device to transfer blood from syringe to vacuum tubes
- Hypoallergenic tape or bandage
- Permanent marking pen or printed labels

- Fluid-impermeable lab coat and disposable gloves
- Biohazard bag
- Sharps container and biohazard waste container

PROCEDURAL STEPS

1. Check the provider's order and/or requisition form to determine the tests ordered. Gather the appropriate tubes and supplies.
   PURPOSE: To collect the specimen properly based on the tube requirements on the requisition.
2. Sanitize your hands and put on the fluid-impermeable lab coat and disposable gloves.
   PURPOSE: To ensure infection control.

PROCEDURE 46-2 *—continued*

3. Verify the patient's identity using two identifiers (e.g., have the person spell his or her last name, state the birth date, and/or show a picture ID). Explain the procedure and obtain permission for the venipuncture.
   PURPOSE: To make sure you have the right patient; explanations help gain the patient's cooperation.

4. Assist the patient to sit with his or her arm well supported and straight in a slightly downward position.
   PURPOSE: The veins of the antecubital fossa are more easily located when the elbow is straight.

5. Assemble the equipment. The choice of syringe barrel size and needle size depends on the amount of blood required for the ordered tests and your inspection of the patient's veins. Attach the needle firmly to the syringe. Pull and depress the plunger several times to loosen it in the barrel while keeping the cover on the needle. The plunger must be pushed in completely after it has been loosened in the barrel.
   PURPOSE: Using the smallest syringe possible minimizes the chance of hemolysis. Engaging the plunger ensures that you will not have to use as much force to pull the blood into the barrel, thereby minimizing the chance of hemolysis.

6. Apply the tourniquet around the patient's arm 3 to 4 inches above the elbow. The tourniquet should never be tied so tightly that it restricts blood flow in the artery (Figure 1). The tourniquet should remain in place no longer than 1 minute.
   PURPOSE: The tourniquet is used to make the veins more prominent. A quick check of the radial pulse ensures that the tourniquet has not been applied too tightly.

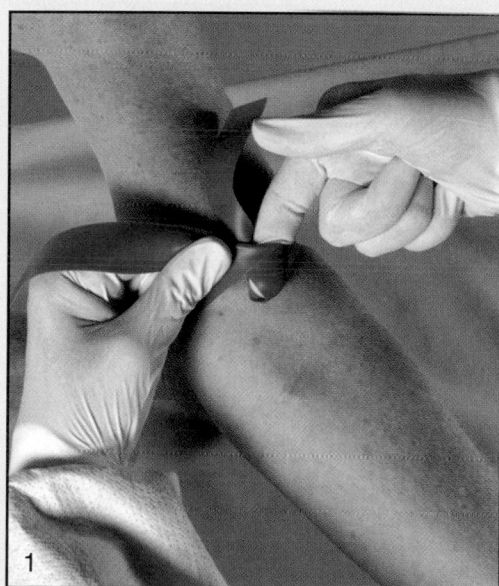

(From Garrels M, Oatis C: *Laboratory and diagnostic testing for ambulatory settings,* ed 3, St Louis, 2015, Saunders.)

7. Ask the patient to make a fist.
   PURPOSE: Clenching the fist produces engorgement of the vein.

8. Select the venipuncture site by palpating the antecubital space (if you have difficulty palpating the vein with gloves, you can remove the gloves,

palpate the vein and visibly mark its location, then put on new gloves before continuing); use your index finger to trace the path of the vein and to judge its depth. The vein most often used is the median cephalic vein, which lies in the middle of the elbow (Figure 2).
PURPOSE: The index finger is most sensitive for palpating. Do not use the thumb because it has a pulse of its own, which may confuse you.

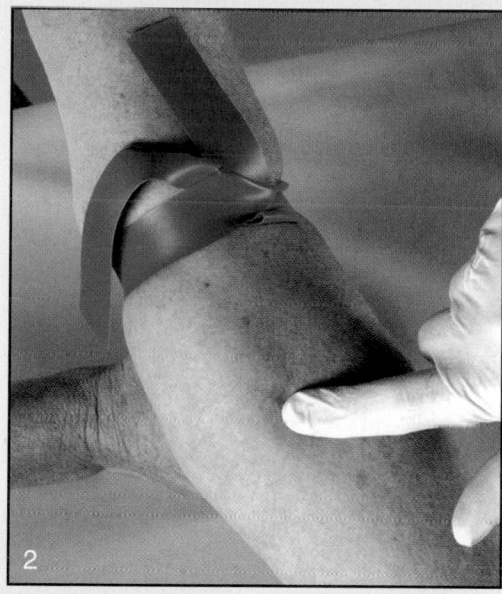

(From Garrels M, Oatis C: *Laboratory and diagnostic testing for ambulatory settings,* ed 3, St Louis, 2015, Saunders.)

9. Cleanse the site, starting in the center of the area and working outward in a circular pattern with the alcohol pad (Figure 3). Allow the area to dry before proceeding.
   PURPOSE: The circular pattern helps prevent recontamination of the area. Puncturing an area that is still wet with alcohol stings and can cause hemolysis of the sample.

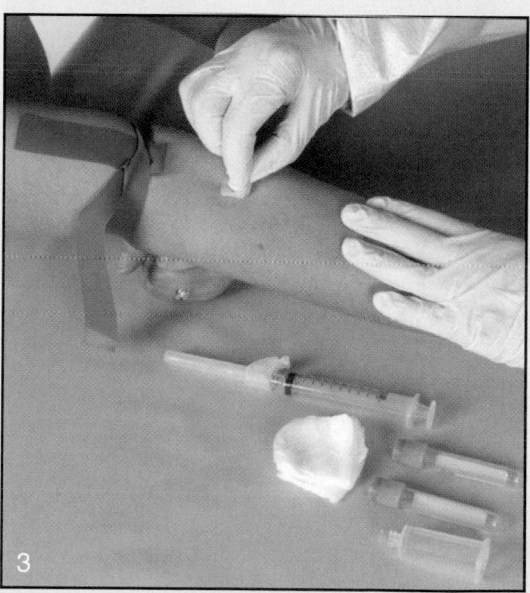

(From Garrels M, Oatis C: *Laboratory and diagnostic testing for ambulatory settings,* ed 3, St Louis, 2015, Saunders.)

PROCEDURE 46-2   *—continued*

10. Hold the syringe in your dominant hand. Your thumb should be on top and your fingers underneath, the same as in the vacuum tube method. Remove the needle sheath.

11. Grasp the patient's arm with the nondominant hand and anchor the vein by stretching the skin downward below the collection site with the thumb of the nondominant hand.
    <u>PURPOSE</u>: Failure to anchor the vein may cause the vein to move away from the needle when it is inserted, resulting in a missed vein.

12. With the bevel up and the needle aligned parallel to the vein, insert the needle at a 15-degree angle through the skin and into the vein rapidly and smoothly (Figure 4). Observe for a "flash" of blood in the hub of the syringe. Ask the patient to release the fist.
    <u>PURPOSE</u>: The sharpest point of the needle is inserted first. The angle ensures that the needle does not penetrate through the vein. The appearance (flash) of blood in the hub ensures that the needle is in the vein.

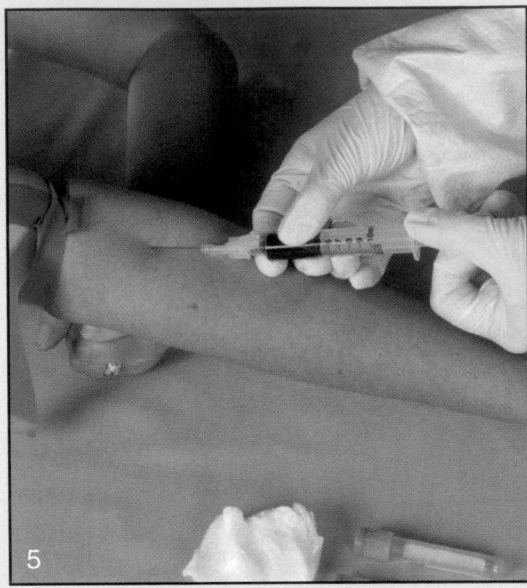

(From Garrels M, Oatis C: *Laboratory and diagnostic testing for ambulatory settings*, ed 3, St Louis, 2015, Saunders.)

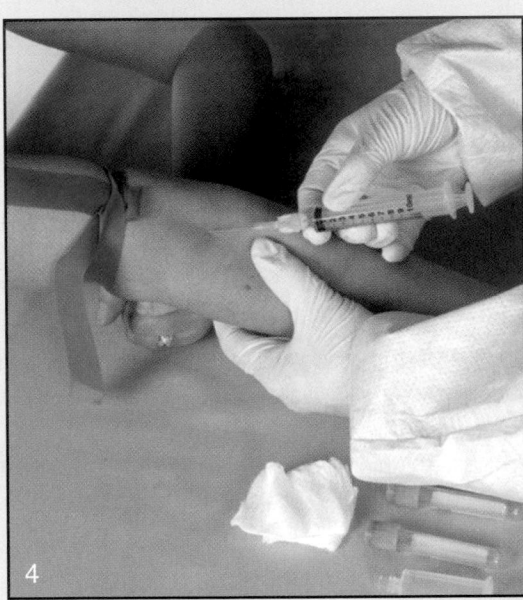

(From Garrels M, Oatis C: *Laboratory and diagnostic testing for ambulatory settings*, ed 3, St Louis, 2015, Saunders.)

13. Slowly pull back the plunger of the syringe with the nondominant hand. Do not allow more than 1 mL of head space between the blood and the top of the plunger. Make sure you do not move the needle after entering the vein. Fill the barrel to the needed volume (Figure 5).

14. Release the tourniquet when the proper volume is reached. The tourniquet must be released before the needle is removed from the arm (Figure 6).
    <u>PURPOSE</u>: Removal of the tourniquet releases pressure on the vein and helps prevent blood from getting into adjacent tissues, causing a hematoma.

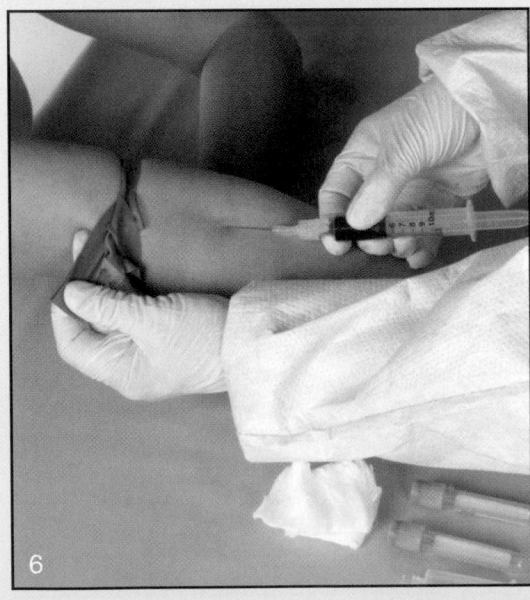

(From Garrels M, Oatis C: *Laboratory and diagnostic testing for ambulatory settings*, ed 3, St Louis, 2015, Saunders.)

PROCEDURE 46-2   *—continued*

15. Place sterile gauze over the puncture site at the time of needle withdrawal (Figure 7). Then, immediately activate the needle safety device using the syringe hand and apply pressure to the site with the nondominant hand.

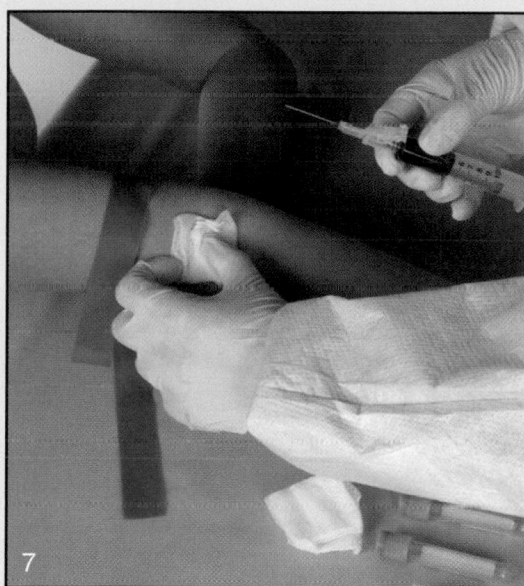

7

(From Garrels M, Oatis C: *Laboratory and diagnostic testing for ambulatory settings,* ed 3, St Louis, 2015, Saunders.)

16. Instruct the patient to apply direct pressure on the puncture site with sterile gauze. The patient may elevate the arm but should not bend it.
    PURPOSE: Direct pressure is the best method to stop bleeding. Elevating the arm above the heart also stops bleeding.
17. Remove the syringe safety needle and transfer the blood immediately to the required tube or tubes using a safety transfer device. Do not push on the syringe plunger during transfer. Discard the entire unit in the sharps container when transfer is complete. Invert the tubes after the addition of blood and label them with the necessary patient information (Figure 8).
    PURPOSE: The safety transfer device protects against accidental needle-sticks and allows the correct amount of blood to be delivered into the tube by vacuum. Pushing the plunger hemolyzes the blood and may alter the amount of blood intended in each tube. Blood begins to clot shortly after collection, so it must be transferred into the vacuum tube and mixed with anticoagulant immediately after collection. Inverting the tubes ensures anticoagulation.

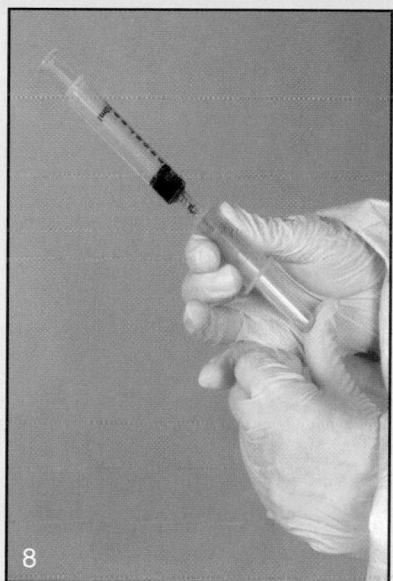

8

(From Garrels M, Oatis C: *Laboratory and diagnostic testing for ambulatory settings,* ed 3, St Louis, 2015, Saundors.)

18. Inspect the puncture site for bleeding or a hematoma.
19. Apply a hypoallergenic pressure bandage (Figure 9).
20. Disinfect the work area. Dispose of blood-contaminated materials (e.g., gauze and gloves) in the biohazard waste container. Remove your lab coat and sanitize your hands.
    PURPOSE: To ensure infection control.

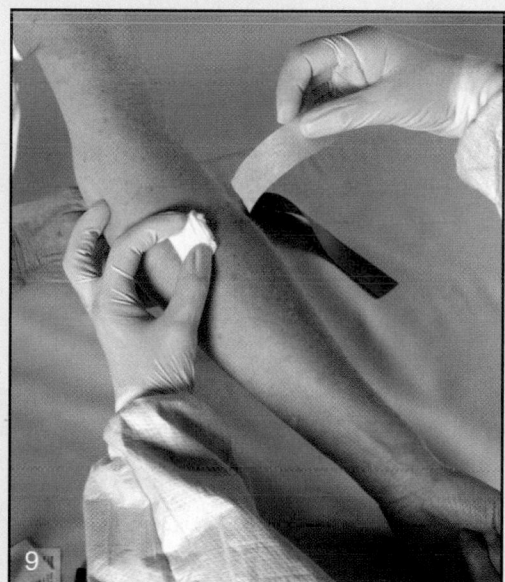

9

(From Garrels M, Oatis C: *Laboratory and diagnostic testing for ambulatory settings,* ed 3, St Louis, 2015, Saunders.)

21. Complete the laboratory requisition form and route it and the specimen to the proper place. Record the procedure in the patient's record.
    PURPOSE: A procedure is not considered complete until it is recorded.

PROCEDURE 46-3	Perform Venipuncture: Obtain a Venous Sample with a Safety Winged Butterfly Needle

Goal: *To obtain a venous sample accurately from a hand or arm vein using a butterfly needle with the vacuum tube method.*

EQUIPMENT and SUPPLIES

- Patient's health record
- Provider's order and/or lab requisition
- Tourniquet
- Alcohol pads or other antiseptic preps
- Gauze pads
- Safety winged (butterfly) needle set
- Appropriate vacuum tubes
- Hypoallergenic bandage
- Permanent marking pen or printed labels
- Fluid-impermeable lab coat and disposable gloves
- Biohazard bag
- Sharps container and biohazard waste container

PROCEDURAL STEPS

1. Check the provider's order and/or requisition form to determine the tests ordered. Gather the appropriate tubes and supplies.
   <u>PURPOSE</u>: For efficiency in preparation
2. Sanitize your hands and put on the fluid-impermeable lab coat and disposable gloves.
   <u>PURPOSE</u>: To ensure infection control.
3. Verify the patient's identity using two identifiers (e.g., have the person spell his or her last name, state the birth date, and/or show a picture ID). Explain the procedure and obtain permission for the venipuncture.
   <u>PURPOSE</u>: To make sure you have the right patient; explanations help gain the patient's cooperation.
4. Remove the butterfly device from the package and stretch the tubing slightly. Take care not to activate the needle-retracting safety device accidentally.
   <u>PURPOSE</u>: To keep the tube from recoiling.
5. Attach the butterfly device firmly to the vacuum tube holder using the sheathed needle at the end of the tubing (Figure 1). *Note:* The sheathed vacuum tube needle is attached to a syringe adapter. Make sure the two are seated firmly together to prevent air from leaking into the vacuum tube when the sheathed needle makes contact with the vacuum.

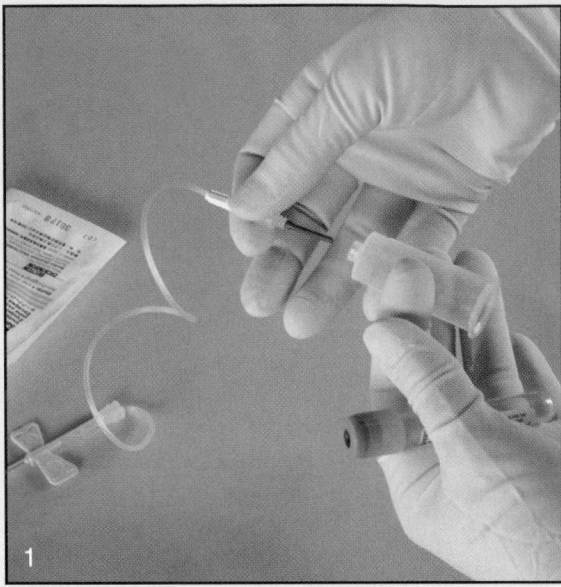

(From Garrels M, Oatis C: *Laboratory and diagnostic testing for ambulatory settings,* ed 3, St Louis, 2015, Saunders.)

6. Seat the first tube in the vacuum tube holder and place the unit carefully where it will not roll away.
7. Apply a tourniquet to the patient's arm or wrist just proximal to the wrist bone. Do not apply the tourniquet so tightly that blood flow in the arteries is impeded.
8. Have the patient place the venipuncture hand over his or her other, fisted hand (or around your nondominant hand) with the fingers lower than the wrist. Or place the patient's arm in the same position as for the previous venipuncture procedures with the arm straight and slightly downward.
   <u>PURPOSE</u>: These positions help blood fill the veins in the hand; this makes it easier for you to identify the veins and choose the draw site.
9. Select a vein and cleanse the site at the bifurcation (forking) of the veins.
10. Using your thumb, pull the patient's skin taut over the knuckles.
    <u>PURPOSE</u>: Stretching the skin prevents the veins from rolling underneath.
11. With the needle bevel up and at a 10- to 15-degree angle, align it with the vein.
12. Insert the needle by holding the wings or the rear of the set. After insertion the wings are never touched again. Make sure the safety device is not activated.
    <u>PURPOSE</u>: Inserting the needle by holding the wings gives a greater sense of control. If the sides are held, the safety shield slides forward over the needle when the point of the needle makes contact with the skin.

PROCEDURE 46-3 —*continued*

13. Push the blood collecting tube into the end of the holder (Figure 2). Note the position of the hands while drawing the blood. When drawing blood into a syringe, make sure the vacuum you create is slow and steady and that no more than 1 mL of head space exists between the blood and the plunger.
    PURPOSE: Drawing blood too forcefully into the syringe may collapse the vein or hemolyze the blood.

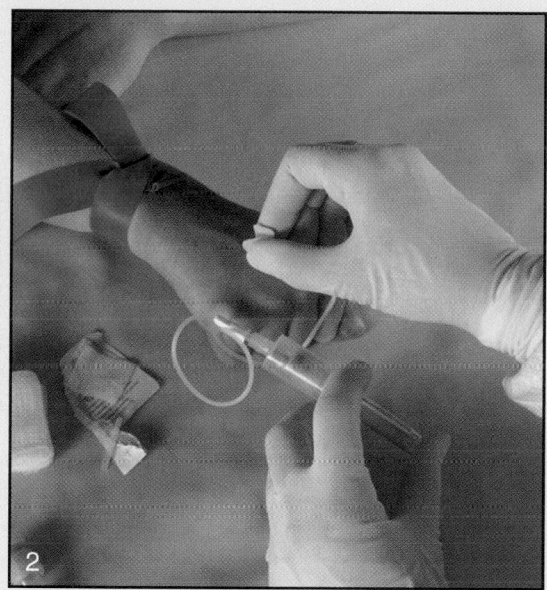

(From Garrels M, Oatis C: *Laboratory and diagnostic testing for ambulatory settings,* ed 3, St Louis, 2015, Saunders.)

14. Release the tourniquet when the blood appears in the tubing or a "flash" of blood is seen in the hub of the syringe.
    PURPOSE: To prevent hemoconcentration, the tourniquet should remain in place no longer than 1 minute.
15. Always keep the tube and the holder in a downward position so that the tube fills from the bottom up.
16. Place a gauze pad over the puncture site and gently remove the needle, engaging the safety device. Dispose of the entire unit in the sharps container (Figure 3).

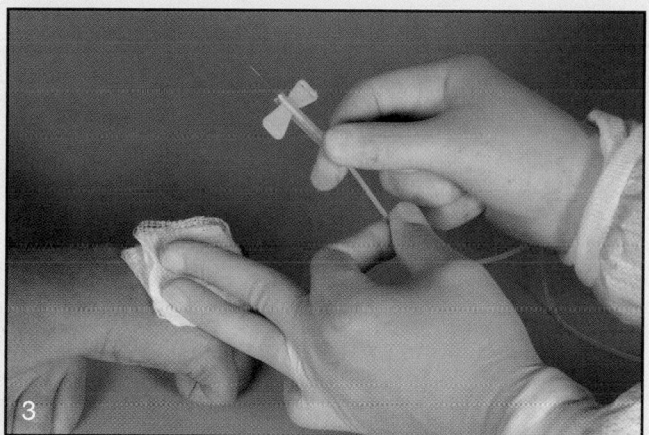

(From Garrels M, Oatis C: *Laboratory and diagnostic testing for ambulatory settings,* ed 3, St Louis, 2015, Saunders.)

17. Complete the procedure as you would for an antecubital draw (see Procedure 46-1, steps 19 through 23).

PROBLEMS ASSOCIATED WITH VENIPUNCTURE

Failure to obtain blood can occur because of a number of factors. Determining the cause of the problem may help you decide whether a second attempt would be successful. The first rule is to remain calm so that you can think clearly and systematically determine the possible cause of the problem.

A *hematoma* is a large, painful, bruised area at the puncture site caused by blood leaking into the tissue, which causes the tissue around the puncture site to swell. The most common causes of hematoma formation during the draw are excessive probing with the needle to locate a vein, failure to insert the needle far enough into the vein, and passing the needle through the vein. A hematoma also can form after a draw if you fail to remove the tourniquet before removing the needle; fail to withdraw the vacuum tube before the needle is withdrawn or fail to apply adequate pressure on the puncture site; or the elbow is bent while pressure is applied. If a hematoma forms, discontinue the procedure STAT, apply pressure to the area for a minimum of 3 minutes, and then apply an ice pack to the area. Notify the provider and observe the site to determine whether the bleeding has stopped. Depending on the facility's policy, an incident report may have to be completed and documented in the

patient's record. A hematoma may also occur if the puncture reopens and bleeds into the tissue due to heavy lifting with the venipuncture arm. Instruct the patient to be careful with the arm for several hours after the procedure.

Fainting, or syncope, can have serious consequences, and the phlebotomist must always be prepared. Securing the patient in a blood collection chair (by turning the armrest pad in front of the patient) prevents bodily injury if the person faints. Constant light conversation with the patient during the procedure can help identify an impending episode, as can observing the patient's face and breathing rate.

Nerve damage can be a consequence of venipuncture, albeit an unlikely one. Preventive measures include avoiding the basilic vein and refraining from blind probing if the vein is missed.

Table 46-4 lists some possible solutions to complications. As a general rule, it is wise to limit yourself to two attempts to obtain blood from a patient. If you fail on the second attempt, ask the patient whether he or she would prefer having someone else try, or whether it would be better to come back at another time. This maneuver lets the patient feel that he or she is in control of the situation. At one time or another, everyone is unsuccessful in obtaining a blood sample, so do not feel that you are a failure.

TABLE 46-4   Managing Possible Blood Draw Complications

COMPLICATION	MANAGEMENT STRATEGIES
Burned area	Choose another site because these areas are prone to infection.
Convulsions	Stay calm. Remove the needle and quickly dispose of it in a sharps container. Then help guide the patient to the floor, protecting him or her from injury. Call for help.
Damaged or scarred veins or infected areas	Look for an alternative site; do not draw blood from scarred or infected areas.
Edema	Avoid the area; look for an alternative site.
Hematoma	Adjust the depth of the needle or remove the needle and apply pressure.
Intravenous (IV) therapy or blood transfusion sites	Blood samples should not be drawn from an arm that is also the site for IV infusion or blood transfusion because of the dilution factor.
Mastectomy	Do not draw blood from the side of the mastectomy, because mastectomy surgery causes lymphostasis, which may produce false results.
Nausea	Place a cold cloth on the patient's forehead, give the patient a basin in case of vomiting, and instruct him or her to take deep breaths. Alert the provider.
No blood	Manipulate the needle slightly or remove the vacuum tube and perform the blood draw again using a syringe or butterfly setup.
Petechiae	Loosen the tourniquet because this complication usually results from the tourniquet being in place longer than 2 minutes.
Syncope	Position the patient's head between the knees (if in a sitting position). Check and record the patient's pulse, blood pressure, and respiration rate, and continue to observe the patient. Never leave the patient unattended.

Fainting

According to the Clinical and Laboratory Standards Institute (CLSI), the procedure for a fainting patient or one who is nonresponsive is as follows:

- If the patient begins to faint, quickly remove the tourniquet and needle from the arm, immediately activate the needle safety device, apply pressure to the site, and dispose of the unit in a sharps container to prevent an accidental exposure.
- Notify staff members for assistance.
- Lay the patient flat or lower the head if the patient is sitting.
- Loosen tight clothing.
- Do not use ammonia inhalants/capsules because these are associated with adverse effects and are no longer recommended.
- Apply a cold compress or washcloth to the patient's forehead and back of the neck.
- Stay with the patient until recovery is complete.
- Document the incident according to facility policies.
- When the patient regains consciousness, he or she must remain in the facility for at least 15 minutes and should not operate a vehicle for at least 30 minutes.

CRITICAL THINKING APPLICATION   46-2

Leah is in her second week at the clinic, and she is confident that she can perform phlebotomy on her own. Melissa has been a good mentor, and Leah has done quite a few successful "sticks" without any problems. Today, however, she is just having a bad day. Mr. Godfrey Lawrence has come to the clinic with numerous problems, and Dr. Gupta has ordered several blood tests. Mr. Lawrence is uncooperative when he sees that Leah must draw four tubes of blood. He angrily tells her that she cannot take that much blood out of him; she is a vampire and she will drain him. How should Leah deal with this problem?

SPECIMEN RE-COLLECTION

Sometimes problems with a sample cannot be determined until the specimen is analyzed in the laboratory. Rejected specimens must be re-collected. The laboratory may reject a specimen for reasons that include the following:

- Unlabeled or mislabeled specimen
- Insufficient quantity
- Defective tube
- Incorrect tube used for the test ordered
- Hemolysis (Table 46-5)
- Clotted blood in an anticoagulated specimen
- Improper handling

TABLE 46-5   Major Causes of Hemolysis during Collection

CAUSE	EXPLANATION	PREVENTION
Alcohol preparation	Transfer of alcohol into the specimen causes hemolysis.	Allow venipuncture site to dry completely.
Incorrect needle size	A high-gauge needle causes the blood to be forced through a small lumen with great force, shearing the cell membranes; a very-low-gauge needle allows a large amount of blood to suddenly enter the tube with great force, causing frothing	Choose the correct needle for the job, aiming for a 19- to 23-gauge needle.
Loose connections on the vacuum tube assembly	If the connection between the needle holder and the double-pointed needle or the syringe and the needle is loose, air can enter the sample and cause frothing.	Make sure all connections are tight before beginning the venipuncture.
Removing the needle from the vein with the tube intact	The remaining vacuum in the tube can cause air to be drawn forcefully into the tube, causing frothing.	Remove the final tube from the needle holder before withdrawing the needle from the patient's vein.
Underfilled tubes	Underfilling tubes leads to an improper blood/additive ratio. Certain additives in disproportionate amounts (e.g., sodium fluoride) can cause hemolysis.	Permit blood to flow into the tubes until no more movement can be seen.
Syringe collections	Pulling back forcibly on the plunger draws blood too quickly through the needle, shearing cell membranes; transferring blood into a vacuum tube further traumatizes red blood cells.	Pump the plunger several times before use to loosen it in the barrel. Use the smallest syringe possible. Pace the aspiration rate so that no more than 1 mL of air space is present at any time. Transfer blood into the vacuum tube immediately, preferably using a transfer device. *Never* push on the plunger when transferring to a vacuum tube. Angle the syringe so that the blood runs gently down the side of the tube, preventing the cells from hitting the bottom of the tube with force.
Mixing tubes too vigorously	All tubes except the red-topped tube must be mixed.	Gently invert tubes immediately after the draw. Anything other than gentle inversion (e.g., shaking) can hemolyze cells.
Temperature and transport problems	Trauma and temperature extremes can damage cells. Freezing results in ice crystals that puncture cell membranes.	Tubes should be transported in the upright position with as little trauma as possible. Temperature should be controlled; neither too hot nor too cold.
Separation of plasma or serum from red blood cells	Removing the serum or plasma from the cells minimizes the risk of contaminating the specimen with red blood cell contents.	Blood samples should be centrifuged, when applicable, as soon as possible and serum or plasma removed from the cells.
Prolonged tourniquet time	While the tourniquet restricts blood flow, interstitial fluid can leak into the veins and hemolyze red blood cells.	Adhere to the 1-minute rule for tourniquet application.
Poor collection; blood flowing too slowly into the tube	The needle lumen may be blocked because it is too close to the inner wall of the vein.	Withdraw the needle slightly to center it within the vein.

Hemolysis is the major cause of specimen rejection. Because it cannot be detected until the blood cells separate from the plasma or serum, it is crucial to take steps to prevent red blood cell damage during collection. Hemolyzed serum or plasma appears rosy to bright red because of the release of hemoglobin from the cells. Some of the more routine tests that are adversely affected by hemolysis are chemistry tests for electrolytes (e.g., potassium, sodium), bilirubin, total protein, and numerous liver enzymes (e.g., alkaline phosphatase, gamma glutamyl transferase).

CAPILLARY PUNCTURE

Capillaries are small blood vessels that connect small arterioles to small venules. A capillary, or dermal, puncture is an efficient means of collecting a blood specimen when only a small amount of blood is required or when a patient's condition makes venipuncture difficult. Because the requisition will not indicate that the collection is to be made in this manner, you must be familiar with the advantages, limitations, and appropriate uses of this technique. Capillary puncture is warranted in the following situations:

- Older patients
- Pediatric patients (especially younger than age 2)
- Patients who require frequent glucose monitoring
- Patients with burns or scars in venipuncture sites
- Obese patients
- Patients receiving intravenous (IV) therapy
- Patients who have had a mastectomy
- Patients at risk for venous thrombosis
- Patients who are severely dehydrated
- Tests that require a small volume of blood (i.e., CLIA-waived tests)

Because capillaries are bridges between arteries and veins, capillary blood is a mixture of the two. Small amounts of tissue fluid also are present in capillary blood, especially in the first drop. Analyte levels are usually the same in capillary and venous blood, with a few exceptions. Hemoglobin and glucose values are higher in capillary blood; potassium, calcium, and total protein are higher in venous blood.

Equipment

Skin Puncture Devices

The device used to perform a dermal puncture is the lancet, which delivers a quick puncture to a predetermined depth (Figure 46-16). OSHA has directed that lancets must have retractable blades; they also must have locks that prevent accidental puncture after use and that prevent the device from being reused. Table 46-6 lists the lancet needles and blades that are used for various testing applications. Skin puncture devices should always be discarded in a sharps container.

Collection Containers

Different types of containers and collection devices are available, and the ones used depend on the test to be performed. Microcollection, or Microtainer tubes (Figure 46-17) are available with a variety of anticoagulants and additives. Their color-coded tops indicate the same additives as evacuated tubes. Blood is collected drop-wise into

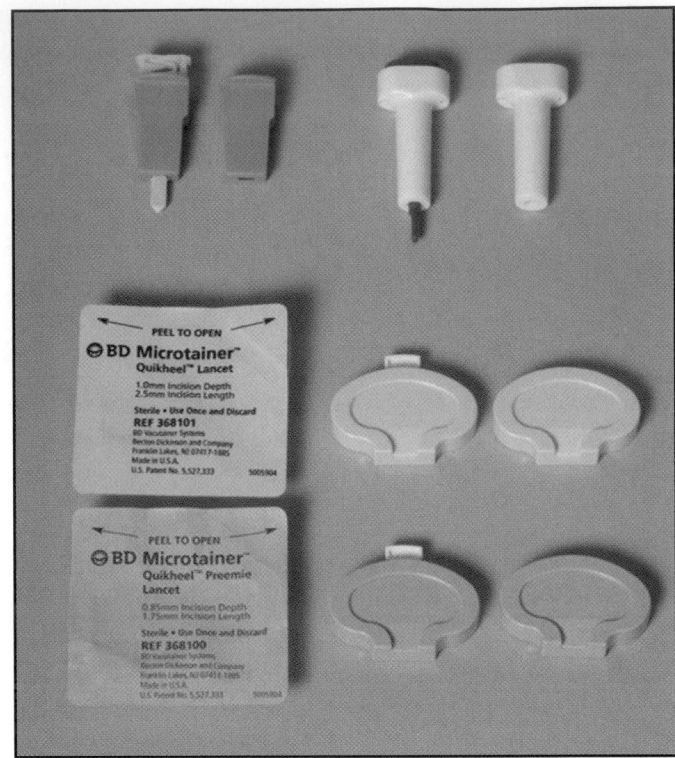

FIGURE 46-16 Skin puncture devices (lancets) include safety needles (blue and white) and safety blades (green and pink) that control the depth and width of the incision. Both types automatically retract after use. (Courtesy Becton, Dickinson, Franklin Lakes, N.J.)

TABLE 46-6	Lancet Blade Recommendations	
DEPTH AND DIMENSION	**BLOOD VOLUME**	**APPLICATION**
2.25-mm, 28-gauge needle	Single drop	Fingersticks
2.25-mm, 23-gauge needle	Single drop	Fingersticks, glucose test
1 × 1.5-mm blade	Low blood flow	Fingersticks, microhematocrit tube, or drop of blood for glucose or cholesterol test
1.5 × 1.5-mm blade	Medium blood flow	Fingersticks; to fill a single Microtainer tube
2 × 1.5-mm blade	High blood flow	Fingersticks; to fill multiple Microtainer tubes

Modified from Beckton, Dickinson. www.bd.com/vacutainer/faqs/#urine_faq. Accessed December 30, 2015.

the Microtainers through a funnel-like device. Capillary tubes are another means of collecting blood from a dermal puncture. These are glass with an exterior protective plastic coating for safety. The blood is drawn into the tube by capillary action; that is, the blood fills into these narrow tubes without the need for suction. If the capillary tube is coated with the anticoagulant heparin, a red band

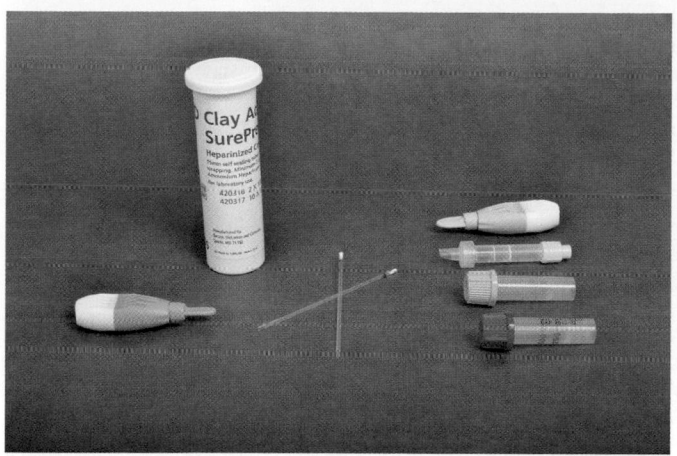

FIGURE 46-17 Pink lancet is to the left of the white container containing self-sealing capillary blood collection tubes (seen in the middle). *Right,* another blue lancet above three color-coded Micro-sample containers.

will be seen at the top. A common, heparin-coated capillary tube is the microhematocrit tube, which is used for determining the percentage of packed red blood cells in the microhematocrit test (discussed in the next chapter). Figure 46-17 also shows a capillary tube being sealed in a clay sealant. Some self-sealing capillary tubes no longer need to be pressed into the sealant.

Manufacturers also provide various collection devices for obtaining small amounts of blood for point-of-care testing, such as for glucose, hemoglobin A$_{1c}$, and cholesterol (see next chapter). The blood is pulled into the collecting device by capillary action after puncture, or it is applied into or onto a reagent strip that has been inserted into the instrument to be analyzed.

Blood from a capillary puncture may also be deposited on paper cards. The Guthrie card (Figure 46-18) is used to test neonates for certain metabolic disorders, such as phenylketonuria (PKU). Blood is deposited into circles on biologically inactive filter paper and is sent to a referral laboratory for analysis within 24 hours of sampling. Federal postal regulations for the mailing of biohazardous material must be followed.

Routine Capillary Puncture

Site Selection

In adults and children, the usual puncture site is the ring finger, but capillary blood can be obtained from the middle finger or heel (Figure 46-19). The thumb usually is too callused, and the index finger has extra nerve endings that make the puncture more painful. The fifth finger has too little tissue for a successful puncture. The puncture is made at the tip and slightly to the side of the finger. Be sure to puncture a fleshy area closer to the center of the finger to prevent damage to underlying bone. Avoid areas that are callused, scarred, burned, infected, cyanotic, or edematous.

For children younger than 1 year, dermal puncture is performed on the medial and lateral areas of the *plantar surface* (bottom) of the heel. Areas other than these are unsafe, and bone or nerve damage to an infant may occur. Blood flow from an infant's heel can be increased as much as sevenfold by applying a warm, moist towel (or other warming device) at a temperature no higher than 42°C

(108°F) for 3 to 5 minutes. Never place bandages on the heel or anywhere on infants younger than age 2, because they may peel off and become a choking hazard.

Patient Preparation

Preparation for a capillary puncture is similar to that for venipuncture. Put on a fluid-impermeable lab coat, sanitize your hands, and put on gloves. Cleanse the finger well with an alcohol prep pad. If the patient's hands are excessively soiled, ask the person to wash them before the procedure. If the patient's hands are cold, warm them in warm water and dry them thoroughly, or ask the person to rub or shake them vigorously.

Generally, you must work very efficiently when performing a capillary puncture because blood flow stops quickly. Be sure to have your supplies organized and within easy reach. Grasp the finger firmly and apply gentle, intermittent pressure, but do not squeeze or "milk" it. Press the puncture device firmly against the skin and quickly depress the plunger.

Collecting the Specimen

After the dermis has been punctured, it is important to wipe away the first drop of blood with sterile gauze. This drop contains tissue fluid that could interfere with test results. Fill the sampling containers according to the manufacturer's directions. Touch the container to the drop of blood as it is released from the puncture site, but do not touch the skin. If blood flow stops, wiping the site with gauze may restart the flow. Be prepared for blood to contaminate your gloves or other surfaces; have spare gloves, extra gauze pads, and disinfectant nearby. After the containers have been filled, ask the patient to apply pressure to the gauze you have placed over the puncture site if he or she is able. Seal and mix the containers by tilting as recommended by the manufacturer if necessary.

Specimen Handling

Capillary collection containers often are too small for a label to be applied. The most efficient way to transport capillary tubes is to remove the stopper from a red-topped tube, insert the capillary tubes, sealed-end down, replace the stopper, and label the tube. Microtainer tubes have plastic plugs that fit over the top. They may be placed in a labeled tube or in a labeled zipper-lock bag for transport. Always decontaminate collection containers before delivering them to the laboratory if blood was deposited on the surface during collection. The procedure for routine capillary collection is outlined in Procedure 46-4.

CRITICAL THINKING APPLICATION   **46-4**

1. Melissa calls Mrs. Cara Miata into the room. Mrs. Miata, who is 88, is seeing the physician today to have a blood glucose test done. She is a pleasant, talkative woman. Melissa begins to organize her supplies. She examines Mrs. Miata's arms and decides that drawing from the hand would be best. Why do you think she made this decision?

2. What supplies will she need to draw from the hand? What tubes and/or testing supplies will she use to collect samples?

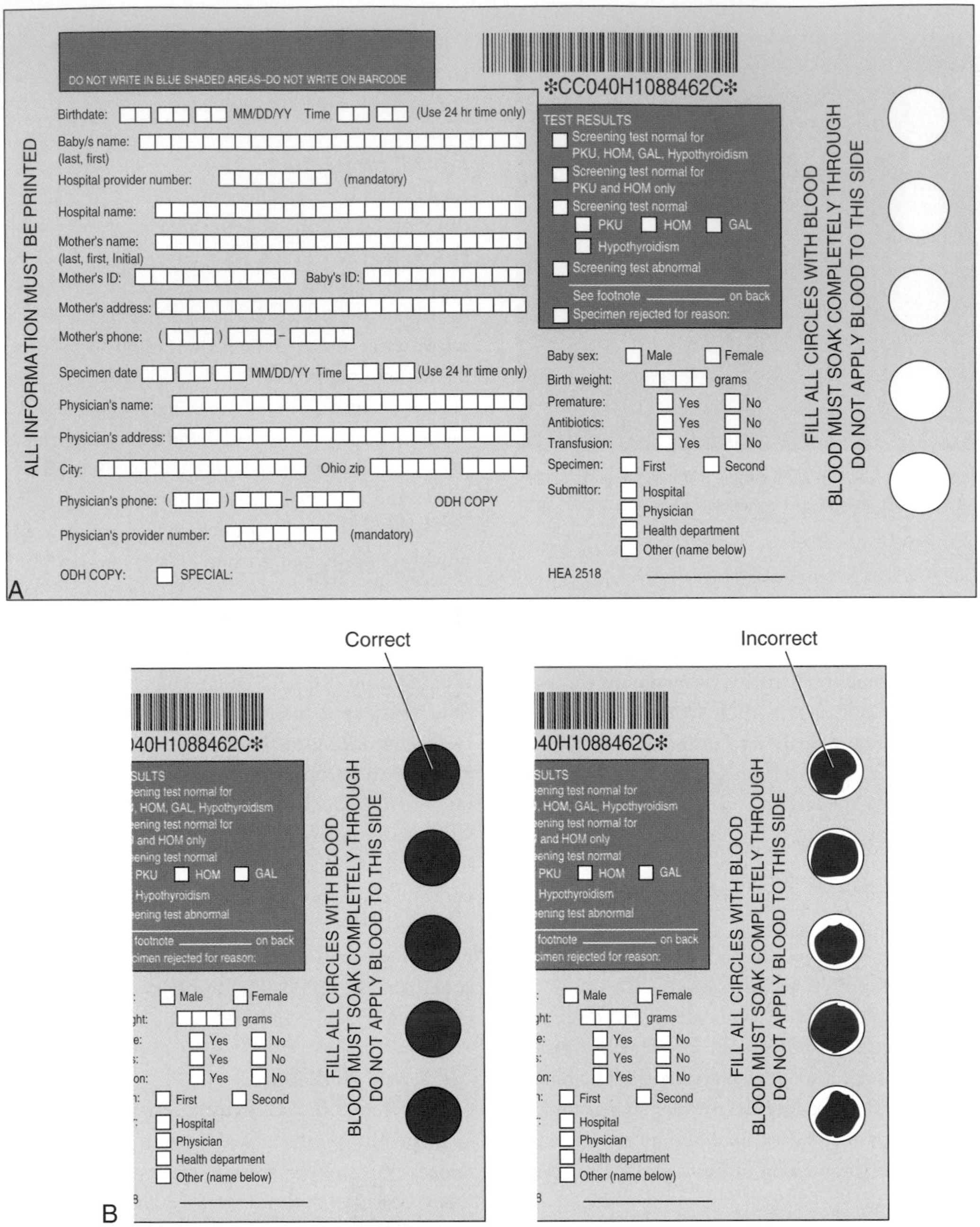

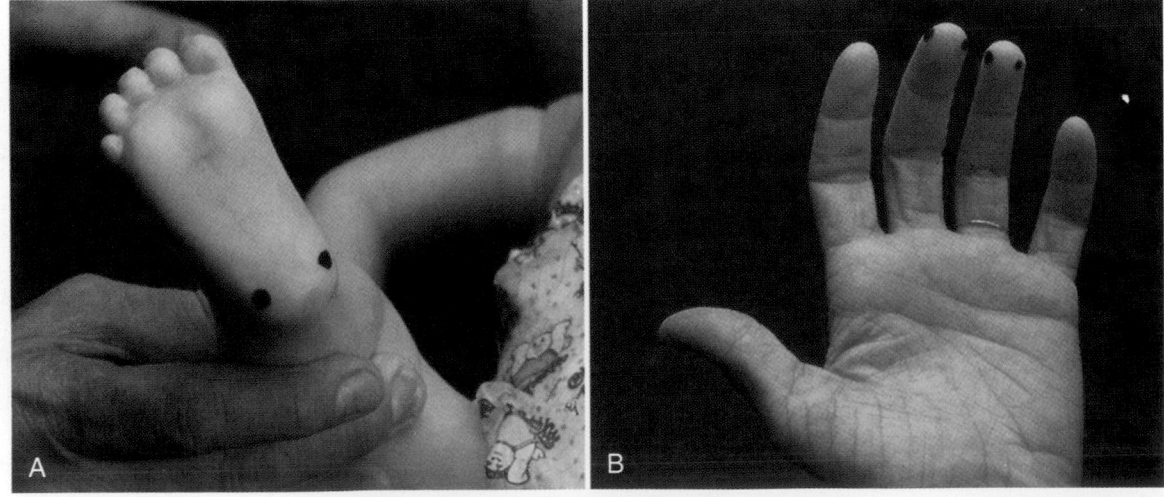

FIGURE 46-18 A, A Guthrie card used in neonatal screening. **B,** Correct and incorrect ways to fill in the circles. (From Warekois RS, Robinson R: *Phlebotomy: worktext and procedures manual,* ed 4, St Louis, 2016, Saunders.)

FIGURE 46-19 Capillary puncture sites on the heel and on the fingers.

| PROCEDURE 46-4 | Instruct and Prepare a Patient for a Procedure and Perform Capillary Puncture: Obtain a Capillary Blood Sample by Fingertip Puncture |

Goal: *To collect a capillary blood specimen suitable for testing using the fingertip puncture technique.*

EQUIPMENT and SUPPLIES

- Patient's health record
- Provider's order and/or lab requisition
- Sterile, disposable safety lancet
- 70% alcohol prep pads
- Gauze pads
- Nonallergenic tape
- Appropriate collection containers (e.g., capillary tubes, Microtainer tubes)
- Sealing clay or caps for capillary tubes
- Permanent marking pen or printed labels
- Fluid-impermeable lab coat and disposable gloves
- Biohazard bag
- Sharps container and biohazard waste container

PROCEDURAL STEPS

1. Check the provider's order and/or requisition form to determine the tests ordered. Gather the appropriate tubes and supplies.
   <u>PURPOSE:</u> To perform the procedure efficiently. Once the skin has been punctured, the collection must proceed as rapidly as possible so that the blood does not clot before the entire specimen has been collected.

2. Sanitize your hands and put on the fluid-impermeable lab coat and disposable gloves.
   <u>PURPOSE:</u> To ensure infection control.

3. Verify the patient's identity using two identifiers (e.g., have the person spell his or her last name, state the birth date, and/or show a picture ID). Explain the procedure and obtain permission for the venipuncture.
   <u>PURPOSE:</u> To make sure you have the right patient; explanations help gain the patient's cooperation.

4. Select a puncture site, depending on the patient's age and the sample to be obtained (e.g., side of middle or ring finger of nondominant hand, medial or lateral curved surface of the heel for an infant).
   <u>PURPOSE:</u> The nondominant hand may have fewer calluses. The side of the finger is less sensitive, and the skin usually is not as thick. Use great caution when performing capillary puncture on infants.

5. Gently rub the finger along the sides.
   <u>PURPOSE:</u> To promote circulation. If the finger is very cold, you may immerse it in warm water or moisten it with warm towels.

6. Clean the site with alcohol, allow it to air dry, or dry it with sterile gauze (Figure 1).
   <u>PURPOSE:</u> Puncturing skin that is wet with alcohol is painful and can hemolyze the specimen.

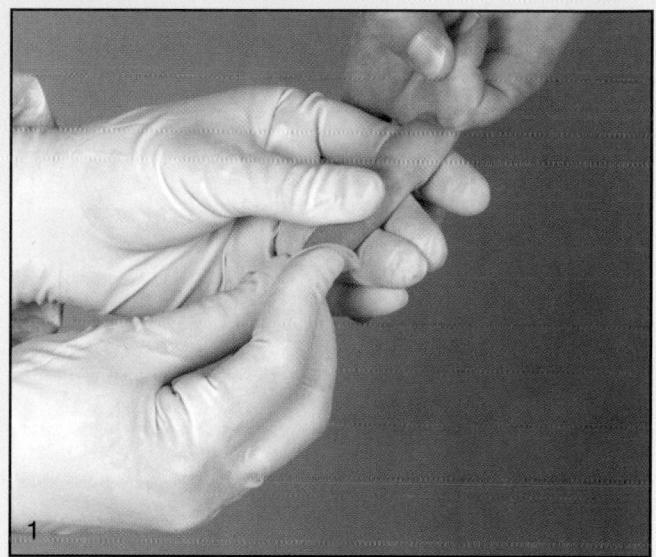

(From Garrels M, Oatis C: *Laboratory and diagnostic testing for ambulatory settings,* ed 3, St Louis, 2015, Saunders.)

7. Grasp the patient's finger on the sides near the puncture site with your nondominant forefinger and thumb.
   <u>PURPOSE:</u> Firmly holding the site allows control of the puncture.

8. Hold the safety lancet against the patient's finger and press down on the button that activates the needle or blade to penetrate the skin and then automatically retract (Figure 2).
   <u>PURPOSE:</u> Lancets are designed to puncture at specific depths that permit the free flow of blood.

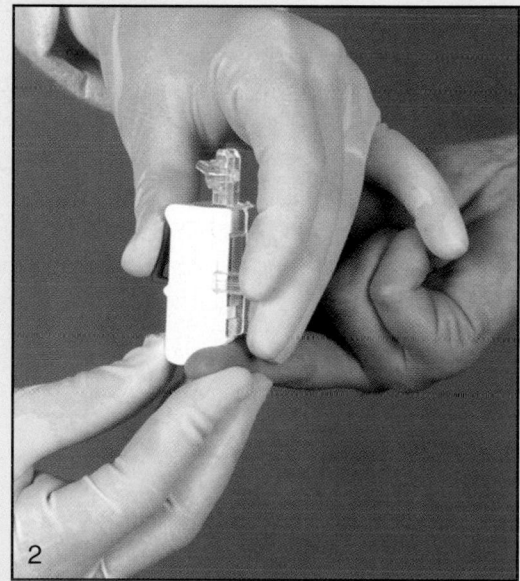

(From Garrels M, Oatis C: *Laboratory and diagnostic testing for ambulatory settings,* ed 3, St Louis, 2015, Saunders.)

9. Dispose of the lancet in the sharps container. Wipe away the first drop of blood with clean, sterile gauze.
PURPOSE: The first drop of blood contains tissue fluid, which may alter test results.

10. Apply gentle, intermittent pressure to cause the blood to flow freely (Figure 3).
PURPOSE: Forceful squeezing liberates fluid that dilutes the blood and causes inaccurate results.

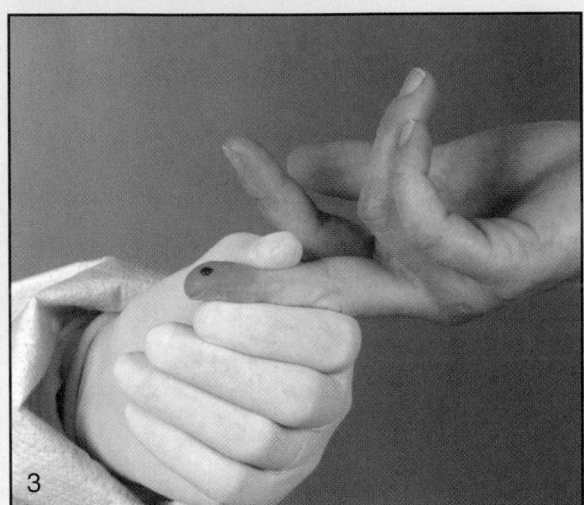

(From Garrels M, Oatis C: *Laboratory and diagnostic testing for ambulatory settings,* ed 3, St Louis, 2015, Saunders.)

11. Collect the blood samples.
(1) Express a large drop of blood. Touch the end of the tube to the drop of blood (not the finger) and fill the capillary to approximately three-fourths full or to the indicated line (Figure 4). Then tip the tube with the presealed end down. When the blood flows down and touches the sealant, hold it for 30 seconds to allow it to seal automatically. Alternatively, place your finger over the blood-free end of the tube and seal the other end of the tube by inserting it into the sealing clay. In both cases, the tube should be approximately three-fourths full before it is sealed.
PURPOSE: The specimen needs to be without air bubbles and then sealed in preparation for centrifuging. Placing your finger over the capillary tube prevents the blood from dripping onto the sealing clay.

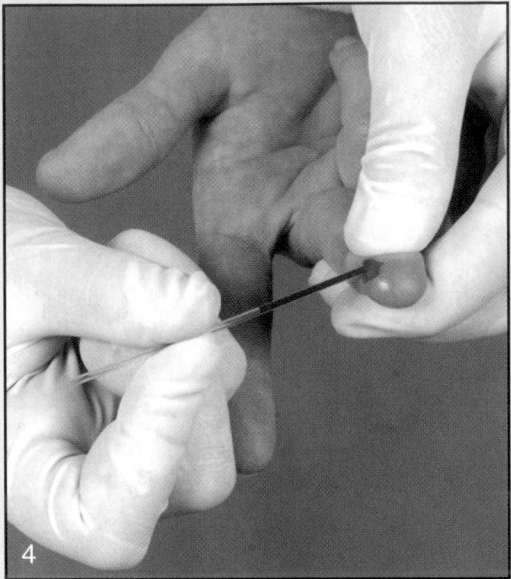

(From Garrels M, Oatis C: *Laboratory and diagnostic testing for ambulatory settings,* ed 3, St Louis, 2015, Saunders.)

(2) Wipe the patient's finger with a clean, sterile gauze pad. Express another large drop of blood and fill a Microtainer (Figure 5). Do not touch the container to the finger. If more blood is needed, wipe the puncture with sterile gauze and gently squeeze another drop. Cap the Microtainer tube when the collection is complete.
PURPOSE: Touching the container to the finger irritates the puncture site and may cause infection.

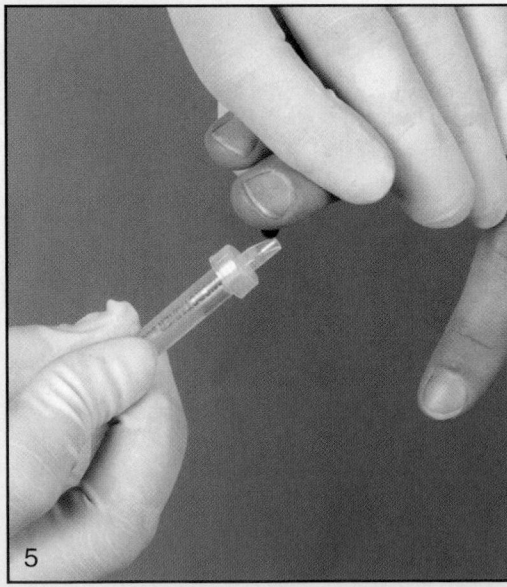

(From Garrels M, Oatis C: *Laboratory and diagnostic testing for ambulatory settings,* ed 3, St Louis, 2015, Saunders.)

12. When collection is complete, apply pressure to the site with clean, sterile gauze (Figure 6). The patient may be able to assist with this step.

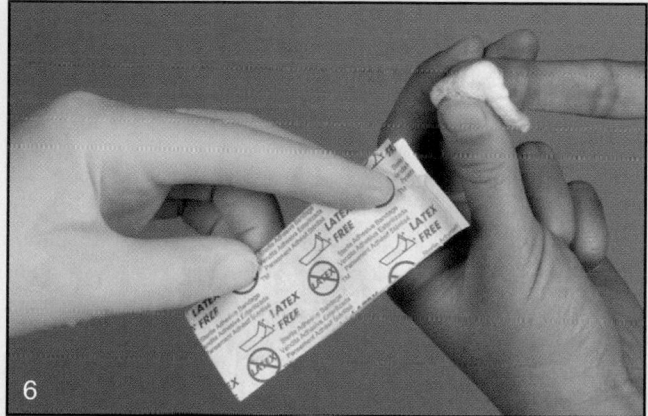

6

(From Garrels M, Oatis C: *Laboratory and diagnostic testing for ambulatory settings*, ed 3, St Louis, 2015, Saunders.)

13. Select an appropriate means of labeling the containers. Sealed capillary tubes can be placed in a red-topped tube, which is then labeled. Microtainers can be placed in zipper-lock biohazard bags that are subsequently labeled.
14. Check the patient for bleeding and clean the site if traces of blood are visible. Apply a nonallergenic bandage if indicated.
15. Disinfect the work area. Dispose of blood-contaminated materials (e.g., gauze and gloves) in the biohazard waste container. Remove your lab coat and sanitize your hands.
   PURPOSE: To ensure infection control.
16. Complete the laboratory requisition form and route the specimen to the proper place. Record the procedure in the patient's record.
   PURPOSE: A procedure is considered not done until it is recorded.

PEDIATRIC PHLEBOTOMY

Obtaining blood from children and infants may be difficult and potentially hazardous. The procedure should be performed only by personnel trained in the techniques for pediatric phlebotomy. Successfully obtaining blood from children requires skill and an understanding of pediatric psychological development, in addition to appropriate communication skills. The phlebotomist must gain the child's confidence and often that of the parent. Parents frequently ask the phlebotomist to explain the tests being done and the reasons for them. You should be very careful when divulging information; never tell the parents what disease or condition a specific blood test detects. Refer questions to the child's provider.

A parent or guardian may or may not be an asset during the procedure. Ask the parent about the child's previous phlebotomy experiences and how cooperative the child is likely to be. Tactfully determine whether the parent is comfortable with assisting in restraining an uncooperative child. Parental behavior greatly influences the child's behavior during the procedure. Children should never be restrained in a way that might cause physical injury. If the parent is unable or unwilling to assist with necessary restraint, always refer to the office or laboratory policy on restraints and procedural holds. Table 46-7 provides information on the typical fears and concerns of children during the procedure and suggested parental involvement.

Removing large amounts of blood, especially from premature infants, may result in anemia (Table 46-8). The amount of blood withdrawn must be recorded in the child's chart. Puncturing deep veins in children may result in cardiac arrest, hemorrhage, venous

TABLE 46-7	Childhood Behavior and Parental Involvement during Phlebotomy	
AGE	**TYPICAL MENTAL STATE**	**SUGGESTED PARENTAL INVOLVEMENT**
Newborns (0-12 months)	Trust that adults will respond to their needs.	Parent should assist by cradling and comforting child.
Infants and toddlers (1-3 years)	Minimal fear of danger but fear of separation; limited language and understanding of procedure.	Parent should assist by holding the child and providing emotional support.
Preschoolers (3-6 years)	Fearful of injury to body; still dependent on parent.	Parent may be present to provide emotional support and to assist in obtaining child's cooperation.
School-aged children (7-12 years)	Less dependent on parent and more willing to cooperate; fear of loss of self-control (crying).	Child may not want parent present.
Teenagers (13-18 years)	Fully engaged in the process; embarrassed to show fear and may show hostility to cover emotions.	Teen may not want parent present.

TABLE 46-8   General Guidelines for Pediatric Venipuncture

WEIGHT (lb)	SINGLE DRAW LIMIT
8-10	3.5 mL
11-15	5 mL
16-40	10 mL
41-60	20 mL
61-65	25 mL
66-80	30 mL

thrombosis, damage to surrounding tissues, or infection. In addition, the child could be harmed during forceful restraint. To prevent these problems, blood should be collected only by dermal puncture from children younger than age 2 unless the procedure warrants venous collection (lead levels or blood culture). Venipuncture on children younger than age 2 should be performed only on surface veins, including the dorsal hand vein, using a 23-gauge winged infusion set coupled to a syringe or a pediatric vacuum tube collection set.

When the medical assistant is required to perform pediatric phlebotomy, wearing a colorful, fluid-impermeable jacket; being truthful about the discomfort the child will feel; and providing tokens and praise for bravery go a long way toward allaying the child's fears. Topical anesthetics (e.g., ethyl chloride [EC] spray or EMLA cream) may be used to reduce pain at the puncture site. A new Buzzy Bee device is very effective in reducing pain during venipunctures and injections. In most cases a calm, professional phlebotomist who understands the developmental needs of the child and relates to the child on that level can gain the acceptance necessary to perform a successful venipuncture or dermal puncture with a minimum of restraint and frustration.

CRITICAL THINKING APPLICATION   46-5

1. As much as Leah likes children, performing capillary puncture on little fingers is not one of her favorite things to do. Mrs. Spix brings in her son, Garrett, for a hemoglobin and hematocrit test. Garrett is 3 years old. Mrs. Spix nervously asks Leah about the procedure and the tests Garrett must have. How can Leah adequately answer Mrs. Spix's questions and make Garrett and his mother feel at ease about this procedure?
2. What supplies will Leah need? Explain how she will perform the capillary puncture and perform the tests.

HANDLING THE SPECIMEN AFTER COLLECTION

It has been said that the results of laboratory testing are only as good as the specimen sent for testing. Specimens handled improperly after collection may provide erroneous results and unnecessarily compromise the patient's health. From the moment the specimen is collected, analytes in the blood begin to decay, and it is a race against time to provide results that accurately represent a patient's condition at the time of the blood collection. After collection, blood may need to be processed before the sample is sent to its final destination. For most samples, this involves separation of the plasma or serum from the red blood cells. If the tube contains no anticoagulant, blood begins to clot when it comes in contact with the red glass tube. The red-topped plastic tubes require the addition of a clot activator; the glass SST red-gray marble-topped tube and the plastic SST gold-topped tube have silica additives to accelerate clotting. All of these "clot" tubes should be allowed to sit upright in a rack for 30 to 60 minutes at room temperature while a solid clot forms. Tubes with clot accelerator should form a dense clot within 30 minutes. The presence of anticoagulants in the patient's blood, such as warfarin (Coumadin) or heparin, may delay clotting. Once the clot has formed, every effort should be made to remove the clot from the serum within 2 hours.

Removal of the clot from the serum requires centrifugation. For the thixotropic gel to form the barrier between the clot and the serum, certain g-force, time, and temperature requirements must be met. The clinical centrifuge instruction manual should provide the appropriate settings for spinning blood specimens. The serum does not have to be removed from the tube after centrifugation because the gel has formed a barrier over the red blood cells. Once a tube with thixotropic gel has been centrifuged, it cannot be centrifuged again. The serum, however, can be decanted and centrifuged in another tube.

For tests that require plasma, the plasma should be removed from the cells as soon as possible. This can be accomplished with centrifugation followed by aspiration of the plasma and transfer to another tube using a disposable pipet. A safer method of obtaining plasma is the use of the glass PST green-gray marble–topped tube or the plastic PST light green–topped tube. Both contain lithium heparin anticoagulant and a thixotropic gel, which forms the necessary barrier when centrifuged as described previously.

Certain blood tests, such as the CBC, require whole blood. It is wise to check the requirements of the laboratory that will perform the test as to how the specimen should be transported and stored. The College of American Pathologists recommends that whole blood for automated blood counts be refrigerated and tested within 72 hours.

Often specimens must be transported by courier to other facilities. The Hazardous Materials Shipping Regulations, established by the Department of Transportation, apply to the packaging or shipping of hazardous materials by ground transportation. Those who ship human specimens must be trained in all aspects of handling, packing, and shipping of biohazardous materials. Reference labs will also send couriers to pick up the specimens. The specimens and their requisitions are typically placed in individual biohazard bags and sorted according to which reference lab is affiliated with the patient's insurance.

CHAIN OF CUSTODY

Blood samples may be collected as evidence in legal proceedings. Blood may be drawn for drug and alcohol testing, DNA analysis, or parentage testing. These samples must be handled according to special procedures to prevent tampering, misidentification, or interference with the test results.

Chain of custody is a legal term that refers to the ability to guarantee the identity and integrity of the specimen from collection to reporting of test results. It is a process used to maintain and document the chronologic history of a specimen. Documents should include the name or initials of the individual collecting the specimen, each person or entity subsequently having custody of it, the date the specimen was collected or transferred, the employer or agency, the specimen number, the patient's or employee's name, and a brief description of the specimen.

Collection kits are available that contain everything needed for the venipuncture, including the tube, the needle, the chain of custody forms and seals, the antiseptic, and even the tourniquet. Familiarize yourself with these kits before you are required to use them. You may be required to testify at a legal proceeding if you are involved in the collection or testing of a sample.

CLOSING COMMENTS

Patient Education

Provide as much explanation as needed to ease the patient's anxiety. Often the patient can help by identifying the site of the last successful blood draw. Follow the patient's suggestion in choosing the site for obtaining a blood specimen. When a patient is allowed to become an active participant in the procedure, he or she remains more relaxed, talkative, and confident in your expertise as a phlebotomist.

Legal and Ethical Issues

Venipuncture and microcapillary blood collection are invasive procedures in which a sterile needle or a lancet is inserted through the skin. Because the skin is penetrated, drawing blood becomes a surgical procedure and is subject to the laws and regulations of surgery. When venipuncture is performed, the rules and regulations must be enforced with no deviations. Be sure to follow the procedures as

written and to become familiar with the regulations and standards established by local and state agencies, in addition to CLSI and OSHA. Deviations leave the medical assistant open to accusations of malpractice. Document any situations that arise in which observation of the standard of care comes into question.

Professional Behaviors

Your appearance and actions reflect your laboratory or facility. A patient's first impression of the facility often comes from you. Clean fluid-impermeable laboratory coats and scrubs tell the patient the facility is clean; sanitizing your hands and wearing gloves tells the patient you will treat him or her with care; and speaking knowledgeably provides the impression that the facility is staffed with professionals.

Medical assistants who perform venous and capillary blood collection must maintain a professional attitude, yet remain sympathetic to the patient's fears and anxiety about being "stuck with a needle." Establishing an environment that encourages the person to relax can minimize the patient's pain and discomfort during the procedure. Always remember to verify your patient's identity and explain what you are going to do. Answer any questions the patient may have, and perform the procedure skillfully before anxiety has time to set in.

The atmosphere can change dramatically if the patient has had an unpleasant experience and associates pain and discomfort with venipuncture. Such a patient usually is ill at ease and apprehensive. In this case, you need to make every effort to perform the procedure quickly, efficiently, and effectively. Once the blood has been drawn and the patient has relaxed, you can help the patient develop a positive attitude.

If your patient has a history of syncope when blood is drawn or if you suspect the patient may faint during the procedure, have the person lie down. Assemble your equipment and alert the provider before beginning the procedure. This type of professional care may help the patient get through the procedure without a traumatic effect.

SUMMARY OF SCENARIO

Leah has learned that phlebotomy is truly an art. Although she was nervous at first, she has become quite proficient with this new skill. She discovered that her nervousness was "contagious," and that if she remains calm and organized, her patients are more likely to feel at ease with the procedure. She has learned that it is necessary to talk with patients before drawing their blood, not only to allay their fears, but also to get clues about past problems or the best site for the draw. She has learned that she is responsible for explaining the tests ordered and how much blood she will draw, but that she is not responsible for explaining the reasons the tests are being done. Effective communication is the most important aspect of phlebotomy.

Through practice and careful attention, Leah has come to recognize the proper equipment to use in phlebotomy, and she never hesitates to call the referral laboratory used by her employer if she has a question about proper collection of a specimen. Communicating with children and adults is as different as the equipment she uses for venipuncture; the small veins of children and the elderly require special care, and she has become proficient in the use of winged infusion sets and syringes to prevent vein collapse. Leah is well aware of the dangers of phlebotomy, and through education and the use of approved safety devices, she is confident that she can provide excellent care for her patients at the Health Alliance Medical Clinic.

SUMMARY OF LEARNING OBJECTIVES

1. **Define, spell, and pronounce the terms listed in the vocabulary.**
   Spelling and pronouncing medical terms correctly reinforce the medical assistant's credibility. Knowing the definitions of these terms promotes confidence in communication with patients and co-workers.

2. **List the equipment needed for venipuncture.**
   Venipuncture requires a double-pointed safety needle, evacuated collection tubes, a needle holder or a syringe fitted with a safety needle, a tourniquet, an alcohol prep pad, gauze or cotton, a sterile bandage, nonlatex gloves, and a biohazard sharps container.

3. **Explain the purpose of a tourniquet, how to apply it, and the consequences of improper tourniquet application.**
   A tourniquet is used to hold back venous flow out of the site, which causes the veins to bulge. The tourniquet makes veins easier to locate and puncture. Tourniquets are applied snugly around the upper arm (or wrist for a hand draw) in a fashion that permits easy release. Leaving the tourniquet on a prolonged time results in hemoconcentration; applying the tourniquet too tightly results in unnecessary discomfort to the patient and the release of tissue fluid into the blood.

4. **Explain why the stopper colors on vacuum tubes differ, and state the correct order of drawing samples for various types of tests.**
   The various colors of vacuum tube stoppers indicate the contents of the tube. Certain additives are compatible with certain laboratory tests. The phlebotomist must be knowledgeable about blood tests and the types of tubes needed. Consulting literature provided by the manufacturer ensures the proper choice of a collection tube. The correct order of draw is (1) pale yellow (sterile or SPS), (2) light blue, (3) red, red-gray marbled, or gold plastic top, (4) green, (5) lavender, and (6) gray. Vacuum tubes are collected in a specific order to prevent carryover of tube additives.

5. **Describe the types of safety needles used in phlebotomy.**
   The venipuncture needle has a shaft with one end cut at an angle (bevel). The other end (the hub) attaches to the syringe or to a needle holder. The inner bore or space in the needle is called the *lumen*. It is measured in gauge numbers (the higher the gauge number, the smaller the lumen). Double-pointed needles are used for the evacuated tube method in which the blood flows directly from the vein into the evacuated tube. Removable safety needles are used with disposable syringes. The collected blood in the syringe is then transferred to the appropriate evacuated tubes using a safety transfer device. Safety lancets are used for dermal puncture.

6. **Explain why a syringe rather than an evacuated tube would be chosen for blood collection.**
   Syringes are more commonly used for blood collection from elderly patients, whose veins tend to be more fragile; from children, whose veins tend to be small; and from obese patients, whose veins tend to be deep. Using a syringe allows a more controlled draw. Syringes commonly are used with winged infusion sets.

7. **Discuss the use of safety-engineered needles and collection devices required for injury protection.**
   OSHA requires that all sharp items (i.e., needles and glass) used for phlebotomy should be engineered with safety devices, such as retractable needles, self-sheathing needles, and blunting devices. Needles should never be recapped with two hands, and in most cases they are not removed from the venipuncture unit. All sharps must be disposed of in an approved biohazard sharps container.

8. **Summarize postexposure management of needlesticks.**
   OSHA requires employers to have a postexposure plan in place for accidental sharps exposures. These plans generally include a means to cleanse the wound with an appropriate antiseptic cleanser; evaluation of the exposure to determine whether the employee is at risk for contracting HBV, HCV, or HIV, depending on the circumstance of the injury; gathering of information about the source of the blood involved; prophylactic care if necessary; confidential counseling for the injured; and follow-up on the exposure.

9. **Do the following related to routine venipuncture:**
   - *Detail patient preparation for venipuncture that shows sensitivity to the patient's rights and feelings.*
     The medical assistant must be sensitive to the needs and concerns of patients both before and during the phlebotomy procedure. The procedure should be explained to the patient, and all questions should be answered. The patient should be observed for any problems during the procedure, and the medical assistant should use therapeutic communication techniques throughout the intervention.
   - *Describe and name the veins that may be used for blood collection.*
     The median cephalic vein is the vein of choice for phlebotomy, but blood can be drawn from the cephalic vein and the median basilic vein. The basilic vein should not be used if possible. The dorsal vein on the hand may be used.
   - *List in order the steps of a routine venipuncture.*
     A routine venipuncture begins with greeting the patient and verifying his or her identity. The medical assistant then sanitizes his or her hands, assembles the equipment and PPE, locates the vein, disinfects the area over the vein, allows the alcohol to dry, draws the blood into the correct vacuum tubes in the proper order of draw, removes and properly disposes of the needle, tends to the puncture site, labels the tubes, and delivers them to the laboratory. Standard Precautions are followed during the procedure.
   - *Perform a venipuncture using the evacuated tube method.*
     Refer to Procedure 46-1.
   - *Perform a venipuncture using the syringe method.*
     Refer to Procedure 46-2.

10. **Do the following related to problems associated with venipuncture and specimen re-collection:**
    - *Discuss various problems associated with venipuncture.*
      Failure to obtain blood can occur because of a variety of factors. Several possible causes, such as hematomas, fainting, and nerve damage, are discussed in the text.
    - *Discuss possible solutions to venipuncture complications.*
      Refer to Table 46-4 for a list of solutions to possible complications.

SUMMARY OF LEARNING OBJECTIVES—*continued*

- *Discuss why a specimen may have to be re-collected.*
Specimens can be rejected by a laboratory for a variety of reasons. Hemolysis is the major cause of specimen re-collection.
- *Describe the major causes of hemolysis during collection.*
Refer to Table 46-5.

11. **Do the following related to capillary puncture:**
    - *Explain why a winged infusion set (butterfly needle) would be chosen over a vacuum tube or syringe needle.*
    A winged infusion set (butterfly needle) is used on blood draws from the hand and from children. The needle is shorter, and the wings assist with holding and guiding the needle. The tubing minimizes the force of the vacuum and prevents collapse of fragile veins. Using a syringe can also control the vacuum to a greater extent than using vacuum tubes.
    - *Perform a venipuncture using a winged infusion set (butterfly needle).*
    Refer to Procedure 46-3.
    - *List situations in which capillary puncture would be preferred over venipuncture.*
    Capillary puncture is preferred over venipuncture for certain point-of-care tests, such as hematocrit or hemoglobin analysis. It is performed routinely on children younger than age 2.
    - *Discuss proper dermal puncture sites.*
    The lateral sides of the tips of the middle two fingers generally are used for capillary puncture. In infants, the medial and lateral sides on the plantar surface of the heel are the sites of choice. The center of the heel must be avoided.
    - *Describe containers that may be used to collect capillary blood.*
    Capillary blood can be collected in or on specific devices related to point-of-care tests. Microtainer tubes, capillary tubes, and paper test cards are also used to send specimens to the lab for testing. The Microtainer tubes may contain anticoagulants and additives and have stopper colors consistent with vacuum tubes.

- *Explain why the first drop of blood is wiped away when a capillary puncture is performed.*
The first drop of blood contains tissue fluid that could affect the test results.
- *Perform a capillary puncture.*
Refer to Procedure 46-4.

12. **Discuss pediatric phlebotomy, including typical childhood behavior and parental involvement during phlebotomy and general guidelines for pediatric venipuncture.**
Obtaining blood from children and infants may be difficult and potentially hazardous. Refer to Table 46-7 for information on typical fears and concerns of children during the procedure and suggested parental involvement. Refer to Table 46-8 for general guidelines for pediatric venipuncture.

13. **Describe handling and transport methods for blood after collection.**
From the moment the specimen is collected, analytes in the blood begin to decay, and it is a race against time to provide results that accurately represent a patient's condition at the time of the blood collection. There are various procedures based on the type of test performed.

14. **Explain chain of custody procedures when blood samples are drawn.**
Chain of custody is a legal term that refers to the ability to guarantee the identity and integrity of the specimen from collection to reporting of the test results. It is a process used to maintain and document the chronologic history of a specimen.

15. **Discuss patient education, in addition to legal and ethical issues, related to assisting in blood collection.**
Provide as much information as needed to ease the patient's anxiety. Document any situations that arise in which observations of the standard of care comes into question.

CONNECTIONS

Study Guide Connection: Go to the Chapter 46 Study Guide. Read and complete the activities.

evolve Evolve Connection: Go to the Chapter 46 link at *evolve.elsevier.com/ kinn* to complete the Chapter Review Quiz. Check out the other resources listed for this chapter to make the most of what you have learned from Assisting in Blood Collection.

47

ASSISTING IN THE ANALYSIS OF BLOOD

SCENARIO

Dana Cummings, CMA (AAMA) is working in the Westhills Family Practice Center. She is preparing to collect blood from Mr. Corrigan, who recently underwent renal transplantation because of complications from diabetes type 1. He has come to the office today for a routine examination. Dr. Fischbach suspects that Mr. Corrigan is anemic and orders an anemia panel in addition to a renal panel; a hemoglobin A_{1c} level; a complete blood count (CBC), including hemoglobin, hematocrit, and differential; prothrombin time/international normalized ratio (PT/INR); and alanine aminotransferase/aspartate aminotransferase (ALT/AST) testing.

While studying this chapter, think about the following questions:
- Why are so many tests being performed for Mr. Corrigan?
- Which of these tests probably will be completed today in the office laboratory?

LEARNING OBJECTIVES

1. Define, spell, and pronounce the terms listed in the vocabulary.
2. Name the main functions of blood.
3. Describe the appearance and function of erythrocytes.
4. Describe the appearance and function of granular and agranular leukocytes.
5. Differentiate between T cells and B cells.
6. Describe the appearance and function of thrombocytes, explain the process of clot formation, and discuss plasma.
7. Do the following related to hematology in the POL:
   - Identify the anticoagulant of choice for hematology testing.
   - Explain the purpose of the microhematocrit test.
   - Perform routine maintenance of a microhematocrit centrifuge.
   - Obtain a specimen and perform a microhematocrit test.
8. Do the following related to hemoglobin:
   - Explain the role of hemoglobin in the body.
   - Obtain a specimen and perform a hemoglobin test.
9. Do the following related to the erythrocyte sedimentation rate:
   - Cite the reasons for performing an erythrocyte sedimentation rate (ESR) test.
   - Describe the sources of error for the erythrocyte sedimentation rate (ESR) test.
   - Perform an erythrocyte sedimentation rate (ESR) test using a modified Westergren method.
10. Do the following related to coagulation testing:
    - Explain how to determine prothrombin time (PT).
    - Obtain a specimen and perform a CLIA-waived PT/INR test.
    - Reassure a patient of the accuracy of the test results.
    - Maintain lab test results using laboratory flow sheets.
11. Identify the tests included in a complete blood count (CBC) and their reference ranges, and differentiate between normal and abnormal test results.
12. Describe the red blood cell (RBC) indices and how they are calculated.
13. Explain the reasons for performing a white blood cell (WBC) count and differential, and discuss preparation of blood smears for the differential.
14. Discuss the identification of normal blood cells and describe the basic appearance of the five different types of leukocytes seen in a normal Wright-stained differential.
15. Discuss red blood cell morphology.
16. Differentiate between the ABO blood groupings and the Rh blood groupings.
17. Describe the medical assistant's responsibility for legally preparing a patient for a blood transfusion.
18. Do the following related to blood chemistry testing:
    - Explain the reasons for testing blood glucose, hemoglobin A_{1c}, cholesterol, liver enzymes, and thyroid hormones.
    - Obtain a specimen and perform a blood glucose, hemoglobin A_{1c}, and cholesterol test using CLIA-waived test methods approved by the U.S. Food and Drug Administration (FDA).
19. Summarize typical chemistry panels, the reason for performing each panel, and the individual tests performed in the panels.
20. Discuss patient education and professionalism related to assisting in the analysis of blood.

VOCABULARY

anemia A condition marked by a deficiency of red blood cells (RBCs).

antibody A specific protein produced by a lymphocytic plasma cell to destroy a specific foreign invader (antigen) in the body.

antigen A foreign invader (e.g., bacterium, virus, toxin, allergen) that generates an immune response with the production of antibodies.

artifacts Structures or features not normally present but visible as a result of an external agent or action.

basophils White blood cells with granules that stain deep blue and play a part in the inflammatory process.

buffy coat The layer of white cells and platelets found between the plasma and the packed RBCs after whole blood is centrifuged.

centrifuge (sen'-trih-fuj) An apparatus consisting essentially of a compartment that spins about a central axis to separate contained materials of different specific gravities or to separate colloidal particles suspended in a liquid.

cuvette A specimen container made of plastic or glass designed to hold samples for laboratory tests using light meter technology (spectrophotometry).

enzymes Complex proteins produced by cells that act as catalysts in specific biochemical reactions.

eosinophils White blood cells with granules that stain red. Their numbers increase during allergic reactions.

leukocytosis An increase in the number of white blood cells (WBCs).

lymphocytes Non-granular small white blood cells with a dense nucleus. Their numbers increase during a viral infection.

monocytes Non-granular large white blood cells with a large lobular nucleus. Their numbers increase during the recovery phase of tissue damage.

neutrophils White blood cells with small granules that stain lavender. They are the most common WBC and fight bacterial infections.

polycythemia vera (pah-le-si-the'-me-uh/vch' rah) A condition marked by an abnormally large number of red blood cells (RBCs) in the circulatory system.

type and cross-match Tests performed to assess the compatibility of blood to be transfused.

urea The major nitrogenous end product of protein metabolism and the chief nitrogenous waste product in the urine.

The average body holds 10 to 12 pints of blood. The heart circulates the blood through the circulatory system more than 1,000 times every day. More than 70,000 miles of passageways, most of which are narrower than a human hair, carry blood throughout the body. The blood is contained in a closed system of vessels; the largest is the aorta, and the smallest are the capillaries. The capillaries are only one cell layer thick, and their thin, permeable walls allow certain substances to move back and forth between blood vessels and surrounding tissue. The circulating blood contains more than 25 trillion cells, and every second the body replaces 8 million old red blood cells (RBCs) with 8 million new RBCs.

The circulating blood supplies the body's cells with nutrients and oxygen. The blood carries away carbon dioxide and **urea**, the waste products of normal cell activity. If the blood did not carry away these waste products, they would accumulate and damage the cells. Carbon dioxide is carried in the blood to the lungs, where it is exhaled as part of normal breathing. The blood carries urea to the kidneys, where it is excreted in the urine along with other body wastes. The blood also distributes **enzymes,** hormones, and other chemicals needed for control and regulation of body activities. In addition, the blood functions to maintain the body at a uniform temperature, to keep other body fluids in a state of pH balance, and to carry hormones from the secreting gland to the tissues where they are needed.

Blood tests are done routinely in the hematology, immunohematology (blood banking), chemistry, and immunology (serology) departments of the laboratory. The degree of blood testing performed by medical assistants depends on the level of service offered by the ambulatory care facility and the regulations established by the Clinical Laboratory Improvement Amendments (CLIA). As a

medical assistant, you are qualified to perform the CLIA-waived procedures described in the physician office laboratory (POL) sections of this chapter. The more highly complex CLIA blood tests are performed at reference and hospital laboratories and are not performed by medical assistants. Nevertheless, this chapter explains these procedures to provide background information critical to an understanding of the analysis of blood, from collection of the specimen, through testing, to recording of the results.

HEMATOLOGY

Whole blood is composed of visible formed elements suspended in *plasma* (a clear, yellow liquid). Plasma makes up approximately 55% of blood by volume. The remaining 45% consists of the following visible cellular elements: erythrocytes (RBCs), leukocytes (WBCs), and thrombocytes (platelets). All these cellular elements have special functions.

Erythrocytes

RBCs, or erythrocytes, are formed in the red bone marrow of the ribs, sternum, pelvis, and skull and in the ends of long bones in adults. The nucleus of the immature RBC disintegrates as the cell matures. Loss of the nucleus results in the familiar shape of the RBC: a biconcave disk that is thicker at the rim than in the middle. Erythrocytes transport oxygen from the lungs to the body cells, and they carry some of the carbon dioxide away from cells back to the lungs to be exhaled. The main constituent of the RBC is the red pigment, hemoglobin, which is composed of iron and protein. Hemoglobin is the carrier of oxygen and some carbon dioxide.

The life span of an erythrocyte is approximately 120 days. As the cell nears the end of its life, it becomes more fragile and eventually ruptures and breaks. The iron is reused for the formation of new RBCs, and the remaining portion is converted into bilirubin, which then becomes bile in the liver.

Leukocytes

WBCs, or leukocytes, have a nucleus and are larger than erythrocytes. The primary function of the leukocytes is to protect the body against infection and disease. The five types of leukocytes are classified into two categories: granular (three types; cells with granules) and agranular (two types; cells without granules).

Granular Leukocytes

The three granular leukocytes are the polymorphonuclear **neutrophils** (PMNs), **eosinophils** (EOs), and **basophils** (BASOs). They are characterized by their heavily granulated cytoplasm and segmented nuclei. The neutrophils are *phagocytic;* that is, they engulf and destroy invading bacteria and viruses. Unlike erythrocytes, leukocytes are found in both the bloodstream and the tissues. During inflammation, the blood carries the PMNs through dilated vessels to the site of injury. Capillary walls become more permeable, and the granular cells squeeze through to the site of infection. Once at the site of infection or injury, the PMNs engulf the invading microorganism, creating pus, which contains dead leukocytes, bacteria, and tissue cells. The eosinophils are associated with allergies, and the basophils play a part in inflammation.

Nongranular Leukocytes

The two nongranular leukocytes are the **monocytes** and **lymphocytes**, both of which have clear cytoplasm (no granules) and a solid nucleus. The large monocytes become *macrophages* (large engulfing) cells when they enter the tissues and engulf pathogens and debris. The small lymphocytes are responsible for immunity and are further classified into T cells and B cells based on their functional characteristics.

T Cells: Cell-Mediated Immunity. T lymphocytes make up about 65% to 80% of the circulating lymphocytes; they have a life span of months to years. This is important for obtaining long-lasting immunity to microbial infections. Four types of T cells mount an immune response to parasites, viruses, fungi, and bacteria:

- *Natural killer cells:* These T cells kill virus-infected cells and tumor cells without previous sensitization.
- *Helper T cells:* These are the most numerous type of T cell. They stimulate the activity of other T cells and help the B cells produce their antibodies. Note: These are the T lymphocytes that are destroyed by the human immunodeficiency virus (HIV), causing the individual to be immunodeficient.
- *Suppressor T cells:* These cells inhibit the activity of other T cells once the invaders are under control.
- *Memory T cells:* These cells, which have a long life span, respond quickly to the presentation of the same antigen at a later date.

B Cells: Humoral Immunity (Antibody-Mediated). B cells are formed in bone marrow and then migrate to other lymph organs (i.e., lymph nodes and the spleen), where they multiply and reside. When stimulated by the T cells, B cells differentiate into plasma cells that produce the specific **antibody** needed to destroy a specific **antigen**. The antibodies circulate in the plasma or are present in secretions.

Antibodies are protein molecules that specifically attach to antigens. Very small antigens, such as toxins and viruses, can be directly neutralized by antibodies. Larger antigens, such as bacteria, require the help of neutrophils to *phagocytize* (engulf) and destroy them.

Three steps are required to activate the B cells to produce their specific antibody that then attacks the particular antigen or the pathogen:

1. *Antigen processing:* When the macrophage (formerly a monocyte) *phagocytizes* (engulfs) bacteria, proteins from the bacteria are broken down into smaller molecules, which are then "displayed" on the surface of the macrophage.
2. *Lymphocyte stimulation:* When a T lymphocyte "sees" the molecules displayed on the macrophage, the T cell brings the message to the B cell which becomes a plasma cell capable of making the specific antibodies to destroy the foreign invader (antigen).
3. *Antibody production:* The stimulated B cell also undergoes repeated cell division, enlargement, and differentiation to form a clone of antibody-secreting plasma cells. The antibodies then bind to the bacteria, making them easier for the white cells to ingest, or the antibodies combine with a plasma component called *complement* that kills the bacteria directly.

Hypersensitivity reactions, such as allergies and autoimmune diseases, are the result of overactive lymphocytic defenses.

Thrombocytes

Thrombocytes are not true cells, but rather cytoplasmic fragments of a megakaryocyte, a large cell in the bone marrow. They are the smallest formed elements of the blood. They typically have a discoid shape; however, when activated, they become globular and form fingerlike cytoplasmic extensions called *pseudopodia.*

Clot Formation

In minor injuries, thrombocytes (platelets) tend to collect and form plugs in blood vessel openings. To control bleeding from vessels larger than capillaries, a clot must form at the point of injury. Coagulation (clotting) of the blood is also initiated by blood platelets. The platelets produce a substance that combines with calcium ions in the blood to form thromboplastin, which in turn converts the protein prothrombin into thrombin through a complex series of reactions. Thrombin, an enzyme, converts fibrinogen, a protein substance, into fibrin, an insoluble protein that forms an intricate network of minute, threadlike structures.. The blood cells and plasma become enmeshed in the network forming a clot.

More than 30 substances in the blood have been found to affect clotting; whether blood will coagulate depends on a balance between the substances that promote coagulation and those that inhibit it *(anticoagulants).* Coagulation of blood within blood vessels in the absence of injury *(thrombosis)* can cause serious illness or death, especially when a clot forms in the coronary arteries, causing heart attacks, or in the cerebral arteries, causing strokes.

Hemophilia, a bleeding disorder, occurs when a person has a mutation in one of the clotting factor genes. It is a hereditary, gender-linked disorder that affects males of all races and ethnic groups. The mutated gene is on the X chromosome inherited from the mother. Approximately one in 5,000 males is born with the disorder; it is rare, but possible, for a female to have hemophilia. People with hemophilia are treated with intravenous (IV) purified clotting factor and/or DDAVP to prevent bleeding episodes. Internal bleeding can affect the joints and the neurologic system. Bleeding within the joints can cause chronic joint disease and pain. Bleeding in the brain can cause seizures, paralysis, and even death.

Plasma

Plasma is the highly complex liquid that is the carrier for the formed elements plus other substances, such as proteins, carbohydrates, fats, hormones, enzymes, mineral salts, gases, and waste products. Plasma is composed of approximately 90% water, 9% protein, and 1% various other chemical substances. When the clotting proteins (prothrombin and fibrinogen) and the other clotting components are used up during the clotting process (e.g. within a "clot" or "SST" specimen), the remaining liquid is called *serum.*

HEMATOLOGY IN THE PHYSICIAN OFFICE LABORATORY (POL)

For most POL hematology tests, an adequate blood sample can be obtained from capillary punctures of the finger. If a larger sample is required, blood can be obtained via venipuncture. For a complete blood count (CBC), venous blood is collected in a lavender-topped tube containing ethylenediaminetetraacetic acid (EDTA), an anticoagulant that prevents clotting. EDTA is the anticoagulant of choice for hematology testing because it also acts as a preservative for the blood cells. It is very important to prevent blood from being hemolyzed during collection for hematology testing.

Hematocrit

The hematocrit (Hct) is a measurement of the percentage of packed RBCs in a volume of blood. The spun microhematocrit test is based on the principle of separating the cellular elements from plasma by centrifugation (Procedures 47-1 and 47-2). Two or three drops of blood are collected from a capillary puncture in two capillary tubes that are placed in a specially designed microhematocrit **centrifuge** (Figure 47-1). Alternatively, the capillary tubes can be filled with EDTA-anticoagulated blood from a lavender-topped vacuum tube. As required by the Occupational Safety and Health Administration (OSHA), capillary tubes must be safe, with plastic-coated glass or all plastic to avoid sharps injuries. They may be either self-sealing at one end or open-ended on both ends. If the tube is self-sealing, it must be tilted upright, causing the blood sample to flow down the tube and come into contact with the seal, and then held in place for 15 seconds. The open-ended tubes must be sealed with special clay before centrifugation.

After centrifugation, the packed RBCs are at the bottom of the tube against the sealant, the WBCs and platelets are in the center **buffy coat**, and plasma is on top (Figure 47-2). The microhematocrit

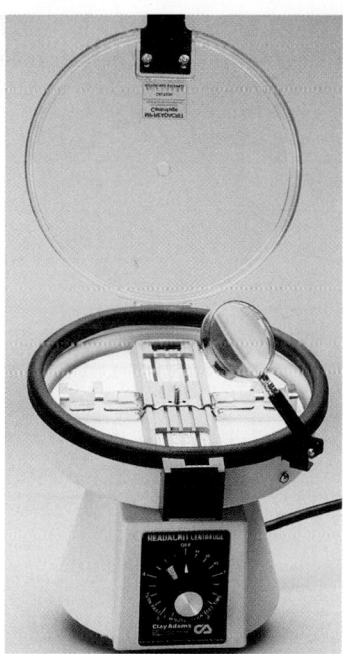

FIGURE 47-1 Centrifuge with indicators for capillary tube placement.

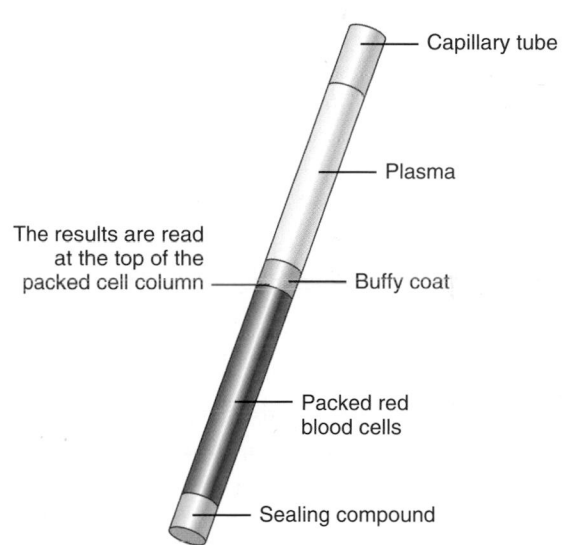

FIGURE 47-2 Hematocrit test results. Cellular elements are separated from plasma by centrifuging an anticoagulated blood specimen, and the results are read at the top of the packed cell column.

is determined by comparing the volume of RBCs to the total volume of the whole blood sample. The percentage is read by placing the tubes on a special microhematocrit reader. Some microhematocrit centrifuges have a built-in reading scale that reads the calibrated capillary tubes. Microhematocrits should be performed in duplicate and the average of the two results reported.

Normal Hct values vary with gender and age (Table 47-1). They range from a low of 36% in women to a high of 52% in men. Low microhematocrit values can indicate **anemia** or the presence of bleeding. High values may be caused by dehydration or by a condition such as **polycythemia vera**. Values can be influenced by physiologic or pathologic factors and by collection

TABLE 47-1 Hematocrit (Hct) Reference Values

AGE/GENDER	Hct VALUE (%)
Neonate (new born-under 1 month)	44-64
Infant (1 month-1 yr)	37-41
Child (1-10 yr)	35-41
Men (greater than 10 yrs)	42-52
Women (greater than 10 yrs)	36-45

techniques. Normal Hct ranges are also affected by geographic location; for example, people living in high altitudes have a higher percentage of RBCs to compensate for the lower oxygen levels in the atmosphere.

The microhematocrit is a commonly performed test requested by providers either separately or as part of the CBC. Because it is a simple procedure that requires only a small amount of blood, it is an ideal screening test and often is part of a routine physical examination. Quality assurance includes care and maintenance of the microhematocrit instrument.

PROCEDURE 47-1 Perform Routine Maintenance of Clinical Equipment: Perform Preventive Maintenance for the Microhematocrit Centrifuge

Goal: *To perform daily, monthly, and quarterly preventive maintenance on a microhematocrit centrifuge.*

EQUIPMENT and SUPPLIES

- Microhematocrit centrifuge
- Maintenance logbook
- Utility gloves
- Disposable gloves
- Face shield, fluid-impermeable gown as needed
- Disinfectant
- Biohazard waste container
- Maintenance logbook

PROCEDURAL STEPS

PPE: Always sanitize your hands; then put on fluid-impermeable gown, face shield, and gloves. In all maintenance procedures, disposable gloves are worn under the utility gloves.

Note: These are generic recommendations. Always check the manufacturer's guidelines for specific instructions.

Always unplug the power cord before cleaning or servicing the centrifuge.

Daily Maintenance

1. Clean the inside of the centrifuge and the gasket with a disinfectant recommended by the manufacturer. Plastic and nonmetal parts may be cleaned with a fresh solution of 5% sodium hypochlorite (bleach) mixed 1 : 10 with water (1 part bleach plus 9 parts water).
   PURPOSE: To remove any dried blood or shattered glass. Do not use bleach on the gasket because it may harden the rubber.

Monthly Maintenance

1. Check the reading device. Misuse and zeroing of the reading devices can result in considerable error. Always use a second, simple reading device as a cross-check. Use a ruler or a flat plastic card specially made for this purpose. To use these cards, lay the spun hematocrit tube on the card and align the red cells with a line on the card to obtain the reading.
2. Check the rotor for cracks or corrosion and check the interior for signs of white powder.

PURPOSE: Cracks, corrosion, or powder may indicate impending rotor failure; these findings require the immediate attention of a service technician.
3. Record all preventive maintenance in the laboratory logbook.
   PURPOSE: Recording maintenance is necessary to maintain warranties and to comply with regulations established by CLIA and other regulatory agencies.

Semiannual Maintenance

1. Check the gasket for cuts and breaks.
   PURPOSE: Cut gaskets allow tubes to leak and must be replaced.
2. Check the timer with a stopwatch.
3. Perform a maximum cell pack to verify the time required for complete packing by reading a sample after centrifugation and then recentrifuging for 1 minute. The results should be the same. If they are not, perform preventive maintenance and/or call the service technician.
   PURPOSE: If the cells compact further during recentrifugation, the centrifuge is not rotating at the proper speed, and hematocrit results will be falsely elevated.
4. Record all preventive measures in the equipment maintenance log.
   PURPOSE: Recording maintenance is necessary to maintain warranties and to comply with regulations established by CLIA and other regulatory agencies.

Annual Maintenance (or Maintenance Performed as Needed)

1. The centrifuge functions and maintenance verification should be performed by qualified personnel. This includes checking the centrifuge mechanism, rotors, timer, speed, and electrical leads.
2. Record all professional service calls in the laboratory logbook.

MICROHEMATOCRIT CENTRIFUGE MAINTENANCE LOG

DATE	SERVICE	INITIALS
10/7/20XX	Performed routine daily and monthly preventive maintenance	DC

PROCEDURE 47-2	Obtain Specimens and Perform CLIA-Waived Hematology Testing: Perform a Microhematocrit Test

Goal: *To perform a microhematocrit test accurately.*

EQUIPMENT and SUPPLIES

- Provider's order and/or lab requisition, microhematocrit lab log, patient's health record
- Fresh sample of blood collected in a tube containing ethylenediaminetetraacetic acid (EDTA) anticoagulant (or equipment for finger stick specimen: lancet, alcohol pad, gauze, bandage)
- Plastic-coated self-sealing capillary tubes, or plain capillary tubes (blue-tipped)
- Sealing clay (if capillary tubes are not self-sealing)
- Gauze
- Hematocrit centrifuge
- Fluid-impermeable lab coat, disposable gloves
- Biohazard waste and sharps containers

PROCEDURAL STEPS

1. Sanitize your hands. Put on disposable gloves, fluid-impermeable lab coat, and protective eyewear.
   PURPOSE: To ensure infection control.
2. Assemble the materials needed.
3. **A)** If the capillary tubes are self-sealing, fill two tubes by inserting the end opposite the sealed end into the well mixed EDTA blood sample. Note: If the capillary tube and the EDTA tube are held almost parallel to the table, the capillary tubes fill easily by capillary action. When the self-sealing capillary tubes are two thirds to three fourths filled, tilt them upright causing the blood sample to flow down the tube and come into contact with the sealant. Continue to hold the tube vertical when the blood makes contact with the sealant for an additional 15 seconds.
   PURPOSE: Duplicates should always be done as a means of quality control. Tubes are not filled completely to provide space for the sealing clay.
   B) Alternatively, fill two plain (blue-tipped) capillary tubes two thirds to three fourths full with the well-mixed EDTA blood by tipping the blood tube slightly and touching the capillary tube into the blood using the tip that is opposite the blue band. When enough blood is in the capillary tube, tip the blue end of the tube down causing the blood to flow towards the blue tip. Then readjust the tube horizontally while inserting the blue tip of the capillary tube into the clay sealant. Insert the tube as many times as needed to achieve a plug up to the blue band.

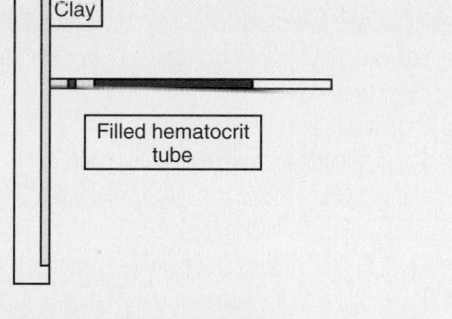

(From Keohane E et al: *Rodak's hematology: clinical principles and applications,* ed 5, St Louis, 2016, Saunders.)

4. Wipe the outside of the tubes with clean gauze without touching the wet open end of the tube.
   PURPOSE: Wiping the outside of the capillary tube removes any blood. Touching the blood inside the capillary tube with absorbent material removes more plasma than blood cells and can alter the hematocrit.
5. Place the tubes opposite each other in the centrifuge with the sealed ends securely against the gasket. (See Figure 47-1).
   PURPOSE: The centrifuge must always be balanced to prevent damage. If the clay ends of the capillary tubes are not outer-most against the gasket, the sample will spin out of the tubes, contaminating the centrifuge.
6. Note the numbers on the centrifuge slots and record the numbers on the log sheet along with the patient's name
   PURPOSE: The sample must be identified throughout the entire procedure.
7. Secure the locking top, fasten the lid down, and lock it.
   PURPOSE: If the locking top is not firmly in place during the spinning cycle, the tubes will come out of their slots and break. The lid is always locked during centrifugation for safety purposes; that is, to prevent ejection of aerosols or broken glass.
8. Set the timer and adjust the speed as needed.
   PURPOSE: The prescribed time is 3 to 5 minutes at 11,000 to 12,000 rpm. Check the manufacturer's instructions for time and speed.
9. Allow the centrifuge to come to a complete stop. Unlock the outer locking top and then remove the inner lid.
   PURPOSE: Opening the centrifuge before it has stopped could result in harm to the user.

PROCEDURE 47-2 —*continued*

10. Remove the tubes immediately and read the results. If this is not possible, store the tubes in an upright position.
    PURPOSE: Tubes left in the centrifuge will show altered results because the red blood cell (RBC) layer will spread out horizontally
11. Determine the microhematocrit values using one of the following methods:
    (1) Centrifuge with built-in reader using calibrated capillary tubes.
    - Position the tubes as directed by the manufacturer's instructions.
    - Read both tubes.
    - The average of the two results is reported.
    - The two values should not vary by more than 2%.
    (2) Centrifuge without a built-in reader.
    - Carefully remove the tubes from the centrifuge.
    - Place a tube on the microhematocrit reader.
    - Align the clay-RBC junction with the zero line on the reader. Align the plasma meniscus with the 100% line. The value is read at the junction of the red cell layer and the buffy coat. The buffy coat is not included in the reading (see the following figure).
    - Read both tubes.
    - The average of the two results is reported.
    - The two values should not vary by more than 2%.
12. Dispose of the capillary tubes in the sharps container.
13. Disinfect the work area and properly dispose of all biohazardous materials. Remove your lab coat, gloves, and eyewear and sanitize your hands.
    PURPOSE: To ensure infection control.

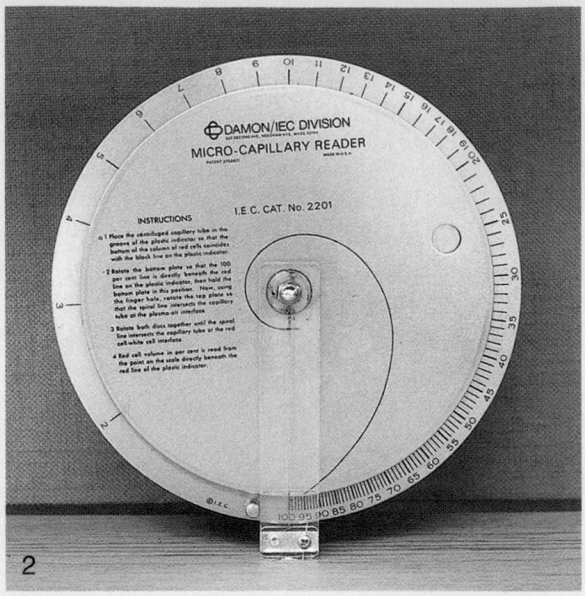

(From Keohane E et al: *Rodak's hematology: clinical principles and applications*, ed 5, St Louis, 2016, Saunders.)

14. Record the results in the Hematocrit Patient Log and document the results in the patient's medical record below..
    PURPOSE: A procedure is not considered done until it is charted.

HEMATOCRIT—PATIENT LOG

Hematocrit expected values:
Adult Males = 42-52 %
Adult Females = 36-48 %
Infants = 32-38 %
Children = increase to adult

DATE	TECH	PATIENT I.D.	SLOT #	RESULT	CHARTED
10/7/20--	dc	#12345	1 & 4	44% & 44%	✓

Documentation in the medical record:

10/7/20— 11:25 AM: Hct 44%. Dana Cummings, CMA (AAMA)

HEMOGLOBIN

The hemoglobin (Hgb) determination is another way to measure the oxygen-carrying capacity of blood. The hemoglobin concentration can be determined as part of the CBC or as an individual test.

CLIA-waived methods include the portable STAT-Site M Hgb, a completely portable, battery-operated hemoglobin analyzer that fits in the palm of the hand (Figure 47-3), and the HemoPointH2 (Procedure 47-3). The HemoPointH2 uses plastic microcuvettes that contain chemicals that lyse (break apart) the erythrocytes in the sample, releasing their hemoglobin. The hemoglobin reacts with chemicals and forms a color, which is detected and measured in the instrument, producing a digital readout. Capillary, venous, or arterial blood can be used in the disposable micro-**cuvette**, and the cuvettes have a long shelf life.

Normal hemoglobin values vary throughout life. They typically are quite high at birth, decline during childhood, and then increase through the teens until adult levels are reached (Table 47-2). Values range from a low of 12 g/dL in women to a high of 17.5 g/dL in men. The various factors that affect the hemoglobin level include age, gender, diet, altitude, and disease.

Hemoglobin and hematocrit tests often are performed together and are referred to as an "H&H." A quick mental calculation should always be done before H&H results are reported: the hemoglobin value × 3 (± 3) should equal the hematocrit value. For example, if the hemoglobin is 15 g/dL, the hematocrit should be 42% to 48%.

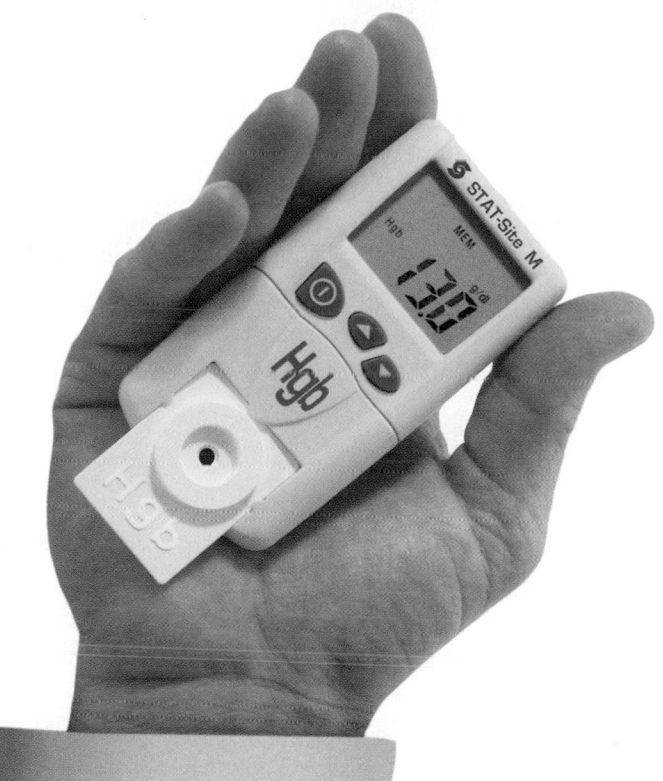

FIGURE 47-3 Handheld instruments, such as the STAT-Site system, can analyze hemoglobin quickly and accurately. (Courtesy Stanbio Laboratory, Boerne, Texas.)

CRITICAL THINKING APPLICATION   **47-1**

Mr. Corrigan's hematocrit value is 37%. What does Dana calculate as the expected hemoglobin value? Does this test confirm the physician's suspicions of anemia?

TABLE 47-2   Hemoglobin (Hgb) Reference Values

AGE/GENDER	HGB LEVEL (g/dL)
Neonate (new born-under 1 month)	17-23
Infant (1 month-1 yr)	9-14
Child (1-10 yr)	10-15
Female (greater than 10 yrs)	12-16
Male (greater than 10 yrs)	14-18

PROCEDURE 47-3   Perform CLIA-Waived Hematology Testing: Perform a Hemoglobin Test

Goal: To determine accurately the level of hemoglobin present in a blood sample using the HemoCue B-Hemoglobin System.

EQUIPMENT and SUPPLIES

- Patient's health record
- Provider's order and/or lab requisition
- Hemoglobin laboratory log
- HemoCue
- HemoCue microcuvette
- Autolet or blood lancet
- Alcohol prep pads
- Gauze squares
- Fluid-impermeable lab coat and disposable gloves
- Biohazard waste and sharps containers

PROCEDURAL STEPS

1. Perform an instrument quality control check by inserting the control cuvette into the instrument. Make sure the reading is within acceptable limits before proceeding.
   PURPOSE: Only instruments that record values within acceptable control limits can be used for patient testing. If the value is outside the control limits, refer to the troubleshooting guide for the instrument or contact the manufacturer.

2. Sanitize your hands. Put on fluid-impermeable lab coat and disposable gloves.
   PURPOSE: To ensure infection control.

PROCEDURE 47-3 —*continued*

3. Assemble all equipment and supplies needed.
4. Greet the patient and verify his or her identity using two identifiers (e.g., have the patient spell the last name, state the birth date, and/or show a picture ID). Explain the procedure to the patient.
   PURPOSE: Explaining the reason for a diagnostic procedure helps gain the patient's compliance and addresses the person's questions and concerns.
5. Examine the patient's fingers and choose the site to be used to obtain the blood sample.
   PURPOSE: The site must be free of trauma, calluses, and scarring.
6. Clean the site with alcohol or another recommended antiseptic preparation.
7. Perform a capillary puncture and wipe away the first drop of blood.
   PURPOSE: This drop may contain tissue fluid.
8. Obtain a large drop blood on the surface of the finger.
9. Touch the microcuvette to the drop of blood. Do not touch the finger. The correct volume is drawn into the cuvette by capillary action. Wipe off any excess blood from the sides of the cuvette (see the following figures).
   PURPOSE: Blood on the cuvette may alter the readings or contaminate the instrument.

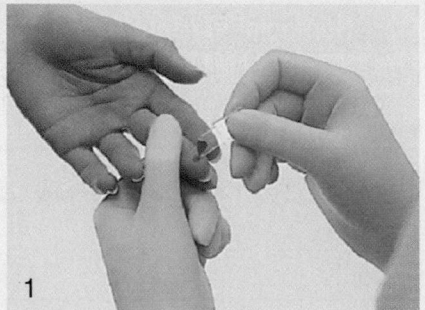

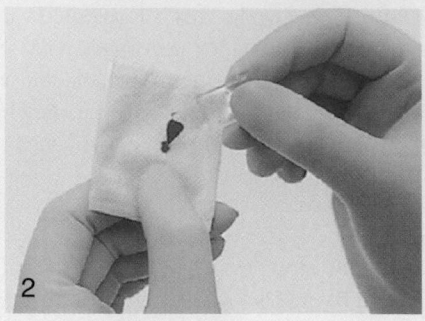

10. Place the cuvette in the cuvette holder and insert it into the instrument (see the following figure).

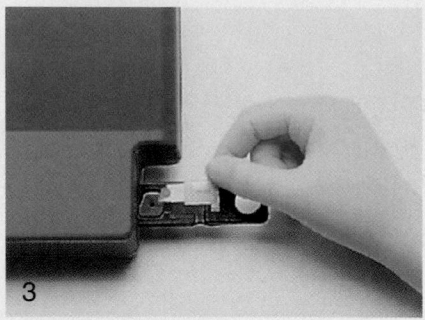

11. Read the result and record it in the lab's hemoglobin log and the patient's health record.
    PURPOSE: A procedure is not completed until the results are recorded.
12. Turn off the instrument. Dispose of biohazardous waste in the correct containers and properly disinfect the work area.
13. Remove gloves and dispose in biohazard waste. Remove lab coat and sanitize your hands.
    PURPOSE: To ensure infection control.

HEMOCUE B HEMOGLOBIN SYSTEM PATIENT LOG

TEST: _____ KIT LOT # _____

Hemoglobin expected values =
Adult Males = 13.0-18.0 g/dL
Adult Females = 12.0-16.0 g/dL
Infants = 10.0-14.0 g/dL
Children = increase to adult

DATE	TECH	PATIENT I.D.	RESULT	CHARTED
10/09/20--	DC	#12345	15.5 g/dL	✔

Documentation in the medical record:

10/9/20–9:30 AM: Hgb 15.5 g/dL. Dana Cummings, CMA (AAMA)

Erythrocyte Sedimentation Rate

The erythrocyte sedimentation rate (ESR) is a laboratory test that measures the rate at which erythrocytes gradually separate from plasma and settle to the bottom of a specially calibrated tube in 1 hour. The test is not specific for a particular disease but is used as a general indication of inflammation. Increases are found in such conditions as acute and chronic infections, rheumatoid arthritis, tuberculosis, hepatitis, cancer, multiple myeloma, rheumatic fever, and lupus erythematosus.

Normal values vary slightly with age and gender (Table 47-3). Only increased ESR rates are significant. Several CLIA-waived methods of measuring the ESR are used, including the Sediplast procedure (Procedure 47-4). This closed system incorporates a pierceable stopper that ensures a leak-proof seal when pierced by a pipet. An automatic self-zeroing cap and reservoir accurately bring the blood level to the zero mark and prevent overfilling. A prefilled vial of sodium citrate diluent is provided for dilution

of blood before testing. A closed-tube *Streck ESR* method utilizes a *Streck* black-topped vacutainer sample of blood that is directly placed in a *Streck* rack that provides results in 30 minute (Figure 47-4).

Many factors can affect the ESR. The tube must be completely filled with blood and must not have air bubbles. The tube must be allowed to sit in a vertical position, undisturbed, for the full designated time; careful timing is important. Minor degrees of tilting may increase the sedimentation rate. Jarring or vibrations from nearby machinery will falsely increase the ESR.

TABLE 47-3 Erythrocyte Sedimentation Rate (ESR) Reference Values

	SEDIPLAST TEST (mm/hr)
Men	≤50 yr: 0-15 >50 yr: 0-20
Women	≤50 yr: 0-20 >50 yr: 0-30

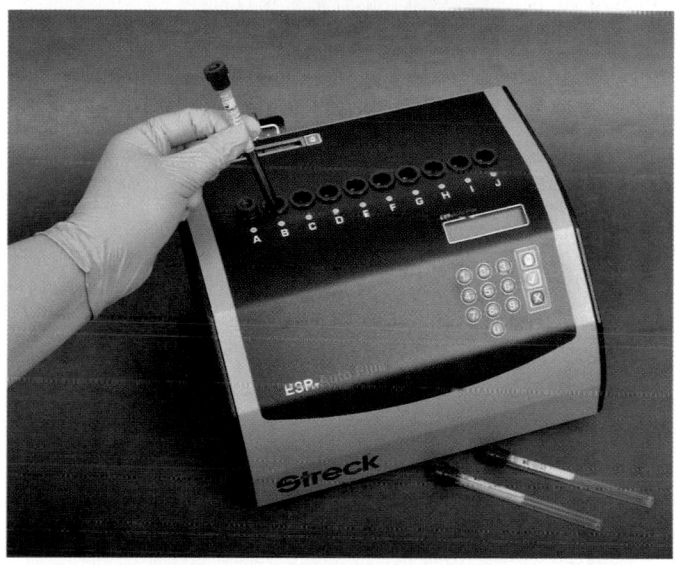

FIGURE 47-4 30-minute Streck ESR CLIA-waived test.

PROCEDURE 47-4 Obtain a Specimen and Perform CLIA-Waived Hematology Testing: Determine the Erythrocyte Sedimentation Rate Using a Modified Westergren Method

Goal: *To fill a Westergren tube properly and to observe and record an erythrocyte sedimentation rate (ESR) obtained by using a modified Westergren method.*

EQUIPMENT and SUPPLIES

- Patient's health record
- Provider's order and/or lab requisition
- Erythrocyte sedimentation rate (ESR) laboratory log
- Ethylenediaminetetraacetic acid (EDTA)—anticoagulated blood specimen
- Safety tube decapper (if tubes do not have a Hemogard plastic top)
- Disposable transfer pipet
- Sediplast ESR system (pre-filled Sediplast vial)
- Sediplast rack
- Timer
- Fluid-impermeable lab coat, disposable gloves, and face protector/shield
- Biohazardous waste container

PROCEDURAL STEPS

1. Sanitize your hands. Put on fluid-impermeable lab coat, face protection, and disposable gloves.
   <u>PURPOSE:</u> To ensure infection control.

2. Assemble the materials needed.
3. Check the leveling bubble of the Sediplast rack.
   <u>PURPOSE:</u> The rack must be horizontal on the table or bench to ensure that the tube is vertical.
4. Bring the blood sample to room temperature if it has been refrigerated and mix the sample well by inverting the tube gently several times, making sure the tube has no bubbles.
   <u>PURPOSE:</u> Cells settle when a specimen stands, and blood must always be well mixed before sampling. Test results will be altered if refrigerated blood is not brought to room temperature.
5. Remove the plastic Hemogard stopper on the blood sample by twisting and slowly pushing up on the stopper with your thumbs (or by using a tube decapper on rubber-stoppered blood tubes). Also remove the stopper on the prefilled Sediplast vial.
   <u>PURPOSE:</u> Using the Hemogard cover or removing the rubber cap with a protective device blocks blood splashes and helps prevent aerosolization of the specimen.

PROCEDURE 47-4   —*continued*

6. Fill the Sediplast vial with blood to the indicated line using a disposable transfer pipet. (See the following figure.) Replace the stopper on the prefilled vial and invert it several times to mix. Recap the blood collection tube with its stopper.
   PURPOSE: This dilutes the blood in accordance with the Westergren procedure.

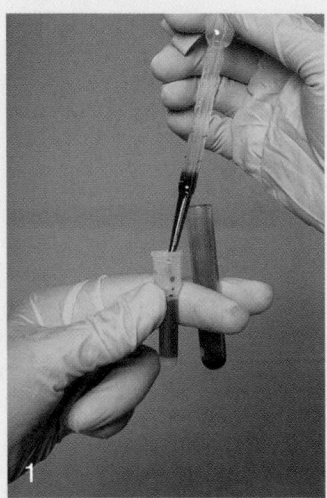

(Courtesy Polymedco, Cortland Manor, N.Y.)

7. Insert a Sediplast pipet through the pierceable stopper on the prefilled vial and push down until the pipet touches the bottom of the vial. The pipet automatically draws the blood up and over the zero mark (see Figure 2).

8. Insert the filled Sediplast pipet and its vial into the Sediplast rack, making sure the vial is vertical.
   PURPOSE: A pipet that is not vertical produces erroneous results.

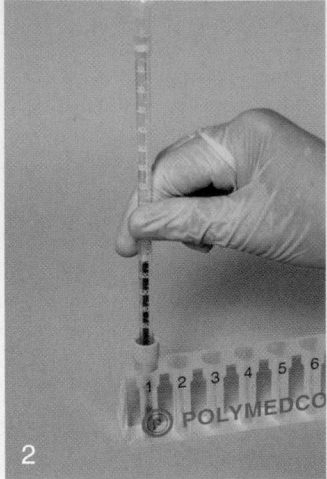

(Courtesy Polymedco, Cortland Manor, N.Y.)

9. Note the start time on the ESR log sheet and allow the vial to stand undisturbed for 60 minutes.
   PURPOSE: Jarring increases the sedimentation rate.

10. After 60 minutes, measure the distance the erythrocytes have fallen at the top of the tube. The scale reads in millimeters; each line is 1 mm.

11. Disinfect the work area and properly dispose of all biohazardous materials. Dispose the plastic Sediplast pipet and its vial into a biohazard container. Remove your gloves, face protection, and lab coat, and sanitize your hands.

12. Record the findings in the lab's ESR log and the patient's health record. Remember—the Westergren ESR is reported in millimeters per hour (mm/hr).
    PURPOSE: A procedure is considered not done until it is recorded.

ESR—SEDIPLAST—PATIENT LOG

ESR expected values:	Adult Males < 50 years = 0-15 mm/hr
	Adult Males > 50 years = 0-20 mm/hr
	Adult Females < 50 years = 0-20 mm/hr
	Adult Females > 50 years = 0-30 mm/hr

DATE	TECH	PATIENT I.D.	SLOT #	TIME	RESULT	CHARTED
10/09/20--	DC	#12345	2	60 min	15 mm	✓

Documentation in the medical record:

10/9/20– 9:30 AM: ESR 15 mm in 60 minutes. Dana Cummings, CMA (AAMA)

Coagulation Testing

The medical assistant may be asked to perform a test to determine prothrombin time (PT) using a handheld, CLIA-waived instrument that uses whole blood from a fingerstick (Figure 47-5). The PT is a method of measuring how long it takes blood to clot. Prothrombin is a protein in the liquid part of blood (plasma) that is converted to thrombin as part of the clotting process. Thrombin then causes fibrinogen to be converted to fibrin during the clotting process.

The PT is often used in combination with the partial thromboplastin time (PTT) to screen for hemophilia and other hereditary clotting disorders. The PT also is used to monitor the condition of patients taking the anticoagulant drug warfarin (Coumadin). Warfarin is given to prevent clots in the deep veins of the legs and to treat pulmonary embolism. It interferes with blood clotting by lowering the liver's production of certain clotting factors.

The CLIA-waived CoaguChek XS PT (Figure 47-6) measures the PT according to the time it takes the blood to form a fibrin clot. A precise amount of blood is dispensed from a fingerstick into the channels in a testing strip, where it is mixed with a thromboplastin reagent (see Figure 47-5). The blood is pumped back and forth in the channel, and a series of light-emitting diodes (LEDs) detect formation of the clot when movement of the blood stops (Procedure 47-5).

PT test results are reported as the number of seconds the blood takes to clot when mixed with the thromboplastin reagent. The international normalized ratio (INR) was created by the World Health Organization (WHO) because PT test results can vary, depending on the thromboplastin reagent used. The INR is a conversion unit that takes into account the different sensitivities of available reagents. It is widely accepted as the standard unit for reporting PT results rather than the time in seconds. Normal PT values are 10 to 13 seconds, or an INR of 1 to 1.4. The warfarin dosage in people treated to prevent the formation of blood clots and in those with artificial heart valves is monitored and adjusted so that the PT is about 1.5 to 2.5 times the normal value (or an INR value of 2 to 3).

It is important that the medical assistant know how to accurately document INR follow-up and related warfarin dosages on a patient flow sheet. The provider will balance repeated INR levels with warfarin doses so the INR is maintained at 2 throughout the anticoagulant treatment period (see Figure 47-6).

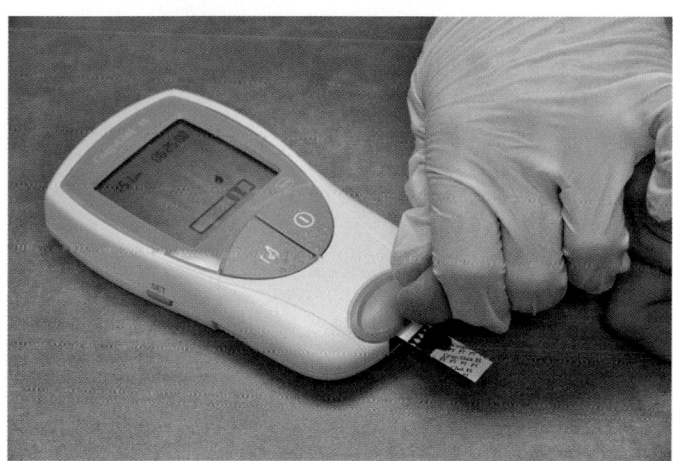

FIGURE 47-5 Applying blood sample to the CoaguChek XS PT Test monitor.

Westhills Family Practice Center
Warfarin Anticoagulant Record

Patient's Name: _____   DOB: _____

Address: _____   SSN: _____

_____

Patient's Phone: _____
Dx for Anticoagulation: _____   ICDM Code: _____
Date Warfarin Started: _____   INR Goal: _____
Phone for Outside Lab: _____

Date	Warfarin Dose Pre-Test	PT	INR	Warfarin Dose Order	Next INR/PT	Signature

FIGURE 47-6 Warfarin flow sheet.

PROCEDURE 47-5   Obtain a Specimen and Perform a CLIA-Waived Protime/INR Test

Goal: *To perform a coagulation test to determine protime/INR using the CoaguChek XS instrument with built-in quality control.*

Order: Perform a protime/INR test on Connie Lange STAT.

EQUIPMENT and SUPPLIES

- Patient's health record or flow chart (see Figure 47-6)
- Provider's order and/or lab requisition
- PT/INR lab log
- gauze, alcohol, bandage for capillary blood specimen
- CoaguChek XS PT Test monitor (see Figure 47-5)
- CoaguChek lancet
- CoaguChek test strip container and code chip
- Package insert or flow chart with directions
- Fluid-impermeable lab coat, gloves, and face protection (if necessary)
- Biohazard waste and sharps containers

PROCEDURAL STEPS

1. Sanitize your hands. Put on fluid-impermeable lab coat, face protection, and disposable gloves.
   PURPOSE: To ensure infection control.
2. Assemble the materials needed.
3. If you are using test strips from a new, unopened container, you must change the test strip code chip. The three-number code on the test strip container must match the three-number code on the code strip. To install the code strip, follow the instructions in the Code Chip section of the *User's Manual*.
   PURPOSE: To ensure that the instrument is calibrated correctly to produce accurate, precise, and reliable results.
4. Place the meter on a flat surface so that it will not vibrate or move during testing.
   PURPOSE: The test results are based on the back-and-forth movement of the blood sample that stops when the clot has formed. Vibrations or other movements will result in an error message, and the test will have to be repeated.
5. Greet the patient and verify his or her identity using two identifiers (e.g., have the patient spell the last name, state the birth date, and/or show a picture ID). Explain the procedure to the patient.
   PURPOSE: Explaining the reason for a diagnostic procedure helps gain the patient's compliance and addresses the person's questions and concerns.
6. Examine the patient's fingers and choose the site to be used to obtain the blood sample.
7. Prepare the site by doing the following before lancing the finger:
   - Warm the hand by placing it under the arm, using a hand warmer, and/or washing the hand in warm water.
   - Have the patient hold his or her arm down to the side so that the hand is below the waist.
   - Massage the palm of the hand toward the base of the finger and toward the tip until the fingertip has increased color.
   - If necessary, immediately after lancing, gently squeeze the finger from its base to encourage blood flow.

PURPOSE: The hanging drop blood sample must be sufficient to travel down the three channels on the test strip. It must be free of contaminants, tissue fluids, and alcohol.

8. When you are ready to test, remove a test strip from the container and immediately close the container. **Make sure it seals tightly. Do not open the container or touch the test strips with wet hands or wet gloves.** PURPOSE: Exposure to moisture damages the test strips.
9. Insert test strip as far as you can into the meter. This powers the meter ON (see the following figure).

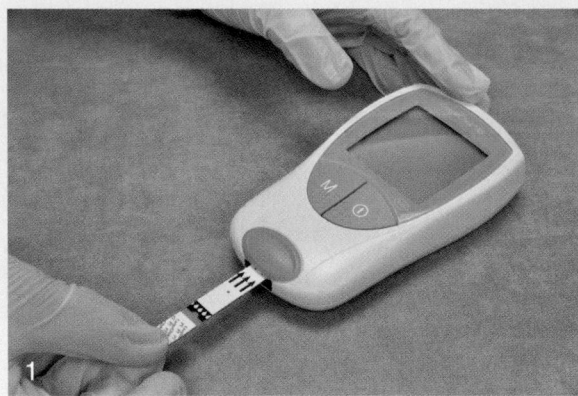

10. Disinfect the finger with alcohol and wipe dry. Perform the fingerstick.
11. Hold the incised finger very close to the target (the clear area of the test strip). Apply 1 drop of blood to the top or side of the target area and wait until you hear the beep. **You must apply a hanging drop of blood to the test strip within 15 seconds of lancing the finger. Do not add more blood. Do not touch or remove the test strip while the test is in progress.** The flashing blood drop symbol changes to an hourglass symbol when the meter detects a sufficient sample (see Figure 47-5).
12. The result appears in approximately 1 minute. It may be displayed in three ways: as the international normalized ratio (INR); as the protime (PT) in seconds; or as %Quick (a unit used mainly in Europe) (see the following figure displaying the INR result of 1.0).

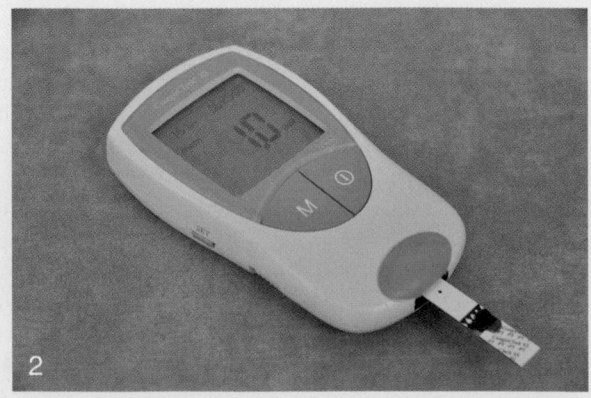

PROCEDURE 47-5 —continued

See the following chart.

PROTIME EXPECTED VALUES FOR NORMAL AND THERAPEUTIC WHOLE BLOOD

	INR	PT (sec)
Normal	0.8-1.2	6.5-11.9*
Low anticoagulation therapy	1.5-2	Varies with method used
Moderate anticoagulation therapy	2-3	Varies with method used
High anticoagulation therapy	3-4	Varies with method used

*Note: Laboratory reports and manufacturers must supply their own reference ranges for PT results along with each patient's results. This is because different methodologies may create different reference ranges and different units of measurement.

13. Record the result in the lab's PT/INR log and in the patient's warfarin therapy flow sheet and/or electronic record. Circle any results that do not fall into the Desirable Ranges column of the preceding table based on a patient who is on "low anticoagulation therapy." You may add comments to the test result about the test conditions or the patient. Identify "critical values" and take appropriate steps to notify the provider.
PURPOSE: The provider needs to know the result while the patient is still in the office, for proper follow-up with the patient.

14. Dispose of all sharps into the biohazard sharps container and regulated medical waste into the biohazard waste container. Disinfect the test area and remove your PPE. Sanitize your hands.
PURPOSE: To ensure infection control.

PROTIME—PATIENT LOG

Protime expected values for both normal and therapeutic whole blood:

	INR	PT seconds (ISI = 1.0)
Normal	0.8-1.2	10.4-15.7 sec
Low anticoagulation	1.5-2.0	19.6-26.1 sec
Moderate anticoagulation	2.0-3.0	26.1-39.2 sec
High anticoagulation	2.5-4.0	32.6-52.2 sec

DATE	TECH	PATIENT I.D.	INR	PT SECONDS	CHARTED
10/09/20--	DC	#12345	1.0	19.7	✓

Documentation in the medical record:

10/9/20– 9:30 AM: INR = 1.0 and PT = 19.7 seconds. Patient is on low anticoagulation therapy. Dana Cummings, CMA (AAMA)

It is also important to educate patients regarding their behaviors when a blood test such as the PT/INR is being monitored. For example, if they are taking the anticoagulant warfarin (Coumadin), they will need to follow up with the required lab work for monitoring their protime/INR. Patients should understand how their vitamin K intake from food directly affects their lab results. Vitamin K can clot the blood faster, thus working against warfarin. Helping patients identify foods high in vitamin K is crucial to maintaining a balance between the warfarin dosage and the lab values. Many providers do not instruct patients to stop eating foods high in vitamin K, but rather stress the importance of eating the same amounts. For instance, during the summer, with all the fresh vegetables available, some patients tend to eat more foods high in vitamin K. This changes their lab results, and they need to take an increased dose of warfarin. If they eat the same amounts of food high in vitamin K and do not overindulge, their lab values remain constant.

Foods high in vitamin K include leafy greens (e.g., kale, collards, spinach, and turnip greens), Brussel sprouts, and broccoli.

HEMATOLOGY IN THE REFERENCE LABORATORY

The CBC is the reference laboratory procedure most frequently ordered for blood specimens and it requires a lavender-topped EDTA tube. It gives a fairly complete look at the cellular components of blood and can provide a wealth of information about a patient's condition. It routinely includes the following:

- RBC count
- Hct
- Hgb
- Red cell indices
- WBC count and differential WBC count
- Estimation of platelet numbers

CBC Laboratory Reports

It is important that medical assistants understand the hematology laboratory reports that arrive from the reference laboratories, and that they are able to distinguish between normal and abnormal levels. Use the following references to complete the Critical Thinking Application exercise that follows:

- **Hematology reference ranges** in Table 47-4
- **The patient report form** (Figure 47-7) is a sample lab report that also identifies the particular lab's reference ranges. Lab reports, both electronic and paper, must supply their own reference ranges along with each patient's results. This is because different methodologies may create different reference ranges and different units of measurement.

Red Blood Cell Count

The RBC count is a commonly performed procedure and is part of the CBC (see Table 47-4). It approximates the number of circulating RBCs. The function of RBCs is to transport oxygen to tissues. The condition in which the oxygen-carrying capacity of blood is below normal is called *anemia*. The RBC count often is decreased in anemia. Increases are found in people with dehydration,

TABLE 47-4	Reference Ranges for Complete Blood Count (CBC) Values*				
TEST	**NEONATES (new born-1 month)**	**INFANTS (1 month-1 yr)**	**CHILDREN (1-10 yr)**	**MEN (>10 yrs)**	**WOMEN (>10 yrs)**
RBCs	4.8-7.1 million/mm³	3.8-5.5 million/mm³	4.5-4.8 million/mm³	4.5-6 million/mm³	4-5.5 million/mm³
Hematocrit (Hct)	44%-64%	30%-40%	35%-41%	42%-52%	36%-45%
Hemoglobin (Hgb)	17-23 g/dL	9-14 g/dL	11-16 g/dL	15-17 g/dL	12-16 g/dL
WBCs	9,000-30,000/mm³	6,000-16,000/mm³	5,000-13,000/mm³	4,000-11,000/mm³	
RBC Indices					
MCV	96-108 fL			82-99 fL	
MCH	32-34 pg			26-34 pg	
MCHC	31-33 g/dL			31-37 g/dL	
WBC Differential					
Neutrophils	≥45% by age 1 wk	32%	60% for children ≥2 yr	50%-65%	
Bands	—	—	—	0%-7%	
Eosinophils	—	—	0%-3%	1%-3%	
Basophils	—	—	1%-3%	0%-1%	
Monocytes	—	—	4%-9%	3%-9%	
Lymphocytes	≥41% by age 1 wk	61%	59% for children ≥2 yr	25%-40%	
Platelets	140,000-300,000/mm³	200,000-473,000/mm³	150,000-450,000/mm³	150,000-400,000/mm³	

fL, Femtoliter; *MCH*, mean corpuscular hemoglobin; *MCHC*, mean corpuscular hemoglobin concentration; *MCV*, mean corpuscular volume; *pg*, picograms; *RBC*, red blood cell; *WBC*, white blood cell.
*Lab reports, both electronic and paper, must supply their own reference ranges along with each patient's results. This is because different methodologies may create different reference ranges and different units of measurement.

		DATE & TIME RECEIVED	ACCESSION NUMBER
		10/ 20/ 2013 20:45	
		LOCATION	DATE REPORTED
			10/ 21/2000

PHYSICIAN		PATIENT INFORMATION	

TEST		RESULTS	REFERENCE RANGE	UNITS
HEMOGRAM	LO	2.9	4. 5-10. 5	CU.MM.
WHITE BLOOD COUNT	LO	2. 39	4.40-5.90	CU.MM.
RED BLOOD COUNT	LO	7.4	14.0-18.0	GM/100ML
HEMOGLOBIN	LO	22.3	40. 0-52.0 %	
MEAN CORPUSCULAR VOLUME		93	80-100	fL
MEAN CORPUSCULAR HGB		31.0	27. 0-32.0	PG
MEAN CORPUSCULAR HgB CONC		33.2	31.0-36.0	%
DIFFERENTIAL, WBC				
SEGMENTED NEUTROPHILS		57	38-80	%
LYMPHOCYTE		29	15-45	%
MONOCYTES		7	1-10	%
EOSINOPHILS		1	0-4	%
BAND NEUTROPHILS	HI	6	0-5	%
ANISOCYTOSIS	ABN	SLIGHT		
HYPOCHROMIA	ABN	SLIGHT		
PLATELET ESTIMATE	ABN	DECREASED		
PARTIAL THROMBOPLASTIN TIME				
PARTIAL THROMBOPLASTIN TIME		31.7	20.0-40.0	SECONDS
CONTROL PTT		30.4	20.0-40.0	SECONDS
PROTHROMBIN TIME				
PROTHROMBIN TIME		12.2	10.0-13.5	SECONDS
CONTROL PT		12.0	11.0-13.0	SECONDS
FINAL Report (Summary)				

FIGURE 47-7 Sample Laboratory Report. Both electronic and paper lab reports must supply their own reference ranges along with each patient's results. This is because different methodologies may create different reference ranges and different units of measurement.

polycythemia vera, or severe burns and in those who live at high altitudes, in whom it reflects an adaptation to the lower oxygen content of the air.

Normal RBC values range from 4 million to 6 million cells/mm³. RBC counts usually are higher in males than in females.

Red Cell Indices

A variety of calculations can be performed using the information obtained from the CBC to produce indices that provide information about RBC disorders. The indices are used to classify anemias and to select additional tests to determine the cause of anemia. They also may be used to monitor the treatment of anemia because they may change in response to treatment. The indices are mathematical ratios of the three red cell tests: Hct, Hgb, and the RBC count.

- *Mean cell volume (MCV):* MCV = (HCT/RBC) × 10. The average size of the RBCs is the most important index for classifying anemias. Abnormally large RBCs are macrocytic and have a higher than normal MCV. Small RBCS are microcytic and have a lower than normal MCV. The normal reference range is 82 to 108 femtoliters (fL).
- *Mean cell hemoglobin (MCH):* MCH = (HGB/RBC) × 10. The MCH is calculated to give the average weight of hemoglobin in the RBC. The reference range is 26 to 34 picograms (pg).
- *Mean cell ratio of Hgb and Hct (MCHC):* MCHC = (HGB × 100)/RBC. The MCHC indicates the average weight of hemoglobin compared with the cell size. The reference range is 32 to 37 g/dL. A decreased MCHC shows pale (or *hypochromic*) RBCs in a stained blood smear. An increased MCHC is rare and probably represents an error in measurement of the Hgb or Hct.

White Blood Cell Count

The WBC count gives an approximation of the total number of leukocytes in circulating blood. The count is performed to help the provider determine whether an infection is present or to aid in the diagnosis of leukemia. It also may be used to follow the course of a disease and as an indication of whether the patient is responding to treatment.

The normal WBC count varies with age. It is higher in newborns and decreases throughout life. The average adult range is 4,000 to 11,000 cells/mm³. Many factors can affect the WBC count.

An increase in the number of normal WBCs is a condition called **leukocytosis**. Physiologic increases in the WBC count are seen with pregnancy, stress, anesthesia, exercise, exposure to temperature extremes, and after treatment with corticosteroids. Pathologic causes of leukocytosis include many bacterial infections, leukemia, appendicitis, and pneumonia.

A decrease in the WBC count is called *leukopenia*. This condition may be caused by viral infection or by exposure to radiation and certain chemicals and drugs.

Differential Cell Count

The purpose of the differential, or "diff," in the CBC is to analyze and quantitate the types of WBCs found in a sample of blood. The differential can be performed manually using a stained blood smear

and a microscope, or with an automated instrument. A number of automated cell counters have integrated differential analyzers that use high-frequency conductivity to gather information about cell size, internal structure, and density.

Preparation of Blood Smears for the Differential

A blood smear enables the examiner to view the cellular components of blood in as natural a state as possible. The morphology of leukocytes, erythrocytes, and platelets can be studied, and their size, shape, and maturity can be evaluated.

A blood smear is prepared by placing a drop of blood from a fingerstick or from an EDTA tube (using a DIFF-SAFE blood dispenser) onto a clean glass slide (Figure 47-8). The slide must be free of dust and grease. The best specimen for a blood smear is capillary blood that has no anticoagulant added. EDTA-anticoagulated blood can be used, provided the smear is made within 2 hours of collection. Because of these time constraints, the medical assistant may be asked to prepare a smear during collection of the CBC specimen.

The wedge smear is used most frequently. It involves placing a small drop of blood ½ inch from the right end of a glass slide. The end of a second glass spreader slide is placed in front (to the left) of the drop of blood at an angle of 30 to 35 degrees. The spreader slide is brought back into the drop with a quick but smooth gliding motion until the blood spreads along the edge of the spreader slide. The spreader slide is then pushed to the left with a quick, steady motion, spreading the blood across the slide. Care should be taken when making a smear because of the sharp glass slides and the possible exposure to blood.

A good wedge smear should cover one half to three fourths of the slide. It should show a gradual transition from a thick to a thin end with a feathered edge (Figure 47-9). It should have a smooth appearance with no ridges, holes, lines, streaks, or clumps. On microscopic examination, the cells should be distributed evenly.

After the smear has been made, it should be allowed to dry. The slide should be propped up to dry with the thick end (heel) down. Do not blow on the slide to dry it. This can cause **artifacts** in the RBCs from the moisture in your breath. Once dry, the patient's name is written on the frosted end of the slide with a pencil or marker.

After it has been labeled, the slide is fixed in methanol, a fixative that preserves and prevents changes or deterioration of the cellular components. Many of the quick stains available on the market contain the fixative in the stain.

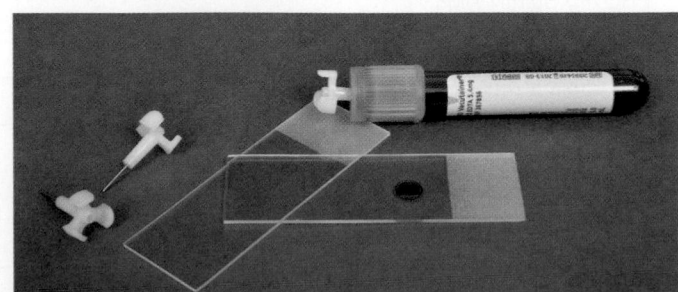

FIGURE 47-8 Note the white DIFF-SAFE device with the needle that will be pushed into the lavender-topped EDTA tube of blood. When the device is inverted and pressed against the slide, a drop of blood is delivered (see slide to the right). (Courtesy Zack Bent)

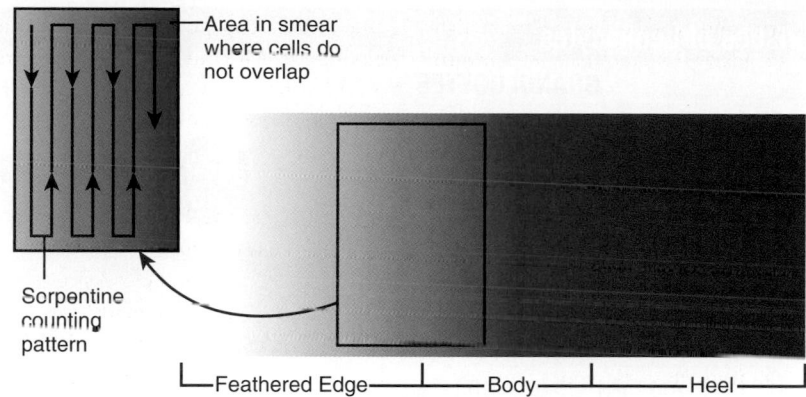

FIGURE 47-9 *Right,* Appearance of a properly prepared wedge smear. *Left,* Serpentine (winding) pattern used to count the cells.

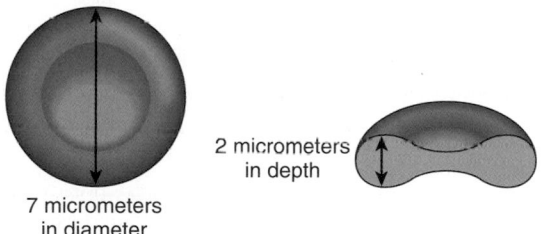

FIGURE 47-10 Red blood cell morphology.

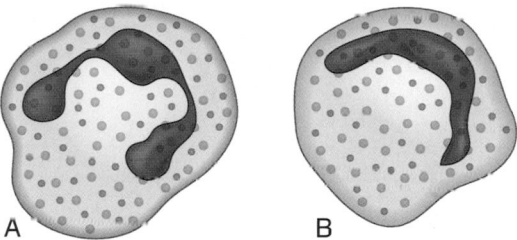

FIGURE 47-11 Neutrophils. **A,** Segmented. **B,** Band.

Staining of Blood Smears

Stains commonly used in the examination of blood cells are described as *polychromatic* because they contain dyes that stain various cell components different colors. These stains are attracted to different parts of the cell, which makes the cells and their structures easier to see and differentiate. The most commonly used differential blood stain is Wright's stain. The traditional Wright's stain dates from the early 1890s; it was an alcoholic solution of methylene blue dye and an eosin red dye. The blue dye attached to the alkaline granules of the basophils, and eosin red dye attached to the acidic eosinophil granules. The granules in neutrophils take up both dyes, appearing as a lavender-pink "neutral" color. Many modifications of the original Wright's stain have been produced, including the Diff-Quick method used in ambulatory facility labs.

Identification of Normal Blood Cells

Much useful information can be gathered from microscopic identification and evaluation of blood cells in a stained smear. A great deal more information can be acquired from observation of these blood cells than from actual cell counts.

The three features hematologists look for in blood cells are *cell size, nuclear appearance,* and *cytoplasm characteristics.*

RBCs are the most numerous of the cellular elements. They are biconcave disks with no nuclei (Figure 47-10).

Thrombocytes, or platelets, the smallest of the cellular elements, may be round or oval. They have no nucleus because a platelet is just a fragment of cytoplasm from a large bone marrow cell.

Leukocytes are the largest of the normal circulating blood cells (Table 47-5). Each of the five types has a characteristic appearance.

As has been mentioned earlier, the granulocytes include neutrophils, eosinophils, and basophils. Granulocytes have distinctive granules in the cytoplasm and may have segmented nuclei.

Neutrophils are known by a variety of names, including PMNs, segmented neutrophils, "polys," and "segs." They are the most numerous WBCs in circulation in adults. Many types of bacterial infections stimulate increased production of neutrophils. The nucleus of a segmented neutrophil (Figure 47-11, *A*) is divided into two to five lobes connected by a strand. An immature form of a neutrophil is called a *band,* or *stab* (Figure 47-11, *B*). Instead of having a segmented nucleus in which the lobes are separated by a thin filament, the band has an unsegmented nucleus shaped like a horseshoe or banana. An increase in bands indicates a recent bacterial infection, such as bacterial meningitis, pneumonia, appendicitis, strep throat, or abscesses. Neutrophils are also increased in chronic granulocytic leukemia.

Eosinophils have large red granules. They are phagocytic and closely associated with allergies (e.g., hay fever) and with asthma, in addition to certain parasitic infestations, such as tapeworm and amebic dysentery.

The *basophil* has large, dark, blue-black granules. It contains histamine, which mediates the inflammatory response, and heparin, which helps prevent excessive clotting of blood.

The agranulocytes include lymphocytes and monocytes. They have few, if any, granules and nonsegmented nuclei.

Lymphocytes are the smallest WBCs and are the second most numerous type of WBC in adults. In children they usually are the most numerous. "Lymphs," as they are commonly called, are responsible for recognizing foreign antigens and producing circulating antibodies for immunity to disease. Increased numbers of lymphocytes are found with most viral diseases; with some bacterial infections,

TABLE 47-5   Characteristics of Leukocytes

	GRANULOCYTES				AGRANULOCYTES	
	NEUTROPHIL, SEGMENTED (MATURE)	NEUTROPHIL, BAND (IMMATURE)	EOSINOPHIL	BASOPHIL	LYMPHOCYTE	MONOCYTE
Cell size	10-15 mcL	10-15 mcL	10-15 mcL	10-15 mcL	6-15 mcL	12-20 mcL
Nucleus shape	Two to five lobes connected by threadlike filaments	Band or U-shaped	Bilobed or band	Slightly segmented, granular, or band	Round or oval	Round, indented, or superimposed lobes
Nucleus structure	Coarse	Coarse	Coarse	Obscured by granules	Smudged, lumpy, or clumped	Brainlike convolutions or folded
Cytoplasm amount	Abundant	Abundant	Abundant	Abundant	Scant	Abundant
Cytoplasm color	Colorless to light pink	Colorless to light pink	Colorless to light pink	Colorless to light pink	Sky blue to dark blue	Dull gray to blue-gray
Cytoplasm inclusions	Many tiny tan, pink, or red-purple granules	Many tiny tan, pink granules, with increased red-purple granules	Large, rounder oval red to red-orange granules	Large, coarse blue-black granules	None to few round red-purple granules	Ground-glass appearance, fine red-purple granules, rare blue granules

such as syphilis and tuberculosis; with agranulocytic leukemias; and in young children who are actively making antibodies. In many viral infections, stimulated or reactive lymphocytes, called *atypical lymphocytes,* are found. These are common in infectious mononucleosis.

Monocytes are the largest type of WBC in circulation. Monocytes are called *macrophages* when they enter tissues and ingest bacteria and debris of cellular breakdown. They are increased in patients with certain viral infections, such as hepatitis and mumps; rickettsial infections, such as Rocky Mountain spotted fever; and bacterial infections, such as tuberculosis and typhoid fever.

Differential Examination

A specific area of a stained smear is examined microscopically when the differential count is done. The slide is examined near the feathered end of the smear, where cells are barely touching one another and are easiest to identify. Cells are examined with the oil immersion objective of the microscope. The light should be bright to facilitate visualization of colors and small structures. The differential examination consists of counting and classifying 100 consecutive WBCs while moving in a specific winding pattern through the smear (see Figure 47-9). A tally of the cells observed is kept on a differential cell counter or a computer (Figure 47-12).

Normal values for a differential vary with age. As mentioned previously, laboratory reports must include the lab's own reference ranges along with each patient's results because different method-

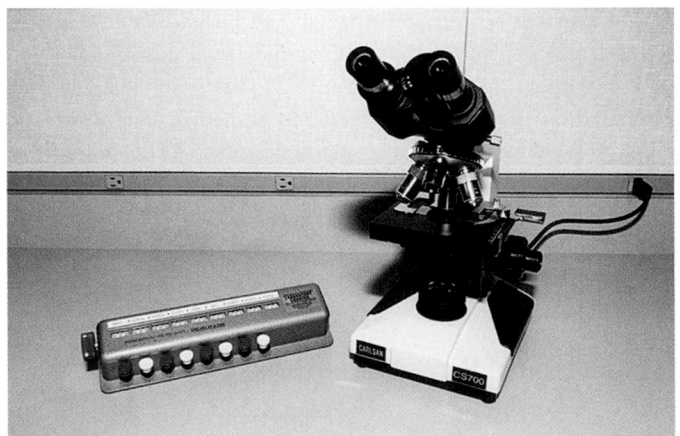

FIGURE 47-12 Microscope with differential cell counter. (Courtesy Cynmar, Carlinville, Ill.)

ologies may create different reference ranges and different units of measurement.

Typical reference ranges for adults are:

- Neutrophils: 40% to 60%
- Lymphocytes: 20% to 40%
- Monocytes: 2% to 8%
- Eosinophils: 1% to 4%
- Basophils: 0.5% to 1%
- Bands: 0% to 3%

Many disease states alter the ratios of the different types of leukocytes, and the differential can be very useful in assisting with the provider's diagnosis. The differential examination typically is performed in a reference laboratory.

Red Blood Cell Morphology

After the differential cell count has been determined, the RBCs are observed and evaluated. Normally, stained RBCs are the same size and shape and are well filled with hemoglobin. Any variations from the normal state are reported (Figure 47-13). The appearance of the RBCs should correlate with the RBC indices.

Size

Normal-sized RBCs are said to be *normocytic*. If the cells are larger than normal, they are *macrocytic;* if smaller than normal, they are *microcytic*. The condition in which different sizes of RBCs are present is known as *anisocytosis*.

Shape

Normal RBCs are round or slightly oval. Cells may be shaped like sickles, targets, crescents, or burs. Poikilocytosis is a significant variation in the shape of RBCs.

Content

An RBC with a normal amount of hemoglobin is said to be *normochromic*. Pale-staining cells are *hypochromic* and have less hemoglobin than normal. Any inclusions in red cells should be reported.

Platelet Analysis

On a stained smear, the morphology of platelets is observed for any abnormalities. Platelets are small and irregularly shaped and may vary considerably in size. The normal platelet count is 150,000 to 400,000/mm³. An increase in platelets is called *thrombocytosis,* and a decrease is called *thrombocytopenia.* Excessive clumping of platelets is also reported in a platelet analysis.

IMMUNOHEMATOLOGY-BLOOD BANK

Formerly called the *blood bank,* the immunohematology division of the laboratory is responsible for blood typing. The major reason for performing immunohematology tests is to prevent problems caused by incompatibility of blood types during blood transfusions. Compatibility testing (cross-matching) is performed to prevent transfusion reactions in patients receiving blood transfusions and to identify potential Rh-incompatibility problems in expectant mothers. Rh incompatibility between an expectant mother and the unborn child may result in hemolytic disease of the newborn.

Blood Grouping

The two major blood antigen systems are the ABO (or Landsteiner) system and the Rh system. The ABO system has four major blood groups: A, B, O, and AB. A person is either Rh positive or Rh negative. Certain blood types are more common in certain countries. For example, in China, more than 99% of the population has Rh-positive blood. In the United States, about 85% of the population is Rh positive. Blood type, like eye color, is inherited. Racial and ethnic differences in blood type and composition exist as a result of inheritance and populations that have migrated and mixed over time. Table 47-6 shows the distribution of blood types of the peoples of the United States for which data are available.

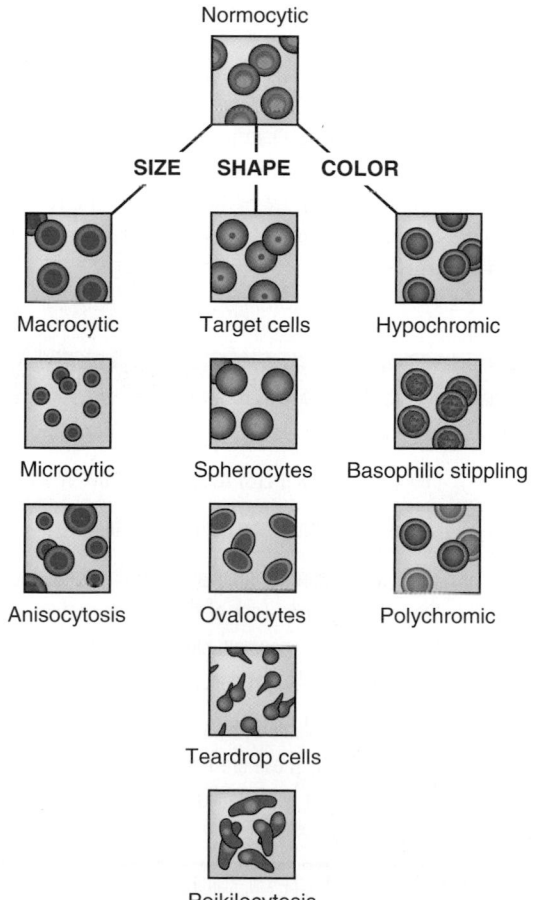

Normocytic

SIZE SHAPE COLOR

Macrocytic	Target cells	Hypochromic
Microcytic	Spherocytes	Basophilic stippling
Anisocytosis	Ovalocytes	Polychromic

Teardrop cells

Poikilocytosis

FIGURE 47-13 Abnormal erythrocytes.

TABLE 47-6 Blood Type Distribution in the United States

TYPE	CAUCASIAN	AFRICAN-AMERICAN	HISPANIC	ASIAN
O+	37%	47%	53%	39%
O−	8%	4%	4%	1%
A+	33%	24%	29%	27%
A−	7%	2%	2%	0.5%
B+	9%	18%	9%	25%
B−	2%	1%	1%	0.4%
AB+	3%	4%	2%	7%
AB−	1%	0.3%	0.2%	0.1%

Data from the American Red Cross. www.redcrossblood.org/learn-about-blood/blood-types. Accessed September 27, 2015.

Determination of ABO Blood Group

Determination of ABO blood groups is a simple test that can easily be performed, but because of the implications of performing the test incorrectly, blood typing is not a CLIA waived. The test detects the presence of A or B antigens on RBCs on the basis of the presence or absence of agglutination with a known antiserum. When the antigen on a patient's RBCs corresponds to the test antibody, agglutination occurs. If the corresponding antigen is not present on the cells, agglutination does not occur.

In addition to the blood antigens found on RBCs, naturally occurring antibodies are found in plasma. These antibodies appear shortly after birth, and the body never produces an antibody that can combine with its own blood antigen. Because of the blood group antibodies, blood transfusions ideally should be specific: Type A blood should receive type A blood in a transfusion. In emergencies, if there is no time for the laboratory to perform a **type and cross-match**, type O negative (O−) blood is administered. Type O negative is referred to as the "universal donor," because there are no circulating antibodies to the ABO antigen, nor are there Rh antigens that might sensitize an Rh-negative recipient. Table 47-7 shows the compatibility among ABO blood types for transfusion.

Determination of Rh Factor

Determination of the Rh type is another simple test (although it is not CLIA waived) that can be performed with a minimum amount of equipment. The Rh factor is so called because it was first discovered in rhesus monkeys. Later this same protein was found on the RBCs of some humans. This test detects the presence of proteins (D antigens) on the surface of RBCs on the basis of the presence or absence of agglutination with anti-D antiserum. When the D antigen is present, agglutination occurs when the anti-D antiserum is mixed with RBCs. If the D antigen is not present, agglutination does not occur. Rh-positive blood agglutinates in the presence of anti-D antiserum but not in the presence of the Rh control (that has no anti-D antibodies). Rh-negative blood does not agglutinate in the presence of anti-D antiserum, nor does it agglutinate in the presence of the Rh control.

There are no naturally occurring antibodies to the Rh factor as there are to the A and B antigens. A person develops antibodies to the D antigen only in the event of exposure to the antigen. This is possible if an incompatible transfusion is administered, or if an Rh-negative mother is exposed to the Rh-positive blood of her infant during pregnancy, a miscarriage, abortion, or delivery. If this occurs, the mother may develop antibodies to the D antigen. This usually does not cause a problem during the first pregnancy. However, in a subsequent pregnancy with an Rh-positive fetus, the woman's immune system begins to produce more antibodies because she was sensitized during the first pregnancy. These antibodies cross the placenta and destroy the RBCs of the fetus, which can lead to anemia, heart failure, or brain damage in the infant and may even cause death. These events are collectively called *hemolytic disease of the newborn* (HDN). The disease may also be called *hydrops fetalis*.

Until 1968 no preventive measure could be taken for this problem. Exchange transfusion, in which all of the infant's blood is replaced, was the only option. Today, however, HDN can be prevented by administration of Rh immune globulin products. Rho(D) immune globulin (rhoGAM) is a protein solution containing large numbers of Rh(D) antibodies. RhoGAM is given at 28 to 30 weeks of gestation to Rh-negative mothers, regardless of the father's Rh type. After delivery, the cord blood is tested, and a dose of rhoGAM is given to the mother only if the baby is Rh positive. rhoGAM is also given for miscarriages or abortions. The immune globulin prevents the infant's Rh-positive cells from stimulating the mother's immune system, thus preventing HDN. The source of Rho(D) immune globulin is plasma from women who have had children affected by HDN or from Rh-negative men who are voluntarily injected with Rh-positive RBCs.

Other Blood Types

In addition to the A and B antigens that characterize the ABO blood grouping, more than 600 antigens and more than 20 other blood type systems are known. Many are named after the person or family in which the blood type system was discovered. Table 47-8 describes other blood systems.

TABLE 47-7 Blood Compatibility

	RECIPIENT BLOOD*	
RBC ANTIGEN	PLASMA ANTIBODIES	COMPATIBLE WITH DONOR TYPES†
Type O (no antigens)	Anti-A and anti-B	O
Type A (type A antigen)	Anti-B	O and A
Type B (type B antigen)	Anti-A	O and B
Type AB (type AB antigen)	None	O, A, B, and AB

RBC, Red blood cell.
*Patients with type AB blood are considered universal recipients.
†Patients with type O blood are considered universal donors.

TABLE 47-8 Other Blood Typing Systems

SYSTEM	REMARKS
Diego	Found only among East Asians and Native Americans.
MNS	Useful in maternity and paternity testing.
Duffy	The malarial parasite requires the Duffy antigen to enter the red blood cells. Lack of the antigen confers resistance to malaria. Duffy-negative blood is found only in descendants of African populations.
Lewis	Antigens are soluble in blood rather than attached to the red blood cells. These are the only blood group antibodies that have never been implicated in hemolytic disease of the newborn.

Other blood group systems include Colton, M, Kell, Kidd, Landsteiner-Wiener, P, Yt or Cartwright, XG, Scianna, Dombrock, Chido/Rodgers, Kx, Gerbich, Cromer, Knops, Indian, Ok, Raph, and JMH.

CRITICAL THINKING APPLICATION 47-4
Before Mr. Corrigan's kidney transplantation, he had a type and cross-match and was determined to be type O+. Explain what antigen/antigens are on his cells. Could he receive blood from a type A+ individual? Why or why not? Could he receive blood from a type O− individual? Why or why not?

LEGAL AND ETHICAL ISSUES RELATED TO BLOOD TRANSFUSIONS

The Blood Safety Act was passed in 1991 to ensure that all donor blood is tested for HIV and other viral diseases. The impact of this law can be seen in the ambulatory care environment. The law requires providers to explain to each elective surgery patient the chances of the need for a blood transfusion. The discussion must include the positive and negative aspects of autologous transfusions (transfusion with a person's own blood) and transfusions of blood from family, friends, or other donors. This discussion must be documented in the patient's health record. Before the surgery, the patient must sign a form giving consent to any needed blood transfusions. The medical assistant should be aware that certain populations (e.g., Jehovah's Witnesses) do not believe in blood transfusions.

If the patient decides to use autologous transfusions, this may require the patient to donate blood several weeks before the procedure. Usually autologous transfusions are performed for stable patients undergoing major orthopedic, vascular, cardiac, or thoracic surgery. The medical assistant might have to assist the patient in making arrangements for the blood donation. Another type of autologous transfusion can occur if the surgeon inserts an autologous drain in the surgical wound. The drain collects the blood from the surgical wound to prevent postoperative hematomas, and the collected blood then is reinfused into the person.

BLOOD CHEMISTRY IN THE PHYSICIAN OFFICE LABORATORY (POL)

CLIA-waived chemistry tests using whole blood from fingersticks have become popular in ambulatory practices because of the increase in diabetes and cardiovascular disease in the United States. Both of these metabolic diseases benefit from early diagnosis and treatment based on continued monitoring of glucose and hemoglobin A_{1c} for diabetes; and cholesterol, lipid panels, and liver enzymes for cardiovascular diseases related to fatty plaque in the arteries.

Blood Glucose Testing

Glucose is used as a fuel by all body cells. Under normal circumstances, it is the only substance used to nourish brain cells. Maintenance of blood glucose levels within a normal range is vital to homeostasis of the human body. Understanding the importance of glucose can help the medical assistant understand why glucose is the most frequently tested chemical analyte in the blood.

Elevated blood glucose levels most often are associated with diabetes mellitus, but they also may indicate pancreatitis, endocrine disorders, or chronic renal failure. Diabetes mellitus is a disorder of carbohydrate metabolism that results in elevated blood and urine glucose levels secondary to the inability of the pancreas to produce sufficient insulin or because of insulin resistance at the cellular level (see Chapter 38).

For initial screening of a patient for diabetes type 2, a fasting blood sample is usually taken in the morning, after a fast of 10 to 14 hours. The patient's fasting blood glucose (FBG) level should be less than 100 mg/dL. If it is higher than 110 mg/dL, the provider may request a blood glucose tolerance test (GTT). For this test, the fasting patient receives a sugary liquid to drink that contains 100 g of glucose. (The amount may be adjusted according to the patient's weight.) A blood sugar level of less than 140 mg/dL after 2 hours is normal. A reading of more than 200 mg/dL after 2 hours may indicate diabetes. A reading between 140 and 199 mg/dL indicates impaired glucose tolerance, or prediabetes.

Self-monitoring of blood glucose levels has become an important part of the management of diabetes. A very small amount of blood from a capillary stick is "sipped" into a strip that turns on the glucose monitor and electronically calibrates the monitor. These rapid-test glucose monitors use an enzymatic method that converts glucose into a product that is measureable and recorded by the monitor.

The medical assistant can screen a patient's blood glucose levels by using a glucometer cleared for home use by the U.S. Food and Drug Administration (FDA). (This procedure is described in Chapter 38.) The blood glucose level is routinely monitored by patients with diabetes mellitus type 1 or type 2. Glucose levels also may be monitored by women with gestational diabetes, a condition seen during pregnancy in which the effect of insulin is partially blocked by a variety of other hormones made in the placenta.

Hemoglobin A_{1c} Testing

Hemoglobin A_{1c} is also described as *glycosylated hemoglobin* (sugar-coated hemoglobin), which is the result of glucose binding irreversibly to the hemoglobin molecules in the RBCs. It is also simply referred to "the A_{1c}."

As mentioned, RBCs have a life span of approximately 120 days. Therefore, measuring the amount of glucose that has been irreversibly bound to hemoglobin provides an assessment of the average blood sugar during the 60 to 90 days preceding the test. The A_{1c} test is performed every 3 months in patients with diabetes to monitor the person's average blood glucose level during those months. An A_{1c} value higher than the normal range indicates that the average blood sugar has been elevated during the past 2-3 months. A normal A_{1c} level for a person without diabetes ranges from 4% to 5.6%. For patients with diabetes, the goal is to maintain the glycosylated hemoglobin level below 7%. Table 47-9 associates glycosylated hemoglobin A_{1c} levels with blood glucose levels. The goal for people with diabetes type 2 is to have A_{1c} levels of 7% or lower. With higher levels, the risk of developing complications from diabetes increases.

Several methods can be used to measure the A_{1c} level, and the medical assistant can perform A_{1c} testing using several CLIA-waived devices. The DCA A1cNOW+ for Professionals (Bayer Diagnostics) provides A_{1c} values in 6 minutes from one drop of capillary

TABLE 47-9   Relationship Between Glycosylated Hemoglobin Levels and Blood Glucose Levels

GLYCOSYLATED HEMOGLOBIN A$_{1c}$ (%)	BLOOD GLUCOSE (mg/dL)
14.0	380
13.0	350
12.0	315
11.0	280
10.0	250
9.0	215
8.0	180
7.0	150
6.0	115
5.0	80
4.0	50

blood obtained from a fingerstick. Patients also can perform A$_{1c}$ testing at home using FDA-approved instruments, such as the A1CNow SelfCheck (Bayer) and the in2it (II) Self-Test A1c System (Bio-Rad).

CRITICAL THINKING APPLICATION   47-5

Mr. Corrigan routinely monitors his blood sugar. Why is Dr. Fischbach also interested in his A$_{1c}$ levels?

CHOLESTEROL TESTING

Cholesterol is a fatlike substance (lipid) present in cell membranes. It is needed to form bile acids and steroid hormones, to name a few of its functions. Cholesterol travels in the blood as distinct particles containing both lipid and proteins. These particles are called *lipoproteins*. The cholesterol level in the blood is determined partly by inheritance and partly by acquired factors, such as diet, calorie balance, and level of physical activity.

Patients often are confused by cholesterol testing. The confusion is caused partly by the way some people use the term *cholesterol*, which often is a catchall term for both the cholesterol a person eats and the cholesterol that is maintained in the body. A high blood level of low-density lipoprotein, or LDL, cholesterol reflects an increased risk of heart disease, which is why LDL cholesterol is often called "bad" or "lousy" cholesterol. Lower levels of LDL cholesterol reflect a lower risk of heart disease. When too much LDL cholesterol circulates in the blood, it can slowly build up in the walls of arteries that feed the heart and brain. Together with other substances, it can

form plaque, a thick, hard deposit that can clog those arteries. This condition is known as *atherosclerosis*. If a clot (thrombus) forms at the site of plaque, blood flow can be blocked in the coronary arteries of the heart muscle, causing a heart attack. If a clot blocks blood flow to part of the brain, a stroke results. LDL results are often interpreted as follows:

- LDL less than 100 mg/dL = Optimal
- LDL 100-129 = Near optimal/above optimal
- LDL 130-159 = Borderline high
- LDL 160-189 = High
- LDL 190 + = Very high

About one third to one fourth of blood cholesterol is carried by high-density lipoprotein (HDL). HDL cholesterol is known as the "good" or "healthy" cholesterol because a high level of HDL cholesterol seems to protect against heart attack. HDL is able to carry cholesterol away from the arteries and back to the liver, where it is passed from the body. It is believed that cholesterol is removed from the lining of the arteries when high levels of HDL exist; in contrast, low levels of HDL cholesterol (i.e., lower than 40 mg/dL) may result in a greater risk of heart disease.

Adults older than 20 years of age should have a cholesterol test at least once every 5 years. Total cholesterol and the combination of LDL and HDL typically are screened and monitored (Procedure 47-6). All three tests are considered screening tests, and elevated results always require additional testing before a diagnosis can be made. In general, total cholesterol levels under 200 mg/dL are considered normal. Results over 240 mg/dL are considered elevated and, on the basis of confirmed testing, place a person in the high-risk category for coronary heart disease. An HDL cholesterol level of 40 mg/dL or higher is considered acceptable for men, and values of 50 or higher are acceptable for women. Conversely, HDL levels below 40 mg/dL for men and below 50 mg/dL for women place a person at risk of coronary heart disease.

Although total cholesterol and HDL cholesterol levels are not significantly affected by food consumption, most providers prefer that patients fast from food and liquids, with the exception of water, for 12 hours before cholesterol levels are checked. If the total cholesterol is elevated, the provider is likely to order a *lipid profile,* which is a series of tests that measures the total cholesterol, HDL and LDL cholesterol levels, and triglyceride levels,. Triglycerides are fat in the blood related to caloric intake. Therefore, the patient must be instructed to fast from all food and alcoholic beverages 12 hours before the triglyceride test and/or lipid profiles. Consistently high triglyceride levels may lead to heart disease, especially in people with low levels of "good" HDL cholesterol and high levels of "bad" LDL cholesterol, and in people with diabetes type 2. Elevated levels of triglycerides are typically stored in the belly and are associated with central obesity.

CLIA-waived cholesterol monitors can measure total cholesterol from a fingerstick. The Cholestech LDX analyzer is capable of measuring a lipid panel of tests and providing a risk assessment using capillary blood from a finger (see Procedure 47-6). This system uses a cassette testing device capable of measuring glucose, total cholesterol, HDL, LDL, VLDL, triglycerides, and the TC/HDL ratio. It uses a combination of enzymatic reactions and reflectance photometry to detect the resulting color changes caused by each of the lipid panel analytes.

PROCEDURE 47-6 · Perform a CLIA-Waived Chemistry Test: Determine the Cholesterol Level or Lipid Profile Using a Cholestech Analyzer

Goal: *To perform a Cholestech test for total cholesterol level and/or a lipid panel and accurately report the results.*

Order: Perform a total blood cholesterol level or lipid panel on Connie Lange STAT.

EQUIPMENT and SUPPLIES

- Patient's health record
- Provider's order and/or lab requisition
- Cholestech analyzer
- Package insert or flow chart with directions
- Optics check cassette
- Test cassettes (provided by Cholestech)
- Level 1 and 2 liquid controls
- Capillary tubes and plungers for fingerstick sample (provided by Cholestech)
- Mini-Pet pipet and pipet tips for venipuncture sample (provided by Cholestech)
- Lancet, gauze, alcohol, bandage for capillary blood, *or* lithium heparin (green-topped) tube for venous blood
- Safety tube decapper (if tubes do not have a Hemogard plastic top)
- Fluid-impermeable lab coat, disposable gloves, and protective eyewear (if needed)
- Biohazard waste and sharps containers

PROCEDURAL STEPS

1. Sanitize your hands. Put on fluid-impermeable lab coat, disposable gloves, and protective eyewear (if needed).
   PURPOSE: To ensure infection control.
2. Assemble the materials needed.
3. Perform quantitative quality control by performing a calibration check with the optics check cassette. (see the following figure). Then test level 1 and level 2 liquid controls if using a new set of cassettes
   PURPOSE: To ensure instrument is reading results accurately, precisely, and reliably.

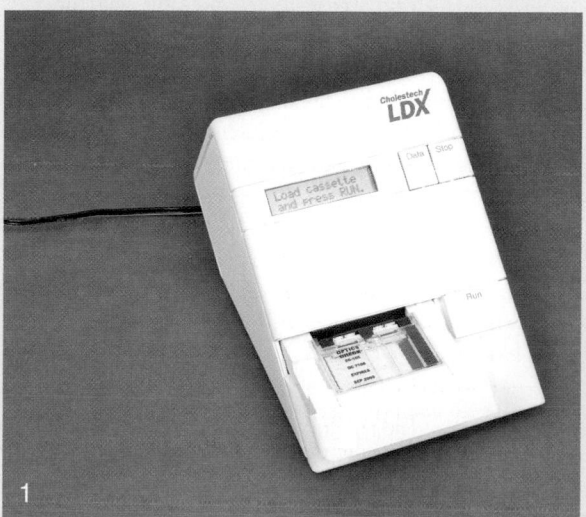

4. Allow refrigerated testing cassettes to come to room temperature (at least 10 minutes before opening).
   PURPOSE: Test is temperature and time sensitive when reading results.
5. Remove cassette from its pouch and place on flat surface without touching the black bar or magnetic strip.
   PURPOSE: The black bar is the testing area, and the magnetic strip must be read by the analyzer. Touching either may interfere with test results
6. Press RUN, allowing the analyzer to do a self-test; this will be followed by OK on the screen, and then the test drawer will open. The drawer will stay open for 4 minutes while the specimen is prepared.
7. Incise the finger, and collect the capillary blood to the black line of the Cholestech capillary tube with its plunger inserted into the red end of the tube. *Or* collect the fresh venous whole blood with the Cholestech Mini-Pet pipet.
   PURPOSE: Both collecting devices are provided by Cholestech to ensure that the exact volume of blood necessary is tested.
8. Place the either whole blood sample into the well of the cassette. Note: The capillary specimen must be in the cassette within 5 minutes of collection. (see the following figure).
   PURPOSE: Fingerstick blood will clot if not tested within 5 minutes.

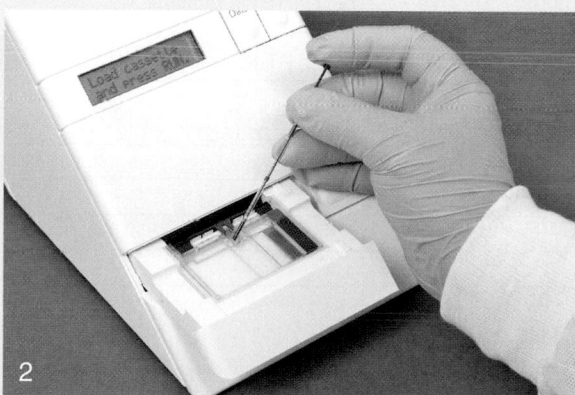

9. Immediately put the cassette into the drawer of the analyzer and press RUN (Note: if the drawer has closed, press RUN again to open the drawer and proceed with loading into the drawer, and then pressing to close the drawer).
   PURPOSE: This is a test with a color reaction that continues to change over time.

10. When the test is complete, the analyzer beeps, and the screen displays and prints out the results (see the following figure).

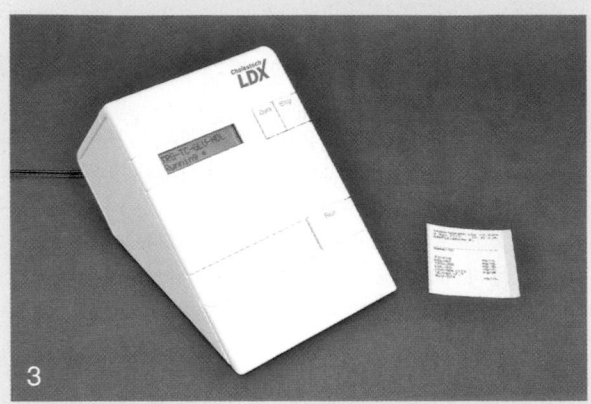

11. Record the findings in the laboratory log and in the patient's health record if they have not been transmitted electronically.
PURPOSE: A procedure is considered not done until it is recorded.

12. Circle the results that do not fall within the Desirable Ranges column of the following table. Identify "critical values" and take appropriate steps to notify the provider.

PURPOSE: The provider needs to know the results while the patient is still in the office, for proper follow-up with the patient.

LIPID PROFILE (CHOLESTECH TEST)

LIPID PROFILE	DESIRABLE RANGES
Total cholesterol	<200 mg/dL
HDL cholesterol	>40 mg/dL
LDL cholesterol	<130 mg/dL
Triglycerides	<150 mg/dL
TC/HDL ratio	4.5 or less
Glucose	Fasting: 60-110 mg/dL
	Nonfasting: <160 mg/dL

Note: Laboratory reports and manufacturers must supply their own reference ranges along with each patient's results. This is because different methodologies may create different reference ranges and different units of measurement.

13. Dispose of all sharps in the biohazard sharps container (i.e. lancet and capillary pipette with plunger). Place all regulated medical waste into the biohazard waste container (i.e. gauze, alcohol pads, and cassettes). Disinfect test area, remove PPE, and dispose gloves in biohazard waste. Sanitize your hands.
PURPOSE: To ensure infection control.

CHOLESTECH LDX PATIENT/CONTROL LOG

Cassette Lot #: _____   Expiration Date: _____   LDX Serial #: _____

DATE	TECH	PT ID	TC	HDL	LDL	TRG	TC/HDL	GLU	CHARTED
10/09/20--	DC	#12345	190	50	120	135	4.3	80	✓

Documentation in the medical record:

Attach printed readout, or record results on the electronic chart:

TEST	RESULTS	DESIRABLE
Total cholesterol (TC)	190	<200 mg/dL
HDL cholesterol	50	>40 mg/dL
LDL cholesterol	120	<130 mg/dL
Triglycerides	135	<150 mg/dL
TC/HDL ratio	4.3	≤4.5
Other		
Glucose	80	Fasting: 60-110 mg/dL
		Nonfasting: <160 mg/dL

ALANINE AMINOTRANSFERASE (ALT) AND ASPARTATE AMINOTRANSFERASE (AST) TESTING

Certain drugs can impair liver function and require the monitoring of two liver enzymes (ALT and AST) that rise in the blood during liver damage. Drugs that cause liver damage include statins and fibrates, pharmaceutical agents used to lower blood cholesterol, and certain antidiabetic and antihypertensive drugs. Liver function tests and panels are ordered by the provider to monitor the liver during therapy with drugs that have the potential to cause liver malfunction.

CLIA-waived liver enzyme testing for ALT and AST may be monitored on the same Cholestech LDX System using ALT/AST test cassettes.

CRITICAL THINKING APPLICATION   47-6

For what reason might Dr. Fischbach want to evaluate Mr. Corrigan's liver enzymes? What clinical chemistry tests might he order from the referral laboratory? What tests for liver enzymes might Dana be able to perform in the POL? What sample will she need for those tests?

THYROID HORMONE TESTING

The thyroid gland is located anterior to the trachea in the throat. It produces the hormones triiodothyronine (T_3) and thyroxine (T_4). These hormones are essential for life and have many effects on body metabolism, growth, and development. The thyroid gland is influenced by hormones produced by two other organs found in the brain, the pituitary gland and the hypothalamus. The pituitary gland produces thyroid-stimulating hormone (TSH), and the hypothalamus produces thyrotropin-releasing hormone (TRH). (Regulation of thyroid hormone production and thyroid disorders are discussed in Chapter 38.)

CLIA-waived rapid diagnostic tests to qualitatively measure TSH are available for point-of-care testing. Using whole blood from a fingerstick, these tests screen patients for hypothyroidism by detecting elevated levels of TSH, which constitutes a sign of hypothyroidism. The tests use lateral flow chromatographic immunoassay technology housed in a plastic cassette. One such commercially available test is the *ThyroTest Whole Blood TSH Test.*

REFERENCE LABORATORY CHEMISTRY PANELS AND SINGLE ANALYTE TESTING AND MONITORING

Automated blood chemistry analyzers often are used to perform blood chemistry testing. It is not uncommon for several analytes to be detected at once. A physician may order a chemistry panel, such as a renal or liver panel, to determine the levels of several related analytes (Figure 47-14). Analytes commonly detected in the chemistry laboratory are listed in Table 47-10. In general, serum from a clotted specimen is needed for these tests. Typical panels are shown in Table 47-11. As noted previously, laboratory reports on patients, both electronic and paper, must provide their own reference ranges along with each patient's results. This is because different methodologies may create different reference ranges and different units of measurement.

CRITICAL THINKING APPLICATION   47-7

What tests are routinely done as part of the renal panel? What information will these tests give Dr. Fischbach about the status of Mr. Corrigan's kidney? What color of rubber stopper or plastic stopper on vacuum tubes would need to be drawn for a serum specimen that will be processed and sent to the reference lab? (*Hint:* There are three colors based on plain "clot" tubes and SST tubes. How will you know which serum tube to use?)

CLOSING COMMENTS

Patient Education

Similar to all other procedures, the test is only as valid as the specimen and the procedure performed on that specimen. You, as the provider's agent, are responsible for that validity when you instruct the patient and when you perform the test.

Legal and Ethical Issues

A medical assistant who is responsible for office laboratory testing must clearly understand the basic concepts of laboratory medicine. Therefore, you must stay current with the rapid technologic advances in laboratory medicine and help establish a protocol of the tests best suited to your provider-employer.

You are responsible for properly collecting specimens and testing them accurately. Patient confidentiality is paramount when testing is performed, as is rigid conformation to all established quality control procedures.

Professional Behaviors

An ever-increasing number of CLIA-waived hematology and chemistry blood tests are relatively simple to perform and require minimal training. This has allowed the provider to share the results with the patient immediately, resulting in greater patient compliance with the prescribed treatment plan. Proper patient care demands attention to detail in all three areas of the testing process:

- *Preanalytic:* Proper care of the testing supplies and equipment, and proper patient identification and specimen collection
- *Analytic:* Running the tests according the specific manufacturer's instructions; recording and analyzing the controls and the patient results
- *Postanalytic:* Proper disposal of biohazardous supplies; routing of test results to the provider and patient.

The medical assistant is the traffic controller for all of these elements. He or she is responsible for the organization and documentation of each performed test on the appropriate lab flow sheet and in the patient's health record.

Physician's Medical Center
77332 E. Capital Drive
Anytown, USA 11123

Ronald J. Haldor, M.D.
Kaye M. Jones, M.D.
Nicholas P. Stepp, M.D.

PATIENT – PLEASE NOTE

If this box is checked, don't eat or drink anything, except water, for 14 hours before going to the lab.

PATIENT NAME _____
                    LAST   FIRST   M.I.
ADDRESS _____ DOB _____

CITY _____ STATE _____ ZIP _____ SEX: M   F

TELEPHONE # _____ SOCIAL SECURITY # ____ – ___ – _____

ORDERING PHYSICIAN _____ DATE _____

BILLING: ☐ HMO ☐ MEDICARE ☐ MEDICAL ☐ OTHER # _____

        GUARANTOR (If other than patient) _____

      ☐ PHONE RESULTS TO _____

      ☐ SEND ADDITIONAL COPIES OF REPORT TO _____
            (Please attach copy of eligibilty card.)

              Patient Diagnosis _____

☐ 906 ARTERIAL BLOOD GASES
        ROOM AIR _____
        RESP. ASSIST _____
☐ 105 BLOOD CELL PROFILE (Hgb + Hct)
☐ 862 BILIRUBIN (NEONATAL)
☐ 868 BILIRUBIN (TOTAL & DIRECT)
☐ 100 CBC (Complete Blood Count & Diff)
☐ 3000 ELECTROLYTES
☐   (NA, K, CO2, Cl)
☐   FANA
☐   GLUCOSE
☐ 915 GLUCOSE, PRE-NATAL DIABETIC SCR.
        (1 Hour Post-Glucola)
☐   GLUCOSE TOLERANCE TEST
        # OF HOURS_____DOSE_____
☐ 3398 HEPATITIS PANEL
        (B-Surf Ag/Ab, B-Core Ab, A-Ab)
☐ 988 LIPID PROFILE
        (Chol, Trig, HDL, LDL, Cardiac Risk)
☐ 3380 LIVER PANEL
        (Alk Phos, Bili, TP, Alb, GGT, SGOT
        (AST) SGPT (ALT), & Consult)
☐ 3006 METABOLIC 7
        (Na, K, CO2, Cl, Glu, Mg)

☐ 3035 PANEL 17
        (Panel 13 + Na + K + Cl + CO2)
☐ 3020 METABOLIC 10
        (Na, K, CO2, Cl, Glu, BUN, Creat)
☐ 3015 METABOLIC 11
        (Met 10 & Phos)
☐ 3160 OBSTETRICAL PANEL 1
        (CBC, UA, ABO/Rh, Antibody
        Screen, Rubella, RPR)
☐ 3172 OBSTETRICAL PANEL 3
        (CBC, ABO/Rh, Antibody Screen,
        Rubella, RPR)
☐ 3445 OBSTETRICAL PANEL 7
        (ABO/Rh, Antibody Screen,
        Rubella, RPR)
☐ 3447 OBSTETRICAL PANEL 7A
        (ABO/Rh, Antibody Screen,
        Rubella, RPR, Hepatitis B Surt Ag)
☐ 3025 PANEL 13
        (Glu, BUN, Creat, Uric Acid, Ca,
        Tp, Alb, Bili, Chol, Alk, Phos,
        SGOT (AST), LDH, Phos)
☐ 3030 PANEL 15
        (Panel 13 + Na + K)

☐ 3010 METABOLIC 8
        (Na, K, CO2, Cl, Glu, BUN)
☐ 3040 PANEL 20 - SMAC
        (Panel 17 + SGPT (ALT) +
        GGT + Osmolality)
☐ 3043 S-1 Panel (Panel 20 + Triglyceride)
☐ 500 PROTHROMBIN TIME (PT)
☐ 505 Partial Thromboplastin Time (PPT)
☐ 7500 RPR
☐ 7515 RUBELLA
☐ 2030 THYROID SCREEN
        (T4, T3, Uptake, Adj T4)
☐ 704 URINALYSIS

              BACTERIOLOGY

        SPECIMEN SOURCE (REQUIRED)
        COLLECTION DATE _____
☐ _____ ROUTINE CULTURE
☐ 8919 AFB CULTURE
☐ 8921 FUNGAL CULTURE

ADDITIONAL LABORATORY TESTS: _____
_____
_____
_____
_____

2804 (4/93)

LABORATORY OUTPATIENT REQUEST

OFFICE USE ONLY

Telephone Order per _____

Order Received by _____

FIGURE 47-14 Panel request form.

TABLE 47-10 Blood Chemistry Tests*

TEST	ABBREVIATION	NORMAL VALUES	DESCRIPTION	PURPOSE
Alanine aminotransferase	ALT (SGPT)	<45 units/L	Enzyme found predominantly in the liver but also in the kidney	To detect liver disease
Albumin		3.5-5 g/dL	Protein	To assess kidney function
Alkaline phosphatase	ALP	20-70 units/L	Enzyme found in several tissues	To detect liver and bone disease
Aspartate aminotransferase	AST (SGOT)	<40 units/L	Enzyme found in several tissues.	To detect tissue damage
Blood urea nitrogen	BUN	7-18 mg/dL *or* 2.5-6.4 mmol/L	Metabolic products of protein catabolism	To detect renal disease
Calcium	Ca	8.4-10.2 mg/dL *or* 2.1-2.6 mmol/L	Mineral	To assess parathyroid function and calcium metabolism
Chloride	Cl	98-106 mmol/L	Electrolyte	To determine acid-base and water balance
Cholesterol	CH, Chol	*Total:* <200 mg/dL *or* <5.18 mmol/L *LDL:* <130 mg/dL *or* <3.37 mmol/L *HDL:* >35 mg/dL *or* >0.91 mmol/L	Lipid	To screen for atherosclerosis related to heart disease
Creatine phosphokinase	CPK	Specific to testing method used	Enzyme found in several tissues	To assess source of muscle damage (myocardial infarct)
Creatinine	creat	0.2-0.8 mg/dL	Metabolic product of protein catabolism	To screen for renal function
Ferritin		20-50 ng/mL	Iron-carrying protein	To detect amount of iron stored in the body
Gamma glutamyl transferase	GGT	0-45 units/L	Enzyme found mainly in liver cells	To detect liver disease
Globulin	glob, Ig	Varies according to type	Protein	To detect abnormalities in protein synthesis and removal
Glucose fasting blood sugar	FBS	70-100 mg/dL *or* 3.9-6.1 mmol/L	Carbohydrate	To detect disorders of glucose metabolism (diabetes)
Glucose tolerance test	GTT	Varies with time	Carbohydrate	To detect disorders of glucose metabolism (diabetes)
Iron	Fe	35-140 mcg/dL	Mineral	To assist in diagnosis of anemia
Lactate dehydrogenase	LDH	<240 units/L	Enzyme found in several tissues	To assist in confirmation of myocardial or pulmonary infarct
pH	pH	7.35-7.45	Measurement of the acid/base (acidity and alkalinity)	To assess acidity or alkalinity of blood
Phosphorus	P	3-4.5 mg/dL *or* 0.97-1.45 mmol/L	Mineral	To assist in proper evaluation of calcium levels and to detect endocrine system disorders

Continued

TABLE 47-10 Blood Chemistry Tests—*continued*

TEST	ABBREVIATION	NORMAL VALUES	DESCRIPTION	PURPOSE
Potassium	K	3.5-5.1 mmol/L	Mineral	To assist in diagnosis of acid-base and water balance
Sodium	Na	135-146 mmol/L	Mineral	To assist in diagnosis of acid-base and water balance
Total bilirubin	TB	0.2-1 mg/dL *or* 3.4-17.1 mmol/L	Metabolic product of hemoglobin catabolism	To evaluate liver function and to aid in diagnosis of anemia
Total iron-binding capacity	TIBC	245-400 mcg/dL		A measure of the potential to transport iron
Total protein	TP	6-8 g/dL; 60-80 g/L		To assess the state of hydration; to screen for diseases that alter protein balance
Troponin I and T		<0.4	Cardiac-specific protein found only with heart muscle damage	To aid in diagnosis of myocardial infarct
Thyroid-stimulating hormone (thyrotropin)	TSH	5-6 milliunits/L	Hormone produced by the pituitary	To assess thyroid and pituitary gland function
Thyroxine	T_4	5-12 mcg/dL *or* 64-155 mmol/L	Hormone produced by the thyroid gland	To assess thyroid function
Triglycerides	Trig	30-190 mg/dL *or* 0.34-2.15 mmol/L		To screen for atherosclerosis related to heart disease
Triiodothyronine	T_3	27%-47%	Hormone produced by the thyroid gland	To assess thyroid function
Uric acid	UA	*Male*: 3.4-7 mg/dL *or* 202-416 mcmol/L *Female*: 2.4-6 mg/dL *or* 143-357 mcmol/L	Metabolic product of protein catabolism	To evaluate renal failure, gout, and leukemia

HDL, High-density lipoprotein cholesterol; *LDL*, low-density lipoprotein cholesterol.
*Lab reports, both electronic and paper, must supply their own reference ranges along with each patient's results. This is because different methodologies may create different reference ranges and different units of measurement.

TABLE 47-11 Typical Chemistry Panels

PANEL	COMPONENT	PANEL	COMPONENT
Liver	Alkaline phosphatase (ALP) Gamma glutamyl transferase (GGT) Aspartate aminotransferase (AST) Alanine aminotransferase (ALT) Lactate dehydrogenase (LDH)	**Cardiac**	Creatine phosphokinase (CPK) Troponin I Troponin T
Anemia	Iron Total iron-binding capacity Ferritin Transferrin	**Electrolyte**	Sodium Potassium Chloride
Thyroid	Thyroid-stimulating hormone (TSH) Thyroxine (T_4) Triiodothyronine (T_3)	**Renal**	Creatinine Blood urea nitrogen (BUN) Uric acid Glucose

Dana knows the important role laboratory analysis of blood plays in patient care. Often many different tests are needed to assess a patient's health. Mr. Corrigan appreciates that he can have many of these tests done during his routine visits with a simple fingerstick, such as the hemoglobin and hematocrit, PT, A₁c level, and ALT/AST testing. The hemoglobin and hematocrit provide Dr. Fischbach with essential information for diagnosing anemia, and the A₁c level

is used to monitor Mr. Corrigan's diabetes. The prothrombin time/international normalized ratio (PT/INR), which monitors coagulation, and the liver enzyme tests (AST/ALT) assure Dr. Fischbach that Mr. Corrigan's liver is functioning properly while he is taking medication to treat his diabetes and to manage the kidney transplant.

SUMMARY OF LEARNING OBJECTIVES

1. **Define, spell, and pronounce the terms listed in the vocabulary.**
   Spelling and pronouncing medical terms correctly reinforce the medical assistant's credibility. Knowing the definitions of these terms promotes confidence in communication with patients and co-workers.

2. **Name the main functions of blood.**
   Blood contains RBCs to deliver oxygen to tissues through hemoglobin, WBCs to fight infections, and platelets to aid in coagulation and the formation of clots. The plasma carries needed nutrients to the cells throughout the body, and removes waste products from the cells and carries them to the lungs and kidneys for elimination.

3. **Describe the appearance and function of erythrocytes.**
   Erythrocytes are also called *red blood cells* because of their red color, which comes from hemoglobin. The biconcave disks lack a nucleus and are responsible for transporting oxygen and carbon dioxide to and from tissues.

4. **Describe the appearance and function of granular and agranular leukocytes.**
   Leukocytes are also called *white blood cells*. Agranular leukocytes lack granules in the cytoplasm, and granular leukocytes have granules. All leukocytes function in fighting infection.

5. **Differentiate between T cells and B cells.**
   T lymphocytes are important in immunity and play roles in killing foreign, virus-infected, and tumor cells; they also assist in antibody production and keep the immune system in check. B cells are responsible for anti-body production.

6. **Describe the appearance and function of thrombocytes, explain the process of clot formation, and discuss plasma.**
   A thrombocyte (platelet) is a fragment of a larger cell (megakaryocyte) found in the bone marrow. Thrombocytes play an important role in clot formation, both physically and chemically. Clot formation begins with the aggregation of thrombocytes, which release a substance that initiates the clotting cascade, resulting in a network of minute threads that trap plasma and blood cells. Plasma is approximately 90% water and is the carrier for the formed elements and other substances.

7. **Do the following related to hematology in the POL:**
   - *Identify the anticoagulant of choice for hematology testing.*
     The anticoagulant required for most hematology testing is ethylene-diaminetetraacetic acid (EDTA). The lavender-topped vacuum tube used in phlebotomy contains this anticoagulant.

   - *Explain the purpose of a microhematocrit test.*
     A microhematocrit (or hematocrit) test is performed to assess the volume of erythrocytes in relation to the total blood volume. The test is performed by centrifuging a small amount of whole blood in a capillary tube. Whole blood normally consists of slightly less than 50% RBCs. Hematocrit is reported as a percentage and is roughly three times the value of hemoglobin in the same specimen.

   - *Perform routine maintenance of a microhematocrit centrifuge.*
     Refer to Procedure 47-1.

   - *Obtain a specimen and perform a microhematocrit test.*
     Refer to Procedure 47-2.

8. **Do the following related to hemoglobin:**
   - *Explain the role of hemoglobin in the body.*
     Hemoglobin is the RBC protein responsible for oxygen transport from the lungs to the tissues. It gives the blood its red color.

   - *Obtain a specimen and perform a hemoglobin test.*
     Refer to Procedure 47-3.

9. **Do the following related to the erythrocyte sedimentation rate:**
   - *Cite the reasons for performing an erythrocyte sedimentation rate (ESR) test.*
     An ESR test is performed to assess inflammation and often is used to monitor rheumatoid arthritis. This test measures the rate at which RBCs fall in a calibrated tube in a 60-minute period.

   - *Describe the sources of error for the erythrocyte sedimentation rate test.*
     An ESR test result may be erroneous if a tube is not standing vertically in the rack; bubbles are present in the Sediplast or Streck ESR tube; dilutions are incorrect; vibrations or jarring occurs; the blood is at a temperature other than room temperature; and the blood has hemolyzed.

   - *Perform an erythrocyte sedimentation rate test using a modified Westergren method.*
     Refer to Procedure 47-4.

10. **Do the following related to coagulation testing:**
    - *Explain how to determine prothrombin time (PT).*
      The PT is a method of measuring how well the blood clots and is used in combination with the partial thromboplastin time (PTT) to screen for hemophilia and other hereditary clotting disorders. It is important

Continued

to educate patients who take warfarin (Coumadin) about the need for follow-up laboratory monitoring of their protime/INR. Helping patients identify foods high in vitamin K is crucial to maintaining a balance between the warfarin dosage and the lab values.

- *Obtain a specimen and perform a CLIA-waived PT/INR test.* Refer to Procedure 47-5.
- *Reassure a patient of the accuracy of the test results.* Refer to Procedure 47-5.
- *Maintain lab test results using laboratory flow sheets.* Refer to Procedure 47-5.

11. **Identify the tests included in a complete blood count (CBC) and their reference ranges, and differentiate between normal and abnormal test results.**

    In the hematology laboratory, blood cells are counted, WBCs are differentiated, and the oxygen-carrying capacity of blood is determined. Hematology testing provides an excellent overview of homeostasis. The CBC involves an erythrocyte count, leukocyte count, thrombocyte count, hemoglobin and hematocrit determination, differential examination of leukocytes, and calculation of red cell indices. Refer to the hematology diagnostic reference ranges in Table 47-4 and Figure 47-7.

12. **Describe the red blood cell (RBC) indices and how they are calculated.**

    RBC indices are calculated using values obtained from the CBC; namely, RBC count, hemoglobin, and hematocrit. They help the provider diagnose blood disorders, such as a variety of anemias.

13. **Explain the reasons for performing a white blood cell (WBC) count and differential, and discuss the preparation of blood smears for the differential.**

    A differential WBC count is performed to assess the percentages of the five types of WBCs in the blood. In addition, the red cells and platelets are examined for distribution and abnormalities. A blood smear is prepared by placing a drop of blood from a fingerstick, or from an EDTA tube using a DIFF-SAFE blood dispenser, onto a clean glass slide that is free of dust and grease. A thin smear of whole blood is spread across the slide, and then stained, typically with Wright's stain, followed by microscopic examination.

14. **Discuss the identification of normal blood cells and describe the basic appearance of the five different types of leukocytes seen in a normal Wright-stained differential.**

    The three features hematologists look for in blood cells are cell size, nuclear appearance, and cytoplasm characteristics. The typical leukocytes seen in the differential examination are (1) the segmented neutrophil, which has a segmented blue nucleus and small lavender granules in the cytoplasm; (2) the eosinophil, resembles the neutrophil but has large red/orange granules; (3) the basophil, which resembles the neutrophil has large blue-black granules; (4) the lymphocyte, which is the smallest WBC, has a light blue cytoplasm (with no granules) and a large dark blue nucleus; and (5) the monocyte, the largest WBC, has an ovulated

blue nucleus and a light blue cytoplasm that appears to have bubble-like inclusions.

15. **Discuss red blood cell morphology.**

    After the differential WBC cell count has been determined, the RBCs are observed and evaluated. The appearance of the RBCs should correlate with the RBC indices.

16. **Differentiate between the ABO blood groupings and the Rh blood groupings.**

    Both the ABO blood type and the Rh type result from antigens on the surfaces of RBCs, and both groups are crucial when it comes to transfusion. There are four different ABO types (A, AB, B, and O), The body produces natural antibodies against the AB antigens that are not present in the blood cells. For example, if a person has type A antigens on the cells, there will be anti-B antibodies in the plasma. A type O blood type would have both anti-A antibodies and anti-B antibodies since they are both foreign to someone with type O blood. There are only two Rh types (positive and negative). Unlike the ABO group, an Rh negative blood type does not have natural antibodies against Rh positive cells. The Rh negative individual must first be exposed to Rh positive cells via transfusion or childbirth which initiates the formation of anti-Rh antibodies that attack and destroy Rh positive cells.

17. **Describe the medical assistant's responsibility for legally preparing a patient for a blood transfusion.**

    The medical practice must comply with the stipulations of the Blood Safety Act if a patient may require a blood transfusion during a procedure. The law requires providers to explain to each elective surgery patient the chances of the need for a blood transfusion. The discussion must include the positive and negative aspects of autologous transfusions (transfusion with a person's own blood) and transfusions of blood from family, friends, or other donors. This discussion must be documented in the patient's health record. Before the surgery, the patient must sign a form giving consent to any needed blood transfusions. The medical assistant may then sign as the witness to the patient's consent.

18. **Do the following related to other blood chemistry testing:**

    - *Explain the reasons for testing blood glucose, hemoglobin A_{1c}, cholesterol, liver enzymes, and thyroid hormones.*

      The *blood glucose* level is monitored routinely in patients with diabetes type 1 or type 2 and in women who have gestational diabetes during pregnancy. *Hemoglobin A_{1c}* levels are measured to determine the average blood glucose level during the 2 to 3 months before the test; this test assists in the management of diabetes. *Cholesterol* testing generally refers to assessing levels of total cholesterol, HDL and LDL; it is done to help determine a patient's susceptibility to coronary artery disease.. *Liver enzyme* testing (ALT and AST) is performed in the POL primarily to monitor the side effects of certain therapeutic drugs, such as those used to treat elevated cholesterol and diabetes. *Thyroid testing* is performed in the POL to detect elevated TSH levels and to assist in the diagnosis of hypothyroidism.. Refer to Table 47-11.

SUMMARY OF LEARNING OBJECTIVES—*continued*

- *Obtain a specimen and perform a cholesterol test using a cholesterol monitor approved by the FDA.*
  Refer to Procedure 47-6.

19. **Summarize typical chemistry panels, the reason for performing each panel, and the individual tests performed in the panels.**
  Certain tests that provide information about a disease or syndrome are grouped together in panels. For example, a liver panel detects abnormalities in a number of different liver enzymes (see Tables 47-10 and 47-11).

20. **Discuss patient education and professionalism related to assisting in the analysis of blood.**
  You, as the provider's agent, are responsible when you instruct the patient and when you perform laboratory tests. A medical assistant who is responsible for office laboratory testing must clearly understand the basic concepts of laboratory medicine. You must stay current and help establish a protocol of the tests best suited to your provider-employer. You are responsible collecting specimens and testing them accurately. Patient confidentiality is paramount when testing is performed, as is rigid conformation to all established quality control procedures.

CONNECTIONS

Study Guide Connection: Go to the Chapter 47 Study Guide. Read and complete the activities.

evolve Evolve Connection: Go to the Chapter 47 link at *evolve.elsevier.com/kinn* to complete the Chapter Review Quiz. Check out the other resources listed for this chapter to make the most of what you have learned from Assisting in the Analysis of Blood.

48

ASSISTING IN MICROBIOLOGY AND IMMUNOLOGY

SCENARIO

Infectious diseases are a continuing threat for everyone. Anna McIntyre, CMA (AAMA), who works in the physician office laboratory (POL) of a local clinic, knows that some diseases have been effectively controlled with the help of modern technology and antibiotics. However, new diseases are constantly appearing, such as the 2014 Ebola epidemic, which affected multiple countries in West Africa; the bird flu (H1N1) pandemic in 2010; and the emergence of the human immunodeficiency virus (HIV) in the 1980s. In addition, other familiar infectious diseases, such as staph infections, tuberculosis, bacterial pneumonia, salmonella poisoning, and malaria, now are appearing in forms that are resistant to drug treatment. Anna knows that it is important to identify pathogens quickly so that proper treatment can begin as soon as possible. Identification of pathogens, she has discovered, can involve several different types of tests, many of which can be performed in the POL.

While studying this chapter, think about the following questions:

- How can Anna protect herself and other patients in the facility from infectious microorganisms?
- How can body fluids or other samples be collected and tested for the presence of pathogenic organisms?
- How are pathogenic organisms differentiated from normal, nonpathogenic species?
- What role do laboratory healthcare workers play in the identification and treatment of infections caused by microorganisms?

LEARNING OBJECTIVES

1. Define, spell, and pronounce the terms listed in the vocabulary.
2. Describe the naming of microorganisms.
3. Describe various bacterial staining characteristics, shapes, oxygen requirements, and physical structures; also, explain the characteristics of common diseases caused by bacteria.
4. Describe the unusual characteristics of *Chlamydia*, *Mycoplasma*, and *Rickettsia* organisms.
5. Do the following related to fungi, protozoa, and parasites:
   - Compare bacteria with fungi, protozoa, and parasites.
   - Identify the characteristics of common diseases caused by fungi, protozoa, and parasites.
   - Perform patient education on the collection of a stool specimen for ova and parasite testing.
6. Compare bacteria with viruses, and describe the characteristics of common viral diseases.
7. Cite the protocols for the collection, transport, and processing of specimens.
8. Explain how pinworm testing is done and when it is recommended.
9. Describe and perform CLIA-waived microbiology tests:
   - Describe three CLIA-waived microbiology tests that use a rapid identification technique.
   - Obtain a specimen and perform the CLIA-waived rapid *Streptococcus* test.
10. Do the following related to CLIA-waived immunology testing:
    - Discuss the purpose of indirect immunology testing.
    - Describe three CLIA-waived immunology tests that could be done in the physician office laboratory.
    - Obtain a specimen and perform the CLIA-waived mononucleosis strep test.
11. Detail the equipment needed in a microbiology reference laboratory, and discuss identification of pathogens in the microbiology laboratory by describing various staining techniques.
12. Describe the reference laboratory assessment of a throat culture and a urine culture.
13. Explain the method used for culture and sensitivity testing.
14. Discuss patient education, in addition to legal and ethical issues, involved in laboratory testing.

VOCABULARY

antibodies Molecular proteins (immunoglobulins) produced by the blood's plasma cells that specifically destroy a foreign invader or substance that has infected the body.

antigens Foreign invaders or substances that cause an immune response in the body in which specific antibodies are produced to attack and destroy it.

antimicrobial agents A general term for drugs, chemicals, or other substances that either kill or slow the growth of microbes. Among the antimicrobial agents are antibacterial drugs, antiviral agents, antifungal agents, and antiparasitic drugs.

arthropods (ahr'-thro-podz) Members of a class of invertebrate animals that includes insects, crustaceans, spiders, scorpions, and others.

broad-spectrum antimicrobial agents Drugs used to treat a wide range of infections.

chromosomes Thread-like molecules that carry hereditary information

cyst A small, capsule-like sac that encloses certain organisms in their dormant or larval stage.

eukaryote (yoo-kar'-e-oht) Single-celled or multicellular organism in which each cell contains a distinct membrane bound nucleus.

genus A classification representing a family of microorganisms and all living beings. The genus is the first name assigned to a microorganism and it is italicized and capitalized.

in vitro A term referring to conditions or tests performed outside a living body.

macromolecules The molecules needed for metabolism: carbohydrates, lipids, proteins, and nucleic acids.

microorganisms Organisms of microscopic or submicroscopic size.

molecule A group of like or different atoms held together by chemical forces.

normal flora Microorganisms normally present on and in our bodies; they perform vital functions and protect the body against infection.

opportunistic organisms Microorganisms normally present in low numbers that are capable of causing disease when the conditions are favorable.

organelles (or-gah-nels') Structures within a cell that perform a specific function.

pathogen An agent that causes disease, especially a living microorganism such as a bacterium or fungus

prokaryote (pro-kar'-e-oht) A unicellular organism that lacks a membrane-bound nucleus.

pure culture A bacterial or fungal culture that contains a single organism.

reagent (re-a'-gent) An ingredient used in a laboratory test to detect or produce a reaction.

species A category of microorganisms below genus in rank; a genetically distinct group. It is the second name given to the microorganism and it is written in all lower case italic letters.

tissue culture The technique or process of keeping tissue alive and growing in a culture medium.

transport medium A medium used to keep an organism alive during transport to the laboratory.

viable Capable of living, developing, or germinating under favorable conditions.

wet mount A slide preparation in which a drop of liquid specimen or the like is covered with a coverslip and observed with a microscope.

Infectious diseases caused by **microorganisms** have gotten a lot of publicity. In 2015 the evening news followed the latest outbreaks of viral influenza and Ebola virus as they swept across particular nations and threatened to spread worldwide. The news also reported on the contaminated water supplies that followed weather catastrophes. Healthcare-associated infections (HAIs), such as methicillin-resistant *Staphylococcus aureus* (MRSA) and *Clostridium difficile* infection, in addition to other intestinal and respiratory diseases, are becoming more and more difficult to control because of the new strains of drug-resistant microorganisms. Bioterrorism became a reality when *Bacillus anthracis* spores were sent through the mail, causing anthrax. Products line the pharmacy shelves, declaring their ability to keep us "germ free." It is no wonder many people have the impression that all microorganisms are harmful. In reality, less than 1% of known microorganisms are **pathogens**.

In fact, without microorganisms we could not survive. Beneficial microorganisms are responsible for the decomposition of waste and natural recycling. The **normal flora** in and on our bodies is needed for the following processes:

- Digesting food
- Forming blood clots properly as a result of vitamin K production by the organisms inhabiting our intestines
- Preventing pathogens from invading our skin, mucous membranes, and gastrointestinal and genitourinary tracts

When the body's normal flora is weakened (e.g., by antibiotic overuse or hormonal changes), certain **opportunistic organisms** that normally are present in low numbers begin to overgrow, causing a superinfection. For example, vulvovaginal candidiasis, a yeast infection of the vaginal tract, is common in women that have taken **broad-spectrum antimicrobial agents**.

As a medical assistant, you need to understand basic microbiology and the role of microorganisms in both health and disease. The main objective in medical microbiology procedures is to identify the organisms responsible for illness so that the provider can properly treat the patient. In addition, your responsibilities will include preventing HAIs by observing infection control in the physician office laboratory (POL) and in the patients the POL serves. Microbiology testing procedures may be performed in the POL or in the microbiology department of a medical referral laboratory.

The study of immunology, or the immune system, is closely tied to microbiology. Invasive microorganisms induce an immune response, leading to the production of a variety of molecular **antibodies** that come to our defense. Often a bacterial or viral infection is diagnosed by testing for the specific antibody that fights the specific infectious agent, rather than by isolating the pathogen itself.

The previous chapters on Infection Control and Assisting in the Clinical Laboratory discussed the chain of infection and how it can be broken through the use of diligent infection control procedures, such as proper hand sanitizing, wearing appropriate personal protective equipment (PPE), observing recommended precautions based on how infectious agents are transmitted, using antiseptics and disinfectants, and performing sterilization procedures.

This chapter covers the major types of infectious agents; the quality control issues related to the collection and handling of microbiologic specimens; and common microbiology and immunology tests that are CLIA waived (i.e., allowed to be performed in the POL under the Clinical Laboratory Improvement Amendments). The chapter concludes with an overview of the more complex microbiology procedures and tests performed in hospitals and reference laboratories.

CLASSIFICATION OF MICROORGANISMS

Although the medical assistant is not responsible for identifying microorganisms, a working knowledge of the terminology used in the classification of microorganisms is essential.

Microorganisms are too small to be seen without magnification. Bacteria are the most prevalent type of microorganism. Other microorganisms include fungi and protozoa. Parasitic worm infections also are identified in the microbiology laboratory because their eggs are seen under the microscope. Viruses are the smallest microorganism and are visible only under the highly magnified electron microscope.

Naming of Microorganisms

Scientists have used the binomial system of nomenclature developed by Swedish botanist Carl Linnaeus to name all living organisms: animals, plants, fungi, protozoa, and bacteria. This binomial system assigns two names; the first name is the **genus** (plural, genera) and the second is the **species**. Both names are either italicized or underlined when written. The genus begins with a capital letter, the species with a lowercase letter. Often the name reveals some characteristic about the organism. For example, *Neisseria gonorrhoeae* is a bacterium that was studied extensively by Albert Neisser, and it causes the sexually transmitted infection gonorrhea. When microbiology laboratory results are reported, it is essential that both the genus and species names be recorded. Different species may cause different symptoms or require different antibiotic treatment. For example, *Neisseria gonorrhoeae* causes disease, whereas *Neisseria sicca* is found in the mouth and does not cause disease under normal conditions.

The genus name of the organism may be represented by a single letter after the organism's full genus and species name has been written once in a report. For example, *Escherichia coli* is commonly referred to as *E. coli*.

CRITICAL THINKING APPLICATION   48-1

Anna receives a telephone call from BioStatLab, the referral laboratory the clinic uses. The results from Ms. Tina Walker's urine culture are ready. The technician says that the organism causing Ms. Walker's urinary tract infection was identified as *Escherichia coli*. How could *E. coli* have infected the urinary tract? (*Hint:* What body part is similar in spelling to "coli"?)

Typical Pathogenic Bacteria

Bacteria are single-celled **prokaryote** organisms that reproduce by binary fission, a process that involves duplication of their genetic **chromosomes** and subsequent fission (splitting in half) of the cell. This process of asexual reproduction results in tremendous numbers of bacteria from a single cell, which explains how bacterial infections can quickly overwhelm a person's immune system. Some bacteria reproduce in as little as 14 minutes, whereas others take days to divide. Theoretically, a single *E. coli* cell, which has a reproduction time of about 30 minutes, produces 351,843, 724,088,831 offspring in 24 hours if it is able to enter the urinary bladder.

Bacteria often are classified according to their staining characteristics, their shapes, and the environmental conditions in which they thrive. Both shape and staining characteristics are direct results of the cell wall composition.

Bacterial Staining Characteristics

Three types of cell wall structures are found among pathogenic bacteria: gram positive, gram negative, and acid fast. These designations are based on reactions in specialized stains used to visualize the bacteria under the microscope. Bacterial cell walls are composed of peptidoglycan (PG), a **molecule** composed of carbohydrate and protein.

- *Gram-positive cells* contain a thick layer of PG with no lipid layer surrounding it; this produces a deep blue/violet when stained with Gram's stain (Figure 48-1, *A*).
- *Gram-negative cells* contain a thin layer of PG with a lipid layer surrounding it; this produces a pinkish red color when stained with Gram's stain (Figure 48-1, *B*).
- *Acid-fast cells* contain a thin layer of PG surrounded by a thick layer of wax-like lipids. Acid-fast bacteria do not stain well with Gram's stain; these cells stain pink with the acid-fast stain (Figure 48-2).

Bacterial Shapes

Pathogenic bacteria assume three different morphologic shapes. Spherical bacteria are called *cocci* (singular, *coccus*); rod-shaped bacteria are *bacilli* (singular, *bacillus*); and spiral bacteria are *spirilla* (singular, *spirillum*). Tightly coiled spirilla are called *spirochetes*. Certain arrangements are also seen in the different genera and species. For example, when bacteria are in a chain formation,

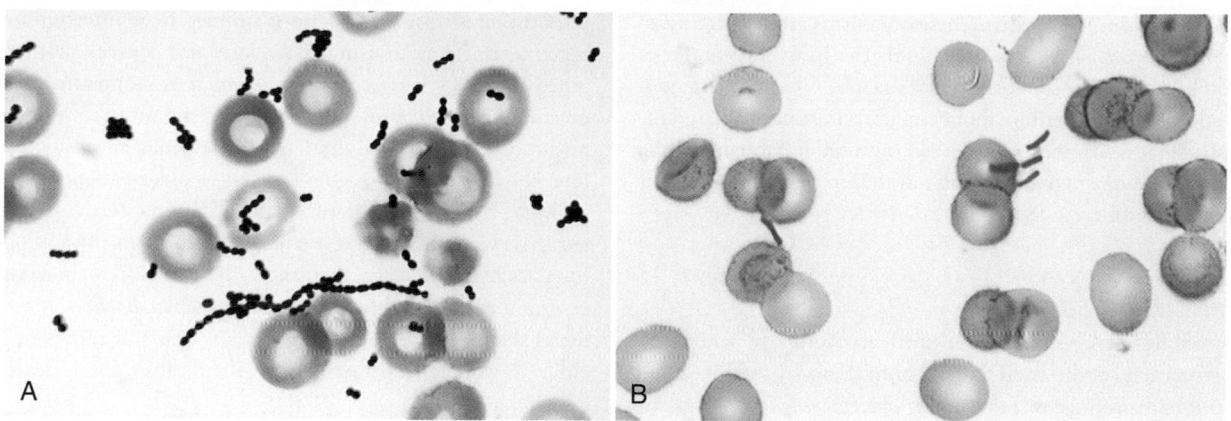

FIGURE 48-1 Gram stain. **A,** Red blood cells (RBCs) and gram-positive cocci. **B,** RBCs with gram-negative bacilli. (From De la Maza LM, Pezzlo MT, Baron EJ: *Color atlas of diagnostic microbiology,* St Louis, 1997, Mosby.)

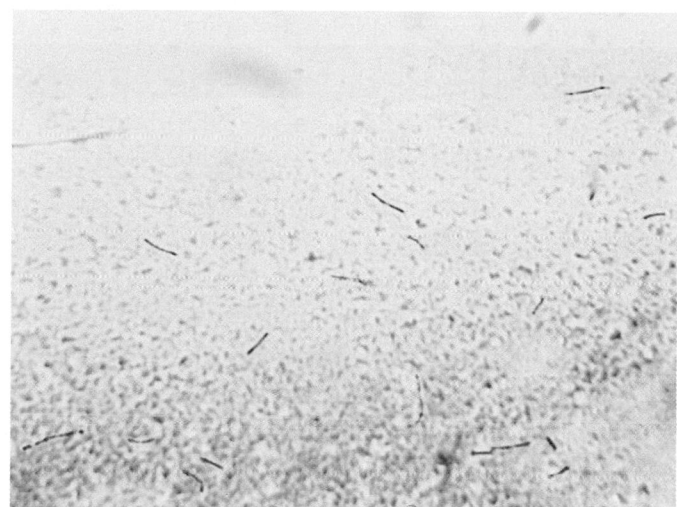

FIGURE 48-2 The acid-fast stain. Pink acid-fast bacilli (AFB) are seen in this smear. (From De la Maza LM, Pezzlo MT, Baron EJ: *Color atlas of diagnostic microbiology,* St Louis, 1997, Mosby.)

the prefix *strepto-* is used. When bacteria are found in pairs, the prefix *diplo-* is used, and when they are found in grapelike clusters, the prefix *staphylo-* is used. Cocci in packets of four are called *tetrads,* and in packets of eight or 16 are called *sarcinae* (Figure 48-3).

CRITICAL THINKING APPLICATION   48-2

Anna knows that impetigo is caused by *Staphylococcus aureus.* Without using a microscope, she knows what the organism's shape looks like. How does she know? (*Hint:* Examine the two parts of the organism's genus.)

Bacterial Oxygen Requirements

Bacteria are also classified according to oxygen requirements. Those that require oxygen to live are called *aerobes*; those that die in the presence of oxygen are *anaerobes.* Some bacteria are flexible concerning oxygen requirements and, although they are anaerobes, can

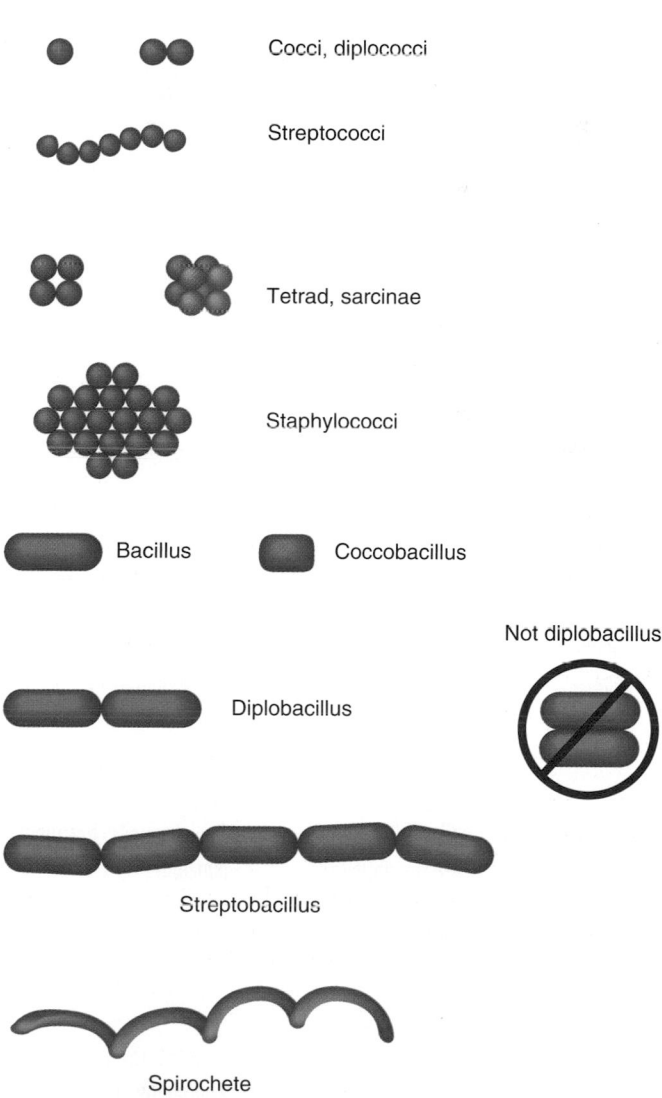

FIGURE 48-3 Typical morphologic arrangements of bacteria.

survive in the presence of oxygen. These organisms are called *facultative anaerobes. Mycobacterium tuberculosis* thrives in white blood cells in the lungs, causing tuberculosis; it is an aerobe. *Bacteroides fragilis* is the predominant bacterium found in the intestines. This gram-negative bacillus is an anaerobe. *E. coli,* also an inhabitant of the intestines and the most common cause of urinary tract infections, is a facultative anaerobe.

Bacterial Physical Structures

Bacteria can be classified and identified according to additional physical structures. Some bacteria have thin, long structures, called *flagella,* that aid propulsion movement. *Proteus vulgaris* is a gram-negative bacillus with many flagella surrounding the cell. It can propel itself into the bladder and is the primary cause of HAI (Healthcare Acquired Infection) urinary tract infections. In some bacteria, thick, gelatinous coats surround the cell wall; these are called *capsules. Streptococcus pneumoniae* is nonpathogenic if it is not producing a capsule; however, it is the most common cause of pneumonia in older adults when it becomes encapsulated. Therefore, the Pneumovax vaccine is given to older patients and to those at high risk for respiratory complications (e.g., patients with asthma). Certain bacteria are also able to form intracellular structures, called *endospores,* that allow the cell to remain **viable** when environmental conditions are not favorable. *Bacillus anthracis* produces such spores, as does *Clostridium tetani.* If spores of *C. tetani* enter a wound and germinate, they cause the disease known as *tetanus.*

Tables 48-1 to 48-3 list some important infectious diseases caused by typical pathogenic bacilli, cocci, and spirilla.

TABLE 48-1   Common Diseases Caused by Bacilli

DISEASE OR CONDITION	ORGANISM	TRANSMISSION	SYMPTOMS	SPECIMENS AND TESTS	PREVENTION AND IMMUNIZATION
Tuberculosis	*Mycobacterium tuberculosis* —Acid-fast branching bacilli	Inhalation	*Pulmonary:* Cough, hemoptysis, sweats, weight loss May affect other systems	Sputum for culture; x-ray films, skin tests	BCG vaccine (not routinely given in the United States); isolation when infection is active
Urinary tract infections	*Escherichia coli, Proteus* spp., *Klebsiella* spp., *Pseudomonas aeruginosa* —Gram-negative bacilli, many flagellated	Ascends urethra; catheterization	*Cystitis:* Frequency, burning, bloody urine *Pyelonephritis:* Flank pain, fever	Clean-catch urine for culture and analysis	Good personal hygiene (always wipe from front to back)
Legionnaires' disease	*Legionella pneumophila* —Gram-negative bacillus (stains poorly with usual methods)	Grows freely in water (air conditioning systems)	Pneumonia-like symptoms	Sputum; blood for culture and analysis	Avoid smoking; patient isolation and proper ventilation to avoid spreading organisms through ducts
Tetanus (lockjaw)	*Clostridium tetani* —Gram-positive spore-forming bacilli, anaerobic	Open wounds, fractures, punctures	Toxin affects motor nerves; muscle spasms, convulsions, rigidity	Blood tests	DTaP in childhood; Tdap is a booster immunization given at age 11 that offers continued protection; it is also routinely given to pregnant women and infant care providers
Botulism	*Clostridium botulinum* —Gram-positive, spore-forming bacilli, anaerobic	Improperly cooked canned foods	Neurotoxin affects speech, swallowing, vision; paralysis of respiratory muscles, death	Contaminated food; blood for culture and analysis	Botulinus antitoxin; boil canned goods 20 min before tasting or eating

TABLE 48-1	Common Diseases Caused by Bacilli—*continued*				
DISEASE OR CONDITION	**ORGANISM**	**TRANSMISSION**	**SYMPTOMS**	**SPECIMENS AND TESTS**	**PREVENTION AND IMMUNIZATION**
Diphtheria (respiratory secretions)	*Corynebacterium diphtheriae* —Gram-positive bacilli, club shaped	Inhalation	Sore throat, fever, headache, gray membrane in the throat	Swabs; Gram stain, culture	DTaP in childhood; Tdap is a booster immunization given at age 11 that offers continued protection; also routinely given to pregnant women and infant care providers
Whooping cough	*Bordetella pertussis* —Gram-negative bacilli	Respiratory secretions	Upper respiratory tract symptoms; high-pitched, crowing whoop	Swabs for culture	DTaP in childhood See Tetanus.
Clostridium difficile infection	*Clostridium difficile* —Gram-positive, spore-forming bacilli	Hospital-acquired infection resistant to antibiotic treatment	Diarrhea, abdominal cramping, blood or pus in the stool, fever, kidney failure	Fecal sample; stool tests, colon examination	Change antibiotic based on *C. diff* culture and sensitivity test results
Salmonella infection	*Salmonella* (multiple species) —Gram-negative	Food-borne illness	Fever, diarrhea, abdominal cramps, headache, possibly nausea, vomiting, and loss of appetite	Fecal sample; stool tests	Wash hands and surfaces when preparing eggs, raw meat; refrigerate meat leftovers; avoid cross-contamination of food

Courtesy Kathleen Moody.
BCG, Bacille Calmette-Guérin vaccine; *DTaP*, diphtheria-tetanus-acellular pertussis vaccine; *T*, tetanus (toxoid).

TABLE 48-2	Common Diseases Caused by Cocci				
DISEASE	**ORGANISM**	**TRANSMISSION**	**SYMPTOMS**	**SPECIMENS AND TESTS**	**PREVENTION**
Pneumonia	*Streptococcus pneumoniae* —Gram-positive encapsulated cocci in pairs	Direct contact, droplets	Productive cough, fever, chest pain	Sputum; bronchoscopy secretions Culture, Gram stain	*Vaccines:* PCV13 recommended for all children <5 yr and adults ≥65 yr PPSV23 recommended for ages ≥65 and for "at risk" individuals age 2-64 yr
Strep throat	*Streptococcus pyogenes* (group A streptococcus) —Gram-positive cocci in chains	Direct contact, droplets, fomites	Severe sore throat, fever, malaise	Direct swab Rapid strep test, throat culture	Good personal hygiene, such as washing hands frequently and not sharing eating and drinking utensils
Wound infection, abscesses, boils	*Staphylococcus aureus* —Gram-positive cocci in clusters	Direct contact, fomites, carriers; poor hand washing	Area red, warm, swollen; pus; pain; ulceration or sinus formation	Deep swab; aspirate of drainage Culture and sensitivity (aerobic and anaerobic)	Good personal hygiene, such as washing hands with soap and water frequently

Continued

TABLE 48-2   Common Diseases Caused by Cocci—*continued*

DISEASE	ORGANISM	TRANSMISSION	SYMPTOMS	SPECIMENS AND TESTS	PREVENTION
Staphylococcal food poisoning	*Staphylococcus aureus* —Gram-positive cocci in clusters	Poor hygiene and improper refrigeration of foods	Vomiting, abdominal cramps, diarrhea	Suspected food, stool Culture of food (organism is not found in stool)	Refrigerate food to prevent toxin production
Gonorrhea	*Neisseria gonorrhoeae* —Gram-negative cocci in pairs; intracellular in white blood cells	Sexually transmitted	*Females:* Pelvic pain, discharge; may be asymptomatic *Males:* Urethral drip, pain on urination	Swab of cervix, urethra; rectal and pharyngeal swabs in men who have sex with men Gram stain; culture	Avoid unprotected sex
Meningococcal meningitis	*Neisseria meningitidis* —Gram-negative diplococci	Respiratory tract secretions	High fever, headache, projectile vomiting, delirium, neck and back rigidity, convulsions, petechial rash	Nasopharyngeal swabs, cerebrospinal fluid, blood Gram stain; culture; cell counts and chemistries	*Vaccination:* MCV4: Menveo for ages 2-55 Menactra for ages 9 mo to 55 yr Prophylactic antibiotics
MRSA infection	Methicillin-resistant *Staphylococcus aureus* —Gram-positive cocci in clusters	Hospital-acquired infection (HAI), transmission via direct contact, fomites, carriers; poor hand washing	Area red, warm, swollen; pus; pain; ulceration or sinus formation	Deep swab; aspirate of drainage Culture and sensitivity (aerobic and anaerobic)	Good personal hygiene, with frequent hand sanitizing and wearing gloves with all patients

TABLE 48-3   Common Diseases Caused by Spirilla

DISEASE	ORGANISM	TRANSMISSION	SYMPTOMS	SPECIMENS AND TESTS	PREVENTION AND IMMUNIZATION
Syphilis	*Treponema pallidum* —Spirochete	Sexually; congenitally	*Primary:* Painless sore (chancre) *Secondary:* Generalized rash involving palms and soles of feet *Congenital:* Birth defects	Blood for serologic tests: VDRL, RPR, FTA-ABS	Avoid unprotected sex; penicillin treatment during pregnancy to prevent congenital infection in fetus
Lyme disease	*Borrelia burgdorferi* —Spirochete	Tick bite	Fever, joint pain, red bull's-eye rash	Blood	Avoid tick-infested areas; report tick bites to practitioner; early treatment with antibiotics
Pyloric ulcers	*Helicobacter pylori* —Gram-negative, spiral shaped	Unknown; possibly food and water	Burning pain in stomach, especially between meals	Stomach biopsy for staining and culture; stool for EIA testing	Use caution with pain relievers Treatment: Antibiotic, antacids; histamine blockers
Food-borne illnesses (most common cause in United States)	*Campylobacter jejuni* —Paired, gram-negative, curved rods forming a seagull shape	Contaminated food, water, and milk	Bloody or watery diarrhea	Stool for darkfield microscopy and culture	Sanitary food preparation and storage; control of water and milk supplies

Courtesy Kathleen Moody.

EIA, Enzyme immunoassay; *FTA-ABS,* fluorescent treponemal antibody absorption (test); *RPR,* rapid plasma reagin (test); *VDRL,* Venereal Disease Research Laboratory.

Unusual Pathogenic Bacteria: Chlamydiae, Mycoplasmas, and Rickettsiae

Typical pathogenic bacteria measure 1,000 to 5,000 nm. Chlamydiae, mycoplasmas, and rickettsiae are tiny, unusual bacteria that fall between the size ranges of typical pathogenic bacteria and viruses (Table 48-4).

Chlamydiae are tiny bacteria that require host cells for growth; they once were considered viruses. Rickettsiae are tiny gram negative bacteria that are transmitted by blood-sucking insects. Rickettsiae cannot multiply outside a living host cell, and once inside the cell,

they are able to perform only some of the life-sustaining metabolic reactions on their own.

Mycoplasmas are unusual in that they have no PG in the cell wall. *Mycoplasma* pneumonia is also referred to as "walking pneumonia."

Pathogenic Fungi

Mycology is the study of fungi and the diseases they cause (Table 48-5). Fungi (singular, *fungus*) are **eukaryotes** that are larger than bacteria and have a nucleus; they include unicellular yeasts and

TABLE 48-4 Diseases Caused by Rickettsiae, Mycoplasmas, and Chlamydiae

DISEASE	ORGANISM	TRANSMISSION	SYMPTOMS	SPECIMENS AND TESTS
Rocky Mountain spotted fever	*Rickettsia rickettsii*	Tick bite	Headache, chills, fever, characteristic rash on extremities and trunk	Blood for serologic tests; skin biopsy for direct fluorescent microscopy
Typhus	*Rickettsia prowazekii*	Tick bite	Fever, rash, confusion	Blood for serology
Atypical (walking) pneumonia	*Mycoplasma pneumoniae*	Respiratory secretions	Fever, cough, chest pain	Blood, sputum for culture
Nongonococcal urethritis and vaginitis	*Chlamydia trachomatis*	Sexual	May be asymptomatic	Swabs for DNA probe and serologic testing
Inclusion conjunctivitis, pneumonia	*Chlamydia trachomatis*	During birth	Severe conjunctivitis or afebrile pneumonia in newborns	Swabs for DNA probe and serologic testing

Courtesy Kathleen Moody.

TABLE 48-5 Common Diseases Caused by Fungi

DISEASE	ORGANISM	PREDISPOSING CONDITIONS AND TRANSMISSION	SYMPTOMS	SPECIMENS AND TESTS
Thrush (oral yeast), vulvovaginal candidiasis, or monilia (vaginal yeast)	*Candida* spp. (yeast)	*Oral:* During birth *Other:* After antibiotic therapy, oral birth control, severe diabetes, AIDS	White, cheesy growth	Swab for KOH prep, culture
Athlete's foot, jock itch, ringworm (tinea)	*Trichophyton* spp., *Microsporum* spp., and others (skin fungi)	Opportunist; direct contact; clothing; prolonged exposure to moist environment	Hair loss, thickening of skin, nails; itching; red, scaly patches	Skin scraping for KOH prep; skin, hair for culture
Histoplasmosis	*Histoplasma capsulatum*	Inhalation of dust contaminated with bird or bat droppings	Mild, flulike to systemic	Serologic; culture of biopsy material
Cryptococcosis	*Cryptococcus neoformans*	Contact with poultry droppings	Cough, fever, malaise; can become systemic	Sputum culture; cerebrospinal fluid culture
Sporotrichosis	*Sporothrix schenckii*	Farmers, florists, people exposed to soil	Skin lesions that spread along lymphatics; can become systemic	Skin scraping for KOH prep; serologic
Pneumocystis pneumonia	*Pneumocystis carinii*	Widely prevalent in animals; occurs in debilitated or immunosuppressed individuals; common in patients with AIDS	Pneumonia-like	Biopsy of lung tissue with microscopic examination

Courtesy Kathleen Moody.
AIDS, Acquired immunodeficiency syndrome; *KOH,* potassium hydroxide.

multicellular molds. Fungi are present in the soil, air, and water, but only a few species cause disease. They are transmitted by direct contact with infected persons, or by prolonged exposure to a moist environment, or by inhalation of contaminated dust or soil. Fungal infections may be superficial, affecting only the skin, hair, or nails. However, some fungi can penetrate the tissues of the internal body structures and cause serious diseases of the mucous membranes, heart, and lungs (e.g., candidiasis in the mouth, fungal endocarditis, and fungal pneumonia). Fungal infections are resistant to bacterial antibiotics and must be treated with specific antifungal medications.

A superficial fungal infection often is referred to as a *tinea* (Latin for "ringworm"). Tinea pedis, for example, is athlete's foot; tinea barbae is a fungal infection of the facial hair follicles. The term *ringworm* arose because the infected area is often circular and appears wrinkled in the center as a result of the healing process. Diagnosis of fungal infections usually is based on culturing or microscopic observation of skin scrapings, hair samples, or samples of sputum or mucous membranes. Usually, before microscopic observation, the samples are treated with potassium hydroxide to dissolve away nonfungal material, making the fungal elements easier to observe.

Pathogenic Protozoa

Protozoa (singular, *protozoon*) are single-celled parasitic eukaryotes that contain a nucleus. They range in size from microscopic to macroscopic (visible to the naked eye) (Table 48-6). They are present in moist environments and in bodies of water, such as lakes and ponds. Protozoa are transmitted through contaminated feces, food, and drink. Some pathogenic protozoa inhabit the bloodstream, whereas others inhabit the intestines and genital tract. Diagnosis usually is based on the patient's signs and symptoms and on microscopic examination of stool and blood.

Pathogenic Parasites

Parasitology includes the study of all parasitic organisms that live on or in the human body (see Table 48-6). In parasitic relationships, the host is harmed as the parasite thrives. Parasites are transmitted by ingestion during the infective stage, direct penetration of the skin by infective larvae, and inoculation by an **arthropod**. A parasite cannot be identified accurately on the basis of a single test or specimen. Most parasites are identified in urine, sputum, tissue fluids, or tissue biopsy samples.

TABLE 48-6   Common Diseases Caused by Protozoa and Parasites

DISEASE	ORGANISM	TRANSMISSION	SYMPTOMS	SPECIMENS AND TESTS
Malaria	*Plasmodium* spp. (protozoa)	Bite of the *Anopheles* mosquito	Chills, fever (cyclic)	Blood: Examination of stained blood for parasites
Toxoplasmosis	*Toxoplasma gondii* (protozoan)	Fecal contamination (cat litter); congenital	Febrile illness, rash; congenital: jaundice, enlarged liver and spleen, brain abnormalities	Skin test for screening blood, fluid, or tissue for confirmation
Amebic dysentery	*Entamoeba histolytica* (protozoan)	Fecal contamination of food and water	Bloody diarrhea, cramping, fever	Stool for ova and parasites (O&P)
Giardiasis	*Giardia lamblia* (protozoan)	Common in intestinal tract, opportunist; contaminated surface water	Asymptomatic to severe diarrhea and abdominal discomfort	Stool for O&P; intestinal biopsy
Trichinosis	*Trichinella spiralis* (roundworm)	Ingestion of undercooked pork, bear meat	Nausea, fever, diarrhea, muscle pain and swelling, edema of face	Biopsy; blood tests
Tapeworm	*Taenia* spp.	Undercooked meat (beef and pork)	Abdominal discomfort, diarrhea, weight loss	Stool for O&P
	Diphyllobothrium latum	Undercooked fish; common among Norwegians, Japanese	As above; may become anemic	Stool for O&P
Pinworm	*Enterobius vermicularis* (roundworm)	Fecal-oral	Severe rectal itching, restlessness, insomnia	Scotch tape applied to perianal region for ova
Scabies	*Sarcoptes scabiei* (itch mite)	Direct contact; clothing, bedding	Nocturnal itching; skin burrows	Skin scrapings for parasites
Lice	*Pediculus humanus; Pthirus pubis* (crabs)	Direct contact; clothing, bedding, furniture (can transmit other diseases via bite)	Intense itching; skin lesions	Finding adult lice or eggs (nits) on body or hair

Courtesy Kathleen Moody.

Helminths (Worms)

Helminths are eukaryote parasites called *worms*. Helminths live on or within another living organism and nourish themselves at the expense of the host organism. They can live in animals or humans and usually are transmitted through the soil, by infected clothing or fingernails, or through contact with infected persons or contaminated food or water. Helminths go through the same life cycle as other worms. The adult worm lays eggs (ova). The ova develop into larvae. Larvae grow into adult worms, which lay eggs, and the cycle begins again. Diagnosis usually is based on microscopic examination of feces for ova and parasites and on the patient's signs and symptoms (Figure 48-4).

Stool specimens commonly are examined for parasitic protozoa and helminths. The specimen is collected and placed into two vials, each with a preservative. Most commonly, sodium acetate acetic acid formalin (SAF) and polyvinyl alcohol (PVA) are used. From these preparations, a **wet mount** is made to observe motile organisms; a stained smear is made to provide contrast to the existing debris in the stool; and the specimen is concentrated either by sedimentation or flotation to allow recovery of protozoal **cysts** and helminth eggs. The medical assistant should always consult the procedure manual provided by the referral laboratory when an ova and parasites stool examination (O&P) is ordered to ensure proper collection and transport of the specimen (Procedure 48-1).

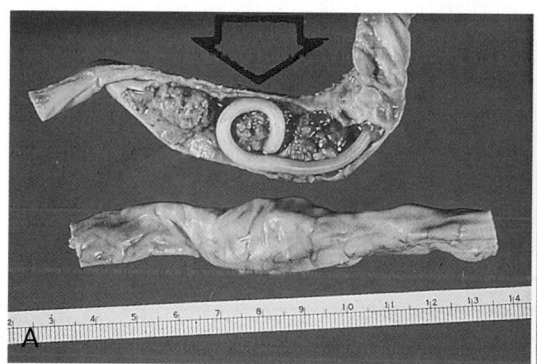 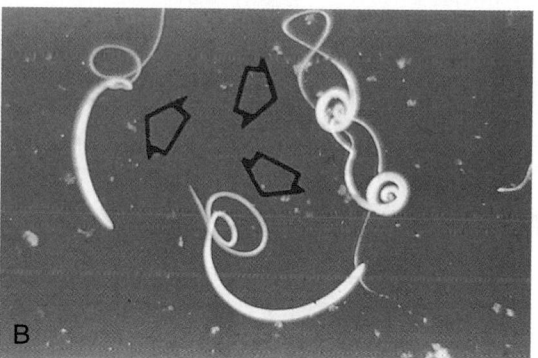

FIGURE 48-4 A, Roundworms. **B,** Whipworms. (From Stepp CA, Woods MA: *Laboratory procedures for medical office personnel,* Philadelphia, 1998, Saunders.)

PROCEDURE 48-1	Instruct and Prepare a Patient for a Procedure: Instruct Patients in the Collection of Fecal Specimens to Be Tested for Ova and Parasites

Goal: *To instruct a patient in the proper collection of stool for an ova and parasite microscopic examination.*

EQUIPMENT and SUPPLIES

- Patient's health record
- Provider's order and/or lab requisition
- Clean, dry container for stool collection
- Two parasitology collection vials*
- Plastic biohazard zipper-lock bag

PROCEDURAL STEPS

1. Greet the patient, introduce yourself, and verify the patient's identity using two identifiers (e.g., have the person spell the last name, state the birth date, and/or show a picture ID).
2. Instruct the patient not to take any antacids, laxatives, or stool softeners before collecting the specimen.

PURPOSE: Laxatives increase fecal transit time and may result in a false-negative test result.

3. Instruct the patient to urinate before collecting the specimen.
   PURPOSE: This eliminates the possibility of the stool becoming contaminated by urine.
4. The patient then collects the specimen.
   - *Adults:* Instruct the patient to defecate into the container. Stool cannot be retrieved from the toilet bowl.
   - *Children:* Loosely drape the toilet rim with plastic wrap and lower the seat. The child should have a bowel movement into the toilet, onto the wrap. Remove the stool using a disposable plastic spoon.
     PURPOSE: The stool cannot be contaminated by or diluted with water.
   - *Infants:* Fasten a "diaper" made of plastic wrap over the child using tape. Remove the plastic wrap immediately after a bowel movement and remove the stool using a plastic spoon. *Never leave the child unattended with the plastic wrap in place because of the risk of suffocation.*
     PURPOSE: Stool cannot be collected in a diaper.

*Several types of preservatives are available. Check with the referral laboratory to make sure the patient is given the proper vials for collection. Preservatives include low-viscosity polyvinyl alcohol (LV-PVA), zinc sulfite polyvinyl alcohol (ZN-PVA), sodium acetate acetic acid formalin (SAF), and 10% neutral buffered formalin.

PROCEDURE 48-1 —*continued*

5. Instruct the patient to add stool to the collection container.
   - If the stool is formed, use the scoop on the lid of the container to add a large, jelly bean–sized piece of stool to the liquid in the containers (Figure 1).

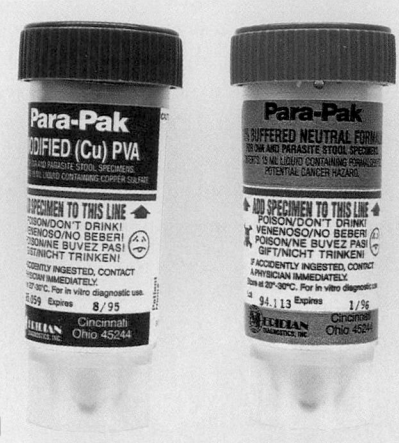

1

(Courtesy Meridian Bioscience, Cincinnati, Ohio.)

   - If the stool is liquid, pour it into the container.
   - In both of the previous cases, keep adding the specimen until the liquid preservative in the vial reaches the indicated level on the containers.
6. Instruct the patient to tighten the caps completely and wipe the outside of the vials with rubbing alcohol or to wash carefully with soap and water. <u>PURPOSE</u>: To ensure infection control.
7. The vials should be labeled, placed in a biohazard bag with a zippered closure, and transported to the laboratory immediately, if possible. The vials should not be refrigerated.
8. Instruct the patient to wash his or her hands after the procedure. <u>PURPOSE</u>: To ensure infection control.

Pathogenic Viruses

Many microbiologists do not consider viruses to be microorganisms, simply because they are not, by definition, alive. Viruses consist of a core of either ribonucleic acid (RNA) or deoxyribonucleic acid (DNA) covered by a protein shell. Alone, they neither metabolize nor reproduce; however, once inside a host cell, viruses use the host cell's **organelles** and **macromolecules** to multiply. Because of this absolute need for a host cell for replication, viruses are called *obligate intracellular parasites,* and they cannot be cultured on artificial media, such as those used to culture bacteria and fungi. Viruses must be cultured in fertilized eggs or in a **tissue culture,** which is done by referral or hospital laboratories.

Often, instead of culturing a specimen for a virus, the patient's blood sample or other body fluids are used to test for the specific antibody related to the suspected viral infection. For example, in the diagnosis of hepatitis B virus infection, the serum is either tested for the specific **antibody** that is produced to fight hepatitis B surface **antigen** (HBsAg), a protein found in the shell of the virus, or the test will detect the hepatitis B surface antigen directly. This form of testing is referred to as *serology* or *immunology testing* (discussed later in the chapter). Table 48-7 lists common diseases caused by viruses.

TABLE 48-7	Common Diseases Caused by Viruses				
DISEASE	**VIRUS**	**TRANSMISSION**	**SYMPTOMS**	**TESTS**	**PREVENTION**
Smallpox	Variola major	Direct contact, fomites	Vesicles on entire body, including soles and palms	N/A	Eradicated (vaccine is still available)
Infectious mononucleosis	Epstein-Barr virus	Direct and airborne	Sore throat, fever, malaise, lymph gland involvement; hepatitis, enlarged spleen	Serology testing for heterophile antibodies; CBC	Avoid direct contact with known cases
Influenza	Myxovirus— influenza A and B	Droplet and fomites	Fever, body aches, cough	Nasopharyngeal swab, nasal wash	Everyone 6 mo or older should receive the annual flu vaccination, with rare exceptions

TABLE 48-7   Common Diseases Caused by Viruses—*continued*

DISEASE	VIRUS	TRANSMISSION	SYMPTOMS	TESTS	PREVENTION
Warts (verruca)	Human papillomavirus (HPV)	Direct and indirect contact	Circumscribed outgrowths on skin; most common on hands and feet	Examination and biopsy	Avoid contact with warts Wash hands carefully after touching warts or surfaces such as shared exercise equipment
Rabies	Rhabdovirus	Contact with saliva of infected animal (dog, cat, skunk, fox, bat are usual)	Fever, uncontrollable excitement, spasms of the throat, profuse salivation	DFA from brain or hair follicle tissue	Vaccine available; vaccinate pets
Mumps	Paramyxovirus— mumps virus	Breathing in infected droplets from sneeze or cough Sharing utensils or cups with infected person	Pain, swelling of salivary glands; fever	Serologic test for mump antibodies and/or virus culture	MMR vaccine: *2* doses are recommended; first between 12 and 15 mo, second between 4 and 6 mo; between 11 and 12 mo if not previously given. *Note:* Young adults with only one dose should receive a booster.
Measles	Paramyxovirus— measles virus	Direct contact, droplets	Fever, nasal discharge, red eyes; Koplik's spots, rash	Serologic titer	MMR vaccine See Mumps regarding booster
Rubella (German measles)		Direct contact, droplets, congenital	Rash, swollen lymph glands; causes severe birth defects	Serologic titer	MMR vaccine See Mumps regarding booster
Common cold	Rhinovirus and many others	Direct contact, droplets, fomites	Headache, fever, runny nose, congestion	N/A	Good hygiene (hand washing)
Polio	Poliovirus	Direct contact (carriers enter via mouth)	Fever, headache, stiff neck and back, paralysis of muscles	N/A	IPV; SC or IM; four doses
Molluscum contagiosum warts	Molluscipox virus	Direct contact with infected individual	Small pink or white domes found in clusters	Microscopic evaluation	Avoid contact with infected individual; have existing warts removed
AIDS	Human immunodeficiency virus (HIV)	Sexual intercourse, sharing needles, risky behavior	Initially flulike; later, if progresses to AIDS: lung disorders, cancers, infections	Home self-test using oral swab, CLIA-waived blood screening test, confirmed with Western blot lab test	Avoid risky behavior (e.g., use condoms, do not share needles)
Ebola hemorrhagic fever	Five identified Ebola virus species	Direct exposure to infected blood and body fluids	Bleeding inside and outside the body	Tests of blood and tissues	Infected individuals must be isolated from the public immediately. Maximum PPE training and practice

Courtesy Kathleen Moody.
CBC, Complete blood count; *DFA*, direct fluorescent antibody; *IM*, intramuscular; *IPV*, inactivated polio vaccine; *MMR*, measles, mumps, rubella; *PPE*, personal protective equipment; *SC*, subcutaneous.

SPECIMEN COLLECTION AND TRANSPORT IN THE POL

Specimen collection and handling are among the most critical considerations in patient care because the results generated by the lab are directly dependent on the quality of the specimen and its condition on arrival in the laboratory. Specimens for microbiology testing must be collected in such a way as to prevent the introduction of any contaminating microorganisms. This means not only using special sterile collection and transport devices, but also taking steps to prevent environmental and patient contamination. Such steps include instructing a patient in the collection of a urine sample using the clean-catch midstream (CCMS) technique as described in the Assisting with Urinalysis chapter, and also antiseptics on the skin to avoid contamination of the site described in the Assisting in Blood Collection chapter.

This chapter teaches you ways to instruct the patient in how to collect a stool specimen for ova and parasites, and you will collect a throat specimen using a sterile swab provided in the testing kit.

Before collecting specimens for microbiologic analysis, you should ask yourself two questions:

1. In what ways can I prevent contamination of this sample?
2. What can I do to protect myself from becoming infected while I collect this sample?

The answers to these questions are:

Question 1:

- Cleanse the area to be sampled with an antiseptic
- Open sterile containers only when necessary
- Never touch a sterile swab or collection device to a nonsterile surface

Question 2:

- Wear gloves, a fluid-impermeable, disposable gown, a surgical mask, and goggles or face shield while collecting a throat or nasal specimen
- Always wear gloves when receiving a fecal or urine specimen from a patient.

Ideally specimens should be collected during the acute phase of an illness and before antibiotics are prescribed. Many types of samples can be collected. Sterile swabs can be used to collect samples from wounds and the upper respiratory tract. Serum or whole blood can be used to test for infectious organisms. Urine and feces can be collected in containers by patients at home. If patients are expected to collect specimens, it is crucial that they receive clear instructions on how to perform the procedure without contaminating the sample. The referral laboratory is responsible for providing a manual of written instructions to the POL, and the POL is responsible for providing clear instructions (preferably written) to the patient, especially if the patient will be collecting the sample in private or at home.

The transport of specimens to referral laboratories is also crucial. Many different types of transport devices are available, and close attention must be given to their proper use. Microorganisms are living organisms; they must be provided with conditions that permit their survival, but do not allow their multiplication. If microorganisms are allowed to multiply after specimen collection, the laboratory's culture results will not reflect the true disease state.

Specialized transport media are often included with the swabbing devices used for specimen collection (Figure 48-5). These collection devices typically consist of a plastic tube that encases a sterile Dacron swab and a sealed vial of **transport medium**. After the specimen has been obtained on the swab, it is placed in the plastic tube and the transport medium is released, usually by crushing the internal vial. It is essential to follow the manufacturer's directions to prevent drying of the swab and specimen. Transport system swabs also have a label that must be filled out completely, indicating the patient's name, the date and time of collection, and the source of the specimen (e.g., deep wound sample from left leg abscess, or throat swab).

If possible, a specimen should be placed on culture media immediately after collection. In most situations, however, this is not possible, and the transport device must be transported to a referral laboratory or held in the POL until it can be cultured. For specimens that will be transported by a courier, make sure the specimen is safely packaged in a leakproof container marked with warning labels (Figure 48-6). The proper temperature and duration of storage are crucial. Most pathogenic organisms prefer

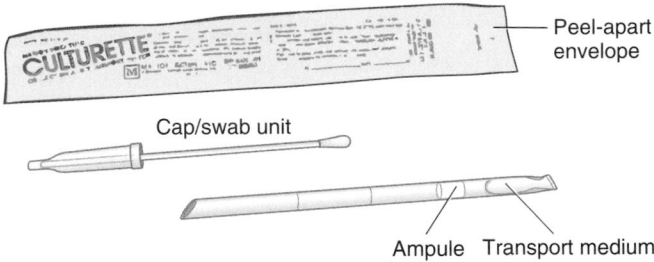

FIGURE 48-5 Culturette collection and transport system.

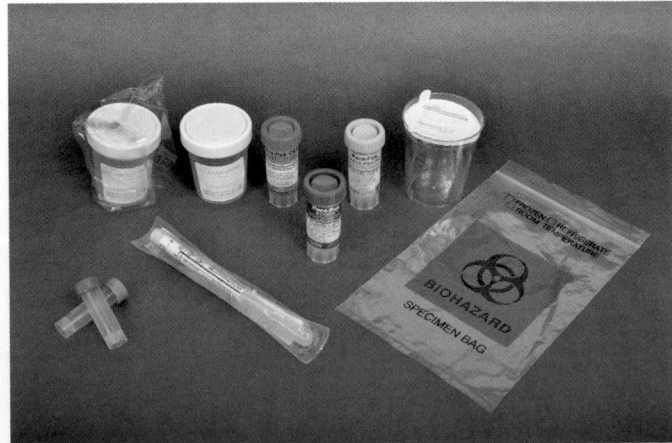

FIGURE 48-6 Microbiology specimen containers. *Top row,* Sterile clean-catch urine kit; sterile sputum container; three containers for fecal ova and parasites; sterile specimen container. *Bottom row,* Two biopsy containers; sterile swabs with transport culture media; biohazard bag for transporting specimens and their requisitions to the reference laboratory.

body temperatures around 37°C (98.6°F); they will remain viable for up to 72 hours if held at room temperature or refrigerator temperature (4°C [39.2°F]). However, some organisms die if exposed to cold temperatures. Always check the referral laboratory's procedure manual for directions on duration and temperature of storage.

Figure 48-7 shows some commonly used microbiology collection devices.

Devices used for both aerobic and anaerobic blood collection are seen in Figure 48-7, *A*, and Bactec blood culture bottles are pictured in Figure 48-7, *B*. Two other commonly used transportation devices are the Jembec plate for transporting *Neisseria gonorrhoeae* (Figure 48-7, *C*), and a viral-chlamydial transport medium (Figure 48-7, *D*).

Table 48-8 shows the specimens, containers, patient preparation, and the storage of specimens commonly collected or handled by medical assistants.

CRITICAL THINKING APPLICATION   **48-3**

Aaron Mitchell, age 9, was brought into the clinic this morning at 9 o'clock with scabbing sores on his upper lip. Dr. Chowdry suspects impetigo (a bacterial infection) and orders a wound culture. How will Anna collect this culture? What device might she use? How should she store this specimen until the courier, who does not come until 3 PM, arrives? Anna knows that impetigo is highly contagious. How can she protect herself from becoming infected?

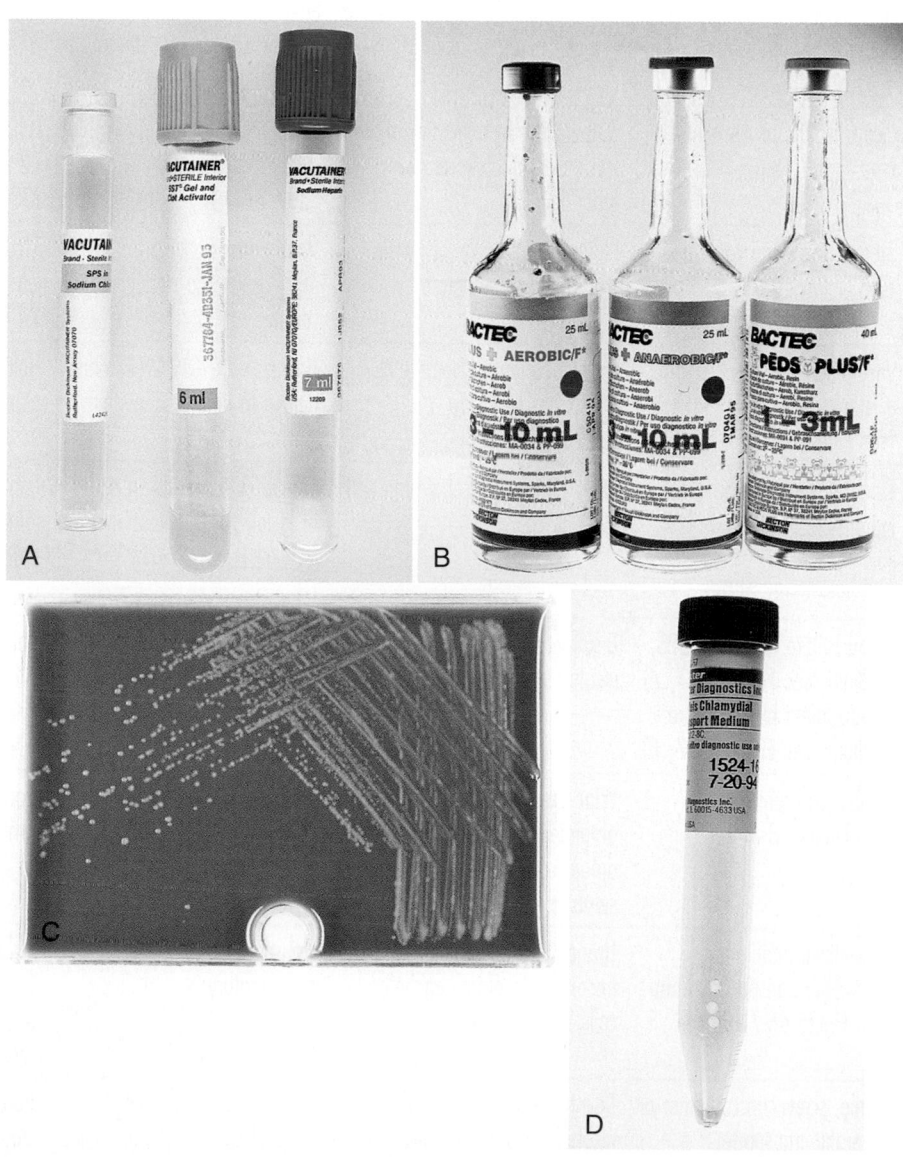

FIGURE 48-7 A, Blood collection Vacutainer tubes, one for aerobic and one for anaerobic growth. **B,** Bactec blood culture bottles. **C,** Jembec plate. **D,** Viral-chlamydial transport medium. (From De la Maza LM, Pezzlo MT, Baron EJ: *Color atlas of diagnostic microbiology,* St Louis, 1997, Mosby.)

TABLE 48-8   Collection, Transport, and Processing of Specimens Commonly Collected in the Physician Office Laboratory*

SPECIMEN	CONTAINER	PATIENT PREPARATION	SPECIAL INSTRUCTIONS	STORAGE BEFORE PROCESSING
Throat	Transport swab (see Figure 48-5)	Have patient sitting with head tilted back	Swab pharynx and tonsils, not mouth, tongue, or teeth	Transport and plate within 24 hr; room-temperature storage
Superficial wound	Aerobic transport swab (see Figure 48-5)	Wipe area with sterile saline before collection	Rotate swab while gently swiping wound	Transport swab stored at room temperature
Eye	Aerobic transport swab (see Figure 48-5)	Pull lower lid down while gently collecting exudate along rim	N/A	Transport swab may be stored up to 24 hr at room temperature
Ova and parasite (O&P)	O&P transport containers (with formalin and PVA) (see Figure 48-6)	See Procedure 48-1 for collection of a stool specimen for ova and parasites	Wait 7-10 days if patient has been taking Pepto-Bismol, Kaopectate, or Milk of Magnesia	Store at room temperature and deliver to laboratory within 24 hr
Stool	Clean, leakproof containers (see Figure 48-6)	Outpatients: At minimum, three specimens are collected every other day	Transport to laboratory within 24 hr if storing at 4°C (39.2°F)	Laboratory must plate within 72 hr if storing at 4°C (39.2°F)
Sputum	Sterile, screw-cap container (see Figure 48-6)	Patient should rinse or gargle with mouthwash before collection	Have patient collect from deep cough; do not collect saliva	Store at 4°C (39.2°F); laboratory must plate within 24 hr
Urine	Vacutainer collection system or sterile, screw-cap container (see Figure 48-6)	Instruct patient in clean-catch midstream collection	Hold at 4°C (39.2°F) and deliver to laboratory within 24 hr	Hold at 4°C (39.2°F) and plate within 24 hr
Skin scraping (fungal culture)	Clean, screw-top tube (see Figure 48-6)	Wipe skin with alcohol prep pad	Scrape skin at leading edge of lesion	Can be held indefinitely at room temperature but best to process within 72 hr of collection
Blood	Blood culture tube with SPS medium (see Figure 48-7, A) or Vacutainer blood culture medium (see Figure 48-7, B)	Disinfect venipuncture site with alcohol swab and Betadine	Draw blood during febrile episodes	Deliver to laboratory within 2 hr; incubate at 37°C (98.6°F) on receipt in the laboratory
Gonorrhea culture	Jembec transport system (see Figure 48-7, C)	Wipe away exudate before obtaining culture specimen, obtain culture specimen with swab	Do not refrigerate	Transport to laboratory within 2 hr
Chlamydia culture	Specialized antibiotic *Chlamydia* transport medium (see Figure 48-7, D)	Urogenital swabs preferred; necessary to obtain epithelial cells, not exudate	Transport immediately on ice to laboratory	Store up to 24 hr at 4°C (39.2°F); inoculate cultures within 15 min of collection if swab is not on ice
Body fluids (e.g., peritoneal, synovial, pleural)	Sterile, screw-cap container or anaerobic transporter	Disinfect aspiration site with alcohol swab and Betadine	Needle aspirations are preferable to swab collections	Transport immediately to laboratory

TABLE 48-8   Collection, Transport, and Processing of Specimens Commonly Collected in the Physician Office Laboratory*—continued

SPECIMEN	CONTAINER	PATIENT PREPARATION	SPECIAL INSTRUCTIONS	STORAGE BEFORE PROCESSING
Rectal swab	Swab placed directly into enteric transport medium	N/A	Insert swab approximately 1 inch past anal sphincter	Store at 4° C (39.2° F), transport within 24 hr to laboratory and plate within 72 hr
Deep wound or abscess	Anaerobic transport device	Wipe area with sterile saline or alcohol prep pad before collection	Aspirate material, excise tissue, or insert swab deep into wound	Store at room temperature; transport to laboratory and plate within 4 hr

Modified from Forbes BA, Sahm DF, Weissfeld AS: *Bailey and Scott's diagnostic microbiology*, ed 11, St Louis, 2002, Mosby.
O&P, Ova and parasites; *PVA*, polyvinyl alcohol, *SPS*, Sodium polyanethol sulfonato.
*Reference laboratories also have specific directions for collecting specimens based on their testing methods.

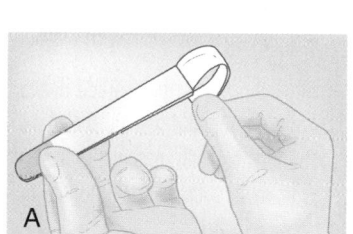 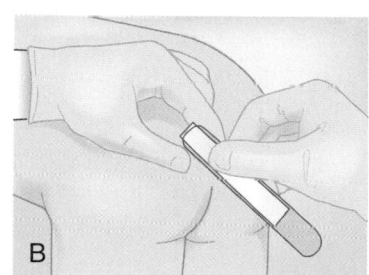 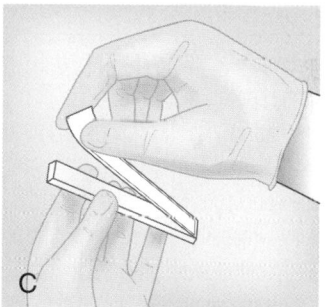

FIGURE 48-8 The three steps for collecting a pinworm specimen from a child. **A,** Place cellulose tape over a tongue depressor with sticky side out. **B,** Press the tape firmly against the right and left anal folds. **C,** Place the tape with adhesive side down on to the microscope slide.

Collection for the Pinworm Parasite

Enterobius vermicularis, commonly called the pinworm, is a species of parasite that infests the colon primarily in young children. Humans are infected by ingesting mature eggs through hand-to-mouth transfers, feces-contaminated fingers, or feces-contaminated foods or liquids or by inhaling eggs in air currents from infected areas. The eggs hatch in the small intestine, and the females migrate out of the anus, usually at night, to deposit the eggs. The eggs adhere to the skin, perianal hairs, sleeping garments, and other clothing. This results in itching of the anal area, which causes the eggs to come in contact with the hands and fingernails of the host.

In children, specimens are best collected late at night or early in the morning before a bowel movement, urination, or bathing. Paraffin swabs impregnated with petroleum jelly or cellulose tape may be used to collect the eggs deposited by the adult worm during the night. The diagnosis is based on laboratory detection of the eggs in fecal smears. If the parent does not feel comfortable about obtaining the needed specimen, instruct the parent to bring the child to the office as soon as he or she awakens in the morning. Instruct the parent not to change the child's clothing or diaper before coming into the office, and bring the child immediately after waking. When the child arrives, have all the needed supplies ready to use and perform the procedure immediately (Figure 48-8).

CLIA-WAIVED MICROBIOLOGY TESTS

Often, growing a pathogen on a culture plate is difficult, and it takes time to grow and isolate the pathogen. A rapid "direct" immunology test demonstrates the presence of the pathogen's antigen in a specimen that is placed in a test kit containing its specific antibody. If the pathogen is present, it produces a colored reaction, indicating a positive result. The rapid strep test detects *Streptococcus pyogenes* and is used in the diagnosis of strep throat. The influenza A and B rapid test detects surface antigens of the viruses that cause influenza. The RSV rapid test detects antigens from RSV, which causes pneumonia and bronchiolitis in young children.

POLs with appropriate CLIA-waived certification can perform many rapid identification tests for a variety of infectious diseases. Rapid tests are designed to give the provider a positive indication of the problem so that treatment can be initiated. For a differential or a specific diagnosis, the provider may need additional referral laboratory tests.

The first step in performing these tests is to review the package insert provided by the manufacturer. This gives valuable information about the test, the principle on which the test is based, the **reagents** and equipment required, proper specimen collection techniques, patient preparation requirements, test procedures, and any precautions or warnings pertaining to the procedure. The insert also provides information about quality control, interpretation of results, limitations of the procedure, and references.

Rapid Strep Testing

Rapid strep testing is commonly performed in the POL and can be completed while the patient waits. The patient's throat is swabbed (see the procedure in the Assisting in Ophthalmology and Otolaryngology chapter). The test swab is placed in an extraction well, and the extract is tested for antigenic proteins found on the surface of *S. pyogenes* (also referred to as strep A). The test kit uses a *lateral flow, direct immunochromatographic assay*; this means that the specimen "flows" into the test area. If the strep A pathogen is present, it will have an "immuno" reaction with the strep A antibodies in the testing area. The reaction of the strep A antigen and the strep A antibodies causes a "chromatic" (color) change that can be seen ("graphic") (Procedure 48-2).

Negative test results should be confirmed with a throat culture performed in the microbiology laboratory (explained later in the chapter). The rapid strep tests are highly specific, but not as highly sensitive. This means that if the test results are positive, there is a high degree of confidence that *S. pyogenes* is in the sample. If the test results are negative, the organism may not have been present in sufficient numbers to be detected, so a transport swab may need to be sent to the microbiology reference laboratory to be cultured.

PROCEDURE 48-2   **Obtain a Specimen and Perform a CLIA-Waived Microbiology Test: Perform a Rapid Strep Test**

Goal: *To perform a rapid strep screening test to assist in the diagnosis of strep throat.*

EQUIPMENT and SUPPLIES

- Patient's health record
- Provider's order and/or lab requisition
- QuickVue In-Line Strep A test kit contents: (Figure 1)
  - 25 Extraction Solution bottles
  - 25 Individually packaged test cassettes
  - 25 Individually wrapped sterile rayon swabs provided in kit
  - 1 Positive (+) control swab provided in kit
  - Visual flow chart outlining the steps of the test
- Rapid Strep Test Log Sheet
- Stopwatch
- Disposable gloves and fluid-impermeable lab coat
- Face protection
- Biohazard waste container

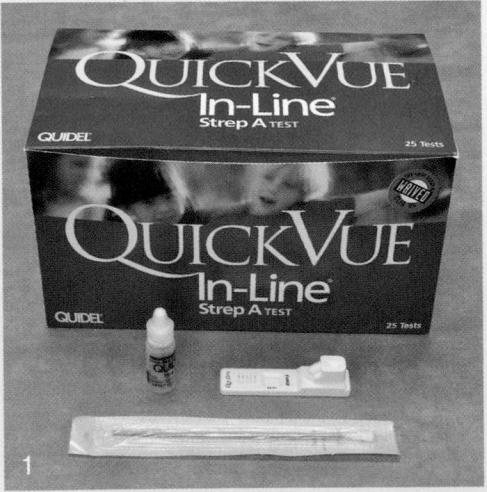

PROCEDURAL STEPS

1. Collect all necessary supplies and equipment. Bring all reagents to room temperature. Check the expiration date on the test kit package.
2. Sanitize your hands.
   PURPOSE: To ensure infection control.

3. NOTE: Before running the first patient test from a new test kit, a positive and negative control test must be run using the control swabs provided in the kit. Confirm that both controls reacted correctly, and record the control results on the log sheet.
   PURPOSE: Both control swabs must be checked before patients are tested. If the controls show the appropriate results, the test kit is reliable.
4. Greet the patient, introduce yourself, and verify the patient's identity using two identifiers (e.g., have the person spell the last name, state the birth date, and/or show a picture ID).
5. Put on gloves and face protection. Collect a throat specimen using the rayon swab provided in the test kit.
   PURPOSE: The test kit provides a rayon swab to avoid the use of cotton swabs, which can kill bacteria, possibly causing a false-negative result.
6. Remove the test cassette from the foil pouch and place it on a clean, dry, level surface. Using the notch at the back of the chamber as a guide, insert the patient's swab completely into the Swab Chamber (Figure 2).

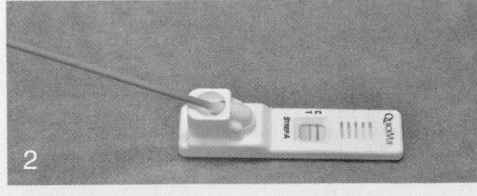

7. Place the extraction bottle between your thumb and forefinger, and squeeze once to break the glass ampule inside the Extraction Solution bottle. Vigorously shake the bottle 5 times to mix the solutions. The solution should turn green.
   PURPOSE: The color change is an indicator of extraction reagent integrity and that the extraction procedure was performed correctly.
8. Immediately remove the cap on the Extraction Solution bottle, hold the bottle vertically over the chamber, and quickly fill the chamber to the rim (approximately 8 drops).
   PURPOSE: The liquid extract reacts with the swab and then flows into the test cassette, passing through the test area (T) and then through the internal control area (C).

PROCEDURE 48-2 —continued

9. Remove your face shield. Wait 5 minutes to read the results, and record them in the lab log.
   - *Positive result:* A pink line shows in the T area, indicating the presence of *Streptococcus pyogenes* antigen; a blue line appears in the C area, indicating that the fluid activated the internal control.
   - *Negative result:* No pink line appears in the T test area; a blue line appears in the C control area, indicating that the internal control worked.
   - *Invalid result:* The blue control line does not appear next to the letter C at 5 minutes. The test result cannot be reported.
10. Discard all the test materials in the appropriate biohazard waste container.
    PURPOSE: Items that come in contact with samples are considered potentially infectious.

11. Disinfect the work area, remove your gloves and fluid-impermeable lab coat, and sanitize your hands.
    PURPOSE: To ensure infection control.
12. Record the test results in the patient's health record.
    PURPOSE: A procedure is considered not done until it is properly recorded.
13. If the test results are negative, a second throat swab should be obtained and sent to the reference laboratory for a throat culture. Often two swabs are used simultaneously when the sample is initially collected from the throat to prevent the need to re-collect a specimen.
    PURPOSE: Negative rapid strep test results should be confirmed with a throat culture.

QUALITATIVE CONTROL/PATIENT LOG SHEET

TEST: __STREP A TEST__

KIT NAME AND MANUFACTURER: QuickVue In-Line Strep A Test — Quidel
LOT # __12345__   EXPIRATION DATE: __11/22/20XX__
STORAGE REQUIREMENTS: __Room Temp__   TEST FLOW CHART __yes__

DATE	SPECIMEN I.D. (CONTROL/PATIENT)	RESULT (+ OR −)	INTERNAL CONTROL PASSED (Y OR N)	CHARTED IN PATIENT RECORD	TECH INITIALS
7/11/20XX	POSITIVE CONTROL	+	Y		DC
7/11/20XX	NEGATIVE CONTROL	−	Y		DC
7/11/20XX	PT ID: 5432	+	Y	✓	DC

Documentation in the medical record:

10/9/20– 9:30 AM: Rapid Strep A Test performed with a positive result. Second swab sent to lab for culture and sensitivity. —————————— Dana Cummings, CMA (AAMA)

Influenza A and B Testing

The influenza virus causes influenza, or "the flu," a highly contagious, acute viral infection of the respiratory tract. The infection is highly communicable through the respiratory route, and outbreaks typically are seen in the fall and winter. Type A viruses usually are more prevalent than type B viruses; type A viruses typically are associated with epidemics, and type B viruses cause a milder infection. Rapid diagnosis of influenza can assist with decisions to administer antiviral medications, which must be given early in the course of the infection if they are to be effective. CLIA-waived rapid lateral flow, direct immunochromatographic assays detect both influenza A and influenza B antigens from nasopharyngeal swabs or nasal washes. If a swab is used, the sample is removed from the swab using a solution provided by the manufacturer. Nasal washings may also be used directly in the test kit if indicated by the manufacturer.

Respiratory Syncytial Virus (RSV) Testing

RSV is a major cause of upper and lower respiratory tract infections and the major cause of bronchiolitis and pneumonia in

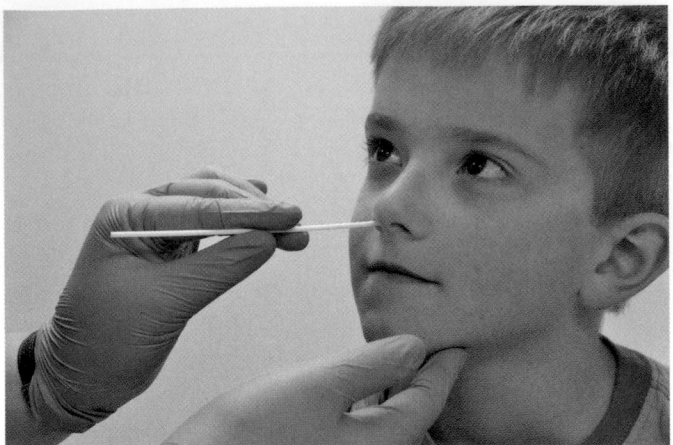

FIGURE 48-9 Note the proper angle of insertion for the foam swab when collecting a nasal specimen. The swab is inserted at least 1 inch along the base of the nostril on the side that has the most discharge. Once inside, the swab is rotated and rocked back and forth gently for 5 to 10 seconds to obtain a sufficient specimen for influenza and respiratory syncytial virus (RSV) testing.

In the "indirect" immunologic tests, the specimen is the patient's blood and/or its separated serum. The blood or serum is tested to see whether the patient has produced the specific antibody for the disease in question. CLIA-waived immunology tests that can be performed by a medical assistant to detect antibodies to a pathogen include infectious mononucleosis, *Helicobacter pylori*, Lyme disease, and human immunodeficiency virus (HIV) tests.

CRITICAL THINKING APPLICATION   **48-4**

Tiffany Warhola, a seventh-grade student, visits Dr. Chowdry complaining of extreme fatigue and a sore throat. Dr. Chowdry orders a rapid strep test and a mononucleosis test. What sample will Anna need for the rapid strep test? (*Hint:* The rapid strep test is a direct test; the test kit provides the antibody to interact directly with strep A if it is in the specimen.) What sample will Anna need for the mononucleosis test? (*Hint:* The mononucleosis test is an indirect test; the examiner checks the specimen for heterophile antibodies that would indicate a mononucleosis infection.)

---

children and infants. Outbreaks typically occur yearly in the fall, winter, and spring and can be severe for very young children. The CLIA-waived rapid direct immunochromatographic assay for RSV uses a nasopharyngeal swab specimen or nasal washings to detect a protein the virus uses to fuse to human cells. Because antiviral agents are available to treat RSV infection, rapid diagnosis can lead to shorter hospital stays, a reduced need for antibiotic therapy to treat secondary bacterial infection, and a lower cost for hospital care. The tests are intended for children under age 5. Figure 48-9 shows the proper placement of the swab when collecting a nasal specimen.

CLIA-WAIVED IMMUNOLOGY TESTING

Immunology testing provides information about past or present infections with bacteria or viruses. It also detects certain types of cancers. Testing done in the immunology laboratory is designed to demonstrate the reaction between an antigen and its specific antibody. Antibodies are formed when the body encounters a foreign agent. In the acute phase of a disease, the antibody level is high; during the convalescent stage, the antibody level declines. Once an antigen has been recognized by the immune system and antibodies have been made, the level of antibody to that particular antigen remains at a low but detectable level indefinitely. The amount of antibody at any given time can be measured with serologic testing and is referred to as the *titer*.

Most serologic/immunologic testing performed in the ambulatory care center is done using individual testing kits (e.g. strep, influenza, mononucleosis, and HIV tests). The difference is the source of the specimen and what is being analyzed.

The "direct" immunologic tests in the previous section (strep test and influenza test) used a throat swab and nasal swab specimen respectively. The test kits provided the specific antibodies to "directly" detect the *S. pyogenes* from the throat swab; and the influenza A and B viruses were directly detected from the nasal swabbed specimen.

Infectious Mononucleosis Testing

Infectious mononucleosis, commonly called "mono," is an acute infectious disease caused by the Epstein-Barr virus (EBV). EBV is one of the most common human viruses, and it occurs worldwide. The virus is especially common in teenagers. It is found most frequently in people 10 to 25 years of age and is seen occasionally in adults. Most people are infected with EBV at some time during their lives. In the United States, as many as 95% of adults between 35 and 40 have already been infected.

In children the infection may pass unrecognized or result in a mild illness lasting only a few days. It is marked by sore throat, fever, swollen tonsils, and enlarged lymph nodes in the neck. These signs and symptoms can be indistinguishable from those of other mild illnesses of childhood. In young people, some of the most common complications include the abrupt onset of fatigue, headaches, aching muscles, faint rash, fever, very swollen tonsils, enlarged lymph glands, and loss of appetite often associated with nausea. There may be a short or prolonged period (days or weeks) after the initial illness when the fatigue continues. Occasionally, complications occur, including the development of a swollen spleen or liver. Heart problems or any involvement of the central nervous system (CNS) is rare, and infectious mononucleosis is almost never fatal.

Testing for mononucleosis involves a complete blood count (CBC) and serology tests. The CBC reveals an increased number of lymphocytes that appear atypical on the blood smear examination. The infected lymphocytes undergo a cellular transformation, causing them to take on an appearance similar to a monocyte (hence the name *mononucleosis*). Most patients exposed to EBV produce a nonspecific "heterophile" antibody response to the virus. These "heterophile" antibodies in the patient's blood react with the heterophile antigens supplied in the test kit, resulting in a positive color reaction in the testing area of the kit (Procedure 48-3).

PROCEDURE 48-3   Obtain a Specimen and Perform a CLIA-Waived Immunology Test: Perform the QuickVue+ Infectious Mononucleosis Test

Goal: *To perform and interpret a rapid CLIA-waived test for infectious mononucleosis.*

EQUIPMENT and SUPPLIES

- Patient's health record
- Provider's order and/or lab requisition
- CLIA-waived QuickVue+ test kit for infectious mononucleosis and blood collecting supplies: (Figure 1)
  - Package with supplies for 20 tests
  - Color-coded bottles of positive and negative controls and the developer
  - Test cassette in its foil-wrapped protective pouch
  - Alcohol prep pad, gauze, and bandage
  - Pipettes supplied in kit with black line indicating amount of capillary blood to collect
  - Lancet
- Timer or wristwatch with sweep second hand
- Disposable gloves and fluid-impermeable lab coat
- Biohazard waste container

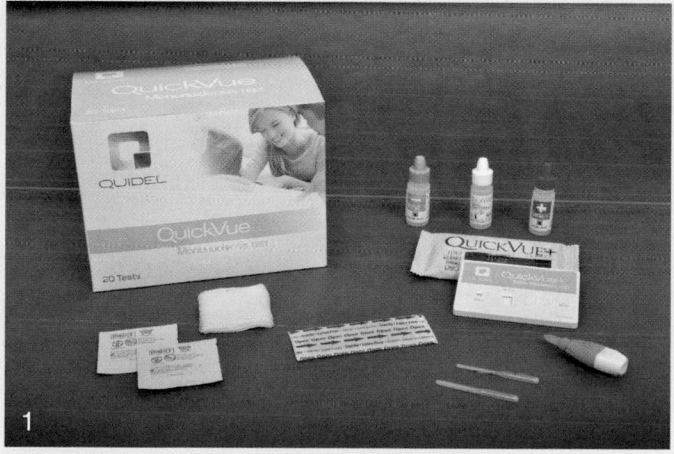

PROCEDURAL STEPS

1. Remove the test kit from the refrigerator and allow the reagents to warm to room temperature. Check the expiration date of the kit.
   PURPOSE: Outdated or cold reagents do not react as expected.
2. Sanitize your hands. Put on the fluid-impermeable lab coat and gloves.
   PURPOSE: To ensure infection control
3. Before running the first patient test from a new test kit, run the positive and negative liquid controls provided in the kit to see whether they react correctly. Record your control results on the log sheet.
   PURPOSE: Both control swabs must be checked before patients are tested. If the controls show the appropriate results, the test kit is reliable.
4. Greet the patient, introduce yourself, and verify the patient's identity using two identifiers (e.g., have the person spell the last name, state the birth date, and/or show a picture ID).

5. Remove the test device from its protective pouch, and label it with the patient's identification.
6. Disinfect the patient's finger with the alcohol swab. Allow it to dry and then perform a capillary puncture.
7. Wipe away the first drop and then fill the disposable pipette provided in the kit to the calibration mark with capillary blood (see the Assisting in Blood Collection chapter for proper blood collection methods) (Figure 2).
   PURPOSE: The plastic capillary tube measures the exact amount of sample, for accurate testing.

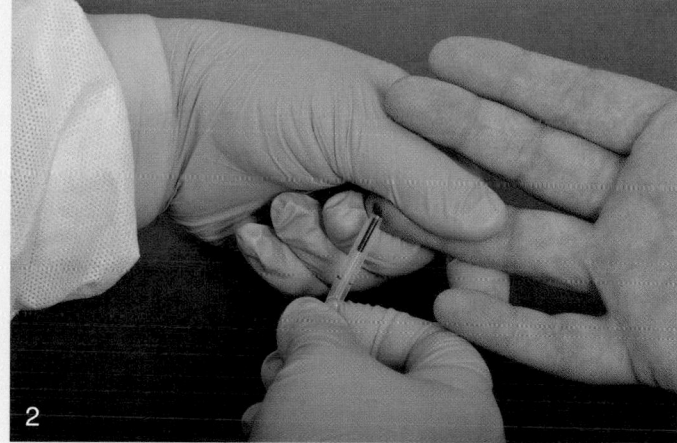

8. Dispense all the blood from the capillary tube into the "Add" well of the testing device. (Or, if you are using venous blood, transfer a large drop from the venous whole blood specimen using the longer capillary pipette provided in the kit).
9. Hold the developer bottle vertically above the "Add" well, and allow 5 drops to fall freely.
   PURPOSE: Holding a dropper vertically ensures delivery of the same-size drop. If the dropper touches other materials, it becomes contaminated and the results will be inaccurate.
10. Read the results at 5 minutes. *Note:* The "Test Complete" box must be visibly colored by 10 minutes.
    - *Positive result:* A vertical line in any shade of blue forms a plus sign in the "Read Result" window, along with a blue "Test Complete" line. Even a faint blue plus sign should be reported as a positive.
    - *Negative result:* No vertical blue line appears, leaving a minus sign in the "Read Result" window, along with a blue "Test Complete" line.
    - *Invalid result:* After 10 minutes, no line is seen in the "Test Complete" window, or a blue color fills the "Read Result" window. If either of these is noted, the test must be repeated with a new testing device. If the problem continues, request technical support.
11. Properly dispose of biohazardous waste material in the proper container, and disinfect the work area.
    PURPOSE: To ensure infection control.

PROCEDURE 48-3   *—continued*

12. Remove your personal protective equipment, and sanitize your hands.
13. Document the patient's and the controls' results in the lab logs and in the patient's health record.
    <u>PURPOSE:</u> A procedure is considered not done until it is properly recorded.

Quality Control Procedures
External positive and negative liquid controls are provided with each new kit. Each new operator of the test should perform liquid positive and negative

external controls once to confirm that his or her testing technique is correct. Also, external controls should be tested and charted when a new kit is used.

The *internal* control occurs in the "Test Complete" window built into each reaction unit. Chart the control results on the control log with the operator's initials.

QUALITATIVE CONTROL/PATIENT LOG SHEET

TEST: <u>**MONONUCLEOSIS RAPID TEST**</u>

KIT NAME & MANUFACTURER: QUICK VUE+ Infectious Mononucleosis Test -QUIDEL
LOT # <u>12345</u>   EXPIRATION DATE: <u>11/22/20XX</u>
STORAGE REQUIREMENTS: <u>REFRIGERATOR</u>   TEST FLOW CHART <u>yes</u>

DATE	SPECIMEN I.D. (CONTROL/PATIENT)	RESULT (+ OR −)	INTERNAL CONTROL PASSED (Y OR N)	CHARTED IN PATIENT RECORD	TECH INITIALS
7/11/20XX	POSITIVE CONTROL	+	Y		DC
7/11/20XX	NEGATIVE CONTROL	−	Y		DC
7/11/20XX	PT ID: 5432	−	Y	✓	DC

Documentation in the medical record:

10/9/20– 9:30 AM: Mononucleosis rapid test performed with a negative result. Lavender-topped EDTA Blood sample sent to lab for CBC and differential. Dana Cummings, CMA (AAMA)

Helicobacter pylori Antibody Testing

H. pylori is a spiral-shaped bacterium that can infect the gastric mucous layer or adhere to the epithelial lining of the stomach. *H. pylori* causes more than 90% of duodenal ulcers and more than 80% of gastric ulcers (see the Assisting in Gastroenterology chapter). Several methods can be used to diagnose *H. pylori* infection. Serologic tests that measure specific *H. pylori* antibodies can determine whether a person has been infected. CLIA-waived rapid qualitative immunochromatographic assay tests use whole blood applied to a well in a test cartridge. The blood migrates from the well through the testing area of the cartridge. The presence of a line in the "test" area of the cartridge indicates the presence of antibodies to the pathogen *H. pylori*.

Lyme Disease Antibody Testing

Lyme disease is the most common insect-borne infectious disease in North America, and it is a significant public health concern. The

spirochete bacterium *Borrelia burgdorferi* is the causative agent in Lyme disease.

The disease is contracted from the bite of a tick whose saliva contains the bacteria. These ticks typically are found on deer, mice, dogs, horses, and birds. Infection occurs when the bacteria enter the wound caused by the tick bite. A characteristic bull's-eye rash, known as *erythema migrans* (EM), develops at the bite site in 60% to 80% of patients. Lyme disease progresses in three stages, which have unclear transition and overlapping symptoms. As the disease progresses, the spirochete bacterium invades the skin, joints, CNS, heart, eyes, bones, spleen, and kidneys. Arthritic or CNS syndromes often accompany late-stage disease and may be the only clinical, symptomatic indications of infection.

Lyme disease can be detected early with a CLIA-waived test, such as the Wampole PreVue *B. burgdorferi* test. This immunochromatographic assay tests for IgG and IgM antibodies in whole blood. A sample of blood is applied to a test cartridge, a diluent is added, and the results are read in 20 minutes. Positive results should be verified by the microbiology reference laboratory.

HIV Antibody Testing

HIV attacks and destroys the T-helper (CD4) lymphocytes. The T-helper lymphocytes play a critical role in protecting the body against infection. They work with the B lymphocytes to produce their specific antibodies that fight infections. As more and more T-helper cells are destroyed by the HIV infection, the body becomes less able to fight off infections and more susceptible to opportunistic infections. If the infection is not treated with antiretroviral (ARV) medications, acquired immunodeficiency syndrome (AIDS) eventually develops. HIV infections become AIDS when life-threatening infections and cancers begin to appear (see the Assisting in Urology and Male Reproduction chapter for more information on HIV and AIDS).

At this time, there is no known cure once someone has an HIV infection. Therefore, in 2013, the Centers for Disease Control and Prevention (CDC) and World Health Organization (WHO) both advised preventive measures to control the disease. This requires early detection and early treatment of individuals infected with HIV. The sooner the virus is detected via immunology testing, the sooner treatment with ARV medications may begin. The current recommended treatment (one or more tablets a day) is able to keep the virus from duplicating and destroying the T cells, thereby reducing the possibility of others becoming infected and halting the progression to AIDS.

Two CLIA-waived HIV tests are readily available to detect the presence of HIV antibodies in blood and in oral specimens. Both immunologic tests are able to detect HIV antibodies after a risk event and/or 3 months later. Risk events were covered in the Urology chapter.

Patients at risk of HIV infection are now strongly encouraged to take the 10- to 20-minute blood test available in POLs or outpatient clinics. *Note:* HIV is a blood-borne pathogen. Therefore, to prevent exposure during the testing process, it is critical that the medical assistant testing for HIV strictly follow the Bloodborne Pathogens Standard established by the Occupational Safety and Health Administration (OSHA).

The patient may also choose to perform an oral self-test from a kit that is available at pharmacies (Figure 48-10). The test kit includes a testing device with a flat pad that is rubbed once over the upper and lower gums. It then is inserted into the test vial, which is placed in a plastic stand that holds the device at the proper angle. The test results are read in 20 minutes. The test includes an internal control band that verifies that a specimen was added and that the test was run correctly.

In both testing methods, it is very important to provide the patient with information and/or counseling regarding HIV infection and its relationship to AIDS. Be aware that patients being tested may be very fearful and that proper knowledge presented in a therapeutic way can help them dispel the fear and take positive action toward preventive behavior and treatment. Positive HIV test results must be verified at a reference laboratory.

MICROBIOLOGY REFERENCE LABORATORY

After receiving the specimens collected in the POL described in "Specimen Collection and Transport" earlier in this chapter, the microbiology laboratory promptly prepares a smear of the specimen on a slide to be stained and then transfers the specimen contents onto culture plates, based on the source of the specimen (Figure 48-11). The equipment and supplies in a microbiology laboratory vary with the size of the facility. Most laboratories have a refrigerator, an autoclave, a safety cabinet, a microscope, and an incubator.

Identification of Pathogens in the Microbiology Laboratory

Staining

Pathogenic microorganisms generally are colorless, and a microscope is needed to see them. Special differential stains (e.g., Gram's stain and acid-fast stain) often are used to differentiate bacteria based on biochemical differences. As discussed previously, Gram's stain differentiates bacteria into two categories according to cell wall thickness, and the acid-fast stain differentiates bacteria into two categories based on the presence or absence of a waxy lipid in the cell wall.

Before staining can be done, the specimen must be applied to a labeled slide. The slide is then air dried and fixed. Either heat or methanol can be used to fix the slide, which results in the material adhering to the slide. Both heat (e.g., from a Bunsen

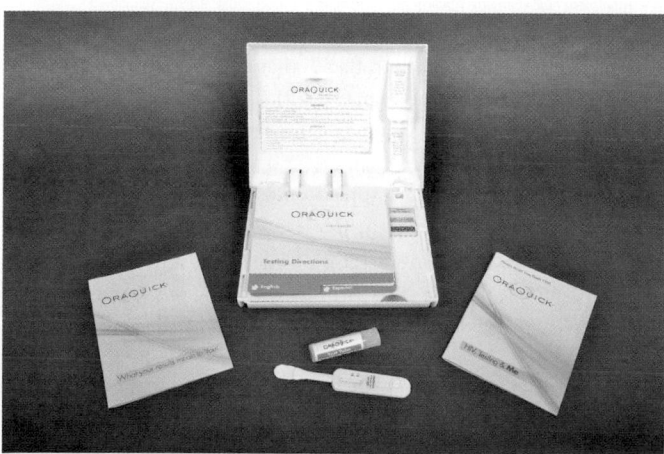

FIGURE 48-10 HIV home testing kit.

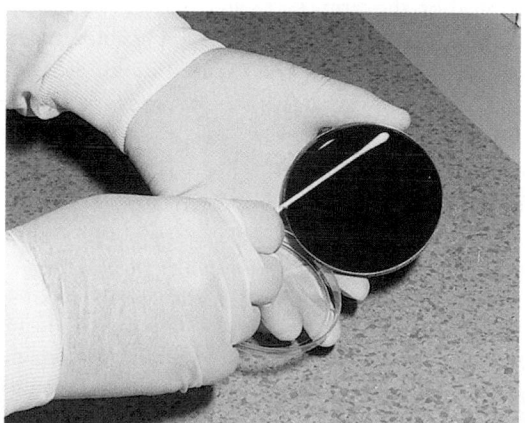

FIGURE 48-11 Inoculating a blood culture plate with a swab. (From Stepp CA, Woods MA: *Laboratory procedures for medical office personnel,* Philadelphia, 1998, Saunders.)

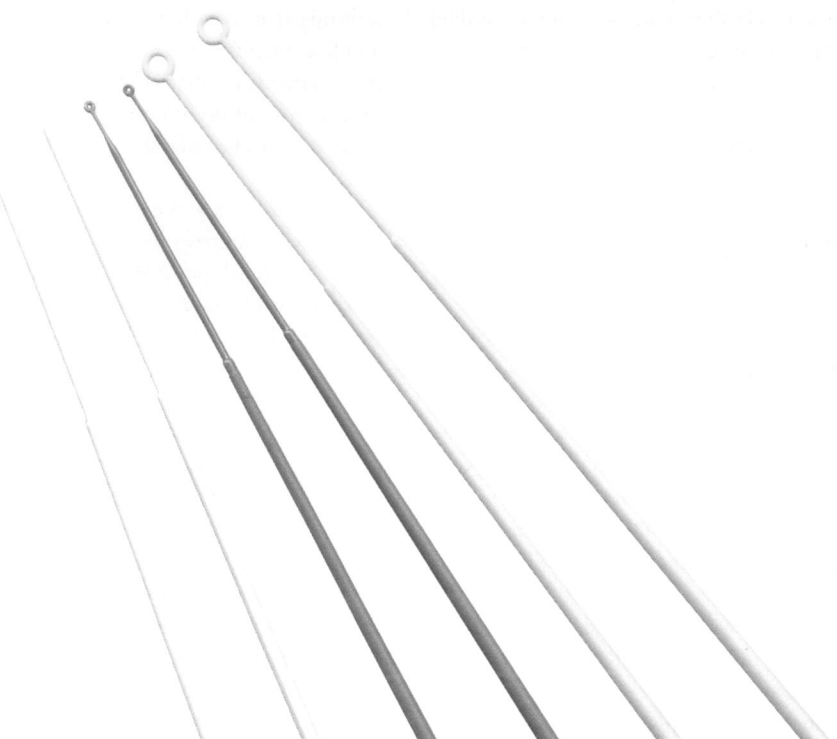

FIGURE 48-12 *Left,* Inoculating needles. *Right,* Loops. (Courtesy Simport Plastics, Beloeil, Quebec, Canada.)

burner or an incinerator) and methanol cause protein in the sample to denature and stick to the slide, much as egg white sticks to a hot frying pan.

Gram's Stain

Gram's stain, developed by Dr. Hans Christian Gram more than 100 years ago, is still the most commonly used stain in the microbiology laboratory. This procedure involves applying a sequence of primary dye, mordant, decolorizer, and counterstain to the slide. The dyes are taken up differently according to the chemical composition of the cell walls. Bacteria react best in the Gram's stain when they are less than 24 hours old. Gram-positive bacteria stain purple, and gram-negative bacteria stain pink or red (see Figure 48-1). It is useful for the medical assistant to understand the procedures and the microscopic results obtained. For example, when a Gram's stain report is called in, the terms *GPCs* and *GNBs* mean "gram-positive cocci" (deeply blue-stained circular cells) and "gram-negative bacilli," (pink/red stained rod-shaped cells) stained pink). See Tables 48-1 and 48-2 for the staining characteristics of various pathogenic bacilli and cocci.

Acid-Fast Stain

The acid-fast stain is used in the identification protocol for *Mycobacterium* species. *M. tuberculosis* and *M. avium* complex (MAC) are two important pathogenic species of mycobacteria. The former causes tuberculosis and can be isolated from sputum or tissue samples from infected patients; the latter is a common soil organism that enters through the respiratory tract and disseminates throughout the body. MAC is one of the causes of death among patients with AIDS. For the acid-fast stain, a red primary dye (carbolfuchsin) is applied first, then the decolorizer (acid-alcohol) is applied, followed by a

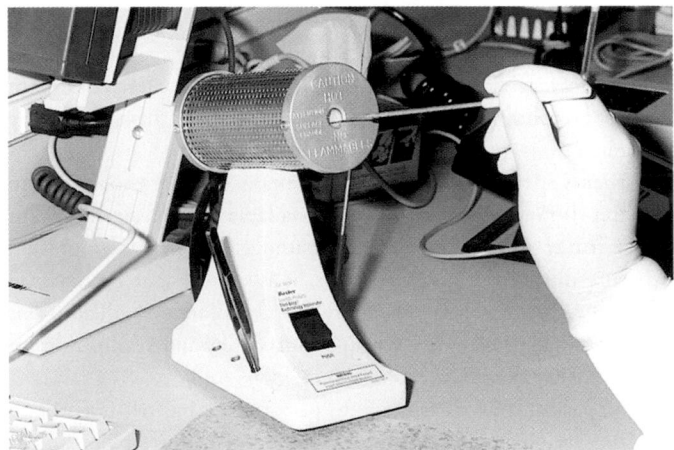

FIGURE 48-13 Loop incinerator for sterilizing wire loops and needles. (From Stepp CA, Woods MA: *Laboratory procedures for medical office personnel,* Philadelphia, 1998, Saunders.)

counterstain (methylene blue). Bacilli that are acid-fast positive often are referred to as *AFB* (see Figure 48-2).

Inoculating Equipment

Next, the specimen must be spread on specific culture plates based on the source of the specimen (see Figure 48-11). The inoculated culture plates are placed in a body temperature incubator to grow overnight. Inoculating needles and loops (Figure 48-12) are used to transfer samples or microbes to culture plates with growth media and/or to slides for staining. Needles and loops may be disposable and presterilized, or they may be made of wire and can be heat sterilized before and after use (Figure 48-13). An inoculating loop is shaped like a bubble wand, and a thin film of liquid adheres to the loop. The amount of fluid held by the loop can be calibrated. For example, a urine culture uses a loop that delivers a 1-mcL sample. The urine in the loop is spread across the culture medium and allowed to grow overnight. The next day, each bacterium becomes a visible colony, and these can then be counted and analyzed to determine the cause of a urinary tract infection.

Assessing a Culture

When the original (primary) culture has incubated at the appropriate temperature for 18 to 24 hours, it is examined for evidence of pathogens. Because normal flora is often present in samples in addition to pathogens, a trained eye is required to spot the organisms that might be causing an infection. Suspicious colonies are subcultured onto the appropriate medium to isolate them in **pure culture**. When the organism is in pure culture, staining and additional biochemical testing can be done to identify it at the genus and species levels. Throat and urine cultures may be performed in POLs that have been CLIA certified to perform moderately complex testing.

Throat Culture

Streptococcus pyogenes, also known as *group A beta hemolytic streptococcus,* causes septic sore throat (strep throat). If not diagnosed and treated promptly, this infection can cause severe complications, including scarlet fever, rheumatic fever, and glomerulonephritis. A swab of the throat is streaked on a sheep's blood agar plate, and then a differentiation disk is placed on the most heavily streaked first quadrant. This disk contains an antibiotic (bacitracin), which inhibits the growth of *S. pyogenes* and is used for differential diagnosis. Complete clearing of the agar around the colonies indicates beta hemolysis as a result of a toxin produced by the pathogenic organism; the toxin lyses the sheep red blood cells in the agar; hence the name *beta hemolytic strep.* The presence of beta hemolytic colonies and a zone of no growth around the disk indicate that the patient has strep throat (Figure 48-14). Additional testing may be needed to confirm the identity of the organism.

Urine Cultures

With urine cultures, the bacterial colonies that appear after incubation are counted. A calibrated inoculating loop is dipped into a

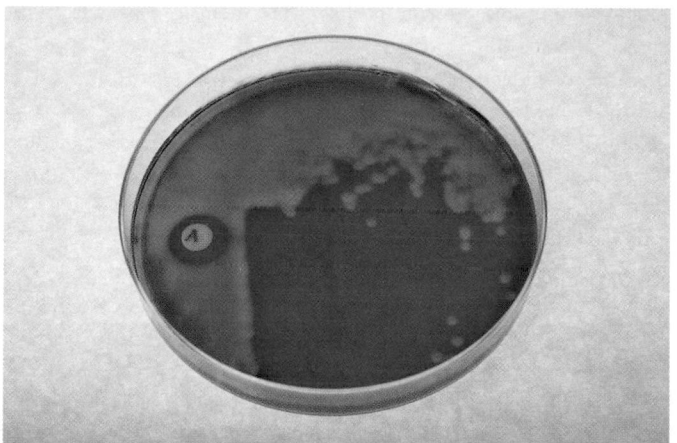

FIGURE 48-14 Positive strep test result on blood agar *(left side of plate)*. The *Streptococcus* group A shows beta hemolysis (clearing) of the blood agar below its growing colonies. Also notice there is no hemolysis or clearing of the blood around the white bacitracin disk. That is because the bacitracin is capable of destroying *Streptococcus* group A.

well-mixed urine sample that was collected by the CCMS method or by catheterization. The urine from the loop is spread on the medium and incubated for 18 to 24 hours at 37°C (98.6°F). Each colony that grows on the plate represents 1,000 colony-forming units (cfu) per milliliter. The final cfu results are interpreted as follows:

- Normal: <10,000 cfu/mL of urine; no urinary tract infection (UTI) present
- Borderline: 10,000 to 100,000 cfu/mL of urine; a chronic or relapsing infection may be present, and the test should be repeated
- Positive: >100,000 cfu/mL of urine; a UTI is likely

Several self-contained, convenient culture systems for urine are also available. These systems are ideal for the smaller laboratory that has been certified to perform moderately complex tests. Examples of these systems include the Diaslide and Uricult. These devices contain culture media either on a paddle or on the walls of a container. The paddle is dipped into the urine, or the urine is poured into the container, swirled, and discarded. The device is then incubated (often at room temperature), and the number of colonies that form on the medium is compared with a colony density chart to determine the level of bacteria.

CRITICAL THINKING APPLICATION   **48-5**

The technician from the referral laboratory indicates that Ms. Walker has a urinary tract infection. Anna records the test results in the patient's record as: >100,000 cfu/mL. What does this mean?

MICROBIOLOGY CULTURE AND SENSITIVITY TESTING

Once a bacterial infection has been identified in the microbiology laboratory or the POL, an additional step is required for successful treatment. When a provider wants to determine the appropriate antibiotic to specifically destroy the pathogen, he or she orders a culture and sensitivity (C&S) test. "Culture" refers to growing or cultivating the organisms, and "sensitivity" refers to a test to determine the organism's susceptibility to certain antibiotics. Most bacteria show resistance to **antimicrobial agents**, and because these patterns of resistance are continuously changing, they cannot be predicted. Shifting patterns of resistance require testing of individual bacteria against a variety of antibiotics.

The healthcare provider must decide which medication to order based on initial test results and the patient's physical examination. C&S test results provide vital information about which antibiotics work best against the particular infective pathogen.

Whenever specimens are collected, asepsis must be strictly observed to ensure safety and good results. The organism being tested must be isolated in pure culture in the microbiology reference laboratory. The antimicrobial test, often referred to as the *Kirby-Bauer antimicrobial susceptibility test,* is performed by inoculating sterile water with the pure culture of bacteria. This suspension is spread with a swab on the surface of the appropriate agar medium. Disks that contain an antimicrobial agent (e.g., penicillin and tetracycline) are placed on the agar with an automatic dispenser. After incubation, the zone of inhibition (area of no growth) around each disk is measured in millimeters and compared with values provided

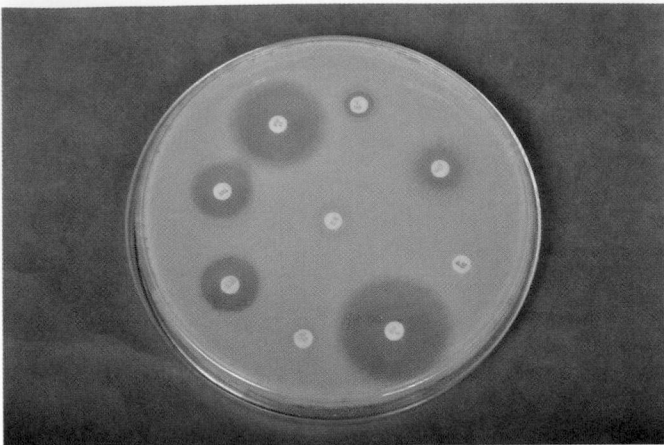

FIGURE 48-15 Reading a culture and sensitivity test to determine whether the bacteria are sensitive (S), intermediate (I), or resistant (R) to the various antibiotics. The cleared areas around four of the disks demonstrate that the bacteria were sensitive to those antibiotics; the disks that did not stop the bacteria from growing indicate that the bacteria were resistant to those antibiotics.

by the manufacturer of the disks (Figure 48-15). Three determinations are possible: S, R, or I.

- **S** means that the pathogen is "susceptible," or that the antibiotic is effective against the organism in that particular concentration **in vitro**.
- **R** means that the organism is "resistant" to the antibiotic.
- **I** means "intermediate"; that is, additional testing must be performed to determine the dosage of antimicrobial necessary for therapeutic treatment.

Choosing an Appropriate Antimicrobial Agent

The appropriate antimicrobial agent meets the following criteria:
- Demonstrates the most activity against the infectious agent
- Has the least toxicity to the patient
- Has the least impact on the normal flora of the body
- Has the desired pharmacologic characteristics
- Is the most economical

CRITICAL THINKING APPLICATION   48-6

Anna is recording the reference lab's results for Ms. Walker's urine culture. On the lab report, she notes that 10 antimicrobial agents had been tested, but the *E. coli* was susceptible to only five of them (similar to the culture and sensitivity plate seen in Figure 48-15). How will Dr. Ling determine which of these five antibiotics would be best for Ms. Walker?

CLOSING COMMENTS

Patient Education

Microorganisms such as bacteria, viruses, fungi, and parasites are responsible for most human infectious diseases. Patient education plays an important role in helping the patient and family control the spread of infection. The teaching topics in the following list can help you educate a patient in infection control:

- An explanation of the patient's type of infection: bacterial, viral, fungal, or parasitic

- How infections spread
- Hand sanitization, proper storage and cleaning of personal items, and disposal of contaminated supplies
- Risk factors for infection, such as poor nutritional habits or poor ventilation with airborne pathogens present
- The patient's role in specimen collection
- Patient preparation for cultures and serologic, hematologic, and imaging tests, as necessary

Explain to the patient that infection does not always occur at the entry site; for example, measles can be transmitted through the respiratory tract. Reinforce the need for strict adherence to the prescribed antimicrobial therapy by pointing out the possible complications of noncompliance, such as relapse or systemic involvement. Explain to the patient that inadequate drug therapy (not taking the medication as prescribed) may result in worsening and spread of the infection.

Above all, always listen to the patient; be sure to answer all questions. However, do not try to answer a question if you are unsure of the answer. Notify the provider of the patient's concerns so that he or she can give further details before the patient leaves the facility.

CRITICAL THINKING APPLICATION   48-7

The culture of the specimen from Aaron Mitchell's infected lip (see Critical Thinking Application 48-3) has confirmed that *Staphylococcus aureus* is the causative agent. What educational information can Anna give Aaron and his mother about the contagiousness of this infection and how to prevent it from spreading to others? (*Hint:* See Table 48-2.)

Legal and Ethical Issues

Maintaining a laboratory in the office increases the physician's liability. By testing patients' specimens in the office, the physician assumes responsibility for the interpretation and accuracy of the results. As the person in the office who runs the tests and notes the results in the patient's record, you are responsible for maintaining optimum accuracy in testing results. A quality assurance (QA) program, including the running, interpreting, and recording of the internal controls supplied in each test kit, must be documented. Both microbiology and immunology tests allow the patient to benefit from the convenience of office testing.

Strict confidentiality is essential. Never release information to anyone other than the patient or legal guardian. Also note that certain infectious diseases must be reported to the CDC or local board of health. Each state legislature determines what diseases must be reported and how the data are to be reported. Additional data for nationally notifiable diseases are published weekly by the CDC in the *Morbidity and Mortality Weekly Report* (MMWR).

Professional Behaviors

This chapter is the fifth and final chapter in this laboratory section. It's time to revisit the Professionalism Evaluation form found in the first laboratory chapter. Your instructor may meet with you one on one to discuss your evaluation results, and/or you may do a self-evaluation of your performance. (See Procedure 48-4 in the study guide.)

Common Notifiable Infectious Conditions

- Anthrax
- Arboviral neuroinvasive and non-neuroinvasive diseases
- Babesiosis
- Botulism
- Brucellosis
- Cancer
- Chancroid
- *Chlamydia trachomatis*, genital infections
- Cholera
- Coccidioidomycosis
- Cryptosporidiosis
- Cyclosporiasis
- Diphtheria
- Ebola virus disease
- Ehrlichiosis/anaplasmosis
- Elevated blood lead levels (child: <16 years; adult: ≥16 years)
- Enterovirus D68
- Food-borne disease outbreak
- Giardiasis
- Gonorrhea
- Granuloma inguinale
- *Haemophilus influenzae*, invasive disease
- Hansen's disease (leprosy)
- Hantavirus pulmonary syndrome
- Hemolytic uremic syndrome, postdiarrheal
- Hepatitis, chronic (B, C)
- Hepatitis, viral, acute (A, B, C, D, E)
- Herpes, genital
- HIV/AIDS infection (acquired immunodeficiency syndrome [AIDS] is now classified as HIV stage III)
- Influenza-associated pediatric mortality
- Legionellosis
- Listeriosis
- Lyme disease
- Lymphogranuloma
- Malaria
- Measles
- Meningococcal disease
- Mumps
- Novel influenza A virus infections
- Pertussis
- Pesticide-related illness, acute
- Plague
- Poliomyelitis, paralytic
- Poliovirus infection, nonparalytic
- Psittacosis
- Q fever (acute and chronic)
- Rabies
- Rocky Mountain spotted fever and spotted fever rickettsioses
- Rubella (German measles)
- Rubella, congenital syndrome
- Salmonellosis
- Severe acute respiratory syndrome–associated coronavirus (SARS)
- Shiga toxin–producing *Escherichia coli* (STEC)
- Shigellosis
- Silicosis
- Streptococcal toxic shock syndrome
- *Streptococcus pneumoniae* invasive disease
- Syphilis (all stages and congenital)
- Tetanus
- Trichinellosis (trichinosis)
- Tuberculosis
- Tularemia
- Typhoid fever
- Vancomycin-intermediate *Staphylococcus aureus* (VISA)
- Vancomycin-resistant *Staphylococcus aureus* (VRSA)
- Varicella (deaths only)
- Varicella (morbidity)
- Vibriosis
- Viral hemorrhagic fever (VHF)
- Water-borne disease outbreak
- West Nile Fever
- Yellow fever

SUMMARY OF SCENARIO

It seems to Anna that she sees something new about harmful bacteria and viruses on the television or in the newspaper every day. Outbreaks on cruise ships, the Ebola virus epidemic in Africa, hepatitis C in baby boomers, new strains of flu epidemics, and healthcare-acquired infections (e.g., MRSA and *C. difficile*) have become common topics. Yet, Anna knows that most microorganisms are harmless. People can protect themselves from infection by using a few simple techniques, such as frequently sanitizing their hands and keeping the hands away from the face. Anna makes a point of explaining this to the patients she sees at the family clinic. Prevention, she knows, is the key to controlling infection.

Anna realizes that the POL can play a vital role in the diagnosis and treatment of infectious disease. She knows that proper specimen collection is of the utmost importance in microbiology testing and that contamination could mean vital time lost in identifying pathogens. Rapid testing allows for quick diagnosis, which is important when dealing with infectious organisms that reproduce quickly. Anna has learned that certain microbiology tests are CLIA waived, and

Continued

as a certified medical assistant (CMA [AAMA]) she is qualified to perform waived tests. Testing, she has discovered, may not always involve detection of the pathogen itself. Sometimes the antibodies made in response to the pathogen must be indirectly detected in the blood to diagnose the disease, such as with the mononucleosis test. The pathogen may also be detected by directly demonstrating its presence in a specimen using an immunochromatographic identification test, such as the rapid strep test.

Anna knows that immunology testing is evolving quickly, and she is aware that she can easily check the website of the U.S. Food and Drug Administration (FDA) for new tests that can be performed in the POL.

SUMMARY OF LEARNING OBJECTIVES

1. **Define, spell, and pronounce the terms listed in the vocabulary.**
   Spelling and pronouncing medical terms correctly reinforce the medical assistant's credibility. Knowing the definitions of these terms promotes confidence in communication with patients and co-workers.

2. **Describe the naming of microorganisms.**
   The naming of all living organisms uses a binomial system consisting of two names; the first "family" name is the *genus,* and the second is the *species.* Both names are either italicized or underlined when written. The genus begins with a capital letter, the species with a lowercase letter. Often the name reveals some characteristic about the organism.

3. **Describe various bacterial staining characteristics, shapes, oxygen requirements, and physical structures; also, explain the characteristics of common diseases caused by bacteria.**
   Identification of bacteria begins with observation of their morphology. Cocci are spherical organisms; bacilli are rod-shaped organisms; and spirilla are spiral-shaped organisms. Staphylococci are cocci in clusters; streptococci and streptobacilli are organisms arranged in chains; and diplococci and diplobacilli are organisms arranged in pairs. Their staining characteristics are gram positive (dark blue), gram negative (pink), and acid-fast (pink). Organisms are classified by oxygen requirements as aerobic (needs oxygen to survive), anaerobic (lives without oxygen), or facultative (anaerobic but able to survive in the presence of oxygen). Tables 48-1 to 48-3 can help explain the characteristics of common diseases caused by bacteria.

4. **Describe the unusual characteristics of *Chlamydia, Mycoplasma,* and *Rickettsia* organisms.**
   Chlamydia and *Rickettsia* organisms are tiny bacteria; however, unlike most bacteria, they require a host cell for replication. *Rickettsia* organisms are transmitted by arthropods. *Mycoplasma* organisms are bacteria without cell walls (see Table 48-4).

5. **Do the following related to fungi, protozoa, and parasites:**
   * *Compare bacteria with fungi, protozoa, and parasites.*
     Bacteria are prokaryotic (containing no nucleus); fungi, protozoa, and parasites are eukaryotic. Bacteria, fungi, and protozoa must be observed microscopically; helminths, or worms, can be seen with the naked eye but their eggs may be microscopic in size.
   * *Identify the characteristics of common diseases caused by fungi, protozoa, and parasites.*

   Tables 48-5 and 48-6 present the characteristics of common diseases caused by fungi and protozoa.
   * *Perform patient education on the collection of a stool specimen for ova and parasite testing.*
     Stool is collected in special transport devices that contain preservatives and fixatives that aid microscopic examination of the specimen. Explicit instructions must be given to the patient to ensure proper collection (see Procedure 48-1).

6. **Compare bacteria with viruses, and describe the characteristics of common viral diseases.**
   Viruses differ from bacteria in that they are not cells. Viruses have a core of nucleic acid surrounded by a protein coat. Unlike bacteria, viruses do not metabolize and cannot replicate on their own. They are called obligate intracellular parasites. Table 48-7 presents the characteristics of various viral diseases.

7. **Cite the protocols for the collection, transport, and processing of specimens.**
   Refer to Table 48-8.

8. **Explain how pinworm testing is done and when it is recommended.**
   Pinworm testing detects the eggs of the pinworm, *E. vermicularis.* The worm deposits eggs in the anal folds at night. The eggs can be retrieved by using a sticky collection device either late in the evening or in the morning before a bowel movement. The diagnosis is made if the eggs are found microscopically.

9. **Describe and perform CLIA-waived microbiology tests:**
   * *Describe three CLIA-waived microbiology tests that use a rapid identification technique.*
     Often growing a pathogen on a culture plate is difficult, and it takes time to grow and isolate the pathogen. A rapid "direct" immunology test demonstrates the presence of the pathogen's antigen in a specimen that is placed in a test kit containing its specific antibody. If the pathogen is present, it produces a colored reaction, indicating a positive result. The **rapid strep test** detects *S. pyogenes* and is used in the diagnosis of strep throat. The **influenza A and B rapid test** detects surface antigens of the viruses that cause influenza. The **RSV rapid test** detects antigens from RSV, which causes pneumonia and bronchiolitis in young children.

SUMMARY OF LEARNING OBJECTIVES—*continued*

- *Obtain and perform the CLIA-waived rapid* Streptococcus *test.*
  Refer to Procedure 48-2.

10. **Do the following related to CLIA-waived immunology testing:**
    - *Discuss the purpose of indirect immunology testing.*
      "Indirect" immunology testing detects antibodies in whole blood, serum, or plasma that react to the specific antigen in the test kit, producing a colored reaction. A positive reaction indicates that the antibodies have been produced and attack the pathogen in question (e.g., heterophile antibodies seen in mononucleosis).
    - *Describe three CLIA-waived indirect immunology tests that could be done in the physician office laboratory.*
      Mononucleosis testing detects the heterophile antibodies made in reaction to an infection of the Epstein-Barr virus. The *H. pylori* **test** detects antibodies to the bacterium that commonly causes stomach ulcers. Early detection of **Lyme disease** can be accomplished using a CLIA-waived test that detects the antibodies that attack the *B. burgdorferi* pathogen. Rapid HIV testing detects the HIV antibodies made in reaction to an HIV infection that could develop into AIDS.
    - *Obtain a specimen and perform the CLIA-waived microbiology strep test.*
      Refer to Procedure 48-3.

11. **Detail the equipment needed in a microbiology laboratory, and discuss identification of pathogens in the microbiology laboratory by describing various staining techniques.**
    Microbiology viewing equipment includes slides, stains, and microscopes. Culturing equipment includes inoculating loops and needles, petri dishes with the appropriate growth media, and incubators. Sterilizing equipment includes incinerators and autoclaves. The Gram stain is the most commonly used stain in the microbiology laboratory. The acid-fast stain is used in the identification protocol for *Mycobacterium* species.

12. **Describe the reference laboratory assessment of a throat culture and a urine culture.**
    The throat culture is observed on the blood agar plate for beta hemolysis and no growth around the bacitracin disk (see Figure 48-14). Urine growth on the urine Culturette strip is assessed after incubation to determine whether a urinary tract infection is present (see Figure 48-15).

13. **Explain the method used for culture and sensitivity testing.**
    Antimicrobial susceptibility testing uses disks impregnated with antimicrobial agents dropped onto the surface of an agar plate inoculated with a pathogen. The pathogen displays susceptibility, resistance, or an intermediate reaction to the antimicrobial agent. These determinations are made by measuring the zone of inhibition around each disk and comparing them with a chart provided by the manufacturer.

14. **Discuss patient education, in addition to legal and ethical issues, involved in laboratory testing.**
    The medical assistant must be aware that patient confidentiality is of utmost importance; however, certain infections must be reported to the CDC and to the local board of health.

CONNECTIONS

Study Guide Connection: Go to the Chapter 48 Study Guide. Read and complete the activities.

evolve Evolve Connection: Go to the Chapter 48 link at *evolve.elsevier.com/kinn* to complete the Chapter Review Quiz. Check out the other resources listed for this chapter to make the most of what you have learned from Assisting in Microbiology and Immunology.

49

SURGICAL SUPPLIES AND INSTRUMENTS

SCENARIO

Tom Anderson, CMA (AAMA), works for Dr. Sheila Samanski, a dermatologist who frequently performs minor surgical procedures in the office. Tom assists Dr. Samanski with procedures and is also responsible for maintaining stock supplies in the minor surgery room, including solutions and medications, and for cleaning, maintaining, and inspecting the surgical instruments. Because no procedures are scheduled for today, Tom plans to compile an inventory of supplies and equipment and perform routine maintenance activities.

While studying this chapter, think about the following questions:

- What solutions and medications should be available in the surgical area of a medical office?
- What are the typical instruments used in minor surgical procedures?
- How are surgical instruments identified and classified?
- How should surgical instruments be cared for and handled before, during, and after a surgical procedure?
- What types of sutures and needles are used in minor surgical procedures?

LEARNING OBJECTIVES

1. Define, spell, and pronounce the terms listed in the vocabulary.
2. Describe typical solutions and medications used in minor surgical procedures.
3. Summarize methods for identifying surgical instruments used in minor office surgery, and then identify some surgical instruments.
4. Outline the general classifications of surgical instruments.
5. Describe the care and handling of surgical instruments.
6. Identify drapes and different types of sutures and surgical needles.
7. Explain the medical assistant's responsibility to help ease patients' concerns about procedures.

VOCABULARY

abscesses Localized collections of pus, which may be under the skin or deep in the body, that cause tissue destruction.

cannula (kan'-yoo-lah) A rigid tube that surrounds a blunt trocar or a sharp, pointed trocar, which is inserted into the body; when the trocar is withdrawn, fluid may escape from the body through the cannula, depending on the insertion site.

curettage (kyur'-eh-tahjz) The act of scraping a body cavity with a surgical instrument, such as a curette.

dilation The opening or widening of the circumference of a body orifice with a dilating instrument.

diluent A fluid that makes a solution less concentrated; it is added to vials of powdered medications to create a solution of the drug for injection.

dissect To cut or separate tissue with a cutting instrument or scissors.

fascia A sheet or band of fibrous tissue deep in the skin that covers muscles and body organs.

fornix A recess in the upper part of the vagina caused by protrusion of the cervix into the vaginal wall.

obturator A metal rod with a smooth, rounded tip that is placed in hollow instruments to reduce injury to body tissues during insertion.

patency Open condition of a body cavity or canal.

stylus A metal probe that is inserted into or passed through a catheter, needle, or tube used for clearing purposes or to facilitate passage into a body orifice.

Office surgery is restricted to the management of minor problems and injuries. The medical assistant is expected to prepare the patient and the sterile field, assist the provider as needed, take care of the patient after the procedure, properly disinfect the area, and document appropriately. Some medical assistants are employed in outpatient surgical facilities and are expected to assist with procedures that once were performed in hospitals. Although these more difficult operations may involve complete gowning and gloving with surgical masks and caps, the two surgical chapters in this text limit discussion and descriptions to the routines necessary to prepare for and assist in minor surgery only. This chapter includes a discussion of surgical supplies and instruments, the care and handling of instruments, and the different types of surgical sutures and needles. The subsequent chapter presents sterilization, preparation of the sterile field, specific minor surgical procedures, and care of the patient.

MINOR SURGERY ROOM

When minor surgery is routinely performed, the medical office is designed to include a minor surgery room that is separate from the other examining rooms. Larger surgery centers have recovery rooms and family waiting areas. The minor surgery room in a physician's office, often called the *procedure room,* should be near a workroom with a sink and an autoclave if the room does not have its own. It should be easy to disinfect and uncluttered to allow easy movement and minimal dust collection. Cabinets with countertops are necessary to serve as a side or back table during surgical procedures. Surgical supplies, wound care equipment, medications, and biopsy containers are stored in these cabinets. The exam table should be easily adjustable. In addition, the room should have bright lighting, a Mayo stand for instruments, vital signs equipment, and possibly an electrocardiograph (ECG) machine as part of the standard equipment for a procedure room (Figure 49-1).

SURGICAL SOLUTIONS AND MEDICATIONS

Treatment room supplies include the standard solutions and medications used in minor surgery and dressing changes. Although the solutions and medications listed here are basic, every physician's office practice has preferred items and methods of applying them. The medical assistant is responsible for their care and for maintaining up-to-date supplies.

Sterile water is kept in two forms. Multiple-dose or single-use vials are used as a **diluent** for medications; larger containers of sterile water are for rinsing instruments that have been in a chemical disinfectant solution.

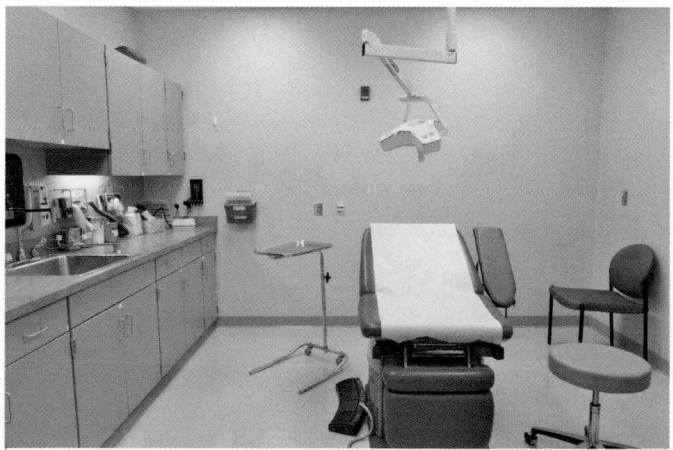

FIGURE 49-1 Surgical procedure room in a typical ambulatory care setting.

Sterile normal saline solution is also stocked in two sizes. The small vial is used for injection (e.g., 0.9% Sodium Chloride Injection USP single-dose vials, Bacteriostatic 0.9% Sodium Chloride Injection USP multiple-dose vials). A larger plastic container of sterile saline (e.g., 0.9% Sodium Chloride Irrigation USP) is used for cleaning, rinsing, and irrigating wounds. These commercially prepared products are ordered from a medical supply company.

Before surgery, the surgical site on the patient must be cleansed with an antiseptic skin cleansing preparation to reduce the number of pathogens. Although it is not possible to remove all microorganisms from the skin, it is important to prepare the surgical site to remove transient and pathogenic microorganisms on the skin's surface and to reduce resident flora. Research indicates that chlorhexidine topical (Hibiclens), Triseptin, gluconate products (Triseptin or Hibiclens), and povidone-iodine (Betadine) are safe and effective antiseptics.

The surgeon's hands and those of the medical assistant also require thorough cleansing to reduce the chances of wound contamination, even though the hands will be covered by sterile gloves. Surgical scrub preparations should have a broad antimicrobial action effective against bacterial spores; they also should work rapidly to reduce transient bacteria, show evidence of persistent activity on the skin, and work despite the presence of organic matter, such as blood or wound drainage. Research has shown that, before sterile gloves are put on, the use of an alcohol-based hand rub can be as effective as an extensive surgical scrub to limit bacterial contamination of the hands during a surgical procedure.

Even minor surgical procedures require the use of anesthetics, which either are injected locally at the site of the procedure or may be applied to the skin as a preinjection anesthetic. For patients who find injections of a local anesthetic painful or traumatic, the provider may first apply a topical anesthetic (e.g., Exactacain), which begins acting in 30 seconds and has a duration of anesthesia of 30 to 60 minutes. Topical anesthetics can be applied in many forms, including sprays, gels, lotions, swabs, and foams. Immediately after applying the topical anesthetic, the provider injects the local anesthetic around the surgical area.

Another topical anesthetic is an ethyl chloride spray, a vapocoolant that controls pain associated with minor surgical procedures (e.g., lancing boils, incision and drainage of small **abscesses**), by causing localized freezing of the affected area. Because ethyl chloride is highly flammable, it should never be used in the presence of electrical cauterizing equipment. In addition, petroleum jelly must be applied to the surrounding areas to protect them from the cooling action of the spray. Ethyl chloride spray has a short duration of action, so all equipment must be prepared and the provider must be ready to perform the procedure before the spray is applied.

Local anesthetics are injected into the subcutaneous tissue. These produce a temporary cessation of feeling at the site of injection by blocking the generation and conduction of nerve impulses. Many different types of local anesthetics are available, but all share the same suffix, *-caine.* Those used most frequently include lidocaine (Xylocaine), chloroprocaine (Nesacaine), and bupivacaine (Sensorcaine). Local anesthetics are purchased in multiple-dose vials of 30 to 50 mL and in various strengths, such as 0.5%, 1%, and 2%. They begin acting relatively quickly, within 5 to 15 minutes; the duration of action depends on the type of anesthetic, but they usually last 1 to 3 hours. When highly vascular areas are involved, local anesthetics containing epinephrine may be used. Epinephrine causes vasoconstriction at the site, which keeps the anesthetic in the tissues longer, prolonging its effect. It also minimizes local bleeding. However, epinephrine is not used in areas where decreased circulation may cause problems with healing, such as fingertips or toes.

All tissues removed, or biopsied, from the patient are sent to the pathology laboratory for analysis. A 10% formalin solution typically is used to preserve excised tissue for specimens. Specimen bottles are purchased with preservatives included and should be part of the supplies prepared for a surgical procedure if a biopsy is to be done. The provider places the specimen in the container, and the medical assistant is responsible for accurately labeling the container with the patient's name and medical history number, the date of collection, and the type of specimen.

Sometimes the provider may want to use topical silver nitrate (AgNO$_3$) solution or coated applicator sticks to stop localized bleeding, such as with epistaxis (nosebleed) or capillary bleeding at the site of a wound. The applicators must be kept in lightproof brown containers; the most commonly used strength is 20%. The applicator sticks are convenient for use in the mouth or nose.

Additional Surgical Supplies

- Sterilized gauze squares or strips saturated with petroleum jelly or petrolatum—used to pack wounds
- Sterilized iodoform gauze strips, $\frac{1}{4}$ inch to 2 inches wide and impregnated with iodoform iodine—used to pack abscesses to act as a wick to draw out the infection; also used as a local antibacterial agent
- Surgical sponges—used to absorb blood and protect tissues during surgery
- Syringes and needles—used to inject local anesthetics and irrigate wounds
- Sterile wound supplies and bandaging materials

CRITICAL THINKING APPLICATION   49-1

Tom is ready to do an inventory of supplies in the minor surgery room. What solutions, medications, and miscellaneous supplies should he make sure are on hand for the busy surgical schedule planned for next week?

SURGICAL INSTRUMENTS

The medical assistant must know which instruments are used for each procedure and should be able to identify and understand the function of the surgical instruments preferred by the provider. Instruments have clearly identifiable parts and can be visually differentiated from one another (Procedure 49-1). The basic

components are the handle, the closing mechanism, and the part that comes in contact with the patient, commonly called the *jaws*. Many instruments can be ordered with either straight or curved tips, depending on the operator's preference and the task to be performed.

Instruments have either ring handles (finger rings; Figure 49-2, *A* and *B*) or spring handles (Figure 49-2, *C*; these sometimes are called *thumb-handled* or *thumb grasp* instruments). Scissors are an example of a ring-handled instrument; tweezers have spring handles. Some instruments have a hinge-type mechanism called a *box lock*.

Ratchets resemble gears and are located just below or next to the ring handle (see Figure 49-2, *A* and *B*). They are used to lock an instrument into position. Most ratchets can be closed at three or more positions, depending on the thickness of the tissue or materials being grasped.

The inner surfaces of the jaws on some instruments have ridged teeth, called *serrations,* and both ring-handled and thumb-type instruments may have them. These serrations may be crisscross, horizontal, or lengthwise (Figure 49-3). Serrations prevent small blood vessels and tissue from slipping out of the jaws of the instrument.

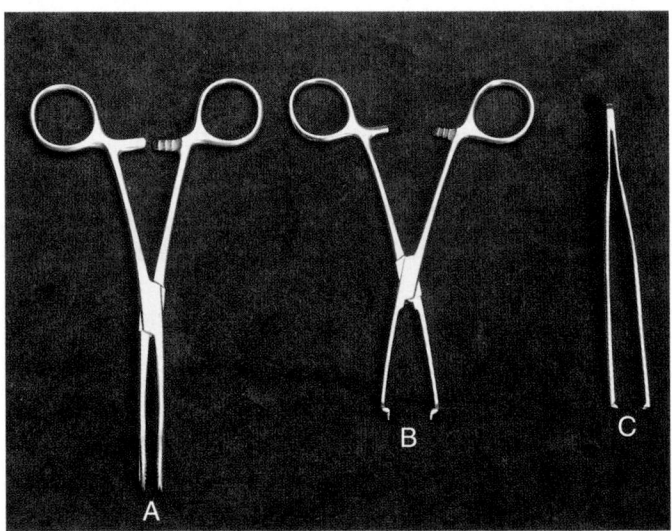

FIGURE 49-2 A and **B,** Ring-handle forceps. **C,** Spring-handle thumb forceps.

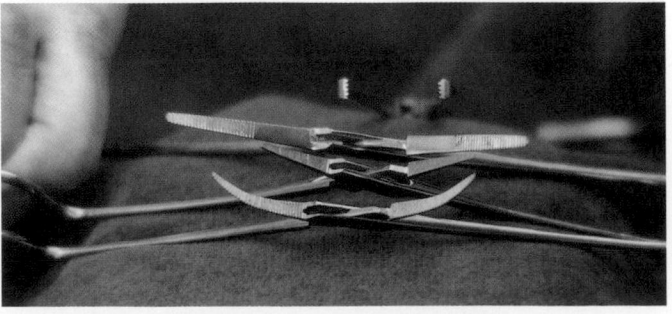

FIGURE 49-3 Instruments with serrations.

Instrument tips or jaws may be plain tipped or mouse toothed (Figure 49-4, *A*). If the tooth is large, the tip is called *rat toothed* (Figure 49-4, *B*). Tissue forceps usually are toothed instruments and are identified by the number of intermeshing teeth (e.g., 1X2,

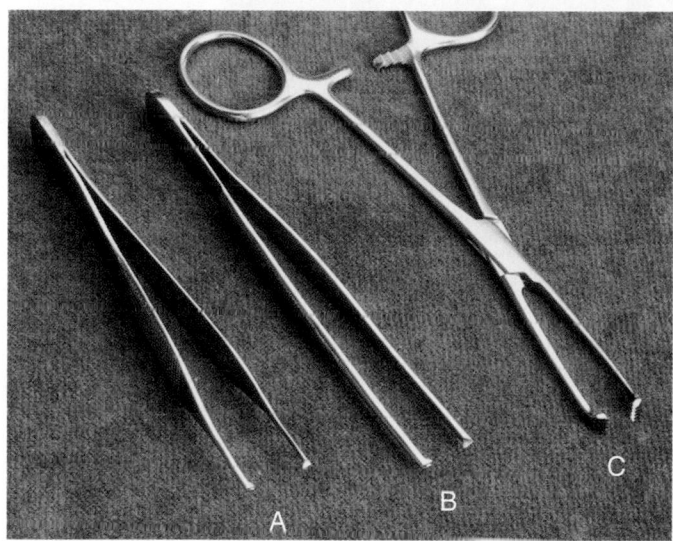

FIGURE 49-4   **A,** Mouse-toothed jaws. **B,** Rat-toothed jaws. **C,** Teeth of Allis tissue forceps.

2X3, 3X4). Allis forceps (Figure 49-4, *C*) are used to grasp delicate, soft tissues, so the teeth are finer, shallower, and more rounded. Other forceps have teeth that are sharper and deeper. Still others have sharp, hooklike, single or double teeth, such as a tenaculum or vulsellum. Usually the tenaculum has a single, sharp hook on each jaw. The vulsellum has a double hook that resembles the fangs of a snake (see Figure 49-17, *F*). Toothed instruments commonly have ratchets for locking into towels or human tissues. Instrument tips may also be either straight or curved, depending on their use.

An instrument is usually named for its use (e.g., splinter forceps, for removing splinters) or after the person or people who developed it (e.g., Mayo-Hegar needle holder). Many general instruments are identified by the part of the body on which they are used (e.g., rectal speculum and nasal speculum).

Thousands of surgical instruments have multiple names. The same instrument may have two or three different names, depending on the provider identifying it or the part of the country in which the practice is located. For example, a provider may ask for a clamp or forceps when he or she wants a Kelly hemostat. It is important to learn the provider's preference in terminology. Learn to recognize the distinctive parts of instruments and the reasons for each part, and you will quickly build a working knowledge of hundreds of instruments.

PROCEDURE 49-1   Identify Surgical Instruments

Goal: *To identify, correctly spell the names of, and determine the use or uses of standard surgical instruments used in the ambulatory care setting.*

EQUIPMENT and SUPPLIES

- Curved hemostat
- Straight hemostat
- Dressing (thumb) forceps
- Paper and pen
- Disposable scalpel and blade
- Dissecting scissors
- Towel clamp
- Vaginal speculum
- Bandage scissors
- Allis tissue forceps

PROCEDURAL STEPS

1. Look for the following parts that determine use: box lock, serrations, finger rings, cutting edge, noncutting edge, thumb type, teeth ratchets, and electric attachments.
   PURPOSE: To determine the combination of features and parts for each instrument.
2. Consider the general classification of the instrument: cutting and dissection, grasping and clamping, retracting, or probing and dilating.

PURPOSE: The clue to the name of the instrument may be found by determining the classification.
3. Carefully examine the teeth and serrations.
   PURPOSE: The clue to the name of the instrument may be found by determining its distinctive parts.
4. Consider the length of the instrument to determine the area of the body for which it is used.
   PURPOSE: The clue to the name of the instrument may be found by determining where it can reach.
5. Try to remember whether the instrument was named for a famous physician, university, or clinic.
   PURPOSE: Many instruments are named for the inventor.
6. If the instrument is a pair of scissors, look at the points and determine whether the tips are sharp-sharp, sharp-blunt, or blunt-blunt.
7. Carefully compare the instrument with similar instruments with which you are familiar to determine whether it is in the same category or has the same name.

Write the complete name of each instrument (using the correct spelling), including its category and use.

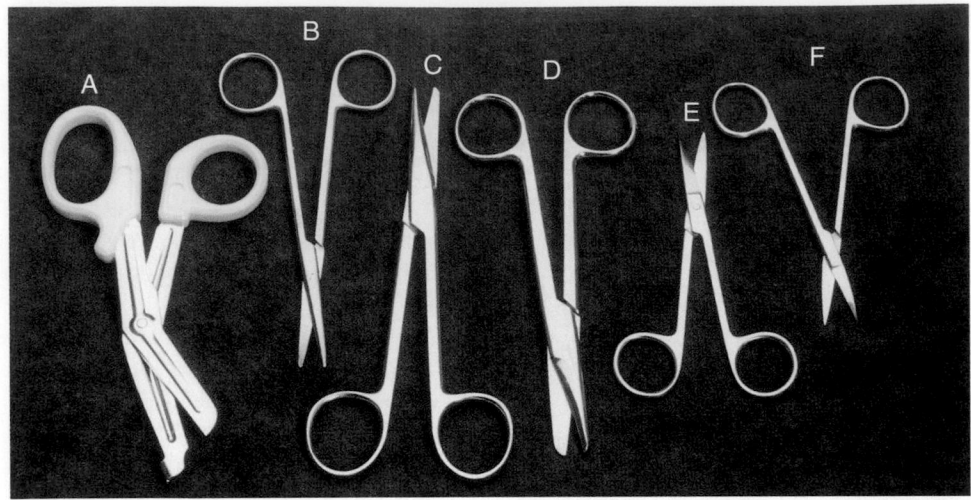

FIGURE 49-5 Operating scissors. **A,** Bandage scissors. **B,** Metzenbaum ("Metz") scissors. **C,** Curved Mayo scissors. **D,** Straight Mayo scissors. **E,** Straight iris scissors. **F,** Curved iris scissors.

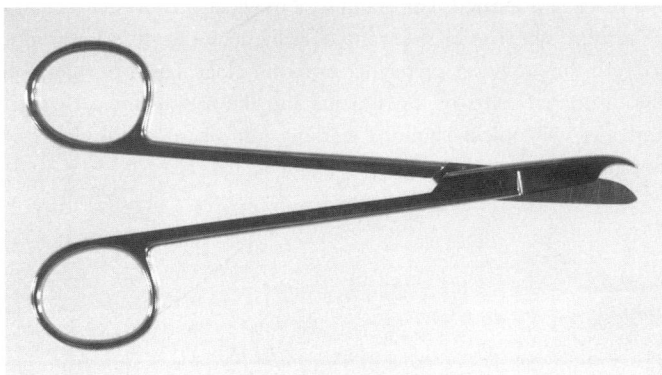

FIGURE 49-6 Suture scissors. (From Wells MP: *Surgical instruments: a pocket guide,* ed 4, St Louis, 2011, Saunders.)

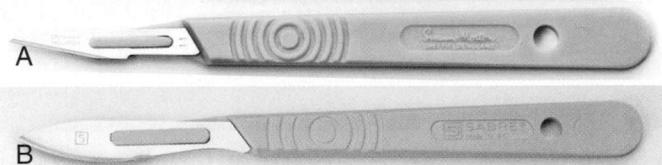

FIGURE 49-7 Disposable scalpels.

CLASSIFICATIONS OF SURGICAL INSTRUMENTS

Surgical instruments generally are classified according to their use, and most belong to one of four groups:

- Cutting
- Grasping
- Retracting
- Probing and dilating

Cutting and Dissecting Instruments

Cutting and dissecting instruments, which are used for cutting, incising, scraping, punching, and puncturing, include scissors, scalpels, chisels, elevators, curettes, punches, drills, and needles. Instruments with a sharp blade or surface can cut, scrape, or **dissect**.

Bandage Scissors (Figure 49-5, A)
- Blunt probe tip
- Easily inserted under bandages with relative safety
- Used to remove bandages and dressings

Operating (Surgical) Scissors
Metzenbaum (Metz) Scissors (Figure 49-5, *B*)
- Most frequently used length is 5¼ inches
- Used to cut and dissect tissue

Mayo Scissors (Figure 49-5, *C* and *D*)
- 5 to 6 inches long
- Curved or straight blade tips
- Used to cut and dissect **fascia** and muscle
- Straight Mayo scissors can be used as suture scissors

Iris Scissors (Figure 49-5, *E* and *F*)
- Usual length is 4 inches
- Curved or straight blade tips
- Straight tips usually are used for suture removal

Littauer Stitch or Suture Scissors (Figure 49-6)
- 4 to 5 inches long
- Blade has beak or hook to slide under sutures
- Used to remove sutures

Disposable Scalpels (Figure 49-7)

Most scalpels used in minor procedures are disposable, with different handle sizes and types of blades already attached to the handles. However, stainless steel, reusable scalpel handles can be ordered. A variety of blades can be used that must be attached to the handle using forceps and sterile technique. After the procedure the handles are sterilized and the blades are discarded in a sharps container. Once used, disposable scalpel/blade units are discarded in a sharps container.

- *Handles:* No. 3 is the standard handle; No. 3L and No. 7 are used in deeper cavities
- *Blades:* No. 15 is commonly used; Nos. 10, 11, and 12 are used for specialty incisions

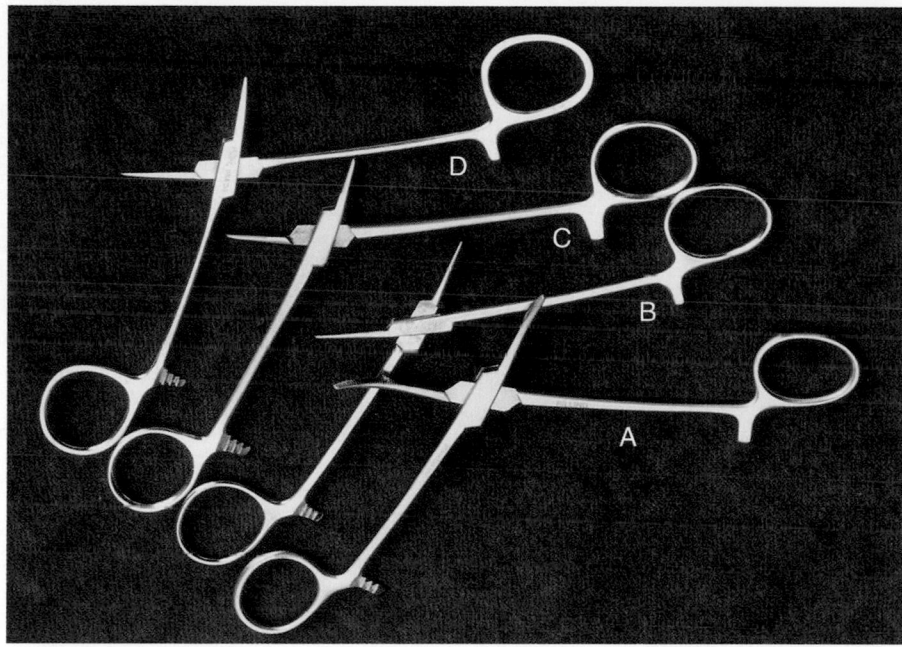

FIGURE 49-8 **A,** Kelly hemostat forceps. **B,** Mosquito hemostat forceps. **C,** Needle holder. **D,** Smooth-tip needle holder.

Grasping and Clamping Instruments

Clamping instruments are used for many different tasks. Many have a sharp tooth or teeth and are used to retract, hold, and manipulate fascia. The most common clamping instruments are hemostats, which originally were designed to stop bleeding or to clamp severed blood vessels. Some clamping instruments are used to grasp other instruments or sterilized materials. Sometimes hemostats and other clamping instruments are used interchangeably.

Hemostat Forceps (Figure 49-8, A and B)
- Jaws may be fully or partly serrated, without teeth
- May be curved or straight
- Used to clamp small vessels or hold tissue
- Mosquito forceps (4 inches) are smaller and used for very small vessels
- Crile forceps (5 inches) are medium-sized
- Kelly forceps (6 to 7 inches) are larger

Needle Holders (Figure 49-8, C and D)
- 4 to 7 inches long
- Jaws are shorter and stronger than hemostat jaws
- Jaws may be serrated or may have a groove in the center
- Used to grasp a suture needle firmly

Splinter Forceps
- Design and construction vary
- Fine tip for foreign object retrieval

Adson Forceps (Figure 49-9)
- Straight or curved jaws, smooth or serrated
- Used to grasp tissue and in suturing

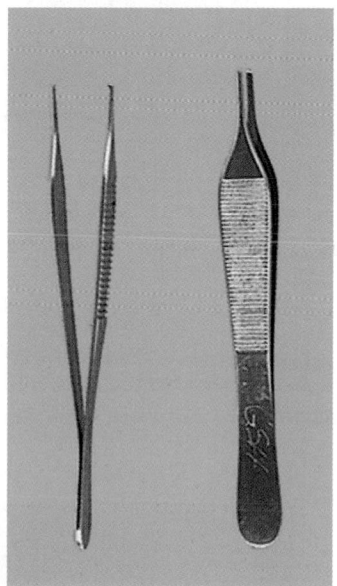

FIGURE 49-9 Adson forceps. (From Tighe SM: *Instrumentation for the operating room: a photographic manual,* ed 9, St Louis, 2016, Mosby.)

Plain Thumb (Dressing) Forceps (Figure 49-10)
- Manufactured in lengths from 4 to 12 inches
- Varying types of serrated jaws but no teeth
- Used to insert packing into or remove objects from deep cavities

Towel Forceps (Towel Clamp) (Figure 49-11)
- Various lengths from 3 to 6½ inches
- May have sharp or atraumatic (dull-edged) tips
- Used to hold drapes in place during surgery

Allis Tissue Forceps (Figure 49-12, A)
- Available in different lengths and jaw widths
- Used to grasp tissue, muscle, or skin surrounding a wound

Foerster Sponge Forceps (Figure 49-12, B)
- Used to hold gauze squares to sponge the surgical site
- Straight or curved, with or without serrations

Transfer Forceps (Figure 49-12, C to E)
- Many sizes and lengths available
- Sterile transfer forceps may be used to arrange items on a sterile tray

Adson Thumb Forceps (Figure 49-13, A and B)
- Usual length is 4 inches
- Manufactured with or without teeth
- Used to grasp tissue and in suturing

Bayonet Forceps (Figure 49-13, C to E)
- Manufactured in different lengths
- Smooth tipped
- Used to insert packing into or remove objects from the nose and ear

Plain-Tip Tissue Forceps (Figure 49-13, F)
- Manufactured in different lengths
- Atraumatic for tissue
- Used to grasp tissue, muscle, or skin surrounding a wound

Toothed Tissue Forceps (Figure 49-13, G)
- Manufactured in 4- to 18-inch lengths
- Pincher grip
- Used to grasp tissue, muscle, or skin surrounding a wound

Retractors

Retracting instruments hold tissue away from the surgical wound (incision). Depending on the provider's preference, handheld skin hooks and Senn retractors are used to retract during most minor surgical procedures.

Senn Retractor (Figure 49-14)
- Flat end is a blunt retractor
- Three-prong end may be sharp or dull
- Used to retract small incisions or to secure a skin edge for suturing

Probes and Dilators

Probes and dilators are used for both surgery and examinations. Probes can be used to search for a foreign body in a wound or to enter a fistula. Dilators are used to stretch a cavity or opening for examination or before inserting another instrument to obtain a tissue specimen.

Probes (Figure 49-15, A to C)
- Lengths range from 4 to 12 inches; available with or without bulbous tip
- May be smooth or may have a grooved director

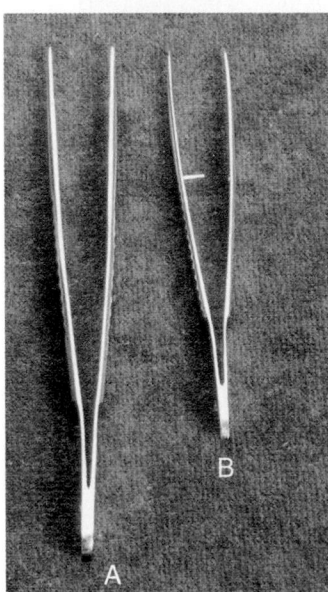

FIGURE 49-10 A, Long plain-tip forceps. **B,** Short plain-tip forceps.

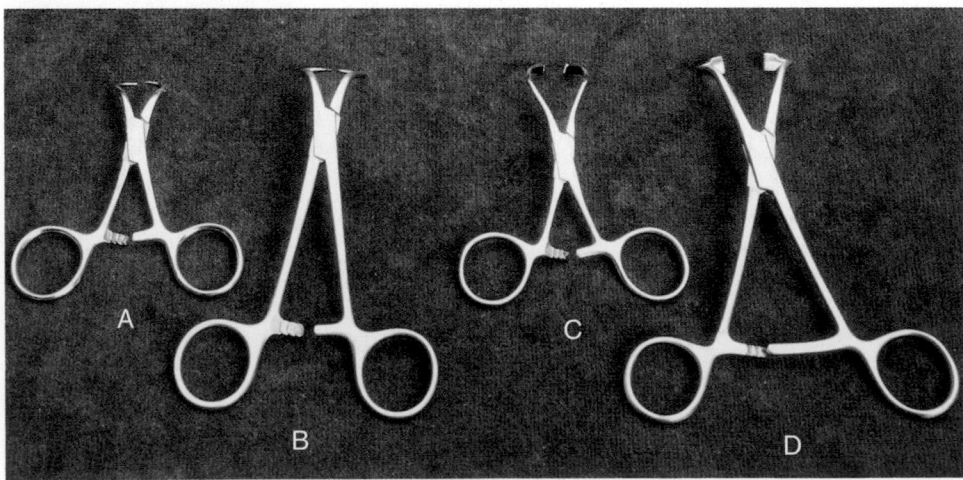

FIGURE 49-11 A, Small sharp towel forceps. **B,** Large sharp towel forceps. **C,** Small atraumatic towel forceps. **D,** Large atraumatic towel forceps.

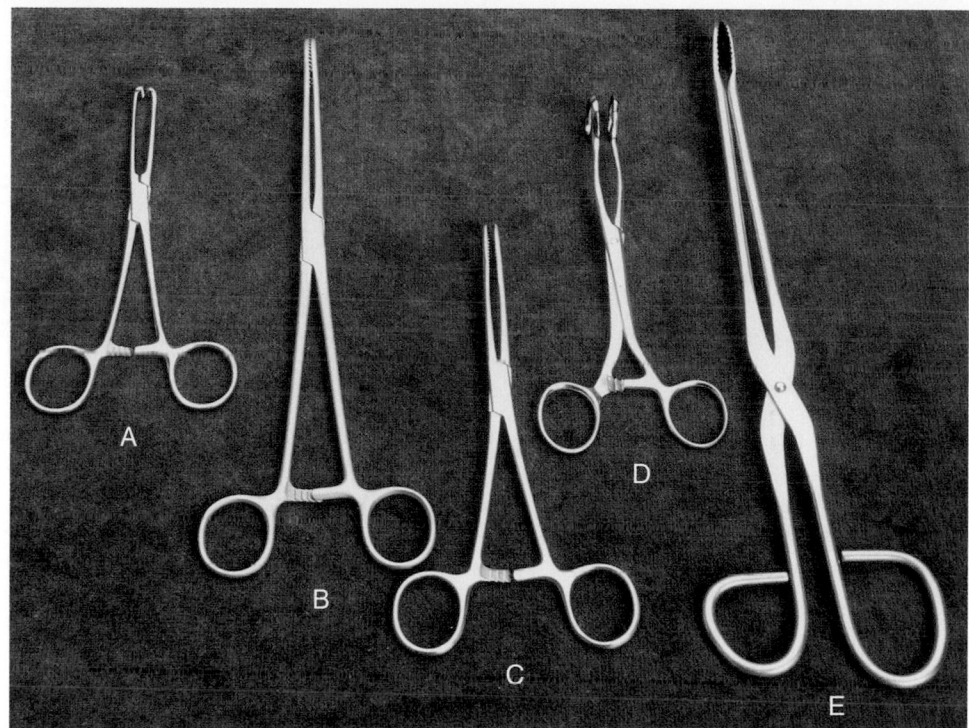

FIGURE 49-12 A, Allis forceps. **B,** Foerster sponge forceps. **C,** Straight transfer forceps. **D,** Short transfer torceps. **E,** Long transfer forceps.

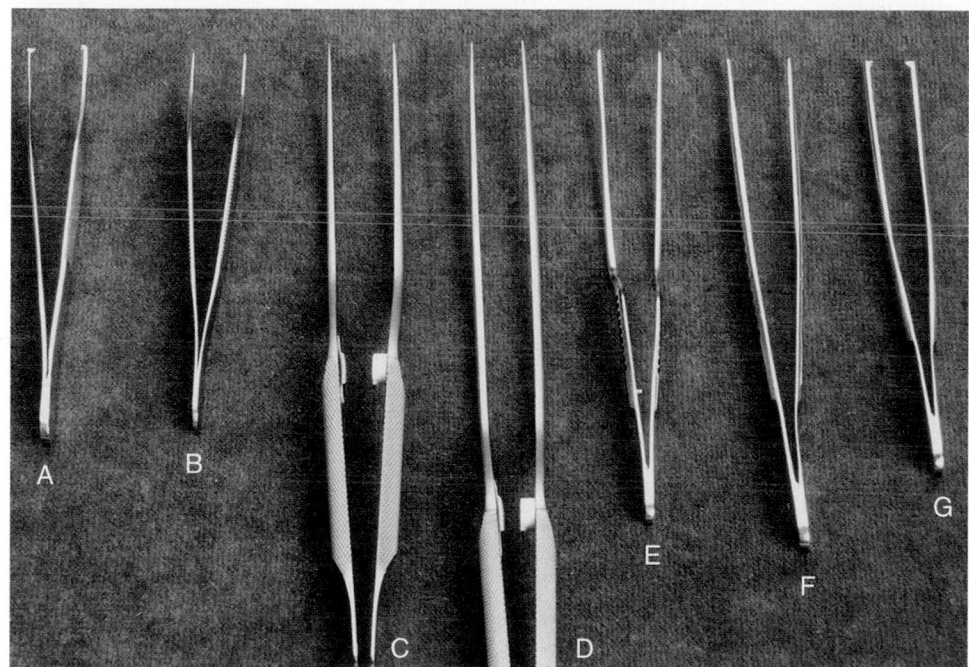

FIGURE 49-13 A, Toothed Adson forceps. **B,** Smooth Adson forceps. **C,** Medium long bayonet forceps. **D,** Long bayonet forceps. **E,** Short bayonet forceps. **F,** Plain-tip tissue forceps. **G,** Toothed tissue forceps.

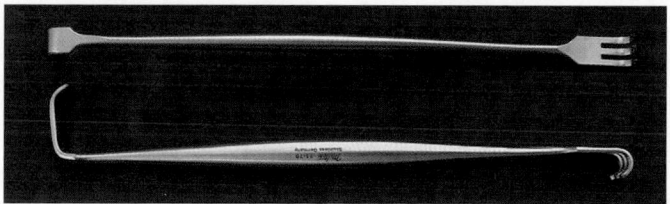

FIGURE 49-14 Senn retractors.

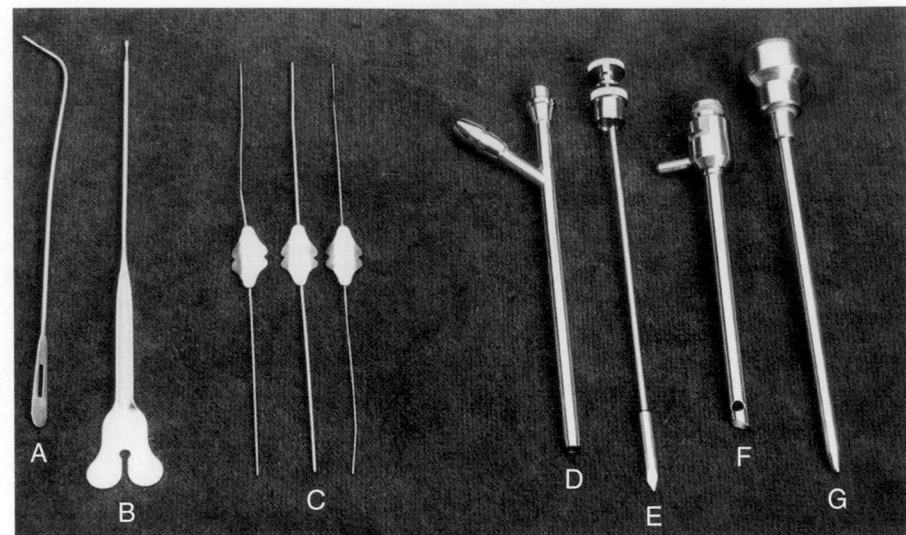

FIGURE 49-15 A, Probe. **B,** Grooved director. **C,** Lacrimal duct probes. **D,** Double-ended cannula. **E,** Sharp trocar. **F,** Cannula. **G,** Blunt-tip obturator.

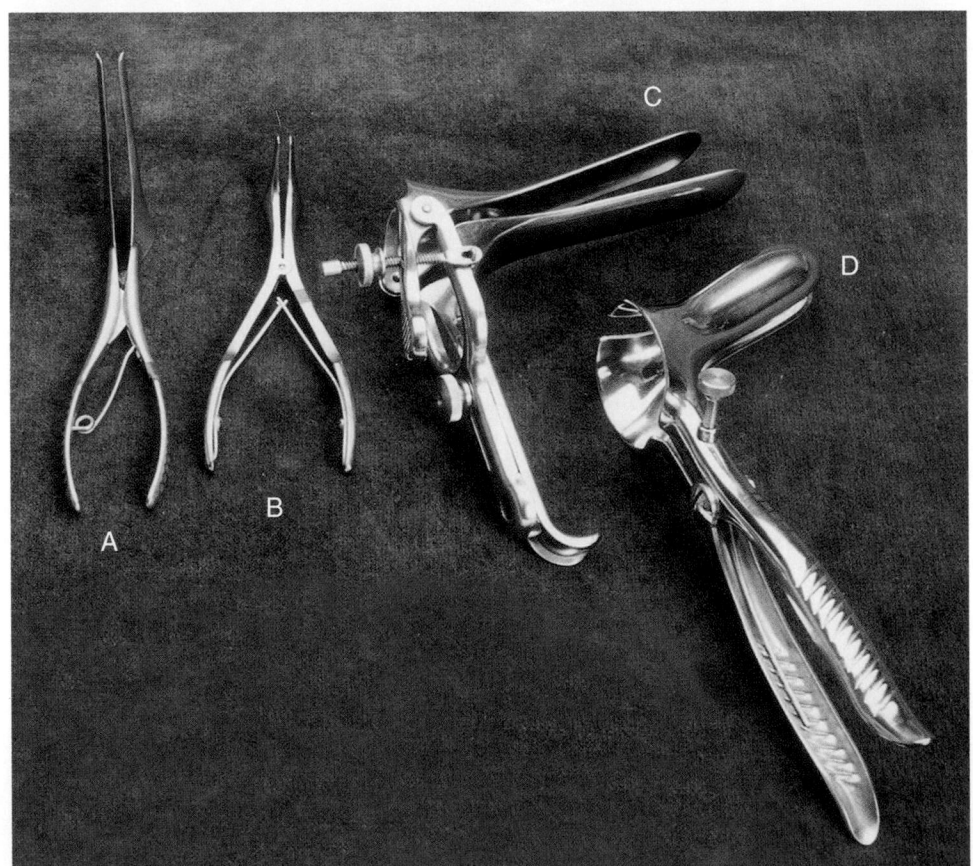

FIGURE 49-16 A, Long nasal speculum. **B,** Short nasal speculum. **C,** Graves vaginal speculum. **D,** Anal speculum, self-retaining.

- Used to find foreign bodies embedded in dermal tissue or muscle or to trace a wound tract

Trocars and Obturators (Figure 49-15, D to G)
- Available in various sizes
- Consist of a sharply pointed **stylus** (**obturator**) contained in a **cannula** (outer tube)

- Used to withdraw fluids from cavities or for draining and irrigating with a catheter

Specula (Figure 49-16)
- Most common dilator used
- Valves are spread apart, dilating the opening
- Used to open or distend a body orifice or cavity

- The most common of these is the vaginal speculum used during gynecologic examinations (Figure 49-16, *C*). Vaginal speculums can be stainless steel (reusable), plastic (disposable), and can also have a light source for illumination.

Nasal Specula (see Figure 49-16, A and B)
- Valves can be spread to facilitate viewing
- Applicator or snare can be introduced through the valves
- Used to spread the nostrils for examination

SPECIALTY INSTRUMENTS

Although all instruments fall into the same four categories as the surgical instruments just discussed, the following instruments are organized into specialty groupings. Presenting the instruments in this manner makes it easy to see how the instruments relate to particular examinations. In addition to recognizing the name and use of each instrument, the medical assistant must organize and set out the instruments needed for each particular examination in what is called a *tray setup.*

Gynecologic Instruments
Foerster Sponge Forceps (Figure 49-17, A)
- Round and serrated tips
- Used in the same way as the dressing forceps

Placenta Forceps (Figure 49-17, B)
- Used to remove tissue from the uterus

Bozeman Uterine Dressing Forceps (Figure 49-17, C)
- Designed to hold sponges or dressings
- Capable of reaching the cervix through the vagina
- Used to swab the area or apply medication

Endocervical Curette (Figure 49-17, D)
- Smaller than the uterine curette
- Used in the same way as the uterine curette

Sims Uterine Curette (Figure 49-17, E)
- Available in several sizes
- Hollow and spoon shaped; used for scraping
- Used to remove polyps, secretions, and bits of placental tissue

Schroeder Uterine Vulsellum Forceps (Figure 49-17, F)
- Used to hold tissue (e.g., the cervix) while a tissue specimen is obtained or to lift the cervix so that the **fornix** can be seen

Long Allis Forceps (Figure 49-17, G)
- Same as Allis forceps
- Used in deeper body cavities

Schroeder Uterine Tenaculum Forceps (Figure 49-17, H)
- Very sharp, pointed tips
- Used to hold tissue (e.g., the cervix) while a tissue specimen is obtained or to lift the cervix so that the fornix can be seen

Hegar Uterine Dilators (Figure 49-18, A)
- Available in sets
- Double or single ended
- Used to dilate the cervix for **dilation** and **curettage**

Sims Uterine Sounds (Figure 49-18, B)
- Used to check the **patency** of the cervical os or the urethral meatus

Ophthalmologic and Otolaryngologic Instruments
Krause Nasal Snare (Figure 49-19, A)
- Wire loop at the tip that can be tightened
- Used to remove polyps from the nares

Metal Tongue Depressor (Figure 49-19, B)
- Used to depress the tongue for oral examinations

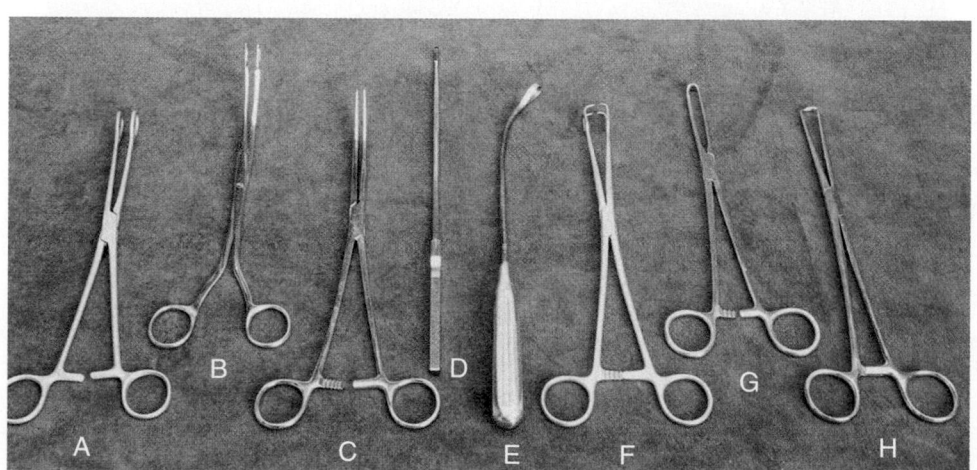

FIGURE 49-17 A, Foerster sponge forceps. **B,** Placenta forceps. **C,** Bozeman uterine dressing forceps. **D,** Endocervical curette. **E,** Sims uterine curette. **F,** Schroeder uterine vulsellum forceps. **G,** Long Allis forceps. **H,** Schroeder uterine tenaculum forceps.

Hartmann "Alligator" Ear Forceps (Figure 49-19, C)

- 3½-inch shaft and is made in a variety of styles
- Action of the jaw similar to that of an alligator's jaws
- Used to remove foreign bodies or polyps

Laryngeal Mirror (Figure 49-19, D)

- Made in various sizes
- May have a nonfogging surface
- Used for examination of the larynx and postnasal area

Ivan Laryngeal Metal Applicator (Figure 49-19, E)

- 6 to 9 inches long with curved end for use in throat or postnasal areas

- Holds cotton in place with its roughened end; used to swab or sponge throat or postnasal tissue
- Used to remove foreign bodies imbedded in the pharynx

"Buck" Ear Curette (Figure 49-19, F)

- Manufactured in various sizes
- Available as disposable curettes in many different sizes
- Has a stainless steel loop at the end
- Made with sharp or blunt scraper ends
- Used to remove foreign matter from the ear canals

Sharp Ear Dissector (Figure 49-19, G)

- Used to remove debris from the ear canal

Biopsy Instruments

Cervical Biopsy Forceps (Figure 49-20, A)

- Available with or without teeth
- Used to obtain cervical specimens for diagnostic examination

Rectal Biopsy Punch (Figure 49-20, B)

- Available in different lengths and styles
- Manufactured with interchangeable stems
- Used through a proctoscope or sigmoidoscope

Silverman Biopsy Needle

- Manufactured with a split cannula
- Stylus is removed, and cannula is inserted to retrieve the specimen
- Needle biopsy can eliminate the need for surgical incision

Genitourinary Instruments

Foley Catheter with Inflated Balloon (Figure 49-21, A)

- Manufactured in sizes 8 to 32 French with a double rubber lining toward the tip (each French unit is equal to 1.32 mm; the higher the number, the larger the lumen)

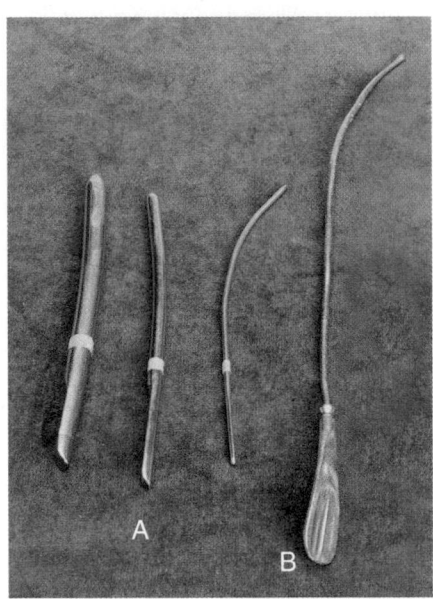

FIGURE 49-18 A, Uterine dilators. **B,** Sims uterine sounds.

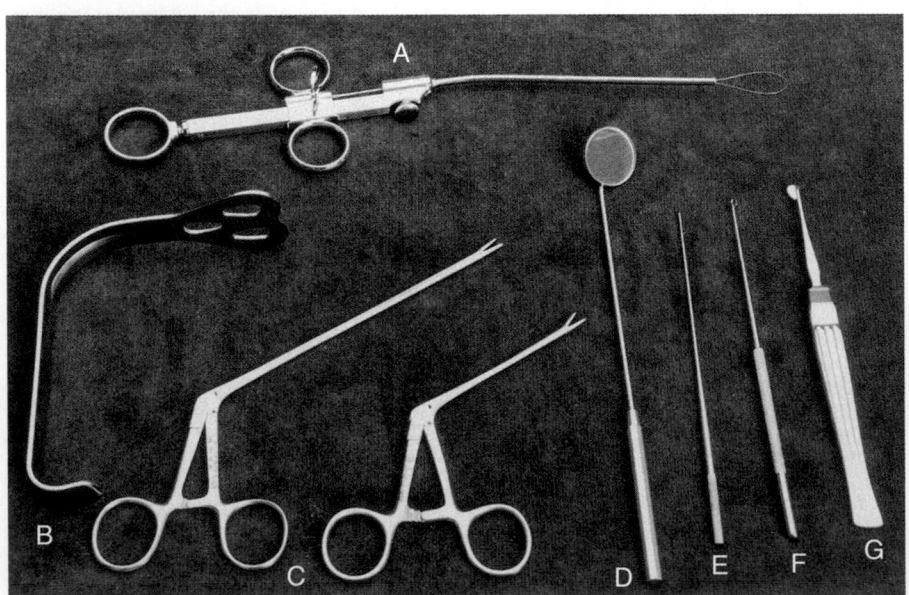

FIGURE 49-19 A, Krause nasal snare. **B,** Metal tongue depressor. **C,** Long and short alligator forceps. **D,** Laryngeal mirror. **E,** Ivan metal applicator. **F,** "Buck" ear curette. **G,** Sharp ear dissector.

- After insertion, sterile solution is injected into the inner lining (inflating the balloon) to hold it in the bladder
- Used as an indwelling catheter

Red Robinson Catheter (Figure 49-21, B)
- Soft rubber urethral catheter in sizes 8 to 32 French
- Inserted temporarily into the bladder for drainage or to obtain a specimen

Coudé-Tip Catheter
- Slightly curved catheter tip
- Designed to allow it to navigate past obstructions in the urinary tract, such as a swollen prostate in men

12-mL Luer-Lok Syringe (Figure 49-21, C)
- Typically used to inject sterile saline into a catheter to inflate the balloon at the tip of an indwelling catheter
- Used for injecting amounts greater than 5 mL

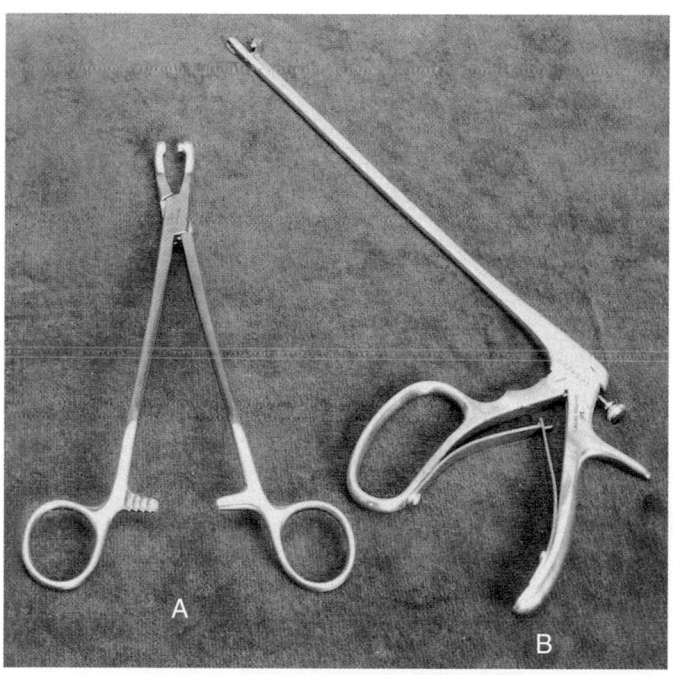

FIGURE 49-20 A, Cervical biopsy forceps. **B,** Rectal biopsy punch.

CRITICAL THINKING APPLICATION   **49-2**

Tom is preparing instrument and supply packs for specific procedures performed by Dr. Samanski. One of the packs he is preparing for the autoclave is for removal of a nasal polyp. Based on your understanding of typical and specialty instruments and supplies, what items should Tom include in the instrument pack?

CARE AND HANDLING OF INSTRUMENTS

Because instruments are expensive and the provider's skill depends on their quality, the medical assistant must properly care for each instrument to maximize its life and ensure that every part is in safe working order.

Instruments that are not disposable are made of fine-grade stainless steel. The term *stainless* usually is taken too literally. Although stainless steel does resist rust and keeps a fine edge and tip longer, even the best stainless steel may develop water spots and stains, especially if water with a high mineral content is used. Proper hardness and flexibility are important. Inexpensive instruments that are chrome plated may be too brittle or too soft. In addition, mistreatment of chrome-plated instruments can cause minute breaks in the finish, which may become a source of contamination or may tear the surgeon's gloves.

All instruments should be carefully examined when they are purchased. Scissors should be tested to see whether they shear the full length of the blades completely to the tip. If the scissors cut a piece of cloth cleanly and do not chew at any point, even at the tip, they are functioning correctly. Teeth and serrations should be checked to see whether they intermesh completely and whether the jaws are even on the sides and tip. Each instrument should be felt over its entire surface for any rough areas that may tear or snag the surgeon's gloves or act as a future source of contamination. Box locks and hinges must work freely but should not be too loose. Thumb- and spring-handled instruments must have the correct tension and meet evenly at the tips. After inspection, instruments should be sanitized and checked again for possible faulty workmanship before sterilization.

Under no circumstances should instruments be bundled together or allowed to become entangled. Do not mix stainless steel instruments with others made of different metals, including chrome-plated instruments, because this may cause electrolysis and result in etching.

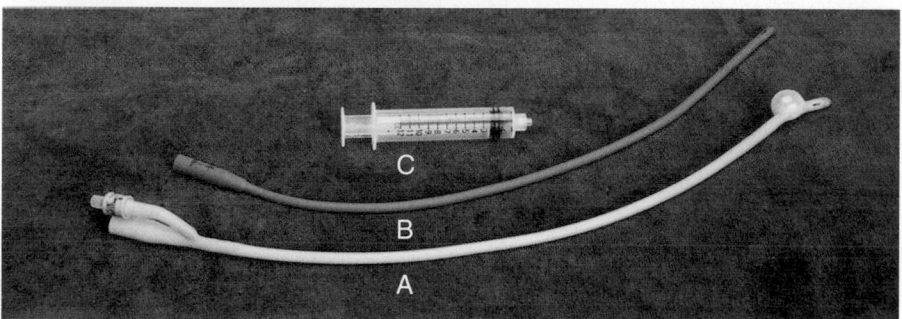

FIGURE 49-21 A, Foley catheter with inflated balloon. **B,** Red Robinson catheter. **C,** 12-mL Luer-Lok syringe.

If an instrument is accidentally dropped, it may be permanently damaged. If scissors are dropped with the blades partly open, there may be a nick at the point where the blades cross. Any damaged or malfunctioning instrument must be disposed of to prevent complications during a surgical procedure.

After a surgical procedure, contaminated instruments should be placed in a basin of disinfectant solution, with heavier instruments on the bottom of the basin and lighter, more delicate instruments on top. Always unlock each instrument before immersing it in the chemical decontaminant to permit sanitization of the entire surface area. Never allow blood or other coagulable substances to dry on an instrument because they will be difficult to remove. If immediate sanitization and disinfection are not possible, the instruments should be rinsed well and placed in a cold water solution with a blood solvent and mild detergent. The detergent increases the wetting ability of the water, giving the instrument surfaces better exposure to the solution. It is best to use a detergent that has a neutral pH and low suds and can be rinsed off easily. The manufacturer's recommendations for the correct dilution and time of immersion of the various sanitizing agents, disinfectants, and blood solvents must be strictly followed for the chemicals to be effective.

When the surgical procedure is completed, the receiving basin for instruments should be transferred from the surgical area to the disinfection and sterilization room. It is important to remove used instruments from the patient's view as soon as possible. After sanitization is complete, instruments should be rinsed thoroughly and either washed by hand or washed mechanically using an ultrasonic device.

Some delicate instruments, such as microsurgical and lensed instruments, should be washed by hand with a mild, low-sudsing, neutral-pH detergent solution and a soft brush. The instruments should be cleaned while submerged to prevent the airborne spread of microorganisms. Throughout the sanitization process, the medical assistant should wear heavy utility gloves to prevent possible exposure to contaminants. Some clinical policies require the medical assistant to wear disposable examination gloves under utility gloves for added protection from contaminants. Instruments then should be rinsed with distilled water, dried with a lint-free cloth, and inspected for proper functioning before they are packed for sterilization.

Mechanical washing, such as with an ultrasonic device, can be used for most instruments and is an especially good method for sanitizing sharp instruments to prevent injuries (Figure 49-22). In an ultrasonic cleaning unit, the instruments are immersed in a cleaning solution and the device produces sound waves that clean contaminants from the instruments' surfaces. The unit then rinses and dries the instruments, leaving them ready for the sterilization process. However, manufacturers' guidelines should be followed for rubber and plastic materials.

After disinfection and inspection, the instruments are ready for the sterilization process. Commercially prepared, disposable packs are available for most minor surgical procedures. They save time and eliminate the need for sanitization, disinfection, and sterilization of reusable stainless steel instruments, but they may be too costly for individual practices.

CRITICAL THINKING APPLICATION   **49-3**

Tom is responsible for inspecting and caring for all the surgical instruments in the minor surgery room and for sanitizing, disinfecting, and preparing contaminated instruments for autoclaving. He is in the process of writing an addition to the office policies and procedures manual on the management of surgical instruments. Based on what you know about the care and handling of surgical instruments, what should Tom include in the policy?

DRAPES, SUTURES, AND NEEDLES

Disposable surgical drapes are available in several different materials and sizes. These typically have an opening (fenestration) for the operative site. The drape is placed over the operative area, using sterile technique, after the patient's skin preparation has been completed (Figure 49-23).

Sutures

The word *suture* is used as both a noun and a verb. As a noun it refers to a surgical stitch or to the material used to close a wound. As a verb it refers to the act of stitching. The primary purpose of a suture is to hold the edges of a wound together until natural healing occurs.

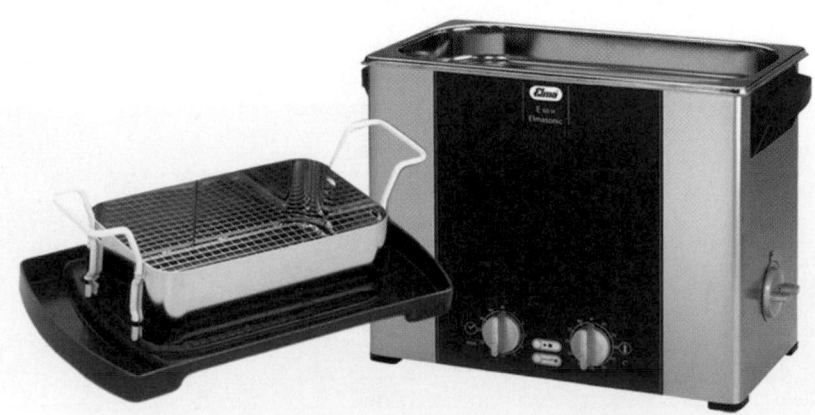

FIGURE 49-22 Elmasonic E ultrasonic cleaner unit. (Courtesy Tovatech, South Orange, N.J.)

A suture may also be used as a *ligature*. This is a strand of suture material used to tie off a blood vessel or to strangulate tissue. If a ligature is used to tie off an internal tubular structure, it must last permanently or long enough for the structure itself to disintegrate. The ideal suture material has certain characteristics:

- Easy to handle and makes a secure knot
- Does not induce a localized tissue reaction and is nonallergenic
- Has adequate strength without cutting through tissue
- Can be sterilized

The provider will request a certain type of suture based on the specific properties of the suture material, the desirable rate of absorption, the size of the suture, and the type of needle the provider prefers. Both natural and synthetic suture materials are available. Sutures may be classified as either absorbable or nonabsorbable. Many different suture materials are available, each having its advantages and disadvantages. Suture materials commonly used in minor

surgical procedures are described in the following paragraphs (Figure 49-24).

Absorbable Sutures

Absorbable sutures are dissolved by the body's enzymes during the healing process. They are used when deep incisions or lacerations require inner layers of sutures to close the wound. Absorbable suture material is also used in areas where suture removal is difficult (e.g., oral surgery). Catgut (sheep, cattle, or pig intestine) once was the absorbable suture material of choice, but it has been replaced in recent years by synthetic absorbable suture material (e.g., Vicryl). Other synthetic absorbable suture materials include Dexon, PDS, and Maxon. These materials remain stable longer than natural catgut (up to 11 weeks), allowing the wound to heal completely before absorption occurs.

Nonabsorbable Sutures and Other Closure Materials

Nonabsorbable suture material is left in the wound site until healing is complete. It frequently is used in minor surgical procedures performed in the medical office because most of the suturing required is superficial, and it can be used in areas where sutures can be removed after healing has taken place. Silk is a common nonabsorbable suture material because it is strong and easy to tie. It is treated with a coating to prevent tissue drag and flaking. Polyester fiber sutures (e.g., Dacron and Prolene) are among the strongest nonabsorbable sutures, along with surgical steel. These fine filaments are braided and have great tensile strength. Nylon suture is strong and has a high degree of elasticity. It is used primarily for skin closure. Owing to its elasticity and stiffness, many knots must be used because the knots tend to untie if placed incorrectly.

Surgical staples can also be used for skin closure. They are made of stainless steel or titanium and are available in different sizes. Surgical staples are applied (Figure 49-25) and removed (Figure 49-26) with specific staple instruments.

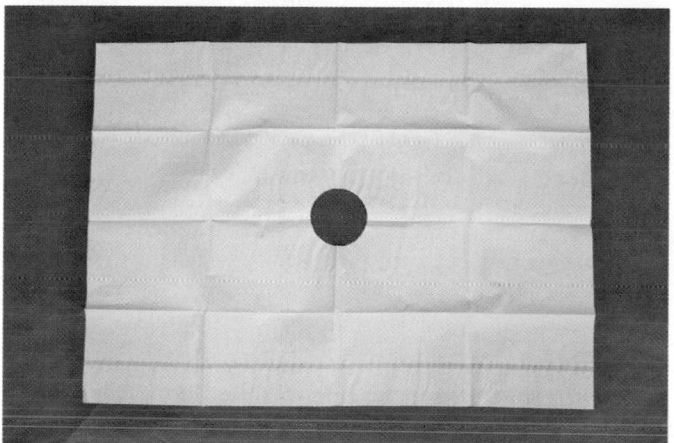

FIGURE 49-23 Fenestrated drape.

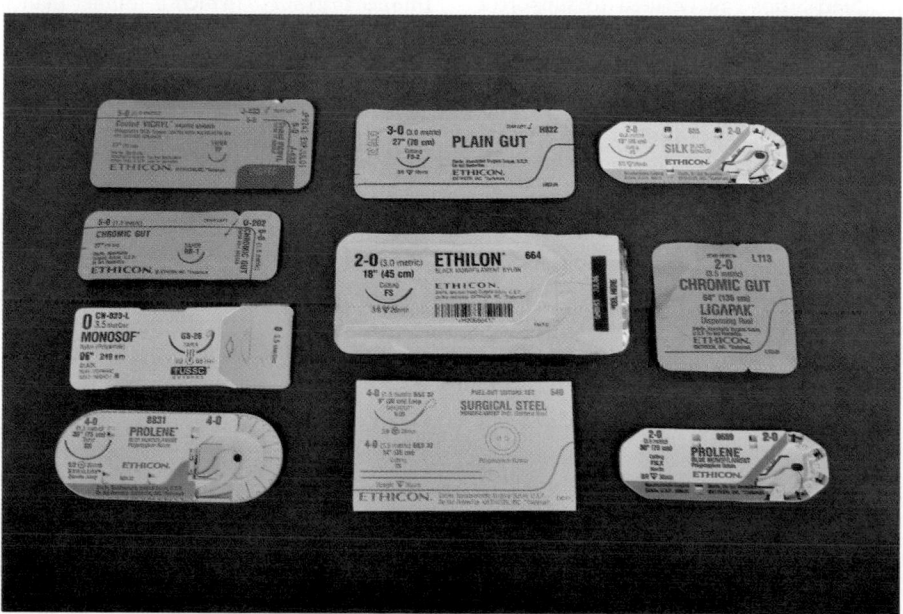

FIGURE 49-24 Suture packets labeled according to size, type, length, and type of needle point and shape.

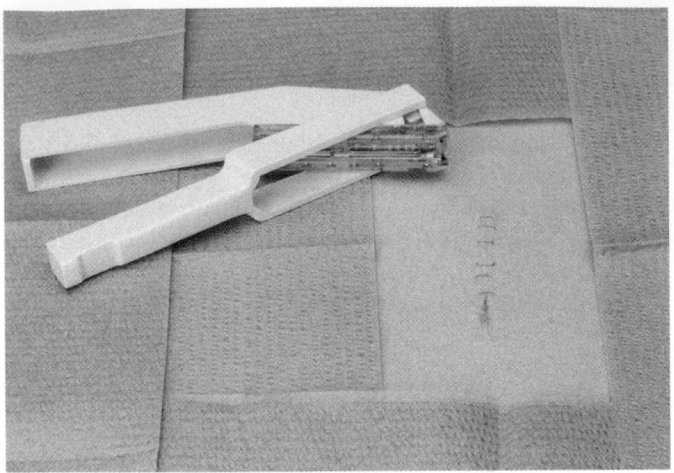

FIGURE 49-25 Disposable skin stapler.

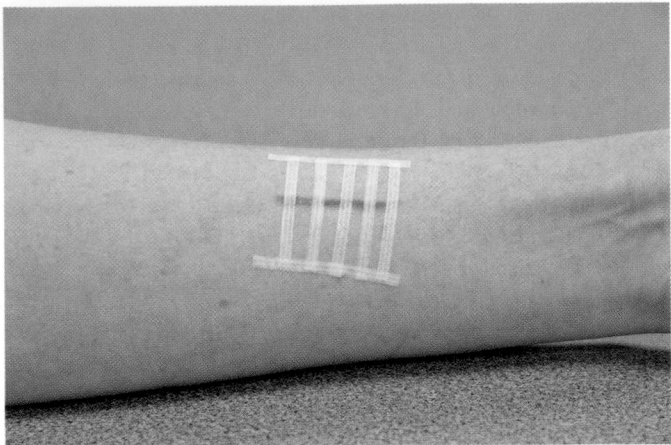

FIGURE 49-27 Wound closed with Steri-Strips.

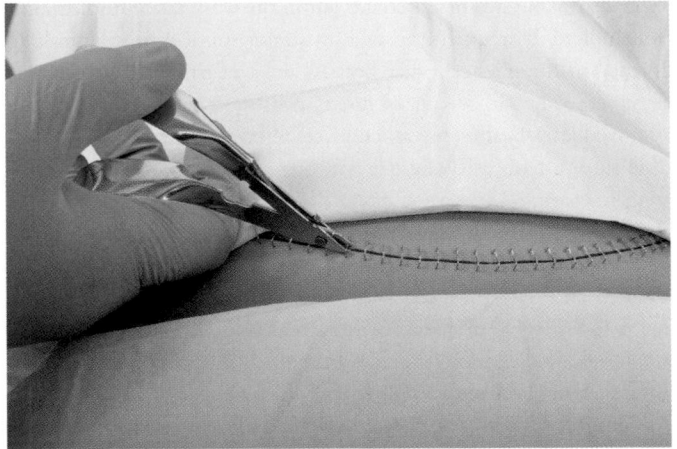

FIGURE 49-26 Surgical staple remover.

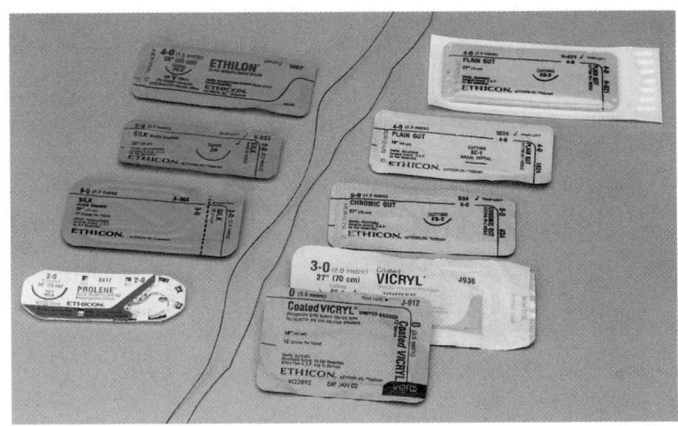

FIGURE 49-28 Suture packets (and opened suture strands) with and without needles.

Another technique for wound closure is the use of Steri-Strips, which are self-adhesive tapes that are placed over the wound, pulling the wound edges together. Steri-Strips can be used to support a wound if there is potential tension at the site or for superficial wounds (Figure 49-27). Tissue adhesives, similar to glue, can also be used for superficial wounds. Examples of tissue adhesives are Histoacryl, Dermabond, and SurgiSeal. Tissue adhesives form a strong bond across wound edges, allowing normal healing to occur below. Some of the advantages of tissue adhesives include the following:

- Saves time during wound repair
- Creates a flexible, water-resistant protective coating for the wound
- Eliminates the need for suture removal
- Results in better cosmetic outcomes because there is no scarring from suture entry
- May also be used on larger wounds for which subcutaneous sutures are needed
- Especially helpful in pediatric patients or individuals afraid of needles

Suture Sizing and Packaging

Suture material is available in a variety of diameters and lengths. The diameter of the suture strand determines its size; the smaller gauges

are numbered below 0 (pronounced *aught*), and the larger gauges are identified with numbers above 0. For instance, 2-0 suture is thinner than size 0, which is thinner than size 2. The sizes from 2-0 to 6-0 are used most frequently in the medical office. The length of the suture material may vary, with strands precut in 18-, 24-, 54-, and 60-inch lengths (Figure 49-28).

Suture Sizes*	
SUTURE SIZE	**DIAMETER**
6-0	0.07 mm
5-0	0.10 mm
4-0	0.15 mm
3-0	0.20 mm
2-0	0.30 mm
0	0.35 mm
1	0.40 mm
2	0.50 mm

*Sutures are sized according to the U.S. Pharmacopoeia (USP) scale.

Needles

Surgical needles are chosen according to the area in which they are to be used and the depth and width of the desired suture. They are classified according to shape, which may be straight or curved. Most sutures are applied with curved needles because they allow the provider to penetrate the surface and then come back up on the other side. The sharper the curve of the needle, the deeper the provider can pass it into the tissue. The point of a needle can be a taper or a cutting edge. A taper is used on delicate tissues. The cutting edge needle is used on the skin. It lacerates the skin as the needle is passed through. This is advantageous on tougher tissues, such as connective tissue.

Needles are manufactured with the suture material attached, or *swaged*, to the needle. These atraumatic needles do not have an eyelet and cause the least amount of trauma as they are passed through the tissue. Manufacturers package suture strands with the suture needle attached in peel-apart sterile, disposable packages. These may be obtained as single, individually packed or as multipack sutures in a variety of needle types and sizes with a wide range of suture materials and lengths. The most common needle type for minor skin repair is the curved, cutting edge, swaged needle (Figure 49-29).

CLOSING COMMENTS

Patient Education

Patients may have questions about the instruments the provider will use, and the medical assistant can help allay patients' fears by answering these questions. Explaining the patient preparation for the procedure, how the procedure will be performed, and what to expect afterward helps make the procedure go more smoothly and encourages the patient to follow the provider's advice and orders.

Legal and Ethical Issues

It is imperative that medical assistants be knowledgeable about their legal responsibilities in surgical procedures done in the ambulatory care center. The medical assistant must know what surgery is planned and whether the patient has been informed about the procedure. In

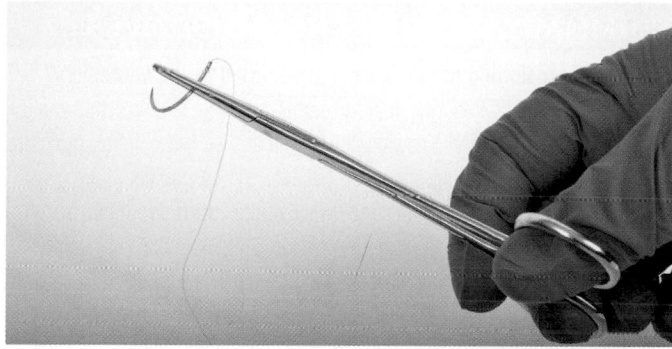

FIGURE 49-29 Suture needle with swaged suture material.

the surgical setting, the medical assistant must realize the full extent of his or her role as the patient's advocate and the provider's agent.

The medical assistant should confirm that the physician has explained the procedure to the patient and that the patient has signed an informed consent. Clarify that the patient understands all aspects of the procedure and has no question before the procedure begins. The better the patient understands the procedure, the greater the likelihood that he or she will comply with presurgical preparations and postsurgical care.

Professional Behaviors

Performing medical assistant duties responsibly and accurately is crucial in the surgical area of the ambulatory care setting. The provider relies on the medical assistant to have the appropriate supplies and instruments available before a procedure begins. To achieve this goal, the medical assistant must have a working knowledge of the typical instruments and supplies used in the facility, in addition to an understanding of the types of instruments needed for each procedure. Medical assistants must make sure tasks are completed according to the facility's policies and procedures so that they are able to assist the provider and protect the patient.

SUMMARY OF SCENARIO

Tom has worked for Dr. Samanski for 2 years and is familiar with her preferences in surgical solutions, local anesthetics, and suture materials, in addition to the typical instruments used in her practice. He also has worked hard to update the policies and procedures manual to include standards for instrument care so that other medical assistants in the office will know how instruments should be sanitized, disinfected, inspected, and prepared for the autoclave. Tom realizes

he needs to continue his education in surgical procedures and takes advantage of professional workshops on the topic. He and Dr. Samanski work well together in the minor surgery area of the office, and Tom consistently attempts to stay up to date on surgical advances and also the medications and instruments Dr. Samanski uses in her practice.

SUMMARY OF LEARNING OBJECTIVES

1. **Define, spell, and pronounce the terms listed in the vocabulary.**
   Spelling and pronouncing medical terms correctly reinforce the medical assistant's credibility. Knowing the definitions of these terms promotes confidence in communication with patients and co-workers.

2. **Describe typical solutions and medications used in minor surgical procedures.**
   Solutions used in minor surgery include sterile water for mixing with medications or rinsing instruments; sterile saline for injection or wound irrigation; antiseptic skin cleansers (e.g., Triseptin, Hibiclens, Betadine) for site preparation; and local anesthetics, including Exactacain topical applications, in addition to lidocaine, Nesacaine, or Sensorcaine injectables. These local anesthetics may come packaged with or without epinephrine. The provider also may use topical silver nitrate to control local bleeding.

3. **Summarize methods for identifying surgical instruments used in minor office surgery, and then identify surgical instruments.**
   Refer to Procedure 49-1.

4. **Outline the general classifications of surgical instruments.**
   Surgical instruments are classified according to their use as cutting, grasping, retracting, probing, or dilating tools. The components of the instrument include the type of handle, the closing mechanism, and the jaws. Instrument tips may be either straight or curved and toothed or not toothed. The instruments used in minor surgical procedures depend on the type of procedure and the provider's preference. Specialty instruments are used in specialty practices (e.g., gynecology, ophthalmology, otolaryngology) and for particular procedures (e.g., biopsies).

5. **Describe the care and handling of surgical instruments.**
   Surgical instruments are expensive and must be cared for properly to maintain function and maximize life. Instruments must be examined when purchased for proper working order and possible faults with mechanisms. Stainless steel instruments should be kept separate from other metal types. Each instrument must be cleaned according to the manufacturer's guidelines, unlocked, and disinfected immediately after use. Most instruments can be cleaned with an ultrasonic washer, which helps prevent injuries.

6. **Identify drapes and different types of sutures and surgical needles.**
   Suture material is available as absorbable (for internal sutures) and nonabsorbable (for skin closure). Dexon, PDS, and Maxon are popular absorbable materials; nonabsorbable sutures can be made of silk or nylon, or staples can be used. Tissue adhesives, similar to glue, can also be used for superficial wounds. Suture materials range in size from smaller gauges (i.e., below 0 [aught] for finer tissues) to thicker gauges (above 0) and are available in various lengths. Surgical needles are either straight or curved. Most needles are manufactured with swaged suture material.

7. **Explain the medical assistant's responsibility to help ease patients' concerns about procedures.**
   The medical assistant can help ease the patient's fears by answering his or her questions. Explaining the patient preparation for a procedure, how the procedure will be performed, and what to expect afterward helps make the procedure go more smoothly and encourages the patient to follow the provider's advice and orders. In the surgical setting, the medical assistant must realize the full extent of his or her role as the patient's advocate and the provider's agent.

CONNECTIONS

📖 Study Guide Connection: Go to the Chapter 49 Study Guide. Read and complete the activities.

ℓVOℓVℓ Evolve Connection: Go to the Chapter 49 link at *evolve.elsevier.com/kinn* to complete the Chapter Review Quiz. Check out the other resources listed for this chapter to make the most of what you have learned from Surgical Supplies and Instruments.

SURGICAL ASEPSIS AND ASSISTING WITH SURGICAL PROCEDURES

50

SCENARIO

Melissa Gelbart, CMA (AAMA), works for a dermatologist, Dr. Susan Armstrong, who frequently performs minor surgical procedures in the office. Melissa was hired to work as an administrative medical assistant at the front desk, but one of the clinical medical assistants has unexpectedly quit, and the office manager has offered Melissa the position. Melissa is excited about this opportunity, but she also is concerned about her skill level in sterile procedures. At least she is familiar with a number of the patients, most of the staff, and the types of outpatient surgeries performed in the facility. Surgical asepsis and assisting with surgery were her favorite topics when she was in medical assisting school. However, before she can assist with surgeries, Melissa must demonstrate her ability to set up a sterile field without contaminating the site. She also must show that she can perform wound care skills, including applying sterile dressings and changing bandages.

While studying this chapter, think about the following questions:

- What are the crucial steps Melissa must follow to set up and maintain a sterile field?
- How does an autoclave work and what are the important rules to remember when preparing surgical trays for the autoclave and correctly operating the machine?
- How will Melissa know whether surgical trays processed in the autoclave are actually sterile?
- What techniques must Melissa follow to prepare for and assist with a surgical procedure?

- What are common surgical procedures performed in an ambulatory care facility?
- What is the medical assistant's role in preparing the patient, equipment, and room for a surgical procedure?
- Why is it important that Melissa understand and be prepared to answer patients' questions about the process of wound healing?
- What bandaging techniques should Melissa be prepared to perform?

LEARNING OBJECTIVES

1. Define, spell, and pronounce the terms listed in the vocabulary.
2. Define the concepts of aseptic technique.
3. Explain the differences between sanitization, disinfection, and sterilization.
4. Summarize tips for improving autoclave techniques; demonstrate how to prepare items for autoclave sterilization.
5. Explain how to wrap materials and discuss the types and uses of sterilization indicators.
6. Summarize the correct methods of loading, operating, and unloading an autoclave.
7. Summarize common minor surgical procedures.
8. Detail the medical assistant's role in minor office surgery.
9. Explain how to perform skin prep for surgery and how to perform a surgical hand scrub.

10. Outline the rules for setting up and maintaining a sterile field; explain how to perform the following procedures related to sterile techniques:
    - Open a sterile pack and create a sterile field.
    - Transfer sterile instruments and pour solutions into a sterile field.
    - Demonstrate how to apply sterile gloves without contaminating them.
11. Discuss how to assist the physician during surgery and demonstrate how to assist with a minor surgical procedure and suturing.
12. Summarize postoperative instructions and explain how to remove sutures and surgical staples.
13. Explain the process of wound healing.
14. Explain how to properly apply dressings and bandages to surgical sites.
15. Conduct patient education in aseptic technique and surgical procedures and discuss the legal and ethical concerns regarding surgical asepsis and infection control.

*A*sepsis is the condition of being free of **infection** or infectious material. *Medical asepsis* is the destruction of organisms after they leave the body. The principles of medical asepsis are implemented to prevent reinfection of a patient and cross-infection of another patient or ourselves. To prevent cross-contamination, potential microorganisms and pathogens must be isolated by following standard blood and body fluid precautions and by sanitizing, disinfecting, and/or sterilizing objects as soon as possible after they become contaminated. Medical asepsis is the process of either reducing the number of pathogens or destroying them; this creates an environment that is clean but not *sterile* (i.e., free of microorganisms).

Surgical asepsis is the complete destruction of organisms on instruments or equipment that will enter the patient's body. This technique is mandatory for any procedure that invades the body's skin or tissues, such as surgery. In surgical asepsis, everything that comes in contact with the surgical site must be sterile, including surgical gowns, drapes, instruments, and the gloved hands of the surgeon and surgical assistants. Anytime the skin or a mucous membrane is punctured or pierced, as in venipunctures or injections, surgical aseptic techniques must be practiced. Urinary catheterizations, biopsies, and dressing changes on open wounds are performed using sterile technique.

A medical assistant must develop an inner sense of sterile procedures. It is important that these techniques be performed on such a routine basis that they become an unbreakable habit. Conscientious attention must be given to sterilizing all items at all times. Frequent checking and rechecking of procedures helps ensure that they are effective and are used without any "breaks" in technique. Single-use, disposable items offer the best method of infection control, and are used frequently in medical facilities. However, when disposable equipment is used, the assistant must know the specific disposal guidelines for contaminated instruments and supplies.

STERILIZATION

Before an instrument or piece of equipment can be used in a surgical procedure, it first must be sanitized, then disinfected, and finally sterilized to remove all forms of microorganisms. It is essential that you understand the concepts of sanitization and disinfection before learning **sterilization** methods. Written sanitization, disinfection, and sterilization procedures should be in place for each workplace.

Utility Room

To ensure proper sterilization for surgical aseptic procedures, an area should be set aside for just this purpose. The area should be divided into two sections, one dirty and one clean. The dirty section is used for receiving contaminated instruments and other materials at the conclusion of surgical procedures. This area should have a sink, receiving basins, proper sanitizing and disinfecting agents, brushes, utility gloves, autoclave wrapping paper or cloth, autoclave envelopes and tape, sterilizer indicators, and disposable gloves. Designated biohazardous waste containers are needed for gloves worn when handling contaminated items. Personal protective equipment (PPE) for sanitization, disinfection, and autoclave procedures includes:

- Fluid-resistant gloves to prevent contact with contaminants
- A laboratory coat or impervious gown, if needed, to protect against splashes
- A face shield and/or goggles if a splash hazard exists
- Heat-resistant autoclave gloves for unloading

The clean section of the utility room should be reserved for receiving the sterile items after they have been removed from the autoclave. Clear, clean plastic bags in which to store sterile packs may be kept in the clean area. Both areas should be spotlessly clean and well organized.

Instruments and other items used in ambulatory surgery, examination, or treatment must be carefully cleaned before proceeding with the steps of disinfection or sterilization. *Sanitization* is the cleansing process that removes organic material and reduces the number of microorganisms to a safe level, as dictated in public health guidelines. This cleansing process removes debris, such as blood and other body fluids, from instruments or equipment. Sanitization should be completed immediately after instruments are used, in a separate workroom or area or on the "dirty" side of the utility room to prevent cross-contamination of clean instruments and equipment. If it is not possible to sanitize instruments immediately after a procedure, rinse them under cold water immediately after their use and place them in a low-sudsing, rust-inhibiting, enzyme-containing detergent solution. Blood and debris must be removed so that later disinfection with chemicals and/or sterilization can penetrate to all the instruments' surfaces. Never allow blood or other substances that can coagulate to dry on an instrument.

The medical assistant should always wear gloves while performing sanitization (thick utility gloves if the instruments have sharp or pointed edges) to prevent possible personal contamination with potentially infectious body fluids that may be present on the articles being cleaned. When you are ready to sanitize instruments, drain off the soaking solution and rinse each instrument in cold, running water.

Clean all sharp instruments at one time, when you can concentrate on preventing injury to yourself. Open all hinges and scrub serrations and ratchets with a small scrub brush or toothbrush.

Rinse the instruments in hot water and then check carefully that they are in proper working order before they are disinfected or sterilized. The items should be hand dried with a towel to prevent spotting.

Disinfection is the process of killing pathogenic organisms or of rendering them inactive. Many types of disinfecting agents are available and have varying degrees of effectiveness. It is important to follow the manufacturer's guidelines on how to use each product properly and to understand its advantages and disadvantages and possible sources of error. Disinfectants are used on equipment that cannot be sterilized (e.g., blood pressure cuffs and stethoscopes); countertops and other physical surfaces in the healthcare facility; and for soaking instruments and equipment before sterilization.

CRITICAL THINKING APPLICATION   **50-1**

The office manager told Melissa she needs to review the office policy and procedures manual on sanitization, disinfection, and sterilization methods. Why is this important to accomplish before Melissa starts performing sterilization procedures? What information in this manual would be most important to Melissa as she starts this new position? Why?

Autoclave

Sterilization can be achieved by moist heat in an autoclave, dry heat, ultraviolet or ionizing radiation, gas, or with chemicals. Medical facilities typically use the autoclave method. Steam under pressure in the autoclave (Figure 50-1) is an excellent method of sterilization because it kills all pathogens and spores.

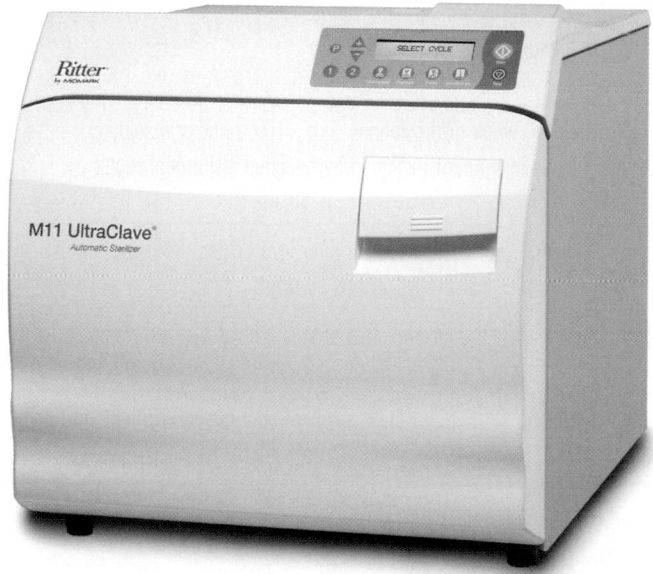

FIGURE 50-1 Steam autoclave. (Courtesy Midmark Corp., Dayton, Ohio.)

Pressurized steam is fast, convenient, and dependable. The pressure allows for heat higher than the boiling point, and when combined with moisture, these two factors create a very effective mechanism for killing all microorganisms. When steam is admitted into the autoclave chamber, it simultaneously heats and wets the object, coagulating the proteins present in all living organisms. When the cycle is complete and the chamber has cooled, the steam condenses and explodes the cells of microorganisms, thus destroying them. To be effective, the steam moisture must come in contact with all surfaces being sterilized. Steam under pressure is capable of much faster penetration of fabrics and textiles than dry heat, but its use has definite limitations if the proper techniques are not followed.

The recommended temperature for sterilization in an autoclave is 121° to 123°C (250° to 255°F). Follow the guidelines that come with the autoclave in use, but in general unwrapped items are sterilized for 20 minutes, small wrapped items for 30 minutes, and large or tightly wrapped items for 40 minutes. Processing time starts *after* the autoclave reaches normal operating conditions of 121°C (250°F) and 15 pounds per square inch (psi) pressure. There are different autoclave cycles for different materials; ambulatory care facilities do not autoclave liquids or dressing material, so the most used will be the gravity cycle, which is used to sterilize stainless steel instruments. In the *gravity* (*"fast exhaust"*) *cycle* the autoclave fills with steam and is held at a set temperature for a set period. When the cycle is complete, a valve opens and the chamber rapidly returns to atmospheric pressure. Drying time may be added to the end of the cycle. Incorrect operation of an autoclave may result in superheated steam. If steam is brought to too high a temperature, it is literally dried out, and the advantage of a higher heat is diminished. Wet steam is another cause of incomplete sterilization. Wet steam results from failing to preheat the chamber, which causes excessive condensation in the interior of the chamber. Condensation is necessary, but too much prevents the sterilization process from being completed properly. It can be compared with taking a hot shower in a cold bathroom, which results in heavily steamed mirrors, walls, and towels. If packs become too saturated to dry during the drying cycle, the packs pick up and absorb bacteria from the air or any surface on which they are placed after removal from the autoclave. Placing cold instruments in a hot chamber also increases condensation. Other causes of wet steam include opening the door too wide at the end of the cycle or allowing a rush of cold air into the chamber. Overfilling the water reservoir may produce this same effect (Table 50-1).

The main cause of incomplete sterilization in the autoclave is the presence of residual air. Without the complete elimination of air, an adequately high temperature cannot be reached. Air and steam do not mix. Because air is heavier than steam, it pools wherever possible. One tenth of 1% (0.1%) residual air trapped around an instrument prevents complete sterilization. This is especially dangerous in older autoclaves that do not have a chamber thermometer separate from the pressure gauge. Adequate chamber pressure does not guarantee a proper chamber temperature. Table 50-2 provides tips for improving autoclave techniques.

Wrapping Materials

Maintenance of sterility depends completely on the wrapper and method of wrapping (Procedure 50-1). The wrapping material

TABLE 50-1   Common Factors Influencing the Effectiveness of Sterilization

CAUSES	POTENTIAL PROBLEM
Improper sanitization of instruments	Protein and salt debris may prevent direct contact with pressurized steam and heat in the autoclave.
Improper packaging	Prevents penetration of the sterilizing agent; packing material may melt.
Wrong packaging material for the method of sterilization	Decreases penetration of the steam and heat.
Excessive packaging material	
Improper loading of the sterilizer Overloading	Increases heat-up time and decreases penetration of pressurized steam and heat to the center of the sterilizer load.
No separation between packages, even without overloading	May prevent or decrease thorough contact of the sterilizing agent with all the items in the chamber.
Improper timing and temperature Incorrect operation of the sterilizer	Insufficient time at proper temperature to kill organisms.

Adapted from CDC: Infection Control. Accessed 2/25/15. http://www.cdc.gov/oralhealth/infectioncontrol/faq/sterilization_monitoring.htm

TABLE 50-2   Tips for Improving Autoclave Techniques

PROBLEM	CAUSES	CORRECTION
Damp autoclave paper	Clogged chamber drain; goods removed from chamber too soon after cycle; improper loading	Remove strainer; free openings of lint. Allow goods to remain in sterilizer an additional 15 min with door slightly open. Place packs on edge; arrange for least possible resistance to flow of steam and air.
Stained autoclave paper	Dirty chamber	Clean chamber with mild detergent solution; never use strong abrasives, such as steel wool; rinse thoroughly after cleaning.
Corroded instruments	Poor cleaning; residual soil; exposure to hard chemicals (e.g., iodine, salt, and acids); inferior instruments	Improve cleaning; do not allow soil to dry on instruments; sanitize first. Do not expose instruments to these chemicals; if exposure occurs, rinse immediately. Use only top-quality instruments.
Spotted or stained instruments	Mineral deposits on instruments; residual detergents from cleaning; mineral deposits from tap water	Wash with soft soap and detergent with good wetting properties. Rinse instruments thoroughly with distilled water.
Instruments with soft hinges or joints	Corrosion or soil in joint; instrument parts out of alignment	Clean with warm, weak acid solutions (e.g., 10% nitric acid solution); rinse thoroughly. Have instrument realigned by qualified instrument repair professional.
Ebullition, or caps that blow off solutions	Too rapid exhausting of chamber	Use slow exhaust, cool liquids, or turn autoclave off and let it cool on its own; that is, let the pressure drop at its own rate.
Steam leakage	Worn gasket; door closes improperly	Replace gasket; reopen door and shut carefully; have serviced if unable to close door properly.
Chamber door does not open	Vacuum in chamber (check chamber pressure gauge)	Turn on controls to start steam pressure; wait until equalized, then vent and open door.

must be permeable to steam but impervious to contaminants. Acceptable wrapping materials for autoclaving should be made of a substance that allows the steam to penetrate and also prevents pathogens from entering during storage and handling. A wrapper should not be used if it is torn or has a hole in it. The types of wrapping material used for instruments that are to be autoclaved are disposable double-ply autoclave paper and peel-apart polypropylene bags (Figure 50-2). Multiple layers of autoclave paper are recommended to maintain the integrity of sterilization during handling and storage of autoclaved instrument packs. Double-layered autoclave paper provides these multiple layers of protection for surgical instruments from contamination and saves time because wrapping is done only once.

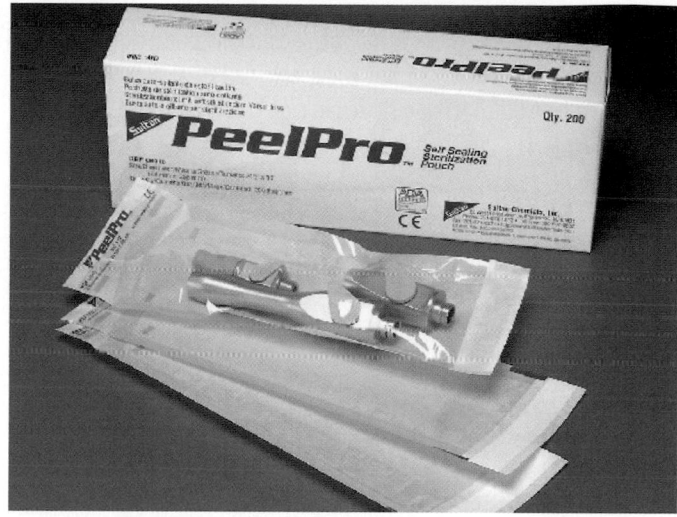

FIGURE 50-2 Sterilization pouches with sterilization indicators on the outside and inside of the envelope. The puncture-resistant, tinted plastic front is safety sealed to an autoclave paper backing. (Courtesy Practicon Dental, Greenville, North Carolina.)

PROCEDURE 50-1	Prepare Items for Autoclaving: Wrap Instruments and Supplies for Sterilization in an Autoclave

Goal: To place dry, inspected, sanitized, and disinfected supplies and instruments inside appropriate wrapping materials for sterilization and storage without contamination.

EQUIPMENT and SUPPLIES

- Dry, inspected, sanitized, and disinfected instruments
- Double-ply autoclave paper
- Autoclave tape
- Sterilization strip
- Biologic sterilization indicator
- Waterproof, felt-tipped pen
- Disposable gloves (if part of office policy)

PROCEDURAL STEPS

1. Sanitize your hands. Collect and assemble already inspected, sanitized instruments to be wrapped. Gloves may be worn.
2. Place the double-ply autoclave paper on a clean, flat surface.
3. Place the instruments diagonally at the approximate center of the double-ply autoclave paper. Make sure the size of the square is large enough for the items (Figure 1).
   <u>PURPOSE:</u> Each of the four corners must fold over and completely cover the instruments, with a few extra inches of overlap for folding.
4. Open any hinged instruments. If the instrument is sharp, its teeth or tip should be shielded with cotton or gauze.
   <u>PURPOSE:</u> To prevent puncture of the package or injury to the operator.

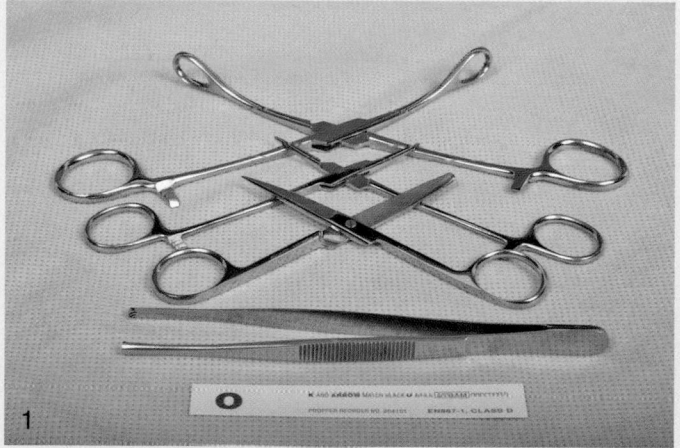

5. Depending on clinic policy, a biologic sterilization indicator or sterilization strip should be placed in the center of the pack to check for sterilization standards.
   <u>PURPOSE:</u> To ensure that the autoclave is reaching effective levels of heat and pressure to destroy all microorganisms.

6. Bring up the bottom corner of the wrap and fold back a portion of it.
PURPOSE: This folded-back flap is the only part of each wrapper corner that can be touched when a sterile package is opened (Figure 2).

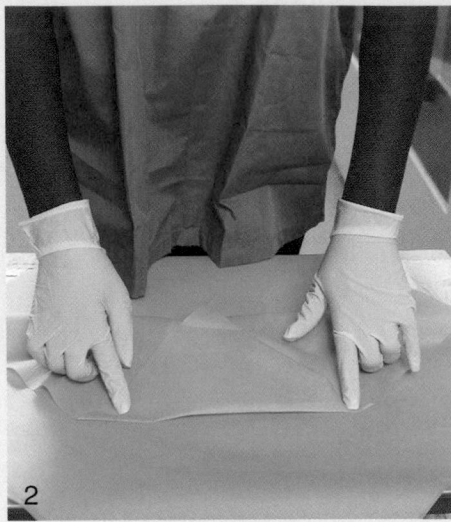

2

7. Repeat the previous step with each corner, making sure to turn back a portion each time (Figures 3 and 4).

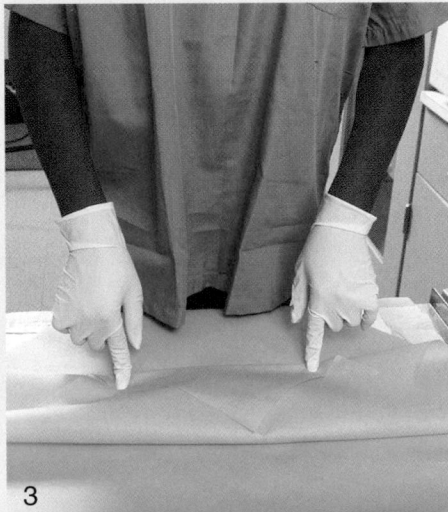

3

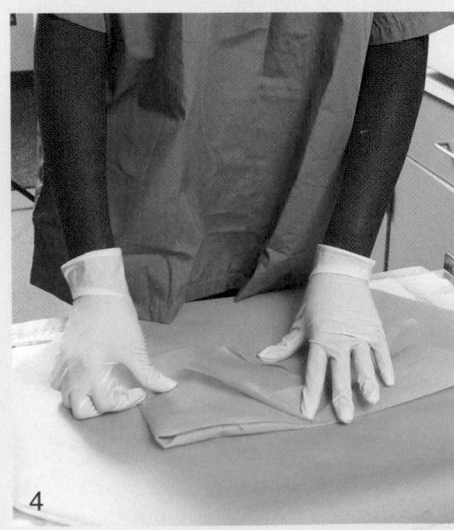

4

8. Fold the last flap over (Figure 5).

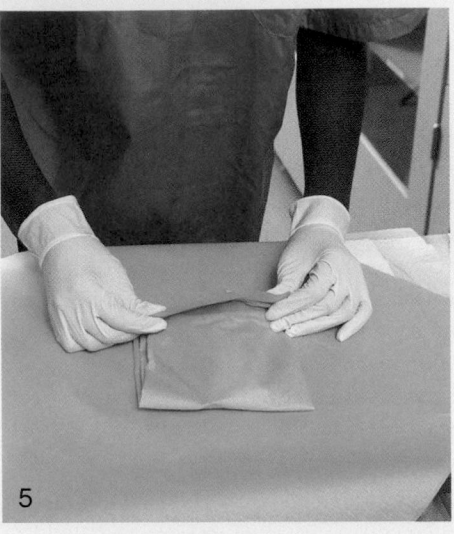

5

9. Secure with autoclave tape (Figure 6) and label the package with the date, including the year, contents, and your initials (Figure 7).
PURPOSE: So that staff members will know what is in the pack, when it was autoclaved, and who performed the task.

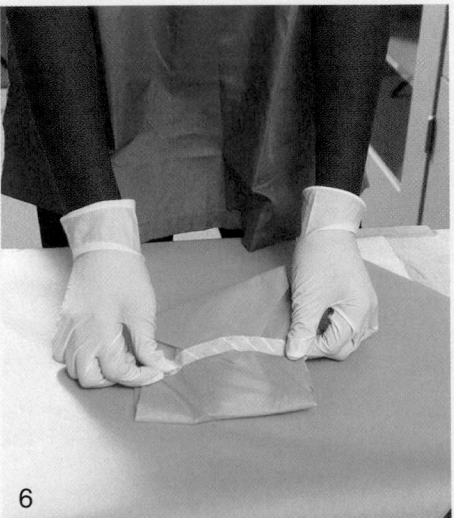

6

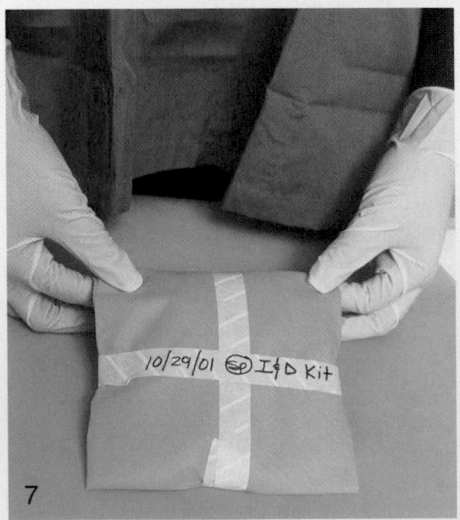

7

Wrapping Instruments

The method used to wrap instruments for autoclave sterilization must allow the pack to be opened without becoming contaminated. The rules for protecting package contents include the following:

- Discard autoclave paper that is torn or has holes.
- Wrap all hinged instruments in the open position to allow full steam penetration of the joint.
- Place a gauze sponge around the tips of sharp instruments to prevent them from piercing the wrapping material.
- If a number of instruments are to be placed on a stainless steel tray for wrapping, first place a double-folded towel on the tray, and then position the instruments. This helps to protect them.
- Polypropylene is a plastic capable of withstanding autoclaving but is resistant to heat transfer. Therefore materials in a polypropylene pan take longer to autoclave than the same materials in a stainless steel pan.
- When using sterilizing bags, insert the handles of the instruments into the end of the bag that will be opened first to ensure that the grasping end of the instrument can be reached easily when the bag is opened.
- When using two-ply autoclave paper, seal the paper with specialized autoclave tape.
- Indicate on the wrapper what is in the package or label it with a code. This code should correspond with a list of instruments that are stored with the pack after sterilization.
- Label each pack according to the instrument contents, sterilization date, and your initials. Use a permanent marker; never use a ballpoint pen.
- Whether you are wrapping one item or many items together on a tray as a surgical pack, the procedure is the same; be sure the wrapper is large enough to cover the items to be sterilized.

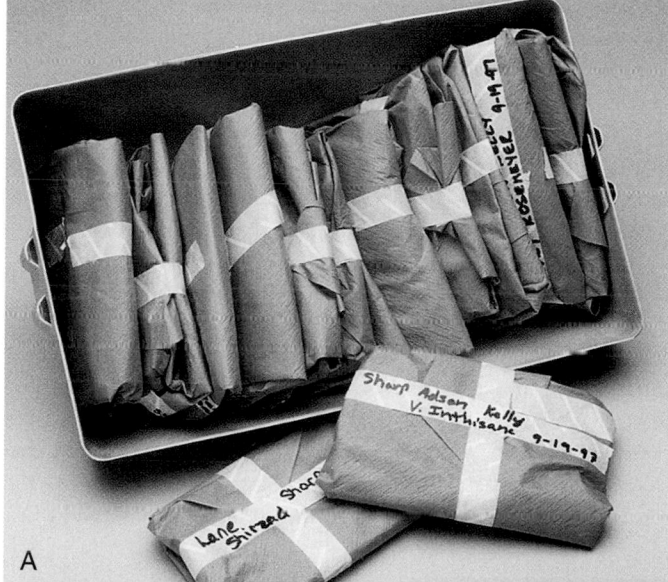

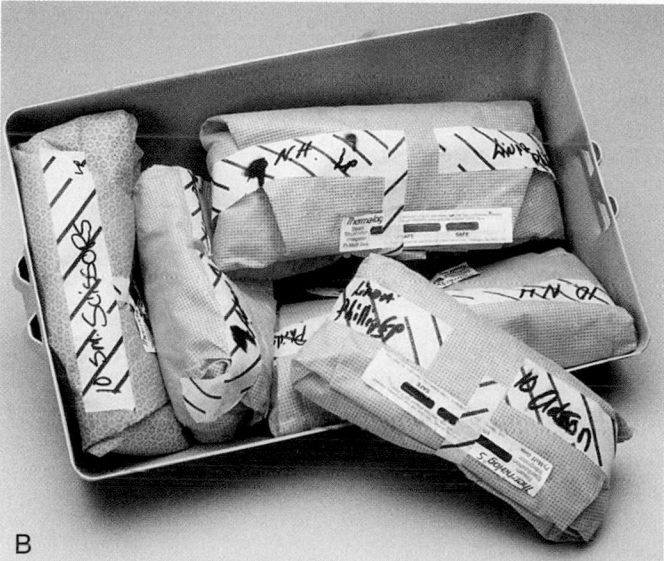

FIGURE 50-3 A, Instrument packs wrapped with autoclave paper and autoclave tape before the autoclave procedure. **B,** Instrument packs after autoclaving. Note the difference in the chemical lines on the autoclave tape.

CRITICAL THINKING APPLICATION   **50-2**

Melissa is processing instruments and trays when she notices that one of her co-workers never places gauze sponge around the tips of sharp instruments before wrapping a pack. She also notices that not all of the packs are labeled properly. What is the significance of Melissa's observation? How should she handle this situation? Why?

Sterilization Indicators

Sterilization is achieved only when steam reaches the optimum temperature for a designated length of time and has penetrated to the center of the articles. Sterilization indicators must be used routinely to determine whether all microorganisms have been destroyed. The two basic types of sterilization indicators are chemical indicators (e.g., autoclave tape) and biologic indicators.

Chemical Sterilization Indicators. Autoclave tape, a commonly used sterilization indicator, contains a chemical dye that changes color when exposed to steam (Figure 50-3). The tape is not an absolute indication that the proper sterilization time, temperature, and steam have been maintained; it merely indicates that a high temperature was reached while the article was in the autoclave. The tape strip must completely change color (colors vary by manufac-

turer) or reveal the word "autoclaved" to ensure effective operation. The main function of autoclave tape, besides holding the wrapping material together or closing a sterilization bag, is to verify at a glance that the package was autoclaved. Internal chemical indicators are placed inside the instrument packages to verify steam and heat penetration of the wrapping. Some instruments are autoclaved unwrapped, such as stainless steel vaginal speculums. A chemical indicator should be placed in the autoclave with unwrapped instruments in an area most difficult for steam to access, such as under the tray or between the instruments.

Biologic Sterilization Indicators. Biologic indicators should be used each day the autoclave is in use. Spore strip indicators have been replaced by rapid-readout biologic indicators that use ampules of *Bacillus stearothermophilus,* which is destroyed at 121°C (250°F). The ampule is placed in the center of the largest pack that is autoclaved in the facility to determine the accuracy of the autoclave and autoclave procedures in destroying all microbes. On completion of the cycle, the ampule is sent to a laboratory for analysis of any type of microbial growth. If tests show that microbes are present in the sample then a report is sent to the facility notifying them that the autoclave, or possibly their sterilization procedures, are not effective in achieving sterilization. Results from the biologic indicator testing must be documented. Failed tests must be investigated and the causes resolved.

Quality-Assurance Records for Office Sterilization

Every office should have specific protocols to follow for quality-assurance evaluations of the autoclave. This is done at specified intervals, depending on the volume and frequency of autoclave use. A log must be kept of the type of control test done, when it was performed, and the testing results. If the testing results indicate that sterilization was inadequate, a report must be made and filed. The report should identify the nature of the problem and how and when

it was corrected. The report also should contain proof of correction by indicating the date and time of a first, subsequent and successful sterilization run.

Loading the Autoclave

Prepare all packs and arrange the load in a way that allows maximum circulation of steam and heat (Procedure 50-2). Articles should be resting on their edges and should not be crowded. Placing the packs in stainless steel racks prevents packing of the autoclave too tightly. Instruments may be autoclaved unwrapped if they do not need to be sterile when used later. For example, although vaginal speculums do not need to be sterilized for use (the vagina is a body cavity that is naturally open to the external environment), they must be sanitized, disinfected, and sterilized to prevent cross-contamination among patients. They can be placed unwrapped on a perforated stainless steel tray in the autoclave and then stored in a clean area for future use.

PROCEDURE 50-2   Perform Sterilization Procedures: Operate the Autoclave

Goal: *To sterilize properly prepared supplies and instruments using the autoclave.*

EQUIPMENT and SUPPLIES

- Autoclave
- Wrapped items ready to be sterilized
- Heat-resistant gloves

PROCEDURAL STEPS

NOTE: The specific instructions for operating an autoclave may vary based on the model number and manufacturer. Refer to the instructions that accompany the autoclave to be sure the appropriate steps are followed.

1. Check the water level in the reservoir and add distilled water as necessary.
PURPOSE: Too much or too little water may alter the effectiveness of the equipment. Tap water leaves lime deposits in the chamber.
2. Turn the control to "Fill" to allow water to flow into the chamber. The water flows until you turn the control to its next position. Do not let the water overflow.
3. Load the chamber with wrapped items, spacing them for maximum circulation and penetration.
PURPOSE: To ensure sterilization of all items.
4. Close and seal the door.
PURPOSE: The door must be closed, or the heated water in the chamber evaporates.

5. Turn the control setting to "On" or "Autoclave" to start the cycle.
6. Watch the gauges until the temperature gauge reaches at least 121°C (250°F) and the pressure gauge reaches 15 lbs. of pressure.
PURPOSE: The proper temperature and pressure must be reached before sterilization can begin.
7. Set the timer for the desired time.
8. At the end of the timed cycle, turn the control setting to "Vent."
PURPOSE: This releases the steam and pressure. The water at the bottom of the chamber drains back into the reservoir. Newer autoclaves automatically perform this step.
9. Wait for the pressure gauge to reach zero.
10. Standing behind the autoclave door, carefully open the chamber door ¼".
PURPOSE: To allow steam to escape faster. Be careful to prevent accidental burns.
11. Leave the autoclave control at "Vent" to continue releasing heat.
PURPOSE: To dry the items faster.
12. Allow complete drying of all articles.
13. Using heat-resistant gloves, remove the items from the chamber and place the sterilized packages on dry, covered shelves or open the autoclave door and allow the items to cool completely before removal and storage.
14. Turn the control knob to "Off" and keep the door slightly ajar.
PURPOSE: To allow the inside of the autoclave to dry completely.

Unloading Guidelines

When the autoclave's sterilization cycle is complete, release the pressure according to the manufacturer's guidelines. Once the pressure gauge reads "0," stand back from the door and, with heat-resistant gloves, open the door approximately ¼". Allow the load to dry for at least 15 minutes (this time varies according to the type of

autoclave and the size of the load). Capillary attraction is the action that draws moisture through the surface of materials. Packs can act like a sponge, attracting outside moisture and microorganisms. Touching a wet pack allows microorganisms on your hands to penetrate the wrappings, making the contents of the pack nonsterile. Dry, wrapped packs may be removed with clean, dry hands, but it is safer to wear heat-resistant gloves to reduce the possibility of burns from the hot instruments inside the packs. If possible, allow all packs to cool in the autoclave with the door open. Place the packs on a dry, dust-free surface inside an enclosed cupboard or drawer for storage. Do not place the packs on cold surfaces, because hot packs may cause condensation, and moisture will contaminate the contents.

Guidelines for unloading an autoclave include the following:

- Stand behind the door when opening it to prevent accidental steam burns.
- Slowly open the door only a crack, allowing the items to cool for 15 to 20 minutes before removing them.
- If for any reason the integrity of the sterilization process is in question, the load should be considered contaminated and autoclaved again. Reasons for concern include the following:
  - Any load that fails to convert a sterilization indicator strip (autoclave tape)
  - Any loads processed after a biologic test indicates that the autoclave is not working properly

Shelf Life of Sterilized Packs. The Centers for Disease Control and Prevention (CDC) no longer identifies specific time limits for the shelf life of sterilized packs. The general recommendation is that as long as the sterilized items are stored so that the packaging material remains intact and undamaged then the pack is considered sterile. All sterile packs should be stored on dry, dust-free, covered shelves or in drawers. Some facilities continue to date every sterilized package and use shelf-life practices such as first in, first out; other facilities have switched to event-related practices. With event-related practices, items remain sterile until some event (e.g., a pack becomes wet or packing material is torn) causes contamination. The quality of the packaging material, storage conditions, and how much the packs are handled all affect the possibility of contamination. Therefore sterile packs should be inspected before they are used to verify the integrity of wrapping material. Any package that is wet, torn, dropped on the floor, or damaged in any way should be sanitized, disinfected, wrapped in new autoclave paper or placed in new autoclave pouches, and autoclaved again.

CRITICAL THINKING APPLICATION   **50-3**

Melissa discovers a number of packages of paper-wrapped sterile instruments that appear to have water marks on them. The indicator tape shows that they have been autoclaved. What should she do with these packs? Why?

Chemical Sterilization

In the medical office, chemical sterilization is used for instruments that cannot be exposed to the high temperatures of steam sterilization. The sterilizing chemical solution must be mixed exactly according to the instructions on the bottle. The solution must be marked with the date of preparation and expiration. Materials to be sterilized must be submerged in this chemical bath with a closed lid for 8 hours or longer. Items are removed with sterile forceps and must be rinsed with water to remove all traces of the chemical before the

items are used on a patient. You must avoid skin contact with the sterilizing solution because it is very caustic.

The use of chemicals for sterilization is not very practical in the ambulatory facility because the instruments or equipment cannot be wrapped during processing in the liquid chemical so once they are removed from the liquid they are no longer considered sterile. In addition, because of the caustic nature of the chemicals, instruments must be rinsed with water after removal from the chemical fluid. This water is typically not sterile. However, high-level chemical disinfectants do have a place in healthcare because they can be used on instruments (e.g., endoscopes) that would be damaged by autoclaving. Therefore because of the inherent limitations of using liquid chemicals for sterilization, their use should be restricted to reprocessing critical devices that are heat-sensitive and incompatible with other sterilization methods.

SURGICAL PROCEDURES

Common surgical procedures that are routinely performed in the primary care facility include suturing, cyst removal, incision and drainage (I&D) of abscesses, and collection of biopsy specimens. The medical assistant should be proficient in explaining each of these procedures to the patient, preparing the patient and the room, assisting the provider with the surgery, and applying a sterile dressing and bandage after the procedure is finished.

Each surgical procedure requires appropriate skin preparation and draping with a *fenestrated* drape. This is a surgical drape with an opening in the center. The size of the opening depends on the size of the surgical field. The opening is placed directly over the surgical site after the site has been suitably prepared (or "prepped," as it is called in healthcare practice). A minor surgery tray is opened, and a sterile field is created on a Mayo instrument stand. Sutures, scalpels, and any other instruments needed are added to the field, according to the provider's preference. Either an injectable and/or spray local anesthetic should also be ready for the provider's use with the needed injection supplies.

After achieving suitable local anesthesia, the physician opens the skin with an incision. If a cyst is being removed, the physician dissects around it and usually tries to "deliver" it from the wound intact. If the procedure is an I&D, foul matter will start oozing from the wound immediately after the skin is incised. The wound is drained completely and flushed with copious amounts of sterile saline solution. If the procedure is a biopsy, a small amount of tissue is removed and placed in a specimen container with preservative. The specimen container must be carefully labeled with the appropriate patient information, the date, and specifics about the specimen type and location. It then is sent to the laboratory, where it is examined microscopically for changes or abnormalities.

Electrosurgery

Electrosurgery is also known as *electrocautery*. An electrosurgical unit (ESU) uses high-frequency current to cut through tissue and coagulate blood vessels. A small probe with an electric current running through it is used to *cauterize* (i.e., burn or destroy) the tissue. When the electric current comes in contact with tissue and blood cells, they are vaporized, producing carbon and steam. This process seals blood vessels, minimizing cellular oozing and bleeding. Electrosurgery may be used to destroy granulations and small polyps or to take a tissue sample for pathology examination. The loop electrosurgical excision procedure (LEEP) uses a wire loop heated by electric current to remove cells and tissue as part of the diagnosis and treatment of abnormal or cancerous conditions of the uterine cervix.

Necessary components are the ESU's power source, the grounding cable and pad, and the active electrode (i.e., a pencil-like instrument with a tip and cord). The grounding pad is a gel-covered adhesive electrode that provides a safe return path for the electrosurgical current. Electrode tips are disposable and are used according to the type of procedure performed. The two most commonly used tips are the needle and flat designs.

Holding the pencil-like instrument, the provider touches the tissue with the tip and activates the electric current with a switch on the instrument. The electric current is delivered to the tissues, and tissue is vaporized at the site of contact or a specimen can be removed for pathology (Figure 50-4).

Important Tips About the Grounding Pad

- Carefully inspect the pad, cable, and skin before the procedure
- Place the pad close to the operative site
- The pad must be tight against the patient's skin
- Apply the pad to a fleshy area, such as the thigh
- Do not place the pad over a bony area
- Do not place the pad over body hair
- Do not place the pad over metal implants or a pacemaker
- Carefully inspect the pad site on the skin after the procedure for signs of burns

---

Laser Surgery

Laser is an acronym for *l*ight *a*mplification by *s*timulated *e*mission of *r*adiation. Because a laser beam is so small and precise, it can be used to safely treat specific tissue with minimal damage to surrounding tissues and limited scar formation. Lasers were first used in medicine to treat diseases of the retina, and they now are used for many procedures, including excision of lesions, cauterization of blood vessels, removal of warts or moles, and cosmetic surgical procedures.

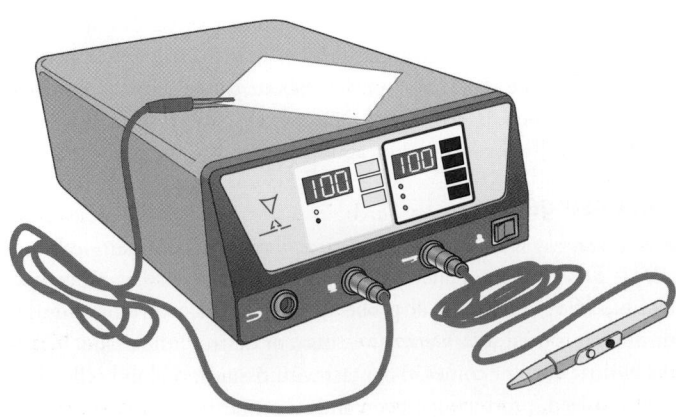

FIGURE 50-4 Electrosurgical unit.

Several types of lasers are used, including the carbon dioxide, yttrium-aluminum-garnet (YAG), and pulsed dye lasers. Each laser has a specific use. The color of the laser light beam is directly related to the type of surgery performed.

A medical assistant must be specially trained to operate a laser before assisting with laser surgery. Laser equipment requires very careful handling, care, and maintenance. Laser light destroys tissue and can harm the patient, the physician, and you if handled improperly. The medical assistant should complete a full laser safety program before assisting in laser procedures. Once trained, the medical assistant's role during laser surgery includes:

- Observing the surgical field through safety goggles for possible contamination and protecting the patient's eyes
- Keeping wet sponges ready
- Removing any flammable item from the laser's path
- Assisting with suctioning of the plume to maintain a clear visual field
- Providing a basin of sterile normal saline solution and a filled irrigating syringe
- Watching each application of the laser beam and anticipating the need for protective supplies, special equipment, or instruments

Microsurgery

Microsurgery involves the use of an operating microscope to perform delicate surgical procedures. One of its major uses is in ophthalmologic surgery. It also is used in otologic, rhinologic and sinus, laryngologic, neurosurgical, microvascular, gynecologic, and genitourinary procedures. A medical assistant must acquire a basic knowledge of the operation and care of a microscope before becoming qualified to assist in these types of procedures.

The basic components of an operating microscope are the light source, eyepieces (also called the *oculars*), lenses, and cord. Accessory pieces include assistant and observer lenses, cameras, video recorders, television monitors, and printers. These are all valuable for documentation and teaching purposes. Disposable sterile drapes and handle covers are used on the microscope during surgical procedures.

Surgical microscopes are expensive, delicate instruments that require extreme care in handling and cleaning. All lenses and cords should be carefully inspected before and after each use.

Endoscopic Procedures

An endoscope is a medical device consisting of a miniature camera mounted on a flexible tube with an optical system and a light source that is used to examine the area inside an organ or cavity. Many types of endoscopes are used, and they are named according to the organs or areas they are used to explore, such as the urinary bladder, bronchus, larynx, colon (Figure 50-5), stomach, uterus, abdomen, and various joints. Small instruments can be used to take samples of suspicious tissues through the endoscope.

Direct visualization with an endoscope is used for diagnostic purposes or to perform surgical procedures. Endoscopes may be rigid (e.g., laparoscope or hysteroscope), semirigid, or flexible (e.g., colonoscopes, bronchoscopes, gastroscopes). All are delicate and expensive and require extreme care in handling to protect them from damage.

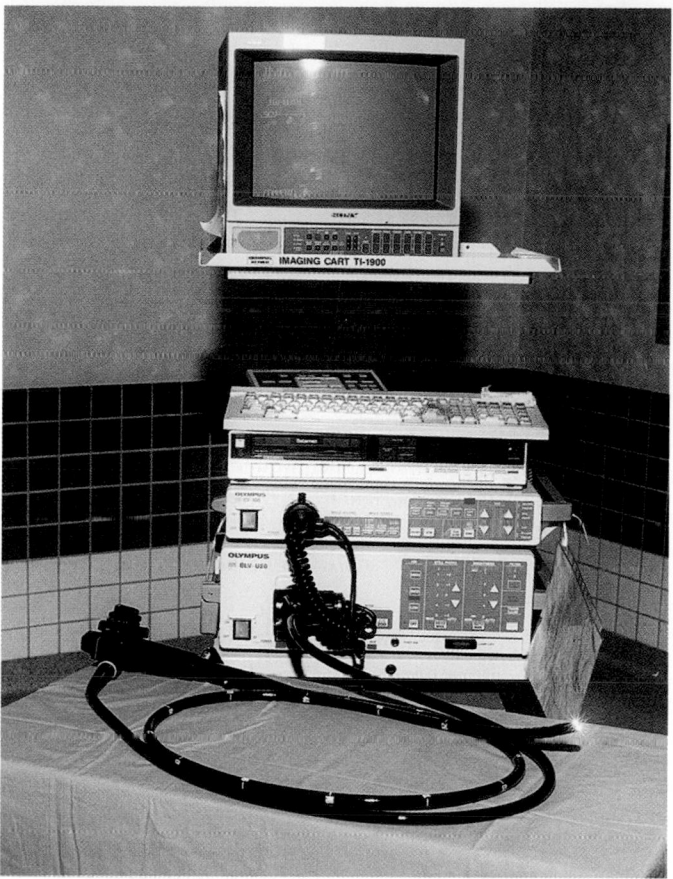

FIGURE 50-5 Flexible colonoscope with monitor and video recorder.

Accessory equipment used with endoscopes includes fiberoptic light cables and light source; irrigators for solution instillation and suction; and a camera, monitor, printer, and video recorder. The fiberoptic light cable consists of hundreds of glass fibers. It is important to protect it from being bent, dropped, kinked, squashed, or smashed. The light source can become very hot and must be kept out of contact with the patient, the physician, the staff, and any flammable material, such as surgical draping. All equipment must be checked before and after use. Always follow the manufacturer's recommendations for use, care, and maintenance of equipment. Endoscopic instruments would be damaged by the high temperature and steam under pressure in autoclaves. Therefore special care must be taken in sanitizing and using high-level disinfectants after each procedure to destroy pathogenic organisms and prevent cross-contamination to subsequent patients.

Cryosurgery

Cryosurgery involves the use of a very-low-temperature probe to destroy tissue by freezing it on contact. The probe's temperature usually is below −20° C (4° F). This cold temperature is achieved by circulating liquid nitrogen through the tip of the probe. A local anesthetic usually is administered before cryosurgery. Cryosurgery is used to treat cancers of the skin and warts. In many situations, cryosurgery is less invasive than traditional surgery and therefore generally has fewer associated complications. Cryosurgery often is

performed in an ambulatory setting or in an outpatient surgery center.

ASSISTING WITH SURGICAL PROCEDURES

Surgery performed in a medical office is restricted to the management of minor problems and injuries. The medical assistant is expected to assist with preparing the patient and setting up the sterile field. The following procedures must be used without exception when assisting with minor surgery. Individual facilities may have specific guidelines for some of these procedures; however, the theory behind sterile technique is universal, regardless of where you work.

Preparation of the Patient

Whether minor surgery is performed because of an unforeseen accident or is a planned, elective procedure, the patient needs both psychological and physical support. A patient facing a surgical procedure may be concerned about pain, disfigurement, and a possible diagnosis of cancer. An injured patient may feel anxious about medical bills or possible loss of employment. Because surgery is a frightening experience, the medical assistant must take the time, both preoperatively and at the time of surgery, to help the patient deal with fears and anxieties. The best way to help is to make sure that the patient understands the details of the procedure, that all questions are answered by the physician, and that the patient has the opportunity to talk about the procedure and voice any concerns.

Questions should be answered directly, but you should answer only the questions that are within your scope of knowledge and the policies of the office. If you cannot answer a question, assure the patient that you will relay it to the provider before the procedure and then be sure to do so. What may seem to be a minor or unimportant question to you may be a very frightening concern to the patient. The minor surgery room can be intimidating, so unless the patient is sedated, try to make conversation with him or her while you prepare for the physician's arrival.

Preoperative preparation may include blood and urine tests, completion of a consent form, and gathering of the current history concerning any recent illnesses, medications, and allergies. Patient preparations before surgery may include a shave prep, cleansing enemas, food intake restrictions, special bathing, and administration of a sedative medication. On the day of surgery, the patient is instructed to empty the bladder and undress and gown as requested. The vital signs are recorded in preparation for the procedure.

Preoperative Instructions

When office surgery is planned, certain procedures are followed before the appointment. These include the following:
- Having the necessary consent forms ready to sign
- Giving the patient the necessary preoperative instructions, such as medications to be used and special skin-cleansing instructions
- Telling the patient to bring a relative or friend to drive him or her home after the surgery
- Instructing the patient to leave jewelry and other valuables at home
- Calling the patient the day before the scheduled surgery to confirm any special instructions

Informed Consent

The provider must have the patient's written informed consent before beginning any surgical procedure. To sign an informed consent form permitting the provider to legally perform the surgery, the patient must understand what procedure will be performed, why it should be done, the potential risks and benefits of the surgery, alternative treatments (including no treatment), and the possible risks of any alternative treatment. This legal requirement is not met simply by having the patient sign an operative permit; a discussion must occur, during which the provider provides the patient or the patient's legal representative with enough information to enable the person to decide whether to proceed with the proposed surgical treatment. After this discussion, the patient either consents to or refuses the surgery. The patient then signs or refuses to sign the consent form. The discussion must be fully documented in the patient's health record. A copy of the signed form must also be included in the patient's record; sometimes the patient will sign the form directly on the electronic record. Treatment may not exceed the scope of the consent form.

The patient must not be under the influence of any sedative medication at the time he or she signs the consent form. This condition must *never* be violated.

CRITICAL THINKING APPLICATION   50-4

Melissa is preparing a patient for a biopsy of a suspected cancer of the skin. The consent form has been signed and is in the chart. While Melissa is chatting with the patient during completion of the final setup for the procedure, it becomes clear the patient thinks she is having a "skin tag" removed from her back. What action should Melissa take, if any? What is the significance of what the patient said in this situation?

Positioning

Have the patient disrobe sufficiently to expose the surgical site completely so that accidental contamination does not occur during the procedure. Clothing may also act as a tourniquet or may make applying a proper dressing or bandage difficult. In addition, the patient's clothing may be stained by the skin prep solution or may interfere with adequate site preparation.

The patient needs to be positioned as comfortably as possible for the procedure. An uncomfortable position can be held for only a limited time, and the patient may have to move, perhaps in the middle of a procedure, if you have not ensured his or her comfort from the beginning. When deciding on the correct position, consider where you and the physician will stand or sit, where the instruments will be placed, and where other needed equipment will be located. If the patient has an open wound, wear nonsterile gloves to assist the patient into position. If there is active and profuse bleeding, wear an impermeable gown and gloves. If there is danger of blood and body fluid contamination to your face or eyes, wear a face shield.

Skin Preparation

The human skin is a reservoir of bacteria, but it cannot be sterilized without the risk of damaging cells and tissues. The goal of adequate skin preparation for a surgical procedure is to reduce the number of transient flora so that transference of harmful organisms at the incision site is limited. Cleansing the patient's skin before surgery with surgical soap and an antiseptic and shaving the area if needed is called a *skin prep* (Procedure 50-3). Sometimes the patient may be instructed to repeatedly cleanse the surgical area with bacteriostatic or antiseptic soap several days before the surgery. Disposable skin prep trays and electric razors should be available in the ambulatory facility.

PROCEDURE 50-3 | Perform Skin Prep for Surgery

Goal: *To prepare the patient's skin and remove hair from the surgical site to reduce the risk of wound contamination.*

EQUIPMENT and SUPPLIES

Disposable skin prep kit, or collect the following:
- Gauze sponges
- Cotton-tipped applicators
- Antiseptic soap
- Disposable gloves
- Electric clippers
- Two small bowls
- Antiseptic or antiseptic swabs (e.g., Betadine swabs)
- Sterile normal saline solution
- Optional: cotton balls, nail pick, scrub brush
- Sterile drape
- Biohazardous sharps container and waste receptacle
- Patient's record

PROCEDURAL STEPS

1. Sanitize your hands.
   PURPOSE: To follow Standard Precautions.
2. Identify and greet the patient. Instruct the patient in the skin preparation procedure, making sure the person understands the procedure and the rationale for it.
   PURPOSE: To ensure cooperation and demonstrate awareness of possible patient concerns.
3. Ask the patient to remove any clothing that might interfere with exposure of the site and provide a gown if needed.
4. Assist the patient into the proper position for site exposure. Provide a drape if necessary to protect the patient's privacy.
5. Expose the site. Use a light if necessary.

PROCEDURE 50-3   *—continued*

6. If hair is present, the area may need to be shaved. Put on disposable gloves and shave the required area with electric clippers.
   PURPOSE: Hair should be removed before any invasive procedure to limit the potential for infection; follow Standard Precautions regarding sharps.
7. While wearing disposable gloves, open the skin prep pack and add the antiseptic soap to the two bowls.
8. Start at the incision site and begin washing with the antiseptic soap on a gauze sponge in a circular motion, moving from the center to the edges of the area to be scrubbed (Figure 1).
   PURPOSE: A circular motion from inside to outside drags contaminants away from the incision site.

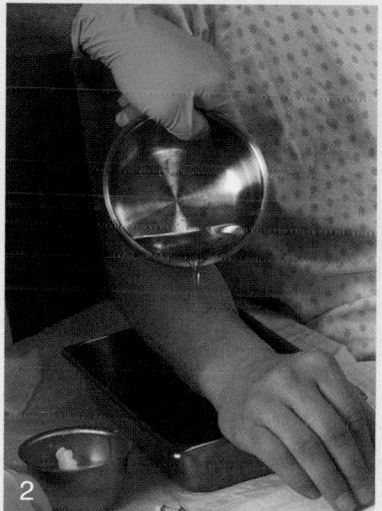

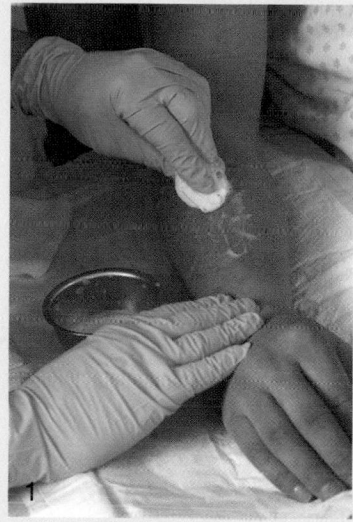

13. Dry the area, using the same circular technique with dry sponges. The area may be dried by blotting with a sterile towel.
14. Paint on the antiseptic with the cotton-tipped applicators or gauze sponges, using the same circular technique and never returning to an area that has already been painted (Figure 3).

9. After one complete wipe, discard the sponge and begin again with a new sponge soaked in the antiseptic solution.
   PURPOSE: After one circular sweep, the sponge is contaminated with skin bacteria and debris.
10. When you return to the incision site for the next circular sweep, you must use clean material.
11. Repeat the process, using sufficient friction for 5 minutes (or follow office policy for the length of time required for a particular prep).
12. Rinse the area with sterile normal saline solution (Figure 2).

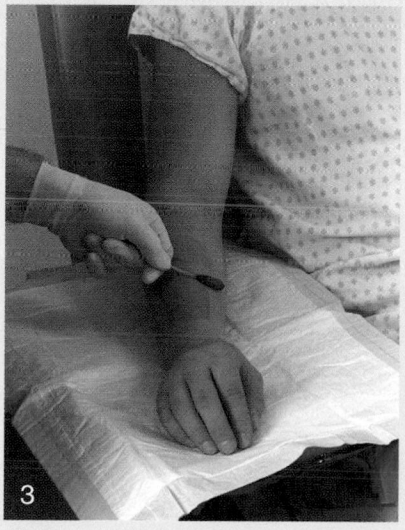

15. Place a sterile drape and/or towel over the area.
16. Answer all the patient's questions to relieve anxiety about the upcoming surgical procedure.
17. Document completion of the skin prep in the patient's health record.

Preparation of the Room

If you are to assist in a minor surgical procedure, study the provider's care preferences, review the procedure, and note the materials needed. Next, prepare the room and gather the supplies to be used. Sterile supplies are opened just before the procedure. Opened materials that have been exposed longer than 1 hour, usually because of a delay, are considered nonsterile. Supplies should not be placed where they can be knocked over or dropped. Wrapped sterile supplies that fall to the floor must not be used. Make sure the patient and family members understand that they should not approach or touch the sterile field.

Sterile Technique

Accurately performing surgical aseptic technique involves a degree of dexterity and vigilance that can come only with practice. It requires a great deal of concentration and planning of all movements and procedural steps. The procedures covered in this chapter are for minor surgery, but they are the same techniques used during major surgery. To develop a sound knowledge of sterility and sterile technique, use the following memory aid: *Everything sterile is white and everything that is not sterile is black. There is no gray!* Sterile surfaces must *never* come in contact with nonsterile surfaces. If this occurs, the sterile surface immediately is considered contaminated or nonsterile. Constant vigilance and absolute honesty are essential for maintaining sterile techniques. When a sterile surface comes in contact with a nonsterile item, this is called a "break" in sterility or a "break" in the sterile field. During any procedure, everything must stop at this point and the "break" must be corrected immediately—which usually means the assistant must start over again at the very beginning of the procedure. Any break could lead to serious wound contamination, postoperative infection, and even death.

Before assisting with minor surgery, the medical assistant must perform a series of procedures to ensure surgical asepsis (Procedures 50-4 to 50-8). These skills must be learned, practiced, and followed precisely to establish and maintain the sterile environment required during a surgical procedure. Surgical asepsis directly affects the health and well-being of the patient, the physician, and the office staff and must be practiced without fail.

CRITICAL THINKING APPLICATION   **50-5**

After completing a surgical scrub before assisting with a minor surgical procedure, Melissa remembers that she forgot to lay out the practitioner's sterile glove package. She opens up the storage cabinet and quickly adds this to the collection of sterile supplies. Can she go ahead with putting on her sterile gloves? Why or why not?

Text continued on p. 1195

PROCEDURE 50-4   Perform Handwashing: Perform a Surgical Hand Scrub

Goal: *To scrub the hands with surgical soap, using friction, running water, and a disposable sterile brush to sanitize the skin before assisting with any procedure that requires surgical asepsis.*

EQUIPMENT and SUPPLIES

- Sink with foot, knee, or arm control for running water
- Surgical soap in a dispenser
- Towels (sterile towels if indicated by office policy)
- Nail file or orange stick
- Sterile disposable brush

PROCEDURAL STEPS

1. Remove all jewelry.
   <u>PURPOSE</u>: Jewelry harbors bacteria and is not permitted in surgical asepsis.
2. Roll long sleeves above the elbows.
3. Inspect your fingernails for length and your hands for skin breaks.
4. Turn on the faucet and regulate the water to a comfortable temperature, being careful to stand away from the sink to prevent contamination of clothing from contact with the sink or counter top.
5. Keep your hands upright and held at or above waist level (Figure 1).
   <u>PURPOSE</u>: Water running from the unscrubbed area above the elbow down to the hands can carry bacteria back onto the hands. All areas below the waist are considered contaminated during all surgical procedures.

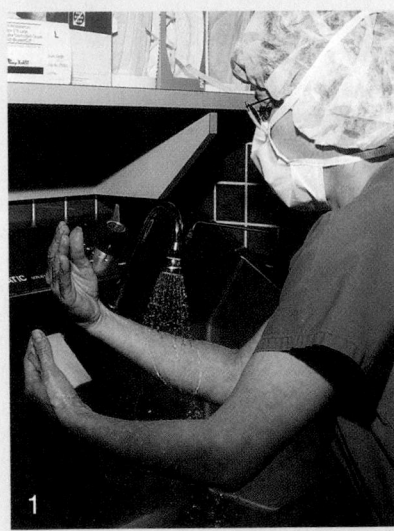

6. Clean your fingernails with a file, discard it (in most situations you will drop the file into the sink and discard it later to prevent contamination by lowering your hands and/or touching a waste receptacle), and rinse your hands under the faucet without touching the faucet or the inside of the sink basin (Figure 2).

PROCEDURE 50-4 —*continued*

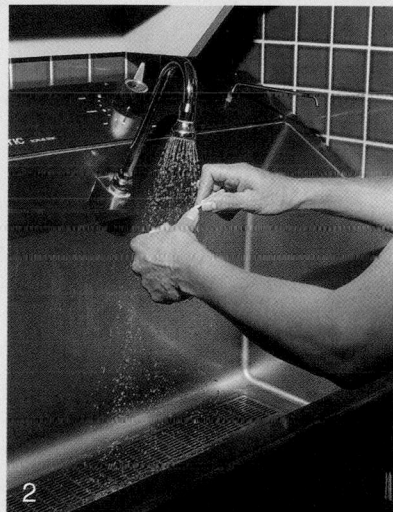

7. Allow the water to run over your hands from the fingertips to the elbows without moving the arm back and forth under the water.
   PURPOSE: Water running from the elbow down to the hands can carry bacteria back onto the hands.

8. Apply surgical soap from the dispenser to the sterile brush (or use a prepared disposable brush) and start the scrub by scrubbing the palm of the hand in a circular fashion.

9. Continue from the palm to the base of the thumb, then move on to the other fingers, scrubbing from the base, along each side, and across the nail, holding the fingertips upward and remembering to rub between the fingers (Figure 3). After the fingers have been completely scrubbed, clean the posterior surface of the hand in a circular fashion and then proceed to the wrist. The scrub process should take at least 5 minutes for each hand and arm.
   PURPOSE: The surfaces of the fingers have four sides that all need to be thoroughly cleaned.

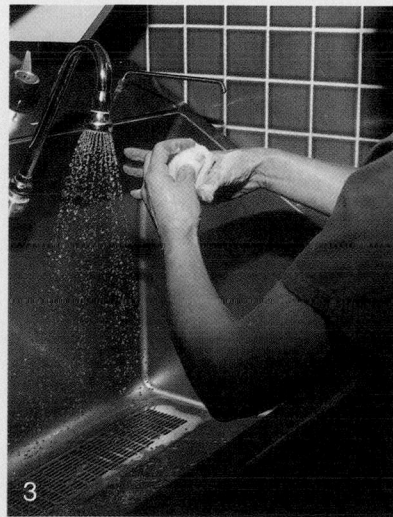

10. Do not return to a clean area after you have moved to the next part of the hand.
    PURPOSE: Once an area has been scrubbed, it is considered surgically clean, and rubbing that area again contaminates it.

11. Wash the wrists and forearms in a circular fashion around the arm while holding your hands above waist level (Figure 4).

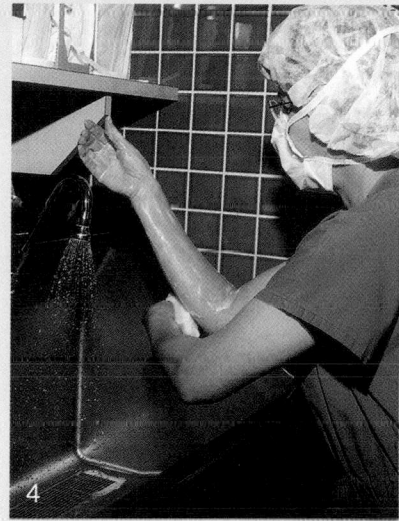

12. Rinse the arms and forearms from the fingertips upward, holding the fingers up, without touching the faucet or the inside of the sink basin (Figure 5).
    PURPOSE: Keep the fingers higher than the rest of the arm to prevent contamination from water running downward from the elbow. Touching the dirty faucet and/or basin causes contamination.

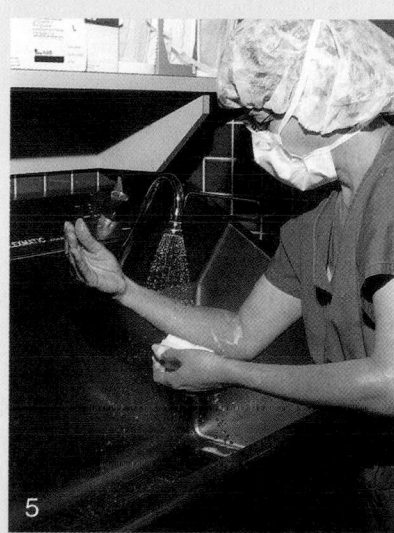

13. Apply more solution without touching any dirty surface and repeat the scrub on the other side, remembering to wash and use friction between each finger with a firm, circular motion.

14. Scrub all surfaces, being careful not to abrade your skin. The second hand and arm should take at least 5 minutes.

PROCEDURE 50-4   *—continued*

15. Rinse thoroughly, keeping your hands up and above waist level. Discard the scrub brush without lowering the arms below the waist (Figures 6 and 7).

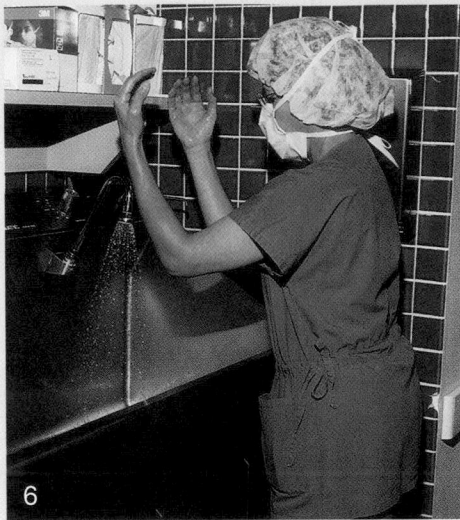

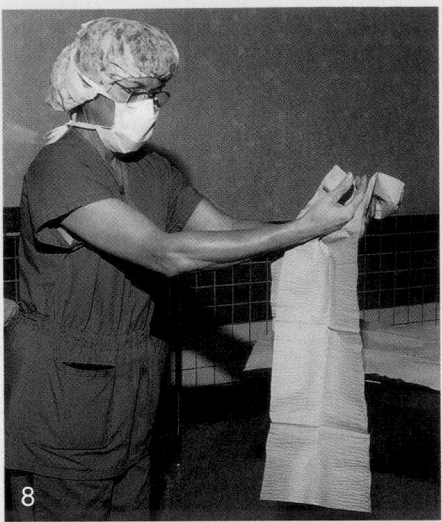

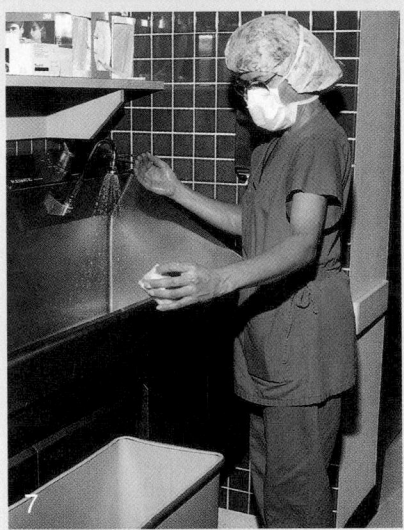

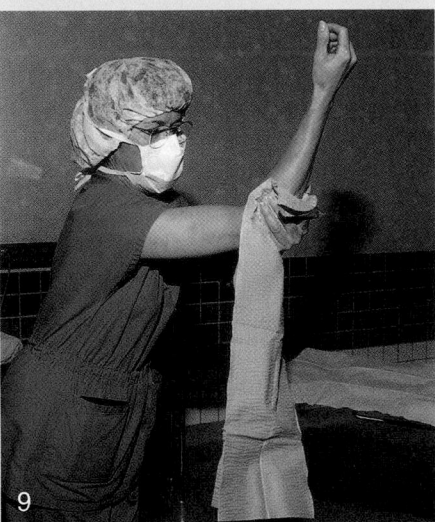

18. Using a patting motion, continue to dry the forearms. Discard the towel and keep your hands up and above waist level (Figure 10).

16. Turn off the faucet with the foot, knee, or forearm lever, if available.
    <u>PURPOSE</u>: To prevent clean hands from touching the contaminated faucet handles.

17. Dry your hands with a sterile towel, being careful to keep the fingers pointing upward and your hands above the waist. Do not rub back and forth, dragging contaminants from the dirtier area of the upper arm down toward the hands (Figures 8 and 9). Use the opposite end of the towel for the other hand.
    <u>PURPOSE</u>: To keep your clean hands from touching the part of the towel that comes in contact with your forearms, which are not as clean as your hands. If you are to gown and glove for a procedure, you must use a sterile towel.

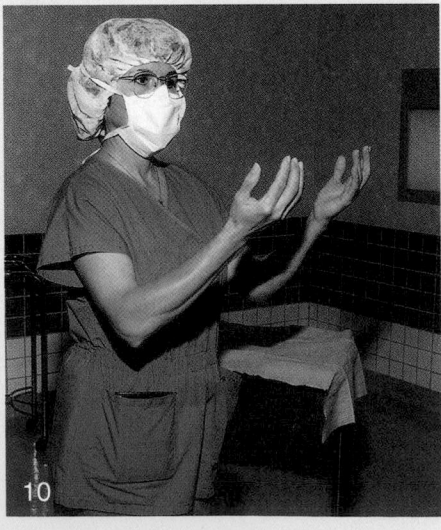

PROCEDURE 50-5 | Prepare a Sterile Field

Goal: *To open a sterile instrument pack using correct aseptic technique and to create a sterile field.*

EQUIPMENT and SUPPLIES

- A sterile instrument pack wrapped with autoclave paper that, when opened, will serve as a sterile table drape or field
- Mayo stand or countertop
- Disinfectant and gauze sponges

PROCEDURAL STEPS

1. Check that the Mayo stand or countertop is dust free and clean. If it is not, clean with 70% alcohol or another disinfectant and allow to air dry.
   PURPOSE: Although some areas cannot be sterile, steps must be taken to keep contamination to a minimum; moisture on a tray contaminates the pack.

2. Sanitize your hands and make sure they are completely dry. If you will be assisting with a surgical procedure immediately after opening the sterile pack, perform the surgical hand scrub as explained in Procedure 50-4.
   PURPOSE: To reduce the number of transient flora on your hands and forearms; moisture on your hands contaminates the pack.

3. Place the sterile pack on the Mayo stand or countertop and read the label.
   PURPOSE: Take care to open the required pack. Most medical offices have a limited supply of autoclaved packs. Opening a wrong package could mean not having enough sterile supplies for a different procedure.

4. If using an autoclaved pack, check the indicator tape for a color change.
   PURPOSE: Autoclave indicator tape changes color after the sterile processing cycle.

5. Open the outside cover (Figure 1). Position the package so that the outer envelope flap is at the top and facing you.
   PURPOSE: This positions the pack for correct opening so that you do not have to cross over the sterile pack to open it.

6. Open the outermost flap (Figure 2). Next, open the first flap away from you. Do not cross over the pack.

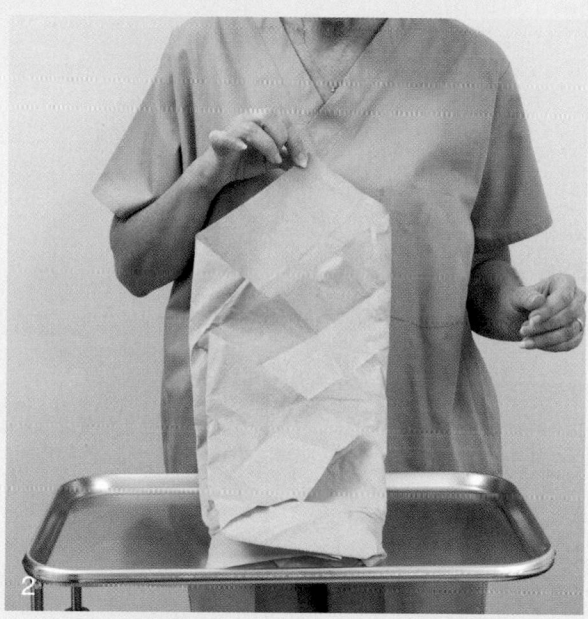

7. Open the second corner, pulling to side (Figure 3).
   PURPOSE: To prevent contamination of the sterile field.

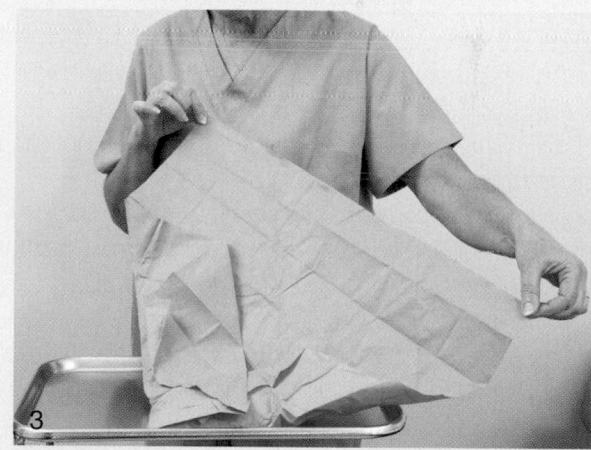

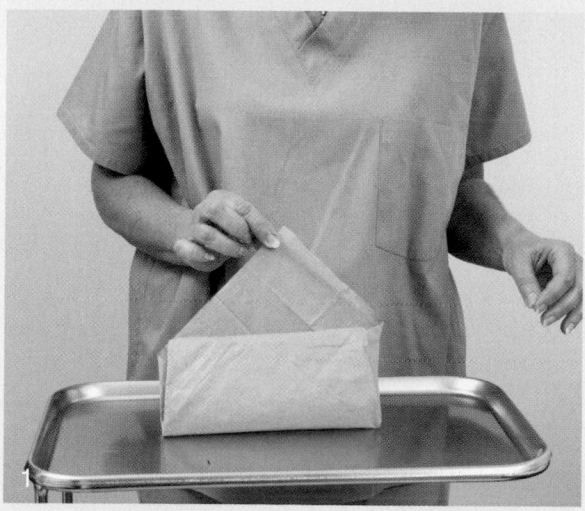

PROCEDURE 50-5 *—continued*

8. Be careful to lift the flaps by touching only the small, folded-back tab and without touching or crossing over the inner surface of the pack or its contents. Open the remaining two corners of the pack (Figure 4).

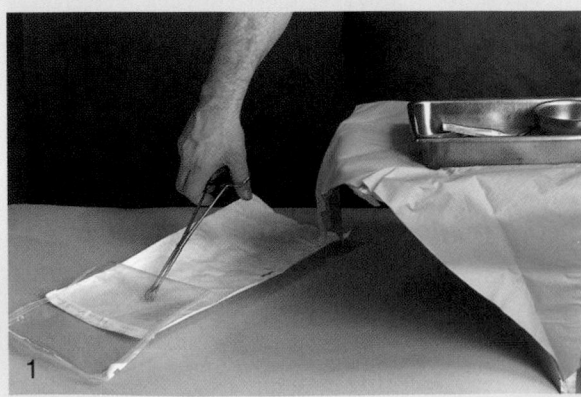

9. You now have a sterile drape as a sterile field from which to work and for the distribution of additional sterile supplies and instruments (Figure 5).

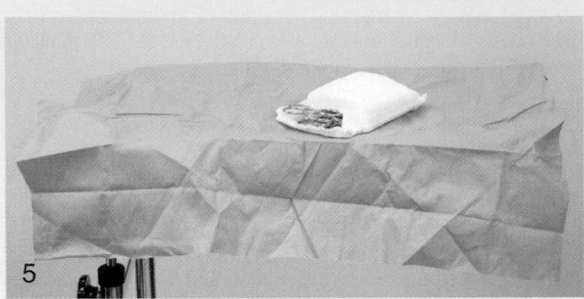

PROCEDURE 50-6   Perform Within a Sterile Field: Use Transfer Forceps

Goal: *To move sterile items on a sterile field or transfer sterile items to a gloved team member.*

EQUIPMENT and SUPPLIES

- Sterile item to move or transfer
- Sterile wrapped transfer forceps
- Mayo stand set up with a sterile field and sterile instruments

PROCEDURAL STEPS

1. Sanitize your hands, making sure they are completely dry. If you will be assisting with a surgical procedure immediately after this procedure, perform the surgical hand scrub as explained in Procedure 50-4.
   <u>PURPOSE:</u> To reduce the number of transient flora on your hands and forearms; moisture on your hands contaminates the pack.
2. Open a package containing sterile transfer forceps (Figure 1).
3. Using sterile technique, handle the sterile forceps by the ring handle only. Always point the forceps tips down.
   <u>PURPOSE:</u> If the tips are turned upward, any solution encountered will run onto the nonsterile area, and then back down over the sterile end when the tips are turned down again, thus contaminating the forceps.

4. Grasp an item on the sterile field with the sterile forceps, points down, and move it to its proper position for the procedure, making sure not to cross the sterile field with the hand or contaminated end of the forceps (Figure 2).

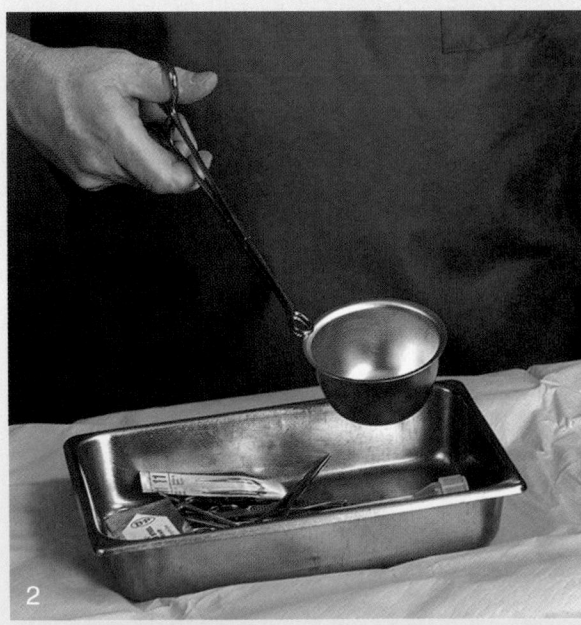

5. Alternatively, transfer an instrument from the autoclave to the sterile field.
6. Remove the transfer forceps after one-time use.

Goal: *To pour a sterile solution into a sterile stainless steel bowl or container sitting at the edge of a sterile field.*

EQUIPMENT and SUPPLIES

- Bottle of sterile solution
- Sterile bowl or container
- Sterile field
- Sink or waste receptacle
  <u>NOTE</u>: The sterile bowl should be placed, using sterile transfer forceps, near one edge of the field and the perimeter of the 1" barrier.

PROCEDURAL STEPS

1. Sanitize your hands, making sure they are completely dry. If you will be assisting with a surgical procedure immediately after this procedure, perform the surgical hand scrub as explained in Procedure 50-4.
   <u>PURPOSE</u>: To reduce the number of transient flora on your hands and forearms; moisture on your hands contaminates the pack.
2. Check the label of the ordered solution.
   <u>PURPOSE</u>: Always perform the three label checks before administering any solution or medication.
3. Place your hand over the label and lift the bottle.
   <u>NOTE</u>: If the container has a double cap, set the outer cap on the counter inside up and then proceed.
4. Lift the lid of the bottle straight up and then slightly to one side; hold the lid in your nondominant hand facing downward.
   <u>PURPOSE</u>: Air currents carry contaminants that could settle on the inside of the lid.
5. Pour away from the label without allowing any part of the bottle to touch the bowl and without crossing over the sterile field (Figure 1).

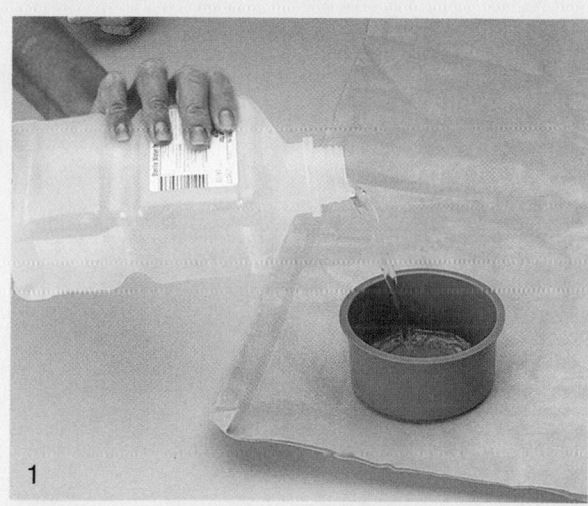

1

<u>PURPOSE</u>: Spills down the side of the bottle can stain the label or make it unreadable. The bottle exterior is not sterile so it cannot pass over the sterile field.

6. If the container does not have a double cap, before pouring the solution into the sterile container, pour off a small amount of the solution into a waste receptacle.
   <u>PURPOSE</u>: To rinse any contaminants off the bottle lip.
7. Tilt the bottle up to stop the pouring while it is still over the bowl.
   <u>PURPOSE</u>: Solutions spilled on the sterile field may contaminate the field.
8. Replace the cap (or caps) off to the side, away from the sterile field, being careful not to touch and therefore contaminate the internal surface of the lid.

Goal: *To put on sterile gloves correctly before performing sterile procedures.*

EQUIPMENT and SUPPLIES

- Pair of packaged sterile gloves in your size

PROCEDURAL STEPS

1. Perform the surgical hand scrub as explained in Procedure 50-4 before putting on sterile gloves.
2. Open the glove pack, being careful not to cross over the open area in the middle of the pack. Remember, a 1" area around the perimeter of the glove wrapper is considered not sterile.
   <u>PURPOSE</u>: The open glove pack is a sterile field.
3. Glove your dominant hand first.
   <u>PURPOSE</u>: This sets up your dominant hand to do the more difficult step, which is to put on the second glove.
4. With your nondominant hand, pick up the glove for your dominant hand with your thumb and forefinger, grabbing the top of the folded cuff, which is the inside of the glove, being careful not to cross over the other sterile glove (Figure 1).

<u>PURPOSE</u>: The inside of the glove will be next to your skin and is considered not sterile.

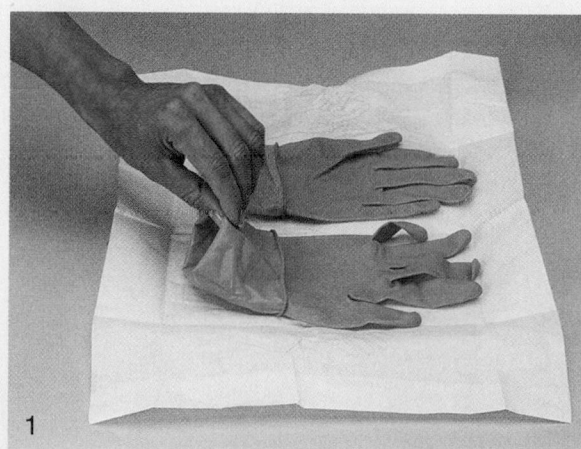

1

PROCEDURE 50-8   *—continued*

5. Lift the glove up and away from the sterile package.
   <u>PURPOSE</u>: To prevent accidental contamination from touching the glove on the 1" area around the perimeter of the glove wrapper.

6. Hold your hands up and away from your body and slide the dominant hand into the glove (Figure 2).

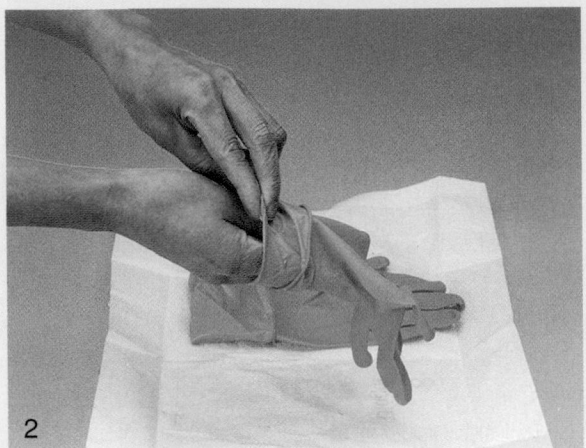

2

7. Leave the cuff folded (Figure 3).
   <u>PURPOSE</u>: You will unfold the cuff later.

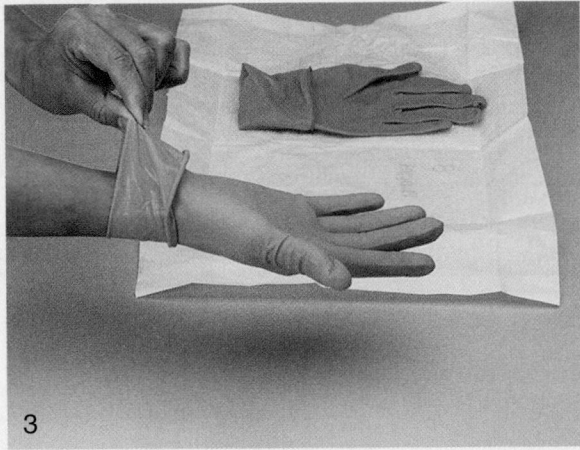

3

8. With your gloved dominant hand, pick up the second glove by slipping your gloved fingers under the cuff, extending the thumb up and away from the glove, so that your gloved fingers touch only the outside of the second glove (Figure 4).
   <u>PURPOSE</u>: Sterile surfaces must always touch sterile surfaces.

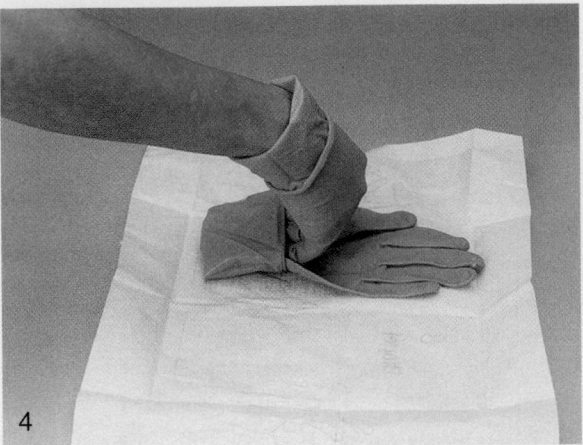

4

9. Slide your nondominant hand into the glove without touching the exterior of the glove or any part of the gloved hand (Figures 5 and 6).

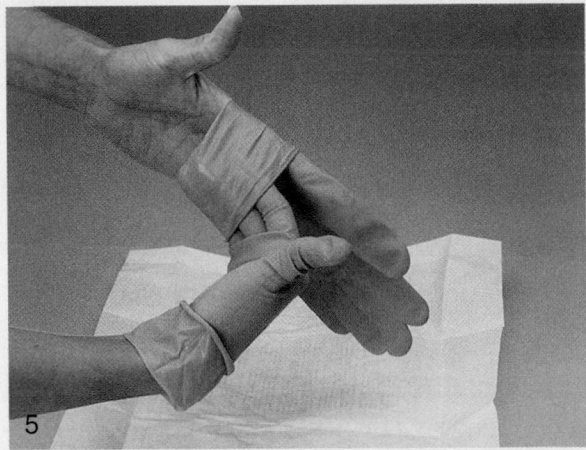

5

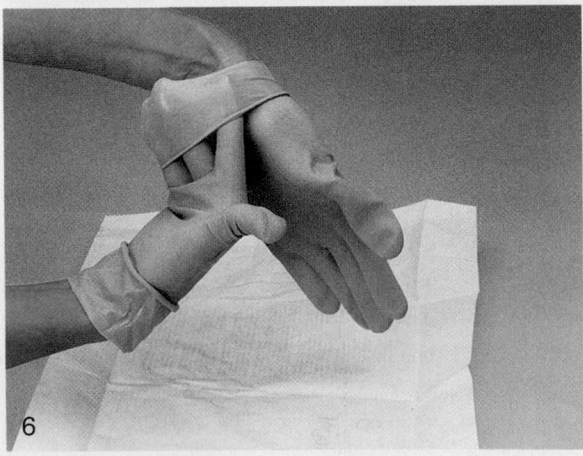

6

PROCEDURE 50-8 —*continued*

10. Still holding your hands away from you, unroll the cuff by slipping the fingers into the cuff and gently pulling up and out. Do not touch your bare arm or the internal surface of the glove with any part of the sterile glove (Figure 7).

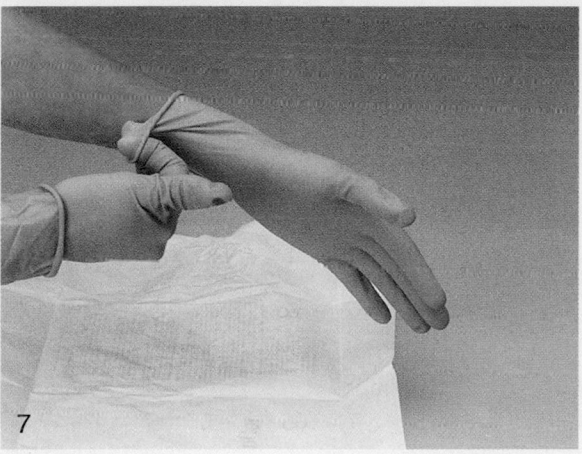

11. Now, slip your gloved fingers up under the first cuff and unroll it, using the same technique (Figure 8).

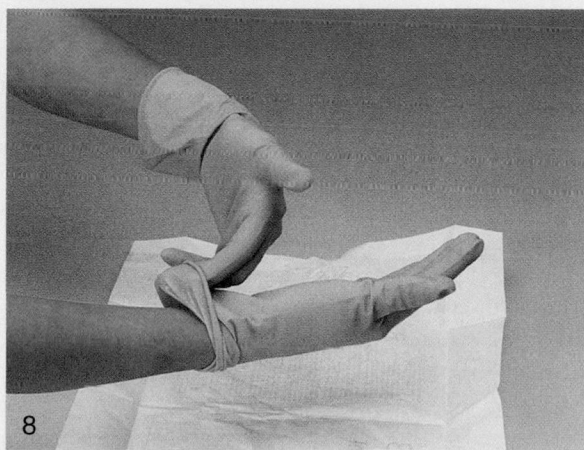

Sterile Field

A sterile field is any sterile surface on which sterile items are placed. In the ambulatory facility, a sterile field most often is set up on a Mayo stand (Figure 50-6). In surgery, a sterile field is created by draping sterile towels (either disposable or from autoclaved packs) over a Mayo stand or table. The surgical site on the patient's skin is prepared and then draped with sterile towels or drapes so that it, also, becomes a sterile field.

Hands and hair are two of the greatest sources of contamination when a sterile field is set up. With practice, you will learn to know what may be touched with your hands and what must be touched only with sterile gloved hands. Hair that falls freely over the shoulders and forward gives off a cloud of bacteria with every movement. It must always be secured back and up, not touching the shoulders.

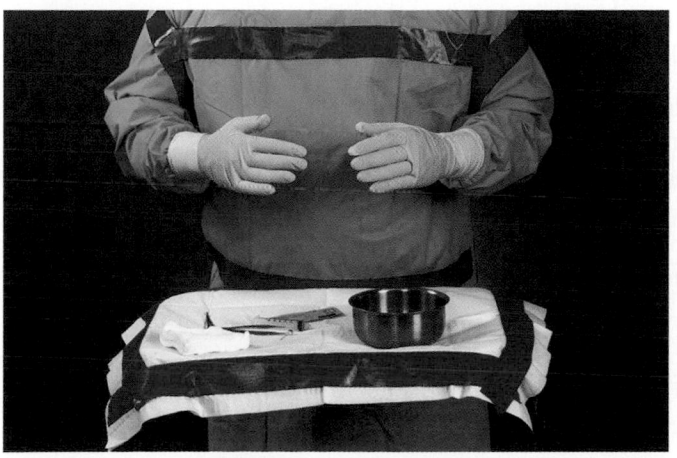

FIGURE 50-6 Sterile field (red outline).

Rules for Maintaining a Sterile Field

- Talking should be kept to a minimum because air currents carry bacteria.
- Sterile team members should always face one another.
- Always keep the sterile field in your view. If you turn your back on a sterile field or lose sight of it, it is considered contaminated.
- Nonsterile body parts (e.g., hands or elbows) and items should never cross over the sterile field.
- Tables and trays are sterile only at table level; anything that falls below the edge of the Mayo tray is considered contaminated. A 1" border around the edge of the tray is considered contaminated, so anything placed on the tray within that 1" border is contaminated.
- Consider a sterile barrier contaminated if it has been wet, cut, or torn.
- Packages placed on a clean surface are contaminated on the outside, but the inside of the sterilized package may be used as a sterile field.
- Keep sterile gloved hands above waist level at all times; do not let hands drop below the waist.
- Never remove and then replace any item in the field (e.g., using sterile forceps to cleanse a wound), or the field is contaminated.
- The inside of a sterile package remains so if the package is peeled open properly; it should be opened the entire way, and the contents then tossed onto the field without crossing over the sterile area; a two-person transfer can be used where one person opens the sterile supplies and another with sterile gloves on removes the contents from the package and places them on the sterile tray.
- If a sterile package falls to the floor, it must be discarded.
- *If you are in doubt about the sterility of anything, consider it contaminated.*

Assisting the Physician during Surgery

The physician ultimately is responsible for the patient; however, the medical assistant is responsible for ensuring that everything the assistant and the physician will use in caring for the surgical patient is accounted for, ready for use, and prepared in a safe and sterile manner (Procedure 50-9). Every team has preferences about the sequence they follow during routine minor surgery. Once a routine has been established, it should be followed in every case. Sample setups for various types of minor surgery are provided in Table 50-3.

The medical assistant sorts and places the scalpels, hemostats, scissors, tissue forceps, and retractors on the sterile field according to their sequence and frequency of use (Figure 50-7). Scalpels and sharp instruments should be conspicuously placed so that they do not accidentally injure a team member. The physician enters the room after scrubbing and then puts on gloves. The physician drapes the patient with towels or a fenestrated drape as the medical assistant hands the drapes, one at a time. Once the site has been draped, the Mayo stand with the sterile field is positioned below the site, and the medical assistant stands opposite the physician over the patient, ready to help as needed.

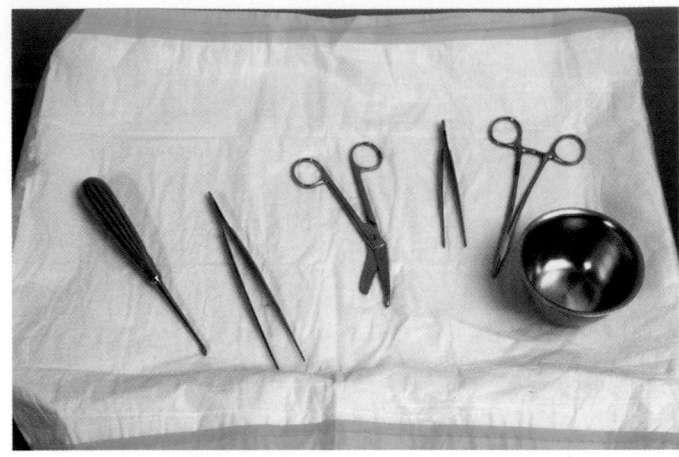

FIGURE 50-7 Mayo stand with surgical setup on sterile field.

TABLE 50-3   Setups for Minor Surgeries

PROCEDURE	SIDE COUNTER	STERILE FIELD	COMMENTS	POSTOPERATIVE CARE
Suture repair	Local anesthetic, dressings and bandages, splints or guards, tape, drape, gloves, sterile normal saline solution	Syringe and needle, hemostats (three), scissors, sponges, suture material and needle, tissue forceps or skin hook, needle holder	If a patient arrives with a pressure dressing over a laceration, follow Standard Precautions. Do not remove the pressure dressing until the physician is ready to suture. If the patient's pressure cloth must be removed, have ample sterile dressings ready to apply immediately. Ask the patient the approximate length, depth, and exact location of the laceration. Follow the physician's directions regarding cleansing of the wound.	Clean lacerations in a moderately protected area; may not require a dressing. The patient is instructed to keep the area clean and dry. Some lacerations may be closed with Steri-Strips or a topical skin adhesive.
Needle biopsy	Specimen container with prepackaged fixative or preserving solution, laboratory form and label, local anesthetic, gloves	Biopsy needle, syringe and needle, sponges	A biopsy is the examination of tissue removed from the living body. Biopsies usually are done to determine whether a growth is malignant or benign; however, a biopsy may be done as a diagnostic aid in other diseases or infections. A needle biopsy may be done by aspiration with a needle and syringe or with a special biopsy needle. The specimen then is sent to a pathologist for either a cytologic or histologic examination.	Usually no special dressing is required after a needle biopsy. An adhesive bandage strip (e.g., Band-Aid) often is sufficient.
Cyst removal	Local anesthetic, disinfectant (skin prep), laboratory form, dressing (size depends on site), gloves, drape, specimen container with prepackaged fixative or preserving solution	Kelly hemostats (two straight and two curved), dressing forceps (two), suture and needle, scissors, dissector (physician's choice), skin hook, syringe and needle, disposable scalpel with No. 11 or No. 15 blade, tissue forceps (two), Allis forceps, needle holder, sponges	A sebaceous cyst is a benign retention cyst of a sebaceous gland containing fatty substance from the gland. The cyst is attached to the skin and moves freely over the underlying tissue. For cosmetic reasons the physician makes the incision on the natural skin crease lines if possible.	See suture repair, earlier, or apply a small sterile dressing, depending on the size of the incision.

Goal: *To maintain the sterile field and to pass instruments in a prescribed sequence during a surgical procedure that involves the making of a surgical incision and the removal of a growth.*

EQUIPMENT and SUPPLIES

- Open patient drape pack on the side counter
- Mayo stand covered with a sterile drape
- Packaged sterile gloves (two pairs)
- Needle and syringe for local anesthetic medication
- Vial of local anesthetic medication
- Sterile drape
- Disposable scalpel with No. 15 blade
- Tissue forceps
- Skin retractor
- Three hemostats
- Supply of sterile gauze sponges
- Biohazardous waste receptacle
- Sharps container
- Needle with suture material
- Specimen cup
- Laboratory requisitions
- Patient's record

PROCEDURAL STEPS

1. Prep the patient's skin with surgical soap and antiseptic solution as explained in Procedure 50-3. Explain the prep procedure to the patient.
   <u>PURPOSE:</u> To ensure infection control and to demonstrate awareness of possible patient concerns.
2. Perform the surgical hand scrub as explained in Procedure 50-4.
3. Set up the sterile field with instruments and supplies in the sequence to be used (Figure 1). If it is necessary to touch sterile supplies, put on sterile gloves (see Procedure 50-8) or use sterile transfer forceps (see Procedure 50-6). After the sterile field has been set up, cover it with a sterile drape.

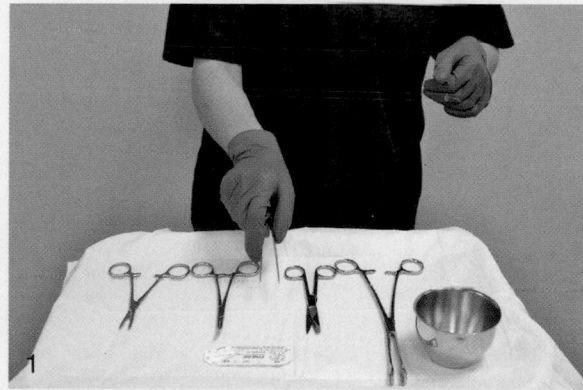

4. Position the Mayo stand near the patient and the operative site, making sure the patient understands not to touch the sterile field (Figure 2).
   <u>PURPOSE:</u> To prevent contamination of supplies and provide easy access for the physician.

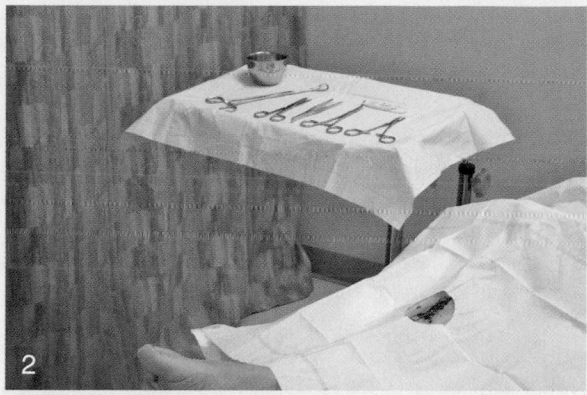

5. Put on sterile gloves using surgical technique.
6. Grasp the patient drape by holding one edge or corner in each hand (Figure 3).

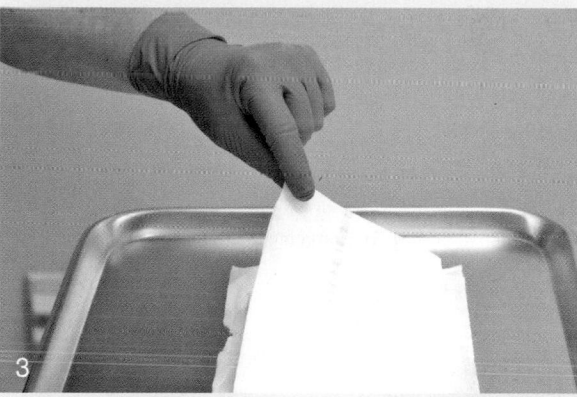

7. Drape the surgical site without touching any part of the patient or the operating area with your gloved hands.
8. If the provider requests medication, such as a local anesthetic, a second circulating assistant holds the vial of local anesthetic so that the provider can read the label. The provider withdraws the desired amount using sterile technique (Figure 4).
   <u>PURPOSE:</u> The vial of local anesthetic medication must be held by the second assistant away from the sterile field to prevent crossing over the field with a nonsterile item. The medication label must be checked before a medication is dispensed or administered.

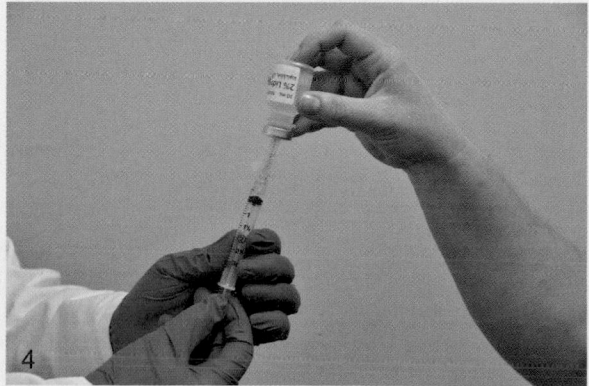

PROCEDURE 50-9   —*continued*

9. The provider injects the local anesthetic and waits a few minutes for it to take effect.

10. Position yourself across from the practitioner. Arrange the sterile field. Check the placement location on the Mayo stand (Figure 5).

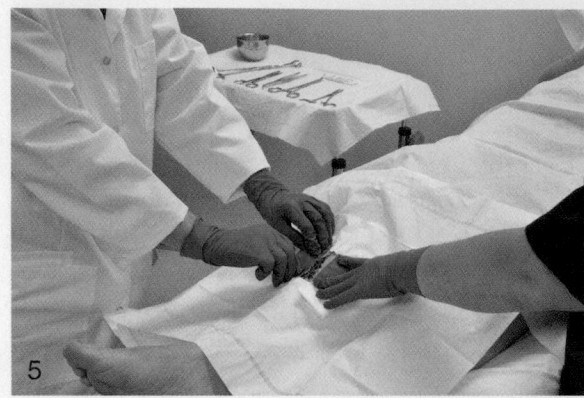

11. Keep all sharp equipment conspicuously placed on the sterile field.
<u>PURPOSE</u>: Sharp instruments that are not clearly visible may injure a team member.

12. Pass the scalpel, blade down and handle first, to the provider, or the provider will reach for it. The provider will take the scalpel with the thumb and forefinger in the position ready for use (Figure 6).
<u>PURPOSE</u>: To protect the practitioner and yourself from injury.

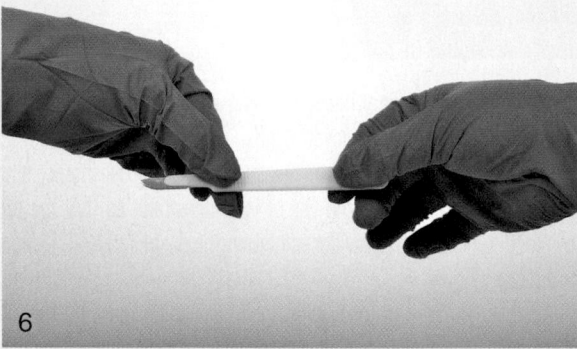

13. Pick up a tissue forceps by the tips and pass it to the provider to grasp a piece of the tissue to be excised (Figure 7).

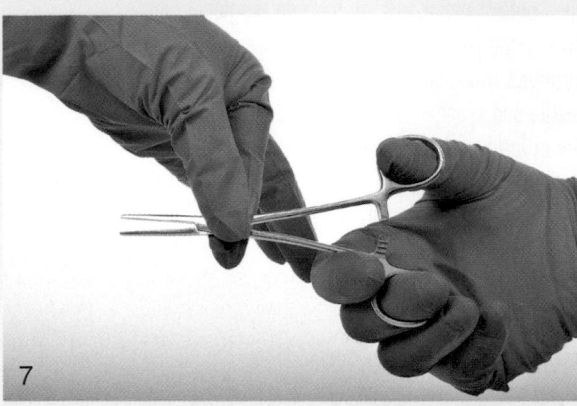

14. Dispose of soiled sponges in the biohazardous waste receptacle, being careful to keep your hands above your waist and to avoid touching any nonsterile items.

15. Hold clean sponges in your hand to pat or sponge the wound as needed

16. Safely position the specimen (if any) where it will not be disturbed in a sterile container on the sterile field.

17. If there is a bleeding vessel or if a hemostat is requested, pass the hemostat in the manner described in step 13.

18. Continue to sponge blood from the wound site.

19. Retract the wound edge, as needed, with a skin retractor.

20. Continue to monitor the sterile field and assist the provider as needed.

21. Pass the needle and suture material to close the wound and apply a sterile dressing as requested (Figure 8).

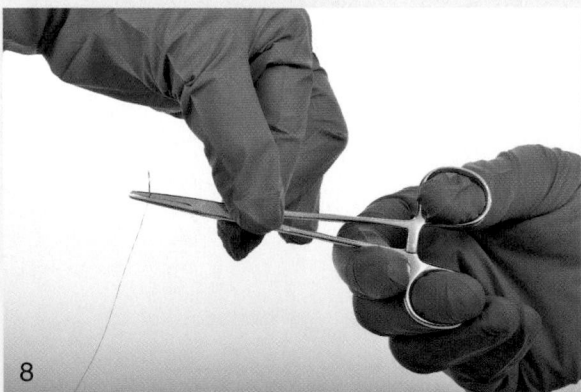

22. Monitor the patient and provide assistance as needed.

23. When the provider is finished, clean the surgical site using sterile technique.

24. Collect the specimen using Universal Standards, place it in a labeled specimen cup, and send it to the laboratory with the proper requisitions.

25. Sanitize your hands. Document the procedure, wound condition, and patient education on wound care.

Passing Instruments

During a procedure, the medical assistant must protect the sterile field from contamination. Notify the provider if a break in sterile technique occurs, dispose of soiled sponges into the biohazardous waste container, and anticipate the provider's need for instruments. The provider may request instruments or may use hand signals (Figure 50-8). As the team works together over time, the physician may not need to give any signals, because the assistant will be able to anticipate the instrument needed next during the procedure.

Instrumentation is logical; if the practitioner requests a suture, scissors will be needed next to cut the suture strand. In the case of sudden hemorrhage from a bleeding vessel, the physician will need an appropriately sized hemostat. While gaining experience, the assistant watches, listens, and learns to judge what will be needed or performed next. Pass instruments with a firm, purposeful motion so that the provider does not have to look up. Wait until you feel the provider grasp the instrument so that it does not drop onto the patient or the floor and be careful that you and the provider are protected from injury. Pass the scalpel with the blade down and present the handle to the provider. Hold all instruments by their tips and pass the handle ends into the provider's palm or fingers.

Specimen Collection

If a specimen is collected during a procedure, it is placed in a sterile specimen cup or basin. Do not remove the specimen from the sterile field until the physician gives the order. The provider may want to examine the specimen again during the procedure. After the procedure is complete, place the specimen in an appropriate container, label it, and send it to the laboratory for analysis.

Completing the Surgical Procedure

At the conclusion of the procedure, the physician begins wound closure (Procedure 50-10). The techniques and methods of tissue

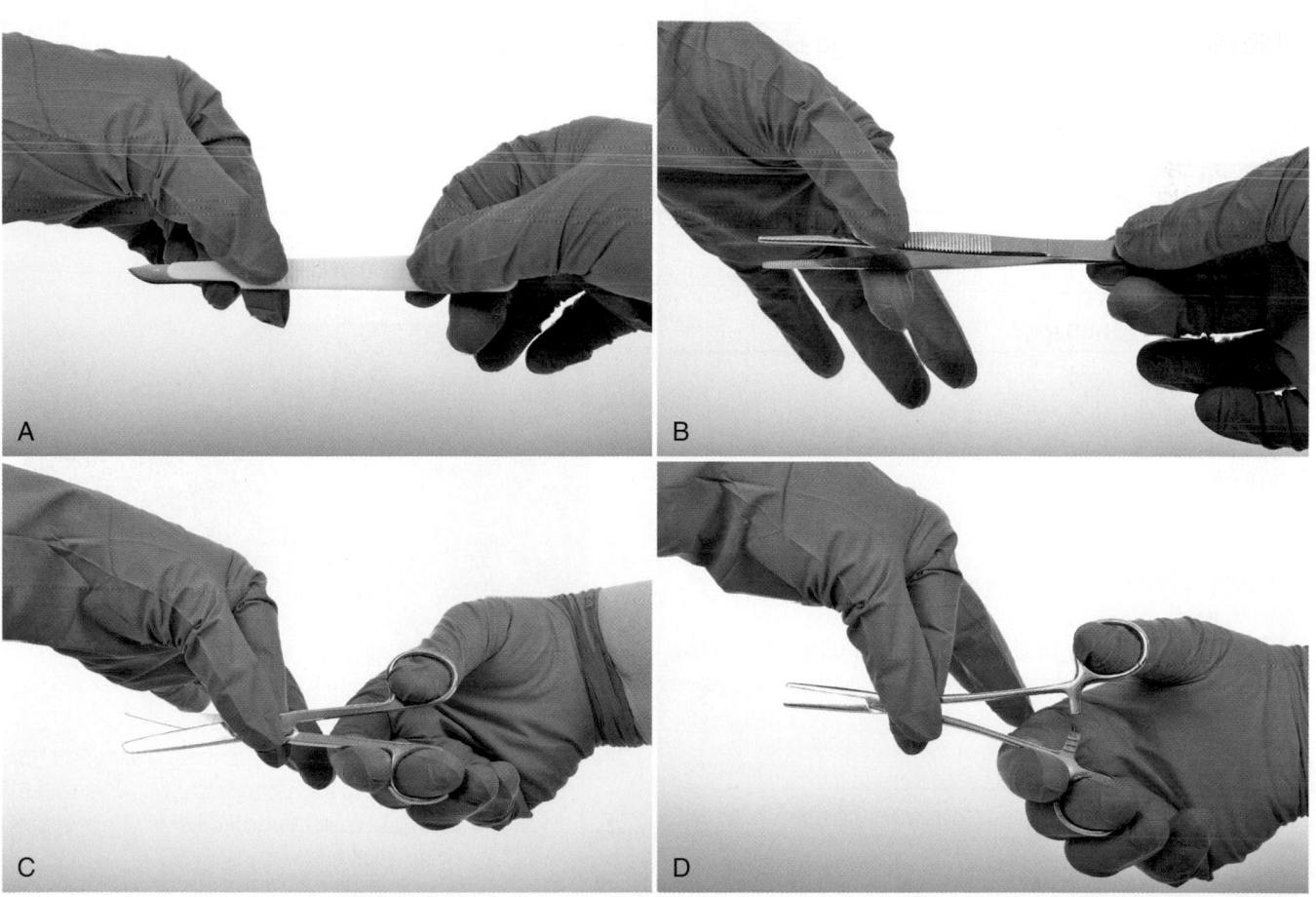

FIGURE 50-8 Passing sterile surgical instruments. **A,** Scalpel. **B,** Forceps. **C,** Scissors. **D,** Clamp.

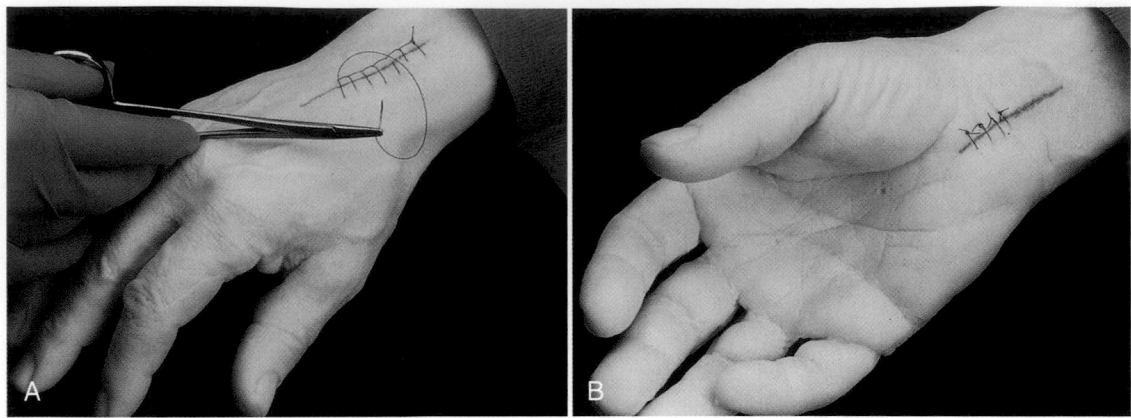

FIGURE 50-9 A, Continuous (i.e., running) suture placement. **B,** Interrupted suture placement.

closure vary; all of them cannot be described or illustrated here. The two basic methods of suturing are the continuous running suture and the interrupted suture, in which each knot is placed and tied one at a time, so that if one breaks, the others keep the wound closure intact (Figure 50-9). The interrupted technique is used for most skin closures in a medical office.

The provider may prefer that the medical assistant place the needle in a needle holder and pass it, handle first. When the wound is closed, you may assist by cutting the suture and sponging the site. If an interrupted suture method is used, the first suture is placed at the midpoint of the incision. Then each side of the first suture is

mentally divided in half again, and the next two sutures are placed at each of these midpoints. The rest of the sutures are placed using the same technique until the wound edges have been completely approximated. The provider may also opt to close a wound with surgical staples.

After the skin closure, sterile normal saline may be poured over the wound area to cleanse it—this process is called a *wound lavage*—or the area is cleansed with an antiseptic and blotted dry using sterile dry sponges. Care must be taken not to disturb the wound edges or sutures. Next a sterile dressing is placed over the incision (Procedure 50-11) and a bandage is applied to support the dressing.

PROCEDURE 50-10   Perform Wound Care: Assist With Suturing

Goal: *To assist the surgeon in wound closure using sterile techniques.*

EQUIPMENT and SUPPLIES

- Sterile field on Mayo stand
- Surgical scissors
- Suture material
- Sterile gloves
- Needle holder
- Sterile gauze sponges
- Biohazardous sharps container and waste receptacle
- Patient's record
  NOTE: This procedure may be a continuation of Procedure 50-9. If done independently, you must perform the surgical scrub and glove before beginning step 1.

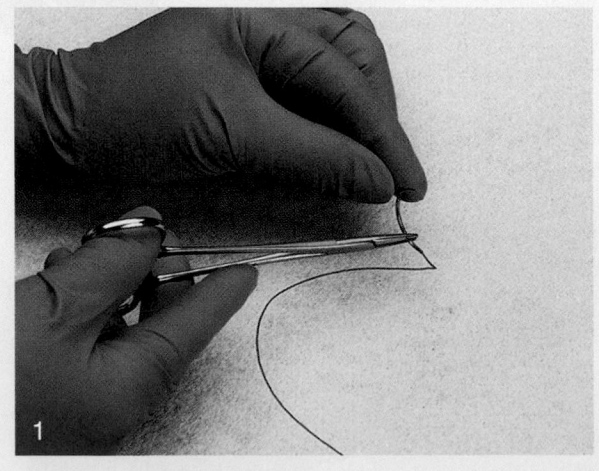

PROCEDURAL STEPS

1. Hold the curved needle point in your nondominant hand, 4 to 5 inches over the sterile field (Figure 1).
   PURPOSE: Always work over a sterile field and take care not to puncture gloves with the sharp needle.

PROCEDURE 50-10 —*continued*

2. With the needle holder, clamp the suture needle at the upper third of its total length (Figure 2).
   PURPOSE: Clamping in the middle weakens and may distort the shape of the needle. Clamping too near the thread may cause the suture to detach from the needle. Clamping at the tip of the needle damages the needle point.

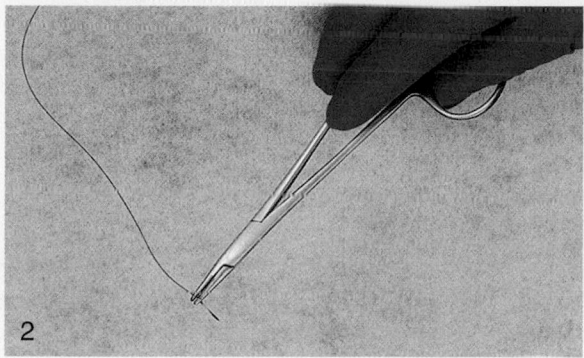

3. With your dominant hand, hold the needle holder halfway down its shaft with the suture needle point up.

4. With your nondominant hand, hold the suture strand and pass the needle holder into the surgeon's hand (Figures 3 and 4).

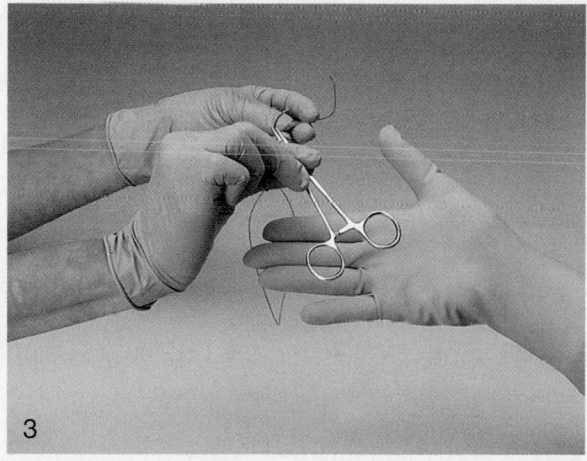

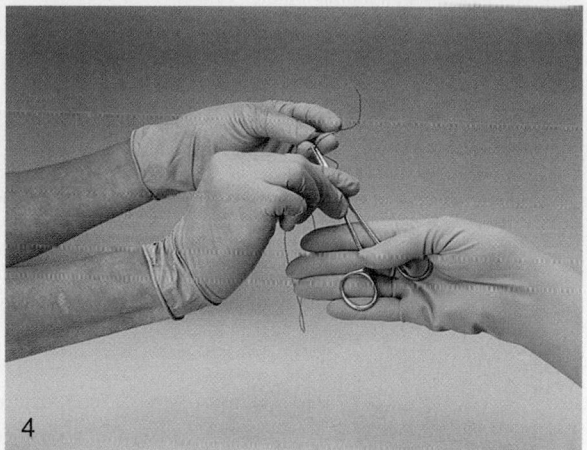

5. Pick up the surgical scissors with your dominant hand and a gauze sponge with your nondominant hand.

6. After the surgeon places a closure suture, knots it, and holds the two strands taut, cut both suture strands in one motion. Cut between the knot and the surgeon, at the length requested, normally approximately $\frac{1}{8}$ inch.
   PURPOSE: Too long a suture may irritate the patient during recovery, and too short a suture may untie during recovery.

7. Gently blot the closure once with the gauze sponge in your nondominant hand.
   PURPOSE: Rubbing or friction may damage the wound edges.

8. If additional strands of suture are needed, repeat the process.

PROCEDURE 50-11 Perform Wound Care and a Dressing Change: Apply or Change a Sterile Dressing

Goal: To apply a sterile dressing properly at the completion of a surgical procedure.

EQUIPMENT and SUPPLIES

- Sterile dressing material or Telfa
- Sterile gloves
- Patient's record

PROCEDURAL STEPS

1. After surgery is complete, lavage or rinse the sutured area with sterile saline.
   PURPOSE: To cleanse the postsurgical site.

2. Before the sterile drape is removed and while you are still wearing sterile gloves, pick up the dressing from the sterile field, place it on the wound, and hold it there.
   PURPOSE: To prevent the introduction of microorganisms into the wound area.

3. Then remove the drape, switching hands to hold the dressing in place.
   PURPOSE: To keep the wound as clean as possible.

PROCEDURE 50-11   —continued

4. Secure the dressing with paper tape and/or an appropriate bandage.
   <u>PURPOSE:</u> To keep the wound covered and protected.
5. Provide patient education as needed for wound care and document the procedure in the patient's health record.
   <u>PURPOSE:</u> A procedure is not completed until it is recorded.

10/12/20XX 2:15 PM Dressing change completed to wound on ⊕ midforearm. Area slightly inflamed, mod amt serosanguineous drainage noted. Site cleansed and sterile dressing applied. Pt instructed on home wound care and to notify physician if drainage changes, inflammation increases, or fever occurs. Melissa Gelbart, CMA (AAMA)

Postoperative Responsibilities

After caring for the patient, the medical assistant clears the sterile field, following Standard Precautions. Wear disposable gloves until all contaminated materials have been properly removed and handled. Place disposable equipment and supplies in biohazardous waste containers and/or sharps containers. The room should be checked for any blood spills or other contamination and disinfected appropri-

ately. After completing this process, remove the contaminated gloves and sanitize your hands.

Use clean gloves to disinfect the room, including the table, Mayo stand, side and back tables, any other equipment in the room, and the floor. Used instruments must be sanitized, disinfected, and resterilized for future use. The provider and the medical assistant both document the procedure in the patient's health record.

Single-Assistant Preparation for Minor Surgery

1. Sanitize your hands and gather all supplies.
   - *Sterile side (Mayo tray):* Two towel packs, skin prep pack, patient drape pack, instrument pack, miscellaneous pack or packs, three glove packs, face shields, impermeable gowns
   - *Nonsterile side (side counter):* Syringes, suture material, anesthesia solutions, additional sponges, sterile dressings, bandages, transfer forceps, waste basin, sharps and biohazard waste containers, nonsterile gloves, face shields, and impermeable gowns
2. Verify that the informed consent is signed and in the patient's health record.
3. Identify the patient and escort him or her into the room.
4. Greet and converse with the patient.
5. Position the patient on the table.
6. Sanitize your hands.
7. Open the first towel pack.
8. Open the skin prep pack.
9. Pour the soap and antiseptic solutions.
10. Expose the site to be prepped.
11. Put on gloves and arrange prep items within the sterile field.
12. Place sterile towels at skin scrub boundaries using sterile technique.
13. Prep the patient's skin.
14. Discard skin prep materials in appropriate sharps/biohazard containers.
15. Discard gloves; sanitize your hands, following the guidelines for a surgical hand scrub (Procedure 50-4) if this procedure is part of the policy of the provider or the facility.
16. Open the table drape pack on the Mayo stand to create a sterile field.
17. Open the instrument pack or packs and transfer the instruments to the sterile field. Add the sterile syringe unit.

18. Add sterile items as requested.
19. The provider joins you and converses with the patient.
20. Open the physician's glove pack (the physician now puts on gloves).
21. Open the patient drape pack (the physician now drapes the surgical site).
22. Cleanse and hold up the anesthesia vial for the physician to withdraw anesthesia with the sterile syringe (the physician now administers the anesthesia).
23. Repeat the surgical hand wash; reglove with a new glove pack.
24. Arrange the sterile field instruments and other materials for safety and in sequence; check the condition of each instrument.
25. Open the suture/needle pack per the physician's choice; load the first suture into the needle holder.
26. Place two gauze sponges at the site.
27. Assist with the procedure.*
    - *For the provider:* Pass the instruments; maintain the field; anticipate his or her needs; and cut sutures.
    - *For the patient:* Retract tissue; sponge blood from the wound; apply the sterile bandage; and care for the specimen.
28. Help the patient sit up and dress if needed and monitor vital signs as instructed.
29. Record and prepare specimens.
30. Sanitize and disinfect the room; clear materials and discard in biohazardous waste containers.
31. Document the procedure in the patient's health record.
32. Help the patient prepare to leave the office.
33. Sanitize, disinfect, and sterilize the equipment at the first available time.

By law, the assistant may not clamp tissues, place sutures, or alter body tissues in any way.

Postoperative Instructions and Care

The patient should be given time to rest after the surgery. If a sedative was administered, make sure the patient has recovered sufficiently to avoid injury after the surgery or during the journey home. If the patient has been given a topical or local anesthetic, explain to the patient that the anesthesia effect will wear off and that some discomfort may be felt at the operative site. Check with the physician whether pain medication needs to be prescribed. If medication has been prescribed, review the purpose of the medication and the directions for its use with the patient and his or her companion. Make a follow-up appointment before the patient leaves the office.

Postoperative care extends for the total recovery period, not just for the time of immediate care before the patient leaves the office. Most medical assistants are responsible for teaching patients to care for themselves at home after surgery. The concentration of a postoperative patient is diminished after the stress of surgery, so all instructions should be given to the patient in writing. They should be simple and easily understood by both the patient and caregivers. These instructions can be preprinted forms for each type of surgery, or a general form with checked boxes for particular postoperative instructions that apply specifically to the individual patient (Figure 50-10).

Warning Signs

Explain to the patient the importance of calling the office if any questions arise or changes occur that cause the person concern. If the patient does not call within the next 24 hours, you should call the patient. Many patients tend to "ride it out" or say they did not want to disturb you. Never allow the postoperative patient to leave the office without the physician's knowledge and approval. Tell the patient to call the office immediately if he or she notes redness around the operative site, bleeding from the wound, fever, swelling, or increasing or severe pain. The wound should be kept clean and dry, and the patient should be taught how to change the dressing if needed.

Follow-Up

If the healing process is a long one or if the wound becomes infected, the patient may return for follow-up care. If the wound requires a new dressing, follow Standard Precautions; wear gloves and other protective barriers as appropriate. If at any time you determine that the wound may be infected, stop and have the physician examine it. Generally, no bandaging material should be reused, including elastic bandage wraps. Tape applied directly to a patient's skin is not a good dressing immobilizer. If tape is used, always keep it to a minimum. If tape is holding a dressing in place, always remove it by pulling toward the wound. If it is adhering to a hairy area of the body, lift the outer tape edge with one hand and slowly and gently separate the underlying hair and skin from the tape with the thumb of your other hand. Peel the skin from the bandage, not the bandage from the skin. Never rapidly "rip" tape from the body, because this may injure the skin. If the tape is not irritating to the patient, it may be advisable to leave the tape in place until total healing has taken place. If the wound has healed, the provider may ask the medical assistant to remove the patient's sutures. If the provider closed the wound with surgical staples, the patient must return to the facility to have the staples removed (Procedure 50-12).

POSTOP INSTRUCTIONS FOR _____

☐ Elevate your arm.
☐ Elevate your leg.
☐ Limit food intake to _____.
☐ Limit activity to _____.
☐ Do not bathe or shower.
☐ Sponge bath only.
☐ Change dressing as instructed.
☐ Call the office for fever, redness, pain, swelling, or bleeding.
☐ Take_____ every 4 hours as needed for pain.
☐ Return to school/work in _____days.
☐ Call the office tomorrow before _____ p.m.
☐ Your next appointment is on M T W Th F S_____ at _____.

FIGURE 50-10 An example of preprinted postoperative patient instructions.

PROCEDURE 50-12 Perform Wound Care: Remove Sutures and/or Surgical Staples

Goal: To remove sutures and/or surgical staples from a healed incision using sterile technique and without injuring the closed wound.

EQUIPMENT and SUPPLIES

Sterile suture removal kit containing the following:
- Suture removal scissors
- Gauze sponges

- Thumb dressing forceps
- Steri-Strips or adhesive bandage strips (e.g., Band-Aids)
- Skin antiseptic swabs (e.g., Betadine swabs)
- Surgical staple remover with 4×4-inch gauze sponges

PROCEDURE 50-12 *—continued*

- Biohazardous waste container
- Sterile gloves
- Patient's record

PROCEDURAL STEPS

1. Assemble the necessary supplies.
2. Sanitize your hands, following Standard Precautions.
3. Identify and greet the patient. Explain the procedure to the patient and instruct the person to lie or sit still during the procedure.
   PURPOSE: To ensure cooperation during the procedure.
4. Position the patient comfortably and support the sutured area.
5. Place dry towels under the site.
6. Check the incision line to make sure the wound edges are approximated and there are no signs of infection, such as inflammation, edema, or drainage.
   PURPOSE: Sutures or staples should not be removed unless the site is completely healed with the wound edges together; infection at the site will interfere with the healing process; removing sutures or staples before the site is completely healed may result in wound **dehiscence**.
7. Put on disposable gloves. Using antiseptic swabs, cleanse the wound to remove exudate and destroy microorganisms around the sutures or staples. Clean the site from the inside out, starting at the top of the wound and working your way down. Use a new swab if the step must be repeated.
   PURPOSE: Dried exudate on sutures or staples may make removing them without traumatizing the wound more difficult. Cleansing the wound reduces the possibility of wound infection.
8. Open the suture or staple removal pack while maintaining the sterility of the contents.
9. Place a sterile gauze sponge next to the wound site.
   PURPOSE: To receive the removed sutures or staples.
10. Put on sterile gloves.
11. Remove the sutures or staples.

To Remove Sutures
a. Grasp the knot of the suture with the dressing forceps without pulling.
b. Cut the suture at skin level.
c. Lift, do not pull, the suture toward the incision and out with the dressing forceps.

d. Place the suture on the sterile gauze sponge and check that the entire suture strand has been removed.
   PURPOSE: Suture fragments left in a wound may cause irritation and/or infection and may prolong the healing process.
e. If any bleeding occurs, blot the area with a sterile gauze sponge before continuing.
f. Continue in the same manner until all sutures have been removed.

To Remove Staples
a. Gently place the bottom jaw of the staple remover (Figure 1) under the first staple.
b. Tightly squeeze the staple handles together.
c. Carefully tilt the staple remover upward until the staple lifts out of the wound.
d. Place the removed staple on a 4×4-inch gauze square.
e. Continue the process until all staples have been removed.

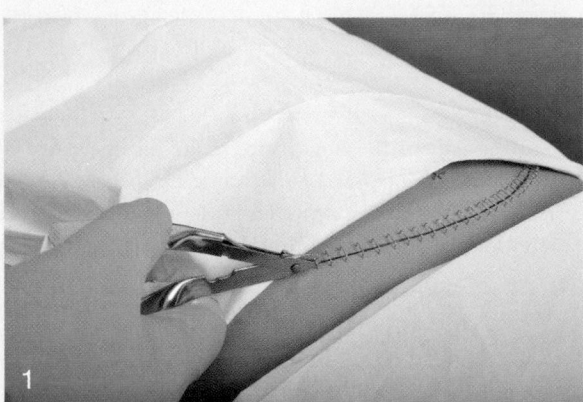

12. Remove the gauze sponge holding the sutures or staples and dispose of contaminated materials in the biohazardous waste container.
13. The surgeon may apply or may have you apply Steri-Strips or an adhesive bandage strip for added support, strength, and protection.
14. Instruct the patient to keep the wound edges clean and dry and not to place excessive strain on the area.
15. Document the procedure, wound condition, number of sutures or staples removed, whether a dressing or bandage was applied, and the instructions on wound care given to the patient.
    PURPOSE: A procedure that is not documented was not done.

WOUND CARE

A wound can be intentional (e.g., from a surgical incision) or accidental, and it may be open or closed (Figure 50-11). An open wound has an outward opening where the skin is broken, exposing the underlying tissues. A closed or nonpenetrating wound does not have an outward opening, but the underlying tissues are damaged, as in a hematoma, contusion, or bruise. Closed wounds usually are the result of some type of blunt trauma to the body. An aseptic (i.e., clean) wound is not infected with pathogens. Septic wounds are infected with pathogens.

Open wounds may be classified according to the appearance of their openings. An incised wound has a clean edge and is made with a cutting instrument. An incised wound may be the result of surgery, an accident, or a knife wound. A lacerated wound has torn or mangled tissues and is made by a dull or blunt instrument. A penetrating or puncture wound is caused by a sharp, slender object, such as a needle or ice pick, and passes through the skin into the underlying tissues. A perforated wound is a penetrating wound that passes through to a body organ or cavity, such as a gunshot wound.

Wound Healing

All wounds go through a healing or repair process that has three phases. The *lag phase* occurs first; the blood vessels contract to control hemorrhage and blood platelets form a network that acts as a glue to plug the wound. After a cascade of chemical reactions, fibrin is released into the wound and clotting begins. Fibrin continues to collect red blood cells (RBCs) and the clot dries into a scab. About 12 hours later special white blood cells (WBCs) called macrophages arrive to clear away bacteria and dead tissue. Within 1 to 4 days the fibrin threads contract and pull the edges of the wound together under the scab.

The second phase, *proliferation*, encompasses wound healing and new growth; this lasts 5 to 20 days. During this phase, the tissues repair themselves. New cells form and the wound continues to contract and seal. If the wound is a clean surgical incision, complete contraction usually takes place and a **cicatrix** forms.

The final phase, the *remodeling phase*, extends from day 21 onward. Clean, shallow wounds may contract in the first two stages; large or mangled wounds require the time and cellular activity of this third phase to build a bridge of new tissue to close the gap of the wound. The cells produce a fibrous protein substance called *collagen* (i.e., connective tissue) that gives the wounded tissues strength and forms scar tissue. Scar tissue is not true skin; it usually is very strong, but it lacks the elasticity of normal skin tissue. Scar tissue also is devoid of a normal blood supply and nerves.

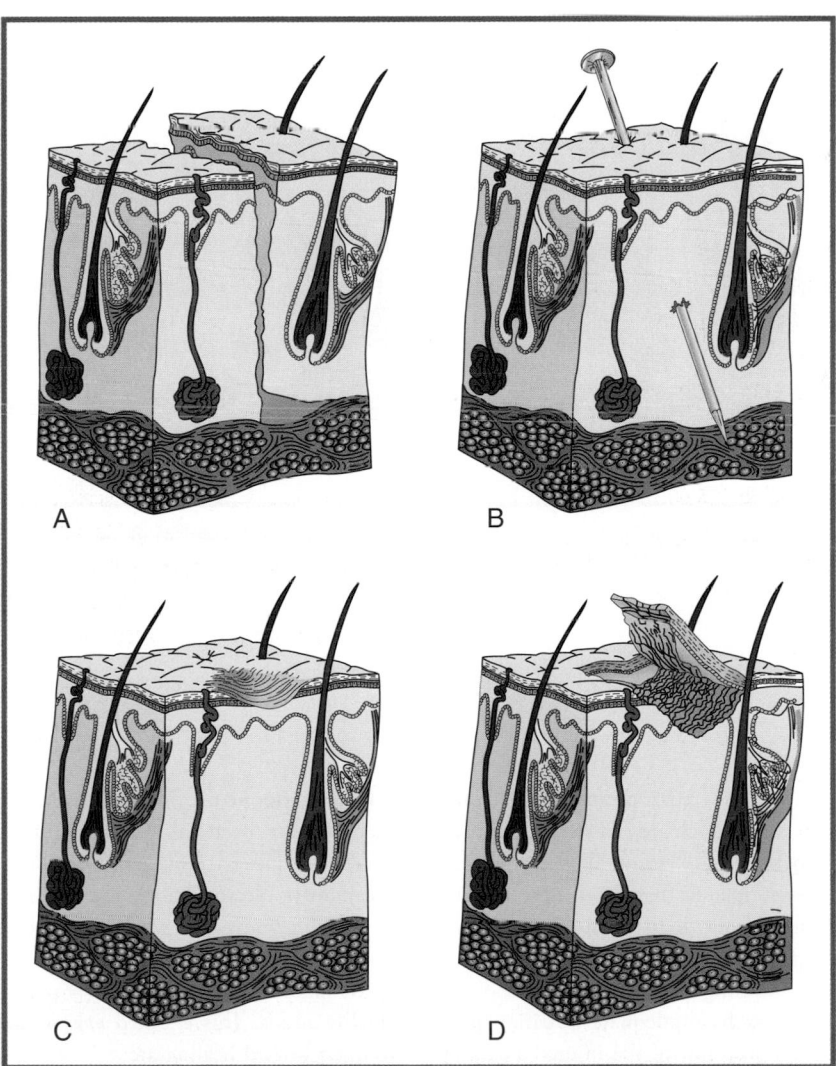

FIGURE 50-11 Types of wounds. **A,** Laceration—a jagged, irregular breaking or tearing of tissues, usually caused by blunt trauma. **B,** Puncture—piercing of the skin by a pointed object, such as a pin, nail, splinter, or bullet. **C,** Abrasion—a superficial wound made by scraping of the skin. **D,** Avulsion—tissue forcibly torn or separated, caused by accidents.

Continued

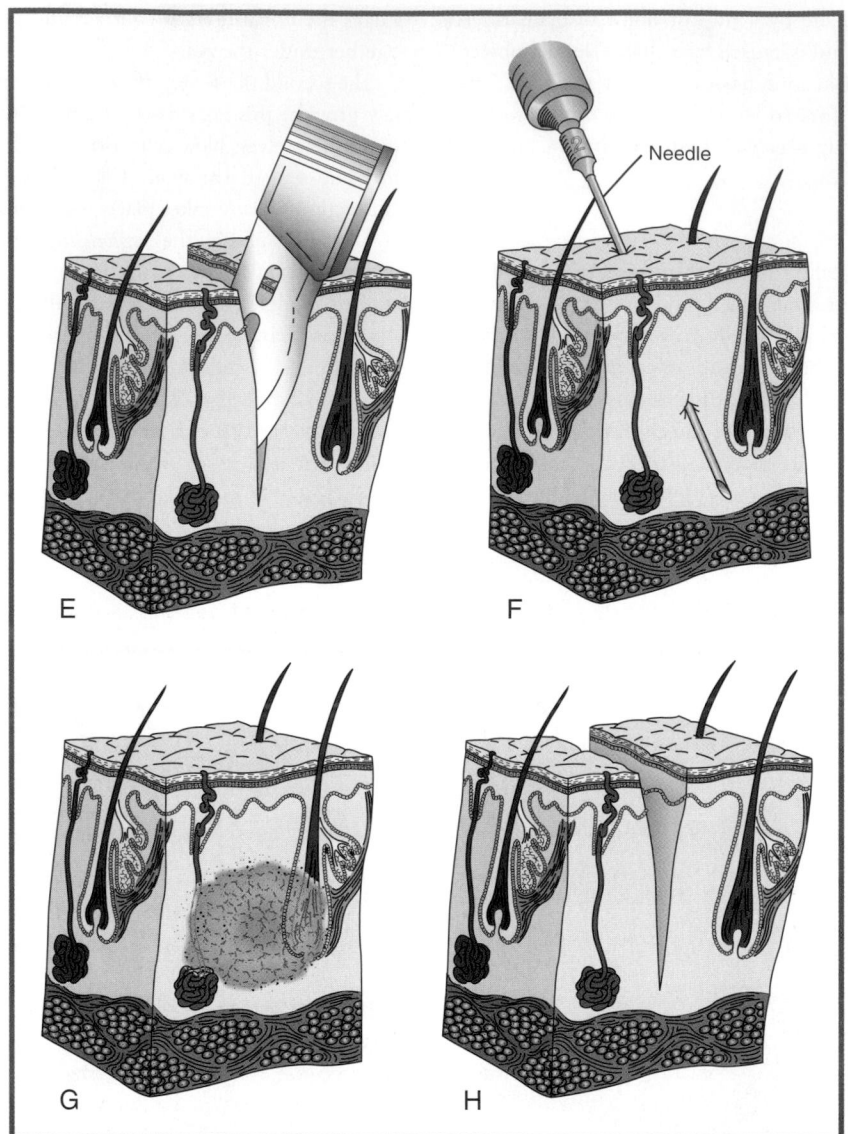

FIGURE 50-11, cont'd **E,** Surgical incision—a neat, clean cut. **F,** Hypodermic puncture—an injection under the skin. **G,** Contusion—a closed, nonpenetrating wound in which blood from broken vessels accumulates in tissues. **H,** Incision—a neat, clean cut from sharp objects, such as glass, knives, or metal.

Wounds are classified by the way they repair themselves. A clean, surgical wound that has been sutured closed and heals quickly without much scarring does so by *first intention.* Tissues that are severely damaged or purposely kept open or that fail to close are said to heal by *granulation* (i.e., healing from the bottom of the wound outward), which is called *second intention.*

Several factors influence the healing process. People who are young, in good general health, and have adequate nutrition heal more rapidly. Adequate protection and rest of the injured area also enhance the healing process. Destruction or reinjury during the second phase can delay healing and increase scarring. Wounds are susceptible to infection because the normal skin barrier is broken. If debris is present in a wound as the result of the breakdown of various cellular components, this dead (i.e., necrotic) tissue acts as a culture medium for bacterial growth. Suppuration (i.e., pus) contains necrotic tissue, bacteria, dead WBCs, and other products of tissue breakdown. Necrotic tissue must be removed; the removal of debris is called *debridement,* which may occur naturally or may be performed surgically.

Sometimes the physician may prefer no dressing or bandage on small wounds. This is called *open wound healing.* Some advantages to open wound healing are:

- Air can circulate freely around the wound.
- The wound is not irritated or rubbed by a dressing.
- The wound stays dry, which inhibits bacterial growth, reducing the chance of infection.

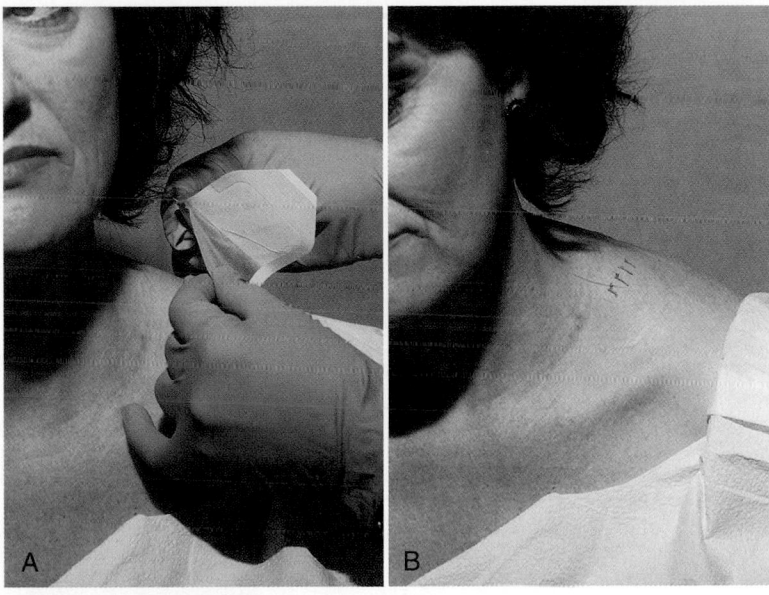

FIGURE 50-12 A, Placing a clear dressing on a sutured wound. **B,** Clear dressing in place over a sutured wound.

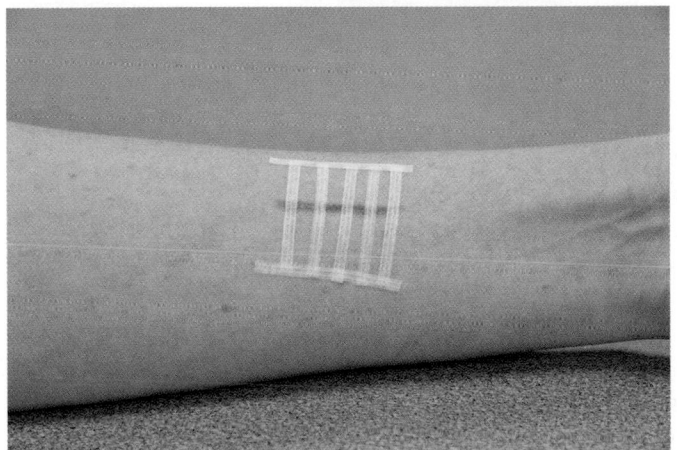

FIGURE 50-13 Steri-Strips on a wound.

material, depending on the provider's preference. Body cavities or wounds that need to remain open for a time are dressed with long, thin packing material that often is impregnated with an antiseptic or a lubricant; this sometimes is called *packing*. A good dressing must be effective and comfortable and must remain in place. If the dressing covers a hairless area, it may be anchored with tape, but no tape should touch the wound.

Frequently, small, clean lacerations may be closed with Steri-Strips (Figure 50-13). These strips reduce the chance of infection and do not leave suture scars. Steri-Strips are used on areas of the body that are protected from movement and stress. They often are used on the face. A medical assistant can place Steri-Strips as ordered by the provider. They are placed on the wound in the same sequence and at the same intervals as interrupted sutures and are left in place until they fall off or the wound heals.

Skin adhesives are also an alternative to sutures. They are frequently used for closure of facial lacerations, especially in pediatric patients, because they are effective for wound closure without requiring the use of needles and sutures.

Bandages

Bandages hold dressings in place and also help maintain even pressure, support the affected part, and help protect the wound from injury and contamination. Bandages can be gauze, cloth, or elastic cloth rolls and are bound by clips, tape, or ties. Dressings and bandages frequently appear easy and simple to apply; however, special skill is required to use different types of bandaging techniques (Procedure 50-13). Bandages that are too loose fall off; those that are too tight may compromise circulation and further harm the patient.

Plain roller gauze is seldom used. It is difficult to handle, has no elasticity, and tends to bind. It also tends to slip because it does not adhere to itself. Wrinkled crepe-type roller bandages (e.g., Kling)

- Sutures stay dry and hold together better.
- Any preexisting infection remains localized and is not spread by the dressing or bandage.

Dressings

A dressing is a sterile covering placed over a wound for the purposes of:
- Protecting the wound from injury and contamination
- Maintaining constant pressure to minimize bleeding and swelling
- Holding the wound edges together
- Absorbing drainage and secretions

A dressing usually consists of a strip of lubricated mesh gauze, a nonstick Telfa pad, or a clear dressing placed over a sutured wound (Figure 50-12). Gauze sponges may be placed over nonadhering

are preferred because they easily conform to various shapes of the body and adhere to themselves (Figure 50-14, *A*). If the bandage is to cover a wound, it should always be applied over a sterile dressing.

Plain elastic cloth (e.g., Ace) bandages or elastic roller cloth with adhesive backing make flexible, secure covers (Figure 50-14, *B*). When an elastic roller bandage is applied as a pressure bandage, especially to the lower limbs, it is essential to keep the bandage consistent in spacing and tension to ensure even pressure. Even, gentle pressure stimulates circulation and healing. Uneven pressure causes constriction points that can create pressure sores, ulcers, or edema. Roller bandages usually are applied from the distal to the proximal part of the area, because it is more even and snug if it is wrapped from a smaller to a larger circumference. Elevate the limb while you are bandaging and work with the roller facing upward, close to the patient's skin. Elastic bandages are excellent for bandaging the hand and wrist (Figure 50-15) and the foot and ankle (Figure 50-16).

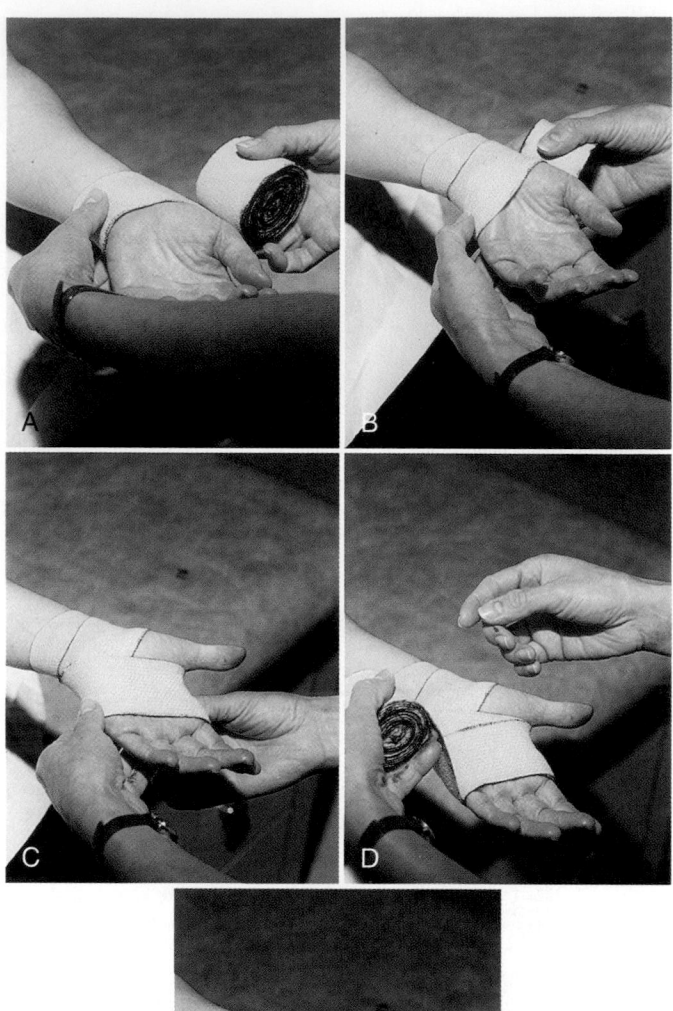

CRITICAL THINKING APPLICATION   **50-7**

Melissa applied a figure-eight elastic bandage to the hand and wrist of a patient who came into the office for suturing. She immediately sent the patient home after applying the bandage. She did not document the procedure in the patient's health record at that time because the office was quite busy. Discuss all of your concerns regarding this situation. In what ways were safe patient practices ignored? What would be the worst-case scenario for the outcome of this situation? How can this potentially serious situation be corrected after the fact?

FIGURE 50-15 A, A combination of recurrent and figure-eight turns are used for the hand. **B,** Bandaging starts at the wrist. **C,** Applying a roller bandage to the hand. **D,** Roller bandage in place on the hand. **E,** Consistent tension is maintained while the bandage is applied.

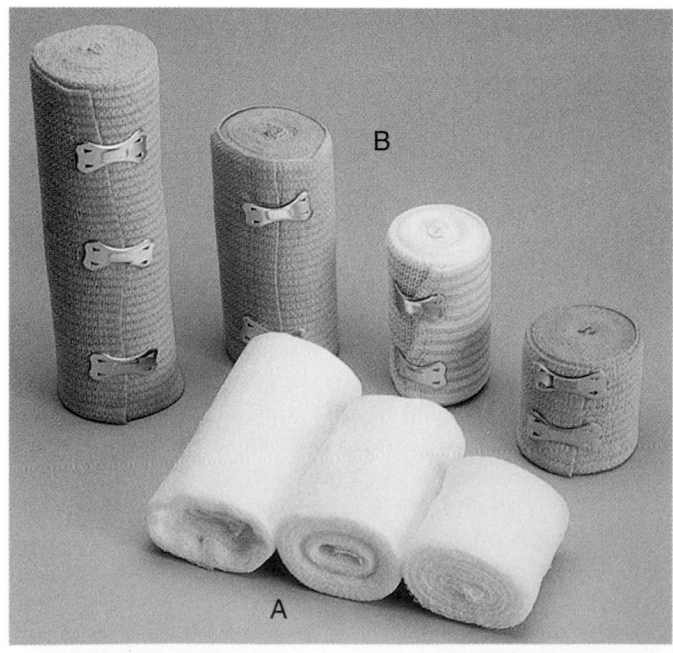

FIGURE 50-14 A, Wrinkled crepe-type roller bandages (e.g., Kling). **B,** Elastic roller bandages (e.g., Ace).

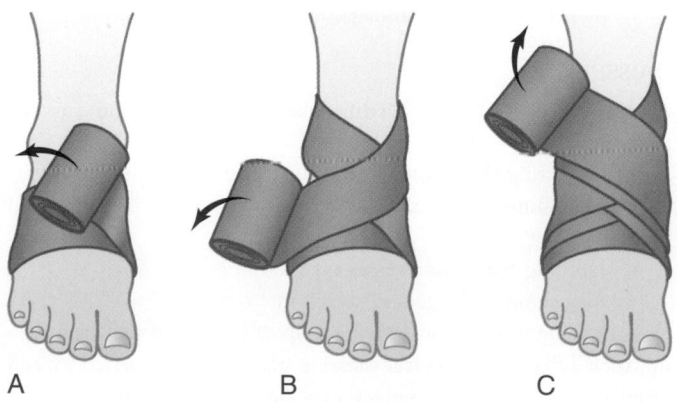

FIGURE 50-16 Using the figure-eight turn for the ankle.

PROCEDURE 50-13	Perform Wound Care: Apply an Elastic Support Bandage Using a Spiral Turn

Goal: *To apply an elastic bandage to the forearm.*

EQUIPMENT and SUPPLIES

- One 3- or 4-inch elastic bandage with clip closures

PROCEDURAL STEPS

1. Choose the proper size bandage for the size of the arm you are bandaging.
   <u>PURPOSE</u>: To provide proper support for the area.
2. Sanitize your hands. Perform a circular turn at the starting point, securing a turneddown corner of the bandage in the first circle around the site.
   <u>PURPOSE</u>: To anchor the bandage at the starting point.
3. Hold the roll so that the bandage can be rolled away from you (Figure 1).
   <u>PURPOSE</u>: To easily and securely apply the bandage.

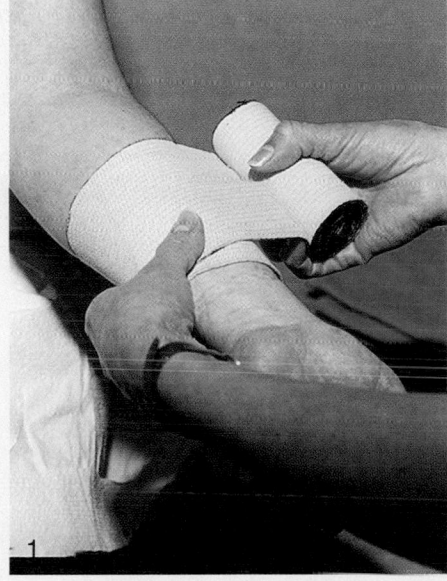

4. Keep the roll close to the patient and keep it facing upward (Figure 2). With each successive turn, overlap the previous bandage turn by half.

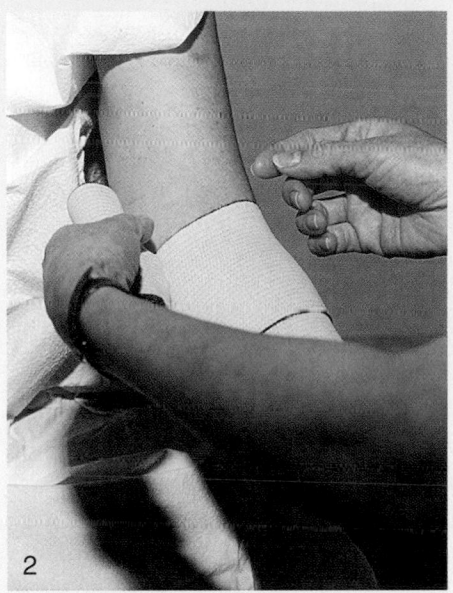

5. Maintain even tension and spacing as you continue to apply the bandage up the forearm.
   <u>PURPOSE</u>: To maintain even, light pressure over the entire area.
6. When crossing a joint, slightly flex the joint (Figure 3).
   <u>PURPOSE</u>: To facilitate patient comfort and maintain normal circulation.

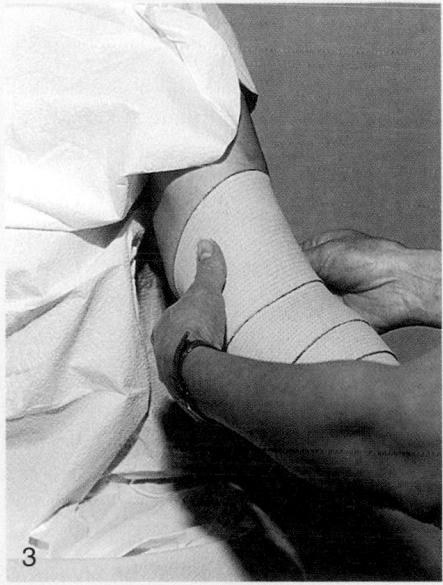

PROCEDURE 50-13   *—continued*

7. Fasten the end of the bandage with clips or tape (Figure 4).

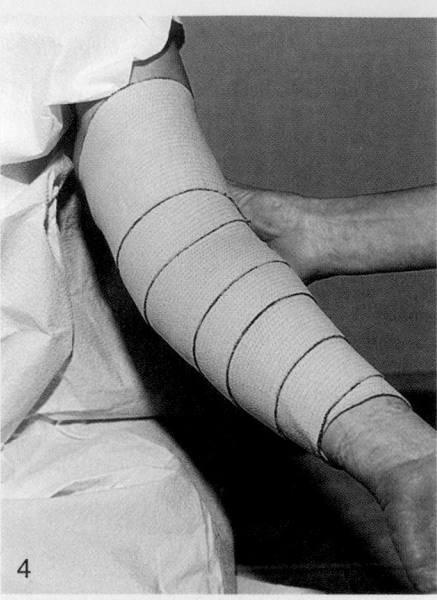

4

8. Check the nail beds for cyanosis; ask the patient whether the bandage is comfortable or feels too tight.
   <u>PURPOSE</u>: To ensure that the bandage is not acting as a tourniquet if applied too tightly.

9. Check the radial pulse on the wrapped arm.
   <u>PURPOSE</u>: To ensure that the bandage is not acting as a tourniquet if applied too tightly.

10. Have the patient move the fingers.
   <u>PURPOSE</u>: To check that nerve function is normal.

11. Document the procedure in the patient's health record; also document instructions given to the patient about bandage care and replacement.
   <u>PURPOSE</u>: The procedure is not completed until it is recorded, dated, and signed.

10/22/20XX 9:40 AM Spiral elastic bandage applied to Ⓡ forearm. Pt denies bandage too tight. Fingers warm to touch. Explained to mother how to replace bandage if needed. No questions. Melissa Gelbart, CMA (AAMA)

Seamless tubular gauze bandage, with or without elastic, is a superior material for covering round narrow surfaces such as fingers or toes. It can be used as a dressing if the gauze material is sterile; it can also be used as a bandage. A tubular gauze bandage is applied with a cagelike applicator (Figure 50-17). Work with the open circle of the applicator toward the patient. Hold the applicator in the dominant hand and control the tension flow with your fingers as the applicator is gradually rotated and the material slides off. Tubular dressing may be applied with or without slight pressure. Beyond the tip of the bandaged part, give the applicator a full half-turn, place the applicator again over the part, and repeat the process, being careful not to create a tourniquet effect when you reverse the applicator. When the desired thickness of the bandage is reached, cut the gauze and anchor the final gauze application with tape or by tying at the wrist.

CLOSING COMMENTS

Patient Education

A medical assistant can help the patient in many ways. The best time to instruct your patient in aseptic techniques to be used at home is while you are performing an aseptic procedure. For example:

- While sanitizing your hands before a procedure or examination, explain to the patient that hands should be washed before meals; after sneezing, coughing, or nose blowing; after using the bathroom; before and after changing a dressing or bandage; and after changing an infant's diaper.
- Instruct the patient about the differences between sterile and clean dressings and bandages. Show the person step by step how to change a dressing properly and then how to dispose of the contaminated items.

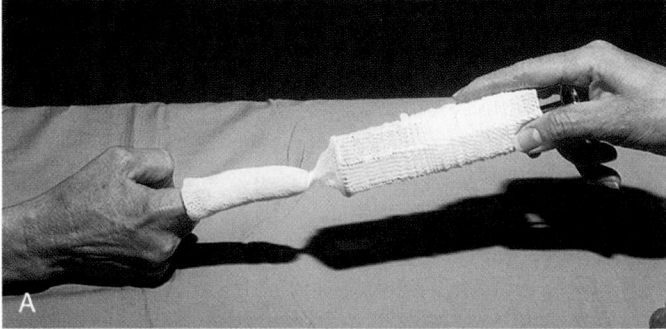

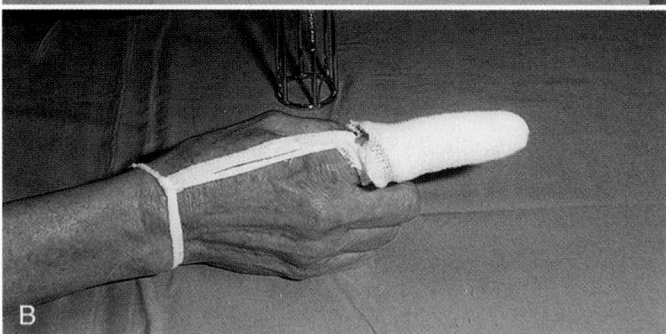

FIGURE 50-17 A, Tube gauze is applied with even tension and is twisted at the fingertip before the next layer is applied. **B,** Tube gauze bandage has been applied and secured by tying at the wrist.

A medical assistant's duty may include calling the patient the day before surgery to confirm the scheduled surgical procedure and appointment time. Explaining the procedure and what to expect during and after surgery prepares the patient and helps calm the person's fears or concerns. Lying still during surgery is important, and eating a light meal the night before should be encouraged.

Bathing before coming to the office helps reduce the number of bacteria on the skin, and comfortable, loose clothing should be worn. Sometimes in the course of general conversation the medical assistant can pick up hints of concerns the patient may have and can direct the conversation into a discussion of these concerns.

Patients should be informed that they may need someone to accompany them home. A bandage is applied after surgery, and it must be kept clean and dry. The patient may have some pain, and the physician probably will prescribe some type of analgesic. After the procedure is complete, make sure the patient makes an appointment for a return visit and examination. Patients should also be encouraged to call the office immediately if they suspect an infection or have a sudden increase in pain at the surgical site.

Legal and Ethical Issues

Many minor surgical procedures previously performed in the hospital are now being done in a medical office, surgery center, or clinic. As insurance companies continue to recognize the cost-effectiveness of performing minor surgical procedures in these settings, the role of the medical assistant continues to expand.

Patients should have absolute assurance that they are being taken care of in an aseptic atmosphere and under the most stringent aseptic conditions. This assurance is just as important for the protection of the office staff as it is for the patient. Allowing the physician to assume that the correct aseptic techniques have been used in the preparation of equipment and allowing him or her to use contaminated equipment on a patient can result in claims of malpractice and charges of battery. Absolute, uncompromising honesty on the part of the assistant builds self-respect and contributes to professional achievement and satisfaction.

To have a good understanding of the subject, you must become familiar with the various techniques of sanitization, disinfection, and sterilization. Ignorance or carelessness can be dangerous and is inexcusable before the law.

The medical assistant must know what procedure is scheduled and whether the patient has been informed about the procedure. In the surgical setting, the medical assistant must realize the full extent of his or her role as the patient's advocate and the physician's agent.

Confirm that the physician has explained the procedure to the patient and that the patient fully understands all aspects of the procedure to be performed. This means that when the patient signs informed consent for surgery, he or she is fully informed. Legal action can result if complications arise because of failure to complete consent forms. The surgical procedure is expedited when the patient is given instructions and knows what to expect. Increasing the patient's understanding ensures greater compliance with presurgical preparations, and the patient is more likely to follow instructions and advice after surgery.

The medical assistant must practice perfect aseptic technique. A break in technique may invite infection and possible legal action. It is the medical assistant's duty to protect the patient. A major responsibility of the medical assistant is to adhere strictly to aseptic technique and to correct immediately any break in technique.

Professional Behaviors

Accountability is a crucial part of the medical assistant's professional responsibilities. An accountable individual recognizes if an error has been committed and does everything possible to correct his or her mistake. Personal accountability and discipline are the primary concerns in surgical asepsis. Often the assistant is alone when performing a surgical aseptic procedure; if contamination occurs, no one may know except the medical assistant. If there is any doubt about the sterility of the surgical field, instruments, or supplies, it is the assistant's responsibility to begin the procedure again. The medical assistant's main responsibilities in this area are performing sanitization, disinfection, and sterilization procedures with precision and with total effectiveness. There is no room for compromise.

SUMMARY OF SCENARIO

Melissa is finding her clinical medical assisting position in Dr. Armstrong's practice rewarding, exciting, and challenging. She enjoys coming to work every day and has learned all aspects of her position much more quickly than most of her peers. Melissa frequently reads the latest information on new developments in minor surgery practice. Her concern for her patient's well-being makes her stand out, and the physician constantly gets positive comments on her level of professionalism.

Melissa has made a few errors in sterile technique since starting the clinical assistant position, but she has learned from each situation and has never covered up a mistake. Whenever she realized that she did not follow procedure, she has discussed the issue with her supervisor and with Dr. Armstrong. In this way, errors can be corrected, if possible, and she most likely will not make the same or similar mistakes again.

Melissa is a team player who consistently tries to anticipate the needs of the physician and patient both before and during surgery. Her cooperative, supportive manner is appreciated by everyone on the clinical staff.

SUMMARY OF LEARNING OBJECTIVES

1. **Define, spell, and pronounce the terms listed in the vocabulary.**
   Spelling and pronouncing medical terms correctly bolster the medical assistant's credibility. Knowing the definitions of these terms promotes confidence in communication with patients and co-workers.

2. **Define the concepts of aseptic technique.**
   Medical asepsis is the process of reducing the number of pathogens; surgical asepsis is the complete destruction of all organisms on instruments or supplies that will enter the patient's body. Surgical asepsis must be followed in all procedures where the skin is broken, such as application of a sterile dressing. Using proper surgical aseptic technique is the primary means of preventing postoperative infections in surgical patients. Everyone on the surgical team is responsible for preventing and correcting breaks in technique.

3. **Explain the differences between sanitization, disinfection, and sterilization.**
   Sanitization is the cleaning of instruments and the environment to reduce the number of pathogens. *Disinfection* is the destruction of pathogens by physical or chemical means. *Sterilization* is the destruction of all microorganisms.

4. **Summarize tips for improving autoclave techniques; demonstrate how to prepare items for autoclave sterilization.**
   Refer to Table 50-2 for tips to improve autoclave techniques and Procedure 50-1 to prepare items for autoclave sterilization.

5. **Explain how to wrap materials and discuss the types and uses of sterilization indicators.**
   The method used to wrap instruments for autoclave sterilization must allow the pack to be opened without being consumed. There are various rules for protecting the package contents when wrapping materials.
   Autoclave tape contains a chemical dye that changes color when exposed to steam.
   Biologic sterilization indicator kits use ampules of *Bacillus stearothermophilus,* which is destroyed at 121° C (250° F). The ampule is placed in the center of the largest pack that is autoclaved in the facility to determine the accuracy of the autoclave and autoclave procedures in destroying all microbes. On completion of the cycle, the ampule is sent to the laboratory for analysis of any type of microbial growth.

6. **Summarize the correct methods of loading, operating, and unloading an autoclave.**
   The load is arranged for maximum circulation of steam and heat. Articles should be resting on edges; jars and bottles should be placed on their sides. When the cycle is complete, the pressure is released according to the manufacturer's guidelines. The medical assistant stands back from the door and, with heat-resistant gloves, opens the door approximately ¼". The load is allowed to dry for at least 15 minutes before removal. Refer to Procedure 50-2.

7. **Summarize common minor surgical procedures.**
   Typical minor surgical procedures include incision and drainage (I&D) of a cyst; electrosurgery, which uses high-frequency current to cut through tissue and coagulate blood vessels; laser surgery, which uses tiny light beams to safely treat specific tissues with minimal damage to surrounding tissues and limited scar formation; microsurgery, which involves the use of an operating microscope to perform delicate surgical procedures; endoscopic procedures, which use a fiberoptic instrument with a miniature camera mounted on a flexible tube to examine the area within an organ or cavity and which are named according to the organs or areas they explore; and cryosurgery, which is the use of extreme cold to destroy tissues such as warts and skin lesions.

8. **Detail the medical assistant's role in minor office surgery.**
   The medical assistant is responsible for preparing the patient for surgery; performing the physician's preoperative orders; confirming that the patient has signed an informed consent form; making sure all the patient's questions and concerns have been addressed; assisting with positioning of the patient; performing skin preparation if ordered; and preparing the room for the procedure.

9. **Explain how to perform a skin prep for surgery and how to perform a surgical hand scrub.**
   Refer to Procedure 50-3 for steps for how to perform a skin prep for surgery.
   A surgical hand scrub is done to lower the number of transient flora on the practitioner's hands so that the risk of wound contamination is reduced (see Procedure 50-4).

10. **Outline the rules for setting up and maintaining a sterile field; explain how to perform the following procedures related to sterile techniques:**
    Sterile surfaces must never come in contact with nonsterile surfaces. If this occurs, the sterile surface immediately is considered contaminated. The rules for maintaining a sterile field include keeping talking to a minimum; maintaining sight of the sterile field; and never crossing over the sterile field. Anything that falls below the edge of the Mayo tray and within a 1" border surrounding the tray is considered contaminated. A sterile barrier that is wet, cut, or torn is contaminated. Sterile gloved hands must be kept above waist level at all times. An item is never removed from and then again put into the field. A sterile package should be opened the entire way and the contents tossed onto the field without crossing over the sterile area. If a sterile package falls to the floor, it must be discarded. If any doubt exists about sterility, the field must be considered contaminated and the process must start all over again.
    - Open a sterile pack and create a sterile field.
    Refer to Procedure 50-5.
    - Transfer sterile instruments and pour solutions into a sterile field.
    Refer to Procedures 50-6 and 50-7.
    - Demonstrate how to apply sterile gloves without contaminating them.
    Refer to Procedure 50-8.

11. **Discuss how to assist the physician during surgery and demonstrate how to assist with a minor surgical procedure and suturing.**
    The physician is responsible for the patient; however, the medical assistant is responsible for ensuring that everything the assistant and the physician will use in caring for the surgical patient is accounted for, ready to use, and prepared in a safe and sterile manner. Refer to Procedures 50-9 through 50-11.

12. Summarize postoperative Instructions and explain how to remove sutures and surgical staples.

If medication is prescribed, review the purpose of the medication and directions for its use with the patient and his or her companion and make a follow-up appointment. The patient should be taught to care for himself or herself at home after surgery and should receive both verbal and written instructions. Explain to the patient the importance of calling the office if any questions arise or if he or she notes redness around the operative site, bleeding from the wound, fever, swelling, or increasing or severe pain. If the patient does not call within the next 24 hours, the medical assistant should call the patient.

Refer to Procedure 50-12 for the steps on how to remove sutures and surgical staples.

13. Explain the process of wound healing.

All wounds go through a healing or repair process that has three phases. The lag phase occurs first when the blood vessels contract to control hemorrhage, platelets form a fibrin network, and a clot dries into a scab. Proliferation is a new growth period during which tissues repair themselves. During the final, or remodeling, phase, a bridge of new tissue is built to close the gap of the wound. Collagen gives the wounded tissues strength and forms scar tissue. Wounds are classified by the way they repair themselves: either by first intention, with clean, straight edges that heal quickly, or by granulation (or second intention), as in tissues that are severely damaged and are left open or fail to close.

14. Explain how to properly apply dressings and bandages to surgical sites.

Refer to Procedure 50-13.

15. Conduct patient education in aseptic technique and surgical procedures and discuss legal and ethical concerns regarding surgical asepsis and infection control.

The best time for a medical assistant to instruct the patient in aseptic techniques to be used at home is during an aseptic procedure. Patient education includes the purpose and importance of hand washing; using disposable tissues to cover the nose and mouth when coughing or sneezing and properly disposing of used tissues; the differences between sterile and clean dressings and bandages; and step-by-step instructions on how to change a dressing properly and dispose of contaminated items.

The medical assistant must know what procedure is to be performed and whether the patient has provided informed consent. The medical assistant must realize the full extent of his or her role as the patient's advocate and the physician's agent. The more patients understand about their procedures, the more they comply with presurgical preparations and the more likely they are to follow instructions and advice after surgery. A major responsibility of the medical assistant is to adhere strictly to aseptic technique and to correct immediately any break in technique.

CONNECTIONS

Study Guide Connection: Go to the Chapter 50 Study Guide. Read and complete the activities.

evolve Evolve Connection: Go to the Chapter 50 link at *evolve.elsevier.com/kinn* to complete the Chapter Review Quiz. Check out the other resources listed for this chapter to make the most of what you have learned from Surgical Asepsis and Assisting with Surgical Procedures.

51

CAREER DEVELOPMENT AND LIFE SKILLS

SCENARIO

Michelle, Krysia, and Zacarias (or Zac to his friends) met during their first semester of college and have developed a great friendship over the last few months. They will be graduating from the medical assistant program in less than 6 weeks. Michelle just graduated from high school a year ago. Krysia entered the military just after her high school graduation and spent 10 years in the Marines. Zac has been out of high school for several years and worked in a factory. He started as a line worker and gradually advanced to supervisory positions, but because of downsizing, his position was eliminated and he went back to school. These friends are looking forward to graduation and getting jobs as medical assistants.

As these three friends discuss finding a job, Michelle is hesitant about the job search experience. Her only work experience is 2 years as a waitress at a local restaurant. She has never created a résumé or a cover letter. She only had a very informal interview with the restaurant owner before she was given the job. Krysia is concerned about her military career. The positions she held were not related to healthcare. She managed inventory, supervised others, and was also deployed to many hot spots around the world. Zac has a lot of experience in the factory setting, but he feels that world is so different from healthcare. As they talk with each other, it is clear that each person has a unique situation and they all must take a closer look at their past experiences as they prepare for their job search adventure.

While studying this chapter, think about the following questions:

- What experience from a medical assistant's background can be utilized in a healthcare position?
- How can a résumé market a medical assistant's characteristics and experiences to potential employers?

- How can the medical assistant organize the job search experience?
- What is considered professional dress for an interview?
- How should a medical assistant prepare for an interview?
- What are appropriate follow-up activities after the interview?

LEARNING OBJECTIVES

1. Define, spell, and pronounce the terms listed in the vocabulary.
2. Describe the four personality traits that are most important to employers.
3. Explain the three areas that need to be examined to determine one's strengths and skills.
4. Discuss career objectives and describe how personal needs affect the job search.
5. Do the following related to finding a job:
   - Explain the two best job search methods.
   - Discuss traditional job search methods.
   - Describe various ways to improve your opportunities.
   - Discuss the importance of being organized in your job search.
6. Discuss the three types of résumé formats, describe how to prepare a chronologic résumé and cover letter, and discuss the importance and format of both the résumé and cover letter.
7. Discuss how to complete an online portfolio and job application.

8. Describe how to create a career portfolio.
9. Do the following related to the job interview:
   - List and describe the four phases of the interview process.
   - List and discuss legal and illegal interview questions.
   - Practice interview skills for a mock interview.
   - Create a thank-you note for an interview.
10. Do the following related to getting a job:
    - Discuss the importance of the probationary period for a new employee.
    - List some common early mistakes of which a new employee should be aware.
    - Discuss how to be a good employee and how to deal with supervisors.
    - Explain why a performance appraisal rating is usually not perfect.
    - Discuss how to pursue a raise and how to leave a job.
11. Discuss various life skills needed in the workplace.

VOCABULARY

counteroffer Return offer made by one who has rejected an offer or a job.

dignity Being worthy of honor and respect from others.

interpersonal skills Ability to communicate and interact with others; sometimes referred to as "soft skills."

job boards Web site that posts jobs submitted by employers and can be used by job seekers to identify open positions.

mock Simulated; intended for imitation or practice.

networking Exchange of information or services among individuals, groups, or institutions; also, meeting and getting to know individuals in the same or similar career fields and sharing information about available opportunities.

proofread To read and mark corrections.

rectify (rek'-tih-fi) To correct by removing errors.

skill set A person's abilities or skills.

vocation The work in which a person is regularly employed.

Each day a person exists is a small portion of a whole—a part of a person's entire lifetime. The events that happen during a day, no matter how small, shape the future. In the same way, the events that happen in the life of a medical assistant play a role in shaping his or her career. Every day, the medical assistant "writes a résumé"— through actions that reveal strengths, highlight skills, and summarize accomplishments—that builds on his or her **vocation**. Each duty performed becomes a part of the medical assistant's sum of experience and is important in the overall growth of the individual. Each action taken can have an effect on the future for the medical assistant. If the actions are professional, accurate, and performed to the individual's utmost ability, the résumé the medical assistant is writing will be one that leads to greater opportunities. If the medical assistant performs poorly, the résumé will be one that does not reflect trustworthiness and dependability. The small decisions made each day greatly affect the overall impression the medical assistant makes in the workplace.

Most people seeking employment have never had any type of formal training in the job search process. A graduating medical assistant student should take advantage of job search training for three reasons:

- It will reduce the amount of time spent searching for a job.
- It will increase the chances of receiving better wages through negotiation.
- It will help reduce the fears of looking for work and interviewing.

MOVING ON TO THE NEXT PHASE OF LIFE

As you move toward graduation, you may be experiencing many emotions. You might be excited about finishing your medical assistant program. You might be scared of the changes that will be occurring over the next months. The thought of finding a job might be overwhelming. These are common feelings of graduates regardless of the career path they have chosen. The important step before graduation is to prepare for the next phase: getting a job.

Preparing for the job-seeking phase is very important. By understanding the characteristics that employers want; identifying your strengths, experiences, and skills; and developing your career objectives, you are ready to market yourself to potential employers through your résumé and interview experiences. Early preparation and marketing yourself to employers, even before graduation, can be the key to landing a job soon after graduation.

UNDERSTANDING PERSONALITY TRAITS IMPORTANT TO EMPLOYERS

As you start with your job search, it is important to understand what employers are looking for in an employee. With the cost and time invested in training new employees, it is crucial employers find the right new employee. Many employers will agree that they can help refine employees' technical skill proficiencies, but it is more difficult to help evolve or change personality traits. The four personality traits that are most important to employers are: collaboration and **interpersonal skills**, professionalism, compassion, and sincere interest in the job.

Collaboration and interpersonal skills are crucial to productivity in today's fast-paced, ever-changing healthcare environment. Employers look for people who can blend well with the current staff. It is important that the new employee is flexible, dependable, supportive of peers, and remains calm under pressure. Employers also look for people who will provide excellent customer service by having outstanding interpersonal skills, which include communication skills and good manners (Figure 51-1). Effective verbal communication involves clear, thoughtful communication. Being focused, calm, polite, and interested in the other person are traits of effective verbal communication. In addition, appropriate nonverbal communication is crucial in the healthcare setting. Your body language relays more to your patients and peers than any words you could use. Eye contact, posture, voice, and gestures provide insights into a person's attitude (Figure 51-2). Listening is also critical when working with peers and patients. For effective communication to occur, listening must occur. Appropriate questions can draw others into the conversation and show others you are listening and care. Using communication techniques such as rephrasing, reflecting, paraphrasing, and asking for clarification are also excellent ways of demonstrating active listening skills. Good manners and a basic understanding of the diversity of other cultures also help facilitate communication.

Professionalism is a trait that employers evaluate from their first contact with interested potential employees. From the application and résumé to the interview, employers are building their perceptions of the candidates' professionalism. Being professional not only encompasses your dress and grooming habits but also your flexibility, punctuality, honesty, attention to detail, and abilities to follow directions, prioritize, and manage time. Employers are looking for loyal employees who provide a professional image

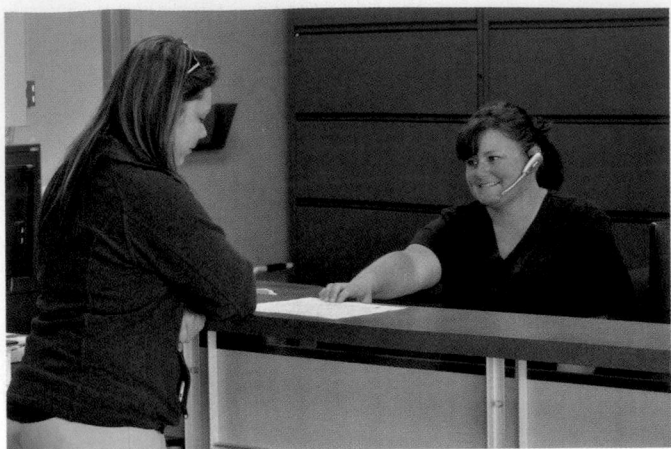

FIGURE 51-1 Having good communication skills and good manners are necessary to provide excellent customer service.

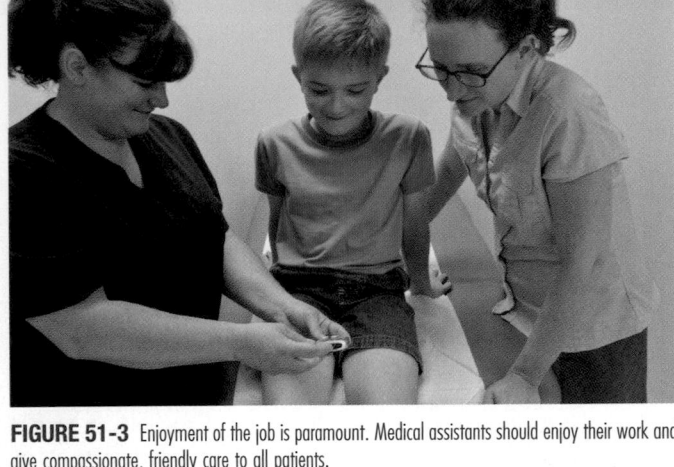

FIGURE 51-3 Enjoyment of the job is paramount. Medical assistants should enjoy their work and give compassionate, friendly care to all patients.

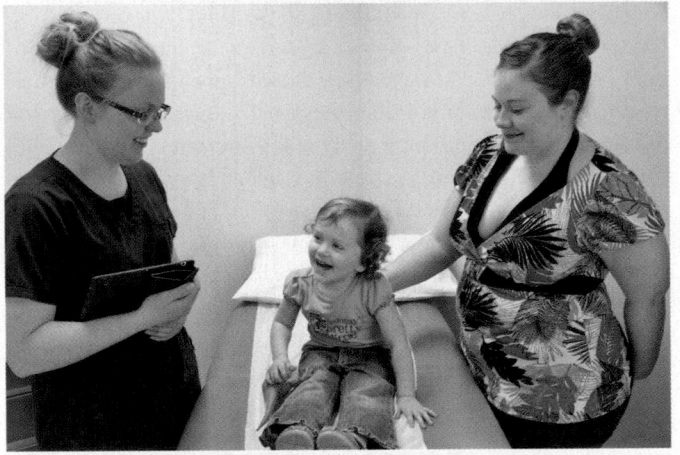

FIGURE 51-2 It is important that medical assistants working in a family practice or pediatric setting have a positive attitude and enjoy working with children.

CRITICAL THINKING APPLICATION   **51-1**

Think of the three friends. Michelle just graduated from high school and has 2 years of waitressing experience. Krysia has ten years in the military, where she managed inventory, supervised others, and was deployed to many hot spots around the world. Zac has been working in a factory, advancing to supervisory positions. Now think about the personality traits that employers want. What personality traits might each friend possess? Explain your answer.

- Create your own list of the personality traits that employers want and you possess.

---

to patients, families, and other customers of the healthcare organization.

Having compassion and providing **dignity** and respect to others is the third trait that is important to employers. Many people go into healthcare to help others, but lack the compassion and respect that is needed when caring for others. Not only do healthcare employees provide technical skills during patient care, they also need to help support and maintain the dignity of the patient. Compassion and respect help healthcare employees connect to patients and their families. Acts of kindness and thoughtfulness that alleviate stress are welcomed by patients.

The last personality trait that employers are looking for is genuine interest in the job. This trait can be seen during the interview when the candidate asks thoughtful questions regarding the position and the agency. Genuine interest in the job extends beyond the hiring phase into the day-to-day operations. Being interested in one's job and looking for ways to improve procedures and provide better patient care are important behaviors to demonstrate to the employer. This genuine interest is reflected in your attitude and performance in the workplace (Figure 51-3). It helps ease your transition into a new job and promotes your success.

Assessing Your Strengths and Skills

As you prepare to market yourself to potential employers, you need to examine your strengths and skills in three different areas. You need to identify the personality traits, technical skills, and transferable job skills that you possess.

As you contemplate the personality traits that employers want, try to honestly identify which of those skills and strengths you have. Many people will tell potential employers what they think the employer wants to hear. They claim to be a "team player," "communicate well," be "dependable," and so on, but employers need more. Words in your résumé or cover letter or voicing these statements in the interview is not enough to convince the potential employer that you truly have those characteristics. Early on in the preparation phase, make a list of the qualities that you believe you possess. Then for each characteristic, provide one or two pieces of "evidence" to support your claims. Your "evidence" may be a past job review or practicum evaluation where the author indicates your strengths and characteristics. These are excellent documents to include in your portfolio, which will be discussed later in the chapter. Using stories of situations where you portrayed those characteristics is another way to illustrate you have the qualities, and you can share these during the interview if pertinent to the questions asked.

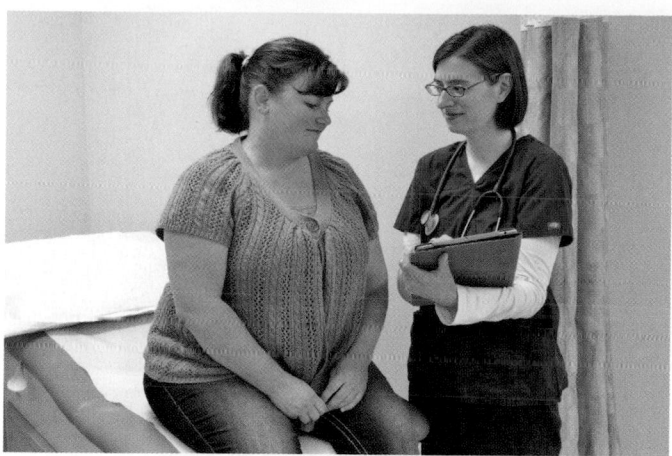

FIGURE 51-4 The potential employer needs to know about the technical skills you have practiced in the classroom and practicum setting.

Employers also need to know about your technical skills. Technical skills for medical assistants can be skills related to clinical procedures, such as phlebotomy, injections, electrocardiograms (ECGs), and obtaining vital signs (Figure 51-4). Technical skills can also be related to administrative procedures and may include software proficiency, keyboard speed, reception duties, and coding procedures. You may be able to provide supporting documentation of your technical skills through the use of practicum skill checklists or through a portfolio. Technical skills might also include skills that you obtained outside of the medical assistant program but still relate to your chosen career. For instance, you worked as a phlebotomist at a local hospital. Many of the technical skills you perform as a phlebotomist may relate to a clinic position.

The last area that needs to be examined during the preparation phase of job seeking is your transferable job skills. These are skills that a person develops in one job or experience that can be transferred to another job. Potential transferable skills include: customer service, compassion and empathy, strong communication and listening, computer skills, teamwork, time management and prioritizing, creativity, leadership, organization, problem solving, and grace under pressure. Many of these skills may sound familiar; they also are characteristics employers are looking for and were discussed in an earlier section.

Identifying transferable job skills can be difficult for many people. Job descriptions for past experiences can be very useful, but many times these are not available. To start, make a list of your past jobs, military experience, and volunteer opportunities. Then ask yourself which of the potential transferable skills you developed and used during that experience. For instance, you have waited on customers in a restaurant. Most wait staff need strong communication and listening skills. Prioritizing and customer service skills are also required. If you worked in a factory setting, communications skills, teamwork, and problem solving might be traits you developed. If you had military experience, strong communication skills, grace under pressure, and prioritizing might be just a few of the skills you developed during your time serving the country. This list of transferable job skills will be utilized as you create your résumé and prepare for your interview.

CRITICAL THINKING APPLICATION   **51-2**

What might be some transferable skills that the three friends, Michelle, Krysia, and Zac, possess? Explain your answer.
- Using the list you have already started, add on the personality traits, technical skills, and transferable job skills that you possess. Also, indicate why you believe you have these skills (e.g., which job or experience helped you develop the skill).

DEVELOPING CAREER OBJECTIVES

Each medical assistant has a reason for entering the healthcare field. This basic desire should influence decisions concerning his or her career choices. Because medical assisting is such a versatile profession, a medical assistant has numerous options after graduation.

Medical assistant students should take some time to think about what they want from their careers. While attending school and subsequently completing the practicum, ideas may surface about the area of healthcare or a specific agency in which the medical assistant most wants to work.

When developing career objectives, the medical assistant should start by asking several questions:
- What areas and skills did I enjoy in practicum?
- Where do I want to be in 5 years?
- Where do I want to be in 10 years?
- What additional skills do I need to get where I want to go?

Write down the questions and answers and go into specific detail. Set realistic goals and develop a plan as to how and when they will be reached. Remember career objectives are reached over time. It is important to know where you want to be, so you can start down the right path to reach your goals. Keep your list of goals available and visible so you can revisit them frequently.

CRITICAL THINKING APPLICATION   **51-3**

For the following four questions, write down your answers and explain them. These answers will help you as you start the job search process.
- What areas and skills did I enjoy in practicum?
- Where do I want to be in 5 years?
- Where do I want to be in 10 years?
- What additional skills do I need to get where I want to go?

KNOWING PERSONAL NEEDS

After evaluating your skills and strengths and developing your career objectives, you need to evaluate your needs. Potential jobs for medical assistants can include different wages, benefits, hours, and locations. Most people have a salary minimum and specific benefits they require to meet their needs and living expenses. Some people have specific hours that work better for them. People with children may need a job that allows them to be home with their children after school. For medical assistants who do not drive or have a reliable mode of transportation, the location of a job will be important to consider. Evaluating your personal needs will help you find a job that matches your requirements.

FINDING A JOB

Many people have misconceptions about the job market that exists today. Fortunately, the medical field is not an industry that sees high levels of unemployment. Usually healthcare employment remains high even in a poor economy. However, graduation from a medical assisting program does not guarantee that the student will obtain employment. Completion of the program gives the medical assistant the job skills needed to work, but a good attitude and positive outlook are essential for success in the job search. In addition, the medical assistant should always be open to new and better opportunities.

Some job seekers assume that potential employers will not interact with students until they graduate and passed a credential examination (i.e., Certified Medical Assistant [CMA] through the American Association of Medical Assistants [AAMA], Registered Medical Assistant [RMA] through the American Medical Technologists [AMT]). However, prospecting before graduation is a smart idea. Some employers do not require credential examinations and others may hire a medical assistant with an understanding that within a period of time the employee needs to obtain the credential. Many employers are interested in hiring new graduates. They consider new graduates "teachable," meaning they can train and "mold" them into the employee they require. Employers recognize that new graduates have more current knowledge and skills in certain healthcare areas including coding and electronic health records (EHRs).

Two Best Job Search Methods

Although there are many ways to find employment, two methods have proved to be the best and most effective: networking and checking job boards.

Networking is the exchange of information or services among individuals, groups, or institutions. When related to a job search, networking involves meeting and getting to know individuals in the same or similar career fields and sharing information about available opportunities. A medical assistant should begin to form a network of friends, business associates, co-workers, and acquaintances early in training, and he or she should stay in contact with these people throughout the job search and beyond (Figure 51-5). E-mail, LinkedIn, Facebook, Twitter, and other electronic advances make staying in touch with former classmates and instructors very easy.

A medical assistant can network through family, friends, and other healthcare professionals. The practicum is the best networking experience. During a practicum, the student meets and works alongside many healthcare professionals. These professionals continually evaluate the student's performance. It is not uncommon that when healthcare professionals find a student who portrays the qualities of a professional medical assistant, they want to assist that student in finding a job. They may offer to provide a future job reference. They may provide the student with insight on potential openings. It is crucial that the medical assistant student looks at the practicum as a constant job interview and strives to do his or her best. As the

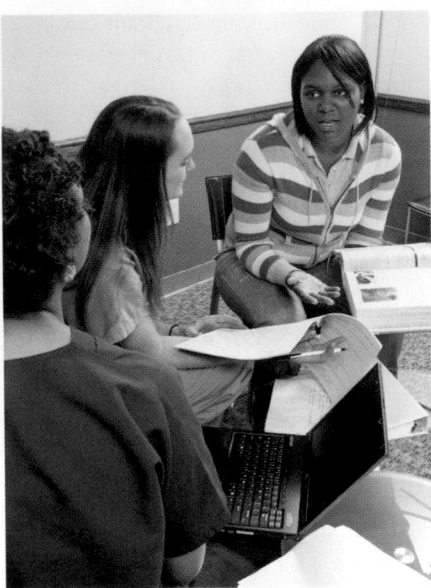

FIGURE 51-5 Stay in touch with classmates. They are excellent networking contacts and may be able to provide job leads.

practicum progresses, students can inquire about potential job openings, either through their mentor, supervisor, or the agency's human resource department. Toward the end of the practicum, the student may want to ask the mentor if he or she would be willing to provide a reference or a letter of recommendation. When the practicum experience concludes, the medical assistant student should formally thank the supervisor, the mentor, and the department with a note and also provide the supervisor with a résumé and cover letter.

Another way to network with professional medical assistants is to join a medical assistant organization. The members who attend regular meetings often know about job leads in the area. Friends and family members can be on the lookout for potential opportunities and may help by asking their friends and personal physicians/ providers if they are aware of positions that will open for applications soon.

Checking **job boards** is the other most common method of identifying job opportunities. Large healthcare organizations usually have their own Web sites and many include an employment or career section that lists available jobs. Some of these larger organizations allow job seekers to register, complete an online application, and upload a résumé and cover letter. These sites will then generate e-mails to job seekers when jobs are posted. By having the online application already completed, the applicant can upload a customized cover letter and résumé, and thus apply for the job very quickly.

Besides healthcare organizations' job boards, there are local, state, and national job boards. Local job boards may include websites from your school or your community's media (i.e., newspaper, television, radio) agencies. Smaller healthcare organizations tend to advertise using these boards because the cost is less than national sites and they are aiming for a local audience. The Department of Workforce in each state addresses unemployment and provides a job board for job seekers. National job boards, like Monster and Indeed, provide job seekers the ability to search for openings across the country. Medical assistant jobs available in the federal government can be found at www.usajobs.gov. National organizations, like the American Association of Medical Assistants (AAMA) or their local chapters, also post jobs.

When looking for a medical assistant position, it is important for job seekers to search beyond "medical assistant" jobs. Many job boards will post medical assistant types of positions under different job titles. It may take a bit of research to identify the local titles used for medical assistants in different regions or with specific employers. A good search method to utilize if unsure of the job title is to look in the allied health positions and review the educational requirements for different positions. Some agencies will use terms such as "technicians" or "coordinator" for medical assistant jobs. Make a list of job titles related to medical assisting and search by those as you identify potential openings.

CRITICAL THINKING APPLICATION 51-6

Michelle, Krysia, and Zac make a list of possible job boards to review frequently for medical assistant postings. They know that sometimes the postings are only available for a short time, so they develop a schedule to review the sites.

- Make a list of five job boards you would like to check for potential jobs.
- What might be other titles that are used for medical assistants in your area?

Traditional Job Search Methods

With the changes in technology, the methods used to find open positions have changed. Networking and checking job boards, as stated in the prior section, are the most effective methods of finding job openings. Mass mailing of résumés to healthcare employers and cold calling to identify opened positions are no longer effective methods. Other methods that remain effective include using the school's placement office resources, newspaper ads (online and print), and employment agencies.

School Career Placement Offices

Students usually have lifetime access to their school placement offices. Take advantage of the opportunities offered, which may include résumé building, job search classes, and interviewing assistance. The school has a vested interest in helping you find employment and the placement office should be the first resource for the student's job search.

Newspaper Ads

Typically, smaller healthcare practices utilize newspaper ads to find potential employees. The ads are run for a set period of time and usually it results in a huge number of applicants for the employer. Many newspaper companies post their ads online, allowing job seekers to look for opened positions.

Applicants need their letter and résumé to stand out from the crowd; people get very creative in how they make this occur. The creative method must stay within the directions given in the ad. For instance, if an employer wants a handwritten cover letter to be included, the applicant needs to follow those directions or the employer may disregard the materials figuring the applicant "can't follow directions." Many employers will provide a mailing address and state no calls or visits will be allowed. If you drop off your materials at the healthcare agency, they may also disregard your documents because the directions were not followed.

Employment Agencies

Employment agencies usually charge a fee for their services. Even when the employer pays the fee, the medical assistant may be offered a lower wage to compensate for the fee. These agencies can be useful, however, especially in salary negotiations. The agency knows the salary range the employer is willing to pay. This means that medical assistants can command a salary within that range and are not shortchanged by asking for a salary that is much lower than the employer is willing to pay.

Improving Your Opportunities

Some students and graduates struggle to find jobs. They may not find postings or they may not have success after applying for jobs. This can be stressful, but it is important not to give up.

For those not having success finding job opportunities, it is important to reevaluate your search methods and ask yourself the following questions:

- Am I looking for a very selective opportunity? For instance, are you looking for a dermatology medical assistant position in a specific facility? Those positions may be very limited. Try to broaden your search to other possible opportunities.
- Am I just looking for the correct job title? Remember employers may use a wide range of titles for a medical assistant.
- Am I looking at all agencies that potentially could hire a person with my skill sets? Depending on your area, medical assistants can be in many agencies besides a medical clinic, including a nursing home, hospital, school, or assisted living facility.
- Can I increase the geographical search area for employment opportunities? Can I relocate to an area with greater employment opportunities?

Those finding and applying for job opportunities, yet not having success obtaining a position, may also have to reevaluate their techniques. The lack of success may be related to the content and presentation of the cover letter and résumé or interviewing skills. One of the first places to start is to meet with the school career placement officer. Many times they will review your letter and résumé and provide you with improvement tips. Cover letters and résumés with misspellings and grammar errors may be discarded by employers and are simple items to fix. Sometimes reformatting or revising content is another way to improve one's résumé and cover letter. Having another party review your documents is highly recommended.

Many employers are also checking out social media sites, such as Facebook. Graduates struggling to find positions may want to review their pictures and postings on social media sites. Depending on the site, tightening up security settings and deleting questionable pictures may be helpful. Refraining from inappropriate postings, tweets, and responses may also be useful when looking for employment.

If you are getting interviews, but no job offers, it may be how you dress, your behavior, or how you answer questions during the interview. Again, the school's career placement office may have interview assistance and **mock** interviews that can help you refine your interview skills and behavior.

If you have heard or feel that your résumé lacks skills needed for specific positions you want to obtain, you may want to increase your **skill set**. This can occur through education and experience. Some people increase their job history and skill sets by obtaining temporary employment through temp agencies. Temporary jobs can provide experience and also help you refine your skills. The other way to increase your skill sets through experience is volunteering at a healthcare agency. Depending on the volunteer position, it may help increase your skill sets and also provide you with potential job leads. Volunteer activities should be added to the résumé, because these valuable experiences often can be used in a healthcare setting. It does not matter that the position was not a paid job; experience counts, whether paid or not.

CRITICAL THINKING APPLICATION   51-7

Michelle, Krysia, and Zac work together to keep an eye on local newspapers for ads that mention a need for medical assistants.

- What current ads in your local papers are interesting and would prompt sending a résumé?
- What factors might the medical assistant consider in choosing ads to which he or she will respond?
- How can the medical assistant determine which are good potential employers?

Being Organized in Your Job Search

As you identify job openings and submit your résumé and cover letter, it is important that you keep organized. Creating résumés and cover letters will be discussed later in the chapter, but it is important for you to customize both documents for each and every job opening. Keeping organized records is critical.

As you create your word processing documents, keep the documents in an organized system on your computer. For instance, if you are sending out materials for five different postings, keep the customized letter and résumé for each posting in a separate folder on your computer and title it with the name of the organization and the position. If you get notified of an interview for one of the five postings, then you have a record of the materials you sent that agency and you can make a copy of them for your interview.

It is also recommended to make a spreadsheet, word processing document, or handwritten log that indicates the postings you have applied for. The following information will help you remember and stay organized:

- Agency's name
- Position title and job number if available
- Date cover letter and résumé was sent to the agency
- Follow-up information (e.g., status of your application)

As you get notified about the interview, add in the interview information (e.g., date, time, location, interview team members) to your log.

One of the most important things to remember with job searching is that it takes time, stamina, and persistence to find a job. Do not expect to get a job with the first résumé and cover letter you send or with the first interview you have. By keeping good records, you will not apply for the same job twice or overlook job opportunities because you thought you applied for them already.

DEVELOPING A RÉSUMÉ

The purpose of a résumé is to get an employer so interested in you that he or she calls you for an interview. A résumé summarizes an applicant's qualifications, education, and experience. Medical assistants must determine what to include in the résumé, remembering that they are "marketing" themselves to an employer (Procedure 51-1). The résumé should be developed before the cover letter is written or job application is completed so that strengths can be identified and highlighted on all job search documents.

PROCEDURE 51-1   Prepare a Chronologic Résumé

Goal: To write an effective résumé for use as a tool in obtaining employment.

EQUIPMENT and SUPPLIES

- Computer with word processing software and a printer
- Current job posting
- Résumé paper
- Paper and pen

PROCEDURAL STEPS

1. Apply critical thinking skills as you create a list of the personality traits (wanted by employers), technical skills, and transfer job skills that you possess. Also write down your career goal(s).
   <u>PURPOSE:</u> To determine the strongest aspects of your abilities so that they can be highlighted on the résumé.

2. Using the current job posting, identify the required and recommended qualifications and credentials needed for the position.
   PURPOSE: Identifying what the employer requires and would like will help you tailor your résumé to address these qualifications and credentials.

3. Using the computer with word processing software, create a professional-looking header in the document's header. Include your name, address, telephone number(s), and e-mail address. Select an appropriate font style for your name and a smaller font size for your contact information.
   PURPOSE: To make sure potential employers have a means of contacting you. Using a font style that is bold and a larger size for your name will help your name stand out. Make sure to have your contact information in a smaller nonbold style so it will not detract from your name.

4. In the body of the document, create a section header for "Objective" and type a concise sentence stating your employment objective or goals. These goals should relate to the position being advertised.
   PURPOSE: To give the prospective employer an idea of what you are looking for in a medical assisting position.

5. Create a section header for "Education." For the learning institution(s) you attended, list the school's name, city and state, degree obtained or coursework successfully completed, and the year. Include any additional educational information, like grade point average (GPA), awards, and practicum information.

6. Create a section header for "Work Experience." Provide details about your work experience, including the agency's name, city and state, title of your position, start and end date (month and year), and job duties. The job duties must start with an active verb using the appropriate tense (e.g., a past job would have past tense verbs and a current job would include present tense verbs).
   NOTE: Typically online profiles and applications gather information about past salaries, reasons for leaving, and supervisors' names and contact information. They will also ask for salary expectations for the new position. This information should not be included on the résumé.

PURPOSE: The potential employer will need to know your employment history and all the details.

7. Create a section header for "Special Skills" and list your special language skills, computer proficiencies, and other unique skills you possess that relate to the position.

8. Create a section header for "Certifications and Credentials" and list the active credentials and certifications you have. Include the title of the certification, awarding agency, and the expiration date.
   NOTE: You may want to consider adding in the date you are taking a credential examination. Employers like to know the status of your credential examination.
   PURPOSE: Employers need to know if you have your medical assistant credential (CMA or RMA) and if you have an active cardiopulmonary resuscitation (CPR) and/or first aid card.

9. All information on the résumé needs to appear in reverse chronologic order (i.e., newest information is on top).

10. The résumé needs to look professional and interesting. Utilize font styles (e.g., bold, underline, italic) to highlight important words and phrases. Use professional-looking bullets to list out job duties and other information. Utilize the key words from the posting throughout the résumé.
    PURPOSE: The more professional and interesting a résumé appears, the better chance that it will be reviewed by the potential employer.

11. Proofread the résumé. Correct any spelling, grammar, punctuation, or sentence structure errors you find. If time allows, have another person review the résumé and use the feedback to revise your résumé.
    PURPOSE: Résumés submitted with errors often are discarded without consideration.

12. Print the résumé on résumé paper and proofread one final time. Any errors should be corrected and the document should be reprinted or e-mailed to the instructor.

Résumé Formats

There are three commonly used résumé formats, which include chronologic, combination, and targeted résumés. The résumé format used will depend on the medical assistant's situation.

A chronologic résumé is the most popular format used. It is useful when a person is seeking employment in the same field as his or her education or prior experience. The chronologic résumé focuses on the person's employment history, bulleting out the job duties for each position (Figure 51-6). See Procedure 51-1 for the steps in creating a chronologic résumé.

The combination résumé has been incorrectly described by many as a functional résumé. A true functional résumé showcases a person's skill sets and does not include a work history. Because employers want to see the person's work history, a combination résumé is

preferred over a pure functional résumé. A combination résumé lists a person's abilities and skill sets like the functional résumé does, but includes the person's employment history like the chronologic résumé (Figure 51-7). A combination résumé may be used if a person is switching careers and has transferable skills that relate to the new position. It can also be used by applicants that have a gap in their work history to put the focus on the person's skills and ability, rather than the employment history.

The third type of résumé is the targeted résumé, which is customized to a unique job posting (Figure 51-8). Key skills required for the new position are detailed in the résumé, indicating how the applicant has demonstrated those skills and is the best person for the position. This résumé takes longer to create, but can be the most effective format.

Michelle Marison

1234 Cedar Way, Mytown, OH 45458
Home phone: 715.555.1899
Cell phone: 715.555.1355
mmarison@elsevier.net

Objective

To find a full-time medical assistant position in a family practice setting, which will utilize my technical and interpersonal skills.

Education

Community College, Mytown, OH
Medical Assistant Diploma, 20XX
- GPA 3.6

Health Care Experience

Family Practice Associates, Mytown, OH
Medical Assistant Practicum, April to May 20XX (220 hours)
- Performed injections, electrocardiograms, wound care, phlebotomy, throat swabs, and waived tests.
- Obtained vital signs and measurements on children and adults.
- Utilized an electronic health record to document patients' histories, test results, and treatments.
- Answered calls, checked in patients, and updated patients' demographic and insurance information.

Mytown Hospital, Mytown, OH
Volunteer, January to May 20XX
- Provided hospital information to visitors.
- Maintained confidentiality of patients.
- Assisted with deliveries of mail and flowers to patients.
- Assisted nursing staff as needed.

Work Experience

Mytown Family Diner, Mytown, OH
Waitress, June 20XX to present
- Provide efficient, accurate, and timely service to customers.
- Prioritize duties to meet customer needs.
- Provide exceptional customer service.

Special Skills

Fluent in Spanish.
Keyboarding speed: 73 wpm.
Proficient in word processing and spreadsheet software.

Credentials

Certified Medical Assistant, American Association of Medical Assistants (expires May 20XX)
BLS for Healthcare Providers, American Heart Association (expires March 20XX)

FIGURE 51-6 Chronologic résumé.

CRITICAL THINKING APPLICATION 51-8

The three friends have very different backgrounds. Michelle has the waitressing experience, Krysia was in the military, and Zac worked in a factory. What type of résumé might each use? Explain your answers.
- What type of résumé would work best for you with your experience and background?

Résumé Content

Between the résumé formats there are similarities and differences in the information presented. The subsequent discussion will describe the content found in the different sections of a résumé. See Procedure 51-1 for the steps in creating a chronologic résumé.

Header

The person's contact information is found in the header of the document. This information or a variation of the information should appear on each sheet if the résumé is more than one page long.

The contact information should include your name, mailing address, professional e-mail address, and phone number. Some applicants will also include their personal websites, such as LinkedIn.

Zacarias Garcia

523 River Way, Mytown OH 45459
Cell phone: 715.555.5472
ZacGarcia@elsevier.net

Objective

To find a full-time medical assistant position in an orthopedic clinic.

Education

Community College, Mytown, OH
Medical Assistant Diploma, 20XX
- Medical Assistant Practicum at Mytown Orthopedic and Massage Center, Mytown, OH
  - Obtained and charted history and vital signs in electronic health record.
  - Assisted providers with tests and treatments.

Credentials

Certified Medical Assistant, American Association of Medical Assistants, expires May 20XX.
BLS for Healthcare Providers, American Heart Association, expires March 20XX.

Skills and Achievement

Strong communication skills
- Supervised 60 employees in a factory setting for over 3 years.
- Initiated procedures to improve communication between employees and management.
- Promoted in union to assist with negotiations with upper management.
- Fluent in Spanish.

Excellent problem-solving skills
- Problem-solved factory issues that delayed shipments to customers.
- Initiated solutions to expedite shipments and increased the profit margin of the company.

Excel in Teamwork
- Assisted team on assembly line, helping fill in when others were absent.
- Promoted to Team Lead within 6 months of hire.
- Received "Outstanding Employee" award in 20XX, 20XX, and 20XX.

Work Experience

Mytown Doors, Mytown, OH
Supervisor (March 20XX – January 20XX)
Team Lead – Door Assembly (January 20XX – March 20XX)
Door Assembler (August 20XX – January 20XX)

FIGURE 51-7 Combination résumé.

Professional e-mail addresses may include your first and last name or first initial and last name. E-mail addresses starting with expressions like: "one_hot_chick" or "party_dude" are not professional and are not used on résumés. If you do not have a professional e-mail, free e-mail sites are available. Like professional e-mails, personal websites should also be professional and contain a professional image of you.

Objective

The objective is a statement indicating to the reader the type of position being sought and the applicant's career goals. The objective should be a concise sentence. "A full-time medical assistant position" is a brief statement, but does not make much of an impression on the reader. A statement like, "To obtain a full-time medical assistant position in a family practice setting, which will utilize my technical and interpersonal skills," is more powerful.

Education

The education section includes information on the schooling the person has received after high school. The information should appear in reverse chronologic order, which means the newest information is on top and the oldest is at the bottom.

If a diploma was obtained, list the school's name, city and state, degree, and the year it was obtained. If a degree was not obtained but coursework was successfully completed, include the earlier mentioned information but summarize the coursework completed in place of the degree information. Additional information that can be included in this section would be academic awards, scholarships, overall GPA if greater than 3.0, and medical assistant practicum information (e.g., location, dates, and duties).

The location of the education section can differ based on the person's situation. If the person is a new graduate, the education section should appear toward the top of the résumé. If the degree is not related to the position or the degree is older, the emphasis would be on the person's achievements or work history; the education section would come toward the end of the résumé.

Work Experience

This section can be titled several different ways, including "Job Experience" and "Related Experience." If people have related

Krysia Debski

111 Mall Drive, Mytown, OH 45457
Cell phone: 715.555.6956
KDebski@elsevier.net

Objective
To find a full-time medical assistant position in an internal medicine clinic, which will utilize my technical and interpersonal skills.

Education
Community College, Mytown, OH
A.S. in Medical Assisting, 20XX
- Medical Assistant Practicum at Mytown Associates, Mytown, OH
  - Obtained and charted history and vital signs in electronic health record.
  - Assisted providers with tests and treatments in a busy internal medicine practice.
  - Performed injections, throat swabs, and phlebotomy.

Skills
ORGANIZATION SKILLS
- Organized supplies to expedite restocking procedures and decrease financial loss.
- Exceptional organizational and filing skills utilized to maintain purchase and delivery records for over 300 suppliers.
- Assisted with the installation and training for inventory tracking software for warehouse.

TEAMWORK
- Refined teamwork skills with over ten years in the US Marines.
- Taught teambuilding courses.
- Promoted teamwork among staff by incorporating incentives.

COMMUNICATION SKILLS
- Assertive when working with suppliers to meet deadlines.
- Utilized excellent listening skills to identify needs of various teams that impact the warehouse.
- Composed frequent emails and letters for supervisors.
- Fluent in Spanish and Polish

Credentials
Certified Medical Assistant, American Association of Medical Assistants (expires May 20XX)
BLS for Healthcare Providers, American Heart Association (expires March 20XX)

Work Experience
United States Marines
Supply Administration and Operations Specialist (May 20XX – September 20XX)
Warehouse Clerk (August 20XX – May 20XX)

FIGURE 51-8 Targeted résumé customized for a medical assistant posting. The medical assistant should possess strong organizational skills, experience with teamwork, and exceptional communication skills. The posting indicated it required a person with a Certified Medical Assistant (CMA) credential and a current Basic Life Support (BLS) certification.

healthcare experience that was either volunteer or part of training, using a broader phrase that does not include the words "job" or "work" may be an option. Applicants may want to use "Related Experience" or "Healthcare Experience," which helps draw the attention of the reader. For additional nonrelated experiences, they may use a section called "Other Work Experience." For those with military experience, it is recommended to add a special section to cover the military experience.

The information in this section should be presented in reverse chronologic order. The three most common formats for résumés require the following elements for each position: name of the agency, city and state, title of position, and dates in that position. Employers prefer to see month and year for the dates instead of just a year. This is especially important if the job only lasted a few months or just over a year. If the person has been in the workforce for ten years or

more, employers want to see ten years of employment information. For those working at the same agency for over ten years, it is important to list changes and advancements in the position over the duration of employment. Any gaps in the employment history should be explained to the potential employer during the interview or in the cover letter.

For the chronologic résumé, the most relevant job duties also need to be listed. For instance, if you worked as a housekeeper in a motel, making beds is not related to medical assisting, but providing customer service would be relevant. The statements regarding the duties should be bulleted and begin with an active verb. For present positions, use active verbs in the present tense (e.g., administer, provide); past positions should use active verbs in the past tense (e.g., administered, provided) (Figure 51-9).

Administered	Copied	Performed
Advocated	Developed	Posted
Aided	Distributed	Prepared
Answered	Documented	Processed
Arranged	Established	Provided
Assigned	Filed	Purchased
Assisted	Guided	Reconciled
Balanced	Helped	Restocked
Calculated	Instructed	Reviewed
Cared	Listened	Scanned
Coded	Logged	Scheduled
Collected	Mailed	Sorted
Compiled	Maintained	Supported
Composed	Monitored	Taught
Computed	Operated	Trained
Contacted	Ordered	Wrote
Coordinated	Organized	

FIGURE 51-9 Action verbs in the past tense.

The position of the education section in the résumé is dependent on the résumé format. Chronologic résumés typically have work experience near the top, whereas combination and targeted résumés list the reverse chronologic employment history toward the end of the résumé.

Summary and Skills

A "Summary" section appears just under the "Objective" section in the targeted résumé. This section summarizes why the applicant is the best candidate for the job. By utilizing key words and phrases found in the job description or job posting, the person can create a customized or targeted résumé. The key words are tied with related statements to help show how the applicant demonstrated the skills required in the new position.

A "Skills" or "Skills and Achievement" section is found in combination résumés and showcases specific transferable skills that relate to the new position. These transferable skills may have been obtained in the military, by a stay-at-home parent, or a person switching careers.

Special Skills

A "Special Skills" section typically only appears in a chronologic résumé. The information in this section would appear in the targeted résumé's "Summary" section and in the combination résumé's "Skills and Achievement" section.

Information that would appear in this section might relate to a fluency in another language, including sign language (e.g., fluent in Spanish). It may also contain the person's computer skills and experiences (e.g., "utilized electronic health records during practicum experience"; "keyboarding speed: 85 wpm").

Certifications

Many employers may require specific certifications or credentials for a job position. Regardless of the résumé format used, it is important to include the certifications and credentials that relate to the job position. When listing the information, include the title of the certification or license, awarding agency, and the expiration date (e.g., "Certified Medical Assistant, American Association of Medical Assistants, expires 10/2020" and "BLS for Healthcare Providers, American Heart Association, expires 10/2020").

Appearance of the Résumé

As you create your résumé, keep in mind the eye appeal or interest the résumé will create in the reader. It is recommended to bold only important information; for instance, a job title should be bold, whereas the agency should not be bold. Simple bullets help organize information and provide a neat appearance to the résumé. Changing the font size in certain areas can emphasize more important elements and help keep content on one page.

Spacing is crucial to the appearance of a résumé. Too much spacing creates too much "white space" and can give the reader a negative impression of the résumé. Too little spacing creates a busy, text-heavy résumé that is difficult to read. It is important to keep the same spacing distance between the sections of the résumé and smaller spacing between subsections (e.g., different employment positions).

It is important to have résumé paper available. Even if you submit your résumé online, you should have copies of your résumé on résumé paper available during the interview. Use a light solid-colored résumé paper (e.g., cream, light gray), which will duplicate better than a pattern or dark-colored paper.

Before submitting your résumé, have another person review it. Obtain the person's initial impression of the résumé's appearance. Is there too much white space? Does the résumé look too wordy? Does it look too plain? Does it look too busy? Then have the person read the content in the résumé and provide you with feedback. Use the feedback to revise your résumé. See Figure 51-10 for additional tips on creating a résumé.

CRITICAL THINKING APPLICATION   **51-9**

Zac, Michelle, and Krysia drafted their résumés. They read each other's and provided feedback. Who else might they give their résumés to for proofreading and feedback?

- Think of your circle of family and friends. List three people who might be great candidates to provide feedback on your résumé.

- Don't add clipart or other pictures

- Don't lie or exaggerate the truth

- Don't add unrelated content, like hobbies and interests.

- Don't include "References available upon request" or a similar statement, since it is understood references will be requested and required.

- Don't use personal pronouns, such as "I".

- Don't repeat content.

- Don't include any pay/salary information.

- Always keep the résumé to one page, unless you have been in the workforce for multiple years. Then use an additional page, but your content must fill both pages.

- Be concise and clear.

- Use key terms found in the job posting or job description in your résumé.

- Put important details first.

- Perform a grammar and spelling check on your résumé.

- Limit abbreviations to only the abbreviations used in the job posting (i.e., BLS for basic life support, CPR for cardiopulmonary resuscitation).

FIGURE 51-10 Tips on creating a résumé.

DEVELOPING A COVER LETTER

A cover letter always must accompany the résumé. The cover letter is a critical tool that gains the reader's attention and interest, thus making the reader want to look at the résumé. The advantage of the cover letter over the résumé is that the applicant can include more expression in it; the résumé tends to be more factual. Much attention to detail must occur to create a cover letter that will fulfill its role.

When developing a powerful cover letter to accompany your résumé, follow these strategies:

- Match the appearance of the cover letter and résumé. This means that your header should be identical, along with your font style and margins. Your contact information in the header should match the résumé's contact information. If you are submitting a paper document, use the same paper for both the résumé and cover letter.

- The inside address and the salutation need to be addressed to a specific person. Address the letter to the person who will be hiring the new employee. Use the person's name and job title in the inside address and be formal in the salutation (e.g., Dear Mr. Jones:) (Figure 51-11). You can contact the healthcare facility or utilize online resources like LinkedIn to gather this information. If you are unable to identify the person's name, use "To whom it may concern," "Dear Sir," "Dear Madam," or some variation. Having a specific name will tell the reader you took the time to find out the details and it may distinguish you over other candidates.

- Start the body of your cover letter off with a bang! In the first paragraph show enthusiasm as you summarize why you believe you are the best candidate for the job. *"Having a strong customer service background and a degree in medical assisting, I am confident that I can fulfill your expectations for the family practice medical assistant position (#123)."* Along with your qualities, it is important to include the job title and number so the reader knows what position you are interested in.

- During the second paragraph, sell yourself to the reader by providing a snapshot of your experiences. Weave in the key "requirement" words that the employer included in the job posting. Address the employer's more important requirements first, followed by the lesser requirements or "would like" qualities. You may want to bold these key words to bring more attention to them. If you bullet out your qualifications and abilities, limit the bullets to four or five points. Be concise, yet clear, but do not repeat the résumé; you want the reader to move onto the résumé for the details.

- Start the final paragraph by reaffirming that you are an excellent match for the job by using such phrases as "I believe I have the qualities you require" or "I am confident I will meet your expectations." You can follow this by stating the action you will take in regards to following up (for instance, "I will call the week of …"). Be careful that your tone is not overly aggressive, which might not sit well with the reader. If you chose not to address how you will follow up, finish the paragraph by expressing your interest and enthusiasm in an interview (e.g., "I am very excited about

Michelle Marison

1234 Cedar Way, Mytown, OH 45458
Home phone: 715.555.1899
Cell phone: 715.555.1355
mmarison@elsevier.net

May 15, 20XX

Ms. Alex Brown
Medical Assistant Supervisor
Mytown Medical Clinic
555 Clover Drive
Mytown OH 45457

Dear Ms. Brown:

I was excited to see the posting on the Mytown Telegram job board for the medical assistant position (#1243) and would like to be considered for that position. I am graduating from Community College on May 30, 20XX and will be taking my AAMA CMA exam June 2, 20XX.

With two years of customer service experience and five months of being a hospital volunteer, I have learned the importance of prioritizing, teamwork, and communication. During my medical assistant practicum, I have utilized these skills along with my attention to detail and my medical assistant knowledge, as I assist providers with procedures and treatments. The knowledge and skills I am learning in practicum combined with the skills I have developed as a waitress and volunteer will help me provide the best care to my future patients.

I have heard excellent things about Mytown Medical Clinic and would love to be a part of the staff of such a caring agency. I am available for interviews whenever it is convenient for you. I am available either by phone or email.

Thank you so much for considering me for this position.

Sincerely,

Michelle Marison

Enclosure: 1

FIGURE 51-11 Basic cover letter.

this opportunity and would enjoy meeting with you to explore how my qualifications could meet your needs."). (See Figure 51-11.)

- Before the closing and signature block, express your thanks to the reader for his or her consideration. Being gracious shows the reader you have good manners.
- When you have completed your letter, review the spelling, punctuation, grammar, and sentence structure. Create a cover letter that is error free and has a professional tone and appearance. Common cover letter weaknesses include:
  - Starting a majority of sentences with "I"
  - Introducing yourself in the first sentence (for instance, "Hi, I am Sally Green.")
  - Spelling, grammar, punctuation, and sentence structure errors
  - Missing parts of the letter (e.g., date, inside address)
  - Missing the position title and posting number
  - Too busy (overuse of font styles), too wordy, or too much "white space"
  - Inappropriate spacing that leads to the body of the letter being too high or too low on the page. Remember the body should be centered vertically on the page.
  - Creating a generic letter that does not contain the key requirement words from the job posting. (Many larger employers utilize software to screen letters and résumés for key words. Those with key words are reviewed closer; those that lack the key words are discarded.)

Use the spell check tool in your word processing software to help identify errors, but do not rely on it solely. **Proofread** your letter and have a few people proofread your letter as well. Use their advice as you make your changes. Refer to the Technology and Written Communication in the Medical Office chapter if you need assistance with composing a business letter. Procedure 51-2 will help guide you in writing a professional cover letter.

PROCEDURE 51-2 Create a Cover Letter

Goal: *To write an effective cover letter that will accompany the résumé.*

EQUIPMENT and SUPPLIES

- Computer with word processing software and a printer
- Current job posting
- Résumé paper
- Pen

PROCEDURAL STEPS

1. Using the job posting, read through the job description. With a pen, circle the position requirements and the key phrases.
   PURPOSE: Your letter should contain the key phrases and position requirements that are found in the job posting.
2. Using the computer with word processing software, create a professional-looking header in the document's header that matches your résumé header. Include your name, address, telephone number(s), and e-mail address.
   PURPOSE: To ensure potential employers have a means of contacting you. You can increase the professional appearance of your documents by having the same header on each document.
3. Type the date in the correct location using the correct format. Have one blank line between the date line and the last line of the letterhead.
   PURPOSE: All letters require a date for legal purposes.
4. Type the inside address using the correct spelling, punctuation, and location for the information. Leave 1 to 9 blank lines between the date and the inside address, depending on the location of the body of the letter.
   PURPOSE: The body of the letter needs to be centered vertically from top to bottom of the document. More blank lines can be added to move the body to the correct location.
5. Starting on the second line below the inside address, type the salutation using the correct professional format, including the individual's name if known.
   PURPOSE: A proper greeting helps set the tone of the letter.

6. Type the message in the body of the letter using the proper location and format. There should be a blank line after the salutation and between each paragraph. The message should be clear, concise, and professional. Use proper grammar, punctuation, capitalization, and sentence structure.
   PURPOSE: Proper grammar usage helps the message be conveyed more accurately and professionally.
7. The first paragraph should contain the title and number of the job posting. The middle paragraph(s) should summarize your strengths and include key phrases from the posting. The final paragraph should discuss your availability for an interview. The body should end with an expression of gratitude to the reader.
   PURPOSE: It is important to thank the reader for considering you for the position.
8. Type a proper closing, leaving one blank line between the last line of the body and the closing. Use the correct format and location.
   PURPOSE: The closing helps end the message with a proper tone.
9. Type the signature block using the correct format and location. There should be four blank lines between the closing and the signature block.
10. Spell check and proofread the document. Check for proper tone, grammar, punctuation, capitalization, and sentence structure. Check for proper spacing between the parts of the letter.
    PURPOSE: The spell check tool will identify only certain errors; proofreading will help to identify incorrect word usage, improper tone, and errors in formatting. The tone of the letter should be professional, but not aggressive.
11. Make any final corrections. Print the document on résumé paper and sign the letter or e-mail the document to your instructor or employer.

COMPLETING ONLINE PROFILES AND JOB APPLICATIONS

With many healthcare agencies utilizing the Internet during the employment process, the human resource software they use may require applicants to create an online profile before applying for open positions. The online profile collects the information that previously was collected by paper applications.

Online profiles have many advantages over paper applications for both the employer and the applicant. An applicant completes the profile once and updates the information as needed. Typically the agencies keep the profiles active for a long period of time, sometimes for years. Employers can track the activities of applicants, easily read a person's information, and advertise new postings to potential applicants whose profiles meet certain requirements.

If a healthcare agency does not utilize online profiles, then the applicant will need to complete a job application (Figure 51-12). Some organizations require the application to be submitted with the cover letter and résumé but others have applicants arriving for interviews complete the application. If you need to complete an application before an interview, come prepared with your information and arrive at least 20 minutes before the interview. See Procedure 51-3 for the steps in completing a job application.

As you complete the online or paper application, you will be required to read important legal statements and add your signature (or electronic signature). This is a legal document; therefore it should be filled out accurately and completely. Regardless of how you complete the application, you will need to provide the same information. Even if you have the information on your résumé, you still need to

APPLICATION FOR EMPLOYMENT

Date:_____

Name: (First, Middle Initial, Last)_____

Social Security No.:_____   Phone: _____

Address:_____

EDUCATION

	Name, City, State	Graduation Date	Degree Obtained
High School:			
College:			
Other:			

LICENSURE/CERTIFICATION/REGISTRATION

Type of Certification, License or Registration	Agency/State	Registration Name

List any special skills or qualifications which you possess and feel are relevant to health care and the position for which you are applying._____

_____

EMPLOYMENT HISTORY

May we contact and communicate with your present employer?   ☐ Yes   ☐ No

Employer:	Phone:
Address:	Supervisor:
Employed	Hourly Pay:
Position title and responsibilities:	
Reason for leaving:	

FIGURE 51-12 Application for employment.

add it to the application. Having the information in a word-processed document will save you time. If you are providing the information online, the copy and paste feature will speed up completion time. Information you should include in the word-processed document includes:

- Education information such as: institution's name and address; dates and titles of coursework or diploma.
- Information related to prior and current employers such as: agency name and address; supervisors' names, titles, and contact information; job title, duties, start and end salary, start and end dates; and reason for leaving.
- Information related to certifications and credentials (e.g., certifying agency's name and address; certification/credential; expiration date). A copy of your certification and BLS card may be required by the employer.

- Information related to your references (e.g., names, contact information, type of reference [co-worker, instructor]).

When filling out the application answer the questions carefully. When addressing your availability date, make sure you know how long you have to give notice at your current position if that is pertinent. Usually, most employers have a 2-week notice policy. If you get hired, your new employer will understand that you need to give a 2-week notice.

When completing the reason why you left prior positions, make sure to write the reason using a positive tone. For instance, *"Obtained a position that would advance my skill set"* or *"Resigned to focus more on my education"* sound more professional than *"I hated the job."* If you have a unique situation (e.g., sick parent, new baby), ask the advice of your school's placement counselor if you are unsure what to say in these sections.

PROCEDURE 51-3   Complete a Job Application

Goal: *To complete an accurate, detailed job application legibly so as to secure a job offer.*

EQUIPMENT and SUPPLIES

- Pen
- Application form
- Information regarding your past education, job experiences, and the skill sets you have obtained (e.g., computer skills, keyboarding speed)
- Contact information for former supervisors and references
- Current résumé

PROCEDURAL STEPS

1. Read the entire job application before completing any part of the document.
   PURPOSE: Reading through the entire application helps prevent errors when filling out the document.
2. Refer to your information on past jobs, education experiences, and skill sets you have obtained as you complete the application. Answers to the questions need to be accurate and honest.
3. Use proper grammar, sentence structure, punctuation, spelling, and capitalization. Handwriting should be legible to the reader.

PURPOSE: Errors on the application or illegible sections may affect whether you are hired.

4. Do not leave any space blank. Answer each question on the document. If the question does not apply, write "not applicable."
   PURPOSE: Leaving a space blank on the application may suggest that the candidate did not want to answer a certain question or accidentally overlooked it. By writing "not applicable" on such questions, the candidate demonstrates competence and attention to detail.
5. Do not write "See résumé" anywhere on the document.
   PURPOSE: Many supervisors view this practice as laziness. Always fill out the job application completely and do not leave blank spaces.
6. Include information on the application that exhibits dependability, punctuality, teamwork, attention to detail, positive work ethics and initiative, the ability to adapt to change, a responsible attitude, and use of technology.
7. Sign the document and date it.
8. Proofread the document and make sure none of the information conflicts with the résumé.
   PURPOSE: Proofreading helps the candidate to catch any errors before submitting the application.

CREATING A CAREER PORTFOLIO

As stated earlier in the chapter, many job seekers claim to have the skill set required by the potential employer, but very few actually show the employer evidence of those qualifications. A career portfolio is a fantastic tool to show a potential employer that you have the skills required for the job. The portfolio should be developed along with the cover letter and résumé. A student may have more than one portfolio if he or she is considering different types of positions (e.g., receptionist, phlebotomist, medical assistant). The portfolio would be customized for each position, highlighting the skills utilized by a person in that position. For a phlebotomist-focused portfolio, evaluations of past venipunctures and related documents would be more useful than content related to coding and billing. The portfolio is utilized during the interview process and shows the interviewer what you have accomplished.

Every career portfolio is unique to the individual. For medical assistants, it is recommended to use a three-ring binder with plastic sheet protectors and divider tabs. (See Procedure 51-4 for the steps in creating a career portfolio.) Typical items found in career portfolios include:

- Cover letter addressed to the interviewer
- Résumé (a copy of what was sent to that facility)
- References document with contact information from three or four people, including one to two instructors, and one to two co-workers or prior supervisors who have given prior consent to be used as references
- Certifications (e.g., copy of BLS card, copy of credentials [e.g., CMA or RMA card])

- Education-related documents:
  - Copy of letters of recommendation
  - Copy of transcripts, awards, and honors
  - A list of the courses successfully completed with a short description of each course (optional, but consider if you are moving to another location where your institution may not be known)
  - Copy of practicum evaluation forms and skill document form
  - Scholarships awarded
  - Copy/details of school-related activities (e.g., officer in student medical assistant group, athlete, volunteer activities)
- Prior employment documents
  - Copy of past employment evaluations
  - Copy of letters of recommendations
  - Documentation showing the student balancing work and education (This can help exhibit a strong work ethic, organizational skills, and prioritizing skills.)
- Examples of work or summary of projects that can provide evidence of abilities and skills
- Criminal background documentation, blood titers, vaccination history, and current tuberculosis (TB) skin test (optional)

The documents placed in the career portfolio binder should be positive and helpful to you in your mission of getting a job. If you have not been very successful in school, you may not want to include your transcript. If you received negative performance evaluations, you should not include those in your portfolio. Be creative as you prepare your portfolio, keeping the appearance professional and neat.

PROCEDURE 51-4   Create a Career Portfolio

Goal: *To create a custom portfolio that provides potential employers evidence of your skills and knowledge as a medical assistant.*

EQUIPMENT and SUPPLIES

- Three-ring binder or folder
- Plastic sleeves for the three-ring binder
- Dividers with tabs for three-ring binder
- Current résumé and cover letter
- Documents providing evidence of your skills and knowledge (e.g., transcripts, job and practicum evaluation forms, practicum skill checklist, projects completed in school, letters of recommendation, copies of certifications [CPR and first aid cards])

PROCEDURAL STEPS

1. Group documents in a logical manner, putting similar documents together. Identify the arrangement for the portfolio. An arrangement could include: cover letter and résumé, education section (e.g., transcript, practicum evaluation form and skills checklist, awards), prior job-related documents (e.g., evaluations), reference letters, and work products (e.g., projects you created in your medical assistant program). Insert a tabbed divider in front of each section. You may want to include a table of contents to identify the tabbed areas.

PURPOSE: Organizing the documents in a logical manner will help the reader identify the important documents. The arrangement will also show the reader your ability to organize content.

2. Neatly write the topic area on the tab of the dividers.
PURPOSE: This will help the reader find the content easier.
3. Insert one document per plastic pocket.
PURPOSE: The plastic pockets will keep the documents clean and neat.
4. Arrange the documents neatly in the binder or folder. Have your cover letter and résumé in the front of all the other documents.
PURPOSE: The reader can review the letter and résumé as needed before looking at the other documents in the portfolio.
5. After the portfolio is assembled, review the entire portfolio to ensure it looks professional and the documents provide positive support of your skill set and knowledge.
PURPOSE: Minimize the negative documents in your portfolio. They will not help you obtain a job as much as the positive, supporting documents.

JOB INTERVIEW

A medical assistant may interview with the office manager, the provider, or both, and other staff members may be brought in for part of the interview. This is especially true in healthcare environments with a cohesive team of employees.

The interview usually is the most stressful of the job search steps. Some individuals dread job interviews and become extremely nervous at the prospect of interviewing. Others are very comfortable and consider the interview to be as much for their own purposes as for the employer's. Either way, the more interviews the medical assistant has, the more comfortable he or she will be with each subsequent interview.

An interview has four phases: preparation for the interview, the interview itself, the follow-up, and the negotiation.

Preparation for the Interview

When preparing for an interview, the medical assistant should learn everything possible about the employer. Look on the Internet for information about the facility. Practice answering possible interview questions. Prepare an outfit to wear to interviews. It is wise to drive to the interview site on a day preceding the interview date if the location is unfamiliar to avoid getting lost on the day of the important event. The better prepared the medical assistant is, the more comfortable he or she will be when interviewing.

The critical part of the interview is the medical assistant's ability to present himself or herself as the best candidate for the job. By preparing to answer interview questions before the interview, the medical assistant will appear much more confident. Although no one can guess exactly what questions will be asked, there are some

standard interview questions (Figure 51-13). Review these questions thoroughly, answer them in writing, and then study them before the interview. Then when the medical assistant is asked, "What are your three greatest strengths?" he or she can confidently answer, "I am professional, reliable, and honest." Expanding on these traits will provide additional information to the interviewers on why these are your greatest strengths. Take time to consider your possible answers to some of the standard interview questions. What perception might you be giving to the interviewers by your answer? Is it the perception you want to be giving?

In addition to preparing to answer interview questions, you should prepare two to three questions to ask the interviewer. The organization's website is an excellent source of information. Be familiar with their mission and value statements, the size of the organization, the size of the department that has the open position, and the number of providers. Possible questions might be:

- "I see that there are two providers in this department. Would I be working with both of them?"
- "There are three locations for your clinic on your website; how will I interact with the other locations?"
- "Given the size of your organization is there an opportunity to interact with the other departments?"
- "When will you be making a decision about this position?"

By having questions that relate to the specific organization and department, you are showing that you are truly interested in the position. Asking about their time frame for making a decision on the position will direct your decision about a thank-you card: for example, if they are deciding later that day or the next, you should send a thank-you e-mail; there would not be time for a card to be delivered.

1. Tell me about yourself.	16. What do you know about this facility and our competitors?
2. Why do you want to work for this company?	17. What has been your most rewarding experience at work?
3. Why should I hire you?	18. What was your single most important accomplishment for the company on your last job?
4. How do you work under pressure?	19. What was the toughest problem you have ever solved and how did you do it?
5. How do you handle criticism?	20. How do you see yourself fitting in with our company?
6. What do you think your co-workers think about you?	21. What skills did you learn on your last job that can be used here?
7. Describe your last supervisor.	22. What immediate contribution could you make if you came to work for us today?
8. What would you like to change about yourself?	23. Do you prefer working with others or by yourself?
9. What is your best asset?	24. Can you take instructions or criticism without being upset?
10. What adjectives would you use to describe yourself?	25. What job in this company would you choose if you could?
11. How would you describe the perfect job?	26. What have you done that shows initiative and willingness to work?
12. Why did you leave your last job?	27. What will previous supervisors say about you?
13. Why did you choose this type of profession?	28. Why would you be successful in this job?
14. What are your strongest and weakest personal qualities?	29. Can you explain the gap in your employment history?
15. What personal characteristics are necessary for success in your chosen field?	30. Are you a member of any professional organizations?

FIGURE 51-13 Top 30 interview questions.

When preparing on the day of the interview, be conservative with wardrobe choices. For women a business suit, or skirt or dress pants and blouse, is appropriate. If you choose to wear a skirt or dress it should be of modest length (i.e., at the knee or longer). Your blouse should not be sheer or show cleavage. For men, a business suit, or dress pants and shirt with a tie, is the best choice. Your tie should be professional. Conservative business suits would always be acceptable in an interview. Be sure clothing is fresh, wrinkle-free, and well-fitting and that shoes are clean and shined. For a medical assistant, scrubs would be acceptable for an interview if you do not have

dress clothes. Take care in washing, pressing, and rolling your scrubs for lint before wearing them on an interview.

Pay particular attention to other aspects of appearance (Figure 51-14). Make sure your hair is clean and styled attractively, your teeth are clean, and your breath is fresh. Nails are also important and should be clean and well groomed, because the medical assistant should give the interviewer a firm handshake. Nails should not be excessively long or painted in highly visible colors. Do not wear perfumes or colognes and do not wear excessive jewelry or makeup. Do not chew gum or smoke in your interview attire. Remember the

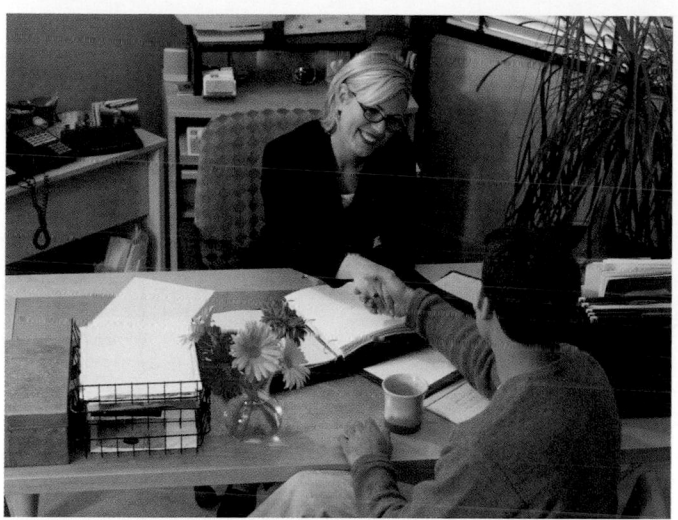

FIGURE 51-14 Present a professional appearance during the job interview and be sure to smile often. (From Yoder-Wise P: *Leading and managing in nursing*, ed 4, 2006, St. Louis, Mosby.)

appearance guidelines that applied to the practicum; some employers will react negatively to tattoos, piercings, extravagant hairstyles, hair colors, or other excessive wardrobe choices. Always dress appropriately and conservatively for an interview. Once hired, the new employee may be allowed to wear more diverse styles that comply with the employee handbook or procedure manual.

Do a test run before the day of the interview to identify the travel time. Always arrive 15 minutes early for the interview. Never take anyone along on a job interview, especially children, even if they are older. Expect to be a little nervous. Any interview can be a stressful situation. The better prepared the medical assistant is, the more of a success the interview will be.

It is a good idea to bring an interview portfolio and a planner or other method of taking notes during the interview; this makes a good impression and indicates interest in the job. The interview portfolio should be reflective of that particular position. It should have a table of contents at the beginning with identified tabbed sections so the interviewer can quickly review materials that he or she finds pertinent. The student should be prepared to leave the portfolio with the interviewer, so no originals should be included. The first items in the portfolio after the table of contents should be a copy of the cover letter and résumé that was sent to the facility; the individual doing the interview may not have received the original documents. A detailed reference list should also be included. Bring a list of questions to ask. If you have not completed an application, bring information regarding former employment (e.g., supervisors' names and contact information, dates of employment, wages, reasons for leaving), education, and any other information that might be needed to accurately complete paperwork; the information could be written down on paper or saved into a document or application in a smart phone. This will help to avoid the embarrassment of asking to look up an address in a phone book or calling to obtain the information while at the interview.

Before the face-to-face interview occurs many organizations will conduct a preliminary phone interview with a human resources representative. This interview is generally done to narrow the applicant pool. It can also give them a very good idea of how you present yourself on the phone. This is an opportunity for you to learn more

about the organization. You have provided this potential employer with your phone number, so you should be prepared to receive a phone call. In anticipation of receiving phone calls from a potential employer you should make sure that your voice mail message is appropriate and professional sounding. You should clearly state your name in this message so that they know they have reached the right person. If you receive the call at a time when it is not appropriate to speak, in a noisy location, or in a quiet location where you should not be speaking, let the call go to voice mail. If you are able to answer the call but it is not a good time to speak to them, it is perfectly all right to explain this and offer to call back at a time convenient for the employer.

During the Interview

Whether the interview is conducted over the phone, face-to-face, or via video conference (e.g., Skype, FaceTime), the interviewer should not ask any illegal questions, including those that are related to age, sex, nationality, religion, marital/family status, affiliations/organizations, and disabilities (Figure 51-15).

Employers may ask illegal questions, whether intentionally or accidentally, and the way that the medical assistant answers the questions can influence the employer's hiring decision. If the medical assistant is openly offended, employers may conclude that the applicant will be offended by abrasive comments from patients and will not be able to handle interaction with patients. If the illegal question is answered, the interviewer may use the information in the answer to weed out the medical assistant as a candidate. The best approach is to politely address the question, either by answering it directly or by redirecting the interviewer back to the job requirements. For example, if the interviewer asks if the candidate plans to put children in day care (which might be a way of determining the age of the dependent children and thus the likelihood of absenteeism because of the children's illnesses), the medical assistant could answer, "I will be able to meet the work schedule and the responsibilities that this job requires." Some questions that might normally be considered illegal, such as "What organizations are you a member of?" might be job related. The employer may be interested in knowing that the medical assistant is a member of various professional organizations, such as the AAMA or the AMT.

Phone Interview

A phone interview may be done to screen applicants and narrow the candidate pool or it may replace a face-to-face interview, especially if the candidate is from out of town. If this interview is replacing a face-to-face interview you will be contacted to set up a time for the interview. You should approach this process with the same preparation that you would do for a face-to-face interview. It is important that you are in a quiet, well-lit room that is free from distractions. You should have a copy of your résumé and cover letter in front of you, as well as your list of questions. It would be a good idea to have a glass of water there, as nerves tend to make your throat dry. Be sure to thank the employer for the opportunity to interview with them.

Face-to-Face Interview

During the actual interview, maintain good eye contact. Many supervisors refuse to hire people who seem uncomfortable looking them directly in the eyes. Never take control of the interview. Allow

Topic	Illegal	Legal
RELIABILITY	How many children do you have? Who is going to babysit? What is your marital status? Do you have a car?	What hours and days can you work? Are there specific times that you cannot work? Do you have responsibilities other than work that will interfere with specific job requirements such as traveling?
CITIZENSHIP	What is your national origin? Where are your parents from?	Are you legally eligible for employment in the United States?
REFERENCES	What is your maiden name? What is your father's surname? What are the names of your relatives?	Have you ever worked under a different name?
ARRESTS AND CONVICTIONS	Have you ever been arrested?	Have you ever been convicted of a crime?
DISABILITIES	Do you have any disabilities?	Can you perform the duties of the job you are applying for?
AGE/DATE OF BIRTH	What is your date of birth?	If hired, can you furnish proof that you are over the age of 18?
RELIGION	What church do you attend?	None
EDUCATION	When did you graduate from high school?	Do you have a high school diploma or equivalent?

FIGURE 51-15 Illegal and legal interview questions.

the supervisor to ask questions at his or her own pace. Do not fidget in the chair. Do not volunteer any negative information; be honest and do not exaggerate experience or lengths of employment. Never speak negatively about former employers.

Be careful when answering questions such as, "Tell me about yourself." Most medical assistants might begin to answer this question with a phrase like, "I'm a recent graduate, and I am married and have two children." The answer to this question should not reflect information about personal issues. Focus all answers on professionalism and the strengths that will be an asset to the healthcare setting. Stating "I am a recent graduate and completed a 6-week practicum in a family practice" opens the door to questions that will allow you to highlight your skills.

Remember that the interview is centered on the medical assistant, so freely discuss the skills and attributes that you would bring to the job. The better prepared the medical assistant is, the smoother the interview will go. Be able to prove the skills you claim and explain how they meet the needs of the company or facility. Utilize your interview portfolio during the interview by referencing past job evaluations or your practicum skill checklist/evaluation. Avoid a "know-it-all" attitude, which indicates overconfidence and reluctance to take direction. Always express an interest in the employer and his or her projects, rather than in what the employer can do for the employee. Ask intelligent questions at the end of the interview if given the opportunity. Your first question should never be, "How much will I be paid?" Money, although important, cannot appear to be your primary concern.

Before the interview ends, the medical assistant should ask when a decision will be made and if it would be acceptable to call to follow up (Procedure 51-5).

Video Interview

A third interview possibility is a video interview using technology such as Skype. As with a phone interview, a video interview works well when the candidate is from out of town. There is a certain amount of technology needed for a video interview. Your school's placement office may be able to help you with that, or the organization may have contacts for you to arrange your end of the interview. The benefit of a video interview over a phone interview is that the interviewers can actually see the interviewee. This allows the interviewers to assess the body language and the verbal message being presented. You should dress as you would for a face-to-face interview and have the same materials ready to access during the interview process.

CRITICAL THINKING APPLICATION   **51-10**

Krysia is enjoying a good interview when the interviewer, a male supervisor, asks her if she is married. When Krysia replies that she is not, he asks if she has a steady boyfriend.

- What might the supervisor's motive be with this line of questioning?
- How should Krysia respond?
- Are these questions inappropriate or do they serve a purpose?

PROCEDURE 51-5   Practice Interview Skills During a Mock Interview

Goal: *To project a professional appearance during a job interview and to be able to express the reasons the medical assistant is the best candidate for the position.*

EQUIPMENT and SUPPLIES

- Current job posting
- Résumé
- Cover letter
- Interview portfolio (optional)
- Application (optional)
- Interviewer
- Mock interview questions

PROCEDURAL STEPS

1. Wear interview-appropriate attire and be groomed professionally.
   PURPOSE: Your appearance will influence the first impression made on this potential employer. Most medical facilities prefer conservative dress.
2. Portray a professional image by shaking hands firmly; bringing a copy of the current résumé and cover letter and copies of earned certificates. Do not engage in visible nervous habits such as tapping your foot, bouncing a crossed leg, or drumming fingers.
3. Answer introductory questions by providing only professional information. For example:

Question: "What can you tell us about yourself?"
Response: "I am a recent graduate of an accredited medical assistant program. I have just completed a 6-week practicum experience where I was able to demonstrate proficiency in a variety of clinical and administrative skills."

4. Answer interview questions with open, honest, and positive responses. Completely answer questions, provide information, and do not answer in single sentences or with limited responses.
5. Utilize key words from the job posting when answering the interview questions.
   PURPOSE: Helps to prove the interviewee has exactly what the organization is looking for.
6. Ask the interviewer two to three appropriate questions about the agency or the position.
   PURPOSE: Demonstrates an interest in the organization and the position.
7. Express interest in the job and politely complete the interview by shaking hands and thanking the interviewer for the opportunity for the interview.

Follow-Up After the Interview

Follow-up is critical after an interview. Always send a written thank-you note or letter to the person who conducted the interview (Procedure 51-6). Many employers wait to see who sends a thank-you letter before making the final hiring decision. Limit follow-up calls to one or two a week. Most employers give an indication of when the hiring decision will be made. The company should notify all those who interviewed once a decision has been made, unless specific protocols were set during the interview about follow-up. For instance, if the office manager says a decision will be made on Friday and the final three candidates will be called for a second interview, the medical assistant knows to continue the job search if a call is not received. Although not all companies provide this type of notification, it is considered professional etiquette to tell the candidates who interviewed for the job if they are no longer under consideration. Never place all your hope in one job; continue to search and interview until an offer is made and accepted. In addition, always be on the watch for the next job opportunity.

PROCEDURE 51-6   Create a Thank-You Note for an Interview

Goal: *To create a meaningful thank-you note to be sent after the interview process.*

EQUIPMENT and SUPPLIES

- Computer with word processing software and a printer
- Job description
- Contact name from interview

PROCEDURAL STEPS

1. Using word processing software compose a professional letter using business letter format. Include all of the required elements in the letter. Use correct spacing between the elements.
2. Highlight the particulars of the interview in the body of the letter.
3. Include positive information you wish you had covered in the interview.
   PURPOSE: Allows you to present any missed skills or details in a professional manner.
4. Create a message that is concise and to the point.
5. Sign and send the thank-you note.

Reasons People Do Not Get Hired

The following is a ranked list of reasons interviewers do not hire job candidates, as expressed by surveyed career consultants and reported on www.workoplis.com:

- Not sufficiently differentiating themselves from others
- Failure to successfully transfer past experience to the current job opportunity
- Not showing enough interest and excitement
- Focusing too much on what they want and too little on what the interviewer is saying
- Feeling they can "wing" the interview without preparation
- Not being able to personally connect with the interviewer
- Appearing over- or under-qualified for the job
- Not asking enough or the right questions
- Not researching a potential employer/interviewer
- Lacking humor, warmth, or personality during the interview process

Negotiation

The negotiation stage of job acceptance can be as stressful as the actual interviews. Salary can no longer be the only consideration when determining whether to accept a position or not. Other benefits can play a crucial role in that decision. When a job offer is made there should also be a discussion of the other benefits. If the salary offered is a bit lower than expected, but the employee share of the health insurance premium is less than expected, the salary offer becomes more attractive. A medical assistant should know the lowest salary/benefit combination he or she can afford and should ask for a little more than that figure. Bracket salary requests are often helpful in this: instead of asking for $13 per hour, ask for a salary in the "mid to high twenties." Let the employer mention a figure or a range of salary first. Usually the person who mentions a salary range first has the disadvantage. If the medical assistant requests $13 per hour and the facility was willing to pay $16 per hour, the medical assistant probably will get $13. The organization may have a starting pay level for new employees. To start at higher than that level you will need to show them why you should: for example, proficiency at the required skills for the job or previous work experience in the field. Having a well-designed interview portfolio will allow you to show the interviewer all that you have accomplished.

Never say "no" to a job offer on the spot. Request at least 24 hours to consider the offer. Before accepting or rejecting a job offer, consider whether the position carries any authority, the benefits, the hours, the distance from home, and the potential for advancement. People accept jobs for reasons other than the salary; remember the value of experience.

CRITICAL THINKING APPLICATION   51-11

Michelle has been on several interviews and likes the prospect of working for three different physicians. If an offer is made at each office, how can Michelle decide which to accept? What will help Michelle make this decision?

YOU GOT THE JOB!

Once the job offer has been made and accepted, a start date will be determined. Before the first day, use the computer, global positioning system (GPS), or smart phone to map several ways to get to work. If you are unsure of the traffic flow, leave home extra-early the first day so that you are guaranteed to arrive on time.

Most employees are placed on a 30- to 90-day probationary period, during which employment may be terminated for unsatisfactory performance. The probationary period also provides the employer and employee an opportunity to learn about each other. The medical assistant will interact with other co-workers, patients, and providers. A new medical assistant should volunteer to help others and efficiently complete the duties assigned. Use the probationary period as a testing ground, carefully observing ways in which the healthcare facility might run more smoothly. However, do not make numerous suggestions for change during this period. Discover why certain methods are used and make an effort to fit in with the rest of the team before suggesting that the office routine be changed. Remember, the people at the office may have been employed for a substantially longer time and may resent suggestions from a new staff member. Learn the office rhythms, procedures, and culture first and demonstrate a team-oriented attitude. After new employees prove their responsibility and positive attitude, other staff members will be open to suggestions about improvements for the office.

Common Early Mistakes

Some medical assistants make mistakes early on in a new job. Never be disruptive to the office by gossiping or complaining. A medical assistant must realize that procedures may be performed in many different ways and that the way he or she was taught in school probably is not the only correct way. Be open to learning new ideas, concepts, and procedures. Although some mistakes are to be expected, make sure that once a mistake has been pointed out, it is corrected. Do not make the same mistakes over and over.

Supervisors may work closely with the medical assistant, or others may expect the medical assistant to carry out orders independently. Although being diligent about your job is commendable you should never hesitate to ask the more experienced medical assistants if you have any doubt about how to perform a task. Finish all assigned duties in a timely manner and avoid procrastination. When significant problems arise, discuss them openly with the supervisor and attempt to find a quick resolution. Limit absences and tardy days to a minimum and miss work only when absolutely necessary, especially during the probationary period.

Being a Good Employee

A medical assistant can be a good employee in several ways. First and foremost, arrive 15 minutes before the scheduled shift and do not leave early. Even the best medical assistant cannot benefit an office if he or she does not come to work. Be honest and demonstrate trustworthiness and professionalism. Get along with co-workers in the facility. A medical assistant should be able to resolve simple problems with others easily without involving the supervisor. Reflect a friendly attitude toward others, even if they are difficult to get along with. Arrive every single day ready to learn. The medical assistant's education does not end upon graduation from school. The medical field is one of constant change, and those who work in it must learn and change along with it. By choosing to work in the healthcare field you are making a commitment to lifelong learning.

A medical assistant should constantly be performing assigned duties and should not expect frequent breaks in the medical office. Most offices are fast paced, and the supervisor expects the medical assistant to keep up with the activity. Even during slow periods, there is always a counter to clean or documents to scan into the EHR. Be supportive of the leadership in the facility and ask for more responsibility if necessary. Take the initiative to perform duties that are cumbersome or repetitive and get them done quickly.

Always treat patients with compassion and empathy. Remember that they are not always at their best when ill, so be kind and courteous to them and their families. The patients are the reason the facility exists. Treat them with great respect and care.

Remember that medical assistants can be held individually responsible for their actions even though they work as an agent of the physician-employer. Although the provider is usually the person against whom professional liability lawsuits are brought, the medical assistant can still be named in a lawsuit.

CRITICAL THINKING APPLICATION   **51-12**

On Zac's second day at the practicum site, he clearly sees a co-worker taking and using a controlled drug from the storage area.
- What should Zac do?
- What potential problems arise with this situation?
- To whom should Zac report this incident, if anyone?

Dealing With Supervisors

Supervisors appreciate employees who come to them when they have questions, but who are able to handle minor decisions on their own. Never hesitate to approach supervisors when an issue at hand needs their attention. Do not allow a situation to go unaddressed and then say, "I didn't want to bother you with that." The office manager is responsible for dealing with difficult issues, and these should be handled immediately when they arise.

A medical assistant should never attempt to cover up a mistake; admitting the error is a much better approach to solving the problem. When talking with the supervisor, do not hesitate to speak and do not avoid the subject. State the problem clearly and explain what routes are available to **rectify** the situation. Assertive communication skills work best in these situations. Work with the supervisor to resolve issues and accept the advice given with a positive attitude.

Performance Appraisals

Performance appraisals usually are done after the initial probationary period and annually thereafter. The performance appraisal is designed to inform the employee of his or her strengths and weaknesses on the job. An appraisal may be done in a 180-degree style, where you are evaluated by your supervisor. Your supervisor uses his or her observations of your performance over the given time period. An appraisal may also be done using the 360-degree style, where the supervisor asks for input from your co-workers and others that you interact with on a regular basis. Do not expect to receive a perfect appraisal, because employees are seldom perfect in all aspects of their jobs. If the supervisor gives perfect scores to an employee, there is no room for growth or improvement. It is the rare employee who completes all duties and meets every expectation without any errors. Take time to review the job description and honestly evaluate your own performance in all areas.

When asked to sit down with your supervisor for a performance appraisal, expect to address areas where you did not receive a perfect score. These are the areas that need improvement from your supervisor's perspective. If you have had an opportunity to see the performance appraisal before your meeting with your supervisor, pay close attention to those areas where you got less than a perfect rating. Come to the meeting with ways to improve that score. You may be asked about the status of your continuing education units (CEUs) needed to maintain your certification or registration. You should also be prepared to discuss your goals for the coming year. These may be goals for improvement or involvement within the organization. Ask questions and work with the supervisor to improve in the areas that may need more effort or a different approach.

If the employee strongly disagrees with any area of the performance appraisal, he or she should discuss this with the supervisor. There may have been a misunderstanding as to the duties involved. Clarify this calmly and patiently and strive to do better next time.

Pursuing a Raise

Most facilities have some type of schedule for pay increases. Some offer a cost of living increase on an annual basis; others use a merit system, offering raises only when earned and deserved based on performance. The requirements are often outlined in the performance review document.

There may come a time when the medical assistant feels the need to ask for a raise. Before doing so, a little self-reflection is important to determine whether a raise is in order. Has attendance been exemplary? How many times was the medical assistant tardy? Does he or she work well with little supervision? Has he or she performed all the expected duties well and in a timely manner? Has he or she gone above and beyond with patients and/or co-workers? Has he or she met the requirements outlined by the organization?

Make an appointment with the supervisor and ask, in private, how a salary raise might be earned in the near future. Do not expect a raise of more than 3% to 5% at any given time, unless the employee is promoted to another position or given additional duties. If the supervisor is unable to grant a raise, determine whether the reasons are valid. Work with the supervisor to determine what steps you need to take to be able to gain a raise. Is there additional education required, is the supervisor looking for more involvement within the organization, such as participation in a committee, or are there additional responsibilities that can be taken on? If the reasons are not valid, the medical assistant may want to pursue other employment options. The medical assistant will find that finding a job is always easier if one already has a job, so do not quit outright unless the work environment is intolerable. Begin networking again and discover the options available.

Leaving a Job

Always offer at least 2 weeks' notice when resigning from a job. Prepare a written notice of resignation and take it to the supervisor in person. Do not just leave it on a desk or place it in the interoffice mail.

Resigning from a job just as an attempt to get a salary increase is a dangerous practice. Once the employer doubts the employee's loyalty, the future usually is not bright for the employee at that facility. Resign only after a final decision has been made. If the medical assistant is resigning to take another position, the current employer may be expected to make a **counteroffer**. However, be wary about accepting counteroffers. What led you to look for a new job in the first place? Has the situation been resolved? Ask yourself these questions before agreeing to stay with the current employer. Often employees who accept a counteroffer and stay at their original job find that few changes are made, and the employee ends up leaving the position in the long run.

LIFE SKILLS

To be successful in the job search, the medical assistant must have the basic entry-level skills needed to perform in the workplace. Even more important, he or she must develop certain life skills that are essential to excel in any profession. If these skills are not developed and refined, the medical assistant may find fewer opportunities and advancements available, as well as less impressive salaries and benefits. Perhaps even more important, the medical assistant who does not have his or her personal life in order will not be able to offer the employer his or her best performance every day. He or she will be expected to give a full day's work for a full day's pay on every single shift. Although personal issues do affect work performance, the medical assistant must make a good effort to put personal problems aside when working.

The most important life skill one can have is the willingness to change. Many employees insist on doing things the same way they have always been done, and they resist any changes in policy or procedure. However, a medical assistant who does not welcome change and work hard to adjust to change is a failure waiting to happen.

Personal Growth

Personal growth is a comprehensive term that applies to many aspects of a person's mental, physical, and spiritual health. This growth is a result of goals that are set for self-improvement. Without clear goals, people rarely experience personal growth that is initiated from within. Growth may happen as a result of some outside influence, but a conscious effort toward personal growth is an innate decision. One goal may be to get more involved with community by helping out at the local food pantry or free clinic. This opportunity not only will help out the community, but also will expose you to things you might not otherwise see. It can also give you a feeling of accomplishment that you were able to in some way help out those less fortunate. Another goal may be to become more physically active. Starting a lunchtime walking team would be one way to become more active and can also foster teamwork and cooperation within the organization.

Steps for Achieving Goals

- Decide what you want.
- Write down the goal.
- Set the date for accomplishment.
- Read the goal three times a day.
- Think of the goal often.
- See yourself accomplishing the goal.
- Develop a plan of action for reaching the goal.
- Do not discuss the plan with others who might be discouraging.
- Be confident.
- Act successful and you will be!

No matter how great the training or how many opportunities are placed in front of a person, fear and doubt can sabotage efforts to improve the self-image, confidence, and future potential of an individual. Personal growth involves such traits as self-control, self-esteem, problem-solving skills, decision-making skills, and stress management.

Self-Control

Self-control is a vital trait in the medical office. Some patients are not at their best because of their illness, and this may make them less than cordial toward the staff. Remember that this is usually a temporary situation. A medical assistant must exercise self-control and must not respond in kind to patients who are disagreeable.

Self-control in your personal life can influence your professional behaviors in your working life. By choosing to stay home on a work night rather than going out with friends, you will be better prepared for the workday. By choosing to manage your money responsibly you will decrease your stress level and make concentrating on your job easier. Self-control is a key piece in having a successful career as a medical assistant.

Self-Esteem

Everyone has certain strengths and weaknesses. Good self-esteem is the result of knowing what those strengths are and overcoming the weaknesses. It is having a positive outlook about oneself and others. A person with good self-esteem is motivated, able to express love, and capable of handling criticism. A person's self-esteem improves if he or she has developed adaptive skills. Especially in the medical profession, one thing that is guaranteed in the workplace is change. Change can be positive or negative; this depends mostly on the way it is viewed by the individual.

A person is not doomed to live with poor self-esteem forever. Take a good look at what you do each day. How have you contributed to taking care of your patients? How have you made things easier for your co-workers? Are you making a difference? With a degree of effort and openmindedness, an individual can work toward better self-esteem, which can make a tremendous difference in the individual's future potential.

Problem-Solving Skills

For individuals to work together, they must have a degree of trust and be willing to make suggestions for the good of the group. The saying "two heads are better than one" is still true when it comes to problem solving. Employees usually want to play a part in solving

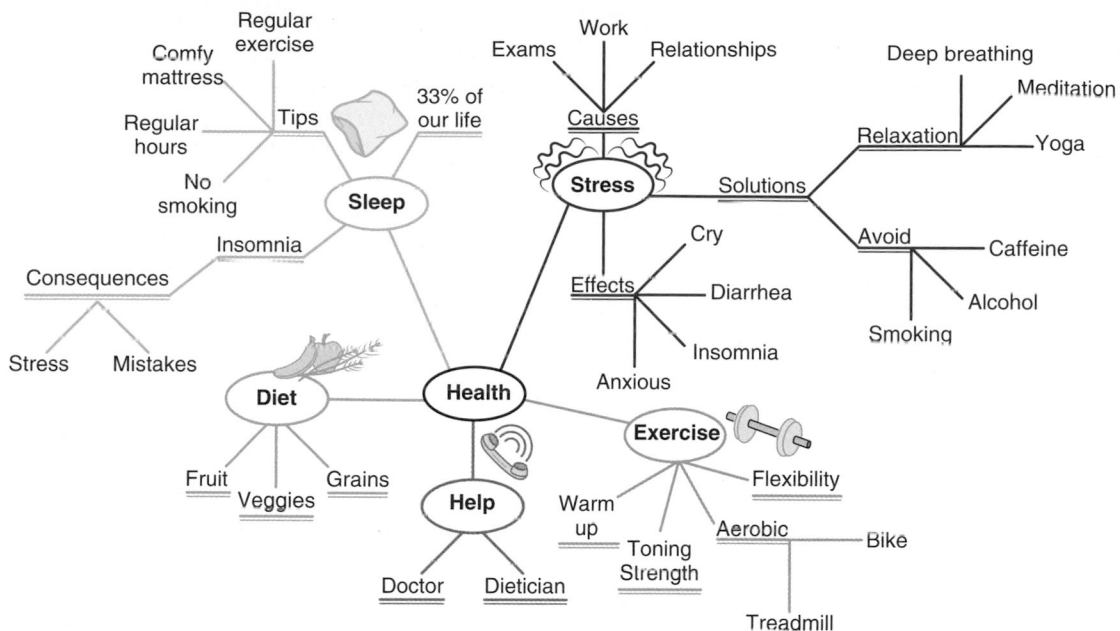

FIGURE 51-16 Mind mapping example.

the problems in the workplace, and they appreciate knowing that their opinions make a difference. Many organizations are looking for the input of their employees. A staff meeting may be called to solicit input when specific issues arise. At this meeting, brainstorming can be a useful problem-solving technique. Everyone should feel free to state his or her ideas, no matter how off-the-wall they are, and participate in the discussion to come up with a solution to the issue. Mind mapping is another problem-solving technique that can help to find a solution to the problem (Figure 51-16). With mind mapping, the problem is shown in the center of a large piece of paper or even on a white board. From this central problem, branches are drawn in all directions with important words or phrases that pertain to the central problem. Additional branches can be added to the important words or phrases until there is a comprehensive diagram of the problem and possible solutions. A medical assistant who can listen to the concerns of others and is willing to give and take will be an excellent problem solver.

Decision-Making Skills

People who know how to make good decisions usually are successful. Thinking through a decision requires logic, and it is best to take some time to think carefully of all the pros and cons. Unfortunately, a medical assistant may not always have time to consider decisions in a leisurely fashion, especially when dealing with emergencies. A good decision maker is honest in identifying the real problems and attempts to keep personal feelings isolated from the process.

There are several steps in making a sound decision. The problem must be specifically defined and evaluated so that the individual understands clearly what needs to happen to resolve the situation. Gather as much information as possible and consider all alternatives. It sometimes is helpful to choose an alternative and consider all the ramifications of making a decision using that alternative. Then, when the best alternative has been determined, the decision should be made and put into action. The last step in this process should be

to evaluate the effectiveness of the decision after a set period of time. Did the decision result in resolution of the problem or should the situation be reevaluated? Care should be taken to avoid making a decision simply because it is easy and comfortable, because more problems could arise later as a result of not addressing the true problem in the beginning.

Professional Development

Many healthcare organizations are looking for credentialed medical assistants. Being credentialed allows you to perform more of the tasks in the organization. If you are a graduate from an accredited program, you are able to take a certification examination. By doing this you are showing a potential or current employer that you are committed to your profession and have been recognized by a national agency for your knowledge about the medical assistant field. The two most common examinations are the CMA credential, given through the AAMA, and the RMA credential, given through the AMT.

Both credentials require that you participate in continuing education to maintain that credential. These CEUs help you to stay current in your field. Both organizations offer many opportunities to earn CEUs in an online format and also through attendance at national, state, or local conventions. Educational opportunities outside of these organizations may also be used for CEU credits if approved by the agency.

Professional development is an ongoing process when working in healthcare. By being committed to continue to learn about your chosen profession you will show your employer that you are a valuable asset to the organization.

Stress Management

The demands of the medical profession make it a stressful environment at times. Stress is not always bad. In fact, some stress is a positive motivator toward a goal. A *stressor* is a stimulus that prompts a reaction from the body. Positive stress, or *eustress,* includes exhilarating activities or success, which often leads to higher expectations from the person experiencing the eustress. The opposite is distress, which includes disappointment, failure, or embarrassment. Stress management is a conscious effort to control the stressors and resulting reactions so that the body and mind operate evenly, even when stress is present in an individual's life.

By learning to recognize the signs of stressful overload, a medical assistant can possibly ward off the negative reactions that are so physically and mentally draining to the body. Many people notice a headache or fatigue when overly stressed. Breathing correctly is one way to reduce stress. Often an accelerated breathing pattern that is quick and shallow is a stress indicator. Breathing from the abdomen at a slower pace, inhaling through the nose, and exhaling through the mouth may help reduce tension. Taking time for relaxing activities and getting plenty of exercise are other methods of stress reduction.

Stress Management Techniques

- Do something you enjoy: gardening, reading, sailing, volunteer work
- Meditate
- Exercise
- Breathe deeply
- Laugh out loud
- Keep a gratitude journal

CLOSING COMMENTS

The period surrounding graduation is a celebration but also a busy time that requires much planning. Cooperate with the school in securing a practicum site and make an effort to obtain a site that will be the most beneficial to the career you want. Do not take a practicum site just because it is close to home. Think about the skills that will be offered and learn as much as possible. Then perform well, so that the staff and providers are happy to offer a good reference to potential employers. Strive to attain goals, and once they are reached, set additional goals to continue moving forward in life.

Even though the medical assistant educational experience ends, remember that there is constantly something new to learn in the medical profession. Join professional associations and participate in as many educational seminars and continuing education classes as possible. Remain in a continual state of learning and be determined to be the best medical assistant you can be.

Legal and Ethical Issues

Always be completely honest when completing a job application and offering information on a résumé. Most facilities stipulate that if an individual is not truthful on these documents, his or her employment can be terminated when the deception is discovered. Employers are more interested in honesty and a forthright explanation than in minor problems that affect the job performance.

If a medical assistant has had some brush with the law that requires disclosure on the job application, the best policy is to be honest and to deal with the ramifications of telling the truth. Most businesses can verify whether a potential employee has any type of criminal record. A solid explanation of the facts, admission of a past mistake, and excellent current references often prompt an employer to have faith and make a positive decision about offering employment.

Professional Behaviors

The development of professional behaviors must begin before the start of a new job. Use your time in school to develop those behaviors that employers are looking for: collaboration and interpersonal skills, professionalism, and compassion. By developing these behaviors in school your teachers and practicum mentors will be able to give a recommendation that stresses those skills. By being on time and prepared for class you are showing that you will be on time and prepared for work. By being diligent and self-directed in the classroom you demonstrate that you have a strong work ethic, which is an important characteristic to employers.

SUMMARY OF SCENARIO

Before graduation, Michelle was offered a job at a family practice clinic working with several physicians. She took her instructor's advice and sent a thank-you note to those who interviewed her. When she was offered the job, the supervisor mentioned how thoughtful the note was. During the call, the supervisor summarized the benefits and the starting salary. She mentioned to Michelle that all medical assistants start at the same wage, but after they pass the CMA certification examination, they get a raise. Michelle took 2 days to consider the position and decided to accept the job offer. The wage was lower than what she was hoping for, but the benefits were much better.

Krysia interviewed for several medical assistant positions over the last few weeks, finding that employers respected her service to her country and valued the skills she learned in the military service. She just received her third job offer within the last few days and has decided to accept the position at the local Veterans Affairs (VA) clinic. It is a full-time position with great benefits and the higher wage will help offset the extra mileage that she will be driving to work. She is very excited to be working with other veterans.

Zac struggled identifying what type of clinic he wanted to work for. With his strong leadership skills, he hopes to find a position where he can advance to a supervisory position. He has interviewed for job positions at small and large clinics. He is finding that he is more interested in working with surgeons than with family practitioners. He likes the complexity involved with surgical patients. He is hoping to receive a job offer shortly after graduation. He has decided that if his "dream job" is not offered to him, he will pursue a position in family medicine or internal medicine to get a solid foundation for his new career and then someday move into orthopedics or surgery.

SUMMARY OF LEARNING OBJECTIVES

1. **Define, spell, and pronounce the terms listed in the vocabulary.**
   Spelling and pronouncing terms correctly bolster the medical assistant's credibility. Knowing the definitions of these terms promotes confidence in communication with patients and co-workers.

2. **Describe the four personality traits that are most important to employers.**
   With the cost of training new employees, employers must find the best person to hire. Many employers struggle with assisting new employees to evolve or change personality traits. Thus employers seek people who already have collaboration and interpersonal skills, professionalism, compassion, and a sincere interest in the job. Collaboration and interpersonal skills allow the new employee to blend well with the current staff. Being flexible, dependable, supportive of peers, remaining calm under pressure, listening, and having good manners are just some of the characteristics of a person with great collaboration and interpersonal skills. Being professional includes proper dress and grooming habits, punctuality, honesty, attention to detail, and the abilities to follow directions, prioritize, and manage time efficiently. Providing compassionate and respectful care and supporting the patient's dignity is crucial to good patient care. Lastly, being genuinely interested in the position positively affects the person's attitude and performance in the job.

3. **Explain the three areas that need to be examined to determine one's strengths and skills.**
   A medical assistant must identify the personality traits, technical skills, and transferable job skills that he or she possesses. Using a portfolio will help the interviewee showcase the qualities that he or she has. Technical skills consist of administrative and clinical skills the person has developed during their medical assistant program. Transferable job skills are skills that were utilized in an unrelated position, but relate or transfer to the new position.

4. **Discuss career objectives and describe how personal needs affect the job search.**
   Medical assistants should take some time to think about what they want from their career and develop a career objective. Your personal needs (e.g., wage, benefits, hours, locations) help you determine what job might be right for you so you can focus your job search.

5. **Do the following related to finding a job:**
   - Explain the two best job search methods.
     The two best methods to identify jobs are through networking and using job boards. Networking involves the medical assistant exchanging information with other professionals and family members in hopes of obtaining possible job leads. Job boards are online sites that list positions posted by employers. They can be specific to the healthcare facilities or they can be managed by local media organizations. National job boards can be very helpful for those who want to relocate to another part of the country.
   - Discuss traditional job search methods.
     Traditional job search methods include school career placement offices, newspaper ads, and employment agencies.
   - Describe various ways to improve your opportunities.
     If you are having trouble finding a job, it is important to reevaluate your search methods and ask yourself some questions. Participating in volunteer activities and temporary employment can help.
   - Discuss the importance of being organized in your job search.
     Keeping organized records is critical. Keep the documents in an organized system on your computer, and make a spreadsheet, word processing document, or handwritten log that indicates the postings you have applied for.

6. **Discuss the three types of résumé formats, describe how to prepare a chronologic résumé and cover letter, and discuss the importance and format of both the résumé and cover letter.**
   The three commonly used résumé formats are chronologic, combination, and targeted résumés. Procedures 51-1 and 51-2 describe the steps involved with preparing a résumé and cover letter. As you create your résumé, keep in mind the eye appeal or interest the résumé will create in the reader. A cover letter should always accompany a résumé and much attention to detail is necessary.

7. **Discuss how to complete an online portfolio and job application.**
   Many healthcare agencies utilize the Internet during the employment process, and online portfolios can have many advantages over paper applications. However, not every employer utilizes online portfolios and students may have to fill out job applications as well. Procedure 51-3 describes the steps involved with completing a job application.

8. **Describe how to create a career portfolio.**
   Procedure 51-4 describes the steps involved with creating a career portfolio.

9. **Do the following related to the job interview:**
   - List and describe the four phases of the interview process.
     The four phases of the interview process are the preparation, the actual interview, the follow-up, and the negotiation. The preparation includes all efforts made before the actual interview in obtaining information about the company, deciding on the wardrobe, and making sure nails are groomed and shoes are shined. The interview itself is designed to help the employer and potential employee get to know each other and discover whether they are compatible. The follow-up is perhaps the most critical stage, wherein the medical assistant should send a thank-you letter and continue to stay in touch with the facility until the job is filled. The negotiation includes discussion of the salary and benefits that will be offered to the new employee.
   - List and discuss legal and illegal interview questions.
     Employers may intentionally or accidentally ask illegal interview questions, and the medical assistant has three choices in this situation: (1) refusing to answer the question, which may indicate that he or she will not tolerate difficult patients; (2) answering the question directly, which may cost the medical assistant the position; or (3) relating the question back to the position, which indicates maturity and the ability to be tactful and polite.

Continued

SUMMARY OF LEARNING OBJECTIVES—*continued*

- Practice interview skills for a mock interview. Refer to Procedure 51-5.
- Create a thank-you note for an interview.
  Writing a thank-you note for an interview is a way to make you stand out from the other people who have interviewed for the same position. It shows that you are a courteous and conscientious person and also gives you another opportunity to show why you are the right person for the job. Refer to Procedure 51-6.

10. **Do the following related to getting a job:**
- Discuss the importance of the probationary period for a new employee.
  The probationary period is a time for the new medical assistant to become oriented to the facility. It also allows the employer to assess whether the medical assistant fits with the team and performs the duties of the job in a satisfactory way. During this time, the medical assistant should demonstrate that he or she is a productive team member with an excellent attitude. There should never be idle time; rather, when all duties are completed, the medical assistant should look for ways to assist others.
- List some common early mistakes of which a new employee should be aware.
  A new employee in the medical office should avoid arriving late or being absent, especially during the probationary period. He or she should never participate in office gossip and should make a good attempt to get along with every employee. A medical assistant should not make excessive supervision necessary and should be open to learning new ways of performing procedures. A new employee who fits in with the team finds the job more rewarding.

- Discuss how to be a good employee and how to deal with supervisors.
  A medical assistant can be a better employee in several ways: arriving early, being honest, getting along with co-workers, consistently performing assigned duties, treating patients with compassion, and being held responsible for his or her actions. Never hesitate to approach supervisors when an issue at hand needs attention.
- Explain why a performance appraisal rating is usually not perfect.
  No employee is perfect, so performance appraisals rarely have perfect ratings. Even an employee who is doing an excellent job has room for improvement in some area. Without comments that suggest improvement, the employee may not feel that the position offers growth potential. Constructive comments help a medical assistant perform better and take on more responsibility.
- Discuss how to pursue a raise and how to leave a job.
  Before asking for a raise, self-reflection is necessary. Make an appointment to talk to your supervisor in private and explain why you think you deserve a raise. Do not expect a raise of more than 3% to 5% at any given time. When leaving a job, always offer at least 2 weeks' notice.

11. **Discuss various life skills needed in the workplace.**
  To be successful in the job search, the medical assistant must have the basic entry-level skills needed to perform in the workplace. Even more important, he or she must develop certain life skills that are essential to any profession. Personal growth, self-control, self-esteem, problem-solving skills, decision-making skills, professional development, and stress management are all important life skills for a medical assistant to attain and continue to develop over time.

CONNECTIONS

Study Guide Connection: Go to the Chapter 51 Study Guide. Read and complete the activities.

evolve Evolve Connection: Go to the Chapter 51 link at *evolve.elsevier.com/kinn* to complete the Chapter Review Quiz. Check out the other resources listed for this chapter to make the most of what you have learned from Career Development and Life Skills.

GLOSSARY

abandonment In medical care, the discontinuation of care without proper notice after a patient has been accepted.

ablation (a-bla′-shun) Amputation or removal of any body part.

abscesses Localized collections of pus, which may be under the skin or deep in the body, that cause tissue destruction.

abstract A summary of the diagnostic statement and/or procedures and services performed.

accepting diversity The practice of accepting every individual, regardless of age, religion, race, disability, and/or gender, in the medical practice.

accommodation The automatic adjustment of the eye that allows a person to see various sizes of objects at different distances.

accounts payable Money owed by a company to other companies for services and goods; pertains to paying the bills of the facility.

accreditation (u-kre-duh-ta′-shun) The process by which an organization is recognized for adherence to a group of standards that meet or exceed the expectations of the accrediting agency.

act The formal action of a legislative body; a decision or determination of a sovereign state, a legislative council, or a court of justice.

acute Having a sudden onset, sharp rise, and short course; providing or requiring short-term medical care.

adhesions (ad-he′-zhuns) Bands of scar tissue that bind together two anatomic surfaces that normally are separate.

adnexal (ad-neks′-uhl) Pertaining to adjacent or accessory parts.

adrenocorticotropic hormone (ACTH) (uh-dren-o-cor-tih-ko-tro′-pik) A hormone released by the anterior pituitary gland that stimulates the production and secretion of glucocorticoids.

advocate (ad′-voh-kat) In medical care, a person who represents the patient when healthcare decisions are made.

affable Pleasant and at ease in talking to others; characterized by ease and friendliness.

age of majority The age at which a person is recognized by law to be an adult; it varies by state.

air kerma Kinetic energy released in matter (Gy$_a$); the SI unit for radiation exposure that represents the amount of radiation in the air that reaches the patient. It is measured in Gray, and a subscript "a" is added to indicate that it is a measurement of the radiation in the air.

albuminuria (al-byoo-muh-nur′-e-uh) The abnormal presence of albumin protein in the urine.

aliquot (al′-ih-kwaht) A portion of a well-mixed sample removed for testing.

allegation (al-eh-ga′-shun) A statement by a party to a legal action of what the party undertakes to prove; an assertion made without proof.

alleviate To partly remove or correct; to relieve or lessen.

allopathic (al-o-path′-ik) A system of medical practice that treats disease by the use of remedies, such as medications and surgery, to produce effects different from those caused by the disease under treatment; medical doctors (MDs) and osteopaths (DOs) practice allopathic medicine; also called conventional medicine.

alopecia (al-o-pe′-se-uh) Partial or complete lack of hair.

alphabetic filing Any system that arranges names or topics according to the sequence of the letters in the alphabet.

alphanumeric Of or relating to systems made up of combinations of letters and numbers.

amblyopia (am-ble o′-pe-uh) Reduction or dimness of vision with no apparent organic cause; often referred to as *lazy eye syndrome*.

amenity (uh-me′-nuh-te) Something conducive to comfort, convenience, or enjoyment.

amino acids The organic compounds that form the chief constituents of protein; they are used by the body to build and repair tissues.

analyte The substance or chemical being analyzed or detected in a specimen.

anaphylaxis (an-uh-fih-lak′-sis) An exaggerated hypersensitivity reaction that in severe cases leads to vascular collapse, bronchospasm, and shock.

anaplastic Relating to an alteration in cells to a more primitive form; a term that describes cancer-producing cells

anastomosis (uh-nas-tuh-mo′-sis) The surgical joining of two normally distinct organs.

anemia A condition marked by a deficiency of red blood cells (RBCs).

angina pectoris (an-ji′-nuh/pek′-tuh-ris) A spasmlike pain in the chest caused by myocardial anoxia.

angiocardiography (an-je-o-kahr-de-og′-ruh-fe) Radiography of both the heart and great vessels using an iodine contrast medium.

angiography (an-je-og′-ruh-fe) The process of producing an image of blood vessels using an iodine contrast medium.

angioplasty (an′-je-o-plas-te) A technique in which a catheter is used to open or widen a blood vessel narrowed by stenoses or occlusions to improve circulation.

anomaly (uh-nom′-uh-le) A congenital malformation that occurs during fetal development.

anorexia (ah-nuh-rek′-se-uh) A lack or loss of appetite for food.

answering service A business that receives and answers telephone calls for the healthcare facility when it is closed.

anterior (an-tuhr′-e-ohr) The front part of the body or body part when a person is in anatomic position.

anteroposterior (AP) projection (an-tuhr-o-pos-ter′-e-ohr) A frontal projection, in which the central ray enters the front of the patient and exits the back to reach the image receptor; the patient is supine or facing the x-ray tube.

anti–kickback statute A criminal law that prohibits the exchange of anything of value in an effort to reward the referral of a patient sponsored by a government insurance plan

antibodies (an′-tih-bah-dees) Molecular proteins (immunoglobulins) produced by the blood's plasma cells that specifically destroy a foreign invader or substance that has infected the body.

anticoagulant Chemicals added to a blood sample after collection to prevent clotting.

antigen (an'-tih-juhn)   A foreign invader (e.g., bacterium, virus, toxin, allergen) that generates an immune response, including the production of antibodies.

antimicrobial agents   A general term for drugs, chemicals, or other substances that either kill or slow the growth of microbes. Among the antimicrobial agents are antibacterial drugs, antiviral agents, antifungal agents, and antiparasitic drugs.

antiseptic (an-tih-sep'-tik)   An agent that inhibits the growth of microorganisms on living tissue (e.g., alcohol and povidone-iodine solution [Betadine]); used to cleanse the skin, wounds, and so on.

anuria   The absence of urine production.

aortogram (a-or'-toh-gram)   An image of the aorta produced using an iodine contrast medium.

apnea (ap'-ne-uh)   Absence or cessation of breathing.

appellate (uh-peh'-lut)   A term referring to courts that have the power to review and change the decisions of a lower court.

aqueous (ak'-we-uhs)   A waterlike substance; a medication prepared with water.

arbitration (ahr-buh-tra'-shun)   A type of alternative dispute resolution that provides parties to a controversy with a choice other than going to court for resolution of a problem. Arbitration is either court-ordered to resolve a conflict, or the two sides select an impartial third party, known as an arbitrator, and agree in advance to comply with the arbitrator's award. The arbitrator's decision is usually final.

arrhythmia   An abnormality or irregularity in the heart rhythm.

arteriography (ahr-ter-e-og'-ruh-fe)   The technique of producing an image of arteries using an iodine contrast medium.

arteriosclerosis (ahr-ter'-e-o-scler-o-sis)   A condition marked by thickening, decreased elasticity, and calcification of arterial walls.

arthritis (ahr-thry'-tis)   Inflammation of a joint.

arthrogram (ahr'-thro-gram)   Fluoroscopic examination of the soft tissue components of joints, in which a contrast medium is injected directly into the joint capsule.

arthropods (ahr'-throh-pods)   A class of invertebrate animals that includes insects, crustaceans, spiders, scorpions, and others.

articular (ahr-tih'-kyuh-luhr)   Pertaining to a joint.

artifacts   Structures or features not normally present but visible as a result of an external agent or action, such as in a microscopic specimen after fixation or in a radiographic image.

ascites (uh-si'-tez)   An abnormal collection of fluid in the peritoneal cavity containing high levels of protein and electrolytes.

assault   An intentional attempt to cause bodily harm to another; a threat to cause harm is an assault if it is combined with a physical action (e.g., a raised fist) so that the victim could reasonably assume there would be an assault.

asymptomatic   Without symptoms of a disease process.

asystole (a-sis'-toh-le)   The absence of a heartbeat.

ataxia (uh-taks'-e-uh)   Failure or irregularity of muscle actions and coordination.

atria   The two upper chambers of the heart.

atrioventricular (AV) node   The part of the cardiac conduction system between the atria and the ventricles.

attenuated (uh-ten'-yoo-wat-ed)   Weakened or changed; refers to the virulence of a pathogenic microorganism in reference to vaccine development.

audiologist (aw-de-ah'-loh-jist)   Allied healthcare professional who specializes in evaluation of hearing function, detection of hearing impairment, and determination of the anatomic site of impairment.

audit   An inspection performed before claims are submitted to examine them for accuracy and completeness.

audit trail   A record of computer activity used to monitor users' actions within software, including additions, deletions, and viewing of electronic records.

augment   To increase in size or amount; to add to so as to improve or complete.

aura   A peculiar sensation that precedes the appearance of a more definite disturbance; commonly seen with migraines or seizure activity.

auscultation   The act of listening to body sounds, typically with a stethoscope, to assess various organs throughout the body.

authorized agent   A person who has written documentation that he or she can accept a shipment for another individual.

autoimmune (aw-to-im-yoon')   Pertaining to a disturbance in the immune system in which the body reacts against its own tissue. Examples of autoimmune disorders include multiple sclerosis, rheumatoid arthritis, and systemic lupus erythematosus.

automatic call routing   A system that distributes incoming calls to a specific group or person based on the caller's need; for example, the individual presses 1 for appointments, 2 for billing questions, and so on.

autonomy (aw-ton'-oh-me)   The ability to function independently.

axial projections   Radiographs taken with a longitudinal angulation of the x-ray beam; sometimes referred to as *semiaxial projections.*

azotemia (a-zo-te'-me-uh)   A condition marked by the retention of excessive quantities of nitrogenous wastes in the blood.

back up   The process of copying and archiving computer data so that the duplicate files can be used to restore the original data if a compromise occurs.

backorder   An order placed for an item that is temporarily out of stock and will be sent at a later time.

bacteriuria   The presence of bacteria in the urine (possible infection).

bailiff   An officer of some U.S. courts who usually serves as a messenger or usher and who keeps order at the request of the judge.

Bartholin's cyst   A fluid-filled cyst in one of the vestibular glands located on either side of the vaginal orifice.

basement membrane   A deep layer of the skin that secures the epithelium to underlying tissue; it separates the epidermis from the dermis.

battery   An intentional act of contact with another that causes harm or offends the individual being touched or injured.

benign   A tumor or tissue growth that is not cancerous; it may require treatment or removal, depending on its location, and/or for cosmetic reasons.

benign   Not cancerous and not recurring.

bevel (bev'-uhl)   The angled tip of a needle.

bifurcates   Divides from one into two branches.

bilirubin (bih-lih-roo'-bin)   An orange pigment in bile; its accumulation leads to jaundice.

bilirubinuria (bi-li-roo-bin-yuhr'-e-uh)   The presence of bilirubin in the urine (possible liver damage).

billable service Assistance (i.e., service) that is provided by a healthcare provider that can be billed to the insurance company and/or patient.

biophysical (bi-o-fih'-zih-kuhl) The science of applying physical laws and theories to biologic problems.

blatant Completely obvious, conspicuous, or obtrusive, especially in a crass or offensive manner; brazen.

blood-brain barrier An anatomic-physiologic structure made up of astrocyte glial cells that prevents or slows the transfer of chemicals into the neurons of the central nervous system (CNS).

bonded Referring to a guarantee obtained by an employer from an insurance company (i.e., a fidelity bond) that the company will cover losses from an employee's dishonest acts (e.g., embezzlement, theft).

bounding A term used to describe a pulse that feels full because of increased power of cardiac contraction or as a result of increased blood volume.

bradycardia (brad-ih-kahr'-de-uh) A slow heartbeat; a pulse below 60 beats per minute.

bradypnea (brad-ip'-ne'-uh) Respirations that are regular in rhythm but slower than normal in rate.

broad-spectrum antimicrobial agents Drugs used to treat a wide range of infections.

bronchiectasis (brong-ke-ek'-tuh-sis) Dilation of the bronchi and bronchioles associated with secondary infection or ciliary dysfunction.

bronchoconstriction Narrowing of the bronchiole tubes.

bronchodilator (brahn-ko-di'-la-tuhr) A drug that relaxes contractions of the smooth muscle of the bronchioles to improve lung ventilation.

bruit (broo'-it) An abnormal sound or murmur heard on auscultation of an organ, vessel (e.g., carotid artery), or gland; it is caused by the flow of blood through a narrowed or partially occluded vessel.

Bucky A moving grid device that holds an image receptor and prevents scatter radiation from fogging the image.

buffy coat The layer of white cells or platelets found between the plasma and the packed red blood cells after whole blood has been centrifuged.

bundle of His Specialized muscle fibers that conduct electrical impulses from the AV node to the ventricular myocardium.

bursae (bur'-say) Fluid-filled, saclike membranes that provide cushioning and allow frictionless motion between two tissues.

buying cycle The frequency with which an item is purchased; it depends on how often the item is used and the storage space available for it.

calibration Determining the accuracy of an instrument by comparing its output with that of a known standard or another instrument known to be accurate.

call forwarding A telephone feature that allows calls made to one number to be forwarded to another specified number.

caller ID A feature that identifies and displays the telephone numbers of incoming calls made to a particular line.

candidiasis (kan-dih-di'-uh-sis) An infection caused by a yeast that typically affects the vaginal mucosa and skin.

cannula (kan'-yoo-lah) A rigid tube that surrounds a blunt trocar or a sharp, pointed trocar, which is inserted into the body; when the trocar is withdrawn, fluid may escape from the body through the cannula, depending on the insertion site.

capitation A contract between the health insurance plan and the provider for which the health insurance plan will pay an agreed-upon monthly fee per patient and the provider agrees to provide medical services on a regular basis.

caption A heading, title, or subtitle under which records are filed.

carcinogens (kar-sih'-noh-juhns) Substances or agents that cause the development of cancer or increase its incidence.

cardiac arrest A condition in which cardiac contractions stop completely

cardioversion The use of electroshock to convert an abnormal cardiac rhythm to a normal one.

cartilage (kahr'-til-ij) A rubbery, smooth, somewhat elastic connective tissue that covers the ends of bones.

cash on hand The amount of money the healthcare practice has in the bank that can be withdrawn as cash.

cassette A special container that holds either film or a phosphorescent screen inside; it is used to transform an x-ray beam into a visible image; also referred to as an *image receptor* when loaded.

cast In kidney disease, a fibrous or protein material molded to the shape of the part in which it has accumulated that is thrown off into the urine. Casts may be identified as hyaline, cellular, granular, or waxy.

cathartics Laxative preparations.

caustic (kos'-tik) A substance that burns or destroys tissue by chemical action.

cell-mediated immunity An immune response that occurs from the action of T lymphocytes rather than from the production of antibodies.

central ray (CR) An imaginary line in the center of the x-ray beam that leaves the tube and reaches the patient.

centrifuge (sen'-trih-fuhj) An apparatus consisting essentially of a compartment that spins about a central axis to separate contained materials of different specific gravities or to separate colloidal particles suspended in a liquid.

Certified Registered Nurse Anesthetist (CRNA) A nursing healthcare professional who is certified to administer anesthesia.

cerumen (seh-room'-en) A waxy secretion in the ear canal; commonly called *ear wax.*

cervical (ser'-vih-kuhl) Pertaining to the neck region containing seven cervical vertebrae.

chain of command A series of executive positions in order of authority.

characteristics Distinguishing traits, qualities, or properties.

Cheyne-Stokes respirations A breathing pattern characterized by rhythmic changes in the depth of respiration. The patient breathes deeply for a short time and then breathes very slightly or stops breathing altogether; the pattern occurs over and over, every 45 seconds to 3 minutes. The Cheyne-Stokes breathing pattern is seen in patients with heart failure or brain damage, but also in healthy individuals who hyperventilate, at high altitudes, and with hypnotic drug or narcotic overdose and sleep apnea.

cholesterol (kuh-les'-tuh-rol) A substance produced by the liver and found in animal fats; it can result in fatty deposits or atherosclerotic plaques in blood vessels.

chordae tendineae (kor'-duh/ten'-din-uh)   The tendons that anchor the cusps of the heart valves to the papillary muscles of the myocardium, preventing valvular prolapse.

chromosomes   Threadlike molecules that carry hereditary information.

chronic   A term describing a disease that manifests over a long period because medical treatment has not been able to resolve it.

chronic bronchitis   Recurrent inflammation of the membranes lining the bronchial tubes.

chronic obstructive pulmonary disease (COPD)   A progressive, irreversible lung condition that results in diminished lung capacity.

cicatrix   Early scar tissue that appears pale, contracted, and firm.

cilia (sil'-e-uh)   Hairlike projections capable of movement; in the lungs, cilia waves move unwanted substances (e.g., mucus, dust, and pus) upward; cilia are destroyed by smoking.

cirrhosis (suh-ro'-sis)   A chronic, degenerative disease of the liver that interferes with normal liver function.

Clinitest   A test tablet commonly used to screen for and confirm glucose and/or to detect other sugars in urine.

clitoris (klih'-tuh-ris)   A small, elongated erectile body above the urinary meatus at the superior point of the labia minora.

clubbing   Abnormal enlargement of the distal phalanges (fingers and toes); it is associated with cyanotic heart disease or advanced chronic pulmonary disease.

coagulate (ko-ag'-yuh-late)   To form into clots.

Coding Clinic   A medical coding industry journal that provides insight into the coding of complex medical cases. The journal is sponsored by the American Hospital Association (AHA), which also supports a website (*www.codingclinicadvisor.com*) that can accept questions from coders on specific cases.

cognitive (kog'-nih-tiv)   Pertaining to the operation of the mind; referring to the process by which we become aware of perceiving, thinking, and remembering.

cohesive   Sticking together tightly; exhibiting or producing cohesion.

coitus   Sexual union of a male and a female; also called *intercourse*.

collagen (kah'-luh-jen)   The protein that forms the inelastic fibers of tendons, ligaments, and fascia.

colloidal (kah-loid'-uhl)   Pertaining to a gluelike substance.

colonoscopy   A procedure in which a fiberoptic scope is used to examine the large intestine.

colostrum (koh-lahs'-trum)   A thin, yellow, milky fluid secreted by the mammary glands a few days before and after delivery.

coma   An unconscious state from which the patient cannot be aroused.

competencies   Mastery of the knowledge, skills, and behaviors that are expected of the entry-level medical assistant.

compliance   In a medical practice, meeting the standards and regulations of the practice's established policies and procedures.

compression   The state of being pressed together.

computed radiography (CR)   A modernized x-ray film technique in which a reusable cassette-plate image receptor stores the image, much as a flash drive functions in household computers.

computed tomography (CT)   A computerized x-ray imaging modality that provides axial and three-dimensional scans.

computer network   A system that links personal computers and peripheral devices to share information and resources.

computer on wheels (COW)   Wireless mobile workstation; also called *workstation on wheels* (WOW).

computerized provider/physician order entry (CPOE)   The process of entering medication orders or other provider instructions into the electronic health record (EHR).

cones   Structures in the retina that make the perception of color possible.

conference call   A telephone call in which a caller can speak with several people at the same time.

congenital (kuhn-jen'-ih-tul)   An anomaly or defect that is present at birth.

congruence (kon-groo'-ents)   Agreement; the state that occurs when the verbal expression of the message matches the sender's nonverbal body language.

contamination (kun-ta-mu-na'-shun)   The process by which something becomes harmful or unusable through contact with something unclean; soiled with pathogens or infectious material; nonsterile.

continuing medical education (CME)   Activities (e.g., conferences, seminars) that promote further education for physicians and providers.

continuity of care   Continuation of care smoothly from one provider to another, so that the patient receives the most benefit and no interruption in care.

contrast media   Substances used to enhance the visibility of soft tissues in imaging studies.

contributory negligence   Instances in which the individual contributes to the injury or condition; the injury is partly due to the individual's own negligence.

control booth   A separated area or room where the radiographer can remain safe from radiation while operating radiography equipment. It is protected by a special wall and/or window lined with lead. This area houses the control console, which contains the settings for the machine.

copulation   Sexual intercourse.

corticosteroids (kawr-tih-koh-ster'-oidz)   Antiinflammatory hormones, which may be natural or synthetic.

costal   Pertaining to the ribs.

counteroffer   A return offer made by a person who has rejected an offer or a job.

CPT Assistant   An online CPT coding journal, supported by the American Medical Association (AMA), that addresses subjects such as appealing insurance denials, validating coding to auditors, training staff members, and answering day-to-day coding questions.

crash carts   Carts stocked with emergency medications and equipment (e.g., oxygen, intravenous [IV], and airway supplies) that are readily available.

creatinine (kre'-a-tuhn-en)   Nitrogenous waste from muscle metabolism that is excreted in urine.

credit   A bookkeeping entry which increases accounts receivable, or what is owed to the provider

crenate   A term describing notched or leaflike, scalloped edges (as seen in shrinking red blood cells).

crepitation (kreh-pih-ta'-shun)   A dry, crackling sound or sensation.

critical thinking   The constant practice of considering all aspects of a situation when deciding what to believe or what to do.

cryosurgery The technique of exposing tissue to extreme cold to produce a well-defined area of cell destruction.

cryptogenic (krip-tuh-jeh'-nik) Pertaining to a disease with an unknown cause.

culpability Meriting condemnation, responsibility, or blame, especially as wrong or harmful.

culture and sensitivity (C&S) A procedure in which a specimen is cultured on artificial media to detect bacterial or fungal growth; this is followed by appropriate screening for antibiotic sensitivity. C&S is performed in the microbiology referral laboratory.

curettage (kyur-eh-tahjz') The act of scraping a body cavity with a surgical instrument, such as a curette.

cuvette A small tube or specimen container made of plastic or glass designed to hold samples for laboratory tests using light-meter technology (spectrophotometry).

cyanosis (si-an-o'-sis) A blue coloration of the mucous membranes and body extremities caused by lack of oxygen.

cyst A small, capsulelike sac that encloses certain organisms in their dormant or larval stage.

cytology (si-tah'-loh-je) The study of cells using microscopic methods.

damages Money awarded by a court to an individual who has been injured through the wrongful conduct of another party. Damages attempt to measure in financial terms the extent of harm the victim has suffered. Harm may be an actual physical injury but can also be damage to property or the individual's reputation.

data server Computer hardware and software that perform data analysis, storage, and archiving; also called a *database server*.

débridement The surgical removal of dead, damaged, or infected tissue to improve the function of healthy tissue.

decedent (dih-se'-dent) A legal term for a deceased person.

decryption The computer process of changing encrypted text to readable or plain text after a user enters a secret key or password.

decubitus ulcer A sore or ulcer that develops over a bony prominence as the result of ischemia from prolonged pressure; also called a *bed sore*.

defendant A person required to answer in a legal action or suit; in criminal cases, the person accused of a crime.

defibrillator A machine that delivers an electroshock to the heart through electrodes placed on the chest wall.

deficiencies (dih-fih'-shun-sees) Conditions that result from below normal intake of particular substances.

dehiscence The separation of wound edges or rupture of a wound closure.

demeanor (dih-me'-nur) Behavior toward others; outward manner.

demographics Statistical data of a population. In healthcare this includes the patient's name, address, date of birth, employment, and other details.

depreciate The decline in the value of an item over a certain period; used for tax purposes.

dermatome (dur'-muh-tohm) An area on the surface of the body that is innervated by nerve fibers from one spinal nerve root.

descendants Family members that take responsibility over the patient's estate after their death.

detrimental (deh-trih-men'-til) Obviously harmful or damaging.

diabetes mellitus type 1 A disease in which the beta cells in the pancreas no longer produce insulin. The individual must rely on daily insulin administration to use glucose for energy and prevent complications.

diabetes mellitus type 2 A disease in which the body is unable to use glucose for energy as a result either of inadequate insulin production in the pancreas or resistance to insulin on the cellular level.

diabetic retinopathy A condition in which microaneurysms and weakness in the capillary wall within the retina result in ischemia and tissue death.

diagnostic statement Information about a patient's diagnosis or diagnoses that has been extracted from the medical documentation, such as the history and physical findings, operative reports, and encounter form.

diaphoresis (di-uh-fuh-re'-sis) The profuse excretion of sweat.

diaphysis (di-ah'-fuh-sis) The midportion of a long bone; it contains the medullary cavity.

diastole The period of relaxation of the chambers of the heart, during which blood enters the heart from the vascular system and the lungs.

dictation (dik-ta'-shun) The act or manner of uttering words to be transcribed.

digestion The process of converting food into chemical substances that can be absorbed and used by the body.

digital radiography (DR) A radiographic technique that does not use cassettes; instead, the radiographic equipment has built-in image receptors that react to radiation and transmit a digital signal directly to the computer.

dignity Being worthy of honor and respect from others.

dilation The opening or widening of the circumference of a body orifice with a dilating instrument; also, the opening of the cervix in the process of labor, measured as 0 to 10 cm.

dilation and curettage (D&C) The widening of the cervix and scraping of the endometrial wall of the uterus.

diluent A fluid that makes a solution less concentrated; it is added to vials of powdered medications to create a solution of the drug for injection.

diplopia (dih-plo'-pe-uh) Double vision.

direct filing system A filing system in which materials can be located without consulting an intermediary source of reference.

discrepancy A lack of correspondence between what is stated and what is found; for instance, when what is stated on the packing slip is different from what is found in the box.

discretionary income Money in a bank account that is not assigned to pay for any office expenses.

disinfectant A liquid chemical that is capable of eliminating many or all pathogens but is not effective against bacterial spores; it cannot be used on the skin.

disinfected The state in which pathogenic organisms have been destroyed or rendered inactive (disinfection procedures do not have this effect on spores, tuberculosis bacilli, and certain viruses).

disparaging Slighting; having a negative or degrading tone.

dispense To prepare a drug for administration.

disruption An unexpected event that throws a plan into disorder; an interruption that prevents a system or process from continuing as usual or as expected.

dissect To cut or separate tissue with a cutting instrument or scissors.

disseminate (dih-se'-muh-na-te)   To disburse; to spread around.

diurnal rhythm (di-ur'-nl)   A pattern of activity or behavior that follows a day-night cycle.

diverticulosis (di-vuhr-tih-kyuh-lo'-sis)   The presence of pouchlike herniations through the muscular layer of the colon.

dosimeter   A badge for monitoring the radiation exposure of personnel.

due process   A fundamental constitutional guarantee that all legal proceedings will be fair; that one will be given notice of the proceedings and an opportunity to be heard before the government acts to take away life, liberty, or property; a constitutional guarantee that a law will not be unreasonable or arbitrary.

dumb terminal   A personal computer that doesn't contain a hard drive and allows the user only limited functions, including access to software, the network, and/or the Internet.

dyspepsia   An uncomfortable feeling of fullness, heartburn, bloating, and nausea.

dysphagia   Difficulty swallowing.

dysplasia   An alteration in cell growth, causing differences in size, shape, and appearance.

dyspnea (disp-ne'-uh)   Difficult or painful breathing.

dysuria   Painful or difficulty urination.

e-prescribing   The use of electronic software to communicate with pharmacies and send prescribing information. It takes the place of writing a prescription by hand and giving it to a patient; most new or refill prescriptions can be submitted electronically, cutting down on fraud and errors.

ecchymosis (eh-kih-moh'-sis)   A hemorrhagic skin discoloration, commonly called *bruising*.

ectopic (ek-top'-ik)   Originating outside the normal tissue.

edema (ih-de'-muh)   An abnormal accumulation of fluid in the interstitial spaces of tissues.

effacement   The thinning of the cervix during labor, measured in percentages from 0% to 100%.

elastin   An essential part of elastic connective tissue; when moist, it is flexible and elastic.

electrocardiogram (ihlek-tro-kar'-de-uh-gram)   A graphic record of electrical conduction through the heart.

electrodesiccation   The destruction of cells and tissue by means of short high-frequency electrical sparks.

electronic health record (EHR)   An electronic record of health-related information about a patient that conforms to nationally recognized interoperability standards and that can be created, managed, and consulted by authorized clinicians and staff members *from more than one healthcare organization.*

electronic medical record (EMR)   An electronic record of health-related information about an individual that can be created, gathered, managed, and consulted by authorized clinicians and staff members *within a single healthcare organization.* An EMR is an electronic version of a paper record.

emancipated minor   A person under the age of majority (usually 18) who has been legally separated from his or her parents by the courts. The person is responsible for his or her own care.

embezzlement   The misuse of a healthcare facility's funds for personal gain.

embolus   A mass of undissolved matter that blocks a blood vessel; frequently a blood clot that has traveled from some other part of the body.

emergency   An unexpected, life-threatening situation that requires immediate action.

emetic (eh-met'-ik)   A substance that causes vomiting.

empathy (em'-puh-the)   Sensitivity to the individual needs and reactions of patients.

emphysema (em-fih-ze'-muh)   The pathologic accumulation of air in the alveoli, which results in alveolar destruction and overall oxygen deprivation; the bronchioles become plugged with mucus and lose elasticity.

empower   To delegate more responsibilities to employees (a management theory).

encounter   Every meeting between a patient and a healthcare provider. The patient's history and chief complaint, in addition to the medical services provided, are documented in the patient's health record.

endemic (en-dem'-ik)   A term describing a disease or microorganism that is specific to a particular geographic area.

endocervical curettage   The scraping of cells from the wall of the uterus.

endorser   The person who signs his or her name on the back of a check for the purpose of transferring all rights in the check to another party.

endoscope (en'-duh-skohp)   An illuminated optic instrument for visualization of the inside of the body; it may be inserted through an incision in minimally invasive surgery.

enteric coated   A term describing an oral medication that is coated to protect the drug against the stomach juices; this design is used to ensure that the medicine is absorbed in the small intestine.

enunciation   The use of articulate, clear sounds when speaking.

enzymatic reaction   A specific chemical reaction controlled by an enzyme.

enzymes   Complex proteins produced by cells that act as catalysts in specific biochemical reactions.

epiphyseal plate (eh-pih-fiz'-e-uhl)   A thin layer of cartilage located at the ends of a long bone where new bone forms.

epiphysis (eh-pih'-fih-sis)   The end of a long bone; it contains the growth (epiphyseal) plates.

eponym   In medical terms, a name of a medical diagnosis or procedure derived from the name of the person who discovered it.

erythropoietin (ih-rith-ruh-poi'-eh-tuhn)   A substance released by the kidneys and liver that promotes red blood cell formation.

eschar   Devitalized skin that forms a scab or a dry crust over a burn area.

esophageal varices (ih-sah-fuh-je'-uhl var'-uh-sez)   Varicose veins of the esophagus that occur as a result of portal hypertension; these vessels can easily hemorrhage.

essential hypertension   Elevated blood pressure of unknown cause that develops for no apparent reason; sometimes called *primary hypertension.*

established patients   Patients who are returning to the office who have previously been seen by the provider.

Ethernet   A communication system for connecting several computers so information can be shared.

etiology The cause of a disorder; a claim may be classified according to the etiology.

eukaryote (yoo-kar'-e-oht) Single-celled or multicellular organism in which each cell contains a distinct membrane-bound nucleus.

evert To turn the eyelid inside out; this typically is done by the provider to inspect the area for foreign bodies.

exacerbation (ig-zas'-er-ba-shun) An increase in the seriousness of a disease, marked by greater intensity of the signs.

exclusions Limitations on an insurance contract for which benefits are not payable.

excoriation (ik-skawr-e-a'-shun) Inflammation and irritation of the skin; abrasions.

executor The individual assigned to make financial decisions for a deceased patient.

expediency (ik-spe'-de-en-se) A means of achieving a particular end, as in a situation requiring haste or caution.

expert witnesses Individuals who provide testimony to a court as experts in certain fields or subjects to verify facts presented by one or both sides in a lawsuit. They typically are compensated and used to refute or disprove the claims of one party.

Explanation of Benefits (EOB) A document sent by the insurance company to the provider and the patient explaining the allowed charge amount, the amount reimbursed for services, and the patient's financial responsibilities.

exposure time The duration of the patient's x-ray exposure, in seconds; the amount of x-rays produced depends on the length of exposure.

extern A student volunteering in the medical office for experience only; externs do not earn any wages for the work they perform.

exudates (ek'-syu-dats) Fluids with high concentrations of protein and cellular debris that have escaped from the blood vessels and have been deposited in tissues or on tissue surfaces.

familial Occurring in or affecting members of a family more than would be expected by chance.

fascia A sheet or band of fibrous tissue deep in the skin that covers muscles and body organs.

febrile (feb'-ril) Pertaining to an elevated body temperature.

fecalith (fe'-kuh-lith) A hard, impacted mass of feces in the colon.

Federal Reserve Bank The central bank of the United States. The Federal Reserve system consists of a seven-member Board of Governors with headquarters in Washington, D.C., and 12 Federal Reserve banks in major cities throughout the country.

fee-for-service A reimbursement model in which the health plan pays the provider's fee for every health insurance claim.

fibrillation Rapid, random, ineffective contractions of the heart.

filtrate The fluid that remains after a liquid is passed through a filter.

firewall A program or hardware that acts as a filter between the network and the Internet.

fissures Narrow slits or clefts in the abdominal wall.

fistula (fis'-chuh-luh) An abnormal, tubelike passage between internal organs or from an internal organ to the body's surface.

flatus Gas expelled through the anus.

flora Microorganisms that live on or within the body; they compete with disease-producing microorganisms and provide a natural immunity against certain infections.

fluoroscopy (floo-ros'-kuh-pe) Direct observation of an x-ray image in motion.

follicle-stimulating hormone (FSH) A hormone secreted by the anterior pituitary; it stimulates oogenesis and spermatogenesis.

follow-up appointment An appointment type used when a patient needs to see the provider after a condition should have been resolved or for monitoring of an ongoing condition, such as hypertension; also known as a *recheck appointment*.

fomites Contaminated, nonliving objects (e.g., examination room equipment) that can transmit infectious organisms.

fontanelle (fon-tan-el') A space covered by thick membranes between the sutures of an infant's skull; called the baby's "soft spots"; there are both anterior and posterior fontanelles.

formulary A list of drugs compiled by a health insurance company that identifies the drugs the insurance company will cover under benefits.

fornix A recess in the upper part of the vagina caused by protrusion of the cervix into the vaginal wall.

fovea centralis (fo'-ve-uh/sen-trah'-lis) A small pit in the center of the retina that is considered the center of clearest vision.

free radicals Compounds with at least one unpaired electron, which makes the compound unstable and highly reactive. Free radicals are believed to damage cell components, ultimately leading to cancer, heart disease, or other diseases.

fundus The curved, top portion of the uterus; the fundal height can be used as a measurement of fetal growth and estimated gestation.

gait The manner or style of walking.

gangrene The death of body tissue as a result of loss of nutritive supply, followed by bacterial invasion and putrefaction.

gantry A doughnut-shaped portion of a scanner that surrounds the patient and functions, at least partly, to gather imaging data.

gatekeeper In medical care, the primary care physician, who can approve or deny when the patient seeks additional care via a referral to a specialist or further medical tests.

generic A medication that is not protected by trademark.

genus A classification representing a family of microorganisms and all living beings. The genus is the first name assigned to a microorganism and it is italicized and capitalized.

germicides (jur'-mih-sides) Agents that destroy pathogenic organisms.

girth The measurement around something; when referring to mail, it is the measurement around the middle of the package that is being shipped.

gleaned Gathered bit by bit (e.g., information or material); picked over in search of relevant material.

global services For purposes of CPT coding, medical services and procedures performed for the patient before, during, and after a surgical procedure that is included with the assigned CPT code.

glomerulonephritis (glo-mer'-yoo-lo-neh-fri'-tis) Inflammation of the glomerulus of the kidney.

gluconeogenesis (glu-kuh-ne-uh-jeh'-nuh-sis) The formation of glucose in the liver from proteins and fats.

glycogen The sugar (starch) formed from glucose; it is stored mainly in the liver.

glycosuria An elevated urinary glucose level (which may be an indicator of diabetes mellitus).

goniometer (goh-ne-om′-ih-ter)   An instrument for measuring the degrees of motion in a joint.

gonioscopy (goh-ne-os′-kuh-pe)   A procedure in which a mirrored optical instrument is used to visualize the filtration angle of the anterior chamber of the eye; the procedure is used to diagnose glaucoma.

government-sponsored health insurance   Health insurance programs that are sponsored by the government and offer coverage for the elderly, disabled, military, and indigent.

gray (Gy)   The international unit of radiation dose.

growth hormone (GH)   A hormone that stimulates tissue growth and restricts tissue glucose dependence when nutrients are not available; also called *somatotropic hormone.*

guarantor   The individual who subscribes to the insurance plan and accepts financial responsibility for the patient.

guardian ad litem   An individual who is assigned by the court to be legally responsible for protecting the well-being and interests of a ward, typically a minor or a person who has been declared legally incompetent.

harmonious   Marked by accord in sentiment or action; having the parts agreeably related.

healthcare clearinghouses   Businesses that receive healthcare transactions from healthcare providers, translate the data from a given format into one acceptable to the intended payer, and forward the processed transaction to designated payers. They include billing services, community health information systems, and private network providers or "value-added" networks that facilitate electronic data interchanges.

hematemesis (hi-mat-uh-me′-sis)   Vomiting of bright red blood, indicating rapid upper gastrointestinal (GI) bleeding. Hematemesis is associated with esophageal varices or a peptic ulcer.

hematocrit   The percentage by volume of packed red blood cells in a given sample of blood after centrifugation.

hematopoiesis (he-ma-tuh-poi-e′-sis)   The formation and development of red blood cells in the bone marrow.

hematuria (he-ma-tuhr′-e-uh)   Blood in the urine (may indicate trauma or infection in the urinary tract).

hemoconcentration   The condition in which the concentration of blood cells is increased in proportion to the plasma.

hemoglobin (he′-muh-glo-bun)   A protein found in erythrocytes that transports molecular oxygen in the blood.

hemoglobinuria   Hemoglobin in the urine (from destruction of red blood cells).

hemolysis (he-mah′-luh-sis)   The destruction or dissolution of red blood cells, with subsequent release of hemoglobin.

hemolyzed   A term used to describe a blood sample in which the red blood cells have ruptured.

hepatomegaly (heh-puh-to-meh′-guh-le)   Abnormal enlargement of the liver.

hereditary (heh-re′-duh-ter-e)   Pertaining to a characteristic, condition, or disease transmitted from parent to offspring on the DNA chain.

hertz   The unit of measurement used in hearing examinations; a wave frequency equal to 1 cycle per second.

holistic (ho-lis′-tik)   A form of healing that considers the whole person (i.e., body, mind, spirit, and emotions) in individual treatment plans.

homeostasis   Internal adaptation and change in response to environmental factors; multiple functions that attempt to keep the body's functions in balance.

hospice (hos′-pis)   A concept of care in which health professionals and volunteers provide medical, psychological, and spiritual support to terminally ill patients and their loved ones.

HR file   The human resource file, which contains all documents related to an individual's employment.

human chorionic gonadotropin (HCG)   A hormone, secreted by the placenta, found in the urine of pregnant females.

hydrocephaly (hi-dro-seh′-fuh-le)   Enlargement of the cranium caused by abnormal accumulation of cerebrospinal fluid in the cerebral system.

hydrogenated (hi-drah′-juh-na-ted)   Combined with, treated with, or exposed to hydrogen.

hypercapnia (hi-per-kap′-ne-uh)   Excess levels of carbon dioxide in the blood.

hypercholesterolemia (hi-per-kuh-les-tuh-ruh-le′-me-uh)   Elevated blood levels of cholesterol.

hyperplasia   An increase in the number of normal cells.

hyperpnea (hy-per-ne′-uh)   An increase in the depth of breathing.

hypertension   High blood pressure.

hyperventilation   Abnormally prolonged and deep breathing, usually associated with acute anxiety or emotional tension.

hypotension   Blood pressure that is below normal (systolic pressure below 90 mm Hg and diastolic pressure below 50 mm Hg).

iatrogenic   A test result or condition caused by medication or treatment.

identity proofing   The process by which a credential service provider validates that a person is who he or she claims to be; the provider must complete this verification before being allowed to e-prescribe controlled substances.

idiopathic   Pertaining to a condition or a disease that has no known cause.

ileostomy   The surgical formation of an opening of the ileum onto the surface of the abdomen, through which fecal material is emptied.

image receptor (IR)   A device used to transform an x-ray beam into a visible image; it may include a cassette (with either film or a phosphorescent screen inside) or a special detector that is built into the table or Bucky.

immune globulin   A substance made from human plasma that contains antibodies to protect the body from disease.

immunosuppressant   A substance that suppresses or prevents an immune system response.

immunotherapy   Administration of repeated injections of diluted extracts of a substance that causes an allergy; also called *desensitization.*

impending   A term used in the diagnosis of a condition that can be imminently threatening. For example, a patient showing signs of prediabetes may in the near future develop diabetes; therefore, in this case, diabetes is an *impending* condition.

implied contract   A contract that lacks a written record or verbal agreement but is assumed to exist. For example, if a patient is being seen in a physician's office for the first time, it is assumed that the patient will provide a comprehensive and accurate health history and that the provider will diagnose and treat the patient in good faith to the best of his or her ability.

in vitro A term referring to conditions or tests performed outside of a living body.

incentives Things that incite or spur to action; rewards or reasons for performing a task.

incidental disclosure A secondary use or disclosure that cannot reasonably be prevented, is limited in nature, and occurs because of another use or disclosure that is permitted.

incompetent A term describing a person who is not able to manage his or her affairs because of mental deficiency (lack of I.Q., deterioration, illness or psychosis) or sometimes physical disability. The individual cannot comprehend the complexities of a situation and therefore cannot provide informed consent.

indicators An important point or group of statistical values that, when evaluated, indicates the quality of care provided in a healthcare facility.

indirect filing system A filing system in which an intermediary source of reference (e.g., a card file) must be consulted to locate specific files.

induration (in-doo-ra′-shuhn) An abnormally hard, inflamed area.

infarction An area of tissue that has died from lack of blood supply.

infection Invasion of body tissues by microorganisms, which then proliferate and damage tissues.

inflammation (in-fluh-ma′-shun) A tissue reaction to trauma or disease that includes redness, heat, swelling, and pain.

informed consent Voluntary agreement, usually written, for treatment after being informed of its purpose, methods, procedures, benefits, and risks. The patient must understand the details of the procedure and give his or her consent without duress or undue influence, and the patient must have the right to refuse treatment or voluntarily withdraw from treatment at any time.

intangible Something of value that cannot be touched physically.

integral (in′-ti-grul) Essential; being an indispensable part of a whole.

interaction A two-way communication; mutual or reciprocal action or influence.

intercellular A term referring to the area between cells.

intercom A two-way communication system with a microphone and loudspeaker at each station for localized use; often a feature of business telephones.

interferon (in-tuhr-fir′-on) A protein formed when a cell is exposed to a virus; the protein blocks viral action on the cell and protects against viral invasion

intermittent claudication Recurring cramping in the calves caused by poor circulation of blood to the muscles of the lower leg.

intermittent pulse A pulse in which beats occasionally are skipped.

interoperability The ability to work with other systems.

interpersonal skills The ability to communicate and interact with others; sometimes referred to as "soft skills."

interval Space of time between events.

intracellular A term referring to the area within the cell membrane.

intravenous urogram (IVU) Radiographic examination of the urinary tract using intravenous injection of an iodine contrast medium; also called an *intravenous pyelogram* (IVP).

inventory The stored medical and administrative supplies used in the medical office; also, the process of counting the supplies in stock.

invoice A billing statement that lists the amount owed for goods or services purchased..

ipsilateral (ips-uh-lah′-tehr-uhl) Pertaining to the same side of the body.

ischemia (is-ke′-me-uh) Decreased blood flow to a body part or organ, caused by constriction or blockage of the supplying artery.

ischemic (ih-ske′-mik) Pertaining to a decreased supply of oxygenated blood to a body part.

jargon The technical terminology or characteristic idioms of a particular group or special activity, as opposed to common, everyday terms.

jaundice Yellowing of the skin and mucous membranes caused by the deposition of bile pigment, which occurs as a result of excess bilirubin in the blood. Jaundice is not a disease, but rather a sign of a number of diseases, especially liver disorders.

job board A website that posts jobs submitted by employers and can be used by job seekers to identify open positions.

Kaposi's sarcoma A malignant tumor of endothelial cells that begins as red, brown, or purple lesions on the ankles or soles.

keloid A raised, firm scar formation caused by overgrowth of collagen at the site of a skin injury.

keratin A very hard, tough protein found in the hair, nails, and epidermal tissue.

keratinocytes The skin cells that synthesize keratin.

ketonuria Ketones in the urine (possible dehydration or diabetic ketoacidosis).

kilovoltage (kVp) The electrical control setting that determines the penetrating power of the x-ray beam; the higher the voltage, the shorter the x-ray wavelengths and the greater the energy of the x-ray beam.

kyphotic (ki-fot′-ik) Relating to the normal convex curvature of the thoracic spine.

lacrimation (lah-krihm-a′-shun) The secretion or discharge of tears.

laryngoscopy (lar-uhn-gahs′-kuh-pe) Visual examination of the voice box area through an endoscope equipped with a light and mirrors for illumination.

lateral position A radiographic position labeled according to which of the patient's sides is facing the image receptor.

law A binding custom or practice of a community; a rule of conduct or action prescribed or formally recognized as binding or enforceable by a controlling authority.

leads Electrical connections attached to the body to record the electrical activity of the heart.

learning style The way an individual perceives and processes information to learn new material.

leukocytosis An abnormal increase in the number of circulating white blood cells (WBCs); it often occurs with bacterial infections, but not with viral infections.

leukoderma Lack of skin pigmentation, especially in patches.

liable (li′-uh-buhl) Obligated according to law or equity; responsible for an act or a circumstance.

liaison An individual assigned to communicate between multiple parties when settling financial responsibilities of a patient's estate after their death.

libel A written remark that injures another's reputation or character.

ligaments (lig'-uh-ments) Tough connective tissue bands that hold joints together by attaching to the bones on either side of the joint.

limited radiography A simplified role in radiography, usually in an outpatient setting; also called *practical radiography*. The limited radiographer may be referred to as a *limited operator* or *basic machine operator*.

litigious (lih-tih'-jus) Prone to engage in lawsuits.

loading dose A large dose administered as the first dose of a medication; it usually is used in antibiotic therapy to quickly achieve therapeutic blood levels of the drug.

lordotic (lor-dah'-tik) Relating to the normal concave curvature of the cervical and lumbar spines.

lower gastrointestinal (LGI) series A fluoroscopic examination of the colon; barium sulfate usually is used as a contrast medium and is administered rectally; also called a *barium enema*.

lumbar (lum'-bahr) Relating to the lower back region that contains the five lumbar vertebrae.

lumen An open space, such as within a blood vessel or the intestine, or within a needle or an examining instrument.

luteinizing hormone (LH) (lu-te-uh-niz'-ing) A hormone produced by the anterior pituitary gland that promotes ovulation.

luxation (luhk-sa'-shun) Dislocation of a bone from its normal anatomic location.

lymphedema (limf-uh-de'-muh) Swelling caused by the accumulation of lymph fluid in soft tissues.

lymphadenopathy (lim-fah-deh-nop'-uh-the) Abnormal enlargement of a lymph gland.

lyse To break open cells (e.g., white or red blood cells).

macromolecules The molecules needed for metabolism: carbohydrates, lipids, proteins, and nucleic acids.

macular degeneration A progressive deterioration of the macula of the eye that causes loss of central vision.

magnetic resonance imaging (MRI) An imaging modality that uses a magnetic field and radiofrequency pulses to create computer images of both bones and soft tissues in multiple planes.

magnetism The attraction of materials to magnets; strong magnets can damage magnetic storage devices, such as hard drives.

malaise (muh-layz') An indefinite feeling of debility or lack of health, often indicating or accompanying the onset of an illness.

malignant A term describing tumor or tissue growth that is cancerous, anaplastic, invasive, and can metastasize.

malpractice A type of negligence in which a licensed professional fails to provide the standard of care, causing harm to a person.

manifestation An indication of the existence, reality, or presence of something, especially an illness; a secondary process.

manipulation Movement or exercise of a body part by means of an externally applied force.

Marfan syndrome An inherited condition characterized by elongation of the bones, joint hypermobility, abnormalities of the eyes, and the development of an aortic aneurysm.

mastication (mas-tih-ka'-shun) Chewing.

matrix Something in which a thing originates, develops, takes shape, or is contained; a base on which to build.

Meaningful Use requirements Requirements established by the Centers for Medicare and Medicaid Services (CMS) as part of the Electronic Health Records (EHRs) Incentives Program. The program provides financial incentives for healthcare organizations that "meaningfully used" their certified EHR technology. The requirements include implementing security measures to ensure the privacy of patients' EHRs.

media A type of communication (e.g., social media sites); with computers, the term refers to data storage devices.

mediastinum (me-de-ast'-uhn-um) The space in the center of the chest under the sternum.

medullary cavity (meh-duhl'-uh-re) The inner portion of the diaphysis; it contains the bone marrow.

Ménière's disease (meyn-yairz') A chronic disease of the inner ear causing recurrent episodes of vertigo, progressive sensorineural hearing loss, and tinnitus.

meniscus (meh-nis'-kus) The curved surface of liquids in a container.

mentor A steady employee whom a new staff member can approach with questions and concerns.

metabolic alkalosis A condition characterized by significant loss of acid in the body or an increased amount of bicarbonate; severe metabolic alkalosis can lead to coma and death.

metabolite The byproduct of the metabolism of a substance, such as a drug.

metastatic (meh-tas-tah'-tik) Pertaining to the process by which cancerous cells spread from the site of origin to a distant site via lymph and blood circulation.

microcephaly (mi-kroh-seh'-fal-e) Small size of the head in relation to the rest of the body.

microfilm A film with a photographic record of printed or other graphic matter on a reduced scale.

microorganisms Organisms of microscopic or submicroscopic size.

milliamperage (mA) The electrical control setting that determines the amount or concentration of the x-rays by controlling how rapidly the radiation is produced; the higher the mA setting, the more x-rays are produced per second.

miotic (mi-ah'-tik) Any substance or medication that causes constriction of the pupil.

mnemonic A learning device (e.g., an image, a rhyme, or a figure of speech) that a person uses to help him or her remember information.

mock Simulated; intended for imitation or practice.

modem A type of peripheral computer hardware that connects to the router to provide Internet access to the network or computer.

molecule A group of like or different atoms held together by chemical forces.

mononuclear white blood cells Leukocytes with an unsegmented nucleus; monocytes and lymphocytes in particular.

monotone A succession of syllables, words, or sentences spoken in an unvaried key or pitch.

mons pubis The fat pad that covers the symphysis pubis.

multiparous Pertaining to women who have had two or more pregnancies.

multiple-line telephone system A business telephone system that allows for more than one telephone line.

murmur In medical care, an abnormal sound heard during auscultation of the heart that may or may not have a pathologic origin; it is associated with valve disease or a congenital heart defect.

mydriatic (mid-re-at′-ik)   A topical ophthalmic medication that dilates the pupil; it is used in diagnostic procedures of the eye and as treatment for glaucoma.

myelomeningocele   A herniation of a portion of the spinal cord and its meninges that protrudes through a congenital opening in the vertebral column.

myelin sheath   A segmented, fatty tissue that wraps around the axon of the nerve cell and acts as an electrical insulator to speed the conduction of nerve impulses.

myelography (mi-uh-log′-ruh-fe)   Fluoroscopic examination of the spinal canal with spinal injection of an iodine contrast medium.

myocardial (mi-o-kar′-de-uhl)   Pertaining to the heart muscle.

myocardium (mi-o-kar′-de-um)   The muscular lining of the heart.

myoglobinuria   The abnormal presence of a hemoglobin-like chemical of muscle tissue in the urine; it is the result of muscle deterioration.

necrosis (neh-kro′-sis)   The death of cells or tissues.

negligence (neh′-glih-jents)   Failure to show the conduct expected of a reasonably prudent person acting under similar circumstances; it falls below the standards of behavior established by law for the protection of others against unreasonable risk of harm.

neoplasm   A growth of uncontrolled, abnormal tissue; a tumor. The ICD-10-CM assigns diagnostic codes for neoplasms based on six criteria, which can be found in a table that follows the Alphabetic Index.

networking   Exchange of information or services among individuals, groups, or institutions; also, meeting and getting to know individuals in the same or similar career fields and sharing information about available opportunities.

neural tube defects   Congenital malformations of the skull and spinal column caused by failure of the neural tube to close during embryonic development; the neural tube is the origin of the brain, spinal cord, and other central nervous system tissue.

no-show   A patient who fails to keep an appointment without giving advance notice.

nocturia   Frequent urination at night.

nodules (nah′-juhls)   Small lumps, lesions, or swellings that are felt when the skin is palpated.

nonallowed amount   The difference (balance) between the provider's charges and the allowed amount. If the provider is a participating provider, he or she cannot bill the patient for the nonallowed amount. If the provider is not participating in the insurance plan contract, he or she can bill the patient for the nonallowed amount.

nonorganic (nahn-awr-gan′-ik)   A term for a disorder that does not have a cause that can be found in the body.

nonstress tests (NSTs)   Fetal monitoring used in combination with maternal reports of fetal movement to evaluate the fetal heart rate response.

normal flora   Microorganisms normally present on and in our bodies; they perform vital functions and protect the body against infection.

nosocomial infections (nos-uh-ko′-me-uhl)   Infections that are acquired in a healthcare setting.

notations   Instructions or guides for assigning classifications, defining category content, or using subdivision codes. Notations are found in both the Alphabetic Index and the Tabular List.

Notice of Privacy Practices (NPP)   A written document describing the healthcare facilities' privacy practices. The patient must be provided with the NPP and sign an acknowledgment of receipt.

NPO   Nothing by mouth, from the Latin *nil per os*.

nuclear medicine   An imaging modality that uses radioactive materials injected or ingested into the body to provide information about the function of organs and tissues.

numeric filing   The filing of records, correspondence, or cards by number.

obesity   An excessive accumulation of body fat; defined as a body mass index (BMI) of 30 or higher.

objective information   Data obtained through physical examination, laboratory and diagnostic testing, and by measurable information.

oblique position   Radiographic position in which the body or part is rotated at an angle that is neither frontal nor lateral.

obliteration (uh-blih-tuh-ra′-shun)   The act of making undecipherable or imperceptible by obscuring or wearing away.

obturator   A metal rod with a smooth, rounded tip that is placed in hollow instruments to reduce injury to body tissues during insertion of the instrument.

occlude   To close off or block (e.g., a blood vessel).

occlusion   Complete obstruction of an opening.

online provider insurance Web portal   An online service provided by various insurance companies for providers to look up patient insurance benefits, eligibility, claims status, and explanation of benefits.

oophorectomy   Surgical removal of the ovaries.

opaque   Not translucent or transparent; murky.

operating system   Software that acts as the computer's administrator by managing, integrating, and controlling application software and hardware.

opportunistic infections   Infections caused by a normally nonpathogenic organism in a host whose resistance has been decreased.

opportunistic organisms   Microorganisms normally present in low numbers that are capable of causing disease when the conditions are favorable.

optic disc   The region at the back of the eye where the optic nerve meets the retina; it is considered the blind spot of the eye because it contains only nerve fibers and no rods or cones and thus is insensitive to light.

optic nerve   Cranial nerve II, which carries impulses for the sense of sight.

ordinance (or′-di-nens)   An authoritative decree or direction; a law set forth by a governmental authority, specifically municipal regulation.

organelles (or-guh-nels′)   Structures within a cell that perform a specific function.

orthopnea (or-thop′-ne-uh)   A condition in which an individual must sit or stand to breathe comfortably.

orthostatic (postural) hypotension   A temporary fall in blood pressure when a person rapidly changes from a recumbent position to a standing position.

osteoporosis (ah-ste-o-puh-ro′-sis)   Loss of bone density; lack of calcium intake is a major factor in its development.

otitis externa   Inflammation or infection of the external auditory canal; commonly called swimmer's ear.

otosclerosis (o-tuh-skleh-ro'-sis) The formation of spongy bone in the labyrinth of the ear, which often causes the auditory ossicles to become fixed and unable to vibrate when sound enters the ears.

ototoxic (o-tuh-tahk'-sik) A medicine or substance capable of damaging cranial nerve VIII or the organs of hearing and balance.

outguide A sturdy cardboard or plastic file-sized card used to replace a folder temporarily removed from the filing space.

output device Computer hardware that displays the processed data from the computer (e.g., monitors and printers).

over-the-counter (OTC) drugs Medications sold without a prescription.

packing slip A document that accompanies purchased merchandise and shows what is in the box or package.

palliative A substance that relieves or alleviates the symptoms of a disease without curing the disease; also, therapy that relieves or reduces symptoms but does not result in a cure.

palpation The use of touch during the physical examination to assess the size, consistency, and location of certain body parts.

palpitations Pounding or racing of the heart; it may or may not indicate a serious heart disorder.

papilledema Swelling of the optic disc as a result of increased intracranial pressure.

parameters Any set of physical properties, the values of which determine characteristics or behavior.

parenteral (puh-ren'-tuh-ruhl) The injection or introduction of substances into the body by any route other than the digestive tract (e.g., subcutaneous, intravenous, or intramuscular administration).

paresthesia (par-uhs-the'-ze-uh) An abnormal sensation of burning, prickling, or stinging.

paroxysmal (par-ek-siz'-muhl) Pertaining to a sudden recurrence of symptoms; a sudden spasm or convulsion of any kind.

participating provider A physician or other healthcare provider who enters into a contract with a specific insurance company or program and by doing so agrees to abide by certain rules and regulations set forth by that particular third-party payer.

parturition (par-too-rih'-shun) The act or process of giving birth to a child.

patency Open condition of a body cavity or canal.

pathogen An agent that causes disease, especially a living microorganism such as a bacterium or fungus.

pathogenic (path-o-jen'-ik) Pertaining to a disease-causing microorganism.

patient portal A secure online website that gives patients 24-hour access to personal health information using a username and password.

pegboard system A manual bookkeeping system that uses a day sheet to record all financial transactions for the date of service and maintains patient account balances by using physical cards.

perceiving (pur-seev'-ing) How an individual looks at information and sees it as real.

perception A quick, acute, and intuitive cognition; a capacity for comprehension.

perinatal (per-uh-nayt'-l) The period between the 28th week of pregnancy and the 28th day after birth.

periosteum (per-e-os'-te-um) The thin, highly innervated, membranous covering of a bone.

peripheral (puh-rif'-er-uhl) A term that refers to an area outside of or away from an organ or structure.

peripheral neuropathy A problem with the function of the nerves outside the spinal cord; symptoms include weakness, burning pain, and loss of reflexes; a frequent complication of diabetes mellitus.

peristalsis (per-uh-stahl'-sis) The rhythmic, involuntary serial contraction of the smooth muscles lining the gastrointestinal tract.

perjured testimony The voluntary violation of an oath or vow, either by swearing to what is untrue or by omission to do what has been promised under oath; false testimony.

permeable (pur'-me-uh-buhl) Allowing a substance to pass or soak through.

personal health record (PHR) An electronic record of health-related information about an individual that conforms to nationally recognized interoperability standards and that can be drawn from multiple sources but that is managed, shared, and controlled by the individual.

petechiae (peh-te'-ke-uh) Small, purplish hemorrhagic spots on the skin.

phenylalanine (fe-nehl-ah'-luh-neen) An essential amino acid found in milk, eggs, and other foods. Children unable to metabolize this amino acid eliminate it in the urine.

phlebotomy The practice of drawing blood from a vein.

phonetic (fuh-neh'-tik) Constituting an alteration of ordinary spelling that better represents the spoken language, uses only characters of the regular alphabet, and is used in a context of conventional spelling.

photophobia An abnormal sensitivity to light.

pitch The depth of a tone or sound; a distinctive quality of sound.

plaintiff The person or group bringing a case or legal action to court.

plaque In medical care, an abnormal accumulation of a fatty substance.

plasma The liquid portion of a centrifuged whole blood specimen that has not clotted and still contains active clotting agents.

pleurisy Inflammation of the parietal pleura of the lungs; it causes dyspnea and stabbing chest pain, which result in restriction of breathing because of the pain.

point of care Something designed to be used at or near where the patient is seen; point-of-care tools and apps are resources for the provider to use when working directly with the patient.

polycythemia vera (pah-le-si-the'-me-uh/veh'-rah) A condition marked by an abnormally large number of red blood cells (RBCs) in the circulatory system.

polydipsia Excessive thirst.

polymorphonuclear (PMN) white blood cells Leukocytes with a segmented nucleus; also known as segmented neutrophils, which appear in the urine during a bacterial infection.

polyphagia (pah-le-faj'-e-uh) Increased appetite.

polyps (pah'-lips) Outgrowths of tissue found in the mucosal lining of the colon. Polyps are considered precancerous.

polyuria (pah-le-yur'-e-uh) Excretion of abnormally large amounts of urine in 24 hours.

portal circulation The pathway of blood flow through the portal vein from the GI system to the liver.

portal hypertension   Increased venous pressure in the portal circulation caused by cirrhosis or compression of the hepatic vascular system.

portrait orientation   The most common layout for a printed page; the height of the paper is greater than its width.

posterior   The back portion of the body or body part.

posteroanterior (PA) projection   A radiographic view in which the central ray enters the back and exits the front of the patient's body; the patient is prone or facing the image receptor.

postherpetic neuralgia   Pain that lasts longer than a month after a shingles infection and is caused by damage to the nerve; the pain may last for months or years.

power of attorney   A legal statement in which a person authorizes another person to act as his or her attorney or agent. The authority may be limited to the handling of specific procedures. The person authorized to act as the agent is known as the *attorney in fact.*

practice management software   A type of software that allows the user to enter demographic information, schedule appointments, maintain lists of insurance payers, perform billing tasks, and generate reports.

preauthorization   A process required by some insurance carriers in which the provider obtains permission to perform certain procedures or services or refers a patient to a specialist.

precedent (preh′-suh-dent)   A person or thing that serves as a model; something done or said that may serve as an example or rule to authorize or justify a subsequent act of the same kind.

precertification   A process required by some insurance carriers in which the provider must prove medical necessity before performing a procedure.

prerequisite (pre-reh′-kwih-zit)   Something that is necessary to an end or to carry out a function.

present illness   The chief complaint, written in chronologic sequence, with dates of onset.

preservatives   Substances added to a specimen to prevent deterioration of cells or chemicals.

pressboard   A strong, highly glazed composition board resembling vulcanized fiber; heavy card stock.

principal   A capital sum of money due as a debt or used as a fund for which interest is either charged or paid.

privacy filters   Devices attached to the monitor that allow visualization of the screen contents only if the user is directly in front of the screen; also called *monitor filters* or *privacy screens.*

privately sponsored health insurance   Health insurance companies that operate for-profit and use managed care plans to reduce the costs of healthcare.

processing (pro′-ses-ing)   How an individual internalizes new information and makes it his or her own.

procurement (pro-kuhr′-ment)   The act of getting possession of, obtaining, or acquiring; in medicine, this term relates to obtaining organs for transplant.

proficiency (pruh-fi′-shun-se)   Competency as a result of training or practice.

profile testing   A series of laboratory tests associated with a particular organ or disease; also referred to as a "panel" of tests.

progress notes   Notes used in the medical record to track the patient's progress and condition.

prokaryote (pro-kar′-e-oht)   A unicellular organism that lacks a membrane-bound nucleus.

prolactin (PRL)   A hormone secreted by the anterior pituitary gland that stimulates the development of the mammary gland; it also stimulates the production of breast milk.

proofread   To read and mark corrections.

proprioception   The sensation of awareness of body movements and posture; nerve impulses that provide the central nervous system with information about the position of body parts.

prosthesis (prahs-the′-sis)   An artificial replacement for a body part.

proteinuria   Protein in the urine (may indicate kidney destruction, especially if casts are present).

provider   An individual or company that provides medical care and services to a patient or the public.

provider's fee schedule   Fees established by the provider for services rendered.

provisional diagnosis   A temporary diagnosis made before all test results have been received.

prudent   Marked by wisdom or judiciousness; shrewd in the management of practical affairs.

psoriasis (suh-ri′-uh-sis)   A usually chronic, recurrent skin disease marked by bright red patches covered with silvery scales.

psychosocial   Pertaining to a combination of psychological and social factors.

psyllium (sih′-le-um)   A grain found in some cereal products, in certain dietary supplements, and in certain bulk fiber laxatives; a water-soluble fiber.

public domain   A classification of information that indicates the information is open for public review; information or technology that is not protected by a patent or copyright and is available to the public for use without charge.

pulmonary consolidation   In pneumonia, the process by which the lungs become solidified as they fill with exudates.

pulse deficit   A condition in which the radial pulse is less than the apical pulse; it may indicate a peripheral vascular abnormality.

pulse pressure   The difference between the systolic and diastolic blood pressures (30 to 50 mm Hg is considered normal).

purchase order number   Unique number assigned by the ordering facility that allows the facility to track or reference the order. Many vendors will add this number to the order documents (e.g., packing slip and statement).

pure culture   A bacterial or fungal culture that contains a single organism.

purging   The process of moving active files to inactive status.

pyemia (pi-em′-e-uh)   The presence of pus-forming organisms in the blood.

pyloric sphincter   A muscular ring at the distal end of the stomach that separates the stomach from the duodenum of the small intestine.

pyrexia (pi-rek′-se-uh)   A febrile condition or fever.

qualified Medicare beneficiaries (QMB)   Low-income Medicare patients who qualify for Medicaid for their secondary insurance.

qualitative   A laboratory test result expressed as positive or negative.

quality assurance   The process of monitoring all the processes involved before, during, and after a laboratory test is performed so as to ensure reliable patient test results.

quality control An aggregate of activities designed to ensure adequate quality, especially in manufactured products or in the service industries; also, manufactured samples with known values used to determine whether a test method is reliable (i.e., consistently produces accurate and precise results).

quantitative A laboratory test result expressed in numeric units of measure.

quantity to reorder The amount of supplies that need to be ordered.

radiograph An x-ray image taken by a radiographer in the process of radiography.

radiographer One who takes x-rays.

radiography The process of creating an x-ray image to examine internal structures of the body.

radiographic position The placement of a body part as seen by the image receptor.

radiographic projection The path of the central ray from the radiographic tube, through the patient, and to the image receptor. The view as seen by the x-ray tube.

radiologist A physician who specializes in medical imaging or therapeutic applications of radiation.

radiopaque A substance that can easily be visualized on an x-ray film.

rales Abnormal or crackling breath sounds during inspiration.

ramifications (ram-ih-fih-ka′-shuns) Consequences produced by a cause or following from a set of conditions.

range of motion (ROM) The extent of movement possible in a joint; the degree of motion depends on the type of joint and whether a disease process is present; ROM exercises are applied actively (independently) or passively (with assistance) to prevent or treat joint problems.

rapport (rah-por′) A relationship of harmony and accord between the patient and the healthcare professional.

reagent (re-a′-gent) A chemical substance used in a test that reacts with the specimen to produce a measurable result.

reagent strips Strips used to test the specific gravity, pH, and chemical analytes in urine.

reasonable cause Circumstances that would make it unreasonable for the covered entity, despite the exercise of ordinary business care and prudence, to comply with the administrative simplification provision (part of Health Information Technology for Economic and Clinical Health Act [HITECH]) that was violated.

reasonable diligence The business care and prudence expected from a person seeking to satisfy a legal requirement under similar circumstances.

recessive Refers to a gene that only produces a particular condition if both the mother and the father carry that particular gene; neither of the parents have the condition.

recheck appointment An appointment type used when a patient needs to see the provider after a condition should have been resolved or to monitor an ongoing condition, such as hypertension. Also known as a *follow-up appointment.*

recourse Turning to something or someone for help or protection.

rectify (rek′-tih-fi) To correct by removing errors.

reduction Return to correct anatomic position, as in reduction of a fracture.

reference range The numeric range of test values for which the general population consistently shows similar results 95% of the time.

referral laboratory A private or hospital-based laboratory that performs a wide variety of tests, many of them specialized; providers often send specimens collected in the office to referral laboratories for testing.

reflection (re-flek′-shun) The process of thinking about new information so as to create new ways of learning. Also, a therapeutic communication technique in which a person responds with a feeling term that indicates how the individual feels about a problem. For example, "You sound angry about being scheduled for this diagnostic test."

registered dietitian (RD) An individual with a minimum of a bachelor's degree in food and nutrition who is concerned with the maintenance and promotion of health and the treatment of diseases through diet; to become an RD, the individual must pass a national examination.

reimbursement The process by which the medical office submits a claim to the insurance company, which then pays the provider for services rendered. All insurance claims must submit diagnoses and procedures as codes, not as descriptions.

relapse The recurrence of the symptoms of a disease after apparent recovery.

release of information A form completed by the patient that authorizes the medical office to release medical records to the insurance company for health insurance reimbursement.

relevant Having significant and demonstrable bearing on the matter at hand.

remission The partial or complete disappearance of the clinical and subjective characteristics of a chronic or malignant disease.

renal threshold The level above which substances cannot be reabsorbed into the blood from the renal tubules and therefore are excreted in the urine (e.g., when glucose reaches its renal threshold, the excess glucose appears in the urine).

renin An enzyme produced and stored in the glomerulus; it is released by a homeostatic response to raise the blood pressure when needed.

reparations (reh-puh-ra′-shuns) Acts of atonement for a wrong or injury.

requisites (reh′-kwih-zitz) Entities considered essential or necessary.

restock Process of replacing the supplies that were used.

retention A term referring to actions taken by management to keep good employees.

retention schedule A method or plan for retaining or keeping health records and for their movement from active to inactive to closed filing.

reverse chronologic order Arranged in order so that the most recent item is on top and older items are filed further back.

rhinitis (rin-i′-tis) Inflammation of the mucous membranes of the nose.

rhinorrhea (ri-no-re′-uh) The discharge of nasal drainage.

rhonchi (ron′-ki) Abnormal sounds heard on auscultation of an airway obstructed by thick secretions; a continuous rumbling sound that is more pronounced on expiration.

rods   Structures in the retina of the eye that form the light-sensitive elements.

Safety Data Sheets (SDSs)   Documents that accompany hazardous chemicals and substances and outline the dangers, composition, safe handling, and disposal of these items. Safety Data Sheets must be formatted to conform to the Globally Harmonized System (GHS), which mandates that SDSs have 16 standardized sections arranged in a strict order.

sanitized   The state of having cleaned equipment and instruments with detergent and water, removing debris, and reducing the number of microorganisms.

sarcoma   A malignant tumor in fibrous, fatty, muscular, synovial, vascular, or neural tissue.

satiety   The state of being satisfied or of feeling full after eating.

sclera   The white part of the eye that forms the orbit.

scleroderma (skleh-rah-der′-muh)   An autoimmune disorder that affects the blood vessels and connective tissue, causing fibrous degeneration of the major organs.

sclerotherapy (skleh-rah-ther′-ah-pe)   The treatment of hemorrhoids, varicose veins, or esophageal varices by means of injection of sclerosing solutions.

scoliosis   An abnormal lateral curvature of the spine.

scored   Referring to a tablet manufactured with an indentation for division through the center.

screening   In medical care, the process of determining the severity of illness that patients experience and prioritizing appointments based on that severity.

seborrhea (seb-uh-re′-uh)   An excessive discharge of sebum from the sebaceous glands, forming greasy scales or cheesy plugs on the body.

secondary hypertension   Elevated blood pressure resulting from another condition, typically kidney disease.

secondary storage devices   Media (e.g., jump drive, hard drive) capable of permanently storing data until it is replaced or deleted by the user.

security risk analysis   Identification of potential threats of computer network breaches, for which action plans are devised.

sediment   Insoluble material that settles to the bottom of a urine specimen and to the bottom of centrifuged urine.

sequentially (sih-kwen′-shuh-le)   Of, relating to, or arranged in a sequence.

serous (seer′-uhs)   A thin, watery, serumlike drainage.

serum   The liquid portion that remains after the blood clot has been removed from a clotted specimen

sievert (Sv) (se′-vuhrt)   The international unit of radiation dose equivalent.

signs   Objective findings determined by a clinician, such as a fever, hypertension, or rash.

sinoatrial (SA) node   The pacemaker of the heart, located in the right atrium.

sinus arrhythmia   An irregular heartbeat that originates in the sinoatrial node (pacemaker).

site map   A list of all Web page links on a website.

skill set   A person's abilities or skills.

slander   An oral defamation or insult; a harmful, false statement made about another person.

small claims court   A last resort option to collect payment from an outstanding patient account in which the healthcare practice can sue the patient for the balance.

social media   Internet-sponsored two-way communication between individuals, individuals and businesses, or businesses to businesses.

sociologic   Oriented or directed toward social needs and problems.

software   A set of electronic instructions to operate and perform different computer tasks.

sonography   A noninvasive procedure used extensively for fetal imaging (often referred to as diagnostic ultrasound); uses high-frequency sound waves to produce echoes in the body, which are used to create images.

source-to-image distance (SID)   The distance between the x-ray tube and the film or other image receptor; the greater the distance, the more widely the x-ray beam is spread and the lower the intensity of the beam.

speakerphone   A telephone with a loudspeaker and a microphone; it can be used without having to pick up and hold the handset.

species   A category of microorganisms below genus in rank; a genetically distinct group. It is the second name given to the microorganism and it is written in all lower case italic letters.

specific gravity   The density of urine compared with an equal volume of water.

specimen   A sample of body fluid, waste product, or tissue collected for analysis.

speed dialing   A telephone function in which a selected stored number can be dialed by pressing only one key.

spermicide (spuhr′-muh-side)   A chemical substance that kills sperm cells.

spirometer   An instrument that measures the volume of air inhaled and exhaled.

spore   A thick-walled, dormant form of bacteria that is very resistant to disinfection measures.

STAT   The medical abbreviation for the Latin term *statum,* meaning immediately; at this moment.

statins   A class of drugs that lowers the level of cholesterol in the blood by reducing the production of cholesterol by the liver; statins block the enzyme in the liver that is responsible for making cholesterol.

stereotactic   Pertaining to an x-ray procedure used to guide the insertion of a needle into a specific area of the breast.

stereotype   Something conforming to a fixed or general pattern; a standardized mental picture that is held in common by many and represents an oversimplified opinion, prejudiced attitude, or uncritical judgment.

sterile (ster′-il)   Free of all microorganisms, pathogenic and nonpathogenic.

sterilization   Complete destruction of all forms of microbial life.

sterilized   The state in which all microorganisms have been removed.

stertorous (stur′-tuh-rus)   A term that describes a strenuous respiratory effort marked by a snoring sound.

stressor   An event, activity, condition, or other stimulus that causes stress.

striated   A muscle that contains fibers divided by bands of cross stripes or striations because of overlapping myofilaments.

stridor (strahy′-dor)   A shrill, harsh respiratory sound heard during inhalation when a laryngeal obstruction is present.

stylus   A metal probe that is inserted into or passed through a catheter, needle, or tube used for clearing purposes or to facilitate passage into a body orifice. Also, a pen-shaped device with a variety of tips that is used on touch screens to write, draw, or input commands.

subjective information   Data or information elicited from the patient, including the patient's feelings, perceptions, and concerns; obtained through interview or questions.

subluxations (suh-bluk-sa′-shuns)   Slight misalignments of the vertebrae or a partial dislocation.

subordinate   Submissive to or controlled by authority; placed in or occupying a lower class, rank, or position.

subpoena duces tecum   A subpoena for the production of records or documents that pertain to a case as evidence.

supernatant   The liquid above the sediment in a centrifuged urine specimen.

suppurative (sup′-yuh-ra-tiv)   Characterized by the formation and/ or discharge of pus.

symptoms   Subjective complaints reported by the patient, such as pain or visual disturbances.

syncope (sing′-kuh-pe)   Fainting; a brief lapse in consciousness.

synovial fluid   A clear fluid found in joint cavities that facilitates smooth movements and nourishes joint structures.

systole   The period of contraction of the heart.

tachycardia (tak-ih-kahr′-de-uh)   A rapid but regular heart rate; one that exceeds 100 beats per minute.

tachypnea (tak-ip-ne′-uh)   A condition marked by rapid, shallow respirations.

tactful   The quality of having a keen sense of what to do or say to maintain good relations with others or to prevent offense.

telemedicine   Healthcare delivered through video conferencing technologies to deliver quality care at a distance.

tendons   Tough bands of connective tissue that connect muscle to bone.

teratogen (teh-rah′-tuh-jen)   Any substance that interferes with normal prenatal development, resulting in a developmental abnormality.

termination letter   A document sent to a patient explaining that the provider is ending the physician-patient relationship and the patient needs to find another provider.

therapeutic range   The blood concentration of a drug that produces the desired effect without toxicity.

third-party administrator (TPA)   The intermediary and administrator who coordinates patients and providers, as well as processes claims, for self-funded plans.

thixotropic gel   A material that appears to be a solid until subjected to a disturbance, such as centrifugation, at which point it becomes a liquid gel that separates blood cells from their serum or plasma.

thready   A term describing a pulse that is scarcely perceptible.

thrombolytics   Agents that dissolve blood clots.

thrombus   A blood clot.

thyroid-stimulating hormone (TSH)   A hormone secreted by the anterior pituitary gland that stimulates the secretion of hormones produced by the thyroid gland.

tickler file   A chronologic file used as a reminder that something must be dealt with on a certain date.

tinea (tin′-e-uh)   Any fungal skin disease that results in scaling, itching, and inflammation.

tinnitus   A noise sensation of ringing heard in one or both ears.

tissue culture   The technique or process of keeping tissue alive and growing in a culture medium.

tonometer (toh-nom′-ih-ter)   An instrument used to measure intraocular pressure.

tracers   Special radioactive materials that are swallowed or injected intravenously, to track the activity of cells and determine the location of fractures.

tracheostomy (tra-ke-os′-tuh-me)   A surgical opening made through the neck into the trachea to allow breathing.

transcription   A written copy of something made either in longhand or by machine.

trans fats   Substances that form from hydrogenation of an unsaturated fatty acid; they make a dietary fat more saturated and solid at room temperature.

transection   Cross section; a division made by cutting across.

transient ischemic attack (TIA)   Temporary neurologic symptoms caused by gradual or partial occlusion of a cerebral blood vessel.

transillumination   Inspection of a cavity or organ by passing light through its walls.

transport medium   A medium used to keep an organism alive during transport to the laboratory.

transvaginal ultrasound   A procedure for examining the vagina, uterus, fallopian tubes, and bladder. An ultrasound transducer (probe) is inserted into the vagina to bounce high-energy sound waves (ultrasound) off internal tissues or organs, resulting in echoes that form a picture (sonogram). The practitioner can identify tumors by looking at the sonogram.

trauma   A physical injury or wound caused by external force or violence.

triage   The process of sorting patients to determine medical need and the priority of care.

triglyceride (tri-glih′-suh-ride)   A fatty acid and glycerol compound that combines with a protein molecule to form high-density or low-density lipoprotein.

trustee   The coordinator of financial resources assigned by the court during a bankruptcy case.

tubercle (too′-buhr-kuhl)   A nodule produced by the tuberculosis bacillus.

turgor   A term referring to normal skin tension; the resistance of the skin to being grasped between the fingers and released. Turgor is decreased with dehydration and increased with edema.

type and cross-match   Tests performed to assess the compatibility of blood to be transfused.

unit dose   Method used by the pharmacy to prepare individual doses of medication.

unsecured debt   Debt that is not guaranteed by something of value; credit card debt is the most common type of unsecured debt.

upcoding   A fraudulent practice in which provider services are billed for higher procedural codes than were actually performed, resulting in a higher payment.

upper gastrointestinal (UGI) series   Fluoroscopic examination of the esophagus, stomach, and duodenum; barium sulfate is used as a contrast medium and is administered orally.

urea The major nitrogenous end product of protein metabolism and the chief nitrogenous component of the urine.

urgency A sudden, compelling desire to urinate and the inability to control the release of urine.

urgent An acute situation that requires immediate attention but is not life-threatening.

urochrome The yellow pigment normally found in urine; it is described as straw, yellow, or amber based on its concentration.

urticaria (uhr-tuh-kar′-e-uh) A skin eruption that creates inflamed wheals; hives.

USB port The most common type of connector device that allows hardware to be plugged into the computer.

utilization management A process of managing healthcare costs by influencing patient care decision making through case-by-case assessments of the appropriateness of care.

Valsalva maneuver The act of attempting to exhale forcibly while keeping the nose and mouth closed, such as occurs when a person strains to defecate or urinate. This causes trapping of blood in the great veins, preventing the blood from entering the chest and right atrium.

vasoconstriction (va-zo-kun-strik′-shun) Contraction of the muscles lining blood vessels, which narrows the lumen.

vasodilation An increase in the diameter of a blood vessel.

vectors Animals or insects (e.g., ticks) that transmit the causative organisms of disease.

vegetations Abnormal growth of tissue surrounding a valve consisting of fibrin, platelets, and bacteria.

vendor A company that sells supplies, equipment, or services to another company or individual.

ventricles The two lower chambers of the heart.

veracity (vuh-rah′-suh-te) A devotion to or conformity with the truth.

verdict The finding or decision of a jury on a matter submitted to it in trial.

vertigo Dizziness; a sensation of spinning or an inability to maintain normal balance.

vested Granted or endowed with a particular authority, right, or property; to have a special interest in.

viable Capable of living, developing, or germinating under favorable conditions.

virulent (vir′-yoo-lent) Exceedingly pathogenic, noxious, or deadly.

viscosity (vis-kos′-ih-te) The degree of thickness; a substance that is viscous is thick and lacks the capability of easy movement.

vocation The work in which a person is regularly employed.

voice mail An electronic system that allows messages from telephone callers to be recorded and stored.

vulva The external female genitalia, which begins at the mons pubis and terminates at the anus.

waiting period The amount of time a patient waits for disability insurance to pay cash payments after the date of injury.

wasting syndrome Physical deterioration resulting in profound weight loss, fatigue, anorexia, and mental confusion.

wet mount A slide preparation in which a drop of liquid specimen or the like is covered with a coverslip and observed with a microscope.

wheal (weel) A localized area of edema or a raised lesion.

wheezing A high-pitched sound heard on expiration; it indicates obstruction or narrowing of respiratory passages.

white noise The sounds from a television or stereo that muffle or mute the conversation of others, thus helping to protect the confidentiality of patients.

willful neglect Conscious, intentional failure or reckless indifference to the obligation to comply with the administrative simplification provision violated.

Zip Software that compresses a file or folder, making it smaller.

zone A region or geographic area used for shipping.

INDEX

Page numbers followed by "*f*" indicate figures, "*b*" indicate boxes, and "*t*" indicate tables.